UHB Trust
U0000000102573

D1458640

UHB TRUST LIBRARY
HOSPITAL
EDGBASTON
BIRMINGHAM B15 2TH

Evidence-Based Medicine Guidelines

Evidence-Based Medicine Guidelines

EDITOR-IN-CHIEF
Ilkka Kunnamo

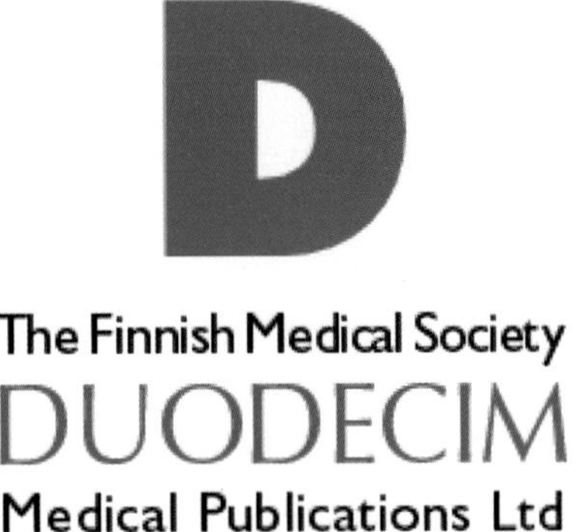

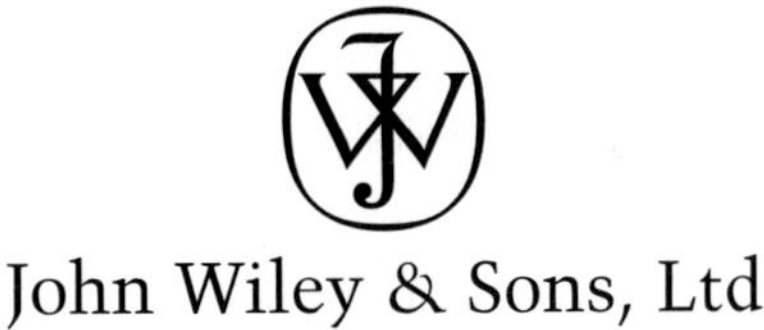

John Wiley & Sons, Ltd

Published by John Wiley & Sons Ltd, The Atrium, Southern Gate, Chichester, West Sussex PO19 8SQ, England

Telephone (+44) 1243 779777

Email (for orders and customer service enquiries): cs-books@wiley.co.uk
Visit our Home Page on www.wileyeurope.com or www.wiley.com

Other Wiley Editorial Offices

John Wiley & Sons Inc., 111 River Street, Hoboken, NJ 07030, USA

Jossey-Bass, 989 Market Street, San Francisco, CA 94103-1741, USA

Wiley-VCH Verlag GmbH, Boschstr. 12, D-69469 Weinheim, Germany

John Wiley & Sons Australia Ltd, 33 Park Road, Milton, Queensland 4064, Australia

John Wiley & Sons (Asia) Pte Ltd, 2 Clementi Loop #02-01, Jin Xing Distripark, Singapore 129809

John Wiley & Sons Canada Ltd, 22 Worcester Road, Etobicoke, Ontario, Canada M9W 1L1

Wiley also publishes its books in a variety of electronic formats. Some content that appears in print may not be available in electronic books.

British Library Cataloguing in Publication Data

A catalogue record for this book is available from the British Library

ISBN 0-470-01184-X

Typeset in 9.5/11pt Times by Laserwords Private Limited, Chennai, India
Printed and bound in Spain by Grafos S.A., Barcelona, Spain
This book is printed on acid-free paper responsibly manufactured from sustainable forestry in which at least two trees are planted for each one used for paper production.

Contents

30 GENETICS

31 PAEDIATRIC INFECTIOUS DISEASES ... 937

32 PAEDIATRICS ... 977

33 PAEDIATRIC PSYCHIATRY 1015

Foreword

Most doctors are uncomfortably aware of the gap between what we know and what we do. We would all like to close this gap, but few know how. One problem is the information flood that faces busy clinicians. With over 1,500 new research articles being indexed in MEDLINE each week, no single doctor can keep up to date by browsing the world literature. A collective effort is needed; and an effort at several levels. This collective effort includes systematic reviews of the evidence, such as those done by the Cochrane Collaboration, and summaries and recommendations from those reviews. Comprehensive, evidence-based, and update guidelines are one way to achieve this. Unfortunately most guidelines fall far short of this. Among the exceptions is the Evidence-Based Medicine (EBM) Guidelines.

These guidelines started decades ago before the birth of evidence-based medicine, largely as the vision of one general practitioner. This vision has transformed primary health care in Finland, where the guidelines are now used widely and on a daily basis. Since their birth they have grown and matured, incorporating the growing demand for guidance to be based on evidence. A singular, and unusual, feature of the EBM Guidelines is the reference to Cochrane reviews whenever appropriate. This is a major step for guidelines, which all too often ignore the available systematic reviews.

Of course, for guidelines to be useable in daily practice, being evidence-based is not enough. Many accurate guidelines are ignored. Good guidelines need to be practical and useable. Again EBM Guidelines achieves this through its friendly format, with its summary of the essentials, and appropriate and helpful pictures and diagrams. And with appropriate indices, contents directories and (in the electronic version) search engines, it is easy to find what is needed. So welcome to the book version of EBM Guidelines. If you find this useful, as I am sure you will, then I also suggest you look at the electronic version.

Can I make a final suggestion on usage? One problem we all have is ignoring the questions that arise in practice. We fail to recognize them or forget them. So I suggest you get a small spiral-bound "questions logbook" to record your questions during clinics. When you get a chance, look up the answers in EBMG (and wherever else you like). As you get comfortable with this process, you'll more often be able to look up questions during clinic. So stay attuned to your uncertainties and enjoy the help that EBM Guidelines can give.

Professor Paul Glasziou
Department of Primary Health Care &
Director, Centre for Evidence-Based Practice, Oxford

Preface

The idea of Evidence-Based Medicine (EBM) Guidelines emerged from the need for a handbook on the wide range of diseases and conditions encountered by the general physician. In 1989 these guidelines were first published as an electronic version, which has existed ever since and experienced several iterative cycles of re-writing and improvement. The concise format of the guidelines aims at high legibility and ease of finding practical guidance. The index is comprehensive, and each chapter has its own list of contents.

These guidelines are primarily intended for the use of GPs and other primary care physicians. They are widely used also by specialists, not in their own field, but as a reference to other specialties. The guidelines have two approaches: problem-based guidelines include a variety of symptoms encountered in primary care, while disease-specific guidelines include even quite rare diseases. Non-invasive primary care technology and minor surgery as well as inpatient care at non-specialist hospitals are all covered. The guidelines also include procedures that are not commonly carried out in general practice but can be performed there after adequate training.

Many authors and editors have contributed to the development of these guidelines. The name of the expert who has supervised the last updating is mentioned at the beginning of each guideline. Many guidelines are authored by the editors, most of whom are practising physicians with research background and training in critical appraisal.

The background in electronic publishing has had a profound effect on the methodology of EBM guidelines. Electronic guidelines are easily updated and linked to the best available evidence. The electronic version is widely used in clinical practice and comments from the clinicians as well as those by external referees have facilitated the continuous updating.

It has also become apparent that a print version of EBM Guidelines is highly desirable for the busy practitioner who wants a quick and handy reference when not at their keyboard.

A specific feature of this textbook is the use of evidence codes (A,B,C,D), (see www.ebm-guidelines.com) that appear in connection with many of the guideline recommendations. The coding corresponds to that proposed by the GRADE Working group (see table) for grading the quality of evidence—they do not indicate the strength of the recommendations. The main sources of evidence, the Cochrane reviews and DARE abstracts, are systematically evaluated as they are published, and if they bear relevance to topics in EBM Guidelines they are abstracted as evidence summaries. Other sources of evidence include Clinical Evidence, original articles and systematic reviews in clinical journals, abstracts in the Health Technology Assessment Database and the NHS Economic Evaluation Database, and clinical guidelines that describe evidence systematically.

In many cases high-quality evidence is not available for the recommendations given in the guidelines, particularly for those concerning diagnosis and non-pharmacological treatment. These recommendations are based on textbooks, review articles, and expert opinion agreed upon by independent referees. Although every effort has been made to ensure that the recommendations are practicable and safe, the clinician should be alert and use his/her own knowledge and judgment in making decisions on individual patients. The information contained includes a significant number of topics; however, it should not be considered complete. The variation in the spectrum of diseases and a number of alternative treatment options cannot be covered by the guidelines.

The production of EBM Guidelines has been built on the fruitful cooperation of hundreds of experts. We would like to thank all of them for their time, enthusiasm and patience. The guidelines were originally created in Finland in close connection with the Finnish Medical Society Duodecim, the scientific society of Finnish physicians. We wish to thank the Society for its support and creative spirit. We are grateful to our colleague editors at Current Care, the National Guidelines project, for their collaboration.

The international version became possible with the support of a number of physicians all over the world many of whom participate in the Cochrane Collaboration. We are grateful to all of those who gave referee comments. We wish to thank the members of the Advisory Board for their assistance. We wish to thank all those who participated in the language revision of these guidelines, especially Ms. Maarit Green and Ms. Maria Kuronen. Last but not least we would like to thank Professor Raimo Suhonen for sharing his excellent collection of dermatological images with us.

Ilkka Kunnamo
Helena Varonen

Grading the quality of evidence*

- **A (high):** Further research is very unlikely to change our confidence in the estimate of effect.
  - — Several high-quality studies with consistent results
  - — In special cases: one large, high-quality multi-centre study
- **B (moderate):** Further research is likely to have an important impact on our confidence in the estimate of effect and may change the estimate.
  - — One high-quality study
  - — Several studies with some limitations
- **C (low):** Further research is very likely to have an important impact on our confidence in the estimate of effect and is likely to change the estimate.
  - — One or more studies with severe limitations
- **D (very low):** Any estimate of effect is very uncertain.
  - — Expert opinion
  - — No direct research evidence
  - — One or more studies with very severe limitations

*(Adapted from the GRADE Working Group (*BMJ* 2004; 328:1490–8))

List of Abbreviations

Units

mm	millimetre
cm	centimetre
m	metre
m^2	square metre
m^3	cubic metre
fl	femtolitre
µl	microlitre
ml	millilitre
cl	centilitre
l	litre
µg	microgram
mg	milligram
g	gram
kg	kilogram
sec.	second
min.	minute
h	hour
J	joule
MJ	megajoule
W	watt
kW	kilowatt
Pa	pascal
kPa	kilopascal
cal	calory
kcal	kilocalory
Hz	hertz
kHz	kilohertz
dB	decibel
mmHg	millimetre of mercury
mmol	millimole
IU	international unit

Pharmacological Abbreviations

Sic!	(Latin); thus, so (not a mistake and is to be read as it stands)
i.d.	intradermal (intracutaneous)
i.m.	intramuscular
i.v.	intravenous
p.o.	per os (Latin), orally, by mouth
s.c.	subcutaneous
o.d.	omni dei (Latin), once a day
b.i.d.	bis in die (Latin), twice a day
b.d.	bis in die (Latin), twice a day
t.i.d.	ter in die (Latin), three times a day
t.d.s.	ter die sumendus (Latin), three times a day
q.i.d.	quater in die (Latin), four times a day
q.d.s.	quarter die sumendus (Latin), four times a day
$1 \times 3 \times 5$	(one tablet 3 times a day for 5 days)
gtt	guttae (Latin), drops

Clinical Abbreviations

ad.	addendum (Latin), to, until
ca.	circa, approximately
e.g.	exempli gratia (Latin), for example
etc.	et cetera (Latin), and so forth
i.e.	id est (Latin), that is, in effect
NB	nota bene (Latin), note well
Ab	antibody
ACE	angiotensin converting enzyme
ACTH	adrenocorticotropic hormone
ADH	antidiuretic hormone
ADHD	attention-deficit hyperactivity disorder
AFP	alphafetoprotein
Ag	antigen
AHA	American Heart Association
AIDS	acquired immunodeficiency syndrome
AIHA	autoimmune haemolytic anemia
ALS	amyotrophic lateral sclerosis
ALT	alanine transaminase (aminotransferase)
ANP	atrial natriuretic peptide
AMI	acute myocardial infarction
AOM	acute otitis media
AP	angina pectoris
APC	activated protein C
ARDS	adult respiratory distress syndrome
ASA	acetylsalicylic acid
ASAT	aspartate transaminase (aminotransferase)
ASD	atrial septal defect
ATII	angiotensin II
AV	atrioventricular
BCG	Calmette–Guérin bacillus (vaccine)
BE	base excess
BMI	body mass index
BNP	brain natriuretic peptide
BP	blood pressure
bpm	beats per minute
CABG	coronary artery bypass grafting
CD4	CD4 cell (helper-inducer T cell)
CHD	coronary heart disease
CIN	cervical intra-epithelial neoplasia
CK	creatine kinase
CK-MB	creatine kinase isoenzyme MB
CMV	cytomegalovirus
CPAP	continuous positive airway pressure
CNS	central nervous system
COPD	chronic obstructive pulmonary disease
COX	cyclooxygenase
CRP	C-reactive protein
CSF	cerebrospinal fluid
CT	compute(rize)d tomography
DIC	disseminated intravascular coagulation

DIP	distal interphalangeal (joint)
DM	diabetes mellitus
DNA	deoxyribonucleic acid
DVT	deep venous thrombosis
EBM	evidence-based medicine
EBV	Epstein-Barr virus
ECG	electrocardiography
EDTA	ethylene diamine tetra-acetic acid
EEG	electroencephalography
EF	ejection fraction
ELISA	enzyme-linked immunosorbent assay
EMG	electromyography
ENMG	electroneuromyography
ENT	ear, nose and throat (specialist)
EPO	erythropoietin
ESR	erythrocyte sedimentation rate
EU	European Union
FDA	The Food and Drug Administration
FSH	follicle-stimulating hormone (follitropin)
FVC	forced vital capacity
FXa	factor Xa (blood coagulation factor)
GAD	glutamic acid decarboxylase (antibody)
GGT	gamma-glutamyl transferase
GI	gastrointestinal
GM	grand mal (epilepsy)
GnRH	gonadotropin-releasing hormone (gonadoliberin)
GP	general practitioner
HbA1c	glyc(osyl)ated haemoglobin
Hb	haemoglobin
HBV	hepatitis B virus
hCG	human chorionic gonadotrophin
HCV	hepatitis C virus
HDL	high-density lipoprotein
Hib	Haemophilus influenzae type b (vaccine)
HIV	human immunodeficiency virus
HLA	human leucocyte antigen
HPV	human papillomavirus
HRT	hormone replacement therapy
HSV	herpes simplex virus
ICD	International Classification of Diseases
ICU	intensive care unit
Ig	immunoglobulin
IHD	ischaemic heart disease
INH	isoniazid (isonicotinic acid hydrazide)
INR	international normalized ratio
ISA	intrinsic sympathomimetic activity
ITP	idiopathic thrombocytopenic purpura
IUD	intrauterine device
IVF	in vitrofertilization
KCl	potassium chloride
KOH	potassium hydroxide
LAD	left anterior descending (artery)
LAFB	left anterior fascicular block (=LAHB)
LAHB	left anterior hemiblock (=LAFB)
LBBB	left bundle brach block
LDL	low-density lipoprotein
LH	luteinizing hormone (lutropin)
LHRH	luteinizing hormone-releasing hormone (luliberin)
LMW	low molecular weight
LMWH	low-molecular-weight heparin
LV	left ventricle
LVH	left ventricular hypertrophy
MAO	monoamine oxidase
MCH	mean cell haemoglobin
MCP	metacarpophalangeal (joint)
MCV	mean cell volume
MI	myocardial infarction
MMR	measles, mumps and rubella (vaccine)
MOF	multi-organ failure
MPA	medroxyprogesterone acetate
MR	magnetic resonance
MRI	magnetic resonance imaging
MS	multiple sclerosis
MTP	metatarsophalangeal (joint)
NMDA	N-methyl-D-aspartate
NNT	number needed to treat
NPH	Neutral Protamine Hagedorn (insulin)
NSAID	non-steroidal anti-inflammatory drug
NYHA	New York Heart Association
Pap	Papanicolaou (classification)
PCOS	polycystic ovary syndrome
PCR	polymerase chain reaction
PDT	diphtheria-pertussis-tetanus (vaccine)
PEF	peak expiratory flow
PID	pelvic inflammatory disease
PIP	proximal interphalangeal (joint)
PM	petit mal (epilepsy)
PMS	premenstrual syndrome
PPI	proton pump inhibitor
PSA	prostate-specific antigen
PTCA	percutaneous transluminal coronary angioplasty
PTH	parathyroid hormone
RAFB	right anterior fascicular block (=RAHB)
RAHB	right anterior hemiblock (=RAFB)
RAST	radioallergosorbent test
RBBB	right bundle branch block
RBC	red blood cell
RDS	respiratory distress syndrome
REM	rapid eye movement
RNA	ribonucleic acid
RVH	right ventricular hypertrophy
SA	sinoatrial (node)
SAH	subarachnoid haemorrhage
SD	standard deviation
SLE	systemic lupus erythematosus
SSRI	selective serotonin reuptake inhibitor
SSS	sick sinus syndrome
ST	sinus tachycardia
STD	sexually transmitted disease
SVT	supraventricular tachycardia
T3	triiodothyronine
T4	thyroxine
tbc	tuberculosis
TENS	transcutaneous electrical nerve stimulation
TIA	transient ischaemic attack
TNF	tumour necrosis factor

TPHA Treponema pallidum haemagglutination test
TSH thyroid-stimulating hormone (thyrotrophin)
TTP thrombotic thrombocytopenic purpura
UV ultraviolet
UVA ultraviolet A
UVB ultraviolet B
VAS visual analogue scale
VC vital capacity
VF ventricular fibrillation
VLDL very low density lipoprotein
VSD ventricular septal defect
VT ventricular tachycardia
WBC white blood cell
WHO World Health Organization
WPW Wolff–Parkinson–White syndrome

Infectious Diseases

Evidence Based Medicine Guidelines. Edited by the Duodecim Editorial Team
© 2005 John Wiley & Sons, Ltd ISBN: 0-470-01184-X

1.10 Prolonged fever in the adult

Ville Valtonen

Principles

- Diagnose common diseases (pneumonia, sinusitis, urinary tract infection) before ordering a large number of tests.
- Decide on the urgency of tests according to the patient's general condition, risk factors (immunosuppression) and local signs.
- Repeat history and physical examination before repeating tests.

Diagnostic strategy

- Exclude the following common diseases before further investigations:
  - Pneumonia (chest x-ray and auscultation)
    - Chest x-ray may also show tuberculosis, sarcoidosis, alveolitis, pulmonary infarction or lymphoma.
  - Urinary tract infection (urine test and culture)
    - Urine test may even also suggest epidemic nephropathy or renal tumour.
  - Maxillary sinusitis (ultrasound or x-ray).
- Important questions on the history include
  - Occurrence (measuring!) and duration of fever
  - Travelling, place (country) of birth, living
  - Past diseases, particularly tuberculosis and valvular defects
  - Drug therapy, including over-the-counter drugs
  - Use of alcohol
  - Systematic review of organ systems for symptoms
- Diagnostic clues and possible aetiologies
  - See Table 1.10.1
- Tests
  - Primary investigations
    - Urine test and culture
    - CRP and ESR
    - Haemoglobin, WBC count (WBC differential and platelet count)
    - AST and ALT
    - Option: serum sample to be frozen for eventual serology
    - Chest x-ray
    - Maxillary sinus ultrasound or x-ray
  - Secondary investigations
    - Abdominal ultrasonography
    - Bone marrow aspiration
    - Serology (Yersinia, tularaemia, HIV, Borrelia burgdorferi, viral antibodies, serum HBs-Ag, serum HCV-Ab, antinuclear antibodies)
    - Blood bacterial culture
- Consider your tactics before continuing with investigations
  - See Table 1.10.2.
- Browse a list of causes for fever to see what may have escaped your notice.

Causes of prolonged fever

- Tuberculosis (any organ)
- Bacterial infections
  - Sinusitis
  - Urinary tract infection
  - Intra-abdominal infections (cholecystitis, appendicitis, abscesses)
  - Perianal abscess
  - Abscesses of the chest cavity (lungs, mediastinum)
  - Bronchiectasis
  - Salmonellosis, Shigellosis
  - Osteomyelitis
- Bacteraemia without focus (more often an acute disease rather than prolonged fever)
- Intravascular infections
  - Endocarditis
  - Infections of vascular prostheses
- Generalized viral or bacterial infections
  - Mononucleosis
  - Adeno-, Cytomegalo- or Coxsackie B viral infections
  - Hepatitis
  - HIV
  - Chlamydial infection (Psittacosis, Ornitosis)
  - Toxoplasmosis
  - Lyme disease
  - Tularaemia
  - Malaria
- Benign temperature elevation after an infectious disease
- Chronic fatigue syndrome
- Sarcoidosis
- Atrial myxoma
- Subacute thyreoiditis
- Thyreotoxicosis
- Hemolytic diseases
- Post-traumatic tissue damage and haematoma
- Vascular thrombosis, pulmonary embolism
- Kawasaki disease
- Erythema nodosum
- Drug fever
- Malignant neuroleptic syndrome
- Allergic alveolitis
  - Farmer's lung
- Connective tissue diseases
  - Polymyalgia rheumatica, temporal arteritis
  - Ankylosing spondylitis
  - Rheumatoid arthritis
  - Systemic lupus erythematosus (SLE)

Table 1.10.1 Prolonged fever in the adult – diagnostic clues

Clue	Possible causes[1)]
Infection parameters (ESR, CRP) are normal	Chronic fatigue syndrome, minor temperature elevation after an infectious disease, drug fever, self-induced fever
Already cured viral or bacterial infection	Mild "vegetative" temperature elevation after an infectious disease lasting for up to 1–2 months is a functional disorder ("thermostatic temperature elevation"). The thermoregulatory system is temporarily reset by high fever, and body temperature remains elevated. Stress and fatigue may contribute to the disorder
Erythema	See 31.3. Meningococcaemia, drug fever
Throat or neck pain	Subacute thyreoiditis, **retropharyngeal abscess**, mononucleosis
Confusion	In elderly confusion is associated with the fever itself, in younger patients remember **encephalitis** and any possible **septic infection (1.70)**
Known valvular defect or murmur suggesting one	**Endocarditis**
GI symptoms	Crohn's disease, ulcerative colitis, **periappendicular abscess**, other peritoneal **abscesses**, yersiniosis
Abnormal urinary findings	UTI, **epidemic nephritis**, renal cancer, endocarditis
History of stay in the tropics	See article on suspected tropical disease 2.30
Farmer	**Farmer's lung**
Suppurative mosquito bite or ulcer	Tularaemia
Lymph nodes felt on palpation	Mononucleosis, Hodgkin's disease, lymphoma
Neuroleptic medication	**Neuroleptic malignant syndrome**
Long-term antimicrobial medication	Drug fever, Clostridium difficile
Immunosuppression patient	See 1.71
Headache	**Temporal arteritis**
Myalgia	Polymyalgia rheumatica (may be associated with the fever itself)
Bone pains	Myeloma, metastasis
Back pain	Ankylosing spondylitis, several infections
Back pain on tapping	Infection focus
Recurring fever	Endocarditis, deep infectious foci
Discrepancy between findings and history	Self-induced fever

1) The diagnosis of diseases marked with bold must not be delayed.

Table 1.10.2 Diagnostic tactics in prolonged fever

Right	Wrong
Take history again	Repeat laboratory and radiologic investigations
Repeat the physical examination	Start drug therapy or increase dosage
Read the journal again	Suggest a surgical intervention
Take time to reflect upon the case	

- Still's disease of the adult
- Rheumatic fever
- Vasculitides
- Periarteritis nodosa
- Wegener's granulomatosis

♦ Inflammatory bowel diseases
- Regional enteritis (Crohn's disease)
- Ulcerative colitis

♦ Cirrhosis of the liver, alcoholic hepatitis

♦ Malignant diseases
- Leukaemia
- Cancer of the pancreatic and biliary ducts
- Renal carcinoma (hypernephroma)
- Sarcomas
- Hodgkin's disease, other lymphomas
- Metastases (renal carcinoma, melanoma, sarcoma)

FUO

♦ The diagnosis Febris e causa ignota (fever of undetermined origin, FUO) is used when a fever above 38°C has lasted longer than 2–3 weeks.

♦ Usually the cause is a serious disease, which can often be treated. An aetiological diagnosis should be pursued intensively, preferably in the hospital.

♦ The final diagnosis is infection in about 35% of the patients, malignant disease in 20%, collagenosis in 15% and some other disease in 15%. In about 15% of the patients the cause remains unknown.

1.20 Yersiniosis

Rauli Leino

Basic rules

- Consider yersiniosis in patients with
  - acute abdominal pain
  - acute diarrhoea
  - fever of unknown origin
  - Reiter's disease
    - arthritis
    - urethritis
    - iritis, conjunctivitis
  - erythema nodosum
  - abnormal results in urine test, liver function tests or tests for pancreatitis
  - hypersedimentation.

Causative agents

- Yersinia enterocolitica 3 and 9, Y. pseudotuberculosis IA and 3.
- The causative agent cannot be identified on the basis of the clinical symptoms.

Symptoms and clinical picture

Symptoms of acute infection

- Fever
- Diarrhoea: children often have blood and mucus in the stools.
- Abdominal pain: in children often in the right lower quadrant. If the patient is operated on, mesenteric lymphadenopathy, terminal ileitis, or true appendicitis may be detected.

Post-infectious symptoms

- Reactive arthritis
  - 1–3 weeks after enteritis
  - The symptoms vary from mild arthralgia to severe polyarthritis, sometimes Reiter's syndrome.
  - A small proportion of the patients develop chronic arthritis.
  - The disease is strongly associated with HLA-B27.
- Ocular symptoms
  - Iritis
  - Conjunctivitis
- Urinary symptoms
  - Urethritis
  - Balanitis
  - Glomerulonephritis
- Skin symptoms
  - Erythema nodosum is the most common skin manifestation (about 10% of cases are caused by Yersinia); it can be the only symptom of yersiniosis.
- Cardiac findings
  - Transient ECG abnormalities
  - Valvular disease is not associated with yersiniosis.
- Other symptoms
  - Hepatitis, pancreatitis or thyroiditis

Diagnosis

Faecal bacterial culture

- Useful in acute disease
- The sensitivity decreases rapidly after the symptoms of enteritis have disappeared.

Serology

- The primary diagnostic method in post-infectious symptoms (arthritis)
- The ELISA method is the most specific.
  - A recent infection can be diagnosed on the basis of one serum sample.
  - Class IgM antibodies appear in a few days and disappear after a few months.
  - Class IgG antibodies can be detected for years.
  - Class IgA antibodies are particularly associated with arthritis.
  - A cross-reaction occurs between Y. enterocolitica 9 and Brucella, but an ELISA inhibition test confirming the diagnosis is automatically performed in positive cases.

Treatment

- The disease is usually cured spontaneously.
- Chronic carriers have not been detected.
- There is little evidence on the effect of antibiotic treatment; its effect on the occurrence of post-infectious symptoms is not known.

Indications for antibiotics

- Septicaemia
- Fulminant disease or severe post-infective symptoms (such as arthritis) are relative indications for antibiotics.

Selection and dosage

- Quinolones, e.g. ciprofloxacin 500 mg × 2 × 7–10 days
- Tetracyclines are a good alternative.
- Trimethoprim-sulpha is the drug of choice for children.

Indications for specialist referral

- Acute appendicitis
- Severe post-infectious symptoms

1.21 Tularaemia

Janne Laine

Aims

- Suspect tularaemia in patients with fever, lymphadenopathy and an ulcerated skin lesion (Figure 1.21.1) at the site of a mosquito bite or a scratch.
- Begin treatment on the basis of the clinical picture if the symptoms are typical. Diagnosis can be confirmed with serology.

Transmission

- The most important reservoir host is the mole.
- The infection is transmitted by
  - mosquitoes (most important)
  - other blood-sucking arthropods (horse-flies, black flies, ticks)
  - bites or scratches of a sick animal
  - inhalation of infected aerosols
  - ingestion of contaminated water or food
  - ingestion of meat from an affected animal (even after freezing the meat)
- Incubation period is 1 to 14 days (mean 4 days)

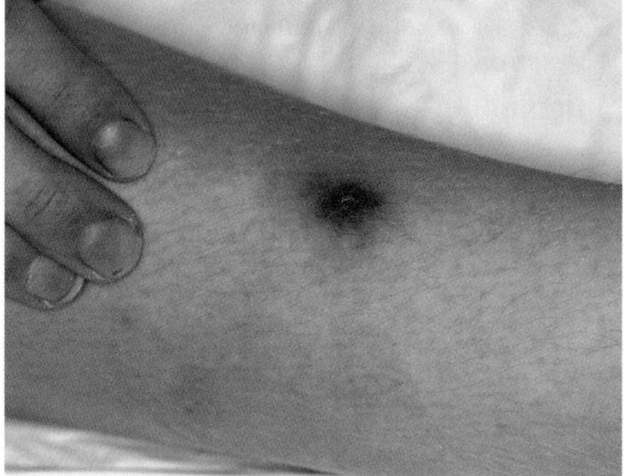

Figure 1.21.1 Francisella tularensis is transmitted to humans by handling an infected animal, but also by mosquito bite, or even by ixodes. Incubation time is usually a few days. In the most common form, ulcero-glandular tularaemia, the inoculation site develops a red papule, which ulcerates. The regional lymph glands enlarge and the patient is febrile. The rising antibody titer is diagnostic. Photo © R. Suhonen.

Symptoms

- Varying clinical manifestations:
  - **The ulceroglandular form** (75–85% of the cases) causes fever, a small infected skin lesion as well as swelling and tenderness of regional lymph nodes.
  - **The glandular form** (5–10% of the cases) causes fever and lymphadenopathy but no skin lesions.
  - **The typhoidal form** (5–15% of the cases) causes severe systemic symptoms (fever, fatigue and weight loss) and possibly enlargement of the liver and spleen.
  - **The oculoglandular form** causes granulomatous conjunctivitis with regional lymphadenopathy.
  - **The oropharyngeal form** (2–4% of the cases) causes tonsillitis, pharyngitis and cervical lymphadenopathy.
- Symptomless infection is common (about 50% of the cases).
- Rash has been reported in up to 20% of the patients.
- Pneumonia is seen in 15% of the ulceroglandular cases and in nearly all patients with other forms of the disease.
- Elevated liver enzyme values, enlarged liver
- Peritonitis, meningitis and osteomyelitis are rare.
- CRP increases moderately, ESR to a lesser extent.
- Anaemia

Diagnosis

- Treatment is begun on the basis of the clinical picture.
- Diagnosis is confirmed by serology. The antibody titre rises first 10–14 days after onset of fever. The blood samples are taken 2–3 times, at 2 week intervals. A rise in the antibody titre is an indication of a recent infection. A 4-fold rise of the titre, or a single clearly elevated titre (1:160 with agglutination technique, 1:128 with microagglutination technique), is considered diagnostic.
- Bacterial culture of the secreting lesion can also be performed.

Treatment

- Fluoroquinolones are the recommended antibiotic therapy in mild and moderate cases (the dose of ciprofloxacin is 500 mg b.d. for adults). Alternatively, doxycycline (100 mg b.d. for 10 to 14 days, or 2–3 weeks after onset of symptoms), or streptomycin or aminoglycosides for 1–2 weeks can be used depending on the severity of the disease.
- If the patient has severe symptoms, an infectious disease physician should be consulted.
- Beta-lactam antibiotics are ineffective.
- Children are managed under the supervision of a paediatrician. Ciprofloxacin has been used for children in verified cases of tularaemia. The dose is 15–20 mg/kg daily divided into two doses.

Prevention

- A live attenuated vaccine has been developed, but is not currently available.
- Recommendations have been issued in the United States for measures to be taken in case tularaemia is used as a biological weapon. Doxycycline and ciprofloxacin are recommended for exposed individuals during an epidemic.

1.22 Erysipeloid

Petteri Carlson

Epidemiology

- The bacterium that causes erysipeloid (Erysipelothrix rhusiopathiae) can be found in many animals (pigs, fish, birds).
- Humans can be infected through skin erosions.
- Occurs as a rare occupational disease among animal farmers, butchers, fishermen, veterinarians etc.

Symptoms

- Swollen, bluish, well-demarcated skin lesions usually in the hands (Figure 1.22.1) . There is no suppuration.
- There is usually intense pain, and itching and a prickling sensations are also common.
- Local lymph nodes often swell, but otherwise systemic symptoms are rare. Septicaemia and endocarditis may sometimes occur.

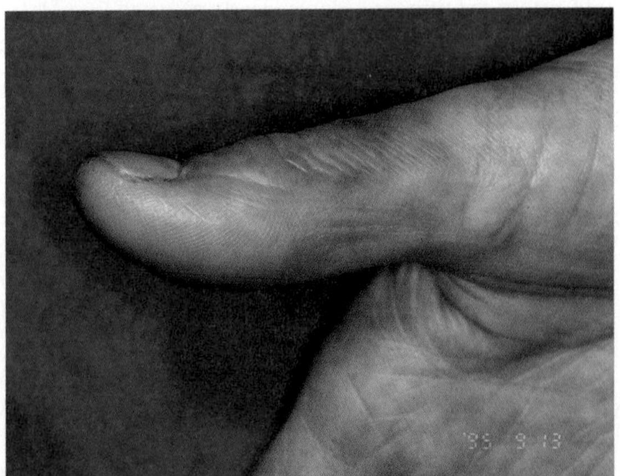

Figure 1.22.1 Erysipeloides is an uncommon infection in humans, mainly in persons working in agriculture and fishing. In this patient Erysipelothrix rhusiopathiae was probably transmitted from poultry. The red, slightly tender area reached the present extent in a couple of weeks. The culture was successful from a small biopsy specimen. Oral penicillin V is curative. Photo © R. Suhonen.

- The disease is self-limiting within a few weeks. The skin remains brown and often scaly.

Diagnosis

- The diagnosis can be made on the basis of history and the typical clinical picture. Staining and culture from a biopsy sample or tissue fluid obtained by aspiration can be performed but is rarely indicated.

Treatment

- Penicillin 1.5 million units × 2 × 10 shortens the duration of the disease. Also cephalosporins, macrolides, and fluoroquinolones are probably effective D [1 2].

Prevention

- Good occupational practice, covering hand wounds and erosions

References

1. Barnett JH, Estes SA, Wirman JA et al. Erysipeloid. J Am Acad Dermatol 1983;9:116–123.
2. Venditti M, Gelfusa V, Tarasi A et al. Antimicrobial susceptibilities of Erysipelothrix rhusiopathiae. Antimicr Agents Chemother 1990;34:2038–2040.

1.23 Listeriosis

Kirsi Skogberg

Epidemiology

- Listeria monocytogenes, a gram-positive rod, has been isolated from soil, animals and stools of asymptomatic individuals; food, dairy products in particular, has also been implicated as a source of infection.
- Pregnant women, foetuses and newborns as well as those with impaired cell-mediated immunity are more susceptible to the infection.

Symptoms

- Sepsis or meningitis are the most common clinical presentations, seen mostly in those with impaired immunity.
- In foetal infection the result is abortion, intrauterine death or sepsis of the newborn (early infection).
- Newborn may also be infected through genital tract or the infection can be hospital born. Meningitis may develop days of weeks after delivery (late infection).

- Listeriosis in individuals with no underlying risk factors may present as a flu like illness or gastroenteritis, rarely as meningitis or sepsis.

Diagnosis

- Bacterial staining and culture. Listeria is grown from normal blood and CSF samples. Special request is needed in order to inform the laboratory of the use of specific conditions for culture from other locations.
- Serology is of little use.

Treatment

- The first drug of choice is ampicillin or G penicillin intravenously in large doses. Synergism with aminoglycosides may prove clinically useful.
- In penicillin allergy, trimethoprim-sulphamethoxazole or in mild cases, erythromycin may be used.
- **Cephalosporins are not effective against listeria.**
- Antimicrobial therapy should continue for at least 2 weeks.

Prevention

- Measures for reducing the risk of listeriosis.
  - General recommendations
    - Cook or roast all meat thoroughly.
    - Wash raw vegetables carefully before eating them.
    - Store uncooked meat away from vegetables, cooked food and convenience foods.
    - Avoid unpasteurized milk and products prepared from such milk.
    - Wash your hands and all knives and chopping boards that you have used for preparing the above-mentioned uncooked foods.
  - Recommendations for persons at risk
    - Avoid soft, (mould-)ripened cheeses.
    - Avoid vacuum-packed raw-pickled or raw-smoked fish products.
    - Before eating leftover foods and convenience foods warm the food until it is steaming hot.

1.24 Tetanus

Janne Mikkola

Aims

- Prevention by vaccination and careful treatment of contaminated wounds
- Early identification of the disease in unvaccinated patients

Definition

- Tetanus is a severe systemic infection in the unvaccinated individual caused by Clostridium tetani, which can be found in high concentrations in the soil and in normal intestinal flora.

Symptoms

- First, a local wound infection in which the bacteria multiply and produce toxin.
- Within days or weeks, a generalized systemic infection with muscle spasms most often beginning at the mandibular joint (trismus)
- Localized tetanus consists of muscle rigidity and painful spasms close to the site of injury.
- In spite of intensive care, mortality is high.

Diagnosis

- Depends mostly on history and clinical features. The usefulness of aspirate gram-stain and culture is limited.

Treatment

- Making the airway secure, supportive care with anticonvulsive medications and sedation require intensive care in most cases.
- Human antitetanus immunoglobulin and debridement of the wound are the cornerstones of treatment.
- Metronidazole orally or i.v. is the drug of choice. The dose for adults is 500 mg × 3 and for children 30 mg/kg daily in three doses. G penicillin is an alternative.
- Active immunization should be initiated during convalescence.

Prevention

- In most developed countries, a universal immunization is effective and the boosters are given every ten years.
  - Td vaccine gives protection also against diphtheria.
- Prevention when treating dirty wounds
  - Booster vaccination
    - A booster is given if it is more than 10 years since the previous vaccination.
    - With a big contaminated wound, the booster is given after 5 years.
    - Patients who have not received the primary series of vaccinations are both immunized and given tetanus immunoglobulin.
  - Frequent vaccinations increase the probability of local reactions.

1.25 Diphtheria

Petri Ruutu

Epidemiology

- An infectious disease with potential for causing serious epidemics, preventable by vaccination.
- The disease spreads via respiratory secretions (nasal secretions, saliva), but also via direct contact with wounds and other secretions.
- The incubation period is 1–7 days.
- A number of cases have been diagnosed in Europe since 1990. Nearly all patients were infected in the countries of the former Soviet Union.
- All new cases should be reported to the WHO.

Symptoms

1. Local inflammation with copious pharyngeal exudates, grey or dark mucosal adhering exudates and soft tissue oedema. In children this phase of the disease may result in the obstruction of the airway.
2. The systemic disease caused by bacterial toxin starts 1–2 weeks after the local symptoms. The toxin affects the heart (myocarditis, arrhythmias particularly during the second week of the disease) and the nervous system (paralyses, neuritis 2–7 weeks after disease onset). If the patient survives the acute phase of the disease he/she usually recovers without sequelae.

Diagnosis

- The need for treatment is decided on the basis of the history and clinical picture (severe, exudative pharyngitis, particularly in a patient who has visited an endemic country 1–7 days before the onset of the disease).
- The diagnosis is confirmed by bacterial culture taken from the exudate into a standard transport tube for bacterial specimens. The specimen should be cultured on special media (inform the laboratory in advance).

Treatment

- Symptomatic patients should be treated in a hospital under the supervision of a specialist in infectious diseases and under isolation to prevent further transmission. Asymptomatic individuals can be treated at home.
- In children, the patency of the airway must be ensured in the initial phase.
- All patients should be treated with antibiotics (penicillin, roxithromycin, erythromycin). The drug should be administered intravenously at first. Diphtheria antitoxin should be administered as early as possible according to the instructions of a specialist in infectious diseases.
- Take throat bacterial cultures from close contacts, treat them with antibiotics (benzathine penicillin, 600 000–1.2 million units as a single dose intramuscularly or erythromycin at a standard dose for 7–10 days), and vaccinate them.

Prevention

- Vaccination prevents complications caused by the toxin but it does not prevent infection.
- If the basic vaccinations have been given, the protection is over 90%. In people over 30 years of age without a booster the protection is not as good. A booster vaccination should be given every 10 years. The booster often contains a combination of tetanus and diphtheria vaccinations.
- Travellers to epidemic areas should be given the basic series of three vaccinations, if they have not been vaccinated previously. A booster vaccination is sufficient in adults if they are over 30 years of age and have previously received a full basic series of three vaccinations.

1.28 Methicillin-resistant Staphylococcus aureus (MRSA)

Jaana Vuopio-Varkila, Pirkko Kotilainen

Definition

- MRSA strains are S. aureus isolates, which are not susceptible to beta-lactamase resistant staphylococcal antibiotics (cloxacillin and dicloxacillin) or other beta-lactam antibiotics (such as cephalosporins and imipenem).
- In addition, MRSA strains are often multi-resistant in which case, for example, clindamycin, aminoglycosides and fluoroquinolones are not effective for treatment.
- This guideline applies in Scandinavia and in other areas where MRSA is not common.

Epidemiology

- The majority of the cases are asymptomatic carriers. Only 10% of the cases are clinical infections.
- In many hospitals in Central and Southern Europe, USA, Asia or Middle East up to 50% of all S. aureus isolates are methicillin-resistant.

Diseases

- MRSA usually causes hospital-acquired surgical site and bone infections or septic systemic infections.

- MRSA infections are rare among outpatients.
- The spectrum and severity of infections caused by MRSA are similar to those caused by methicillin-susceptible S. aureus.

Why is prevention important?

- Treatment of MRSA is difficult as the only drugs of choice for severe systemic infections are intravenously administered vancomycin or teicoplanin. Increased use of vancomycin may lead to bacterial strains resistant to vancomycin. This has already been shown to be the case with enterococci.
- It is important to prevent MRSA epidemics and the spread of MRSA by blocking the route of transmission.
- Each new MRSA case means significant cost for the hospital.
  - Isolation precautions
  - Wide-scale screening for MRSA colonization
  - Prolonged hospitalization of patients with MRSA
  - Increased work load of healthcare personnel

Diagnostics

- In order to prevent spread of MRSA, patients who are infected or colonized by MRSA should be identified as soon as possible after admission to the hospital.
  - **A patient, who has been hospitalized in an area where MRSA is common, should be treated in contact isolation**, until his/her MRSA screening culture has been shown to be negative.
  - The clinical microbiology laboratory should be requested to screen specifically for MRSA from the samples.
- Bacterial cultures for MRSA screening and follow-up are performed on an individual basis. It is recommendable to consult a specialist in infectious diseases or a clinical microbiologist about the timing and technique of taking the MRSA cultures.
  - Nasal swab is performed by rotating a cotton swab in both nostrils, and applying the swab directly in to enrichment broth or into a transportation culture tube.

Ways of transmission

- The most important way of transmission is through MRSA-infected or colonized patients.
- In the hospital, patient-to-patient transmission of MRSA strains may occur rapidly through direct contact, often via healthcare personnel.
- Healthcare workers may become colonized with MRSA while taking care of MRSA-positive patients. This type of colonization is a significant source of transmission only when the person has a skin disease or a defective skin area.
- Among hospitalized patients MRSA acquisition usually first leads to asymptomatic colonization. The most common areas of colonization are the nostrils, throat, perineum, groins, armpits and skin lesions (for example skin eruptions).

Prevention of transmission

- Careful hand disinfection after all contact with patients is the most important means of preventing the spread of MRSA in hospitals.
- An MRSA patient must be isolated from other patients. Type of isolation may vary, depending on the situation. In hospital settings the patients should be placed in contact isolation.
- When a patient is found to be MRSA-culture positive, it is advisable to screen at least his/her roommates for MRSA colonization.
- If a second MRSA case is detected from the same hospital ward within a short time period, it is necessary to consider screening also other patients or healthcare personnel for MRSA colonization. If resources available for surveillance cultures are limited, it is better to direct them for detection of colonized patients.
- The patient records of those patients who are known to have been colonized or infected by MRSA previously, should be labelled accordingly.
- In case a patient is transferred to another healthcare facility, it is necessary to inform the receiving unit of his/her MRSA-status.

Treatment and follow-up

- During hospitalization, patients who are infected or colonized by MRSA are treated in contact isolation.
- MRSA acquisition often prolongs hospitalization. The patient should be discharged from the hospital as soon as it is possible without compromising patient care.
- Treatment of MRSA infections and MRSA colonization is performed in collaboration with a physician responsible for infection control or an infectious diseases specialist. MRSA must not prevent the patient from receiving any care or treatment he/she needs.

Colonization

- MRSA colonization of an outpatient is not treated.
- Among hospitalized patients treatment of asymptomatic MRSA colonization may be indicated.
- An MRSA-colonized healthcare worker is usually treated.
- If colonization is restricted for example to the nostrils, the bacterium can be eradicated by local treatment D [1].
  - A small amount of ointment containing mupirocin is applied three times daily to the nostrils during 5 days.
- If colonization is widespread or the patient has a severe skin disease, eradication of the bacterium will usually not be successful. Also foreign bodies (a urinary catheter, a tracheotomy tube, a nasogastric tube and different drainage tubes) may prevent successful eradication.
- Systemic antimicrobial agents have little effect on colonization D [1], because they are secreted to the mucosal surfaces only in a limited degree. Their usage should be considered if MRSA colonization is very large-scale or affects areas of the body where local treatment cannot be administered. Systemic treatment of colonization is reasonable only in exceptional cases.

- Washing the patient with disinfectants (for example liquid soaps containing chlorhexidine) aims at diminishing the amount of bacteria on the skin and mucosal surfaces. There is no definite proof of its effect on treatment of colonization.
- The patient is considered cleared from colonization if three consecutive MRSA-surveillance cultures taken at 1-week intervals are negative.
- Relapses are, however, common especially if the patient has received antimicrobial treatment because of an infection. As relapses are possible even after several years, it is advisable to perform MRSA cultures from previously colonized patients every time they are readmitted to hospital.
- The decision of whether MRSA carrier personnel should be removed from patient care is made by the Infection Control Doctor of the hospital or medical district. Staff who are solely nasal carriers are commonly allowed to continue work whilst being treated with mupirocin. Staff who are employed in intensive care units or on wards, where immunocompromised patients are cared for, are usually removed from duty until the MRSA colonization has been successfully treated.

Infections

- At present, the only drug of choice is vancomycin, which is used for treatment of all severe MRSA infections.
- Rifampin, fluoroquinolones, fusidic acid and sulphatrimethoprim can be used on the basis of susceptibility pattern for the treatment of less severe infections.
- Apart from the choice of the antimicrobial treatment, MRSA infections are treated following the common principles of treatment of staphylococcal infections.

National guidelines for prevention of MRSA

- Many countries have developed national guidelines for control of MRSA.

Reference

1. Loeb M, Main C, Walker-Dilks C, Eady A. Antimicrobial drugs for treating methicillin-resistant Staphylococcus aureus colonization. Cochrane Database Syst Rev 2003(4):CD003340.

1.29 Lyme borreliosis (LB)

Dag Nyman, Peter Wahlberg

Aims

- To recognize the primary stage of the disease and to treat it with antibiotics in order to prevent later manifestations.
- To remain alert to the late symptoms and signs of Lyme disease as a diagnostic possibility, and to avoid overdiagnosis.

Causative agent

- The disease is caused by the tick-borne spirochete **Borrelia burgdorferi sensu lato** including at least three human-pathogenic species. The borrelia species causing human disease in Europe are **B. afzelii**, **B. garinii** and **B. burgdorferi sensu stricto**. In USA, **B. burgdorferi s.s.** is almost the sole cause of Lyme disease.
- Spirochetes may be transmitted by all stages of the tick, also the small larvae and nymphs, which may be difficult to observe.

Geographical distribution

- The tick **Ixodes ricinus** is the common vector of the disease in Europe. In Eastern Europe and in Asia, **Ixodes persulcatus** has also been reported to function as a vector. Lyme disease was originally observed in the USA, and has now been diagnosed all over Europe and in parts of Asia.
- The infection has now been reported from all parts of Europe. The spectrum of Borrelia species and subspecies and incidence of infection varies from country to country, from region to region and even between local areas within the same region. In heavily endemic regions, the incidence of infection may be as high as 1500/100 000, whereas in other areas it may be below 1/100 000. Because of travelling and the sometimes long latency period of the late stages of the disease, doctors almost everywhere may see patients with Lyme borreliosis.
- In Northern Europe, the risk of a tick bite is greatest in moist, grassy terrain.
- The seroconversion rate in healthy inhabitants of a highly endemic area may be over 1000/100 000/year, and the prevalence of seropositivity in the population of such highly endemic regions varies between 15% and 45% increasing with age.

Symptoms and Signs

Primary Infection (Stage I)

- The most common form of primary LB is Erythema migrans (EM) (Figures 1.29.1 and 1.29.2) at the site of the tick bite. It begins at or continues for about 1 week after the bite, and if untreated, disappears within 2–4 weeks, but may also stay on for a much longer time. The erythema varies in appearance. Often, but not always, it spreads centrifugally as a ring around the bite ("bull's eye lesion"), but it may also form an enlarging patch or even become multiple. Multiple erythemata are usually regarded to belong to disseminated borreliosis.
- The lesion must not be confused with the common small erythema around the bite that is caused by irritants and subsides within a few days.

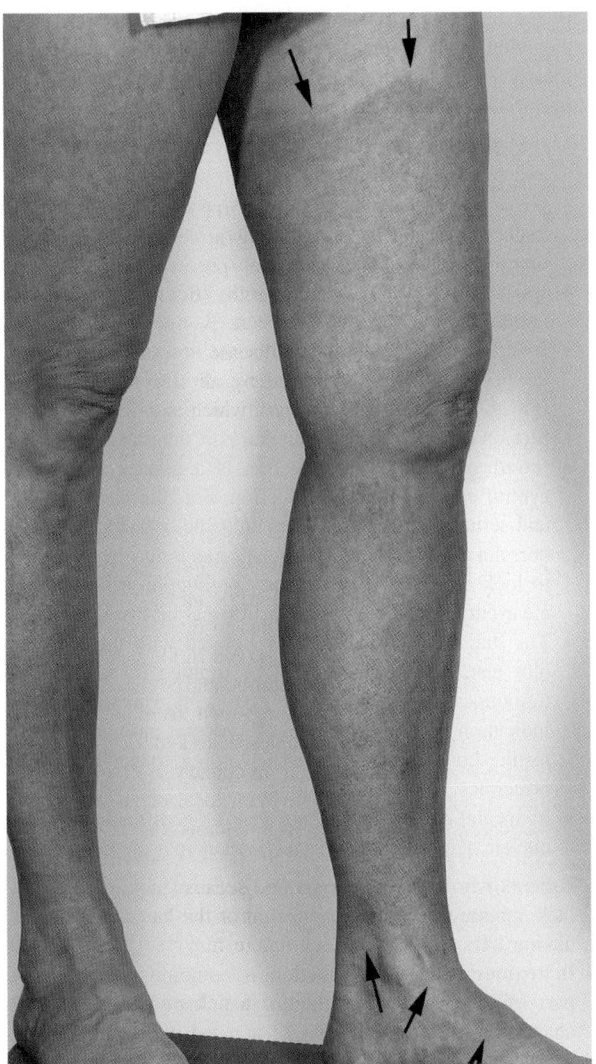

Figure 1.29.1 An unusually wide Erythema migrans, affecting almost the whole left lower extremity. The positive IgG- serology, positive PCR to Borrelia and rapid and complete response to amoxycillin therapy confirmed the diagnosis. Photo © R. Suhonen.

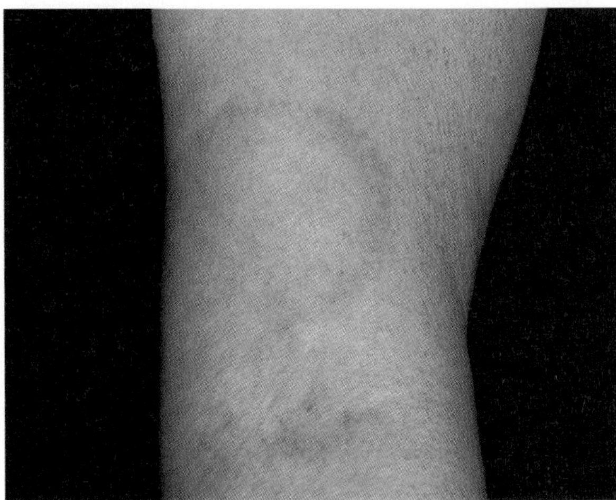

Figure 1.29.2 Erythema (chronicum) migrans, primary borrelial infection in the skin, has a variable outlook. The central skin may be normal, and only the margin is red and spreads peripherally. The whole area may be red, even bullous. IgG antibodies may be negative in early phase. Photo © R. Suhonen.

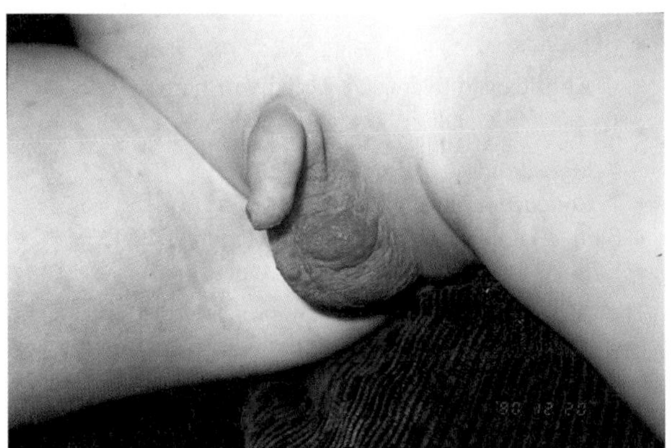

Figure 1.29.3 Lymphocytoma, induced by infection with Borrelia. The borrelial IgG serum antibody titre was high, but it returned to normal after antibiotic therapy. The patient is a boy of pre-school age. Photo © R. Suhonen.

- As a rule, if an erythema around a tick bite is more than 5 cm in diameter and starts or persists for more than a week after the bite, it should be regarded as EM.
- During the primary stage the patient usually feels well. Sometimes there may be malaise and fatigue, or the patient may run a slight temperature.
- Even in the presence of a borrelia infection, the primary lesion may be absent, or it may not be observed because the bite has been on the patient's back or in a skin fold.
- Borrelial lymphocytoma (Figure 1.29.3), or lymphadenosis benigna cutis, is a rarer form of primary borreliosis. It may occur at a tick bite in very soft tissue, often an ear lobe, and consists of a soft local non-tender, often bluish or reddish swelling. It follows approximately the same timetable as EM.

Disseminated Lyme borreliosis

- If the primary infection is not treated, up to 50% of patients may have later manifestations, which may develop weeks, months and even years after the primary lesion.
- Some common symptoms and signs of later borreliosis are
  - Paresis
    - Cranial nerve pareses, particularly facial nerve paresis, occur frequently. Borrelia antibodies in the serum or CSF should be assayed in all patients with facial nerve paresis if there is the slightest suspicion of borreliosis.
  - Central nervous system
    - Lymphocytic meningitis, meningoencephalitis
    - Meningoradiculitis (Bannwarth's syndrome)
    - Chronic progressive encephalomyelitis

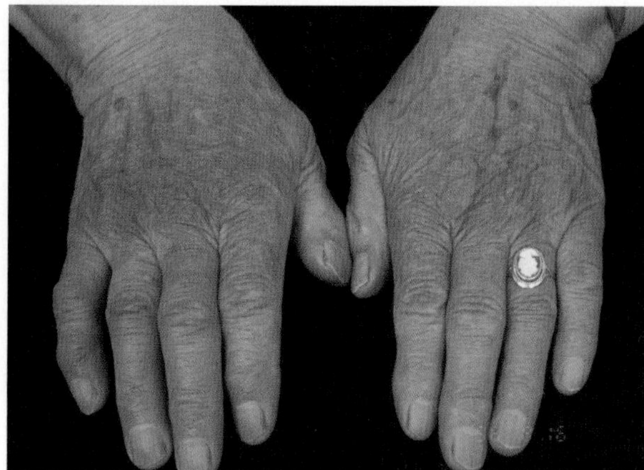

Figure 1.29.4 Acrodermatitis chronica atrophicans (ACA) is a skin manifestation in the late phase of borrelial infection. This elderly female patient had skin atrophy on the back of her right hand. The patient had typical histopathological features and positive IgG borrelial serum antibodies, and borrelial DNA was found in a PCR study of the lesional biopsy specimen. Atrophy was reversed to some degree after appropriate antibiotic therapy. Photo © R. Suhonen.

- Big joints
  - Arthritis and hydrops, especially of big joints
- Heart
  - Myocarditis
  - Conduction disturbances
- Skin: Acrodermatitis atrophicans (Figure 1.29.4)
- Eyes: Ocular inflammatory syndromes

♦ The manifestations of late LB are protean, and this disease must be kept in mind as a possibility if a patient has otherwise unexplained symptoms and signs and the history includes moving about in terrain where ticks may thrive.

Diagnosis

Primary Stage

♦ Laboratory tests are usually not carried out in primary Lyme borreliosis. If an erythema of more than 5 cm in diameter is still present at the bite site 1 week after the tick bite, the patient is regarded as having EM. Lymphocytoma at the tick bite is diagnostic for primary LB.

Disseminated Lyme borreliosis

♦ The diagnosis starts from clinical symptoms and signs and a history of tick bite or of having moved about in areas where ticks have been found (B) [1 2]. Lymphocytic pleocytosis of the CSF is a helpful corroborative sign.

♦ The principal laboratory test is the determination of specific antibodies to borrelia antigens (B) [1 2]. As a screening test, in order to rule out disease, an ELISA-based test is mostly used. In nervous system involvement, elevated titres of antibody and intrathecal antibody production are found in the CSF, sometimes even in the absence of significant elevation of serum antibody. The serological method should ideally be tested and adapted for the local spectrum of borrelia species and antigens.

- IgM antibodies rise within ca. 3 weeks after the infection and remain high for ca. 6 weeks, after which the titres go down. Not all patients revert to normal levels but expression of IgM antibodies may be seen for a longer time even without active disease.
- IgG antibody titres rise ca. 6 weeks after the infection and remain high, sometimes for years.
- A repeated test one month after the first one may help if the first result is borderline or negative. Conversion from IgM to IgG antibody, or a significant rise of IgG antibody titre on repeated testing may support the diagnosis.
- Intrathecal antibody production is a good criterion for central nervous borrelia infection. For this purpose CSF and serum from the same day must be obtained. Thus, if borrelia infection is strongly suspected it may be advisable to look for intrathecal antibody production even without clear-cut clinical signs of neurological involvement.
- The diagnosis is usually corroborated with the aid of a blot test. The blot test may be omitted by using such immunoassay methods that give a statistically proven indication of the presence of specific antibodies. The result should be interpreted according to the EUCALB principles.
- In special cases, where the diagnosis is difficult to reach, nucleic acid amplification techniques may be helpful.

♦ Patients who have symptoms and signs of possible LB but lack laboratory confirmation should not be diagnosed as having LB.

♦ In regions where LB infection is common, a substantial part of the healthy population may have elevated titres against borrelia. A diagnosis of active LB in symptomless people who have elevated borrelia antibodies in the serum is therefore not appropriate.

♦ Culture of the spirochete would be the best laboratory investigation but is difficult to perform and thus restricted to specialized laboratories.

♦ The most appropriate approach to the interpretation of a positive serology would be the application of Bayesian principles of analysis to the positive respectively the negative predictive values of the test, taking into account both the level of background seropositivity and the pre-test likelihood of disease (Table 1.29).

Treatment

Tick bite without any symptoms or signs of primary borreliosis

♦ A tick bite without erythema does not call for treatment with antimicrobial agents (C) [3 4]. In pregnancy, prophylaxis with antimicrobial drugs may be considered (consult a specialist in infectious diseases).

Table 1.29 Bayesian analysis of the post-test probability of disease in relation to the pre-test probability and the endemic serological situation

	Pre-test probability		
	> 80%[1)]	20–80%[2)]	<20%[3)]
Background seropositivity		Post-test probability	
5%	**> 96%**	**61–96%**	**< 61%**
15%	**> 94%**	**49–94%**	**< 49%**
30%	**> 90%**	**37–90%**	**< 37%**
45%	**> 87%**	**30–87%**	**< 30%**

- The basis of reasoning is that a serological test with a sensitivity of 0.95 and a specificity of 0.90 is applied on groups of patients with different grades of clinical suspicion of borreliosis (= pre-test probability) and coming from regions with various degrees of background seropositivity.

1. A pre-test probability of disease > 80% represents a situation where an observed tick bite is followed by an erythema and lymphocytic meningitis.
2. A 20–80% pre-test probability of disease exists in patients from endemic areas showing lymphocytic meningitis or monoarthritis.
3. Patients from non-endemic regions without observed tick bites presenting with non-specific symptoms, for example fatigue and diffuse myofascial pain, have a disease probability below 20%.

- In the case of a background seropositivity of 5–15% a positive serology is associated with a moderately positive likelihood for disease whereas higher background seropositivity gives lower likelihood values.

Primary stage (Erythema migrans or lymphocytoma)

- The treatment time is usually 15 days. It may be extended to 3 weeks if signs are still present after the first 15 days.
- The drug of choice is amoxicillin **B** [5 6].
    - adults 1 g b.i.d.
    - children, 50 mg/kg body weight divided into 2 daily doses
- If amoxicillin cannot be given because of confirmed allergy, the drug is
    - for adults, doxycycline **B** [5 6] 100 mg b.i.d.
    - for children, cefuroxime axetil 30 mg/kg body weight divided into 3 or 4 daily doses (for children a paediatrician should be consulted if doxycycline were to be given).
- Doxycycline is not recommended as the first choice because of its side-effects, especially sensitivity to sunlight, as the infection usually occurs during summertime when people often live an outdoor-life and are exposed to sunlight for long periods of time.
- Pregnancy: The general view is that the infection in pregnant women should be treated. LB has however not been shown to cause damage to the foetus.
    - The recommended treatment for primary LB in pregnancy is amoxicillin 500 mg q.i.d. for 30 days. A specialist in infectious diseases should be consulted when a pregnant woman has any form of LB.

Late stages

- The treatment is time-consuming and demanding. Treatment recommendations from USA cannot be directly followed in Europe because of the difference in the spectrum of borrelia subspecies. The choice of treatment, and especially its duration, is a subject of controversy.
- If the attending physician is unfamiliar with patients with LB, the advice of a specialist in infectious diseases or LB should always be sought.
- Reported results vary from country to country, possibly because of differences in borrelia species, but in some cases also because of insufficient follow-up time.
- There are so far no randomized prospective double-blind studies on the treatment of late LB in Europe, and even some semi-official recommendations for treatment are based merely on subjective clinical experience.
- A frequent suggestion for treatment is a 2–3-week course of i.v. ceftriaxone 2 g daily, for children 100 mg/kg daily. Many authors recommend adding a course of an oral antibiotic after the ceftriaxone.
- In Finland, good results have been reported with a regimen of i.v. ceftriaxone 2 g daily for 14 days, followed by either amoxicillin or cephadroxil, for 100 days.
- In Sweden, oral doxycycline 200 mg daily for 8–20 days has been recommended nationally, however without organized trials.
- Clinical experience indicates that early neuroborreliosis tends to react more favourably to antibacterial treatment than other forms of the disease.
- One should distinguish between failure of treatment because the bacteria have not been eradicated, and persistent symptoms and signs due to permanent damage of tissues by the bacteria. This differentiation would require reliable objective laboratory criteria for eradicated infection vs. persistent infection. Such criteria that would be constantly reliable have not been found. A sharp decline in antibodies may serve as indicator of eradication, or the continued presence of borrelia DNA as shown by PCR technique may be an indicator of persistent infection.
- It has been shown that in some patients borrelial proteins may cross-react with human proteins, which helps to explain persistent arthritis after treatment of Lyme borreliosis.
- There is still no totally reliable laboratory method for assessing the success of therapy. Clinical treatment results should be interpreted cautiously, as the disease can flare several months after an apparently successful therapy.

Prevention of Lyme borreliosis

- Obviously, the best prevention is to avoid being bitten by ticks when moving about terrain where ticks thrive.
- There is no danger in rocky and dry terrain. The ticks thrive in moist terrain, especially in grass. Use the centre of the footpath when walking in the woods.
- Long trousers (light-coloured to help identifying the ticks), tucked into the socks hamper the ticks' access to the skin.
- Every day after moving about in terrain where ticks thrive, the skin should be inspected and any ticks removed. An embedded tick is easily removed by rolling it under a moistened finger tip or by pulling the tick out with pliers. There are special pliers for this purpose for sale in most pharmacies. One should avoid pulling hard on the tick, as its head may remain in the skin and cause local purulent infection. If this should happen, the dislodged tick head will eventually come out spontaneously.
- The method of removal of the tick does not influence the possible risk for borrelia infection. An embedded tick should preferably be removed within the first day, as the risk for infection increases with time.
- Experiments has been done for developing a vaccine against Lyme borreliosis. Such a vaccine must be tailored to fit the local spectrum of borrelia subspecies. Vaccines based on the outer surface protein A of borrelia burgdorferi sensu stricto were for some time used in the United States but are no longer manufactured. The spectrum of borrelia subspecies and the antigenic composition in Europe are quite different from those in the United States.

References

1. Tugwell P, Dennis DT, Weinstein A, Wells G, Shea B, Nickol G, Hayward R, Lightfoot R, Baker P, Steere A. Laboratory diagnosis of Lyme disease: clinical guideline, part 2. Ann Intern Med 1997;127:1109–1123.
2. The Database of Abstracts of Reviews of Effectiveness (University of York), Database no.: DARE-988128. In: The Cochrane Library, Issue 4, 1999. Oxford: Update Software.
3. Warschafsky S, Nowakowski J, Nadelmann RB, Kamer RS, Peterson SJ, Wormser GP. Efficacy of antibiotic prophylaxis for prevention of Lyme disease. J Gen Int Med 1996;11: 329–333.
4. The Database of Abstracts of Reviews of Effectiveness (University of York), Database no.: DARE-961130. In: The Cochrane Library, Issue 4, 1999. Oxford: Update Software.
5. Loewen PS, Marra CA, Marra F. Systematic review of the treatment of early Lyme disease. Drugs 1999;57:157–173.
6. The Database of Abstracts of Reviews of Effectiveness (University of York), Database no.: DARE-990609. In: The Cochrane Library, Issue 4, 2000. Oxford: Update Software.

1.40 Influenza

Terho Heikkinen

Basic rules

- Influenza vaccination is recommended to all persons with high-risk medical conditions and the elderly population.
- The vaccine should be administered well before the expected influenza epidemic.
- It is important to be aware of the local epidemiological situation in the community.
- Updated web-based information about the epidemiology of influenza is available in most developed countries.

Cause

- Influenza viruses are classified into three distinct types (A, B, and C), of which influenza A viruses are clinically most important.
- During the past decades, influenza outbreaks have been caused by subtypes A/H3N2 and A/H1N1 as well as B viruses.
- Other subtypes of influenza A viruses (e.g. H5N1 and H7N7) have also caused severe illnesses in humans during the recent years. Extensive preventive measures have so far been successful in preventing large-scale transmission of these "new" subtypes into human population. However, the risk of an influenza pandemic exists all the time.

Epidemiology

- Influenza epidemics occur usually during wintertime in temperate regions of the northern hemisphere.
- The severity of influenza outbreaks varies between different years depending on the antigenic variation of the circulating virus strains.
- Influenza viruses spread mainly via small-particle aerosols, but transmission can also occur through direct contact.
- The incubation period ranges between 1 to 7 days, but is most often 2–3 days.
- Excretion of the virus may begin already 1–2 days prior to the onset of clinical symptoms.

Clinical presentation

- Varies from asymptomatic infection to severe lethal illness (multiple organ failure).
- The duration of illness is usually 3–8 days.
- Typical initial symptoms in adults include sudden onset of illness, fever, chills, headache, myalgia, malaise, and cough. Rhinitis is not common in the early phase.

- In children, the symptoms often overlap with those of other viral respiratory infections. Rhinitis is present in most children already in the early phase of the illness. Also febrile convulsions may occur in young children.
- The most frequent complications of influenza in adults are pneumonia, sinusitis, and exacerbation of asthma or chronic bronchitis. Pneumonia is usually caused by bacteria (pneumococci, staphylococci or haemophilus). However, influenza viruses may also cause primary viral pneumonia which is often very severe.
- Acute otitis media is the most common complication in children.

Diagnosis

- During a verified local influenza outbreak, the sudden onset of fever and a dry hacking cough are indicative of influenza in adults, although distinguishing influenza is usually very difficult on clinical grounds alone.
- Several rapid tests are available for the detection of influenza in clinical specimens within 15–30 minutes, but the sensitivity and specificity of these tests vary substantially.

Treatment

- Treatment is mainly symptomatic: rest and anti-inflammatory drugs or paracetamol (not acetylsalicylic acid).
- Specific antiviral drugs available for the treatment of influenza include oseltamivir B [1 2 3 4 5], zanamivir A [6 7 8 9 10 11] and amantadine (plus rimantadine in some countries).
  - Oseltamivir and zanamivir are effective against both influenza A and B viruses whereas amantadine is only effective against influenza A viruses.
  - Oseltamivir and amantadine are administered orally. Zanamivir is administered by inhalation with the use of a special device.
  - All drugs shorten the duration of clinical illness by 1.0–1.5 days when the treatment is initiated within 48 h of the onset of symptoms.
  - The effect is inversely correlated with the time lag between the onset of symptoms and treatment initiation.
  - Oseltamivir treatment started within 48 h of the onset of symptoms decreases the rate of development of acute otitis media as a complication of influenza by 40% in children.
  - Elderly persons may find it difficult to use the inhalation device that is necessary to administer zanamivir into the airways.
  - The most important limitation to the use of amantadine is the rapid emergence of resistance to the drug. Resistant viral strains have been isolated from a substantial proportion of patients within 2–3 days of treatment initiation.
- Salicylates should not be used for influenza especially in children and adolescents because of increased risk of Reye's syndrome.

Prevention

- Influenza vaccination is the cornerstone of the prevention of influenza B [12 13 14 15].
- The antigenic composition of the vaccine is changed every year. Therefore, to maximise the preventive efficacy, the vaccine should be administered annually.
- The vaccine is administered intramuscularly. The inactivated vaccine currently available is safe and well-tolerated but local reactions at the injection site are possible.
- Influenza vaccine can be administered to any person older than 6 months of age to decrease the likelihood of contracting influenza.
- Oseltamivir and amantadine can also be used to prevent influenza. However, the preventive efficacy can only be expected during the medication period, whereby seasonal prevention of influenza with these drugs is rarely a reasonable option.

References

1. Nicholson KG, Aoki FY, Osterhaus ADME, Trottier S, Carewicz C, Rode A, Kinnersley N, Ward P on behalf of the Neuraminidase Inhibitor Flu Treatment Investigator Group. Lancet 2000;355:1845–1850.
2. Canadian Coordinating Office for Health Technology Assessment. Oseltamivir for the treatment of suspected influenza: a clinical and economic assessment. Ottawa: Canadian Coordinating Office for Health Technology Assessment (CCOHTA). 2001. 90. Canadian Coordinating Office for Health Technology Assessment (CCOHTA).
3. Husereau DR, Brady B, McGeer A. An assessment of oseltamivir for the treatment of suspected influenza. Ottawa: Canadian Coordinating Office for Health Technology Assessment (CCOHTA). 2002. 12. Canadian Coordinating Office for Health Technology Assessment (CCOHTA).
4. Health Technology Assessment Database: HTA-20020468. The Cochrane Library, Issue 1, 2004. Chichester, UK: John Wiley & Sons, Ltd.
5. Health Technology Assessment Database: HTA-20020370. The Cochrane Library, Issue 1, 2004. Chichester, UK: John Wiley & Sons, Ltd.
6. Management of Influenza in the Southern Hemisphere Trialists Study Group. Randomised trial of efficacy and safety of inhaled zanamivir in treatment of influenza A and B virus infection. Lancet 1998;352:1877–1881.
7. Zanamivir for the treatment of influenza in adults: a systematic review and economic evaluation Burls A, Clark W, Stewart T, Preston C, Bryan S, Jefferson T, Fry-Smith A. Zanamivir for the treatment of influenza in adults: a systematic review and economic evaluation. Health Technology Assessment. 2002. 6(9). 1–87.
8. The Database of Abstracts of Reviews of Effectiveness: DARE-20028442. The Cochrane Library, Issue 1, 2004. Chichester, UK: John Wiley & Sons, Ltd.
9. Health Technology Assessment Database: HTA-20020527. The Cochrane Library, Issue 1, 2004. Chichester, UK: John Wiley & Sons, Ltd.
10. Brady B, McAuley L, Shukla V K. Economic evaluation of zanamivir (Relenza) for the treatment of influenza. Ottawa:

Canadian Coordinating Office for Health Technology Assessment/Office Canadien de Coordination de l'Evaluation des Technologies de la Sante. 2001. 63. Canadian Coordinating Office for Health Technology Assessment (CCOHTA).
11. Health Technology Assessment Database: HTA-20010045. The Cochrane Library, Issue 1, 2004. Chichester, UK: John Wiley & Sons, Ltd.
12. Efectividad de la vacunacion antigripal en los ancianos. Una revision critica de la bibliografia. Medicina Clinica 1995;105:645–648.
13. The Database of Abstracts of Reviews of Effectiveness (University of York), Database no.: DARE-960136. In: The Cochrane Library, Issue 4, 1999. Oxford: Update Software.
14. Gross PA, Hermogenes AW, Sacks HS, Lau J, Levandowski RA. The efficacy of influenza vaccine in elderly persons: a meta-analysis and review of the literature. Ann Intern Med 1995;123:518–527.
15. The Database of Abstracts of Reviews of Effectiveness (University of York), Database no.: DARE-952722. In: The Cochrane Library, Issue 4, 1999. Oxford: Update Software.

1.41 Herpes zoster

Jaakko Karvonen

Basic rules

- Aim at identifying herpes zoster at an early stage to avoid unnecessary diagnostic investigations.
- Start antiviral medication immediately for immunosuppressed patients and if the disease is localized in the trigeminus area.
- Treat other patients with antiviral drugs if the symptoms are severe and if no more than 3 days have elapsed since the appearance of the rash. For immunosuppressed patients the antiviral medication should be started even if more time has elapsed.

Aetiology

- Herpes zoster is caused by the varicella-zoster virus that has remained in the paraspinal ganglia after a varicella infection. Recurrence is not common.

Symptoms and signs

- A linear bullous rash is confined to one side of the midline and occurs most often on the trunk or face (Figure 1.41.1), rarely on the extremities.
- Local pain may begin days before the rash erupts.
  - Remember herpes zoster in the differential diagnosis of chest pain and examine the patient's skin.

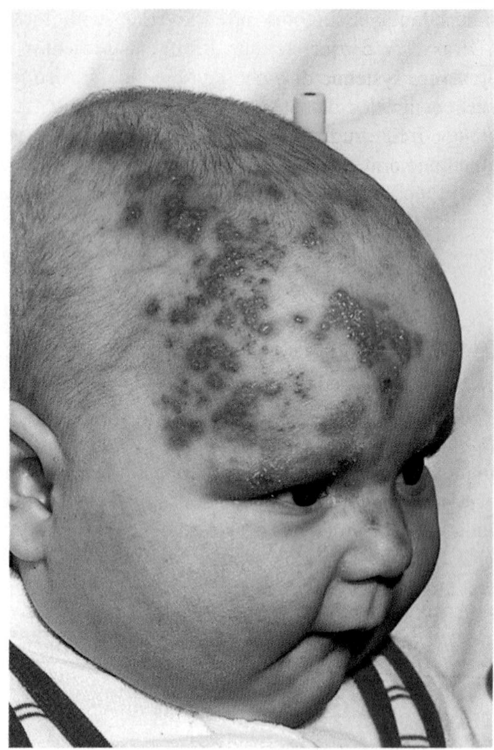

Figure 1.41.1 Herpes zoster in a young child is very unusual. This 7-month-old boy was born during an epidemic of varicella in his family. He had no signs of varicella, and the serum sample taken at the onset of HZ was negative. Two weeks later the level of antibodies to VZ virus was positive. Probably he was infected during the first days of his life, but was protected at that moment by the antibodies received from his mother. Because of nasociliary nerve affection he was treated with parenteral acyclovir. No ocular complications developed. Photo © R. Suhonen.

- If the patient has fever and the rash is not situated in one or two dermatomes on one side of the body, the cause may be primary herpes simplex infection.

Antiviral medication

Effect of antiviral drugs on herpes zoster

- Antiviral therapy started early
  - shortens the duration of the disease
  - limits ulceration
  - alleviates pain in the acute phase
  - reduces need for analgesics
  - reduces the number of ocular complications
  - probably prevents and alleviates postherpetic neuralgia B [1 2 3 4].

Absolute indications

- Patients who are immunosuppressed because of the following diseases or medications should always be treated with antiviral drugs:
  - bone marrow depression (leukaemia, granulocytopenia)

- immunodeficiency
- AIDS or HIV carrier
- any severe systemic disease
- poorly controlled diabetes
- antineoplastic drugs
- continuous oral corticosteroid medication.

♦ Herpes zoster in the trigeminus area should always be treated because of the risk for ocular complications.

- The risk is present if the rash is situated on one side of the nose.
- If the eye is clearly red, the sensation of the cornea is impaired when tested with a cotton wool probe or visual acuity is decreased (possible iridocyclitis) the patient should be referred to an ophthalmologist. The referral should not delay the start of antiviral medication.

Relative indications

♦ Persons over 60 years of age frequently need antiviral therapy, because the clinical course is more severe.

♦ Young patients should be given antiviral drugs if the disease is severe enough to warrant hospitalization.

Dosage

♦ Acyclovir 800 mg × 5 × 7 p.o.

♦ Famciclovir 250 mg × 3 × 7 or 500 mg × 2 × 7 p.o.

- The effective agent is pencyclovir

♦ Valacyclovir 1 g × 3 × 7 p.o.

- Valacyclovir is metabolized into acyclovir and valine in the gastrointestinal tract
- Absorption is superior to that of acyclovir.

♦ Immunosuppressed patients should be treated with intravenous acyclovir.

♦ Local acyclovir creams have limited efficacy in the treatment of herpes zoster.

Adverse effects

♦ Acyclovir, famciclovir and valacyclovir are well tolerated. Serious adverse effects are rare, but some patients may have

- gastrointestinal symptoms
- rashes
- headache
- transient increases in liver transaminase concentrations.

Contagiousness and need for isolation

♦ Varicella-zoster virus may be transmitted during the bullous phase.

♦ The patient should avoid contact with children on antineoplastic drug therapy, as the consequences of a herpes infection may be serious for them. If a contact has already occurred, the child should receive zoster-hyperimmunoglobulin.

Postherpetic neuralgia

♦ Nearly all patients have pain or skin hyperaesthesia after the rash has disappeared. In the elderly the neuralgia may last for years.

♦ Antiviral treatment given in the acute phase probably prevents and alleviates postherpetic neuralgia (A) [5].

♦ NSAIDs should first be tried against postherpetic pain. If they are not effective

- tricyclic antidepressants (e.g. amitriptyline 25–50 mg × 1 in the evening) should be prescribed to patients whose skin is sensitive to contact with clothes (hyperaesthesia) or who are in continuous pain (A) [5].
- carbamazepine can be prescribed for stabbing pain sensations. The initial dose is 100 mg × 2. The dose can be increased to 200 mg × 3 over 2 weeks. If no response is obtained within one week on the full dose, the medication should be discontinued.

References

1. Lancaster T, Silagy C, Gray S. Primary care management of acute herpes zoster: systematic review of evidence from randomized controlled trials. British Journal of General Practice 1995;45:39–45.
2. Jackson JL, Gibbons R, Meyer G, Inouye L. The effect of treating herpes zoster with oral acyclovir in preventing postherpetic neuralgia: a meta-analysis. Arch Intern Med 1997;157:909–912.
3. The Database of Abstracts of Reviews of Effectiveness (University of York), Database no.: DARE-978103. In: The Cochrane Library, Issue 4, 1999. Oxford: Update Software.
4. Tyring S, Barbarash RA, Nahlik JE, Cunningham A, Marley J, Heng M, Jones T, Rea T, Boon R, Saltzman R. Famciclovir for the treatment of acute herpes zoster: effects on acute disease and postherpetic neuralgia. A randomized, double-blind, placebo-controlled trial. Annals Of Internal Medicine 1995;123:89–96.
5. Volmink J, Lancaster T, Gray S, Silagy C. 1996. Treatments for postherpetic neuralgia: a systematic review of randomized controlled trials. Family Practice 1996;13:84–91.

1.42 Mononucleosis

Jukka Lumio

Aims

♦ To recognize the disease and differentiate it from streptococcal tonsillitis.

♦ To avoid antibiotic treatment, for it does not help, even if the pharyngitis is severe.

Epidemiology

- Caused by Epstein–Barr virus (EBV) which spreads by the transfer of saliva ("kissing disease").
- Incubation time varies from 7 to 50 days.
- In Northern Europe, half of the children under 5 years of age, and nearly all adults have serum antibodies to EBV as a sign of earlier infection or subclinical exposure to the virus.

Symptoms and clinical manifestations

- Symptomless or mild fever in pre-school-aged children and therefore rarely diagnosed
- In older patients the symptoms are more pronounced: high fever, tonsillitis, generally enlarged lymph nodes or spleen, hepatitis; oedema of the eyelids (in 15%) may be a prodromal symptom.
- About one out of ten patients gets a rash with small erythematous macules. It will also be provoked in nearly all patients treated with amoxicillin.
- Spontaneous recovery is often seen within 2 weeks, even though fever may persist for 4–6 weeks.
- Hospitalization may be required in cases with severe symptoms or complications, which are rare: myocarditis, autoimmune haemolytic anaemia (AIHA), bleeding (thrombocytopenia), glomerulonephritis, arthritis, meningitis or encephalitis, neuropathies and polyradiculitis, psychic disturbances, and spontaneous rupture of the spleen, which is the most common serious complication sometimes resulting in death (1/3000 of hospitalized patients).
- NSAIDs can be used to relieve the throat pain and swelling, if the patient is able to swallow the medicine. Severe swelling (which impairs eating and breathing) can safely be treated with corticosteroids. These patients belong in hospital care.
- The symptoms of mononucleosis may reoccur or become chronic.

Laboratory diagnosis

- Clinical manifestations, blood picture (including differential white cell count) and a quick test for mononucleosis (several commercial alternatives) are sufficient for making a reliable diagnosis.
- If the clinical suspicion is strong but the immediate test is negative, IgM class antibodies to EBV can be detected from a single serum sample.
- A typical finding in the blood picture is an increase of mononuclear cells (over 50% of white blood cells are lymphocytes). Over 10% of all the lymphocytes in peripheral blood are atypical. Thrombocytopenia and granulocytopenia are fairly common.
- Other laboratory tests are needed only for differential diagnosis. Erythrocyte sedimentation rate is slightly elevated, CRP remains nearly normal, liver function tests, such as transaminases, are clearly elevated (by as much as several hundred IU/ml) and the patient may even be icteric. Bacterial culture from the throat should be taken from those with tonsillitis; simultaneous streptococcal colonization (20–30%) or infection is common in mononucleosis.

Mononucleosis in outpatient setting

- In adults the illness often manifests with a vast number of long lasting symptoms; 1 to 2 weeks of sick leave from work to start with.
- Streptococcal tonsillitis, other fevers, hepatitis and even lymphoma have to be remembered in differential diagnosis.
- Spleen and liver should be palpated; the patient has to be warned to avoid physical exercise if the spleen is enlarged (i.e. the spleen can be felt upon palpation or it is larger than 10–12 cm by ultrasonography; risk of spleen rupture).
- In case of throat symptoms along with group A streptococcus in the culture or antigen test, treatment with penicillin is indicated; there is a risk of peritonsillar abscess.
- Isolation of the patient is not necessary (even symptomless persons have generous loads of viruses). One out of ten patients has a symptomatic secondary infection case in the immediate surroundings. It is advisable not to donate blood for 6 months following the infection.

1.43 Nephropathia epidemica (NE)

Jukka Mustonen

Epidemiology

- A mild form of haemorrhagic fever with renal syndrome (HFRS).
- Caused in Northern Europe by Puumala (PUU) hantavirus spread by a bank vole (Clethrionomys glareolus).
- The bank vole exhibits in 3–4-year population cycles. Most human NE cases occur in the peaks of the population cycle.
- 2/3 of the patients are men. NE rarely occurs in children.
- The risk groups are farmers, forestry workers, animal trappers and soldiers.

Clinical picture

- Symptoms and signs found in more than 30% of the patients:
    - High fever with rapid onset
    - Nausea and vomiting
    - Headache
    - Back pains
    - Abdominal pains
    - Decreased diuresis

- Symptoms and signs found in less than 30% of the patients:
  - Transient visual disturbances
  - Clinical bleedings: conjunctivae, mucous membranes, skin, nose
  - Visible haematuria
  - Vertigo
  - Hypotension, even shock
  - Diarrhoea, obstipation
  - Cough
  - Throat pain
  - Arthralgias
  - Oedemas

Laboratory findings

- Blood samples
  - Elevated serum creatinine in 90% of hospital-treated patients
  - Thrombocytopenia in 75% of the patients in the acute phase
  - Leucocytosis in 50% of the patients (11.0×10^9/l)
  - Elevated ESR 80% of the patients (mean ESR, 40 mm/h)
  - Elevated CRP level in 90% of the patients (mean CRP, 50 mg/l)
  - Elevated haemoglobin or haematocrit in some patients (haemoconcentration) due to drying; later on anaemia is common.
  - Hypoproteinaemia, hypokalaemia, hyponatraemia, hypocalcaemia
  - Slightly elevated liver function tests, e.g. ALT in 80% of the patients
- Urinary findings
  - Proteinuria (albuminuria) in most patients during the acute phase
  - Haematuria is common as well; usually microscopic
  - Pyuria or glucosuria are uncommon.
- Chest x-ray
  - Normal in most patients
  - Abnormal findings are caused by increased capillary permeability and fluid retention: pleural effusion, atelectasis, parenchymal infiltrates, venous congestion and pulmonary oedema.
- Ultrasonography
  - Enlarged kidneys with abnormal echoes are observed.
- ECG
  - Nonspecific findings, ST-depression or T-wave inversion, are rather common. Findings are transient.

Investigations

- Clinical picture
- Laboratory studies
  - First-line studies in an outpatient unit include haemoglobin or haematocrit, CRP or ESR, serum creatinine and urinalysis (clearly voided urine).
  - Antibodies to Puumala hantavirus
    - Often one serum sample is enough because of the rapid increase in antibodies. The result is found out the same day or the day after that.
    - If the symptoms have lasted less than 6 days and the finding is negative it should be confirmed by another sample.

Differential diagnosis

- Other viral infections
- Acute bacterial infections (septicaemias, urinary infection)
- Other types of acute nephritis
- Meningitis
- Acute abdomen

Course of the disease

- There are typical phases in the clinical course; however, they are not seen in all patients.
  - Febrile phase (high fever, pains, general symptoms)
  - Hypotensive phase (haemoconcentration, shock)
  - Oliguric phase (renal failure, fluid retention)
  - Polyuric phase (weight loss–on average 3 kg)
  - Convalescence phase (days, weeks, or even months)
- About 5% of hospitalized patients need dialysis.

Treatment

- In mild cases the patient does not need hospitalization, if differential diagnosis has been considered adequately.
  - Fluid therapy
  - Analgesics
- Send the patient for hospital care, if he/she has
  - Poor general condition
  - Obvious dehydration
  - Fluid retention
  - Renal failure (serum creatinine > 150 μmol/l), anuria
  - Uncertain diagnosis
- Transient dialysis therapy is needed in less than 10% of hospital treated patients. The most severe cases must be treated in an intensive care unit.

Follow-up

- About one month after the acute phase the clinical picture and the laboratory findings are usually normal or near normal.

Prognosis

- NE is not known to causes chronic renal disease.
- For most patients, good
- Lifelong immunity

- Fatal cases are rare. Causes of death have been severe dehydration or shock associated with increased capillary permeability and severe renal failure on admission.

1.44 Pogosta disease

Satu Kurkela, Olli Vapalahti

Basic rule

- The disease should be identified on the basis of the clinical picture and serology in order to avoid unnecessary investigations and treatment attempts.
- Chronic joint manifestations of Pogosta disease should be considered in the differential diagnosis of undefined joint symptoms.

Epidemiology

- The etiological agent is Sindbis-virus (family Togaviridae, genus Alphavirus), which is spread by late summer mosquito species. The disease can be found in most of Finland in August-September.
- Outbreaks of hundreds or thousands of patients have occurred every seventh year in Finland (the last outbreak was in 2002). During the years in between, there are some dozens (up to couple of hundreds) of cases diagnosed.
- Clinically similar diseases in nearby geographical areas are called Ockelbo disease in Sweden and Karelian Fever in Russian Karelia.

Symptoms

- The typical clinical manifestation consists of arthritis, itching maculopapular rash in the trunk and limbs (Figure 1.44.1), fatigue, and mild fever.
- Other possible symptoms are headache, muscle pain and nausea.
- Usually polyarthritis (typically 3–5 joints), especially affecting ankle, finger, wrist and knee joints. The joint symptoms usually co-occur with other symptoms.
- Arthritis typically manifests as tenderness in movement, ache and oedema.

Diagnosis

- When Pogosta disease is clinically suspected, the diagnosis should be confirmed with serology.
- Serodiagnosis is based on measuring antibodies to Sindbis virus (SINV) using IgG-EIA, IgM-EIA and/or hemagglutination inhibition from a serum sample.

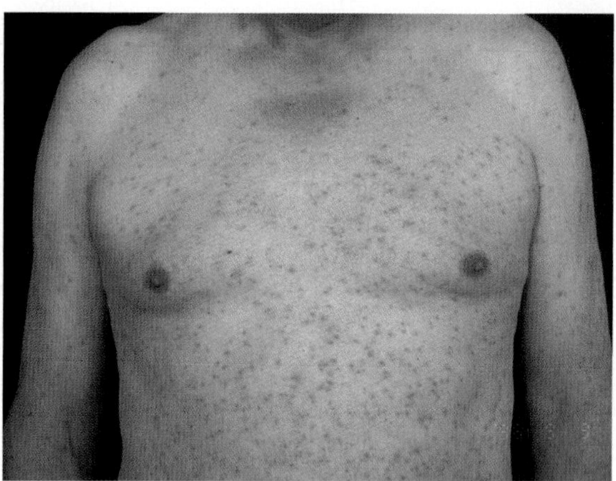

Figure 1.44.1 Arbovirus arthritis, a viral eruption commonly with transient joint symptoms, caused by arbovirus, transmitted in late summer in Finland (Pogosta disease), in Sweden (Ockelbosjukan), and in Russian Karelia (Karelian fever) by otherwise harmless mosquitos. Therapy is symptomatic. Photo © R. Suhonen.

- Positive IgM-result and/or a four-fold rise in SINV antibody titer is decisive for the diagnosis.
- If there is less than a week from the onset of symptoms, a negative antibody result does not rule out the infection, and a second sample is required.
- The majority of cells in synovial fluid are mononuclear – or polynuclear; the total white blood cell count is usually $< 10\ 000$.
- Basic blood picture and CRP are usually normal.
- Differential diagnosis: parvovirus infection, rubella, varicella, rheumatoid arthritis.

Treatment and prognosis

- Symptomatic treatment. NSAIDs can be prescribed when necessary.
- Rash and fever usually disappear within a few days.
- Joint symptoms generally last for some weeks. However, a considerable proportion of patients feature arthritis for several months or even years.

1.45 HIV infection

Janne Laine, Janne Mikkola

In general

- Suspect HIV infection on clinical grounds
  - in patients with a history of high-risk behaviour and who present with symptoms suggesting primary HIV infection

- in patients with unexplained immunosuppression and in young individuals with weight loss, dementia or oesophageal candidiasis, thrombocytopenia or anaemia without a clear cause.

- Serology will become positive 1–4 months after contracting the infection. The patient may manifest primary symptoms 2–6 weeks after infection. Serological diagnosis is usually possible 2–4 weeks after symptom onset or 4–8 weeks after contracting the infection. To exclude the possibility of HIV infection antibody testing should be carried out until four months have elapsed.
- There is no cure for HIV infection, but a combination therapy (HAART – highly active antiretroviral therapy) has greatly improved the patients' outlook **A** [1 2].

Epidemiology

- In 2003, an estimated 5 million new infections with HIV were diagnosed worldwide, a total of 3 million people died of HIV/AIDS-related causes and there were 40 million people living with HIV/AIDS.

Natural course of HIV infection

Primary infection

- Primary HIV infection develops in 30–50% of infected patients, 2–6 weeks after contracting the virus.
- The symptoms may include: fever, tiredness, sore throat, headache, diarrhoea, myalgia, arthralgia and occasionally enlarged lymph nodes as well as an eruption of small papules on the body (Figure 1.45.1). Primary infection often resembles mononucleosis.
- The symptoms resolve within a month.
- Diagnosis is made difficult by the fact that during primary infection over 50% of the patients will be HIV antibody negative when tested with ELISA serology. The HIV antigen test and PCR assay become positive at an earlier stage. A positive PCR assay warrants confirmation with other test methods at a later stage **C** [3 4].

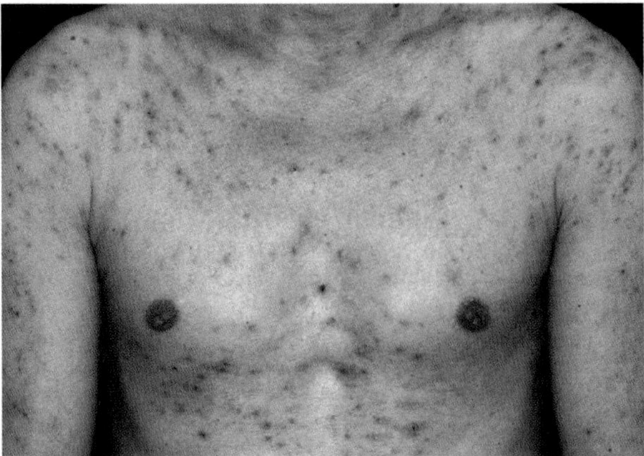

Figure 1.45.1 Eosinophilic folliculitis belongs to the skin symptoms of the late phase of HIV infection. Diagnosis is based on histopathology. The mechanism is probably an immunoinflammatory reaction to the normal skin flora, in a situation of severe immunologic depression. In most cases the HIV infection has caused other symptoms in an earlier phase. Photo © R. Suhonen.

Asymptomatic phase

- Lasts for several years, in some cases over 10 years.
- A high viral load will hasten the disease progression.

Symptomatic HIV infection

- CD4 cell count has often decreased to below 0.35×10^9/l.
- An increasing viral load is often predictive of symptom emergence.
- Symptoms are non-specific, such as weight loss, fever and persistent diarrhoea.
- Herpes zoster (shingles), oropharyngeal candidiasis and seborrhoeic eczema are also indicative of reduced immune response, but do not warrant the diagnosis of AIDS.

AIDS

- AIDS is defined as an HIV infection with at least one of the officially listed opportunistic diseases.
- The introduction of HAART has significantly reduced the occurrence of opportunistic diseases.
- The most common opportunistic diseases in Western Europe are:
  - fungal oesophagitis or stomatitis
  - infections caused by atypical mycobacteria (M. avium-intracellulare)
  - Pneumocystis carinii pneumonia
  - Kaposi's sarcoma.
- Tuberculosis is common in the rest of the world.

Indications for an HIV test

- An HIV test may be indicated particularly in the following clinical conditions:
  - fever, diarrhoea, weight loss or dementia of unknown origin
  - history of intravenous drug use
  - unexplained thrombocytopenia
  - sexually transmitted diseases
  - tuberculosis in a young or middle-aged person
  - atypical pneumonia or fever with exertional dyspnoea (Pneumocystis carinii)
  - widespread oral candidiasis associated with dysphagia or pain on swallowing (oesophageal candidiasis)
  - Kaposi's sarcoma (wine-red or violet spots or tumours in the palate, gums or skin)
  - HIV serology should always be tested on the patient's request.
- The need to test the HIV status must be discussed with the patient. If the patient declines the test, the problems and possible harm caused by the delayed diagnosis, both for the patient himself/herself, the treating personnel (extra

investigations and prolonged treatment time) and other people (infection risk), should be further explored with the patient.

Diagnosis

- HIV antibody test. A positive sample is retested; if it remains positive the laboratory will request a further sample before submitting a result.
- The test will become positive 2–4 weeks after symptom onset or 1–4 months after contracting the virus.
- HIV nucleic acid test should be considered when strong suspicion of the infection exists in a patient with primary symptoms and if urgent diagnosis is required and the antibody test is negative.

Investigations and patient education in primary care

- Adequate time must be allocated for breaking the news of a positive test result. The patient should also be given contact details of how to obtain more information or moral support (AIDS help lines are available 24 hours a day).
- If the result is negative the patient should be given advice regarding high-risk behaviour and the possible need of a repeat test.
- Any unit carrying out HIV testing should be able to provide a patient whose HIV test result is positive with general information regarding the mode of HIV transmission, course of the disease and the treatment choices available. The unit should also be prepared to answer any questions relating to daily hygiene needs etc. (B) [5 6].
- The disease staging and the assessment of an individual patient's prognosis, as well as the decision on specific drug therapies, are carried out by a specialist team.
- As soon as a positive test result is obtained every effort should be made to identify and inform the patient's past contacts, who should be encouraged to agree to be tested.
- An official notification of an infectious disease should be made.
- If the patient is an intravenous drug user the following blood tests should be carried out: HCVAb, HBsAg, HBcAb. A hepatitis B vaccination programme should also be instigated, unless the patient has had the disease.
- The follow-up of the patient is usually undertaken by an infectious disease team.

Treatment

Specific treatment with HIV drugs

- Treatment of an HIV infection requires specialist skills, and the prescription and implementation of drug therapies should be undertaken only by those experienced in their use.
- The development of HIV drugs has significantly improved the prognosis of an HIV infection. No cure exists, but it may be possible to add several tens of years to the life expectancy of an HIV positive patient (A) [1 2]. Quality of life has also improved significantly as has the patients' ability to continue in working life.
- Indications for starting drug therapy for an HIV infection are:
  - symptomatic disease (particularly if AIDS is diagnosed)
  - asymptomatic disease, if CD4 cell count falls below 0.35×10^9/l.
  - an HIV positive pregnant mother (to prevent vertical transmission) (A) [7].
- The treatment is carried out with the combination of at least three antiviral drugs (HAART) (A) [8].
- The drugs that are available today are divided into four groups:
  - nucleoside reverse transcriptase inhibitors (NRTI)
  - non-nucleoside reverse transcriptase inhibitors (NNRTI)
  - protease inhibitors (PI)
  - HIV entry inhibitors.
- Once antiviral drug therapy has been started, its uninterrupted continuation is of vital importance.
  - Development of drug resistance and loss of efficacy may follow irregular adherence to therapy.
  - The treatment must not be interrupted without prior consultation with the treating physician.
  - HIV drugs interact with several other drugs. There is potential for too high or too low concentrations of either drug. Specialist consultation should always be sought in unclear cases.
- Patient compliance is the most important factor in successful drug therapy for HIV infection.
  - The patient is expected to take a large number of tablets and adverse effects are common, particularly in the beginning.
  - To facilitate dosing at the same time every day may involve some lifestyle changes.
- In some countries all pregnant mothers are tested for HIV antibodies. An HIV positive pregnant mother should be referred to the care of a specialist team with expertise in HIV management.

HIV and the general practitioner

- The asymptomatic phase lasts for a long time, and the correct timing of the specific antiviral drugs effectively reduces the occurrence of opportunistic diseases. These patients will visit their GP more often than before with common infections, skin or dental problems or with problems totally unrelated to their positive HIV status.
  - When an HIV positive patient presents with a febrile illness the treating specialist unit should be consulted over the telephone in all unclear cases, particularly if antiretroviral medication has been introduced.
  - Abnormal headache, paralysis, impaired consciousness or visual disturbances in an HIV positive patient always

warrant an immediate referral to specialist care for further investigations.

- HIV is not curable with current drug therapies and the introduction of terminal care may have to be broached at some stage. The options include home nursing services, hospices or general hospital wards. The situation should be anticipated in good time to allow the appropriate staff time to undertake any additional training.

The working capacity of HIV carriers

- During the asymptomatic phase the working capacity of the patient remains normal in most occupations.
- The decreased working capacity during primary infection is transient. AIDS often causes permanent loss of working capacity, but its degree varies according to the occurrence of opportunistic diseases. Working capacity may be restored by antiviral treatment. In some cases the patient can continue to work even after AIDS has been diagnosed.
- Infection risk does not usually contribute towards the patient's inability to work.

Guidelines for health care professionals

- When exposure to blood is a possibility, gloves and a facial shield should be worn.
- Gloves should be worn when taking blood samples, but there is no need to wear a facial shield (if vacuum tubes are used).
- Particular attention should be paid to following recommended procedures in order to avoid needle stick injuries.

Post-exposure prophylaxis in an occupational setting

- In percutaneous exposure, where the source patient is known to be HIV positive, prophylaxis is recommended with a combination of three drugs for four weeks. The treatment should be started within two hours of the exposure. Post-exposure prophylaxis has been found to be highly effective but should be reserved for cases where the potential for infection transmission exists. Prophylaxis after mucous membrane exposure is discretionary. An infectious disease physician should be consulted in uncertain cases and in order to obtain assistance in risk assessment.
- The decision about initiating post-exposure prophylaxis must be made by a physician with HIV experience. Health care staff must have access to post-exposure prophylaxis 24 hours a day.
- An HIV antibody test should be taken without delay and again after (1), 3 and 6 months.
- If antiviral medication was prescribed for prophylaxis, antibody testing may be continued for even longer.
- Official notification must always be made of a needle stick injury.
- During the follow-up period, a condom must be used during sexual intercourse (B) [9].

References

1. HIV Trialists' Collaboration Group. Zidovudine, didanosine, and zalcitabine in the treatment of HIV infection: meta-analyses of the randomized evidence. Lancet 1999;353:2014–2015.
2. The Database of Abstracts of Reviews of Effectiveness (University of York), Database no.: DARE-999298. In: The Cochrane Library, Issue 4, 2000. Oxford: Update Software.
3. Polymerase chain reaction for the diagnosis of HIV infection in adults: a meta-analysis with recommendations for clinical practice and study design. Ann Intern Med 1996;124:803–815.
4. The Database of Abstracts of Reviews of Effectiveness (University of York), Database no.: DARE-968203. In: The Cochrane Library, Issue 4, 1999. Oxford: Update Software.
5. Wolitski RJ, MacGowan RJ, Higgins DL, Jorgensen CM. The effects of HIV counseling and testing (HIV CT) on risk-related practices and help-seeking behaviour. AIDS Educ Prevent 1997;(suppl B):52–67.
6. The Database of Abstracts of Reviews of Effectiveness (University of York), Database no.: DARE-973563. In: The Cochrane Library, Issue 4, 1999. Oxford: Update Software.
7. Brocklehurst P. Interventions for reducing the risk of mother-to-child transmission of HIV infection. Cochrane Database Syst Rev. 2004;(2):CD000102.
8. Rutherford GW, Sangani PR, Kennedy, GE. Three- or four-versus two-drug antiretroviral maintenance regimens for HIV infection. Cochrane Database Syst Rev. 2004;(2):CD002037.
9. Weller S, Davis, K. Condom effectiveness in reducing heterosexual HIV transmission. Cochrane Database Syst Rev. 2004;(2):CD003255.

1.46 Suspicion of rabies

Juha Vuorte

Aims

- Always start vaccine therapy in all suspected cases (see Indication for vaccination therapy)
- Always include rabies immunoglobulin in the treatment regime if
  - the animal responsible for the exposure is suspected to be rabid or
  - the nature of contact is considered to be in the high risk category (see Indication for both vaccination therapy and rabies immunoglobulin).

General

- Rabies is a mammalian, neurotrophic viral infection which
  - is distributed worldwide

- is spread via saliva (either from a bite or through mucous membrane contact)
- will lead, after an average incubation period of 20–90 days, to encephalomyelitis which is always fatal unless early prophylactic treatment has been administered
- causes an estimated 100 000 human deaths annually, mostly in underdeveloped countries.

♦ Treatment with vaccine and rabies immunoglobulin will always prevent the development of clinical disease, provided that
- it is started early (< 24 hours) after exposure
- it is carried out appropriately.

Human infection

♦ Rabies is transmitted via saliva. A rabid animal can transmit the disease to a human through
- a bite or
- a lick on mucous membrane or broken skin

♦ Species of possible reservoir include:
- Wild animals: fox, wolf, raccoon, badger and bat
- Domestic animals: dog, cat and cattle.

Establish the following

1. When and where the exposure occurred?
2. Was the contact a bite, a lick or other type of contact (nibbling, scratching etc.)?
3. What type of animal was involved?
4. Does the animal appear rabid, for example abnormal aggressiveness or other symptoms suggesting central nervous system involvement?
5. If the animal is a domestic animal, what is the vaccination status?
6. Was the animal caught and will it be possible to keep it for observation?
7. Has a veterinarian been consulted regarding the rabies status of the animal?

Post-exposure treatment

Local treatment of the wound

♦ The following measures should be undertaken as soon as possible, preferably at the scene of exposure:
- Remove any dirt or debris from the wound.
- Rinse the wound with running water. Wash the wound with soap and water.

♦ At a Health Centre
- Repeat the cleaning if necessary.
- Disinfect the wound, for example with an alcohol solution.
- Remove any dead tissue, but leave the wound open, i.e. no suturing.

♦ Early, effective local treatment can reduce the risk of rabies by 90%.

Vaccination therapy

♦ Should be started as soon as possible, preferably within 24 hours of exposure.
- In some cases it may be justified to initiate vaccination therapy even after a considerable time delay.

♦ Administered at a Health Centre or hospital.

♦ The dose for individuals not previously vaccinated (unimmunized)
- consists of five 1 ml (2.5 IU/ml) injections on days 0, 3, 7, 14 and 28
- should be injected into the deltoid muscle. In infants, into the upper region of the outer thigh muscle.

Rabies immunoglobulin

♦ Rabies immunoglobulin is usually available from specialist microbiology laboratories; check the availability in your country.

♦ When immunoglobulin administration is indicated it should be administered
- preferably within 24 hours of exposure
- no later than on the day of the third injection (on day 7).

♦ The dose is 20 IU/kg (150 IU/ml) and it is administered as a single dose. Rabies immunoglobulin should be infiltrated into the depth of the wound(s) and injected into surrounding tissues.

♦ Both the vaccine and immunoglobulin may be administered at the same time provided that the injection sites are not anatomically adjacent;
- i.e., if immunoglobulin is infiltrated into the left upper arm give the vaccine into the right upper arm.

Note

♦ Always consider consulting the appropriate rabies advisory centre of your country.

♦ Rabies is a notifiable disease.

♦ Remember the need for tetanus prophylaxis. Prophylactic antibiotic treatment is often warranted in cases of animal bites (for example oral amoxicillin + clavulanic acid orally).

Indication for vaccine therapy and rabies immunoglobulin

No indication for vaccination therapy or rabies immunoglobulin

♦ The contact only involved touching the animal or minor scratches.

♦ The animal has only licked unbroken skin and no animal saliva has been in contact with broken skin or mucous membranes.

♦ A bite or mucous membrane exposure caused by a vaccinated domestic animal

- with no direct signs of rabies
- the health status of which can be monitored.
- Note. The animal must be observed for 10 days! If it shows any signs of rabies, the exposed individual should be treated with vaccine therapy and rabies immunoglobulin.

Indication for vaccination therapy

- A wild animal or a (possibly) non-vaccinated domestic animal
  - has licked broken skin or
  - has caused a small superficial cut to body parts other than the head, neck or a peripheral part of a limb.
- Treatment can be interrupted if the animal does not show any signs of rabies during the 10-day observation period.
- If the animal shows signs of rabies at the time of contact or during the observation period, the treatment of the exposed individual should consist of both vaccination therapy and rabies immunoglobulin.

Indication for both vaccination therapy and rabies immunoglobulin

- A wild animal or a (possibly) non-vaccinated domestic animal has caused one of the following (high risk exposure):
  - a serious and deep bite
  - several bites
  - a bite to the head, neck or a peripheral part of a limb
  - a mucous membrane exposure.
- In cases where it is possible to observe the animal clinically, or to carry out laboratory examination of the brain tissue of a dead animal, it is possible to withdraw the vaccination therapy if
  - the animal shows no clinical symptoms signs of rabies during the 10-day observation period or
  - the brain reveals no histopathological changes consistent with rabies.

1.50 Schistosomal dermatitis

Editors

Causative agent and source of infection

- Schistosomal dermatitis is caused by a worm with aquatic birds serving as the principal host and molluscs as the intermediate host.
- Humans cannot serve as hosts but the cercarias may penetrate the skin and cause a hypersensitivity reaction.

Symptoms

- A papular, itching rash particularly on the feet (after wading).

Diagnosis

- Based on a typical history.
- A cercaria may sometimes be detected from a papule by microscopy.
- No serological test is available.

Treatment

- Itching can be alleviated with ointments and oral antihistamines. The disease is cured spontaneously.

Prevention

- Drying the skin thoroughly after swimming.

1.51 Echinococcosis

Kirsi Skogberg

Basic rules

- Cystic echinococcosis is caused by Echinococcus granulosus, a canine helmint parasite. Alveolar echinococcosis, a less frequent form of echinococcosis, is caused by Echinococcus multilocularis.

Course of the disease

- Echinococci (Echinococcus granulosus and the more rare Echinococcus multilocularis) are tapeworms. The adult worm is 3–9 mm long. Dogs and other canines act as the final host and the eggs are excreted in their faeces. Intermediate hosts include humans, sheep, reindeer and moose.
- Infection to humans is transmitted by ingestion of food that has been contaminated with faeces of the final host. The parasite eggs are transported through the intestinal wall, usually into the liver and lungs, where they form a hydatid cyst. The cyst is filled with infectious larvae and may grow to a diameter of several centimetres. Symptoms usually reflect the size of the cyst and may become evident only several years after infestation.

Symptoms

- The cysts cause no symptoms for a long time and are often found accidentally, e.g. in ultrasonography of the liver.
- The cysts may cause compression symptoms depending on their location (most often in the liver or lungs but also in the central nervous system, bones etc.)
- A cyst rupture may result in anaphylactic reaction or haemoptysis (pulmonary cyst).

Diagnosis

- The diagnosis is based on finding a typical echinococcus cyst with radiographic imaging (ultrasound, chest radiograph, CT or MRI) in a patient with a history of exposure.
- The presence of echinococcus antibodies confirms the diagnosis, but does not rule out echinococcosis. Even false positive antibodies can be present.
- If a suspected cyst is removed, the diagnosis of echinococcosis can be made in a parasitologic laboratory. Even puncture with albendazole protection (to prevent spreading) is a possible, but rarely used, procedure.
- Inspection of a faecal sample for the presence of parasites is of no value.

Treatment

- Surgical excision of the intact cyst
- Albendazole 10 mg/kg/day for 28 days is the drug of choice. The course is repeated after an interval of 2 weeks.

Prevention

- Dogs must be wormed (praziquantel).
- Dogs and predators must not be allowed access to offal and carcasses.

1.52 Tapeworm disease

Sakari Jokiranta

The infectious agents

Diphyllobothrium sp.

- Caused most frequently by Diphyllobothrium latum, D. dendriticum, or D. ursi.
- Crustaceans and fish are intermediate hosts.
- The larvae that infest fish are frequently found in muscles and a coiled larva can be seen as a white mass.
- An adult tapeworm infesting the small bowel is 0.5–2 cm wide and may be more than 10 m long.
- Endemic in Scandinavia, North America, Russia, Eastern Europe, Uganda, and Chile.

Taenia sp.

- Intestinal taeniasis can be caused by Taenia saginata and T. solium. In addition to the intestinal infestation T. solium may cause more severe disease, cysticercosis, characterised by tissue larvae.
- The larvae are acquired from poorly cooked beef (T. saginata) or pork (T. solium).
- An adult Taenia worm is 2–7 m long and 5–7 mm wide.
- Both Taenia species are worldwide in distribution. T. saginata is common in parts of the Middle East, Central Africa, and South America while T. solium is rare in muslim countries.

Other tapeworms

- Hymenolepis nana, H. diminuta, and Dipylidium caninum are tapeworms of mouse, rat, and dog, respectively, but may also cause human tapeworm disease.
- The infections are obtained by accidental ingestion of beetles (Hymenolepis) or fleas (Dipylidium).

Clinical picture

- Infestations are usually asymptomatic but mild intestinal discomfort, abdominal pain, and nausea may occur. Intestinal obstruction is a rare complication.
- Due to vitamin B12 adsorbtion by Diphyllobothrium, B12 deficiency may develop and is characterised by
  - macrocytic anaemia (15.24)
  - smooth tongue
  - neurological abnormalities (paraesthesias of the limbs, ataxia).
- Patients often become aware of the infestation when worm segments are passed in faeces.

Diagnosis

- Identification of eggs or worm segments from a faecal sample is diagnostic.
- Due to sequential release of ova from proglottids several faecal samples may be necessary for diagnosis. Sensitivity of the faecal ova analysis can be enhanced by concentration methods.
- Eosinophilia may occur in taeniasis but does not help in diagnosis.

Treatment

- The drug of choice is Praziquantel as a single dose of 5–10 mg/kg. For treatment of Hymenolepis nana higher dose is used (25 mg/kg).

- Niclosamide is an alternative as a single dose of 2 g for adults. The pediatric dose is 50 mg/kg.
- Niclosamide can be administered in conjunction with a laxative to facilitate expulsion of the worms.
- To verify treatment efficacy the stools are re-examined for eggs three months after the treatment.

Prevention

- Fish, roe and meat should be well cooked, salted or frozen (for a minimum of 24 hours at −18C or −0.4F).
- Meat inspection helps to prevent Taenia infections.

1.53 Trichinosis

Editors

The infectious agent

- The trichin is a parasite of predators. Humans are infected from uninspected, infested meat. The most common sources of infection are poorly cooked pork, sausage, or bear meat.
- The larvae are released in the gut and invade muscles via the bloodstream.
- Once inside a muscle the larvae develop into a cyst that becomes calcified and remains viable for years.

Symptoms

- In the intestinal phase symptoms are mild or non-existent.
- One week after inoculation, in the migration phase, the patient has fever, eosinophilia, myalgia, vasculitis, oedema around the eyes, urticaria, increased blood concentrations of aminotransferases and occasionally a cough.
- During the third week, in the muscle-infestation phase, the patient has myalgia, ocular pain, and haemorrhages under the nails and in the conjunctivae.

Diagnosis

- The diagnosis is based on history and the clinical picture.
- Consumption of uninspected meat (home-slaughtered pork, bear meat) is usually disclosed by history.
- **Eosinophilia** can be observed about 10 days after inoculation, and antibody levels rise after 2–3 weeks. The concentrations of muscle enzymes creatine kinase and lactate dehydrogenase may be increased.
- Larvae can be found in muscle biopsy samples (deltoid, gastrocnemius) most easily on the fourth week after inoculation.

Treatment

- Consult a specialist on infectious diseases.
- If ingestion of infected meat is strongly suspected, give the patient thiabendazole 25 mg × 2 × 7, starting within 24 hours. In later stages of the disease give large doses of mebendazole as a long course (e.g. 400 mg × 3 × 14).
- Initial treatment of the acute phase also consists of rest, NSAIDs, and (for severe symptoms) corticosteroids.

Prevention

- Inspection of meat (regular, thorough).
- Cooking (over 77°C) or freezing meat (−15°C for at last 20 days). Smoking fish or meat is not sufficient.

1.54 Ascariasis

Sakari Jokiranta

The infectious agent

- **Ascaris lumbricoides** is a 15–35 cm long and 0.3-0.6 cm wide intestinal roundworm.
- Ascariasis is worldwide in distribution and is very common in developing countries (estimated 1–1.5 × 10^9 cases).
- The inoculation occurs by ingestion of eggs from the soil. The larvae hatch in the gastrointestinal tract and invade the bloodstream. They migrate through lungs to the pharynx from where they are again swallowed into the gut where the adult cream-coloured worms live.
- The eggs are transported to soil with faeces. They then mature in the soil for a couple of weeks until they are infective. A female worm produces massive amounts of eggs (2 × 10^5–10^6 per day) and this explains the wide distribution of ascariasis.

Clinical picture

- Most infestations are asymptomatic or the symptoms are very mild.
- Vague abdominal discomfort or pain is the most usual intestinal symptom followed by nausea and colic.
- During the migratory stage of the larvae cough and fever may occur in association with pneumonitis; urticaria may also develop.
- Large amounts of worms cause malnutrition and may cause intestinal obstruction.
- Since the adults are actively motile nematodes they may enter the biliary tract followed by symptoms of biliary

obstruction or may even penetrate the intestinal wall and cause peritonitis.

Diagnosis

- Identification of eggs or a worm from a faecal sample is diagnostic.
- Sensitivity of the faecal ova analysis can be enhanced by concentration methods.
- During the migratory stage of the larvae eosinophilia and an increase in the serum IgE concentration can be detected and occasionally the larvae can be detected in sputum.

Treatment

- Ascariasis should always be treated. Treatment for ascariasis should precede treatment of other intestinal worms.
- The drug of choice is a single dose of albendazole 400 mg (for children < 2 years 200 mg). Alternatively, for adults and children > 2 years, mebendazole 100 mg b.i.d for three days (or as a 500 mg single dose) can be used. Also pyrantel pamoate (11 mg/kg single dose) can be used.
- In intestinal or biliary duct obstruction piperazine citrate is given as a single daily dose of 50–75 mg/kg (maximum of 3.5 g) on two consecutive days to cause flaccid paralysis of the worms.
- During pregnancy piperazine or pyrantel pamoate is usually given.

1.55 Pinworm (enterobiasis)

Sakari Jokiranta

The infectious agent

- The causative agent, **Enterobius vermicularis** (pinworm, threadworm), is a white nematode worm. It is exclusively a human parasite.
- The infestation is obtained by ingestion of mature eggs. The adults live in colon and are frequently found in coecum.
- The female worms (8–13 mm long and less than 1 mm wide) come out through the anus, often during sleep, to lay eggs onto the perianal skin.
- Distribution is worldwide and pinworm is the most common helminthic infection in several industrialized countries. The infections are mostly found in children at the age of 3 to 10.

Clinical picture

- The most usual symptom is perianal pruritus, particularly at night.
- Secondary bacterial dermatitis of the perianal region may develop.
- Anorexia or irritability may occur.
- Rarely, the worms invade the female genital tract followed by vulvovaginitis, peritoneal granulomas, or urethritis.

Diagnosis

- For diagnostic detection of eggs, samples should be taken from the perianal skin in the morning before defecation or shower.
- The most frequently used methods for sampling are adhesive tape and a cotton swab.
- Sensitivity of the perianal sampling is increased by taking several samples over a few days.
- Adult worms are diagnostic when visible on the perianal skin or motile on the surface of the stools.
- The eggs can sometimes be identified from faecal samples (successful only in 10% of cases).

Treatment

- The drug of choice is a single dose of pyrantel pamoate (11 mg/kg, max. 1 g), mebendazole (100 mg, 50 mg for children under 2 years of age), or albendazole (400 mg).
- Pyrvine as a single dose (7.5–10 mg/kg) is also effective.
- The treatment should be repeated after 2 weeks.
- The bedlinen are usually changed on the day after the treatment and children's fingernails are trimmed.
- The whole family is often treated at the same time, including asymptomatic family members.
- If many children in a day care facility are infected it should be considered if the whole group needs to be sampled or treated.

Prevention

- The most effective preventive act seems to be more careful hand washing and improved toilet hygiene.
- It might be beneficial to keep children's fingernails short.
- Sleeping in the same bedlinen as a pinworm carrier should be avoided.

1.60 Giardiasis

Sakari Jokiranta

The infectious agent

- Giardia lamblia (G. intestinalis, G. duodenalis) is a protozoan flagellate that lives attached to the mucosa of the duodenum and jejunum.

- Transmission
  - from stools of an infected individual by ingestion of cysts in food or water or through hand contact
  - adding chlorine to water does not reduce infection risk; however, filtering does
  - cysts can remain viable in cold water for 2 to 3 months
  - several species of wild animals may transmit the disease
  - high risk of transmission among children for example in day-care centers
- Giardia is found worldwide with prevalence varying from abundant (5 to 50% in developing countries) to moderate (0.5 to 7% in industrialized areas).

Clinical picture

- Varies from symptomless cases to severe acute gastroenteritis and chronic malabsorption. Abdominal cramps and diarrhoea are dominant features.
- Specific diagnosis cannot be based on clinical picture.
- Symptoms of acute giardiasis
  - Symptoms usually begin 1–3 weeks from infection.
  - Epigastric cramps, nausea.
  - Stools may vary from watery to more solid, and they may be profuse, foul smelling, pale and may float.
  - Tenesmus is present especially in the mornings and after meals.
  - Bloating, flatulence, anorexia, weight loss.
- Symptoms of chronic giardiasis
  - Similar to the acute form but milder and periodical.
  - Recurrent diarrhoea and abdominal discomfort and distention are dominant features.
- The following complications are possible: secondary malabsorption, for example lactose intolerance, even subtotal villus atrophia, pancreatitis, cholangitis, rarely growth retardation in children and possibly also reactive arthritis, urticaria and uveitis.
- Differential diagnosis

Diagnosis

- Based on detection of protozoa cysts, antigen or trophozoites.
- Stool is preserved in formalin, concentrated and microscoped for cysts.
- Usually at least three stool samples are collected 2 to 3 days apart for faecal parasite examination.
- If the laboratory test for faecal parasites is repeatedly negative, the more sensitive method of antigen detection (ELISA or immunofluorescence assay) can be used to reveal Giardia. Unlike the faecal microscopy test, antigen detection does not reveal other faecal parasites.
- Giardiasis is characterized by a so-called prepatental period, which means that the protozoa may be detected in stools rather late after the transmission. Incubation period is often shorter which may lead to false negative stool samples at the onset of the disease.
- In chronic giardiasis the protozoa are few, and detection of cysts or Giardia antigens in stools is sporadic.
- Trophozoites may be searched from duodenal mucus or intestinal wash. Mucosal biopsies should be the so-called touch preps, i.e. a clean microscopic slide is touched with the villus biopsy and allowed to dry before subjecting to staining of the trophozoites.
- Differential diagnosis
  - Other intestinal infections–finding one does not rule out another.
  - Bile disorders, ulcus, gastritis, lactose intolerance
  - Coeliac disease, impairment of pancreatic function and other causes of malabsorption

Treatment, follow-up, prognosis

- The aim is to eradicate both symptoms and the protozoa. Treating symptomless individuals is indicated in order
  - to eliminate the source of transmission
  - to prevent development of further disorders associated with giardiasis.
- The most effective drugs are metronidazole as a 5-day course (the usual dose is 250 mg × 3 for adults and for children 15 mg/kg/day divided into three doses) and tinidazole Ⓐ [1], taken as a single dose of 1.5–2 g; these drugs provide cure for over 90% of the patients.
- Alternatively albendazole (po 400 mg daily, for 5 days) or quinacrine (po 100 mg × 3 after meals, for 5 days) may be used. Recently the Food and Drug Administration (FDA) has approved nitazoxanide for treatment of giardiasis in 1–11 year-old patients.
- In relapses a longer course of metronidazole with a higher dose is often efficient (up to 750 mg × 3, for 2 to 3 weeks). That can be combined with quinacrine (100 mg × 3, for 2 to 3 weeks) in refractory patients.
- During pregnancy, a case of giardiasis with mild symptoms may be temporally left untreated; in an infection with severe symptoms non-absorbable paromomycin po (25–35 mg/kg/day) divided into four doses for 7 days is preferable. There is, however, no evidence of any relationship between metronidazole exposure during the first trimester of pregnancy and birth defects Ⓑ [2,3].
- Relapses occur in most cases 2 weeks after treatment, although they may be seen even after 2 months.
- Relapses can also be symptomless. Control specimens are useful at least 1 and 2 months after treatment.
- It is useful to examine and, if necessary, treat all persons living in the same household with the patient, particularly in case of relapse.
- Prognosis is good, and after the protozoan is eliminated, all the complications will also be cured, with perhaps the exception of reactive arthritis.

References

1. Zaat JOM, Mank ThG, Assendelft WJJ. Drugs for treating giardiasis. Cochrane Database Syst Rev. 2004;(2):CD000217.

2. Caro-Paton T, Carvajal A, de Diego IM, Martin-Arias LH, Requejo AA, Pinilla ER. Is metronidazole teratogenic: a meta-analysis. Br J Clin Pharmacol 1997;44:179–182.
3. The Database of Abstracts of Reviews of Effectiveness (University of York), Database no.: DARE-971056. In: The Cochrane Library, Issue 1, 2000. Oxford: Update Software.

1.61 Cryptosporidiosis

Sakari Jokiranta

The infectious agent

- **Cryptosporidium parvum** is a protozoan of the Apicomplexa phylum and it can infect many animal species (e.g. pigs, calves, sheep, horses, mice, chickens, dogs, cats) in addition to man.
- Transmission occurs readily by ingestion of oocysts in food or water or via fecal-oral route; as low as 10–100 oocysts can cause an infection.
- The parasite lives in the intestinal epithelial cells in small bowel and the infection leads to excretion of oocysts in faeces. The whole life cycle is completed in one individual causing an autoinfective stage and huge production of oocysts.
- Cryptosporidium infects both immunocompetent and immunocompromised individuals and is found worldwide.
- Cryptosporidium infection has been estimated to account for 2 to 6% of cases of diarrhoea.
- Several local and large outbreaks have been reported, largest being an outbreak in Milwaukee and Georgia in 1993 with estimated 403 000 affected persons.
- Two other protozoans, Cyclospora cayetanensis and Isospora belli, can cause Cryptosporidium-like infections.

Clinical picture

- The incubation period is 7 to 10 days.
- In immunocompetent patients
  - more than 90% of infected patients present with watery diarrhoea and epigastric cramps.
  - one third of the patients have a short fever period.
  - nausea is common, vomiting less frequent.
  - symptoms last on average 12 days, varying from 2 days to 1 month.
  - the disease is cured spontaneously.
  - asymptomatic carriage occurs.
- In immunocompromised patients
  - severe watery diarrhoea develops (up to 6 litres/day).
  - the disease persist for several weeks to years and may even be fatal.
  - in HIV patients the infection may be self-limiting if CD4 cell count is 180 mm^3 or more.
- Cryptosporidium can infect epithelial cells of biliary tree and respiratory tract, mainly in patients with AIDS.

Diagnosis

- Cryptosporidium should be considered as the cause of prolonged or acute diarrhoea, especially in immunocompromised patients.
- The diagnosis is based on detection of the causative organism.
- Oocysts are excreted most abundantly and are thus best detected in the early phase of the disease, which is when two samples may be sufficient.
- After the symptoms have disappeared oocysts continue to be excreted in the faeces for about 1 week, sometimes for up to 2 weeks.
- Cryptosporidium can be identified from stool samples using modified acid-fast stains or immunoassay reagents. The acid-fast stain can be performed from the same formalin-fixed stool sample as the routine parasitological examination ("ova and parasites") or from non-fixed faeces.
- Sometimes Cryptosporidium is detected accidentally when faeces is examined for other parasites; however, when Cryptosporidium is suspected the more sensitive acid-fast staining or an antigen detection assay should be used. The staining is also sensitive for the oocysts of the diarrhoea-causing protozoans, Cyclospora cayetanensis and Isospora belli.
- Antigen detection assay (ELISA or immunofluorescence technique) is an alternative for the traditional acid-fast staining. At least most of the commercially available immunoassays are more sensitive in detecting Cryptosporidium. They fail, however, to detect Cyclospora and Isospora.

Treatment and prevention

- Because the disease is self-limiting in immunocompetent patients, the treatment is usually symptomatic.
- In immunocompromised patients no therapy has been proven efficacious. Cryptosporidiosis may be treated p.o. with a long course of oral roxithromycin D [1], azithromycin (600 mg × 1, for 4 weeks), and/or paromomycin (500–750 mg × 3–4, for at least 4 weeks). There is, however, only limited and partly controversial scientific evidence on the benefits of these drugs.
- In treatment of cryptosporidiosis in immunocompetent or malnourished pediatric patients nitazoxanide (2000 mg/day) has been shown to be effective. The Food and Drug Administration (FDA) has approved nitazoxanide for the treatment of diarrhea caused by cryptosporidiosis in 1–11 year-old patients.
- Prevention is based on avoiding contamination, which requires identification of the possible sources of infection, i.e. diagnosing Cryptosporidium infections in human and domestic animals.

- Cryptosporidium is easily transmitted and can, therefore, cause epidemics spread by water, food or person-to-person contact.
- Cyclospora cayetanensis and Isospora belli infections that cause Cryptosporidium-like manifestations can be treated with trimethoprim-sulfamethoxazole. In addition, pyrimethamine can be used in Isospora infections.

Reference

1. Uip DE, Lima AL, Amato VS, Boulos M, Neto VA, Bem David A. Roxithromycin treatment for diarrhoea caused by Cryptosporidium spp in patients with AIDS. J Antimicr Chemother 1998;41(suppl B):93–97.

1.62 Toxoplasmosis

Maija Lappalainen, Klaus Hedman

Causative agent

- The most common latent protozoan infection
- The transmission is usually from cat faeces, soil, or inadequately cooked meat.
- Symptomatic disease is the consequence of a primary infection or the reactivation of a latent infection.

Epidemiology

- The seroprevalence increases with age, and there is no significant difference between men and women.
- There are considerable geographic differences. The reasons are explained by differences in the cat population, climatic conditions, farming methods, hygiene, and cultural habits in regard to cooking food.
- In the Nordic countries and the USA, approximately 80% of fertile-aged women are seronegative and thus at risk for primary toxoplasma infection during pregnancy. In countries with a high number of seronegative women and a low infection rate the actual number of primary infections might be the same as in a country with a low number of seronegative women and a high infection rate.
- Estimates of incidences of primary toxoplasma infection during pregnancy and congenital toxoplasma infection in various parts of the world are presented in Table 1.62.

Source of infection

- Tissue cysts
  - Food (uncooked or inadequately cooked meat) C [1]
  - Organ transplantation
- Oocysts occur in the intestines of members of the cat family. It is estimated that approximately 1% of cats in Central and Northern Europe excrete oocysts.
  - Cat faeces
  - Soil
  - Unwashed and unpeeled fruit and vegetables
  - The oocysts may remain viable for months in warm and moist surroundings.
- Tachyzoites
  - Blood and tissue transplantation
  - Infected secretions
- The tachyzoite form may traverse the placenta during parasitaemia so that the foetus becomes infected. Primary infection in the mother poses a danger to the foetus, but a reactivation does not.

Table 1.62 The seroprevalence of toxoplasma-specific antibodies, incidence of primary toxoplasma infections among seronegative pregnant women, and congenital toxoplasma infections in different countries.

Country	Seroprevalence (%)	Incidence per 1000 seronegative pregnancies	Incidence of congenital toxoplasma infections
Austria	37	1–2	<1/1000
France[1)]	71	2.3	no data
Belgium	56	9.5	2/1000
Germany	68	2.5	0.7/1000
UK [1)]	13	1–5	1/13 000[2)]
Sweden	21	4–6	1.4/1000
Norway	13	2	1/1000
Denmark	27	6.5	3.3/1000
Japan	30	no data	no data
USA	15	1–6	< 1/1000
Australia	35	0.3–0.5	2.3/1000
Finland	20	2.4	0.3–0.5/1000
Slovenia	no data	no data	3/1000
Scotland	no data	no data	0.5/1000

1 seroprevalence among native born inhabitants
2 only manifest cases included

Symptoms and signs

- Acquired infection is often either asymptomatic or the symptoms are ignored.
- The usual incubation period is 10–14 days.
- When symptoms exist, lymphadenopathy is the most common manifestation in non-pregnant and pregnant individuals, causing 3–7% of cases of clinically significant lymphadenopathy.
- Fever, fatigue, muscle pain and dermatologic manifestations may also occur.
- Even without known immune defects, patients with primary toxoplasma infection can develop severe manifestations, such as encephalitis, pneumonia or myocarditis.
- The term **chronic active toxoplasmosis** refers to patients whose symptoms and signs have persisted for months or years. In these patients the parasite or its DNA can be detected in blood.
- **Immunocompromised patients** have often serious sequelae: encephalitis, pneumonia or myocarditis. Antiparasitic treatment is indicated in these patients.
- **Congenital toxoplasma infection** results from primary infection of the mother during pregnancy, but as a rule, not from reactivation of her latent infection.
  - The rate of transmission from mother to foetus increases from less than 10% to 80% with gestational age.
  - Infection early in pregnancy usually results in severe disease, while foetal infection following third-trimester infection is usually subclinical.
  - Most children with intrauterine infection are initially asymptomatic. However, by early adulthood 80–90% develop late manifestations such as retinochoroiditis or neurologic defects. The clinical manifestations of congenital toxoplasmosis range extremely widely from a normal appearance to encephalitis.
- Retinochoroiditis is the most common lesion in **ocular toxoplasmosis**.
- Toxoplasmic retinochoroiditis is usually considered to be the result of congenital infection rather than of acquired infection, although retinochoroiditis related to acquired infection has been reported.

Diagnosis

- The diagnosis of primary infection is usually serological.
  - Toxoplasma-specific IgG and IgM antibodies are first determined from one serum sample.
  - According to the result of the IgM test the avidity of IgG may be determined, and in infants also IgA.
- PCR examinations from the blood, cerebrospinal fluid, amniotic fluid or tissues can be determined if there are special indications.
- Diagnosis of congenital toxoplasmosis after birth requires several serum samples.

Diagnosis of primary toxoplasma infection during pregnancy

- Irrespective of the toxoplasma-IgM result, high avidity of specific IgG during the first trimester is a strong indicator against maternal primary infection; the foetuses of such women are at a very low risk for congenital toxoplasmosis.
- Low avidity of IgG, on the other hand, suggests recent primary infection, and further investigations are indicated.
- Follow-up of the seronegative women could be based primarily on IgG serology. The mothers with verified primary infection during pregnancy should be referred to the central hospital for further investigations and treatment.

Treatment

- Treatment of the immunocompetent patients is in most cases unnecessary.
- Treatment is indicated in
  - patients with severe infection
  - immunocompromised patients
  - pregnant women
  - infants with congenital toxoplasma infection.
- Spiramycin or a combination of pyrimethamine and sulphonamide is the treatment of choice in toxoplasmosis during pregnancy.
- Pregnancy need not be interrupted if repeated foetal ultrasound is normal, toxoplasma-PCR from amniotic fluid is negative and antiparasitic treatment is given.

Prevention

Advice for pregnant women on avoiding toxoplasma infection

- Clean cat litter trays daily (if it is you who has to do it) and wear gloves and wash hands afterwards.
- Wear gloves when gardening, and wash hands afterwards, as well as after contact with children's sandpits.
- Peel or at least wash vegetables that have been in contact with soil. Peel fruit.
- Do not eat undercooked meat (especially on holidays abroad) and wash hands after handling raw meat.
- Do not drink unpasteurized milk or eat raw eggs.
- A common piece of advice for tourists is valid also in this context: "Peel it, boil it, cook it–or forget it".

Screening for primary toxoplasmosis during pregnancy

- Arguments for and against the screening of pregnant women have been voiced.

Reference

1. Cook AJC, Gilbert RE, Buffolano W, Zufferey J, Petersen E, Jenum PA, Foulon F, Semprini AE, Dunn DT on behalf of

the European Research Network on Congenital Toxoplasmosis. Sources of toxoplasma infection in pregnant women: European multicentre case-control study. BMJ 2000;321:142–147.

1.63 Amoebiasis

Sakari Jokiranta

The infectious agent

- The causative agent of amoebiasis is a pathogenic protozoa (amoeba) called Entamoeba histolytica. Entamoeba histolytica is now recognized as a separate species from the closely related non-pathogenic Entamoeba dispar.
- E. histolytica invades the large intestine and feeds on the host's dead cells, red blood cells and bacteria.
- E. histolytica may penetrate the intestinal mucous layer, destroy epithelial cells, cause crater-shaped ulcers, invade the peritoneum via the intestinal wall and disseminate through the venous circulation into the liver and other organs leading to development of amoebic abscesses.
- Contamination occurs when cysts are ingested via faecally contaminated food or drink.
- Adding chlorine to drinking water does not destroy the cysts of E. histolytica, but good filtering systems, treating water with iodine tablets, freezing it to −20°C or heating it (5 min +50°C) will eliminate the cysts.
- Its distribution is worldwide with a higher prevalence in tropical and subtropical regions. The WHO estimates that the annual number of patients with amoebic colitis or amoebic abscesses is approximately 40–50 million, with associated mortality around 0.1%.

Clinical picture

- The most common manifestations of the pathogenic E. histolytica are amoebic colitis and liver abscesses. Other manifestations include:
  - intestinal region: peritonitis, toxic megacolon, amoeboma
  - extraintestinal: skin fistula and amoebiasis cutis, amoebic abscess in the spleen/lungs/brain, pericarditis, amoebic empyema.
- Specific diagnosis is not possible on clinical manifestation alone.
- The incubation period from contracting the infection until symptom onset is from 1 week to 4 months.
- It was previously thought that 90% of patients with E. histolytica cysts in their faeces were asymptomatic carriers. However, over the past few years differentiation has been made between E. histolytica and the non-pathogenic E. dispar which, according to current knowledge, does not induce symptomatic illness. Of the combined E. histolytica/dispar laboratory findings up to 90% are in fact positive to E. dispar only. It appears that most of the patients previously considered to be asymptomatic carriers of E. histolytica are in fact infected with the non-pathogenic E. dispar. Nevertheless, some patients infected with E. histolytica still appear to remain asymptomatic or only have mild symptoms.

Amoebic colitis

- The clinical picture varies from very slight diarrhoea to bloody diarrhoea, i.e. dysentery, which, if left untreated, may be life threatening.
- In addition to diarrhoea, the symptoms may include abdominal pain, cramps, lethargy, low grade fever, loss of appetite, headache and lower back pain.
- On examination the patient usually has a tender abdomen and fever (38%).
- Complications include intestinal bleeding as well as peritonitis or amoeboma following intestinal perforation. Amoeboma is a granulomatous colonic tumour-resembling lesion which may cause local intestinal obstruction.

Amoebic abscess

- The most common is a liver abscess which manifests itself as upper abdominal pain, diarrhoea (in recent past) and weight loss.
- On examination the patient usually has a tender upper abdomen, fever and enlarged liver.
- Leucocytosis as well as increased alkaline phosphatase and CRP values are common.

Differential diagnosis

- In amoebic colitis: other intestinal infections, particularly those causing bloody diarrhoea, as well as ulcerative colitis and irritable bowel syndrome
- Sometimes a stool or intestinal sample for E. histolytica may reveal the presence of other amoebae. Entamoeba coli, E. hartmanni, E. dispar, Endolimax nana and Iodamoeba bütschlii are all non-pathogenic and do not therefore require treatment with antibiotics.
- In amoebic abscess: bacterial abscesses, tumours, echinococcosis, cysts.
- Dientamoeba fragilis is an amoeba flagellate, which may cause an intestinal infection with associated diarrhoea. It can only be detected from a stool sample with the use of trichrome staining or another amoeba staining.

Specific diagnosis

- Diagnosis is based on detecting the protozoa from a stool sample or a colonic biopsy.

- The stool sample may be examined after it has been fixed with formalin or with polyvinyl alcohol (PVA), or Schaudinn's fixative. An untreated sample may also be used. Only the cysts may be isolated from samples fixed with formalin whereas, in addition to the cysts, trophozoites may be isolated from samples fixed with the other fixatives. These morphological studies are not sufficient to distinguish between the pathogenic E. histolytica and non-pathogenic E. dispar.
- Antigen detection may be carried out on untreated stool samples to distinguish between the pathogenic E. histolytica and non-pathogenic E. dispar. Differentiation may also be carried out using methods based on a polymerase chain reaction (PCR).
- In severe diarrhoea, no cysts are formed but the majority of the amoebae will be shed as trophozoites. Therefore, a PVA-fixed sample or an untreated sample (for antigen testing) are recommended for diagnosis. In cases of suspected chronic amoebiasis or suspected amoebic abscess a formalin-fixed sample can be used. A minimum of three samples should be collected with an interval of 2–3 days to accommodate for the periodic shedding of cysts.
- Samples (biopsies) taken during colonoscopy can be examined either immediately for the presence of characteristically moving trophozoites or the samples can be subsequently stained and examined for the presence of trophozoites.
- The significance of stool and colonic samples is small in the diagnosis of amoebic abscess, since in most cases the amoebae are no longer present in the intestines. In these cases, the detection of amoebic antibodies in the serum, imaging of the abdominal and hepatic regions and, where necessary, the examination of percutaneous aspirates of suspicious abscesses are beneficial. A specific diagnosis is usually achieved with antigen detection studies or microscopic examination of the aspirate. However, due to the associated complications this procedure cannot always be recommended.

Treatment, monitoring, prognosis

- The aim of the treatment is to eliminate both the symptoms and the amoebae.
- The most effective treatment of amoebic colitis and extraintestinal amoebiasis is metronidazole 750–800 mg t.d.s., for 7–10 days (children: 10–16 mg/kg t.d.s.). For the elimination of the intestinal cysts diloxanide furoate should be administered 500 mg t.d.s., for 10 days (children: 6.5 mg/kg t.d.s.) or iodoquinol 650 mg t.d.s., for 20 days (children: 10–13 mg/kg t.d.s., up to 2 g/day).
- In amoebic abscesses, percutaneous aspiration of the abscess could be attempted as an adjunct to the metronidazole treatment. Metronidazole may also be substituted with chloroquine.
- During pregnancy, if the illness is asymptomatic or the patient only has mild symptoms, it is recommended that paromomycin (8–12 mg/kg t.d.s., for 7 days) is used rather than metronidazole.
- The aim of treating asymptomatic carriers of E. histolytica is to eliminate the source of infection and to prevent the development of a subsequent symptomatic illness. The first line treatment of asymptomatic infection is usually metronidazole. However, if diloxanide furoate or iodoquinol are available they might be better justified for the eradication of an asymptomatic infection since they both are effective against the cysts. Carriers of E. dispar do not need to be treated.
- Relapses do sometimes occur and 2–3 repeat stool samples should therefore be submitted 3–12 weeks after the treatment.

1.70 Septicaemia

Veli-Jukka Anttila

Basic rules

- A severe microbe-induced systemic infection with usually, but not always, positive blood culture results
- Suspect septicaemia in all patients who are very unwell and manifest severe symptoms.
- Check serum CRP without delay in patients who are not to be admitted to hospital immediately.
- Consider the possibility of streptococcal and staphylococcal sepsis in patients with a skin infection.
- Petechiae and extensive haematoma: meningococcus, pneumococcus or Capnocytophaga canimorsus (for example, following a dog bite)
- Check for nuchal rigidity, and assess the level of consciousness, to diagnose meningitis in all suspected cases of severe infection.

Symptoms suggesting septicaemia

- General malaise
- Fever
- Generalized or local pain
- Chills
- Fatigue, weakness
- Nausea
- Vomiting
- Rapid pulse rate
- Increased respiratory rate
- Skin symptoms (often petechiae, haematoma)
- Low blood pressure
- Confusion
- Unexplained worsening of an underlying illness

Investigations

- Clinical examination: vital signs, auscultate heart and lungs, examine skin, auscultate and palpate abdomen, examine mouth and throat, palpate lymph nodes, inspect anal area.

- A high serum CRP is a good indicator of a septic infection provided that the symptoms have lasted for at least 12 hours, before which time CRP may be normal even in the presence of septicaemia.
- Leucocyte count may increase earlier than the CRP concentration (and should therefore be measured if the symptoms have been present for less than 12 hours). However, a low leucocyte count does not exclude a septic infection.
- A low platelet count supports the diagnosis of septicaemia or other severe infectious disease (consider the possibility of epidemic nephropathia, see 1.73).
- Blood cultures should be taken **twice** before antibiotic treatment is instigated. In septic shock, samples are taken simultaneously from both arms. The samples need not be taken during a peak in the patient's temperature. If high temperature persists, blood cultures should be repeated during antibiotic treatment.

The most common causative agents of septicaemia in a previously healthy individual

- Staphylococcus aureus
- Pneumococcus
- Meningococcus
- Group A beta-haemolytic streptococcus
- E.coli

Treatment

- Intravenous fluids (normal saline) should be started as soon as possible (before transportation to the hospital) to treat the shock. The patient may need several litres. If hypotension cannot be corrected, plasma expanders and gradually increasing doses of dopamine can be attempted.
- If the clinical picture suggests meningococcal sepsis or if the patient's general condition is poor and transportation to an intensive care unit will take more than one hour:
  - start antibiotics (e.g. penicillin G, cefuroxime or a third generation cephalosporin)
  - consult the hospital and take blood cultures before starting antibiotics (if blood culture bottles are not available transport a syringe full of blood in a warm place, e.g. jacket pocket along with the patient). A delay in antibiotic therapy will worsen the patient's prognosis.
- In patients with granulocytopenia (receiving cytostatic drugs) a third generation cephalosporin (e.g. cefepime, ceftazidime) or antipseudomonas penicillin (piperacillin/tazobactam) or carbapenem (imipenem, meropenem) with or without aminoglycoside should always be started after blood cultures have been taken. Ceftriaxone as a betalactam with aminoglycoside can be used, if the risk of Pseudomonas septicaemia is low. Please follow the antibiotic instructions given by your own institution.
- A doctor should accompany the patient during transportation.

1.71 Infections in immunosuppressed and cancer patients

Juha Salonen

Diseases and drugs causing immunosuppression

- Malignant haematological diseases
- HIV infection
- Congenital immunodeficiencies (hypogammaglobulinaemia, impaired phagocytosis, disorders of cell-mediated immunity)
- Organ transplantations
- Prematurity (infants)
- Cytotoxic drugs (including azathioprine and methotrexate prescribed for rheumatoid arthritis)
- Cyclosporin, mycophenolate, tacrolimus
- Prednisolone in doses exceeding 0.3 mg/kg
- TNF-α inhibitors
- Antilymphocyte globuline

Fever in the immunosuppressed patient

- The blood granulocyte count is determined immediately. If the count exceeds 1×10^9/l and the general condition is good or fair, the patient can be treated as a normal patient with fever, but if the count is below 1×10^9/l the patient should be admitted to hospital and a septic infection should be suspected. In severely immunodeficient patients an empiric broad-spectrum antibiotic should always be started immediately after taking blood culture samples because the course of the disease is often violent and difficult to predict. The antibiotic therapy can later be changed after receiving answers from blood culture and sensitivity studies.
- Serum CRP concentration is usually high in immunosuppressed patients with a bacterial infection, but can be near normal right at the very beginning of the infection. High fever is therefore the only certain sign of infection in a neutropenic patient, because e.g. imaging findings are often scarce during severe neutropenia. If the fever has lasted at least for 12 hours a normal serum CRP concentration almost rules out a serious bacterial infection.
- The blood granulocyte count is more important than serum CRP for the decision on hospital admission.

Causes of infection in patients with cancer

- Neutropenia (after cytostatic therapy)
  - Gram-negative rod bacteria (enterobacteria, Pseudomonas)

- Staphylococcus aureus
- Staphylococcus epidermidis (central venous catheter)
- Yeasts (Candida species)
- Aspergillus moulds (especially in severe and prolonged, i.e. lasting for several weeks, neutropenia)

♦ Disorders of humoral immunity (myeloma, chronic lymphocytic leukaemia)

- Bacteria with a capsule (pneumococci, Haemophilus influenzae, meningococcus)

♦ Splenectomized patients

- Pneumococci, Haemophilus influenzae, meningococcus

♦ Disorders of cell-mediated immunity (HIV infection, lymphomas, organ transplantations)

- Mycobacteria
- Listeria
- Salmonella
- Herpes
- Cytomegalovirus
- Toxoplasma
- Pneumocystis carinii
- Cryptococcus
- Candida yeasts
- Aspergillus moulds

Infections in cancer patients without severe granulocytopenia

♦ The granulocyte count is above 1.0×10^9/l.

♦ The infections are often associated with obstruction, interruption of anatomical borders caused by tumours, invasive procedures, and tumour necroses.

♦ The causative agents are ordinary virulent bacteria.

♦ Longlasting hospitalization exposes the patient to colonization caused especially by intestinal bacteria and therefore exposes the patient to severe infections.

♦ The infections should be treated like infections in other immunosuppressed hospital patients.

♦ Local radiation can increase the risk of infection by damaging the mucosal lining of the gastrointestinal tract.

Prevention of bacterial infections in neutropenic patients or patients who have received stem cell transplantation

♦ The key to preventing hospital-acquired infections is properly functioning hospital hygiene which prevents the transmission of infections via hands. In addition, it is important to shorten the duration of neutropenia (leucocyte growth factors).

♦ Even though prophylactic antimicrobial treatments have in some studies been shown to reduce the occurrence of bacterial infections, most experts find the routine use of prophylactic treatment to bring more harm than benefit.

Herpes zoster

♦ Acyclovir treatment (1.41) is indicated in patients with cancer with the exception of cases where more than 3 days has elapsed since the emergence of the first vesicles and several days since the emergence of new skin lesions.

♦ Herpes zoster may be more violent and widespread in severely immunodeficient patients (especially during severe neutropenia) than normal, so it is important to begin antiviral therapy (acyclovir or valaciclovir) immediately after emergence of the first vesicles.

Cytomegalovirus (CMV)

♦ CMV is a significant cause of infection in patients who have received stem cell or organ transplantation. The virus may reactivate during longlasting immunosuppressive therapy in patients who are themselves positive for CMV antibodies and those who are negative for CMV antibodies, but who have received a transplant from a CMV antibody positive person. These patients are given either prophylactic or pre-emptive therapy with canciclovir or foscarnet. The initiation of pre-emptive treatment is based on follow-up of CMV-pp65-antigen or CMV-DNA-PCR.

♦ CMV infection can be treated with ganciclovir, foscarnet or cidofovir.

♦ The mortality rate of CMV pneumonia is especially high. It is treated with antiviral drugs combined with intravenous immunoglobulin.

Tuberculosis

♦ Remember the possibility of reactivation of tuberculosis in immunosuppressed patients.

♦ Prophylactic treatment is considered if

- earlier tuberculosis has not been treated by chemotherapy
- tuberculosis was treated before the year 1970 (before the time of effective combination chemotherapy)
- the patient was exposed to a case of pulmonary tuberculosis in the family as a child.

Pneumocystis carinii

♦ Secondary or primary prevention is indicated according to the aetiology of immunosuppression. Prophylactic medication is given to all patients who have received allogeneic stem cell transplantation and patients with HIV whose CD4 level is below 0.2×10^9/l.

♦ Prophylactic therapy consists of either sulphatrimethoprim, given three times a week, or inhaled pentamidine, given once a month. The prophylactic therapy is continued for 6 months after allogeneic stem cell transplantation, even longer if the patient receives other potently immunosuppressant drugs e.g. corticosteroids or ciclosporin. In patients with HIV the prophylaxis is continued until the CD4 level has permanently risen to 0.2×10^9/l.

- The drug of choice for treatment of Pneumocystis carinii infection is intravenous sulphatrimethoprim in large doses. For allergic patients the alternative drug is intravenous pentamidine. In severe infections corticosteroids are added to the regimen.

Fungal infections

- During prolonged and severe neutropenia patients are usually given empiric antifungal medication, if they still have fever after 3–5 days of broad-spectrum antibacterial medication. The drug of first choice is amphotericin B. There are also newer and better tolerated drugs, e.g. liposomal amphotericin B, caspofungin and voriconazole. These new drugs have been shown to be at least as effective as traditional amphotericin B in empiric antifungal treatment, but their high treatment costs limit their extensive use. Fluconazole may in some cases be appropriate for empiric antifungal therapy, but its problems include poor effect in mould fungal infections and the increasing resistance of yeast fungi.
- Antifungal prophylaxis has been shown to reduce superficial oropharyngeal yeast infections (A) [1]. The prevention of deep fungal infections is most effective in patients who have received allogenic stem cell transplantation. According to current opinion, routine antifungal prophylaxis is therefore indicated only for these patients. The dose of fluconazole is 400 mg/day. Extensive prophylaxis with fluconazole in other immunodeficient patients may lead to increase of resistant yeast species.

Chickenpox and measles

- Chickenpox can be prevented by administering varicella-zoster hyperimmunoglobulin within 3 days from exposure.
- Measles can be prevented by administering ordinary immunoglobulin intramuscularly soon after exposure.

Reference

1. Worthington HV, Clarkson JE, Eden OB. Interventions for preventing oral candidiasis for patients with cancer receiving treatment. Cochrane Database Syst Rev. 2004;(2):CD003807.

1.72 Prevention and treatment of infections in splenectomized patients

Juha Salonen

- Splenectomy increases the risk of serious infections for the rest of the patient's life. The infections are associated with high mortality (as high as 60% in pneumococcal septicaemia).
- The most common causative agents in serious infections are encapsulated bacterias, pneumococci, Haemophilus influenzae B, and meningococci.
- The risk of infection is also increased in patients with splenic insufficiency, including those with sickle cell anaemia, thalassaemia, essential thrombocytopenia, stem cell transplantation, and lymphoproliferative diseases.

Vaccinations

- Absence of the spleen is not a contraindication for vaccinations.
- Pneumococcal vaccine
  - Recommended for all splenectomized patients.
  - The vaccination should be performed 2 weeks before elective splenectomy.
  - A booster is indicated every 5 years.
- Vaccine against Haemophilus influenzae B
  - Recommended for patients who have not been vaccinated when they were children.
  - The vaccine is given only once.
- Meningococcal vaccine
  - The vaccine does not protect from infections caused by type B meningococci. The protective effect against meningococci types A and C is rather short-lived. According to British guidelines meningococcal vaccination should be given to all patients after splenectomy, and before travelling to epidemic areas.
- Influenza vaccine
  - Vaccination against influenza should be performed annually because the vaccination decreases the risk of secondary bacterial infections.

Guidelines in suspected infections

- The patients should carry a note about their splenectomy to inform health care personnel in emergencies.
- In case of fever and chills or nausea the patient should contact a doctor immediately.
- A 5-day course of amoxicillin is indicated after animal bites.
- If a serious infection is suspected in a splenectomized patient a parenteral dose of penicillin can be administered before transportation to a hospital. A blood sample for culture should be taken before giving penicillin if this can be carried out without delay.
- People travelling to areas where malaria is endemic should be informed about the increased risk of severe malaria, and they should be provided with proper proplylaxis.

1.80 Ecology of the use of antimicrobial drugs

Pentti Huovinen

Introduction

- The first true antimicrobial drugs were introduced in 1935 (sulphonamides) and 1942 (penicillin). Since then, hundreds of new antimicrobials have been launched into the market.
- Most antibiotics are prescribed in outpatient care. Some 80% of the antimicrobials used in outpatient care are prescribed for the treatment of respiratory tract infections, e.g otitis media and sinusitis. The next most common indications for antimicrobial drug therapy are infections of the urinary tract and skin. In hospitals, the most frequent indication is surgical prophylaxis.

Development of resistance

- Bacteria have been present on the earth for 3.8 billion years. Depending on the manner of calculation, the human species is a few million years old. Bacteria are able to multiply every 20 minutes in optimal circumstances, and they have an excellent capacity of adaptation to changes in their environment. Some bacteria are known to withstand temperatures of several hundred degrees or survive the hydrostatic pressure at thousands of meters below the sea surface. Thanks to their DNA repair mechanism, some bacteria are even resistant to radioactive radiation.
- During the past 60 years, man's own bacteria and those in his immediate surroundings have been subjected to an unparalleled selection pressure. The use of antimicrobial drugs favours bacteria with a natural resistance to drugs. Susceptible bacteria die and the most resistant ones survive, whereby man may already have altered the species composition or relative frequencies of species in his bacterial flora. As the composition of man's normal microbial flora has so far been beyond study, it is impossible to estimate the changes that may have taken place, let alone appraise their consequences for human health.
- Hundreds of different resistance genes have been discovered in bacteria. They have been surmised to originate from within or without the normal bacterial flora, but bacteria are also able to compile new resistance genes. The pneumococcal penicillin resistance genes, for instance, are a compilation from other bacteria of the oral flora.
- The most worrying feature of bacteria is multiple resistance, i.e. the ability to withstand several antimicrobial drugs at the same time. Many resistant bacteria of clinical relevance possess multiple resistance. Bacteria are able to collect resistance-coding genes into gene cassettes that are transferred from one bacterium to another. On the other hand, resistance may also be encoded by mutations in chromosomal genes.

Control of resistance

- Resistance poses problems for everyday clinical work within primary care and especially in hospitals. As the use of antimicrobial drugs is a necessity, bacterial resistance will remain a permanent problem. Although there is a constant effort to reduce the use of antimicrobial drugs, it appears instead that their use is increasing all the time, resulting in further aggravation of the resistance problem.
- New antimicrobial drugs do not present a solution to the problem. Although there is continual drug development, new drugs are likely to offer only short-term remediation. The development of a new drug takes at least 5–12 years.
- Bacterial resistance can be controlled by reducing the use of antimicrobials and by preventing bacteria from spreading.
    - Always try to reach a precise diagnosis. Use laboratory tests and radiography according to recommendations.
    - Use antimicrobial drugs only when needed. Do not deviate from the therapeutic recommendations for the various indications, unless you have a valid reason for doing so.
    - If you decide not to start antimicrobial drug therapy, ensure careful follow-up of the patient.
    - Adhere to stringent hand hygiene. Alcohol-based hand rubs are clearly better than regular soap in reducing hand contamination (B) [1].
- It is probable that the level of hygiene influences the spread of resistant bacteria. In hospitals the hands of staff and patients are the most important factor in spreading microbes. In many countries, an optimal climate maintains an abundant flora, which in turn contributes to the problem of resistance.
- In the future, in all countries and especially in ambulatory care there is a need to improve hygiene. For example, day care centres are important in spreading infections among children.

The importance of normal flora increases

- It is in the patient's interest that antimicrobial drugs be used only when clearly necessary. Several studies have found that antimicrobial treatment increases the patient's risk of being colonised by new resistant bacteria. Animal experiments have shown that 1000 to 100 000 times less bacteria are needed for colonisation during antimicrobial treatment than without such treatment.
- Antimicrobial drugs destroy bacteria of the normal flora, and the resultant vacuum is easily occupied by foreign resistant bacteria that now have room to proliferate. The patient then starts shedding these resistant bacteria, thereby facilitating their spreading.
- In young women, antimicrobial treatment of any infection involves a two- to fivefold risk of urinary infection. This is probably due to the suppression of normal bacterial flora, which favours colonisation by pathogenic bacteria two to four weeks after the treatment.
- Preliminary studies suggest that correction of the disturbance in bacterial flora by means of oral and oropharyngeal alpha-haemolytic streptococci after antimicrobial treatment affords

a statistically significant protection against the recurrence of otitis media and pharyngitis.

Diarrhoea caused by antibiotics

- Suppression of the normal intestinal flora allows Clostridium difficile to grow in the intestine. C. difficile produces diarrhoeagenic toxins. Its significance has increased, especially with the increased use of cephalosporins. Wide-spectrum antibiotics together with repeated treatments are important risk factors for antibiotic-associated diarrhoea.
- Prevention of antibiotic-associated diarrhoea: Avoid unnecessary use of antimicrobial drugs. Isolate patients with antibiotic-associated diarrhoea in hospitals. Adhere to good hand hygiene. In children, the administration of Lactobacillus GG capsules brings about a statistically significant prevention of antibiotic-associated diarrhoea. In addition, Saccharomyces boulardii yeast product can help to reduce recurrent episodes of antibiotic-associated diarrhoea.

Successful and safe treatment

- Preserving the efficacy in the future requires the avoidance of unnecessary use of antimicrobic drugs and the correction of biased treatment practices.
- Efficacy and safety are not independent of each other. The use of new broad-spectrum antimicrobial drugs in outpatient care is very rarely justified in the changed resistance situation. On the contrary, over-enthusiastic use of wide-spectrum drugs causes unnecessary suppression of normal flora and promotes development of resistance to these drugs that are not intended for first-line therapy.
- By following up the development of bacterial resistance situation and the consumption of antimicrobial drugs, guidelines promoting efficient and safe antimicrobial treatment can be drafted and issued.

Reference

1. Girou E, Loyeau S, Legrand P, Oppein F, Brun-Boisson C. Efficacy of handrubbing with alcohol based solution versus standard handwashing with antiseptic soap: randomised clinical trial. BMJ 2002;325:362.

1.81 Guidelines for antimicrobial therapy

Editors

- These guidelines (Table 1.81) have been collected from other guidelines in the EBMG. The numbers indicate priority of the drugs. Careful clinical and laboratory investigations are essential to proper diagnosis. Local resistance patterns should always be considered before making decisions on individual patients.

Table 1.81 Recommendations for antimicrobial treatment (the numbers indicate priority)

Indication, drug	Dosage	Remarks
Tonsillitis		
1. Penicillin V	adults: 1–1.5 million IU × 2 × 10 children: 50 000–100 000 IU/kg/day/2 × 10	
2. Cephalexin/Cefadroxil	adults: 750/500 mg × 2–3 × 10 children: 50 mg/kg/day/2 × 10	In penicillin allergy without anaphylaxis
3. Clindamycin	adults: 150 mg × 4 or 300 mg × 2–3 × 10 children: 20 mg/kg/day/3 × 10	For patients with anaphylactic penicillin allergy
Sinusitis or otitis media in the adult		
1. Amoxicillin	500–750 mg × 2 × 5–7	
2. Doxycycline	150 mg × 1 × 5–7 or 100 mg × 2 one day, then 100 mg × 1× 5–7	
3. Amoxicillin clavulanate	750 mg × 2 × 5–7	
4. Cefaclor	500 mg × 2 × 7	Only if allergic to other drugs
Azithtromycin	500 mg, 250 mg × 1 × 4	Only if allergic to other drugs
Roxithromycin	150 mg × 2 × 7	Only if allergic to other drugs
Otitis media or sinusitis in the child		
1. Amoxicillin	40 mg/kg/day/2 × 5–7	
Penicillin V	100 000 IU/kg/day/2 × 5–7	
2. Amoxicillin clavulanate	40–45 mg/kg/day/2 × 7	
3. Cefaclor	40 mg/kg/day/2 × 7	Only if allergic to other drugs
Cefuroxime axetil	40 mg/kg/day/2 × 7	Only if allergic to other drugs

Table 1.81 (*continued*)

Indication, drug	Dosage	Remarks
Pneumonia in ambulatory care		
1. Penicillin V	1 mill. IU × 4 × 10	Suspected pneumococcal pneumonia: rapid onset, chills, increased blood leucocyte count and serum CRP, consider hospital care
Roxithromycin	150 mg × 2 × 10	Or some other macrolide
2. Doxycycline	100 mg × 2 × 10	
Community-acquired pneumonia in the hospital		
1. Penicillin G	1–2 mill. IU × 4 i.v.	Strong suspicion of pneumococcal pneumonia
2. Cefuroxime	1.5 g × 3 i.v.	Severe pneumonia (respirations > 30/min, hypoxia), unknown aetiology. Consider also in combination with macrolide drugs.
Pneumonia in children		
1. Amoxicillin	40 mg/kg/day/2 × 7–10	Children under 4 years of age
Erythromycin	40 mg/kg/day/3 × 10	Children above 4 years of age, and in penicillin allergy
Urinary tract infection in the adult in ambulatory care (the local resistance pattern should guide the choice of drug)		
1. Trimethoprim	160 mg × 2 × 5 or 300 mg × 1 × 5	Varying resistance especially in aged patients
Nitrofurantoin	75 mg × 2 × 5	Not in renal insufficiency
Pivmecillinam	200 mg × 3 × 5	Not effective against Staphylococcus saprophyticus
2. Norfloxacin	400 mg × 2 × 3–7	
Ciprofloxacin	100–250 mg × 2 × 3	Complicated infections and pyelonephritis: 250–500 mg × 2 × 7–14
Levofloxacin	250 mg × 1 × 3–7	
Cephalexin	500 mg × 2 × 5–7	
Cefadroxil	500 mg × 1 × 5–7	
Fosfomycin	3 g × 1 × 1	
Renal insufficiency:		
3. Cephalexin, cefadroxil, amoxicillin, pivmecillinam		
Pregnancy:		
Pivmecillinam, nitrofurantoin, cephalexin, cefadroxil, amoxicillin according to the antibiogram		
Urinary tract infection with fever in the hospital		
1. Cefuroxime	1.5 g × 3 i.v.	
Urinary tract infection in a child (treat infants for 10 days, cystitis in older children for 5 days)		
1. Nitrofurantoin	5 mg/kg/day/2	
2. Cephalexin	40 mg/kg/day/2	
3. Trimethoprim	8 mg/kg/day/2	
4. Pivmecillinam	20–40 mg/kg/day/3	
Mastitis		
1. Cephalexin	500 mg × 3 × 7	
Cefadroxil		
2. Roxithromycin	150 mg × 2 × 7	Or some other macrolide
Erysipelas		
1. Penicillin G	1–3 mill. IU × 4 i.v.	Followed by penicillin V orally for at least three weeks
Procaine penicillin	1.2–1.5 (–2.4) mill. IU × 1	Followed by penicillin V orally for at least three weeks

(*continued overleaf*)

Table 1.81 (*continued*)

Indication, drug	Dosage	Remarks
2. Cefuroxime	750–1 500 mg × 3 i.v.	
Clindamycin	300–600 mg × 4 i.v.	For patients with allergy for penicillin
Further treatment: Penicillin V 1.5 mill. IU × 2 or cephalexin 750 mg × 2 or cefadroxil 1 g × 1		
Prophylactic medication: Penicillin V 1.5 mill. IU × 1 (–2) perorally or benzatine penicillin 1.2–1.4 mill. IU i.m. every 3rd-4th week		
Impetigo in children		
Cephalexin	50 mg/kg/day/3 × 7	
Cefadroxil	50 mg/kg/day/3 × 7	
Purulent skin infection caused by staphylococci in adults		
Cephalexin	500 mg × 3 × 7	
Cefadroxil	500 mg × 2 × 7	
Eradication of Helicobacter pylori		
Amoxicillin **and**	1000 mg × 2 × 7	Recurrent infection, see 8.32.
Clarithromycin **and**	500 mg × 2 × 7	
Proton pump inhibitor	Normal doses	
Campylobacter		
Roxithromycin	150 mg × 2 × 10 (or some other macrolide)	
Salmonella gastroenteritis		
Ciprofloxacin (or some other fluoroquinolone)	500–750 mg × 2 × 14	Always assess the need for antimicrobial treatment individually
Gonorrhoea		
1. Ciprofloxacin	500 mg as a single dose	
2. Ceftriaxone	250 mg i.m. single dose	
Chlamydial urethritis or cervicitis		
1. Azithromycin	1000 mg as a single dose	
Doxycycline	100 mg × 2 × 7–10, 100–150 mg × 2 × 21	Complicated or recurrent disease
Erythromycin	500 mg × 3 × 10	During pregnancy

1.93 Streptococcal epidemics

Marjukka Mäkelä

Basic rule

- Identify and control epidemics quickly.

Aetiology

- Group A streptococci are the most common cause of epidemics, but group C and G may also cause them.
- The epidemics can be food-borne (particularly if the epidemic is severe).

Diagnosis

- Epidemics commonly occur in day-care institutions, schools and military units.
- Suspect an epidemic if
  - several patients come from one family or other unit in a short time, or
  - the same patient has recurrent streptococcal disease.

Treatment

- A nurse should visit the site of the epidemic and take streptococcal culture both from symptomatic and asymptomatic people.
- All persons with positive cultures are treated simultaneously, and kept away from day care, school or work for one day after starting treatment whether they have symptoms or not. Symptomatic patients may need a longer sick leave. Control samples need not be taken after treatment.
- Consider also taking cultures from and treating family members of symptomatic patients.
- Food-borne epidemics
  - The disease usually manifests as tonsillitis.
  - All kitchen personnel should be cultured and treated as usual.
- Treat with penicillin V or a first generation cephalosporin for ten days (38.20).

Travelling and Tropical Diseases

Evidence Based Medicine Guidelines. Edited by the Duodecim Editorial Team
 ISBN: 0-470-01184-X

2.1 Traveller's infection prophylaxis

Terhi Heinäsmäki

Aims

- To ensure adequate and specific protection against certain diseases.
- To inform about other measures of health protection.
- To start prophylaxis and protection early enough, no later than 3 months before travel, for those who will stay in the tropics for a long time and for chronically ill persons.

Grouping of patients

- Destination
  - Europe and North America
  - Charter flights to tourist destinations
  - Other
- Duration and type of trip
  - Short (less than one month) or longer
  - Holiday or business
  - In cities or also in the countryside (jungle)

Specific protection according to the infectious agent

- Europe and North America
  - Routine vaccinations
  - Consider Hepatitis A vaccination or gammaglobulin when Eastern Europe is the destination
- Charter flights to tourist destinations
  - Routine vaccinations
  - Other vaccinations depending on the destination
  - Malaria prophylaxis, if indicated (rarely)
  - Consider hepatitis A vaccination or gammaglobulin
- Other
  - Individual prophylaxis depending on the destination and type of the trip

Routine vaccinations

- Tetanus, diphtheria
- A polio booster is recommended every 5–10 years, even for short trips, when travelling in areas where the risk of infection is considerable.
- For children; also pertussis and haemophilus
- Always for children over 6 months of age, for adults if particularly indicated: measles, mumps, rubella
- Diphtheria vaccination is recommended for persons over 30 years of age travelling to high-risk areas in Russia, former Soviet states or the Baltic.

Hepatitis A vaccination or gammaglobulin

- Recommended for following destinations: Africa, Asia, South and Central America, Pacific islands, Middle East and repeated trips to Baltic countries, Russia, and other Eastern European countries and North Mediterranean countries.
- Vaccination is nowadays the primary method of protection against hepatitis A. Two vaccinations are available. Havrix® R 1440 ELISA-U/ml vaccine is given for persons over 15 years; children aged 1–15 years are given half the dose. For the Epaxal® vaccine the dose is the same for both adults and children from 2 years of age onwards. The vaccination should be given 2 weeks before travelling. A booster vaccination given 6 to 12 months later gives protection for 10–20 years.
- Twinrix Adult and Twinrix Paediatric vaccines protect against both Hepatitis A and B. The first is for immunization of over 15-year-olds and the latter for 1–15-year-olds. The vaccination series includes three doses at 0, 1 and 6 months.
- Gammaglobulin is an alternative on short trips when vaccination is not desired. It gives an 80–90% protection against hepatitis A for 2 to 4 months. The dose is 2 ml for adults and 0.02–0.04 ml/kg i.m. for children under 12 years of age. Gammaglobulin should be given at least a week before the trip.

Malaria prophylaxis

- Is initiated as a rule a week before the journey and continued, depending on the medication, for 1 to 4 weeks after the journey (2.2).

Additional vaccinations

- There are more than 20 different vaccinations–**choose only those that are necessary for the individual traveller**.
- To be considered:
  - Yellow fever is endemic in Africa and South America, but not in Asia. In many countries near the equator vaccination is obligatory for those who come from endemic areas. One injection of the vaccine (Stamaril®) is given at least 10 days before the journey. The only acceptable vaccination certificate is the one issued by the WHO, which must include the date of vaccination, signature of the physician, and name and batch number of the vaccine as well as the official status of a vaccination clinic authorized to give yellow fever immunization. The certificate becomes effective 10 days after the first vaccination and immediately after a booster. The certificate is valid for 10 years.
  - Japanese encephalitis (Far East, countryside). The endemic area reaches from Japan and Korea to India and Nepal. Inactivated vaccine (Je-VAX*) is given in three subcutaneous 1 ml doses (to children from 1 to 3 years, 0.5 ml) on days 0, 7 and 30 (or 0, 7 and 14, if necessary because of

time schedule). The third dose should be given at least 10 days before the journey. A booster is necessary at 3-year intervals if the person stays in endemic areas. Immunization is recommended for persons staying in endemic areas for more than a month during normal times of occurrence and even for shorter stays during epidemics.

- Hepatitis B is endemic in large areas around the world. Vaccination (Engerix-B®) is given in three doses at months 0, 1 and 6. Immunization is recommended for persons staying in endemic areas for longer than 6 months and for those whose work contains the risk of blood contact or other risk of acquiring hepatitis B (small child, sexual contacts, use of i.v. drugs). About 10% of the vaccinated persons do not obtain sufficient immunity. If the risk of exposure to the virus is high and long-lasting, the presence of immunity should be confirmed serologically about 2 months after the third dose. If there is no antibody response, the risk of exposure should be decreased by e.g. job arrangements.
- Vaccination against meningococci (Meningovax A+C®, Mencevax ACWY®) is recommended for persons staying for longer periods in the country or in small cities outside tourist regions in Asia, Africa or South America. ACWY vaccination is obligatory for pilgrims in Saudi Arabia.
- Oral cholera vaccination is recommended only to people who are going to spend long times in endemic areas in bad hygiene conditions. A special permit is required for the vaccination. A cholera vaccination certificate may be "unofficially obligatory" in some countries, although WHO does not recommend it in international travelling.
- Typhoid vaccination (Vivotif® orally, Typherix® intramuscularly) is recommended for persons staying for longer periods in the country or in small cities outside tourist regions in Asia, Africa or South America. Typhoid is best avoided with good hand and food hygiene.
- Rabies vaccination (for those who work among wild animals in endemic areas, possibly for small children in countries where stray dogs are abundant). WHO has founded an information and mapping system for rabies, where updated information can be found, www.rabnet.who.int
- Tick encephalitis vaccination (TBE) for persons over 7 years of age staying for longer periods in endemic areas in Siberia, Baltic countries or Central Europe. In children younger than 7 years the infection rarely leads to more serious complications.

- If necessary, all vaccinations can be given at the same time. Two live vaccines must be given either at the same time or with at least a 1-month interval (yellow fever, oral typhoid vaccination, MMR).

Other protective measures

- Written instructions on sensible eating and hygiene
- Suitable clothing and footwear
- Mosquito repellents and nets
- Condom protects against STDs and HIV
- Diarrhoea prophylaxis (2.3)–alcohol is not beneficial
- Protection against UV radiation

2.2 Diagnosis and prevention of malaria in travellers

Heli Siikamäki

Basic rules

- **Fever in a traveller returning from the tropics should be regarded as malaria until proven otherwise.**
- **The diagnosis must be made and treatment started urgently**.
- Incubation time is usually 7–30 days, but may also be months or even years from infection.
- In addition to fever, the patient may have diarrhoea, icterus or may suffer from confusion; blood count may show reduced amounts of leukocytes and platelets.
- It is recommended to consult a specialist when malaria is suspected.
- Prevention of malaria is vital when travelling in the tropics.
- Travellers should always be reminded that there is no perfect protection against malaria, and that fever after returning home is always a reason to see a doctor.

Epidemiology

- Malaria is globally the most serious infectious disease. Yearly 300–400 million people are affected, and it is estimated that 1.5–2.5 million people, mostly children, die of it every year.
- Malaria is an increasing problem in those Western countries where travelling to the tropics has become more common.
- Increasing resistance to drugs of the malaria parasite makes prevention and treatment difficult.
- Doctors giving advice to travellers should keep their skills up-to-date by following reports on the prevalence and resistance as well as recommendations on prophylaxis. WHO publishes yearly a handbook on vaccinations and prophylaxis (International Travel and Health. Vaccination Requirements and Health Advice www.who.int).

Diagnosis of malaria

- **Always an urgent measure**
- Capillary sample from fingertip, preferably during a fever peak (several if necessary)
    - **3–4 thin smear preparations** at least one of which should be fixed, stained and examined immediately under magnification of 1:1000. The usual May–Grunwald–Giemsa stain can be used, plain Giemsa is usually better.

- **3–4 thick smear preparations**. Drop 2–3 drops of capillary blood on a slide, spread it out to a 2 × 2 cm patch by rubbing with a glass rod for about 30 s, allow to dry thoroughly, do not fix.

- Preparations are sent to a laboratory without being fixed or stained. Remember to include a travel history and information on malaria prophylaxis or treatment in the referral.
- One negative sample does not exclude malaria. Sampling should be repeated after 3–4 hours and during a fever peak.

Treatment of malaria

- Following drugs can be used for treatment of malaria:
  - Plasmodium falciparum
    - quinine alone or in combination with doxycycline
    - mefloquine
    - combination of atovaquone and proquanil
    - artemisin derivates B [5] [6] either alone or in combination.
  - Plasmodium ovale, P. vivax, P. malariae
    - chloroquine
    - primaquine for eradication of hypnozoite forms of Plasmodium vivax and ovale after chloroquine treatment.

Avoiding mosquito stings in endemic areas

- Mechanical avoidance
  - Mosquito nets on windows and at doors, bed net (preferably one impregnated with permethrin A [1]) that can be folded under the mattress.
  - Insecticides to kill mosquitoes, inside dwelling quarters, particularly in the bedroom
  - Wearing light-coloured clothes that cover the skin well between dusk and dawn. Clothes can be treated with permethrin, which stays on for a few washings and does not ruin them.
  - Mosquito repellents (diethyltoluamide) should be used on bare skin when outdoors in the dark.

Recommended malaria prophylaxis in short-term exposure

For updated recommendation for specific area consult international Travel and Health (www.who.int)

Dosage of prophylatic drugs in adults

- Mefloquine A [2]
  - 250 mg tablet: 1 tablet/week
  - start one week before, continue 4 weeks after exposure.
- Malarone®
  - atovaquone 250 mg, proguanil 100 mg: 1 tablet/day
  - start one day before, continue one week after exposure.
- Doxycycline
  - 100 mg: 1 tablet/day
  - start one day before, continue 4 weeks after exposure.
- Proguanil
  - only with chloroquine
  - 100 mg tablet: 2 tablets/day
  - start one day before, continue 1–4 weeks after exposure.
- Chloroquine
  - 250 mg tablet: 2 tablets/week
  - start one week before, continue 4 weeks after exposure.
- Safe drugs during pregnancy are chloroquine and a combination of chloroquine and proguanil C [3] [4]. According to WHO, mefloquine can also be used C [3] [4], but only starting from the 4th month of pregnancy.
- Mefloquine should not be prescribed to persons with a history of depression or convulsions.

Prophylaxis in children

- See Table 2.2
- Prophylaxis is especially important for children as the infection can become complicated more quickly than in adults.
- Mosquito repellents may irritate the skin and are therefore not recommended for children under the age of 3 years.
- Chloroquine and proguanil can be used for prophylaxis from the age on 1 month onwards.

Table 2.2 Malaria prophylaxis dose (tablets)

Drug	Dose (mg)	Adults	Children < 1-year-old	1–4 years	5–8 years	9–15 years
Chloroquine phosphate	250	2 /week	1/4 /week	1/2 /week	1 /week	1.5
Proguanil	100	2 /week	1/4 /day	1/2 /day	1 /day	1.5
Mefloquine (per week)	250	1 /week	1/6–1/8 (=crumb) (not for children under 3 months or weighing under 5 kg)	1/4 /week	1/2 /week	3/4
Doxycycline	100	1 /day	—			
Atovaquone + proguanil	Atovaquone 250 mg, proguanil 100 mg	1 /day	—			

Children weighing over 45 kg are given the doses of an adult.

- Mefloquine can be used for children weighing at least 5 kg.
- Bad-tasting malaria tablets should be crushed and mixed in strongly flavoured juice and be given with a syringe. Chloroquine syrups for children are available in some countries.

References

1. Lengeler C. Insecticide-treated bed nets and curtains for preventing malaria. Cochrane Database Syst Rev. 2004;(2): CD000363.
2. Croft AMJ, Garner P. Mefloquine for preventing malaria in non-immune adult travellers. Cochrane Database Syst Rev. 2004;(2):CD000138.
3. Phillips-Howard PA, Wood D. The safety of antimalarial drugs in pregnancy. Drug Safety 1996;14:131–145.
4. The Database of Abstracts of Reviews of Effectiveness (University of York), Database no.: DARE-960563. In: The Cochrane Library, Issue 4, 1999. Oxford: Update Software.
5. Pittler MH, Ernst E. Artemether for severe malaria: a meta-analysis of randomized clinical trials. Clinical Infectious Diseases 1999;28:597–601.
6. The Database of Abstracts of Reviews of Effectiveness (University of York), Database no.: DARE-990625. In: The Cochrane Library, Issue 1, 2001. Oxford: Update Software.

2.3 Prevention and first aid treatment of traveller's diarrhoea

Tapio Pitkänen

Dietary advice

- In suspect situations one should eat only foods that are well cooked, fruits that are peeled by oneself and use drinks that are boiled or bottled.
- Often it is advised to avoid salad. If one eats salad as a first course, some pathogens may be destroyed by stomach acid.
- Individuals on antacids should select their food with special caution.
- Uncooked or half-cooked crustaceans may spread hepatitis A, salmonella, cholera, or calicivirus, especially if they are cultivated or captured near sewer pipes.

How to disinfect water

- Boiling for five minutes is the most certain way to decontaminate drinking water. It destroys common bacteria that cause diarrhoea, hepatitis A virus, and parasites, even at high altitude, where water boils at temperatures below 100°C.
- A litre of water may be chemically disinfected in half an hour by adding two drops of 2% iodine solution. Very cold water needs two hours.
- Chloramine tablets tend to become lumpy in humid air. Disinfection of water takes half an hour, and to improve the taste thiosulphate should be added.
- Filtration alone is an insufficient method of making safe drinking water if the quality of water is poor.

Prophylactic treatment with antibiotics

Travellers who may use prophylactic treatment

- Persons with gastric non-acidity
  - Patients who use histamine H_2-blockers, proton pump inhibitors or antacids
  - Patients with gastrectomy
- Cancer patients
- Patients with severe diabetes
- Patients with severe cardiac insufficiency
- Patients with severe immunodeficiency
  - Hypogammaglobulinaemia, treatment with antineoplastic drugs
  - Treatment with prednisolone at daily doses higher than 20 mg
- Patients with active intestinal disease (Crohn's disease, ulcerative colitis)
- Patients with reactive arthritis, Reiter's disease (HLA B27)
- A traveller may benefit from prophylactic antibiotics on a trip (duration 4 to 14 days) to countries with a high risk of diarrhoea.
- Norfloxacin at a daily dose of 200 mg is a suitable prophylactic treatment of diarrhoea. It does not prevent diarrhoea caused by Giardia lamblia or amoebas. During the last few years, one out of two Campylobacter strains found in travellers has been resistant to fluoroquinolones. Doxycycline is an alternative drug in a selected group of travellers (it may even serve as malarial prophylaxis). Macrolides may also be used, preferably for less than two weeks.

First aid

- Hydration is the primary treatment.
- In the absence of fever, symptomatic drug therapy may be used, e.g. loperamide.
- If diarrhoea with fever has continued for more than 6 to 24 hours, treat an adult with antibiotics (A) [1].
  - Norfloxacin, 400 mg twice daily or
  - Siprofloxacin, 500 mg twice daily.
  - Duration of the treatment is three days, or even less if symptoms subside.
- One may consider including the antibiotic in the traveller's first aid kit, if the journey lasts more than two weeks and the risk of diarrhoea is high.

Reference

1. De Bruyn G, Hahn S, Borwick A. Antibiotic treatment for travellers' diarrhoea. Cochrane Database Syst Rev. 2004;(2): CD002242.

2.4 Air travel and illness

Pekka J. Oksanen

Background

- The cabin altitude of a modern passenger aircraft varies between sea level and 2100 meters depending on the type of aircraft and its actual flight altitude. The oxygen content of the cabin air is always 21%, but when the cabin altitude increases, the alveolar oxygen partial pressure decreases.
- The arterial oxygen partial pressure (pO_2) of a healthy individual at sea level is approximately 13 kPa, and at 2100 m altitude still about 8 kPa. Hypoxia symptoms appear only above 3000 m when the arterial oxygen partial pressure falls below 7 kPa. The respective haemoglobin oxygen saturation values are 98% at sea level, 92% at 2100 m and 87% at 3000 m.
- The cabin air is re-circulated so that it is changed 6–12 times in an hour. The cabin air is very dry with the relative humidity varying between 10% and 20% during the flight.
- Cabin pressure changes cause pressure changes in the closed cavities of the body unless the pressure can be equalized. The most common symptoms are due to infective or allergic conditions of the middle air or sinus cavity.

Absolute contraindications for air travel

- Recent heart or brain infarct (2–4 weeks from onset)
- Uncompensated heart failure
- Stenocardia at rest
- Pneumothorax
- Severe anaemia (Hb $<$ 75 g/l)
- Recent postoperative conditions (air inside a closed body cavity, ileus)
- Dangerous contagious infections (diphtheria, untreated lung tuberculosis, anthrax, plague, cholera, Ebola fever, Lassa fever)

Precautions

- Mild angina pectoris
  - If the patient can walk on ground level for 100 meters or climb stairs, he/she is fit to travel by air.
- Chronic obstructive lung disease
  - If pO_2 at sea level is below 9 kPa, the patient needs extra oxygen on flights that last for more than one hour.
- Psychosis
  - A medically qualified escort and pre-notification of the airline are compulsory.
- Diabetes
  - During long flights follow the local time of the country of departure, taking meals and medications accordingly. Apply new meal times and medication schedules only after arrival (23.21).
- Trauma patients
  - A patient with a limb plaster may not be able to fit into an aircraft seat; during take-off and landing a normal sitting posture must be maintained with the seat in an upright position and the safety belt fastened. The limb must not extend into the corridor of the aircraft.
- Operated otosclerosis
  - The patient may experience severe vertigo due to pressure changes.
- Communicable diseases in children
  - No restrictions. The possibility of infecting other passengers is minimal because of the outflow direction of cabin ventilation.
- Pregnancy
  - Flight travel is allowed until the end of the 36th week if there are no pregnancy complications and no signs of imminent labour. On short domestic and intra-Scandinavian routes, travel is allowed until end of the 38th week.
- Post-delivery
  - No restrictions apply to the mother or the newborn child.

MEDIF form

- Airlines may request medical information using a standard MEDIF (Medical Information) form before issuing medical clearance for transport of the sick. The form is available from airline ticket offices and medical departments.
- A MEDIF form is required always when the patient is transported on a stretcher, and when there is uncertainty concerning a passenger's ability to travel alone.

Aircraft medical equipment

- Medical oxygen
- MediBox
  - Contents
    - Bandages
    - Dressings
    - Adhesive dressings
    - Antiseptic wound cleaner
    - Ear drops

- Over-the-counter medicines
  - Acetylsalicylic acid
  - Paracetamol
  - Nasal decongestant
  - Antacid
  - Antidiarrhoeal medication
- First Aid Kit (FAK)
  - Contents
    - Bandages
    - Burn dressings
    - Large and small wound dressing
    - Adhesive dressings
    - Adhesive tape, safety pins, scissors
    - Sterile wound closures
    - Antiseptic wound cleaner
    - Adhesive wound closures
    - Splints for upper and lower limbs
    - Sling for the arm
    - Thermoblanket
    - First-aid handbook
    - Ground/air visual signal code book
    - Disposable gloves
    - Fresh-up towels
    - Leatherman multi-purpose tool
- Emergency Medical Kit (EMK)
  - Contents
    - Blood pressure meter (non-mercury)
    - Stethoscope
    - Tourniquet
    - Syringes, 1 ml, 2 ml, 5 ml
    - Injection needles
    - Tracheal tube
    - Alcohol-containing sterile towels
    - Urinary catheter
    - Ventilation mask
    - Disposable gloves
    - Needle disposal box
    - List of contents/indications
- Drugs
  - Adrenocortical steroid (hydrocortisone)
  - Antispasmodic (scopolamine butylbromide)
  - Adrenaline
  - Major analgesic (buprenorphin)
  - Diuretic (furosemide)
  - Antihistamine
  - Anxiolytic (diazepam)
  - Antiemetic (metoclopramide hydrochloride)
  - Atropine
  - Digoxin
  - Uterine contractant (methylergometrine)
  - Bronchodilator (inhaler and injectable)
  - Hypoglycaemic medication
  - Coronary vasodilator

2.30 Fever in returning traveller

Heli Siikamäki

Basic rules

- Fever in a traveller arriving from the tropics should be considered as malaria until proven otherwise. Like-threatening diseases such as sepsis and malaria have to be diagnosed and treated immediately
- The general practitioner should raise the suspicion of a tropical disease on the basis of the patient's history and refer the patient if necessary diagnostics for tropical diseases are performed in specialized units.
- When travelling, people can acquire diseases that are common also in their home country. Specially when arriving from the tropics, the differential diagnosis spectrum is wider and requires accuracy. Do not prescribe antibiotics without performing diagnostic tests. Arrange proper follow-up of the patient if treatment is carried out in ambulatory care.

Diagnostic workup for disease in travellers

- The first thing to assess is the possibility of malaria, septic infection, severe dehydration, or impaired general condition requiring immediate referral. Intravenous fluids may be indicated as first aid.
- Ask about
  - Exact travelling history (destinations and schedule) from the preceding 2 months, or even years if symptoms are prolonged
  - prophylactic drugs and vaccinations taken
  - all symptoms and their temporal relationship with the travel
  - symptoms in travelling companions.
- The primary investigations of a febrile traveller include
  - Peripheral blood thin smear and thick smear to detect malaria. At least one blood smear should be examined immediately. Both samples (2–3 slides each) should be sent immediately to the nearest parasitological laboratory.
  - Haemoglobin, leucocytes, differential count, thrombocytes, and serum CRP
  - Blood culture × 2
  - Urine test
  - Faecal bacterial cultures and examination for faecal parasites are indicated in patients with gastrointestinal symptoms.
  - Chest x-ray
- Table 2.30.1 presents diseases to be remembered according to symptoms. The most probable cause (often not a tropical disease) is presented in italic type.
- See also tables 2.30.2, 2.30.3, 2.30.4

Table 2.30.1 Clues to the aetiology of a tropical disease based on the clinical presentation

Clues from the clinical presentation	Findings supporting the diagnosis
Skin changes	
Insect bites	Single papules/skin lesions
Cutaneous leishmaniasis	Chronic ulcer
Trypanosomiasis	Chancre
Leprosy	Pale insensitive skin areas
Lung infection with severe symptoms	
Pneumonia	
Legionellosis	
Q fever	Fever, headache, myalgia, and elevated liver enzyme values
Pulmonary anthrax	Mediastinitis
Plague	
General symptoms, malaise	
Brucellosis	Lymphadenopathy, hepatomegaly
Visceral leishmaniasis	Lymphadenopathy, hepatomegaly, pancytopenia
2nd phase of trypanosomiasis	History of tsetse fly sting and a chancre
Acute schistosomiasis	History of contact with fresh water, eosinophilia
Fever, poor general condition	
Malaria	History of staying in an endemic area
Typhus	
Spotted fever	Rash, eschar, tache noire
Dengue fever	Thrombopenia, leukopenia, elevated liver enzymes
Recurrent fever	
Meningitis/encephalitis	
Herpes encephalitis	
Leptospirosis	
Japanese encephalitis	
Haematuria	
Schistosomiasis	
Diarrhoea	
Gastrointestinal infections: Salmonella, Shigella, Campylobacter, Yersinia, etc.	
Malaria	
Hepatitis, particularly hepatitis A and E	
Amoebiasis, giardiasis, cryptosporidiosis	
Jaundice	
Hepatitis	
Malaria	
Delirium	
Any septic infection	
Malaria	
Japanese encephalitis (the Far East)	
Other encephalitis or meningitis	
Mefloquine used as prophylaxis against malaria	
Bleeding diathesis	
Dengue haemorrhagic fever	
Yellow fever (Africa, Middle and South America)	History of residing in Africa and South America
Tropical haemorrhagic fevers (Crimean-Congo haemorrhagic fever)	

Table 2.30.2 Fevers occurring in the tropics.

Common and endemic in large areas
♦ Dengue fever
♦ Typhoid fever
♦ Viral hepatitis
♦ HIV infection
♦ Tuberculosis
Rarer diseases that occur in large areas
♦ Amoebic liver abscess
♦ Brucellosis
♦ Schistosomiasis
♦ Toxoplasmosis
♦ Leptospirosis
♦ Rickettsioses
♦ Filariasis
Rarer diseases that occur in limited areas
♦ Visceral leishmaniasis
♦ Relapsing fever
♦ Trypanosomiasis
♦ Polio
♦ Plague
♦ Melioidosis
♦ Haemorrhagic fevers
♦ Yellow fever

Table 2.30.3 Incubation times of some of the fevers possibly acquired by travellers.

Incubation time	Duration
Short incubation time	(less than 7 days)
	Traveller's diarrhoea
	Dengue fever and other arbovirus infections
Medium long incubation time	(less than 21 days)
	Malaria
	Hepatitis A
	Rickettsioses[1]
	Typhoid fever
	Leptospirosis
	Haemorrhagic fevers
Long incubation time	(more than 21 days)
	Malaria[2]
	Viral hepatitis (A, B, C, D, E)
	Amoebic liver abscess
	Acute HIV infection
	Secondary syphilis
	Brucellosis
	Tuberculosis[2]
	Acute schistosomiasis
	Visceral leishmaniasis

1. Usually less than 10 days
2. Symptoms may appear months or even years from infection

Table 2.30.4 Skin findings in some infections.

The appearance of the skin change	Possible diagnoses
Maculopapular rash	Dengue fever
	Acute HIV infection
	Leptospirosis
	Haemorrhagic fevers
Erythema chronicum migrans	Lyme disease
Rose spots	Typhoid fever
Pustules	Generalized gonococcal infection
Petechiae, ecchymoses, haemorrhages	Meningococcaemia
	Dengue fever
	Haemorrhagic fevers
	Yellow fever
	Rickettsioses
	Leptospirosis
Necrotic papule ("eschar", "tache noire")	Rickettsioses
	Anthrax
	Congo-Crimean haemorrhagic fever
Ulcer	Tularemia
	Cutaneous diphtheria
Urticaria	Infections caused by worms

2.31 Bacterial diseases in warm climates

Heli Siikamäki

Anthrax

Causative agent

- ♦ Bacillus anthracis (a gram positive rod)

Epidemiology

- ♦ Animal anthrax occurs, for example, in South and North America, the Caribbean, Eastern and Southern Europe, Middle East, Asia and Africa.

Route of infection

- ♦ Anthrax is not transmitted from person to person.
- ♦ The disease occurs in herbivores and is occasionally transmitted to humans.
- ♦ Cattle, sheep, goats, horses and pigs serve as reservoirs.
- ♦ Bacterial spore remain viable in dried or otherwise processed leather and remain in the soil for years.

- Human cutaneous anthrax infection may be mediated by animal tissue, wool, leather, hair, or any product made of these or by contaminated soil or bone. Pulmonary anthrax is acquired by inhaling spores, for example, when handling goat wool (wool-sorter's disease).
- Intestinal anthrax may be acquired by eating contaminated meat.
- In biological warfare or terrorism the bacteria would most likely be spread as an aerosol and the main manifestation would be pulmonary anthrax.

Global importance

- An animal disease, human infections are rare.
- A potential agent for biological warfare and terrorism.

Symptoms

- Cutaneous anthrax is the most common form. Incubation time is 1–7 (usually 2–5) days. The disease starts as a papule that widens and turns into a vesicle. The vesicles spread and rupture and 7–10 days from the onset a black painless ulcer a few centimetres in diameter develops. The ulcer develops a crust that falls in 1–2 weeks leaving a scar. If untreated, the infection may spread and become generalized.
- Inhalation of germs results in a biphasic disease that begins after an incubation time of 1–5 days with flu-like symptoms. In 2–5 days these are followed by severe, often fatal mediastinitis.
- Intestinal anthrax is rare. Symptoms include vomiting, fever, and at a later stage, abdominal pain, haematemesis and melena, which may resemble acute bleeding.

Diagnosis

- Suspicion
  - Acute febrile disease in a person arriving from endemic areas who has been in contact with animals or animal products and has the above-mentioned clinical symptoms.
  - When intentional spreading of anthrax bacteria is suspected, look for symptoms of pulmonary or cutaneous anthrax.
- Blood culture × 2, bacterial staining and culture, PCR from a skin lesion, sputum sample or stool depending on the form of the disease.
- Antibody determination
- All samples must contain information about anthrax suspicion and be marked with a yellow triangle for indicating contagiousness.
- A patient with suspected anthrax does not need to be isolated, standard precautions are sufficient. Wastes are handled as contagious material.
- Antibiotics must be started as soon as possible. Intravenous ciprofloxacin 400 mg × 2 is the drug of choice. Dose for children is 20–30 mg/kg/day. Treatment is adjusted when the diagnosis is verified and bacterial sensitivity is known. The duration of treatment is around 60 days, in cutaneous anthrax 7–10 days.
- Differential diagnosis: staphylococcus infection, plague, tularaemia
- All verified cases of anthrax and strong suspicions must be reported to national authorities.

Prognosis

- Cutaneous anthrax
  - Mortality is 5–20% in untreated cases, and extremely low with antibiotic therapy
- Pulmonary anthrax
  - Mortality is 90–100% even with treatment
- Intestinal anthrax
  - Without treatment mortality is 25–100%

Exposure (suspicion of intentional spreading of anthrax)

- Evaluate the probability of exposure: decision on taking samples and treating exposed persons is made in cooperation with health authorities and authorities in charge of national safety issues.
- Any space that is suspected of being contaminated by bacteria is closed. All persons who have resided in that space are listed and officials ensure that samples are taken from suspected sources of infection.
- Exposed persons should undress, wash carefully in a shower and dress in clean clothes.
- Exposed persons are not infectious and need not be isolated.
- If authorities evaluate the exposure to be real, start prophylactic antibiotics, primarily ciprofloxacin 500 mg × 2 orally, for children 20–30 mg/kg daily divided into two doses (not over 1 g/day). If exposure is verified, continue antibiotics for 60 days.

Prevention

- Surveillance of infections in animals. Corpses of sick animals should be cremated.
- A vaccine is available in some countries A [1].

Plague

Causative agent

- Yersinia pestis

Epidemiology

- All over the world rather rare, around 200 cases are reported annually from Africa, Asia and South America. Plague occurs also in the USA.

Route of infection

- Rodents, particularly rats, are carriers.
- Infection spreads through fleabites.

- Pneumonic plague may be transmitted from person to person as an aerosol-borne infection.

Global importance

- In the past the disease caused large pandemics.
- Could in principle be used as a weapon in biological terrorism. The most likely method of spreading the disease would be aerosol form.

Symptoms

- In bubonic plague, lymph node enlargement in the inguinal region, armpits or the neck and a high fever develop after an incubation period of 2–8 days.
- Inhalation of the bacteria may cause pneumonia, which is often fatal (pneumonic plague: may also develop as a complication of bubonic plague).

Diagnosis

- Clinical suspicion of plague is an indication for immediate treatment.
- Bacterial staining and culture is the traditional method. A new rapid dipstick test for F1 antigen of Yersinia pestis is both sensitive and specific.

Treatment

- Streptomycin is the drug of choice.
- Tetracyclines and probably also fluoroquinolones are effective.

Prognosis

- If left untreated, mortality is about 50% in the patients with bubonic plague and up to 100% in those with pneumonic or septicaemic plague.
- Antibiotics are effective only when initiated in the early stages of the disease. Mortality is then approx. 5%.

Prevention

- Extinction of rodent vectors.
- No effective vaccine exists D [2].

Brucellosis

Causative agent

- The Brucellae are Gram-negative rods.

Epidemiology

- Occurs in the Mediterranean countries, Arabian peninsula, India, Central and South America and Africa.

Route of infection

- Milk is the most common source of human infection, in particular, unpasteurized goat's milk.

Global importance

- The infection was common earlier, but pasteurization of milk has lowered the incidence.

Symptoms

- The symptoms are varied and differentiation from other prolonged systemic infections is difficult. Some cases are subclinical.
- Fever, sweating, headache, backache and nausea develop after an incubation period of 2–8 weeks. Some patients have a strange taste in the mouth. Depression, lymphadenopathy and enlargement of the spleen and liver may occur. The patient may have symptoms affecting the gastrointestinal tract, skeleton, joints, central nervous system, heart, lungs and the urinary tract.

Diagnosis

- The diagnosis is made on the basis of clinical suspicion and history of exposure
- Brucellae can be cultured from the blood, bone marrow and tissues. Brucella antibodies can be determined.

Treatment

- A combination of doxycycline and gentamycin or streptomycin, or of doxycycline and rifampicin (6 weeks), in children trimethoprim-sulpha (6 weeks) and gentamycin (2 weeks).

Prognosis

- The mortality is about 2%, if untreated.

Prevention

- Mass immunization of animals in endemic areas

Relapsing fever

Causative agent

- Epidemic recurrent fever is caused by Borrelia recurrentis.
- Endemic recurrent fever is caused by other Borrelia species.

Epidemiology

- Epidemic recurrent fever occurs in Africa and South America, and in any part of the world where people live in squalor but are clothed. Endemic disease occurs in most parts of the world.

Route of infection

- Borreliae are transmitted by blood. Louse transmits the disease from person to person in the epidemic form. In the endemic form ticks transmit the disease from small mammals to humans.

Global importance

- The disease is rather common. Louse-borne epidemic relapsing fever causes epidemics during war, famine and man population movements.

Symptoms

- Fever with shivering, severe headache, myalgia, arthralgia, photophobia and cough develop after an incubation period of one week. The first phase of the fever lasts 3–6 days.
- After an afebrile period of one week the patient has relapses lasting 2–3 days. In the epidemic form of the disease, 1–5 relapses are usual, in the endemic form there are more relapses.
- At the end of the febrile period the following symptoms or findings are the most common: enlargement of the spleen and liver, jaundice, rashes, cranial nerve palsies, meningitis, hemiplegia, epileptic seizures.

Diagnosis

- From a blood smear during a febrile period (malaria slide).

Treatment

- The epidemic form can be treated with a single 500 mg dose of tetracycline; the endemic form requires 500 mg × 4 for 5–10 days.
- Herxheimer reaction often follows treatment in epidemic relapsing fever with a rise in temperature, confusion, tachycardia and transient hypertension followed by hypotension.

Prognosis

- Mortality in the epidemic form is 4–40% and that in the endemic form is 5%.

Prevention

- Improving general hygiene, delousing, avoidance of tick bites

Leptospirosis

Causative agent

- Spirochetes of the Leptospira genus
- Leptospira interrogans is the most common.

Epidemiology

- The disease occurs worldwide.

Route of infection

- The disease is transmitted into humans by soil or water contaminated by the urine of an infected animal.
- The bite of an infected animal or handling of infected tissue or eating it are more rare routes of infection.

Global importance

- Fairly common

Symptoms

- Incubation time is 2–30 days.
- Symptoms usually resemble those of influenza, meningitis or hepatitis.
- Other symptoms include vomiting, myalgia, headache, photophobia, subconjunctival haemorrhage, lymphadenopathy, splenomegaly and carditis.
- The concentration of creatine kinase may be high when muscles are affected.
- The complications include renal failure, which sometimes requires dialysis and cardiogenic shock.

Diagnosis

- Suspicion
  - Febrile disease with symptoms or influenza, hepatitis or meningitis and a history of possible exposure.
- The diagnosis is based on serology.

Treatment

- Severe forms of the disease should be treated with intravenous penicillin, milder forms with oral doxycycline B [3], which can also be used prophylactically if the risk of exposure is high C [4].

Prognosis

- The mortality is 5–10% in the icteric form of the disease.

Prevention

- 200 mg of doxycycline once a week in endemic areas if the risk of exposure is high. Does not necessarily prevent the disease, but makes it milder.
- Vaccination is available in some countries. Is used to protect people living in endemic areas who are exposed to leptospira in their work.

Leprosy

Causative agent

- Mycobacterium leprae

Epidemiology

- Endemic in the tropics and subtropics

Route of infection

- A prolonged contact with a disease carrier is required.

Global importance

- A rather important health problem in endemic areas

Symptoms

- Tuberculoid leprosy (small amounts of bacteria on the skin)
  - Benign course
  - Insensitive pale areas on the skin, mononeuropathies
- Lepromatous leprosy
  - Wide areas of thickened skin and nodules
  - Injuries of the fingers and toes resulting from neuropathy

Diagnosis

- Staining for mycobacteria from skin smears

Treatment

- Dapsone, clofazimine, rifampicin as combination therapy

Prognosis

- The prognosis is good if treatment is started early.
- Treatment prevents spread of the disease and infectiousness, but the cosmetic problems remain.

Prevention

- All infectious patients should be treated.

Rickettsioses or spotted fevers

Causative agent

- Rickettsia are intracellular microbes that invade the intima of blood vessels causing vasculitis. Sixteen species of rickettsia are known to cause human disease. R. prowazekii causes epidemic or louse born typhus, R. typhi (moseri) causes endemic or murine or flea-borne typhus, R. conorii causes Mediterranean spotted fever, R. africae causes African tickbite fever, R. ricketsii causes Rocky Mountain spotted fever and R. tsutsugamushi causes scrub typhus.

Epidemiology

- Epidemic typhus occurs particularly in Africa, South and Central America and Asia. It is spread, for example, in refugee camps and anywhere where people live crowded and wear clothes. Epidemics usually appear in the winter. Minor epidemics have been reported in the recent years from Burundi and Russia. Endemic typhus occurs in Africa, Asia and Europe. Rocky Mountain spotted fever occurs in North, Central and South America. Other rickettsioses occur in more restricted endemic areas. Mediterranean spotted fever occurs in countries around the Mediterranean, Africa, India, around the Black Sea and Russia. African spotted fever occurs on the African continent and scrub typhus in Far East.

Route of infection

- The infection is spread by the following arthropods depending on the species of rickettsia: louse (R. prowazekii), flea (R. typhi) or tick (the spotted fever group: R. ricketsii, R. conorii, R. africae, R. Helvetica, etc.).

Global importance

- Epidemic spotted fever spreads in conditions where hygiene is poor, and it has been estimated to have killed more people in the course of history than all the wars in the world.

Symptoms

- Incubation time is usually less than 2 weeks.
- Acute high fever, myalgia, nausea and severe headache are typical symptoms.
- Typical maculopapular eczema and/or purpura appears in most rickettsioses in 3–7 days. However, it can also be absent. In some rickettsioses the rash may be vesicular, resembling chickenpox.
- In some tick-borne spotted fevers (e.g. African and Mediterranean spotted fevers) and scrub typhus, the patient may have a necrotic lesion on the skin (eschar, tache noire) at the site of the arthropod bite (resembles a cigarette burn).
- Other possible symptoms
  - lymphadenopathy, cough, lung infiltrates, conjunctivitis, pharyngitis, nausea, vomiting, abdominal pain, elevated liver enzyme levels, hepatosplenomegaly, CNS syndromes, arrhythmias, myocarditis, proteinuria, renal failure.

Diagnosis

- Febrile illness and eczema and/or an eschar in a person who is suspected of having been exposed to a tick, flea or louse bite in endemic areas. Treatment is initiated on the basis of clinical picture, as rapid diagnostic methods are not available in routine use. If malaria is possible, it must be excluded before treatment is started.
- Specific antibodies (R. conorii antibodies cross react with rickettsias of the spotted fever group, R. typhi cross react with R. prowazekii and B. Quintana) are often elevated not until after 4–12 weeks of the onset of the disease.
- Positive PCR from a biopsy of the eschar (sometimes also from blood during fever).

Treatment

- Doxycycline 100 mg × 2–3 days after fever has disappeared, usually for 7 days.

Prognosis

- Varies with different species, usually good.

- Epidemic typhus, Rocky Mountain spotted fever, Mediterranean spotted fever and scrub typhus may be life threatening, particularly if the diagnosis is delayed.

Prevention

- Avoidance of arthropod bites

Q fever

Causative agent

- Coxiella burnetii, an intracytoplasmic microbe which, unlike Rickettsias, can survive outside the cell and remain viable in spore form in dry dust for long times.

Epidemiology

- Occurs globally, especially in cattle rearing areas.

Route of infection

- Transmitted to humans mainly as an aerosol either in contact with cattle, goat or sheep excrement or air borne. May be acquired from contaminated wool, unpasteurized milk or from the afterbirth of domestic animals such as cats.

Global significance

- Common febrile disease

Symptoms

- Most infections are asymptomatic or mild and self-limiting febrile diseases.
- Symptomatic patient develop high, long lasting fever, headache and myalgia after an incubation time of about 20 days (1–5 weeks).
- Some patients have pneumonia and/or elevated liver enzyme levels.
- Severe cases may involve renal complications, myocarditis and aseptic meningoencephalitis.
- May cause chronic endocarditis.

Diagnosis

- History of residing in cattle rearing areas where the disease is endemic and contact with unpasteurized milk, cattle excrement, slaughtering remains or animal afterbirth.
- Antibody determination

Treatment

- Doxycycline

Prognosis

- Rarely fatal

Prevention

- Avoidance of contact with animals

References

1. Jefferson T, Demicheli V, Deeks J, Graves P, Pratt M, Rivetti D. Vaccines for preventing anthrax. Cochrane Database Syst Rev. 2004;(2):CD000975.
2. Jefferson T, Demicheli V, Pratt M. Vaccines for preventing plague. Cochrane Database Syst Rev. 2004;(2):CD000976.
3. Guidugli F, Castro AA, Atallah AN. Antibiotics for preventing leptospirosis. Cochrane Database Syst Rev. 2004;(2): CD001305.
4. Guidugli F, Castro AA, Atallah AN. Antibiotics for leptospirosis. The Cochrane Database of Systematic Reviews, Cochrane Library number: CD 001306. In: The Cochrane Library, Issue 2, 2002. Oxford: Update software. Updated frequently.

2.32 Viral diseases in warm climates

Heli Siikamäki

- For infectious hepatitis see article 9.20.

Yellow fever

Causative agent

- A flavivirus

Epidemiology

- Yellow fever is endemic in South America and Sub-Saharan Africa, but not in Asia.

Route of infection

- The infection is transmitted by mosquitoes.

Global importance

- Large epidemics occur at times.

Symptoms

- The incubation period of yellow fever is 3–6 days. The clinical picture varies from a mild febrile disease to a severe form with headache, myalgia, hepatic and renal dysfunction and haemorrhages.

Diagnosis

- Antibody determination

Treatment

- No specific treatment exists.

Prognosis

- The mortality in yellow fever is about 5%, 20–50% in the icteric form.

Prevention

- An effective and safe vaccination against yellow fever is available. One shot gives protection for 10 years. It is highly recommended for people travelling to endemic areas. Yellow fever vaccination is the only vaccination that may be officially required by border authority. Official vaccination certificate is usually required of all persons arriving from endemic areas.
- Avoidance of mosquito bites

Dengue

Causative agent

- A flavivirus, 4 different serotypes

Epidemiology

- Dengue occurs in many tropical and subtropical areas mainly in urban and semiurban areas.
- Haemorrhagic dengue fever occurs in Southeast Asia and the Caribbean, not in Africa.

Route of infection

- The infection is transmitted from person to person by mosquitoes (Aedes aegypti, stings in the daytime).

Global importance

- Incidence is rising, large epidemics occur occasionally.
- 50–100 million cases/year, 25 000 deaths/year of severe dengue
- 40% of world population are of risk from dengue.

Symptoms

- Incubation period
  - short, 2–7 days
- Symptoms
  - Fever (often biphasic), headache, myalgia and arthralgia, nausea, respiratory symptoms, enlarged lymph nodes, rash
  - Symptoms resolve in two weeks, often followed by weeks of fatigue and depression
- Laboratory findings
  - Leucopenia, thrombopenia, elevated liver enzyme levels

Dengue haemorrhagic fever

- A person with a previous dengue infection becomes infected within a short time with a dengue virus of another serotype.
- Begins like the ordinary dengue fever, but after 2–5 days petechiae and bleeding appear followed by shock.

Diagnosis

- Antibody determination
- Exclusion of malaria

Treatment

- No specific treatment exists.

Prognosis

- Good, mortality is under 1% in ordinary dengue.
- In the dengue haemorrhagic fever mortality is about 20% without treatment, with supportive treatment in a hospital the mortality can be lowered to under 1%.

Prevention

- Prevention of mosquito bites

Japanese encephalitis

Causative agent

- A flavivirus

Epidemiology

- Occurs in a wide area in Asia, from India to Korea.
- The disease is most prevalent in India and Southeast Asia.

Route of infection

- Transmitted by mosquitoes

Global importance

- Important cause of viral meningitis in children in endemic areas
- For example, the incidence in Thailand in an endemic area is 3–5 cases/100 000 inhabitants/year.

Symptoms

- The incubation period is 4–15 days.
- The severity varies from a febrile illness with headache to meningitis or encephalitis.

Diagnosis

- Antibody determination

Treatment

- No specific treatment exists.

Prognosis

- Mortality 30–40% in encephalitis
- Most survivors (50–80%) have various neuropsychiatric symptoms.

Prevention

- An effective inactivated whole-virus vaccine exists.
- The vaccination is associated with hypersensitivity reactions with an incidence of 1–100/10 000 persons vaccinated.

Haemorrhagic fevers: Lassa fever, Ebola fever, Marburg disease, Crimean-Congo haemorrhagic fever

Causative agents

- Viruses carrying the names of the diseases

Epidemiology

- Lassa fever has been observed in Nigeria, Sierra Leone and Liberia.
- Marburg disease is known from a single epidemic that occurred in Germany and Yugoslavia and was transmitted by imported monkeys.
- Ebola fever has emerged as limited epidemics in Central and Eastern Africa, for instance in Sudan and Zaire in 1995 and 2000–2001 in Uganda.
- The Crimean-Congo haemorrhagic fever occurs in a wide area in Eastern Europe, Middle and Western Asia and Africa.

Route of infection

- The Lassa virus resides in the rat. Infection is transmitted by dust, foodstuffs and excretions contaminated by rat urine. The Marburg virus resides apparently in monkeys. The host of the Ebola virus is not known. It may be transmitted from person to person in close contact with the blood or secretions of an infected person. The Congo-Crimean virus resides in many domestic and wild animals, the tick serving as the vector.

Global importance

- The diseases have not big public health importance; however, because of its contagiousness and high fatality rate the Ebola virus has aroused attention in the media during epidemics.

Symptoms

- Haemorrhagic fever should be suspected if a patient has fever of unknown origin and/or an unexplained tendency for bleeding and within the last three weeks one of the following is known to have occurred:
  - close contact with a person with verified haemorrhagic fever
  - blood contact with a laboratory sample taken from a patient with haemorrhagic fever
  - contact with an animal with haemorrhagic fever
  - working in health care in an area where haemorrhagic fever occurs.

Diagnosis

- Clinical picture
- Viral culture, antibodies, PCR analysis (require a special safety laboratory)

Prognosis

- Lassa fever is usually a mild febrile disease with aches. The mortality is about 2%.
- The Ebola fever and Marburg disease have a case fatality rate in the range of several tens of per cent.
- The case fatality rate of the Crimean-Congo haemorrhagic fever is about 10–15%.

Treatment

- Symptomatic
- Ribavirine in Lassa fever

Prevention

- Avoiding areas with epidemics
- Avoidance of contact with blood and excretions
- Special isolation measures are needed in handling patients and laboratory specimens.

2.33 Parasitic diseases in warm climates: protozoa and worms

Heli Siikamäki

- See separate guidelines for malaria 2.2, giardiasis 1.60, cryptosporidiosis 1.61, toxoplasmosis 1.62, and amebiasis 1.63.

Leishmaniasis

Causative agent

- The flagellate Leishmaniae

Epidemiology

- Visceral leishmaniasis (kala azar)
  - The Mediterranean (endemic on the eastern coast of Spain), the Near East, Middle Asia, India, China, Africa, South America
- Cutaneous leishmaniasis
  - Countries surrounding the Mediterranean, Turkey, India, Africa, Middle and South America
- Mucocutaneous leishmaniasis
  - South America

Route of infection

- The infection is spread by sand flies from rodents and dogs into humans.

Global importance

- The global prevalence is 12 million, and the annual incidence is 600 000.

Symptoms

- The usual incubation period for visceral leishmaniasis is 3–8 months, but may vary from 3 weeks to 2 years. Many cases are asymptomatic. Typical symptoms in visceral leishmaniasis include fever, weight loss and lymphadenopathy. Hepatomegaly, splenomegaly, and diarrhoea are common. Dark pigmentation may occur on the skin, and the patient may have haemorrhages.
- Cutaneous leishmaniasis manifests as a crust after an incubation period of several months. The crust develops into an ulcer. The ulcer heals in a few years, but the skin remains unpigmented.
- Mucocutaneous leishmaniasis starts from the face as a skin lesion that heals spontaneously. After months or years ulcers develop. They may totally destroy the nasal septum and the soft tissues of the mouth and nose.

Diagnosis

- Leishmanias are detected from tissue samples: a bone marrow specimen is usually taken if visceral leishmaniasis is suspected, and a skin biopsy or smear from the lesion if cutaneous leishmaniasis is suspected.
- Antibodies can be found in serum in visceral leishmaniasis.

Treatment

- Small skin lesions can be cured surgically.
- Parenteral antimony pentavalent.
- Amphotericin B is alternative treatment in visceral leishmaniasis.

Prognosis

- Cutaneous leishmaniasis heals spontaneously. If necessary, local surgery or drugs are used.
- Visceral leishmaniasis often results in death if left untreated. The response to treatment is good.
- Mucocutaneous leishmaniasis is more difficult to cure.

Prevention

- No vaccination or prophylactic medication exists.
- Avoidance of sand fly bites

Trypanosomiasis

Causative agent

- Trypanosomas are flagellates infesting the blood and tissues.

Epidemiology

- African trypanosomiasis (sleeping sickness) is endemic in tropical Africa. There are two forms: chronic West African (Gambian) and acute East African (Rhodesian) forms.
- American trypanosomiasis (Chagas' disease) occurs in the countryside and slums in Central and South America.

Route of infection

- African trypanosomiasis is transmitted by tsetse fly sting and American form by reduvid bug. The source of infection is another human or mammal.

Global importance

- 20 000 cases of African trypanosomiasis occur annually.
- Chagas' disease affects 16–18 million people and is the most important cause of death in young and middle-aged people in some areas.

Symptoms

- African trypanosomiasis
    - Chronic African trypanosomiasis develops in three phases.
        - Chancre, a painful, red papule develops about one week after the sting, and disappears in a few weeks.
        - Fever, lymphadenopathy, rash, and oedema develop after weeks or months. Carditis may occur.
        - CNS symptoms: irritability, apathy (sleeping sickness) appear after months or years.
    - The East African form has a similar clinical course, but develops more quickly.
- Chagas' disease
    - A wheal develops at the site of the sting.
    - Fever and lymphadenopathy follow after 1–2 weeks. Myocarditis or meningoencephalitis may develop.
    - The disease often subsides spontaneously, but may become chronic and cause heart failure. Other complications include dilatation of the oesophagus and the colon as a result of autonomic nerve injury.

Diagnosis

- In acute disease the diagnosis is made by isolation of trypanosomae from a chancroid lesion (wheal) or the blood.
- Serological diagnosis at a later phase is more inaccurate.

Treatment

- Early African trypanosomiasis can be treated with drugs (suramin, pentamidine, eflornithine). Eflornithine is also effective when the disease has affected the CNS in chronic West African trypanosomiasis.
- Drugs used for Chagas' disease probably do not prevent the chronic form of the disease and they have adverse effects.

Prognosis

- In the early stages of disease African trypanosomiasis can be managed with drugs. The disease may be lethal if left untreated. When the central nervous system is involved, the disease has a mortality of 10% despite treatment.
- Mortality in Chagas' disease is 5–10% in the acute phase, and 20–30% of the patients are affected by late complications.

Prevention

- No vaccination exists.
- Avoidance of insect stings and bites

Parasitic worms

- Parasitic worms occur on all continents. About one fifth of the world population is infested by at least one species of worms. One person often carries several species of worms.
- The worms identified as human parasites include nematodes, trematodes, and cestodes.
- Most infections caused by worms are chronic and they give few symptoms. Symptoms only develop after a long stay in an endemic area when the number of infesting worms is high.

Epidemiology

- The nematodes **Enterobius vermicularis** (pinworm) (1.55) and **Ascaris lumbricoides** (1.54) occur world wide. **Trichuriasis, ancylostomiasis** (hookworm) and **strongyloidiasis** are common in the tropics and subtropics. The hookworm and strongyloides also occur in Southern Europe.
- **Trichinosis** (1.53) occurs world wide where pork is consumed. **Dracunculiasis** occurs in Africa, the Near East, and India. **Lymphatic filariasis** occurs widely in the tropics and subtropics. **Onchocerciasis** occurs in tropical Africa, Central and South America, and Yemen. **Loiasis** is endemic in the rain forests of West and Central Africa.
- **Schistosomiasis** occurs in Africa and the Near East, Central and South America, and in East and Southeast Asia. Liver flukes occur in China and all over the world in sheep rearing areas.
- Diphyllobotrium latum or the **fish tapeworm** (1.52) occurs in Northern Europe and other areas where uncooked fresh water fish is consumed. **Echinococcosis** (1.51) or hydotid disease occurs world wide in cattle and sheep raising areas. **Hymenolepiasis** occurs in warm climate. **Cysticercosis** is endemic in areas where a lot of pork is consumed: Mexico, South America, Indonesia, and South Africa.
- **Larva migrans** denotes infestation of the skin by worms that do not develop into adult worms in the human body. **Toxocariasis** or visceral larva migrans occurs world wide.
- **Myiasis** denotes infestation of the skin by the larvae of flies. Typically a wheal develops in the skin that subsequently erupts and a living larva emerges.

Route of infection

- Humans are infected by mouth (the most common route), through the skin (ancylostomiasis, strongyloidiasis, and schistosomiasis), or by an insect sting (loiasis, onchocerciasis, lymphatic filariasis).
- Usually the worms do not spread from person to person (with the exception of pinworms, Strongyloides, Hymenolepis and Cysticercus). Only Strongyloides and Echinococcus can breed in the human body.

Global importance

- Ascariasis and hookworm affect about one billion, schistosomiasis affects 200 million, and filariasis 90 million people. The prevalence of river blindness (caused by onchocerciasis) is about 300 000 in Africa.

Examples of Symptoms

- Anaemia
  - Hookworm, wide tapeworm (pernicious anaemia)
- Upper abdominal pains
  - Strongyloidiasis, hookworm
- Pruritus ani
  - Pinworm
- Lung symptoms (when the larvae migrate)
  - Ascariasis, strongyloidiasis
- Myalgia
  - Trichinosis
- Larvae migrating under the skin
  - Larva migrans
- Larvae emerging from the skin
  - Myiasis, dracunculiasis (above the ankle, up to one meter long)
- Obstruction of lymphatic drainage (elephantiasis)
  - Lymphatic filariasis
- Itching of the skin
  - Loiasis, larva migrans, onchocerciasis
- Intestinal and biliary symptoms, hepato- and splenomegaly
  - Ascariasis, liver flukes, schistosomiasis
- Haematuria
  - Schistosomiasis
- Epilepsy and other central nervous system symptoms
  - Cysticercosis, schistosomiasis
- Liver and lung cysts
  - Echinococcosis

Diagnosis

- Eosinophilia and a high concentration for IgE are typical of most worm diseases.
- The diagnosis of intestinal worms is based on the detection of worm eggs or larvae in the stools.

- Schistosoma eggs can be detected from the stools, urine, or tissue biopsy.
- Microfilaria can be detected from a thick blood smear in lymphatic filarias, and from a skin snip sample in onchocerciasis.
- Cysticercosis is often detected on brain CT or MRI examination, and a hydatid cyst caused by Echinococcus can be seen on liver ultrasonography, CT or MRI.

Treatment

- Nematode diseases can be treated with mebendazole or albendazole, strongyloidiasis is best treated with ivermectine or albendazole.
- Lymphatic filariasis is treated with diethylcarbamazepine C [1] [2] and onchocerciasis with ivermectin D [3].
- Schistosomiasis and infestation by other trematodes as well as cestodes are treated with praziquantel A [4], echinococci with albendazole and surgery.
  - In schistosomia haematobium single-dose praziquantel is more effective than split-dose metrifonate B [5].
  - In schistosomiasis mansoni both praziquantel and oxamniquine are effective A [4].
- In neurocysticercosis albendazole and praziquantel are used as therapy. There is, however, only weak evidence of benefit C [6] of cysticidal therapy.

Prognosis

- The prognosis of worm infections is good with treatment.
- Untreated strongyloidiasis can cause lethal systemic infection in immunocompromised patients.
- Lymphatic filariasis, if left untreated, may cause swelling of the limbs and genitals resulting in malformations.
- Cysticercosis and schistosomiasis are important causes of epilepsy in some areas.
- River blindness caused by onchocerciasis is a major health problem in some areas.

Prevention

- Improvement of general hygiene, avoidance of vectors, inspection of meat, and avoidance of contact with water in endemic areas.

References

1. Ivermectin for the chemotherapy of bancroftian filariasis: a meta-analysis of the effect of single treatment. Trop Med Internat Health 1997;2:393–403.
2. The Database of Abstracts of Reviews of Effectiveness (University of York), Database no.: DARE-970744. In: The Cochrane Library, Issue 4, 1999. Oxford: Update Software.
3. Ejere H, Schwartz E, Wormald R. Ivermectin for onchocercal eye disease (river blindness). Cochrane Database Syst Rev. 2004;(2):CD002219.
4. Saconato H, Atallah A. Interventions for treating schistosomiasis mansoni. Cochrane Database Syst Rev. 2004;(2):CD000528.
5. Squires N. Interventions for treating schistosomiasis haematobium. Cochrane Database Syst Rev. 2004;(2):CD000053.
6. Salinas R, Prasad K. Drugs for treating neurocysticercosis (tapeworm infection of the brain). Cochrane Database Syst Rev. 2004;(2):CD000215.

Vaccinations

Evidence Based Medicine Guidelines. Edited by the Duodecim Editorial Team
 ISBN: 0-470-01184-X

3.1 Vaccinations

Hanna Nohynek, Satu Rapola, Ville Postila

Basic rule

- Protect the whole population or defined risk groups from important infectious diseases.

Problems

- Complete protection cannot be provided for everybody.
- Adverse effects may occur, but the benefit at the population level is always greater than the harm.

Schedule

Basic rules

- Early protection
- Immunization is performed as soon as the child has the capacity to develop immunity.
- The risk of adverse effects varies with age, which has been taken into account in the vaccination schedules.
- Either the whole population or the population at high risk is targeted.

Deviations from schedule

- If vaccination series has been interrupted it is continued, not restarted.
- Intervals between vaccinations should not be shortened.
- If the child has clearly passed the recommended age for vaccination the second dose (booster) can be given after an interval shorter than usual.
- The minimum interval between 2 vaccinations is, however, always 1 month.
- Several vaccinations can be given at a time:
  - Use different vaccination sites–record local reactions.
  - No immunoglobulin simultaneously with the MMR vaccination: immunoglobulin–6 weeks–vaccination

Hepatitis B

- Newborn infants of HBsAg carriers (both mothers and fathers) soon after birth. If the mother is a carrier, one dose of HB immunoglobulin must also be given (125 IU) B [1 2].
- People living in the same household as those with an acute HBV infection or HBsAg carriers
- Regular sex partners of people with acute HBV infections and HBsAg carriers
- Haemophiliacs on frequent substitution therapy
- Users of intravenous drugs, and their regular sex partners, and people living in the same household. The most important group to be vaccinated are the newborn children of drug-addict mothers.
- Professional prostitutes
- People at risk of needle stick injuries
- Health care students and trainees who are required to receive HBV vaccination when working abroad

Influenza

- Patients with chronic cardiac or pulmonary disease D [3] or diabetes
- Patients with renal insufficiency (serum creatinine permanently above 150 µg/l)
- People on peroral steroids
- People with immunodeficiency or immunosuppression. The vaccination should be given between treatment courses or at least 1–2 weeks before a course of cytostatics.
- People receiving steroid replacement therapy or those suffering from immunodeficiency. Vaccination is not given in hypogammaglobulinaemia that requires immunoglobulin replacement therapy.
- Children and adolescents on long-term aspirin treatment (in order to prevent Reye's syndrome).
- Vaccination reduces the rate of hospitalization in the elderly B [4 5 6 7].
- Pregnant women belonging to any of the above risk groups can be vaccinated regardless of the phase of pregnancy.

Pneumococcal and polysaccharide vaccine

- The vaccine is not included in the general vaccination schedule but the effectiveness of the vaccine is proven C [8 9 10 11].
- The protective effect is 50–80% .
- The vaccination should be repeated after 5 years only once.
- The vaccine is not effective in children under 2 years of age because of poor effect.
- The vaccine can be given simultaneously with the influenza vaccine but at a different site.

Primary target groups

- Splenectomized patients and patients with splenic dysfunction (either 2 weeks before splenectomy or immediately after)
- Patients with a CSF fistula
- Patients with lymphoma
- Patients with multiple myeloma
- Patients with nephrotic syndrome
- HIV infected patients
- Patients with congenital or acquired immunodeficiency (but not those with agammaglobulinaemia). The vaccination should be given 2 weeks before immunosuppressive therapy.

Other target groups (consider vaccination)

- Patients with
  - heart failure
  - chronic pulmonary disease
  - diabetes
  - hepatic insufficiency
  - renal insufficiency
- Persons aged 65 or above
- Alcoholics

Pneumococcal conjugate vaccines

- Pneumococcal conjugate vaccine is recommended in children under 5 years of age in the following high-risk groups:
  - Splenectomized children and children with splenic dysfunction (e.g. sickle cell anaemia)
  - Children with HIV infection
  - Other children with immunodeficiencies (congenital immunodeficiencies, nephrotic syndrome, children on antineoplastic drugs or high-dose steroids, or receiving radiotherapy)

Recommendations for vaccinations not included in the general vaccination schedule

Hib

- Splenectomized patients

Hepatitis A

- Travellers to endemic and epidemic areas (duration of travel >1 month, or recurrent travel) (9.20)

Japanese encephalitis

- Travellers to endemic areas (South-East Asia, including India), particularly if the duration of the travel exceeds 1 month and includes visits to the countryside.

Yellow fever

- Equatorial Africa, Central and South America

Tick-borne encephalitis

- People travelling to endemic areas (Northern, Central and Eastern Europe) if the probability of exposure to ticks is considered high.

Typhoid fever

- People travelling to endemic areas, particularly if food hygiene is poor.

Cholera

- Travellers to endemic areas, particularly if food hygiene is poor. Cholera killed cell vaccines are relatively safe and effective (A) [12].

Meningococci

- Meningococcal polysaccharide vaccines are used in
  - Splenectomized patients
  - People travelling to endemic and epidemic areas
- A meningococcal conjugate vaccine is included in the national vaccination schemes of several EU countries.

Rabies

- People exposed to wild animals at work in endemic areas, or working in developing countries for long periods.
- As a part of treatment after being bitten by an infected animal (1.46).

Chickenpox (Herpes varicella-zoster)

- Contains attenuated viruses
- One vaccination is effective in healthy seronegative children.
- Some vaccinated individuals develop mild signs of chickenpox (a few vesicles or papules that do not develop into vesicles). Usually there is no fever.
- The target groups include
  - Patients with high risk of complications from chickenpox: children with leukaemia or cancer, organ transplant recipients, systemic steroids, or severe chronic diseases.
  - Healthy near contacts of the above-mentioned patients at risk, including health personnel treating immunosuppressed children, and the family of those children if they have not had chickenpox.
  - According to physician's consideration for healthy children aged 12 months or above who have not had chickenpox. In the USA chickenpox vaccination is recommended for all children aged 12–18 months. The vaccine is usually administered simultaneously with the MMR vaccination in the arm.

Vaccination techniques

- **S.c. (subcutaneously)**
  - Outer aspect of the thigh or upper arm
- **I.m. (intramuscularly)**
  - The femoral muscle, outer upper quadrant of the buttock, trapezius muscle
  - Use a 25-mm needle (B) [13]
- **I.d. (intracutaneous)** (BCG)
  - Outer upper aspect of the left thigh (BCG)
  - A pale wheal should be raised.

Vaccines in general use

- Information on immunization coverage in different countries is available from the WHO (www.who.int/country/en)
- See Table 3.1.

Adverse effects

Local reactions

- Erythema, tenderness at the site of vaccination
- The reactions are usually toxic. The most common causative vaccine is pertussis-diphtheria-tetanus.
- Treatment: immobilization of the site of vaccination
- Symptomatic medication (analgesics, antihistamines)

Generalized reactions

- Fever, itching rash, irritability
  - Symptomatic treatment
- Anaphylactic reaction
  - Adrenaline 1:1 000 i.m. **0.1 ml/10 kg**
  - Adequate follow-up

Avoidance of adverse effects

- Record severe adverse reactions carefully.
- Ask about allergies to antimicrobial agents, eggs, or vaccine components (14.3).
- Give diphtheria-tetanus after an adverse reaction to pertussis-diphtheria-tetanus vaccine.
- For contraindications see below.
- Inform health authorities about severe adverse reactions.

The following conditions are NOT contraindications for vaccination

- A history of the disease against which the vaccination is aimed at
- Incubation period of an infectious disease
- A mild infectious disease (flu or diarrhoea without fever)
- Antimicrobial medication
- Local steroids or a small dose of systemic steroids
- Atopic diseases (atopic rhinitis, asthma, dermatitis)
- Dermatites, limited skin infections
- History of convulsions in the family
- Stabile neurological disease
- Down's syndrome
- Chronic cardiac, liver, lung, or renal disease, rheumatoid arthritis or diabetes
- Neonatal jaundice
- Pre-term infant, small for date
- Undernourishment
- Breast-feeding
- Pregnancy of the mother (the child of a pregnant woman can be vaccinated)

Contraindications for vaccination

- An infection with fever: **all vaccinations**
  - Vaccination is given as soon as the patient has recovered.
  - If the vaccination is being given because of an ongoing epidemic, fever is not a contraindication.
- Disorders of the immunological system: **live vaccines**

Table 3.1 Vaccines in common use in Finland 2003

Vaccine	Type	Dose (ml)	Site
BCG	live bacteria	0.05 (<3 months) 0.1 for older children	i.d.
DTP	inactivated bacteria and toxoid	0.5	i.m.
Hib	component vaccine	0.5	i.m./s.c.
Polio	inactivated virus	dose depends on the (strength of the) preparation	s.c.
MMR	live virus	0.5	s.c.
Td	toxoid	0.5	i.m.
Influenza	component	0.5	s.c.
Pneumococci	component	0.5	i.m./s.c.
Meningococci	component	0.5	s.c.
Hepatitis B	component	0.5 (0–15 years) 1.0 (>15 years)	i.m.
Hepatitis A	inactivated virus	dose depends on the (strength of the) preparation	i.m.
Tick-borne encephalitis	inactivated virus	0.5	i.m.
Japanese encephalitis	inactivated virus	• 0.5 (1–3 years) • 1.0 (>3 years)	s.c.
Rabies	inactivated virus	1.0	i.m.
Typhoid fever	• live bacteria • component	• 3 capsules • 0.5	• p.o. • i.m./s.c.
Yellow fever	live virus	0.5	s.c.
Cholera	inactivated bacteria	2 doses	p.o.
	live bacteria	1 dose	p.o.

- Immunosuppressive diseases
  - Immunosuppression caused by cancer
  - Immunosuppressive treatment (cytostatics, irradiation, systemic corticosteroids, e.g. prednisolone > 60 mg/day for adults, > 2 mg/kg/day for children for 7 days or more
- **HIV infected patients**
  - MMR can be given to symptomatic HIV infected patients
  - BCG vaccination must not be given to any patients with HIV infection.

♦ Severe adverse reaction from an earlier vaccination: **the same vaccine**

- Anaphylaxis, shock, encephalitis, encephalopathy, convulsions
- **Febrile convulsions** are not a contraindication: provide antipyretics after the vaccination

♦ A convulsive disorder that has not been investigated is a contraindication for the **pertussis vaccine**

- Vaccinations are continued after the investigations have ruled out a progressive central nervous system disease.

♦ Pregnancy: **all vaccinations**

- No vaccinations during the first trimester of pregnancy
- Vaccines other than live vaccines can be given if the epidemiological situation requires them (tetanus, influenza, and pneumococcal vaccinations are used in many countries). See instructions on influenza above.
- Adverse effects have not been observed even with live vaccines (including at least oral polio and MMR).
- An accidental MMR vaccination is not an indication for termination of pregnancy.

♦ Severe allergy to vaccine constituents

- Severe egg allergy: if food containing eggs causes urticaria, dyspnoea, itching in the throat, or severe generalized symptoms, the following vaccines should not be given: **influenza, yellow fever, tick-borne encephalitis.**
- Mild hypersensitivity to eggs: the vaccine can be given with precautions (facilities to treat eventual reactions)
- Hypersensitivity to antibiotics
  - neomycin: **do not give MMR, yellow fever or rabies vaccines**
  - polymyxin: **do not give yellow fever vaccine**

References

1. Andre FE, Zuckerman AJ. Review: protective efficacy of hepatitis B vaccines in neonates. J Med Virol 1994;44:144–151.
2. The Database of Abstracts of Reviews of Effectiveness (University of York), Database no.: DARE-940807. In: The Cochrane Library, Issue 4, 1999. Oxford: Update Software.
3. Cates CJ, Jefferson TO, Bara AI, Rowe BH. Vaccines for preventing influenza in people with asthma. Cochrane Database Syst Rev. 2004;(2):CD000364.
4. Efectividad de la vacunacion antigripal en los ancianos. Una revision critica de la bibliografia. Medicina Clinica 1995;105:645–648.
5. The Database of Abstracts of Reviews of Effectiveness (University of York), Database no.: DARE-960136. In: The Cochrane Library, Issue 4, 1999. Oxford: Update Software.
6. Gross PA, Hermogenes AW, Sacks HS, Lau J, Levandowski RA. The efficacy of influenza vaccine in elderly persons: a meta-analysis and review of the literature. Ann Intern Med 1995;123:518–527.
7. The Database of Abstracts of Reviews of Effectiveness (University of York), Database no.: DARE-952722. In: The Cochrane Library, Issue 4, 1999. Oxford: Update Software.
8. Hutchison BG, Oxman AD, Shannon HS, Lloyd S, Altmayer CA, Thomas K. Clinical effectiveness of pneumococcal vaccine: meta-analysis. Canadian Family Physician 1999:45; 2381–2393.
9. The Database of Abstracts of Reviews of Effectiveness (University of York), Database no.: DARE-992110. In: The Cochrane Library, Issue 1, 2002. Oxford: Update Software.
10. Fine MJ, Smith MJ, Carson CA, Meffe F, Sankey SS, Weissfeld LA, Detsky AS, Kapoor WN. Efficacy of pneumococcal vaccination in adults: a meta-analysis of randomized controlled trials. Arch Intern Med 1994;154:2666–2677.
11. The Database of Abstracts of Reviews of Effectiveness (University of York), Database no.: DARE-941119. In: The Cochrane Library, Issue 4, 1999. Oxford: Update Software.
12. Graves P, Deeks J, Demicheli V, Pratt M, Jefferson T. Vaccines for preventing cholera. Cochrane Database Syst Rev. 2004;(2):CD000974.
13. Diggle L, Deeks J. Effect of needle length on incidence of local reactions to routine immunisation in infants aged 4 months: randomised controlled trial. BMJ 2000;321:931–933.

Cardiovascular Diseases

Evidence Based Medicine Guidelines. Edited by the Duodecim Editorial Team
 ISBN: 0-470-01184-X

4.1 Interpretation of adult ECG

Markku Ellonen

Overview and heart rate

- Essential pathology is often revealed at a glance; however, a **systematic interpretation** is also required. QT-interval is often missed.

QRS axis

- Electrical axis in the frontal plane can be approximated:
  - left axis deviation if QRS is negative in limb lead II
  - right axis deviation if QRS is negative in limb lead I
- A computer measures the axis from surface areas of positive and negative deflections of QRS (not from the amplitude). A computer also measures the atrial axis.
- For interpretation, see article on ventricular hypertrophies 4.2.

PR (PQ) interval

- Normal PR interval is up to 0.20 seconds
- PR interval in **Wolff-Parkinson-White (WPW) syndrome** is often below 0.12 seconds (4.39).
- PR interval is considered **prolonged** when it is longer than 0.20 seconds. Slightly prolonged PR interval is **very common and usually a harmless variation of a normal ECG**. It is often associated with coronary artery disease and hypertension, and if very minor (<0.24 s) does not prevent the use of beta-blockers or digoxin. However, since these drugs have the potential of further prolonging the PR interval, the patient's ECG should be checked a few days after the instigation of such medication.
- Vagotonic functional prolongation of the PR interval is seen at rest, for example in athletes. The PR interval normalises during exercise. The PR interval varies, therefore, according to heart rate, as does the QT interval.
- A more prolonged PR interval is regarded as evidence of a first-degree AV block. The conduction delay occurs in the AV node or further down the conduction pathway, or in both. If the conduction pathway shows other abnormalities (e.g. RBBB, LAHB, LPHB), a prolonged PR interval may be more serious and herald total AV block.
- **Mobitz I (Wenckebach)**-type second-degree AV block is characterized by sequential increase in the length of the PR interval until a QRS complex is missed after a P wave. The conduction disturbance occurs almost invariably in the AV node. The disturbance is a functional and transient sequel of inferior myocardial infarction.
- **Mobitz II**: The PR interval does not gradually increase in length, but a QRS complex is occasionally missed (randomly or regularly). The block is frequently located in the bundle of His. The disturbance is usually serious and predicts a total AV block (Note! Not to be confused with sinoatrial block where the P wave is occasionally absent; this is not serious).
- In AV dissociation the ventricular rhythm (rate 30–50) is completely dissociated from the more rapid atrial rhythm. In this **third-degree AV block** QRS may be narrow or wide **(Note! In tachycardia some QRS complexes may be missed without an underlying AV block.)**

P wave

- Most easily seen in lead V1.
- When P waves are difficult to detect, marking the visible P waves on a bit of paper with a pen helps to work out the atrial rate and to detect P waves hidden in the QRS complex and T waves.
- PTF (P terminal force) is calculated from the P wave in lead V1: the duration of the negative terminal deflection of the P wave in seconds is multiplied by its depth in millimetres. PTF is pathological if the result is higher than 0.03 mms. In practice, an estimation will suffice: PTF is positive when the negative terminal deflection of the P wave is deeper and longer than the positive initial deflection. Left atrial strain increases PTF. The change may become evident quite rapidly in LV failure. PTF is a fairly specific but not a sensitive sign.
- P wave is negative in the so-called coronary sinus rhythm (low atrial rhythm) where the pacemaker is, exceptionally, located in the lower part of the atrium.
- Computers have difficulties recognising small P waves leading to difficulties in arrhythmia diagnosis.

QRS complex

- The direction of the QRS deflection in limb leads indicates the electrical axis in the frontal plane (see QRS axis above).
- Broad QRS (>0.12 s) is indicative of a bundle branch block or another abnormal intraventricular conduction.
- A pathological Q wave is a sign of a myocardial infarction, but it is not specific (4.60).
- High amplitude of a QRS complex is the voltage criterion of ventricular hypertrophy (4.27).

QT interval and QTc

- QT interval is measured from the beginning of the QRS complex to the end of the T wave. Lead II is usually used for the measurement. QT is corrected for heart rate using the formula: QTc = measured QT time (ms) × square root (heart rate/60). The result will be the corrected QT interval, i.e. QTc. QT is corrected to HR 60/min.
- A lengthening of a QT time over 10% of the reference value given on an ECG ruler is usually pathological. A QTc time over 440–480 ms is usually abnormal.
- A prolonged QT interval increases the patient's risk of the arrhythmia "torsade de pointes". The risk is further increased

by hypokalaemia, hypomagnesaemia and hypocalcaemia. An episode of unconsciousness may be a warning sign of a self-limiting run of torsade de pointes ("subsided sudden death").

- The following can cause prolongation of the QT interval
  - Inherited long QT syndrome (Romano–Ward). The QTc may be normal in a resting ECG. A QTc > 480 ms and a history of syncope during exercise or fright are suggestive of the condition. A QTc < 480 ms does not rule out the diagnosis. The patient must be warned against all medication which may prolong the QT interval.
  - Quinidine, disopyramide and sotalol when used at therapeutic doses. Prescribing these drugs necessitates measurement of the QT interval within two days of the introduction of medication. The prolongation of the QT interval more than 10%, or above 500 ms, is not acceptable. Sotalol and quinidine may be a dangerous combination in atrial fibrillation.
  - Tricyclic antidepressants and phenothiazines (particularly thioridazine, but also haloperidol) at high doses, particularly if the patient has a history of myocardial disease.
- The interaction of some drugs may cause prolongation of the QT interval and put the patient at risk of arrhythmias. These drugs include certain antifungal drugs (itraconazole and ketokonazole), antihistamines (terfenadine), cisapride and erythromycin. These drugs must not be used concomitantly with each other or with any cardiac drugs which have the potential of prolonging the QT interval. With recent discoveries the list of such drugs is growing.
- An illness which damages the myocardium may itself prolong the QT time. The effects of quinidine, disopyramide and sotalol are therefore more serious and severe in the presence of damaged myocardium. Other antiarrhythmic drugs of Class Ia and Class III may also prolong the QT interval.
- **A short QT interval** may denote hypercalcaemia and **a long QT interval** may denote severe hypocalcaemia.
- **QT dispersion** is present if the lengthening of the QT interval varies greatly in the different leads of a 12-lead ECG. The effects of QT interval lengthening drugs might be potentiated in the presence of QT dispersion. QT dispersion measured from an ECG at rest does not give sufficiently accurate information to assess an individual patient's arrhythmia risk.
- For more information see 4.7.

ST segment and T wave

- An elevation of the ST segment is associated with acute ischaemia and is the most important sign of imminent myocardial injury. The localization of the injury is identifiable from the ST elevations overlying the site of injury and from the reciprocal ST segment depression on the opposite site of the injury.
- In myocarditis ST elevation appears in all leads (except V1 and aVR), whereas in infarction the ST elevation is evident only in the leads overlying the infarcted area.
- ST elevation of 1–3 mm may be a normal finding in anterior chest leads (V1–V3) (early repolarization, particularly in an "athlete's heart" (19.10)). A benign ST elevation is often followed by a T wave, the peak of which is higher than the initial part of the ST segment.
- Digoxin may cause a gradual down slope ST segment depression. This effect is normal and does not indicate an overdose.
- ST depression is often a sign of chronic ischaemia and/or LVH.
- ST segment elevation may persist after an extensive anterior myocardial infarction, in which case it often is suggestive of an aneurysm.
- Sympathicotonia, particularly in women, may cause inferior or anterior/lateral ST-T changes, which mimic ischaemic changes. The changes will resolve with beta-blockade when HR slows down to 60/min (give e.g. 40 mg of propranolol and ask the patient to masticate the tablet).
- Negative T wave is a very non-specific sign and can accompany several conditions:
  - numerous factors with heart damaging or straining properties
  - ventricular hypertrophy
  - intoxication
  - recovery from long standing episode of tachycardia
  - subarachnoid haemorrhage or elevated intracranial pressure

U wave

- QT(U) syndrome
- Evident in severe hypokalaemia (24.10)

Arrythmias

- See 4.39, 4.42.

4.2 Ventricular hypertrophies (RVH, LVH) in ECG

Markku Ellonen

General

- The most important criterion of hypertrophy is an increase in QRS amplitude (voltage criterion). Other criteria are axis deviation, QRS widening (VAT), repolarization abnormality (ST-T strain pattern) and concomitant atrial hypertrophy.
- The amplitude correlates with muscle mass. It changes with body build and temporary sympathicotonia. Amplitudes are

lower in women and are decreased with age and by obesity, pulmonary emphysema and myocardial damage. Amplitudes increase with heavy labour and exercise, and are higher at young age and in men. These factors should be taken into consideration when the ECG is interpreted.

- ST-T strain (ST segment depression and asymmetric T wave inversion) does not result from increased muscle mass, but rather from its slow relaxation. A repolarization disturbance can also be caused by branch blocks and other types of myocardial damage.
- Sophisticated computer programs modify the statements according to the age and gender of the patient. Computers state the certainty of hypertrophy giving the rationale for it. However, the program does not take into account the patient's physical properties. To improve sensitivity, the "universal" highly specific voltage criteria have been lowered in many programs.
- Echocardiography is more sensitive and accurate than ECG in the investigation of hypertrophies.

Right ventricular hypertrophy, RVH

- The criteria for RVH are not as obvious as those for LVH, as the aetiology includes a wide range of diseases causing changes in ECG. RVH is not always visible in ECG because the greater muscle mass of the LV dominates.
- The most common cause of acquired RVH ("cor pulmonale") is chronic obstructive pulmonary disease (COPD). Emphysema reduces sensitivity by lowering QRS amplitudes. ECG is more sensitive when RVH is caused by right heart valvular defects or congenital heart defects. Assessment of RVH is difficult in concomitant RBBB and often impossible because of LBBB.

RVH is probable if one or more of the following ECG changes is present:

1. QRS axis > +100(110)° (in the absence of RBBB); QRS negative in lead I.
2. R/S > 1 in lead V1 (and V2) (no RBBB)
3. R/S < 1 in leads V5–6 (in the absence of LAHB and anterior infarction)
   - Additional criteria are right atrial hypertrophy presenting as a prominent p-wave ("p-pulmonale"), ST-T strain in V1–V2, and incomplete RBBB.

Acute "cor pulmonale" caused by massive embolia may present as:

- incomplete RBBB
- septal q-waves in V1–4 resembling anteroseptal infarction
- minor axis change to the right
- anterior ST segment depression (V1–4) and/or and reciprocal inferior ST elevation mimicking inferior myocardial injury.
- Remember: moderate pulmonary embolism does not cause definite changes in ECG (often no ECG abnormalities at all)!

Left ventricular hypertrophy, LVH

- The most common causes of LVH are hypertension, aortic stenosis and/or regurgitation, and mitral regurgitation. The patient's body build and other characteristics must always be taken into account as they have a great effect on LVH voltage criteria.

LVH is probable if even one of the following voltage criteria is fulfilled:

1. SV1 + RV5–6 > 3,5 mV (over 35 mm) (Sokolow, Lyon)
2. RaVL > 1,1 mV
3. R in any limb lead > 2.0 mV (1.8 mV)
4. SV1 > 2.5 mV
5. RV5–6 > 2.5 mV
6. RaVL + SV3 > 2.8 mV
   - Additional criteria:
     - Left atrial hypertrophy (= PTF+).
     - ST-T strain in leads V5–6, I, aVL (= repolarization abnormality)
     - QRS axis < −30 (LAHB not present)
     - QRS widening > 100 ms.
   - Voltage criteria are often too low for young people, particularly for men. Correspondingly, they are too high for women. The above given voltage criteria are unspecific, which is why computer programs that aim at better sensitivity tend to lower them. Many computer programs automatically modify the criteria according to age and gender. LBBB is a strong evidence (90%) of LVH. Repolarization disorder is a sign of severe and often irreversible hypertrophy.
   - Estes' scoring criteria for LVH, see 4.27.
   - In the LIFE and ASCOT studies LVH was defined by using the Sokolow-Lyon criterion of 3.8 mV or, alternatively, by using the Cornell product which takes into account, in addition to voltage criteria, also the width of the QRS axis and the patient's gender: the patient has LVH if the voltage duration product > 2.44 mm × s
     - Men (RaVL + SV3) × duration of QRS
     - Women (RaVL + SV3 + 6 mm) × duration of QRS

4.3 Bundle branch blocks in the ECG

Editors

General

- RBBB and LBBB are blocks of the main branches of the bundle of His. In addition to these main branches, functional (pulse rate-dependent) and structural (permanent) conduction disturbances appear in subdivisions (hemiblocks) and in the periphery.

- Injuries at various sites (or at several sites concomitantly) may cause similar changes in the ECG. The exact localization of a conduction defect is often difficult and classification is always artificial.
- WHO has given recommendations for diagnostic criteria (1985). In this chapter only the most common conduction disturbances (with the criteria in brief) are summarized, and focus is directed at their clinical significance.

RBBB

- See Figures 4.3.1, 4.3.2, 4.3.3 and 4.3.5

ECG features

1. QRS interval at least 0.12 s

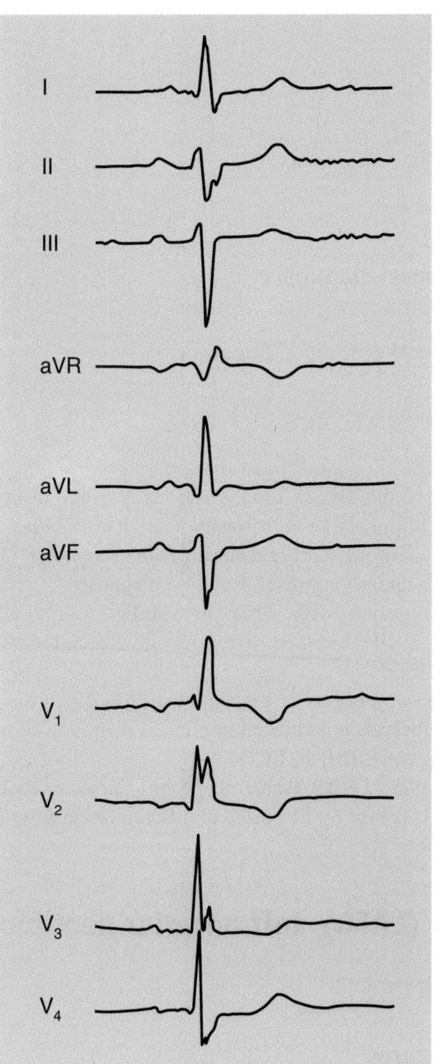

Figure 4.3.1 RBBB + LAHB and normal PQ time. Bifascicular block. Voltage criteria for LVH are also fulfilled.

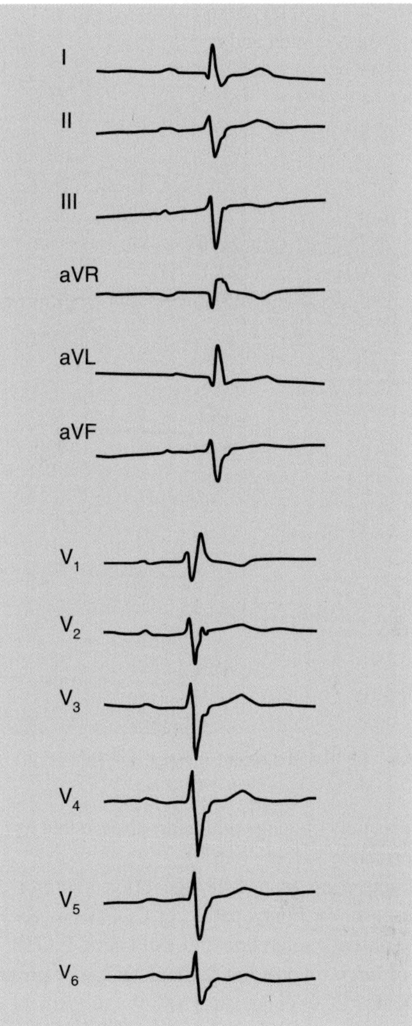

Figure 4.3.2 RBBB + LAHB and long PQ time (0.26 sec.). A trifascicular block forebodes an AV block.

2. QRS positive (M-shaped, "rabbit's ear", or RSR) in right chest leads (V1–V2), often of the shape rsR, rSR or rR
3. Repolarization disturbance in leads V1–V2 (ST segment depression, T wave inversion)
4. Wide S waves in left leads I, V5 and V6
5. The shape of QRS varies greatly and is dependent on the underlying disease.

Differential diagnosis

- Right ventricular hypertrophy (RVH)
- Wolff-Parkinson-White syndrome (WPW)
- Peripheral conduction disturbances

Clinical significance

- Commonly seen without serious heart disease.
- Clinical significance depends on the possible underlying disease, which may be myocardial infarction, myocarditis, pulmonary embolism, COPD (cor pulmonale).

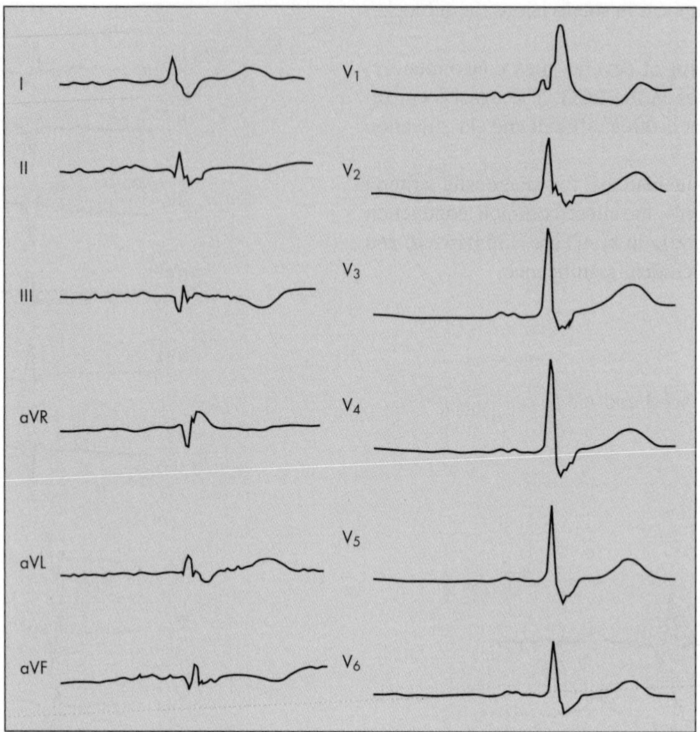

Figure 4.3.3 RBBB and a recent inferior wall infarction: Q III, aVF and T wave inversion.

- Often a sequela of congenital heart disease that remains even after corrective surgery (ASD)
- RBBB appearing in middle age often signifies ischaemic heart disease, cardiomyopathy, or COPD (= RVH).
- In acute anterior infarction and associated LAHB, RBBB is a sign of large myocardial damage and poor prognosis.
- Complicates ECG diagnostics and the judgement of:
  - posterior infarction
  - LVH and RVH
- Incomplete RBBB (same shape but duration < 0.12 s) is a common and innocent ECG change in young endurance athletes. The aetiology of the rSR' in these cases is not a conduction defect.

LBBB

- See Figure 4.3.4

ECG features

1. QRS duration at least 0.12 s
2. M-shaped broad R wave in leads I, aVL, V5–V6 and without Q wave
3. ST deviation and T wave directed away from the QRS complex (repolarization disturbance)
4. Broad and deep S shaped rS or QS in leads V1–V2
5. Variations in shape depend on simultaneous LVH, infarction etc. The axis is often to the left.

Differential diagnosis

- WPW
- Peripheral conduction disturbances

Clinical significance

- Frequently a sign of heart disease
- LBBB at middle age usually reflects acquired heart disease, most commonly LVH, coronary heart disease or myocarditis. The underlying disease determines the prognosis. Occasionally no underlying disease can be diagnosed.
- In connection with acute myocardial infarction (AMI), recent LBBB predicts extensive myocardial damage and poor prognosis.
- LBBB complicates or prevents the ECG diagnosis of AMI. Thrombolysis is indicated in clinical diagnosis of infarction and recent LBBB in ECG.
- Incomplete LBBB (same shape but duration < 0.12 s) is usually caused by LVH. Exact differentiation from LBBB is not necessary.

LAHB (LAFB), left anterior hemiblock

- See Figure 4.3.6

ECG features

1. Frontal axis deviation to the left (−30°– −90°)
2. Deep S wave of the shape rS in leads II, III and aVF

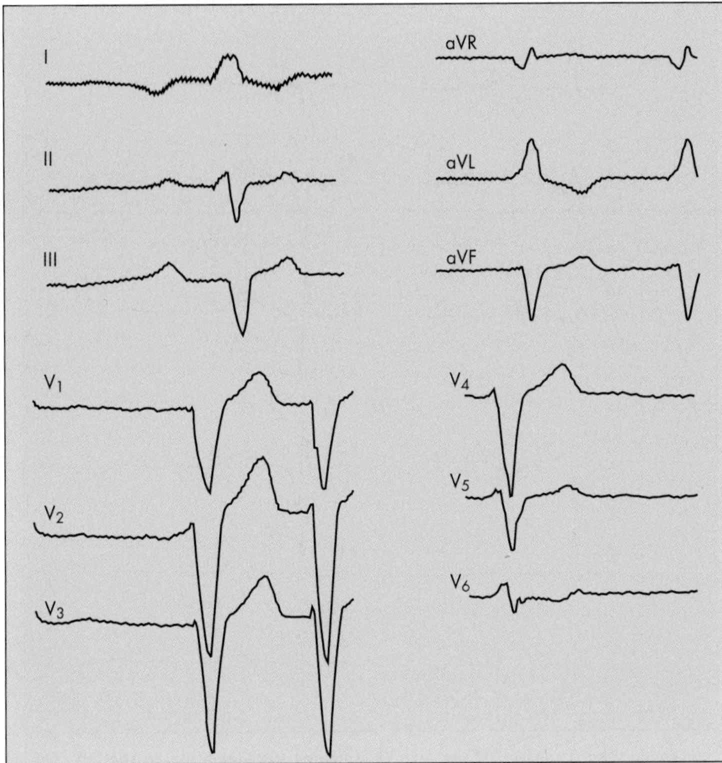

Figure 4.3.4 LBBB and atrial fibrillation.

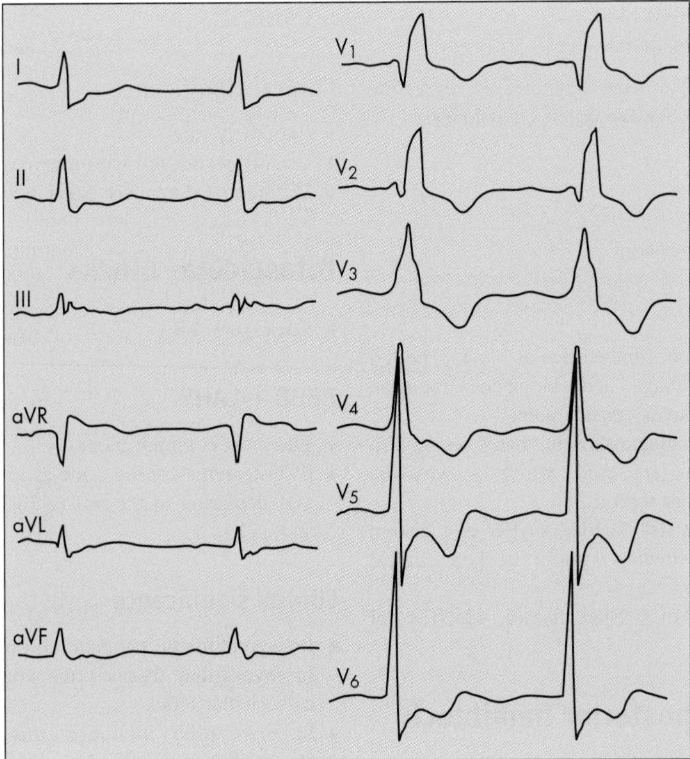

Figure 4.3.5 RBBB + LVH. The ST-T change in left chest leads is caused by LVH. A high RV5 is associated with hypertrophy.

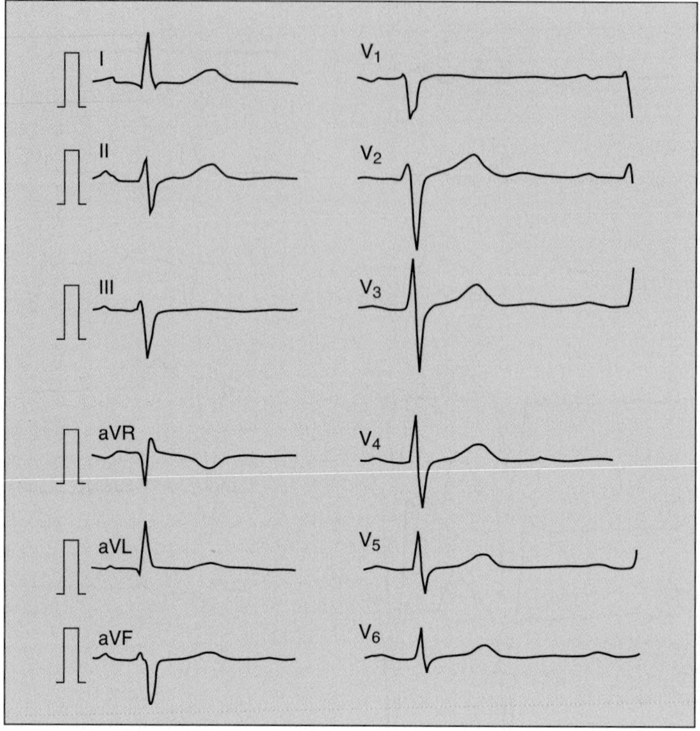

Figure 4.3.6 LAHB in a healthy person. The negative QRS on lead II indicates axis deviation to the left. The most common reasons for this are LAHB, LVH or both.

3. qR in leads I and aVL
4. Minor widening of QRS (<0.12 s)
5. Repolarization disturbance absent

- Additional criteria that support the diagnosis are regression of the R wave and a deep S wave in left chest leads.

Differential diagnosis

- LVH (left axis deviation)
- Anterior infarction (R regression)

Clinical significance

- LAHB is the most common intraventricular block. The left anterior branch is easily damaged and a block does not mean that the damage to the heart is considerable.
- LAHB complicates ECG diagnostics in many ways, also when computer programs are used, which is why the physician should be familiar with it.
- In young patients without risk factors, LAHB is a benign and innocent ECG abnormality without marked clinical significance.
- At middle age, LAHB predicts heart disease, which is not necessarily severe.

LPHB (LPFB), left posterior hemiblock

ECG features

- Axis to the right
- QRS complexes to opposite directions compared with LAHB

Clinical significance

- Extremely rare
- Usually associated with massive posterior infarction
- Differential diagnosis: RVH

Bifascicular blocks

- See Figure 4.3.1

RBBB + LAHB

- The most common block
- ECG features are the same as in RBBB. In addition, frontal axis deviation to the left (−30°–−90°): rS in leads II, III and aVF.

Clinical significance

- In asymptomatic patients the prognosis is frequently good. In myocardial diseases the condition may progress to a trifascicular block.
- In myocardial infarction this is a sign of extensive myocardial damage and predicts total AV block.
- A pacemaker often necessary if the condition is associated with AMI. When a long PQ time is associated with the

conduction disturbance, the condition is called trifascicular block (see later), which is always an indication for a pacemaker in AMI.

Trifascicular blocks: RBBB + LAHB + AV block

- See Figure 4.3.2
- A bifascicular block with grade I or II AV block. The condition is more severe if the PQ time is long, suggesting a defect in the bundle of His. Caution with drugs that prolong PQ time is necessary.
- The most common type is RBBB + LAHB + prolonged PQ time.
- The risk of total AV block is high, which is why pacemaker is often necessary. The prognosis is rather poor even with a pacemaker.

4.5 Ambulatory ECG monitoring

Markku Ellonen

Principles

- ECG monitoring during the patient's normal daily activities. The principal aim is to detect rhythm and conduction disturbances.
- A patient activated event recorder only registers episodes specified by the patient.
- The most commonly used devices are a Holter monitor (1–2 days), an event recorder (3–7 days) and a new implantable loop recorder (up to 1 year or more).

Indications

- Unexplained disturbances of consciousness
- Severe symptoms suggestive of arrhythmias: attacks of palpitations associated with disturbed conscious level
- Assessment of the efficacy on antiarrhythmic drugs
- Investigation into functional problems of a pacemaker. Assessment of the need of a pacemaker, for example, in sick sinus syndrome.
- Only in exceptional cases, for diagnosis and monitoring of ischaemia: a 12 lead ECG recording is needed instead of the usual 3 lead.
- A "therapeutic" investigation of a patient disabled by presyncope or palpitations is a relative indication. An event recorder is the optimal choice for this purpose.

Interpretation

- Computerised interpretation in particular is hindered by technical artefacts; arrhythmias and the ST segment are affected most.
- The "attack" being looked for might not appear during the monitoring period. In such cases, monitoring may be extended for a longer period or an event recorder could be used. The patient activates the monitor at the moment the symptoms occur (memory Holter). Monitoring may be continued for up to several weeks.
- Implantable loop recorder is a new device. It is implanted in the same way as a pacemaker. The main indications for its use are infrequently occurring syncope attacks of cardiac origin, which are often serious and require medical attention.
- Healthy, asymptomatic persons are frequently found to have ventricular ectopics, self-limiting episodes of ventricular tachycardia, bradyarrhythmias and AV conduction disturbances. Computerized programmes interpret any broad complex beats as ventricular ectopics. These symptoms must be interpreted with the patient's age and any existing heart disease in mind.
- Assessing ST segment depression is technically demanding and often difficult. An asymptomatic ST depression less than 2 mm is not diagnostic and thus not a sign of "silent" ischaemia.
- Asymptomatic ischaemia recorded during ambulatory ECG monitoring does not warrant further measures in a patient whose coronary artery disease shows no signs of sudden deterioration.
- Ambulatory ECG monitoring is more suitable for the monitoring of a symptomatic patient with coronary artery disease.
    - The condition of a patient with unstable angina can be assessed with 12-lead monitoring.
    - If a patient is diagnosed with an acute coronary syndrome and has associated asymptomatic ischaemia during ambulatory ECG monitoring, urgent angiography is warranted.
- An event register records only the events specified by the patient. The arrhythmias found are in most cases clinically insignificant (atrial fibrillation, paroxysmal supraventricular tachycardia, bradycardia). However, such rhythms may explain the patient's symptoms. A normal rhythm whilst the symptoms are present, on the other hand, excludes arrhythmias as the cause, and investigations must be directed to other causes.
- In the assessment of dizziness and syncope the most common findings of clinical importance are sinus arrest or slow atrial fibrillation, AV block, ventricular tachycardia and fast supraventricular arrhythmia.
- The information obtained by ambulatory ECG monitoring should be weighed against the patient's overall condition in order to evaluate if the findings are of clinical significance, irrespective of whether the patient is sick or healthy. Such an assessment requires specialist skills, and in some cases some

uncertainty about the pathology of the monitoring results may still remain.

4.6 Computerised ECG interpretation

Markku Ellonen

- A computer programme interprets an ECG recording systematically, taking into account the various intervals, deflections and complex amplitudes. These programmes should, however, mainly be used to ensure that no abnormalities have inadvertently been missed by the treating physician.
- The programmes are designed to be highly sensitive, which may lead to over-diagnosis. The evaluation standards of the programmes often allow some latitude for the interpretation, and the programmes often state the predicted degree of accuracy of the interpretation. False positive anterior infarctions are reported, for example, on the basis of R-regression in leads V2, V3 and V4 (Minnesota code 1-2-8). The regression may also result from LAHB, hypertrophic cardiomyopathy, RV hypertrophy or a wrongly placed electrode. A narrow Q wave (less than 0.03 s) in leads III and aVF may give rise to a suspicion of old inferior infarction.
- The diagnosis of an acute infarction is based on ST segment changes. Because the programmes have been made extra sensitive for the sake of safety, and ST segment changes are common and often non-specific, the computer interpretation may be vague and not of great value when support is sought for quick decision making in cases of possible acute infarction. The computer does not "see" the shape of an ST segment as a human eye would. Nevertheless, it does calculate the ST:T ratio. If the ratio is high, myocardial damage is a more likely diagnosis than early repolarisation. Before interpreting the significance of any ST elevation the computer, like the physician, looks for reciprocal ST depression and, if present, will suggest myocardial damage. If ST elevation is present in several leads, perimyocarditis should be suspected. On the other hand, the computer might ignore a finding and merely report it as "non-specific ST elevation". The clinical significance of such a finding must then be decided by the physician
- Programmes cannot interpret the shape of the P wave reliably. This causes problems in arrhythmia diagnosis which remains the main weakness of computerised ECG interpretation.
- The "deterministic" programmes base their interpretation on sensitized adaptations of traditional criteria.
- The latest "intelligent" programmes do not use traditional criteria for the interpretation. These programmes have been "taught" to identify abnormalities with the aid of thousands of ECG recordings.
- A computerised programme often gives an approximate evaluation of the accuracy of its interpretation (probable, may be a normal variant). A programme also gives a brief report of the reasons behind its diagnosis. An ECG machine is usually delivered complete with a description of the evaluation criteria used by the software programme.
- The statement "normal ECG" is usually reliable.
- A programme may give several suggestions, the relevance of which the physician must decide. The patient's clinical presentation and findings must also be taken into account. A computer programme is not responsible for any incorrect interpretations.

4.7 Long QT syndrome (LQT)

Markku Ellonen

Introduction

- Consider long QT syndrome (LQT) as a cause of syncope in a child or adolescent.
- Acquired LQT may result from the use of certain drugs and, more often, from the use of several drug combinations. The QT interval should be measured when these drugs are prescribed.
- LQT is a complicated syndrome: the QT interval may be normal at the time of measurement. Reference values are to be used only as a guide. QT dispersion further complicates the matter.
- The QT interval should be measured with an ECG ruler; "a glance" is not enough to interpret abnormal QT interval (Figure 4.7.1).
- Patients with LQT must not be administered drugs that prolong the QT interval. Such administration increases the patient's risk for the arrhythmia "torsade de pointes".
- Severe hypocalcaemia prolongs the QT interval without the concomitant risk of torsade de pointes.

Congenital long QT syndrome (congenitally weakened repolarization)

- Onset at school age: symptom onset in boys almost always by the age of 15. In female patients symptom onset in some cases (20%) after this age (15–30 years).
- The most common first symptom is loss of consciousness during exercise or fright. Loss of consciousness is caused by a run of torsade de pointes which usually, but not always, is self-limiting and lasts a few second or minutes ("subsided sudden death"). The episode of tachycardia may be so brief that no unconsciousness due to cerebral ischaemia develops and the patient gives a history of palpitations or blurred vision. LQT might be the partial reason behind some cot

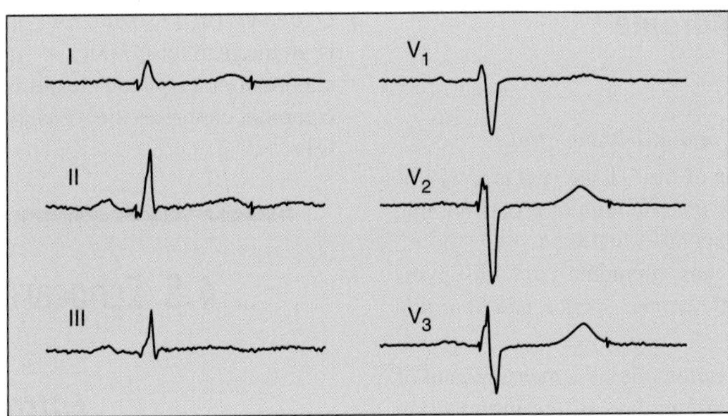

Figure 4.7.1 Long QT syndrome (LQT) in a young woman, who repeatedly fainted during physical exercise. The ECG appears to be normal, if the QT interval is not measured: in lead II 0.44 sec. and V3 0.48 sec., which for this pulse rate (60/min.) is prolonged. A normal QT interval at a pulse rate of 60/min. would be 0.39 sec.

deaths; QTc greater than 440 ms has been considered to be the risk limit.

- Some carriers may not manifest any symptoms of the illness. Several affected families have been identified. The most common is the Romano–Ward syndrome which is inherited as an autosomal dominant trait, i.e. 50% of the affected person's offspring will inherit the faulty gene.
- The syndrome involves an ion channel defect in the cell membrane leading to impaired flow of potassium out of the cells. This in turn will prolong repolarization. At least five faulty genes have been identified so far (LQT 1–5).
  - The most common is LQT1. The QT interval becomes prolonged during exercise or a few minutes thereafter.
  - LQT2 and 3 manifest themselves as nocturnal episodes which are often initially suspected to be epileptic in origin.
  - The heart of a patient with LQT is of normal structure.
- Suspect inherited LQT if
  - the patient gives a history of syncope or presyncope particularly during exercise or intense emotions or soon thereafter. A seizure of a short duration is possible but, unlike during an epileptic fit, the seizure is preceded by the patient lying still for 5-10 seconds.
  - the patient suffers from vague nocturnal epilepsy
  - the QTc is prolonged (more than 440–480 ms is usually abnormal). T wave is often abnormal, i.e. bifid.
  - there is a family history of LQT.

Diagnosis

- Criteria based on the QT interval are nonsensitive and defective. Nevertheless if the QT interval corrected for heart rate (QTc) is greater than 480 ms, and the patient has suffered an episode of unconsciousness, the diagnosis of LQT is likely.
  - Conventionally the upper limit of normal QT interval has been considered to be 440 ms with heart rate of 60/min.
  - Corrected QT interval exceeding 440 ms, in a patient with an episode of unconsciousness, is suspicious.
  - The QT interval of some patients with LQT may be within the normal reference range.
  - Positive family history is an important additional criteria.
  - An abnormal T wave morphology and bradycardia in a child are suggestive of LQT.
- A prolonged QT interval is present in the resting ECG of 70% of affected individuals.
  - First degree relatives of affected individuals should be investigated.
  - Exercise ECG increases the sensitivity; the QT interval usually becomes prolonged after the exercise. QT dispersion may be greater than normal.
- Diagnosis should be confirmed with DNA studies. Population screening is not feasible due to the multitude of faulty genes.
- A negative DNA result does not definitely exclude LQT. 30% of carriers have a normal QT interval.
- The differential diagnosis in children and adolescents should take into account normal vasodepressive syncope, epilepsy, inherited polymorphic ventricular tachycardia and hypertrophic cardiomyopathy.

Treatment

- If the cause of symptoms is suspected to be LQT, a cardiologist should be consulted.
- The treatment usually consists of permanent beta-blockade. Sustained-release propranolol is the most popular choice.
- The patient must not take part in competitive sports, and swimming in particular should be banned.
- The same bans and instructions also apply to asymptomatic carriers, but no medication is usually required. However, children are often started on a beta-blocker.
- An internal cardioverter defibrillator (ICD) is warranted for patients who do not respond to medication.
- The avoidance of medication with the potential of prolonging the QT interval is of utmost importance. The patient must be given a list of such medication. The dose of beta-agonists, which cause tachycardia, should be minimized.
- Situations with the potential to lead to electrolyte imbalances should be avoided.

Acquired long QT syndrome

Causes

- Potassium-channel blocking anti-arrhythmic drugs.
  - However, the prolongation of the QT interval is a sign of their therapeutic effect, but the safe limit of proarrhythmic prolongation of the QT interval is not fixed.
  - The most well known are quinidine and disopyramide (Class IA) and amiodarone, sotalol and ibutilide (Class III).
    - Prescribing these drugs necessitates the measurement of the QT interval within a few days of the introduction of medication. The prolongation of more than 25% is alarming. Sotalol should be replaced by another beta-blocker.
  - Many other drugs also prolong the QT interval and increase the risk of torsade de pointes. The mechanism is often unknown.
    - These drugs include conventional phenothiazides (particularly thioridazine), haloperidol, tricyclic antidepressants and doxepin. The risk is increased if the psychiatric patient has a co-existing heart disease.
  - Some cases of prolonged QT interval are due to latent defects of the ion channels.
    - Of antibiotics, intravenous erythromycin is the most well known inducer of torsade de pointes.
  - The combined use of two common drugs, which are safe when used alone, may predispose the patient to the risk of torsade de pointes. A shared metabolic route with a drug that prolongs QT interval raises the concentration to a dangerous level increasing the risk of torsade de pointes even in a healthy heart. Another possible mechanism is a minor inherited ion channel defect which is not usually evident.
    - The list of these drugs is long and new drugs are constantly added.
    - The most common ones are the antihistamines terfenadine and astemizole, conazoles, macrolides, cisapride, ciprofloxacin etc. Many have been withdrawn from the market or are only sold with accompanied warnings.

Measuring QT interval

- The QT interval is measured from the beginning of the QRS complex to the end of the T wave.
- Abnormal morphology of the T wave, or the presence of a U wave, may impede the measurement.
- An ECG ruler will provide the normal, heart rate calibrated, QTc intervals. A variation of 10% is common and acceptable.
- Lead II is usually used for the measurement. Different leads may yield a QT interval of varying duration. This is called QT dispersion, and it increases the risk of arrhythmias, particularly in patients with co-existing heart disease. Significant QT dispersion indicates disparity in repolarization between the different parts of the heart.
- QTc = QT(ms) / square root of R-R (s). The Bazett formula is an alternative: QT(ms) × square root (heart rate/60). An abnormal or suspicious result is a value over 440 ms. ECG-computer calibrates the measured QT-interval to HR 60/min: QTc.

4.8 Echocardiography

Editors

Basic rule

- Any anatomical abnormality and functional disturbance can be detected with different modifications of echocardiography.

Transthoracic method

- Heart failure of unknown aetiology; systolic, diastolic or asymptomatic heart failure.
- Determining the ejection fraction
  - The formula for calculating ejection fraction: left ventricular volume (V) is obtained by the formula $V = (7 \times D^3)/(D + 2.4)$, where D is the diameter of the left ventricle measured immediately from the distal side at the level of the mitral valve. To calculate ejection fraction (EF) first subtract left ventricular systolic (V_s) volume from the diastolic (V_d) volume and then calculate the percentage of this difference from the diastolic volume:
  - $EF = (V_d - V_s) \times 100/V_d$
- Determining the extent and anatomical complications of myocardial infarction (papillary muscle rupture, septum perforation, aneurysm, mural thrombus).
- Assessing the extent, and viability, of ischaemic myocardium.
- Hypertrophies; echocardiography is more sensitive and specific than an ECG. Left ventricular hypertrophy suggests the need to start antihypertensive medication.
- Cardiomyopathies
- Pericardial effusion and marked myocarditis.
- Mitral valve and tricuspid valve. Diagnosis and assessment of the clinical significance of mitral valve prolapse are only possible by echocardiography, and even then overdiagnosis remains a possibility.
- Aortic and pulmonary valves (complemented by Doppler) It is not possible to differentiate between a calcified aortic valve and aortic stenosis by a heart murmur alone. Valve diameter of 1–1.5 cm^2 is indicative of moderate stenosis and pressure gradient of 50–100 mmHg.
- Function of valvular prostheses.
- Massive pulmonary embolism: right ventricular strain

- Pulmonary hypertension
- Suspicion of a congenital heart defect

Doppler cardiography (Doppler, colour Doppler)

- More accurate information of the degree of valve stenosis or regurgitation (pressure gradient).
- More accurate information of congenital heart diseases and follow-up of patients who have undergone surgery.
- Coronary artery stenosis, particularly LAD

Transoesophageal echocardiography

- Valvular vegetation (endocarditis)
- Atrial thrombus; young patient with cerebral infarction
- Valvular prostheses
- Aortic dissection
- Atrial septal defect (ASD)

Exercise echocardiography

- An alternative to exercise tolerance test and isotope scanning in the diagnosis of coronary heart disease when exercise test is not diagnostic because of the following reasons:
  - chest pain without ECG changes
  - ECG changes without symptoms
  - ECG not diagnostic due to concomitant LVH, LBBB, WPW, etc.
- Dobutamine stress echocardiography can be carried out to predict the viability of akinetic myocardium prior to coronary artery by-pass surgery.

4.11 The most common acquired adult valvular heart diseases and associated murmurs

Markku Ellonen

Aims

- Assess the significance of a murmur: valvular disease or an innocent systolic murmur.
- Estimate the severity of the valvular disease and consider the need for echocardiography.
- Remember the possibility of valvular disease in any patient with dyspnoea or ventricular hypertrophy on the ECG.
- Endocarditis prophylaxis should be given to all patients with valvular disease or a congenital heart defect (with the exception of ASD).

In general

- The loudness of a murmur does not always correlate to the severity of the stenosis. As the ejection fraction (EF) decreases, the murmur may become softer or even disappear totally (aortic stenosis).
- In severe aortic regurgitation the regurgitant murmur becomes weaker and a systolic flow murmur, caused by the increased flow is heard, without coexisting stenosis. A combined valvular disease is characterised by stenosis and regurgitation.
- Only the most common valvular diseases are described here. The rare adult ventricular septal defect (VSD), pulmonary stenosis, mitral stenosis or adult congenital heart defects are not included.

Systolic murmurs

Aortic stenosis (AS)

- The most important valvular disease in adults, incidence increases with age.
- In patients under the age of 60, the deterioration and calcification of the aortic valve is slow, often associated with bicuspid anomaly (in 1–2%).
- In patients over the age of 60, the valvular defect is caused by atherosclerotic changes the risk factors being the same as for coronary artery disease
- The symptoms progress gradually and are non-specific. The classic triad of AS symptoms consists of dyspnoea, angina pectoris and syncope on exertion. The pressure overload may impair coronary circulation leading to myocardial ischaemia without coexisting coronary artery disease.
- Early detection of symptoms is important. When the valvular orifice is <1 cm^2 and the pressure gradient >50 mmHg, the stenotic valve becomes symptomatic.
- After the appearance of the symptoms, the prognosis worsens rapidly; without surgery life expectancy is 2–5 years.
- The outcome of surgery is poor if heart failure has already developed. However, low EF is not a contraindication for surgery.
- Murmur (Figure 4.11.3)
  - Harsh or rough, peak in mid-systole or late systole. An early systolic ejection suggests mild stenosis whereas an ejection murmur of a longer duration suggests more severe stenosis.
  - Area of transmission from the aortic area to the neck and apex. Apical transmission may be difficult to differentiate from the murmur of mitral regurgitation, which is transmitted towards the axilla.
  - As the valve becomes more stenotic, the opening and closing sounds (S2) become weaker and disappear

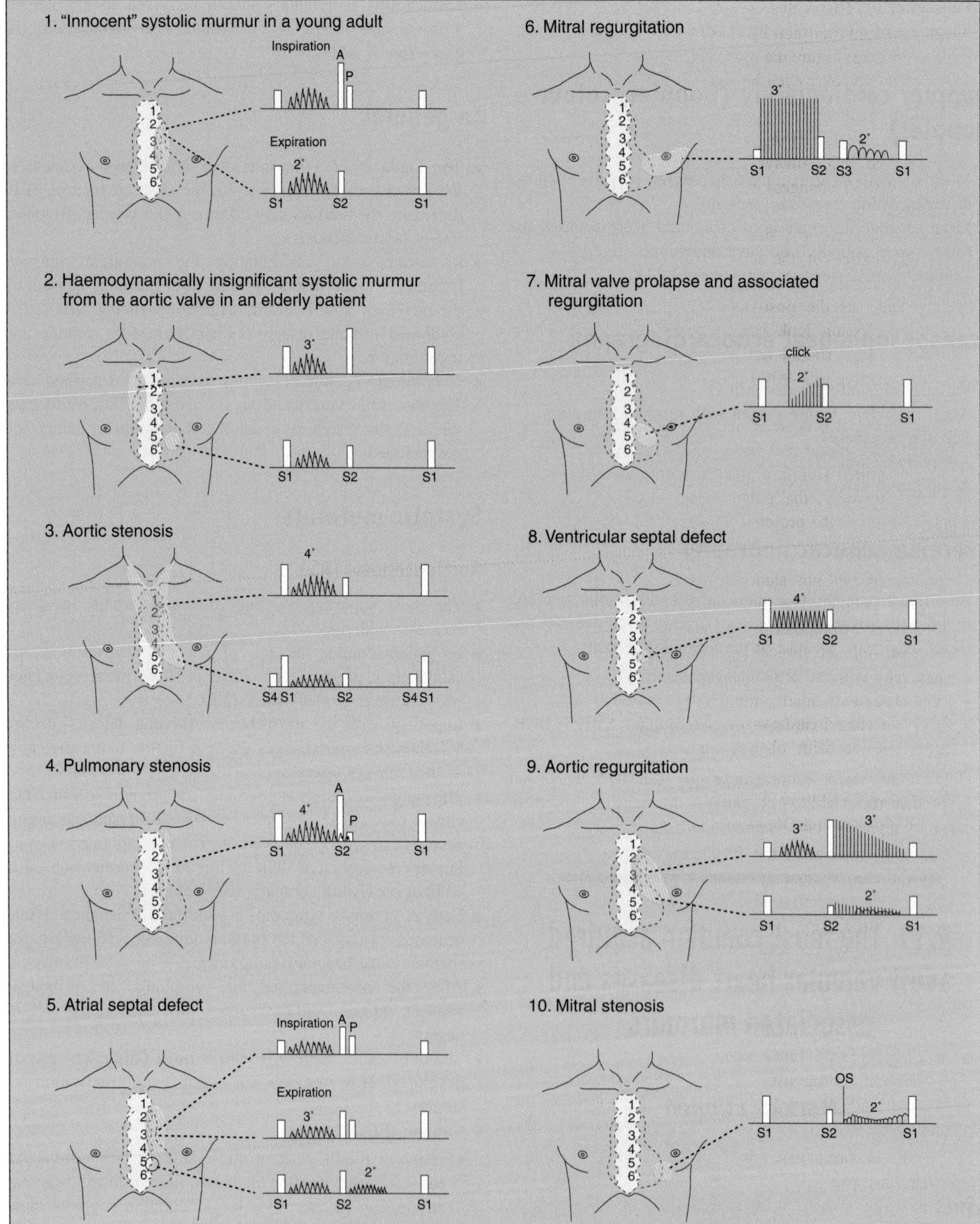

Figure 4.11 Cardiac murmurs.

completely. The valve begins to leak and diastolic regurgitant murmur can be heard.
  - In severe heart failure the murmur may decrease markedly in loudness or may even become inaudible.
- Other signs
  - Palpation reveals a strong apical beat of long duration.
  - In principle, ECG always shows LVH (and the presence of QRS and ST changes) with the exception of the elderly patients.
  - On a chest x-ray, the size of the heart is often normal and the outline of the left ventricle rounded. This is why the diagnosis of AS is often delayed. On the chest x-ray look for the post-stenotic dilatation, and in the lateral projection look for calcified aortic cusps. This important sign should not be overlooked because it is both a sensitive (80–90%) and a specific (60–70%) sign of AS.
  - The carotid pulse is weak and slowly rising ("parvus et tardus"), and blood pressure readings manifest a narrow pulse pressure. This is a sign of severe stenosis. In the elderly, however, the pulse pressure may be over 50 mmHg even in the presence of significant AS.
- Differential diagnosis
  - A calcified but not stenosed aortic valve is common in older people. The murmur resembles AS and is difficult to differentiate by means of auscultation only. Other above-listed clinical signs of stenosis (LVH, narrow pulse pressure) are absent. An echocardiogram is often necessary! Mere calcification of the valve may also be a sign of increased cardiovascular risk C [1]. Calcification not associated with obstruction might represent early stages of AS.
  - Hypertrophic cardiomyopathy (4.86)
- Echocardiography and Doppler examination
  - Will reveal the size of the orifice, the surface area of the cusp and the pressure gradient as well as the thickness of the walls, and thus also the degree of stenosis and the need for surgery. If the pressure gradient exceeds 50 mmHg or the surface area is less than 1 cm^2 the condition is considered to be serious and is usually symptomatic.
- Treatment
  - Patients with symptomatic stenosis should be considered for surgery, even those over 80 years of age (valve replacement). Prognosis is poor without surgery but improves with surgery.
  - Asymptomatic patients must be closely monitored
    - Some asymptomatic patients with severe stenosis warrant surgery.
    - Moderate symptoms and coexisting coronary artery disease is an indication for surgery.
    - The emergence of symptoms or worsening of the ECG changes are indications for an echocardiogram and the consideration for urgent surgery.
  - Physical exertion and exercise tolerance testing may be hazardous for AS patients due to the risk of ischaemia and arrhythmias.
  - The use of nitrates and other vasodilators has traditionally been avoided because of the risk of syncope. However, they are suitable for most patients and constitute an important part of their treatment (particularly ACE inhibitors) since the patients often have coexisting hypertension, coronary artery disease as well as valvular insufficiency.
  - Antibiotic prophylaxis for endocarditis

Mitral regurgitation (mitral insufficiency) (MR)

- The most common valve disease in adults.
- Aetiologies include recent or old myocardial infarction (MI), cusp insufficiency resulting from the dilatation of the left ventricle and the mitral valve ring (dilated cardiomyopathy), papillary muscle dysfunction, or degeneration of the valvular connective tissue.
- The aetiology of a suddenly worsening regurgitation, or regurgitation of a sudden onset, might be ruptured chordae tendineae, papillary muscle rupture or cardiac trauma.
- Murmur (Figure 4.11.6)
  - The high frequency, pansystolic blowing murmur is loudest in the area between the apex and midaxillary line. In mild regurgitation only a short ejection murmur may be heard.
  - In posterior cusp regurgitation the murmur is transmitted towards the upper sternum and mimics AS. A common problem in clinical practice is the differentiation between AS and MR. In the anterior cusp regurgitation the murmur is transmitted towards the axilla.
  - The closing of the valve (S1) is often soft and S3 often audible.
  - Loudness of the murmur does not relate to the degree of mitral regurgitation. If the function of the left ventricle has remained good, the regurgitant murmur will also be strong. As the left ventricle becomes weaker so will the murmur. In severe regurgitation a soft diastolic inflow murmur may be heard. A regurgitant murmur caused by papillary muscle damage, resulting from MI, is usually soft even when the regurgitant volume is large. In dilated cardiomyopathy the degree of regurgitation, and associated murmur, vary depending on the size of the mitral valve ring. The character of the murmur changes according to the size of the ventricle and EF. As the heart size diminishes the murmur may become inaudible.
- Other signs
  - The apex of the dilated left ventricle is felt on palpation as lifting, extending into the parasternal area, and it may mimic the dilatation of the right ventricle.
  - In significant regurgitation, an ECG will show signs of both left ventricular (LVH) and left atrial (PTF) strain. The rhythm is often atrial fibrillation.
  - A chest x-ray shows an enlarged left atrium and left ventricle with pulmonary vascular congestion.
- Echocardiography and Doppler examination
  - The most important investigation in the evaluation of the severity of MR. Can be used to assess the need and timing for surgery before the LV is damaged irreversibly.

- Treatment
  - The drugs of choice are diuretics or vasodilators (ACE inhibitors and nitrates), which are used to treat possible hypertension or heart failure. Atrial fibrillation is also often treated (digoxin, beta-blocker and anticoagulant). In many cases the appearance of atrial fibrillation aggravates the condition acutely, leading to heart failure.
  - A continuously decreasing EF(<60%) progressive left ventricular dilatation (end-systolic dimension >45 mm), and worsening of symptoms are indications for valvular surgery. Note that the patient compensates for the regurgitation, and may have only mild symptoms when the time is optimal for surgery.
  - A left ventricle that has been damaged by volume loading does not recover even with surgery.
  - The operation is either valve repair or valve replacement.
  - Remember antibiotic prophylaxis against endocarditis.

Mitral valve prolapse (Barlow syndrome) (MVP)

- Common and often innocent (in up to 10%) auscultatory finding. Its prevalence is approximately only 2.4% (USA) according to current echocardiography criteria.
- A classic auscultation sign is a high-frequency mid-systolic click and a blowing late systolic MR murmur or both (Figure 4.11.7). Such a finding does not always mean that the patient meets the current echocardiographic criteria for MVP. In significant regurgitation the murmur is lengthened and may even be pan-systolic.
- Mitral valve prolapse is not an independent disease but a heterogenic phenomenon, at the one end of which is a totally healthy (incidental auscultation finding) individual and at the other end is the patient with a distinct illness where the degenerated cusp is causing a significant and progressing regurgitation.
- The condition needs no treatment unless there is significant mitral regurgitation.
- Many patients complain of ectopic beats, which is often the reason for seeing a doctor. A typical patient is a symphaticotonic young, slim female who can be prescribed a beta-blocker if necessary.
- The murmur is often found incidentally in a healthy person. Haemodynamically non-significant MVP is not associated with a stroke or TIA as was previously thought
- Echocardiography can be carried out to evaluate the degree of regurgitation, and thickening and degeneration of the cusps, when significant regurgitation is suspected.
- Prophylaxis against endocarditis is given only to patients with significant regurgitation. These patients should be monitored. Atrial fibrillation or TIA usually warrant a prescription for an anticoagulant.

Tricuspid regurgitation (TR)

- TR is almost always a consequence of pulmonary hypertension.
- Murmur
  - A pansystolic murmur which resembles mitral regurgitation. It is best heard parasternally at the fourth intercostal space. The murmur is augmented by inspiration.
  - Often soft and difficult to hear, even when the regurgitation is gross on echocardiogram.
- Other signs
  - Signs and symptoms of increased venous pressure
  - Venous pulse waves (v waves) in the neck are a typical sign.
  - Ascites, oedema, enlarged and pulsatile liver
  - Other secondary signs of pulmonary hypertension; right atrial lift on palpation
  - Minor regurgitation without clinical significance is often found by colour Doppler echocardiography.
  - ECG and chest x-ray: hypertrophy and enlargement of the right ventricle and atrium

Diastolic murmurs

- May be regurgitatant murmurs (AR) or diastolic flow murmurs (MS).
- Invariably pathological, even if not haemodynamically significant.
- Often soft and easily missed. Examine the patient in a quiet room. Pay attention to the diastole.

Aortic regurgitation (AR)

- Valvular lesions (degeneration, endocarditis, rheumatic fever, bicuspidal anomaly of the valve)
- Dilatation of the fibrous valve ring (degeneration, dissection, Marfan's syndrome, syphilis etc.)
- Murmur (Figure 4.11.9)
  - A diastolic, decrescendo, blowing murmur is best heard with the diaphragm of the stethoscope.
  - The murmur is heard best at the aortic area and towards the apex, with the patient sitting up and leaning forward and holding his breath after expiration. The pitch of the regurgitant murmur and the breath sounds is similar.
  - As the regurgitation worsens, a systolic ejection murmur is present even without stenosis as a result of increased stroke volume. A systolic murmur may also be heard if there is concurrent MR resulting from the dilating ventricle.
  - An early diastolic murmur usually signifies mild regurgitation and a late diastolic murmur severe regurgitation.
  - Difficult to separate from normal breath sounds because of the high frequency.
  - In severe regurgitation with accompanying heart failure, the murmur becomes softer.
- Symptoms
  - Asymptomatic for a long time because the left ventricle adapts to the volume loading (cf. aortic stenosis and pressure overloading!)
  - Dyspnoea on exertion and other signs of heart failure
- Other signs
  - Pulse pressure is wide, diastolic pressure is low (can be 0 mmHg).

- The pulse has a rapid rise with a large volume.
- Left ventricular bulge with laterally displaced apex beat.
- ECG shows LVH.
- In chest x-ray the heart is markedly enlarged (cf. aortic stenosis, in which the heart size remains normal for a long time)

♦ An echocardiogram and Doppler examination
- The width of the aorta
- The size of the LV and the thickness of the LV walls
- The amount of regurgitation

♦ Treatment
- ACE inhibitor, vasodilating calcium-channel blocker and diuretics
- Surgery should be considered before the functional capacity deteriorates and when there are signs of systolic dysfunction (EF reduction < 50–55%).
- Markedly impaired systolic function of a long duration (6-12 months) cannot be corrected by surgery.

Systolic and diastolic murmur (continuous murmur)

Combined valvular diseases (stenosis and regurgitation within the same valve)

♦ Aortic and mitral stenoses do not usually exist alone. A diseased stenosed valve will also leak to some extent with a resultant murmur during both systole and diastole.

♦ In aortic regurgitation, a systolic ejection murmur caused by increased stroke volume is heard in addition to the diastolic murmur even if the valve is not stenotic.

♦ A common problem in practice is to decide which of the components is haemodynamically more important: the stenosis or the regurgitation. Auscultation alone is not often a sufficient method for determining this issue.

Murmurs of valve prostheses

♦ Aortic valve prosthesis
- Usually an early systolic, grade 1–3 aortic ejection murmur (the valvular ring obstructs the outflow tract). May be accentuated in anaemia, and by fever and exercise. When the valve opens, 2–3 soft snaps (at short intervals) are audible.
- The "metallic" closing "bang" of a the valve is audible even without a stethoscope

♦ Mitral valve prosthesis
- The murmur is a diastolic, soft, short, low-pitched mitral flow murmur (the prosthesis obstructs the mitral orifice).
- The coupled opening sounds are heard in early diastole just as in aortic valve prosthesis.
- The closing sound is a single bang that mostly makes up the S1.

♦ Aortic paraprosthetic leak mimics aortic regurgitation. Might be indicative of endocarditis or valve dehiscence.

♦ Thrombotic obstruction of the prosthesis reduces the movements of the valves and diminishes the intensity of the closure click (or even abolishes it).
- In an aortic valve prosthesis the systolic murmur may be accentuated when a thrombosis blocks the outward flow, and correspondingly, an immobile valve may produce a new aortic regurgitant murmur.
- A thrombotic mitral valve accentuates and prolongs the diastolic mitral flow murmur.
- In both states, the patient usually has pulmonary oedema and hypotension. Valve clicks are totally absent.
- A weak and short mitral regurgitant murmur is an unusual finding. Paraprosthetic mitral leak may be severe even in the absence of a murmur.

Other investigations for the estimation of murmur

♦ Pulse, blood pressure, venous pressure, cardiac palpation and a history of exertion tolerance.

♦ ECG and chest x-ray

♦ If necessary, echocardiography and Doppler examinations are performed as these almost invariably resolve the need for surgery.

Reference

1. Otto Cm, Lind BK, Kitzman DW et al. Association of aortic-valve sclerosis with cardiovascular mortality and morbidity in the elderly. N Engl J Med 1999;341:142–147.

4.12 Heart valve replacement: patient follow-up

Editors

Goals

♦ Prophylaxis of valve obstruction and thromboembolism by careful anticoagulation

♦ Early detection of mechanical valve complications (pannus or thrombosis of the valve and paraprosthetic regurgitation). Refer the patient to the correct unit for treatment.

♦ Endocarditis prophylaxis

♦ Careful treatment of the underlying diseases: hypertension, congestive heart failure

♦ Cooperation with hospital cardiologist

Basic rules

♦ Annually, about 4–8% of heart valve replacement patients have serious complications (A) [1 2]. Half of these are associated with the underlying disease and are therefore difficult to prevent. However, the other half may be prevented by careful follow-up of the patients.

- Most problems occur in the first few months after surgery, when the cardiologist still has responsibility for the patient. Follow-up visits are usually scheduled at 3 months and 1 year from the operation.
- Later follow-up at a health centre may take place at 1-year intervals if the patient is otherwise healthy and has no major risk factors.
- Thrombosis of the valve may occur any time as a consequence of failure of anticoagulation. All emboli cannot be prevented by anticoagulation.
- Pregnancy presents many problems and challenges to both the mother and the foetus. A cardiologist should evaluate the risks before conception. Whenever possible, valve replacement should be scheduled after pregnancy. Warfarin is teratogenic and should be replaced by heparin at least during the first trimester and also before delivery to avoid bleeding complications. In Europe, the recommendations concerning the two latter trimesters are not as strict as they are in the United States.
- For instructions on warfarin therapy in scheduled surgery and procedures, see 5.44.

Complications

- Postpericardiotomy syndrome (4.65)
- Thrombotic obstruction of the valve and arterial emboli
- Adverse effects of anticoagulation (5.44)
- Endocarditis (4.81)
- Occult haemolysis (15.25)

Thrombosis of the mechanical valve in the aortic or mitral position

General observations

- A mechanical prosthesis is more liable to thrombosis in the mitral position than in the aortic position. The risk also depends on the type of prosthesis.
    - Patients with biological valves (both aortic and mitral) need anticoagulation therapy for three months after valve surgery after which they often need only aspirin (100–250 mg/day), unless there are other indications for anticoagulation (atrial fibrillation, impaired pumping function of the left ventricle, a high gradient in the valve, a large atrium or a perioperatively detected thrombus in the atrium).
- The target level of anticoagulation may vary somewhat depending on the risk of thrombosis. It is also affected by other risk factors, such as atrial fibrillation, cardiac enlargement and congestive heart failure. The target is set at a level on which the sum of the risks of thromboembolic and bleeding complications is lowest.
- Most cases of valve thrombosis are caused by failure of anticoagulant therapy.
    - The target level of anticoagulation should be precise, and the medication may not be reduced or stopped for a common surgical procedure with a low bleeding risk. Surgery with a high risk of bleeding requires the relief or cessation of anticoagulation for a few days (INR 1.5). Severe intestinal or cerebral haemorrhage necessitates temporary cessation of anticoagulant therapy for 3 days or longer.
    - If the INR falls below target level, warfarin therapy should temporarily be complemented with a LMW heparin with a therapeutic dose, at least for patients with a mitral valve prosthesis and atrial fibrillation.
    - Successful anticoagulation therapy requires adequate patient information. The patient must be aware of the defined target level and the rules of management when the target is not achieved. The target should be set by a cardiologist.
    - INR is usually set at 2.5–3.5 for patients with a mitral valve (and preferably also with a tricuspid valve) prosthesis and at 2.0–3.0 for patients with aortic valve prosthesis.
    - The patient must be aware of the influence of accessory medications and diet on the anticoagulant level. The level of vitamin K intake should be kept constant. Patient self-monitoring of anticoagulation is possible and has been carried out successfully. A monitoring device for this purpose is available.
    - In some patients with a prosthesis in the mitral position and other risk factors for thrombosis (AF, CHD or LV-dysfunction, decreased ejection fraction, two valve prostheses), warfarin therapy should be supplemented with additional aspirin (A) [3 4 5] and/or dipyridamole (C) [6 7].

Symptoms of valvular thrombosis

- Symptoms of arterial thromboembolism (cerebral insult)
- Impairment of exercise tolerance, fatigue
- Dyspnoea, syncope, angina pectoris
- Symptoms may last from days to weeks.

Clinical signs

- Weak or missing clicks of prosthesis
- Louder ejection or flow murmur, new regurgitation murmur
- Hypotension, narrow pulse-pressure, tachycardia
- Dilatation of the heart or heart failure
- The sounds and murmurs or the heart should be recorded in the patient's chart when the valve prosthesis functions normally. This allows to compare the sounds and to detect possible changes.

Diagnosis

- Echocardiography is the main method of investigation and is of particular value if an earlier recording exists for comparison.

Therapy

- A patient with a suspected valve thrombosis must be referred without any delay to the cardiology unit where he/she has been treated earlier.
- The therapeutic alternatives are thrombolysis or valve replacement.
- If the anticoagulation of an asymptomatic patient is insufficient, rapid correction should be performed and the thromboplastin time controlled after 2 days.
- If emergency surgery is necessary, anticoagulation can be reversed quickly by giving fresh frozen plasma or coagulation factors. The effect of vitamin K begins only after 8 hours. The dose of vitamin K in patients with prosthetic valves is only 1 mg i.m. or i.v.

References

1. Cannegieter SC, Rosendaal FR, Briet E. Thromboembolic and bleeding complications in patients with mechanical heart valve prostheses. Circulation 1994;89:635–641.
2. The Database of Abstracts of Reviews of Effectiveness (University of York), Database no.: DARE-940039. In: The Cochrane Library, Issue 4, 1999. Oxford: Update Software.
3. Little SH, Massel DR. Antiplatelet and anticoagulation for patients with prosthetic heart valves. Cochrane Database Syst Rev 2003(4):CD003464.
4. Pouleur H, Buyse M. Dipyridamole in combination of anticoagulant therapy in patients with prosthetic heart valves. J Thor Cardiovasc Surg 1995;110:463–472.
5. The Database of Abstracts of Reviews of Effectiveness (University of York), Database no.: DARE-952416. In: The Cochrane Library, Issue 4, 1999. Oxford: Update Software.
6. Pouleur H, Buyse M. Dipyridamole in combination of anticoagulant therapy in patients with prosthetic heart valves. J Thor Cardiovasc Surg 1995;110:463–472.
7. The Database of Abstracts of Reviews of Effectiveness (University of York), Database no.: DARE-952416. In: The Cochrane Library, Issue 4, 1999. Oxford: Update Software.

4.20 Hypertension: definition, prevalence and classification

Matti Nikkilä

Definition of hypertension

- In the earlier recommendation given by WHO blood pressure exceeding 160/95 mmHg was considered elevated.
- Stricter criteria should be applied to younger persons, as a slightly elevated diastolic blood pressure (>90 mmHg) predicts the development of hypertension. According to the current recommendation by WHO and the International Society of Hypertension the upper limits of normal systolic and diastolic blood pressure should be set at 140/90 mmHg. This corresponds to 135/85 in home measurements and to an average of 135/85 in Holter monitoring.
- According to international recommendations three grades of hypertension can be defined:
  - Mild: 140–159/90–99 mmHg
  - Moderate: 160–179/100–109 mmHg
  - Severe: ⩾180/110 mmHg
- The patient has isolated systolic hypertension when systolic BP ⩾160 mmHg, but diastolic BP < 90 mmHg.
- The target BP is 130/85, and an acceptable BP level is 130–139/85–89 mmHg. In young adults the target pressure is 120/80 mmHg.

Prevalence of hypertension

- At point measurements, 15–25% of the adult population have an elevated BP (>160/90). In half of them hypertension persists during follow-up.
- The prevalence of hypertension increases after the age of 40 years.

The WHO classification

- **WHO class I**: Repeatedly elevated BP without signs of cardiovascular complications
- **WHO class II**: Persistent hypertension with signs of left ventricular hypertrophy
- **WHO class III**: Persistent hypertension with signs of other end-organ damage
- The benefits of therapy are greatest in patients with grade II and grade III hypertension.
- **Essential** (without apparent cause) hypertension is diagnosed in 90–95% of hypertensive patients.
- **Secondary** hypertension is detected in 5–10% of hypertensive patients.

End-organ damage caused by hypertension

- Heart
  - Left ventricular hypertrophy
  - Ischaemic heart disease
- Brain
  - Infarction
  - Haemorrhage
  - Encephalopathy
- Kidneys
  - Nephrosclerosis
  - Kidney failure
- Retina
  - Arterial narrowing
  - Intersection signs
  - Haemorrhage

- Exudates
- Papillar oedema (grades 1–4)

4.21 Risk factors for hypertension

Matti Nikkilä

Risk factors that can be influenced by health education

- Smoking
- Obesity **C** [1]
- Diet rich in salt
- Consumption of saturated fatty acids
- Stress
- Ample consumption of liquorice
- Use of oral contraceptives
- Use of non-steroidal anti-inflammatory drugs **A** [2,3]
- Low physical activity
- Alcohol

Risk factors and comorbidity favouring early antihypertensive medication

- Heredity
  - Myocardial infarction or stroke
    - in father or brother below the age of 55
    - in mother or sister below age of 65
- Age below 40 years
- Male sex
- Ischaemic heart disease
- Hyperlipidaemia
- Diabetes

References

1. Mulrow CD, Chiquette E, Angel L, Cornell J, Summerbell C, Anagnostelis B, Brand M, Grimm R Jr. Dieting to reduce body weight for controlling hypertension in adults. Cochrane Database Syst Rev. 2004;(2):CD000484.
2. Johnson AG, Ngyen TV, Day RO. Do non-steroidal anti-inflammatory drugs affect blood pressure: a meta-analysis. Ann Intern Med 1994;121:289–300.
3. The Database of Abstracts of Reviews of Effectiveness (University of York), Database no.: DARE-948074. In: The Cochrane Library, Issue 4, 1999. Oxford: Update Software.

4.22 Diagnosis of and initial investigations for hypertension

Matti Nikkilä

Aims

- Ensure that all adults below 50 years of age have their blood pressure (BP) measured at 5-year intervals; this is achieved by measuring BP opportunistically during normal patient encounters. In over 50-year-olds, blood pressure should be measured annually.
- Arrange sufficient follow-up of patients with elevated BP before starting medication.
- Rule out secondary hypertension at an early stage by laboratory investigations, and by referring young patients with markedly elevated BP and all patients with therapy-resistant hypertension.
- Assess risk factors (4.21) and comorbidity.

Measuring blood pressure

- BP is measured on the right arm of a sitting patient using the cup of the stethoscope.
- Choose the cuff size according to the circumference of the arm: a 12-cm cuff when the arm is 26–32 cm, a 15-cm cuff when the arm is 33–41 cm. For thicker arms use the cuff intended for thighs (18 cm). For children, see 28.3.
- The patient should rest for 5 minutes with the cuff around his arm before the measurement.
- The cuff pressure is elevated well above the systolic pressure and is then lowered by 2 mmHg per second.
- Korotkoff's sounds
  - The first sound is the systolic pressure and the fifth sound the diastolic pressure. (In some patients the sounds may disappear in the middle range between the systolic and diastolic pressures).
  - If the sounds do not disappear, the pressure at which they become muffled is recorded (e.g. 120/80/0). This is common in pregnant women and children and in patients with atherosclerosis.
- The measurement is repeated after a couple of minutes, and the lowest reading is recorded as the blood pressure (if the recorded levels are close to each other).
- Readings are recorded at an accuracy of 2 mmHg. In patients with atrial fibrillation, the appearance or disappearance of repetitive sounds is recorded as the BP. A digital manometer is not reliable if the patient has atrial fibrillation or frequently occurring ectopic beats.
- If the BP is elevated, the reading is controlled after the patient has rested for 5 min in a supine position. Before starting drug therapy, the pressure should be measured with the patient lying, sitting and standing. During drug therapy,

it is important to take readings while the patient is standing, particularly in the elderly, in diabetic patients, and if the patient has had orthostatic symptoms.
- On the first visit BP is measured from both arms.

Initial investigations in primary care

- Establish the patient's history, in particular heredity, smoking, consumption of salt and alcohol, physical condition, amount of exercise, and other diseases and risk factors (4.21).
- Take the following tests when planning drug therapy:
  - serum creatinine
  - fasting blood glucose
  - serum potassium (hypokalaemia–Conn's syndrome (24.41), renal hypertension)
  - serum cholesterol, high density cholesterol, and triglyserides
  - urine test
  - ECG
  - Chest x-ray (in suspicion of heart failure)
- Echocardiography is performed if the ECG is difficult to interpret (LBBB), heart failure is suspected but not verified or the patient has a valvular defect.

Clinical examination

- Cardiac palpation (LVH) and auscultation
- Arteries (femoral, carotid, abdominal)
- Oedemas, liver, midbody
- Fundus of the eye, if diastolic BP exceed 120 or the patient has headache.

Hospital investigations

- See 4.28
- Indications
  - Therapy-resistant hypertension
  - A young patient with marked hypertension
  - Moderately severe or severe hypertension with acute onset
- Laboratory investigations (see 4.28)
  - Plasma renine (rest/exercise)
  - Plasma aldosterone (rest/exercise)
  - 24-h urine aldosterone
  - Captopril test has been used for screening
    - 24-h urine metanephrine and normetanephrine if feochromocytoma is suspected
- Radiological investigations
  - Renal ultrasonography (difference in size?)
  - Captopril renography (unilateral finding?)
  - Renal MR angiography
  - Renal angiography, if necessary (selective renine samples from the renal veins during the examination)
  - Computed tomography of the adrenal glands, if an adrenal tumour or hyperplasia is suspected. Scintigraphy of the adrenal glands may be performed if CT is equivocal or negative.
- Retinal examination (especially if the pressure is high or the patient has headache)

Measuring blood pressure at home

- The results of home measurements can be used when deciding on the initiation of therapy and for follow up when the patient is well motivated. The results are evaluated as any single measurements. Values measured at home are on average 5 mmHg lower than those measured in the office.
- The reliability increases when the mean of two similar results is counted.
- The measurements are performed in a standardized fashion at rest and in a normal state (physical and mental).
- Having a blood pressure meter at home improves compliance and treatment balance.
- Home measurements reduce the workload of the health care personnel and are thus economical. They are recommended always when the need for therapy continues for long.

Continuous ambulatory blood pressure monitoring (ABPM)

- Used both as a diagnostic and a follow-up investigation D [1 2 3 4 5 6].
- Rather inexpensive oscillometric devices can be used in primary care.
- In essential hypertension, the nightly readings are often normal, but in secondary hypertension they are often elevated and diurnal variation is absent. The significance of the absence of diurnal variation is, however, uncertain and it is not always associated with secondary hypertension.
- In hypertension more than 50% of the readings exceed 140/90 mmHg.

Indications for ambulatory monitoring

- Large variation in the results of measurements
- Suspicion of "white coat hypertension" (occurs in 20–30%)
- Poor response to drug therapy
- Side effects of drugs, particularly orthostatic hypotension
- Not recommended for routine use (unlike home BP meters)

Problems with ambulatory monitoring

- Cost (equipment and personnel)
- Availability. The measurement is performed by a laboratory nurse and takes about a half an hour per patient.
- Technical malfunction is fairly common.
- Difficulty of interpreting results (established reference values have been published lately; the levels are approximately 5 mmHg lower that the results obtained in the office). Blood pressure levels measured by ambulatory monitoring correlate better with LVH and microalbuminuria than levels from one-time measurements.
- Therapy is often recommended in the average ABPM level exceeds 140/90.

References

1. Australian Health Technology Advisory Committee. Ambulatory blood pressure monitoring: a literature review. Canberra: Australian Health Technology Advisory Committee. Australian Health Technology Advisory Committee (AHTAC). 0642367086. 1997. 28.
2. The Health Technology Assessment Database, Database no.: HTA-988692. In: The Cochrane Library, Issue 1, 2001. Oxford: Update Software.
3. Norderhaug P I. Ambulatory blood pressure measurement. A review of international studies. Oslo: The Norwegian Centre for Health Technology Assessment (SMM). 2000. The Norwegian Centre for Health Technology Assessment (SMM). (www.sintef.no/smm/).
4. Health Technology Assessment Database: HTA-20001787. The Cochrane Library, Issue 1, 2004. Chichester, UK: John Wiley & Sons, Ltd.
5. Canadian Coordinating Office for Health Technology Assessment. 24-hour ambulatory blood pressure monitoring. Preassessment No. 15 Jan 2003. Canadian Coordinating Office for Health Technology Assessment (CCOHTA) 2003. (www.ccohta.ca).
6. Health Technology Assessment Database: HTA-20030836. The Cochrane Library, Issue 1, 2004. Chichester, UK: John Wiley & Sons, Ltd.

4.23 Thresholds for starting therapy and targets for treatment of hypertension

Matti Nikkilä

- Recommendations of the Finnish National Guidelines committee
  - If systolic pressure exceeds 160 mmHg or diastolic pressure exceeds 100 mmHg in repeated measurements, pharmacotherapy should be started for all patients.
  - If the patient has diabetes, renal disease, signs of organ damage or a clinically significant cardiovascular disease, pharmacotherapy is indicated already at the level >140/90 mmHg.
  - Actions to be taken after the first blood pressure measurement, see Table 4.23

Diastolic blood pressure 90–99 mmHg

- No symptoms, no complications: nonpharmacological therapy, yearly follow-up
- Drug therapy is indicated after a follow-up if:
  - the patient has diabetes, a kidney disease or diabetic nephropathy (microalbuminuria or an elevated serum creatinine level), signs of organ damage or a clinically significant cardiovascular disease, and the diastolic blood pressure is repeatedly at least 90 mmHg.
- Drug therapy should be considered if blood pressure continues to be over 140/90 mmHg despite lifestyle modifications and other actions targeted at risk factors, and if the risk of coronary heart disease is high (SCORE: over 5%; Framingham: risk for myocardial infarction 20% per 10 years).

Organ damage

- Left ventricular hypertrophy (LVH) (4.27)
- Ischaemic heart disease
- Heart failure
- Cerebral vascular disease
- Renal insufficiency
- Disorder of peripheral circulation or claudication
- Hypertensive retinopathy

Risk factors favouring antihypertensive medication

- Myocardial infarction
- Diabetes
- Hyperlipidemia
- Male sex
- Myocardial infarction, atherosclerotic disease or hypertension in a relative under 60 years of age
- Other risk factors, see 4.21

Table 4.23 Classification of blood pressure levels based on the first measurement of systolic (SBP) and diastolic (DBP) pressures, with a scheme for follow-up.

Class	SBP (mmHg)		DBP (mmHg)	Actions
Optimal	< 120	and	< 80	Follow-up measurement after 5 years
Normal	< 130	and	< 85	Follow-up measurement after 2 years
Satisfactory	130–139	and	85–89	Follow-up measurement after 1 year, lifestyle counselling
Hypertension				
Slightly elevated	140–159	or	90–99	Assessment of blood pressure level[1)] during 2 months, lifestyle counselling
Moderately elevated	160–179	or	100–109	Assessment of blood pressure level[1)] during 1 month, lifestyle counselling
Markedly elevated	≥180	or	≥110	Assessment of blood pressure level[1)] during 1–2 weeks, lifestyle counselling

– Mean value of double measurements from at least four different days.

Diastolic blood pressure 100–109 mmHg

- Follow-up measurements for 1 month. Start medication, if the patient has organ damage, signs of LVH, and if the diastolic pressure is persistently above 100 mmHg A [1 2 3 4 5 6].
- Start medication after 3–6 months of follow-up if there is no organ damage or LVH.

Diastolic blood pressure 110–119 mmHg

- Follow-up measurements for two weeks. Start medication if the pressure does not fall below 110 mmHg A [1 2 3 4 5 6]. If the patient has organ damage, medication should be started earlier.

Diastolic blood pressure > 120 mmHg

- In symptomless patients medication is started immediately after a maximum follow-up of a few days if the pressure does not fall.
- **Symptoms of hypertensive crisis** (headache, disturbances of consciousness, convulsions) or of a cardiovascular complication are indications for immediate hospitalization in an internal medicine ward.
  - The condition is nowadays rare.
  - Examine the fundi of the eyes.

Systolic hypertension

- Results of medication trials are favourable in the age group 60–85 years A [7 8 9]. In younger patients isolated systolic hypertension is rare, and nonpharmacological treatment is recommended. Remember that aortic regurgitation and coarctation cause elevated systolic pressure.
- A systolic pressure of 180 mmHg or higher is lowered by medication if the pressure does not fall spontaneously with nonpharmacological treatment in 1–3 months. During long-term follow-up a systolic pressure exceeding 160 mmHg is an indication for drug treatment.
- A systolic pressure of 140–159 mmHg should be treated by lifestyle changes, and their effect should be monitored for 3–6 months. Medication is then considered, particularly if the patient has organ damage, a clinically significant cardiovascular disease, a renal disease or diabetes.
- The systolic pressure should not fall too low in patients with cerebral vascular disease or at an advanced age.

Follow-up and target level

- The general treatment target is below 140/85 mmHg, in diabetics < 140/80 mmHg and in patient with a renal disease or significant proteinuria <130/80 mmHg.
- Follow-up measurement by a nurse using a sphyghmomanometer is recommended; the physician is informed of the results.
- The blood pressure of elderly patients should not be lowered too effectively. The aim should be a graded fall over a period of months to 160/90 mmHg.
- Orthostatic hypotension may be a complication of excessive medication in the elderly.

References

1. Hoes AW, Grobbee DE, Lubsen J. Improvement of survival with antihypertensive drugs in mild-to-moderate hypertension. J Hypertens 1995;13:805–811.
2. The Database of Abstracts of Reviews of Effectiveness (University of York), Database no.: DARE-952543. In: The Cochrane Library, Issue 4, 1999. Oxford: Update Software.
3. The Swedish Council on Technology Assessment in Health Care. Moderately elevated blood pressure. J Intern Med 1995;238(suppl 737):1–255.
4. The Database of Abstracts of Reviews of Effectiveness (University of York), Database no.: DARE-978053. In: The Cochrane Library, Issue 4, 1999. Oxford: Update Software.
5. Gueyffier F, Froment A, Gouton M. New meta-analysis of treatment trials of hypertension: improving the estimate of therapeutic benefit. J Human Hypertens 1996;10:1–8.
6. The Database of Abstracts of Reviews of Effectiveness (University of York), Database no.: DARE-960514. In: The Cochrane Library, Issue 4, 1999. Oxford: Update Software.
7. Mulrow C, Lau J, Cornell J, Brand M. Pharmacotherapy for hypertension in the elderly. Cochrane Database Syst Rev. 2004;(2):CD000028.
8. Insua JT, Sacks HS, Lau TS et al. Drug treatment of hypertension in the elderly: a meta-analysis. Ann Intern Med 1994;121:355–362.
9. The Database of Abstracts of Reviews of Effectiveness (University of York), Database no.: DARE-948064. In: The Cochrane Library, Issue 4, 1999. Oxford: Update Software.

4.24 Non-pharmacological therapy for hypertension

Matti Nikkilä

- Cessation of smoking (the most important measure in reducing cardiovascular risk) (40.20)
- Lowering excessive body weight (24.2)
  - A 5-kg reduction of body weight lowers blood pressure on average by 5.4/2.4 mmHg C [1]
  - Central obesity associated with hypertension and hyperlipidaemia suggests metabolic syndrome.

- Limitation of alcohol consumption B [2].
  - In women weekly consumption of 160 g or more of alcohol (corresponding to 14 standard servings) and in men 240 g (21 standard servings) raises blood pressure significantly.
- Reducing salt intake A [3 4 5]
  - The target is below 5 g daily
- Keeping a low-fat diet
  - Body weight and blood cholesterol are lowered.
  - The risk of cardiovascular disease is decreased.
- Regular physical exercise A [6 7 8 9 10 11 12 13 14 15]
  - Brisk walking or corresponding exercise for 30–45 min at least 3–4 times a week, preferably daily
- Reducing psychosocial stress
- Relaxation therapy
- Cessation of liquorice product consumption and discontinuing combined oral contraceptives.
- According to some studies, increased intake of potassium A [16 17] and magnesium C [18 19] lowers blood pressure. The effect of increased intake of calcium has yielded conflicting results but may also be beneficial B [20 21 22 23 24 25].

References

1. Mulrow CD, Chiquette E, Angel L, Cornell J, Summerbell C, Anagnostelis B, Brand M, Grimm R Jr. Dieting to reduce body weight for controlling hypertension in adults. Cochrane Database Syst Rev. 2004;(2):CD000484.
2. Mulrow C, Pignone M. What are the effects of lifestyle changes in asymptomatic people with primary hypertension? In: Primary prevention. Clinical Evidence 2002;7:91–123.
3. Midgley JP, Matthew AG, Greenwood CM, Logan AG. Effect of reduced dietary sodium on blood pressure: a meta-analysis. JAMA 1996;275:1590–1597.
4. The Database of Abstracts of Reviews of Effectiveness (University of York), Database no.: DARE-968221. In: The Cochrane Library, Issue 4, 1999. Oxford: Update Software.
5. Jürgens G, Graudal NA. Effects of low sodium diet versus high sodium diet on blood pressure, renin, aldosterone, catecholamines, cholesterols, and triglyceride. Cochrane Database Syst Rev. 2004;(2):CD004022.
6. Fagard RH. Prescription and results of physical activity. J Cardiovasc Pharmacol 1995;25(suppl 1):20–27.
7. The Database of Abstracts of Reviews of Effectiveness (University of York), Database no.: DARE-950039. In: The Cochrane Library, Issue 4, 1999. Oxford: Update Software.
8. Kelley GA. Effect of aerobic exercise in normotensive adults: a brief meta-analytical review of controlled clinical trials. South Med J 1995;88:42–46.
9. The Database of Abstracts of Reviews of Effectiveness (University of York), Database no.: DARE-951240. In: The Cochrane Library, Issue 4, 1999. Oxford: Update Software.
10. Halbert JA, Silagy CA, Finucane P, Withers RT, Hamdorf PA, Andrews GR. The effectiveness of exercise training in lowering blood pressure: a meta-analysis of randomised controlled trials of 4 weeks or longer. Journal of Human Hypertension 1997;11:641–649.
11. The Database of Abstracts of Reviews of Effectiveness (University of York), Database no.: DARE-980039. In: The Cochrane Library, Issue 1, 2000. Oxford: Update Software.
12. Kelley G. Effects of aerobic exercise on ambulatory blood pressure: a meta-analysis. Sports Medicine Training and Rehabilitation 1996;7:115–131.
13. The Database of Abstracts of Reviews of Effectiveness (University of York), Database no.: DARE-988195. In: The Cochrane Library, Issue 1, 2000. Oxford: Update Software.
14. Kelley GA. Aerobic exercise and resting blood pressure among women: a meta-analysis. Preventive Medicine 1999;28:264–275.
15. The Database of Abstracts of Reviews of Effectiveness (University of York), Database no.: DARE-998457. In: The Cochrane Library, Issue 1, 2001. Oxford: Update Software.
16. Whelton PK, He J, Cutler JA, Brancati FL, Appel LJ, Follman D, Klag MJ. Effect of oral potassium on blood pressure: meta-analysis of randomised controlled trials. JAMA 1997;277:1624–1632.
17. The Database of Abstracts of Reviews of Effectiveness (University of York), Database no.: DARE-978171. In: The Cochrane Library, Issue 4, 1999. Oxford: Update Software.
18. Mizushima S, Cappuccio FP, Nichols R, Elliott P. Dietary magnesium intake and blood pressure: a qualitative overview of the observational studies. Journal of Human Hypertension 1998;12:447–453.
19. The Database of Abstracts of Reviews of Effectiveness (University of York), Database no.: DARE-981430. In: The Cochrane Library, Issue 4, 2000. Oxford: Update Software.
20. Allender PS, Cutler JA, Follmann D, Cappuccio FP, Pryer J, Elliott P. Dietary calcium and blood pressure. A meta-analysis of randomised clinical trials. Ann Intern Med 1996;124:825–831.
21. The Database of Abstracts of Reviews of Effectiveness (University of York), Database no.: DARE-968202. In: The Cochrane Library, Issue 4, 1999. Oxford: Update Software.
22. Bucher H, Cook RJ, Guyatt GH, Lang JD, Cook DJ, Hatala R, Hunt DL. Effects of dietary calcium supplementation on blood pressure: a meta-analysis of randomized controlled trials. JAMA 1996;275:1016–1022.
23. The Database of Abstracts of Reviews of Effectiveness (University of York), Database no.: DARE-968182. In: The Cochrane Library, Issue 4, 1999. Oxford: Update Software.
24. Griffith LE, Guyatt GH, Cook RJ, Bucher HC, Cook DJ. The influence of dietary and nondietary calcium supplementation on blood pressure: an updated metaanalysis of randomized controlled trials. American Journal of Hypertension 1999;12:84–92.
25. The Database of Abstracts of Reviews of Effectiveness (University of York), Database no.: DARE-990635. In: The Cochrane Library, Issue 4, 2000. Oxford: Update Software.

4.25 Pharmacotherapy of hypertension

Matti Nikkilä

- Remember the benefits of nonpharmacological treatments (4.24).

Diuretics

- Diuretics are the primary choice of medication for most patient groups. They are especially suitable for women and the elderly, and in combination therapy.

Drugs and dosage

- **Hydrochlorothiazide** 12.5–25 mg daily, initial dose 12.5 mg for the elderly
- **Amiloride** in combination with hydrochlorothiazide when serum creatinine is in normal range and there is no risk of hyperkalaemia. Hypokalaemia should be avoided especially in patients with cardiac disease or digitalis medication C [1 2].
- **Indapamide** 2.5 mg × 1 is an alternative to hydrochlorothiazide. It has no advantages over small doses of thiazides, is more expensive and causes severe electrolyte disturbances in some patients.
- **Furosemide** should be used only in patients with renal insufficiency (serum creatinine > 150 μmol/l).

Adverse effects

- Hypokalaemia, hyponatraemia
- Hypomagnesaemia
- Hyperuricaemia
- Hyperglycaemia
- Increase in serum triglycerides, decrease in serum HDL cholesterol, and increase in serum total cholesterol. In practice the effects on lipids are small and do not affect the choice of drugs.

Contraindications

- Potassium-sparing diuretics should be avoided in renal failure because of the risk of hyperkalaemia.

Precautions

- Serum potassium and sodium should be determined at 3 months from the beginning of treatment. If the findings are normal, yearly controls are sufficient thereafter.

Beta-blockers

- Beta-blockers are suitable for young, hyperkinetic patients, for patients with ischaemic heart disease, and in combination therapy.
- Carvedilol and labetalol may cause orthostatic hypotension.
- Selective beta-blockers are preferable to the non-selective ones.

Drugs and dosage

- The superselective beta-blockers are best tolerated and have no effect on lipid metabolism
  - Betaxolol 10–20 mg × 1
  - Bisoprolol 5–10 mg × 1
- Selective beta-blockers are superior to non-selective ones in efficacy and tolerance.
  - Atenolol 50–100 mg × 1
  - Metoprolol 100–200 mg daily
  - Acebutolol 400–800 mg daily
- Vasodilating effect (alpha-antagonist and $beta_2$-agonist)
  - Seliprolol 200–400 mg × 1
    - Suitable for patients with dyslipidemia as it decreases the triglyceride concentration significantly.
  - Carvedilol 25 mg × 1
  - Labetalol 200–800 mg daily

Adverse effects

- Bradycardia
- Heart failure
  - However, when combined with an ACE inhibitor and a diuretic, beta-blockers (bisoprolol, carvedilol, metoprolol) reduce cardiac deaths and need for hospitalization in patients with heart failure. Heart failure is therefore an indication for beta-blocker therapy. The initial dose for heart failure patients should be small and increased cautiously.
- Conduction disturbances, sick sinus syndrome
- Beta-blockers may aggravate the symptoms of severe obstructing arterial disease of the lower limbs; however, in mild or moderate peripheral arterial disease these drugs can be used.
- Asthma (when no alternative exists, a hyperselective beta1-selective blocking agent or one that also has a beta2-agonist effect may be tried cautiously).
- Sleep disturbances
- Hypoglycaemia in diabetics (masking of hypoglycaemic symptoms!)
- Only selective beta-blockers are suitable for patients with increased triglyceride concentration and a decreased HDL cholesterol concentration.

Contraindications

- See adverse effects above.
- Non-selective beta-blockers without intrinsic sympatomimetic activity (ISA) are unsuitable for men with dyslipidaemia.
- All beta-blockers affect unfavourably the maximum physical performance of athletics.

Calcium antagonists

- Calcium antagonists are suitable in cases where beta-blockers are contraindicated, e.g. for the physically active.

Drugs and dosage

- **Amlodipine** 5–10 mg daily
- **Diltiazem** 180–360 mg daily
- **Felodipine** 5–10 mg daily
- **Isradipine** 5–10 mg daily
- **Levcanidipine** 10 mg daily
- **Nifedipine** 20–60 mg daily
- **Nilvadipine** 8–16 mg daily
- **Nisoldipine** 10–40 mg daily
- **Verapamil** 120–240 mg daily

Adverse effects

- Headache A [3 4]
- Dizziness
- Oedema of the legs A [3 4]
- Flushing A [3 4]
- Obstipation
- Cardiac conduction disorders

Contraindications

- Verapamil should not be used in combination with beta-blockers.
- Heart failure and atrioventricular block are contraindications for verapamil and diltiazem.
- In some studies nifedipine used without betablockers have been associated with increased risk for cardiac events in patients with ischaemic heart disease.

ACE inhibitors

- ACE inhibitors are suitable for all grades of hypertension. Their efficacy is enhanced by a high renine concentration.

Drugs and dosage

- **Captopril** 50–150 mg daily
- **Enalapril** 10–40 mg daily
- **Lisinopril** 10–40 mg daily
- **Ramipril** 1.25–10 mg daily
- **Kinapril** 10–40 mg daily
- **Silazapril** 1.25–10 mg daily
- **Perindopril** (2 -) 4 mg daily
- **Trandolapril** 1–4 mg daily

Adverse effects

- Cough in 20% of the patients
- Rash
- Dyspeptic symptoms
- Dizziness
- Headache
- Taste disturbances
- Angio-oedema

Contraindications

- Bilateral renal artery stenosis or stenosis of the renal artery for a solitary kidney
- Renal insufficiency in the elderly
- Severe stenosis of the aortic or mitral valve

Precautions

- Serum potassium and creatinine should be determined one month after ACE inhibitor therapy is started. If the patient has symptoms of peripheral atherosclerosis, the levels should be determined after one week of treatment. The use of the drug and the dosing must be followed up and the drug must be stopped if serum creatinine rises to a level that is more than 150 μmol/l above the normal range, or by more than 180 μmol/l in the elderly (4.28).

Angiotensin-receptor blockers

- **Candesartan** 4–16 mg × 1
- **Losartan** 50 mg × 1 A [5 6]
- **Valsartan** 80–160 mg × 1
- The drugs are equally effective A [7 8], well tolerated, with minimal side effects.
- Suitable for patients who get a cough from ACE inhibitors.
- The contraindications are the same as for ACE inhibitors.

Vasodilators

- Use of these drugs has declined, because of the vasodilating effects of calcium antagonists and ACE inhibitors. They can be used as reserve drugs when other drugs are unsuitable.

Drugs

- Prazozine and minoxidil

Adverse effects

- Prazozine: orthostatic hypotension, oedema, increased urinary frequency, priapism, palpitation
- Minoxidil: hirsutism, fluid retention

Sympathetic blocking agents

- Use has declined markedly because of the number of adverse effects. Can be used as reserve drugs when other drugs are unsuitable.

Old drugs

- Methyldopa, clonidine, reserpine

New drugs

- Moxonidine 0.2–0.6 mg daily

Combination of antihypertensive agents

- See Figure 4.26.1

Aims

- To promote additive effects of different antihypertensive drugs
- To reduce adverse effects
- To improve blood pressure control

Recommended combinations

- ACE inhibitor or angiotensin-receptor blockers, and diuretic (or reduction of salt intake to below 5 g daily)
- Beta-blocker and diuretic (or the reduction of salt intake to below 5 g daily)
- Beta-blocker and vasodilating calcium antagonist (felodipine, isradipine, nifedipine or nilvadipine)
- ACE inhibitor or angiotensin-receptor blocker and calcium antagonist (diltiazem, amlodipine)

Possible combinations

- Beta-blocker and ACE inhibitor
  - Beneficial in patients with tachycardia or concomitant angina pectoris
- Calcium antagonist and thiazide

Combinations to be avoided

- Beta-blocker and verapamil or diltiazem
  - May cause excessive bradycardia, hypotension or heart failure, particularly in the elderly and in patients with impaired cardiac function.

Combinations of three drugs

- ACE inhibitor, calcium antagonist and diuretic
- Beta-blocker, vasodilating calcium antagonist and diuretic

Combinations of four drugs

- Beta-blocker, diuretic, ACE inhibitor and calcium antagonist. A centrally acting drug (clonidine, methyldopa, reserpine) can be substituted for any of the former.

Reducing or stopping antihypertensive medication

Principles

- May be feasible in cases of mild, uncomplicated hypertension (WHO I) if the blood pressure has remained normal for 1–3 years with medical therapy and modification of life-style.
- Blood pressure should be monitored monthly when the dose is reduced. After medication is stopped, blood pressure should be monitored monthly for 6 months, and thereafter at 3–4 month intervals continuously, as hypertension often recurs after a few years. The dangers of stopping medication are minimal if follow-up is not neglected. The need to restart therapy usually becomes apparent within 2–3 months, but sometimes only after several years.
- Permanent modifications of life-style are essential.

Reasons for a diminished need for drugs

- Retirement or alleviation of stress
- Reduction in body weight
- Positive changes in other factors causing high blood pressure
- Inappropriate start of drug therapy
- Ageing and admittance to long-term institutional care (often "cures" uncomplicated hypertension. Diuretics in particular can cause orthostatic hypotension, and other adverse effects affecting the quality of life.)
- Heart failure following myocardial infarction

References

1. Hoes AW, Grobbee DE, Peet TM, Lubsen J. Do non-potassium sparing diuretics increase the risk of sudden cardiac death in hypertensive patients? Recent evidence. Drugs 1994;47: 711–733.
2. The Database of Abstracts of Reviews of Effectiveness (University of York), Database no.: DARE-940120. In: The Cochrane Library, Issue 4, 1999. Oxford: Update Software.
3. Sakai H, Hayashi K, Origasa H, Kusunoki T. An application of meta-analysis techniques in the evaluation of adverse experiences with antihypertensive agents. Pharmacoepidemiology and Drug Safety 1999;8:169–177.
4. The Database of Abstracts of Reviews of Effectiveness (University of York), Database no.: DARE-991294. In: The Cochrane Library, Issue 2, 2001. Oxford: Update Software.
5. Simpson KL, McClellan KJ. Losartan: a review of its use, with special focus on elderly patients. Drugs and Aging 2000, 16(3), 227–250.
6. The Database of Abstracts of Effectiveness (University of York), Database no.: DARE-20000710. In: The Cochrane Library, Issue 3, 2002. Oxford: Update Software.
7. Colin PR, Spence JD, Williams B, Ribeirao AB, Saito I, Benedict C, Bunt AM. Angiotensin II antagonists for hypertension: are there differences in efficacy. American Journal of Hypertension 2000:13; 418–426.
8. The Database of Abstracts of Reviews of Effectiveness (University of York), Database no.: DARE-20001051. In: The Cochrane Library, Issue 1, 2002. Oxford: Update Software.

4.26 Antihypertensive drug choice for different patient groups

Matti Nikkilä

Principles

- When choosing antihypertensive drugs the following should be considered:
  - the degree of hypertension
  - any associated end-organ damage
  - comorbidites and other medication
  - the cost of the treatment.
- Despite the potent new drugs available, significant blood pressure reduction from baseline is achieved with monotherapy in only 40–60% of the patients.
- **An ineffective drug** should be changed to another drug.
- **In combination therapies** (4.25), the efficacy of each added drug must be ascertained by follow-up.
- The possibility of secondary hypertension should be considered in **treatment-resistant cases.**
- The effect of conventional (diuretics, beta-blockers) and newer (ACE inhibitors, new calcium channel blockers) antihypertensive drugs on the prevention of cardiovascular mortality and end events appears to be similar, at least in the elderly. Drug choices must be based on tolerability, co-existing illnesses and price.
- According to the ALLHAT trial, thiazides are the first-line drug choice for most patient groups (B) [1 2 3]. Thiazides also prevent osteoporosis and are, therefore, a good choice for post-menopausal women (C) [4 5].

Factors affecting drug choices

Uncomplicated essential hypertension

- In uncomplicated essential hypertension the treatment is started with a low-dose thiazide (hydrochlorothiazide 12.5–25 mg per day), an ACE inhibitor or a beta-blocker.
- Calcium-channel blockers can be used as the first-line treatment if the systolic pressure is high.
- Angiotensin-II receptor antagonists should be considered when the adverse effects of ACE inhibitors or other drugs have proven problematic.
- If no response is achieved, or adverse effects emerge, a product of another drug group should be prescribed.
- Combination therapy is started if desired blood pressure reduction is not achieved with monotherapy (Figure 4.26.1).
- The reasons behind poor response must be established.

Uncomplicated isolated systolic hypertension

- In uncomplicated isolated systolic hypertension the treatment is started with
  - a low dose thiazide or
  - a long-acting dihydropyridine calcium-channel blocker.
- Since the thiazide is a more economical choice, it is recommended as the first-line treatment.
- If the thiazide or calcium-channel blocker cause adverse effects, an ACE inhibitor should be prescribed.

Dyslipidaemias

- The effect of antihypertensive drugs on serum lipids is slight (C) [6 7 8 9], and their clinical significance is poorly understood.
- Dyslipidaemia plays no role in drug choices.

Combination of antihypertensive drugs

	Diuretics	Beta-blockers	ACE inhibitors	ARB	CCB	Alpha-blockers
Alpha-blockers	++	+	±	±	–	–
CCB	±	+**	++	++	–	
ARB	+++	±	–	–		
ACE inhibitors	+++	±	–			
Beta-blockers	++	–				
Diuretics	++*					

+++ Excellent combination
++ Good combination
+ Possible combination
+/– Possible combination in special situations
– Unsuitable combination

* Combination of hydrochlorothiazide and potassium-sparing diuretic (amiloride, triamterene)
** Do not combine beta-blockers and calcium channel blockers that slow the heart rate (diltiazem, verapamil)
ARB = Angiotensin receptor blockers
CCB = Calcium channel blockers

Figure 4.26.1 Suitable and less suitable combinations of antihypertensive drugs.

Diabetes

- The main aim in the treatment of diabetic patients with hypertension is good blood pressure control (B) [10].
- Treatment of hypertension with ACE inhibitors, diuretics, beta-blockers and calcium-channel blockers improves the prognosis of a diabetic patient.
- The reduction achieved in the incidence of cardiac events and deaths in diabetic patients may be more significant with an ACE inhibitor than with a calcium-channel blocker.
- In diabetic nephropathy, ACE inhibitors and angiotensin-II receptor antagonists are the first-line treatment since they reduce proteinuria and slow down the renal deterioration.
- Thiazides and beta-blockers, which lack intrinsic sympathomimetic activity (ISA), might increase blood glucose concentrations slightly, but the accompanying blood pressure reduction will improve the prognosis of the diabetic patient.
- When ACE inhibitors have been used as antihypertensive agents, the emergence of diabetes has been noted to be either lower, or similar, as compared with diuretics or beta-blockers.

Left ventricular hypertrophy

- Antihypertensive medication usually reduces left ventricular mass and wall thickness.
- The reduction of left ventricular mass appears to improve the patient's prognosis. The significance of the drug choice on the prognosis is not established. Most studies have been carried out on ACE inhibitors (B) [11 12 13 14].

Coronary artery disease

- In myocardial infarction survivors, beta-blockers reduce the incidence of recurring infarction and cardiac death by approximately 25% (A) [15].
- Beta-blockers are the first-line choice when treating hypertension in a patient with coronary artery disease.
- If needed, a beta-blocker can be combined with a low-dose combination diuretic.
- Verapamil and diltiazem may reduce, and short-acting nifedipine may increase, ischaemia and the risk of infarction.
- ACE inhibitors reduce the incidence of myocardial infarction and sudden death in about 20% of the patients with arteriosclerotic disease or diabetes and another cardiovascular risk factor.

Heart failure

- In heart failure, ACE inhibitors and diuretics are the first-line treatment for hypertension (4.72).
- ACE inhibitors improve the prognosis of patients with heart failure or left ventricular dysfunction (A) [16 17 18 19 20].
- Diuretics alleviate the symptoms of heart failure.
- Spironolactone has been shown to improve the prognosis in severe heart failure (B) [21].
- Beta-blockers (bisoprolol, carvedilol, metoprolol), combined with ACE inhibitors and diuretics, reduce the incidence of cardiac death (A) [22 23 24 25] and the need for hospitalisation in heart failure.
- A beta-blocker should be introduced gradually after the failure is brought under control.
- Angiotensin-II receptor antagonists are warranted when ACE inhibitors cause adverse effects.

Arrhythmias and conduction disturbances

- Beta-blockers, diltiazem and verapamil may prevent the occurrence of atrial arrhythmias in hypertensive patients, and reduce the ventricular response rate in fast AF.
- However, these drugs must be avoided if the AV conduction is delayed.
- Clonidine must not be used in sick sinus syndrome.

Peripheral arterial disease

- Vasodilating drugs (alpha-blockers, calcium-channel blockers, ACE inhibitors and angiotensin-II receptor blockers) may alleviate the symptoms of Raynaud's disease.
- Beta-blockers may impair the circulation of the lower limbs and thus worsen the symptoms of severe arterial disease. However, their use is acceptable, if necessary, in mild to moderate peripheral arterial disease.

Disorders of cerebral circulation

- Blood pressure lowering drug interventions reduce the risk of stroke recurrence in hypertensive stroke survivors.
- The treatment of hypertension following a stroke should be instigated with the risk of orthostatic hypotension in mind.

Renal impairment

- ACE inhibitors are recommended as the first-line treatment for hypertension in renal impairment since they have been shown to slow down renal deterioration more effectively than conventional antihypertensive therapy and beta-blockers.
- A diuretic is often also needed to correct hypervolaemia.
- Thiazides loose their antihypertensive effect in marked renal impairment. A loop diuretic (furosemide) should be chosen when serum creatinine is > 150 micromol/l.
- Due to the risk of hyperkalaemia, potassium-sparing diuretics should be avoided in renal impairment.
- ACE inhibitors must be used with care in moderate to severe renal impairment, and in renovascular hypertension, with constant monitoring of serum creatinine and potassium concentrations.
- In renovascular hypertension the need and potential benefit gained from balloon dilatation or surgery should be evaluated.

Asthma or chronic obstructive pulmonary disease

- Diuretics, calcium-channel blockers and ACE inhibitors are suitable for the treatment of hypertension in asthma or chronic obstructive pulmonary disease.
- The recommended diuretic treatment is a fixed combination of a potassium-sparing diuretic and another diuretic, since $beta_2$-receptor agonists and cortisone may cause hypokalaemia.

- ACE inhibitors may cause dry cough, and increase the hyperreactivity of the airways, which in turn may either worsen or trigger asthma.
- Beta-blockers are usually contraindicated.
- If the use of beta-blockers is imperative the blocker with the most $beta_1$-selective effect, or a blocker with an additive $beta_2$-agonist effect, should be chosen.

References

1. Psaty BM, Smith NL, SIskovick DS, Koepsell TD, Weiss NS, Heckbert SR, Lemaitre RN, Wagner EH, Furberg CD. Health outcomes associated with antihypertensive therapies used as first-line agents: a systematic review and meta-analysis. JAMA 1997;277:739–745.
2. The Database of Abstracts of Reviews of Effectiveness (University of York), Database no.: DARE-978068. In: The Cochrane Library, Issue 4, 1999. Oxford: Update Software.
3. The ALLHAT Officers and Coordinators for the ALLHAT Collaborative Research Group. The Antihypertensive and Lipid-Lowering Treatment to Prevent Heart Attack Trial. Major outcomes in high-risk hypertensive patients randomized to angiotensin-converting enzyme inhibitor or calcium channel blocker vs diuretic: The Antihypertensive and Lipid-Lowering Treatment to Prevent Heart Attack Trial (ALLHAT). JAMA 2002;288:2981–2997.
4. Jones G, Nguyen T, Sambrook PN, Eisman JA. Thiazide diuretics and fractures: can meta-analysis help? J Bone Mineral Res 1995;10:106–111.
5. The Database of Abstracts of Reviews of Effectiveness (University of York), Database no.: DARE-988096. In: The Cochrane Library, Issue 4, 1999. Oxford: Update Software.
6. Howes LG, Lykos D, Rennie GC. Effects of antihypertensive drugs on coronary artery disease: a meta-analysis. Clin Exp Pharm Physiol 1996;23:555–558.
7. The Database of Abstracts of Reviews of Effectiveness (University of York), Database no.: DARE-973026. In: The Cochrane Library, Issue 4, 1999. Oxford: Update Software.
8. Kasiske BL, Ma JZ, Kalil SN, Louis TA. Effects of antihypertensive therapy on serum lipids. Ann Intern Med 1995;122:133–141.
9. The Database of Abstracts of Reviews of Effectiveness (University of York), Database no.: DARE-950295. In: The Cochrane Library, Issue 4, 1999. Oxford: Update Software.
10. Adler AI, Stratton IM, Neil HAW, Yudkin JS, Matthews DR, Cull CA, Wright AD, Turner RC, Holman RR on behalf of the UK Prospective Diabetes Study Group. Association of systolic blood pressure with macrovascular and microvascular complications of type 2 diabetes (UKDPS 36): prospective observational study. BMJ 2000;321:412–419.
11. Schmieder RE, Schlaich MP, Klingbeil AU, Martus P.Reversal of left ventricular hypertrophy in essential hypertension: a meta-analysis of randomized double-blind studies. JAMA 1996;275:1507–1513.
12. The Database of Abstracts of Reviews of Effectiveness (University of York), Database no.: DARE-968208. In: The Cochrane Library, Issue 4, 1999. Oxford: Update Software.
13. Schmieder RE, Schlaich MP, Klingbeil AU, Martus P. Update on reversal of left ventricular hypertrophy in essential hypertension (a meta-analysis of all randomized double-blind studies until December 1996). Nephrology, Dialysis, Transplantation 1998;13:564–569.
14. The Database of Abstracts of Reviews of Effectiveness (University of York), Database no.: DARE-980602. In: The Cochrane Library, Issue 1, 2000. Oxford: Update Software.
15. Lonn E. What are the effects of other drug treatments. In: Secondary prevention of ischaemic cardiac event. Clinical Evidence 2002;7:124–160.
16. Flather MD, Yusuf S, Kober L, Pfeffer M, Hall A, Murray G, Torp-Pedersen C, Ball S, Pogue J, MoyeL, Braunwald E, for the ACE-Inhibitor Myocardial Infarction Collaborative. Long-term ACE inhibitor therapy in patients with heart failure or left-ventricular dysfunction: a systematic overview of data from individual patients. Lancet 2000;355:1575–1581.
17. Garg R, Yusuf S. Overview of randomized trials of angiotensin-converting enzyme inhibitors on mortality and morbidity in patients with heart failure. JAMA 1995;273: 1450–1456.
18. The Database of Abstracts of Reviews of Effectiveness (University of York), Database no.: DARE-950776. In: The Cochrane Library, Issue 4, 1999. Oxford: Update Software.
19. Lubsen J, Chadha DR, Yotof YT, Swedberg K. Meta-analysis of morbidity and mortality in five exercise capacity trials evaluating ramipril in chronic congestive cardiac failure. Am J Cardiol 1996;77:1191–1196.
20. The Database of Abstracts of Reviews of Effectiveness (University of York), Database no.: DARE-961103. In: The Cochrane Library, Issue 4, 1999. Oxford: Update Software.
21. Pitt B, Zannad F, Remme WJ et al. The effect of spironolactone on morbidity and mortality in patients with severe heart failure. N Engl J Med 1999;341:709–717.
22. Heidenreich PA, Lee TT, Massie BM. Beta-blockers and mortality in patients with heart failure. J Am Coll Cardiol 1997;30:27–34.
23. The Database of Abstracts of Reviews of Effectiveness (University of York), Database no.: DARE-970828. In: The Cochrane Library, Issue 4, 1999. Oxford: Update Software.
24. Doughty RN, Rodgers A, Sharpe N, MacMahon S. Effects of beta-blocker therapy on mortality in patients with heart failure: a systematic overview of randomized controlled trials. Eur Heart J 1997;18:560–565.
25. The Database of Abstracts of Reviews of Effectiveness (University of York), Database no.: DARE-978097. In: The Cochrane Library, Issue 4, 1999. Oxford: Update Software.

4.27 Left ventricular hypertrophy (LVH) in hypertensive patients

Markku Ellonen

- See also, Ventricular hypertrophies (RVH, LVH) in ECG 4.2.

- In patients with hypertension LVH may also result from aortic valve disease or mitral valve regurgitation. Mild LVH is common in obese and elderly persons. LVH is an independent and high risk factor for coronary disease. LVH, verified by ECG, is associated with a 6–8-fold increase in the risk of coronary disease or sudden death. An ST–T change ("strain") doubles the risk. LVH should be prevented with effective therapy of hypertension.
- Many of the classic ECG criteria are insensitive, and LVH is detected on the basis of these criteria in only a minority of those hypertensive patients in whom it is seen on echocardiography. Voltage criteria appear first, after that QRS becomes wider, and in severe hypertrophy ST–T strain appears.
- LVH causes thickening of the left ventricular wall, resulting in diastolic dysfunction. LVH increases the demand for oxygen and simultaneously compromises the coronary flow, which leads to ischaemia even without pathological changes in coronary arteries. These factors may explain the increased risk of ischaemic events. Sudden deaths are caused by severe ventricular arrhythmias.
- Hypertension associated with LVH is traditionally classified as WHO stage II hypertension. Antihypertensive medication is initiated at lower blood pressure level and after shorter follow-up in such patients. LBBB strongly (90%) suggests LVH.
- In addition to the WHO classification (WHO I–III), the Glasgow classification (1–4) is now used: normal ECG, voltage criteria, voltage criteria + ST–T and infarction ECG.
- Regression of hypertrophic changes B [1 2 3 4] indicates that blood pressure is well controlled, which improves the prognosis of the disease. No drug is preferred over other drugs. According to recent studies, ACE inhibitors and angiotensin blockers are proving more effective than calcium-blockers, beta-blockers or diuretics, particularly in patients with several risk factors. LVH regression occurs if the pressure decreases. Drugs are chosen individually on the basis of other diseases and patient's characteristics. In the LIFE study losartan was slightly superior to atenolol in preventing cardiovascular morbidity B [5]. "High voltage" is the most quickly resolving condition. A significant ST-T change (repolarization disturbance) is caused by permanent damage to the heart and is thus usually irreversible.
- LVH is often associated with systolic hypertension, especially in elderly women 20% of whom may have LVH related to old age without any other cause. The decrease in elasticity of the vessels causes a rise in systolic pressure and a decrease in diastolic pressure.

Estimation of LVH

- Precordial palpation reveals a sustained thrust of apical beat lateral to its normal position and in a wider area than normally. A sturdy or emphysematous chest impedes palpation but percussion may succeed. Atrial gallop S4 may be heard and it may signify diastolic failure.
- ECG is the most important diagnostic procedure. Echocardiography is, however, more sensitive. In cases of abnormal anatomy echocardiography has limitations. There are various recommendations regarding the estimation of the left ventricle mass by echocardiography. Echocardiography should be used in cases of a discrepancy between clinical findings and ECG. When the patient has had an elevated blood pressure for long and ECG is normal, echocardiography is often necessary for deciding whether drug treatment should be initiated. If LVH is evident by ECG or hypertension is complicated, echocardiography is not necessary: the ECG criteria are quite specific. On the basis of echography, 20–50% of patients with hypertension have LVH.
- The use of echocardiography in the estimation of LVH should be promoted. Dilatation of the ventricles can also be assessed by echocardiography.
- Chest x-ray is insensitive. A prominent LV contour may be the only radiological abnormality. Another common and important finding is elongation of the aorta.

Sokolow and Cornell criteria

- In assessment of LVH, the voltage criteria (high R wave) are essential. The Sokolow–Lyon criteria are among the most commonly used: SV1 + RV5–6 > 3.5 mV.
- The Cornell criteria include voltage criteria, width of the QRS and sex. Cornell QRS voltage-duration product criteria at baseline (LIFE)
  - man (RaVL + SV3) × QRS > 2.44 mm × s
  - woman (RaVL + SV3 + 6 mm) × QRS >2.44 × s
  - The above-mentioned criteria are currently used in LIFE and other ongoing large LVH studies. By manipulating the criteria the sensitivity and specificity can be modified.
- A common practice for judging the ECG is to use the grading by Estes. In addition to voltage criteria, Estes criteria include ST–T change, axis, widening of the QRS complex and LVH. The classic Estes voltage criteria are insensitive but specific and therefore not applicable in clinical medicine. Several computer-based assessment methods have lowered the voltage criteria to increase the sensitivity. The physician must then consider whether the patient has characteristics that may induce "high voltage" (heavy work, sport, young age, male gender, slenderness) or diminish it (obesity, pulmonary emphysema, old age, female gender, previous myocardial infarction). New computer-based programmes for estimation of LVH give the criteria and confidence intervals; they can even take into account the age and gender of the patient.
- LBBB in particular disturbs computer programs and also the physician in the estimation of LVH. The probability of LVH in LBBB is 90%.

Estes criteria for assessing LVH

- See Table 4.27

Table 4.27 Romhilt and Estes criteria for assessing LVH

ECG criteria		Score
1.	R or S in limb leads −20 mV or R or S in chest leads V1 V2 V5 V6 −30 mV	3
2.	ST change without digitalis	3
	ST-T change with digitalis	1
3.	QRS axis more than −30°to the left	2
4.	QRS duration over 90 ms or activation time (VAT) V5–V6 over 50 ms	1
5.	P-terminal force over 0.04 mms (absolute value) (= left ventricle hypertrophy)	3

Interpretation: certain LVH 5, possible 4. Sensitivity ca. 50% and specificity 97%.

References

1. Schmieder RE, Schlaich MP, Klingbeil AU, Martus P.Reversal of left ventricular hypertrophy in essential hypertension: a meta-analysis of randomized double-blind studies. JAMA 1996;275:1507–1513.
2. The Database of Abstracts of Reviews of Effectiveness (University of York), Database no.: DARE-968208. In: The Cochrane Library, Issue 4, 1999. Oxford: Update Software.
3. Schmieder RE, Schlaich MP, Klingbeil AU, Martus P. Update on reversal of left ventricular hypertrophy in essential hypertension (a meta-analysis of all randomized double-blind studies until December 1996). Nephrology, Dialysis, Transplantation 1998;13:564–569.
4. The Database of Abstracts of Reviews of Effectiveness (University of York), Database no.: DARE-980602. In: The Cochrane Library, Issue 1, 2000. Oxford: Update Software.
5. Dahlöf B, Devereux R, Kjeldsen SE et al. for the LIFE study group. Cardiovascular morbidity and mortality in the Losartan Intervention For Endpoint reduction in hypertension (LIFE): a randomised trial against atenolol. Lancet 2002;359:995–1003.

4.28 Secondary hypertension

Editors

Aim

- Suspect secondary hypertension if the condition is associated with any of the following:
  - onset before the age of 30–40 years
  - systolic blood pressure over 220 mmHg or diastolic blood pressure over 120 mmHg
  - rapidly increasing blood pressure (BP) at an older age
  - poor response to therapy (therapy goals not reached with three medications)
  - no hereditary predisposition
  - abnormal laboratory results and other clinical findings (urine sediment, serum potassium, serum creatinine, left ventricular hypertrophy)

Epidemiology

- Of new patients with hypertension
  - 95% have essential hypertension
  - 4% have renal hypertension
  - 1% has hypertension caused by other factors

Renal hypertension

- On one hand, renal damage predisposes to hypertension on the other hand elevated blood pressure may lead to hypertensive renal damage.

Renovascular hypertension

- The most common form of secondary hypertension
- Suspect renovascular hypertension when
  - the patient has therapy-resistant hypertension or the response to therapy declines
  - the patient has clinical signs of arteriosclerosis, e.g. claudication or weak or absent peripheral pulses
  - a renal artery hum is audible on the upper abdomen (in one in three patients with renovascular hypertension)
  - a systolic murmur is audible on the abdomen (uncommon)
- Urine sediment and serum creatinine may be normal if one kidney functions normally.
- All patients with suspected renal artery stenosis should be referred for renal artery imaging.
- Surgery or angioplasty is possible in selected cases. The result of treatment is particularly good in young patients with fibromuscular hypertrophy, but also in other patients treatment with angioplasty may result in fewer cardiovascular and renovascular complications and less use of antihypertensive drugs than medical therapy C [1].

Renal hypertension due to renal parenchymal disease

- Consider renal disease as the cause of hypertension in patients with increased serum creatinine, proteinuria, or haematuria (4.42). Normal results do not rule out renal hypertension. Only one kidney may be affected.
- The cause of renal disease is often evident at outset: diabetic nephropathy, nephritis, chronic pyelonephritis, or amyloidosis (uncommon), bilateral hydronephrosis and polycystic renal disease.
- If the cause of renal disease is known, it should be treated optimally, and antihypertensive drug should be selected accordingly (4.26).
- The diagnostic assessment of renal disease of unknown aetiology should be performed on an internal medicine ward or outpatient clinic.
- Secondary renal disease due to hypertension may further aggravate hypertension.

Principles of hypertension management in a renal patient

- Limitation of salt intake is vital (<3–5 g/day)
- NSAIDs should be avoided.
- ACE inhibitors or angiotensin antagonists are the primary drugs that slow the progression of the renal disease (reduce proteinuria). In specialist care ACE inhibitors are used to reduce proteinuria at serum creatinine levels of 250–300 μmol/l.
- For starting doses, see article on chronic renal failure 10.21.
- An excessive rise in serum creatinine or hyperkalaemia may pose a problem. Creatinine level must be checked already within one week: if the value has risen by more than 90 μmol/l from the baseline, discontinuation of ACE therapy should be considered. Concomitant hyperkalaemia is alarming.
- When creatinine level exceeds 150–200 replace thiazide by furosemide. Remember that creatinine level is dependent on muscle mass.
- Calcium-sparing diuretics and spironolactone should be avoided.
- Calcium antagonists and beta-blockers are frequently used in combination therapy and do not cause problems.
- In many cases, a four-drug combination is needed.
- Potassium, sodium and creatinine levels must be checked already one week from the initiation of therapy. Follow-up must be regular if a tendency for elevation is detected. Remember that excessive medication with diuretics and dehydration elevates creatinine level.

When should endocrine hypertension be suspected

- Suspect an endocrine cause for hypertension when
  - the patient has unexplained symptoms
  - the patient has a very high BP
  - response to therapy is poor
  - response to spironolactone is good (Conn's syndrome)

Causes of endocrine hypertension and initial investigations

- Oral contraceptives
  - Always ask the method of contraception from women under 40 years of age (27.3). BP above 140/90 mmHg is a cause for changing from a combination pill to a progesterone pill or other method of contraception.
  - Hormone replacement therapy does not elevate blood pressure.
- Primary aldosteronism (Conn's syndrome (27.3))
  - Consider the diagnosis if the patient has a low serum potassium concentration at onset (<3.5 mmol/l) or persistent hypokalaemia on a small dose of diuretics (serum potassium <3 mmol/l).
  - Investigations (medication must be discontinued)
    - Serum potassium and sodium, 24-h urine potassium and sodium
    - Plasma aldosterone elevated, plasma renin decreased
    - 24-h urine aldosterone increased
    - Low serum potassium may also be observed in renal hypertension caused by secondary hyperaldosteronism. In this case, renin concentration is also increased.
  - If an adenoma is visible in a CT scan, it is usually treated surgically. In other cases the patient is treated conservatively with spironolactone.
- Hyperparathyroidism
  - Consider the diagnosis when a middle-aged woman presents with renal impairment, fractures, abdominal colics, or psychological disturbances (24.21).
  - Investigations
    - Initially, serum calcium and albumin
    - In the next phase, serum PTH (elevated serum PTH level is usually secondary and associated with renal failure or malabsorption that cause a decline in serum calcium)
  - The hypertension of a patient with mild hypercalcaemia is treated with drugs and followed up. In more severe cases the treatment is surgical.
- Cushing's syndrome (24.40)
  - Typical clinical manifestations are the most important diagnostic clue.
  - Do not forget to ask about the patient's use of corticosteroids.
  - Investigations
    - Short dexamethason test ((24.40))
  - The treatment is surgical.
- Pheochromocytoma (24.68)
  - Typical clinical manifestations are the most important diagnostic clue. Blood pressure rises paroxysmally (40%) or permanently.
  - Rare (<1% of all cases of secondary hypertension)
  - Differential diagnosis: panic disorder
  - Investigation
    - 24-h urine metanephrines
  - The treatment is usually surgical.
- Hyperthyroidism

Other causes of secondary hypertension

- Coarctation of the aorta
  - Palpation of the femoral artery: weak or absent pulse
  - Difference in BP between upper and lower limbs (in young hypertensive patients both upper and lower limb BPs should always be recorded)
- Sleep apnoea
- Cyclosporin therapy

Reference

1. Nordmann AJ, Logan AG. Balloon angioplasty versus medical therapy for hypertensive patients with renal artery obstruction. Cochrane Database Syst Rev. 2004;(2):CD002944.

4.35 Symptoms of arrhythmia and examination of an arrhythmia patient

Editors

Basic rules and aims

- Symptoms of arrhythmia, such as palpitation, are very common.
- Most cases of arrhythmia are harmless.
- If the patient's family history does not include incidences of sudden deaths, if no pathological changes in either structure or function of the heart can be found, if the functional capacity is normal and the arrhythmia does not cause syncopal symptoms, arrhythmia is generally benign.
- A careful medical history is the basis for all treatment. A family history is always indicated for identification of rare dominantly inherited serious arrhythmias requires taking a family history.
- **Syncopal and presyncopal attacks in particular must be investigated** because an attack of arrhythmia should always be considered dangerous if it causes a serious haemodynamic disturbance C [1] [2]. Investigating **arrhythmia that causes haemodynamic symptoms** demands cardiological expertise and often extensive examinations.
- The objective of the diagnostics and treatment of **ventricular arrhythmias that affect haemodynamics** is to prevent their recurrence (ventricular tachycardia and fibrillation). Ensuring the effectiveness of treatment generally requires an electrophysiological examination, but sometimes an extended period of ambulatory electrocardiographic recording is sufficient (Holter).
- **Making a distinction between atrial and ventricular arrhythmia** is also essential for both the prognosis and choice of medication.
- Ventricular arrhythmias (also temporary short ventricular tachycardia) that cause **sensations of palpation in people with healthy hearts** are benign.
- Even symptomless **atrial fibrillation** increases the risk of thromboembolism, and functional capacity is often poorer than with sinus rhythm.

Disturbances in consciousness

- The reason for a loss of consciousness should always be clarified.
- The symptoms of **cardiac arrest** and vasovagal syncope are similar: black out, loss of muscle control, and collapse.
  - If blood pressure decreases slowly, the patient is sometimes capable of grabbing hold of something and avoids hurting himself/herself; however, in the case of a cardiological syncope most the patients notices only afterwards that they "fainted" and fell (that is, if the patient did not die!).
  - Afterwards, it is often possible to identify "nitroglycerin collapse" and also collapses that are related to nauseating situations (vomiting, coughing and urinating) by gathering information on the patient's past.
  - The identification of an epileptic seizure may be difficult, but afterwards the patient is often sleepy and tired, while a patient waking up from a cardiological collapse is perky.

Sensations of palpitation

- The patients often describe **extrasystoles** as the feeling of a sudden jerk, as pauses in the heartbeat ("the heart stops") that are followed by a strong beat (after a long diastole).
- **Supraventricular tachycardia (SVT)** generally starts and ends suddenly, like on the turn of a switch.
- **Sinus tachycardia** starts and ends slowly, first increasing and then decreasing.

Other symptoms

- The symptoms of **atrial fibrillation** usually include the "mix-up" of rhythm, pulsation and a sensation of irregular rhythm. It may well be, however, that the only symptoms are a feeling of weakness and a shortness of breath caused by cardiac failure.

Description of the arrhythmic symptom

- An exact description and history of the symptom
  - Is it extrasystolic
  - Is the rhythm completely "mixed-up" (atrial fibrillation)?
  - Does it start suddenly and is it rapid and regular (SVT)?
  - Has the patient had arrhythmias ever since childhood or have the symptoms started, for example, after a myocardial infarction?
  - Teach the patient to feel his or her pulse (for example, from the carotid artery) during the arrhythmia
  - The sensations during a rise in heart rate, e.g. when the conduction changes to a left bundle branch block (LBBB) at certain levels of strain.
  - Does the arrhythmia cause attacks of syncope or momentary inertness?

Basic examinations

- Family history
  - CV history
    - risk factors, smoking, lipids, hypertension
    - prior CV diseases: MI, hypertension, etc.
  - Other illnesses present and past

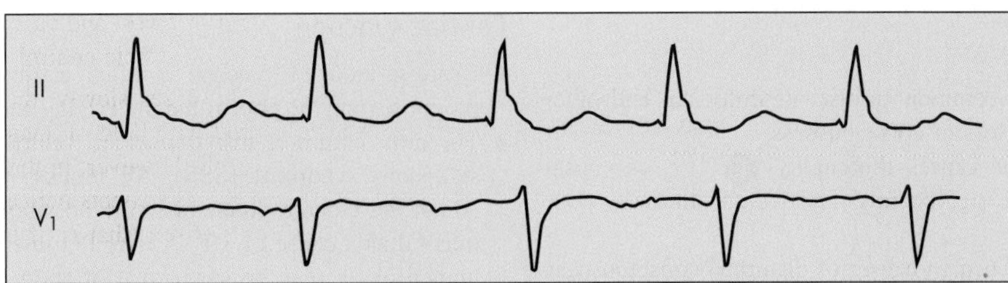

Figure 4.35.1 Paroxysmal atrial fibrillation. There are no P waves (look for them in leads II and V1). The ventricular response (140/min.) is deceivingly regular. The patient is an otherwise healthy 50-year-old woman.

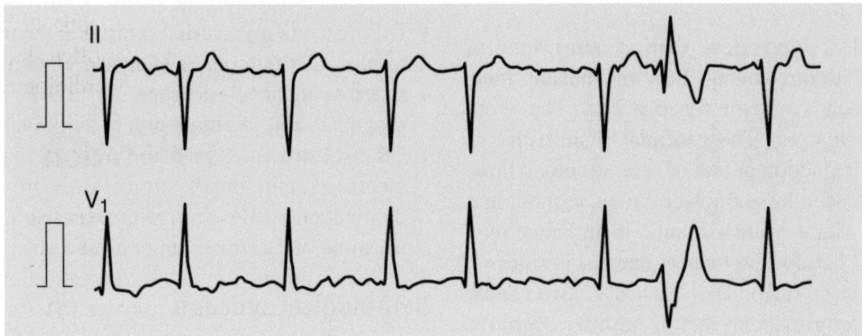

Figure 4.35.2 Atrial fibrillation. Ventricular response 103/min. A wide-complex "extra beat" is not a ventricular ectopic beat, but an aberrant atrial ectopic beat with a transient RBBB. The R-R-interval preceding the beat is longer than the others (Ashmann's phenomenon).

- Clinical examination
  - Murmurs
  - Blood pressure
  - Palpation of the carotid artery pulse (slowly rising–aortic stenosis)
  - Electrocardiography (ECG) (Figures 4.35.1 and 4.35.2)
    - Conduction times (PQ time, QT time), hypertrophies, pathological Q waves, repolarization disturbances)
- Consider a chest x-ray (decrease in functional performance, pathological findings)
- Basic blood count according to the patient's clinical condition
- Thyroid-stimulating hormone (TSH) from patients with atrial fibrillations

Extensive investigations

- Clinical exercise test, especially if the symptoms occur during strain or functional performance is decreased.
- Consider a 24-hour ambulatory ECG recording if the patient has
  - attacks of syncope
  - other disabling attacks
  - in the investigation of difficult cases of sensations of palpation a "therapeutic" examination is a relative indication
  - Alternatively an event ECG can be used (the patient registers the ECG recording during symptoms)
- Echocardiography if the patient
  - has had an infarction
  - has a suspicious murmur
  - has a decrease in performance
  - has pathological Q waves (septum hypertrophy?)
  - has an unusually enlarged heart on chest x-ray
- Tests made according to a cardiologist's decision include perfusion tests, coronary angiography, magnetic resonance imaging.

References

1. Linzer M, Yang EH, Estes M, Wang P, Vorperian VR, Kapoor WN. Diagnosing syncope part 1: value of history, physical examination, and electrocardiography. Ann Intern Med 1997;126:989–996.
2. The Database of Abstracts of Reviews of Effectiveness (University of York), Database no.: DARE-978219. In: The Cochrane Library, Issue 4, 1999. Oxford: Update Software.

4.36 Syncope: causes and investigations

Markku Ellonen

- See also article on Differential diagnosis of paroxysmal loss of consciousness 36.4

Aims

- Identify the most common cardiac, neurological and other causes of sudden loss of consciousness.
- Investigate cardiac causes thoroughly C [1 2], as causal therapy may often significantly improve an otherwise poor prognosis.
- Identify common, benign causes of disturbed consciousness in order to avoid unnecessary extensive investigations.

Definition

- **Syncope** is a sudden, brief (less than 3 min) loss of consciousness with accompanying loss of muscle tone. Fainting is a common synonym for syncope. The word collapse is also often used. The essential disturbance is always a momentary reduction or loss of cerebral blood flow.
- A **drop attack** is a sudden loss of postural tone, without loss of consciousness. A slight haemodynamic disturbance may make the patient fall but does not cause unconsciousness.
- Syncope and collapse (fall) are basically two separate diagnoses. Elderly patients with normal cognitive function are rarely able to report of disturbances of consciousness. Instead of syncope they have often experienced dizziness when falling. The underlying cause of unexplained falling may be serious (but treatable) cardiac syncope.

Causes and presentation

Vasovagal syncope (neurocardiogenic syncope), simple faint

- Most common
- Precipitated by
  - standing in an upright position, particularly if the calf muscle pump is not used
  - pain, fright, unpleasant experiences (vaccination or blood test, sight of blood)
  - nausea and vomiting
  - micturition (micturition syncope)
  - coughing (cough syncope)
- Prodromal symptoms are helpful when making a diagnosis of a simple faint
  - unsteadiness when standing (swaying, motor restlessness, restless eye movements)
  - pallor
  - nausea or sweating
  - closing in of visual field or blurred vision
- As a first aid, lie the patient down (supine position) with the legs elevated. Check the pulse and breathing. After vagal syncope the pulse is slow and weak and the faint can be easily mistaken for cardiac arrest. The skin is sweaty and pale. On regaining consciousness, the patient is tired and appears frightened.
- Consciousness is restored rapidly.

Cardiac syncope

- Exercise-induced syncope is often cardiac in origin. The prognosis may be poor if the underlying cause is not treated.
- The most common arrhythmias are ventricular tachycardia, sick-sinus syndrome (SSS), AV blocks, WPW, SVT, and AF in the elderly. Remember the possibility of a long QT interval as a cause of VT. A long PQ interval and a bundle branch block may be suggestive of short runs of complete heart block.
- Vasodepressive syndrome (neurocardiogenic syncope) and hypersensitivity of the carotid sinus; the patient usually has no cardiac disease. The patient is often an elderly man.
- During acute myocardial infarction the patient may faint due to brady-arrhythmia or tachyarrhythmia.
- Exercise-induced syncope in aortic stenosis has poor prognosis and warrants urgent surgery.
- Other obstructions of blood flow are pulmonary embolism, increased pulmonary artery pressure, hypertrophic cardiomyopathy, some congenital cardiac diseases, intracardiac myxoma and cardiac tamponade.

Neurological syncope

- See 36.4
- Epileptic seizures
- Vertebro-basilar ischaemia
- Autonomic neuropathy

Drug-induced syncope

- Nitroglycerin-induced syncope is common in the elderly, particularly as the drug is often taken for vague symptoms of malaise or weakness when the blood pressure is already low.
- Quinidine, disopyramide and other drugs of the same group with QT interval prolonging properties can be hazardous, especially to a patient with cardiac disease.
- Interaction of terfenadine, itraconazole and ketoconazole with other drugs can induce prolongation of the QT interval and torsade de pointes. Phenothiazines and tricyclic antidepressives may also have similar effects (4.1).
- Beta-blockers may cause severe bradycardia or an AV block in patients with a previously damaged conduction system (SSS, AV blocks).
- The mechanism of syncope induced by diuretics, phenothiazines and antiparkinson drugs is usually orthostatic. Vasodilators have the same effect, especially if the patient is dehydrated due to a prior diuretic therapy.

Syncope caused by hypovolaemia

- Diuretics
- Sweating
- Vomiting or diarrhoea
- Acute intestinal bleeding and extrauterine pregnancy may present with a low BP and syncope.

Orthostatic hypotension

- Long-standing bed rest
- Fever and dehydration

- Drugs: diuretics, phenothiazines, nitrates and beta-blockers
- Diabetic autonomic neuropathy
- Parkinsonism and drugs used for its treatment
- Carry out a brief orthostatic test (3 min) in the acute phase as the condition may normalise itself quickly.
  - Significant findings include weakness, dizziness, swaying and decreased muscle tone associated with a decrease of >20 mmHg in systolic blood pressure.
  - Loss of muscle tone, collapse and syncope, in particular, are suggestive of orthostatic hypotension.

Psychogenic causes

- A psychogenic cause should be considered when no other cause is found for recurring syncope.

Syncope of unknown aetiology

- The aetiology of a single syncopal attack is not always established even after comprehensive investigations. In such cases the cause is probably vasovagal, and the prognosis is good provided that the patient has no cardiac problems.

Diagnostic clues

- See also 36.4
- Serious symptoms and signs are chest pain, tachycardia (>160/min), bradycardia (<40/min), hypotension, even whilst lying down, dyspnoea, headache and neurological signs.
- The clinical history of a syncope attack is often diagnostic. Eyewitness evidence is often useful: convulsions, pallor, pulse, regaining of consciousness, position and predisposing factors. Remember that convulsions of a short duration are often associated with cardiac syncope.
- Syncope in a young and healthy person is usually benign, particularly if associated with an unpleasant situation or emotion. A routine medical examination, with an ECG and Hb, will suffice.
- With cardiac illness, and advanced age, the probability of serious syncope increases, and more detailed investigations are warranted. The first syncope attack in a man over 54 years of age, with risk factors, is a serious symptom! An ECG of a cardiac patient will often reveal LVH, an old infarction, various degrees of AV conduction disturbances and/or ventricular conduction disturbances (bi- or trifascicular block).
- The history may include palpitations before the loss of consciousness. If the duration of palpitations is less than 5 seconds, the condition is serious. The onset of cardiac syncope is sudden.
- Aural symptoms and convulsions suggest epilepsy. However, tonic-clonic convulsions of a short duration may also precede cardiac, or even vasovagal, syncope as a result of temporary cerebral ischaemia. When patients diagnosed as being epileptics fail to respond to antiepileptic medication and further investigations are carried out, they are often found to be, in fact, suffering from attacks of cardiac syncope.
- Exercise-induced syncope, and syncope in a cardiac patient, should be considered serious and requires thorough cardiac investigation (aortic stenosis, serious arrhythmias, coronary artery disease etc.) In young persons, or even children, a long QT syndrome may be the underlying cause of exertional syncope.
- Syncope whilst lying down suggests epilepsy, or, rarely, serious arrhythmia.
- Syncope when turning the head, or one induced by a tight collar, suggest carotid sinus hypersensitivity.
- Neurological hemilateral symptoms suggest TIA.
- Repeated episodes of syncope require extensive investigation, unless the patient is a young and healthy so-called "easy fainter". This group also includes the neurocardiogenic syncope patients who should be examined by tilt testing. A recurrence of syncope may be an innocent sign in a healthy young person.

Clinical examination

- Auscultation of the heart and carotid arteries. Measure blood pressure also with the patient standing up.
- A short 2–3-minute orthostatic testing is often indicated, as is nitrate tolerance test in some patients. (However, the test result may be false negative if the patient has already recovered.)
- A per rectum examination should be carried out for the presence of melaena when hypovolaemia, due to intestinal bleeding, is suspected as the cause.

Laboratory investigations

- ECG, haemoglobin, pO_2 (or pulse oximetry), serum CK-MB, serum troponin.
- If the ECG is normal, cardiac origin for the syncope is unlikely (vagal attack possible).
- Based on the history of palpitations and the ECG findings, the patient may warrant 24-hour monitoring in a cardiac care unit or with a Holter monitor C [1,2]. An event ECG monitor (activated by the patient during symptoms) often reveals arrhythmias that cause presyncopal symptoms. The underlying cause of syncope is seldom found.
- An exercise tolerance test is indicated in exertional syncope or if the patient has coronary artery disease.
- Suspected valvular dysfunction should be further evaluated by echocardiography.
- Carotid sinus massage with concurrent ECG and blood pressure monitoring may reveal carotid sinus hypersensitivity. The test can also be performed with the patient standing up. Press first for 5 sec on one side then on the other. Significant bradycardia, 3 sec asystole or a decrease in systolic pressure suggest hypersensitivity.
- Tilt testing must be considered as a further investigation in cases of recurring syncope without diagnosis C [1,2]. Electrophysiological studies are indicated for cardiac patients.
- EPS, an electrophysiological study, is performed on patients with an organic cardiac disease when the cause of syncope is not otherwise found.

- An implantable loop recorder is a new study method. The device is placed like a pacemaker under the skin for up to a year. The patient activates the device himself. It is used to assess severe attacks of suspected cardiac syncope when the cause is not found otherwise.
- In old persons, identifying and treating the precipitating factors is the primary target of the treatment. It is often difficult to distinguish a 'fall' from syncope. In the elderly syncope is often a drop attack during which the patient falls but does not lose consciousness. Orthostatic hypertension is a common ailment, but often other causes are present concomitantly.

Treatment

- Treatment is aimed at the underlying cause when it has been found.
- Beta-blocker (atenolol) has been tried in patients with an abnormal result in tilt testing; the response may be varying and appear only after a longer use. The drug cannot be used "as needed".
- Etilefrine is not beneficial in vagal syncope; apparently some patients with orthostatic hypotension benefit from it.
- Simple pacemakers that keep the ventricular frequency steady have been used for patients who often fall because of recurrent bradycardia; results have been promising in small unblinded trials, but negative in a larger blinded trial C [3].
- Long and trying standing exercises that are performed daily have helped some patients.

References

1. Linzer M, Yang EH, Estes M, Wang P, Vorperian VR, Kapoor WN. Diagnosing syncope part 1: value of history, physical examination, and electrocardiography. Ann Intern Med 1997;126:989–996.
2. The Database of Abstracts of Reviews of Effectiveness (University of York), Database no.: DARE-978219. In: The Cochrane Library, Issue 4, 1999. Oxford: Update Software.
3. Connolly SJ, Sheldon R, Thorpe KE, Roberts RS, Ellenbogen KA, Wilkoff BL, Morillo C, Gent M,. Pacemaker therapy for prevention of syncope in patients with recurrent severe vasovagal syncope: Second Vasovagal Pacemaker Study (VPS II): a randomized trial. JAMA 2003;289(17):2224–2229.

4.37 Supraventricular ectopic beats

Editors

Epidemiology and clinical significance

- Supraventricular ectopic beats occur both in healthy persons and in patients with heart disease. Supraventricular ectopic beats are common in the normal population, increasingly in the elderly. In the age group over 60 years 20% of the population have more than 100 ectopic beats per 24 hours and 5% have more than 1000 ectopic beats per 24 hours.
- Supraventricular ectopic beats have only minor clinical importance, even if the patient has heart disease.

Treatment

- Thorough examination of the patient is not only a part of the diagnostics but also a part of the treatment.
- Patients with palpitations should be told that the symptom is benign; the annoyance caused by the symptoms should not be disregarded. If the patient does not have any other significant problems with heart, the physician should reassure that the symptoms are not dangerous.
- If the patient has **symptoms or signs of heart failure, drug therapy is indicated**. Particularly hypertension should be treated carefully. Beta blockers can be used if antiarrhythmic medication is considered necessary.

4.38 Sinus tachycardia

Editors

Definition

- Heart rate is >100 beats/min.

Aetiology

- Shock
- Fever
- Anxiety
- Nervousness
- Hyperthyroidism
- Anaemia
- Myocarditis
- Heart failure
- Pulmonary embolism
- Respiratory insufficiency (obstructive pulmonary disease)

Differential diagnosis

- **Atrial tachycardia and flutter, associated with a 2:1 atrioventricular (AV) block**, may simulate sinus tachycardia (Figure 4.38.1). In this case the ventricular rate is 110–150 beats/min. Vagus stimulation does not decrease ventricular rate, but it prevents AV conduction so that F waves become visible. Adenosine can be used for the same purpose.
- If the ventricular rate is more than 150 beats/min, sinus tachycardia resembles **supraventricular tachycardia** (and vice versa), because the P wave is hidden in the preceding T wave.

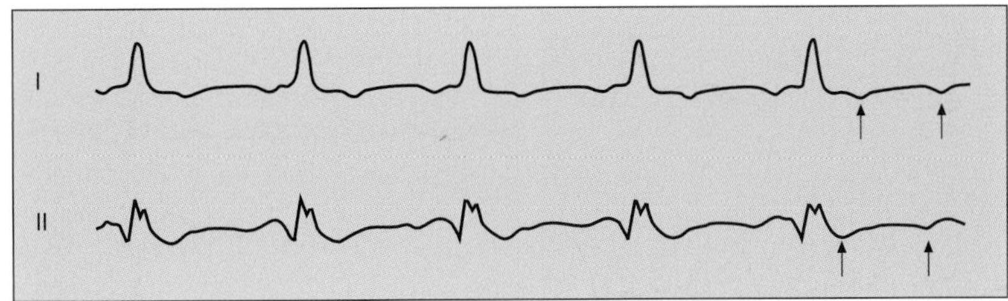

Figure 4.38.1 Atrial tachycardia with a 2:1 block. The P wave is clearly visible. In addition there is an inferior wall infarction. The atrial rate is 240/min and the ventricular response is 120/min.

- Sympathicotonia or fever does not usually cause sinus tachycardia over 120 beats/min. In shock or in hypoxia the heart rate may be quite rapid (as high as 160/min) and sinus tachycardia may be misdiagnosed as supraventricular tachycardia.

Treatment

- The cause of sinus tachycardia should be identified and treated. Remember especially **hyperthyroidism, anaemia, myocarditis and pulmonary embolism**.
- The patient can be treated symptomatically with beta-blockers or verapamil starting with the lowest recommended doses.

4.39 Supraventricular tachycardia (PSVT)

Editors

Principles

- The aim is to treat haemodynamically threatening SVT in the first possible emergency service. Transferring the patient involves the risk of haemodynamical crisis (e.g. pulmonary oedema).
- Vagal stimulation is always attempted prior to other treatment alternatives.
- Wolff-Parkinson-White (WPW) syndrome must be identified. Digoxin, verapamil and lidocaine are always avoided when QRS complexes are wide or the patient has atrial fibrillation with high ventricular frequency (>200). The treatment of choice in this case is electric cardioversion.
- In a narrow-complex SVT, adenosine given intravenously is the treatment of choice.

Mechanism

- Re-entry causes **paroxysmal supraventricular tachycardia (PSVT)** with a frequency ranging from 150 to 220 bpm. These re-entry tachycardias may start in childhood or adolescence. (Paroxysmal tachycardias starting at a later age are usually atrial fibrillation or atrial flutter or 2:1 atrial tachycardia.)
  - In two thirds of the patients, re-entry occurs at the AV node (AV junctional SVT) (Figure 4.39.1).
  - One third of the patients have an accessory conduction pathway (WPW syndrome) (Figure 4.39.2).
  - Few patients have an activation centre either in the sinus node or in atrial muscle (automatic atrial tachycardia) (Figure 4.39.3).

Diagnosis

- The PSVT usually starts and ends suddenly. Its duration varies from a moment to several days.

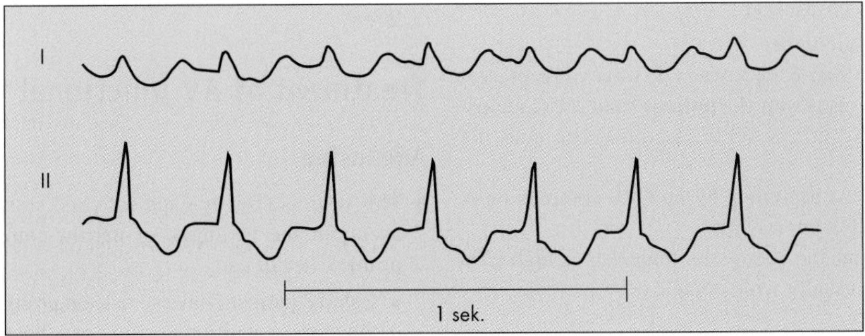

Figure 4.39.1 An intranodal, re-entry-type tachycardia with a rate of 205/min. This is a narrow-complex paroxysmal tachycardia, where the P wave is often indistinguishable at the end of the QRS complex.

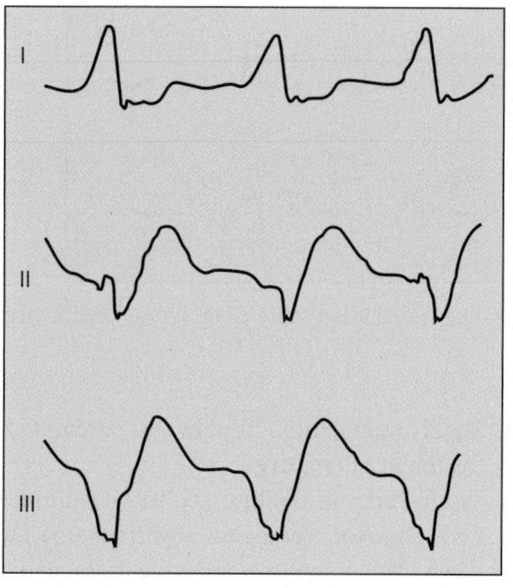

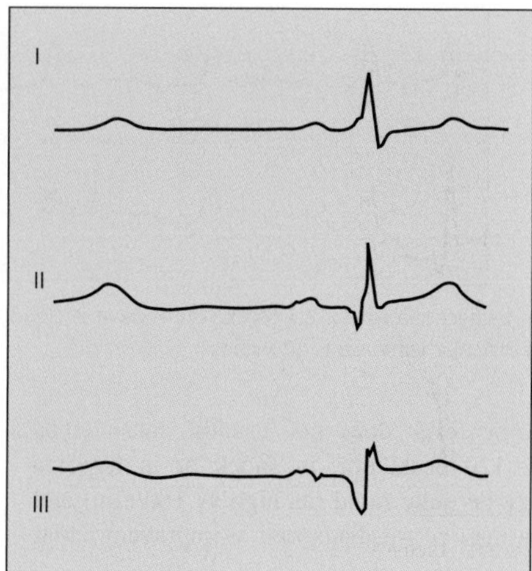

Figure 4.39.2 WPW and atrial fibrillation. The rate is 160/min. The stimulus is conducted from the atria to the ventricles via an accessory conducting pathway. A wide QRS complex is present during tachycardia. During sinus rhythm a delta wave can be seen in leads I and aVL. In leads II, III and aVF the delta wave mimics infarction.

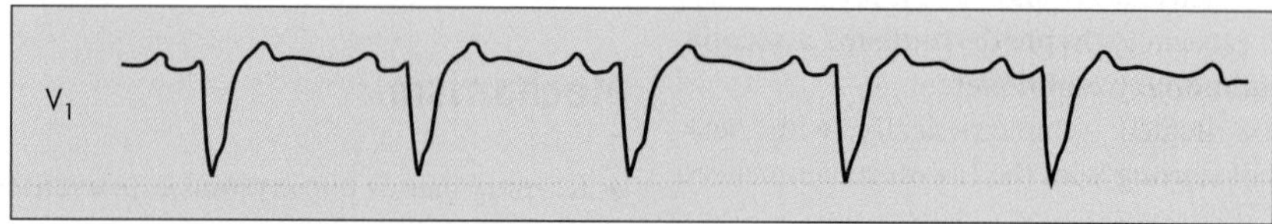

Figure 4.39.3 Atrial tachycardia, that is either classic or a variant of atrial flutter. The condition is associated with an organic heart disease and is rare. The atrial rate is 290/min. and the ventricular response is 145/min.

- The rhythm is regular, 150 to 220 bpm. Vagal stimulus either ends the attack or has no effect on the heart rate (this helps distinguishing from sinus tachycardia). Recognize SVT + 2:1 conduction (HR 110 to 120, conduction of every second P wave).

AV junctional SVT (hidden WPW)

- Activation of an accessory conduction pathway from the ventricle to the atrium is probable if
  - QRS complexes are narrow
  - no P waves are visible
  - the QRS complex does not begin with a delta.

WPW syndrome

- WPW syndrome is probable if
  - QRS complexes are wide
  - PQ time is less than 0.10 s when P waves are present (**check PQ time also from the patient's old ECG strips**: a short PQ time confirms WPW, a normal one does not exclude it)
  - A delta wave at the beginning of the QRS complex on at least two leads (Figure 4.39.4)
  - In atrial fibrillation, the ventricular frequency is high (200 to 300 bpm and usually wide-complex).

Automatic atrial tachycardia

- Automatic atrial tachycardia is probable if
  - P wave morphology differs from the one during sinus rhythm (comparison with earlier ECG strips)
  - PQ time is normal or prolonged
  - Tachycardia usually starts slowly after a few atrial extrasystoles.

Vagal stimulation as the first treatment

- Increasing vagal tone should always be attempted by using primarily the Valsalva method involving blowing against closed epiglottis. Induced vomiting can also be used. Carotid sinus massage increases vagal tone and may stop the tachycardia. If vagal stimulation does not help immediately, it can be repeated after giving the first dose of medication. Electric cardioversion may be followed by a short asystolic phase.

Treatment of AV junctional tachycardia

Adenosine

- This drug is effective and safe and suitable as the first-line agent for the treatment of narrow-complex tachycardia in primary health care.
  - Elderly patients have a risk of prolonged AV block and they are treated more safely at a hospital.
  - Adenosine influences only the AV node by slowing conduction and is metabolized completely within a few

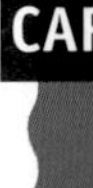

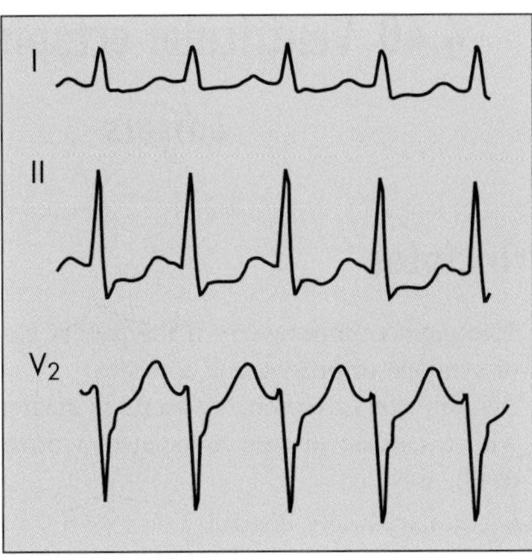

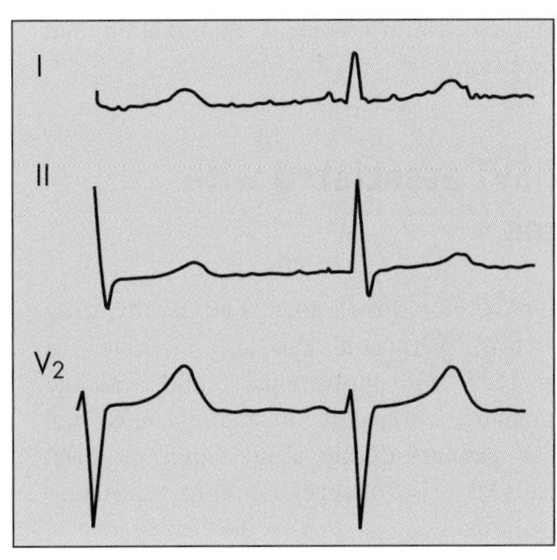

Figure 4.39.4 Paroxysmal tachycardia with a rate of 240/min. The patient is young and healthy. There are no P waves, but they can be interpreted to be present in lead V2. In the right-hand picture there is a sinus rhythm, without an associated delta wave. This is a hard-to-diagnose variant of WPW. Valsalva's maneuver may end the attack.

minutes (half-life 10 seconds). The rhythm is converted within 20 to 30 seconds following the injection.
- The drug has no effect on ventricular tachycardia, i.e. it can be used in hospitals for differential diagnosis of wide-complex SVT and VT.
- Adenosine is also safe in the treatment of WPW.
- Adenosine does not convert atrial fibrillation or atrial flutter into sinus rhythm, but slows down the ventricular response temporarily.

♦ Contraindications
- II and III degree AV block and sick sinus syndrome without a functioning pacemaker

♦ Caution is necessary
- Should be given at lower doses to patients on dipyridamole (potentiates the effect by up to 4-fold).
- Should be given at higher doses to patients on theophyllamine. Short-term exacerbation of asthma is possible.
- Severe coronary heart disease involves a risk of bradycardia and AV block.
- Heart transplant patients are highly sensitive to adenosine: very low doses!

♦ Preparation
- Adenocor®, 2-ml ampoules of 6 mg.

♦ Dosage
- Before the use of adenosine, conventional vagal stimulation is performed.
- (3 to) 6 mg is given as a rapid intravenous bolus under monitor observation; a sufficiently large-bore infusion cannula in the antecubital vein, elevation of the limb, rapid infusion following the bolus.
- If necessary, another (6 to) 12 mg is given after 2 min and another again after 2 min.

♦ Advantages of adenosine over verapamil
- Does not induce fall of blood pressure and can be used in connection with ventricular tachycardia, myocardial infarction and cardiac insufficiency.
- Beta-blockade is not a contraindication for use.
- Adenosine is safer in the treatment of antidromic SVT tachycardia where activation passes in the conduction pathway from the ventricles to the atria and via an accessory pathway from the atrium to the ventricle.

♦ Side-effects
- Facial flushing, dyspnoea, compression of the chest, nausea and dizziness are normal after the injection; the patient should be warned about them.
- Bradycardia that does not respond to atropine, short-term sinus bradycardia, AV block, atrial extrasystoles, sinus tachycardia. These usually last for a few seconds only.
- Adenosine may accelerate conduction in the accessory conduction pathway in WPW patients during atrial fibrillation.

Verapamil and digoxin

♦ Verapamil very efficiently slows down atrioventricular conduction, digoxin also increases the tonus of vagal nervous system.

♦ The intravenous dose of verapamil is 5 mg and it should be given as a slow injection over a few minutes because of the risk of hypotension. The dose can be repeated after 5 min according to blood pressure and pulse.

♦ Alternatively, to a patient not on digitalis, 0.25 mg digoxin can be given slowly intravenously. **These medicines may never be given to a patient with ventricular tachycardia**.

Electric cardioversion

♦ Is used as the first choice or after the above means if they have not been effective or if the patient has a severe haemodynamic disturbance or if polypharmacy should be avoided in patients using several cardiovascular medicines.

Prophylactic treatment

♦ If arrhythmia recurs repeatedly, consulting a specialist is necessary in these cases concerning the suitability of the medication, electrophysiological examination and consideration of ablation.

Treatment of SVT associated with WPW syndrome

- If the QRS complex is narrow, adenosine is the drug of choice (see above). Verapamil can also be given as a slow injection of 5 mg intravenously, and repeated after 5 to 10 minutes. Verapamil or digoxin must not be given to WPW patients during atrial flutter or atrial fibrillation because of the risk of acceleration of ventricular response.
- If the QRS is wide, the evoked potential may be conducted from the atrium to the ventricle via an accessory pathway. Verapamil, digoxin and lidocaine do not slow AV conduction but may even accelerate it fatally, particularly in connection with atrial fibrillation. The patient can be given adenosine, amiodarone (300 mg or 5 mg/kg over 10 minutes i.v.) or flecainide (2 mg/kg, maximally 150 mg as an infusion over 20 to 30 minutes). **Electric cardioversion is a reliable and safe way of terminating the arrhythmia.**
- Atrial fibrillation in connection with WPW is a life-threatening arrhythmia: the accessory pathway may accelerate the ventricular response to the extent that ventricular fibrillation results. WPW patients should always be treated in consultation with a cardiologist. **Cardioversion is the primary treatment of atrial fibrillation in a WPW patient.**
- A specialist should be consulted on the treatment of symptomatic WPW patients, as ablation performed in connection with electrophysiological examination is an appropriate curative treatment. In some WPW patients the extra conduction pathway has a short refractory period that may lead to a fatally high frequency of ventricular contractions. Ablation of the pathway reduces the risk of death, and the patient is rendered asymptomatic with this low-risk procedure.

Treatment of automatic (ectopic) atrial tachycardia

- Ventricular response is slowed down by inhibition of AV conduction with digitalis, beta-blocking agent, verapamil or diltiazem.
- Flecainide, propefenone or quinidine or class 3 antiarrhythmic agents (amiodarone) may be used for prevention of arrhythmia.
- In a heart with pathological changes, arrhythmias tend to recur after cardioversion. If the disturbance is resistant to other forms of treatment, ablation of the arrhythmia focus can be performed in connection with electrophysiological examination.

4.40 Ventricular ectopic beats

Editors

Principles

- Treatment is unnecessary if the patient has no heart disease or syncope or presyncope episodes.
- Beta-blockers are probably useful in the treatment of patients with a cardiac disease associated with the risk of sudden death, such as
  - coronary artery disease
  - recent myocardial infarction
  - hypertrophic or dilating cardiomyopathy
  - aortic valve disease
  - hypertension and heart disease
  - congenital long QT time
  - heart failure.
- Hypokalaemia is a risk factor in patients with organic cardiac pathology and a tendency for ventricular ectopic beats.

Occurrence and symptoms

- According to long-term ECG recordings, ventricular ectopic beats occur in more than half of the general population.
- The incidence (or perception) of arrhythmias varies.
- Palpitation is the most common and often an annoying symptom.
- Stress increases the tendency for ventricular ectopic beats.
- Syncope or presyncope episodes must be looked for in the patient's history as they are symptoms of severe arrhythmias.
- Whether the ectopic beats are uni- or multifocal has no effect on the prognosis.

Treatment

- Avoiding precipitating factors (coffee, alcohol, smoking, late bedtime) is recommended if they cause more harm than pleasure.
- Patients with coronary disease or hypertrophic or dilating cardiomyopathy and ventricular ectopic beats have an increased risk of death. Antiarrhythmic drugs do not, however, improve the prognosis if the arrhythmias are symptomless or palpitation is the only symptom. Patients with hypertrophic cardiomyopathy who are at risk, need an implanted pacemaker. Beta-blockers improve the prognosis of patients who have had a myocardial infarction.
- Patients with severe symptoms require drug therapy.
  - Beta-blockers may benefit patients with stress and high sympathetic tone.
  - Antiarrhythmic drugs should be used only in exceptional cases. Initiation and control of the therapy belongs to a cardiologists.

4.41 Ventricular tachycardia

Editors

Definition

- **Ventricular tachycardia** is defined as an arrhythmia with three or more repetitive ventricular extrasystoles at a rate exceeding 100 (or 120) beats/min.

Main types

- **Sustained monomorphic ventricular tachycardia** causes haemodynamic dysfunction or lasts for more than 30 s. The QRS complexes are uniform.
- The QRS complexes in **polymorphic and torsade de pointes ventricular tachycardias** have variable shapes, and differentiation between this type of tachycardia and coarse ventricular fibrillation may be difficult. Ventricular fibrillation very rarely returns to sinus rhythm, but polymorphic ventricular tachycardia may do so.

Diagnosis

- The ECG diagnosis of ventricular tachycardia may be difficult because supraventricular tachycardia associated with a bundle branch block or aberrant conduction may resemble ventricular tachycardia
  - However, ventricular tachycardia is often mistakenly diagnosed as supraventricular tachycardia and considered more benign than what it really is.
  - **Wide-complex tachycardia (QRS > 0.14 s) in a patient who has had a myocardial infarction must not be considered supraventricular before the diagnosis has been confirmed by ECG analysis or atrial ECG (4.42) (Figure 4.41.1).**
  - If the patient has an irregular, rapid, wide-complex tachycardia the diagnosis can be atrial fibrillation associated with the WPW syndrome.
- If the condition of the patient allows, the aetiology of the tachycardia should be investigated carefully. A 12-channel ECG and carotid massage can be used (with simultaneous recording on paper).
- Because of the risk of recurrence of ventricular tachycardia and ventricular fibrillation, the patients should be examined with an exercise test, ambulatory (Holter) ECG monitoring, isotope scanning, coronary angiography, and electrophysiological examination.

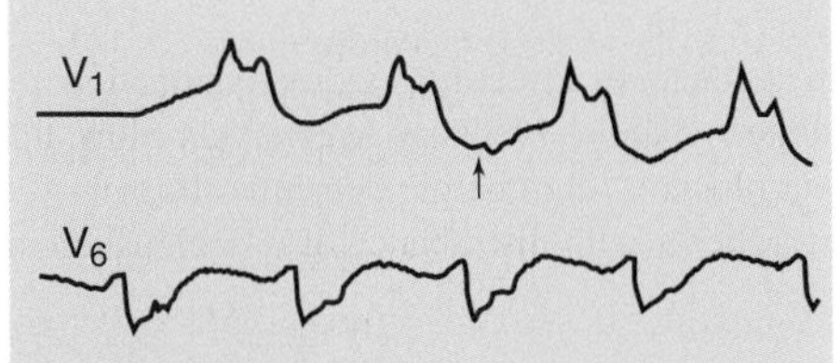

Figure 4.41.1 Wide-complex tachycardia which resembles RBBB. The shape of the QRS complex in lead V1 strongly indicates ventricular tachycardia. Also the width of the QRS complex, which exceeds 0.14 sec., is indicative. The rate (150/min.) fits both ventricular and supraventricular tachycardia.

Prognosis and treatment

- A haemodynamic dysfunction (syncope, presyncope, symptomatic hypotension) associated with the arrhythmia is an indicator of a poor prognosis if the cause of the arrhythmia cannot be treated (acute infarction, recurrent ischaemia, metabolic disturbance, electrolyte imbalance, arrhythmogenic medication).
- Short-lived ventricular tachycardia associated with the early hours of acute myocardial infarction has no prognostic significance. It needs no treatment unless it recurs frequently or affects haemodynamics. In the late phase of infarction, even a short, asymptomatic ventricular tachycardia indicates increased risk of sudden death. Beta-blockers have a positive effect on the prognosis (A) [1 2].
- If the patient has no cardiac disease, a short-lived, asymptomatic tachycardia (or a tachycardia causing only palpitations) is not dangerous. **Drug treatment must not be started empirically (by trial and error) because it may be more dangerous than the arrhythmia**. The patient should be referred to a specialist.

References

1. McAlister FA, Teo KK. Antiarrhythmic therapies for the prevention of sudden cardiac death. Drugs 1997;54: 235–252.
2. The Database of Abstracts of Reviews of Effectiveness (University of York), Database no.: DARE-970958. In: The Cochrane Library, Issue 4, 1999. Oxford: Update Software.

4.42 Differential diagnosis of broad complex tachycardia

Markku Ellonen

Basic rules

- Some broad complex tachycardias are supraventricular of origin, with aberrant conduction.

- In cardiac patients, broad complex tachycardia is almost invariably ventricular of origin.
- Distinguish ventricular tachycardia (VT), supraventricular tachycardia (SVT) and Wolff-Parkinson-White (WPW) syndrome from each other, as their acute drug therapy, prognosis and need for further investigation differ considerably.
- Intra-atrial ECG, oesophageal ECG and electrophysiological studies are often indicated.

In general

- Broad complex tachycardia may be sustained VT or paroxysmal supraventricular tachycardia (PSVT, atrial fibrillation or flutter) with aberrant conduction
  - QRS complex might be broad in SVT due to aberrant conduction (temporary BBB); usually conduction through the right bundle branch is interrupted. An accessory pathway (WPW) or permanent BBB may also result in a broad QRS complex.
  - **Any broad complex tachycardia should be considered VT until proved otherwise.**
    - If the patient has ischaemic heart disease, or the attacks appear at an advanced age, a broad (regular, sustained) complex tachycardia is most likely to be VT (90 probability).
    - Treating VT erroneously with verapamil might be dangerous. Adenosine is harmless and, furthermore, helpful in diagnostics: it slows down or stops SVT, but only rarely VT.

Clinical differences

- Sustained VT is almost always caused by structural heart disease. Sustained VT has, however, also been encountered in a "healthy" heart.
- PSVT, is a reentrant circuit tachycardia, and WPW is associated with accessory conduction pathways. The attacks usually begin at a young age. In most cases the heart is otherwise healthy. Atrial flutter and tachycardia are acquired arrhythmias seen in the diseased heart of an older person.
- Vagotonic manoeuvres (carotid massage or Valsalva) or adenosine may reduce the heart rate or terminate PSVT, but rarely have any effect on VT. Continuous ECG recording should be carried out during carotid massage.
- SVT is often, but not always, more rapid than sustained VT, which usually has a rate of 130–170/min. There are exceptions to this rule. A HR over 200/min suggests WPW syndrome or PSVT.
- AV dissociation during VT may be seen in the neck as periodical cannon waves in the jugular vein as the atrium contracts against the closed tricuspid valve.
- Ventricular arrhythmia with a rate below 100/min, seen in association with an acute MI, is termed "accelerated idioventricular rhythm". It is usually benign and needs no treatment.

ECG differences between VT and broad complex SVT

- A 12-lead ECG is usually fairly indicative and sometimes verifies the diagnosis. Intracavital ECG is decisive. Misdiagnosing SVT as VT carries little risk, but the reverse may be dangerous.
  - In VT, QRS is usually >140–160 msec; in SVT 120–140 msec.
  - In VT, the direction of the initial deflection of the QRS is different from that of a normal beat; in SVT the direction is normal.
  - In VT, the frontal axis is directed upwards (over $-45°$) and the direction of the QRS is the same in V1–V6.
  - Independent P waves may occur in VT. They are difficult to distinguish and are a sign of AV dissociation. When present, P waves are specific (>90) to VT. However, they are absent in about half of the patients and thus have low sensitivity.
  - In VT, the QRS pattern does not usually resemble that of typical RBBB or LBBB. In SVT, the QRS pattern often follows a typical RBBB or LBBB pattern. Unfortunately, some VTs originating from the bundle of His may also resemble typical BBBs.
  - Fusion beats are typical to VT. In SVT they are absent.
  - The broad complex tachycardia seen in WPW is caused by atrial fibrillation being conducted to the ventricles via an accessory pathway. The ventricular response rate may be very high (>200/min). However, RR intervals vary slightly. ECG during sinus rhythm may show a delta wave.

4.43 Bradycardia

Markku Ellonen

Objectives

- To identify symptomatic bradycardia and to determine the underlying cause.
- To stop medication affecting cardiac conduction (digitalis and calcium channel blocking agents that slow the pulse rate, beta blockers, cholinergic dementia drugs)
- To refer patients with disturbance of consciousness or heart failure.

General

- Bradycardia is often benign unless it causes disturbance of consciousness, presyncope or heart failure.

- The cause of bradycardia (<50 beats/min) may be sinus bradycardia, dysfunction of the sinus node SA block or sinus arrest or an atrioventricular (AV) conduction disturbance.
- If the pulse is only palpated in a patient with atrial fibrillation or ectopic beats, the weakest beats are not felt and there is an erroneous impression of bradycardia. A bigeminy of 80 bpm can be palpated as 40 bpm.

Sinus bradycardia

- In sinus bradycardia the P, QRS and T waves are normal and the heart rate is below 50. Physiological conditions, general diseases or temporary or chronic heart disease can cause sinus bradycardia. These causes include
  - increased vagal activity, nausea, sleep
  - physical fitness, e.g. in endurance athletes
  - vasodepressive syndrome (4.36)
  - hypersensitivity of carotid sinus
  - increased intracranial pressure
  - hypothermia
  - hypothyroidism
  - beta-blockade (in patients with heart disease, also conduction disturbances) dementia drugs etc.
  - acute phase of myocardial infarction, especially low posterior infarction (conduction disturbances are common)
  - sick sinus syndrome (4.47)

Bradyarrhythmias

- Disturbance of the activation of the sinus node or its atrial or AV conduction (sinus arrest, sinoatrial block).
  - Sick sinus syndrome (SSS) manifests most often as sinus bradycardia and/or breaks in the function of the sinus node (4.47) and often also as tachyarrhythmias. The patients are very sensitive to all drugs that slow the function of the sinus node or block conduction: digoxin, beta blockers, most antiarrhythmic drugs, cholinergic dementia drugs. These medications must be discontinued unless patient safety can be guaranteed with a pacemaker.
  - hypersensitivity of carotid sinus causes SA block or AV block. See syncope 4.36
  - AV conduction disturbances (AV block). A complete AV block may be congenital. Usually it is acquired, resulting from damage or degeneration of the conduction pathway. The heart rate is 60–20 bpm, depending where the substituting rhythm originates. Digitalis poisoning is the most common drug-related cause of AV block.

Treatment

- Not always necessary (depends of the severity of the haemodynamic disturbance).
- Treat the underlying cause.
- Atropine 0.5 mg i.v., repeated at 5-min intervals, is the first-line therapy for acute bradycardia of various origins.
- Adjustment of medication: digoxin, beta-blockers (also eyedrops!) several antiarrhythmic drugs. The medications must be stopped.
- Possible antagonists: in case of beta-blockers the antagonist is beta-1-agonist and glucagon; in case of calcium channel blockers the antagonist is i.v. calcium gluconate.
- Pacemaker temporary or permanent (4.48). The need for a pacemaker often rises from difficult attacks of bradycardia. The attacks cause dizziness or syncope.

4.45 Atrial fibrillation: drug treatment and electric cardioversion

Editors

- Anticoagulant therapy, see 4.46.

Principles

- In acute atrial fibrillation (AF), a beta-blocker is used to control the heart rate.
- In chronic atrial fibrillation, or before an elective cardioversion, digoxin, a beta-blocker, verapamil or diltiazem may be used: a ventricular rate of 60–80 bpm is usually optimal. Do not give calcium channel blockers if the patient has cardiac insufficiency.
- The indications for, and timing of, electric cardioversion must be considered carefully.
- Acute AF (duration less than two days) can be treated with i.v. or oral flecainide if the patient does not have cardiac insufficiency, hypotension or bradycardia and has not taken other drugs that block either the function of the sinus node or atrioventricular conduction.
- Electric cardioversion is indicated if the situation is urgent, if the patient has Wolff-Parkinson-White-syndrome, or is on medication that modifies the conduction system of the heart.

Digitalization

- The patient with heart failure and acute AF is primarily digitalized, if electric cardioversion has not been planned, if the ventricular rate is >80–100 beats/min, and if the patient has not used digitalis or has severe heart failure.
- Digitalization either intravenously or orally:
  - Initially, a slow **intravenous** injection of 0.25 mg digoxin. A dose of 0.125 mg is given at one-hour intervals, until the total dose is maximally 0.75 mg (three 0.25-mg ampoules).
  - **In oral therapy**, maintenance doses are usually administered, but if a more rapid action is needed, a loading dose of 0.75–1.0 mg of digoxin can be given.

Optimizing the ventricular rate

- A rapid ventricular rate must be slowed down to attain an appropriate heart rate. A ventricular rate of 60–90 bpm is appropriate for most patients.
- **The ventricular rate can be slowed down** with an intravenous beta-blocker (e.g. metoprolol 5 mg, repeated twice at 5-min intervals and in case of fast AF with stable haemodynamics the total dose can be increased to up to 30 mg. Short-acting esmolol, or 5 mg of verapamil are alternatives). If slowing the rate is not urgent, the drugs can be given orally (atenolol 25–50 mg × 1 or metoprolol 50–100 mg × 2, or verapamil 40 mg × 3) A [1 2].
- In cardiac insufficiency, verapamil and diltiazem may worsen heart failure. Therefore digoxin A [3] is preferred. A beta-blocker can be used in small doses while carefully observing the response.
- **If the ventricular response rate is slow and the patient is symptomatic**, reduce the doses of drugs that have negative chronotropic action, or stop the medication completely. If the patient continues to have bradycardia and symptoms, implanting a pacemaker should be considered.
- Digitalis optimizes the ventricular response rate during rest, and often digitalization is all that is needed in elderly patients. During exercise, however, the heart rate can increase too much, impairing exercise capacity. To prevent this, younger patients may need, instead of digitalis, a beta-blocker or a calcium channel blocker in exercise and mental stress as well as at rest.
- An increase in ventricular response rate in AF may be a sign of aggravated heart failure. In this case merely slowing down the ventricular response rate is not sufficient.

Restoration of sinus rhythm

- Measures to convert AF to sinus rhythm should be undertaken if the sinus rhythm has not been restored after the reduction of heart rate and correction of possible heart failure. However, in patients over 65 years of age, repeated cardioversion to maintain sinus rhythm does not improve survival or quality of life compared to rate control of AF B [4 5 6 7].
- **Electric cardioversion** is recommended if the patient
  - has used several antiarrhythmic drugs
  - is hypotensive
  - is in a critical condition because of the arrhythmia
  - has chronic AF.
- Drugs used for this indication include flecainide and propafenone; previously, quinidine 0.2 g 3 times at 2-hour intervals was often used in some countries. Monitoring the patient during the conversion of the rhythm, and for at least 3 hours after it, is recommended because of the risk of ventricular tachycardia.

Conversion of the rhythm with flecainide

- Note the following contraindications
  - Dysfunction of the sinus node should be considered if acute AF with ventricular rate <80 bpm when the patient has not taken any medication that slows the ventricular response rate.
  - Second- or third-degree AV block
  - Severe cardiac insufficiency
  - Use of a class I antiarrhythmic drug or sotalol more than 160 mg/day, or less than 8 hours since the ingestion of the last sotalol tablet. If the patient is not in a hospital with special care facilities, it may be advisable not to use pharmacological cardioversion in patients on antiarrhythmic medication.
- Mix flecainide in 100 ml of 5% glucose. The dose is 2 mg/kg, maximally 150 mg as an infusion over 30 minutes. Discontinue the infusion if the sinus rhythm is restored.
- Monitor the patient for at least one hour after the restoration of the sinus rhythm; after that the patient is allowed to stand up. The patient may not leave the premises during the first three hours after restoration of the rhythm.
- If sinus rhythm has not been restored in three hours, perform electric cardioversion.

Treatment of atrial flutter

- See Figure 4.46.1
- Electric cardioversion is the optimal treatment.
- Verapamil and digoxin slow the ventricular response rate.
- With sufficient digitalization, the rhythm usually reverts to atrial fibrillation, which is better tolerated than an atrial flutter.
- I.v. ibutilide restores sinus rhythm in 60% of patients who have had AF or flutter for less than 30 days. The patient should be monitored for a few hours because of the risk of proarrhythmia (about 2%).

Maintenance of sinus rhythm

- Rule out hyperthyroidism as the cause of AF.
- **Digoxin** does not prevent the recurrence of AF. However, in heart failure digoxin prevents the recurrence of supraventricular arrhythmia.
- Sodium channel blockers (**quinidine, disopyramide, flecainide and propafenone**) must not be used if the left ventricular ejection fraction is below 40%, e.g. after myocardial infarction, because they increase the likelihood of serious proarrhythmia. If therapy with sodium channel blockers is initiated, left ventricular function must be estimated. The therapy should be initiated in a hospital, unless arrhythmia is primary and not caused by cardiac pathology.
- Beta-blockers (metoprolol 50–100 mg × 1 B [8], bisoprolol 5 mg × 1 and sotalol 80–160 mg × 2) prevent recurrence of AF, and are especially suitable for patients with ischaemic heart disease or high blood pressure. Heart failure does not prevent the use of beta blockers but is an indication for it. The treatment should be started cautiously with a small dosage. Because sotalol lengthens the QT interval it is being discarded. C [9 10]

- Beta-blockers are suitable for the prevention of arrhythmias associated with physical exercise.
- **Flecainide** (C) [11 12], **propafenone** (A) [13 14] and **amiodarone** (C) [11 12] are effective in preventing atrial fibrillation, but the therapy should be initiated only after consultation of a specialist in cardiology or internal medicine or cardiology. These antiarrhythmic agents are often combined with a selective beta-blocker. Amiodarone is also used as a short-course prophylactic medication in association with surgical procedures.

Anticoagulant therapy after conversion

- **Anticoagulation** is usually continued for 4 weeks after the conversion of the rhythm. Embolic risk is high after restoration of sinus rhythm, e.g. in patients with hyperthyroidism. The mechanical function of the atria begins slowly, and formation of thrombi may continue even during electrical sinus rhythm. Continuation of anticoagulation also offers the possibility of repeating electric cardioversion during the follow-up visit, if the fibrillation has recurred. This is possible in patients who have not started a prophylactic medication after the first electric cardioversion.
- See article on Indications and contraindications of anticoagulant therapy 4.46.

Consultation about prophylactic treatment

- Prophylaxis of AF with antiarrhythmic drugs requires knowledge of cardiology, as sodium channel blockers (e.g. quinidine, disopyramide, flecainide, propafenone) may be a greater risk to the cardiac patient than AF as such.

References

1. Segal JB, McNamara RL, Miller MR, Kim N, Goodman SN, Powe NR, Robinson K, Yu D, Bass EB. The evidence regarding the drugs used for ventricular rate control. Journal of Family Practice 2000, 49(1), 47–59.
2. The Database of Abstracts of Reviews of Effectiveness (University of York), Database no.: DARE-20003312. In: The Cochrane Library, Issue 2, 2002. Oxford: Update Software.
3. Lip GYH, Kamath S, Freestone B. Effects of treatments for acute atrial fibrillation. Clinical Evidence 2002;7:1–10.
4. Golzari H, Cebul R, Bahler R. Atrial fibrillation: restoration and maintenance of sinus rhythm and indications for anticoagulant therapy. Ann Intern Med 1996;125:311–323.
5. The Database of Abstracts of Reviews of Effectiveness (University of York), Database no.: DARE-968388. In: The Cochrane Library, Issue 4, 1999. Oxford: Update Software.
6. Van Gelder IC, Hagens VE, Bosker HA, Kingma JH, Kamp O, Kingma T, Said SA, Darmanata JI, Timmermans AJ, Tijssen JG, Crijns HJ; Rate Control versus Electrical Cardioversion for Persistent Atrial Fibrillation Study Group. A comparison of rate control and rhythm control in patients with recurrent persistent atrial fibrillation. N Engl J Med 2002;347:1834–1840.
7. Wyse DG, Waldo AL, DiMarco JP, Domanski MJ, Rosenberg Y, Schron EB, Kellen JC, Greene HL, Mickel MC, Dalquist JE, Corley SD; The Atrial Fibrillation Follow-up Investigation of Rhythm Management (AFFIRM) Investigators. A comparison of rate control and rhythm control in patients with atrial fibrillation. N Engl J Med 2002;347:1825–1833.
8. Kuhlkamp V, Schirdewan A, Stangl K, Homberg M, Ploch M, Beck OA. Use of metoprolol CR/XL to maintain sinus rhythm after conversion from persistent atrial fibrillation: a randomized, double-blind, placebo-controlled study. J Am Coll Cardiol 2000;36:147–180.
9. Southworth MR, Zarembski D, Viana M, Bauman J. Comparison of sotalol versus quinidine for maintenance of normal sinus rhythm in patients with chronic atrial fibrillation. American Journal of Cardiology 1999;83:1629–1632.
10. The Database of Abstracts of Reviews of Effectiveness (University of York), Database no.: DARE-991282. In: The Cochrane Library, Issue 1, 2001. Oxford: Update Software.
11. Zarembski DG, Nolan PE Jr, Slack MK, Caruso AC. Treatment of resistant atrial fibrillation: a meta-analysis comparing amiodarone and flecainide. Arch Intern Med 1995;155:1885–1891.
12. The Database of Abstracts of Reviews of Effectiveness (University of York), Database no.: DARE-988075. In: The Cochrane Library, Issue 4, 1999. Oxford: Update Software.
13. Reimold SC, Maisel WH, Antman EM. Propafenone for the treatment of supraventricular tachycardia and atrial fibrillation: a meta-analysis. American Journal of Cardiology 1998;82:N66–N71.
14. The Database of Abstracts of Reviews of Effectiveness (University of York), Database no.: DARE-981970. In: The Cochrane Library, Issue 4, 2000. Oxford: Update Software.

4.46 Indications and contraindications for anticoagulation in atrial fibrillation

Editors

Objective

- To find and treat patients with an increased risk of embolism, who would benefit from long-term anticoagulation (A) [1 2].

Background

- Chronic atrial fibrillation increases the risk of arterial embolism. The emboli increase morbidity and mortality and result in long-lasting disability.

- Antithrombotic therapy prevents 60% of strokes that otherwise annually affect 5% of patients with atrial fibrillation A [3]. Treatment with aspirin is significantly less effective A [4 5] providing only a small benefit.
- The risk of stroke in a patient with a previous TIA is 4/100 patient years during anticoagulation A [1 2]; 10/100 patient years during aspirin therapy C [6 7]; and 12/100 patient years during placebo treatment.

Indications for anticoagulation in atrial fibrillation

- See Figure 4.46.1
- **In mitral stenosis, heart failure and dilated cardiomyopathy**, the risk of embolism is high and anticoagulation is indicated.
- Factors that increase the risk of stroke in patients with atrial fibrillation include:
  - old age
  - hypertension
  - heart failure (low left ventricular function)
  - enlarged left atrium
  - previous stroke or arterial embolism elsewhere in the system
  - mitral stenosis, valvular calcification.
- Anticoagulant therapy should be given to these patients B [8 9]. (On the other hand, old age associates with factors that increase bleeding risk during anticoagulation.)
- **In paroxysmal atrial fibrillation**, complications occur less often than in sustained fibrillation. The initiation of anticoagulant therapy depends on the relapse rate and other factors predisposing to embolism.
- **Lone fibrillation** that by definition occurs without any cardiac or systemic diseases rarely causes complications, at least in patients younger than 60 years. Anticoagulation is probably not beneficial, but treatment with aspirin may be considered.
- Cardioversion includes a small but undeniable risk of embolism. Anticoagulation for at least three weeks is indicated if the duration of fibrillation is unknown, or fibrillation has lasted more than 2 days. Anticoagulation is continued for 4 weeks after cardioversion, even when it was successful.
- Echocardiography helps to identify the cause of atrial fibrillation and to measure the left ventricular function and the size of the atria. However, it is not necessary for all patients with atrial fibrillation.

Contraindications

- Anticoagulation unavoidably involves a risk of major haemorrhage, especially in elderly patients who have other diseases and therapies that increase the risk of bleeding.
- Contraindications include
  - memory problems and irregular drug use (compliance)
  - alcohol abuse
  - previous brain haemorrhage

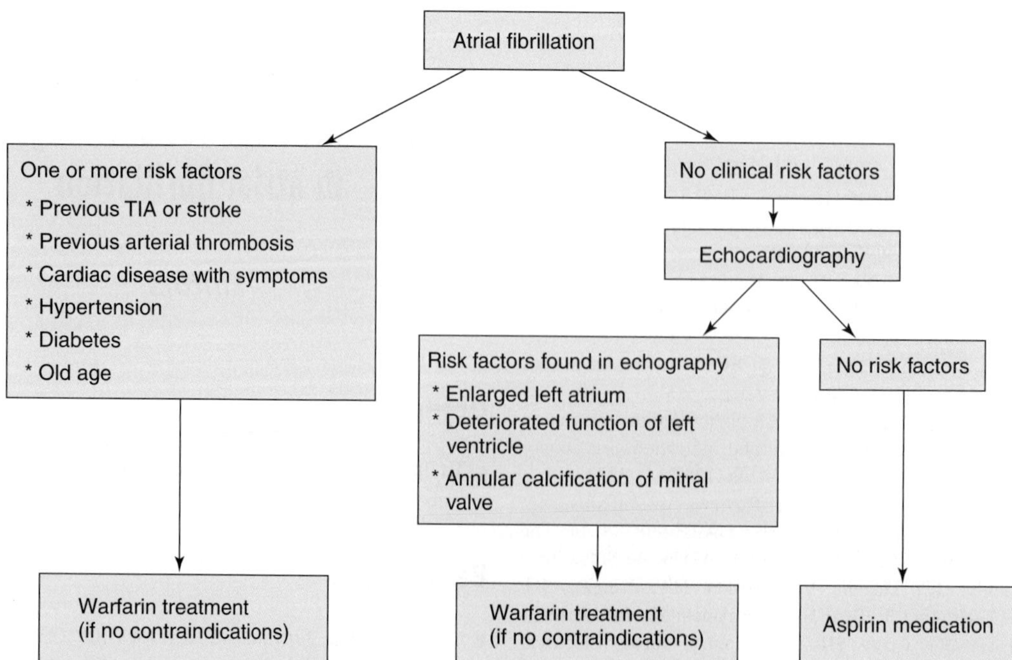

Figure 4.46.1 Treatment of atrial fibrillation.

- recent ulcer, or a previous bleeding ulcer
- tumour in the gastrointestinal or urogenital system
- use of non-steroid anti-inflammatory drugs (NSAID) increases the risk of gastrointestinal bleeding
- other conditions predisposing to bleeding.

- The risk to patients with a previous ulcer must be estimated individually. After successful eradication of Helicobacter pylori, for example, the risk of duodenal ulcer and bleeding is rather small.

The required therapeutic level

- In antithrombotic therapy the recommended INR is 2.0–3.0 during oral antithrombotic therapy.

Acetylsalicylic acid (aspirin)

- Aspirin may be indicated in patients in whom anticoagulation is problematic or contraindicated, or if the indications for anticoagulation are relative C [6] [7].
- If the risk of thromboembolism is very high, aspirin at 100 mg/day may be added to antithrombotic therapy B [10] [11] [12] [13] [14] [15]. These cases include, for example, patients with mitral valve prostheses and atrial fibrillation, and patients with two valvular prostheses. A specialist will make the decision about medication.

Modifying warfarin therapy when an operation or an invasive procedure is performed

- If the procedure is minor and carries a small risk of haemorrhage, anticoagulant therapy may be continued if considered necessary.
- If the risk of haemorrhage is high and the indications of anticoagulant therapy are relative (atrial fibrillation), the therapy is discontinued before the procedure.
- If the indications of anticoagulant therapy are evident (two valvular prostheses, mitral valve prosthesis + atrial fibrillation) and bleeding risk is high, oral anticoagulation should be discontinued before operation and heparin should be used instead.
  - Determine INR one week before the planned operation.
  - Decide whether discontinuing anticoagulant therapy is necessary (see above).
  - If anticoagulant therapy is discontinued, stop warfarin 1–5 days before surgery.
    - If the patient has a particularly high risk of thromboembolism, give low-molecular-weight (LMW) heparin subcutaneously in treatment doses. In very particular cases the effect of heparin can be followed up by measuring FXa inhibition, where the target treatment level is 0.3–0.7 anti-FXa activity units/ml.
    - The pause in warfarin therapy depends on the INR value. Discontinue warfarin before an operation:
      - 5 days earlier if INR > 4
      - 3–4 days earlier if INR = 3–4
      - 2 days earlier if INR = 2–3.
  - INR should be determined in the evening prior to a major operation. If the value is over 1.8, give 0.5–1.0 mg of phytomenadione (vitamin K1).
    - On the day of the operation, consider whether an infusion of unfractionated heparin or a prophylactic dose of LMW heparin is necessary.
    - If the patient has received heparin subcutaneously, continue the treatment for 5–7 days simultaneously with warfarin therapy.
  - Start warfarin therapy at the maintenance dose after minor surgery in the evening of the day of operation, and after major surgery on the day when the patient receives nutrition orally.

References

1. Green CJ, Hadorn D, Kazanjian A. Anticoagulation for stroke prevention in chronic non-valvular atrial fibrillation. Vancouver: B.C. Office of Health Technology Assessment, Centre for Health Services and Policy Research, University of British Columbia, VII, 89, 1995.
2. The Database of Abstracts of Reviews of Effectiveness (University of York), Database no.: DARE-950385. In: The Cochrane Library, Issue 4, 1999. Oxford: Update Software.
3. Benavente O, Hart R, Koudstaal P, Laupacis A, McBride R. Oral anticoagulants for preventing stroke in patients with non-valvular atrial fibrillation and no previous history of stroke or transient ischemic attack. The Cochrane Database of Systematic Reviews, Cochrane Library number: CD001927. In: The Cochrane Library, Issue 2, 2002. Oxford: Update Software. Updated frequently.
4. Segal JB, McNamara RL, Miller MR, Powe NR, Goodman SN, Robinson KA, Bass EB. Anticoagulants or antiplatelet therapy for non-rheumatic atrial fibrillation and flutter. Cochrane Database Syst Rev. 2004;(2):CD001938.
5. Benavente O, Hart R, Koudstaal P, Laupacis A, McBride R. Antiplatelet therapy for preventing stroke in patients with non-valvular atrial fibrillation and no previous history of stroke or transient ischemic attacks. Cochrane Database Syst Rev. 2004;(2):CD001925.
6. Koudstaal PJ. Antiplatelet therapy for preventing stroke in patients with nonrheumatic atrial fibrillation and a history of stroke or transient ischemic attacks. Cochrane Database Syst Rev. 2004;(2):CD000186.
7. EAFT Study Group. Secondary prevention in nonrheumatic atrial fibrillation after transient ischaemic attack or minor stroke. Lancet 1993;342:1255–1262.
8. Ezekowitz MD, Levine JA. Preventing stroke in patients with atrial fibrillation. JAMA 1999;281:1830–1835.
9. The Database of Abstracts of Reviews of Effectiveness (University of York), Database no.: DARE-999256.

In: The Cochrane Library, Issue 1, 2001. Oxford: Update Software.

10. Cappelleri JC, Fiore LD, Brophy MT, Deykin D, Lau J. Efficacy and safety of combined anticoagulant and antiplatelet therapy in patient with mechanical heart-valve replacement. A meta-analysis.
11. The Database of Abstracts of Reviews of Effectiveness (University of York), Database no.: DARE-952502. In: The Cochrane Library, Issue 4, 1999. Oxford: Update Software.
12. Loewen P, Sunderji R, Gin K. The efficacy and safety of combination warfarin and ASA therapy: a systematic review of the literature and update of guidelines. Can J Cardiol 1998;14:717–726.
13. The Database of Abstracts of Reviews of Effectiveness (University of York), Database no.: DARE-981006. In: The Cochrane Library, Issue 1, 2000. Oxford: Update Software.
14. Hart RG, Benavente O, Pearce LA. Increased risk of intracranial hemorrhage when aspirin is combined with warfarin: a meta-analysis and hypothesis. Cerebrovascular Diseases 1999;9:215–217.
15. The Database of Abstracts of Reviews of Effectiveness (University of York), Database no.: DARE-991428. In: The Cochrane Library, Issue 1, 2001. Oxford: Update Software.

4.47 Sick sinus syndrome

Editors

Diagnosis

- The diagnosis of sick sinus requires ECG-verified sinus dysfunction of the sinus node or impulse conduction disturbance (sinoatrial block).
- If the patient also has rapid atrial arrhythmias, the condition is called "brady-tachy syndrome".

Treatment

- If the patient is symptomatic because of the bradycardia, any drugs that depress sinus node action or prevent conductance must not be used (digoxin, beta-blockers, rate-slowing calcium blockers, antiarrhythmic drugs).
- If bradycardia causes severe symptoms, a pacemaker is needed. If the patient also has episodes of tachycardia antiarrhythmic drug therapy is indicated with a pacemaker for prevention of symptomatic bradycardia.

4.48 Cardiac pacemakers: follow-up of patients and surveillance of pacemaker function

Editors

Aims

- To recognize pacemaker malfunctions and signs of end of battery life
- To recognize local complications caused by pacemakers
- To understand the significance of arrhythmias in pacemaker therapy
- To master the terminology used on pacemaker cards

Principles of pacemaker function

- In a unipolar pacemaker, the distal tip of the pacing lead serves as the negative pole and the pulse generator casing as the positive pole.
- In a bipolar pacemaker, both poles are in the pacing lead: the negative pole at the extreme tip and the positive pole some 2 cm proximal to it. Bipolar pacemakers are superior to unipolar ones in monitoring the intrinsic activity of the heart during electrical interference from muscles or extraneous electromagnetic interference. Persons who are exposed to strong electromagnetic fields at work are usually fitted with a bipolar pacemaker. With no current flow at the pulse generator casing, bipolar pacemakers are less prone to cause twitching of the surrounding muscle tissue.
- The electrical pacing stimulus is often 0.3–1.5 ms in duration and 2.5–5 V in amplitude. The stimulation threshold of a lead is the minimum pacing impulse that consistently elicits a heartbeat. The output stimulus is adjusted to the stimulation threshold one to three months after the implantation of the pacemaker.
- Pacemakers are either single-chamber devices (with the pacing lead placed in either the right atrium or right ventricle) or dual-chamber devices (with leads placed in both the right atrium and right ventricle). Dual-chamber pacemakers are also known as physiological pacemakers. In cases of complete atrioventricular block, a dual-chamber pacemaker can pace the ventricles according to the normal sinus rhythm of the atria, allowing natural variation in heart rate.
- Rate-modulating pacemakers contain a sensor that detects increases in physical activity and respond by accelerating the pacing rate.
- Pacemaker programming involves setting the pacing rate, amplitude and width of the output stimulus, sensitivity to intrinsic depolarization signals from the heart, and pacing mode. The pacemaker settings have to be adjusted if the

patient's heart failure worsens or the patient develops atrial arrhythmia.

Selection of pacing mode

- See Table 4.48.
- In patients with sick sinus syndrome, the atrial rate is set sufficiently high whereafter the intact atrioventricular conduction takes care of ventricular rate (AAI pacing). In patients with atrioventricular block, the lost conduction is restored by pacing the ventricles in synchrony with atrial activity (DDD or VDD pacing).
- Traditional ventricular pacing (VVI) is used for atrial fibrillation and bradycardia.
- Ventricular pacing (VVI) dilates the atria, causes atrial fibrillation and predisposes the patient to brain embolism. As atrial function is lost, it also aggravates or causes heart failure. VVI pacemakers are inexpensive and simple to use but nonphysiological in their effects.
- In cases where the intrinsic heart rhythm is intact and there is only an occasional need for cardiac pacing, the simple ventricular pacemaker (VVI) will usually suffice. Old people are often treated by merely ensuring a sufficient heart rate at rest by means of ventricular pacing. If the patient develops pacemaker syndrome, physiological or atrial pacing may be required instead of ventricular pacing.

Frequency of follow-up

- Annual follow-up visits are usually sufficient.
- More frequent follow-up may be needed with physiological pacemakers if alteration of intrinsic rhythm is suspected.
- When the power source shows signs of depletion, the patient should be seen more often.
- Pacemaker check-ups can be arranged within primary care, with (magnet-mode) electrocardiograms being sent for a specialist's opinion.

Issues to be addressed in pacemaker surveillance

- Symptoms
    - Syncopal symptoms: inadequate pacemaker function or pacemaker syndrome (see below). Syncope is always an indication for immediate examination of pacemaker function and referral for further investigations.
    - Any signs of infection around the pulse generator casing require urgent referral to hospital.
    - Twitching in the diaphragm or around the pulse generator casing suggests a fault or (if the twitching occurs in the apex of the diaphragm) wrong placing of the tip of the lead. Twitching always requires referral to a specialized outpatient clinic for investigation of the underlying cause.
    - Physiological pacing may be associated with pacemaker-mediated tachycardia through impulse reentry, atrial flutter or atrial fibrillation.
- Electrocardiography (ECG) with and without a magnet
    - It is advisable to always perform ECG both in magnet mode and without magnet application.
    - The start and end of magnet application should always be carefully marked on the ECG tracing!
    - The preparation for magnet-mode ECG starts with palpation of the location of the pacemaker.
    - A normal 12-lead electrocardiogram is then obtained, in the course of which the magnet is placed on top of the pacemaker during recording of precordial leads V1–V3.
- Battery life
    - The service life of the power source is 6–10 years.
    - The magnet makes the pacemaker send impulses at a constant frequency. A reduction in pulse frequency down to a certain limit indicates that the power source is weakening and the time for pacemaker replacement is approaching. As there are various indicators of the impending end of battery life, there is no general rule on the procedure to follow.
- Stimulation threshold
    - The stimulation threshold may increase because of migration of the tip of the lead (soon after implantation) or development of fibrosis around the tip or breakage of the lead.
    - The stimulation threshold may be measured using a magnet in some pacemaker models but most models require a programming device for threshold determination.
- Condition of leads

Table 4.48 Pacing modes

Pacing mode	Code[1]	Function	Disadvantages
Atrial pacing	AAI, AAIR	Paces the atria, requires normal atrioventricular conduction	Does not react to ventricular asystole
Ventricular pacing	VVI, VVIR	Paces only the ventricles	Does not restore atrio-ventricular synchrony
Pacing with atrial tracking	VDD, VDDR	Paces the ventricles according to the atrial rate	Does not pace the atria
Atrioventricular sequential pacing	DDI, DDIR	Paces both the atria and ventricles	Does not correct atrio-ventricular block
Universal pacing	DDD, DDDR	Both atrial tracking and atrioventricular sequential pacing	

1. R: The pacing rate is modulated according to the patient's physiological status. No letter R: pacing at a constant rate.

- Faults are more common in leads than in pulse generators.
- Suspected disturbance is examined by x-ray or by measuring the electrical resistance with a programming device.

♦ Detection of intrinsic cardiac events (P waves and QRS complexes)
- The pacemaker's ability to sense atrial depolarization (P waves) is prone to change and therefore has to be checked in conjunction with every follow-up visit concerning pacemakers with atrial pacing.

♦ Underlying intrinsic rhythm
- The heart's intrinsic rhythm is important in cases where the pacing rate has been set low to account for occasional bradycardia, as well as in patients with a physiological pacemaker who develop permanent atrial fibrillation and have to be converted to plain ventricular pacing.

♦ The relevance of the pacing modes and pacemaker settings should be reviewed whenever the patient's circumstances may have changed and he/she has symptoms suspected to originate with the pacemaker.

Pacing failures apparent on ECG

♦ The electrocardiogram should be inspected to determine whether the pacemaker is pacing and sensing properly.

Observations requiring consultation with an outpatient clinic or hospital specialized in cardiac pacing

♦ The pacemaker rate is slower than the set minimum rate according to the pacemaker card.
♦ The pacing impulse does not reach its target (exit block).
♦ There is no pacing.
♦ Oversensing (events such as muscle activity or T waves are sensed)
♦ Undersensing (events such as QRS complexes or P waves fail to be sensed), resulting in asynchronous pacing
♦ The polarity (direction) of the pacemaker spike has changed. (This is pathological if present in more than one ECG lead; it may also be a sign of electrode migration.)

Harmless phenomena

♦ If an intrinsic heartbeat falls within the refractory period (generally approx. 1/3 of a second) of the pulse generator, one may get the erroneous impression that the pacemaker is out of order.
♦ A spike known as a fusion beat occurs when an intrinsic heartbeat and a pacemaker-triggered beat coincide in time. Both the above phenomena are harmless.

Pacemaker syndrome

♦ In ventricular pacing (VVI), the atria may contract simultaneously with the ventricles, unless the patient has atrial fibrillation. This may cause atrial distension, hypotension, chronic fatigue and a tendency to syncope.
♦ Factors predisposing to pacemaker syndrome are sick sinus syndrome and retrograde conduction of ventricular pacing over to the atria. The conduction can be examined and any pacing-induced hypotension measured at the time of pacemaker implantation. ECG tracing shows a P deviation on top of the ST-T wave (transoesophageal ECG).
♦ Pacemaker syndrome is treated by reducing the rate of VVI pacing or by converting to another pacing mode.
♦ Sometimes pacemaker syndrome occurs without retrograde conduction. It gives rise to unspecific symptoms which are often wrongly attributed to the patient's underlying disease.

Electrical and magnetic fields in the environment

♦ Electromagnetic fields may interfere with the sensor function of the pacemaker.
♦ Pacemakers have an escape function which makes them pace at a predetermined rate irrespective of the heart's intrinsic rhythm.
♦ Appliances in homes, offices and public venues, as well as security detection devices at airports are usually harmless to pacemakers.
♦ Electrical fields in power stations and industrial premises have field strengths (1–10 kV/m) that may interfere with pacemaker function.
♦ Electric arc welding is not permitted for persons with pacemakers.
♦ Power transmission lines (110–400 kV) generate strong fields, and **patients with pacemakers should therefore avoid staying in the vicinity of power lines up to a distance of 40 m**. Brief stays in such areas are permitted, for instance when passing under power lines by car.
♦ **Prohibited medical procedures** comprise magnetic resonance imaging (MRI), as well as radiotherapy to the proximity of the pulse generator casing. Among the physiotherapeutic procedures, short-wave diathermy is not permitted, and transcutaneous electrical nerve stimulation is not recommended without simultaneous ECG monitoring. In surgical diathermy, bipolar diathermy must be employed, and the diathermy circuit must be conducted as far away from the cardiac pacemaker as possible.

Arrhythmias in pacemaker patients

♦ Atrial fibrillation occurring during atrial or physiological pacing calls for restoration of sinus rhythm. Plain ventricular pacing is sufficient in atrial fibrillation.
♦ If spontaneous beats emerge, bradycardiac agents should be avoided (except in situations where antiarrhythmic drugs are specifically needed and cardiac pacing ensures their sufficient dosage).
♦ The presence of a pacemaker does not alter the indications for anticoagulant therapy in atrial fibrillation.

- ♦ If the patient requires electrical cardioversion, the line connecting the electrodes must be transverse to the direction of the pacemaker lead (sternal and dorsal placement of the electrodes is recommended; no electrode should be placed at the apex of the heart).

Instructions for the pacemaker patient

- ♦ Always carry your pacemaker card with you.
- ♦ Measure your heart rate about once a month. If your heart rate falls below the agreed limit by more than three beats per minute, contact your doctor.

4.55 Differential diagnosis of chest pain

Editors

Objectives

- ♦ Pain caused by myocardial ischaemia or impending infarction must be differentiated from non-ischaemic chest pain. Non-ischaemic pain may be caused by other severe conditions that require acute treatment, such as pericarditis, aortic dissection and pulmonary embolism.
- ♦ Remember that patients at risk can have ischaemic chest pain in addition to non-ischaemic chest pain.
- ♦ Differentiate between stable and unstable angina (4.58).

Myocardial ischaemic pain

- ♦ The main feature of myocardial ischaemia (impending infarction) is usually prolonged chest pain. Typical characteristics of the pain include:
  - Duration usually over 20 minutes.
  - Located in the retrosternal area, possibly radiating to the arms (usually to the left arm), back, neck or the lower jaw.
  - The pain is described as pressing or heavy or as a sensation of a tight band around the chest; breathing or changing posture does not notably influence the severity of the pain.
  - The pain is continuous and its intensity does not alter.
  - The symptoms (pain beginning in the upper abdomen, nausea) may resemble the symptoms of acute abdomen. Nausea and vomiting are sometimes the main symptoms, especially in inferoposterior wall ischaemia.
  - In inferoposterior wall ischaemia, vagal reflexes may cause bradycardia and hypotension, presenting as dizziness or fainting.

Table 4.55.1 Minor ECG changes of an MI, and MI with left bundle branch block (LBBB)

Minor ECG changes suggestive of an MI	Diagnosis of an MI in the presence of LBBB
Poor R wave progression	ST elevation in the acute phase
Even a small Q wave in V2–V4 and no anterior fascicular block	New Q wave in V5–V6
Notching of both the initial and terminal portion of the QRS complex	QS or R depression in V1–V6
Acute bundle branch block or fascicular block	Low amplitude QRS complex
Disappearance of old changes of an infarction	QR morphology in ventricular ectopic beats
Q wave less than 30 ms in III, aVF	

- ♦ ECG is the key examination during the first 4 hours after pain onset, but a normal ECG does not rule out an imminent infarction.
- ♦ Markers of myocardial injury (cardiac troponins T and I, CK-MB mass) start to rise about 4 hours after pain onset. An increase of these markers is diagnostic of myocardial infarction irrespective of ECG findings (4.60).
- ♦ Minor signs of myocardial infarction in ECG, see Table 4.55.1.

Non-ischaemic causes of chest pain

- ♦ For non-ischaemic causes of chest pain, see Table 4.55.2.
- ♦ For ECG changes resembling those of an MI, see Table 4.55.3.

Table 4.55.2 Non-ischaemic causes of chest pain

Illness/condition	Differentiating signs and symptoms
Reflux oesophagitis, oesophageal spasm	♦ No ECG changes ♦ Heartburn ♦ Worse in recumbent position, and also whilst straining, like angina pectoris ♦ The most common cause of chest pain
Pulmonary embolism	♦ Tachypnoea, hypoxaemia, hypocarbia ♦ No pulmonary congestion on chest x-ray ♦ Clinical presentation may resemble hyperventilation ♦ Both PaO_2 and $PaCO_2$ decreased ♦ Pain is not often marked ♦ D-dimer assay positive

Table 4.55.2 (*continued*)

Hyperventilation	Hyperventilation syndrome ♦ The main symptom is dyspnoea, as in pulmonary embolism ♦ Often a young patient ♦ Tingling and numbness of the limbs, dizziness ♦ $PaCO_2$ decreased, PaO_2 increased or normal Secondary hyperventilation ♦ Attributable to an organic illness/cause; acidosis, pulmonary embolism, pneumothorax, asthma, infarction etc.
Spontaneous pneumothorax	♦ Dyspnoea is the main symptom. ♦ Auscultation and chest x-ray
Aortic dissection	♦ Severe pain with changing localization ♦ Type A dissection sometimes obstructs the origin of a coronary artery (usually the right) with signs of impending inferoposterior infarction ♦ Pulses may be asymmetrical ♦ Sometimes broad mediastinum on chest x-ray ♦ New aortic valve regurgitation
Pericarditis	♦ Change of posture and breathing influence the pain. ♦ A friction sound may be heard. ♦ ST elevation but no reciprocal ST depression
Pleuritis	♦ A stabbing pain when breathing. The most common cause of stabbing chest pain is, however, caused by prolonged cough
Costochondral pain	♦ Palpation tenderness, movements of chest influence the pain ♦ Might also be an insignificant incidental finding
Early herpes zoster	♦ No ECG changes, rash ♦ Localized paraesthesia before rash
Ectopic beats	♦ Transient, in the area of the apex
Peptic ulcer, cholecystitis, pancreatitis	♦ Clinical examination (inferior wall ischaemia may resemble acute abdomen)
Depression	♦ Continuous feeling of heaviness in the chest, no correlation to exercise ♦ ECG normal
Alcohol-related	♦ A young male patient in a casualty department, inebriated

Table 4.55.3 ECG changes resembling those of an MI

ST changes resembling those of acute ischaemia	
ST segment elevation	Early repolarization in V1–V3. Seen particularly in athletic men ("athlete's heart") Acute myopericarditis in all leads except V1, aVR. Not resolved with a beta-blocker. Pulmonary embolism –in inferior leads Hyperkalaemia Hypertrophic cardiomyopathy
ST segment depression	Sympathicotonia Hyperventilation Pulmonary embolism Hypokalaemia Digoxin Antiarrhythmics Psychiatric medication Hypertrophic cardiomyopathy Reciprocal ST depression of an inferior infarction in leads V2–V3–V4 Circulatory shock
QRS changes resembling those of Q wave infarction	Hypertrophic cardiomyopathy WPW syndrome Myocarditis Blunt cardiac injury Massive pulmonary embolism (QS in leads V1–V3) Pneumothorax Cardiac amyloidosis Cardiac tumours Progressing muscular dystrophy Friedreich's ataxia
ST changes resembling those of a non-Q wave infarction	Increased intracranial pressure – subarachnoid bleed –skull injury Hyperventilation syndrome Post-tachyarrhythmia state Circulatory shock–haemorrhage–sepsis Acute pancreatitis Myopericarditis

4.58 Unstable angina pectoris

Editors

Objective

♦ To recognize angina pectoris that may be prodromal to acute infarction (acute coronary syndrome ACS) and to accompany the patient to a cardiac monitoring unit for active drug treatment or rapid revascularization (B) [1].

Definition

1. Recent (less than 1–2 months) angina pectoris,
2. Accelerated angina pectoris
3. Angina pectoris at rest

Risk groups and clinical signs

- The presence of a marker (cardiac troponin T and I, CK-MBm) is the single most important predictor for future coronary events
  - Marker-positive patients are referred to angiography and revascularization
  - Marker-negatives are referred to exercise tolerance test.
- Unstable angina pectoris (UAP) is a heterogeneous group of diseases covering the range between stable AP and acute myocardial infarction (AMI).
- New (sudden) AP in a high-risk patient is always a serious condition.
- An aggravation in stable AP to unstable AP always necessitates a reassessment of risk and often a change in the line of treatment.
- There may not always be pain rather the main symptom is a decrease in exercise tolerance (sudden decrease in physical fitness) or acute left ventricle failure.
- In the ECG a ST segment depression precedes the pain. Symptomless (silent) ischaemia in a patient at risk is a significant finding. Ischaemia may not always be visible in ECG. An ECG registered while the patient has pain is invariably valuable.
- The border between UAP and T-wave infarction (non-Q infarction) is shifting. For example, very proximal occlusion in the left anterior descending artery (LAD) causes a symmetric T inversion in chest leads. Elevation of myocardial markers indicates that the patient has an infarction.

Treatment

- Treatment is normally carried out in a cardiac monitoring unit.
- Pharmacological treatment should be started in the first point of care.
- The mildest form (recent angina) can be treated in a health care centre ward under careful monitoring. Remember the risk of MI. The risk diminishes with time as the angina stabilizes.

Anti-ischaemic and antithrombotic treatment

- All patients with suspected unstable angina (no changes in ECG or myocardial markers)
  - Aspirin 250 mg (chewable) first. Thereafter 100 mg/day, unless there are contraindications **A** [2 3].
  - Oxygen
  - Nitrate infusion **D** [4] for 24–36 hours (4.59). Systolic blood pressure should be lowered by 10–15 mmHg and always to a level below 150 mmHg.
  - Beta-blocker **C** [5] (metoprolol or atenolol). Heart rate should be 50–70 beats/min and systolic pressure below 150 mmHg.
  - Low-molecular-weight (LMW) heparin **A** [6 7 8 9] (e.g. dalteparin 100–120 IU/kg × 2 daily for one week) is given simultaneously with aspirin. The treatment can be continued with half the dose for about 1 month. UAP patients with an elevated troponin T concentration derive the greatest benefit from the treatment (LMWH + aspirin). Pharmacotherapy and invasive treatment do not exclude one another.
- High-risk patients: Unstable angina and ischaemia on ECG or elevated myocardial markers **A** [10 11], acute left ventricle failure (lung oedema, mitral regurgitation, hypotension)
  - Immediate angiography and revascularization. While waiting for the procedure the thrombosis should be stabilized with clopidogrel (an initial dose of 300 mg before transportation, thereafter 75 mg daily) and an i.v. GPIIb/IIIa inhibitor **B** [12] in addition to aspirin and LMW heparin. (Fibrinolytic treatment has no effect on a vessel obstruction caused by aggregated platelets).
- Thrombolytic therapy or immediate percutaneous transluminal angioplasty (PTA) (during which a stent can be inserted) is indicated if ECG reveals a transmural injury. See article on revascularization 4.63. After the insertion of a stent, clopidogrel is used in combination with aspirin at least one month.
- Further treatment of patients with symptoms or signs of ischaemia on ECG and normal myocardial markers
  - Symptom-limited exercise test performed within 2–4 days
  - If the patient has symptoms or signs of ischaemia during the exercise test or signs in ECG at a low pulse-pressure product, refer immediately to angiography.
  - In case of no symptoms or signs of ischaemia during light exercise or no signs in ECG, or if they occur only with a high pulse-pressure product, begin conservative treatment and elimination of risk factors. Prophylaxis can be intensified by adding clopidogrel to aspirin.

Organizing treatment

- UAP is a serious but often curable syndrome. A well-organized care pathway ensures that the appropriate treatment can be given rapidly.

References

1. Wallentin L, Lagerqvist B, Husted S, Kontny F, Ståhle E, Swahn E, for the FRISC II invasive randomised trial. Lancet 2000;356:9–16.
2. Natarajan M. Unstable angina. Clinical Evidence 2002;7: 214–226.

3. Antithrombotic Trialists´ Collaboration: Collaborative overview of randomised trials of antiplatelet therapy - I: prevention of death, myocardial infarction, and stroke by prolonged antiplatelet therapy in various categories of patients. BMJ 1994;308:81–106.
4. Natarajan M. Nitrates in unstable angina. Clinical Evidence 2000;4:159–160.
5. Natarajan M. Unstable angina. Clinical Evidence 2002;7: 214–226.
6. Zed PJ, Tisdale JE, Borzak S. Low-molecular weight heparins in the management of acute coronary syndromes. Archives of Internal Medicine 1999;159:1849–1857.
7. The Database of Abstracts of Reviews of Effectiveness (University of York), Database no.:DARE-999714. In: The Cochrane Library, Issue 1, 2001. Oxford: Update Software.
8. Nicholson T, Milne R, Stein K. Dalteparin and enoxaparin for unstable angina and non-Q-wave myocardial infarction: update. Southampton: Wessex Institute for Health Research and Development. DEC Report No. 108. 2000. 53.
9. The Health Technology Assessment Database, Database no.:HTA-20000891. In: The Cochrane Library, Issue 1, 2001. Oxford: Update Software.
10. Olatidoye AG, Wu AH, Fent YJ, Waters D. Prognostic role of troponin T versus troponin I in unstable angina pectoris for cardiac events with meta-analysis comparing published studies. Am J Cardiol 1998;81:1405–1410.
11. The Database of Abstracts of Reviews of Effectiveness (University of York), Database no.:DARE-981100. In: The Cochrane Library, Issue 2, 2000. Oxford: Update Software.
12. Natarajan M. Unstable angina. Clinical Evidence 2002;7: 214–226.

4.59 Nitrate infusion in angina pectoris and myocardial infarction

John Melin

Indications

- Given to all patients with angina pectoris or myocardial infarction, if the pain is not relieved with nitrates administered as a spray or sublingually.
    - The treatment improves oxygenation by alleviating coronary spasm and reduces oxygen consumption by decreasing the preload of the ventricles.
    - Nitrates in combination with beta-blockers and antithrombotic medication continue to be the drug of choice in unstable angina pectoris, although evidence on the impact of this therapy on mortality or the incidence of myocardial infarction is lacking (D) [1].
- Intravenously administered nitrate is a safe method for treating pain in myocardial infarction (A) [2].

Table 4.59 Dosing with 0.1 mg/ml nitrate solution

Drop counter (drops/min)	Volume pump (ml/h)	Dos (mg/h)
3	10	1
7	20	2
10	30	3
13	40	4
17	50	5
20	60	6
23	70	7
27	80	8
30	90	9
33	100	10
37	110	11
40	120	12

Contraindications

- Hypovolaemia
- Severe hypotension (systolic blood pressure below 90 mm Hg)
- Right ventricle infarction (V4R lead!)
- Shock without inotropic medication.

Use of isosorbide dinitrate

1. Dilute 50 mg of nitrate concentrate with 500 ml of 0.45% NaCl solution (concentration 0.1 mg/ml) or use a commercial 0.2-mg/ml infusion solution.
2. Initial dosage of infusion is usually 2 mg/h (7 drops/min, if the solution is 0.1 mg/ml) using a volume pump or a drop counter.
3. The dose is increased every 10 min depending on the response (pain relief) and blood pressure, 1–2 drops at a time (3–6 ml/h in a volume pump, if the solution is 0.1 mg/ml). See Table 4.59.
    - Increasing the dose is interrupted, if
        - systolic blood pressure is below 90 mm Hg or diastolic blood pressure is below 60 mm Hg.
        - the patient does not feel better and systolic blood pressure decreases by more than 10% in a normotensive patient or by more than 30% in a hypertensive patient, or if heart rate increases by more than 10%.
4. Potential hypovolaemia must be identified (empty jugular and peripheral veins, cold extremities) and corrected with fluid infusion while nitrate infusion is continued. Rapid lowering of blood pressure must be avoided.
5. Oral therapy is usually initiated at 12–48 hours, when the effective anti-anginal dose is 2 mg/h = 7 drops/min at the most.
6. Longer-acting oral treatment with nitrates is a safe and efficient symptomatic treatment.

References

1. Natarajan M. Nitrates in unstable angina. Clinical Evidence 2000;4:159–160.

2. Mehta S, Yusuf S. Nitrates in myocardial infarction. Clinical Evidence 2000;4:7–8.

4.60 Myocardial infarction

Editors

Objectives

- If a person at risk of a myocardial infarction has an acute coronary syndrome lasting over 20 minutes, imminent myocardial infarction must be suspected. Instead of chest pain, acute dyspnoea may be the primary symptom.
- An acute coronary syndrome without myocardial damage is often unstable angina, which calls for active treatment.
- The diagnosis should be made without delay since early therapy improves the prognosis decisively.
- Thrombolytic therapy is given as early as possible in all cases with a clinical picture of imminent myocardial infarction and corresponding ECG changes (4.61).
- Acute angioplasty (PTCA, PCI) is an alternative or a complementary procedure to thrombolytic therapy (A) [1 2 3]. Angioplasty is probably preferred, at least in ST elevation MI.
- If there are no contraindications, aspirin and a beta-blocker should be started for all patients and for most patients also an ACE inhibitor and a statin on the first days of treatment.
- Health care system should include a planned care pathway for coronary patients.

Diagnosis

- See Figures 4.60.1–4.60.4
- The diagnostic criteria change in the course of treatment.
  - During first aid, pain is the primary symptom in younger patients. Presentation in the elderly is often atypical.
  - When thrombolytic therapy is considered, an ST elevation on the ECG or a recent left bundle branch block (LBBB) should be taken into account (4.61).
  - In addition to pain and ECG findings, myocardial enzyme levels are needed for definite clinical diagnosis.
- For differential diagnosis of chest pain, see 4.55.
- The pain in myocardial infarction lasts over 20 minutes and is localized widely in the retrosternal area, transfers to the arms, back, neck or lower jaw. The pain is squeezing, is experienced as tightness, heaviness and pressure or pressing. Breathing or changing posture does not influence the intensity of pain. The pain is usually severe and consistent. It may be localized in the upper abdomen, in which case, if nausea and vomiting are also present, it simulates acute abdominal disease. The patient is often pale, in a cold sweat and anxious.

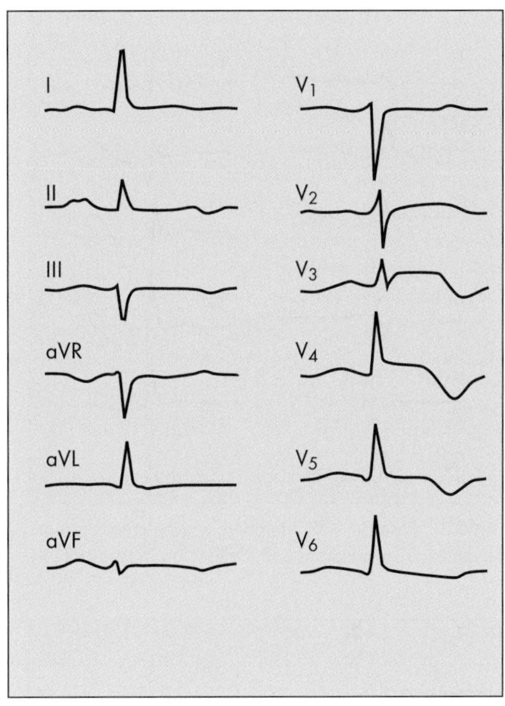

Figure 4.60.1 An incipient infarction: ST elevation in leads V3–V5. The Q wave has not yet developed, so thrombolytic therapy is strongly indicated.

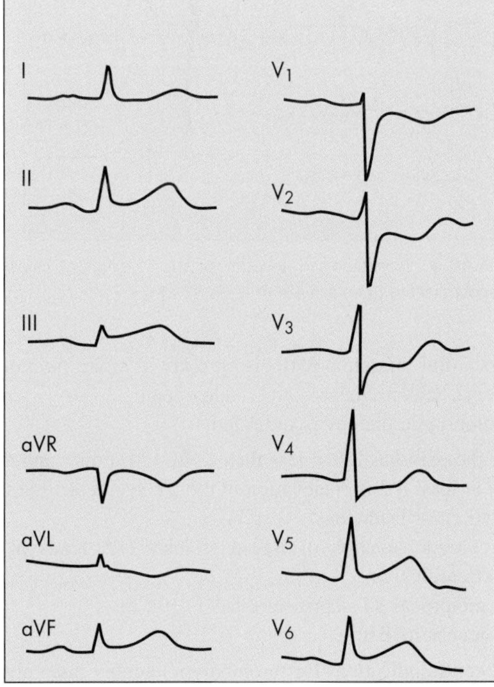

Figure 4.60.2 A recent inferoposterior wall infarction. The Q wave (=R elevation in leads V2–V3) has not yet developed, so thrombolytic therapy is indicated. Reciprocal ST depressions in leads V2–V3 correlate with ST elevations in anterior wall infarction. ST elevations in inferior leads, leads II, III and aVF.

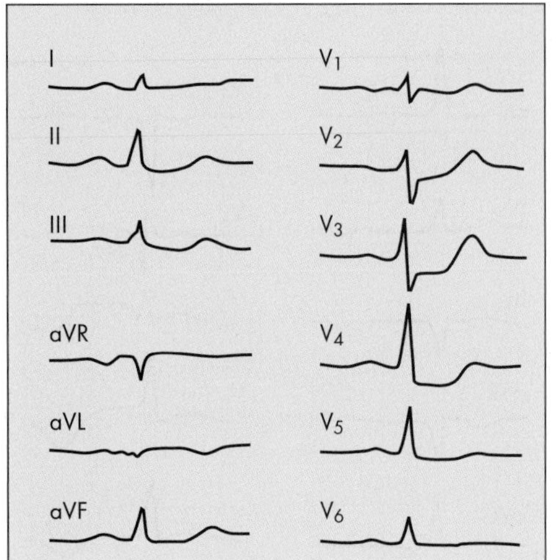

Figure 4.60.3 Posterior wall infarction, which extends laterally (lead aVL). Reciprocal ST depressions and R elevation in leads V2–V4.

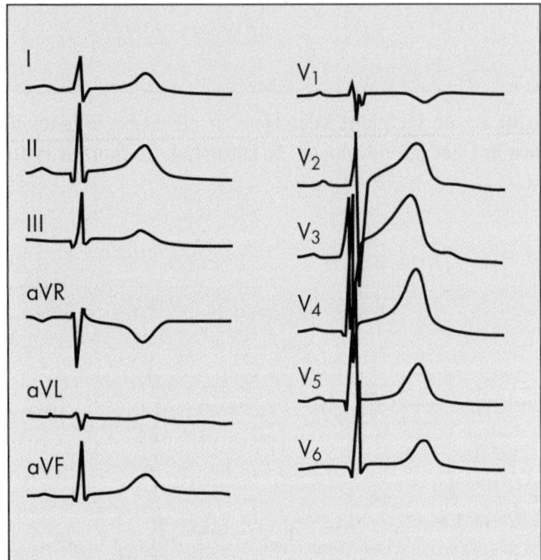

Figure 4.60.4 Physiological elevation of the ST segment caused by early repolarization in an athlete in leads V2–V4.

- Myocardial infarction may also present as acute pulmonary oedema, unconsciousness or sudden death.
- Thrombolytic therapy is indicated
    - if the pain has lasted less than 6–12 (24) hours and there is at least a 2-mm elevation in the ST segment in at least two chest leads, or
    - a 1-mm elevation of ST in at least two leads in the extremities, or
    - a reciprocal ST depression in V1–V4, or
    - a recent LBBB.
- The contraindications for thrombolytic therapy must always be considered (4.61).
- In clinical investigation, remember that the ECG and myocardial markers change with the course of the disease: first there is an ST elevation, after that development of the Q wave, and finally T-wave inversion. Complications must also be recognized. In a T-wave infarction (non-Q-wave infarction), no classical Q waves are present, but the diagnosis is based on an increase of myocardial enzymes, chest pain, or ST-T changes. Classical Q-wave changes, ST elevations and T inversions may be caused by various other diseases, which should be remembered in the differential diagnosis. An old infarction, BBB and early repolarization make the diagnosis difficult, in which case the change in ECG is important and an old ECG recording valuable. When added to other criteria, "minor" signs of infarction are also important.
- The European Society of Cardiology and the American College of Cardiology have agreed on a new definition of myocardial infarction:
    - Typical increase in the concentration of serum cardiac troponins or CK-MB associated with at least one of the following:
        - symptoms of cardiac ischaemia
        - recent pathological Q waves in the ECG
        - ischaemic ST segment changes in the ECG
        - coronary artery revascularization.

ECG diagnosis

- Points for taking an ECG: acute care, emergency room, 12 hours later, on day 2, upon discharge from hospital and thereafter as deemed necessary.
- ECG is the most important diagnostic procedure. To start with, the positions of the chest leads must be marked on the skin to allow detection of significant changes on the ECG. By monitoring the ECG, the efficacy of the treatment can be assessed. However, in the early stages there may be no changes in ECG, and the changes may be first evident after hours or even days. An ECG diagnosis is made more difficult by an old infarction, LBBB or posterior infarction.
- In posterior wall infarction, a reciprocal ST segment depression in V1–V4 simulates ischaemia. A posterior infarction is, however, often inferoposterior and, in addition to ST segment depression, ST segment elevations are found in leads III and aVF.
- ST depression is suggestive of ischaemia and/or unstable angina pectoris. Extensive ST depressions in connection with a clinical picture of myocardial infarction can indicate subendocardial damage.

Tests following the ECG

- Troponin is the most important new marker and is replacing CK.
- CK and CK-MB or CK-MB mass
- A negative troponin T, troponin I or CK-MBm result 9–12 hours after the onset of symptoms practically rules out myocardial infarction.
- Troponin T test is also valuable, if the time lapse since the beginning of the symptoms is more than 24 hours (the concentration remains elevated longer than that of CK).

An elevated troponin T or troponin I concentration predicts adverse events irrespective of ECG findings (A) [4,5].

- The tests should be performed 3 times in case of suspected infarction: on arrival of the patient and 12 and 24 hours after arrival.
- Blood haemoglobin, leukocytes, ESR and CRP
- Serum sodium and potassium, and chest x-ray if needed

Troponin-T or troponin-I

- Principal indicators of myocardial damage, which can also be determined by means of rapid testing methods suited for primary health care. A reading device facilitates the interpretation.
- Troponin is more myocardium-specific than CK-MB and is also very sensitive.
- The concentration increases rapidly (in 4–6 hours) after myocardial damage, and the elevated levels persist for at least one week.
- Indications:
  - To verify or exclude myocardial infarction (or myocarditis) when at least 6 hours have elapsed from the onset of pain. Unstable angina pectoris may give positive results, indicating slight myocardial damage, which means that the prognosis is serious regardless of the ECG findings and active treatment is necessary. The normal reference concentration is zero, or the method-dependent threshold is often given as <0.5 µg/l.
  - A negative result within 12 hours after the onset of pain excludes infarction.
  - Also used for the diagnosis of infarction when the patient's arrival for treatment is delayed, and CK has returned to normal.
  - Troponin verifies myocardial infarction in cases where high CK concentration from skeletal muscle increases the CK-MB concentration over normal limits.
- Mild elevations in the concentration that exceed the threshold are often seen in cardiac surgery. The threshold level that would verify the diagnosis of myocardial infarction has not been defined for the situations. Mild elevations may also occur in connection when prolonged tachycardia causes a strain on the sick heart.

Serum CK-MB mass

- More specific and sensitive than CK-MB
- Abnormal within 6–8 hours from the beginning of the pain, and remains abnormal for 1–2 days.
- Slightly positive values may indicate mild myocardial damage that requires active treatment. Unlike with troponin, the normal concentration of CK-MB is not zero. There is an uncertain borderline area of 5–10 µg/l between the positive and negative result.

Myoglobin

- Reacts most rapidly to myocardial damage and is positive from the first hours onward.
- Not a specific indicator of myocardial damage. Negative myoglobin is valuable in exclusion diagnosis.
- Lack of reference values limits use.

Differential diagnosis

- The most important differential diagnoses include
  - myopericarditis (4.82)
  - aortic dissection (5.63)
  - pulmonary embolism (5.43)
  - unstable angina pectoris (4.58)
  - oesophageal pain (8.30).
- See also article on differential diagnosis of chest pain 4.55.

Treatment

- Oxygen, if there are problems in oxygenation (pulmonary oedema).
- For treating pain
  - Glyceryl nitrate: mouth spray or sublingual tablet
  - Morphine 4–6 mg i.v., additionally 4 mg 1–3 times at 5 min intervals, if necessary. Oxycodone 3–5 mg i.v. is an alternative.
  - A beta-blocker (metoprolol, atenolol, practolol) 2–5 mg i.v. may sometimes ease the pain.
- Aspirin 250 mg, chewable tablet or dissolved in water, unless there are contraindications (active ulcer, hypersensitivity to aspirin, anticoagulation) (A) [6,7]
- A beta-blocker (A) [8] is always instituted, unless there are contraindications (asthma, hypotension, heart insufficiency, conduction disturbance, bradycardia). The first dose can be given intravenously if the patient is in pain, or orally if the patient is pain-free and time has passed since the infarction. Beta-blockers are useful especially in patients who are tachycardic and hypertensive but do not have heart failure.
  - i.v. dose: metoprolol or atenolol 5 mg.
  - Orally, metoprolol or atenolol 25–50 mg × 2
- Thrombolytic therapy, unless there are contraindications (4.61) (A) [9,10].
- **Immediate PTCA** (A) [1,2,3] if available. May be performed when thrombolytic therapy is contraindicated. The effect is better than that of thrombolysis in the acute phase (B) [11,12,13,14,15] and also in long-term follow-up. Stenting probably improves the outcome (A) [16,17]. Further treatment with clopidogrel for 3 months.
- An ACE inhibitor to all patients with signs or symptoms of heart failure or EF < 40, anterior wall infarction or reinfarction (A) [18,19,20]. Therapy is not usually started on the first day.
  - E.g. captopril. Start with 6.25 mg and increase the dose rapidly.
- Continuous nitrate therapy (A) [21]
  - Administered as an infusion, if the patient has ischaemic pain and pain medication has no effect. Nitrate infusion (4.59).
  - Orally, e.g. isosorbide dinitrate 10–20 mg × 2–3.

- Heparinization is often indicated, if the patient
  - needs prolonged bed rest and is clearly obese (thrombosis prophylaxis)
  - has atrial fibrillation (also permanent warfarin therapy)
  - has ventricular aneurysm (also permanent warfarin therapy)
  - has unstable angina pectoris
  - has embolic complications
- Anticoagulation with warfarin is often started in massive anterior infarction and when TIA or stroke (mural thrombosis) occurs with MI.

Arrhythmias in myocardial infarction

Objectives

- To prevent sudden death and to treat severe arrhythmias immediately.
- To prevent arrhythmias by treating the underlying conditions.

Causes of arrhythmias

- Myocardial damage, ischaemia and sympathetic stimulation are associated with ventricular arrhythmias.
- Ejection failure causes supraventricular tachyarrhythmias and atrial fibrillation.
- Vagal stimulation causes bradyarrhythmias and AV conduction disturbances, especially in cases of inferior-posterior wall infarction.
- Reperfusion often causes benign ventricular rhythm; however, it also causes severe ventricular arrhythmias.

Ventricular fibrillation

- Often occurs within 2–4 hours of infarction. After 12 hours, primary ventricular fibrillation is rare.
- An early ectopic beat may initiate ventricular fibrillation in an ischaemic myocardium. Ectopic beats are not treated if cardiac monitoring is effective.
- Treatment
  - Acute ventricular fibrillation is treated by immediate defibrillation starting with 200 joules. Prolonged ventricular fibrillation frequently calls for cardiopulmonary resuscitation (CPR).
  - To prevent recurrence of fibrillation, lidocaine is given: initially as bolus of 100 mg, which can be repeated if necessary. Thereafter, a continuous infusion of 3–4 mg/min is given. Amiodarone is a modern and more effective alternative to lidocaine: infuse a 150–300 mg bolus in 20 minutes. Thereafter infusion at 800–1200 mg/24 hours.
  - A beta-blocker is usually added to the therapy.

Ventricular tachycardia

- More than three ectopic beats and a heart rate over 120 beats/min.
- Brief, spontaneously ending bursts are seen in over 50% of patients with infarction during the first two days. They occur mainly 8–14 hours after, not immediately after the infarction, as does ventricular fibrillation.
- Ventricular tachycardia leads to haemodynamic collapse or ventricular fibrillation. The severity depends on the duration, variability, frequency and timing of tachycardia.
- VT may be monomorphic or polymorphic.
- Treatment
  - Beta-blocker
  - Lidocaine boluses and infusion as in ventricular fibrillation, if haemodynamics compromise. Amiodarone may be a better alternative.
  - If necessary, synchronized cardioversion shock with 50 joules is performed.
  - Late in infarction, ventricular tachycardia is, like ventricular fibrillation, a serious problem that requires further examination.

Ventricular ectopic beats

- Occur in nearly all patients with painful myocardial infarction.
- May cause complications if they are frequent (more than 5/min), are variable or occur concomitantly with an early T wave.
- Treatment is usually not necessary if cardiac monitoring is effective. A beta-blocker may be indicated. Potassium level should be kept above 4.0.

Idioventricular rhythm

- Idioventricular rhythm is an arrhythmia often associated with myocardial infarction. In the reperfusion phase, it may even indicate that thrombolysis has been successful. The frequency is often 70–80 bpm and drug therapy is not necessary.

Supraventricular tachyarrhythmias

- Atrial fibrillation in a patient with infarction is often associated with cardiac insufficiency and it worsens the prognosis. Atrial fibrillation increases the risk of stroke, which is why LMW heparin and warfarin therapy are indicated.
- Atrial fibrillation is often associated with the thrombosis of the right coronary artery or the circumflex branch: reperfusion also often restores the rhythm.
- Atrial function is important in myocardial infarction. In cardiac insufficiency, rapid atrial fibrillation requires active direct current (DC) cardioversion. Often, the achieved sinus rhythm does not remain. In such a case, haemodynamics must be stabilized (oxygenation, treatment of pulmonary oedema, controlling of ventricular response with a beta-blocker and digitalis) after which spontaneous reversal of the rhythm is waited for. The effect of the beta-blocker is seen rapidly but that of digitalis not before several hours. Rapid ventricular response may be controlled even if cardiac insufficiency is present: the benefit often outweighs the disadvantage.

- Selective beta-blockers are best suited for maintaining the achieved sinus rhythm.
- Intravenous amiodarone will not reduce the contraction of the myocardium. It is effective in prophylaxis of atrial fibrillation (together with a beta-blocker) and it may be used in cardioversion of atrial fibrillation and/or slowing down the ventricular response.
- Ibutilide is a new class III drug with a single indication: treatment of atrial fibrillation and flutter. There are limited data on its use in patients with infarction.
- Note! A broad QRS complex tachycardia in a patient with infarction must always be treated as a ventricular tachycardia.

Bradyarrhythmias

- A strong vagal reaction in the early stages of infarction may lead to a circulatory collapse.
- Postero-inferior wall infarction is often associated with a functional AV block. The QRS complex is narrow and the heart rhythm is 50–60 even in cases of a total block. A pacemaker is rarely needed.
- In anterior wall infarction, the proximal conduction system may be blocked: the QRS complex is wide, the substituting rhythm is slow (30–40), the patient is in a poor condition and pacing is necessary. Prognosis is poor even with pacing.
- Drug treatment
    - atropine 0.5 mg i.v., repeated as necessary, for treatment of functional bradycardia.

Pacemaker

- In anterior wall infarction pacing is indicated if there is a 2nd or 3rd degree block. Pacing should be anticipated in case of a trifascicular block, alternating right and left bundle branch block, or if an extensive infarction is associated with LAFB or LPFB.
- Postero-inferior wall infarction associated with a 3rd degree AV block requires pacing if bradycardia is detrimental to haemodynamics and not responsive to treatment with atropine.
- Sinus bradycardia may be temporarily controlled with i.v. atropine.

Circulatory conditions and their treatment after myocardial infarction

- Table 4.60.1

Table 4.60.1 Circulatory conditions and their treatment in myocardial infarction

Condition and treatment	Symptoms and signs
Normal circulation ♦ monitoring ♦ i.v. line (saline drop)	♦ heart rate and blood pressure normal ♦ no arrhythmias ♦ no heart insufficiency
Hyperdynamic state ♦ beta-blocker (metoprolol, atenolol, practolol 2–5 mg i.v.)	♦ increased heart rate, high blood pressure
Neurovascular reflex (bradycardia-hypotension) ♦ atropine 0.5 mg i.v., repeated ad 2 mg ♦ dopamine infusion, if necessary	♦ usually in connection with postero-inferior infarction ♦ bradycardia, hypotension
Hypovolaemia ♦ 0.9% saline 200 ml in 5–0 min according to the response	♦ low blood pressure, low CVP, tachycardia ♦ cold extremities ♦ decreased venous distension (also jugular veins)
Severe heart failure ♦ nitrate infusion ♦ dopamine infusion ♦ CPAP ♦ treatment of pulmonary oedema	♦ low blood pressure ♦ cold extremities ♦ engorged neck veins ♦ chest crackles ♦ chest x-ray

Treatment in hospital

Follow-up and treatment

- Pain: morphine, nitro, beta-blocker
- Blood pressure
- Skin, peripheral circulation
- Increased respiratory rate suggests cardiac insufficiency.
- Monitoring of arrhythmias
- ST segment changes
- Oxygen saturation; oxygen or CPAP
- A comfortable posture
- Informing and reassuring the patient
- Nicotine replacement therapy is started already in the hospital. Nicotine addiction may be evaluated by using the Fagerstrom test, and the planning of further treatment may be based on it.
- In an uncomplicated infarction, patients are allowed to sit as soon as they want, they can eat unassisted, and they can be helped to a portable toilet at the bedside. Intensive monitoring is usually needed for 1–2 days.
- The infarction is complicated and treatment lasts longer if the patient has had
    - shock
    - hypotension
    - obvious cardiac insufficiency (usually requires thrombosis prophylaxis or anticoagulation, especially if in connection with atrial fibrillation)
    - prolonged chest pain
    - serious ventricular arrhythmias
    - thromboembolic complications
    - anatomical complications (papillary muscle dysfunction or rupture)
    - pericarditis on days 2–4.
- Treatment of the patient in primary health care (in a primary health care hospital) is justifiable if the patient's prognosis is otherwise poor: those who are permanent inpatients

or otherwise severely disabled and for whom invasive treatment has not been planned.

Assessment of risk factors in a patient with myocardial infarction

- The most important causes of mortality are
  - reinfarction
  - cardiac insufficiency
  - arrhythmias.
- During hospitalization, a poor prognosis is indicated by
  - cardiac insufficiency and extensive infarction (EF < 25%)
  - chest pain and ischaemic ST changes (send to angiography)
  - In connection with non-Q-wave infarction, risk factors for CHD and especially diabetes mellitus.
- Evaluation of ischaemia and need for active treatment
  - Risk is highest during the first few weeks and months after infarction. Therefore, at the end of the hospital treatment, an early symptom-limited exercise test is performed on many patients to estimate the need for angioplasty and coronary surgery in particular (see Table 4.60.2).
- For indications of coronary angiography see also 4.64.

Care after myocardial infarction

Drug treatment

- Aspirin, beta-blocker Ⓐ [22 23 24], ACE inhibitors and statins have been shown to improve the prognosis. Glycaemic control is also important.
- Unnecessary drugs instituted during the initial phase should be discontinued already towards the end of hospital treatment, or when the patient comes to the first check-up, not on the last day in hospital.
- Only those with cardiac insufficiency or poorly controlled blood pressure need a diuretic.
- Aspirin 50–100 (–250) mg is given unless there are contraindications Ⓐ [6 7].
- Patients with hypertension, angina pectoris, ventricular arrhythmias, ischaemia during an exercise test, previous infarction, an enlarged heart, low ejection fraction or a cardiac insufficiency need a beta-blocker. In practice, these drugs are given to all patients who have no contraindications. Adequate beta-blockade is achieved when the heart rate at rest is about 60 bpm.
- Nitrate plus a beta-blocker are given to all patients with angina pectoris or ischaemia during an exercise test. Nitrate is a drug used for symptom relief that can often be discontinued.
- An ACE inhibitor is given to all patients with clear systolic dysfunction (ejection fraction <40%) Ⓐ [25]. A milder systolic dysfunction is treated with an ACE inhibitor if the patient has cardiac insufficiency (symptomatic or asymptomatic), valvular regurgitation, hypertension, or diabetic nephropathy. The indications of ACE inhibitors have been constantly extended, and they are now given to almost every patient who has had an infarction. So-called "asymptomatic cardiac insufficiency" and even secondary prevention (according to the HOPE study) in high-risk patients have become indications. ACE inhibitor therapy may be more difficult if the patient has a valvular obstruction, hypotension or uraemia. Patients on diuretics have a risk of hypotension, especially when treatment with an ACE inhibitor is started. The ACE inhibitor dose should not remain at the level of the initial dose unless hypotension and creatinine elevation prevent the titration.
- A lipid-lowering drug (a statin) is given to all patients with serum LDL cholesterol >3.0 mmol in spite of the diet Ⓐ [26 27].
- An anticoagulant is given if the patient has atrial fibrillation, an embolic complication or ventricular aneurysm verified by

Table 4.60.2 Assessment of risk of reinfarction and patient's prognosis

	Ejection fraction		Performance		Symptoms and findings
Low risk	>40%	and	>100 W[1] or > 2 W/kg	and	No ischaemia or arrhythmia in exertion, blood pressure rises > 10%
Moderate risk	25–40%	and/or	ca. 100 W[1] or 1.5–2 W/kg	and/or	a) In moderate exertion chest pain or some ischaemia, but no cardiac failure or arrhythmia b) Severe ischaemia or low ejection fraction, but no symptoms in moderate exertion c) Successive ventricular ectopic beats, symptomless ventricular tachycardia
High risk	<25%	and/or	<100 W[1] or <1 W/kg	and/or	a) Enlarged and failing heart and/or chest pain or ischaemia with low exertion and pulse (<120/min) or blood pressure doesn't rise with exertion b) Low ejection fraction and symptomatic cardiac failure requiring medication c) Stenosis of left main coronary artery or three arteries in angiography

1. Mean workload of last 4 minutes

echocardiography, often also short-term in the treatment of an extensive anterior wall infarction.

- Elevated serum homocystein concentration is associated with cardiovascular diseases, but it does not appear to predict arterial disease in healthy persons C [28 29 30]. See 4.63.
- A quiet moment should be reserved for discussing life after MI and living with CAD while the patient is still in the hospital.
  - Such a discussion helps to reduce psychological problems and disability.
  - Give instructions for dealing with possible exacerbation of the disease.
  - The motivation to quit smoking is highest after an infarction:
    - Nicotine replacement therapy according to individual evaluation (Fagerstrom test)
  - A cholesterol and saturated fatty acid-restriction diet and/or drug treatment.
  - Exercise counselling according to individual evaluation: the patient must be able to talk while exercising.
  - Rehabilitation course
  - Secondary prevention

Sick leave

- Duration 2–3 months.
- Re-examination after about one month, usually within specialist health care.
  - History of symptoms: if the patient has had angina pectoris symptoms, consider testing exercise capacity, if the test has not been performed yet.
  - Remind the patient of the principles of healthy life style.
  - Serum lipids should be measured if they were high on an earlier measurement.
  - Control the adequacy of beta-blockade: target heart rate 50–60 bpm.
  - Possible depression should be diagnosed.
- The ability to work is evaluated before the end of the sick leave. If necessary, an exercise test is carried out to assess working ability.

References

1. Sim I, Gupta M, McDonald K. Bourassa MG, Hlatky MA. A meta-analysis of randomised trials comparing coronary artery bypass grafting with percutaneous transluminal coronary angioplasty in multivessel coronary artery disease. Am J Cardiol 1995;76:1025–1029.
2. The Database of Abstracts of Reviews of Effectiveness (University of York), Database no.: DARE-953385. In: The Cochrane Library, Issue 4, 1999. Oxford: Update Software.
3. Grines CL, Cox DA, Stone GW, Garcia E, Mattos LA, Giambartolomei, et al. Coronary angioplasty with or without stent implantation for acute myocardial infarction. N Engl J Med 1999;341:1949–1956.
4. Olatidoye AG, Wu AH, Fent YJ, Waters D. Prognostic role of troponin T versus troponin I in unstable angina pectoris for cardiac events with meta-analysis comparing published studies. Am J Cardiol 1998;81:1405–1410.
5. The Database of Abstracts of Reviews of Effectiveness (University of York), Database no.: DARE-981100. In: The Cochrane Library, Issue 2, 2000. Oxford: Update Software.
6. Antiplatelet Trialists' Collaboration. Collaborative review of randomised trials of antiplatelet therapy - I: Prevention of death, myocardial infarction, and stroke by prolonged antiplatelet therapy in various groups of patients. BMJ 1994;308:81–106.
7. The Database of Abstracts of Reviews of Effectiveness (University of York), Database no.: DARE-948032. In: The Cochrane Library, Issue 4, 1999. Oxford: Update Software.
8. Danchin N, De Benedetti E, Urban P. How to improve outcomes in acute myocardial infarction. Clinical Evidence 2002;7:11–35.
9. Fibrinolytic Therapy Trialists' (FTT) Collaborative Group. Indications for fibrinolytic therapy in suspected myocardial infarction; collaborative overview of early mortality and major morbidity results from all randomised trials of more than 1000 patients. Lancet 1994;343:311–322.
10. The Database of Abstracts of Reviews of Effectiveness (University of York), Database no.: DARE-948029. In: The Cochrane Library, Issue 4, 1999. Oxford: Update Software.
11. Vaitkus PT. Percutaneous transluminal coronary angioplasty versus thrombolysis in acute myocardial infarction: a meta-analysis. Clin Cardiol 1995;18:35–38.
12. The Database of Abstracts of Reviews of Effectiveness (University of York), Database no.: DARE-988078. In: The Cochrane Library, Issue 4, 1999. Oxford: Update Software.
13. Cucherat M, Bonnefoy E, Tremeau G. Primary angioplasty versus intravenous thrombolysis for acute myocardial infarction. Cochrane Database Syst Rev. 2004;(2):CD001560.
14. Weaver WD, Simes RJ, Betriu A, Grines CL, Zijlstra F, Garcia E, Grinfeld L, Gibbons RJ, Ribeiro EE, DeWood MA, Ribichini F. Primary coronary angioplasty vs intravenous thrombolytic therapy for acute myocardial infarction. JAMA 1997;278:2093–2098.
15. The Database of Abstracts of Reviews of Effectiveness (University of York), Database no.: DARE-988115. In: The Cochrane Library, Issue 4, 1999. Oxford: Update Software.
16. Meads C, Cummins C, Jolly K, Stevens A, Burls A, Hyde C. Coronary artery stents in the treatment of ischaemic heart disease: a rapid and systematic review. Health Technology Assessment 2000, 4(23), 1–153.
17. The Database of Abstracts of Reviews of Effectiveness (University of York), Database no.: DARE-20018012. In: The Cochrane Library, Issue 2, 2002. Oxford: Update Software.
18. Domanski MJ, Exner DV, Borkowf CB, Geller NL, Rosenberg Y, Pfeffer MA. Effect of angiotensin converting enzyme inhibition on sudden cardiac death in patients following acute myocardial infarction: a meta-analysis of randomized clinical trials. Journal of the American College of Cardiology 1999;33:598–604.
19. The Database of Abstracts of Reviews of Effectiveness (University of York), Database no.: DARE-990660. In: The Cochrane Library, Issue 4, 2000. Oxford: Update Software.

20. Danchin N, De Benedetti E, Urban P. How to improve outcomes in acute myocardial infarction. Clinical Evidence 2002;7:11–35.
21. Mehta S, Yusuf S. Nitrates in myocardial infarction. Clinical Evidence 2000;4:7–8.
22. Freemantle N, Cleland J, Young P, Mason J, Harrison J. B blockade after myocardial infarction: a systematic review and regression analysis. BMJ 1999;318:1730–1737.
23. The Database of Abstracts of Reviews of Effectiveness (University of York), Database no.: DARE-999336. In: The Cochrane Library, Issue 1, 2001. Oxford: Update Software.
24. Lonn E. What are the effects of other drug treatments. In: Secondary prevention of ischaemic cardiac event. Clinical Evidence 2002;7:124–160.
25. Lonn E. What are the effects of other drug treatments. In: Secondary prevention of ischaemic cardiac event. Clinical Evidence 2002;7:124–160.
26. Rembold CM. Number-needed-to-treat analysis of the prevention of myocardial infarction and death by antidyslipemic therapy. J Fam Pract 1996;42:577–586.
27. The Database of Abstracts of Reviews of Effectiveness (University of York), Database no.: DARE-961089. In: The Cochrane Library, Issue 4, 1999. Oxford: Update Software.
28. Knekt P, Alfthan G, Aromaa A, Heliövaara M, Marniemi J, Rissanen H, Reunanen A. Homocysteine and major coronary events: a prospective population study amongst women. J Intern Med 2001;249(5):461–465.
29. Biochemical markers of cardiovascular disease risk. Bloomington, MN: Institute for Clinical Systems Improvement (ICSI). 2003. Institute for Clinical Systems Improvement (ICSI).
30. Health Technology Assessment Database: HTA-20030537. The Cochrane Library, Issue 1, 2004. Chichester, UK: John Wiley & Sons, Ltd.

4.61 Thrombolytic therapy and PTCA in acute ST elevation myocardial infarction (STEMI)

Editors

Basic rules

- The earlier the thrombolytic therapy is started, the better the outcome. Time is more crucial than the agent used. "One hundred minutes from the onset of pain".
- All patients fulfilling the criteria should be offered treatment. Delays must be prevented at all treatment phases. Treating an imminent major acute myocardial infarction (MI) with thrombolytic therapy is as urgent as the treatment of multiple trauma!
- ECG recordings of acute angina patient must be repeated if the first one is non-diagnostic.

Indications

- All the criteria 1-4 must be met.
  - Clinical picture of imminent MI (note that the main symptom is sometimes dyspnoea, not pain).
  - Pain lasting more than 20 minutes but less than 12–24 h. Treatment might be indicated even if the symptoms have lasted for longer, especially if the pain and ST segment persist. Treatment outcome worsens sharply when treatment delay exceeds four hours.
  - ECG shows new signs of imminent myocardial damage:
    - 2mm ST segment elevation in at least two chest leads or
    - 1mm ST segment elevation in at least two limb leads or
    - left bundle branch block (that prevents the evaluation of ECG) or
    - reciprocal ST segment depression (V1–V3,4) due to posterior wall damage.
  - No contraindications
- If previous ECGs are available, check that the changes are new. Most interpretation errors occur with early repolarisation (ST segment elevations in chest leads V1–V4) and myocarditis.
- A small Q wave does not prevent thrombolysis, although it indicates that myocardial damage has already occurred.
- Thrombolytic therapy is particularly important for patients with high ST segment elevations in chest leads and no deep Q waves.

Possible indications

- There is no consensus on whether a true posterior wall infarction manifesting with reciprocal anterior ST segment depression (V1–V3, 4) should be treated with thrombolysis because anterior ischaemia may cause similar changes. If the clinical picture is suggestive of an acute MI, thrombolysis is recommended. Thrombolysis is recommended particularly if the ST segment changes persist after the administration of nitrates, aspirin and beta-blockers. A posterior infarction is often associated with a more extensive inferior-posterior infarction with accompanying inferior ST segment elevation (II, III, aVF) and/or ST segment elevation in V4R suggestive of right ventricular involvement. If a posterior infarction is associated with a lateral infarction, ST segment elevation will be seen in the lateral leads (aVL, I, V6).
- If the ECG is distorted by a bundle branch block or paced rhythm, the need for thrombolysis must be based on the clinical picture.
- Thrombolysis is not effective in a non-Q wave infarction (ST depression + increased cardiac enzymes) nor in unstable angina, where the pain is caused by a partially occluded artery blocked by a platelet-rich clot originating from a plaque rupture. Medication to inhibit platelet aggregation

is recommended for these patients (aspirin, clopidogrel, GP IIb/IIIa inhibitors).

- T wave inversion, for example with a diseased LAD, is usually indicative of a recanalized coronary artery. Due to the risk of reocclusion, angiography should be carried out during the same admission.

Contraindications

- If thrombolysis is contraindicated the patient must be referred urgently to a hospital where the occluded artery can be opened with a PTCA.

Absolute

- Strong suspicion of dissection of the aorta
- Pericarditis (a rare problem)
- Active gastrointestinal or urogenital bleeding (within the last 2–4 weeks)
- Recent surgery or significant trauma (within the last 2 weeks)
- Intracranial tumour, arteriovenous malformation or aneurysm
- Recent ischaemic stroke (within the last 1–2 months; a verified TIA is an exception)
- Recent intracerebral haemorrhage (within the last 6 months) or subarachnoid haemorrhage
- Recent intracranial procedure or trauma (within the last 2 months)
- Severe bleeding disorder or severe hepatic disease

Relative

- Treatment may be indicated if the onset of pain is within three hours, a large (anterior) infarction is imminent and no deep Q-waves have developed yet, in patients with the following relative contraindications.
    - Active ulcer (<6 months)
    - Recent operation or significant trauma (2–4 weeks)
    - Hypertension systolic over 180–200, diastolic over 110 mmHg. The blood pressure should be lowered before thrombolysis with a nitrate infusion
    - Prolonged resuscitation with rib fractures
    - Previous intracerebral haemorrhage or trauma
    - Other life-threatening illness
    - In patients over 75 years of age who are receiving anticoagulant therapy, the risk of intracerebral haemorrhage is increased.

Procedure before treatment

1. Continuous ECG monitoring, readiness to defibrillate.
2. Administer glyceryl trinitrate – two sublingual tablets or two doses of a spray – and oxygen: observe ST segment changes. (If the changes are reversible, reconsider the need for the thrombolytic treatment.)
3. Aspirin 100 mg orally (not if the patient is on warfarin or allergic to aspirin).
4. Insert two intravenous cannulas and connect them to a NaCl infusion (0.45% or 0.9%).
5. Take the following blood samples (preferably from the i.v. cannula before connecting the infusion): haemoglobin, leucocytes, Na, K, creatinine, CK, CK-MB or troponin. (Do not wait for the results.)
6. Beta-blocker (atenolol, metoprolol) 5 mg i.v. over 5 min.; repeat after 10 min. if heart rate is over 50 beats/min. and there are no other contraindications (severe heart failure, asthma).
7. If blood pressure exceeds 180–200/110, it should be reduced with a nitrate infusion.

Carrying out thrombolytic treatment

- Thrombolysis can be carried out using streptokinase, the traditional treatment, or a tissue plasminogen activator (TPA) (tenecteplase, reteplase or alteplase). The price difference is considerable but the effect on mortality is small. Streptokinase therapy is more difficult to carry out as it requires vigorous monitoring of blood pressure and continuous infusion.
- Every effort must be made to minimize treatment delays.

Administering streptokinase

1. Rapid infusion of 200–300 ml of 0.9% NaCl if the patient is hypotensive. Give prophylactically, unless the patient has pulmonary oedema.
2. Streptokinase (Streptase®) 1.5 million U over one hour as a continuos infusion
    - Streptokinase 1.5 million units dry substance is dissolved first into 5 ml 0.9% NaCl, or into another suitable diluent, and then further into 100 ml of 0.9% NaCl.
    - Streptokinase infusion often causes hypotension. Should hypotension occur elevate the patient's legs and discontinue any nitrate infusions. If hypotension persists, slow down or discontinue the streptokinase infusion. If necessary, infuse 0.9% NaCl or, in very severe hypotension, dopamine.
    - Reperfusion, like acute infarction itself, is often accompanied by arrhythmias (ventricular ectopic beats, idioventricular rhythm). Isolated ventricular ectopic beats or short runs of ventricular tachyarrhythmias can be observed only. Lidocaine or electric cardioversion (30–100 J) is indicated in long-lasting ventricular tachyarrhythmias and when haemodynamic complications become apparent.

Special indications for streptokinase administration

- Increased risk of intracerebral haemorrhage (age over 75 years, high blood pressure, previous cerebral infarction)
- Little benefit expected from thrombolytic therapy (small infusion infarction, time lag over 6 h).
- Reasons of cost.

Special indications for TPA administration

- Streptokinase allergy
- Previous streptokinase treatment (5 days–2 years)
- Hypotension
- Large anterior wall damage A [1 2 3 4]
- New thrombus after streptokinase therapy (in 10–15% of patients, usually within a few hours–days after thrombolysis)
- Right ventricle infarction with haemodynamic dysfunction

Reteplase treatment

- Give two bolus injections (10 + 10 U) or reteplase (Rapilysin®) at a 30 min. interval.
- Heparinization B [5 6], e.g. enoxaparin 30–40 mg bolus intravenously at the beginning of thrombolysis, 1 mg/kg subcutaneously at the end of thrombolysis and 1 mg/kg b.d. subcutaneously during the next 3 days.

Tenecteplase treatment

- Give tenecteplase (Metalyse®) according to body weight (Table 4.61; maximum dose is 10 000 units = 50 mg).
- Give as a single bolus over 10 s.
- Heparinization as described above.

Alteplase treatment

1. Dilute the two 50 mg bottles of alteplase (Actilyse®).
2. Give 15mg (15 ml) by intravenous injection over 1–2 min.
3. This is followed by intravenous infusion of:
   - 0.75 mg/kg over the next 30 min. (maximum 50 mg = 50 ml) and then
   - 0.5 mg/kg over the next 60 min. (maximum 35 mg) A [1 2 3 4]
   - The total duration of the treatment is 90 minutes. An infusion pump must be used for the administration.
   - Heparinization B [5 6] as described above for reteplase treatment.

Transfer to hospital

- The patient can be transported to a hospital accompanied by a doctor or by a competent paramedic crew.
- The patient should be monitored continuously and a defibrillator must be ready for use. Adrenaline (epinephrine), atropine and lidocaine (for a bolus and infusion) must be readily available.
- A patient with an MI can be treated on a general ward, with adequate facilities, if invasive treatment is not an option.

Table 4.61 Administration of tenecteplase

Patient's weight (kg)	Tenecteplase (U)	Tenecteplase (mg)	Amount of reconstituted solution (ml)
<60	6000	30	6
60–69	7000	35	7
70–79	8000	40	8
80–89	9000	45	9
90–	10 000	50	10

Treatment of complications

- If bleeding is not severe, thrombolytic therapy is continued and bleeding is stopped by applying compression if possible.
- In severe bleeding, thrombolysis is discontinued and Ringer's solution or 0.9% NaCl is rapidly infused along with tranexamic acid (Cyclocapron® 2 × 5 ml i.v.). Cryoprecipitated anti-haemophilic factor (800 IU) is an alternative. If the patient is heparinized, also give protamine.
- If there are symptoms of cerebral stroke the thrombolytic treatment must be stopped.
- In case of an anaphylactic shock, administer 1–3 ml of adrenaline (epinephrine) 1:10 000 i.v. over 5–10 min. or 0.4–0.8 ml of adrenaline 1:1000 i.m. See also 14.1.

Assessment of coronary artery patency

- Chest pain improves
- ST segments normalize rapidly
- Reperfusion arrhythmias
- Early but short lasting rise in cardiac enzymes (8–12 h).

Primary percutaneous transluminal angioplasty (PTCA)

- PTCA has been shown in several studies to be more effective than thrombolytic therapy in the treatment of STEMI. The availability of PTCA and the provision of cardiologist cover remains a problem for many centres. According to the Danish DANAMI2 study the outcome after PTCA is superior to that achieved with thrombolysis provided that the PTCA can be carried out within a 150 km radius. It is likely that the use of PTCA as a treatment for acute STEMI will increase as the facilities of treating centres improve.
- Primary PTCA may be considered at present for patients at high risk, i.e. with extensive infarction + contraindication to thrombolysis, extensive anterior infarction, inferior infarction with significant right ventricular involvement, acute failure or cardiogenic shock.
- If the patency of the artery was not achieved with thrombolysis a so-called rescue PTCA can be considered. The results of a PTCA carried out after thrombolysis are not as good as those of a primary PTCA, but with modern equipment the procedure does, however, improve the patient's prognosis.

Thrombolysis as first aid

- The delay in treatment is shortened if the members of the emergency services start thrombolytic therapy. Motivated and trained personnel of an emergency service unit are able to interpret ECGs and make the diagnosis of an MI even better than an untrained doctor.

- Legal implications must be considered if a non-medical person initiates a potentially dangerous treatment. Therefore, the aim should be for a consulting physician to make the decision on initiating thrombolysis. Telemetry ECG makes such consultation possible.
- The hallmarks of the diagnosis are typical chest pain and ECG changes. Risk stratification should always be carefully carried out to avoid adverse treatment decisions. The current contraindications are not difficult to comply with.
- An international recommendation has been issued for the administration of pre-hospital thrombolysis, which should be adjusted to local conditions. The AHA recommendation is available on the Internet. Tenecteplase (single bolus) is the easiest to administer, while streptokinase is the most difficult.

References

1. Granger CB, White HD, Bates ER, Ohman EM, Califf RM. A pooled analysis of coronary artery patency and left ventricular function after intravenous thrombolysis for acute myocardial infarction. Am J Cardiol 1994;74:1220–1228.
2. The Database of Abstracts of Reviews of Effectiveness (University of York), Database no.: DARE-988081. In: The Cochrane Library, Issue 4, 1999. Oxford: Update Software.
3. Barbagelata NA, Granger CB, Oqueli E, Suarez LD, Boerruel M, Topol EJ, Califf RM. TIMI grade 3 flow and reocclusion after intravenous thrombolytic therapy - a pooled analysis. Am Heart J 1997;133:273–282.
4. The Database of Abstracts of Reviews of Effectiveness (University of York), Database no.: DARE-970352. In: The Cochrane Library, Issue 4, 1999. Oxford: Update Software.
5. The Database of Abstracts of Reviews of Effectiveness (University of York), Database no.: DARE-988072. In: The Cochrane Library, Issue 4, 1999. Oxford: Update Software.
6. Antman EM, Louwerenburg HW, Baars HF, Wesdorp JC, Hamer B, Bassand JP, Bigonzi F, Pisapia G, Gibson CM, Heidbuchel H, Braunwald E, Van de Werf F. Enoxaparin as adjunctive antithrombin therapy for ST-elevation myocardial infarction: results of the ENTIRE-Thrombolysis in Myocardial Infarction (TIMI) 23 Trial. Circulation 2002;105(14):1642–9.

4.62 Right ventricle infarction

Markku Ellonen

Aims

- To recognize right ventricle infarction as a cause of hypotension in cases of inferior wall infarction.
- Verified in lead V4R on the ECG.
- Treated with hydration, even if venous pressure is high.

Occurrence

- Occurs in connection with extensive inferoposterior infarction (occlusion of the stem of the right coronary artery).

Symptoms and signs

- Hypotension, bradycardia and high venous pressure without pulmonary oedema and cold limbs are characteristic symptoms.
- The lead V4R on the ECG gives a conclusive diagnosis: a 1-mm elevation is sensitive (70%) and specific (nearly 100%) (Figure 4.62.1). ECG usually shows a concomitant left ventricular inferoposterior wall infarction.

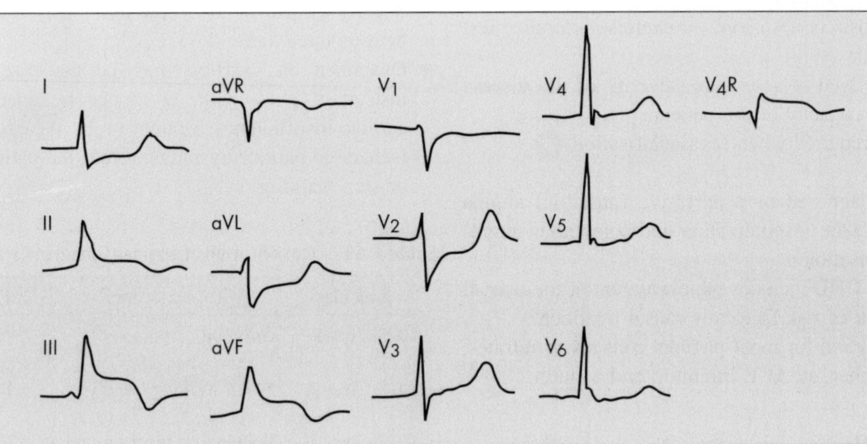

Figure 4.62.1 Extensive inferoposterior wall damage which has extended to the right ventricle (can be assessed by the ST elevation in lead V4R). Keep in mind that posterior wall damage is seen as reciprocal ST depression and T elevation in lead V2. The Q wave is not yet visible in posterior wall leads III and aVF, so it is possible to repair the condition with thrombolysis.

- The tricuspidal valve is insufficient, but regurgitation is usually not audible (detected on echocardiography).
- As the right coronary artery usually (90%) supplies blood to the AV node, a partial or complete AV block is often present.

Differential diagnosis

- All diseases that cause hypotension, pulmonary embolism being the most important.

Treatment

- Thrombolytic therapy with tissue plasminogen activator (TPA), which does not cause hypotension (4.61).
- Rapid correction of the hypotension by hydration is essential.
- Hypotensive drugs (nitrates) must be avoided.
- Atropine for bradycardia
- If pacing is required, a sequential pacemaker is preferable.

4.63 Coronary heart disease (CHD): symptoms, diagnosis and treatment

Editors

Basic rules

- A history, clinical examination and some basic tests are usually sufficient for clinical diagnosis of stable angina (pectoris).
- The diagnosis is often confirmed when prescribed drug therapies alleviate symptoms.
- When the diagnosis is not clear, an exercise tolerance test (ETT) is required.
- An ETT can be used to assess the severity of the disease and the working capacity of the patient.
- An ETT is also required when revascularisation (A) [1 2 3 4] is considered.
- Severe, newly-diagnosed or progressive (unstable) angina often requires urgent hospitalization and sometimes angioplasty revascularisation.
- The treatment of CHD includes the evaluation of the overall risk. Management of risk factors is causal treatment.
- The basic medication for most patients consists of nitrates, aspirin, beta-blocker, an ACE inhibitor, and a statin.

Epidemiology

- Under the age of 65, CHD mortality in men is three times that of women. In the older age group, the mortality of both genders is equal. After the age of 80 the CHD mortality of women is twice that of men.
- Total CHD mortality remains unchanged but mortality under the age of 65 has fallen by 50% over the past two decades (Finland).

Clinical manifestations of CHD

- Chest pain is the most common presentation.
- Other disease manifestations are dyspnoea or collapse on exertion, arrhythmias, unstable angina, acute or chronic heart failure, myocardial infarction and sudden death.

Symptoms and clinical diagnosis

- For differential diagnosis of chest pain, see 4.55.
- Stable angina is a clinical diagnosis which indicates the repeated occurrence of chest pain, induced by an exercise level typical for the patient. The pain is relieved by rest and shows no great daily variation; variation is typical for nonischaemic chest pain.
- Typical angina pain
  - is precipitated on exertion
  - becomes worse as the exertion continues
  - is felt across a wide area in the middle of the chest (not in the cardiac apex) and is tight and constrictive in nature
  - may be transmitted to the neck, jaw, arms, epigastric region or back
  - may become worse in cold weather, after a heavy meal or during static work
  - is relieved in a few minutes by rest or glyceryl trinitrate.
- However, only about half of all patients have a typical presentation of the symptoms.
- The patients history of pain is more reliable for diagnosis in men than in women aged less than 50 years. The probability of CHD in males over 55 with typical symptoms is 90%.
- Classification of chest pain (CCS, Canadian Cardiovascular Society –corresponds to the previously used NYHA classification), see Table 4.63.
- Dyspnoea on exertion may be the presenting symptom instead of chest pain. Dyspnoea is caused by temporary cardiac insufficiency brought on by the exertion.
- Ischaemic pain or dyspnoea forces the patient to slow down or stop walking.

Table 4.63 Classification of angina (Canadian Cardiovascular Society)

Angina class	Angina occurs	Exercise tolerance
CCS-Class1	Only with strenuous exercise	120 W or more
CCS-Class 2	When walking briskly or uphill	80–120 W
CCS-Class 3	Walking on level ground at normal pace	20–80 W
CCS-Class 4	At rest, whilst talking or dressing	below 20 W

- Nocturnal chest pain is in most cases a symptom of gastro-oesophageal reflux.
- Some patients describe the pain as burning, which might be misinterpreted as oesophageal pain.
- The pain is usually induced by predictable levels of exercise when the rate-pressure product exceeds the patient's individual threshold. However, in some patients exercise tolerance may vary to some degree but, in general, totally asymptomatic days are rare. Large variations are typical of non-ischaemic pain.
- The pain may also be precipitated by mental stress as the causes rate-pressure product increases.
- The pain may be triggered by rapid onset of walking. After warming up the patient can continue to "walk through his angina".
- The transmission of pain does not vary.
- After more intense exercise the pain may persist for over 15 minutes. More prolonged pain should be considered as myocardial infarction or delayed recovery from an ischaemic insult (stunning).
- The above text refers to stable angina, for unstable angina see 4.58.

Atypical chest pain not suggestive of coronary heart disease

- Appears at rest.
- Exercise tolerance is good despite pain.
- Continues for hours or days.
- Is associated with breathing or chest wall movements.
- Is sharp in character.
- Is displaced laterally towards the apex.
- May be felt on palpation.
- Is experienced as palpitations or occasional ectopic beats.
- Is felt in the upper abdominal region or below the left costal arch.
- Is not relieved with glyceryl trinitrate within a few minutes.

Investigations

Physical examination

- In most patients, physical examination is totally normal!
- Check blood pressure and heart rate (might be elevated due to pain).
- Listen for systolic bruit: CHD patients often have concomitant carotid disease or generalized arteriosclerotic disease.
- Aortic stenosis is frequently associated with CHD.
- S3 and a soft mitral regurgitant murmur are signs of impaired cardiac function. They may also be a transient functional effect of prolonged ischaemia or only be audible during exercise.
- Cardiac palpation may reveal LVH. A patient with LVH will experience angina even in mild coronary heart disease.
- Pallor may suggest anaemia.
- Transient signs of heart failure may appear after a prolonged ischaemic attack.

ECG

- The ECG is normal at rest in 30–50% of the patients.
- ST-T changes are a sensitive finding but non-specific.
- Slightly prolonged (<0.24 sec) PR interval is common.
- Patients with LVH often suffer from ischaemia and angina.
- LBBB is suggestive of CHD or hypertrophy or both.
- A previous infarction is a definite sign of CHD.
- A reversible ST segment depression, which appears during pain, is strong evidence for CHD.
- Continuous monitoring in the CCU or by the Holter method may reveal silent ischaemia (ST depression). Silent ischaemia is more common than symptomatic ischaemia but it is not harmless, and its diagnosis is dependent on the Holter technique **B** [5] [6]. The assessment of silent ischaemia with Holter monitoring is difficult and technically demanding. In the diagnosis of ischaemia its significance is limited to risk stratification of a patient with unstable angina.

Laboratory investigations

- Risk factor investigations: serum lipids **A** [7] [8] and blood glucose
- Haemoglobin
- Chest x-ray: heart failure, valvular calcification, and other causes of chest pain
- A small rise in cardiac enzymes or markers is possible after a prolonged angina attack, even in the absence of actual infarction. Such a rise is often a serious sign and is predictive of future infarction. Further investigations are necessary (see 4.58).

Exercise stress test

- Exercise stress test or exercise tolerance test (ETT) is the most common test carried out in angina patients. However, it does have limitations and interpretation problems.
- ETT will assist in determining the severity of the disease (See Table 4.63).

Radionuclide imaging

- The sensitivity is higher than, but the specificity is equal to, that of the ETT.
- Should be considered when ETT is normal but the disease is highly likely.
- Valuable for patients with mobility problems.
- First-line choice when an abnormal ECG impairs the interpretation of ETT.

Exercise echocardiography

- Ischaemia induces myocardial wall motion abnormalities, which can be detected with sensitive imaging equipment. When carried out by an experienced operator the test is considered to be even more sensitive and accurate than ETT. Particularly good around the anterior wall area.
- Useful when ECG is non-diagnostic because of abnormalities.

Coronary angiography

- The gold standard for preoperative investigation and CHD diagnostics. Nowadays used increasingly for diagnostic purposes.

Special diagnostic problems in women

- The diagnostic specificity of "typical angina pain" in premenopausal women is low.
  - Only about half of the women with typical angina pain have a significant CHD.
  - Premenopausal women complain of chest pain more often than men. The pain is usually atypical.
  - In old age, the diagnostic specificity of the symptoms becomes as high as in males (90%).
- The predictive value of ETT is worse in women because of ST changes due to sympathicotonic response. The number of false-positive test results is high in premenopausal women.
- An ST change resembling ischaemia with normal angiography finding (syndromeX) is much more common in premenopausal women than in men.
- Under the age of 50, the specificity of radionuclide imaging and exercise echocardiography is higher than that of the conventional ETT.

Treatment of CHD risk factors

- It is difficult to obtain firm evidence, based on extensive follow-up studies, on the benefits of modifying a single risk factor. The conclusions are based on epidemiological observations and pathophysiology.
- To improve prognosis, minimizing all risk factors to slow down atherosclerosis and prevent MI is valuable. Efficient secondary prevention usually includes aspirin, a beta-blocker, a statin and discontinuation of smoking.
- Smoking should be stopped A [9]. The risk of an MI is 3-fold in smokers and even higher in women. Alcohol consumption should be limited to moderate amounts.
- Hypertension should be treated. The target level of below 140/90 mmHg should be achieved. According to the latest study the optimal level is 138/83mmHg. Further is neither more beneficial (except for diabetics) nor harmful.
- Effective reduction of hyperlipidaemia often requires the prescription of a statin. Target levels below are only meant as a guideline. According to the HPS study in particular, hyperlipidaemia should be treated in high-risk patients, who will benefit from a statin even when their initial cholesterol level is nearly normal. Statins have an effect on endothelial dysfunction of coronary arteries, as well as on the inflammatory reaction and thrombosis
- Recommendations:
  - Serum cholesterol concentration below 5.0 mmol/l
  - LDL concentration below 3.0 mmol/l. Optimal level below 2.5mmol/l.
  - Serum triglyceride concentration below 2 mmol/l
  - Serum cholesterol/serum HDL below 4 mmol/l. Serum HDL in men >0.9 mmol/l and in women >1.1 mmol/l.
  - See article 24.56 for details on relevant drug therapy.
- Treating obesity
  - Weight should be reduced to achieve a BMI < 28.
  - Recognize metabolic syndrome and consider starting combination therapy with a statin and fibrate. Such treatment warrants the monitoring of liver enzyme and CK values.
- Physical exercise
  - Regular exercise improves the sense of well being as well as prognosis, by reducing many risk factors A [10] [11] [12] [13] [14] [15] [16] [17] [18] [19] (19.1) . Physical activity also plays a part in primary prevention C [20] .
  - Intense physical strain should be avoided.
- Based on a randomized secondary prevention study (HERS) and a primary prevention study (WHI A [21]), hormone replacement therapy offers no benefit.
- Antioxidant therapy with vitamin E had no beneficial effect in the HPS study, and neither did vitamins A and C.
- Elevated serum homocysteine concentration is associated with vascular diseases; however, it does not appear to act as a predictor of arterial disease in healthy individuals C [22] [23] [24]. Nevertheless, homocysteine concentration correlates positively with blood pressure, cholesterol concentration and smoking, and is thus an indicator of the severity of the atherosclerotic process. The correlation has been explained by atherosclerosis-induced renal insufficiency leading to reduced homocysteine clearance, which, in turn, will increase its plasma concentration. Folic acid (and vitamins B_6 and B_{12}) lower serum homocysteine concentration, but evidence on its effect in slowing down the progression of vascular disease is scant (only one study in which the administration of vitamins after PTCA lowered the incidence of restenosis B [25]). Several studies on secondary prevention are ongoing, but so far there is no evidence that vitamin substitution would reduce the incidence of cardiovascular diseases.
- Age, male gender and family history of CHD are non-modifiable risk factors. They must be included in the stratification of overall risk.

Pharmacotherapy: modes of action and aims

- Myocardial ischaemia is reduced by lowering blood pressure and heart rate. Beta-blockade is sufficient when heart rate is down to 60–50 bpm. The treatment of hypertension aims at an optimal pressure, which according to the HOT study (1998) is 138/83 mmHg.
- Aspirin is not prescribed for symptom relief. It reduces the thrombosis of coronary arteries. Aspirin is recommended for all patients with CHD at the dose of 75–150 mg/day, unless it is contraindicated. However, aspirin is ineffective in approximately 20% of the patients, and clopidogrel should be prescribed.

- The treatment of unstable angina (pre-infarction angina) requires clopidogrel in addition to aspirin, as well as the consideration of LMW heparin and revascularisation.
- In primary prevention, aspirin can prevent myocardial infarctions but increases the risk of gastrointestinal bleeding and appears to increase the risk of hemorrhagic stroke. The net benefit of aspirin increases with increasing cardiovascular risk **A** [26 27].

Choosing the medication

- Sublingual or aerosol nitrates that are classically used for acute episodes should also be used for prophylaxis.
- A selective beta-blocker reduces both the heart rate and blood pressure. It will also have a beneficial effect on tremor and migraine. Intermittent claudication is not a contraindication, unless the ischaemia is critical. The target heart rate is about 60 bpm at rest and below 120 bpm during exercise. With advancing age the dose can usually be reduced. Beta-blockers are also the first-line drugs for the treatment of arrhythmias of CHD patients. Heart failure is not a contraindication. Carvedilol might be the best choice in these cases. In heart failure an ACE inhibitor is usually combined with a beta-blocker. Beta-blockers are not only for symptomatic therapy; they also reduce the risk of reinfarctions and sudden deaths in MI survivors by 10–30%. The prognosis is also improved in CHD patients who have not suffered an MI.
- Calcium-channel blockers may be considered if beta-blockers are unsuitable **B** [28 29]. Of the older classic-calcium channel blockers, diltiazem is often chosen. Angina after a non-Q-wave infarction has been considered as its special indication. New dihydropyridine derivatives (amlodipine, felodipine, isradipine, nisoldipine) can be combined with beta-blockers in the treatment of stable angina particularly if the patient is hypertensive. The effect of calcium-channel blockers on the prognosis is not as well documented as that of beta-blockers **B** [30 31].
- A long-acting nitrate can be combined with a beta-blocker when the latter is not sufficient alone, or used instead of a beta-blocker, when it is not tolerated. The nitrate is administered at the time when symptoms occur most often, which is often during the daytime. The usual dose is 20–40 (–60) mg/day. A nitrate patch can be used to treat nocturnal angina. The patch should be removed in the morning to avoid the development of nitrate tolerance. For the same reason a pause should be kept in the administration of long-acting nitrates, for example in the evening or at night. Nitrates are symptomatic therapy and are not needed if the patient is asymptomatic. They improve exercise tolerance but probably not the prognosis.
- The combination of beta-blockers, calcium-channel blockers and long-acting nitrates (triple therapy) is usually more harmful than beneficial.

Revascularisation

- Coronary angiography is warranted if the patient, whilst receiving appropriate medication, has troublesome ischaemic chest pain, and myocardial ischaemia has been verified, e.g. by exercise tolerance test. The method of revascularisation is defined by coronary anatomy and the location and number of stenoses as confirmed by the coronary angiography.
- Coronary artery bypass grafting (CABG) **A** [32 33]
  - Stenosis of the left main coronary artery (LCA) or three-vessel disease, which is of equal significance, are established indications for surgery
  - CABG is often a better option if the patient has several total occlusions, the coronary anatomy is unfavourable for PTCA, or if the patient has diabetes, uraemia, significant left ventricular dysfunction or a significant valvular disease.
- Minimally invasive off-pump bypass grafting **C** [34 35]. OP-CAB is a new surgical method that does not require the use of the heart-lung machine and thoracotomy is not needed.
- Percutaneous transluminal coronary angioplasty (PTCA)
  - 1–2 vessel coronary artery disease is an established indication for PTCA.
  - If the operative risks are high (difficult pulmonary disease, age, etc.) PTCA can also be performed in LCA stenosis and in three-vessel disease.
  - A post CABG patient with symptomatic coronary stenosis is primarily treated with PTCA.
  - Insertion of a stent is an important part of PTCA. Approximately 80% of patients are fitted with stents. This has greatly diminished the number of complications and risk of restenosis. In selected cases a drug-eluting stent, which is impregnated with a smooth muscle growth inhibitor, is inserted in the stenosed artery. The preliminary results are promising and the use of drug-eluting stents will extend the indications for PTCA.
  - Acute MI: a large infarction that does not respond to thrombolysis (rescue PTCA) or the patient has a contraindication to thrombolysis and is at risk of an extensive anterior infarction. Primary PTCA is increasingly replacing thrombolysis **A** [36 37 38 39], which is clearly not as efficient as PTCA in achieving patency of the vessels. Long-term outcomes also favour PTCA, largely due to stenting **B** [40 41 42 43].

References

1. Effect of coronary artery bypass graft surgery on survival: overview of 10-year results from randomised trials by the Coronary Artery Bypass Graft Surgery Trialists Collaboration. Lancet 1994;344:563–570.
2. The Database of Abstracts of Reviews of Effectiveness (University of York), Database no.: DARE-920031. In: The Cochrane Library, Issue 4, 1999. Oxford: Update Software.
3. Rihal C. What are the effects of surgical treatments. In: Secondary prevention of ischaemic cardiac event. Clinical Evidence 2002;7:124–160.
4. Davies RF, Goldberg AD, Forman S, et al. Asymptomatic Cardiac Ischemia Pilot (ACIP) study two-year follow-up: outcomes of patients randomized to initial strategies of medical therapy versus revascularization. Circulation 1997;95: 2037–2043.

5. Tresch DD. Diagnostic and prognostic value of ambulatory electrocardiographic monitoring in older patients. J Am Ger Soc 1995;43:66–70.
6. The Database of Abstracts of Reviews of Effectiveness (University of York), Database no.: DARE-951202. In: The Cochrane Library, Issue 4, 1999. Oxford: Update Software.
7. Biochemical markers of cardiovascular disease risk. Bloomington, MN: Institute for Clinical Systems Improvement (ICSI). 2003. Institute for Clinical Systems Improvement (ICSI).
8. Health Technology Assessment Database: HTA-20030537. The Cochrane Library, Issue 1, 2004. Chichester, UK: John Wiley & Sons, Ltd.
9. Critchley J, Capewell S. Smoking cessation for the secondary prevention of coronary heart disease. Cochrane Database Syst Rev 2003(4):CD003041.
10. U.S. Department of Health and Human Services. Cardiac rehabilitation. Clinical practice guideline 1995;17:1–202.
11. The Database of Abstracts of Reviews of Effectiveness (University of York), Database no.: DARE-968500. In: The Cochrane Library, Issue 4, 1999. Oxford: Update Software.
12. Effects of rehabilitation programmes on anxiety and depression in coronary patients: a meta-analysis. Br J Clin Psychol 1994;33:401–410.
13. The Database of Abstracts of Reviews of Effectiveness (University of York), Database no.: DARE-955057. In: The Cochrane Library, Issue 4, 1999. Oxford: Update Software.
14. Scottish Health Purchasing Information Centre. Cardiac rehabilitation. Aberdeen: Scottish Health Purchasing Information Centre. 1998. 11. Scottish Health Purchasing Information Centre (SHPIC).
15. NHS Centre for Reviews, Dissemination. Cardiac rehabilitation. York: Centre for Reviews and Dissemination. 1998. 12. Centre for Reviews and Dissemination (CRD).
16. Cardiac rehabilitation. Bloomington, MN: Institute for Clinical Systems Improvement (ICSI). 2002. Institute for Clinical Systems Improvement (ICSI).
17. Health Technology Assessment Database: HTA-989125. The Cochrane Library, Issue 1, 2004. Chichester, UK: John Wiley & Sons, Ltd.
18. Health Technology Assessment Database: HTA-998327. The Cochrane Library, Issue 1, 2004. Chichester, UK: John Wiley & Sons, Ltd.
19. Health Technology Assessment Database: HTA-20030540. The Cochrane Library, Issue 1, 2004. Chichester, UK: John Wiley & Sons, Ltd.
20. Foster C, Murphy M. Effects of physical activity on coronary heart disease. In: Primary prevention. Clinical Evidence 2002;7:91–123.
21. Writing Group for the Women's Health Initiative Investigators. Risks and benefits of estrogen plus progestin in healthy postmenopausal women. Principal results from the Women's Health Initiative Randomized controlled trial. JAMA 2002;288:321–333.
22. Knekt P, Alfthan G, Aromaa A, Heliövaara M, Marniemi J, Rissanen H, Reunanen A. Homocysteine and major coronary events: a prospective population study amongst women. J Intern Med 2001;249(5):461–465.
23. Biochemical markers of cardiovascular disease risk. Bloomington, MN: Institute for Clinical Systems Improvement (ICSI). 2003. Institute for Clinical Systems Improvement (ICSI).
24. Health Technology Assessment Database: HTA-20030537. The Cochrane Library, Issue 1, 2004. Chichester, UK: John Wiley & Sons, Ltd.
25. Schnyder G, Roffi M, Flammer Y, Pin R, Hess OM. Effect of homocysteine-lowering therapy with folic acid, vitamin B(12), and vitamin B(6) on clinical outcome after percutaneous coronary intervention: the Swiss Heart study: a randomized controlled trial. JAMA 2002;288(8):973–979.
26. Hayden M, Pignone M, Phillips C, Mulrow C. Aspirin for the primary prevention of cardiovascular events. Rockville, MD: Agency for Healthcare Research and Quality (AHRQ). 2002. Agency for Healthcare Research and Quality (AHRQ). (www.ahrq.gov).
27. Health Technology Assessment Database: HTA-20031099. The Cochrane Library, Issue 1, 2004. Chichester, UK: John Wiley & Sons, Ltd.
28. Heidenreich PA, McDonald KM, Hastie T, Fabel B, Hagan B, Lee BK, Klatky MA. Meta-analysis of trials comparing beta-blockers, calcium antagonists, and nitrates for stable angina. JAMA 1999;281:1927–1936.
29. The Database of Abstracts of Reviews of Effectiveness (University of York), Database no.: DARE-999257. In: The Cochrane Library, Issue 4, 2000. Oxford: Update Software.
30. Held PH, Yusuf S. Calcium antagonists in the treatment of ischaemic heart disease: myocardial infarction. Coronary Artery Disease 1994;5:21–26.
31. The Database of Abstracts of Reviews of Effectiveness (University of York), Database no.: DARE-940073. In: The Cochrane Library, Issue 4, 1999. Oxford: Update Software.
32. Sim I, Gupta M, McDonald K. Bourassa MG, Hlatky MA. A meta-analysis of randomised trials comparing coronary artery bypass grafting with percutaneous transluminal coronary angioplasty in multivessel coronary artery disease. Am J Cardiol 1995;76:1025–1029.
33. The Database of Abstracts of Reviews of Effectiveness (University of York), Database no.: DARE-953385. In: The Cochrane Library, Issue 4, 1999. Oxford: Update Software.
34. Mack MJ, Osborne JA, Shennib H. Arterial graft patency in coronary artery bypass grafting: what do we really know. Annals of Thoracic Surgery 1998;66:1055–1059.
35. The Database of Abstracts of Reviews of Effectiveness (University of York), Database no.: DARE-981734. In: The Cochrane Library, Issue 3, 2000. Oxford: Update Software.
36. Cucherat M, Bonnefoy E, Tremeau G. Primary angioplasty versus intravenous thrombolysis for acute myocardial infarction. The Cochrane Database of Systematic Reviews, Cochrane Library number: CD001560. In: The Cochrane Library, Issue 2, 2002. Oxford: Update Software. Updated frequently.
37. Sim I, Gupta M, McDonald K. Bourassa MG, Hlatky MA. A meta-analysis of randomised trials comparing coronary artery bypass grafting with percutaneous transluminal coronary angioplasty in multivessel coronary artery disease. Am J Cardiol 1995;76:1025–1029.
38. The Database of Abstracts of Reviews of Effectiveness (University of York), Database no.: DARE-953385. In: The Cochrane Library, Issue 4, 1999. Oxford: Update Software.
39. Grines CL, Cox DA, Stone GW, Garcia E, Mattos LA, Giambartolomei, et al. Coronary angioplasty with or without stent implantation for acute myocardial infarction. N Engl J Med 1999;341:1949–1956.

40. The Wessex Institute for Health Research and Development. Stents for coronary artery disease (CAD). Development and Evaluation Committee Report 1998;87:1–33.
41. The Database of Abstracts of Reviews of Effectiveness (University of York), Database no.: DARE-989742. In: The Cochrane Library, Issue 3, 2000. Oxford: Update Software.
42. Meads C, Cummings C, Stevens A. Coronary artery stents. West Midlands Development and Evaluation Committee Report. 9. 1998:1–76.
43. The Database of Abstracts of Reviews of Effectiveness (University of York), Database no.: DARE-999268. In: The Cochrane Library, Issue 1, 2001. Oxford: Update Software.

4.64 Coronary angiography and indications for CABG or angioplasty

Editors

Aims

- To determine the extent of anatomic coronary artery obstruction when coronary artery bypass grafting (CABG) **A** [1 2 3 4] or percutaneous transluminal coronary angioplasty (PTCA) **A** [5 6] is considered.
- To evaluate difficult diagnostic problems in patients with unstable angina, survival of sudden death, atypical chest pain.

Indications in patients with angina pectoris (AP)

- Severe stable AP resistant to medication
- Occlusion of left anterior descending artery (LAD) or a 3-vessel disease is suspected on the basis of an exercise tolerance test (also when the symptoms are mild)
  - Ischaemic ST (>2 mm) with minimal load and low heart rate.
  - Deficient rise in BP during exercise test.
- AP after acute myocardial infarction
  - Pain at rest or when walking, while the patient is still in the hospital.
  - AP and severe heart failure (myocardial stunning).
  - ST-depression outside the infarction area during exercise.
- Unstable AP resistant to medication.
- AP following PTCA.
- In cases of rapidly recurring AP after CABG, PTCA may be considered.

Indications in patients without AP

- Angiography may be indicated or considered:
  - in patients accepted for heart surgery (e.g. valve prosthesis)
  - in survivors of ventricular fibrillation without MI
  - when the exercise ECG changes are clearly pathological
  - in acute pulmonary oedema without cause.
  - When ECG after a T-wave infarction (non-Q-wave infarction) shows long lasting and wide T inversions in anterior wall leads.
  - As a diagnostic method in special situations, e.g. LBBB and LVH disturb the interpretation of the exercise test.

Management of acute imminent myocardial damage

- Acute PTCA is preferred to thrombolysis whenever available: the results are better and the price is lower.
- Acute PTCA may be an alternative to thrombolysis **B** [7 8 9 10] when the latter is contraindicated because of the risk of bleeding or shows no effect.

References

1. Effect of coronary artery bypass graft surgery on survival: overview of 10-year results from randomised trials by the Coronary Artery Bypass Graft Surgery Trialists Collaboration. Lancet 1994;344:563–570.
2. The Database of Abstracts of Reviews of Effectiveness (University of York), Database no.: DARE-920031. In: The Cochrane Library, Issue 4, 1999. Oxford: Update Software.
3. Rihal C. What are the effects of surgical treatments. In: Secondary prevention of ischaemic cardiac event. Clinical Evidence 2002;7:124–160.
4. Davies RF, Goldberg AD, Forman S, et al. Asymptomatic Cardiac Ischemia Pilot (ACIP) study two-year follow-up: outcomes of patients randomized to initial strategies of medical therapy versus revascularization. Circulation 1997;95:2037–2043.
5. Sim I, Gupta M, McDonald K. Bourassa MG, Hlatky MA. A meta-analysis of randomised trials comparing coronary artery bypass grafting with percutaneous transluminal coronary angioplasty in multivessel coronary artery disease. Am J Cardiol 1995;76:1025–1029.
6. The Database of Abstracts of Reviews of Effectiveness (University of York), Database no.: DARE-953385. In: The Cochrane Library, Issue 4, 1999. Oxford: Update Software.
7. Vaitkus PT. Percutaneous transluminal coronary angioplasty versus thrombolysis in acute myocardial infarction: a meta-analysis. Clin Cardiol 1995;18:35–38.
8. The Database of Abstracts of Reviews of Effectiveness (University of York), Database no.: DARE-988078. In: The Cochrane Library, Issue 4, 1999. Oxford: Update Software.

9. Weaver WD, Simes RJ, Betriu A, Grines CL, Zijlstra F, Garcia E, Grinfeld L, Gibbons RJ, Ribeiro EE, DeWood MA, Ribichini F. Primary coronary angioplasty vs intravenous thrombolytic therapy for acute myocardial infarction. JAMA 1997;278:2093–2098.
10. The Database of Abstracts of Reviews of Effectiveness (University of York), Database no.: DARE-988115. In: The Cochrane Library, Issue 4, 1999. Oxford: Update Software.

4.65 Follow-up of a revascularized patient

Markku Ikäheimo

First visit

- To the outpatient department of the operating hospital 1–3 months after bypass surgery or to a cardiologist at the local central hospital.
  - Clinical examination, chest x-ray, ECG, serum lipids
  - Assess
    - Symptoms of angina pectoris
    - Operation cuts
    - Cardiovascular status
    - Medication and risk factors
    - Need for further sick leave
    - If the patient's condition is satisfactory, the next follow-up visit should be to his/her own physician.

First year

- Follow-up visits to the physician in charge of the treatment at 3–6 months and 12 months after surgery.
- Investigations
  - ECG
  - Chest x-ray if required
  - Serum total cholesterol, HDL cholesterol and triglycerides
  - Blood ESR and CRP if symptoms of postpericardiotomy syndrome are present

Aims of the follow-up visits

- To recognize postpericardiotomy syndrome (frequency 10–20% with varying severity). The syndrome most commonly presents several weeks after surgery, but sometimes after a longer period, up to one year.
  - Symptoms
    - Fatigue
    - Mild fever
    - Pain resembling pericarditis
    - Arrhythmias
  - Signs
    - Friction rub: pericardial or pleural
    - Supraventricular arrhythmias present on ECG
    - Blood ESR and CRP usually elevated
    - Chest x-ray may reveal an enlarged heart and pericardial effusion
    - Effusion can be diagnosed by echocardiography
  - The diagnosis is defined and the treatment initiated by a cardiologist
    - NSAID drugs
    - Steroids: initial dose of prednisolone 40–60 mg/day, reduced later. Steroid therapy is effective, with few recurrences after stopping medication.
    - Drainage of the pericardium is seldom necessary.
- If chest pain occurs after surgery, it is important to distinguish ischaemic pain from non-ischaemic pain.
  - Non-ischaemic causes of pain include tenderness of the cut and chest wall pain of costochondral origin.
    - Avoid prescribing nitroglycerin automatically as this may cause the patient to become depressed about the poor result of surgery and may thereby increase the pain.
    - Use NSAID drugs.
  - If the pain is ischaemic pain typical of angina pectoris (typically relieved by nitroglycerin) the patient must be referred to exercise tolerance test.
- Reduce the risk factors for coronary artery disease.
  - Smoking must be stopped.
  - Hypertension should be lowered to an optimal level.
  - Lipids should be lowered: serum cholesterol <5.0 mmol/l, LDL <3.0 mmol/l (preferably <2.5 mmol/l), HDL >1.0 mmol/l.
  - Proper treatment of diabetes.
  - Encourage physical exercise and weight loss.
- Discontinue unnecessary medication
  - Aspirin is indicated for all patients if there are no contraindications. The usual long-term dosage is 100–250 mg/day. For hypersensitive patients clopidogrel 75mg/day.
  - A beta-blocker is indicated if the patient has had myocardial infarction before the bypass surgery or during the operation. The drug may be discontinued in asymptomatic patients who do not have tachycardia or hypertension.
  - Prophylactic antiarrhythmic medication can usually be discontinued.
  - The need for digoxin should be considered.
  - Arrhythmias
    - Treatment of ventricular ectopic beats with proper antiarrhythmic drug therapy should be avoided. The patient is advised to avoid smoking, and drinking excess alcohol and coffee. Troubling ectopy may be treated with small doses of beta-blocking agents. A

cardiologist should prescribe more potent antiarrhythmic drugs.
   - Attacks of syncope or ventricular tachycardia must be evaluated urgently. Electrophysiological investigations are often relevant.

- Assess all aspects of the patient's psychosocial condition.
  - Problems continuing at work
  - Unnecessary restrictions originating from the preoperative time
  - Investigate possible symptoms of depression.

Further follow-up visits

- Annual follow-up visits: more often if the patient has symptoms or risk factors.
- Goals
  - To control for risk factors and keep the patient informed.
  - Recurring angina pectoris must be evaluated by an exercise tolerance test.
- Investigations
  - ECG
  - Other investigations depending on risk factors and medication.

4.70 Acute pulmonary oedema

Editors

Aims

- Oxygen, morphine, nitrate spray and furosemide should be available at every first aid station. Prone position is beneficial.
- A CPAP mask and i.v. nitrate should be available at every health care unit responsible for early treatment of cardiac emergencies.
- The drugs of choice are
  - nitrate in infarction
  - diuretic in aggravation of chronic heart failure
  - and digitalis and/or a beta-blocker in atrial fibrillation or supraventricular tachycardia.

Causes

- The systolic function of the left ventricle (ejection fraction, EF) collapses as a result of infarction, ischaemia or acute mitral regurgitation.
- In hypertension-induced pulmonary oedema EF remains and the condition results from diastolic dysfunction.
- Acute left ventricular failure (ischaemia, infarction, hypertension, aggravation of chronic failure) or valvular failures resulting in elevated pulmonary capillary pressure and consequent alveolar oedema.
- Toxins, pneumonias, aspirations and pancreatitis may increase the permeability of alveolar membranes, resulting in adult respiratory distress syndrome (ARDS).
- Atrial fibrillation and other tachyarrhythmias; in rare cases bradyarrhythmia.
- Cardiogenic shock (low output syndrome: hypotension, collapsed peripheral veins and cold skin) is a form of acute circulatory failure and is treated differently from pulmonary oedema, by correcting hypovolaemia and giving inotropic medication.

Symptoms and diagnosis

- Severe dyspnoea, cough, tachypnoea, anxiety, fear and confusion.
- Bronchospasm ("cardiac asthma") may be the presenting symptom.
- Sinus tachycardia, atrial fibrillation, other tachyarrhythmias
- Pulmonary oedema rales
- Cyanosis, pallor and sweating.
- The chest x-ray is characteristic revealing many signs of decompensated chronic heart failure or, in a newly developed acute case, only the "bat's wing" at the pulmonary hilum.
- The ECG may reveal LVH, ischaemia, infarction, tachyarrhythmias.
- Arterial pO_2 is below 8 kPa and/or oxygen saturation is below 90%.
- Echocardiography shows the regions of the ventricular wall that move poorly as well as the function of the valves.
- Differential diagnoses include pneumonia, aspiration, embolism, asthma and COPD with or without chronic heart failure.

First aid for acute heart failure

- Optimize:
  - heart rate: pain and anxiety relieved by morphine
  - oxygenation: CPAP whenever possible (keep saturation > 90%)
  - left ventricle filling pressure (preload): oedema in chest x-ray is not a reliable sign of fluid overload. A pulmonary artery wedge pressure (PAWP) catheter (Swan-Ganz) is reliable.
  - Blood haemoglobin 120–130 g/l
  - Reduce BP (afterload) with i.v. nitrate (or nitroprusside).
  - Slow down rapid atrial fibrillation with digitalis and beta-blockers or, in critical cases, by electric cardioversion.
  - In severe cases reduce the work of breathing by a respirator.
  - Contractile function can be improved by giving e.g. dopamine or levosimendan.

Treatment

1. Position
   - A half-sitting position is best if the patient is not in shock.
2. Sedation
   - Morphine 6–8 mg i.v. If required, give additional doses of 4–6 mg at 5 min. intervals up to a total dose of 16–20 mg. Watch the respiration, especially in elderly and COPD patients. Shallow and slow respiration is a sign of excessive sedation.
3. Breathing
   - Oxygen by ventimask 8 l/min.
   - A cooperating patient is managed by CPAP (4.71).
   - Bronchospasm is relieved by a slow 200 mg theophylline infusion over 5 minutes.
4. Nitrate infusion
   - At first, repeated oral spray while the infusion is being prepared.
   - I.v. nitrate (4.59) is particularly useful in oedema caused hypertension or acute myocardial infarction: it reduces both preload and afterload. The infusion must be monitored with an infusion pump.
   - Systolic blood pressure must be over 100 mmHg. If not, consider dopamine (dobutamine) infusion. The risk of a sudden fall in blood pressure is greatest in dehydrated patients. Manage with a rapid infusion of fluids.
   - Initial dose is low: 4 gtt/min. (= 12 ml/h) with a solution of 10 mg/100 ml. Administer at 5–10 min. intervals, maintaining systolic BP above 90 mmHg. Lower the pressure by about 20 mmHg in patients with initially normal BP.
   - If i.v. infusion is not available, use an oral spray repeatedly.
5. Diuretics
   - Indicated especially in an acute worsening of chronic heart failure with lung oedema. Diuretics are safe in patients with sufficient blood pressure.
   - Furosemide 20 mg i.v. If no response is seen, repeat dosing: maximum dose is 60 mg.
   - Symptomatic relief is quick in patients with acute pulmonary oedema. However, pulmonary oedema on chest radiograph is not a reliable sign of total body fluid overload. Excessive diuretics may result in hypovolaemia, tachycardia and a fall in cardiac output. Chest x-ray does not "improve" as quickly as the patient.
6. Digitalis and a beta-blocker to optimize heart rate
   - In patients with rapid atrial fibrillation or supraventricular tachycardia
   - Doses: initially digoxin 0.25 mg i.v., followed by 0.125 mg at one hour intervals up to 0.75 mg, if no digitalis medication has been given earlier.
   - Digitalis has a slow mode of action. For a rapid normalization of heart rate use an additional beta-blocker: metoprolol 5 mg + 5mg + 5mg at 10 min. intervals (4.45). Esmolol with its ultra-short half-life is the alternative.
7. Dopamine infusion
   - May be used for severely hypotensive patients. Often gives a temporary relief. Disadvantage is that it increases cardiac workload.
   - The initial dose of dopamine is 4 µg/kg/min. This is 6 gtt/min. (18 ml/h) for a 70-kg adult patient.
   - Increase the dose at 5 min. interval to 15 gtt/min. if required.
8. Levosimendan (Simdax®)
   - A new (expensive) i.v. drug for use in hospitals. Alleviates symptoms and improves prognosis. Is also suitable for treating heart failure associated with acute ischaemia.

Further treatment

- After first aid the patient is moved to a cardiac unit. This is important especially if the treatment is prolonged or the patient does not have an exact diagnosis.
- Echocardiography is always indicated if the aetiology of lung oedema is not apparent.
- Treatment of the cause of the heart failure is always the goal: coronary bypass or balloon dilatation and valvular surgery (4.63).
- Hypertension is treated primarily with ACE inhibitors.
- Loop diuretics given as continuous infusion in acutely decompensated heart failure seem to provide greater diuresis and a better safety profile as compared to single intravenous bolus administration, but good quality evidence is lacking C [1].

Reference

1. Salvador DRK, Rey NR, Ramos GC, Punzalan FER. Continuous infusion versus bolus injection of loop diuretics in congestive heart failure. The Cochrane Database of Systematic Reviews, Cochrane Library Number: CD003178. In: Cochrane Library, Issue 1, 2004. Chichester, UK: John Wiley & Sons, Ltd.

4.71 CPAP treatment in pulmonary oedema

Editors

Basic rules

- Elevation of the airways pressure is an effective treatment of pulmonary oedema that in most cases substitutes for intubation and respirator therapy. A pressure of 10 cmH_2O and a 40% oxygen mixture are sufficient to

correct hypoxaemia in two-thirds of patients with pulmonary oedema within 10 minutes from the start of the treatment.

- CPAP treatment is the most important and urgent treatment of pulmonary oedema B [1 2] and must be started immediately in the emergency room before infusion or medication.
- CPAP equipment should be available at health centres giving first aid to cardiac patients or treating them at bed wards, and also in emergency transport vehicles.

Indications and contraindications for treatment

- Respiratory insufficiency of cardiac origin (pulmonary oedema) when pharmacotherapy and oxygen therapy are not sufficient B [1 2].
- Dyspnoea at rest caused by cardiac insufficiency when respiratory frequency is increased, stasis rales from the lungs are audible and pulmonary congestion is clearly pronounced in chest x-ray (interstitial oedema). Restlessness of the patient is often a sign of hypoxaemia that requires treatment measures.
- Treatment is contraindicated if the patient cannot maintain patent airways because of blurred consciousness or if the respiratory rate and efficacy of a patient in critical condition are impaired. Manual ventilation and intubation are indicated if the overall situation of the patient requires them.

Implementation

1. Help the patient into a half-sitting position.
2. Place the mask over the face without the pressure valve and tighten the support straps.
3. Open the flow meter and connect the patient tube to the mask.
4. Adjust the flow so that the expiratory valve is maintained open both during expiration and inspiration.
5. Check that the mask fits tightly.
6. Give additional oxygen, adjust for humidification.
7. The initial pressure is 7.5 (−10) cmH_2O. If the patient's condition does not improve within a few minutes, increase the airways pressure up to 15 cmH_2O (caution is necessary if the patient is clearly hypovolaemic). If increasing the pressure does not help, oxygen concentration is increased.
8. During the treatment, monitor
   - respiratory rate (should decrease)
   - use of auxiliary respiratory muscles
   - subjective condition
   - oxygen saturation (should rise)
   - patency of the expiratory valve of the mask (if the valve does not stay open, increase flow and check mask tightness).
9. Even short-term removal of the mask should be avoided, as it immediately increases respiratory work and hypoxaemia recurs. If the patient is transported to a hospital, CPAP treatment should be continued during transportation.
10. CPAP treatment is terminated when the patient's condition has become alleviated and respiratory rate is below 25/min. Positive pressure is decreased stepwise and oxygen administration is continued.

References

1. Pang D, Keenan SP, Cook JD, Sibbald WJ. The effect of positive pressure airway support on mortality and the need for intubation in cardiogenic pulmonary edema: a systematic review. Chest 1998;114:1185–1192.
2. The Database of Abstracts of Reviews of Effectiveness (University of York), Database no.: DARE-981920. In: The Cochrane Library, Issue 2, 2000. Oxford: Update Software.

4.72 Chronic heart failure

Markku Ellonen

- Acute heart failure, see 4.70.

Aims

- Avoid making false positive diagnoses on the basis of non-specific symptoms.
- Diagnose the underlying cause and treat it.
- Assess the severity of disease, and identify exacerbating factors.
- Identify patients who must be referred for echocardiography.
- Be aware of drugs and interventions that improve prognosis.

General principles

- Heart failure is a symptom of a severe heart disease, (not a diagnosis in its own right). Recognize the underlying disease and exacerbating factors.
- Systolic heart failure is caused by the lack of functioning myocardium, and the prognosis of severe heart failure (NYHA III–IV) is poor without treatment.
- Heart failure after an MI may be asymptomatic and only detectable by echocardiography (EF $< 40\%$). Even in such cases treatment with an ACE inhibitor and/or a beta-blocker may be indicated and improve prognosis.
- The treatment should always be targeted at underlying causes: hypertension, ischaemia, valvular surgery etc. Echocardiography is often indicated for the determination of the underlying cause and the severity of the disease. Several diseases may coexist, which might complicate diagnosis and treatment.

- Treatment of hypertension and coronary heart disease are of importance in primary prevention. In secondary prevention ACE inhibitors are the most important drug group, and then can also be used for asymptomatic patients (A) [1 2 3 4 5] and high-risk patients.

Common causes of heart failure

- Coronary heart disease and/or hypertension are the cause in 80% of the cases.
- Systolic dysfunction
  - Ischaemic heart disease
  - Hypertension (a more common cause of diastolic dysfunction)
  - Valvular regurgitation
  - Dilated cardiomyopathy
  - Other causes: fast atrial fibrillation, sustained tachycardia (tachycardia–cardiomyopathy), hyper- and hypothyroidism, myocarditis.
- Diastolic dysfunction
  - Left ventricular hypertrophy associated with hypertension and advanced age
  - Amyloidosis, pericarditis, and other rare restrictive conditions
- Right heart failure
  - True right heart failure is often caused by pulmonary disease which elevates pulmonary arterial pressure. Patients with COPD often have concurrent CHD.
  - Left heart failure may gradually lead to pulmonary hypertension and right heart failure.

Exacerbating or triggering factors

- Severe infections, particularly in the lungs
- Anaemia
- Hyper- or hypothyroidism
- Tachy- and bradyarrhythmias (atrial fibrillation)
- High-volume infusion (crystalloid solutions or blood)
- NSAIDs, particularly if renal function is impaired
- Drugs, which reduce myocardial contractility (verapamil, beta-blockers and their combinations)
- Noncompliance with medication
- Excess body weight
- Excessive alcohol and salt consumption
- Hypertension
- Silent MI, unstable angina
- Pulmonary embolism

Symptoms

- General fatigue, shortness of breath and diminished physical capacity.
- Dyspnoea during normal exertion (NYHA II) is an unspecific symptom the reason for which might be CHD, excess body weight or the patient being physically unfit.
- Dyspnoea and cough in the supine position (orthopnoea) occurs only in moderate or severe heart failure.
- Weight gain and pitting oedema are sensitive signs but non-specific if they occur independently. However, when they are both present they are of clinical importance, particularly in the monitoring of treatment response.
- Loss of appetite is associated only with advanced heart failure (cardiac cachexia).

Findings

- Tachycardia (>90/min), if no beta-blockade
- Tachypnoea (>20/min)
- Significantly raised jugular venous pressure (JVP), i.e. jugular pulsation can be seen with the patient sitting up. The sign is specific if the patient does not have a pulmonary disease. It is associated with severe heart failure. A more modestly risen JVP (8 cm) is seen with the patient slightly reclined. A positive hepatojugular reflex is helpful in making the final decision; however, great inter-observer variability exists, and the test is underused.
- S3 in a patient above 40 years of age is a specific sign suggestive of decompensated heart failure.
- Mitral regurgitation without valvular disease
- Enlarged heart (palpation)
- Liver enlargement, a positive hepatojugular reflex.
- Rales, which, suggest pulmonary congestion are a non-specific sign, and they are also associated with several pulmonary diseases.
- Pitting oedema of the leg may also be caused by several other conditions (5.10).
- Because the signs and symptoms are non-specific, the diagnosis should be based on an objective test, usually echocardiography.

Further investigations

- Chest x-ray
  - Cardiomegaly (systolic dysfunction). Calculated in ml/m^2 or by the CT-ratio (cardio-thoracic ratio over 0.5 is abnormal). The size of the heart and the function of the left ventricle usually correlate poorly with each other. The variation in size is more indicative of the status of the right ventricle. Especially in acute heart failure the heart is of normal size.
  - Pulmonary venous congestion, interstitial oedema, Kerley B lines, bilateral pleural effusions. The interpretation of mild vascular congestion on isolated x-rays is often difficult and does not suffice for the diagnosis. In mild failure, chest x-rays are not sensitive and their interpretation is susceptible to error. Questionable x-ray changes must be viewed in the context of the entire clinical picture.
- ECG
  - Might have signs of infarction or ischaemia, which also indicate the reason for the failure.

- Hypertrophy (LVH, LAH), and LBBB
- Arrhythmias and atrial fibrillation, could act as exacerbating factors.
- A normal ECG suggest that the diagnosis of heart failure is highly unlikely.
- A normal ECG and a normal exercise test rule out heart failure.

♦ Laboratory tests

- Check basic haematology, serum K, Na, creatinine, ALT, glucose, CRP, urine sediment and serum free T4 or serum TSH for differential diagnosis. Hyponatraemia and renal failure indicate a poor prognosis. Atrial fibrillation and heart failure may be the only symptoms of thyrotoxicosis in an elderly person. Elevated ALT suggests hepatic congestion. Cardiac enzymes are often slightly elevated in decompensated failure.
- Spirometry is a basic investigation for dyspnoea. A clearly abnormal result suggests pulmonary disease. Patients with COPD often also have CHD and heart failure.

Diagnostic criteria

1. Dyspnoea or fatigue or both whilst walking on the flat.
2. Ventricular gallop or heart rate above 90 bpm or both (if the heart rate is not slowed down by medication)
3. Raised jugular venous pressure or venous congestion on chest x-ray, or both.
4. Markedly enlarged heart on chest x-ray.

♦ If an untreated patient presents with three out of the four above findings, heart failure is highly probable. The underlying disease, contributing towards the failure, should also be identified.

Criteria supplied by the European Society of Cardiology

♦ See Table 4.72.1.

Problems with diagnostics

♦ The above mentioned four criteria are specific and prevent false positive diagnosis, which is common. Inter-observer agreement on the presence of S3, and on the assessment of JVP, is low, which lessens their clinical value and use of these observations. The absence of a single symptom or sign does not imply that the patient does not have heart failure; the most specific signs are not sensitive and occur only in advanced and untreated heart failure. Heart failure that calls for treatment can be asymptomatic and detectable only by an ultrasound.

♦ For the assessment of the efficacy of the treatment more sensitive (and simultaneously more non-specific) criteria can be used, particularly with regard to any changes:

- exertional dyspnoea, nocturnal cough
- pulmonary rales, weight gain, leg oedema, hepatic congestion

♦ Problems in differential diagnosis are caused by:

- excess weight, especially in women, also makes the interpretation of the chest x-ray more difficult
- physical inactivity and poor fitness
- venous insufficiency, working in standing position and immobilization can all cause swelling of legs (positive effect of diuretic therapy does not confirm the diagnosis of heart failure)
- pulmonary diseases: COPD and exercise–induced asthma
- silent CHD, with exertional dyspnoea as the main symptom (important!)
- several exacerbating factors listed earlier
- diastolic dysfunction with exertional dyspnoea as the main symptom, with normal sized heart on chest x-ray.
- recurrent pulmonary embolism.

♦ If the diagnosis is uncertain, consider

- consulting a cardiologist
- echocardiography
- a trial of stopping medication
- determining of ANP or BNP.

Further investigations

♦ Echocardiography

- An essential and objective investigation for the assessment of the presence and severity of heart failure. It also often indicates the cause of the failure (see 4.8). In practice echocardiography cannot be offered to all patients with suspected heart failure. The examination should be

Table 4.72.1 Diagnosis of heart failure–a simplified chart

Required	Does not support	Supports	Must be excluded
Signs and symptoms of heart failure	Normal ECG	Response to therapy	Renal disease, anaemia
Cardiac dysfunction (usually detected by echocardiography)	Normal chest x-ray	Cardiomegaly on chest x-ray	Pulmonary diseases (chest x-ray, pulmonary function tests)
	Normal exercise tolerance in ETT	Decreased exercise tolerance in ETT	
	Normal concentration of plasma ANP, BNP	Increased concentration of plasma ANP, BNP	

offered to patients who have a clinically established heart failure and whose treatment could be affected by echocardiography findings.

- Echocardiography also differentiates between systolic and diastolic heart failure: in systolic dysfunction EF is under 40%, in diastolic dysfunction EF is normal. Interpreting the diastolic dysfunction with echocardiography can be problematic. An asymptomatic heart failure that calls for treatment can be detected with echocardiography.
- The systolic pressure of the right ventricle can be assessed with echocardiography. Systolic pressure reflects the pressure in the pulmonary arteries, which is valuable for the diagnosis of pulmonary embolism.
- Echocardiography should be performed on all younger patients with heart failure as well as on all patients with uncertain diagnosis or aetiology. Even when the diagnosis is confirmed an echocardiography can be performed in order to determine the degree of systolic function of the heart. (NYHA classification depicts the patient's overall functional capacity).

♦ Natriuretic peptides (ANP, BNP)

- Atrial natriuretic peptide (ANP) and brain natriuretic peptide (BNP) are released in response to atrial and ventricular stretch, respectively. Increased plasma concentrations are suggestive of untreated heart failure.
- BNP, which is synthesized in the ventricles, is more suitable for heart failure diagnostics since it is more stable and specific than ANP, which is synthesized in the atria.
- If heart failure is the suspected aetiology behind dyspnoea, natriuretic peptides are clinically useful in the diagnostic work-up and as a "rule out" test.
- A normal BNP has a very high negative prediction value (heart failure ruled out with 95% certainty). A markedly elevated concentration is suggestive of heart failure. Various other causes may induce slightly elevated values.
- Slightly elevated BNP values are seen in asthma, pulmonary embolism and COPD which all increase left ventricular pressure. Slight increases are also induced by aortic stenosis, LVH, renal impairment, hepatic cirrhosis, aging and the female gender. Atrial fibrillation particularly increases ANP.
- Increased BNP and ANP concentrations indicate severe failure and poor prognosis.
- In addition to diagnosis, BNP has also been used for the monitoring of the disease progress. BNP concentration falls rapidly as the failure is treated. A normalized BNP does not necessarily prove the optimal treatment.
- When the BNP test is elevated the patient should usually be referred for echocardiography.

Diastolic dysfunction

♦ Diastolic dysfunction belongs to aging. It occurs mainly in association with systolic dysfunction, but it may exist alone. EF remains nearly normal but diastole is impaired.

♦ Suspect diastolic dysfunction, when dyspnoea is the main symptom and

- the size of the heart is normal or nearly normal
- ECG shows LVH
- the patient is elderly (>75 years), and has ischaemic heart disease or hypertension.
- The main differential diagnosis for diastolic dysfunction is ischaemia which is also its main cause.

♦ Treatment is determined according to the underlying cause. Medication is prescribed according to general guidelines.

- Diuretics for hypervolaemia
- Lower rapid pulse with a beta-blocker in order to prolong diastole.

The severity of heart failure

♦ Clinical examination and symptoms correlate poorly with EF which, in turn, determines the patient's prognosis. Echocardiography is an objective investigation of the systolic capacity of the heart.

♦ NYHA classification describes the overall functional capacity.

- NYHA I: No symptoms although left ventricular dysfunction can be detected by echocardiography.
- NYHA II: Symptoms appear with brisk walking or whilst working.
- NYHA III: Dyspnoea appears with minimal exertion or at rest.
- NYHA IV: Symptoms appear with light exercise or at rest. The prognosis is poor in III–IV and all forms of causal treatment should be considered.
- Also verbal counterparts are used: no symptoms, mild, moderate, severe.

♦ Ejection fraction

- An ejection fraction below 25% usually signifies severe dysfunction (corresponds to NYHA classes III and IV). The alleviation of symptoms, pulmonary oedema in particular, is the main goal of therapy.
- An ejection fraction above 40% usually rules out systolic dysfunction, but not diastolic dysfunction.

Principles of treatment

♦ Behaviour modifications: regular exercise **C** [6 7], avoidance of excess weight, reduction of salt intake, moderate alcohol consumption. In severe heart failure fluid intake should be restricted (1.5–2 l), as should the level of exercise taken.

♦ Effective treatment of hypertension and myocardial infarction, secondary prevention of CHD.

♦ Whenever possible the underlying cause of heart failure must be treated, i.e.: revascularization, valvular surgery etc. Cardiac transplantation should be considered in the most severe cases for patients below 60 years of age.

♦ Factors exacerbating and triggering heart failure should be recognized and treated.

- Other coexisting diseases must be taken into consideration; the most common of which is renal insufficiency.
- Aspirin is prescribed to all patients with CHD or type 2 diabetes.
- Anticoagulant therapy is prescribed in severe systolic heart failure.
- ACE inhibitors A [1 2 3 4 5] and beta-blockers A [8 9 10 11] improve prognosis in systolic heart failure. Most of these patients have suffered from myocardial infarction. Even in asymptomatic patients the prognosis will be improved and the manifestation of the disease reduced.
- Nurse-led caring should be planned together with a cardiac nurse.

Drug therapy

- An ACE inhibitor and an adequate dose of a beta-blocker should be prescribed to all patients in order to improve prognosis.
- **A diuretic** is the first-line symptomatic treatment of pulmonary and peripheral oedema. The response to therapy is rapid. The initial dose is often higher than the maintenance dose.
- **ACE inhibitors** improve the prognosis in mild, moderate and severe heart failure, as well as in heart failure due to myocardial infarction, even in asymptomatic patients. Salt restriction or diuretics enhance the effect of ACE inhibitors. The response to therapy is slow.
- **Digoxin** is not likely to significantly improve the prognosis of a patient in sinus rhythm. Special indications for digoxin include atrial fibrillation with rapid ventricular response rate and systolic dysfunction with tachycardia.
- **Beta-blockers** improve the prognosis.
- **Nitrates** can be combined with the other drugs if the patient has symptomatic CHD.
- **Calcium-channel blockers** amlodipine or felodipine can be used if the patient has coexisting hypertension.
- The above mentioned drugs can be prescribed in various combinations.

Drug therapy for heart failure

Diuretics and spironolactone

- Start with a combination of a thiazide and an ACE inhibitor, if fluid retention is slight. If serum creatinine is above 180–200 μmol/l, furosemide should be used. The maximum dose of hydrochlorothiazide is 50 mg and it should not be exceeded. If a higher dose is needed, furosemide should be prescribed. The dose of furosemide can be increased as needed.
- In severe fluid retention thiazide and furosemide can be combined. In such a case an ACE inhibitor or an angiotensin-II receptor antagonist (which also prevents hypokalaemia), is usually added.
- Spironolactone may also be added B [12], with a dose of 12.5–50 mg, if serum potassium is monitored for hyperkalaemia. Potassium-sparing diuretics or potassium supplements should not usually be used as the combination of spironolactone and an ACE inhibitor inhibits hypokalaemia and may even cause hyperkalaemia. The risk of hyperkalaemia remains low if the daily dose does not exceed 25 mg. An early introduction of spironolactone probably improves prognosis.
- All diuretics tend to slightly elevate serum creatinine and urate concentrations. A more significant increase may indicate dehydration caused by an excessive dose. In this case the patient will complain of tiredness and has orthostatic hypotension, which is the most important adverse effect of diuretic therapy. A cardiac patient often feels better when slightly hypervolaemic. This is why patients often decrease the dose of diuretics themselves.
    - A large dose of diuretics, and its adverse effects, can be reduced by adding an ACE inhibitor to the treatment.
    - The patient can be instructed to monitor his/her condition and self-manage the dose of the diuretic by adjusting it to variations in weight. Leg oedema is not a reliable indicator.
- Adverse effects
    - Check serum potassium at 2 weeks, 3 months, and one year.
    - Hyponatraemia. Severe heart failure is often associated with mild hyponatraemia (about 130 mmol/l), which is a sign of poor prognosis. It should not be corrected by salt supplementation. Severe hyponatraemia may be caused by a thiazide, or in particular, by a combination of a thiazide and amiloride. The mechanism behind this condition is inappropriate ADH secretion (24.12).
    - Hyperuricaemia and gout principally affect obese men, and women with renal failure, particularly when the dose of the diuretics is too large.
    - Increased creatinine concentration; particularly if the patient has coexisting renal failure and an ACE inhibitor is added (see ACE inhibitors).

ACE inhibitors and angiotensin-II receptor antagonists

- ACE inhibitors are effective drugs which improve the prognosis. They should be prescribed to all patients with heart failure A [1 2 3 4 5]. Remember to increase the dose from the starting dose to the maintenance dose. The target dose should be in accordance with the latest trial results, unless not limited by adverse effects.
- Initially ACE inhibitors were used only in severe heart failure, but nowadays they are also used to treat patients belonging to NYHA classes I and II, particularly if the patient is hypertensive and has had myocardial infarction. These drugs are currently also used prophylactically in asymptomatic heart failure when the patient has cardiovascular risk factors.
- Diuretics enhance the effect of ACE inhibitors. Beta-blockers or nitrates are often added depending on the underlying disease. Patients with NYHA III-IV heart failure, who are on ACE inhibitor and furosemide, should also

be prescribed spironolactone at 25 mg/day to improve prognosis B [12].

- During treatment, serum potassium concentration should remain below 5.5 mmol/l and creatinine below 220–250 µmol/l. Systolic pressure can be allowed to drop down to 90 mmHg provided that the patient remains asymptomatic.
- Patients on diuretics are sensitive to ACE inhibitors and may experience an initial hypotensive reaction. The treatment should begin with a small dose (25% of the maintenance dose) and the patient's condition should be monitored daily. In severe heart failure the maintenance dose in clinical trials has been rather high: 100–150 mg daily for captopril and 20 mg daily for enalapril (often even higher). However, smaller doses can also be beneficial. See Table 4.72.2 for dose recommendations.
- Serum creatinine and potassium should be checked frequently at the beginning of therapy; in severe heart failure within one week after starting the medication. A small increase (<20%) in serum creatinine concentration is to be expected and is insignificant. Renal failure and an increase in serum creatinine are special indications, but may also be contraindications, for ACE inhibitors. In these cases, the electrolyte balance and serum creatinine must be monitored in a hospital or under similar conditions. A marked increase in serum creatinine concentration may be caused by either diuretics or an ACE inhibitor, and particularly by a combination of these two drugs. If severe heart disease requires ACE inhibitor therapy, and serum creatinine increases markedly (200–250 µmol/l), the dose of the diuretic should be reduced first. A large increase in serum creatinine may sometimes indicate renal artery stenosis. Renal failure, potassium-sparing diuretics and spironolactone, in particular, increase the risk of hyperkalaemia. The risk of diuretic-induced hypokalaemia is reduced with a concomitant administration of an ACE inhibitor.
- Special indications for ACE inhibitors include valvular insufficiency and hypertension, even with normal EF. Valvular stenosis is a conventional contraindication. However, most patients with aortic stenosis can tolerate an ACE inhibitor if the medication is started at a low dose and the patient is monitored for orthostatic problems.
- Angiotensin-II receptor antagonists (losartan, valsartan, candesartan and eprosartan) can be prescribed in heart failure instead of ACE inhibitors, particularly when a cough prevents the use of ACE inhibitors. Some of the drugs in this group may prove to be even better than ACE inhibitors.

Table 4.72.2 Dose recommendations for ACE inhibitors–initial and maintenance doses

ACE inhibitor	Starting dose/day	Maintenance dose /day
Captopril	6.25 mg t.d.s.	25–50 mg t.d.s.
Enalapril	2.5 mg	10 mg b.d.
Lisinopril	2.5 mg	5–20 mg
Quinapril	2.5–5 mg	5–10 mg
Perindopril	2 mg	4 mg
Ramipril	1.25–2.5 mg	2.5–5 mg b.d.
Trandolapril	1 mg	4 mg

However, evidence is so far limited C [13 14]. According to the CHARM study the combination of an ACE inhibitor and candesartan improves the prognosis in patients with an EF < 40%.

Digoxin

- Digoxin is an important drug for patients in atrial fibrillation with a rapid ventricular response rate. A beta-blocker may also be prescribed. The dose of digoxin is determined by the ventricular rate and is generally higher than required in sinus rhythm (0.125 mg). During sinus rhythm the use of digoxin should be restricted mainly to systolic dysfunction with cardiomegaly and a small ejection fraction. In addition to digoxin, a diuretic is often prescribed for these patients, and always an ACE inhibitor and a beta-blocker.
- Digoxin has a minor or neutral effect on prognosis. Digoxin alleviates symptoms and reduces the number of hospital admissions A [15].
- For elderly persons in sinus rhythm, 0.125 mg of digoxin daily is usually sufficient. The dose is lower in renal insufficiency, and serum digoxin levels should be checked as necessary.
- Adverse effects include atrioventricular block and bradycardia. A slightly prolonged PR interval (0.20–0.24 s) is very common in cardiac patients and is not a contraindication for digitalization; however, the length of the PR interval should be monitored.
- The symptoms of digoxin toxicity include loss of appetite, nausea and bradyarrhythmias. Serum creatinine and digoxin level should be determined if toxicity is suspected (dixogin levels do not need to be monitored in routine use). Digoxin is not prescribed in accordance with blood concentration, but small doses are recommended.

Beta-blockers

- Prescribed to all patients despite the aetiology of heart failure. Adequate doses must be used.
- Contraindications include bradycardia (<60 bpm), hypotension (<100 mmHg) and a significant AV block.
- Excessive sympathetic activity is harmful to the heart and therefore its decrease alleviates symptoms and improves long-term prognosis. Patients with ischaemic heart disease and hypertension benefit most; a beta-blocker is to be added to other heart failure treatment. A beta-blocker is started with a very small dose when the patient's condition is stable. Recommended starting doses:
    - metoprolol 10 mg
    - carvedilol 6.25 mg
    - bisoprolol 1.25 mg.
- The dose is increased at an interval of a few weeks, and the patient should be monitored by medical personnel. The use of quite high doses has improved prognosis, but in practice, high doses often lead to problems with bradycardia.
- The symptoms will alleviate slowly, over 1–2 months. At the beginning, the need for a diuretic may even increase.
- There is evidence on the effect of metoprolol, bisoprolol and carvedilol (at doses of 200 mg, 10 mg and 50 mg,

respectively). There is no evidence on the effect of the other beta-blockers. Carvedilol may be the most beneficial. It decreases both morbidity and mortality irrespective of whether the underlying disorder is an ischaemic or a non-ischaemic heart disease (A) [8 9 10 11]. As a non-selective beta-blocker, carvedilol may worsen the symptoms of asthma.

Anticoagulants and aspirin

- Cardiomegaly with atrial fibrillation is an indication for anticoagulation.
- Even without atrial fibrillation, the risk for arterial embolism is increased in patients with cardiomegaly and poor EF. However, no consensus exists on its treatment with warfarin (D) [16 17 18].
- Patients who are generally unwell and have limited activity level, have an increased risk of venous thrombosis. The risk can be reduced with prophylactic LMWH.

Treatment of resistant heart failure

- Determine whether treatment-resistant heart failure results from fluid retention (skin moist and warm) or inadequate minute volume (skin cold and dry). A large intravenous dose of a loop diuretic is needed to resolve fluid retention. In low output states (cold and dry), there often is no fluid retention and a diuretic would therefore be of no benefit. The patient's pulse is weak, the limbs are cold and the patient is restless or confused.
- Can the underlying cause be treated? Revascularization, transplantation.
- Identify exacerbating factors and treat them: anaemia, infection, NSAID, etc.
- Organize nurse-led care that responds readily to the need for a loop diuretic. Add a thiazide and spironolactone. Do not add salt to correct mild hyponatraemia, which is characteristic for this condition. Salt restriction is always needed, often also fluid restriction.
- Ensure that the dose of the ACE inhibitor is sufficient.
- Keep the patient on a beta-blocker if the effect has originally been beneficial.
- Discuss the severity of the condition, the limited treatment choices available and the poor prognosis with the patient's family.
- Levosimendan is an inotropic, vasodilating calcium sensitizer (i.v. inodilator), which can be used for a short time to treat severe heart failure. It is safer than dobutamine. It requires adequate filling pressures and is not suitable in hypotension.

Follow-up

- The possibility of the symptoms worsening, and also the possibility of dehydration, must be discussed with the patient. Rapid weight gain is an important and easily detected sign. The patient can be advised to increase the dose of diuretics if the symptoms become worse.
- The patients often reduce the dose of diuretics because they feel better with slight hypervolaemia. A chest x-ray might show mild congestion, which needs no treatment. Hypovolaemia causes fatigue and orthostatic hypotension.
- Frequent follow-up visits are indicated at the beginning of therapy. Later on, the patient's condition and problems determine the frequency of follow-up visits.
- At the follow-up visits ask the patient about symptoms, but remember the poor specificity of the sensitive symptoms. Chest x-ray, and particularly a lateral projection, is not indicated at every visit. History and clinical examination may indicate treatment response better than an x-ray. BNP can be used to monitor the disease progress (B) [19 20].
- A cardiologist consultation and echocardiography are indicated if there is no response to treatment or if the underlying diagnosis is uncertain.
- Nurse-led care by a cardiac nurse is an important part of the treatment, particularly for patients with severe heart failure.

References

1. Flather MD, Yusuf S, Kober L, Pfeffer M, Hall A, Murray G, Torp-Pedersen C, Ball S, Pogue J, MoyeL, Braunwald E, for the ACE-Inhibitor Myocardial Infarction Collaborative. Long-term ACE inhibitor therapy in patients with heart failure or left-ventricular dysfunction: a systematic overview of data from individual patients. Lancet 2000;355:1575–1581.
2. Garg R, Yusuf S. Overview of randomized trials of angiotensin-converting enzyme inhibitors on mortality and morbidity in patients with heart failure. JAMA 1995;273: 1450–1456.
3. The Database of Abstracts of Reviews of Effectiveness (University of York), Database no.: DARE-950776. In: The Cochrane Library, Issue 4, 1999. Oxford: Update Software.
4. Lubsen J, Chadha DR, Yotof YT, Swedberg K. Meta-analysis of morbidity and mortality in five exercise capacity trials evaluating ramipril in chronic congestive cardiac failure. Am J Cardiol 1996;77:1191–1196.
5. The Database of Abstracts of Reviews of Effectiveness (University of York), Database no.: DARE-961103. In: The Cochrane Library, Issue 4, 1999. Oxford: Update Software.
6. McKelvie RS, Teo KK, McCartney N, Humen D, Montaque T, Yusuf S. Exercise training in patients with congestive heart failure. J Am Coll Cardiol 1995;25:789–796.
7. The Database of Abstracts of Reviews of Effectiveness (University of York), Database no.: DARE-951171. In: The Cochrane Library, Issue 4, 1999. Oxford: Update Software.
8. Heidenreich PA, Lee TT, Massie BM. Beta-blockers and mortality in patients with heart failure. J Am Coll Cardiol 1997;30:27–34.
9. The Database of Abstracts of Reviews of Effectiveness (University of York), Database no.: DARE-970828. In: The Cochrane Library, Issue 4, 1999. Oxford: Update Software.
10. Doughty RN, Rodgers A, Sharpe N, MacMahon S. Effects of beta-blocker therapy on mortality in patients with heart failure: a systematic overview of randomized controlled trials. Eur Heart J 1997;18:560–565.
11. The Database of Abstracts of Reviews of Effectiveness (University of York), Database no.: DARE-978097.

In: The Cochrane Library, Issue 4, 1999. Oxford: Update Software.
12. Pitt B, Zannad F, Remme WJ et al. The effect of spironolactone on morbidity and mortality in patients with severe heart failure. N Engl J Med 1999;341:709–717.
13. Boucher M, Ma J. Heart failure: is there a role for angiotensin II receptor blockers? Ottawa: Canadian Coordinating Office for Health Technology Assessment (CCOHTA). 2002. 4. Canadian Coordinating Office for Health Technology Assessment (CCOHTA). www.ccohta.ca.
14. Health Technology Assessment Database: HTA-20020902. The Cochrane Library, Issue 1, 2004. Chichester, UK: John Wiley & Sons, Ltd.
15. Hood WB Jr, Dans AL, Guyatt GH, Jaeschke R, McMurray JJV. Digitalis for treatment of congestive heart failure in patients in sinus rhythm. Cochrane Database Syst Rev. 2004;(2):CD002901.
16. Lip GYH, Gibbs CR. Anticoagulation for heart failure in sinus rhythm. The Cochrane Database of Systematic Reviews, Cochrane Library number: CD003336. In: The Cochrane Library, Issue 2, 2002. Oxford: Update Software. Updated frequently.
17. Baker DW, Wright RF. Management of heart failure IV: anticoagulation of patients with heart failure due to left ventricular systolic dysfunction. JAMA 1994;272:1614–1618.
18. The Database of Abstracts of Reviews of Effectiveness (University of York), Database no.: DARE-941150. In: The Cochrane Library, Issue 4, 1999. Oxford: Update Software.
19. Thoughton RW, Frampton CM, Yandle TG, Espiner EA, Nicholls MG, Richards AM. Treatment of heart failure guided by plasma aminoterminal brain natriuretic peptide (N-BNP) concentrations. Lancet 2000;355:1126–1130.
20. Lip GYH, Gibbs CR. Anticoagulation for heart failure in sinus rhythm. The Cochrane Database of Systematic Reviews, Cochrane Library number: CD003336. In: The Cochrane Library, Issue 2, 2002. Oxford: Update Software. Updated frequently.

4.81 Prevention of bacterial endocarditis

Editors

Heart diseases that require prophylactic treatment with antimicrobial drugs

- ♦ Congenital heart diseases (also after surgery, except in cases of operated patent ductus arteriosus and atrial septal defect where prophylactic treatment is not necessary)
- ♦ Acquired valvular disease (e.g. in association with ankylosing spondylitis or following rheumatic fever)
- ♦ Mitral prolapse with significant regurgitation
- ♦ After heart or pulmonary transplantation
- ♦ Artificial valve (also homografts)
- ♦ Previous endocarditis

Heart diseases that do not require prophylactic treatment

- ♦ Prophylactic use of antimicrobial drugs is unnecessary in cases of
  - atrial septum defect
  - after 6 months have elapsed from surgery for patent ductus arteriosus (applies to both surgical and "umbrella" occlusion)
  - mitral prolapse without regurgitation
  - postoperative state after bypass surgery
  - Kawasaki disease
  - pacemaker; operations should be avoided for 3–6 months after implanting the pacemaker
  - presumably innocent heart murmur.
- ♦ Prophylactic treatment is not recommended for patients with joint prosthesis, arterial or venous grafts or CSF shunts. (Exception: immunodeficient rheumatic patients with joint prosthesis.) However, during the first 6 months after implanting a prosthesis or a graft, before the formation of the pseudointima, operations causing bacteremia should be avoided.

Procedures that require antimicrobial prophylaxis of endocarditis

- ♦ Prophylactic treatment is indicated before operations where the disruption of the skin, epithelium or mucous membranes will possibly or probably cause bacteremia.
  - Gum or tooth operations commonly causing gum bleeding
  - Drainage of maxillary sinuses
  - Tonsillectomy, adenoidectomy
  - Bronchoscopy with a rigid bronchoscope
  - Bronchoscopy in which biopsies are taken
  - Biliary tract surgery
  - Gastrointestinal endoscopy with biopsies
  - Dilatation of oesophagus and sclerotherapy
  - Cystoscopy and dilatation procedures, if the patient has bacteriuria
  - Prostate surgery
  - Transvaginal hysterectomy

Procedures where prophylactic treatment with antimicrobial drugs is not recommended

- ♦ Dental treatment with no bleeding (dental filling, root canal filling)
- ♦ Local anaesthesia in the mouth

- Fitting of a dental prosthesis
- Intubation
- Tympanocentesis
- Insertion and removal of tympanostomy tubes
- Flexible fibre-optic bronchoscopy when no biopsies are taken
- Echocardiography via the oesophagus
- Catheterization of the heart
- Gastrointestinal endoscopy where no biopsies are taken
- Gastrointestinal lavage and imaging with contrast media
- Surgery and catheterization of the urinary tract when the patient has no bacteriuria
- Insertion and removal of an IUD
- Labour and delivery
- Caesarean section
- Hysterectomy
- Curettage of the uterus
- Dilatation of the cervix
- Change of temporary urethral catheter

Antimicrobial prophylaxis of endocarditis

Oral

- First-line therapy
  - Amoxicillin, a single dose of 3 g 1 hour before an operation (children 50 mg/kg).
- Alternative treatment for patients allergic to penicillin
  - Roxithromycin, a single dose of 300 mg (children 8–10 mg/kg), or
  - Erythromycin, a single dose of 800 mg (children 30 mg/kg), or
  - Clindamycin, a single dose of 600 mg (children 20 mg/kg).

Intravenous

- Operations above the diaphragm
  - Ampicillin, 2 g infusion (children 50 mg/kg), or
  - Vancomycin, 1 g infusion for 1 hour (children 20 mg/kg)
- Operations below the diaphragm
  - Ampicillin or vancomycin as above, plus
  - Tobramycin, 120 mg infusion (children 3 mg/kg), or
  - Netilmycin, 150 mg infusion (children 3 mg/kg).

Operation in an infected area

- Drug treatment is chosen according to the probable causative bacteria. If, for example, a soft tissue abscess is treated surgically, prophylactic medication must be effective against staphylococci (e.g. dicloxacillin 1 g orally as a single dose, or vancomycin intravenously).

4.82 Myocarditis

Jouko Karjalainen

Objective

- Myocarditis must be differentiated from myocardial infarction and harmless ECG changes caused by increased sympathetic tone.

Definition

- As myocarditis and pericarditis often are concomitant diseases, the term myopericarditis (perimyocarditis) may also be used.
- Myocarditis is usually caused by microbial infection, sometimes also by other systemic disease; the cause may also remain unknown.
- Possible causes include
  - viral infection (Coxsackie B4 and B5, influenza, EBV, cytomegalovirus, parvovirus and adenovirus)
  - rheumatic fever
  - mycoplasma, chlamydia and streptococcus infection
  - borreliosis (Lyme disease)
  - connective tissue diseases (SLE, mixed connective tissue disease, arthritis, systemic type of juvenile arthritis)
  - septic conditions
  - eosinophilic conditions
  - use of cytostatic drugs or phenothiazines
  - heart transplantation
  - radiation therapy.
- Myocarditis may be acute or chronic. Acute myocarditis may be part of an infection, or it may be the only sign of a general infection. Chronic myocarditis may manifest as dilating cardiomyopathy.

Symptoms of myocarditis

- Chest pain, arrhythmias, respiratory distress or acute cardiac insufficiency, especially in the case of current or recent infection.
- Excessive fatigability, tachycardia, arrhythmias.
- Mild cases occur without cardiac symptoms.

Signs

- Often insignificant and non-specific.
- Pericardial friction rub may be heard.
- Ventricular gallop is common.
- In severe cases, cardiac insufficiency.

ECG

- Changes in the ST-T segment (wide increases in the ST segment, followed by T wave inversions, or T inversions only)
- Ventricular arrhythmias
- Conduction disturbances
- The ECG may be normal.

Chest x-ray

- In severe myocarditis, the heart is enlarged and vascular markings are increased.

Laboratory tests

- Cardiac enzymes and troponins are often increased in the acute phase B [1 2] along with ECG changes, especially ST segment elevations. The concentrations of these markers usually normalize within one week.

Echocardiography

- Left ventricular dilatation and decrease in contractility.
- Local hypokinesia, in the early phases possibly local swelling.
- In severe myocarditis, symptoms and signs of dilating cardiomyopathy. When mild, the findings may be insignificant.
- Pericardial effusion if pericardial involvement.
- During recovery, signs of hyperkinesia.

Other diagnostic procedures

- Indium-111 antimyosin scintigraphy
  - In selected cases, negative finding excludes myocarditis.
  - Confirms myocarditis even after several months
- Biopsy of endomyocardium
  - Severe myocarditis
  - Suspected eosinophilic syndrome
  - Negative findings do not exclude myocarditis.

Differential diagnosis

- Chest pain, elevated cardiac markers, and ST elevation often simulate myocardial infarction. Thrombolytic therapy has seldom caused severe complications, even if used in cases of myocarditis. If thrombolytic drugs are used in the treatment of pericarditis, a risk of haemopericardium exists. Differentiating myocarditis from infarction:
  - The patient is often a young man.
  - There is no history of symptoms of ischaemic heart disease.
  - Q waves are seldom present.
  - ST elevations are always found also in leads V4–V6.
  - No reciprocal depression of the ST segment (except aVR and V1).
- Increased sympathetic tone is often associated with tachycardia and T wave changes in ECG. A beta-blocker abolishes these only if they are not caused by myocarditis or any other organic disease.
  - Test with a beta-blocker: an ECG is recorded in a recumbent position and again 3 minutes later standing in an upright position. The same procedure is repeated 2 hours after oral administration of atenolol 100 mg. An alternative is to record an ECG after a 10-minute rest, then give e.g. metoprolol 5 mg intravenously (to a patient weighing 70 kg), and repeat the recording after 5 minutes.
  - Changes resulting from increased sympathetic tone are exaggerated by standing position, a beta-blocker normalizes the T waves on the ECG at rest, and the orthostatic changes diminish.
  - The beta-blocker has almost no effect on the T wave changes if they are caused by organic disease.
- The athletic heart or early repolarization on the ECG may simulate the signs of myocarditis; echocardiography and follow-up of the ECG will confirm the diagnosis.

Treatment

Acute phase

- Immediate hospital observation is needed if the patient with symptoms has clear ECG changes, elevated cardiac enzymes, or signs of cardiac insufficiency. The risk of severe ventricular arrhythmias is highest in the first days of the disease.
- Pain is treated with anti-inflammatory analgesics or opioids if necessary.
- Causative treatment of the infection is initiated.
- A patient with no or only mild symptoms or signs and minor ECG changes may be followed in outpatient care. The condition is monitored every 1–2 weeks for 2 months, and always if cardiac symptoms appear.

Recovery phase

- Vigorous physical exercise should be avoided until the resting ECG has normalized, which in a typical case of myocarditis takes about two months. In athletes, an exercise test is recommended at this stage.
- The hyperkinetic state can be treated with beta-blockers.
- In case of infection myocarditis, recovery is usually complete, except in the most severe cases that may lead to dilating cardiomyopathy.

References

1. Smith S C, Landenson J H, Mason J W, Jaffe A S. Elevations of cardiac troponin I associated with myocarditis. Experimental and clinical correlates. Circulation 1997; 95: 163–168.
2. Bonnefoy E, Godon P, Kirkorian G, et al. Serum cardiac troponin I and ST-segment elevation in patients with acute pericarditis. Eur Heart J 2000; 21: 832–836.

4.85 Dilated cardiomyopathy

Editors

Pathophysiology and predisposing factors

- Hereditary causes (cover 10–30% of the cases)
    - Familial autosomal: in some cases a conduction disturbance is present. Family history may be negative.
    - Muscular dystrophy-related, chromosome X-linked (Duchenne, Becker)
    - Mitochondrial disorders
- Consequence of myocarditis: viruses and immunological response induced by them.
- Systemic connective tissue disease (arthritis, SLE, polymyositis)
- Alcoholism: dilated cardiomyopathy is rare in alcoholics. The so-called "drinker's heart" with a thick-walled left ventricle and associated diastolic insufficiency and tendency for arrhythmias is much more common.
- Metabolic causes: hyperthyroidism, hypothyroidism, diabetes and obesity. Some storage diseases (haemochromatosis, amyloidosis and sarcoidosis) often lead to restrictive cardiomyopathy, with diastolic dysfunction as the main symptom.
- Cardiotoxic drugs: doxorubicin, cyclophosphamide, fluorouracil
    - The delay in the appearance of symptoms is frequently several years or longer.
    - Predisposing factors include other heart diseases and age
- Long-lasting (up to years) tachycardia: atrial fibrillation, etc.
- So-called peripartum cardiomyopathy of late pregnancy and puerperium. In many cases some other cause is also present.
- Idiopathic or primary: no cause is found.
- Note! The diagnosis of cardiomyopathy requires the exclusion of other heart diseases with similar clinical manifestations: hypertension, coronary artery disease, valvular diseases and congenital heart diseases. Coronary artery disease may lead to a extensive ischaemic cardiomyopathy that is revealed only by isotope examination or positron emission tomography.

Symptoms and findings

- In the early stages, only minor symptoms; cardiomegaly on chest x-ray or abnormal ECG.
- Exertional dyspnoea caused by left ventricular failure. At a later stage, right ventricular failure is also found.
- Most common in middle-aged men. Prevalence < 1:1 000
- Blood pressure is normal or low.
- Tachycardia is common
- Gallop: always S3, often also S4
- Often a murmur of functional mitral regurgitation
- ST and T changes, left ventricle hypertrophy, left bundle branch block, P terminal force, Q waves are found. ECG is always pathological.
- Persistent atrial fibrillation develops in 15–20% of the cases.
- Recurring ventricular arrhythmias develop in 40–50% of the cases (syncope, sudden death). Long-term ECG monitoring!
- On the chest x-ray, cardiomegaly and signs of cardiac failure

Diagnosis

- Depends on exclusion of other diseases causing heart failure and cardiac hypertrophy (4.72). The most important of these are ischaemic heart disease and hypertensive cardiomyopathy.
- Echocardiography is always indicated if cardiomyopathy is suspected: ejection fraction and differential diagnoses.
- Echocardiography reveals: aneurysm of the left ventricle, severe aortic stenosis, primary mitral insufficiency, chronic effusive pericarditis and pulmonary heart disease.
- Consider the need to examine first-degree relatives.

Treatment

- Directed against the underlying cause!
- The patient must stop drinking alcohol and smoking, and lose weight, if obese.
- The patient should exercise as much as he/she tolerates.
- Good response to treatment is probable in cardiac insufficiency.
    - primarily with an ACE inhibitor and an angiotensin II antagonist
    - with a diuretic, if there is congestion
    - with a beta-blocker: remember to start with a small dose.
    - with digoxin, if the failure is not compensated with the above drugs (even with a sinus rhythm), and always if the patient has atrial fibrillation.
- Anticoagulant therapy is always in place, if there are no contraindications.
- Symptomatic arrhythmias are treated: beta-blockers and amiodarone are the safest drugs.
- Heart transplantation is performed when
    - heart failure causes severe symptoms and deteriorates continuously
    - the patient is under 60 years of age and otherwise healthy.

Prognosis

- Five-year survival after the diagnosis is 60–80%.

4.86 Hypertrophic cardiomyopathy

Editors

Definition and pathophysiology

- The left ventricle, or a part of it, hypertrophies without known cause. The disease is rare (prevalence in adult population 2/1000) and in about half of the cases the condition is congenital. Degree of severity varies greatly.
- In cases of a hypertrophic obstructive cardiomyopathy (HOCM), the interventricular septum is hypertrophied, causing an increase in the outflow tract gradient. Haemodynamically, the narrowing of the left ventricular outflow tract resembles aortic coarctation, or mitral stenosis if the left ventricular filling is impeded.
- Onset often in early adulthood, but sometimes first in middle age.

Symptoms and signs

- A decrease in exercise tolerance is often the first sign: exertion dyspnoea? May lead to investigation of pulmonary diseases.
- Other symptoms include angina pectoris, dyspnoea, arrhythmias, syncope, or sudden death during exercise. In mild cases the symptoms are diffuse and are associated with diastolic dysfunction.
- A harsh end-systolic murmur at the left sternal edge and often simultaneous mitral regurgitation murmur. In mild cases, the murmur is an "innocent" sounding left ventricle outflow tract ejection
- The ECG shows signs of left ventricle loading, often also pathological Q waves. The ECG findings resemble those of infarction, Wolff-Parkinson-White syndrome (WPW) and athlete's heart. ECG is always pathologic!
- Chest x-ray shows a normal or globular cardiac silhouette.
- The condition may be asymptomatic and be revealed accidentally by abnormal findings on ECG.
- Family history includes cases of this disease, or sudden deaths at a young age. Several underlying gene defects have been identified. The severity of the disease varies greatly even within a family. Inherited autosomally dominantly.

Diagnosis

- Clinical manifestations vary from asymptomatic disease to severe cardiac insufficiency, which is mainly diastolic in the early stages.
- The diagnosis is based on echocardiography, exclusion of other diseases, and family history: a suspicion is always an indication to send the patient to a specialist hospital. The objective is early diagnosis and treatment. First-degree relatives are also examined.
- The most important differential diagnosis is athlete's heart. Others are hypertension and aortic stenosis.

Treatment

- Aims at a symptom-free life and avoidance of sudden death.
- Alcohol and heavy exercise must be avoided.
- A beta-blocker or verapamil (calcium channel blocker) prolongs diastole and reduces ischaemia.
- A tendency to ventricular tachycardia is treated according to findings on ECG Holter monitoring: implanted defibrillator, amiodarone.
- Antimicrobial prophylaxis to prevent endocarditis is indicated if the patient has had mitral regurgitation.
- In some cases, septal myectomy, mitral valve prostheses or heart transplantation.

4.90 Primary pulmonary hypertension

Markku Ellonen

Aetiology

- Primary (idiopathic) pulmonary hypertension is a rare disease (incidence 1–3/million per year). The patients are usually 30–40-year-old women.
- Aetiology is heterogeneous, and generally difficult to confirm (genetic defect in a minority of cases). The use of appetite suppressing medications may increase the risk of disease C [1]. In some patients the disease is secondary, resulting from chronic pulmonary embolism.
- The right ventricle of the heart begins to hypertrophy. Tricuspidal valve fails, and the right atrium is dilated resulting in right heart failure.

Symptoms

- Dyspnoea on exertion is the only symptom at first.
- Many patients adapt to it or the underlying cause remains unrecognized, which often results in delayed diagnosis.
- Syncope attacks during exertion and cor pulmonale are late symptoms and signs.

Diagnosis

- ECG and chest x-ray are insensitive examinations in the early stages. In ECG the frontal QRS axis gradually deviates to the right: R1 < S1, RV1 > SV1, P-pulmonale.

- Echocardiography is a sensitive diagnostic method.
- No abnormalities are seen in the pulmonary scan.
- Diagnosis is made by exclusion of all other causes of secondary pulmonary hypertension (of which chronic pulmonary embolism is the most important).

Treatment

- Options are presently very limited and prognosis is poor.
- Intravenous prostacyclin is beneficial B [2] and inhaled prostaglandin derivatives are under research C [3]
- Sildenafil may be beneficial.
- Anticoagulant therapy is started when pulmonary embolism is suspected. The diagnosis is difficult to reach which is why the treatment is started just in case.
- Some patients benefit from calcium antagonists.
- Cautious treatment with diuretics may relieve oedema resulting from right ventricle failure.
- Oxygen concentrator relieves symptoms.
- Heart-lung transplantation may be the only option.

References

1. Abenhaim L, Moride Y, Brenot F et al. Appetite-suppressant drugs and the risk of primary pulmonary hypertension. N Engl J Med 1996;335:609–616.
2. Paramothayan NS, Lasserson TJ, Wells AU, Walters EH. Prostacyclin for pulmonary hypertension. Cochrane Database Syst Rev. 2004;(2):CD002994.
3. Hoeper MM, Schwarze M, Ehlerding S, Adler-Schuermeyer A, Spiekerkoetter E, Niedermeyer J, Hamm M, Fabel H. Long-term treatment of primary pulmonary hypertension with aerosolized iloprost, a prostacyclin analogue. N Engl J Med 2000;342:1866–1870.

Vascular Diseases

Evidence Based Medicine Guidelines. Edited by the Duodecim Editorial Team
 ISBN: 0-470-01184-X

5.10 Leg oedema

Ilkka Kunnamo

Aims

- To recognize indications for urgent care: **deep venous thrombosis and cardiac insufficiency**.
- To treat oedema caused by deep venous insufficiency with **compression** (compression stockings or devices).
- To consider surgical intervention in case of perforating vein insufficiency.
- To recognize oedema caused by medications (especially calcium channel blockers).
- To avoid excessive diuretic treatment when the swelling is caused by immobilization, phlebostasis, or lymphostasis.

Initial examination of the patient

- Usually, the presenting case has **pitting oedema**, in which an indentation created by finger pressure remains for a time, most easily on the tibia.
- **Firm** (non-pitting) oedema that persists overnight is rare, and malfunction of the lymph circulation should be investigated as the possible underlying cause.
- Determine any **asymmetry** of the oedema by measuring the circumference of both calves at their fullest point.
- **Skin discoloration** (stasis eczema) and visible **varicose veins**.
- Erysipelas frequently includes local oedema in addition to skin redness and tenderness.

Differential diagnostics and basic rules

- **Unilateral oedema** indicates a **local cause**: in acute oedema, rule out thrombosis; in chronic oedema, look for deep venous insufficiency. Remember the possibility of a ruptured Baker's cyst, particularly in patients with persistent knee hydrops.
- **Bilateral oedema** is usually caused either by cardiac insufficiency, deep venous insufficiency, or the standing position.
  - Cardiac-related oedema is always accompanied by other symptoms or findings of cardiac insufficiency (4.72).
  - Postthrombotic syndrome is accompanied by stasis eczema or by varicose veins.
  - Overweight, or work requiring standing, are the most frequent causes for pitting oedema in the evening.
- When the oedema does not appear to be either cardiac- or vein-related, look for kidney or liver disease. If a cause is not found, refer the patient to a hospital for further tests. Bilateral pitting oedema occurring in the evenings in a woman under 40 years of age, however, may be considered benign with no further extensive tests.

Clinical manifestations

Thrombosis

- See 5.40
- Commonly **unilateral**, with relatively acute onset of swelling (rarely more than a week before visiting a physician)
- The calf is often sensitive to walking and pressure. There may also be some pain.
- The absence of calf pain at passive dorsiflexion of the ankle (positive Homans' sign) does not rule out the possibility of thrombosis.
- Increased skin temperature in the area of the thrombus is a typical finding. It may be observed best by feeling each calf alternately with the backs of the fingers.
- The most important factors in the history, which suggest the presence of a thrombus, are earlier deep-seated phlebitis, illness requiring bed rest, or a recent limb immobilization (do not forget to ask about travel by air).
- A deep thrombus in a bedridden patient is usually not painful, and even the swelling is less pronounced.
- The Doppler stethoscope is a useful tool in the diagnosis of thrombosis (5.20).

Ruptured Baker's cyst

- Possible to diagnose clinically, if the patient describes having had a lump behind the knee and having pain with a sudden onset.
- An ultrasound usually confirms the diagnosis

Cardiac insufficiency

- Bilateral oedema with a relatively rapid onset (days–weeks).
- The patient is often known to suffer from severe heart disease.
- The insufficiency causing the oedema is almost invariably accompanied by shortness of breath under stress and night-time orthopnoea.
- Ask the patient about rapid weight gain.
- Tachycardia is common.
- The liver may be swollen and tender.
- Chest x-ray reveals an enlarged heart. The ECG is almost invariably pathological.
- Neglect in taking medications, a recent change in medication (such as adding a calcium channel blocker), or a fresh atrial fibrillation frequently exacerbate the insufficiency (4.72).

Valvular venous insufficiency

- The best diagnostic indicator is stasis eczema—a thinning and browning of the skin on the inner side of the ankle and loss of skin hair C [1 2].

- Frequently superficial varicose veins are also seen. Perforating vein ends may bulge out from the inner side of the ankle and lower leg when the patient is standing, and they may be tender to the touch.
- Swelling usually develops more slowly than in cardiac insufficiency and is accompanied by pain in the ankles, especially in the evening.
- Diagnosis may be made on the basis of the above-mentioned findings, if no symptoms pointing to cardiac insufficiency are present.
- A completely unilateral insufficiency of the deep veins can be found in the **postphlebitic syndrome**. In such a case, the past history includes deep venous thrombosis C [1] [2] or a fracture requiring casting.

Orthostatic oedema

- In older individuals who often sit with their knees bent, emptying of the veins may weaken to the extent that pitting oedema may develop.
- The history and the absence of findings of cardiac and venous insufficiency suffice for the diagnosis.
- In the treatment, avoid excessive diuretic therapy not directed at the basic cause.
- In women under 40 years of age, mild pitting oedema occurring only in the evening with no other symptoms or findings is usually harmless.

Other causes

- Venous compression **caused by a tumour** in the region of the hip or abdomen is an extremely rare cause of leg oedema. Abdominal palpation and a gynaecological examination for women are therefore part of the investigation of an anomalous oedema.
- Use of **medications causing oedema** should be checked. The most common oedema-inducing medications are
  - calcium channel blockers
  - pain medications (prostaglandin blockers)
  - steroids
  - beta-blockers (rarely).

Refining the diagnostics and hospital referral

- If **deep venous thrombosis** is suspected, the patient should be referred readily to the hospital for venography or compression echography.
- If the patient does not have any risk factors for deep venous thrombosis, a negative D-dimer result rules out thrombosis in practice. The patient does not need to be referred.
- In borderline cases, the necessity of referral may be decided with the Doppler stethoscope (5.20) or compression echography performed by a general practitioner familiar with the procedure.

Laboratory tests

- When the cause of bilateral oedema does not appear to be either cardiac insufficiency or venous stasis, for test
  - Urine protein and serum creatinine
  - Serum ALT or GGT (liver-generated oedema is common in alcoholics)
  - Serum TSH, particularly if the oedema extends beyond the legs and is impossible to eliminate by compression.

Treating leg oedema

Cardiac insufficiency

- The efficacy of treatment can be seen in a few days as a reduction of weight and swelling and palliation of dyspnoea symptoms.
- A normal serum N-peptide concentration will rule out untreated cardiac insufficiency (4.72).

Deep venous insufficiency

- A symptomatic deep vein insufficiency should be treated with compression in order to prevent the development of a leg ulcer.
- Regular work with the calf muscle pump and elevating the legs whenever feasible can go a long way in alleviating the symptoms.
- For patients in good health, with the exception of the very old, venous surgery or endoscopic ligation, accompanied by valvuloplasty C [3], is well worthwhile.
- The primary compression treatment method, the **compression stocking**, is a good treatment for motivated patients. (Note: NOT the so-called support stocking.) The stocking is individually selected by measuring the length and circumference of the leg and by determining the required degree of compression (for venous insufficiency patients the degree is usually 2). A physical therapist is generally responsible for the measurement and provision of the stocking. The stocking is put on in the morning and removed in the evening. Its anti-oedema effect is based on continuous compression, which is strongest around the foot and diminishes proximally. Problems with this treatment include the fairly high price of the stocking, stretching (a stocking in continuous use will last around 6 months), and the difficulty of pulling it on.
- A very effective means of treatment for even severe leg or foot oedema is **cyclic compression** (5.53) C [4]. For example, a home-care nurse can give this treatment. The treatment is also applicable to patients with open leg ulcers.
- **Oedema of venous origin should generally not be treated with diuretics** because the results are poor and the adverse effects of the medication may easily exceed its benefits, especially in older individuals. Sometimes in annoying oedema a trial of diuretic therapy is indicated. During the trial, the patient's weight and the occurrence of oedema must be monitored closely, and diuretics should be stopped if weight loss or clear improvement of the oedema is not observed.

References

1. Kurz X, Kahn SR, Abenhaim L, Clement D, Norgren L, Baccaglini U, Berard A, Cooke JP, Cornu-Thenard A, Depairon M, Formandy JA, Durand-Zaleski I, Fowkes GR, Lampling DL, Partsch H, Scurr JH, Zuccarelli F. Chronic venous disorders of the leg: epidemiology, outcomes, diagnosis and management: summary of an evidence-based report of the VEINES task force. International Angiology 1999;18: 83–102.
2. The Database of Abstracts of Reviews of Effectiveness (University of York), Database no.: DARE-991266. In: The Cochrane Library, Issue 1, 2001. Oxford: Update Software.
3. Abidia A, Hardy SC. Surgery for deep venous incompetence. Cochrane Database Syst Rev. 2004;(2):CD001097.
4. Kolbach DN, Sandbrink MWC, Neumann HAM, Prins MH. Compression therapy for treating stage I and II (Widmer) post-thrombotic syndrome. Cochrane Database Syst Rev 2003(4):CD004177.

5.11 Calf pain

Editors

- See also leg oedema 5.10.

Basic rules

- Diagnose acute arterial occlusion, deep venous thrombosis and erysipelas immediately.
- Recognize critical ischaemia and refer the patient urgently.
- Recognize compartment syndrome and stress fracture (which are particularly common in military conscripts and athletes).

Symptoms, signs, and diagnostic clues

- See Table 5.11

Clinical examination

- Localize the pain by history, palpation, and straight leg raising test.
- Recognize pitting oedema of the ankle by pressing with a finger for long enough.
- Palpate the peripheral pulses (only a strong pulse is definitely normal)
- Examine the arteries (and veins) with a doppler stethoscope if available (5.20).
- Deep vein thrombosis can be excluded in low-risk patients with d-dimer test in primary health care.

Table 5.11 Symptoms, signs, and diagnostic clues in calf pain

Symptom or sign	Diagnostic clue
Calf or ankle oedema (5.10)	Deep venous thrombosis (5.40) Insufficient valves in deep veins (5.10) (stasis eczema) Ruptured Baker's cyst (history of a mass in the popliteal fossa)
Erythema of the skin	Erysipelas (13.20)
Local pain in the skin	Superficial thrombophlebitis
Intermittent claudication	Lower limb ischaemia (5.60) (weak or absent pulses) Spinal stenosis (20.33)
Back pain exacerbated by bending forwards	Radicular syndrome due to herniated intervertebral disk (20.30)
Military conscripts or athletes	Stress fracture (local tenderness on the tibia) Compartment syndrome
Sudden onset	Muscle injury Ruptured Baker's cyst Arterial embolism (coldness, pulselessness, paleness)

5.20 Doppler stethoscopy in diagnostics

Ilkka Kunnamo

- The Doppler stethoscope has several uses.
- Arterial diagnostics is technically rather easy with a high degree of certainty in interpretation.
- Venous diagnostics requires careful study and longer training, and includes difficulties in interpretation. Making a fairly rough diagnosis of deep vein insufficiency is rather easy.

Ischaemia of the lower extremities

- Arterial obstructions in lower extremities (5.60) can nearly always be detected or ruled out with an examination with the Doppler stethoscopy by comparing the blood pressure of the lower with the upper extremity. Indications include
  - claudication pain
  - acute pain in the lower extremity (suspected embolism or thrombosis)
  - distal ulcers in lower extremity
  - coldness in the feet
  - fear of gangrene.
- Examination with a Doppler stethoscope makes the selection of patients to be referred for vascular surgery more reliable.
- Fear of gangrene is a common reason for a medical visit. Doppler stethoscopy performed so that the patient

him/herself can hear the arterial pulse sound from his/her foot is effective "therapy" for this condition.

Examination procedure

- The patient is in a supine position.
- Palpate the pulses and the temperature of the limb. Detection of peripheral pulses or a weak pulse does not rule out mild arterial occlusive (ASO) disease, and their absence, especially in an elderly individual, is insufficient for a diagnosis of vascular obstruction. The detection of a temperature boundary is significant in the diagnosis of embolism.
- With the Doppler stethoscope, find the pulse sounds of the posterior tibial artery behind the medial malleolus, and the dorsal artery on top of the foot. The sound is best located by moving the sensor of the Doppler stethoscope slowly across the direction of the artery. Occasionally, instead of the dorsal artery it is easier to hear the lateral tarsal artery, which is more laterally situated. The quality of the sound itself will point to a possible occlusion.
  - Normally, the sound is as sharp as a whipslash and has at least two phases (first a rapid forward flow, then a short backflow caused by the elasticity of the artery). Often a third phase is also heard, in which the blood flows slowly forward during the diastole.
  - Below an arterial obstruction the flow sound is a soft hiss and has only one phase (collateral flow).
  - If the obstruction is severe, the sound can be found only by searching carefully for it, and sometimes earphones are needed.
- Place a sphygmomanometer cuff around the ankle, increase the pressure gradually while concurrently auscultating the artery with the Doppler stethoscope. The pressure reading at the point when the sound disappears is the systolic arterial pressure. Auscultate both the posterior tibial artery and the dorsal foot artery, and record the readings for both.
- Measure the upper extremity pressure from the upper arm. Auscultate the wrist for the pulse sound preferably with a Doppler stethoscope (measurement with an ordinary stethoscope is valid).
  - **Pressure index (ABI) = lower extremity/upper extremity pressure**
  - Calculating the index is required in order to determine the extent of the obstruction and to monitor the condition (the ankle pressure will vary from one measurement to another, as will the blood pressure measured from the upper extremity).
- If the aim of the diagnostics is merely to confirm or rule out an arterial obstruction and to determine its extent, the ankle measurement is sufficient. Segmental pressure measurement may be performed later at a hospital.

Interpretation

- If the ankle pressure is lower than the upper limb pressure, there is a high likelihood of an arterial obstruction.
- Ankle pressure below 50 mmHg and an ulcer in the foot or pain at rest are signs of **critical ischaemia**, which requires urgent care.
- Segmental pressure readings taken above the ankle are usually higher than those at the ankle because of the dampening effect of thicker tissues on the cuff pressure (thigh/ankle = 1.2, equal pressure in the upper arm and thigh usually indicates a proximal obstruction at the iliac level or in the femoral artery). It is important to note bilateral differences.
- **In diabetics, the inelasticity of vessel walls may cause too high readings in ankle pressure**. In such a case, low-pitched pulsation and the absence of a two-phase pulse sound indicate an obstruction.

Deep venous thrombosis

- See 5.40. The examination aims at establishing unobstructed blood flow in the posterior tibial and popliteal veins. It is advisable to perform the examination first on the healthy limb.

Technique and interpretation of results

- Auscultate **posterior tibial vein** with the patient supine. The auscultation area is behind the medial malleolus next to the artery. The flowing blood becomes audible by compressing the calf steadily by hand and letting go suddenly. If the vein is unobstructed, the flow is audible immediately after the grip is released.
- Auscultate the **popliteal vein** from behind the knee with the patient lying prone. Pressing the calf lightly with a flat palm will make the flow audible. At first, press the upper part of the calf. If the flow is audible, repeat the pressure at the lower part of the calf.
  - **Absence of an audible flow or unmistakable dampening of the sound in either vein compared with the healthy side indicates venous thrombosis and calls for venographic or compression echography tests.**
  - The unilateral absence of respiratory arrhythmia is another indication of an obstruction.
  - Occasionally, an unusually clear continuous sound is audible in an obstructed vein, which will respond to pressure and release with delay or not at all.
- **The femoral vein** is auscultated at the groin, medial to the artery. Normally, the flow sounds like a wailing wind, varying in synchrony with the patient's breathing (respiratory arrhythmia). The absence of respiratory arrhythmia indicates obstruction. If the lower abdomen is pressed by hand and the pressure is released suddenly, a rapid forward flow is audible, when the blood in the compressed interior vena cava begins to flow. The absence of this forward flow indicates a large thrombus at a site higher up.

Sources of error

- An obstruction at a lower site, not in the venous trunk of the posterior tibial vein and not reaching up to the knee, often remains undetected with the Doppler stethoscope.

- When the calf is pressed, the popliteal vein generates an audible flow if the vein is even partially open or if the obstruction does not reach the knee. A quiet sound and its lower, whispery (not whipping) tone compared with the other side indicate an obstruction.
- With a careful examination technique, the proportion of false negative findings is a few percentage points. False positive findings are more common than false negative ones.
- **In addition to Doppler stethoscopy, pay attention to patient history and symptoms when determining the need for venography.** Venography or echography should be performed on all patients whose Doppler findings are abnormal. It should also be performed when the Doppler finding is normal but the patient has obvious risk factors for deep thrombosis (previous thrombi, surgery or other immobilization, injury of the lower extremities, known coagulation problems, polycytaemia vera, contraceptive pills in case of a smoker), and no other explanation for the oedema in the limbs can be found. Along with the D-dimer assay, Doppler stethoscopy is useful, particularly in situations where the physician, for other reasons, has difficulty deciding whether or not to refer the patient for venography.

Deep venous insufficiency

- See 5.10
- Normal valves prevent the backflow of blood in the deep veins. In the Doppler stethoscope, the blood flow in the posterior tibial vein, behind the medial malleolus, sounds like a howling wind. The sound is interrupted for a moment if the calf is pressed by hand, and becomes stronger as soon as the grip is released and the flow increases.
- In deep venous insufficiency, as the calf is pressed, a clear hiss caused by the backflow can be heard. The severity of the venous insufficiency can be determined if the thigh is also pressed and the backflow then heard again. This examination also serves as a concrete demonstration of the cause of the swelling.

Measuring blood pressure in children's limbs

- Measuring blood pressure in the upper and lower extremities in order to rule out coarctation is necessary in children whose femoral pulses are weak or who have a systolic murmur (28.3) (28.4).
- Measuring the ankle pressure with a Doppler stethoscope does not usually frighten a child, and the measurement can be taken while the child is calm. The child is not required to lie down, but may sit on the parent's lap. Blood pressure in the upper extremity is also worth measuring while auscultating the wrist with a Doppler stethoscope.
- Interpretation
    - Normally, a pressure reading taken from the ankle of a sitting child is at least 10 mmHg higher than the pressure from the upper extremity.
    - If the readings are equal, the measurement should be repeated later.
    - If the upper extremity pressure is higher than the lower extremity pressure, the child should generally be referred to a specialist for ruling out coarctation.

Measuring blood pressure in a patient in shock

- Doppler stethoscopy may be used to measure systolic blood pressure even in a situation where measurement with an ordinary stethoscope is unsuccessful.
    - Place the cuff around the upper arm and auscultate the pulse at the antecubital fossa.
    - This measurement is usually successful even during ambulance transport. If the Doppler stethoscope includes earphones, they are worth using in a noisy environment.

Diagnosis of testis torsion

- Blood circulation in the testes is copious. In the normal state, a distinct arterial pulse is audible when the sensor is placed against the lower pole of the testis. In epididymitis and torsion the pulse sounds behave differently.
    - In epididymitis, circulation on the side of the swollen testis is accelerated or at least as copious as on the healthy side.
    - In torsion, the flow on the side of the painful testis is weaker.
- A carefully performed examination is reliable. However, swollen testes and pain in a child or youth who is not sexually active is, independent of Doppler findings, a sufficient cause to send the patient to hospital because epididymitis in this group is rare.

5.35 Superficial venous thrombosis

Juha Sinisalo

Basic rules

- Superficial venous thrombosis is a common and usually benign condition.
- If the clinical picture is not obvious or if something suggests deep venous thrombosis, ultrasound examination allows to verify the diagnosis and to exclude the possibility of deep venous thrombosis.
- Treatment is symptomatic when the superficial venous thrombosis is the first one the patient has and if an underlying cause can be identified, e.g. trauma, varices or venous insufficiency.

- In 5–10% of the cases deep venous thrombosis occurs concurrently with a superficial one in either the same or the other (!) extremity. Deep venous thrombosis may also develop with a delay (weeks from the diagnosis of a superficial thrombosis). Pulmonary embolisms are rare (approx. 1%). D-dimer is not useful in the differential diagnosis between superficial and deep venous thrombosis.
- If a venous thrombosis recurs, restoration of the superficial veins is indicated. If the patient does not have venous insufficiency, possible systemic diseases must be ruled out.

Predisposing factors

- Chronic venous insufficiency
- Superficial trauma
- Medicinal infusion or use of i.v. narcotics
- Pregnancy
- Coagulation disorders (particularly protein S and C deficiencies)
- Hormone replacement therapy
- Malignant neoplastic diseases, for example,
  - myeloproliferative diseases (polycythaemia vera and essential thrombocytaemia)
  - migrating thrombophlebitis (short venous cord, often in the upper extremity is initially blocked and then cured but recurs in another part) may be associated with GI carcinomas.
- Collagenous diseases, for example,
  - Behcet's disease
  - Buerger's disease (i.e. thromboangiitis obliterans), usually affects the small and medium-sized arteries in smokers. Approximately one third of these patients also have superficial venous thrombi. Recurring superficial venous thrombi in a young person who smokes may suggest Buerger's disease.

Symptoms

- The affected vein is painful, the area around is reddish and hot and swollen with a palpable resistance. The patient may have fever.
- The inflammation may take 2–6 weeks to subside, however, the obstructed vein may give symptoms for months.

Treatment

- Symptomatic: the leg is held up, the patient wears compressive stockings, and uses cold compresses.
- Pain medication: pain is usually alleviated within 3–5 days, redness and swelling disappear in 2–3 weeks, for which time NSAID medication (not COX_2 selective) is beneficial.
- Topically applied anticoagulant cream may accelerate the healing of a superficial venous thrombus.
- Surgery is indicated for recurring thrombophlebitis of the lower extremity after conservative therapy has failed. Ultrasound and/or consultation with a specialist are indicated in the following acute phase conditions:
  - thrombophlebitis appears above the mid-thigh (the risk of deep venous thrombosis is increased)
  - thrombophebilits in the vena saphena parva (calf) region predisposes to deep venous thrombosis (because of the perforating veins).
- I.v. low-molecular-weight heparin in prophylactic dosage is indicated in extensive phlebitis and during pregnancy. The treatment is continued during pregnancy and 6 weeks after delivery.

5.40 Deep venous thrombosis

Editors

Aims

- To prevent pulmonary embolism and post-thrombotic syndrome.
- To suspect thrombosis in high risk patients.
- Plasma D-dimer test can be used in primary care as the first-line test to rule out deep-vein thrombosis (DVT). If the D-dimer concentration is increased, or DVT is clinically apparent, the patient should be referred for diagnostic imaging investigations.
- A suspected DVT is verified by venography or compression ultrasonography.
- To prevent DVT in immobilized patients: calf muscle exercises, compression stockings, and, if necessary, prophylactic treatment with subcutaneous low-molecular-weight heparin (LMWH).
- When the diagnosis has been confirmed, DVT can be treated at home or in a general hospital ward. A distal deep calf thrombosis does not cause emboli, and only about 25% of the thrombi reach the femoral level.
- Idiopathic venous thrombosis may be a sign of malignancy.

Risk factors for deep venous thrombosis

- Immobilisation due to an acute illness, especially if the circulation is simultaneously impaired (e.g. heart failure, paralysis, surgery, infection, long flight)
- Trauma to the lower limbs (fractures in plaster cast in particular)
- Hereditary or acquired coagulation disorder (5.10) (always suspect these aetiologies when no external cause is evident)
- Polycythaemia, essential thrombocytosis
- Use of oral contraceptives, hormone replacement therapy particularly in smokers
- Previous venous thrombosis
- Pregnancy and the postpartum period (6 weeks), caesarean section, the age of the mother
- Cancer in an active phase
- Central venous catheters, often located in an upper limb.

Symptoms

- Oedema of the entire leg or calf (for differential diagnosis, see 5.10)
- Tenderness or ache at rest
- Pain in the calf while walking
- Concurrent pain, tenderness and oedema are strongly suggestive of DVT (59%). Each sign alone indicates thrombosis in only 11–22% of the cases.
- Often completely asymptomatic, particularly in bed bound patients in whom the first symptom may be pulmonary embolism. In patients with a hip fracture the thrombosis often only occurs in the femoral and pelvic areas.
- Almost half of proximal DVTs are associated with either symptomatic or asymptomatic pulmonary embolism.

Diagnosis

- The probability of a patient having DVT is influenced by his/her predisposition to thrombotic events and whether there is a history of previous venous thrombosis.
- Clinical findings
  - Oedema of the ankle and lower leg; in iliac vein thrombosis oedema of the entire leg
  - Deep calf tenderness on palpation along the involved vein
  - Positive Homans' sign (not always, especially if the patient is in bed rest)
  - Warmth of the skin when compared with the other leg and prominent superficial collateral veins
- Doppler ultrasound examination (5.20) to assist diagnosis:
  - Impaired or slowed flow in the popliteal vein when the calf is compressed.
  - Slowed flow in the posterior tibial vein when the compression is released.
  - In iliac vein thrombosis there is an absence of phasic respiratory signals or a weakened flow sound from the femoral vein when listened to at the groin.
- For differential diagnosis, see 5.10.

Care guidelines in suspected deep venous thrombosis

- The probability of venous thrombosis can be estimated and scored using the below list of signs and conditions. (Give 1 point for each finding or condition which is likely to increase the pretest probability of DVT. If a diagnosis other than DVT is highly likely for other reasons, subtract 2 points from the final sum.)
  - Cancer that is being actively treated or that has metastasised
  - Paralysis or recent immobilisation of a lower limb
  - Bed rest of more than 3 days' duration
  - A major operation within 1 month
  - Local tenderness in the calf, or in the thigh, around the deep venous trunk. Often indicated as the reason for referral, but when presents alone has poor prognostic value for DVT.
  - More than a 3-cm difference in the circumference of the calves.
  - Strong familial predisposition (at least 2 first-degree relatives with a history of venous thrombosis).
  - Even though the studies evaluating the value of risk scoring did not take the use of oral contraceptives and a personal history of a previous DVT into consideration, a point could be allocated for both in clinical adaptations of the scoring system.
- **Plasma D-dimer test** is used for the exclusion of DVT (the test is very sensitive, but not as specific. A positive result does not therefore always indicate thrombosis).
  - If the D-dimer test is negative in a low-risk patient (0 risk points), no further investigations are needed. In clinical practice, a negative D-dimer test is also sufficient to exclude DVT in patients who only score one point for palpation tenderness in the calf or thigh.
  - If the first ultrasonographic result and plasma D-dimer test are both normal in a patient at a higher risk, repeated ultrasonography is not necessary.
  - D-dimer concentration may also be increased during normal pregnancy.
- Initial treatment with LMWH can often be started on the basis of suspicion alone. Any delay in imaging investigations will thus not pose extra risk for the patient.
- **Compression ultrasonography** is used currently as an early phase investigation. It is sensitive (90%) particularly in proximal thrombosis, but less so (50%) in distal thrombosis. Compression ultrasonography is replacing venography, which is useful in the diagnosis of recurrent DVTs.
  - An abnormal ultrasonography finding is an indication for treatment. A normal result in a low-risk patient (0 risk points) excludes venous thrombosis. A normal result with a positive D-dimer in a moderate-risk patient (1–2 risk points) warrants a repeat ultrasonography in 7 days, and in a high-risk patient (3 or more risk points) venography should be performed immediately.
  - An abnormal venography (a persistent intravenous filling deficit in at least two projections) is an indication for treatment. A normal result excludes venous thrombosis.

Treatment

Basic rules

- Compression bandaging (see below)
- In proximal thrombosis, early mobilisation is recommended after a few days of heparin therapy.
- Distal, and often also proximal, thrombosis can be treated at a general hospital ward or at home either by a district nurse or the patient him/herself. Based on individual situations, the treating physician will decide where the treatment should be carried out. Obese patients will need two injections because of the large doses needed. An underweight patient or one with multiple illnesses is not usually suitable for home care. The patient will need written instructions for home care.

- Hospital treatment is indicated if there is
  - severe oedema of the entire leg
  - thrombosis above the groin
  - other coexisting illnesses requiring hospital treatment.
- If the treatment is carried out at home, ensure that
  - the injection technique and drug doses are correct
  - the follow-up of the anticoagulation therapy is adequate
  - the patient has instructions regarding compression bandages and stockings
  - the patient is monitored for possible complications (bleeding, emboli).

Treatment according to the location and duration of thrombosis

- A high, ileofemoral thrombus, or thrombus in the upper extremities, with onset within the last 7 days
  - Systemic fibrinolytic therapy, similar to the one given in myocardial infarction, is used in some centres. Its efficacy against post-thrombotic syndrome has not been established. Local fibrinolysis is implemented by introducing a catheter into the thrombus mass. The success of fibrinolysis is monitored by venography. The currently used agent for fibrinolysis is tissue plasminogen activator (tPA). Treatment time is 1–3 days, and the aim is to minimize the time because of the risk of bleeding.
  - The contraindications are the same as for fibrinolytic therapy in myocardial infarction (4.61). The aim is to decrease the risk of post-thrombotic syndrome. The use is limited to young patients with recent, extensive ileofemoral thrombosis or pulmonary emboli with potentially hazardous haemodynamic consequences. Total lysis is rarely achieved because venous thrombi are often old and organised.
  - LMWH A [1 2 3 4 5 6 7 8 9 10 11] has replaced i.v. heparin. Begin warfarin therapy concomitantly. Heparin may be stopped when INR has been within the target range (usually 2.0–3.0) for at least 2 days.
  - Thrombectomy may be indicated if the viability of the leg is threatened or when the aim is to reduce the severity of post-thrombotic syndrome.
- Distal thrombosis in a leg or any other thrombosis with onset more than 7 days ago
  - LMWH (e.g. dalteparin 200 IU/kg once daily, enoxaparin 1.5 mg/kg once daily or 1 mg/kg twice daily) A [1 2 3 4 5 6 7 8 9 10 11]. In patients with increased tendency for thrombosis, the twice daily regimen is recommended. Heparin may be stopped when INR has been within the target range for at least 2 days. The treatment does not necessitate laboratory follow-up, provided that haemostasis is stable. In pregnant women and in patients with renal insufficiency, thrombophilia or haemophilia, the concentration of active heparin must be monitored. LMWH is at least as effective as standard heparin A [1 2 3 4 5 6 7 8 9 10 11] and causes less thrombocytopenia and paradoxical embolism.

Table 5.40 Duration of anticoagulant therapy is determined individually with the anticipated success of therapy, the patient's other illnesses and age as well as the risk of recurrence being the decisive factors.

Indication	Duration of therapy
First episode of thrombosis and a transient or modifiable predisposing factor (surgery, trauma, bed rest, oestrogen therapy)	3–6 months
First episode of thrombosis without a predisposing factor	At least 6 months
First episode of thrombosis in a patient with cancer, cardiolipin antibodies, combined coagulation disorder, homozygous Factor V Leiden or prothrombin gene mutation.	12 months to lifetime
Recurring thrombosis without a predisposing factor or in association with increased coagulability of blood.	Lifetime

  - Start warfarin therapy concomitantly with heparin (see 5.44 for instructions) and continue it according to Table 5.40.
  - Bandage the leg from the foot up to the upper thigh. The patient can start to walk when the leg has been bandaged.
  - Only about 25% of untreated distal thrombi progress to above the knee. Heparin–warfarin therapy is implemented only if there are no contraindications. Distal thrombosis may often receive no anticoagulant treatment; it may remain subclinical, or occur whilst the leg is immobilized within a plaster.
- For the duration of warfarin therapy, see 5.44, and Table 5.40.
- Prevention of deep venous thrombosis, see 5.42.

Treatment of heparin-induced bleeding

- If heparin induced severe bleeding occurs, the missing blood products must be replaced (fresh frozen plasma, thrombocytes). Protamine is administered if unfractionated heparin had been used. Protamine is not as effective in counteracting the action of LMWH.
- In 1% of the patients, heparin causes thrombocytopenia (HIT), which is a prothrombotic condition.

Prognosis

- The risk of recurrence depends primarily on the underlying cause and its possible elimination. The duration of anticoagulation therapy is determined by the severity of the thrombosis and the risk of its recurrence. In idiopathic thrombosis, the risk of recurrence is high, the treatment time is often long, sometimes even lifelong. Recurrence during well-implemented therapy may suggest malignancy or phospholipid antibody syndrome.

- The condition of the venous valves is the decisive factor when assessing the risk for post-thrombotic syndrome. Anticoagulation therapy prevents the recurrence of the thrombus but does not offer protection for the valves. On the other hand, a recurrence increases the risk of post-thrombotic syndrome manyfold.
- The extent and, particularly, high location (above the groin) of a thrombus have been considered as risk factors for post-thrombotic syndrome, and in these cases fibrinolytic therapy is aimed at protecting the valves. This may be achieved by local fibrinolytic therapy administered by catheterisation. However, this therapy is not readily available and may lead to complications, and each case must be assessed individually.
- **An elastic compression stocking reduces the risk of post-thrombotic syndrome and should always be worn** Ⓐ[12].
  - The leg is bandaged using an elastic bandage starting from the foot, with greater pressure near the ankle and reduced pressure higher up. The bandage is worn for two weeks day and night and is changed at 2–3 day intervals. After this, a compression stocking is fitted. It reduces the risk of post-thrombotic syndrome by approximately 50%. The knee-length stocking is usually used. Compression class 2 is the most commonly used. The stocking is worn from 6 months to 2 years, sometimes permanently.

References

1. van den Belt AGM, Prins MH, Lensing AWA, Castro AA, Clark OAC, Atallah AN, Burihan E. Fixed dose subcutaneous low molecular weight heparins versus adjusted dose unfractionated heparin for venous thromboembolism. Cochrane Database Syst Rev. 2004;(2):CD001100.
2. Leizorovicz A, Simonneau G, Decousus H, Boissel JP. Comparison of the efficacy and safety of low molecular weight heparins and unfractionated heparin in the initial treatment of deep venous thrombosis a meta-analysis. BMJ 1994;309:299–304.
3. The Database of Abstracts of Reviews of Effectiveness (University of York), Database no.: DARE-948053. In: The Cochrane Library, Issue 4, 1999. Oxford: Update Software.
4. Leizorovicz A. Comparison of the efficacy and safety of low molecular weight heparins and unfractionated heparin in the initial treatment of deep venous thrombosisan updated meta-analysis. Drugs 1996;52(suppl 7):30–37.
5. The Database of Abstracts of Reviews of Effectiveness (University of York), Database no.: DARE-970245. In: The Cochrane Library, Issue 4, 1999. Oxford: Update Software.
6. Martineau P, Tawil N. Low-molecular weight heparins in the treatment of deep-vein thrombosis. Ann Pharmacother 1998;32:588–601.
7. The Database of Abstracts of Reviews of Effectiveness (University of York), Database no.: DARE-980950. In: The Cochrane Library, Issue 2, 2000. Oxford: Update Software.
8. Hirsh J, Siragusa S, Cosmi B, Ginsberg JS. Low molecular weight heparins (LMWH) in the treatment of patients with acute venous thromboembolism. Thrombosis & Haemostasis 1995;74:360–363.
9. The Database of Abstracts of Reviews of Effectiveness (University of York), Database no.: DARE-963681. In: The Cochrane Library, Issue 4, 1999. Oxford: Update Software.
10. Gould MK, Dembitzer AD, Doyle R, Hastie TJ, Garber AM. Low-molecular weight heparins compared with unfractionated heparin for treatment of acute deep venous thrombosis. Ann Intern Med 1999;130:800–809.
11. The Database of Abstracts of Reviews of Effectiveness (University of York), Database no.: DARE-999249. In: The Cochrane Library, Issue 4, 2000. Oxford: Update Software.
12. Kolbach DN, Sandbrink MWC, Hamulyak K, Neumann HAM, Prins MH. Non-pharmaceutical measures for prevention of post-thrombotic syndrome. The Cochrane Database of Systematic Reviews, Cochrane Library Number: CD004174. In: Cochrane Library, Issue 1, 2004. Chichester, UK: John Wiley & Sons, Ltd.

5.41 Thrombophilia (inherited)

Editors

Aims

- Diagnosis of thrombophilia is important
  - for implementing anticoagulation therapy, when required
  - for thrombose prophylaxis during pregnancy, labour and puerperium
  - for investigating close relatives and informing them about the risks of thrombosis.

Causes of inherited thrombophilias

- Patients with hereditary abnormalities in the coagulation or fibrinolytic system are predisposed to deep-vein thrombosis.
- Thrombophilias are inherited dominantly. They are not sex-linked. Most patients are heterozygous. Causes in descending order of frequency:
  - Resistance to activated protein C (APC resistance)
    - Found in 20% of young patients with venous thromboembolism, but only in 4% of the general population. This gene mutation is 5–10 times as common as the others put together.
    - This mutation affects coagulation factor V and results in resistance to activated protein C.
  - Protein C deficiency
  - Antithrombin III deficiency (in 0.2% of the general population)
  - Protein S deficiency

- The three last-mentioned count for about 10% of thrombophilias. All four mutations have a dominant inheritance.
- Disorders of the fibrinolytic system (possibly not predisposing to thrombosis)
- Others
  - Prothrombin mutation G20210A polymorphism in 1% of general population and 5–7% of patients with venous thromboembolism
  - Dysfibrinogenaemia
  - Lupus anticoagulant (acquired antiphospholipid antibody syndrome) is not an inherited thrombophilia.
  - Hyperhomocystinemia

Indications for investigation of thrombophilia

- Deep vein thrombosis with the following characteristics:
  - spontaneous thrombosis in a young and healthy person
  - patient on contraceptives or pregnant
  - recurrence at young age (under 45 yr)
  - exceptional location
  - spontaneous thrombosis in close relatives
- Arterial thrombosis with following characteristics:
  - young age (<30 yr)
  - both arterial and venous thromboses
- A first-degree relative with inherited thrombophilia. The problem may become current if the patient is exposed to risks of venous thrombosis (surgery, pregnancy, contraceptives). The diagnosis of thrombophilia in a healthy person is not a cause for anticoagulant therapy; however, prophylaxis should be emphasized.
  - Widespread genetic screening to detect the most common thrombophilia (APC resistance or factor V Leiden) from young healthy women has been suggested in order to select a safe contraceptive method. The viewpoint, however, is commercial and so far not clinical practice.
  - The close relatives of young patients with spontaneous venous thrombosis can at first be examined only for Factor V Leiden and FII G20210A. If the mutation has been defined, the patient can at first be examined only for the same mutation. If not defined, the patient should be examined for the other most common causes of thrombophilia.

Blood specimen

- If possible the specimen should be taken before initiation of treatment. A special specimen tube is required.
- The specimen should be taken before anticoagulation or after stopping it for 3–4 weeks. Examining the parents of the patient is another possibility if anticoagulation cannot be stopped.
- Factor V Leiden can be measured with a DNA technique without stopping anticoagulant therapy.

Treatment of thrombophilia patients

- F V Leiden increases the risk of venous thrombosis during oral contraceptives by 35-fold. The increase in the risk during pregnancy is not known.

Table 5.41 Treatment guideline for APC resistance (FV mutation) (Nordic coagulation meeting, Uppsala 24.–26.4.1997)

Advising the patient	Duration of peroral anticoagulant therapy	Prophylaxis in connection with surgery or immobilization	Prophylaxis during pregnancy	Prophylaxis during delivery and puerperiumin
No thrombosis, not even in 1-degree relatives	—	Normal prophylaxis given in connection with high-risk procedures	None, unless the patient is immobilized	None, except in cases of caesarean section or immobilization
No thrombosis in the patient, but a 1-degree relative has suffered from thrombosis	—	See above	Consider each case individually, most often not needed	Consider each case individually, most often not needed
The patient has had thrombosis, but none of his 1-degree relatives have suffered from it	Temporarily on diagnosing the thrombus[1)]	Yes	Consider the need individually, often necessary	Yes
Thrombosis in the patient and in a 1-degree relative	Temporarily on diagnosing the thrombus[1)]	Yes	Most often necessary	Yes
Two thrombi	Until otherwise decided	Yes	Yes	Yes

1) Duration of therapy: (a) Transient triggering factor: in distal thrombosis continue therapy for a minimum of 6 weeks, in proximal thrombosis for 3 months; (b) Spontaneous thrombosis: distal thrombosis continue for 3–6 months, in proximal thrombosis for (3 -) 6 months.

- Antithrombin III deficiency increases the risk of venous thrombosis by up to 2–4% annually.
- Anticoagulation therapy prevents the thromboses.
- Surgery can be carried out with prophylactic heparin or warfarin.
- Trombophilia is common (4%) in the general population. Anticoagulation therapy is not used if the patient has not had a thrombosis. The duration of anticoagulation depends on the seriousness of the consequences and on the causes of deep vein thrombosis. Its spontaneous origin often requires long-term therapy. The decision to start long-term anticoagulation must be made individually. If the patient has two hereditary defects (double heterozygote) anticoagulant treatment should be started more easily. Note also family history and other factors predisposing to thrombosis. A suggestion by a Nordic group for anticoagulation time in F V Leiden patients after thrombosis is given in Table 5.41.
- Heparin prophylaxis during pregnancy is always necessary in antithrombin III deficiency patients. In the case of other thrombophilias, therapy during pregnancy is carried out only in patients with an earlier thrombosis and even then after individual assessment.
- Oral contraceptives are contraindicated. Hormone replacement therapy is usually allowed.

5.42 Prevention of venous thrombosis

Markku Ellonen

Basic rules

- Venous thrombosis is a common and dangerous disease that can, however, be treated and often prevented.
- Venous thrombosis of a bedridden patient can be asymptomatic–the first symptom may be pulmonary embolism.
- Early mobilisation, antiembolism stockings, low molecular weight heparin and warfarin is used for primary prevention. ASA is primarily used for the prevention of arterial occlusion.
- If the patient is under 40 years of age and has a venous thrombosis without any causative factors, consider the possibility of a hereditary coagulation disorder.
- In addition to hereditary (intrinsic) factors there are extrinsic factors and conditions that contribute to venous thrombosis:
    - previous venous thrombosis
    - oral contraceptives
    - pregnancy and labour
    - surgery and tissue trauma
    - varicose veins
    - obesity
    - polycythaemia
    - heart insufficiency and immobilisation
    - paralysis, inactivity
    - malignant diseases
    - immobilization (cast, long flights).

Prevention of venous thrombosis in surgery

- Low risk (risk of venous thrombosis 2–3%)
    - Minor surgery (<30 min), no risk factors
    - Age < 40, no risk factors
- Moderate risk (risk of venous thrombosis 10–30%)
    - Minor surgery, risk factors
    - Nonmajor surgery, no risk factors, age 40–60
    - Major surgery, age under 40, no risk factors
- High risk (risk of venous thrombosis 50–80%)
    - Major surgery, age > 40 years and earlier deep venous thrombosis or pulmonary embolism or cancer
    - thrombophilia
    - knee or hip arthroplasty, hip fracture
    - major trauma, injury of the spinal cord
- The estimated risk of venous thrombosis in the above-mentioned risk groups is about 10%, 30% and 60%, respectively. In classifying patients into risk groups, take into account both the type of surgery and personal predisposing factors. Give prophylactic medication against thrombosis to patients belonging to the moderate or high-risk groups. Low-molecular-weight heparin (LMWH) is safe and easily administered at home. It should be used more often for the low-risk patients and the course of medication should be prolonged in high-risk patients.
- Immobilization increases the risk of thrombosis: e.g. an ankle fracture in a cast involves a 20% risk, and a fractured tibia in a cast a 60% risk.

How to prevent thrombosis in surgical patients

- Avoid immobilization before and after surgery, avoid general anaesthetics and prefer spinal or epidural anaesthetics, optimize the fluid balance.
- Start preventive therapy before the operation, if possible **C** [1 2].
- Among the available physical measures the most common and easiest are compression dressings or a surgical stocking **A** [3 4 5 6 7], which in low-risk patients suffice as the only methods of prevention. Their usefulness has been shown in surgical and obstetric patients.
- Early mobilization does not mean that the patient is placed in a sitting position: mere sitting may even increase the risk of thrombosis.
- Warfarin can also be used for prophylaxis, as it is practical and inexpensive, and can be used when long-term prophylaxis is needed (e.g. a fractured pelvis and long immobilization). The use of warfarin involves the risk of bleeding and requires regular monitoring.

- Heparin is effective in reducing the incidence of deep vein thrombosis (A) [8 9 10 11 12]. LMWHs have displaced ordinary heparin because of their higher efficacy and easy administration (once daily). If the immobilization is prolonged, continue heparin treatment until the patient is able to get up again. The most common treatment period is 1–2 weeks. Prophylactic treatment with LMWH is safe and often possible to carry out at home. Treatment should be prolonged in hip and knee prosthesis surgery (A) [13], during pregnancy and puerperium and probably in cancer surgery (B) [14]. In a high-risk group the treatment can be continued with warfarin for 6–12 weeks. LMWH could also be administered to high-risk patients for 3–4-weeks by a nurse making home visits.
- The usual prophylactic treatment scheme with LMWH
  - Moderate risk patients
    - Enoxaparin 20 (–40) mg s.c. 2 hours before surgery and then the same amount once daily.
    - Dalteparin 2500 IU 2 hours before surgery and then the same amount once daily.
  - High risk patients
    - Enoxaparin 40 mg s.c. 12 hours before surgery and then the same amount once daily.
    - Dalteparin 5000 IU 12 hours before surgery and then the same amount once daily.
- Adverse effects: postoperative and post-traumatic bleeding. The antidote is protamine.
- Also aspirin reduces the incidence of venous thrombosis (A) [15 16].
- On long flights it is recommended that high risk patients wear antiembolism stockings, possibly also LMWH (one dose of prophylaxis half an hour prior to flight).
- Fondaparinux is an inhibitor of coagulation factor X, that may prevent venous thrombosis more efficiently during orthopedic surgery than enoxaparin (A) [17 18 19 20].

Prevention of venous thrombosis in internal medicine

Risk factors for venous thrombosis

- Heart failure and other non–surgical high risk patients
- Heart failure and myocardial infarction
- Pulmonary embolism is a common cause of death of patients with infarction of the brain. The risk can be lowered with early mobilisation, antiembolism stockings and LMWH. Haemorrhage complications diminish the benefits.
- Cancer
- Severe infection

How to prevent thrombosis in medical patients

- LMW heparin has replaced ordinary heparin. LMWH therapy should be considered for all patients who are at bed rest for more than 3 days and who have one or more of the above-mentioned risk factors. The efficacy of this prophylactic treatment has not been documented as well as in surgical patients.

Prevention of venous thrombosis during pregnancy

- Carried out in special care units

High risk of thromboembolism

- A venous thrombus above the knee, or pulmonary embolism during an earlier pregnancy.
- Patients with a hereditary blood coagulation disorder and a previous venous thrombosis. (In antithrombin III deficiency the risk is so high that prophylactic treatment must always be given, even if the patient has no history of thrombosis).

Treatment is planned in special care units

- Start prophylactic treatment with LMWH after confirming the pregnancy, or at the latest on weeks 16–18, following up the activated partial thromboplastin time (APTT). Mini-heparin treatment is not sufficient! Continue antithrombotic therapy for 6 weeks after parturition; however, at the time of delivery the drug can be changed to oral warfarin, which is contraindicated during pregnancy. The risk of thrombosis is highest at the end of the pregnancy, and higher doses of LMWH are often used.
- The initiation of heparin treatment depends on the risk: in women who have had thromboembolism during an earlier pregnancy or on oral contraceptives the treatment should always be started on week 24 at the latest.
- Prophylactic treatment in patients with Factor V deficiency (APC resistance):
  - Heterozygotes who have not had a thrombosis: prophylactic treatment is recommended only in cases of caesarean section or immobilization.
  - Heterozygotes who have had a thrombosis: prophylactic treatment is recommended during pregnancy and puerperium
  - Homozygotes: prophylactic treatment is recommended regardless of whether the patient has had a thrombosis or not.

Thrombocytopenia and thrombosis as complications of heparin treatment

- Early thrombocytopenia is benign and caused by aggregation of thrombocytes.
- Severe immunologically mediated thrombocytopenia leads to activation of thrombocytes and endothelial damage, causing arterial thrombi. This complication occurs more often with ordinary heparin than with LMW heparin.
- Symptoms are caused by arterial thrombosis during weeks 1–3 of the treatment.
- The laboratory finding is a clear decrease in the thrombocyte count (or a value below 100 in one measurement).

- In the follow-up of heparin treatment, haemoglobin and thrombocyte values should be taken at 1-week intervals for 4 weeks.

References

1. Hull RD, Brant RF, Pineo GF, Stein PD, Raskob GE, Valentine KA. Preoperative vs postoperative initiation of low-molecular-weight hepatin prophylaxis against venous thromboembolism in patients undergoing elective hip replacement. Archives of Internal Medicine 1999;159:137–141.
2. The Database of Abstracts of Reviews of Effectiveness (University of York), Database no.: DARE-998406. In: The Cochrane Library, Issue 3, 2000. Oxford: Update Software.
3. Amaragiri SV, Lees TA. Elastic compression stockings for prevention of deep vein thrombosis. Cochrane Database Syst Rev. 2004;(2):CD001484.
4. Wells PS, Lensing AW, Hirsh J. Graduated compression stockings in the prevention of postoperative venous thromboembolism: a meta-analysis. Arch Intern Med 1994;154:67–72.
5. The Database of Abstracts of Reviews of Effectiveness (University of York), Database no.: DARE-948033. In: The Cochrane Library, Issue 4, 1999. Oxford: Update Software.
6. Agu O, Hamilton G, Baker D. Graduated compression stockings in the prevention of venous thromboembolism. British Journal of Surgery 1999;86:992–1004.
7. The Database of Abstracts of Reviews of Effectiveness (University of York), Database no.: DARE-991642. In: The Cochrane Library, Issue 1, 2001. Oxford: Update Software.
8. Handoll HHG, Farrar MJ, McBirnie J, Tytherleigh-Strong G, Awal KA, Milne AA, Gillespie WJ. Prophylaxis using heparin, low molecular weight heparin and physical methods against deep vein thrombosis (DVT) and pulmonary embolism (PE) in hip fracture surgery. The Cochrane Database of Systematic Reviews, Cochrane Library number: CD000305. In: The Cochrane Library, Issue 2, 2002. Oxford: Update Software. Updated frequently.
9. Efficacy and safety of low molecular weight heparin, unfractionated heparin and warfarin for thrombo-embolism prophylaxis in orthopaedic surgery: a meta-analysis of randomised clinical trials. Haemostasis 1997;27:75–84.
10. The Database of Abstracts of Reviews of Effectiveness (University of York), Database no.: DARE-973598. In: The Cochrane Library, Issue 4, 1999. Oxford: Update Software.
11. Howard AW, Aaron SD. Low molecular weight heparin decreases proximal and distal deep venous thrombosis following total knee arthroplasty: a meta-analysis of randomized trials. Thrombosis and Haemostasis 1998;79:902–906.
12. The Database of Abstracts of Reviews of Effectiveness (University of York), Database no.: DARE-983696. In: The Cochrane Library, Issue 2, 2000. Oxford: Update Software.
13. Hull RD et al. Extended out-of-hospital low-molecular-weight heparin prophylaxis against deep venous thrombosis in patients after elective hip arthroplasty. Ann Intern Med 2001;135:858–869.
14. Berqvist D, Agnelli G, Cohen A, Eldor A, Nilsson PE, Le Moigne-Amrani A, Dietrich-Neto F for the ENOXAN II Investigators. Duration of prophylaxis against venous thromboembolism with enoxaparin after surgery for cancer. N Engl J Med 2002;346:975–980.
15. Antiplatelet Trialists' Collaboration. Collaborative review of randomised trials of antiplatelet therapy - III: Reduction in venous thrombosis and pulmonary embolism by antiplatelet prophylaxis among surgical and medical patients. BMJ 1994;308:235–246.
16. The Database of Abstracts of Reviews of Effectiveness (University of York), Database no.: DARE-948030. In: The Cochrane Library, Issue 4, 1999. Oxford: Update Software.
17. Garces K, Mamdani M. Fondaparinux for post-operative venous thrombosis prophylaxis. Ottawa: Canadian Coordinating Office for Health Technology Assessment (CCOHTA). 2002. 4. Canadian Coordinating Office for Health Technology Assessment (CCOHTA). www.ccohta.ca.
18. Health Technology Assessment Database: HTA-20020900. The Cochrane Library, Issue 1, 2004. Chichester, UK: John Wiley & Sons, Ltd.
19. Fondaparinux for venous thromboembolism. Birmingham: National Horizon Scanning Centre (NHSC). 2001. 5. National Horizon Scanning Centre (NHSC).
20. Health Technology Assessment Database: HTA-20020849. The Cochrane Library, Issue 1, 2004. Chichester, UK: John Wiley & Sons, Ltd.

5.43 Pulmonary embolism (PE)

Markku Ellonen

Aims

- Suspect PE readily and make the diagnosis rapidly as this is a common, insidious and severe condition that requires treatment.
- Recognize the different clinical patterns of PE: acute massive and sub-acute embolism.
- Identifying patients at risk is important for both diagnosis and prophylaxis.
- Use the D-dimer test to exclude PE (in low-risk patients this is the only test needed).
- Start anticoagulation with low-molecular-weight heparin (LMWH) readily on the basis of clinical suspicion. Verify the diagnosis and avoid over-diagnosis

Predisposing factors for PE and deep venous thrombosis (DVT)

- One or more **important** predisposing factors are found in 80–90% of patients with PE. The presence of risk factors aids the clinician in making a correct diagnosis. Risk factors may also guide decision-making when the results of tests are contradictory or difficult to interpret. PE occurs seldom without a predisposing cause:

- Immobilization from different causes: surgery, severe cardiac disease, disabling diseases. Risk increases with age.
- Pelvic and abdominal surgery. Hip and knee surgery. Obesity and age increase the risk. Prophylaxis is often indicated.
- Myocardial infarction and heart failure
- Malignant diseases: particularly abdominal and pelvic neoplasms but also others when metastatic
- Pregnancy, early puerperium and operative delivery
- Lower limb problems: fractures, varicose veins, paralysis or plastercast. Even a compression bandage around the knee may cause distal DVT
- Previous DVT and PE
- Thrombophilia

♦ Minor risk factors include
- Oral contraception in an otherwise healthy under 40-year-old woman has been shown to be a smaller risk than what has been suspected. Thrombophilia increases the risk slightly, but not enough to warrant systematic screening.
- Hormone replacement therapy in an otherwise healthy woman
- Long flights when no other risk factors are present.

Clinical features

♦ The diagnosis of acute and massive PE is often obvious in the absence of other diseases and in the presence of risk factors.
- The diagnosis is made easier by the presence of the following symptoms: hypotension, syncope, shock, anoxia, elevated venous pressure

♦ Embolism presenting as isolated dyspnoea is more difficult to diagnose.
- The initial dyspnoea subsides rapidly, and exertion dyspnoea is common and unspecific.

♦ In elderly patients with several diseases even a small embolus may aggravate the symptoms of the underlying disease.
- Diagnosis is difficult to reach if the symptoms match the underlying disease: e.g. chronic heart failure, aggravation of coronary artery disease, or even worsening of dementia as the result of cerebral ischaemia.

Symptoms and signs

♦ The most common clinical features in descending frequency (from 70% to 10%) are: dyspnoea, tachypnoea (over 20/min), pleuritic pain, fearfulness, tachycardia, cough, haemoptysis, and clinical DVT. Unfortunately, the findings with high specificity have low sensitivity and vice versa. The symptoms, even in combination, are of limited value in making a positive diagnosis. However, PE is very unlikely in the absence of the first three common symptoms: dyspnoea, tachypnoea (over 20/min) and pleuritic pain (3%). If chest x-ray and pO_2 are also normal, the diagnosis of PE is virtually excluded.

♦ Dyspnoea of varying severity is the most important clinical sign. In mild cases it is present at first transiently during rest and later on only during exercise. The patient may describe it as a dramatic fall in fitness. Sudden-onset dyspnoea in patients at risk should always be suspected as PE.

♦ Dyspnoea is often associated with tachypnoea and tachycardia.

♦ Chest pain may simulate myocardial infarction, pericarditis, pneumothorax and pleuropneumonia. However, the pain may be mild or even absent.

♦ Cough and mild fever simulate pulmonary infections.

♦ Haemoptysis is uncommon (approx. 10%).

♦ Clinical DVT is often absent, especially in bedridden patients. Venography has been normal in up to 30% of patients with angiographically verified PE. Nor does a normal ultrasound finding exclude embolism.

♦ Auscultation of lungs and chest x-ray are usually normal. Tachypnoea may be present. Atelectasis is often seen in the lower parts of the lungs after surgery of the upper abdomen.

♦ Jugular vein engorgement is associated with massive PE. The patient is hypotensive and may faint in the sitting position.

♦ Worsening of the basic severe cardiopulmonary disease may be the only apparent symptom of PE. Here correct diagnosis is difficult.

Clinical probability of pulmonary embolism

♦ In the evaluation of probability the clinician should consider predisposing factors, possibility of different clinical manifestations and found or absent symptoms. The **basic tests** listed below are non-specific and are often performed to exclude other conditions with similar symptoms. After their exclusion the probability of PE can be classified as high, moderate or low. This information should be used when the results of the **perfusion scan** are interpreted, particularly when the result of the scan is not obvious.

D-dimer in plasma

♦ D-dimer in plasma is used for exclusion of venous thrombosis and PE.
- D-dimer depicts fibrinolysis and due to its unspecific nature it is useful only when it is negative C [1 2].
- The test can be used for exclusion. Its sensitivity in pulmonary embolism is 97–99% but for hospitalised patients its sensitivity may not be as good.
  - A thrombus that is small in size or fresh does not release measurable amounts of degradation products. This may sometimes cause false negative test results.
  - If D-dimer is positive or the clinical probability of PE is high, referral to hospital is necessary.
- D-dimer is suitable for use in primary care health centres (requires centrifugation of blood sample quickly). A point of care test is also available.

Basic tests

- The chest x-ray is normal in simple PE. However, it is extremely valuable in excluding other diseases such as pneumonia, pneumothorax, heart failure, etc. The chest x-ray is needed for interpretation of subsequent pulmonary scans. More common (but non-specific) findings in PE are focal infiltration, atelectasis, a raised diaphragm and pleural effusion. The classic wedge-shaped opacity is rare, but significant when present. The x-ray is often of poor quality in acutely dyspnoeic patients. A normal chest x-ray in a breathless and hypoxic patient should always arouse suspicion of PE! The x-ray is necessary for the interpretation of the perfusion scan.
- The ECG is in most cases normal or reveals abnormalities due to other concurrent disease. The ECG is important in excluding myocardial infarction, myopericarditis, etc. Severe right heart strain may cause non-specific changes in the ST-segment and/or T-wave and long-term embolism may turn the axis to the right. Hypoxia may worsen myocardial ischaemia and the ECG may resemble coronary artery disease (Figure 5.43.1).
- Arterial pO_2 is a quick and easy initial test when available. p_aO_2 is lowered and p_aCO_2 is lowered as the result of hyperventilation. (When these findings are present together, they strongly suggest PE). $p_aO_2 < 9$ kPa is a significant finding. Remember that obesity commonly reduces pO_2. Giving oxygen affects the result for 15 min after discontinuation. A normal result means that a massive embolus is unlikely. However, blood gas values may be normal in otherwise healthy patients even with a moderate embolus. Normal values do therefore not exclude PE or remove the need for further investigations. Oxygen saturation below 90–92% measured by pulse oximetry supports the diagnosis of PE (and suggests severe embolism).

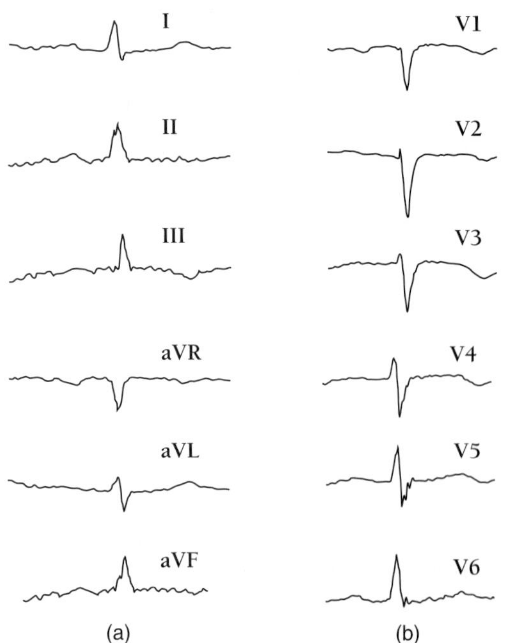

Figure 5.43.1 Massive pulmonary embolism in an orthopaedic patient despite LMWH-prophylaxis. Systolic blood pressure barely 100 mmHg and PSO2 < 90%. ECG shows tachycardia, T inversions in leads V1–V4 and s1 Q3 T3.

Spiral tomography

- Shows pulmonary arteries more directly and is more specific than perfusion scanning
- Does not reveal (and thus does not exclude) small peripheral emboli.
- Requires patient cooperation.

Perfusion scanning

- Perfusion scanning is the most important non-invasive investigation, which should be available in acute hospitals. Normal finding excludes PE.
- It should be performed within 24 hours which makes it an emergency investigation.
- Ventilation imaging may improve the diagnostic accuracy of perfusion scanning. The additional benefit is limited, which is why perfusion scan alone is acceptable.
- A current, good quality chest x-ray is necessary for interpretation.
- Direct communication between clinician and radiologist is important as the scan often contains findings that are unspecific and difficult to interpret. The clinical significance of these findings is determined by the probability of PE. An uncertain finding on the perfusion scan warrants further investigations (ultrasonography, spiral tomography).
- Interpretation of lung scans may be difficult for several reasons: previous PE, heart failure, atelectases, COPD, lung fibrosis, scars or tumour.

Pulmonary angiography

- Used only rarely as the examination is invasive and not widely available and the interpretation requires special skills.
- Angiography is indicated if reaching the correct diagnosis is urgent and the other investigations fail to provide a diagnosis.
- Considered the golden standard of PE diagnostics. Yet, interpretation is difficult and even between experienced specialists the discrepancy can be up to 20%.

Other investigations

- Leg vein imaging is a first-line investigation in decision-making when PE is suspected. When positive it confirms venous thromboembolism. However, 30% of patients with PE have normal venograms.
- Echocardiography can confirm the diagnosis of massive PE and at the same time exclude cardiac diseases in differential

diagnosis. Signs of elevated pulmonary pressure are found: enlarged right ventricle and tricuspid valve regurgitation.

Differential diagnosis

- Symptoms of PE are non-specific and similar features are seen in myocardial infarction, heart failure, myopericarditis, pneumothorax, pleuropneumonia, septic shock and other hypotensive conditions.
- Atelectases seen in the lower fields of the lungs, which are common after upper abdominal surgery, may cause difficulties in interpreting chest x-rays and pulmonary scans.
- In practice it is important to distinguish primary hyperventilation syndrome (HVS) from pulmonary embolism, as PE easily causes secondary hyperventilation. In HVS oxygen concentration is high and CO_2 is low. In PE the concentrations of both oxygen and CO_2 are lowered. With smaller emboli the PaO_2 is often normal.

Management of suspected pulmonary embolism

- A negative D-dimer practically excludes PE and is nowadays the primary screening method.
- If the D-dimer test is positive, the next investigations are usually ultrasonography of the lower limb veins or venography.
    - If the result is positive, treatment is started.
    - If the result is negative, the next investigations are spiral tomography or perfusion scan.
- If the perfusion scan is normal or near normal massive PE is excluded. If the scan contains several wedge-like areas of low perfusion, heparinization and anticoagulation is indicated without further examination.
- About half of all scans are interpreted as non-diagnostic or low-probability. The scan shows basal areas of low perfusion and the chest x-ray shows minor opacity or venous congestion. The reliability of the scan can be improved by combining ventilation scanning to it. This is done automatically if the x-ray shows opacity. The finding suggests PE, if the low perfusion area of the perfusion scan is not seen in the ventilation scan.
- If perfusion scan is the first investigation and the result is uncertain, continue by compression ultrasound or venography. If a thrombus is found, PE is probable and anticoagulation is started. If a thrombus is not found and PE is still suspected, spiral tomography is indicated. If this investigation is not available, the patient can be followed up and perfusion scan and compression ultrasound or venography can be repeated. If compression ultrasound or venography is normal, the risk of re-embolism is small.
- If the patient initially presents with a cardiovascular collapse, begin investigations with echocardiography (RV dilatation suggests severe PE).
- Instead of a perfusion scan, start investigations with venography or ultrasound when the suspicion of a thrombus is strong. If the findings are obvious, begin anticoagulation.

Treatment

- Important and absolutely necessary. Untreated embolism often recurs and may be fatal. There is no international concensus of the treatment of DVT limited to the calf that usually does not release an embolus, although 25% of these distal emboli rise to the level of the thigh. In practice many smaller emboli and distal DVT remain without diagnosis and without therapy and cause no damage.
- In the treatment of PE low-molecular weight (LMW) heparin has taken the place of i.v. heparin.
    - Enoxaparin 1 mg/kg twice daily, dalteparin 100 IU/kg twice daily.
- Warfarin is started at the same time with heparin. Heparin is discontinued in most cases after five days when the INR (TT, SA) has been in the therapeutic range for a few days. Anticoagulation does not dissolve emboli, but it prevents recurrences.
- Thrombolytic therapy is used in life-threatening massive PE. Recently thrombolytic therapy has been used also for submassive embolism when haemodynamics is still normal. The therapy accelerates the clearing of emboli and may reduce mortality. The risk of bleeding must be taken into consideration. If the patient does not show signs of right ventricular dysfunction thrombolysis should not be given unless haemodynamics are impaired due to existing heart or lung disease. Thrombolysis has replaced embolectomy; however, embolectomy may be indicated if thrombolysis fails or is contraindicated. Thrombolytic therapy does not require angiography or a central catheter. The treatment time is longer than in myocardial infarction (alteplase 100 mg/2 hours i.v.).
- The duration of anticoagulation is 3 months or less (5.44) if the risk factor is temporary. If the cause of PE remains unidentified, the therapy is continued for at least 6 months. In recurrences and when the underlying cause persists, anticoagulation therapy is long-term or lifelong.
- In pregnancy, warfarin is usually contraindicated and can be replaced with heparin (LMWH).
- The patient must have a personal anticoagulation card stating the diagnosis, INR range and duration of therapy.

Prophylaxis

- See 5.42
- Inferior vena cava (IVC) filters may be used in acute situations where anticoagulation fails or is contraindicated.

References

1. Becker D, Philbrick J, Bachhuber T, Humphries J. D-dimer testing and acute venous thromboembolism. Arch Intern Med 1996;156:939–946.

2. The Database of Abstracts of Reviews of Effectiveness (University of York), Database no.: DARE-968209. In: The Cochrane Library, Issue 4, 1999. Oxford: Update Software.

5.44 Oral anticoagulation therapy

Editors

Basic rules

- Anticoagulants act by interfering with various coagulation factors. However, in the follow-up, mainly factor VII is measured.
- Factor VII decreases to the therapeutic level in 2 days, although a real therapeutic response is obtained only after 5–7 days. Therefore, when anticoagulant therapy is acutely required, heparin and warfarin must be used concomitantly.
- Heparin is discontinued when warfarin has been at the therapeutic level for 2 days.

How to begin warfarin treatment

- See Table 5.44.1.
- Starting dose of warfarin treatment can be chosen from two alternatives
  - In an acute thrombosis give the patient heparin concomitantly with 10 mg of warfarin daily for 3 days (for the aged, small-sized and patients with a liver disease 5 mg). An estimate of the maintenance dose of warfarin should be made on the 4th day by defining INR which gives directions for the dosage of warfarin for days 4, 5 and 6.
  - It is recommended, especially in outpatient care, to start the treatment with the estimated maintenance dose (3–6 mg /day according to age, condition of the liver, diet etc.).
- A small starting dose (5 mg) is safe also in outpatient care, as it does not decrease the protein C concentration of the natural anticoagulant as rapidly as the 10 mg dose. The risk of skin necrosis, which is a rare condition associated with the onset of warfarin therapy, is lower when a small starting dose is used. Achieving efficient anticoagulation does not take significantly longer than with the above-given higher doses.

Table 5.44.1 Starting, maintaining and adjusting anticoagulant treatment according to INR values in average-sized adults (target: INR 2.0–3.0) without diseases or medications affecting the anticoagulant dose. However, the response to anticoagulant treatment varies individually and must be adjusted individually according to repeated INR measurements (sources: Andrew et al. 1994 and Dartnell et al. 1995).

Day	INR	Dose[1]
1	–	10 (5)[2]
2	–	10 (5)
3	<2.0	10 (5)
	2.0–2.4	5 (2.5)
	2.5–2.9	3 (1.5)
	3.0–3.4	2.5 (interval day or 1.5)
	3.5–4.0	1.5 (interval day)
	>4.0	Interval day (interval day)
4–6	<1.4	10 (5)
	1.4–1.9	7.5 (3)
	2.0–2.4	5 (2.5)
	2.5–2.9	4.5 (1.5)
	3.0–3.9	3 (1.5)
	4.0–4.5	Interval day, then 1.5 mg (Interval day, then 1.5 mg)
	>4.5	2 interval days, then 1.5 mg (2 interval days, then 1.5 mg)
7–	1.1–1.4	Increase weekly dose by 20%
	1.5–1.9	Increase weekly dose by 10%
	2.0–3.0	Same weekly dose
	3.1–4.0	Decrease weekly dose by 10%
	>4.5	Interval, until INR < 4.5, continue with a dose reduced by 20%

1. In elderly and frail patients and patients with INR spontaneously > 1.2, the starting dose is 5 mg and INR is measured already on the 3rd day. (This is why INR is mentioned also for day 3.)
2. Treatment is currently often started with 5 mg instead of 10 mg. This halved dosing is shown in parentheses.

Interactions

- Resins (cholestyramine, colestipol) interfere with the absorption of oral anticoagulants.
- The bleeding risk increases with concomitant use of acetylsalicylic acid (ASA) that has an irreversible effect on thrombocyte function; the effect of other non-steroidal anti-inflammatory drugs is reversible and they may be used concomitantly. Usually, ASA is contraindicated during warfarin therapy, but in certain situations the combination is used when intensive anticoagulation is needed (valvular prostheses, pulmonary embolism that recurs during anticoagulant therapy).
- Enzyme induction, inhibition and binding to plasma proteins cause various interactions that warrant follow-up of the therapeutic level of anticoagulation. The most common drugs and diseases that affect the anticoagulant therapy are mentioned in the following list.

Increased anticoagulation

- Aspirin (thrombocyte inhibition)
- Temporary heavy use of alcohol
- Allopurinol
- Quinidine, amiodarone
- Clofibrate, gemfibrozil and some statins
- Metronidazole, and several other antibiotics together with the illness connected to their use.
- Tamoxifen, toremifen
- Trimethoprim-sulfamethoxazole, wide-spectrum antibiotics, miconazole

- Infections, traumas, liver disease, heart failure, malabsorption, catabolism, frail elderly patient.

Decreased anticoagulation

- Cholestyramine
- Carbamazepine, phenytoin
- Rifampicin
- Vitamin K and a vegetarian diet

Indications for oral anticoagulation

- Deep venous thrombosis, prevention of deep venous thrombosis in selected cases (5.42)
- Pulmonary embolism
- Atrial fibrillation in selected cases (4.46) A [1,2,3].
- Cardioversion when atrial fibrillation has lasted over 2 days
- Valvular prostheses (4.12)
- Mitral stenosis
- Acute (anterior wall) myocardial infarction (3 months)
- Severe heart failure D [4]
- TIA in selected cases, if aspirin (dipyridamole) is not effective enough (36.30)
- Hereditary predisposition to thrombosis and previous thrombosis (5.41)
- In progressive stroke (36.30), unstable angina pectoris (4.58) and prevention of deep venous thrombosis low-molecular-weight heparin is used. In long-term prevention of venous thrombosis heparin can be replaced by warfarin.

Contraindications for anticoagulation

- Recent massive stroke (unless it is an indication!)  [5], (36.31)
- Uncontrolled hypertension
- Hepatic cirrhosis, oesophageal varices
- Recent ulcer, colitis, cancer in the gastrointestinal tract
- Pregnancy. The highest risk is during weeks 6–12. Thereafter the contraindication is not absolute. Pregnancy must not begin during warfarin therapy.
- Bleeding tendency; thrombocytopenia.
- Low patient compliance (e.g. alcoholism, dementia)
- In an elderly patient: tendency to fall.

Duration of the treatment

- See Table 5.44.2.
- The above recommendations do not deal with the intensity of the anticoagulant therapy, which has a major impact on the risk of complications.
- In recurrent thromboembolism the duration of the treatment may be shorter than those listed above if there is a clear predisposing factor: surgery, trauma, childbirth, immobilization, etc. If there were no predisposing factors, the treatment should be long lasting (or even permanent).

Table 5.44.2 Duration of anticoagulant therapy is determined individually with the anticipated success of therapy, the patient's other illnesses and age as well as the risk of recurrence being the decisive factors.

Indication	Duration of therapy
First episode of thrombosis and a transient or modifiable predisposing factor (surgery, trauma, bed rest, oestrogen therapy)	3–6 months
First episode of thrombosis without a predisposing factor	At least 6 months
First episode of thrombosis in a patient with cancer, cardiolipin antibodies, combined coagulation disorder, homozygous Factor V Leiden or prothrombin gene mutation.	12 months to lifetime
Recurring thrombosis without a predisposing factor or in association with increased coagulability of blood.	Lifetime

Intensity of the treatment

- See Table 5.44.3.
- An intensive therapeutic level (INR 4.5–3) is warranted in patients with valvular prostheses (especially mitral valve). The alternative is normal therapy (INR 3–2) and aspirin 100 mg daily.
- Intensive therapy is indicated when the treatment of pulmonary embolism or venous thrombus above the knee is initiated.
- An intensive therapeutic level is maintained for a long time in recurrent venous thrombosis.
- The normal therapeutic level is sufficient in atrial fibrillation (Table 5.44.3). Patients with lower risk (no heart insufficiency, no valvular diseases, no previous emboli) have traditionally had a lower therapeutic level, but its efficacy has not been established. Instead of warfarin, low-risk patients can be treated with aspirin (4.46).

Controls

- Initiation, maintenance and corrections, see Table 5.44.1.
- First at 2–3 day intervals, then once a week until a steady therapeutic level has been reached.

Table 5.44.3 Therapeutic INR range

Indication	INR range
Prevention and treatment of venous thrombosis or pulmonary embolism	2.0–3.0
Prevention of systemic embolism	
- Chronic atrial fibrillation	2.0–3.0
- Mechanical prosthetic valve	2.5–3.5

- Later on once every 1–2 months, unless a new medication is added to the therapy or there are significant changes in the medication or health of the patient. Follow-up is needed in situations where the liver function changes. The amount of vitamin K in diet should not vary much.
- If the indication for the treatment is important, low-molecular-weight heparin (LMWH) should be added to warfarin temporarily if the treatment level can not be maintained; fresh pulmonary embolism and mitral valve prosthesis.

Temporary reduction of anticoagulant dosage

- During surgery or biopsies the dosage is often reduced (to the upper limits of the therapeutic range, INR around 1.5) according to the extent of surgery and indication for anticoagulant therapy. Note in the referral the indication for anticoagulation, and the possibility and method of reducing the medication. Reduction of the dose is not necessary if haemostasis is easily accomplished, e.g. in cases of tooth extraction.
- In major surgery, warfarin is discontinued 4 days before the operation which results is an INR level of <1.5 during the operation. If the risk of thrombosis is high, LMWH in treatment doses is given after surgery.
- Warfarin treatment in scheduled surgery and endoscopic biopsies
  - Determine INR one week before the planned operation.
  - Decide whether discontinuing anticoagulant therapy is necessary (see above).
  - If anticoagulant therapy is discontinued, stop warfarin 1–5 days before surgery.
    - If the patient has a particularly high risk of thromboembolism, give LMWH subcutaneously at therapeutic doses. The effect of heparin can be followed up by measuring FXa inhibition where the target treatment level is 0.3–0.7 anti-FXa activity units/ml.
    - The pause in warfarin therapy depends on the INR value. Discontinue warfarin before an operation:
      - 5 days earlier if INR > 4
      - 3–4 days earlier if INR = 3–4
      - 2 days earlier if INR = 2–3.
  - INR should be determined in the evening prior to a major operation. If the value is over 1.8, give 0.5–1.0 mg of phytomenadione (vitamin K1).
    - On the day of the operation, consider whether an infusion of unfractionated heparin or a prophylactic dose of LMW heparin is necessary.
    - If the patient has received heparin subcutaneously, continue the treatment for 5–7 days simultaneously with warfarin therapy.
  - Start warfarin therapy at the maintenance dose after minor surgery in the evening of the day of operation, and after major surgery on the day when the patient receives nutrition orally.
- **In patients with valvular prostheses, do not interrupt anticoagulant therapy or even reduce the dose in normal cases!**
- During pregnancy use heparin at least during the first trimester. In mid- and end-pregnancy warfarin may be used when considered necessary, particularly in patients with a valve prosthesis. Warfarin is teratogenic. Its use varies in different countries. Before delivery, warfarin is replaced by heparin.

Thrombosis despite warfarin treatment

- The most common cause (30%) is a too small dose (INR below treatment level).
- Cancers can cause such strong predisposition to thrombosis that warfarin may not be effective. Treatment in such cases is LMWH in two injections.
- Antiphospholipid antibody syndrome does not respond to warfarin.
- Idiopathic thromboses that have occurred for no reason are more likely to recur. Antiphospholipid antibody syndrome or cancer can be the cause. LMWH is an option to warfarin in such cases.

Complications

- The risk of bleeding is at least fivefold higher during warfarin therapy. The risk is greatest in the beginning of the treatment.
- Intensive treatment, old age, other diseases, and drugs that cause gastrointestinal haemorrhage increase the risk of bleeding.
- When the indication for anticoagulation is relative (e.g. benign atrial fibrillation with no embolism) the therapeutic level can be maintained at the upper limit of the therapeutic range.

Treatment of bleeding complications

- Local haemostasis
- Vitamin K: small dose for patients with valvular prosthesis: 1 mg, i.m. Effect begins only after 8 hours.
- Fresh frozen plasma or a coagulation factor.

References

1. Koudstaal P. Anticoagulants for preventing stroke in patients with nonrheumatic atrial fibrillation and a history of stroke or transient ischemic attacks. The Cochrane Database of Systematic Reviews, Cochrane Library number: CD000185. In: The Cochrane Library, Issue 2, 2002. Oxford: Update Software. Updated frequently.
2. EAFT Study Group. Secondary prevention in nonrheumatic atrial fibrillation after transient ischaemic attack or minor stroke. Lancet 1993;342:1255–1262.
3. Koudstaal PJ. Anticoagulants versus antiplatelet therapy for preventing stroke in patients with nonrheumatic atrial

fibrillation and a history of stroke or transient ischemic attacks. Cochrane Database Syst Rev. 2004;(2):CD000187.
4. Lip GYH, Gibbs CR. Anticoagulation for heart failure in sinus rhythm. Cochrane Database Syst Rev. 2004;(2): CD003336.
5. Sandercock P, Mielke O, Liu M, Counsell C. Anticoagulants for preventing recurrence following presumed non-cardioembolic ischaemic stroke or transient ischaemic attack. Cochrane Database Syst Rev. 2004;(2):CD000248.

5.50 Conservative treatment of leg ulcers

Ken Malanin

Differential diagnosis

- About 90% of leg ulcers are caused by vascular diseases:
  - Venous
  - Venous and arterial
  - Arterial
  - Diabetic
  - Vasculitic
  - Hypertensive
- The venous and arterial circulation of lower extremities should be evaluated: If the pulses of dorsal pedal and posterior tibial arteries cannot be felt, record the ankle-brachial systolic blood pressure index (ABI) of these arteries. ABI is normally 1 or more. ABI less than 0.8 is clearly reduced. The ABI might be misleadingly high, especially in diabetics, because of sclerosis of the arteries. There are dozens of rare causes of ulcers. For example, do not forget e.g. skin malignancies.
- Compression therapy is the most important treatment of venous leg ulcers A [1 2 3 4 5].
- Ulcers caused by arterial insufficiency should be referred to a vascular surgeon.

Reduction of leg oedema in venous ulcer

- Elevation of leg
- Compression bandages and stockings A [1 2 3 4 5]
  - Short-stretch elastic bandages can be worn 24 hours a day. They are only removed for dressing changes.
  - Compression stockings (compression class 2 to 3)
- Intermittent pneumatic compression treatment (5.53)
- After the ulcer has healed, compression stockings should be used permanently if the underlying venous disease cannot be corrected C [6].

General management

- Correction of anaemia
- Proper treatment of diabetes
- Proper treatment of cardiac insufficiency
- Improvement of peripheral circulation (pentoxifyllin may be effective B [7])
- Deep infections and ulcers infected by beta haemolytic streptococci should be treated by systemic antibiotics (13.20) (23.44)

Topical treatment

- The aim is to remove any dead tissue and purulent exudate to create optimal healing conditions for the ulcer.

Ulcers with black necrosis

- Bathing to soften necrosis
- Surgical debridement D [8 9]
- Topical enzyme therapy D [8 9]
  - streptokinase/streptodornase solution or gel
  - clostridiopeptidase ointment
- Softening gels

Ulcers with slough

- Bathing to soften slough
- Mechanical cleansing D [8 9]
- Hydrocolloid paste + sheet
- Topical enzyme therapy
- Softening gels

Ulcers which are infected and suppurate

- Antiseptic baths
- Mechanical cleansing D [8 9]
- Moist dressings: Physiological saline, silver nitrate solution of 0.01 to 0.1%, zinc sulphate solution of 0.25%
- Iodine containing polysaccharide products
- Activated charcoal dressings
- Alginates

To be remembered in local treatment

- Use products with low sensitizing potential, because the development of allergic contact dermatitis is common among leg ulcer patients.
- Before mechanical cleansing, a painful ulcer can be anaesthetized using lidocaine gel or lidocain/prilocain cream B [10].

References

1. Cullum N, Nelson EA, Fletcher AW, Sheldon TA. Compression for venous leg ulcers. Cochrane Database Syst Rev. 2004;(2):CD000265.

2. Palfreyman SJ, Lochiel R, Michaels JA. A systematic review of compression therapy for venous leg ulcers. Vascular Medicine 1998;3:301–313.
3. The Database of Abstracts of Reviews of Effectiveness (University of York), Database no.: DARE-993749. In: The Cochrane Library, Issue 1, 2001. Oxford: Update Software.
4. Peters J. A review of the factors influencing nonrecurrence of venous leg ulcers. J Clin Nurs 1998;7:3–9.
5. The Database of Abstracts of Reviews of Effectiveness (University of York), Database no.: DARE-985381. In: The Cochrane Library, Issue 2, 2000. Oxford: Update Software.
6. Nelson EA, Bell-Syer SEM, Cullum NA. Compression for preventing recurrence of venous ulcers. Cochrane Database Syst Rev. 2004;(2):CD002303.
7. Jull AB, Waters J, Arroll B. Pentoxifylline for treating venous leg ulcers. Cochrane Database Syst Rev. 2004;(2): CD001733.
8. Bradley M, Cullum N, Sheldon T. The debridement of chronic wounds: a systematic review. Health Technology Assessment 1999;3:1–78.
9. The Database of Abstracts of Reviews of Effectiveness (University of York), Database no.: DARE-999770. In: The Cochrane Library, Issue 2, 2001. Oxford: Update Software.
10. Briggs M, Nelson EA. Topical agents or dressings for pain in venous leg ulcers. Cochrane Database Syst Rev. 2004;(2):CD001177.

5.52 Pinch grafting of the skin

Editors

Basic rules

- Pinch grafting is defined as the grafting of small pieces of superficial skin on a wound. It is a simple and effective treatment for venous leg ulcers, provided that the leg can be prevented from swelling by using compression stockings after the grafting.
- Other physicians in addition to surgeons can use this technique. It is suitable for patients who fail to respond to conservative treatment but who are not eligible for plastic surgery.
- The procedure is not difficult to perform; however, the physician should have seen how the procedure is carried out and how the wound is dressed.
- The procedure can be performed on ambulatory patients if aftercare can be given at home.

Technique

1. Clean the wound and the donor site (usually on the thigh) with antiseptic dressings (e.g. chlorhexidine).
2. Infiltrate the skin with an adrenaline-containing local anaesthetic.
3. Pinch the skin with an injection needle and cut a small piece intradermally with a straight scalpel using sawing movements. An assistant places the grafts on the wound (Figure 5.52.1).
4. Place a greasy mesh dressing on the grafts and apply an antibacterial ointment on the dressing, simultaneously compressing the grafts gently. The next layer should be a piece of cotton cloth, then polyester wool, a bandage, tube gauze, and a tension bandage. Cover the donor site with a greasy mesh dressing, gauze, and adhesive dressing.
5. The patient should stay mostly in bed with the leg raised for 2–3 days. The dressings on the grafting site should be removed on day 7 and those of the donor site on day 14. The epithelialization of the wound is complete in about one month if the treatment was successful.

Further treatment

- Because pinch grafting does not cure the underlying cause of leg ulcers it is mandatory that the swelling of the leg is treated before the procedure and that the patient is able to prevent swelling until venous surgery has been performed surgically. If surgery is not performed the patient must wear compressive dressings or stockings for the rest of his/her life.

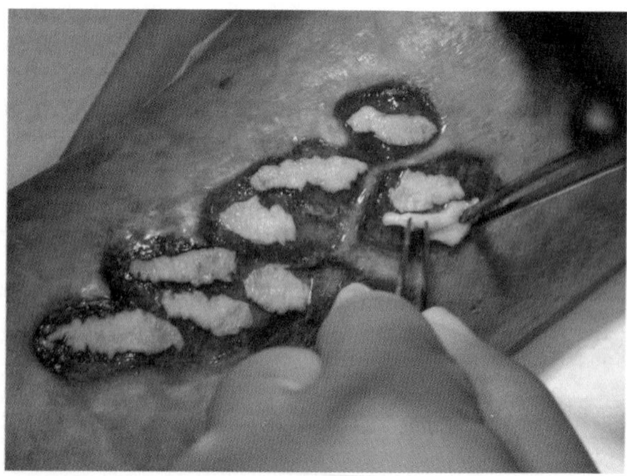

Figure 5.52.1 The swellings associated with a venous leg ulcer have been treated with compression bandages and the ulcerations have been cleaned. Whole-thickness skin grafts taken from the thigh are placed sparsely on the ulcer surface and fixed with a combination of greasy gauze, padding, zinc oxide ointment and bandaging. All the grafts were vital after one week. The swelling were later controlled with custom-made compression stockings. Neglecting this would destroy the whole treatment. Photo © R. Suhonen.

5.53 Intermittent compression for leg swelling

Editors

Basic rules

- Intermittent compression is a suitable treatment for
  - leg swelling and ulcers of venous origin D [1]
  - lymphatic swelling
  - post-traumatic or postoperative swelling.
- A compressive bandage or stocking is usually necessary for a favourable outcome.
- Be careful when treating an ischaemic limb (short compression, low pressure, the patient may not have pain at rest).
- The outcome of treatment can be evaluated by measuring the circumference of the leg and by observing the increase in urine output during treatment.

Lymphatic swelling

- Swelling of the arm in a patient with breast cancer is the most common indication for treatment.
- The duration of treatment is 1–2 hours.
- The maximum pressure is 70–80 mmHg.
- The duration of the filling phase is under 20 s (optimum 12–15 s).
- After treatment, a compression bandage or stocking is placed on the arm.
- Lymphatic massage is an alternative. Proximal lymphatic massage before intermittent compression may be helpful in the treatment of massive lymphatic swelling.

Venous swelling

- Increased venous pressure is caused by valvular insufficiency that raises the capillary pressure and increases capillary filtration, resulting in oedema.
- The duration of treatment is 45–60 min (shorter than for lymphatic swelling).
- The pressure is 50–70 mmHg (lower than for lymphatic swelling).
- The pulse frequency is about 1/s.
- After treatment, a compression bandage or stocking should be applied on the extremity and kept always when the patient is in an upright position. The bandage or stocking can be removed at bedtime.

Post-traumatic or postoperative swelling

- The treatment is the same as for venous swelling.
- If cooling of the extremity is desired simultaneously with intermittent compression, the incoming air tube can be submerged in cold water.

Leg ulcers

- The ulcer should be clean before the treatment is started.
- Treatment can be considered (with systemic antibiotics) even in discharging or necrotic ulcers if the swelling is massive.
- If absorbing gel dressings have been applied on the ulcer they need not be removed during compression treatment.
- If the ulcer is not dressed before the treatment, it should be covered with gauze moistened with saline (not a dry gauze).
- The duration of treatment and the pressure are the same as in venous swelling.
- The treatment is given daily at first, then 5 times a week for the second week, 3 times a week for the next two weeks, and twice during the fourth week.
- After the treatment a compression bandage should be applied or the leg should be kept in a raised position.
- A compression stocking should be used in the meantime. Intermittent compression can be repeated at 1-week intervals at first, and later at 2–4 week intervals or even more frequently if the condition of the skin is impaired.

Atherosclerotic and diabetic ulcers

- The severity of arterial occlusion should be determined before the treatment is started (the ankle pressure, measured with a doppler stethoscope, should exceed 80 mmHg, and the patient should not have ischaemic pain at rest).
- Use a short compression phase (about 12 s) and low pressure (50 mmHg).
- It is important to cover the skin with smooth saline gauze.

Reference

1. Mani R, Vowden K, Nelson EA. Intermittent pneumatic compression for treating venous leg ulcers. Cochrane Database Syst Rev. 2004;(2):CD001899.

5.60 Ischaemic disease of the lower limb

Markku Ellonen

Goals

- Recognize acute limb-threatening ischaemia and refer the patient to hospital immediately.

- Diagnose chronic and critical limb ischaemia. Organize adequate further investigations without delay.
- Confirm the suspicion of peripheral arterial occlusive disease (PAOD) by doppler measurement (5.20).
- Treat co-existing coronary heart disease and prevent stroke. PAOD patients are usually comorbid with generalized atherosclerosis. Their prognosis is not determined by limb ischaemia. Lipid-lowering pharmacotherapy may be useful C [1].

Symptoms and signs of chronic ischaemia

- Intermittent claudication can be defined as limb pain and fatigue on exertion, subsiding at rest after a couple of minutes. Then the patient is able to walk the same distance again.
- Cold feet.
- Pain at night at rest, relieved by walking or by hanging the feet down over the end of the bed.
- Loss of peripheral hair.
- Leriche's syndrome: occlusion of the distal aorta causes weakness of both lower limbs, buttock–thigh claudication and impotence.
- Occlusion of the iliac artery results in thigh–calf claudication. Femoral occlusion leads to calf claudication, and popliteal occlusion to foot claudication.
- Palpation of foot and ankle pulses
  - Explore the dorsalis pedis artery (ADP) and posterior tibial artery (ATP) C [2 3].
  - Oedema may hinder the examination.
  - The physician's own capillar pulse may complicate palpation.
  - Evident pulses in both arteries (ADP and ATP) make significant occlusion improbable.
  - Confirm your findings by doppler measurement (5.20).
- Femoral bruit C [2 3]

Noninvasive management of claudication (chronic ischaemia)

- Smoking cessation C [4 5]
  - The most important single intervention.
  - The symptoms are relieved in 85% of patients and the progression of the disease is delayed.
- Physical exercise A [6 7 8]
  - Inform the patient to walk at least one hour every day.
  - When pain occurs the patient may rest for a moment and then continue walking.
  - Relief of symptoms may be expected in three months.
  - Marked improvement is often not expected in a patient with a claudication who is able to walk less than 50m or with arterial occlusion at iliac level.
- Pharmacological therapy
  - Aspirin 100–250 mg daily. There is no evidence of effect of aspirin in preventing the progression of peripheral vascular disease. But its effect on associated coronary arterial disease is documented. The effect of aspirin after peripheral revascularization is documented A [9 10 11 12 13].
  - Lipid-lowering drugs C [1]. Statins reverse simultaneous coronary artery disease and probably also prevent the progression of PAOD.
  - Clopidogrel or dipyrimadole may replace aspirin in case of allergy or aspirin resistance.
  - Pentoxyfylline is debated. A therapeutic trial at a dose of 400mg three times daily may be justified for several weeks C [14 15].
  - A selective beta blocking agent may not cause adverse effects except in critical ischaemia. A beta blocking agent is often indicated for co-existing coronary artery disease and/or hypertension.
- Local therapy of the feet
  - Especially important in diabetes patients.
  - Injuries and hot or cold baths should be avoided.

Invasive management of chronic ischaemia

- Intermittent claudication is a troublesome complaint but seldom a serious risk. Risks arise from co-existent coronary and cerebral vascular diseases. They determine survival.
- Management of PAOD is at first noninvasive: "stop smoking and keep walking" A [6 7 8].
- Angioplasty is simple and usually effective. Vascular surgery C [16] should be consulted if symptoms worsen. Even minimally symptomatic proximal occlusions may be worth finding and treating by balloon dilatation with C [17 18 19] or without stent replacement. Proximal occlusions are often associated with smoking and distal occlusions with diabetes.
- An aortofemoral Y-prosthesis is efficient and the patency rate over 5 years is above 80% C [20 21].
- About half of femoropopliteal bypasses remain patent after 5 years. The rate is somewhat less in femorotibial bypasses.
- Distal reconstructions are complicated and the patency rate is lower.

Acute limb-threatening ischaemia: symptoms and diagnosis

- The condition may be caused by exacerbation of chronic ischaemia when an atherosclerotic vessel becomes trombotic, by occlusion of an earlier vascular reconstruction or by an embolus, which is in most cases of cardiac origin.

Symptoms and signs

- The rule of the 5 Ps: "pain, pallor, pulselessness, paraesthesia and paralysis"
- In addition, the temperature of the limb may be compared with the other limb. A border between cold and warm may even be evident.

Diagnosis

- Embolic occlusion has acute onset. The primary cause is often atrial fibrillation or myocardial infarction.
- The onset is slower in accelerating chronic ischaemia. There is a history of claudication and PAOD also in the other leg.
- The differential diagnosis includes massive ileofemoral venous thrombosis: additional signs are oedema, cyanosis and venous congestion.
- Ischaemic occlusion with paralysis may sometimes simulate stroke.

Critical limb ischaemia

- Critical ischaemia is defined as a threat of gangrene.
- Suspect critical ischaemia if distal ulcer does not recover in two weeks. Distal gangrene ("toe infarct") is typical of ischaemia as well as an ulcer outside the decubital area (heel and ball of the foot belong to decubital areas).
- The limb feels cool or cold and looks pale and/or cyanotic.
- Often associated with diabetic microangiopathy.
- Patient may feel the ischaemia as numbness.
- Venous insufficiency and a venous ulcer may make the diagnosis difficult.
- Ischaemia be considered critical if:
    - there is aching at rest, usually at night
    - foot ulcer or gangrene is not recovering and the ankle-brachial index (ABI) is <0.85. Doppler measurement may be falsely normal in diabetes patients. A weak and monotonous ejection sound reveals ischaemia.

Vascular surgery of acute and critical ischaemia

- Acute ischaemia requires urgent and immediate hospitalization.
- Embolectomy is a simple operation and possible during local anaesthesia even in old patients in poor condition. If a differential diagnosis cannot be made, thrombosis should be considered as the underlying cause in acute ischaemia.
- The thrombotic event of chronic ischaemia with acute onset may sometimes be reversed with intra-arterial infusion of a thrombolytic drug.
- In addition, critical ischaemia often requires endovascular procedures or peripheral bypass surgery.
- Non-operative management is possible initially if the patient has normal limb motion, the sense of touch, and an ankle blood pressure of >30 mmHg. Cyanosis and muscular pain must be excluded.
- Critical ischaemia is often associated with long stenoses in small vessels. Patients are often aged and have multiple diseases with poor life expectancy. However, amputations should be avoided by vascular surgery in walking patients.
- Primary amputation is the alternative for patients in poor general condition who cannot move independently. Amputation is obligatory when half of the foot is gangrenous.
- After amputation for ischaemia, patients seldom learn to walk with a prosthesis. Therapeutic bypass surgery is the goal whenever possible.

References

1. Leng GC, Price JF, Jepson RG. Lipid-lowering for lower limb atherosclerosis. Cochrane Database Syst Rev. 2004;(2): CD000123.
2. McGee SR, Boyko EJ. Physical examination of chronic lower-extremity ischemia: a critical review. Archives of Internal Medicine 1998;158:1397–1364.
3. The Database of Abstracts of Reviews of Effectiveness (University of York), Database no.: DARE-999281. In: The Cochrane Library, Issue 2, 2001. Oxford: Update Software.
4. Girolami B, Bernardi E, Prins MH, Ten Cate JW, Hettiarachchi R, Prandoni P, Girolami A, Buller HR. Treatment of intermittent claudication with physical training, smoking cessation, pentoxifylline and nafronyl. Archives of Internal Medicine 1999;159:337–345.
5. The Database of Abstracts of Reviews of Effectiveness (University of York), Database no.: DARE-998439. In: The Cochrane Library, Issue 4, 2000. Oxford: Update Software.
6. Leng GC, Fowler B, Ernst E. Exercise for intermittent claudication. Cochrane Database Syst Rev. 2004;(2):CD000990.
7. Gardner AW, Poehlman ET. Exercise rehabilitation programs for the treatment of claudication pain: a meta-analysis. JAMA 1995;274:975–980.
8. The Database of Abstracts of Reviews of Effectiveness (University of York), Database no.: DARE-952716. In: The Cochrane Library, Issue 4, 1999. Oxford: Update Software.
9. Tangelder MJ, Lawson JA, Algra A, Eikelboom BC. Systematic review of randomized controlled trials of aspirin and oral anticoagulants in the prevention of graft occlusion and ischemic events after infrainguinal bypass surgery. Journal of Vascular Surgery 1999;30:701–6709.
10. The Database of Abstracts of Reviews of Effectiveness (University of York), Database no.: DARE-992060. In: The Cochrane Library, Issue 2, 2001. Oxford: Update Software.
11. Collaborative overview of randomised trials of antiplatelet therapy-II: Maintenance of vascular graft or arterial patency by antiplatelet therapy. BMJ 1994;308:159–168.
12. The Database of Abstracts of Reviews of Effectiveness (University of York), Database no.: DARE-948031. In: The Cochrane Library, Issue 4, 1999. Oxford: Update Software.
13. Anand S, Creager M. Peripheral arterial disease. Clinical Evidence 2002;7:79–90.
14. Ernst E. Pentoxifyllin for intermittent claudication: a critical review. Angiology 1994;45:339–345.
15. The Database of Abstracts of Reviews of Effectiveness (University of York), Database no.: DARE-940251. In: The Cochrane Library, Issue 4, 1999. Oxford: Update Software.
16. Leng GC, Davis M, Baker D. Bypass surgery for chronic lower limb ischaemia. Cochrane Database Syst Rev. 2004;(2): CD002000.
17. Bosch JL, Hunink MG. Meta-analysis of the results of percutaneous transluminal angioplasty and stent placement for aortoiliac occlusive disease. Radiology 1997;204:87–96.
18. The Database of Abstracts of Reviews of Effectiveness (University of York), Database no.: DARE-970844.

In: The Cochrane Library, Issue 4, 1999. Oxford: Update Software.
19. Bachoo P, Thorpe P. Endovascular stents for intermittent claudication. Cochrane Database Syst Rev. 2004;(2):CD003228.
20. de Vries SO, Hunink MG. Results of aortic bifurcation grafts for aortoiliac occlusive disease: a meta-analysis. J Vasc Surg 1997;26:1–12.
21. The Database of Abstracts of Reviews of Effectiveness (University of York), Database no.: DARE-978276. In: The Cochrane Library, Issue 4, 1999. Oxford: Update Software.

5.61 Cholesterol embolization

Tom Pettersson

Aim

- Cholesterol embolization has to be taken into account as a cause of vascular occlusive or systemic symptoms, particularly if a patient with atherosclerosis has undergone angiography or aortic surgery.

General

- In cholesterol embolization syndrome cholesterol crystals are released from the arterial wall and dispersed in the circulation. The crystals may block small vessels and cause local ischaemia or a syndrome mimicking systemic vasculitis.

Occurrence

- Most patients are men in their 60s or 70s with risk factors for cardiovascular disease.
- There is often a preceding interventive diagnostic or therapeutic procedure, e.g. angiography or aortic surgery.
- Anticoagulants are regarded as risk factors for cholesterol embolization.

The clinical picture

- The clinical picture is highly variable and depends on the extent of dissemination of cholesterol emboli.
- Skin symptoms
  - Blue toes, distal ulcers and gangrenes
  - The peripheral pulses can usually be felt.
  - Purpura, livedo reticularis
- Renal symptoms
  - Hypertension, proteinuria, haematuria, renal failure
- Amaurosis fugax and other transient neurological symptoms
- Myocardial infarction
- Intestinal haemorrhage
- Pancreatitis
- Myalgia
- In a hospital-based patient population, mortality approaches 80%.

Laboratory findings

- Elevated ESR and high serum CRP level in up to 80% of patients
- Leucocytosis in 40%
- Eosinophilia in 80%
- Thrombocytopenia
- Hypocomplementaemia

Diagnosis

- Histological evidence of cholesterol crystals in a biopsy specimen.
- Ophthalmoscopy may reveal cholesterol emboli in retinal vessels.
- Many milder cases probably remain undiagnosed.

Differential diagnosis

- Cholesterol embolization syndrome is a "great masquerader" that can mimic a number of other clinical syndromes, including systemic vasculitis.
- Recognition of cholesterol embolization syndrome is important in order to avoid unnecessary immunosuppressive treatment.

Therapy

- There is no specific therapy.
- Hypertension should be treated actively.
- Anticoagulants should be avoided or withdrawn.

5.62 Vibration syndrome (vibration-induced white fingers)

Editors

General

- Local vibration of the hands causes white finger attacks (Raynaud's syndrome).
- Vibration may also cause peripheral neuropathy D [1 2 3] with or without white fingers.
- Vibration is suspected to predispose to or worsen carpal tunnel syndrome D [4 5].

Sources of exposure

- Hand-held vibrating tools, such as chain saws, rock drills, hand tools driven by motor, electricity or compressed air (e.g. compressed-air hammers, grinding machines and concrete vibrators) may cause vibration syndrome. As chain saws have improved technically, the prevalence and severity of vibration syndrome have decreased among forest workers. New cases have been found among metal workers, for example, tool grinders.
- Vibration syndrome is generally preceded by many years of exposure to hand-arm vibration. Pedestal grinders may get white fingers after exposure for less than one year C [6]. Vibrations occurring in impulses and large muscle force used at work probably explain the rapid development of symptoms.

Diagnosis

- Symptoms
  - Attacks of white fingers
  - Neurological symptoms such as numbness, clumsiness and weakened hand force
- Finger plethysmography
- Differential diagnosis
  - Primary Raynaud's disease (21.4)
  - Collagenoses
  - Traumas
  - Stenoses in proximal vessels
  - Obstructive angiopathy
  - Dysglobulinaemia
  - Drugs and chemicals (ergot alkaloids, beta-blockers)
  - Neurogenic diseases

Treatment

- Exposure to vibration should be stopped or restricted or exposure time should be limited C [7 8 9]
- Other working conditions (coldness, noise) should be improved.
- Smoking should be reduced
- Pharmacological treatment, e.g. nifedipine (see Raynaud's syndrome)

Prognosis

- Vibration syndrome does not cause necrosis or atrophic changes in the skin.
- Diminishing exposure to vibration usually leads to reduction or disappearance of symptoms C [7 8 9].

References

1. Seppäläinen AM. Peripheral neuropathy in forest workers. A field study. Work environ health 1972;9:106–111.
2. Alaranta H, Seppäläinen AM. Neuropathy and the automatic analysis of electromyographic signals from vibration exposed workers. Scand J Work Environ Health 1977;3:128–134.
3. Aatola S, Färkkilä M, Pyykkö I et al. Measuring method for vibration perception threshold of fingers and its application to vibration exposed workers. Int Arch Occup Environ Health 1990;62:239–424.
4. Färkkilä M, Pyykkö I, Jäntti V et al. Forestry workers exposed to vibration: a neurological study. Brit J Ind Med 1988;45:188–192.
5. Koskimies K, Färkkilä M, Pyykkö I. Carpal tunnel syndrome in vibration disease. Brit J Ind Med 1990;47:411–416.
6. Starck J, Färkkilä M, Aatola S, Korhonen O. Vibration syndrome and vibration in pedestal grinding. Brit J Ind Med 1983;40:426–433.
7. Pyykkö I, Sairanen E, Korhonen O et al. A decrease in the prevalence and severity of vibration-induced white fingers among lumberjacks in Finland. Scand J work & Health 1978;4:246–254.
8. Futatsuka M, Ueno T, Sakurai T. Follow up study of vibration induced white finger in chain saw operators. Brit J Ind Med 1985;42:267–271.
9. Koskimies K, Pyykkö I, Starck J et al. Vibration syndrome among Finnish forest workers between 1972 and 1990. Int Arch Occup Environ Health 1992;64:251–256.

5.63 Aortic aneurysm and dissection

Editors

Basic rules

- Diagnose aortic aneurysm before rupture: nearly all aneurysms can be treated surgically. Monitor a small aneurysm, found incidentally or through screening, until it reaches a size where the benefit of surgical repair outweighs the risks associated with such surgery.
- It is easy for a general practitioner to learn the diagnosis of abdominal aortic aneurysm with ultrasonography.
- Remember the possibility of aortic dissection in a patient with severe pain suggestive of acute myocardial infarction (AMI) but without clear ECG findings.
- Patients with aortic dissection must be referred to a hospital immediately.

Aortic aneurysms

Abdominal aortic aneurysm

- Atherosclerosis is the most important causative factor.
- 85% of the patients are men. An aneurysm is found in 10% of men aged 75 years or more.

- A palpable, pulsating mass in the upper or middle abdominal region is a typical finding Most aneurysms are found accidentally.
- The patient may complain of pain which may resemble pain originating from the ureter or spinal cord. The pain often radiates to the back. Pain indicates an expanding aneurysm that needs surgery.
- Sometimes a calcified aneurysm can be recognised on plain abdominal x-rays or urography films.
- The diagnosis is confirmed by ultrasonography (which can be performed by a general practitioner familiar with the examination).
- Treatment
  - Hypertension and other cardiovascular risk factors should be treated effectively.
  - An aneurysm with a diameter of over 3 cm is **monitored with ultrasonography** every 12 months. When the diameter of the aneurysm has reached 5 cm in a man or 4.5 cm in a woman the ultrasonographic checks are carried out every 6 months.
  - **Surgery** is indicated when the diameter of the aneurysm exceeds 5.5 cm B [1].
    - About 1% of aneurysms with diameter of 4 cm rupture annually compared with 10% of aneurysms with a diameter of 6 cm or more. The mortality from a ruptured aneurysm is 90%.
  - Aneurysms extending into the chest cavity should be operated on.
  - Elderly brothers of patients with known aneurysms should be screened with ultrasonography C [2].

Aneurysm of the thoracic aorta

- Usually asymptomatic. Pain suggests expansion.
- Aortic regurgitation (with symptoms related to it) (4.11).
- Tracheal or bronchial compression or phrenic nerve paralysis.
- Sometimes the neck veins are dilated due to the compression caused by the aneurysm.
- May be visible as an incidental finding on a chest x-ray.
- Treatment is either surgical or conservative.

Aortic dissection

- The typical locations are the ascending (type I and II) and descending thoracic aorta (type III). Type I is confined to the ascending aorta. Dissections of the other types may extend into the abdominal aorta.
- As the tunica interna ruptures the blood rushes into the layers of the tunica media. The aorta is often (but not always) dilated and may be visible on a chest x-ray.
- Marfan's syndrome is often associated with dissection or annuloaortic ectasia and aortic regurgitation.
- The incidence of aortic dissection is about 10/million inhabitants/year.

Symptoms

- **Suspect aortic dissection** in a patient with sudden excruciating pain without ECG findings suggestive of AMI.
- The patient is usually a hypertensive male.
- The location of the pain may change as the dissection advances.
- The pain radiates in the same way as pain associated with AMI, including the jaw and sometimes the palate. Pain is often also felt in the back.
- The associated symptoms include those resulting from the occlusion of aortic branches, i.e. ischaemic symptoms of the brain, heart, kidneys and intestines.
- Acute aortic regurgitation may occur (a new murmur).

Findings

- Even though pulse asymmetry is presented only in a minority of patients it is worth checking for. A murmur from aortic regurgitation or bruits may be heard.
- Blood pressure is high, particularly in distal dissection.
- ECG will not be indicative of AMI but may show left ventricular hypertrophy, an old infarction or ischaemia (AMI is sometimes possible when the dissection occludes a coronary artery).
- A chest x-ray may show a dilated aortic arch, but often the x-ray is nearly normal.
- Transoesophageal echocardiography is a good primary investigation. Computed tomography, MRI or angiography is often needed for final diagnosis.

Treatment

- The systolic blood pressure should be lowered quickly to around 100–120 mmHg. First aid treatment includes nifedipine 10 mg chewed, nitrate (or nitroprusside) infusion, a beta-blocker and effective analgesia.
- Dissection of the ascending aorta should be operated on immediately. Prognosis without surgery is very poor.
- The immediate treatment of a dissection of the descending aorta is conservative, i.e. reduction of blood pressure and heart rate.
- Thrombolysis is contraindicated.

References

1. The UK Small Aneurysm Trial Participants. Mortality results for randomized trial of early elective surgery or ultrasonographic surveillance for small abdominal aortic aneurysms. Lancet 1998;352:1649–1655.
2. Salo JA, Soisalon-Soininen S, Bondestam S, Mattila PS. Familial occurrence of abdominal aortic aneurysms. Ann Intern Med 1999;130:637–642.

Pulmonary Diseases

Evidence Based Medicine Guidelines. Edited by the Duodecim Editorial Team
 ISBN: 0-470-01184-X

6.1 Haemoptysis

Pentti Tukiainen

Aetiology

- In young patients: various infections
- In older patients: chronic bronchitis, tumours and tuberculosis
- The aetiology remains unknown in about 20% of patients with a normal chest radiograph.

Infections

- Bronchitis (sometimes acute, usually chronic)
- Pneumonia
- Abscess
- Tuberculosis
- Bronchiectasis

Tumours

- Cancer
- Carcinoid

Cardiovascular diseases

- Pulmonary embolism, pulmonary infarction
- Mitral stenosis (and other diseases that increase pulmonary pressure)
- Left ventricular failure – pulmonary oedema
- Pulmonary arteriovenous malformation
- Aortic aneurysm (leakage into the pulmonary parenchyma)

Traumas

- Thorax injury
- Postoperative condition
- Biopsies, catheterizations

Miscellaneous

- Haematological diseases, coagulation disorders
- Anticoagulant therapy
- A foreign object
- Vasculitis (21.44)

Differential diagnosis

- Patient history, clinical examination and chest radiograph are essential for the differential diagnosis.
- Find out first whether the haemoptysis originates from the lungs or is associated with sinusitis, previous nose bleeding or gum bleeding.
- **If there is no shadowy area** on the chest x-ray, the cause of haemoptysis is usually chronic bronchitis or bronchiectasis. Mitral stenosis, pulmonary embolism, an endobronchial tumour and a coagulation disorder must be kept in mind.
- **A local shadow** is usually caused by pneumonia, tuberculosis, carcinoma, or pulmonary infarction.
- **A diffuse shadow** is usually caused by left ventricular failure or pneumonia.
- Further investigations or bronchoscopy are not necessary if the patient is under 50 years of age, does not smoke, has a normal chest x-ray, and haemoptysis is clearly associated with an infection.

Treatment

- According to the aetiology.
- Peroral tranexamic acid 1 g three times daily may be used as a symptomatic treatment.

6.2 Prolonged cough in adults

Vuokko Kinnula

Aims

- To recognize as a cause of a prolonged cough
  - asthma
  - chronic bronchitis (and incipient COPD)
  - chronic pulmonary infections, especially tuberculosis
  - sinusitis (mucus draining down the back of the throat)
  - sarcoidosis
  - pulmonary fibrosis
  - a cough associated with connective tissue disorders and their treatment
  - asbestosis, (silicosis)
  - farmer's lung
  - adverse drug reaction (ACE inhibitors, beta-blockers, nitrofurantoin)
  - lung tumours
  - pleural effusion
  - cardiac insufficiency.

Definition

- A cough that lasts more than 4–8 weeks is defined as prolonged. Coughs of shorter duration are usually caused by pulmonary infections and hyper-reactivity of the airways as the infection subsides.
- It is common that after certain infections (e.g. mycoplasma or chlamydia pneumonia, pertussis) the cough may last for a few months.

Prolonged cough that begins with symptoms of infection

- **Prolonged respiratory infection** (sinusitis) and **early asthma** are common causes of a prolonged cough.
- Primary tests include chest x-ray and echo- or x-ray imaging of the sinuses.
- Basic blood tests may be taken if considered necessary (CRP, basic blood parameters and cell count)
- First-line therapy
  - Treatment of sinusitis: antimicrobial drugs, vasoconstrictor nasal drops, possibly lavage (38.31).
  - Antimicrobial treatment (amoxicillin, doxycycline, erythromycin) is indicated for a patient with fever or purulent sputum. Treatment of dry cough with no fever includes bronchodilators, possibly in combination with antitussives. Need for antibiotics must be evaluated individually.
- If the cough does not improve in 2 months, or continues despite antimicrobial treatment, there may be other causes than the coincident infection. Especially in the early stages of asthma, a dry prolonged cough may be the only symptom. At this point, at the latest, a bronchodilator test should be performed and PEF measurements started at home (without and with bronchodilating medication) and spirometry should be considered. It is also possible to test the response to treatment with inhaled steroids (but this may delay asthma diagnosis if the pulmonary function tests have not been performed).
  - If the response is poor, the cough probably is not caused by early asthma.
  - If the response is good, the patient may have mild asthma that requires further examination (6.30).

Prolonged cough in patients with hypertension and cardiac disease

- If the patient uses an **ACE inhibitor**, it is the most probable cause of the cough. Treatment alternatives are selection of another ACE inhibitor, or rather an angiotensin II receptor antagonist, which does not usually cause a cough. If the patient has diabetes, consider whether the harm caused by a dry cough outweighs the beneficial effect of ACE inhibitors on kidney function.
- **Beta-blockers**, even beta1-selective ones, may also cause a cough, especially in patients with an atopic constitution or bronchial hyper-reactivity.
- Examine for possible signs of **cardiac insufficiency**. The first sign of mild insufficiency is often a cough at night. The primary test is a chest x-ray.

Prolonged cough in patients with connective tissue disorders

- **Pulmonary fibrosis** is one possible cause of cough and dyspnoea. This may be in connection with rheumatoid arthritis or scleroderma but may also be an **adverse effect** of drug therapy for these diseases (gold, sulphasalazine, penicillamine, methotrexate).
- A chest x-ray is the primary examination. Pulmonary fibrosis is a typical finding, but in early stages the picture may be normal, although diffusion capacity – which reflects oxygen exchange through the alveoli–may already be decreased, and there may be restriction in dynamic spirometry.
- Consult a specialist in internal medicine or pulmonary diseases.

Prolonged cough in smokers

- The most probable diagnoses are **prolonged acute bronchitis** and **chronic bronchitis**. Remember the possibility of **cancer** in middle-aged patients, especially in those over 50 years of age. Ask if the patient has had haemoptysis.
- A chest x-ray especially if the patient is over 40 years of age, unless it has been taken during the past 6 months. Sinus radiograph is taken simultaneously if echography has not been carried out. If pneumonia infiltration is found and the cough is treated as pneumonia, control the chest x-ray after 5 to 6 weeks.
- If **COPD** is suspected, perform spirometry.
- Treat a prolonged purulent cough with antibiotics. First-line therapy includes amoxicillin, doxycycline or trimethoprime sulfamethoxazole. Haemophilus influenzae or gram-positive cocci are often the causative bacteria.

Prolonged cough in certain risk occupations

- Always keep in mind the possibility of **asbestosis** (6.55) if the patient has been exposed to asbestos (workers on construction sites or in small car repair shops).
  - The primary tests are a chest radiograph and spirometry (restriction).
  - If you suspect asbestosis, consult a special clinic for pulmonary diseases.
- In a farmer, suspect **farmer's lung** (6.41) (hypersensitivity pneumonitis caused by mouldy hay) or **asthma**.
  - The primary tests are a chest x-ray, PEF measured at home, and spirometry (and a bronchodilator test).
  - If you suspect farmer's lung, consult a special clinic for pulmonary diseases.
- Occupational asthma that begins with a cough is possible in various occupations where the patient has been exposed to chemicals, solvents (isocyanates, formaldehyde, acrylates, etc.) (in car repair shops, the plastics industry, the cleaning business, dental laboratories and dentists' offices, etc.).

Prolonged cough in atopic, allergic or ASA-sensitive patients

- The most probable diagnosis is **asthma**.

- Symptoms often include transient dyspnoea and secretion of mucus.
- Primary tests
  - PEF measurements at home
  - Spirometry and a bronchodilator test
  - Exercise test (particularly in young persons)
  - Testing of bronchial hyper-reactivity (provocation with inhaled histamine or metacholine) in unclear cases if considered appropriate.
  - Testing the response to inhaled corticosteroids

Prolonged cough and fever, purulent sputum

- If a patient with pneumonia has multiple other diseases or is elderly the recovery may be prolonged for several reasons (22.7). Suspect **tuberculosis**; in patients with pulmonary disease also suspect atypical **pulmonary infection caused by atypical mycobacteria** or **bronchiectasis** (6.24). **Vasculitis** (e.g. polyarteritis nodosa, Wegener's granulomatosis) or **eosinophilic pneumonia** may begin with these symptoms (21.31).
- Primary tests
  - Chest x-ray
  - Smear and culture of sputum
  - Blood count and sedimentation rate, CRP (may also be increased in vasculitis)
- Remember also **eosinophilic pneumonias (6.42)**.
- Consult a pulmonologist if symptoms continue.

Other causes of a prolonged cough

- Chronic cough may be the only symptom in **pulmonary sarcoidosis (6.43)**.
- Primary tests
  - Chest x-ray (hilar hyperplasia, parenchymal infiltrations)
  - Serum angiotensin converting enzyme (may be normal)
- **Subacute pulmonary reaction to nitrofurantoin**
  - Ask if the patient uses nitrofurantoin for prevention of urinary tract infections.
  - In a subacute case, eosinophilia may not be present.
- A cough may be the only sign of **pleural effusion** (6.80). To resolve the aetiology, carry out
  - a thorough general examination
  - punction and biopsy of the pleura.
- Prolonged cough or bronchial irritation may sometimes be associated with gastro-oesophageal reflux.

Conclusion

- Because prolonged cough is not always caused by asthma or infection, bear in mind that, especially in adults, a chest x-ray must be taken to exclude cancer. A normal or abnormal x-ray picture helps in making decisions about further investigations or treatment.

6.3 Dyspnoea

Editors

Basic rules

- Diagnose **immediately** a foreign body in the airways and anaphylaxis, and **on first consultation** spontaneous pneumothorax, pulmonary embolism, pulmonary oedema and an exacerbation of asthma.
- Identify asthma or heart failure as the cause of recurrent or chronic dyspnoea; both can be treated effectively with drugs.
- Diagnose psychogenic hyperventilation syndrome and explain its cause and benign nature to the patient.
- Dyspnoea is a subjective feeling of obstructed breathing. Acute respiratory failure (6.5) is a disturbance of blood gas exchange: $PO_2 < 8.0$ or $PCO_2 > 6.7$.

Dyspnoea with acute onset

- Foreign body in the airways (6.60)
  - Inspiratory wheezing
- Asthma attack, the disease is usually known
- Anaphylaxis (14.1)
  - Acute dyspnoea starts after the administration of a (parenteral) drug, vaccination, or insect sting.
  - Expiratory wheezing
- Spontaneous pneumothorax (6.61)
  - Pain is often felt at the onset of the symptoms. The patient adapts quickly to the dyspnoea.
  - Respiratory sounds are weak on the side of the pneumothorax; listen for a difference between the lungs.
  - Young smoking adults and patients with COPD are most frequently affected.
- Pulmonary embolism (5.43)
  - The patient has several risk factors.
  - Chest pain and cough are often present.
  - A smallish embolism can cause few symptoms in a basically healthy person, but may be critical in a person with poor health.
  - A large pulmonary embolism causes shock and poor oxygenation.
  - The findings at auscultation are variable: normal, rales, wheezing, or both. Tachypnoea.
  - PO_2 is lowered or normal, PCO_2 is lowered. ECG and chest x-ray are often normal or may show pleural effusion, atelectasis and right heart ST-T changes.
- Acute pulmonary oedema (4.70)
  - Congestive rales can usually be heard.
  - Foam may be visible when the patient coughs.
  - The neck veins are filled with blood. The extremities are cold.
  - The patient usually has a history of heart failure.

- Cardiac ischaemia (4.58) or infarction (4.60), are the most common causes.
  - Chest pain is the dominant symptom; however, in many patients dyspnoea is the most annoying symptom.
  - ECG and chest x-ray invariably show pathology.
- Non-cardiac pulmonary oedema
  - ARDS in an adult = smoke, toxic chemicals, several serious diseases
  - Irritant gases (6.44)
  - ECG is often normal
- Arrhythmia
  - Atrial fibrillation, atrial flutter or supraventricular tachycardia (4.39) in a cardiac patient may lead to acute heart failure that is sometimes difficult to distinguish from the physiological sinus tachycardia caused by respiratory failure.
- Carbon monoxide poisoning: pulse oximetry reading is normal even though the patient has severe hypoxaemia.
- Hyperventilation syndrome or panic disorder (35.29)
  - The patient is a young adult with a tendency for the condition.
  - The patient feels short of air; however, PO_2 is high and $PCO_2$is low.
  - The patient has paraesthesia of the hands and dizziness.
  - Lung auscultation is normal. The patient is often slightly tachycardic, and ECG shows several ST depressions.
  - The condition may be associated with preceding misuse of alcohol.
  - Secondary hyperventilation syndrome with a normal or only slightly lower PO_2 is often associated with pulmonary embolism, asthma, pneumothorax and metabolic acidosis

Dyspnoea that has lasted from a few hours to one day

- Exacerbation of asthma or COPD (6.32)
  - Wheezing
  - A respiratory tract infection (sinusitis!) or exposure to dust is often the cause of the exacerbation. The symptoms are aggravated by infection, allergen and/or physical exertion.
  - The onset of obstructive pulmonary disease is often slow.
  - In COPD patients dyspnoea does not always correlate with pulmonary function: "blue bloaters" adapt to CO_2 retention dangerously well; "pink puffers" suffer from severe dyspnoea even when PCO_2 is normal and PO_2 only slightly lowered.
- Aggravation of chronic heart failure
- Pneumonia; bacterium or virus
  - Particularly in cases with underlying severe pulmonary disease
- Allergic alveolitis (6.41)
  - Farmer's lung: fever and dyspnoea after handling hay
  - Crepitation on auscultation (basal rales)
  - Fever and cough
- Pleural effusion (6.80)
  - Silent respiratory sounds basally, dull percussion note
- Recurrent small pulmonary emboli (5.43)
  - Young adults with a predisposition to thromboses may also be affected (users of oral contraceptives)
  - The clinical course is insidious, quite unlike the acute form of the disease.
  - Shortness of breath and tachycardia, and tachypnoea
- Anaemia; usually caused by GI bleeding, tendency for syncopes
- Unstable angina pectoris; for many patients with supraventricular tachycardia dyspnoea is the most annoying symptom.

Dyspnoea that has developed over weeks or months

- Chronic left heart failure (4.72)
- Obstructive pulmonary diseases
  - Asthma (6.30)
  - COPD (6.34)
- Diseases causing pulmonary fibrosis
  - Fibrosing alveolitis (6.40)
  - Sarcoidosis (6.43)
  - Pulmonary damage caused by medications
    - Cytotoxic reaction
    - Immunological reactions: intersitial pneumonia or alveolitis
    - A reaction caused by a drug can manifest very differently between individuals.
    - Cytostatic drugs are often the cause of cytotoxic reactions (primarily methotrexate).
    - The most significant immunological reactions are nitrofurantoin lung and gold lung.
    - Long-term use of amiodarone causes pulmonary damage in 5–7%.
  - Pneumonitis caused by radiotherapy
- Structural disorders of the thorax
  - e.g. ankylosing spondylitis, cyphosis; particularly if the patient has central adiposity (metabolic syndrome)
- Obesity and lack of physical activity cause most problems in the differential diagnosis of chronic heart failure.
- Neuromuscular diseases
  - Multiple sclerosis (36.75), ALS (36.84)
  - Paralysis of the diaphragm; bilateral condition is rare.

The most important diagnostic investigations

- The patient's history and a thorough clinical examination reveal the cause of dyspnoea in most cases. The key questions are:
  - Do you have diagnosed asthma, COPD or cardiac disease?
  - Do you have dyspnoea at rest?
  - Do you have chest pain or a feeling of suffocation in the throat?
  - Do you have a cough or (bloody) sputum, cough at nights or orthopnoea?
  - What did you do before the symptoms commenced?
  - What is your present medication? Any changes in medication? Drugs that can cause pulmonary damage?
  - Do you have symptoms of infection? Does physical activity alleviate symptoms? Do you feel dizzy?
  - Remember that the manifestations of a disease vary between individuals.
- Chest x-ray
  - is usually indicated
  - is most often normal (e.g. in asthma, pulmonary embolism, laryngotracheitis, bronchitis, hyperventilation, anaemia).
- ECG
  - Should be recorded from all middle-aged or elderly patients if a non-cardiac cause is not evident.
- Peak expiratory flow (PEF) and spirometry
  - are easy and useful examinations if obstruction is suspected; the result is often slightly pathological also in restrictive conditions.
- Blood gas analysis
  - Informative, but rarely available in primary care. The patient has respiratory failure when $PO_2 < 8.0$ and/or $PCO_2 > 6.7$ (6.5).
- Pulse oximetry and interpretation of the result (17.11)
- Serum N-peptide concentrations if heart failure is suspected

Pitfalls

- Obesity and poor physical condition are often misdiagnosed as heart failure.
- Slow pulmonary embolism gives initially few symptoms; remember thrombosis susceptibility.
- Clinical signs of pneumothorax are not easily detected unless they are searched for intentionally.
- The main symptom of unstable angina pectoris is often dyspnoea on exertion; remember the risk factors.
- The diagnosis of carbon monoxide poisoning is often missed; pulse oximetry does not reveal anoxia!
- Physiological tachycardia resulting from respiratory failure is sometimes difficult to distinguish from primary arrhythmia.

6.4 Hyperventilation

Editors

Aims

- To recognize and treat non-psychogenic causes of hyperventilation, especially in elderly patients.
- To recognize psychogenic hyperventilation as a cause of chest pain or undefined neurological findings, and to be able to explain the benign character of the symptoms to the patient.

Definitions

- Hyperventilation means increased alveolar ventilation causing a decrease in arterial blood pCO_2, which in turn causes neurological symptoms and manifestations induced by vasoconstriction.
- In practice hyperventilation syndrome means psychogenic hyperventilation which often is connected with panic disorder. The definition of panic disorder in DSM-III includes many signs of hyperventilation (35.29). Hyperventilation may, however, also be a symptom in many somatic diseases.

Pathophysiology

- Pulmonary causes
  - Pneumonia
  - Pneumothorax
  - Pulmonary embolism (5.43)
  - Asthma and chronic obstructive pulmonary disease (COPD)
  - Pulmonary fibrosis, alveolitis
- Other causes
  - Psychological distress, panic disorder (35.29)
  - Drugs that stimulate respiration (aspirin, beta-sympathomimetics)
  - Cardiac insufficiency
  - Metabolic acidosis
  - Hepatic insufficiency
  - Neurological diseases (tumours of the brain stem)

Symptoms

- Chest pain
  - Often a stabbing pain on the left side
  - Hyperventilation may cause coronary spasm and thus typical exercise angina pectoris, including ST- and T-wave changes on the ECG.
- Tachycardia

- Neurological symptoms
  - Dizziness, fainting
  - Weakness
  - Paraesthesias
  - Clumsiness
  - Concentration difficulties, memory disturbances
  - Tetany
- Psychological symptoms
  - Anxiety, panic attack
  - Hallucinations
  - Euphoria, depersonalization

Diagnosis of psychogenic hyperventilation

- Patient history
- If you suspect pulmonary embolism, check D-dimer and blood gas analysis
  - Low arterial blood pCO_2, but normal or increased arterial blood pO_2
- Hyperventilation test
  - If voluntary hyperventilation causes the familiar symptoms, the diagnosis is supported and the patient can better understand the pathophysiology of the symptoms.

Treatment

- Causative treatment
- Treatment of acute psychogenic hyperventilation
  - Calming the patient and making the patient talk is often helpful.
  - If necessary, the patient breathes into a paper bag.
  - Rectal diazepam is given if needed.
  - Try to identify the triggering factor and make a plan of treatment for the patient (observing one's own respiration, holding the breath when necessary).
- Treatment of panic disorder: see 35.29.

6.5 Acute respiratory failure

Editors

Aims

- To achieve sufficient elimination of carbon dioxide, satisfactory tissue oxygenation and adequate ventilatory workload.
- To avoid excessive oxygen administration that can lead to further respiratory depression in patients with chronic pulmonary disease.
- To avoid toxic effects of oxygen.

Definition

- Respiratory failure usually means disturbance in gas exchange between ambient air and arterial blood (arterial blood $pO_2 < 8$ kPa, arterial blood $pCO_2 > 6.7$ kPa) (17.10) (17.11).
- It can be divided into three subgroups:
  - disturbance of gas exchange at the alveolar level (hypoxaemia as the primary problem)
  - impaired ventilation (hypercapnia as the primary problem)
  - exacerbation of a pulmonary disease (obstruction as the primary problem).

Aetiology

- Respiratory centre depression
  - Overdose of drugs (opioids!), intoxications
  - Incautious oxygen therapy in a patient with pulmonary disease
  - Unconsciousness (various causes)
- Nerve impulse is not transmitted to respiratory muscles
  - Spinal neck injury
  - Neurological diseases (myasthenia gravis, botulism, polyradiculitis)
  - Muscular dystrophies
- Impaired ventilation mechanics
  - Crush injury of the thorax
  - (Pressure) pneumothorax (6.61), haemothorax
- Airway obstruction
  - Foreign object (6.60)
  - Obstructing tumour or mucus
  - Asthma or chronic obstructive pulmonary disease (6.32)
- Alveolar hypoventilation
  - Severe pneumonia
  - Adult respiratory distress syndrome
  - Pulmonary oedema (4.70)
- Insufficient pulmonary circulation
  - Pulmonary embolism (5.43)
- Decreased oxygen saturation in blood
  - Severe anaemia
  - Carbon monoxide poisoning
- Prolonged convulsions

Basic principles of treatment

- The primary therapeutic aim is to maintain adequate tissue oxygenation. Keep in mind all the following aspects: oxygenation of arterial blood, cardiac output and the oxygen carrying capacity of the blood (haemoglobin concentration).
- Prone position C [1 2]
- Oxygen treatment
  - E.g. Ventimask 40%

- Be careful while treating patients with chronic pulmonary disease (Ventimask 28%) because excessive correction of hypoxaemia may lead to respiratory depression (pO_2, not pCO_2, regulates respiration in patients with chronic hypoxaemia).
- Note: Oxygen therapy does not improve ventilation, and it must be used carefully in the treatment of impaired ventilation.

♦ Treatment with continuous positive airways pressure (CPAP) A [3 4]
- Increases lung volume, opens collapsed airways, does not assist respiration mechanically.

♦ Treatment with ventilator
- Increases lung volume, opens collapsed airways, mechanically assists respiration.
- Mild cases
  - Non-invasive positive pressure ventilation A [3 4]. BiPAP can be used e.g. in acute exacerbations of COPD causing respiratory insufficiency, with face mask and initial pressure support (6 cm H_2O, IPAP–EPAP)
  - Using e.g. Bennet or Bird ventilators, 10–15 cm overpressure for 15 minutes at 1–2 hours intervals, in milder cases every fourth hour.
- More severe cases
  - Respirator treatment in an intensive care unit is necessary.

♦ Remember the toxicity of oxygen.
- 80–100% oxygen is safe for hours.
- 50–80% oxygen is safe for days.
- <50% oxygen is safe in continuous use.
- Arterial blood pO_2 should not exceed 17–18 kPa (130–135 mmHg; risk of eye damage).

References

1. Ball C. Use of the prone position in the management of acute respiratory distress syndrome. Clinical Effectiveness in Nursing 1999;3:36–46.
2. The Database of Abstracts of Reviews of Effectiveness (University of York), Database no.: DARE-999301. In: The Cochrane Library, Issue 1, 2001. Oxford: Update Software.
3. Keenan SP, Kernerman PD, Cook DJ, Martin CM, McCormack D, Sibbald WJ. Effect of noninvasive positive pressure ventilation on mortality in patients admitted with acute respiratory failure: a meta-analysis. Crit Care Med 1997;25:1685–1692.
4. The Database of Abstracts of Reviews of Effectiveness (University of York), Database no.: DARE-971294. In: The Cochrane Library, Issue 4, 1999. Oxford: Update Software.
5. Wunsch H, Mapstone J. High-frequency ventilation versus conventional ventilation for treatment of acute lung injury and acute respiratory distress syndrome. The Cochrane Database of Systematic Reviews, Cochrane Library Number: CD004085. In: Cochrane Library, Issue 1, 2004. Chichester, UK: John Wiley & Sons, Ltd.

6.7 Pulmonary function tests

Vuokko Kinnula

Peak expiratory flow (PEF, PEFR)

Basic rule

♦ PEF records (Figure 6.7.1) the airflow in large airways. It is not a very sensitive or specific test, but cheap and easy to conduct.

♦ Spirometry is more sensitive in the diagnosis of asthma.

♦ Lowered PEF may suggest chronic obstructive pulmonary disease (COPD) in smokers.

Indications

♦ Screening of pulmonary function

♦ Diagnosis of asthma
- Monitoring diurnal variation in airway obstruction
- Monitoring response to bronchodilators at home
- Monitoring respiratory function at work
- Bronchial provocation tests

♦ Follow-up of asthma

♦ Suspicion of COPD

♦ Differential diagnosis between asthma and COPD

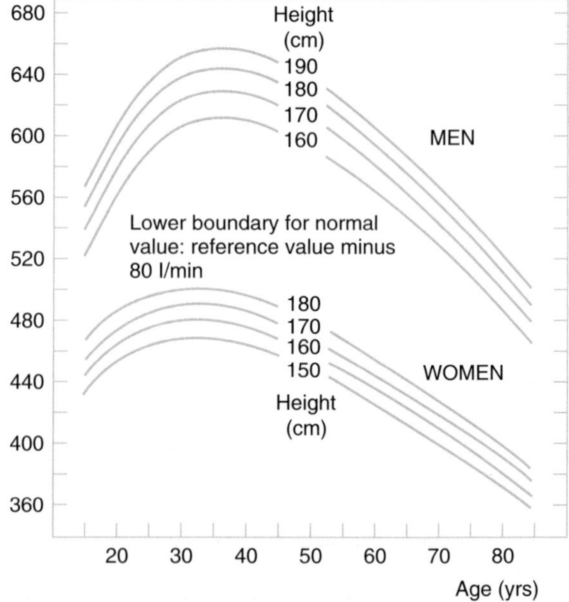

Figure 6.7.1 Reference values for PEF in men and women aged 15–85 years (Nunn A J, Greg I. BMJ 1989; 298: 1068–1070).

Recording PEF

- The patient stands.
- A maximal short expiration is performed after maximal inspiration.
- The patient closes his/her lips tightly around the mouthpiece.
- The test is repeated at least three times, or even more often if the difference between the best two readings is more than 20 l/min.
- The best reading is recorded.
- The results are compared to age-, sex- and length-adjusted reference values (Figure 6.7.1).

Diagnostic PEF monitoring at home

- First week
  - PEF is recorded in the morning and in the afternoon/evening (always at the same time of day), and during episodes of dyspnoea or coughing.
  - Bronchodilators are used only if necessary.
- Second week
  - PEF is recorded in the morning and in the afternoon/evening before the inhalation of a bronchodilator (usually a betasympathomimetic), and 15 minutes thereafter.
- Interpretation
  - If the difference between the highest and lowest values divided by their mean exceeds 20% (and is at least 60 l/min) the diagnosis of asthma is strongly supported.
  - If the readings improve by 15% or more from the baseline value on at least 3 occasions, and are at least 60 l/min above the baseline value, the improvement is significant and suggests asthma.
  - Lowered PEF values without diurnal variation may suggest COPD, but the finding is not specific.
  - The morning and evening recordings should always be made at the same time of the day. The greatest difference in the 24-hour variation is shown between the blows performed early in the morning and late in the afternoon.

Spirometry

Basic rule

- Spirometry is used to record lung volumes (static spirometry) or changes in lung volumes on a time or flow axis (dynamic spirometry) (Figure 6.7.2).

Indications

- Diagnosis and follow-up of obstructive lung diseases (asthma, COPD)
- Diagnosis and follow-up of restrictive lung diseases (e.g., lung tissue diseases)
- Assessment of working capability

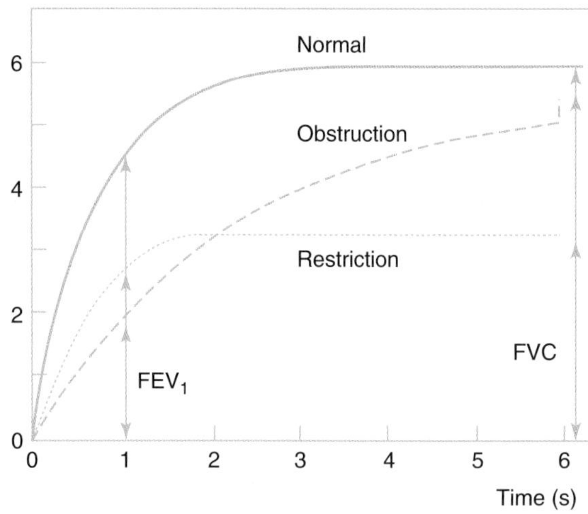

Figure 6.7.2 Normal spirometry and an obstructive and restrictive finding on a volume-time-axis.

- Assessment of suitability for surgical procedures
- Monitoring of the effect of radiotherapy, operations, or drug treatment

Preparation for the examination

- No smoking for at least 4 hours before the examination
- No heavy meals, coffee or cola drinks for at least 2 hours before the examination
- Avoidance of physical exercise and inhaling cold air for at least 2 hours before the examination
- At least 15 minutes of rest
- Medications should be discontinued if the examination is to be diagnostic.
  - Betasympathomimetics, anticholinergics, chromoglycate, nedocromil, and leukotriene receptor antagonists for 1–3 days.
  - Theophyllin, combination preparations, antitussives for 3 days.
  - Corticosteroids: the effect is long-term and difficult to estimate (weeks). Regular corticosteroid medication should not be started before the diagnosis of asthma has been confirmed.
  - Antihistamines need not be discontinued before diagnostic spirometry.
- Because of diurnal variation, a follow-up examination should always be performed at the same time of the day if possible.

Contraindications

- Acute respiratory infection within the preceding 2 weeks
- Severe ischaemic heart disease
- Severe arrhythmias (which can be provoked by the bronchodilator test)

A. Obstruction of small airways

V̇
PEF
Normal
Obstruction
MEF50
MEF25
V
FVC
FEV1

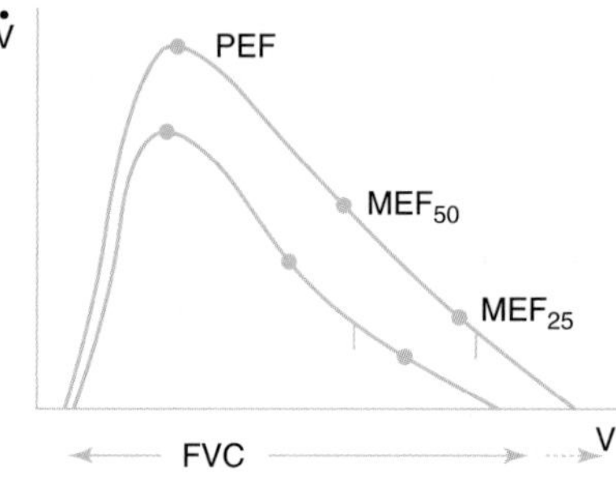

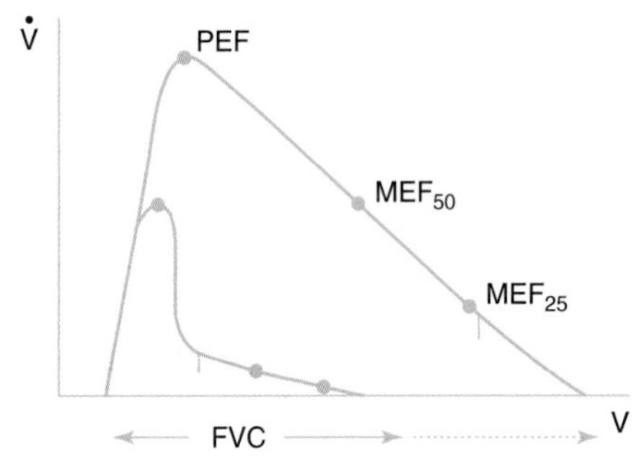

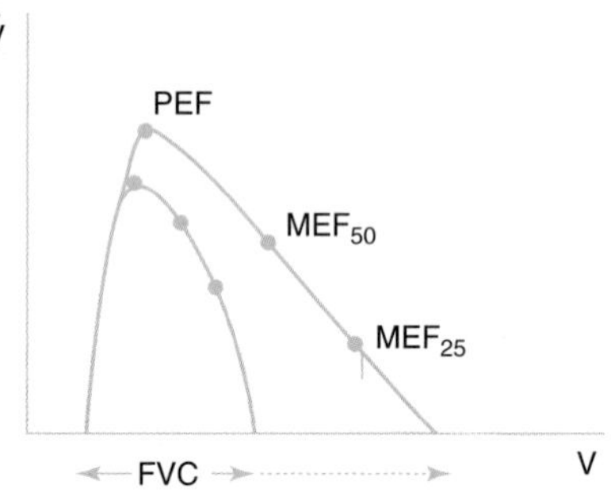

Figure 6.7.3 Typical findings in a flow-volume spirometry. The normal curve is pointed with an arrow in picture A.

Equipment

- Spirometers for laboratory-use and pocket-sized turbine spirometers.
- The equipment should fulfil the quality standards of the European Respiratory Society.
- Pay particular attention to quality control
  - Education (and advanced training) of the personnel
  - Calibration of equipment and scheduled maintenance
  - Reference values adjusted for sex, age, and height

Methods and parameters

- Static spirometry
  - The most important parameter is vital capacity (VC).
  - Preferably the inspiratory vital capacity should be recorded (maximal slow inspiration after maximal expiration).
  - The largest of three readings is recorded.
  - The difference of the two highest values must not exceed 0.2 l.
- Dynamic spirometry (volume–time recording, Figure 6.7.2)
  - Rapid and complete expiration after maximal inspiration
  - Parameters
    - Forced vital capacity (FVC)
    - Forced expiration in one second (FEV_1)
    - Percentage of FEV_1 from FVC (FEV%)
  - The results are adjusted according to body temperature (body temperature standard pressure saturated, BTPS) because expired air is cooled on its way to the spirometer.
  - The largest and the second largest FEV_1 and FVC must not differ by more than 4% from each other. An unreliable recording should not be printed.
- Dynamic spirometry (flow–volume recording, Figure 6.7.3)
  - Performed in the same way as volume–time recording
  - Parameters
    - FVC, FEV_1, FEV%
    - Peak expiratory flow (PEF)
    - Flow at volumes of 75, 50, and 25 percent of the FVC (MEF_{75}, MEF_{50}, MEF_{25})
  - PEF and MEF_{75} are dependent on the calibre of large airways, the muscular force used during expiration, and the compliance of the lungs.
  - MEF_{50} and MEF_{25} are more dependent on the calibre of the medium and small airways, compliance and muscular force.
  - The readings of several respiratory cycles are recorded one over the other. Graphs differing from the majority are not included.

The bronchodilator test

Indications

- Detection of reversible obstruction in the diagnosis of asthma

- Assessment of the adequacy of drug therapy for asthma: the patient should use his/her normal medication (ascertain the use of the drug and record the timing of the administration in the report.)

Performing the test

- Spirometry or PEF is recorded before and after inhalation of a betasympathomimetic, e.g., 0.4 mg salbutamol.
- Doses and timing of peak response
  - Rimiterol 3 × 0.2 mg: 5 min
  - Salbutamol 2 × 0.2 mg: 10 min
  - Terbutaline 3 × 0.5 mg: 10 min

Interpretation

- Changes from the initial value and minimum changes suggesting asthma
  - FEV_1 15% (0.20 l)
  - VC and FVC 15% (0.25 l)
  - PEF 15% (at least 60 l/min, measured with a PEF meter).

Typical profiles

Asthma

- FEV_1, FEV%, PEF, MEF_{50} or MEF_{25} is
  - decreased
  - or temporarily normal in mild or well-controlled asthma.
- VC, FVC are
  - usually normal.
  - FVC may be decreased ("dynamic restriction") in severe asthma where VC may be clearly larger than FVC, and the FEV% may be normal.
- A significant response is recorded in the bronchodilator test.
- MEF_{50} and MEF_{25} are very sensitive to technical variations in expiration. Pathological results in MEF_{50} or MEF_{25} without significant abnormalities in FEV_1, FEV% and PEF are not diagnostic.

Chronic obstructive pulmonary disease (COPD)

- FEV_1, FEV% or PEF is
  - continuously decreased, or normal in mild COPD.
- MEF_{50} and MEF_{25}
  - are often decreased in the early stage of the disease, even before clinical symptoms (obstruction of small airways).
  - Particularly in emphysema, MEF_{50} and MEF_{25} may be very low ("collapse").
- FVC is often decreased ("dynamic restriction").
- No significant response is observed in the bronchodilator test.

Restrictive pulmonary disease

- Causes
  - Pulmonary parenchymal disease (alveolitis, fibrosis)
  - Extrapulmonary causes (pleural thickening, pleural effusion, chest or thoracic spine deformities, obesity)
- VC and FVC are
  - decreased.
- FEV_1 and PEF are
  - decreased (but FEV% is normal).
- No significant response is observed in the bronchodilator test.

Assessment of suitability for surgery

- Rule of thumb: FEV_1 should exceed 1 litre for elective surgery.
- The values need to be compared to the reference values (i.e. sex and age of the patient)

6.10 Acute bronchitis

Editors

Basic rules

- Bronchitis is usually a viral infection that does not require antibiotic therapy (A) [1 2 3 4].
- Bronchitis and pneumonia are often impossible to distinguish clinically. Therefore, the patient's general condition and duration of symptoms determine whether laboratory tests and radiographs are required.
- A condition diagnosed as acute bronchitis should be treated like pneumonia if the patient's general condition is impaired, respiratory rate accelerated or CRP clearly elevated.

Aetiology and clinical picture

- Viral and bacterial aetiologies usually cannot be told apart on the basis of the clinical picture.
- Bronchitis and pneumonia are often caused by the same microbes – these diagnoses constitute differences in severity of the same disease.
- The Table 6.10.1 may provide valuable clues.

Indications for chest x-ray

- The patient has fever but no upper respiratory symptoms.
- Impaired general condition.
- The patient has an underlying disease predisposing to pneumonia: COPD, bronchiectasia, diabetes, or chronic cardiac, hepatic or kidney disease.
- A recent (<1 year) history of pneumonia.
- Prolonged or unusual course of illness.

Table 6.10.1 Aetiologies of acute bronchitis

Causative organism	Characteristic features
Influenza A virus	Epidemics affecting all age groups
Influenza B virus	Often endemic affecting all age groups
Parainfluenza 1–3	Isolated cases, epidemics uncommon
Adenovirus	
Pneumococcus (6.41)	♦ In middle-aged or older people ♦ Sudden onset ♦ Upper respiratory symptoms
Mycoplasma (6.30)	♦ Epidemics in the under-30 age group ♦ Upper respiratory symptoms in the early stages ♦ Dry cough
Bordetella pertussis	Prolonged cough
Haemophilus influenzae	Smokers and individuals with chronic bronchitis
Moraxella catarrhalis	Chronic bronchitis, immunodeficiency

Other investigations and differential diagnosis

- Bronchitis may be difficult to discern from pneumonia.
  - Auscultation findings of the lungs such as vesicular rales, decreased breath sounds and shallow and accelerated breathing are suggestive of pneumonia.
  - If the patient is seriously ill or the symptoms persist, a chest x-ray should be taken.
- Serum-CRP is low (less than 50 mg/l) in a significant proportion of patients with viral bronchitis or pneumonia B [5 6 7 8 9 10].
- The possibility of sinusitis should be excluded by ultrasound examination or x-ray in patients with persisting symptoms or local signs of sinusitis.
- The following conditions that sometimes resemble bronchitis should be borne in mind
  - farmer's lung (6.41)
  - pulmonary toxicity of nitrofurantoin
  - other medicine-related (tolfenamic acid, parenteral gold, methotrexate) pulmonary symptoms.
- Recurrent and prolonged episodes of "bronchitis" can be a sign of early asthma (6.30).

Treatment

- Supportive care
- Antitussive medication as required.
  - Cough remedies can be used only if the cough disturbs normal life (e.g. sleep). They may help the patient to cope with the symptoms and prevent unnecessary use of antibiotics.
  - Inhaled betasympathomimetics may be more effective than cough remedies in controlling wheezing and dry cough in patients with bronchial obstruction C [11].

Table 6.10.2 Antimicrobial drugs in acute bronchitis

Drug	Dose
Penicillin V[1)]	1–1.5 million units × 3
Doxycycline	100–150 mg × 1
Roxithromycin[2)]	150 mg × 2

1. For patients allergic to penicillin, use first-generation cephalosporins, e.g., cephalexin or cefadroxil.
2. Even other macrolides are possible. If roxithromycin is dosed 300 mg × 1, its gastric adverse effects increase.

- **Antimicrobial drugs should not be used for acute bronchitis in patients who are otherwise healthy and in good general condition.**
  - If the patient is in good general condition despite symptoms that have lasted for several days, CRP determination can be used to support a decision not to administer antibiotics B [5 6 7 8 9 10]. However, low CRP value does not exclude the possibility of a serious bacterial disease in patients with severe symptoms.
- Pneumococcal pneumonia is the most important serious infection of the lower respiratory tract, and it is justified to treat very ill patients with this condition in mind 6.11. However, if mycoplasma or chlamydia are suspected doxycycline or macrolides are drugs of choice. Patients with COPD should be treated with doxycycline, amoxicillin or cotrimazole because Haemophilus influenzae is often the causative agent. The recommended duration of treatment is 5–7 days (see Table 6.10.2).
- Antimicrobial therapy should be considered if
  - serum CRP is above 50 mg/l
  - the patient's general condition is impaired or worsening
  - fever continues for more than one week
  - fever starts again after already having settled
  - mycoplasma, chlamydia or pertussis is suspected on the basis of the epidemiological situation
  - the patient is immunocompromized.

References

1. Mackay DN. Treatment of acute bronchitis in adults without underlying lung disease. J Gen Int Med 1996;11:557–562.
2. The Database of Abstracts of Reviews of Effectiveness (University of York), Database no.: DARE-961823. In: The Cochrane Library, Issue 4, 1999. Oxford: Update Software.
3. Bent S, Saint S, Vittinghoff E, Grady D. Antibiotics in acute bronchitis: a meta-analysis. American Journal of Medicine 1999;107:6267.
4. The Database of Abstracts of Reviews of Effectiveness (University of York), Database no.: DARE-991491. In: The Cochrane Library, Issue 2, 2001. Oxford: Update Software.
5. Chest 1995;107:1028–1031.
6. Chest 1995;108:1288–1291.
7. Scand J Infect Dis 1990;22:537–545.
8. Tidsskr Nor Lägeforen 1991;111:2249–2252.
9. Scand J Prim Health Care 1992;10:234–240.

10. Scand J Infect Dis 1995;27:457–462.
11. Smucny J, Flynn C, Becker L, Glazier R. Beta2-agonists for acute bronchitis. Cochrane Database Syst Rev. 2004;(2): CD001726.

6.11 Pneumonia

Pekka Honkanen

Basic rules

- Take a chest x-ray to diagnose or exclude pneumonia if the patient has a cough or fever and his or her general condition has deteriorated **B** [1 2].
- Treatment must be effective against pneumococcus. Other causative agents must be considered if there are clinical or epidemiological implications suggesting them.
- Parenteral antibiotics are given to patients whose general condition is poor or who have any other disease that impairs the immune defence system.
- Cephalosporins are not indicated for ordinary pneumonia because their spectrum is too wide and they cause ecological problems (1.80). Quinolones are not suitable in pneumonia that has begun at home as they are not effective enough against pneumococcus. Ten per cent of pneumococci are resistant to macrolides. The response to therapy must be monitored closely.

Aetiology and diagnostic tips

- Microbial aetiology depends essentially on
  - whether the patient caught the disease in or out of hospital
  - whether there are predisposing aetiological factors, e.g. aspiration, chronic pulmonary disease, immunosuppressive drug therapy or surgery.
  - See Table 6.11.

Signs and symptoms

- Fever and chills, a cough, dyspnoea and stabbing chest pain are common.
- In the elderly, confusion, abdominal symptoms or worsening of the symptoms of an underlying disease may sometimes be the most prominent symptoms. Many (30% of the patients) may not have fever.
- Vesicular crackles are usually heard, but the auscultation finding may be normal (in one third of patients).
- Respiratory frequency > 26/min, leukocytes > 12×10^9/l, and CRP level > 110 mg/l indicate a severe clinical picture.

Diagnosis

- Clinical status **B** [1 2]
  - General condition, dyspnoea, pulmonary auscultation, heart, abdomen
  - respiratory frequency
  - state of hydration
- Chest x-ray
  - Not absolutely necessary if the patient is young and in good condition and is not treated in hospital.
  - Define the nature and localization of infiltrations.
  - Is there heart failure?
  - Lack of infiltrates does not exclude pneumonia if the clinical picture and laboratory findings suggest it.
  - A follow-up radiograph should usually be taken after treatment.
- Laboratory tests
  - Serum CRP and blood count reflect tissue damage better than microbial aetiology. A CRP of > 80 mg/l usually indicates bacterial infection, and a very high CRP pneumococcus infection.
  - If the patient's condition is poor, take serum potassium, sodium, creatinine and arterial acid-base balance (or pulse oximetry, if acid-base balance is not available).
  - In establishing a differential diagnosis, ECG, urine culture and blood glucose are often necessary.
  - If legionellosis or pulmonary chlamydia is suspected, also determine serum ALT and serum alkaline phosphatase.
- Aetiological tests
  - Usually not necessary in non-institutional care.
  - Take blood culture twice from patients whose general condition is poor.
  - If the response to treatment is poor, consider other aetiological tests selectively: antibodies against viruses, mycoplasma, Chlamydia pneumoniae, Legionella pneumophila
  - In case of an epidemic examine a few patients.
- Sinusitis often accompanies pneumonia (echography, maxillary sinus x-ray if necessary).
- In problem cases consult a specialist in pulmonary diseases (for bronchoscopy or bronchoalveolar lavage, especially in immunodeficient patients or in severe pneumonia in non-institutional care) and a specialist in infectious diseases.

Differential diagnosis

- Heart failure
- Tuberculosis (6.21)
- Pulmonary infarction
- Lung cancer
- Eosinophilic infiltration (6.42)
- Sarcoidosis (6.43)
- Atelectasis
- Old shadowed area
- Radiation reaction, adverse reaction to a drug and other rare causes
- See also opacity in chest radiograph 42.1

Table 6.11 Aetiology of pneumonia and diagnostic tips.

Aetiology	Diagnostic tips
Pneumonia acquired outside hospital	
Pneumococcus	♦ Most common (half of pneumonias in adults requiring hospitalization ♦ Rapid onset, high fever, sometimes confusion ♦ Often lobular pneumonia ♦ Very high CRP level suggests pneumococcus
Mycoplasma and chlamydia	♦ More common than pneumococcus in under 45-year-old patients in non-institutional care ♦ Slow onset ♦ Dry cough, mild fever ♦ Occurs in epidemics
Viruses	♦ Common in children and adolescents in particular ♦ E.g. influenza virus occurs as epidemics in the winter, adenovirus ♦ Many viruses can cause isolated cases of pneumonia ♦ Chest radiograph often shows a diffuse shadow
Mycobacterium tuberculosis	♦ Tuberculosis can have a sudden onset and may resemble common pneumonia
Legionellae	♦ Travellers ♦ Spread by colonized water pipes or air conditioning systems
Chlamydia psittaci	♦ A history of bird contact
Coxiella burnetii	♦ Q fever is a globally significant cause of pneumonia
Francisella tularensis	♦ Epidemiological situation, other symptoms of tularaemia?
Staphylococcus aureus	♦ A young patient, sequela of influenza ♦ Sometimes shadows with cavities on chest radiograph
Klebsiella pneumoniae	♦ Occurs often in alcoholics ♦ Sometimes shadows with cavities on chest radiograph
Hemofilus, Branhamella and enterobacteria	♦ Frequently associated with, e.g., chronic bronchitis and diabetes
Anaerobes	♦ Frequently associated with aspiration
Pneumocystis carinii	♦ HIV ♦ Immunodeficient patients
Mixed infections	♦ Common
Pneumonia acquired in hospital (on ward)	
Gram-negative bacilli	♦ Often caused by a tumour or other underlying immunodeficiency
Staphylococcus aureus	♦ Often severe, septicaemic course of infection
Cytomegalovirus, mycoplasma, Pneumocystis carinii	♦ In transplant recipients
Legionella	♦ In immunosuppression patients

Almost all microbes can cause pneumonia in a patient in poor condition

Antimicrobial treatment of pneumonia contracted outside hospital

Unknown aetiology

- Clinical suspicion of pneumococcus
  - Mild clinical picture: peroral **penicillin V** 1 million IU four times daily for 10 days
  - Deteriorated general condition or clear lobular pneumonia: intravenous **penicillin G** 2 million IU 4 times daily
- Suspected mycoplasma, chlamydia or Legionella or penicillin allergy
  - Macrolide, e.g. **erythromycin** 500 mg 3–4 times daily for 10 days, or **roxithromycin** 150 mg twice daily for 10 days. In poor general condition erythromycin 0.75–1 g four times daily i.v. Pneumococcal resistance to macrolides has increased, and therefore response must be carefully monitored.
  - As a reserve medication to erythromycin and its derivates, **tetracyclines** can be used. They are effective against mycoplasma, but the effect against Chlamydia pneumoniae is uncertain.
- Acute pneumonia in a patient with chronic bronchitis
  - Amoxicillin 500 mg three times daily for 10 days when the patient is in good condition
  - In poor general condition, cefuroxime 750 mg–1.5 g i.m. or i.v.
- Severe pneumonia in non-institutional care
  - Cefuroxime 750 mg–1.5 g three times daily i.v.
- Aspiration in non-institutional care
  - Penicillin G 1–2 million IU six times daily i.v.
  - If there is a good and rapid response to treatment in uncomplicated pneumonia in non-institutional care, intravenous treatment can be changed to oral therapy in a couple of days. **If the aetiology is verified, e.g. with blood culture, the drug must immediately be changed**

to an antibiotic with the narrowest effective spectrum (always penicillin in pneumococcal pneumonia).

Known aetiology

- Pneumococcus
  - Penicillin G or V
- Mycoplasma or chlamydia
  - Erythromycin or roxithromycin
- Legionella
  - Erythromycin + rifampicin 300 mg three times daily p.o.
- Haemophilus
  - Amoxicillin or third generation cephalosporine
- Staphylococcus aureus
  - Cloxacillin
- Aerobic gram-negative rod
  - Beta-lactam (e.g. wide-spectrum penicillin or third-generation cephalosporin) + aminoglycoside (note! blood level determination)
- Pneumocystis carinii
  - Sulphamethoxazole 25 mg/kg + trimethoprim 5 mg/kg four times daily i.v., or pentamidine 4 mg/kg once daily i.v.

Antimicrobial treatment of pneumonia contracted in hospital

Patients who are not immunodeficient

- Moderate general condition, no need for oxygen therapy or respirator.
  - Cefuroxime 750 mg–1.5 g three times daily i.v., or ceftriaxone 1–2 g once daily i.v. or i.m.
- Severely deteriorated general condition, or the patient needs oxygen therapy or a respirator
  - Erythromycin 0.75–1 g four times daily i.v. + ceftazidime 2 g three times daily i.v.
- After aspiration in hospital
  - Penicillin G 2 million IU six times daily i.v. + aminoglycoside (blood level determination!)

Immunodeficient patients

- Consult a specialist in infectious diseases

Other therapy

- If there is no response to therapy in 2–3 days, specify the aetiology, try to exclude complications in hospital patients and in patients in a poor condition (pleural effusion, empyema, pulmonary abscess) and consult a specialist whenever necessary.
- Estimate the need for oxygen therapy (pulse oximetry, acid-base balance).
- Treat dehydration.
- Avoid unnecessary antipyretic and antitussive medication.
- Treat other existing diseases (heart failure, diabetes).

Indications for hospital treatment

- Pneumonia can usually be treated at home. Indications for hospital treatment include
  - poor general condition
  - vomiting
  - dyspnoea and other respiratory complications
  - problems with differential diagnosis
  - severe primary disease
  - immunosuppression
  - poor conditions at home.

Follow-up

- Antibiotic treatment can usually be discontinued after 10 days of treatment, or at the latest when CRP has normalized.
- Follow up the chest radiograph readily, always if the patient is a smoker or over 40 years of age.
- Recovery often takes a long time, which means that sick leave must readily be extended if necessary.

Prevention

- Risk groups must receive influenza vaccination.
- Pneumococcus vaccination is indicated at least for patients who have had splenectomy or who have a significant primary disease (3.1).

References

1. Metlay JP, Kapoor WN, Fine MJ. Does this patient have community-acquired pneumonia? Diagnosing pneumonia by history and physical examination. JAMA 1997;278:1440–1445.
2. The Database of Abstracts of Reviews of Effectiveness (University of York), Database no.: DARE-978377. In: The Cochrane Library, Issue 4, 1999. Oxford: Update Software.

6.12 Mycoplasma pneumoniae infections

Marjaana Kleemola

- Mycoplasma pneumoniae, a minute bacterium, is a common cause of community-acquired pneumonia especially in children and young adults.

Diagnosis

- Suspect Mycoplasma pneumoniae as the cause of a respiratory infection if
  - an epidemic is known to be present
  - other confirmed cases have occurred in the surroundings
  - the patient is a child or a young adult.
- ESR, CRP, blood leucocytes, and chest x-ray are not helpful in the differential diagnosis: the findings are variable and nonspecific.

Laboratory investigations

- No accurate rapid test is available, and serology has its limitations. Serological tests are indicated in at least two situations:
  - In the initial stage of an epidemic, serology should be examined in a few "typical" cases.
  - In severe and complicated pneumonia.
- The following tests are available:

Mycoplasma antibodies from paired serum samples (complement fixation or EIA method)

- The main problems are the delay of the result and occasional nonspecific reactions. These tests are routine in most virological laboratories.
- Serum samples
  - Sample I in the initial stage of the disease
  - Sample II 10–20 days later
- Interpretation
  - A significant increase in titre is diagnostic.
  - At least two classes of antibodies (IgG + IgM or IgG + IgA or all three) should be examined with the EIA method to improve diagnostic accuracy.

Specific IgM

- Most commercial kits are satisfactory, when following facts are kept in mind:
  - The antibody level rises in about 1 week, and may remain high for months. The test is most useful when the infection is primary, as is usually the case in (small) children.
  - In reinfections the IgM titre does not usually change.

Cold agglutinins

- The test is nonspecific and insensitive, and it should be abandoned.

Other tests

- Culture is only suitable for research purposes.
- The role of PCR is still unclear.

Treatment of M. pneumoniae infection

- Adequate antibiotic treatment shortens the duration of the symptoms even if the mycoplasma is not always eradicated from the pharynx. The drugs of choice are
  - erythromycin or tetracycline 30–50 mg/kg/day for 10 days (up to 1 500–2 000 mg/day), or
  - doxycycline 100–150 mg/day (adult dose) for 10 days C [1 2].
  - Newer macrolides (which may be better tolerated A [3 4]) can also be used, e.g. roxithromycin 150 mg × 2 for 10 days, or azithromycin for 3–5 days C [5 6].

Prognosis

- M. pneumoniae infections are usually cured fairly easily, even without antibiotics.
- After M. pneumoniae pneumonia the general condition may be affected for a long time, and the cough may last for weeks. The chest x-ray may normalize slowly. Sometimes pulmonary function may be impaired for months.
- Fatal infections caused by M. pneumoniae are extremely rare.

References

1. Ahonen A, Koskinen R, Rantanen P ym. Atypical pneumonia in the Nordic countries: Aetiology and clinical results of a trial comparing fleroxacin and doxycycline. J Antimicr Chemother 1997;39:499–508.
2. Foy HM et al. Mycoplasma pneumoniae pneumonia in an urban area. Five years of surveillance. JAMA 1970;214:1666–1672.
3. Milne R, Olney RW, Gamble GD, Turnidge J. Tolerability of roxithromycin versus erythromycin in comparative clinical trials in patients with lower respiratory tract infections. Clin Drug Invest 1997;14:405–417.
4. The Database of Abstracts of Reviews of Effectiveness (University of York), Database no.: DARE-971501. In: The Cochrane Library, Issue 2, 2000. Oxford: Update Software.
5. Schonwald S, Barsic B, Klinar I, Gunjaca M. Three-day azithromycin compared with ten-day roxithromycin treatment of atypical pneumonia. Scand J Infect Dis 1994;26:706–710.
6. Lode H, Schaberg T. Azithromycin in lower respiratory tract infections. Scand J Infect Dis 1992 (suppl);83:26–33.

6.20 Exposure to tuberculous infection

Editors

Contagiousness

- In practice, only pulmonary tuberculosis is infectious.

- The infection is spread by a coughing patient who sheds such high numbers of bacilli in the sputum that they can be demonstrated by staining of a sputum smear. This requires 10 000–100 000 bacilli per ml of sputum.
- On the other hand, a culture of tubercle bacilli is positive at concentrations as low as 10–100 bacilli per ml. Such low concentrations carry only minimal risk of spreading the infection.

Exposure

- Persons in the same household and in the close contact with the patient are most exposed to the infection. The more bacilli are shed and the longer the period of exposure, the greater is the risk of being infected. Maintenance of a good coughing hygiene by the patient reduces the amount of bacillus aerosol in the environment.
- Effective chemotherapy reduces the number of bacilli essentially within a few days, and the risk of infection is practically over in a few weeks.

Contact tracing

- Every infectious patient should be enquired about close contacts, and examinations should at first concentrate on these persons. If new cases are found, the investigations should be expanded to include the patient's casual contacts, for example fellow workers, etc.
- Tracing of the patient's contacts befalls the general practitioner even if an initial survey of the patient's contacts has been carried out at the hospital.

Examination of exposed persons

- All exposed persons should be examined immediately. The nature of the exposure of each contact should be recorded, and they should all receive information about the possibility of infection. In the case of children, the information should be given to parents. Each contact should also be reminded to mention the possibility of tuberculous infection whenever he/she sees a doctor.
- This guideline is based on the assumption that BCG vaccination is included in the national vaccination program.

Infants

- The date of BCG vaccination and the presence of vaccination scar should be confirmed. If deemed appropriate, the physician may perform a Mantoux test with 2 TU. If an induration of 10 mm or more is observed, a chest radiograph may be taken and, if necessary, the child may be referred to a paediatrician for evaluation (see prophylactic therapy).

Older children

- Examination as above. Chest x-ray has a place in screening school-age children as many healthy vaccinated school-aged children exhibit a Mantoux reaction exceeding 10 mm.

Adults

- Examinations are performed according to the physician's judgement. Tuberculin tests are of limited usefulness. Chest radiographs can be used for screening, and bacteriological tests are recommended in suspect cases. Patients may also be referred to a pulmonary outpatient clinic for further investigations.

Follow-up of exposed persons

- Sound judgement should be used in repeating tuberculin tests, as previous test may have a booster effect on a subsequent test, making conclusions difficult.
- In healthy children and adults, follow-up visits after 6, 12 and 24 months are sufficient. On these visits, examinations are performed according to the physician's judgement.

Prophylactic chemotherapy

- If BCG vaccination coverage is good, chemoprophylaxis is very rarely used. In latent tuberculosis, one drug is sufficient. In all cases, clinical tuberculosis must be excluded, as it requires an effective combination therapy.
  - If the sputum staining is positive, the close contacts of the patient are susceptible to infection. All exposed children should preferably be seen by a paediatrician. After initial investigations, exposed persons are followed up for 2 years, and chest x-ray and tuberculin test are performed as deemed necessary. The decision to start prophylactic chemotherapy must be justified. The smaller the child, the more readily the therapy is started (A) [1]; strong and long-term exposure and an induration exceeding 10 mm in the tuberculin test are indications for chemotherapy. Pre-school-aged children are treated with a six-month course of INH 10 mg/kg daily (maximum dose is 300 mg daily).
- Chemoprophylaxis is rarely indicated in adults.

Risk of disease

- The risk of an infected person to later develop tuberculosis is greater during the first two years. About 10% of all exposed fall ill, but if there is simultaneous tuberculous and HIV infection, the risk of manifest tuberculosis is manifold, about 10% per each year.

Special situations

- If tuberculosis is contracted in an institution, such as a kindergarten or a school, it is advisable to consult with a specialist from the outset and plan together a strategy to deal with the situation.
- If the person spreading the tuberculous infection has drug-resistant bacilli, instructions should be sought from a clinic of pulmonary medicine or infectious diseases.

- If the tuberculous patient also has HIV, the contacts are examined in the same manner as contacts of a sputum staining-positive patient.

Health care workers

- The staff risk of exposure to tuberculous infection may be especially high in connection with bronchoscopy and autopsy of patients with unexpected tuberculosis. Infection has been reported to have occurred in 10 minutes during an autopsy.

Reference

1. Smieja MJ, Marchetti CA, Cook DJ, Smaill FM. Isoniazid for preventing tuberculosis in non-HIV infected persons. Cochrane Database Syst Rev. 2004;(2):CD001363.

6.21 Diagnosing tuberculosis

Paula Maasilta

Risk groups for tuberculosis

- Unvaccinated children
- People whose tuberculosis has been treated inadequately in the past
- Patients on immunosuppressive drugs
- Alcohol misusers
- Drug addicts
- Prisoners
- People with HIV infection
- Refugees, immigrants
- Health care personnel

Bacteriological investigations

- Staining and culture from repeated, consecutive specimens, usually on three consecutive days.
- The specimens may include
  - Body excretions and fluids: sputum, urine, blood, CSF, pleural fluid, bone marrow, wound discharge
  - Needle and aspiration samples
  - Tissue samples (in a clean tube without formaldehyde)
- The culture takes 4–6 weeks.
- Routine use of PCR-techniques is increasing.

Findings in tissue samples

- Epithelioid cells
- Langhans' giant cells
- Caseous necrosis

Pulmonary tuberculosis

Symptoms

- Asymptomatic
- General symptoms
  - Fatigue
  - Poor appetite
  - Weight loss
  - Fever
- Pulmonary symptoms
  - Cough
  - Discharge of sputum
  - Bloody sputum
  - Pleurisy
  - Dyspnoea

Investigations

- All cases of suspected tuberculosis should be referred to a specialist.
- Staining and culture samples can be taken in primary care.
- History
- Tuberculin tests
- Chest x-ray
- Bacteriological samples (the culture takes 4–6 weeks)
- There is no immediate test (PCR) for routine use C [1].

Differential diagnosis

- Nonspecific pneumonias (consider tuberculosis if the response to treatment is poor)
- Primary or secondary tumours of the lung
- Sarcoidosis (6.43)
- Eosinophilic pulmonary infiltrates (6.42)
- Pneumoconiosis (6.55)
- Fungal diseases
- Atypical mycobacteria (6.23)

Extrapulmonary visceral tuberculosis

Common sites

- Lymph nodes
- Urogenital region
- Central nervous system (the drug treatment differs from standard treatment and must be started urgently!) (36.56)
- Bones and joints
- Pleura
- Pericardium

Miliary tuberculosis

- A disseminated blood-borne form of tuberculosis
- The chest x-ray may be normal at the initial stage. Computed axial tomography may be diagnostic in such cases.
- A negative tuberculin test may be a sign of severe tuberculosis.
- Consider miliary tuberculosis in elderly institutionalized patients with prolonged fever and an elevated serum alkaline phosphatase concentration.
- **In patients with AIDS** a mycobacterial infection may have special features. Tuberculosis may be the first manifestation of an HIV infection.

Causes of misdiagnosis

- The diagnosis is not considered.
- Tuberculosis is treated as an other disease.
- The symptoms of tuberculosis are thought to be an exacerbation of an underlying disease.

Infectiousness

- Mycobacteria-containing aerosol is most infective (coughing, suction of the airways).
- In practice only pulmonary tuberculosis is infectious.
- The disease is never transmitted by contaminated objects.
- The infectiousness depends on the amount of mycobacteria in the sputum (6.20). If the bacteria are detected by staining, the risk of transmission is considerable. If bacteria are only detected by culture the risk of transmission is negligible, and no special measures are indicated (with the exception of organ transplant recipients, childcarers, etc.)

Reference

1. Schluger NW, Kinney D, Harkin TJ, Rom WN. Clinical utility of the polymerase chain reaction in the diagnosis of infections due to Mycobacterium tuberculosis. Chest 1994;105: 1116–1121.

6.22 Antituberculous medication in ambulatory care

Paula Maasilta

Basic rules

- The standard treatment regimen consists of rifampicin (RMP) and isoniazid (INH) for 6 months, combined with pyrazinamide (PZA) during the first 2 months. Sometimes ethambutol is used as the third drug.
- The normal daily dose for RMP is 600 mg (450 mg for patients under 60 kg), 300 mg for INH, and 2000 mg for PZA (1500 mg for patients under 60 kg) A [1].
- Quinolones should not be used as primary drugs for tuberculosis.
- All drugs are taken in the morning.
- It is mandatory that all drugs are taken regularly C [2]. Patient's adherence to treatment should be supported B [3] [4]. If there is a suspicion of poor compliance the patient should take the drugs under the supervision of a nurse D [5] (the tablets for weekends can be dispensed to the patient on Fridays). A next of kin or other reliable person can serve as a supervisor.

Adverse effects of antituberculous drugs

Rifampicin

- Stains all excretions red (may stain contact lenses).
- Liver function abnormalities
- Gastrointestinal symptoms
- Skin symptoms
- Immunologically mediated symptoms
  - Flu-like syndrome
  - Thrombocytopenia
  - Haemolytic anaemia
- Anuria
- Shock, dyspnoea
- Rifampicin may decrease the effect of a number of drugs, including
  - oral contraceptives
  - anticoagulants
  - corticosteroids
  - tolbutamide
  - barbiturates
  - cyclosporin.

Isoniazid

- Liver function abnormalities
- Rash
- Fever
- Neurological symptoms
  - Peripheral neuropathy
  - Convulsions, psychological symptoms

Pyrazinamide

- Liver function abnormalities
- Arthralgias (an asymptomatic increase in serum urate concentration is more common)
- Gastrointestinal symptoms
- Sensitization to sunlight

Investigations during treatment

- Laboratory examinations
  - ESR, blood count, platelet count, AST, ALT, bilirubin, GGT, creatinine, urine test, CRP (and urate if the patient is on PZA)

    - The tests are performed before starting medication. Follow-up tests are performed after 2 weeks and 1, 2, 4, and 6 months on medication, and at any time if indicated by symptoms.
- Chest x-rays for follow-up of pulmonary tuberculosis
    - Before the treatment, 2 and 6 months after starting treatment, and always if indicated on clinical grounds (suspicion of poor response to treatment).
- Staining of smear and culture from sputum in pulmonary tuberculosis
    - Before treatment, including determination of resistance to drugs
    - If the staining is initially positive, the staining samples should be examined every 2 weeks until they turn negative.
    - If the culture is initially positive, the culture samples should be taken every month until they turn negative.
    - Other samples are taken if clinically indicated.
- The patient is considered cured after adequate chemotherapy (provided that he/she does not have AIDS etc.), and no routine follow-up examinations are indicated.

Treatment of multiresistant tuberculosis

- Effective and regular chemotherapy prevents the development of drug resistance. Multiresistant tuberculosis (MDR) occurs in countries where treatment is inadequate.
- If the bacteria are resistant to only one drug, the treatment is usually successful, but if resistance develops to both isoniazid and rifampicin (MDR) the mortality may be as high as before antituberculous drugs were developed (50–60%).
- If the patient has received antituberculous drugs in the past, if there is no reliable record of the treatment, if the medication has been discontinued, or if the patient arrives from a region where drug resistance is common, the treatment should be started with four drugs, and the treatment regimen should be revised when the results of the sensitivity tests are available. Never add one drug if the disease has responded poorly to the used combination of drugs!
- Multiresistant tuberculosis should be treated in strict isolation. The treatment is long and expensive.

Treatment of latent infection

- In high risk patients isoniazid for 6 months is effective in preventing tuberculosis (A) [6].
    - The daily INH dose is 300 mg or 5–15 mg/kg
    - Treatment of latent infection can be considered in patients with
        - recent skin conversion
        - chronic renal or respiratory disease and risk of TB reactivation
        - recent household contact with skin positive test
        - residency in endemic areas
        - otherwise suspected high risk patients
    - For the prevention of tuberculosis with HIV-infected persons (A) [7 8 9], see 1.45.

References

1. Joint Tuberculosis Committee of the British Thoracic Society. Chemotherapy and management of tuberculosis in the United Kingdom: recommendations 1998. Thorax 1998, Vol 53, 7: 536–548.
2. Mwandumba HC, Squire SB. Fully intermittent dosing with drugs for treating tuberculosis in adults. Cochrane Database Syst Rev. 2004;(2):CD000970.
3. Chaulk CP, Kazandjian VA. Directly observed therapy for treatment completion of pulmonary tuberculosis: consensus statement of the public health tuberculosis guidelines panel. JAMA 1998;279:943–948.
4. The Database of Abstracts of Reviews of Effectiveness (University of York), Database no.: DARE-988440. In: The Cochrane Library, Issue 1, 2000. Oxford: Update Software.
5. Volmink J, Garner P. Directly observed therapy for treating tuberculosis. Cochrane Database Syst Rev. 2004;(2): CD003343.
6. Smieja MJ, Marchetti CA, Cook DJ, Smaill FM. Isoniazid for preventing tuberculosis in non-HIV infected persons. Cochrane Database Syst Rev. 2004;(2):CD001363.
7. Woldehanna S, Volmink J. Treatment of latent tuberculosis infection in HIV infected persons. Cochrane Database Syst Rev. 2004;(2):CD000171.
8. Bucher HC, Griffith LE, Guyatt GH, Sudre P, Naef M, Sendi P, Battegay M. Isoniazid prophylaxis for tuberculosis in HIV infection: a meta-analysis of randomized controlled trials. AIDD 1999;13:501–507.
9. The Database of Abstracts of Reviews of Effectiveness (University of York), Database no.: DARE-993945. In: The Cochrane Library, Issue 2, 2001. Oxford: Update Software.

6.23 Atypical mycobacterial infections

Paula Maasilta

Basic rules

- Consider atypical mycobacterial infection in patients with
    - persistent pulmonary infection and chronic pulmonary disease or immunosuppression
    - suspected pulmonary tuberculosis that responds poorly to treatment.

Epidemiology

- The incidence of infections caused by atypical mycobacteria is probably increasing.
- The infection is mostly acquired from water or soil.
- Human-to-human transmission has not been reported.

Causative agent

- The following species cause pulmonary infections: M. avium-intracellulare, M. kansasii, M. xenopi, M. malmoense, M. scrofulaceum, M. simiae, M. szulgai, M. chelonae, and M. fortuitum.

Symptoms

- Cough
- Sputum
- Dyspnoea
- Weight loss
- Fever and bloody sputum are rare.
- The disease may have special features in patients with AIDS.
- The clinical picture may resemble that of ordinary tuberculosis. Sometimes an atypical mycobacterial infection is the cause of a poor response to antituberculous treatment.

Investigations

Bacterial culture

- Atypical mycobacteria are more difficult to culture than M. tuberculosis.
- Repeated ample growth of the same species of Mycobacteria is significant.
- Pulmonary disease caused by atypical mycobacteria must be differentiated from mere colonization (or contamination of the specimen).

Radiology

- In subacute disease the parenchymal infiltrates and caverns are situated unilaterally in the upper lobe.
- In chronic forms the patient often has bilateral fibrotic changes.

Skin tests

- Not generally available.

Treatment

- The treatment is clearly more difficult than the treatment of ordinary tuberculosis.
- Antituberculous medication, other antibiotics, and occasionally surgery.
- Eradication of the causative agent is not always possible.

6.24 Bronchiectasias

Olli Säynäjäkangas

PUL

Aim

- To recognize bronchiectasias as a cause of prolonged or repeated respiratory infections.

Aetiology

- Pulmonary infections in childhood (pneumonia, pertussis)
- Severe pneumonia even at a later age
- Several other conditions, such as ciliary dysfunction and immunoglobulin deficiencies.

Symptoms and signs

- Symptoms
  - Symptoms of chronic bronchitis (especially if the patient is not, nor has been, a smoker), cough, dyspnoea, haemoptysis
  - Episodes of bronchitis
  - Repeated pneumonia
- Signs
  - Coarse crackles, or normal auscultation findings
  - Sometimes expiratory wheezing

Diagnosis

- Chest x-ray
  - Peribronchial striae
  - Honeycomb pattern
  - Sometimes normal
- High-resolution computed tomography
  - Verifies the diagnosis
- Laboratory findings
  - In exacerbation phase leukocytosis, increased sedimentation rate and CRP

Treatment

Conservative

- Physical therapy C [1]
  - According to clinical experience, postural drainage at home and active exercising C [1] until breathlessness (the most effective way to remove mucus) may be beneficial.
  - Use of expiratory resistance in sputum clearance (6.34). Bronchopulmonary hygiene physical therapy (BHPT)

does clear sputum in patients with bronchiectasies but does not have any significant effects on pulmonary function D [2].

- Antimicrobial treatment, if the patient has fever and ample mucous sputum production: amoxicillin, doxycycline, trimethoprim-sulpha, cephalosporins, ciprofloxacillin. Quinolones are effective but should not be used without taking bacteriological samples to rule out possible problems with resistance.
  - There is not enough evidence for routine use of mucolytics in bronchiectasies D [3].
- Inhalation bronchodilators, if there is secondary bronchial obstruction (6.34).

Surgical treatment

- Lobectomy/pulmectomy
- Indications
  - Despite conservative treatment the patient's symptoms remain.
  - The changes are restricted to one lobe.
- Even in these cases, surgery is seldom indicated D [4].

References

1. Bradley J, Moran F, Greenstone M. Physical training for bronchiectasis. Cochrane Database Syst Rev. 2004;(2):CD002166.
2. Jones AP, Rowe BH. Bronchopulmonary hygiene physical therapy for chronic obstructive pulmonary disease and bronchiectasis. Cochrane Database Syst Rev. 2004;(2):CD000045.
3. Crockett AJ, Cranston JM, Latimer KM, Alpers JH. Mucolytics for bronchiectasis. Cochrane Database Syst Rev. 2004;(2):CD001289.
4. Corless JA, Warburton CJ. Surgery versus non-surgical treatment for bronchiectasis. Cochrane Database Syst Rev. 2004;(2):CD002180.

6.30 Asthma: symptoms and diagnosis

Timo Keistinen

Pathophysiology

- Asthma is an inflammatory disease of the airways.
- Persons susceptible to asthma get symptoms associated with the inflammation. The symptoms usually include an airway obstruction of variable degree, which is relieved spontaneously or with treatment.
- The inflammation increases the sensitivity of the airways to many irritants.

Epidemiology

- The cumulative prevalence of asthma in the population is 2–6%, but there may be up to 15-fold differences in the prevalence of asthma symptoms between countries. According to several studies the prevalence is increasing, especially among younger age groups.
- Asthma affects especially two population groups: young children and those aged 40 years or over.
- Annually about 20–30 persons out of one million die of asthma. Only 10% of them are under 40 years of age.
- A general practitioner with a list size of 2000 has about 80 asthmatic patients. Half of the patients know they have asthma, and half of these patients see their doctor regularly at least once a year. The resting 25 patients manage their disease by themselves. Most patients with asthma have mild symptoms, but an average GP encounters one death from asthma every 10 years.

Symptoms

- The symptoms of asthma are variable, and differ greatly between patients. The symptoms may even vary in one single patient from month to month.
- Common symptoms of asthma include
  - Dyspnoea
    - in the early morning hours
    - after exercise (especially in cold weather)
    - in association with upper respiratory tract infections
    - in association with exposure to allergens such as pollen and animal dander.
  - wheezing
    - simultaneously with dyspnoea
  - prolonged cough
    - in the early morning hours
    - in association with irritating factors
    - For about one-third of patients with persistent cough an asthma diagnosis is set later.
    - The cough may be dry, but often clear mucus is excreted from the lower respiratory tract.
- For differences between asthma and COPD, see Table 6.30.

Diagnostic approach

- The diagnosis of asthma may sometimes be made on the basis of history and auscultation.
- The extent of the necessary examinations needed and the location where they are performed depends on the case and regional practices.
- If continuous medication is considered, the baseline situation should be assessed thoroughly and the diagnosis should be certain. This enables the doctor to compare the later course of the disease with the baseline situation (which is the requirement in some countries for the patient to get reimbursement for the medication).
- The diagnostic investigations are listed below in the order of importance. Auscultation of the lungs and peak expiratory

Table 6.30 Differences between asthma and COPD

Disease characteristics	Asthma	COPD
Aetiology	Unknown, atopy	Smoking
Onset	Often rapid	Slow
Dyspnoea	Paroxysmal	On physical exertion
Obstruction	Variable	Progressive, constant
Diffusion of respiratory gases	Normal	Often impaired
Eosinophilic leukocytes in sputum	Often present	Rarely present
Response to bronchodilating drugs	Strong	Weak
Course of the disease	Variable	Progressive

flow (PEF) measurement should always be performed. Other examinations may be needed in uncertain cases, as well as in cases where a more exact classification of the disease is pursued (intrinsic/extrinsic, predisposing factors).

Auscultation of the lungs

- End-expiratory wheezing is nearly always a sign of an obstructive disease such as asthma.
- In mild incipient asthma the auscultation is nearly always normal when the patient is asymptomatic.
- The auscultation may be normal even in patients with excessive symptoms.

PEF measurement

- The result is usually normal in incipient asthma during an asymptomatic phase.
- A 15% improvement from baseline (and more than 60 l/min) in the bronchodilatation test is significant (6.7).

Spirometry

- Gives more accurate information on pulmonary function than PEF.
- Forced vital capacity (FVC), forced expiratory flow in one second (FEV1) and the ratio of the two (FEV%) are the most important measurements (6.7)
- The examination is rather easy to perform and inexpensive.

PEF monitoring at home

- PEF monitoring at home is a good examination in the confirmation of asthma diagnosis (6.7).
- The patient measures the PEF value in the morning and later in the afternoon for one week without medications.
  - Three consecutive, forceful, brief blows are performed, and the best result is recorded.
  - A difference of at least 20% (calculated as the difference between the highest and the lowest value within a 24-h period divided by their mean), or a difference over 60 l/min, occurring at least three times during the follow-up period, strongly supports an asthma diagnosis.
- The following week the PEF recordings are repeated with a bronchodilating medication.
  - Three consecutive blows in the morning after wake-up; the best value is recorded.
  - Bronchodilating medication is taken with a dose inhaler.
  - After 15 minutes, the three blows are repeated and the best value is again recorded.
  - The same procedure is repeated in the afternoon.

Exercise test

- Running in the open air, especially in cold weather often triggers bronchoconstriction is asthmatic patients.
  - After PEF recording, the patient runs out of doors for 6 min.
  - Auscultate the lungs and record PEF value immediately after the exercise and repeatedly after 5, 10 and 15 min. A decrease of more than 15% in the PEF value is a significant finding.
- The examination is particularly suitable for young asthmatics in whom coronary heart disease is not suspected.

Laboratory tests

- The number of eosinophil leukocytes in blood and sputum is sometimes increased, but seldom in the elderly.
- Specific serum IgE may be determined if skin prick tests are not available.

Radiological examinations

- Chest x-ray
  - A differential diagnostic examination (heart failure, lung tumour)
  - Usually normal in patients with asthma
  - Not needed in the follow-up without specific reason.
- Sinus x-ray or ultrasonography
  - Sinusitis may be the cause of prolonged cough.
  - Persons with asthma often have sinusitis.

Skin prick tests

- May be indicated in suspected pollen or animal dander allergy

Allergen provocation tests

- Performed only in specialized clinics

6.31 Long-term management of asthma

Timo Keistinen

Aims

- Teach the patient self-management in the follow-up and treatment A [1].
- The patient's own primary care physician checks the adequacy of the treatment regularly.
  - Minimal symptoms
  - Normal functional ability
  - Minimal need for an inhaled sympathomimetic drug
  - Minimal daily variation in the peak expiratory flow (PEF) values (maximum 10–20%)
  - No side effects of drugs
  - Normal pulmonary function at least after inhaled sympathomimetic
- Diagnose sinusitis as a potential cause of an exacerbation.

Principles of long-term management

- Anti-inflammatory drugs (corticosteroids) are an essential part of the treatment A [2 3 4 5 6].
- Teaching and monitoring the inhalation technique of drugs is important.
- The treatment should be tailored for each patient according to the severity of the disease and modified flexibly step-by-step. Self-management of drug dosing is encouraged (written instructions!).
- Short courses of oral corticosteroids are occasionally needed.
- All persons with asthma should avoid exposure to high allergen concentrations D [7] and, e.g., sensitizing chemicals at work.
- Aspirin and other NSAIDs should be used cautiously, as 10–20% of patients with asthma are allergic to these drugs.
- Beta-blockers often exacerbate the symptoms of asthma.
- Smoking may wreck the results of asthma care.
- Desensitisation therapy may help some patients A [8 9 10].

Implementation of long-term management

- The patient has symptoms only occasionally (not every week), and they do not disturb sleep
  - Allergy proofing of the environment D [7] and cessation of smoking
  - Inhaled short-acting beta-sympathomimetic as needed B [11] (salbutamol, terbutalin or fenoterol)
- If inhaled sympathomimetics are needed several times a week or if sleep is disturbed by asthma, adding regular anti-inflammatory medication is indicated.
  - Inhaled B [12] corticosteroid (beclomethasone, budesonide A [13], or fluticasone A [14 15]) 100–400 μg twice daily
    - The most effective anti-inflammatory medication A [2 3 4 5 6]
    - Pressurized aerosols should not be used without an inhalation chamber.
    - Inhalation powders are usually well tolerated; however, patients with weakened respiratory muscles or lowered vital capacity should preferably take their drugs as dose aerosols using a spacer.
  - A leukotriene antagonist (e.g. montelukast 10 mg daily, or zafirlukast 20 mg twice daily A [16 17]) may be used as an alternative, but the effect in usual licensed doses is inferior to inhaled corticosteroids A [18].
  - Inhaled chromoglycate 5–20 mg four times daily or nedochromil 4 mg 2–4 times daily are alternatives
    - These drugs are usually not as effective as inhaled corticosteroids.
  - There is no evidence that antileukotrienes would have an inhaled steroid-sparing effect. Evidence on the benefit from doubling the dose of inhaled corticosteroids is insufficient. Antileukotrienes at high doses (2–4 times those recommended) used as add-on therapy to inhaled corticosteroids reduce exacerbations that require systemic steroids C [19].
- If the symptoms continue daily, if the need for an inhaled sympathomimetic is frequent, and obstruction is present according to PEF monitoring
  - Check the inhalation techniques, recognize any factors that might worsen the asthma and verify the patient's compliance.
  - Add a long-acting inhaled sympathomimetic A [20] (salmeterol 50 μg twice daily, formoterol 12–24 μg twice daily) without omitting the necessary anti-inflammatory medication.
- If the long-acting beta-sympathomimetic drug is not effective or is not tolerated, discontinue it and make a therapeutical trial with leukotriene antagonist B [21], or theophylline 200–300 mg at night.
- If the symptoms are not controlled adequately with a combination of a 800 μg daily dose of inhaled steroid and a long-acting beta-sympathomimetic drug, added with a short-acting sympathomimetic when needed, add one or more of the following:
  - Daily dose of inhaled steroid up to 2 mg
  - Leukotriene antagonist C [19], montelukast or zafirlukast
  - Long-acting theophylline 200–300 mg at night
  - Beta-sympathomimetic in liquid form administered with a nebulizer
  - Inhaled anticholinergic drug, if symptoms of COPD are present (ipratropium 80 μg or oxytropium 200 μg four times daily) A [22 23]
  - Chromoglycate or nedochromil (effect often quite limited)

- Assess the effect of the added drug. If a favourable response is not observed within 3–4 weeks the drug should be discontinued.
- If the symptoms are not adequately controlled with the above-mentioned treatments add
  - oral corticosteroids (prednisolone, methylprednisolone). Use the smallest dose that controls the symptoms. Corticosteroid taken every other day is usually not enough to control severe asthma in adults.

Tapering down of medication

- With regard to systemic adverse effects, the doses of inhaled corticosteroids that are considered safe in maintenance therapy are in adults 800 μg (beclomethasone, budesonide) and 400 μg (fluticasone).
- As the symptoms alleviate, the medication can be tapered down gradually.
- If the symptoms are minimal, if the need for inhaled bronchodilating medication is small, if the PEF values are normal, and if there is no diurnal variation, the dose of anti-inflammatory medication can be halved about 6 months after the disease has stabilized. PEF values and diurnal variation should be monitored.
- In chronic asthma it is often not possible to stop all anti-inflammatory medication.

Other treatments for asthma

Antihistamines

- Antihistamines have a very limited role in the treatment of asthma **B** [24 25]. They may mainly be used to alleviate other allergic symptoms.

Antibiotics

- Only clear signs of bacterial infection are an indication for antibiotics.
- Infections associated with acute exacerbations of asthma are often of viral origin. Remember sinusitis, but avoid unnecessary antibiotics.

Cough medicines

- Cough and sputum are usually signs of poor asthma control. Intensification of the treatment, or a short course of oral corticosteroids may be more effective than cough medicines.

Course of oral corticosteroids

Indications

- Increasing symptoms and decreasing PEF values over consecutive days
- The effect duration of inhaled bronchodilating medication is shortening.
- PEF values are less than 50–70% of the patient's best values.
- Sleep is disturbed by asthma.
- Morning symptoms persist until noon.
- Maximal medication without oral corticosteroids shows no sufficient effect.
- An acute exacerbation for which the patient has received nebulised or intravenous bronchodilating medication in an emergency setting **A** [26].

Dosage

- Prednisolon is given 30 (–40) mg daily until the symptoms are alleviated and the PEF values are normalised, and still for 3 days thereafter (usually 30–40 mg for 5–10 days).
- The drug may usually be stopped at once without tapering the dose gradually.

Self-management of asthma

- The patient should have good knowledge of self-management.
- The components of successful self-management are
  - acceptance and understanding of asthma and its treatment
  - effective and compliant use of drugs
  - a PEF meter and follow-up sheets at home
  - written instructions for different problems.
- As a part of guided self-management the patient may receive a PEF follow-up sheet with individually determined alarm thresholds and the following instructions **B** [27]:
  - If the morning PEF values are 85% of the patient's earlier optimal value, the dose of the inhaled corticosteroid should be doubled for two weeks.
  - If the morning PEF values are less than 50–70% of the optimal value, the patient starts a course of oral prednisolone 40 mg daily for one week and contacts the doctor or asthma nurse by telephone.

Indications for specialist consultation

- The indications for consultation are relative and they depend on the services available and the experience of the patient's primary care doctor in the treatment of asthma.
  - Newly diagnosed patients
  - Suspected cases of occupational asthma
  - Recurrent exacerbations
  - Assessment of working ability
  - Severe exacerbation
  - Symptoms in spite of a large dose of inhaled corticosteroids
  - Nebuliser for home use is considered
  - Pregnant women with increased symptoms
  - Asthma interferes with the patient's way of living (e.g. sports activities)

Follow-up

- Because asthma is a common disease it should be mainly treated and followed up by a general practitioner.
- A patient on medication should meet his/her own doctor regularly.
- In mild cases one follow-up appointment yearly is sufficient.
- In addition to symptom history and lung auscultation, a two-week recording of PEF values at home is often sufficient

as follow-up, eventually complemented by a simple spirometry (6.7).

References

1. Gibson PG, Powell H, Coughlan J, Wilson AJ, Abramson M, Haywood P, Bauman A, Hensley MJ, Walters EH. Self-management education and regular practitioner review for adults with asthma. Cochrane Database Syst Rev. 2004;(2):CD001117.
2. Adams NP, Bestall JB, Jones PW. Inhaled beclomethasone versus placebo for chronic asthma. Cochrane Database Syst Rev. 2004;(2):CD002738.
3. van Grunsven PM, van Schayck CP, Molema J, Akkermans RP, van Weel C. Effect of inhaled corticosteroids on bronchial responsiveness in patients with "corticosteroid naive" mild asthma: a meta-analysis. Thorax 1999;54:316–322.
4. The Database of Abstracts of Reviews of Effectiveness (University of York), Database no.: DARE-990806. In: The Cochrane Library, Issue 3, 2000. Oxford: Update Software.
5. Haahtela T, Herrala J, Kava T ym. Comparison of a $\beta 2$-agonist, terbutaline, with an inhaled corticosteroid, budesonide, in newly detected asthma. N Engl J Med 1991;325: 388–392.
6. Reed CE; Offord KP; Nelson HS; Li JT; Tinkelman DG. Aerosol beclomethasone dipropionate spray compared with theophylline as primary treatment for chronic mild-to-moderate asthma. The American Academy of Allergy, Asthma and Immunology Beclomethasone Dipropionate-Theophylline Study Group. J Allergy Clin Immunol 1998;101:14–23.
7. Gøtzsche PC, Johansen HK, Burr ML, Hammarquist C. House dust mite control measures for asthma. Cochrane Database Syst Rev. 2004;(2):CD001187.
8. Abramson MJ, Puy RM, Weiner JM. Allergen immunotherapy for asthma. Cochrane Database Syst Rev. 2004;(2):CD001186.
9. Malling HJ. Immunotherapy as an effective tool in allergy treatment. Allergy 1998;53:461–472.
10. The Database of Abstracts of Reviews of Effectiveness (University of York), Database no.: DARE-981030. In: The Cochrane Library, Issue 2, 2000. Oxford: Update Software.
11. Walters EH, Walters J. Inhaled short acting beta2-agonist use in chronic asthma: regular versus as needed treatment. Cochrane Database Syst Rev. 2004;(2):CD001285.
12. Mash B, Bheekie A, Jones PW. Inhaled vs oral steroids for adults with bronchial asthma. The Cochrane Database of Systematic Reviews, Cochrane Library number: CD002160. In: The Cochrane Library, Issue 2, 2002. Oxford: Update Software.
13. Adams N, Bestall J, Jones PW. Budesonide for chronic asthma in children and adults. Cochrane Database Syst Rev. 2004;(2):CD003274.
14. Adams N, Bestall J, Jones PW. Inhaled fluticasone propionate for asthma. The Cochrane Database of Systematic Reviews, Cochrane Library number: CD003135. In: The Cochrane Library, Issue 2, 2002. Oxford: Update Software. Updated frequently.
15. Adams N, Bestall JM, Jones PW. Inhaled fluticasone at different doses for chronic asthma. Cochrane Database Syst Rev. 2004;(2):CD003534.
16. Kelloway JS. Zafirlukast: the first leukotriene-receptor antagonist approved for the treatment of asthma. Ann Pharmacother 1997;31:1012–1021.
17. The Database of Abstracts of Reviews of Effectiveness (University of York), Database no.: DARE-971168. In: The Cochrane Library, Issue 4, 1999. Oxford: Update Software.
18. Ng D, Di Salvio F, Hicks G. Anti-leukotriene agents compared to inhaled corticosteroids in the management of recurrent and/or chronic asthma in adults and children. Cochrane Database Syst Rev. 2004;(2):CD002314.
19. Ducharme F, Schwartz Z, Hicks G, Kakuma R. Addition of anti-leukotriene agents to inhaled corticosteroids for chronic asthma. Cochrane Database Syst Rev. 2004;(2):CD003133.
20. Walters EH, Walters JAE, Gibson, MDP. Inhaled long acting beta agonists for stable chronic asthma. Cochrane Database Syst Rev 2003(4):CD00001385.
21. Bjermer L, Bisgaard H, Bousquet J, Fabbri LM, Greening AP, Haahtela T, Holgate ST, Picado C, Menten J, Dass SB, Leff JA, Polos PG. Montelukast and fluticasone compared with salmeterol and fluticasone in protecting against asthma exacerbation in adults: one year, double blind, randomised, comparative trial. BMJ 2003;327(7420):891.
22. Rodrigo G, Rodrigo C, Burschtin O. A meta-analysis of the effects of ipratropium bromide in adults with acute asthma. American Journal of Medicine 1999, 107(4), 363–370.
23. The Database of Abstracts of Reviews of Effectiveness (University of York), Database no.: DARE-992129. In: The Cochrane Library, Issue 3, 2002. Oxford: Update Software.
24. Van Ganse E, Kaufman L, Derde MP, Yernault JC, Delaunois L, Vincken W. Effects of antihistamines in adult asthma: a meta-analysis of clinical trials. Eur Resp J 1997;10:2216–2224.
25. The Database of Abstracts of Reviews of Effectiveness (University of York), Database no.: DARE-971348. In: The Cochrane Library, Issue 4, 1999. Oxford: Update Software.
26. Rowe BH, Spooner CH, Ducharme FM, Bretzlaff JA, Bota GW. Corticosteroids for preventing relapse following acute exacerbations of asthma. Cochrane Database Syst Rev. 2004;(2):CD000195.
27. Lahdensuo A, Haahtela T, Herrala J ym. Randomised comparison of guided self-management and traditional treatment of asthma over one year. BMJ 1996;312:748–752.

6.32 Treatment of acute exacerbation of asthma

Timo Keistinen

Basic rules

- The patient, family members, and the physician often underestimate the severity of an acute exacerbation of asthma.

- The aim of the treatment is
  - to prevent asthma deaths
  - to restore the condition and the pulmonary functions of the patient to a satisfactory level as soon as possible
  - to maintain an optimal functional status and to prevent a recurrence of the exacerbation.

Recognition of an acute exacerbation of asthma

- Occurrence of even one of the following signs means that the attack is severe:
  - Wheezing and dyspnoea have increased so that the patient cannot finish one sentence without stopping for breath, or cannot stand up from a chair.
  - Respiratory frequency is constantly 25/min or more.
  - Heart rate is constantly 110/min or more (>30 minutes after salbutamol inhalation).
  - PEF is less than 40% of the best previous value, or below 200 l/min, if the best previous value is not known.
  - Oxygen saturation is below 92%.
  - The condition of the patient deteriorates despite treatment.

Signs indicating a life-threatening attack

- Silent respiration sounds in auscultation
- Cyanosis
- Bradycardia or hypotension
- Exhaustion, confusion or unconsciousness
- Arterial blood $pO_2 < 8$ kPa even after breathing extra oxygen, and arterial $pCO_2 > 6$ kPa.

Immediate treatment

1. Put the patient in a **comfortable sitting position**, legs down if possible, so that he/she can bend forward if needed and have support for the hands and legs.
2. Give **oxygen** (usually 35% concentration is enough; in resuscitation, maximal concentration and flow) at the rate of 4–5 l/min either through mask or nasal cannulas.
3. Give **salbutamol aerosol** 0.1 mg/dose 4–8 puffs with a spacer B [1 2 3], or 2.5–10 mg with a nebulizer (or fenoterol 1.25 mg), and ipratropium bromide 0.5 mg A [4 5] nebulized (e.g. Bennet, Bird, Spira), with or without oxygen. Repeat the treatment every 20–30 minutes 2–4 times when necessary. Theophylline is not recommended anymore for routine use in the treatment of an exacerbation of asthma B [6] because its effectiveness is questionable and it has adverse effects. In a severe attack, however, when intensive care should be considered, theophylline may be tried: 5 mg per kg of weight intravenously over 20–30 minutes, to be continued with an infusion (400 mg theophylline is diluted in 1,000 ml of 0.9% NaCl or 5% glucose solution; infusion rate is 0.6 mg/kg/h for patients under 50 years of age and 0.4–0.5 mg/kg/h to patients over 50).
4. Give a high dose of **corticosteroid** intravenously or orally (e.g. 40–80 mg methyl prednisolone or 125–250 mg hydrocortisone) A [7 8 9 10]. Oral corticosteroids (e.g. 30–40 mg prednisolone) are given independent of the intravenous steroids as soon as the patient is able to swallow.
5. Continue with oral corticosteroids (e.g. prednisolone 30–40 mg in the morning) for several days. If the patient has continuous corticosteroid medication at home he/she may require a higher dose.
6. In a life-threatening and severe acute asthma attack, when the bronchodilating medication does not show sufficient effect, consider magnesium sulphate 1.2–2 g as a slow intravenous infusion over 20 minutes C [11 12 13].
7. If the attack is prolonged, the patient may be dehydrated because dyspnoea prevents drinking. The patient may need **fluids** 2000–3000 ml in excess of normal diurnal need. Caution is needed with old patients and those with heart disease!

Further treatment

- The patient should not be left alone until the condition has clearly improved.
- Continue oxygen therapy as needed.
- Continue oral corticosteroid therapy (e.g. 30–40 mg prednisolone/day) A [14].
- If the condition has improved, continue nebulisation treatment at 4-hour intervals.
- If the condition has not improved, repeat nebulisation treatment in 15–30 minutes.
- **Sedative drugs** must not be used in exacerbation of asthma, except in intensive care units.
- **Antimicrobial drugs** are not indicated if there are no signs of a bacterial infection. Patting physiotherapy is contraindicated.

Tests and investigations

- PEF in the beginning of the treatment and in the follow-up
- Arterial blood gas analysis in severe conditions; repeated as needed
- Pulse oximetry (reveals hypoxia, but not hypercapnia)
- Heart rate
- Theophylline concentration in prolonged infusion
- Serum potassium and blood glucose
- ECG in elderly patients
- Chest x-ray in severe and poorly responding cases to exclude pneumothorax, pulmonary infiltrates and pulmonary oedema
- Serum haematocrit, if necessary, to estimate dehydration

Indications for intensive care

- Persistent severe dyspnoea despite beta2-sympathomimetics given repeatedly 3–4 times at 20–30 min intervals.
- Arterial blood pO_2 is below 8 kPa despite breathing of extra oxygen
- Arterial blood pCO_2 is over 6 kPa

- Exhaustion
- Confusion, drowsiness
- Unconsciousness
- Respiratory arrest

Hospital discharge after acute exacerbation of asthma

- Pulmonary functions must be normalised before the patient is discharged
  - PEF value must be over 75% of reference value or of previous maximal value.
  - Diurnal variation in PEF must be less than 25%.
  - Nightly symptoms must be absent.
- Upon discharge, make sure that the patient has
  - an oral steroid (prednisolone 20–40 mg/day) for 1–2 weeks A [14]
  - an inhalable anti-inflammatory drug (usually steroid)
  - an inhalable beta sympathomimetic drug
  - had the long-term maintenance therapy re-evaluated
  - preferably an own PEF meter at home
  - knowledge of the correct inhalation technique
  - an appointment for the next follow-up visit.

References

1. Cates CJ, Bara A, Crilly JA, Rowe BH. Holding chambers versus nebulisers for beta-agonist treatment of acute asthma. Cochrane Database Syst Rev. 2004;(2):CD000052.
2. Turner MO, Patel A, Ginsburg S, Fitzgerald JM. Bronchodilator delivery in acute airflow obstruction. Arch Intern Med 1997;157:1736–1744.
3. The Database of Abstracts of Reviews of Effectiveness (University of York), Database no.: DARE-978301. In: The Cochrane Library, Issue 4, 1999. Oxford: Update Software.
4. Stoodley RG, Aaron SD, Dales RE. The role of ipratropium bromide in the emergency management of acute asthma exacerbation; a metaanalysis of randomized clinical trials. Annals of Emergency Medicine 1999;34:8–18.
5. The Database of Abstracts of Reviews of Effectiveness (University of York), Database no.: DARE-991385 In: The Cochrane Library, Issue 2, 2001. Oxford: Update Software.
6. Parameswaran K, Belda J Rowe BH. Addition of intravenous aminophylline to beta2-agonists in adults with acute asthma. Cochrane Database Syst Rev. 2004;(2):CD002742.
7. Rowe BH, Spooner C, Ducharme FM, Bretzlaff JA, Bota GW. Early emergency department treatment of acute asthma with systemic corticosteroids. Cochrane Database Syst Rev. 2004;(2):CD002178.
8. Manser R, Reid D, Abramson M. Corticosteroids for acute severe asthma in hospitalised patients. The Cochrane Database of Systematic Reviews, Cochrane Library number: CD001740. In: The Cochrane Library, Issue 2, 2002. Oxford: Update Software. Updated frequently.
9. Rodrigo G, Godrigo C. Corticosteroids in the emergency department therapy of acute adult asthma: an evidence-based evaluation. Chest 1999;116:285–295.
10. The Database of Abstracts of Reviews of Effectiveness (University of York), Database no.: DARE-991636. In: The Cochrane Library, Issue 1, 2001. Oxford: Update Software.
11. Rodrigo G, Rodrigo C, Burschtin O. Efficacy of magnesium sulfate in acute adult asthma: a meta-analysis of randomized trials. American Journal of Emergency Medicine 2000, 18(2), 216–221.
12. The Database of Abstracts of Reviews of Effectiveness (University of York), Database no.: DARE-20000726. In: The Cochrane Library, Issue 2, 2002. Oxford: Update Software.
13. Rowe BH, Bretzlaff JA, Bourdon C, Bota GW, Camargo CA Jr. Magnesium sulfate for treating exacerbations of acute asthma in the emergency department. The Cochrane Database of Systematic Reviews, Cochrane Library number: CD001490. In: The Cochrane Library, Issue 2, 2002. Oxford: Update Software. Updated frequently.
14. Rowe BH, Spooner CH, Ducharme FM, Bretzlaff JA, Bota GW. Corticosteroids for preventing relapse following acute exacerbations of asthma. Cochrane Database Syst Rev. 2004;(2):CD000195.

6.33 Occupational asthma

Henrik Nordman

Introduction

- Consider occupational irritants and sensitizers as well as work conditions in cases of adult onset asthma.
- Familiarize yourself with the diagnostic investigations of asthma, to be carried out either in primary or specialist care.
- Remember that you may be under a statutory obligation to report clinically diagnosed cases of occupational asthma.
- Work-related asthma does not always fulfil the statutory criteria of an occupational asthma.

Occurrence

- Epidemiological studies carried out during recent years suggest that occupational asthma is likely to be underreported. According to several epidemiological studies, the proportion of adult asthma attributable to work is as high as 15–30%. The significance of occupational agents in the multifactorial etiology of asthma thus appears to be much greater than was previously thought.

Common causes of occupational asthma

- In agriculture, the most common causative agents include animal epithelium (cow dander being the most significant), animal secretions, flour, grain, animal feed and laboratory storage mite. In bakeries, flour as well as spices and bread improvers, such as various enzymes, are sensitizers.

- Moulds in damp buildings increase the risk of asthma and can also act as specific sensitizers.
- In woodwork, several hard woods (e.g. apache, cedar) may sensitize.
- Of chemicals, di-isocyanates remain an important cause of occupational asthma. Latex rubber, organic acid anhydrides, epoxy resins and plastics as well as formaldehyde are further examples of other small molecular weight agents causing asthma.
- Welding fumes, particularly of stainless steel, and cutting fluids should be borne in mind.

Symptoms

- Asthma-like symptoms occur on work days or during a work shift, i.e. cough (often nocturnal), dyspnoea, wheezing shortness of breath.
- At the beginning there is a clear distinction between days at work and days off work. As the exposure continues the symptoms may persist over the weekend and only clear after a prolonged exposure-free period.
- The symptoms may not emerge until after a work shift, or at night, particularly when the causative agent is a chemical.
- Upper respiratory tract and eye symptoms often precede the asthmatic symptoms.

Diagnostic work-up

- A detailed occupational history is important. Valuable data can be obtained from the patient's subjective observations, workplace studies carried out by the occupational health department and relevant operational safety instructions.
- The symptoms should be consistent with those of occupational asthma.
- Asthma should be properly diagnosed.
  - The diagnostics of asthma is the same as that for asthma (see 6.30) to the causative agent in general.
  - Sometimes asthma can be demonstrated only in conjunction with exposure.
- Demonstration of sensitization to specific work-related agents aids the diagnosis.
  - Skin prick tests
  - If possible, measurement of specific IgE antibodies
  - The presence of IgG antibodies merely demonstrates exposure, not sensitization, and are therefore not diagnostic.
- Demonstration of a work-related asthmatic reaction
  - PEF recordings at work (organised by the occupational health department or specialist centres, see below)
  - Specific challenge tests (specialist centres only)

PEF recordings at the workplace

- An important part of the diagnosis of occupational asthma. Should always be carried out if occupational asthma is suspected.
- Differs from the PEF (peak expiratory flow) measurements carried out to diagnose ordinary asthma, see 6.30
- Should not be carried out in acute or severe asthma.
- Serial measurements must be carried out for a sufficient length of time, preferably for three weeks including two weekends (or other time off work).
- PEF measurements should be made every two hours when awake, both at work and at home.
- The patient must be motivated to carry out the recordings, and adequate instructions must be provided. If carried out incorrectly, PEF recordings at the workplace cannot be interpreted.
- The information obtained from recordings taken at the workplace may be augmented by monitoring bronchial reactivity at work and during holidays.
- The occupational health personnel should be aware that investigations should be initiated without delay. It is also worth carrying on with the PEF recordings during sick leave; the monitoring should continue when the employee returns to work.

Specific challenge tests

- Challenge tests should be carried out only by specialist centres with sufficient expertise.
- The most reliable method to establish a causal relationship between an occupational agent and asthma.
- Challenge tests may be carried out in a variety of ways:
  - Commercial allergen extracts may be used, e.g. in cases of suspected allergy to cow dander.
  - Specific challenge tests may be carried out in challenge chambers (specialist facilities only) using for example flour, wood dust, glue, paint and chemicals, such as formaldehyde, isocyanates and acid anhydrides.
  - A challenge test may also be carried out at the workplace if the causative agent has not been isolated or commercial extracts are not available. A hospitalized patient will go to work with an accompanying nurse, who will monitor the patient at work. The monitoring continues when the patient returns to hospital.
- A positive result is reliable. However, a negative result does not exclude the possibility of occupational asthma. Reasons for a negative result may include the following: wrong substance was used for testing, the extract did not contain a sufficient amount of the allergen, the time period away from exposure was too long and the reaction had subsided, or the short exposure time does not correspond to fulltime exposure five days a week.

Treatment and rehabilitation

- Medical treatment does not differ from that of other types of asthma.
- The most important consideration is the total avoidance, or significant reduction, of exposure to the causative agent. This can be achieved by

- setting restrictions to the work environment
- relocating the patient within the previous workplace
- retraining
- using a breathing mask, useful mainly in temporary exposure
- considering the options of early retirement/disability pensions etc.

♦ If the patient is relocated within the previous workplace, the occupational health team must be involved in monitoring the patient's condition.

♦ If the relocation is unsuccessful, other forms of rehabilitation should be considered.

Prognosis

♦ The symptoms usually resolve when exposure to the causative agent is either totally avoided or significantly reduced. The sooner the exposure is eliminated after the onset of symptoms the better the prognosis.

♦ Occupational asthma may remain symptomatic for several years and, in some cases, may become permanent. The recovery from asthma caused by chemicals is often poor. In particular, the prognosis of asthma caused by isocyanates is known to be poor.

♦ When occupational asthma is diagnosed the monitoring of the patient and optimal medication are of utmost importance.

Other symptoms resembling asthma

♦ Some patients may suffer from work-related asthma-like symptoms but lack changes in pulmonary function. In these cases asthma cannot be diagnosed.

♦ A third of these patients are likely to develop clinical asthma within a year or two.

♦ These patients should be treated in the same way as those with work-related exacerbation of asthma. Restrictions should be set on the patient's work environment, and anti-inflammatory medication should be prescribed to prevent the emergence of clinical asthma.

♦ The occupational health department should be in charge of monitoring the condition of these patients.

♦ If the symptoms become worse, the investigations for an occupational illness should be repeated.

Work-related exacerbation of asthma

♦ All types of asthma may often be exacerbated by dust and other irritants encountered at workplaces.

♦ Work-related exacerbation can be demonstrated using PEF measurements.

♦ Patients with conventional asthma may often return to work after their medication has been optimised.

♦ Return to work should be supervised by the occupational health department.

6.34 Chronic obstructive pulmonary disease (COPD)

Vuokko Kinnula

Basic rules

♦ Consider the diagnosis of COPD in any smoker who has the following: symptoms of cough, sputum production or dyspnoea.

♦ Make an early diagnosis by spirometry and promote smoking cessation.

♦ In mild COPD, FEV_1/FVC is below 0.7 and FEV% > 80% predicted (GOLD criteria).

♦ A trial of steroids must be performed if long-term steroid treatment is considered.

♦ Most important differential diagnostic problem is asthma. Also many asthmatics smoke.

Definitions

♦ Chronic bronchitis: sputum for at least 3 months in 2 consecutive years.

♦ Pulmonary emphysema (is a pathologic anatomic diagnosis): terminal air spaces widen and alveolar walls rupture.

♦ Chronic obstructive pulmonary disease (COPD): the patient has chronic, mainly progressive airway obstruction, with no significant response to treatment.

Aetiology

♦ Most COPD patients (>95%) are smokers. Half of those who smoke have symptoms of chronic bronchitis. At least in 15–20% of smokers a slowly aggravating airway obstruction is detected.

♦ Deficiency of alpha-1-antitrypsin is a rare cause of emphysema in young patients.

Symptoms

♦ Cough and sputum excretion are common symptoms of chronic bronchitis.

♦ Patients with progressive disease suffer from slowly increasing dyspnoea during exercise.

♦ The symptoms are aggravated by respiratory infection.

Signs

♦ Most patients consult a doctor late, when the disease is already moderate to severe. In mild disease auscultation may be normal and no auscultatory signs for obstruction can be detected.

- Absence of the following signs of severe COPD does not exclude the existence of mild COPD.
- Because of airway obstruction, wheezing rattles may be heard at the end of forced expiration.
- The patient with advanced emphysema has a barrel-chested appearance, on auscultation silent respiratory sounds are heard and on percussion the sound is hypersonor.
- Cyanosis is associated with hypoxaemia.

Complications

- Acute
  - Repeated and prolonged lower respiratory infections
  - Acute respiratory failure
  - Pneumothorax (disruption of emphysematic bullae)
- Chronic
  - Cardiopulmonary disease

Diagnosis

- Early diagnosis by spirometry combined with active promotion of smoking cessation is essential.
- Test with a bronchodilating drug (6.7)
  - The objective response to a bronchodilator (increase >15%) is measured with spirometry and bronchodilator dose (e.g. inhaled salbutamol 400 µg twice daily), or PEF follow-up for two weeks.
- Evaluate the effectiveness of anti-inflammatory treatment with a trial of steroids.
  - Oral prednisolone, initially 30–40 mg/day (if necessary, give protection against ulcers, e.g. a PPI), or inhaled steroid (e.g. budesonide 800 µg twice daily). In oral administration the duration of the trial is 2 weeks, with an inhaled steroid 6 weeks.
  - If there is an objective response (PEF or FEV_1 increase >15% and at least 200 ml), continue with inhalation steroid (the patient may also have asthma).
- Diffusion capacity
  - Decreased in COPD, normal in asthma.
- Blood gas analysis
  - In late stages of COPD arterial blood pO_2 decreases and pCO_2 may increase
- Chest x-ray is of limited value in COPD diagnosis.

Treatment

Cessation of smoking

- The most essential factor regarding the prognosis.
- Does not normalize lung function, but the progressive deterioration of FEV_1 slows down and proceeds at the same pace as in non-smokers.
- According to present knowledge, there is no drug therapy available that could delay the deterioration of lung function if the patient continues smoking. Drugs are useful only for relieving subjective symptoms and in the treatment of acute exacerbations.

Basic rules of drug therapy

- Mild disease
  - Asymptomatic patients
    - No drug therapy
  - Patients with occasional symptoms (generally FEV_1 > 50% predicted)
    - Anticholinergics or short-acting beta-2-agonists according to clinical response
    - Trial of steroids if asthma is suspected
- Continuous symptoms (generally FEV_1 < 50% predicted)
  - Anticholinergics and short-acting beta-2-agonists (combined) according to clinical response or
  - Long acting anticholinergic or beta-2-agonist, or their combination.
  - In selected cases inhaled glucocorticoid if frequent exacerbations.
  - Trial of theophylline (A) [1]
  - Surgery (bullectomy, lung transplantation, lung volume reduction) can be recommended only to a small subset of the patients after careful evaluation

Bronchodilating medication

- Inhaled short acting (ipratropium, oxytropium bromide) or long acting (tiotropium) anticholinergic drug (C) [2]
  - First line treatment
  - The dose must be high enough; administration 4–6 times daily with the short acting drug, once a day with the long acting tiotropium.
- Inhaled beta-sympathomimetic (salbutamol, terbutaline, fenoterol) (A) [3]
  - May be combined with an anticholinergic drug
  - Long-acting beta-sympathomimetics (formoterol, salmeterol) may improve quality of life and reduce symptoms (C) [4].
- Oral, long-acting theophylline (A) [1]
  - adverse effects (central nervous system, gastrointestinal symptoms) are common (follow-up of serum concentrations is necessary!)
  - Arrhythmias and convulsions are signs of toxicity.
  - Keep in mind the various interactions with other drugs (e.g. antibiotics)!

Anti-inflammatory medication

- Inhaled steroids are only prescribed for patients who objectively benefit from a trial of steroids. The benefit in terms of lung function is very limited. Selected patients with frequent exacerbations may benefit from inhaled corticosteroid (B) [5 6].

Treatment of mucous excretion

- If production of mucus is a problem, the patient may empty the lungs (D) [7] at home

- by performing forced expiration with the upper body tilted downwards (on the edge of the bed)
- by using expiration resistance (PEP mouthpiece) or blowing air through a straw into a bottle filled with water, combined with effective coughing

♦ Mucolytic agents should be used only temporarily B [8].

Treatment of acute exacerbation

♦ Oxygen by nasal catheter or by venturi mask. Caution should be exercised when dosing (if the result of an arterial blood gas analysis is not available, the concentration of mask oxygen should not exceed 28%, or nasal catheter flow should not exceed more than 2 l/min in patients above the age of 50 years).

♦ Non-invasive ventilation has improved the recovery in severe acute exacerbation of COPD A [9].

♦ An inhaled sympathomimetic (salbutamol 2.5–5 mg or terbutaline 5–10 mg) by a dosing device or a spray. Inhaled ipratropium bromide 0.5 mg can be added to it.

♦ There is no evidence of a significant effect of theophylline infusion C [10] and its usage is not recommended. It may sometimes be used at a dose of 0.5 mg/kg/h if response to other treatments is poor. Serum theophylline concentration should be monitored if possible.

♦ Methyl prednisolone 0.5 mg/kg every 6 hours is probably beneficial. Also oral corticosteroids (prednisolone 30–40 mg/day) are used empirically for 7–14 days.

Acute infection

♦ Antimicrobial treatment in an exacerbation of COPD is controversial B [11] [12] [13]. Factors that indicate starting antimicrobial treatment include

- increased dyspnoea
- increased sputum
- purulent sputum.

♦ If the patient exhibits two of the three symptoms listed above, an antimicrobial drug is usually indicated B [11] [12] [13].

♦ Alternatives in antimicrobial treatment:

- Amoxicillin 500 mg three times daily for 10 days
- Doxycycline 150 mg once daily for 10 days
- Sulpha-trimethoprim, dose of trimethoprim 160 mg twice daily for 10 days.

♦ Antibiotics have no place in the basic maintenance therapy of COPD.

Improvement of exercise capacity

♦ Long-lasting, regular, and moderate exercise 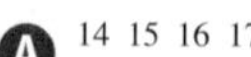 A [14] [15] [16] [17]

Vaccinations

♦ Influenza vaccination should be given yearly to all patients with clearly decreased ventilatory function C [18].

♦ Pneumococcal vaccination is recommended.

♦ Haemophilus influenzae vaccination may also be beneficial B [19]

Oxygen therapy at home

Basics

♦ Oxygen therapy at home can be used to prevent elevation of pulmonary arterial pressure in advanced COPD and to extend the life of the patient.

♦ The effect of oxygen therapy on symptoms (e.g. shortness of breath) is quite limited.

♦ Oxygen therapy at home is meant only for patients with chronic hypoxaemia, i.e. arterial desaturation.

♦ Treatment decisions should be made after critical consideration.

♦ When initiating oxygen therapy at home, appropriate monitoring of the treatment must be ensured. Treatment decisions and implementation of treatment should be the responsibility of the local pulmonary clinic.

Initiation criteria for oxygen therapy

♦ Chronic, advanced pulmonary disease ($FEV_1 < 1.5$ l)

♦ The partial pressure of oxygen in arterial blood, measured with the patient in a stable phase of the disease breathing room air is < 7.3 kPa in two samples taken with an interval of at least three weeks.

♦ Partial pressure of oxygen can also be 7.3–8.0 kPa if one of the following criteria is involved:

- signs of increased pulmonary arterial pressure (e.g. oedema)
- secondary polycythaemia (haematocrit > 55)
- significant nocturnal hypoxaemia established by oximetry and reversible by oxygen therapy and not caused by concomitant sleep apnoea syndrome
- significant neuropsychological symptoms reversible by oxygen therapy.

♦ Oxygen therapy gives the desired response ($PaO_2 > 8.0$ kPa) without unfavourable increase in the partial pressure of carbon dioxide in arterial blood.

♦ The patient does not smoke and is sufficiently co-operative.

Implementation of treatment

♦ Oxygen therapy at home is currently implemented in most cases using an electric oxygen concentrator. The oxygen concentrator eliminates nitrogen from room air and provides the patient with over 90%-proof oxygen. Compressed tanks can still be used in places with no electricity.

♦ Portable liquid oxygen is suitable for a minority of patients. Primarily these are patients who are still working or who for some other reason have special needs for mobility.

♦ All oxygen therapy necessitates good co-operation by the patient and willingness for long-term co-operation with the treating unit.

♦ Home calls made by a rehabilitation instructor are an essential part of the monitoring of patients receiving oxygen therapy at home.

References

1. Ram FSF, Jones PW, Castro AA, de Brito Jardim JR, Atallah AN, Lacasse Y, Mazzini R, Goldstein R, Cendon S. Oral theophylline for chronic obstructive pulmonary disease. Cochrane Database Syst Rev. 2004;(2):CD003902.
2. Brown CD, McCrory D, White J. Inhaled short-acting beta2-agonists versus ipratropium for acute exacerbations of chronic obstructive pulmonary disease. Cochrane Database Syst Rev. 2004;(2):CD002984.
3. Sestini P, Renzoni E, Robinson S, Poole P, Ram FSF. Short-acting beta 2 agonists for stable chronic obstructive pulmonary disease. Cochrane Database Syst Rev. 2004;(2):CD001495.
4. Appleton S, Poole P, Smith B, Veale A, Bara A. Long-acting beta2-agonists for chronic obstructive pulmonary disease patients with poorly reversible airflow limitation. Cochrane Database Syst Rev. 2004;(2):CD001104.
5. van Grunsven PM, van Schayck CP, Derenne JP, Kerstjens HA, Renkema TE, Postma DS, Similowski T, Akkermans RP, Pasker-de Jong PC, Dekhuijzen PN, van Herwaarden CL, van Weel C. Long-term effects of inhaled corticosteroids in chronic obstructive pulmonary disease: a meta-analysis. Thorax 1999;54:7–14.
6. The Database of Abstracts of Reviews of Effectiveness (University of York), Database no.: DARE-990281. In: The Cochrane Library, Issue 1, 2001. Oxford: Update Software.
7. Jones AP, Rowe BH. Bronchopulmonary hygiene physical therapy for chronic obstructive pulmonary disease and bronchiectasis. Cochrane Database Syst Rev. 2004;(2):CD000045.
8. Poole PJ, Black PN. Mucolytic agents for chronic bronchitis or chronic obstructive pulmonary disease. Cochrane Database Syst Rev. 2004;(2):CD001287.
9. Ram FSF, Picot J, Lightowler J, Wedzicha JA. Non-invasive positive pressure ventilation for treatment of respiratory failure due to exacerbations of chronic obstructive pulmonary disease. Cochrane Database Syst Rev. 2004;(2):CD004104.
10. Barr RG, Rowe BH, Camargo CA Jr. Methylxanthines for exacerbations of chronic obstructive pulmonary disease. Cochrane Database Syst Rev. 2004;(2):CD002168.
11. Saint S, Bent S, Vittinghaoff E, Grady D. Antibiotics in chronic obstructive pulmonary disease exacerbations: a meta-analysis. JAMA 1995;273:957–960.
12. The Database of Abstracts of Reviews of Effectiveness (University of York), Database no.: DARE-950358. In: The Cochrane Library, Issue 4, 1999. Oxford: Update Software.
13. Staykova T, Black P, Chacko E, Ram FSF, Poole P. Prophylactic antibiotic therapy for chronic bronchitis. Cochrane Database Syst Rev. 2004;(2):CD004105.
14. Lacasse Y, Wong E, Guyatt GH, King D, Cook DJ, Goldstein RS. Meta-analysis of respiratory rehabilitation in chronic obstructive pulmonary disease. Lancet 1996;348:1115–1119.
15. The Database of Abstracts of Reviews of Effectiveness (University of York), Database no.: DARE-968413. In: The Cochrane Library, Issue 4, 1999. Oxford: Update Software.
16. Cambach W, Wagenaar RC, Koelman TW, Ton van Keimpema AR, Kemper HC. The long-term effects of pulmonary rehabilitation in patients with asthma and chronic obstructive pulmonary disease: a research synthesis. Arch Phys Med Rehab 1999;80:103–111.
17. The Database of Abstracts of Reviews of Effectiveness (University of York), Database no.: DARE-990269. In: The Cochrane Library, Issue 2, 2000. Oxford: Update Software.
18. Poole PJ, Chacko E, Wood-Baker RWB, Cates CJ. Influenza vaccine for patients with chronic obstructive pulmonary disease. Cochrane Database Syst Rev. 2004;(2):CD002733.
19. Foxwell AR, Cripps AW, Dear KBG. Haemophilus influenzae oral whole cell vaccination for preventing acute exacerbations of chronic bronchitis. Cochrane Database Syst Rev. 2004;(2):CD001958.

6.40 Pulmonary fibrosis

Pentti Tukiainen

Incidence

- Idiopathic pulmonary fibrosis (IPF), about 16–18 patients/100 000 population/year

Symptoms

- Dry cough or progressive exertional dyspnoea
- Pulmonary fibrosis may occur in association with rheumatoid arthritis, scleroderma or other connective tissue disorders (1/4 of patients). Some patients also have additionally obscure joint complaints or Raynaud's phenomenon.

Physical signs

- End-inspiratory fine rales in >90%
- Hippocratic nails and clubbed fingers in about 50%
- Advanced disease is associated with signs of right ventricular cardiac stress

Laboratory findings

- ESR elevated, but CRP often normal.
- Tests for rheumatoid factor or antinuclear antibodies are often positive.

Radiological findings

- Chest x-ray
  - Linear markings or honeycomb-type of infiltrations are seen in the basal parts of the lungs.
- High-resolution computed tomography (HRCT)
  - A typical subpleural honeycomb pattern posteroinferiorly and anterosuperiorly.

Pulmonary function

- Blood gas analysis shows hypoxaemia, first on exertion, later even at rest.
- Spirometry shows restriction (in 50%) and reduced diffusing capacity (in all patients).

Diagnosis

- Clinical picture and HRCT
- Exclusion of other causes
  - Extrinsic alveolites: allergic alveolitis (6.41), eosinophilic pneumonia (6.42), chlamydial and mycoplasmal pneumonia (6.11), pneumoconioses (6.55)
  - Intrinsic alveolites: sarcoidosis (6.43), connective tissue disorders, and malignancies
- Lung biopsy
  - Thoracoscopy or open biopsy

Treatment

- Steroid in decreasing doses, e.g. prednisolone or equivalent starting with 30–50 mg/day
- Therapeutic response is obtained within six months.
- Maintenance therapy, e.g., with prednisolone 15 mg every other day.
- Azathioprine or cyclophosphamide should be instituted if no response is obtained with a steroid **C** [1].

Prognosis

- Objective therapeutic response very uncommon
- Unfavourable prognosis (five-year mortality 50%)

Reference

1. Davies HR, Richeldi L, Walters EH. Immunomodulatory agents for idiopathic pulmonary fibrosis. Cochrane Database Syst Rev. 2004;(2):CD003134.

6.41 Allergic alveolitis (farmer's lung, etc.)

Pentti Tukiainen

Aim

- To recognize allergic alveolitis as a cause of recurrent fever and dyspnoea in farmers.

Aetiology

- Sensitization to mouldy plant matter (hay, litter, straw, sawdust, chips, mushroom culture medium) (= farmer's lung) or the droppings of cage birds (= bird breeder's lung)

Symptoms

- The symptoms of acute alveolitis begin about four to eight hours after exposure to the allergen.
  - Exertional dyspnoea, chest tightness and cough
  - Fever, chills, muscle and joint pain, headache
  - Often also nausea, vomiting, sweating, loss of appetite and weight loss
- The symptoms generally appear after the working day or at night, and they abate within a few days. With repeated exposure, the attacks recur and become more severe.
- In its insidious, subacute form (the most common form!), allergic alveolitis may manifest as febrile episodes, various degrees of bronchitic symptoms, a feeling of malaise, loss of appetite, weight loss and development of exertional dyspnoea. The cause often remains undetected.
- The symptoms usually appear during the indoor feeding season.

Signs

- Fine inspiratory rales from the basal lung segments

Chest x-ray

- A normal finding or diffuse, micronodular ("milk-glass") shadowing

Laboratory findings

- Early stages often show ESR elevation and leukocytosis.
- Precipitating antibodies to mould spores. The presence of antibodies indicates exposure, not necessarily a disease.
- Bronchoalveolar lavage shows a strong accumulation of lymphocytes.

Pulmonary function tests

- Blood gases: reduced partial pressure of oxygen (pO_2) in arterial blood.
- Reduced diffusing capacity.
- Spirometry
  - Restriction
  - Some patients exhibit concurrent asthma-induced reversible obstruction.

Diagnosis

- Based on a typical clinical picture.

- In suspected new cases, it is advisable to contact a pulmonary medicine unit by phone to arrange for diagnostic investigations (spirometry and measurement of diffusing capacity) to be done without delay while the patient still has symptoms (if the investigations are done after the patient's sick leave, all findings may be normal).

Differential diagnoses

- Respiratory tract infections, other alveolites and obstructive pulmonary diseases

Treatment

- Exposure should be avoided.
- The patient should be prescribed a sick leave until recovery.
- Recurrence of the illness is prevented by use of personal protective equipment systems (face-masks and air-purifying respirator).
- Farmers may be entitled to compensation for the disease as an occupational illness.

Prognosis

- Long-term, untreated illness can develop into pulmonary fibrosis.
- Generally, pulmonary function will more or less normalize if the disease is diagnosed promptly.

6.42 Eosinophilic pneumonia

Olli Säynäjäkangas

Basic rule

- Consider a diagnosis of eosinophilic pneumonia if
  - pneumonia does not respond to treatment
  - pneumonia is associated with eosinophilia
  - the patient has systemic symptoms.

Aetiology

- Drugs (nitrofurantoin, penicillin, sulphonamides, tetracycline, tolfenamic acid, aspirin, naproxen, injectable gold etc.)
- Infection caused by Aspergillus fumigatus (bronchopulmonary aspergillosis, usually in patients with asthma)
- Intestinal parasites
- Inhalation of vaporized narcotics
- In most cases no specific aetiology is detected.

Symptoms and signs

- Symptoms
  - 60% of the patients have a history of allergic dermatitis, rhinitis, or asthma
  - cough, pleurisy, dyspnoea (asthma)
  - fever
- Signs
  - Expiratory wheezing (asthma)
  - Fine inspiratory rales (rather seldom)

Diagnostics

- Laboratory findings
  - Leucocytosis, blood eosinophilia (in 2/3 of patients)
  - Increased ESR and CRP
  - Eosinophilia in bronchoalveolar lavage sample
- Chest x-ray
  - Diffuse infiltration in 1/3 of the patients
  - One or more patchy infiltrates that may shift position (in 1/3 of the patients)
- Pulmonary function tests
  - Bronchoconstriction (asthma)
  - Restriction and decreased diffusion capacity (widespread affection of the lungs)
- Rapid response to steroids

Treatment

- A course of steroids with decreasing dose, e.g., prednisolone 30 mg, 20 mg, 15 mg, 10 mg and 5 mg, each dose for one week.

Prognosis

- More than 1/3 of the patients have only one episode of the disease.
- 1/3 of the patients have one or more relapses after the treatment is stopped.
- Less than 1/3 of the patients need continuous steroid treatment because the disease relapses recurrently after the treatment is stopped.

6.43 Sarcoidosis

Anne Pietinalho

Basic rules

- Suspect sarcoidosis in patients with symptoms from the lungs, skin, eyes or lymph nodes, and take a chest x-ray.

- Monitor pulmonary function and chest x-ray in patients with sarcoidosis and prevent the development of complications.

Epidemiology

- Sarcoidosis is a systemic granulomatous disease of unknown aetiology.
- The annual incidence in Scandinavia is 10–30/100 000, and the prevalence is 30–100/100 000.
- The onset of the disease most commonly occurs between the ages of 20 and 40 years, and very rarely in childhood.

Symptoms

- May occur in any organ, most commonly in the lungs (cough, dyspnoea), eyes (uveitis, iritis), skin (erythema nodosum, maculopapular lesions, scar reactions), and lymph nodes.
- About 50% of cases are diagnosed incidentally in an asymptomatic stage during investigations for some other disease or during routine check-ups.

Acute sarcoidosis

- For some patients, the disease may appear with symptoms of so-called acute sarcoidosis:
  - Erythema nodosum (particularly in women)
  - Arthralgia, swelling of joints
  - Elevated body temperature
  - Iritis or uveitis
  - Salivary gland oedema
  - Scar sarcoidosis (old scars become erythematous, swollen, and tender)
  - Cough and dyspnoea
  - Enlarged lymph nodes

Chronic sarcoidosis

- Dyspnoea
- Variable papulous skin lesions
- Chronic uveitis, glaucoma
- Symptoms of hypercalcaemia
- Renal insufficiency as a result of nephrocalcinosis
- Arrhythmias and conduction abnormalities (also in the acute stage)
- Hypersplenism
- Neurological symptoms

Initial investigations in primary health care

Chest x-ray

- Ask for a consultation by a radiologist and mention the suspicion of sarcoidosis.
- Classification of radiological findings
  - Type I: enlarged hilar lymph nodes
  - Type II: as above + symmetrical parenchymal infiltrates
  - Type III: Only parenchymal abnormalities
  - Type IV: Pulmonary fibrosis
- In erythema nodosum the initial chest radiograph may be normal: repeat the chest x-ray after one month.

Laboratory investigations

- For some patients all tests may be normal
- Blood count (leuco- and thrombocytopenia may occur)
- ESR (often increased at the onset of the disease)
- Serum and 24-hour urinary calcium (sometimes increased)
- Serum ACE (may be elevated in about 2/3 of patients at the onset and active stages of the disease)

Differential diagnosis

- Consider other differential diagnostic alternatives
  - Tuberculosis
  - Rheumatoid arthritis or collagenosis
  - Bacterial or viral infection

Further investigations

- If sarcoidosis is strongly suspected on the basis of radiographs or other tests, serum ACE and serum lysozyme can be determined as confirmatory tests. Increased concentrations suggest sarcoidosis. These tests are also valuable measures of disease activity during follow-up.
- The diagnosis should finally be confirmed by biopsy (consult a pulmonologist or an internist).

Treatment

- The aim of the treatment is to prevent pulmonary or other fibrosis.
- The treatment should be started by a specialist. Follow-up of the patient can be arranged jointly with the primary care physician and the specialist.
- Acute sarcoidosis is usually cured spontaneously.
- NSAIDs can be prescribed for arthralgia.
- If necessary, corticosteroids **A** [1] can be administered for 12 to 18 months, or sometimes much longer.
- In maintenance treatment of pulmonary sarcoidosis, also inhaled steroids **A** [1] are beneficial and with less adverse effects for some patients.

Follow-up

- Upon agreement may be performed in primary care in co-operation with specialised care.
- If the disease is mainly in the lungs, chest radiography, pulmonary function tests (vital capacity) are monitored at 3 to 6 month intervals. Serum ACE, serum lysozyme and serum calcium are measured when needed.

- If the disease is primarily in extra-pulmonary organs, the follow-up is aimed at the target organ's symptoms and findings.

Prognosis

- More than 50% of all patients with sarcoidosis are cured spontaneously.
- 50% are left with radiological pulmonary changes.
- Respiratory insufficiency develops rarely.
- 15% develop chronic sarcoidosis.
  - The prognosis of chronic sarcoidosis is variable and depends on the extent of the disease.
  - Mortality is around 1%.

Reference

1. Paramothayan NS, Jones PW. Corticosteroids for pulmonary sarcoidosis. Cochrane Database Syst Rev. 2004;(2): CD001114.

6.44 Acute pulmonary reactions to irritant gases

Pentti Tukiainen

Aims

- Pulmonary oedema in persons exposed to certain irritant gases (e.g. nitrogen dioxide, chlorine) is prevented by immediate administration of inhaled corticosteroid.
- Workplaces where irritant gases are handled should keep inhaled corticosteroid available.

Exposure

- Fires
  - Mixtures of various gases and particulate substances
  - E.g., acrolein is released from burning oil products and plastics.
- Industrial exposure
  - Gases released in industrial processes
  - Gas leaks in industrial plants and during transportation

Affected organs and symptoms

- **Highly water-soluble gases** (ammonia, hydrochloric acid, sulphuric acid, formaldehyde, acetaldehyde, acetic acid) are absorbed through the mucous membranes of the upper respiratory tract, causing
  - intensive coughing
  - a burning sensation
  - oedema of the epiglottis or larynx.
- **Moderately water-soluble gases** (hydrofluoric acid, sulphur dioxide, chlorine, chlorine dioxide, iodine, bromine, fluorine) affects also the bronchi, causing
  - coughing
  - increased mucus production
  - bronchial obstruction.
- **Poorly water-soluble gases** (phosgene, ozone, nitrogen dioxide, methyl bromide, acrolein, dimethyl sulphate, zinc chloride) reach the alveolar level, potentially causing pulmonary oedema that can develop immediately or after a delay of more than 24 hours. For example, nitrogen dioxide typically leads to pulmonary oedema within 3 to 30 hours after exposure. The symptoms of pulmonary oedema caused by irritant gases comprise
  - dry cough or blood-stained sputum
  - dyspnoea, wheezing
  - nausea, vomiting
  - possibly fever, symptoms of hypotension.
- Any irritant gas can cause life-threatening alveolar injury if the exposure is very intensive or lasts long.

Treatment

Prevention of pulmonary oedema

- It is always safer to administer a corticosteroid with the aim of preventing pulmonary oedema than to refrain from it.
- Prophylactic procedures
  - First 24 hours: the patient is given as soon as possible after the exposure (preferably within 15 minutes) 800 μg budesonide or 1000 μg beclomethasone by inhalation, using an inhalation chamber. The dose is repeated at four-hour intervals.
  - Following four days: the same dose is administered 4 times daily during the patient's waking hours.
  - After five days: The treatment is withdrawn unless there are pulmonary findings in which case the treatment will be continued until recovery.
- Very intensive exposures call for high-dose intravenous corticosteroid therapy. Such therapy or established pulmonary oedema requires intensive care in hospital.

Treatment of bronchial obstruction

- A beta-sympathomimetic every three hours, e.g.
  - Salbutamol 0.4 mg
  - Terbutaline 0.5 mg
  - Fenoterol 0.4 mg

Treatment of epiglottic and laryngeal oedema

- Adrenaline inhalation

• Up to three inhalations within 30 minutes
• At least one minute between inhalations

Treatment of cough

♦ E.g. clobutinol hydrochloride 20 mg (= 2 ml 10 mg/ml) i.m. or i.v.
♦ Beta-sympathomimetics also have an effect on cough.

6.50 Lung cancer

Karin Mattson

Aims

♦ To actively disseminate information about such risk factors of lung cancer which are within the patient's control, including the importance of giving up smoking and adhering to occupational safety regulations in certain industries.
♦ To make patients aware of risk factors and to inform them about the possibilities and methods for reducing them.
♦ To identify groups at risk:
  • middle-aged and older (over 45 years) smokers with
    – altered characteristics of unusual cough;
    – haemoptysis;
    – recurrent pneumonia;
    – weight loss and impaired general condition.
♦ To achieve early diagnosis.
♦ To recognise lung cancers of occupational origin, e.g. asbestos exposure-related lung cancer which are compensated as an occupational disease.

Aetiology

♦ Smoking
  • Smoking causes 90% of cases of lung cancer.
  • **Passive smoking** is also a risk factor for lung cancer.
  • Lung cancers in non-smokers are usually adenocarcinomas.
♦ Asbestos
  • About 10% of lung cancers are caused by asbestos.
  • A smoker exposed to asbestos has an almost 100-fold risk of lung cancer compared with a non-exposed non-smoker.
♦ Other
  • inter alia, arsenic, chromium and nickel (occupational exposure).
  • Radiation (radon).

Classification

♦ Non-small cell carcinomas
  • Squamous cell carcinoma (35%); on the decline.
  • Adenocarcinoma (40%) and its subtype, bronchoalveolar carcinoma; on the increase.
  • Large cell anaplastic carcinoma (5%).
♦ Small cell carcinoma (20%).

Dissemination

♦ Dissemination to extrathoracic sites
  • To brain, bones, liver and adrenals.
♦ Local and regional dissemination
  • To another lobe of the same lung, to the other lung
  • To hilar, mediastinal, clavicular or axillary lymph nodes
  • Direct invasion into the mediastinum, great vessels of the chest wall, pericardium, pleura, vertebrae or ribs, and brachial plexus.
♦ Small cell lung carcinoma spreads at a very early stage to both local and extrathoracic sites. Exclusively local treatment is therefore rarely possible. The primary treatment is chemotherapy Ⓐ [1 2 3].

Symptoms and findings

♦ Principal early symptoms and their prevalence
  • Cough or altered cough 60%.
  • Haemoptysis 27%.
  • Pain (thoracic or extrathoracic) 34%.
  • Dyspnoea 46%.
  • Loss of appetite, weight loss 56%.
♦ Findings
  • An opacity in the lung on a chest x-ray with or without enlarged lymph nodes in the hilum and/or mediastinum.
  • Enlarged lymph nodes in the neck, clavicular fossae and/or axillae.
  • Metastases (brain, bones, lungs, liver, adrenals).

Diagnostics

♦ The most important examination at the early stage is plain **chest x-ray**.
♦ Even if the chest x-ray finding is interpreted as normal, the patient should be sent to a pulmonary medicine unit for **endoscopy** and **computed tomography** if there is a strong suspicion of lung cancer (e.g., haemoptysis in a smoker with no apparent infection).
♦ The most important **differential diagnoses** with respect to haemoptysis are bronchiectases and pulmonary embolism, as well as tuberculosis and atypical mycobacterial infections (6.21), which may resemble lung cancer both clinically and radiologically.

Prevention

- Young people should not start smoking.
- Smokers must quit smoking.
- Protection against asbestos exposure and other known occupational carcinogers.
- Warn the population about passive smoking

Treatment

- The choice of therapy is based on cell type and clinical extent of the disease (TNM stage).
- The patient's general condition (WHO 0–5) and compliance also influence the choice of therapy.
- The primary treatment for unspread **non-small cell** lung cancer (25% of cases) is surgery: resection of a pulmonary lobe or an entire lung. Radical surgery is possible only in 25% of patients. In the case of loco-regional involvement (25%), the patient is given new combined modality regimes that combine all forms of therapy; (e.g., chemotherapy A [4 5 6 7 8 9 10 11] may be given before surgery B [12 13] or simultaneously with radiotherapy A [14 15]). In disseminated disease (50%) both first- and second-line chemotherapy A [4 5 6 7 8 9 10 11] are used in patients who are in good condition.
- The primary treatment for **small cell** lung cancer limited to the thoracic area is chemotherapy in combination with radiotherapy. Patients with disseminated disease are given chemotherapy. Prophylactic radiotherapy to the brain is given to those patients in whom an almost complete response to primary therapy has been obtained. Small cell lung cancer is operable only if it is detected at a very early stage (4% of cases), in which case chemotherapy should be administered after surgery (4–6 courses).
- Symptomatic treatment for patients with lung cancer, see 6.51.

Follow-up

- Systematic (25% of cases) follow-up in specialized health care is recommended for the first 5 years. Follow-up is justified since treatment is available should relapse occur.
- The most important parameters to be monitored:
  - Auscultation of the lungs, palpation of lymph node areas;
  - Chest x-ray, chest and upper abdomen CT;
  - Liver enzymes, ESR, blood count;
  - General status, weight loss.
- The carcinoembryonic antigen (serum CEA) can be used as a tumour marker in non-small cell lung cancer (adenocarcinoma). The marker for small cell lung cancer is neurone-specific enolase (serum NSE). These markers are relevant only if their concentration has been found to be elevated at the time of diagnosis of the disease.

Prognosis

- Non-small cell lung cancer
  - The five-year survival rate for all patients is 12%;
  - The five-year survival rate for those treated exclusively by surgery (25%) is 65%.
- Small cell lung cancer
  - The two-year survival rate is 20%.

References

1. Frodin JE, for Swedish Council on Technology Assessment in Health Care. Lung cancer. Acta Oncologica 1996;35:46–53.
2. The Database of Abstracts of Reviews of Effectiveness (University of York), Database no.: DARE-978125. In: The Cochrane Library, Issue 4, 1999. Oxford: Update Software.
3. The Prophylactic Cranial Irradiation Overview Collaborative Group. Cranial irradiation for preventing brain metastases of small cell lung cancer in patients in complete remission. Cochrane Database Syst Rev. 2004;(2):CD002805.
4. Walling J. Chemotherapy for advanced non-small-cell lung cancer. Respiratory Medicine 1994;88:649–657.
5. The Database of Abstracts of Reviews of Effectiveness (University of York), Database no.: DARE-953438. In: The Cochrane Library, Issue 4, 1999. Oxford: Update Software.
6. Non-small Cell Lung Cancer Collaborative Group. Chemotherapy in non-small cell lung cancer: a meta-analysis using updated data on individual patients from 52 randomized trials. BMJ 1995;311:899–909.
7. The Database of Abstracts of Reviews of Effectiveness (University of York), Database no.: DARE-952726. In: The Cochrane Library, Issue 4, 1999. Oxford: Update Software.
8. Marino P, Preatoni A, Cantoni A, Buccheri G. Single-agent chemotherapy versus combination chemotherapy in advanced non-small cell lung cancer: a quality and meta-analysis study. Lung Cancer 1995;13:1–12.
9. The Database of Abstracts of Reviews of Effectiveness (University of York), Database no.: DARE-952578. In: The Cochrane Library, Issue 4, 1999. Oxford: Update Software.
10. Lilenbaum RC, Langenbrg P, Dickersin K. Single agent versus combination chemotherapy in patients with advanced non-small-cell lung carcinoma: a meta-analysis of response, toxicity, and survival. Cancer 1998;82:116–126.
11. The Database of Abstracts of Reviews of Effectiveness (University of York), Database no.: DARE-980209. In: The Cochrane Library, Issue 4, 2000. Oxford: Update Software.
12. Goss G, Paszat L, Newman TE, Evand WK, Browman G. Use of preoperative chemotherapy with or without postoperative radiotherapy in technically resectable stage IIA non-small-cell lung cancer. Cancer Prevention and Control 1998;2:32–39.
13. The Database of Abstracts of Reviews of Effectiveness (University of York), Database no.: DARE-983999. In: The Cochrane Library, Issue 4, 2000. Oxford: Update Software.
14. Arriagada R, Pignon JP, Ihde DC et al. Effect of thoracic radiotherapy on mortality in limited small-cell lung cancer. A meta-analysis of 13 randomized trials among 2,140 patients. Anticancer Research 1994;14:333–335.
15. The Database of Abstracts of Reviews of Effectiveness (University of York), Database no.: DARE-955090. In: The Cochrane Library, Issue 4, 1999. Oxford: Update Software.

6.51 Palliative treatment of a patient with lung cancer

Paula Maasilta

Basic rules

- The quality of life of the patient with lung cancer can often be improved even if curative treatment is not possible.
- As a rule, palliative treatment in lung cancer is not very different from palliative treatment in any type of cancer (16.11).

Pain

- Pain in lung cancer is managed in the same way as pain in any cancer (16.10). There are, for example, no particular restrictions concerning medication. Morphine has a favourable effect also on dyspnoea.

Cough

- Codeine-containing cough remedies
- Codeine tablets (today tablets containing a combination of codeine and aspirin or paracetamol are available)

Haemoptysis

- Tranexamic acid in sufficiently high doses
- Palliative radiotherapy usually brings effective relief.

Dyspnoea

- If the tumour obstructs the trachea (or a main bronchus), causing severe dyspnoea
  - A steroid orally or intramuscularly (also useful in lymphangitis carcinomatosa)
  - Bronchodilators (theophylline and, e.g., inhaled salbutamol)
  - Prevention or treatment of infections
  - Palliative radiotherapy occasionally yields a good therapeutic response for a while.
  - Bronchoscopic laser treatment offers effective palliation to some patients but this treatment may not be available in all hospitals.
- If there is no specific treatable cause
  - Small dose of (oral) morphine (A) [1]
  - Benzodiazepines, e.g., diazepam, if the symptoms include mental distress
  - In the literature, low-dose chlorpromazine combined with atropine has been proposed if other therapies fail to bring adequate relief.

Lung infections

- This is a common problem, with anaerobes often involved.
- Adequate treatment will improve the patient's quality of life. Fluoroquinolones are very often effective against secondary infections in patients with lung cancer.
- An atelectatic lung is in a constant state of infection.
- If the patient continues to have fever despite antibiotics, it may be tumour-induced and can be controlled with regular use of a NSAID.

Malignant pleural effusion

- Drainage (no more than 1 litre at a time) is advisable only if the fluid clearly causes dyspnoea (6.80). The best pleurodesis results have been obtained by early thoracoscopic insufflation of talc (C) [2].

Oxygen therapy

- Can be administered either from an oxygen bottle or from a concentrator. Open fire carries a risk of explosion (smoking). Oxygen therapy may have a dyspnoea-relieving effect.

Smoking

- To forbid a patient with incurable lung cancer to smoke is unnecessary and actually cruel.

References

1. Jennings AL, Davies AN, Higgins JPT, Broadley K. Opioids for the palliation of breathlessness in terminal illness. Cochrane Database Syst Rev. 2004;(2):CD002066.
2. Hartman DL, Gaither JM, Kesler KA, Mylet DM, Brown JW, Mathur PN. Comparison of insufflated talc under thoracoscopic guidance with standard tetracycline and bleomycin pleurodesis for control of malignant pleural effusions. J Thoracic Cardiovasc Surg 1993;105:743–747.

6.55 Asbestos-related diseases

Matti S. Huuskonen

Aims

- The primary aim is to prevent the exposure of humans to asbestos dust.
- The new imaging methods used in the diagnosis of asbestos-related diseases, high-resolution computed tomography (HRCT) in particular, have proven far superior to conventional chest x-rays.

- Early diagnosis of occupational diseases and close monitoring of patients who have developed such a disease aims to improve the prognosis of occupational diseases and, at the same time, will secure the patients with the benefits offered by insurance systems.
- Asbestos-related diseases have a latency period of many years, and surveillance must therefore be continued even when the exposure has been eliminated.

Exposure to asbestos dust

- Asbestos is the generic name used for a group of naturally occurring fibrous silicate minerals (crocidolite, actinolite, amosite, anthophyllite, tremolite and chrysotile).
- In many countries the use of asbestos has been banned.
- The exposure to asbestos may be especially high in building renovation work when the old structures are demolished, particularly if protection guidelines and recommended techniques are not followed.
- Before the introduction of current legislation asbestos exposure was possible when working under the following circumstances: asbestos spraying, asbestos mines, manufacture of asbestos products, brake and clutch work, service and maintenance work, shipyards, installation of boilers, lining or dismantling stoves, lagging of pipes, other insulating work, production of building materials, building construction and property maintenance.

Asbestos-related diseases

- Asbestos may cause lung cancer, mesothelioma (malignancy of the pleura and peritoneum), fibrosis of the lung parenchyma (asbestosis) as well as pleural changes such as fibrosis of the parietal pleura (plaques), diffuse fibrosis of the visceral pleura, exudative pleurisy and retroperitoneal fibrosis. Asbestos also increases the risk of laryngeal cancer.
- The threshold exposure level, below which the risk of asbestos-related diseases is not increased, has not been established.
- On the other hand, the higher the exposure the higher the risk of asbestos-related cancers.
- The latent phase from exposure to disease emergence usually lasts over 10 years; in the case of asbestos-related cancers the phase may often last 10–40 years or even longer.
- Asbestos-induced cancers attributable to earlier asbestos exposure will peak in 2010–2015.

Lung cancer

- The combination of smoking and asbestos carries a very high risk of cancer.
- Asbestos-induced lung cancer does not differ from ordinary lung cancer in location or histology, but it tends to occur at a younger age.
- Early diagnosis of incipient, small and operable lesions is possible with low-dose spiral computed tomography.
- The employment history of each lung cancer patient must be mapped out and the possibility of an occupational aetiology must be considered.
- In unclear cases, specialists in pneumoconiosis may be consulted.

Mesothelioma (a neoplasm of the pleura and peritoneum)

- The only established causes of mesothelioma are asbestos and the naturally occurring erionite fibre.
- Occupational aetiology should be suspected in all cases of mesothelioma, for which purpose a detailed employment history is usually sufficient.
- Due to the difficulties encountered in diagnosis, mesothelioma, peritoneal mesothelioma in particular, is underdiagnosed.

Asbestosis (a pneumoconiotic disease)

- Accumulation of asbestos dust in the lungs can cause pulmonary fibrosis.
- Owing to the long latency period (20–40 years), those who today develop asbestosis have usually been exposed to asbestos in the 1970s.
- A diagnosis of asbestosis is based on the demonstration of significant occupational exposure to asbestos and radiological findings, usually on HRCT of the lungs.
- The interpretation of a chest x-ray for incipient diffuse pulmonary fibrosis requires a highly skilled radiologist. HRCT will detect changes in lung tissue earlier than chest radiography, particularly where pleural changes mask any parenchymal lesions.
- Asbestosis diagnosis is also supported by clinical signs and symptoms as well as findings of pulmonary function tests. Typical findings of such tests are indicative of restricted pulmonary function or impaired gas exchange. Lung biopsy is sometimes required for differential diagnosis.

Pleural changes

- HRCT is clearly superior in identifying pleural disease compared with chest x-ray.
- Pleural plaques
  - Pleural plaques usually occur on the parietal pleura between the fifth and tenth rib on the posterolateral aspect. They may also be found over the mid diaphragm and on the mediastinal pleura. The plaques are fairly well defined, elevated nodules that become calcified with time.
  - If the pleural plaques occur without other asbestos-induced disorders, the patient is usually asymptomatic. Sometimes mildly restrictive pulmonary function has been noted.
  - Bilateral thickening of the outer pleura is a reliable sign of asbestos exposure. Often the thickening is first detected unilaterally but with continued monitoring plaques appear on both sides.
- Lesions of the visceral pleura
  - The visceral pleura thickens because of fibrosis and becomes attached to the parietal layer. At least in some

patients this is due to exudative pleurisy. The early stages of the disease are symptom-free but in more advanced cases the patient presents with symptoms suggestive of asbestosis. Differential diagnosis should take into account the accumulation of fat in the pleural space in obese persons.
  - In the absence of asbestos exposure, diffuse pleural fibrosis may be present in connective tissue disorders or as an adverse effect of pharmaceuticals.
- Round atelectasis
  - Can occur in any part of the lungs. The atelectatic lung tissue beneath the fibrotic pleura becomes twisted, producing a rounded shadow. The spiral structure of a round atelectasis is readily apparent on tomography.
  - Unless the investigations reveal unequivocally a structure typical to spiral atelectasis, the non-malignant nature of the finding should be verified, for example by needle biopsy.
- Exudative pleurisy
  - Asbestos exposure can lead to exudative pleurisy within as little as 10 years of the first exposure. There is no specific sign indicative of this condition. The association with asbestos exposure is often uncertain, and the association can only be confirmed during subsequent follow-up.
- Visceral pleural lesions usually indicate heavier exposure to asbestos than plaques alone, and are indicative of an increased risk of lung cancer.

Retroperitoneal fibrosis (RPF)

- RPF is an uncommon disease. The pathognomonic finding is a fibrous mass covering the abdominal aorta and the ureters. Occupational asbestos exposure may be an important causal factor for RPF. For patients with work-related asbestos exposure, RPF should be considered an occupational disease.

Surveillance and diagnostics of asbestos-exposed persons

- The health of individuals who have been subjected to occupational exposure to asbestos should be monitored at regular intervals.
- If signs or symptoms consistent with, or suggestive of, asbestos-related diseases occur, it is advisable to have any clinical diagnostic investigations carried out either at a lung hospital or at a unit specialising in occupational medicine.

Procedures to be followed in cases of occupational disease

- Mesotheliomas, lung cancers and pleural and parenchymal fibroses in asbestos-exposed individuals are investigated, and all such diagnoses are reported to an appropriate insurance company.
- This ensures that the affected persons will receive due compensation for their occupational diseases. The compensation paid out to diseased persons and the survivors' family pension payable to the next-of-kin of a deceased individual, can be substantial, particularly in cases of occupational cancer.
- Whenever there is reason to suspect that an illness resulting from occupational exposure to asbestos has caused or hastened a patient's death, a medicolegal autopsy has to be performed. This also applies to cases where the suspicion arises during medical autopsy.
- The surveillance of the health of a patient with asbestos-related disease must be consistent and well-organized.

Guidelines

- According to regulations in many countries, the presence of asbestos in indoor air is unacceptable.
- If the concentration of asbestos fibres (>5 μm in length) in indoor air exceeds 0.01 fibres/cm^3, the authorities should stipulate measures for removing asbestos from the indoor air.
- The use and handling of asbestos-containing materials in residential buildings must be avoided in all circumstances.

6.56 Silicosis

Matti S. Huuskonen

Exposure

- Exposure to crystalline silica (silicon dioxide) dust (quartz, cristobalite or tridymite) may cause silicosis. Silicosis is caused by exposure to almost pure crystalline silica dust. Simultaneous exposure to a mixture of mineral dusts may cause more irregular pulmonary fibrosis (mixed dust pneumoconiosis).
- Exposure to crystalline silica dust and contracting silicosis predispose the individual to pulmonary tuberculosis. Pulmonary tuberculosis in a patient with silicosis may be considered as an occupational disease. The patients with silicosis usually give a history of continuous silica dust exposure over a time period generally exceeding 10 years. The latency period of silicosis is also long, averaging over 20 years.
- Exposure to crystalline silica dust increases the risk of lung cancer.
- IARC (International Agency for Research on Cancer/WHO) classifies crystalline silica dust as a Group 1 substance (carcinogenic to humans).
- Exposure may occur in the following occupations:
  - mining, quarrying, stone work, construction, and foundry work

- manufacture of glass, porcelain, enamel, clay and stone products
- sand blasting and grinding
- production and dismantling of refractory material
- in the construction industry: demolishing old structures for renovation work, dry grinding and clearance. In addition to siliceous earth, asbestos has been used for example in the manufacture of pipe lagging (exposure to mixed dust).

Pathogenesis

- Particles under 5 μm in diameter cause an alveolar and bronchiolar reaction, gradually resulting in fibrosis.

Clinical picture

- Silicosis presents as nodular fibrosis of the lung tissue particularly in the upper lung fields, and in mixed dust exposure as a more widespread irregular fibrosis.
- Even when radiological findings are visible on HRCT of the lungs or on the chest x-ray the patient may remain asymptomatic.
- The symptoms may include an irritative cough and dyspnoea. The symptoms do not correlate with the x-ray findings.
- Fine mid- and end-inspiratory rales can be heard on auscultation.
- Lung function tests initially show a decrease in vital capacity. As the disease progresses, restrictive pulmonary function is often observed, with slightly impaired gas exchange. Even in advanced cases the abnormalities in gas exchange are never severe.
- Silicosis is know to predispose the patient to pulmonary tuberculosis.
- Silicosis is also associated with an increased risk of lung cancer.
- Lung cancer patients with a history of considerable exposure to crystalline silica dust in their work should always be considered as suspected cases of occupational disease.

Diagnosis

- Significant exposure to quartz dust
- Even when abnormalities on radiological findings are visible the patient may remain asymptomatic.
- Sometimes lung biopsy
- Pulmonary function tests help to determine the degree of disability.

Surveillance

- The health of individuals who have been subjected to occupational exposure to crystalline silica dust or mixed dust should be monitored at regular intervals.
- The surveillance of the health of a patient with an occupational disease must be consistent and well-organized.

PUL

6.60 Foreign body in the respiratory passages

Editors

Basic rules

- Personnel at emergency telephone service and health care facilities should know simple measures to remove foreign bodies from the upper respiratory passages.
- Mouth-to-mask or mouth-to-mouth ventilation should always be tried after unsuccessful removal of a foreign body, as increased pressure in the respiratory passages may lead air past the foreign body.

Removing a foreign body

Hanging down by the feet

- A child with obvious breathing difficulties and a suspicion of a foreign body in the respiratory passages should first be held upside down by the feet and tapped forcefully on the back with the palm.
- Try Heimlich's manoeuvre if hanging down by the feet and tapping prove unsuccessful (Figure 6.60.1)

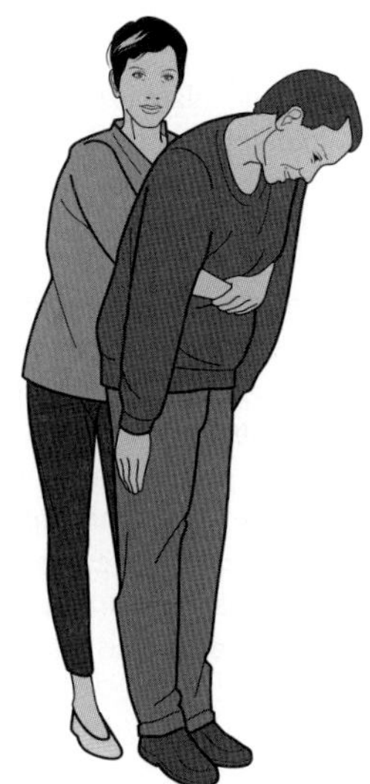

Figure 6.60.1 Grasp the patient from behind by putting your hands on the upper abdomen above the navel and thrush forcefully upwards and inwards so that the intra-abdominal pressure rises, the diaphragm is elevated and pushes the air out of the lungs. Photo © R. Suhonen.

Heimlich's manoeuvre

- The method of choice for adults and the second method for children who cannot be helped by hanging down by the feet.
- Grasp the patient's upper abdomen from the back by crossing your hands above the navel and thrust upwards and backwards so that the intra-abdominal pressure rises, the diaphragm is elevated, and air is blown from the lungs.

Laryngoscopy or bronchoscopy

- Should be used if the aforementioned methods are unsuccessful.

Opening an airway with a needle

- If the **upper airway** has been blocked, e.g., by facial trauma and intubation is unsuccessful, the trachea can be cannulated with a thick Viggo® needle just below the thyroid cartilage. This method is easier and quicker than emergency tracheostomy.
  - If quickly available, attach a syringe with saline to a needle.
  - Insert the needle into the trachea in the midline aspirating continuously. Bubbling of air in the syringe indicates that the needle is in the trachea.
  - Remove the mandrine and attach the cannula to a breathing bag using e.g. a 2-ml syringe.
  - Ensure that the cannula remains in the trachea by keeping it in place manually (do not bend the cannula).
  - If necessary, place another cannula next to the first one to hasten expiration.

Foreign body in lower respiratory passages

- Most common in children, especially in 1 to 2-year-olds
  - A nut from hazelnut chocolate is the most common cause, also other foods and small objects

Symptoms

- Often begin with a forceful coughing spell. The initial phase often also includes wheezing and even cyanosis.
- The symptoms continue for a few minutes and then stop, even though the foreign body remains in the bronchus.
- An asymptomatic phase will then follow, lasting hours or even days, before the pneumonia phase; at this point the initial event may already have been forgotten, which delays and complicates diagnosis. The physician should therefore actively ask about the early history of the condition.

Diagnosis

- An acute coughing spell with accompanying symptoms in a child of a certain age should be considered a suspected aspiration.
- The significance of a chest x-ray is limited: it can be normal, show atelectasis, and possibly emphysema, later pneumonia.
- The final diagnosis is based on bronchoscopy.

6.61 Pneumothorax

Editors

Basic rules

- Tension pneumothorax must be identified and treated immediately.
- Consider spontaneous pneumothorax as a cause for acute chest pain and dyspnoea in young smokers and patients with chronic obstructive pulmonary disease.

Classification

- Primary spontaneous pneumothorax
  - More than 90% of the patients are smokers.
  - Occurs most frequently in men aged 20–40 years.
  - The patients are often tall and thin.
- Secondary pneumothorax
  - A complication of a pulmonary disease
  - The condition is often severe, even life-threatening, because pulmonary function is already affected by pulmonary disease.
- Traumatic pneumothorax
  - Iatrogenic or other aetiology
- Tension pneumothorax
  - A one-way valve is formed in the pleural cavity. The intrathoracal conditions change rapidly, and ventilation is suddenly impaired.
  - Usually seen in trauma patients and in connection with mechanical ventilation and resuscitation.
  - Urgent treatment is essential.

Symptoms

- Chest pain and dyspnoea are the main symptoms.
  - The onset is rapid.
  - The symptoms are exacerbated by breathing and physical exertion.
  - The pain radiates to the ipsilateral shoulder.
- Cough irritation

Clinical signs

- The clinical findings can be normal in a small pneumothorax.
- Suppressed respiratory sounds, impaired chest mobility, and hypersonoric percussion sounds are often observed.
- Tachycardia, cyanosis, and hypotension can be observed in tension pneumothorax.
- Subcutaneous emphysema may be present (a crepitation on pressing the skin).
- Signs of injury (haematoma, crepitation from a broken rib, etc.) may be visible on the chest.

Diagnosis

- A chest x-ray is necessary to confirm the diagnosis.
  - A small pneumothorax may be difficult to detect. A radiograph taken during expiration may be helpful.
  - A large emphysematous bulla may resemble pneumothorax.

Conservative treatment

- Conservative treatment (follow-up by chest x-ray every 1–3 days) is feasible in **spontaneous pneumothorax** if the following conditions are fulfilled:
  - The patient is otherwise healthy.
  - The patient does not have dyspnoea, the air-filled space is less than half of the pleural cavity (the maximum width is less than 3 cm), and it does not become larger during follow-up.
- The pneumothorax should decrease in size in 3–4 days and disappear in two weeks at the latest.
- The follow-up can be performed in ambulatory care. The patient should contact the doctor immediately if the symptoms get worse.
- If conservative treatment is carried out in hospital, oxygen therapy may hasten the resorption of air from the pleural cavity. (The nitrogen content of pulmonary capillary blood decreases, resulting in as much as a 10-fold increase in the gradient necessary for resorption).

Active treatment

- **Tension pneumothorax** is always an indication for immediate treatment. Thoracocentesis is indicated in a trauma victim or resuscitated patient with difficulty in breathing and signs suggesting tension pneumothorax even if a confirmatory chest radiograph cannot be obtained. Any needle (e.g. a large vein cannula) can be used.
- **Active treatment** (drainage or aspiration) is indicated in other types of pneumothorax if one of the following conditions is fulfilled:
  - The lung is markedly or completely collapsed.
  - The patient has a chronic pulmonary disease.
  - The patient has significant dyspnoea (e.g. a previously healthy patient has dyspnoea on slight exercise such as walking).
- **Aspiration** as the only treatment is feasible, at least in conditions where it would be difficult to refer the patient to a hospital for pleural suction. Aspiration has even been recommended as the treatment of choice for all types of pneumothorax. The outcome of aspiration is good in 70% of patients. The procedure is carried out as follows:
  - Puncture the pleural space after local anaesthesia between the second and third ribs (the second rib is on the level of angulus sterni) at the midclavicular line with a needle (minimum length 3 cm) and catheter (e.g. a thick Viggo® catheter).
  - Remove the needle from the catheter and connect the catheter to a 50–100 ml syringe (Luer lock).
  - Aspirate air until resistance is felt or the patient gets a heavy cough, or until more than 2.5 l of air has been aspirated.
- **Pleural suction** is recommended in traumatic pneumothorax, collapsed lung, and in patients with severe dyspnoea. The procedure is performed as follows:
  - Use a small pleural puncture catheter (French 9–12) with a trocar if there is no fluid in the pleural space. Other catheters can be used if they have several holes in the last 10 cm of the catheter tip.
  - A local anaesthetic is infiltrated under the second or third rib. The tissue near the rib periost must be anaesthetized particularly well.
  - Incise the skin and subcutaneous tissue with a lancet as far as the upper margin of the rib. Make the way to the pleural space with a blunt instrument (crile), not forcefully with the catheter trocar.
  - Insert the trocar in to the pleural space without force.
  - Connect the catheter with suction (10–20 cm H_2O) immediately or use a Heimlich valve. Do not close the catheter.
  - Traumatic pneumothorax is often associated with haemothorax. In such cases the pleural space should be drained at the mid- or posterior axillary line in the sixth intercostal space (the nipple is usually situated on the fifth intercostal space) with a larger (French 20–24) catheter. It is safest to make an incision with a lancet and then use the finger to make the way to the pleural space. Usually it is not necessary to drain a haemothorax before transportation to a hospital.
  - If the lung is not inflated insert another drain.
- If an air leak continues despite the suction, the leak should be treated surgically, nowadays usually **endoscopically**. Open thoracotomy is rarely needed.
- After treatment the patient should avoid physical exercise for 2–4 weeks and travelling by air for 2 weeks.

Prognosis

- Both primary and secondary pneumothorax tend to recur in 50% of patients.
- Surgical treatment should be considered after the second episode at the latest.

6.62 Pneumomediastinum

Editors

Definition

- Air or other gas is collected in the mediastinum

Causes

- Valsalva manoeuvre or other change in normal respiration
    - Singing, shouting
    - Pulmonary function tests
    - Playing wind instruments
    - Smoking marijuana
    - Delivery
    - Vomiting, defecation
    - Coughing, blowing the nose, hiccup
    - Convulsions
    - Lifting heavy objects
- Airway obstruction
    - Asthma, COPD
    - Respiratory infection
    - Foreign body, tumour
- Decompression
    - Flying
    - Decompression sickness in a diver (pressure chamber treatment)
- Increased intrathoracic pressure for an external reason
    - Mechanical ventilation, oxygen therapy
    - CPAP
    - Heimlich's manoeuvre (6.60)
    - Traffic accidents
- Rupture of the oesophagus
    - For example, as a complication of gastroscopy

Symptoms

- Pain
    - Retrosternal
    - Associated with respiration and changes of posture
    - Radiating to the back, shoulder and arm
- Difficulty in swallowing, lump in the throat
- Nasal voice
- Dyspnoea Findings
- Subcutaneous emphysema in the neck and supraclavicular fossa
- Hamman's sign: a typical precordial auscultation finding ("crackling", synchronous with heartbeat)
- Raised body temperature

Diagnosis

- Chest x-ray
    - Retrosternal air is best seen in the lateral projection.
    - Diagnosing pneumomediastinum and differentiating it from a small pneumothorax can be difficult.

Prognosis and treatment

- Usually the gas finds it way to subcutaneous tissue and is resorbed within a few days after the gas leak has stopped.
- Removing the cause is usually sufficient.
- Pneumomediastinum associated with mechanical ventilation may cause pressure pneumothorax that needs immediate treatment (6.61).

6.71 Sleep apnoea

Jaakko Herrala

Aims

- Remember the role of sleep-related breathing disorders in the aetiology of poor sleep and daytime sleepiness.
- The treatment of the overweight patient with suspected sleep apnoea should be started (with instructions for losing weight, weight loss groups) before any further referrals (24.2). By the time of further investigations, the patient may already have lost enough weight, yielding a normal finding upon somnography.
- Patients with sleep apnoea are examined and treated primarily at units of pulmonary medicine.

Sleep apnoea syndrome

Definitions

- **Sleep apnoea**: a pause of more than 10 seconds in breathing during sleep
- **Hypopnoea**: significant depression (>50% reduction in the amplitude of respiratory movements) of more than 10 seconds in breathing
- **Obstructive sleep apnoea** (or hypopnoea): apnoea/hypopnoea caused by obstruction of the upper respiratory tract during sleep. Respiratory movements continue during this type of apnoea/hypopnoea.
- **Central sleep apnoea** (or hypopnoea): apnoea/hypopnoea caused by a disturbance of central respiratory control. No respiratory movements take place during this type of apnoea/hypopnoea.
- **Mixed sleep apnoea**: a combination of the above

- **AI** = apnoea index: number of apnoea episodes per hour of sleep
- **AHI** = apnoea/hypopnoea index: total number of apnoea and hypopnoea episodes per hour of sleep. An AHI value >15 is generally considered as abnormal and AHI < 5 as normal.
- **ARI** = arousal index: number of EEG-recorded arousals per hour of sleep
- **ODI_4** = oxygen desaturation index: number of episodes of oxygen saturation (SaO_2) reduction exceeding 4% per hour of sleep
- **Sleep apnoea syndrome**: clinical symptoms or findings resulting from repeated episodes of apnoea during sleep
- **UARS = upper airway resistance syndrome**: repeated arousal from sleep by increased flow resistance in the upper respiratory tract, with symptoms similar to those of sleep apnoea syndrome

Background

- About 4% of working-age men and about 2% of women suffer from obstructive sleep apnoea syndrome. The syndrome is encountered at any age but most patients are middle-aged men or postmenopausal women.
- Sleep apnoea appears to be associated with an increased risk of traffic accidents and accidents at work C [1].
- Sleep apnoea is the most common organic cause of abnormal daytime sleepiness.
- **Pickwickian syndrome** manifests as chronic respiratory insufficiency in addition to repeated episodes of sleep apnoea.
- Central sleep apnoea syndrome is rare and is usually associated with central nervous system disorders or heart failure (Cheyne-Stokes respiration).

Symptoms of obstructive sleep apnoea syndrome

- Loud intermittent snoring
- Episodes of apnoea during sleep
- Excessive daytime sleepiness, narcolepsy
- Nocturia, nocturnal sweating, disturbed sleep at night, impotence, insomnia, irritability and rashness, impaired memory and concentration
- Nocturnal arrhythmias, nocturnal attacks of chest pain
- Morning headache
- Bed-wetting (children)

Signs

- Overweight (50–70% of patients are overweight)
- Narrow pharynx; slack, low-reaching soft palate; swollen, large uvula that reaches the tongue; large tonsils; narrow nose; small or backward-sloping lower jaw; large tongue; large adenoids in children; short and thick neck
- Leg oedema
- Elevated blood pressure

Differential diagnoses

- Other diseases causing daytime sleepiness (36.9)

Examinations

- History, physical examination, weight, body mass index, blood pressure, blood count, blood glucose, thyroid function tests, chest radiography, electrocardiography

Further investigations

- Overnight polysomnography is the most reliable method. Less extensive sleep studies (the following are generally recorded simultaneously: air flow with a thermistor, respiratory movements with a static charge-sensitive bed, oxygen saturation with an oximeter, sometimes even sleep position with a body position sensor and snoring sounds with a microphone) are carried out within specialized medical care at most departments of pulmonary medicine and at some neurological departments. These are usually sufficient for demonstrating clinically significant sleep apnoea and reaching a treatment decision C [2].
- Extensive overnight polysomnography also includes concurrent electroencephalographic recording of sleep phases.
- Extensive polysomnography is required for differential diagnosis in difficult cases where less extensive recording is insufficient to reach a diagnosis. Such cases include various parasomnias, hypersomnias, UARS and forms of mild sleep apnoea.

Conservative treatment

- Weight reduction is the first and foremost method of treatment of sleep apnoea in patients who are overweight.
- In mild sleep apnoea which is dependent on sleeping position, "tennis ball treatment" may be helpful: sleeping on one's back is prevented by fastening a tennis ball on the back of one's pyjamas or nightgown between the scapulas. The same effect may be achieved also by pillow arrangement.
- Hypnotics and sedatives, as well as taking alcohol before going to bed, must be avoided (these tend to increase the frequency and duration of apnoea episodes).
- Treatment of nasal congestion
- Optimal treatment of underlying diseases such as diabetes mellitus, hypertension and obstructive pulmonary disease
- Avoidance of high altitudes

Mechanical aids

- Treatment by **nasal continuous positive airway pressure** (nasal CPAP) is effective. It is currently the first-line treatment of clinically significant obstructive sleep apnoea B [3 4 5].
  - In nasal CPAP, a slight positive pressure preventing the collapse of the airways during sleep is maintained with a nasal mask.
  - This treatment is usually available at units of pulmonary medicine.
  - Some 60–80% of patients comply well with long-term nasal CPAP treatment. Problems related to the treatment include nasal congestion, runny nose, noise from

the pressure apparatus, epistaxis, and mouth dryness C [4 6 7].

- The patient's symptoms, other diseases, risks associated with sleep apnoea and polysomnographic findings must be considered when evaluating the benefit of starting a patient on nasal CPAP.
- The degree of daytime sleepiness can be assessed with the Epworth Sleepiness Scale.
- The patient should have follow-up examinations at one- to two-year intervals. The CPAP apparatus should nevertheless be serviced annually or more often, as required. CPAP apparatuses are classified as rehabilitation aids.
- The indications for nasal CPAP should be re-evaluated if the patient loses weight or undergoes surgery for sleep apnoea.

♦ Use of a **nose plaster** at night dampens the snoring sounds slightly in some patients but has no effect on apnoeas.

♦ Aids such as **mandibular advancers** that influence the positions of the mandible and tongue reduce apnoeas and daytime sleepiness significantly in some patients, especially those with mild sleep apnoea. Referrals for treatment with these aids are provided by dentists.

Surgical treatment

♦ Surgical treatment is indicated in some 5–10% of patients with sleep apnoea.

♦ Controlled clinical trials on surgical treatment are scarce, and there are no long-term follow-up studies C [4 6 7]. The decision on surgical treatment is usually made by a panel consisting of an oral and maxillofacial surgeon, an otorhinolaryngologist, and a specialist in pulmonary medicine.

♦ Dilative pharyngeal surgery

- **UPPP = uvulopalatopharyngoplasty; UPP = uvulopalatoplasty (LUPP = laser uvulopalatoplasty)**
  - effective against apnoea in the long term in less than 50% of patients C [4 6 7]
  - **not** suitable for treatment of severe sleep apnoea or in overweight patients
  - **N.B.** If the operation is desired solely for the treatment of socially annoying snoring, sleep apnoea should be ruled out by overnight somnography before surgery!
- **Tonsillectomy/adenoidectomy**
  - especially in children

♦ **Dilative nasal surgery**

- Septoplasty, removal of polyps
- Although these operations reduce snoring and improve the effect of nasal CPAP treatment, they seldom suffice as treatment for sleep apnoea.

♦ **Maxillofacial operations**

- Applicable in cases where narrowness of the upper airway is related to bony structures of the face
- The mode of surgery is based on cephalometric radiography and dynamic nasopharyngeal fiberoscopy.
- The most common method is box surgery whereby the root of the tongue is brought forward, thus enlarging the air space behind the base of the tongue.
- The mandible alone or together with the maxilla can be moved forward surgically.
- So far there is no evidence from controlled studies of the efficacy of maxillofacial surgery.

♦ **Tracheostomy**

- Needed only in life-threatening sleep apnoea when nasal CPAP treatment is not feasible.

References

1. Wright J, Johns R, Watt I, Melville A, Sheldon T. Health effects of obstructive sleep apnoea and the effectiveness of continuous positive airways pressure: a systematic review of the research evidence. BMJ 1997;314:851–860.
2. Systematic review of the literature regarding the diagnosis of sleep apnea. Evid Rep Technol Assess (Summ) 1999 Feb;(1):i-viii, 1–154.
3. Wright J, White J. Continuous positive airways pressure for obstructive sleep apnoea. The Cochrane Database of Systematic Reviews, Cochrane Library number: CD001106. In: The Cochrane Library, Issue 4, 2001. Oxford: Update Software. Updated frequently.
4. Lojander J, Maasilta P, Partinen M, Brander PE, Salmi T, Lehtonen H. Nasal-CPAP, surgery, and conservative management for treatment of obstructive sleep apnea syndrome. A randomized study. Chest 1996;110:114–119.
5. Sher AE, Schechtman KB, Piccirillo JF. The efficacy of surgical modifications of the upper airways in adults with obstructive sleep apnea syndrome. Sleep 1996;19:156–177.
6. Sher AE, Schechtman KB, Piccirillo JF. The efficacy of surgical modifications of the upper airways in adults with obstructive sleep apnea syndrome. Sleep 1996;19:156–177.
7. The Database of Abstracts of Reviews of Effectiveness (University of York), Database no.: DARE-973082. In: The Cochrane Library, Issue 4, 1999. Oxford: Update Software.

6.80 Pleural effusions; thoracentesis

Editors

Definition

♦ Pleurisy means inflammation of the pleura.

♦ There are other causes of pleural effusion besides inflammation.

Aetiology of pleural effusion

Transudates

- Heart failure
- Constrictive pericarditis
- Liver cirrhosis
- Nephrotic syndrome

Exudates

- Infections
  - Bacterial pneumonia
  - Tuberculosis
  - Viral infections
  - Fungal infections
- Cancers
  - Lung cancer
  - Lymphoma
  - Mesothelioma
  - Other
- Connective tissue disorders
  - Systemic lupus erythematosus (SLE)
  - Rheumatoid arthritis
- Other reasons, i.a.
  - Pulmonary infarction (pulmonary embolism)
  - Pancreatitis
  - Subphrenic abscess
  - Asbestos
  - Trauma
  - Medicines (bromocriptine)
- Post-thoracotomy state

Symptoms and signs

- Dyspnoea
- Flank pain
- Often cough and fever
- Dull percussion note
- Friction rub on auscultation

Investigations in patients with pleural effusions

- Detailed examination of the patient
  - Particular emphasis is placed on searching for a cause of pulmonary embolism (atrial fibrillation, deep venous thrombosis of the leg).
- Indices of inflammation
  - ESR, serum CRP, blood count
- Thoracentesis
  - Unless the reason is self-evident

Differential diagnosis

- In practice there are three stages in investigating the cause of pleural effusion.
  - The first question to ask is whether the effusion is transudate or exudate by nature.
  - In the case of exudate, the question is whether it is due to a malignant or non-malignant condition.
  - In the case of a probably non-malignant condition, a search for indications of bacterial pneumonia, tuberculosis and connective tissue disorders will be made.
- Diagnosis of cancer and tuberculosis often require pleural biopsy.

Indications for thoracentesis

- **Diagnostic** thoracentesis in connection with pleural effusions of uncertain aetiology
- **Therapeutic** thoracentesis if a large amount of pleural fluid causes symptoms
- Thoracentesis is usually unnecessary in cases of right-sided or bilateral pleural effusion in connection with evident heart failure. Such accumulation of pleural fluid is reversed when pulmonary circulation is normalized (pleural effusion that is limited to the left side is not considered to be due to heart failure).

Performance of thoracentesis

- Before the procedure, the presence of excess fluid in the pleural cavity should be established. This can be demonstrated by chest x-ray showing rounding of the lateral and posterior costodiaphragmatic recess. Sometimes rounding of the recess is not seen with infrapulmonary pleural effusions. Ultrasound examination can be used to confirm the presence of pleural effusion and to locate a suitable puncture site (it is advisable to perform an ultrasound examination whenever the apparatus is easily available).
- The patient should sit leaning slightly forward with forearms on the examination table and with his/her forehead resting on the forearms.
- The area of dull percussion caused by pleural fluid is located by comparing the percussion sound with that obtained from the healthy lung. The diaphragmatic margin is marked on the side of the healthy lung. The upper border of dull percussion on the affected side should be at least two intercostal spaces higher than the diaphragmatic margin on the healthy side.
- The site of puncture is one or two intercostal spaces below the upper border of percussion dullness along the posterior axillary line (or a site determined by echography). The site is anaesthetized over the upper border of a rib by 1% lidocaine. At the end of administration of anaesthetic, some pleural fluid is withdrawn to confirm the presence of excess fluid. In general, pleural aspiration is best performed using a disposable needle, syringe, three-way stopcock and tubing connected to a collection bag. If a small amount of sample

is needed (e.g. for protein determination when suspecting transudate), the sample may be aspirated with a thin needle into a 20 ml syringe.

- When performing therapeutic thoracentesis, no more than 1500–2000 ml fluid (depending on the patient's weight) should be aspirated at a time to avoid pulmonary oedema.
- With diagnostic thoracentesis, attention is paid to the smell and appearance of the pleural fluid. Empyema has a putrid smell. Blood-stained pleural fluid is probably caused by trauma, cancer or pulmonary infarction. Milky pleural effusion (chylothorax) is related to a trauma or a mediastinal malignancy.

Samples of pleural fluid

- Protein: 1 ml in a test tube
- Differential cell count: e.g. a 10 ml EDTA tube
- Bacterial culture is necessary only if the fluid is turbid or purulent: about 5 ml in a blood culture bottle or 1 ml in a Transpocult® tube, e.g., with a tuberculin syringe.
- Mycobacterial culture in a 5 ml test tube or preferably directly in a culture medium, e.g., a Bactec® bottle
- A cytology sample is shipped to the laboratory for example in two 50 ml plastic bottles. If the sample cannot be analysed right away, 5 ml of pleural fluid and 5 ml of 96% alcohol may be placed in three clean test tubes.
- No other investigations are necessary in primary care.

Interpretation of the results

- If the protein concentration is less than 30 g/l, the sample is a transudate.
- A predominance of neutrophils (over 50%) suggests bacterial pneumonia.
- The sensitivity of a cytology sample is in the order of 30–50% in cancer.
- Mycobacterial culture is positive in about 30% of patients with tuberculosis.

Oral Medicine

Evidence Based Medicine Guidelines. Edited by the Duodecim Editorial Team
© 2005 John Wiley & Sons, Ltd ISBN: 0-470-01184-X

7.10 Dryness of the mouth

Aira Lahtinen

Goals

- To identify or diagnose possible systemic disease(s) or medication causing dry mouth.
- To prevent, by using up-to-date treatment and information, the development of dental caries and mucosal infections caused by reduced salivary flow rate.

Symptoms of dryness of the mouth

- Hyposalivation (reduced salivary flow rate) enhances and often leads, for example, to
  - rapid decay of the teeth
  - mucosal irritation (e.g. candidosis)
  - foul-smelling breath
  - soreness of the tongue ("burning mouth syndrome")
  - unusual taste sensations (e.g. metallic taste)
  - difficulty in wearing removable dentures
  - difficulties with speech and swallowing.

Diagnosis of dry mouth

- Diagnostically relevant questions include:
  - Is it difficult to swallow dry food (biscuits, bread) without drinking simultaneously?
  - Does the mouth feel dry when speaking?
  - Do you also need to moisten your mouth at night?

Measurement of salivary flow rate

- Can be performed by a dentist or an oral hygienist. The easiest and most common method to measure salivary flow rate is to quantify the amount of saliva produced during 5 min chewing on a piece of paraffin wax. Normally this amount exceeds 5 ml. Subjective feelings of a dry mouth (xerostomia) usually appear if the stimulated flow rate is less than 2.5 ml in 5 minutes.
- The base rate of saliva flow should be at least 0.5 ml in 5 minutes. The resting salivary flow rate is measured in the same manner, only without chewing.

Aetiology of the dryness of the mouth

- Medication, especially multiple medicines at the same time
- Rheumatic diseases, in particular Sjögren's syndrome (21.43)
- Diseases of the salivary glands
- Irradiation to the head and neck region (7.25)
- Mouth breathing
- Hormonal changes, e.g. climacteric
- Anorexia nervosa, fasting
- Labile juvenile (type 1) diabetes mellitus

How to relieve or treat dryness of the mouth

Chewing

- The 5–6 daily normal, regular meals and snacks should contain food that requires extensive chewing. Ending a meal by eating vegetables, nuts or cheese, which all neutralize bacterial acids, is beneficial.
- Rinsing the mouth or drinking water after each meal is recommended.
- Sugar-containing snacks, and acidic fruits or drinks should be avoided between meals. Plain water or mineral water are both safe for the teeth.

Xylitol-containing chewing gum, tablets and lozenges

- Chewing gum flavoured with xylitol is the best way to enhance salivary flow rate between and immediately after meals or snacks.
- If chewing capability is poor, the use of xylitol-sweetened tablets or lozenges or lozenges containing xylitol, calcium and fluoride, is recommended.

Saliva substitutes and moisturizing gels

- Saliva substitutes relieve the symptoms of dry mouth longer than any drinks. They can be used regularly if needed.
- Commercial saliva substitutes are available. Pharmacies can also prepare saliva substitutes.
- Saliva substitutes can be replaced by moisturizing gel that contains antimicrobial agents, or vegetable or olive oil.
- Mouth breathing can be avoided with oil-containing nasal sprays or drops.

Medication

- Assess the patient's medication; may any medicines safely be changed to others that cause less drying of the mouth?
- For patients who suffer from severe dryness of the mouth, e.g. after head and neck irradiation or in Sjögren's syndrome, pilocarpine tablets 5 mg × 3–4 can be used.

Treatment of the mouth

- Cleaning the teeth and interdental spaces daily is essential. In addition to fluoride dentifrice the use of some other local fluoride supplement, such as fluoride-containing tablets or fluoride chewing gum, is recommended.
- Dentures should be cleaned especially well. If there is inflammation under the prostheses, the dentures should not be kept in the mouth at night but instead in a dry and airy container.
- Mouthwashes containing alcohol should be avoided.

♦ A patient who suffers from dryness of the mouth needs expert advice on how to clean his/her teeth and dentures and on daily preventive dental care. The patient should visit the dentist every 3–6 months, i.e. more frequently than usual.

7.11 Cheilitis

Tuula Salo, Maria Siponen

Angular cheilitis in the elderly

♦ Often associated with edentulousness, dentures and over-closing of the mouth leading to an increased skin fold at the angle of the mouth (Figure 7.11.1). Constantly pooling saliva at the skin fold creates an ideal environment for fungal and bacterial infections.

♦ In 20% of cases the causative agent is Candida albicans, in 60% a mixture of C. albicans and Staphylococcus aureus and in 20% S. aureus alone.

♦ Deficiency of iron or vitamin B may predispose a person to cheilitis.

♦ Treatment

- Treatment of predisposing factors (correction of poor dental occlusion, correction of iron or vitamin B deficiency).
- A combination ointment of hydrocortisone, natamycin and neomycin sulphate, a combination of hydrocortisone and chlorhexidine, chlorhexidine gel, or emollient.

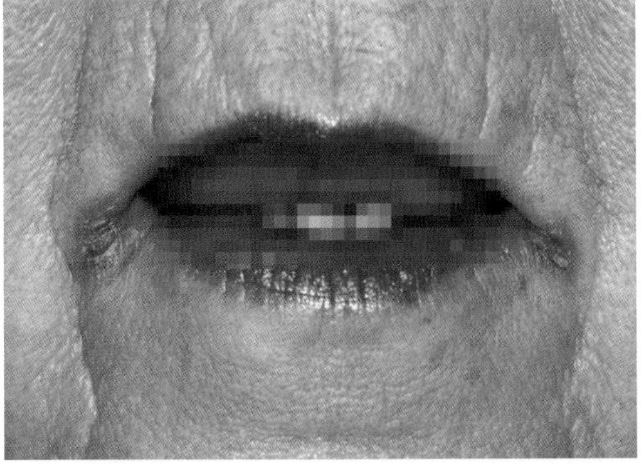

Figure 7.11.1 Angular cheilitis in the elderly is mostly associated with the use of dentures. Malocclusion resulting from worn teeth leaves the angular region wet and the elastotic old skin deepens the furrow at the angular region. Moisture C. albicans and/or S. aureus form the combined aetiology leading to painful fissures at the worst. Combinations of antifungals and corticosteroids often give relief. Photo © R. Suhonen.

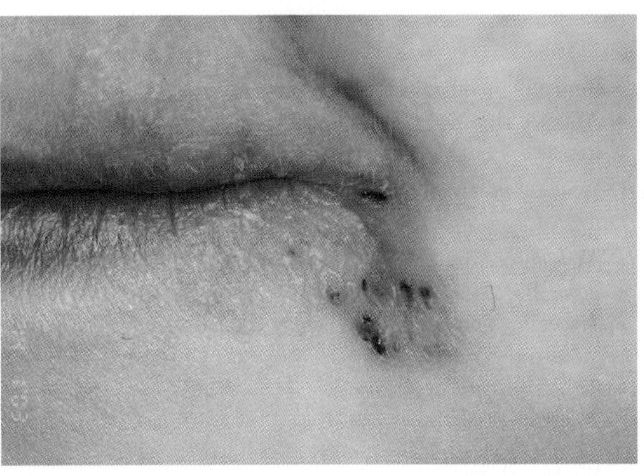

Figure 7.11.2 Angular cheilitis is common in atopic dermatitis, especially in children as shown here. Therapy follows the general rules of dermatitis in facial skin. Vitamins and antifungals seldom are helpful. In birch pollen allergic patients, contact with fruit and vegetables may provoke the symptoms. Photo © R. Suhonen.

Angular cheilitis in children

♦ Usually caused by atopic dermatitis, hardly ever by a fungal infection (Figure 7.11.2).

♦ Cheilitis may persist if the skin of a child, predisposed to allergies, is in repeated contact with food allergens, e.g. vegetables or fruit. It is also advisable to go without sweets for a week or two.

Other forms of cheilitis

♦ Actinic (solar) cheilitis is a skin change which increases the risk of cancer of the lower lip. It can be treated with liquid nitrogen cryotherapy or laser.

♦ Crohn's disease and HIV infection are also associated with cheilitis.

♦ See also perioral dermatitis 13.62.

7.12 Disturbances of taste

Editors

Basic rule

♦ Determine first whether the patient actually has a disturbed sense of smell (38.6).

Weakened sense of taste

♦ Dry mouth (7.10)

- Mouth breathing
- Drugs

- Disturbances in the sense of smell influence the sense of taste (38.6).
  - Sinusitis or other acute infection
  - Allergic rhinitis
  - Injuries
- Deficiency of vitamin B_{12} (15.24)
- Drugs
  - ACE inhibitors
  - Penicillamin
  - Tricyclic antidepressants (may cause dryness of the mouth)
  - Lithium

Taste of metal

- Parenteral gold (taste of metal may be the first symptom of stomatitis)
- Metronidazole
- Metformin
- Zopiclone
- Lead or mercury poisoning

Neurological causes

- If the patient complains of a disturbance of taste he may have a neurological disease affecting the sense of smell (e.g. a brain tumour).
- A unilateral disturbance of taste may be associated with other unilateral sensory symptoms.
- Peripheral facial nerve palsy may cause a disturbance of taste in the anterior part of the tongue.

7.13 Bad breath

Editors

Basic rules

- Neglecting oral hygiene is the most important reason for bad breath, and in 80% of the cases the cause is found in the mouth.
- The sense of smell adapts quickly even to a strong smell, and the patient is often unaware of the problem.
- When inspecting the mouth and the pharynx the physician can take up the subject discreetly and instruct the patient to see a dentist.
- Patients consulting a doctor because of bad breath have usually been encouraged to do so by their spouse or another family member after they have first seen a dentist.

Causes of bad breath

- Poor oral hygiene, dental caries (7.31), periodontal diseases (7.32), and difficulty in cleaning prostheses.
- Reduced salivation and drying of the mouth
  - Sjögren's syndrome (21.43)
  - Radiotherapy and post-operative conditions
  - Anticholinergic drugs
- Some systemic diseases
  - Diabetes
  - Renal and hepatic failure
- Bad-smelling nutrients, drugs, and stimulants and their degradation products
  - Garlic
  - Tobacco
  - Alcohol
  - Isosorbide nitrate
  - Disulfiram
- Infection and putrefaction
  - Salivary glands, tongue (7.24), ulcers and lesions of the oral mucosa.
- Infection of the tonsils, adenoids or lingual tonsil (38.24)
- Retropharyngeal or nasopharyngeal accumulation of mucus and pus, adenoids (cause mouth breathing, particularly in children)
- Nasal tumours, foreign bodies, atrophic rhinitis and ozaena (38.56), maxillary sinusitis
- Oesophageal diverticles, achalasia, reflux disease
- Bronchitis, bronchiectasis, pulmonary empyema

Treatment

- Treatment is symptomatic
- Good oral hygiene, the surface of the tongue is brushed
- Stimulation of salivation (pastilles, chewing gum, artificial saliva)
- Refreshening mouth rinses

A comatose patient with abnormal odour of breath

- Alcohol poisoning
- Diabetic coma (acetone)
- Hepatic coma (ammonia)
- Uraemia

7.14 Swelling of the salivary glands

Editors

Goals

- To diagnose parotitis as either a uni- or bilateral cause of swelling of the parotid glands.

- Antibiotic treatment is necessary if purulent suppuration is secreted from the orifice of the gland ducts or there are other signs of bacterial infection.
- Fluctuating and painful unilateral swelling could be a sign of sialolithiasis.
- If swelling is bilateral and almost asymptomatic, rheumatic diseases or other systemic diseases should be considered as a possible cause.
- If the patient is over 50 years of age and the swelling is slowly developing and unilateral, the possibility of malignancy is to be considered. **Do not** take a biopsy but send the patient to a specialist.

Examination of the salivary glands

- In case of symptoms affecting the salivary glands take into account the patient's age and gender.
  - Women have rheumatic diseases affecting the salivary glands more often than men.
  - Young people usually have viral infections.
  - Middle-aged people may suffer from calcifications in the ducts of the salivary glands or from sialadenosis (sialosis).
  - Elderly persons may have tumours of the salivary glands.
- The examination consists of bimanual palpation of the salivary glands (also intraorally!). Note that healthy parotid glands cannot be felt upon palpation, whereas pain upon palpation of the glands usually suggests inflammation.

Differential diagnosis of salivary gland swelling

Purulent parotitis

- Painful, usually unilateral swelling with redness of the skin area outside the gland. Severe general symptoms.
- Inflammation in the submandibular gland causes a similar clinical condition.
- Diagnosis
  - Often elevated leukocyte count and CRP
  - Under pressure by finger, the parotid ducts may secrete purulent suppuration that should be studied bacteriologically.
- Treatment
  - In cases of severe symptoms, cephalosporin 750 mg–1.5 g × 3 for one week i.v. plus anti-inflammatory medication. If the symptoms are less severe or slowly disappearing, cephalosporin can be administered orally.

Chronic bacterial parotitis

- Fluctuating fever; the gland may feel hard on palpation and remain swollen between periods of acute infection.
- Should be treated by a specialist.
- The most prevalent causes are staphylococci and streptococci, but in persistent cases the possibility of tuberculosis should also be considered. An infection of the submandibular glands can have a similar clinical picture.
- Diagnosis
  - CRP and leukocyte count rise during fever
  - If the gland remains permanently swollen, it is advisable to take a biopsy at a hospital outpatient clinic to exclude the possibility of a tumour or tuberculosis.
- Treatment
  - Antibiotics for 1–2 months (amoxicillin or doxycycline)
  - Gentle massage of the gland can be helpful
  - Other treatments according to the aetiology.

Mumps (Epidemic parotitis)

- See 31.83.
- Rare among patients who have been vaccinated
- Uni- or bilateral
- Symptoms include fever, rapid onset of a soft swelling of the parotid gland(s), pain on palpation, spontaneous pain, and secretion of mucous fluid from the parotid duct(s). The symptoms usually disappear in 1–2 weeks.
- Diagnosis is made from paired serum sample.

Sialolithiasis (calcifications in salivary gland ducts)

- The calcifications usually develop in the ducts of the submandibular glands or (less frequently) in the ducts of the parotid glands, and only unilaterally.
- Pain and swelling of the gland and duct appear rapidly, particularly after eating, and may last from a few hours to several days.
- Diagnosis
  - Upon inspection, the yellow sialolith can be seen at the opening of the duct.
  - Ultrasonography, if necessary
- Treatment
  - If the calcifications, which can often be palpated or can be seen in radiographs, are not removed, they may cause chronic inflammation of the glands. The calcifications are removed either by enlarging the duct or by incision at hospital.
  - Episodes of infection are treated with antibiotics.

Sialadenosis (sialosis)

- Non-neoplastic or inflammatory bilateral, diffuse and slowly developing swelling of the salivary gland(s) (most often parotid). There is no pain on palpation. This condition gradually leads to hyposalivation (7.10).
- Sialadenosis may have different aetiologies, most often
  - rheumatic sialadenosis (for example in Sjögren's syndrome)
  - sialadenosis related to sarcoidosis
  - hormonal reasons
  - diabetes.
- Treatment is focused on the systemic disease, not on the gland(s) itself.

Diagnostic strategy in detecting the cause for swelling of the salivary glands

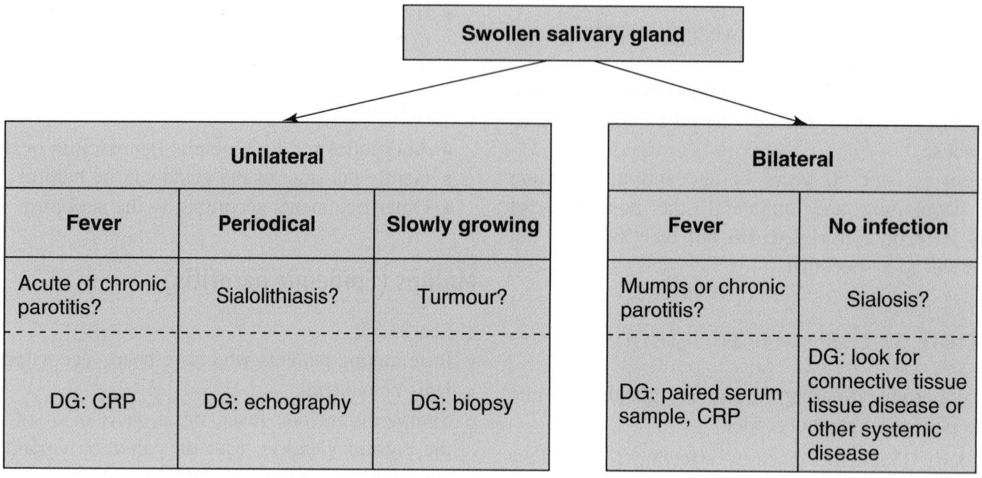

Swollen salivary gland				
Unilateral			Bilateral	
Fever	Periodical	Slowly growing	Fever	No infection
Acute of chronic parotitis?	Sialolithiasis?	Turmour?	Mumps or chronic parotitis?	Sialosis?
DG: CRP	DG: echography	DG: biopsy	DG: paired serum sample, CRP	DG: look for connective tissue tissue disease or other systemic disease

(DG = diagnostic method, CRP = C-reactive protein)

Figure 7.14.1 Diagnosis of swollen salivary glands

Tumours of the salivary glands

- Usually painless or causing minor symptoms. Tumours in the region of the parotid glands can be felt immediately under the skin.
- From the point of view of differential diagnosis the most notable differences from parotitis and sialosis are unilaterality and distinct borderline with other tissue, as well as hardness of the lump.
- The swelling may also occur close to the tonsillar region behind the angle of the mandible.
- If the swelling is suspected to be caused by a tumour, biopsy is not indicated: the patient should be referred to a hospital clinic for a more detailed examination, either to the department of otorhinolaryngology or oral diseases.
- Approximately 80% of salivary gland tumours are benign.
- See Figure 7.14.1

7.15 Burning mouth and glossalgia

Arja Kullaa

- See also Viral diseases of the oral mucosa 7.21, Oral manifestations of skin diseases 7.23.

Aims

- Local aetiology is determined by careful inspection of the oral mucosa, tongue and teeth.
- Treatable systemic diseases are diagnosed (vitamin B_{12} deficiency, diabetes).
- Dryness of the mouth is identified (causes include pharmaceuticals, such as anticholinergics and tricyclic antidepressants, and Sjögren's syndrome).
- Burning mouth often has a psychiatric cause that should be treated.

Epidemiology

- Burning mouth usually originates from areas where the mucosa is mobile, such as the buccal mucosa and tongue. In addition, there may be taste disturbances.
- Nearly 3% of the population may suffer from burning mouth. Mouth symptoms are five times as common among middle-aged women as among other people.
- Burning mouth mostly occurs in association with clinically evident lesions. Stomatitis caused by dentures is the most common lesion of the oral mucosa. Up to every second person with dentures may have oral inflammation. Almost one half of patients seeking medical attention because of glossalgia or burning mouth may have some lesion of the tongue.

Causes of burning mouth

- A specific cause of burning mouth is not always found, and the problem can be very complex. Both local and systemic factors may be involved.

Local causes

- Ulcers (e.g. aphthous stomatitis)
- Dental calculus, carious teeth
- Inflammation caused by dentures or other factors (e.g. yeasts)

- Smoking, use of alcohol
- Dietary habits: very hot, strongly spiced foods
- Continual use of mouth rinses
- Dry mouth (mouth breathing, xerostomia-inducing drugs, sometimes pregnancy, menopause)
- Malocclusion
- Mouth tumours
- Sometimes even lichenoid oral lesions, leukoplakia, erythroplakia and specific glossal lesions such as fissured tongue, geographic tongue and atrophy of filiform papillae (7.24)
- Allergy to dental materials
- Certain jaw disorders

Systemic causes

- Dermal and mucosal diseases (lichen planus, erythema multiforme, pemphigus, etc.)
- Pernicious anaemia
- Iron-deficiency anaemia
- Deficiency of group B vitamins
- Diabetes
- Sjögren's syndrome
- Acute leukaemia
- Agranulocytosis
- Multiple sclerosis

Psychiatric causes

- Burning mouth or facial pain can be a psychiatric symptom related to a number of mental disturbances, such as depression, anxiety and even incipient psychosis.
- Examination of patients suffering from persistent atypical facial pain will often reveal an underlying psychiatric disturbance.
- Psychiatric consultation is advisable when dealing with persistent intractable oral or facial pain.

Examination of the patient with burning mouth

History and clinical examination

- The patient history is essential.
- **Smoking**. Clinical examination reveals small reddish dots on the palate, i.e. inflammation of minor salivary glands. Sometimes there may be a reddened area with loss of filiform papillae along the midline of the tongue (central papillary atrophy = CPA).
- **Dietary habits**. Very hot, strongly spiced food can cause a burning sensation in the tongue. On the other hand, strong taste stimuli sometimes give rise to a burning sensation on the mucosa. No clinical lesions are encountered.
- Continual use of **mouth rinses** irritates the oral mucosa. In some cases, the oral mucosa exhibits small reddish areas that change their location daily. Continual taste stimulation can cause taste disturbances.
- A **dry mouth** (7.10) is susceptible to various forms of irritation and inflammation. Dryness of the oral mucosa can be due to mouth breathing, salivary gland disorders or pharmaceuticals that reduce the secretion of saliva. Menopausal symptoms may be aggravated by changes in the secretion and composition of saliva. Reduced saliva secretion is usually accompanied by taste disturbances.
- **Carious teeth or fillings**, heavy dental calculus and large diastemata can cause glossalgia, which is often localized to the tip of the tongue.
- Pain associated with **malocclusion** is localized in the tongue and the sites of insertion of masticatory muscles. The patient also has headache. Probable causes of malocclusion problems include a low denture, incomplete dentition and extensively filled teeth.
- **Angular cheilitis** and associated denture stomatitis suggest a fungal infection of the mouth. Clinical symptoms include redness and pain of the mucosa underneath the denture. The most severe cases also present with atrophy of filiform papillae on the surface of the tongue. Reduced secretion of saliva makes the mouth susceptible to fungal infections, which should be taken into account in planning therapy. In addition to pharmacological therapy, appropriate treatment of oral fungal infections includes examination and eventual replacement of old dentures (dentist's assessment).
- **Alveolar ridge pain** in persons with dentures is generally due to resorption of the bony crest, which renders the alveolar bone sharp as a knife. In such cases, it is advisable to assess potential bone lesions by means of orthopantomography. Treatment consists of ridge remodelling by an oral surgeon.
- Denture-related pain is very rarely allergic in origin, whereas **allergy to filling materials** is more common. Clinically, contact allergy is characterized by lichenoid lesions on the oral mucosa, with the lesions being in contact with the filling material. A biopsy should be taken of the lichenoid lesions. Based on the clinical finding and the histopathological diagnosis, the patient may be referred for allergy testing, as required.
- The most significant **drug-induced adverse effect** is the reduction of saliva secretion, which brings all sorts of discomfort, including mouth irritation and increased incidence of inflammations and dental diseases. Many different types of pharmaceuticals have been reported to cause oral mucosal symptoms resembling oral lichen. Since burning sensations in the mouth as well as disturbances of the senses of taste and touch may also be drug-related, it is important to enquire about the patient's use of medicines as part of the assessment of oral symptoms.
- A **burning sensation** on the oral mucosa may be accompanied by reddish, erosive patches. This is an absolute indication for determining blood count to assess the presence of anaemias.
- **Pain limited to a specific site** must always be taken seriously. Especially pain in the lateral side of the tongue can be a sign of a malignant tumour.
- **Neurological disorders** (multiple sclerosis, bulbar palsy, ALS, diabetic neuropathy). Other neurological findings may provide clues.

Laboratory tests

- Blood count (+ differential cell count by cell analyser) and blood glucose are the first tests.
- Any leucoplakia or tumour-like changes on the oral mucosa should always be biopsied.

Follow-up

- Clinical lesions on the oral mucosa must be monitored initially at three- to six-month intervals.

7.17 Malocclusions

Olli Rönning

- Dental malocclusions are generally developmental disturbances.

Malpositions of teeth related to health disturbances in the mouth and jaws

- Deep bite, which occurs when the lower anterior teeth, incisors, are completely covered by the upper incisors when biting the posterior teeth together, can give rise to repeated irritation of the mucosa posterior to the upper incisors. This is caused by the lower incisors, and sometimes leads to tissue lesions.
- Chronic infection of the gingiva, or gums, can force the teeth apart.
- Some malpositioned teeth may guide the lower jaw off its normal closing path, which often disturbs the functioning of the temporomandibular joint. This may cause a mild but harmful developmental disorder in children.

The most common disturbances associated with malpositions of the teeth and disproportionate relations between the jaws

Oropharyngeal adenoid tissue

- Enlarged adenoids may be associated with excessive mouth breathing. As a result, the upper incisors are proclined, and their gingivae become dry and inflamed. Removal of the adenoid tissue is not necessarily followed by cessation of this breathing habit.

Speech disturbances

- The relationship between malpositioned teeth and speech disorders is incompletely understood. The most common problems concern the sounds "r" and "s". The difficulty with "s" has been found to be related to anterior open bite, in which the upper and lower anterior teeth do not come into contact when the posterior teeth are occluded.
- Sagittal malrelation of the jaws, especially in combination with a narrow upper jaw, increases the risk of speech disorders. There is no definite information on the effect of orthodontic treatment on speech.

Rheumatoid arthritis

- About 60% of children afflicted with rheumatoid arthritis have lesions of the temporomandibular joint by the age of 16 years.
  - Opening of the mouth and protrusion of the lower jaw may be difficult and hamper, for example, dental treatment.
  - In the case of unilateral involvement, the jaw deviates to the affected side upon opening the mouth.
  - Bilateral involvement may lead to a slowing down of the growth of the lower jaw, development of a convex profile ("bird face"), a clearly noticeable impression in the posterior part of the lower jaw ("antegonial notch"), and open bite.
  - Changes of a similar nature have also been observed in adults with rheumatoid arthritis, and are not necessarily pathognomonic.

Cleft lip and palate

- See 7.26.
- This developmental disturbance is characterized by the congenital missing or mild deformation of some anterior teeth. As a result of disturbed growth of the upper jaw, the anterior teeth may bite edge-to-edge or be in crossbite, in which the upper anterior teeth are situated posterior to the lower ones.
- Middle ear infections are common, and speech has a nasal twang.

Scoliosis

- Malpositioning of the teeth seems to be associated with scoliosis as such, and particularly with treatment using a Milwaukee brace, which often leads to proclination of the anterior teeth and a reduction in the height of the lower face. The malpositioning of the teeth may be corrected spontaneously after termination of treatment with the brace.

Torticollis

- The teeth in the side regions in particular, the premolars and molars, are in faulty positions.

Multiple developmental disturbances

- Early treatment of the Pierre Robin syndrome (small lower jaw, cleft palate, disturbed respiration in the neonatal phase) is important. Tracheotomy is one of the many treatment methods recommended in the literature. With an improvement in respiration the discrepancy between the jaws undergoes spontaneous correction within some months.

- Cleidocranial dysplasia (cleidocranial synostosis) is typically associated with supernumerary teeth and their eruption disturbances.

Malnutrition and endocrinological disturbances

- Some health disturbances that are rare or nowadays generally treated early (e.g. rickets, cretinism, hypopituitarism) involve developmental disturbances in the dentition.

Treatment

- Malocclusions (malpositioning of teeth) can be treated by specialists in orthodontics.
- Complicated anomalies are sometimes treated by a team including an orthodontist, an oral or plastic surgeon, a specialist in dental prosthetics, a phoniatrician, a speech therapist and a psychologist.

7.20 Oral mucosal ulcers

Editors

Principles

- Always check the condition of any dental prosthesis.
- Always keep in mind the possibility of oral cancer. Any ulcer that has not healed in 2 weeks warrants biopsy.
- Consult a dentist; patients in whom biopsy and excision are indicated are, in most cases, referred to an oral surgeon.

Aetiology

- Oral mucosal ulcers can be classified into the following categories according to their aetiology:
  - **Mechanical trauma**
    - Usually heals without suture; however, ulcers on the lip mucosa or fissurating ulcers of the skin should be closed by suture with resorbing material.
  - **Neoplasia**
  - **Aphthous ulcers**
    - These are usually small, painful blisters localized in the gingiva, which resolve leaving painful, grey ulcers.
    - This is a common disorder, and usually a completely innocent lesion.
    - Treatment consists of mouth rinses, local corticosteroids, and topical lidocaine solution for the soreness. In severe cases, topical application of tetracycline solution might be indicated. Topical therapy with triamcinolone tablets is also an option.
    - Recurrent aphthous ulcers may be a sign of coeliac disease (8.84). Test for antibodies to gliadin, endomysium or transglutaminase or consider gastroscopy if the patient has other symptoms suggestive of coeliac disease.
    - Whenever symptoms in the joints or mucous membranes occur in association with aphthous ulcers, the possibility of Behçet's syndrome should be seriously considered.
  - **Systemic disorders**
    - Haematological deficiency syndromes (iron, folic acid, vitamin B_{12} deficiency).
    - Cyclic neutropenia
    - Gastrointestinal diseases (Crohn's disease, ulcerative colitis)
    - Skin diseases (lichen ruber, see Figure 7.23.2; pemphigus, pemphigoid, erythema multiforme, dermatitis herpetiformis, epidermolysis bullosa, SLE, Reiter's syndrome 7.23)
    - Infections (HSV, Coxsackie virus, syphilis, tuberculosis 7.21, HIV, gonorrhoea)
    - Drugs (cytostatics, antihypertensives, antidiabetics, gold salts, anti-inflammatory agents, antimalarial drugs)

7.21 Viral infections of the oral mucosa

Editors

Herpes simplex virus (HSV)

- Herpes simplex virus (HSV) type 1 is usually responsible for symptoms in the oral mucosa and the lip skin.

Primary infection

- In almost 99% of the cases the primary infection is asymptomatic or mildly symptomatic.
- Primary infection is usually contracted in childhood, rarely after the age of 20 years.
- In 1% of patients, primary oral HSV infection presents with a fulminant febrile stomatitis, in which painful blisters appear in both the gingival region and elsewhere in the oral mucosa.

Recurrent HSV infection

- Recurrence begins as a reddish itching area where clear, small and rapidly rupturing blisters develop. These result in superficial ulcers, which, however, heal spontaneously in a week.

- Among the factors activating HSV-1 are common cold, exposure to excessive sunlight, stress or even menstruation. Impaired immunity (e.g. HIV infection, blood transfusion, cancer patients on cytostatic treatment) predisposes to frequent recurrence of HSV and to increased duration of the symptomatic phase. Around 10–15% of recurrent oral HSV infections are caused by HSV-2.

Diagnosis

- The diagnosis of oral HSV infection is easily made on the basis of the clinical appearance, or by demonstrating the virus in the scrape from the base of the ulcer, either immunohistochemically or by using gene technology (hybridization).
- Examination of serum antibodies is useful only for demonstrating primary HSV infection.

Treatment

- **Primary infection**: Rest is recommended, supplemented with the application of lidocaine gel on the painful blisters or chlorhexidine mouth rinse (2 mg/ml) 10 ml twice daily for 1 minute. The mouth rinse is spat out. Aciclovir therapy may be used: for patients above 2 years of age, give 200 mg as a tablet or 5 ml as a mixture (40 mg/ml), 5 times daily for 5 days. For children aged 3 months to 2 years, give 2.5 ml of the mixture 5 times daily for 5 days.
- **Recurrent infection**: Aciclovir cream, five times a day for 5 days or as a mixture, 5 ml five times a day for 5 days, is recommended. Preventive treatment (200 mg four times a day or 400 mg twice daily for 6–12 months) should be given only in special cases.
- It is noteworthy that aciclovir-resistant strains of HSV are currently emerging.

Varicella zoster virus (VZV)

- In **varicella**, in addition to the generalized rash with small pustules all over the body, small, yellowish blisters that rupture easily are found on the oral mucosa.
- Of all **herpes zoster infections** (1.41), 20% appear in the head and neck region. In the area of the nerves innervating the maxilla and the mandible, herpes zoster usually starts with pain localized in the teeth (simulating the pain of inflammatory dental pulpitis). After 3–4 days this is followed by the appearance of blisters both inside and outside the oral cavity. As in zoster elsewhere, the blisters do not cross the middle line of the body (except the anterior part of the maxilla).

Diagnosis

- The clinical picture is typical enough to enable a correct diagnosis.

Treatment

- See 1.41 for treatment.

Coxsackie virus infections

- These infections have a fairly mild course.

Herpangina

- This disorder appears as epidemics, usually among children.
- Symptoms include fever, malaise, abdominal pains, headache and muscular pain. The generalized symptoms appear before the oral symptoms.
- Oral symptoms include blisters on the palatal arch, soft and hard palate, uvula and tonsils. At the onset, the blisters are small and surrounded by a clear halo. They gradually increase in size and heal spontaneously in 2–10 days.
- **Differential diagnosis**: In herpangina, no bullae appear in the gingival area, unlike in HSV infections. HSV lesions also last markedly longer and are painful in contrast to those of herpangina.

Hand-foot-and-mouth disease

- Synonym: vesicular stomatitis with exanthema
- The incubation period is usually 3–5 days.
- Painless blisters appear on the dorsum of the hands, on the soles and on oral mucosa, usually in the buccal region. The general symptoms are usually minor and resolve in 5 days.
- **Diagnosis** is clinical or is made by demonstrating Coxsackie viruses by culture.

Papillomaviruses (HPV)

- Currently, over 100 different types of human papillomavirus (HPV) are recognized, of which some cause infections only on the skin and other types exclusively at mucosal sites. The oral mucosa is special in that it is capable of harbouring HPV infections of both the genital types (e.g. HPV 6, 11, 16, 18) and the skin types (e.g. HPV 2, 4, 7).
- Exophytic, cauliflower-like warts (papillomas, condylomas) are encountered on the oral mucosa of some 0.4% of the population. In children, common hand warts can be transmitted to the oral mucosa, following sucking of the fingers.
- The aetiological agent of another characteristic HPV lesion, focal epithelial hyperplasia (FEH) is HPV 13 or HPV 32. These lesions are smooth and resemble a small fibroma. In addition to these well-defined clinical lesions, HPVs can also appear on the oral mucosa as latent infections (in around 15% of subjects). The full significance of oral mucosal HPV infections remains to be elucidated. HPVs seem to have a clear association with carcinomas of the uterine cervix, but their implication in the aetiology of oral cancer is not straightforward.
- **Diagnosis** is based on the clinical appearance, or on characteristic morphological changes (HPV-induced cytopathic changes) detected in the cytological scrape or by histological biopsy. However, detection of HPV DNA is the only reliable means of diagnosing HPV infection. With these methods, the specific HPV type can also be identified.
- **Treatment**: A large proportion of these lesions resolve spontaneously. When appropriate, surgical excision may be

carried out, or the lesions can be eradicated by using laser or cryotherapy. Whenever dysplastic changes are detected in the biopsy, careful follow-up of the patient is warranted.

Epstein-Barr virus (EBV)

Infectious mononucleosis (kissing disease)

- In typical cases, the symptoms include fever, enlarged cervical and axillary lymph nodes (due to lymphadenitis), and an exudative, diphtheria-like tonsillitis that does not respond to penicillin. Sometimes, painful ulcers appear in the gingival area or on the palate.
- **Diagnosis**: The peripheral blood is characterized by leukocytosis and lymphocytosis as well as elevation of EBV antibodies. EBV can be demonstrated directly from the pharyngeal swab by using immunohistochemistry or DNA techniques (hybridization methods or PCR).
- **Treatment**: Oral changes due to mononucleosis do not require any active treatment.

Hairy leukoplakia

- This is characteristically a lesion with a whitish covering on the tongue that in most cases affects both sides of the tongue symmetrically, starting from its posterior third.
- This lesion clearly associates with immunosuppressive states (of any cause), and is quite common in HIV-infected subjects. The aetiological factor has been confirmed to be EBV.
- The clinical hairy leukoplakia lesion is asymptomatic and according to current understanding it is completely harmless because, for example, no dysplastic changes are detected in biopsy. In HIV patients, however, the appearance of hairy leukoplakia is considered a sign of a poor outcome.
- The **differential diagnosis** should take into account hyperkeratotic lesions due to mechanical irritation, fungal infections and lichen planus lesions.
- **Diagnosis**: The clinical picture and histological presentation are typical.
- **Treatment**: The lesion does not require any treatment. In some cases, aciclovir has been administered according to the scheme used in the treatment of HSV infections.

7.22 Oral fungal infections

Editors

General

- Candida albicans is a normal parasite of the oral cavity. The prevalence of symptom-free oral carriage of candida organisms in a clinically normal mouth ranges from 20 to 50% in healthy adults.
- Clinical candida infections occur when the host defence is compromized and the balance of oral bacteria and fungi is disturbed. Fungal infection is thus a sign of either locally or generally weakened defence.
- Factors that predispose to candidiasis are age, hormonal status, endocrinological factors and uncontrolled diabetes. Predisposing factors also include smoking, reduced salivation, and ill-fitting dentures.

Clinical manifestation

- The infection has three different manifestations. Fungal infection can be acute or chronic.
  - **Atrophic** (erythematous) candidiasis is the most common infection with ill-defined, painful and red areas, on buccal mucosa.
  - **Pseudomembranous** candidiasis (thrush) is characterized by white patches on the surface of the buccal mucosa that reveal a raw, erythematous and sometimes bleeding base when they are scraped.
  - **Hyperplastic** candidiasis presents thick whitish plaques, hard and rough to the touch and cannot be scraped off. Hyperplastic candidiasis is the most common change on the oral mucosa in HIV-infected patients.
- **Angular stomatitis** (perlèche, angular cheilitis) (7.11) is usually caused by Candida albicans (occasionally by Staphylococcus aureus), poorly fitting dentures, iron or vitamin B_{12} deficiency, Crohn's disease or HIV infection.

Differential diagnosis

- Geographic tongue (7.24), hairy leukoplakia (7.21), leukoplakias and other hyperkeratotic lesions of the oral mucosa.

Diagnosis

- A culture sample, smear or biopsy can be used for culture or microscopy.

Treatment

- Treatment is always targeted at the cause of the infection. Predisposing factors are elimininated, wherever possible.
- Pharmacotherapy
  - Amphotericin lozenge (amphotericin B) 10 mg × 4 for 4 weeks or
  - Nystatin mixture (100 000 IU/ml), 1 ml × 4 for 4 weeks or
  - Natamycin drops (2.5%) for adults and over 6-year-old children 1 ml × 4–6 after a meal; for infants 0.5 ml × 4 after breastfeeding
  - Miconazole 2% gel, 2.5 ml at 6-hour intervals for 4 weeks, mainly for topical treatment of candidiasis.
  - Fluconazole, 50 mg per day (single dose therapy) for 2 weeks.

- Dentures should always be rebased by boiling in water or changed to new ones. If the denture is new and not in need of repair, a local infection can be managed by applying miconazole denture lacquer (50 mg/g) at 3-week intervals.
- The primary disease should be managed appropriately (e.g. diabetes)

7.23 Skin diseases and the mouth

Tuula Salo, Maria Siponen

- Table 7.23 lists possible clinical findings on the oral mucosa and their possible causes.

Erythema multiforme

- Erythema multiforme is an acute, inflammatory bullous disease that causes exudative lesions on the oral mucosa and the lips. Skin changes occur usually in the extremities; they are erythematous, fairly well defined with cocentric rings (bull's eye lesions).
- The disease is self-limiting but may recur several times.
- The aetiology is unknown, but in about 50% of the cases it is possible to identify a provoking factor. Such factors include: infections (particularly HSV or mycoplasma), drugs, pregnancy, chemicals, foods, malignancies, systemic illness, stress or irradiation.
- In the generalized form of the disease (Stevens–Johnson syndrome) severe exfoliative lesions occur both on the skin and on at least two mucosal areas. The most serious form of the disease is Lyell's syndrome (toxic epidermal necrolysis) with over 30% of skin surface area involvement.
- **Diagnosis** is usually based on the clinical picture and history to identify possible provoking factors. Diagnosis can be verified with provocation tests.
- **Treatment** consists of elimination of the cause, sufficient hydration and antihistamines when necessary. Topical corticosteroid preparations are usually effective in relieving symptoms caused by oral lesions. Chlorhexidine (2 mg/ml) mouthwashes 2–3 times daily will prevent the emergence of complications and maintain good oral hygiene. If the disease was triggered by herpes simplex virus, aciclovir may be beneficial. Severe forms of the disease warrant hospitalization and systemic corticosteroids.

Pemphigus vulgaris

- Rare, chronic autoimmune bullous disease.
- In approximately 75% of cases the disease first manifests itself as blistering in the oral mucosa. The blisters rupture easily causing painful erosions. Intact blisters are rarely encountered in the oral cavity. Typical sites for lesions are the palate, buccal mucosa and the lower lip. Pressing uninvolved mucosa around a blister with a blunt instrument for one minute will cause blister formation or the epithelium will separate from the lower layers (positive Nikolsky's test).
- Skin lesions appear as thin walled flaccid blisters filled with clear fluid. They remain on one site for a few months and will then spread to other skin areas.
- **Diagnosis** is based on the clinical picture, histopathology (intraepithelial vesicle), and both on direct and indirect immunofluorescence (IF) methods. A sample for the direct IF examination should be collected from unaffected mucous membrane or skin next to a lesion. The sample must be delivered to a laboratory whilst it is fresh (either immediately, wrapped in saline soaked gauze, or in special medium, supplied by the laboratory, which will maintain the freshness of the sample for three days).
- **Treatment** consists of systemic corticosteroids, either alone or combined with methotrexate, azathioprine, cyclophosphamide or gold. Corticosteroid creams can be used topically.

Pemphigoid

- Chronic, autoimmune bullous disease. The two main forms are bullous pemphigoid and benign mucous membrane pemphigoid. In bullous pemphigoid, oral symptoms occur in approximately 15–30% of cases. In benign mucous membrane pemphigoid oral symptoms are always present, and in 95% of cases the primary lesion is within the oral cavity.
- The blisters in the mouth are filled with clear fluid or blood, and rupture readily. The mucous membrane surrounding the blisters is erythematous. After the blisters rupture the wound surface is slow to heal and may leave a scar. The most common clinical manifestation of benign mucous membrane pemphigoid in the mouth is gingival erythema and ulceration, i.e. desquamative gingivitis. Lesions are typically also seen on the palate, the buccal mucous membrane and the tongue.
- **Diagnosis.** Age (usually 60–70 years), clinical picture, histopathology (subepithelial vesicle), IF studies, positive Nikolsky's test (see pemphigus vulgaris).
- **Treatment** of lesions on oral mucosa consists of topical corticosteroids. More severe cases should be treated with systemic corticosteroids and/or with other immunosuppressive medication. The patient should also be advised to avoid any trauma to the skin and mucous membranes which may provoke bullae formation (e.g. food of hard consistency).

Lichen planus (lichen ruber planus)

- Aetiology is unknown; cell-mediated immune response to either an external or allogenic antigen.
- Not an uncommon condition, in about 2% of the population.
- Approximately two thirds of the patients are female, incidence is highest at middle-age.

Table 7.23 Clinical findings on the oral mucosa and their possible causes.

Clinical picture of the finding	Possible cause
Light coloured	
♦ Can be scraped off	Candidosis, fibrin coated ulcer (chemical/thermal trauma), toothpaste-induced peeling of the mucosal surface layer
♦ Cannot be scraped off	Irritative hyperplasia, lichenoid reaction, drug reaction, lichen planus, hyperplastic candidosis, leukoplakia, leukoedema, white sponge naevus, hereditary benign intraepithelial dyskeratosis, Darier's disease, chewing tobacco-induced changes, nicotine stomatitis, solar cheilitis, hairy leukoplakia, hairy tongue, geographic tongue, submucous fibrosis, Fordyce's granules, ectopic lymphatic tissue, gingival cyst, gingival abscess, lipoma
Erythematous	Atrophic candidosis, lichen planus, drug reaction, contact allergy, pemphigoid, iron or vitamin B deficiency, measles (Koplik's spots), haemangioma, pyogenic granuloma, peripheral giant cell granuloma, median rhomboid glossitis, erythroplakia, Kaposi's sarcoma, geographic tongue, psoriasis, scarlet fever, plasma cell gingivitis, petechiae and bruising (trauma, blood disorder)
Ulcerous	Trauma, aphtha, syphilis, gonorrhoea, tuberculosis, leprosy, aktinomycosis, noma, fungal infection, Behçet's disease, Reiter's syndrome, lichen planus, erythema multiforme, lupus erythematosus, drug reaction, contact allergy, Wegener's granulomatosis, midline granuloma, chronic granulomatous disease, cyclic neutropenia, epidermoid carcinoma, maxillary sinus carcinoma
Bullous	Herpes simplex infection, varicella zoster infection, enterovirus, herpangina, pemphigoid, pemphigus, dermatitis herpetiformis, epidermolysis bullosa, drug reaction, contact allergy
Verrucous	Palatal papillomatosis, squamous papilloma, condyloma acuminatum, condyloma latum, oral verruca vulgaris, focal epithelial hyperplasia, keratoacanthoma, verrucous leukoplakia, verrucous carcinoma, pyostomatitis vegetans, verrucous xanthoma
Hyperpigmentation	Amalgam tattoo, melanotic macule, physiological pigmentation, tobacco, inflammation, drugs, heavy metals, Addison's disease, Peutz-Jeghers syndrome, Laugier-Hunziker syndrome, naevus, melanoma, childhood neuroectodermal tumour
Submucosal swelling	
♦ gums	Pyogenic granuloma, peripheral giant cell granuloma, peripheral fibroma, gingival abscess, exostosis, gingival cyst, eruption cyst, congenital epulis of a newborn, generalized gingival hyperplasia
♦ floor of the mouth	Ranula, dermoid cyst, lymphoepithelial cyst, salivary gland tumour, mesenchymal tumour
♦ buccal and labial mucosa	Salivary gland tumour, mucocoele, traumatic fibroma, mesenchymal tumour
♦ tongue	Traumatic fibroma, pyogenic granuloma, granular cell tumour, neurofibroma, mucosal neuroma, salivary gland tumour, lingual thyroid
♦ palate	mucocoele, salivary gland tumour, dental abscess, lymphoma, torus, tumour of upper jaw or maxillary sinus

- Lichen planus affecting the oral mucosa is divided into the following types, according to its clinical manifestation: papular, reticular, plaquelike, atrophic, erosive and bullous. The reticular type, with pale Wickham's striae on the mucous membranes (Figures 7.23.1, 7.23.2), is the most common form of the disease. Changes of different types may co-exist. The lichen planus lesions usually show symmetrical distribution over the buccal mucosa, the tongue and/or the gums.
- Approximately 30–40% of patients with oral lichen planus also manifest skin lesions. On the other hand, 70% of patients with skin lesions have co-existing oral lesions.
- Skin changes are intermittent in character whereas oral lesions are persistent.
- The disease is often (in approximately 50% of cases) accompanied by secondary oral fungal infection.
- **Diagnosis** is based on the clinical picture and histopathology.
- **Treatment** consists of the elimination of any possible aggravating factors (dental calculus, sharp edges of dental

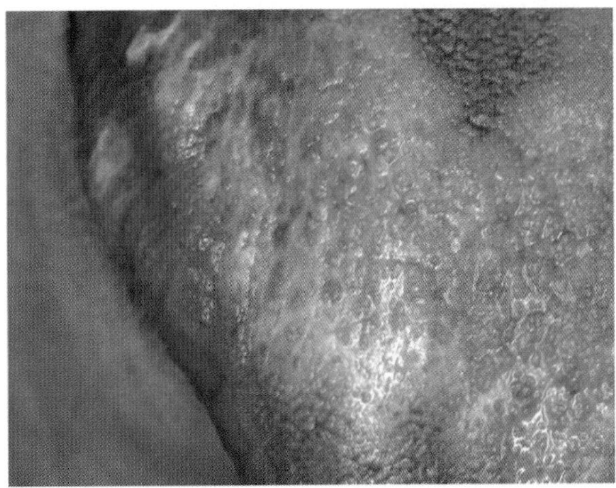

Figure 7.23.1 Lichen planus can affect the surface of the tongue. The whitish, patchy lichen on the surface of the tongue is often misinterpreted as a Candida infection. Analogous findings are regularly found (e.g. in buccal mucosa and typical skin areas). Photo © R. Suhonen.

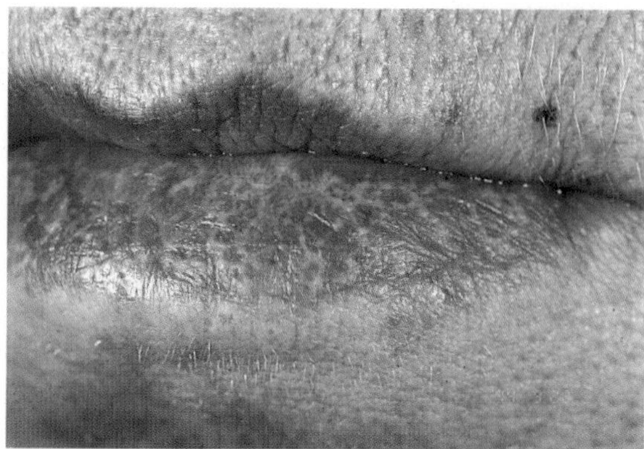

Figure 7.23.2 Lichen planus may affect also the lower lip, where typical Wickham's striae can be seen - in this picture unusually clearly. Topical potent corticosteroid for a limited period is usually curative, but recurrence is possible. Photo © R. Suhonen.

fillings, rubbing prosthesis), good oral hygiene and treatment of fungal infections (confirm diagnosis with a fungal culture). Furthermore, any symptomatic and/or erythematous lesions should be treated locally with corticosteroid preparations (triamcinolone acetonide ointment or nasal spray, betamethasone ointment 0.1%, clobetasol propionate ointment 0.1%). A good method to apply hydrocortisone cream (betamethasone cream 0.1%) to lesions situated predominantly on the gums is the use of medicinal trays. In severe cases lesions may also be injected directly with corticosteroids. Good preliminary results have been achieved from the use of topical tacrolimus in the treatment of lichen planus of the oral mucosa; however, its use is limited to specialist care settings.

- N.B. Approximately 1% of lichen planus lesions become malignant. Follow-up is important, and a repeat biopsy may be needed.

Lichenoid reactions

- Lichenoid reactions do not totally fulfil the criteria for lichen planus, either clinically or histologically.
- Often a single, localized lesion (compare with lichen planus)
- Lichenoid reactions can be provoked by:
  - **Drugs** (ACE inhibitors, allopurinol, beta-blockers, carbamazepine, chlorpromazine, chloroquine, cytostatic agents, furosemide, gold salts, ketoconazole, lithium, levomepromazine, methyldopa, NSAIDs, penicillamine, penicillin, phenothiazines, quinidine, salazopyrine, sulphonylureas, tetracyclines, thalidomide, thiazides, zidovudine)
  - **Autoimmune diseases** (myasthenia gravis, SLE, ulcerative colitis, alopecia areata, vitiligo, hepatic dysfunction)
  - **Dental filling materials**
- An aetiological factor cannot always be identified.

Discoid lupus erythematosus (DLE)

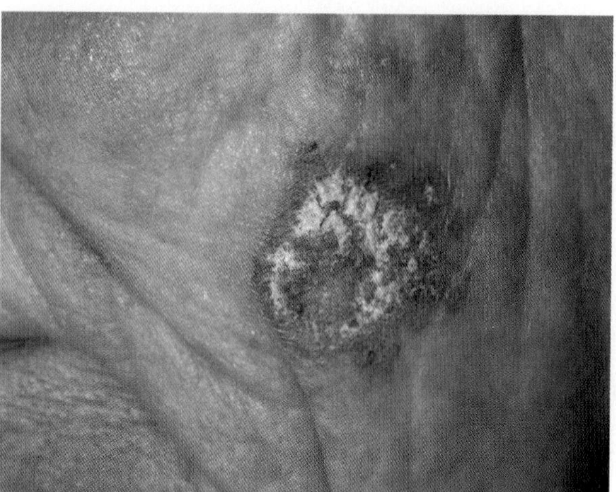

Figure 7.23.3 Discoid lupus erythematosus, DLE, is a collagenosis limited to the skin and mucous membranes. Characteristically the skin lesions are red, sometimes moderately painful and the hyperkeratotic scales may even mimic a psoriatic plaque. Photo © R. Suhonen.

- Chronic, inflammatory, photosensitive autoimmune disease limited to the skin and oral mucosa (Figure 7.23.3) of unknown aetiology. SLE is the systemic manifestation of the same condition.
- The majority of the patients are female.
- DLE causes fairly defined reddened skin lesions. As the lesions heal they become scaly in the centre, which is followed by atrophy and scar formation as well as discolouration. The mouth lesions are round, non-defined reddish areas encircled by a radial white rim, and may be associated with white spotting. The most common sites are the buccal areas, palate and the lower lip. The mouth lesions are usually painfree.
- **Diagnosis** is based on the clinical picture and histological findings of a biopsy. If DLE is suspected a biopsy should be taken of a lesion, and half of the sample should be sent for IF examination (fresh tissue required). The systemic form of the disease can be diagnosed of a biopsy taken from an unaffected area.
- Less than 5% of patients with DLE will go on to develop SLE.
- **Treatment** consists of topical corticosteroids and antirheumatic medication. Sun screens are also recommended. It is considered that DLE lesions, particularly those involving the lips, might increase the risk of cancer.

Recurrent aphthous stomatitis (ulcers)

- Recurrent aphthous stomatitis is a common condition affecting 20–60% of the population (Figure 7.23.4).
- The aetiology is unknown; however, sometimes they are clearly associated with stress, mechanical irritation, certain foods, haematological abnormalities (deficiency of iron, folic acid, vitamin B or zinc) and hormonal changes.
- They are classified according to their presentation as minor, major and herpetiform.
- The ulcers usually occur on the labial and buccal mucous membranes, more rarely on the tongue and gums. They are

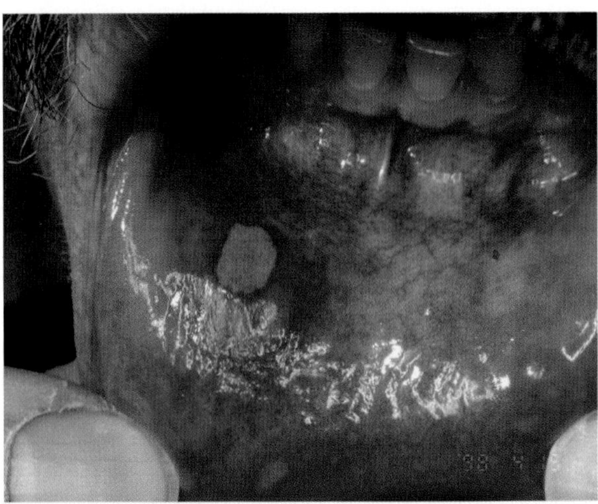

Figure 7.23.4 Aphthous stomatitis is a painful condition of unknown aetiology. One or several whitish ulcerations 1 mm to 1 cm in size appear periodically in oral mucosa. Topical corticoids give relief. In severe cases and in multiorgan affection Behçet's syndrome should be considered as a differential diagnosis. Photo © R. Suhonen.

usually painful and will heal within 1–6 weeks, depending on the size of the ulcer.

- **Diagnosis** is based on the clinical picture and history.
- **Treatment.** If necessary, topical corticosteroid products could be tried (oromucosal tablets or oral paste) as well as chlorhexidine mouthwashes. Recurring major ulcers may be treated with tetracycline mouthwashes. Some patients have benefited from the use of certain herbal and vitamin products ("Longo Vital"). The use of toothpaste without sodium lauryl sulphate is recommended.

Leukoplakia and erythroplakia

- Leukoplakia is a clinical concept signifying a light-coloured well-defined patch or area on the oral mucosa that cannot be scraped off and cannot be diagnosed as any other specific disease.
- Erythroplakia denotes a reddish mucous membrane lesion that cannot be diagnosed as any other specific disease.
- Leukoplakias can be classified according to their aetiology either as being idiopathic or induced by tobacco use or spirits (alcohol) intake.
- Leukoplakias can be clinically homogenous or non-homogenous (nodular, verrucous, proliferative verrucous leukoplakia or erythroleukoplakia). The mean risk of a malignant change is 4% in homogenous leukoplakia, but considerably higher in non-homogenous leukoplakia. Proliferative verrucous leukoplakia, in particular, will almost always develop into a carcinoma.
- Statistically the most dangerous area is the floor of the mouth and the underside of the tongue (50% will become malignant).
- Erythroplakia is always associated with dysplasia and 90% of the cases will develop into a cancer, regardless of the site of occurrence.
- **Diagnosis** is based on the clinical picture and histology.
- **Treatment** involves surgical excision, if a biopsy shows moderate to severe dysplasia, and clinical follow-up at 6 monthly intervals. It has been noted that the removal or non-removal of a leukoplakia does not correlate with the prognosis of the lesion. Follow-up is most important!

Pigmentation of the oral mucosa

- Physiological pigmentation is usually symmetrical over the gums. Inflammatory diseases, such as lichen planus, may cause pigmentation of the mucous membranes.
- Smoking-induced melanosis usually occurs in the gums at the front of the mouth.
- Amalgam tattoo is the most common pigmented lesion of the oral mucosa. It is caused by amalgam particles invading the mucous membranes. Amalgam tattoo is usually a greyish dark spot on the gums, close to a dental filling (Figure 7.23.5).
- Some cases of pigmentation are drug-induced (e.g. antimalarials, cytostatic medication, zidovudine).
- A widespread pigmentation may be attributable to a systemic illness, such as Addison's disease, Peutz-Jeghers syndrome, Albright's syndrome or neurofibromatosis. If the patient presents with diffuse pigmentation of the oral mucosa and the lips without a systemic illness, the possibility of Laugier-Hunziker syndrome should be considered.
- Melanotic macule refers to a local pigmented lesion. It may be idiopathic or caused by one of the aforementioned factors.
- Naevi and melanoma are rare but possible on the oral mucosa.
- If in doubt the diagnosis must be confirmed with a biopsy.

Venous lake

- Venous lake is a thick-walled dilatation of a vein that can be treated with liquid nitrogen freezing (Figure 7.23.6).

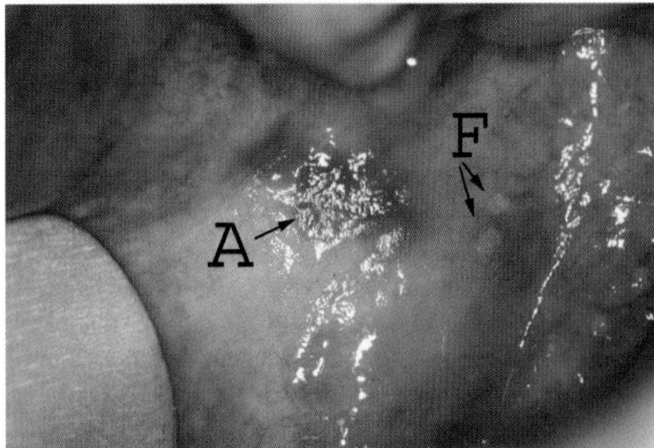

Figure 7.23.5 Dark, even black colour in the buccal mucous membrane is most commonly due to amalgam tattoo (A). The yellowish spots (F) seen in the picture are normal variants of sebaceous glands (Fordyce spots). Photo © R. Suhonen.

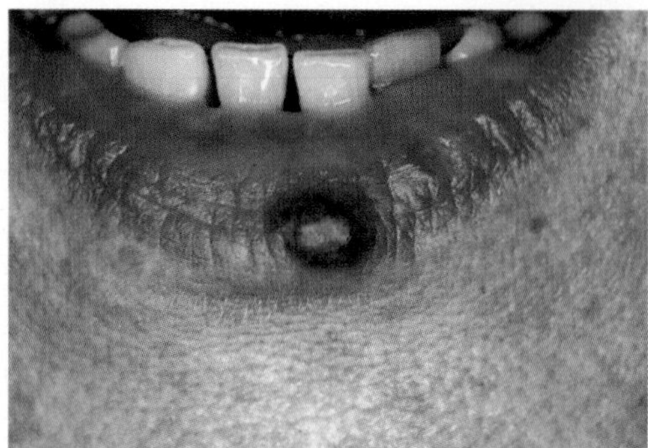

Figure 7.23.6 A venous lake at the most usual location - at the vermilion margin of the lower lip. The easiest and most reliable method of treatment is liquid nitrogen cryotherapy. Usually the result is cosmetically excellent. The blood-filled lesion is compressed during freezing by using a closed probe. Photo © R. Suhonen.

7.24 Benign lesions of the tongue

Tuula Salo, Maria Siponen

Geographic tongue (benign migratory glossitis)

- Unknown aetiology. Might be associated with stress, fungal infection, atopy (HLA B15ag), asthma, psoriasis or Reiter's syndrome.
- Prevalence is about 2–3% of population.
- Irregular, red lesions on the surface of the tongue surrounded by a pale yellow marginal zone (desquamated filiform papillae within the lesions with normal papillary structure in the surrounding tissue; Figure 7.24). The lesions change shape, sometimes from day to day.
- Often associated with furrowed tongue.
- Lesions on other sites within the oral cavity are called erythema migrans.
- The condition is usually asymptomatic but a burning sensation may occur particularly on contact with irritant substances (citrus fruit, spices, alcohol, tobacco). Secondary yeast infection may also cause a burning sensation.
- Treatment
    - Reassure the patient about the benign nature of the lesions, and encourage avoidance of irritant substances. Symptomatic lesions may be treated with corticosteroid/antifungal ointment or with 7% salicylic acid solution in 70% ethanol which is painted on for 3 seconds twice daily for up to 4 days.

Hairy tongue

- Caused by hypertrophy and defective desquamation of the filiform papillae of the tongue.

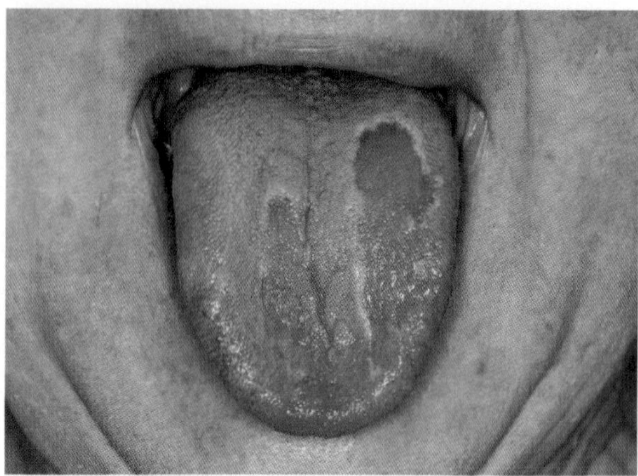

Figure 7.24 Lingua geographica, geographic tongue, is a benign condition of unknown origin. Its course is variable. There is no need to treat it - also because there is no effective therapy. This is one of the most common non-diseases, "treated" with oral antifungal agents. Photo © R. Suhonen.

- Usually idiopathic, but may be provoked by antibiotics, systemic corticosteroids, smoking, poor oral hygiene, chlorhexidine-hydrogen peroxide mouthwashes, radiotherapy.
- The surface of the tongue is covered by white, pale brown or dark brown "hair".
- Usually asymptomatic, but secondary fungal infection may cause a burning sensation. Associated halitosis may be present.
- Might disappear spontaneously.
- Treatment:
    - avoidance of predisposing factors, good oral hygiene, cleaning the tongue with a brush or special cleaning tool (available from a chemist). If necessary, topical antifungal medication.

Furrowed tongue (fissured tongue, scrotal tongue)

- In about 1% of the newborn, mucosal furrows divide the surface of the tongue into several sections making the tongue appear redder than normal. The finding becomes more common with age (up to 7% of population).
- Furrowed tongue is a familial condition, and may sometimes be associated with Down's syndrome or Melkersson-Rosenthal syndrome. About 20% of patients with geographic tongue also have furrowed tongue.
- Due to the furrowing the tongue may become infected and symptomatic. Treatment consists of brushing the tongue with a soft toothbrush or cleaning it with a special cleaning tool.

Median rhomboid glossitis

- Prevalence about 0.01–1% in adult population, not usually seen in children.

- A red, usually smooth-surfaced, lesion on the midline of the dorsum of the tongue anterior to the vallate papillae, with rhomboid or oval shape.
- Chronic candida infection is considered currently as the most likely aetiological factor.
- Usually asymptomatic. If associated with tenderness, treat with topical antifungal medication.
- Differential diagnosis: ectopic thyroid tissue, an ulcer attributable to tertiary syphilis or tuberculosis or deep fungal infection. Oral cancer is rarely seen in the midline of the dorsum of the tongue.

Lingual varices

- Varicosities on the ventral surface of the tongue
- Common in the elderly (prevalence over 50%)

7.25 Cancer and oral health

Editors

Effect of antineoplastic drugs on oral health

- Because the turnover rate of the oral epithelium is rapid, antineoplastic drugs may be often associated with transient oral complications such as
  - stomatitis
  - ulcerations
  - gingivitis
  - transient xerostomia.
- The ulcerations may become secondarily infected (for example by Candida albicans or Herpes simplex).
- Sometimes patients with leukaemia may also have pain in healthy teeth.
- Antineoplastic drugs may have permanent effects on teeth such as
  - increased caries
  - mild developmental defects of teeth in children.

Effect of irradiation therapy on oral health

- Irradiation of dental arches and/or teeth may disturb developing teeth and cause temporomandibular joint (TMJ) disorders.
- In adults, radiation therapy of the jaws and/or salivary glands reduces salivary flow. Hyposalivation or xerostomia may cause
  - caries
  - gingivitis
  - difficulties in wearing dentures.

Dental treatment of cancer patients

- Dental examination should be carried out as soon as possible after cancer diagnosis. Teeth with a focus require urgent treatment if the patient is scheduled to receive irradiation therapy to the dental arches and/or salivary glands. These patients are at risk of tooth loss for the rest of their lives because of osteoradionecrosis. The treatment plan should be made in a hospital dental clinic.
- Ordinary dental treatment can be performed at any dental clinic or private practice.
- Regular appointments at an interval of 3–6 months and fluoride prophylaxis are very important for cancer patients. Children with cancer can use fluoride tablets normally.
- During the cancer therapy it is important to avoid plaque accumulation. If a child has fixed orthodontic appliances, these must be removed before cancer therapy. Orthodontic therapy may sometimes be restarted when the patient is in remission and cancer therapy is less intensive. In patients requiring prosthetic therapy, the therapy can be planned only after remission is achieved.
- In case of periodontitis, root canal therapy, extractions, and operations in the mouth, prophylactic antibiotic therapy is often recommended. Blood count must also be checked if the dental procedures involve connection to circulation. Pulpotomies and root canal treatments are not recommended in primary teeth, because of poor prognosis. It is safer to extract these teeth. Cooperation between the dental surgeon and the physician is very important.
- Transient acute complications in the mouth can be treated for example by using mucosal anaesthetics during food intake. In cases of decreased salivary flow, artificial saliva, xylitol chewing gum, gel or lozenges can be used (7.10).

7.26 Cleft palate

Reijo Ranta

Aims

- To provide counsel and support to children with oral clefts and to their parents when they visit their primary care physician or a child health clinic.
- To pay special attention to recognition and treatment of glue ear which is a common condition in these children.

Prevalence

- Cleft lip or palate is one of the most common congenital malformations.
- The prevalence is approximately 1/500–700.

Clinical picture of cleft lip and/or palate

- There are two main groups of clefts:
  - **Cleft lip, gingiva and palate** may be unilateral or bilateral, and it may involve only the lip or both the lip and the alveolar ridge, or it may extend from the lip and gingiva to the pharynx.
  - **Cleft palate** is in the midline and limited either to the soft palate or both the soft and hard palates. Sometimes cleft palate involves only muscles and some bone, leaving the mucosa intact. Such submucous clefts often become apparent only later when the child's speech is characterized by open rhinolalia.
- 15–20% of patients with oral clefts have other associated malformations. Often there is an extensive array of malformations of various origins, of which the oral cleft is only one. Congenital oral clefts are usually not associated with mental retardation.

Aetiology

- **Genetic factors** play a part in the aetiology of oral clefts. About 25% of children with oral clefts are born into families with one or more previous cases of oral clefts.
- During the **foetal period**, extrinsic adverse influences in the first trimester of pregnancy clearly promote the development of oral clefts.

Organization of treatment

- The treatment of all patients with cleft lip and/or palate is concentrated in the cleft centres. The treatment uses a team approach, the core specialities being reconstructive surgery, dentistry and speech therapy. Other specialities are also involved.
- An oral cleft is usually diagnosed at the maternity hospital.
- Current methods allow the clefts, speech, teeth and occlusion of all patients to be rendered close to normal. The prerequisites for successful management are co-operation of the entire team and correct timing of the interventions by the various specialities. For a favourable outcome, the patient should also have regular check-ups from infancy until early adulthood.

Surgical treatment

- Primary corrective surgery of the cleft lip is usually undertaken at the age of 3 months and cleft palate at the age of 9 months.
- To improve the child's speech, corrective surgery is usually undertaken around the age of three to six years.
- Any remaining opening in the palate and bone defects of the alveolar ridge are corrected around the age of eight to ten years.
- Cosmetic surgery on the nose and lip takes place at the age of 15–16 years.

Orthodontics

- Children with oral clefts have several abnormalities in the size, shape and number of teeth. Development of the upper jaw is often incomplete. The ensuing defects in tooth position and occlusion are managed with orthodontic devices between the ages of eight and fourteen years according to individual requirements.
- Gross developmental anomalies of the jaws require surgical correction of their occlusal relationship. These operations are undertaken between the ages of 16 and 20 years.
- Many patients with a cleft lip, gingiva and/or palate need dental prosthetic treatment because of congenitally missing teeth.

Speech therapy

- All children with cleft palate should be seen by a phoniatrician, reconstructive surgeon, dentist and otologist around the age of three to eight years and later on according to individual requirement.
- On the basis of examinations at the age of three years, the child may be referred for speech monitoring or speech therapy.

Hearing

- Without palatal surgery, the palatal muscles inserting in the vicinity of the eustachian tube cannot function normally, and the middle ear tends to develop a negative pressure and accumulate viscous glue-like secretion, which causes auditory impairment. Nevertheless, normal hearing can be restored by tympanostomy tube placement. These ventilation tubes are inserted in conjunction with the first operation around the age of nine months.
- The child with an oral cleft may experience frequent ear inflammations while the palate is still patent, as food has free access to the eustachian tube orifice. With closure of the palatal cleft, these problems usually subside after a while. If otites start to occur before the age of six months, prophylactic antibiotic therapy may be considered.

7.30 Developmental defects in teeth

Irma Thesleff

Basic rules

- The first teeth usually erupt at the age of six months. If no teeth have erupted by the age of 1.5 years, further examination is warranted.

- Complete loss of teeth (anodontia) (extremely rare) is usually associated with some syndrome and requires paediatric consultations.
- Many teeth are usually missing in ectodermal dysplasia syndromes. The most common of these, hypohidrotic ectodermal dysplasia (HED) may be diagnosed early when only few (conically) peg shaped teeth erupt (this is important since the hyperthermia caused by lacking sweat glands may be fatal).
- Severe familial tooth agenesis may be associated with colorectal cancer when the gene AXIN2 is mutated. Therefore, genetic consultation is indicated in patients with many missing teeth who have colorectal cancer in the family.
- Of the minor dental defects the following require attention:
    - a supernumerary tooth, especially in the midline of the maxilla
    - aesthetically disturbing enamel defects
    - missing teeth.
- Tetracyclines may cause discolouration and other permanent defects in the developing teeth. They should be used neither by mothers during the latter half of pregnancy nor by children during the first seven years of life. If there is no special indication for the use of tetracyclines, they should be avoided throughout pregnancy and in children until puberty. (Tetracyclines are hardly ever used in Europe today).
- APECED (autoimmune polyendocrinopathy-candidiasis-ectodermal dystrophy) syndrome (24.63) and coeliac disease (8.84) may be diagnosed early by identification of enamel hypoplasias in children.

Tooth development

- The part of the tooth that is visible in the oral cavity, the tooth crown, is completely developed inside the jaw-bone.
- The development of most teeth starts prenatally.
- The development of the roots of teeth is completed after eruption of the teeth into the oral cavity.
- The calcification of permanent teeth starts several years before their eruption, and their development can be followed by radiographs.

Missing and supernumerary teeth

- The number, size and shape of teeth are almost completely genetically regulated.
- The lack of a single tooth is common. One or more wisdom teeth are missing in 25% and other teeth in 5–10% of the population.
- Small or (conically) peg shaped teeth are typically seen in association with missing teeth.
- The lack of several teeth or complete lack of teeth is usually associated with some syndrome. These are often conditions where also hair and other ectodermal organs are affected. The most common of these is ectodermal dysplasia (HED). The remaining teeth may be smaller than normal and have an abnormal conical shape. Female carriers of the gene mutation in X-linked HED have usually some missing and conical teeth. Missing teeth are also seen, for example, in Down's syndrome.
- Severe familial tooth agenesis may be associated with colorectal cancer when the gene AXIN2 is mutated. The lack of teeth may be an indication of predisposition of cancer in these patients and their relatives and therefore genetic consultation is indicated in patients with many missing teeth who have colorectal cancer in the family.
- Supernumerary teeth are seen in less than 4% of individuals.
- Mild abnormalities in tooth shape are common. Extra cusps on the occlusal surfaces of teeth represent these abnormalities.
- Sometimes the crowns or roots of neighbouring teeth fuse during development.
- Missing or abnormally shaped anterior teeth in the upper jaw may be associated with cleft lip and palate.

Enamel hypoplasia

- Defects in the mineralization of tooth crowns, enamel hypoplasias, are relatively common. They are seen as structural changes of the tooth surface. Structural changes often cause secondary discoloration.
- Enamel hypoplasias are usually caused by environmental factors (e.g. infections) that disturb the functions of enamel-producing cells.
- Exposure to high concentrations of fluoride causes hypomineralization, but this is rare in countries where the groundwater does not contain much fluoride. Fluoride deficiency is not visible in the structure of teeth, however, the enamel is more susceptible to caries.
- Genetic conditions affecting the structure of the enamel or the dentin are rare. They always affect both the deciduous teeth and the permanent teeth.

Developmental defects requiring treatment

- Most developmental defects in teeth do not need treatment.
- **A supernumerary tooth,** particularly in the midline of the maxilla, may prevent the eruption of other teeth. It should therefore be extracted.
- **Missing teeth** should ideally be diagnosed early (8–10 years of age) when growth-adapted measures can be used to minimize the need for treatment.
- **Missing teeth** can usually be corrected by moving teeth orthodontically or surgically or by prosthetic treatment including implants (usually placed when growth is completed.)
- Aesthetically disturbing **enamel defects** can be corrected by modern composite materials making them almost invisible.

7.31 Dental caries and other diseases of the hard tissues of the teeth and dental pulp

Markku Larmas

Dental caries

- Caries is a disease of the hard dental tissues. It has a high prevalence; it concerns almost everyone in industrialized countries.
- The first stage of carious attack is the formation of dental plaque on certain surfaces of the tooth. The micro-organisms of normal oral microbial flora accumulate on the pellicle (formed from saliva) on tooth surfaces, and the formation of dental plaque starts.
- The first locations of carious attack are the occlusal fissures and fossae of molar teeth, then the interproximal surfaces of the teeth and finally the gingival margin area. Normally the development of caries in the gingival margin area requires the occurrence of dental plaque on that site for years. In persons with reduced salivary flow, the incidence of caries in the gingival margin area and even in the gingival sulcal area is very high.
- The first sign of carious attack on the enamel surface is the disappearance of the shine of the tooth. The active form of dental caries is seen as whitening and softening of the enamel surface. When the carious attack is slow or even if progression stops, the carious area turns grey, brownish or even black and the lesion is leatherly.

Diseases of dental pulp and periapical tissues

Pulpitis and its complications

- Pulpitis is the inflammation of dental pulp due to the invasion of microbial toxins, normally through the carious lesion, into the pulp.
- When the microbes invade the pulpal cavity, it results in necrosis of the pulpal tissue.
- When the microbes invade deeper into the dental pulp, the tissue remnants of the necrotic pulp induce an inflammatory reaction in the periodontium and bone around the tooth root apex, resulting in an acute apical periodontitis of pulpal origin. This disease may lead to chronic apical periodontitis and further to a periapical abcess with a sinus if the disease is left untreated.
- The treatment of all these diseases is endodontal removal of the necrotic pulp tissue and infected dentin around the pulp cavum and replacement by a root filling material. In some cases removal of the necrotic pulp material requires extraction of the whole tooth.

Abnormal wearing of teeth

Excessive attrition of teeth

- Wearing of the tooth material due to grinding of the teeth against each other.
- Seen on occlusal surfaces as well as on interproximal surfaces of teeth.
- It also results in so-called mesial wandering of teeth, which means that all the teeth move in a mesial direction during the lifetime of the subject.
- It is classified as a disease only in excessive cases when the wearing exceeds the so-called physiological attrition.
- The reason for pathological attrition might be an imbalanced occlusion of the dentition, teeth grinding, especially during night-time (bruxism) and dentofacial anomalies.
- Attrition has special diagnostic significance when the wearing is particularly concentrated on the occlusal surfaces of molar teeth. This type of wearing is typical in users of ecstasy.

Abrasion of teeth

- Wearing of the tooth caused by an external material.
- The reasons might be, for example, dentifrice, tooth brushes, or too aggressive tooth brushing in general.
- Even tooth-restoration materials might be a reason for tooth abrasion.

Erosion of teeth

- Erosion means the chemical dissolution of tooth material by acids that are not produced by the dental plaque micro-organisms.
- The first sign of erosion is the disappearance of the shine on the tooth surface. Thereafter the process leads to the disappearance of enamel minerals.
- Erosion normally starts on the lingual side of the upper incisors, resulting in very thin enamel on the incisal edge that leads to enamel fractures. This results in a rugged incisor edge and shortening of the crowns.
- Reasons
  - External causes are drinking acidic sport drinks, soft drinks and sometimes a vegetarian diet.
  - The most important internal reason is heartburn or gastro-oesophagial reflux (GER) resulting in gastric acid reflux into the oral cavity.
  - Erosion of teeth has significance in the diagnosis of persistent regurgitation in cases of bulimia and anorexia nervosa, because these patients are often reluctant to reveal vomiting.
- When salivary secretion is normal (or there is hyperfunction of the salivary glands) even persistent vomiting or gastro-oesophageal reflux does not lead to dental erosion.
- Treatment
  - A dentist replaces the eroded tooth material with a restoration material. If the erosion is extensive, the teeth may have to be crowned.

7.32 Periodontal diseases (gingival inflammation and dental calculus)

Jukka Ainamo

Incipient gingival inflammation and its treatment

- Inflammation of the marginal gingiva is called gingivitis. Oral microbes have a tendency to attach to originally clean tooth surfaces where they gradually colonize and develop into increasingly thick layers of plaque bacteria. If bacterial deposits are not regularly removed from the surfaces of the teeth, gingival inflammation may develop. Hormonal and drug-induced risk factors can aggravate previously existing gingivitis.
- The typical sign of gingival inflammation is bleeding from the gums, for example when brushing the teeth. At an early stage it may be possible to stop the bleeding (reverse the gingivitis) by careful daily cleaning of the teeth with a soft toothbrush and, if necessary, by using soft triangular toothpicks and/or dental floss for cleaning between the teeth.
- If the patient is unable to maintain adequate oral hygiene, mouthwashes containing chlorhexidine can be used to prevent plaque formation and gingivitis. Of the local antiseptic products available, 0.1% aqueous chlorhexidine solution gives excellent results. On the other hand, side effects associated with chlorhexidine rinses can reduce patient compliance due to disagreeable staining and discolouration of the teeth and white fillings. This staining can be removed with dental instruments. Optimal treatment of gingivitis therefore includes both mechanical and chemical approaches.

Chronic inflammation

- Bacterial deposits may also grow into the space of the gingival pocket, between the hard surface of the tooth and the soft tissue of the gingiva. This results in widening of the inflammated area. As plaque growth proceeds deeper into the gingival pockets, the bacterial flora will consist of increasing amounts of Gram-negative anaerobic microbes. With time, the chronic gingival inflammation may advance to a stage where the connective tissue, attaching the tooth to the jaw bone, starts to break down. Breakdown of tooth attachment is irreversible.

Dental calculus

- The bacterial deposits on the tooth surfaces often show a tendency to mineralize gradually. This change results in the formation of so called dental calculus, the surface of which is covered with living bacteria. The mechanical removal of dental calculus by a dentist or a dental hygienist, together with careful daily cleaning of all tooth surfaces, are the means by which the chronic inflammation can be cured.

7.33 Dental traumas

Kyösti Oikarinen

General principles in cases of avulsed teeth

- An avulsed permanent tooth should be replanted if the tooth is intact and alveolar socket is uninjured. Even if replantation later fails, it improves the outcome of a later final replacement and, in case of children, postpones the procedure until the child or teenager has stopped growing.
- Avulsed primary teeth should never be replanted.

First aid for an avulsed tooth

- The patient is advised to preserve the tooth in, for example, milk or in the mouth during transportation to a dentist.
- In the dental chair the tooth is polished gently with saline and gauze.
- The root surface must not be damaged mechanically during the cleaning procedure.
- Replantation can sometimes be performed without local anaesthesia in a normal doctor's office. The alveolar socket can be cleaned of dirt and blood clot by rinsing with physiological saline before the tooth is pressed gently in place.
- The positions of the neighbouring teeth help to align the tooth correctly. After replantation the tooth should be fixed to the neighbouring teeth by a dentist. According to current understanding, one-week fixation may be sufficient. The fixation device must be vertically flexible.
- Systemic antibiotics decrease the risk of late inflammatory complications.
- A tetanus booster is needed.

Crown fractures and injuries to primary teeth

- Exposed dentin surfaces in crown fractures can be covered with an isolating varnish as first aid. This can be done out of the dental chair.
- All crown fractures can be treated with conventional fillings or artificial crowns.
- Sharp edges on the crowns of fractured primary teeth can be rounded, but luxated primary teeth should be extracted in order to avoid damage to the growing permanent tooth underneath.

- Intrusively luxated primary teeth should be left and followed-up to observe whether they erupt spontaneously or need to be extracted.

Root fractures

- The diagnosis is made by dental radiography.
- Depending on the location of the fracture line root fractures may go unnoticed and heal spontaneously or they may require long-term (up to 3 months) fixation, or result in the loss of the tooth.

Luxations

- Do not attempt to reposition luxated teeth in the doctor's office as they require local anaesthesia and immediate fixation.
- During transportation to the dentist the patient can bite a gauze dressing that stabilized the luxated teeth and reduces bleeding.
- Mild forms of luxation include concussion and subluxation, in which the tooth is loose, but not dislocated. The dislocation may be palatinal, buccal, extrusive or intrusive, or the tooth may be totally avulsed.
- Usually more than one tooth is injured even if clinical signs of injury are visible in only one tooth. Late complications reveal damage to neighbouring teeth.
- Fracture of the alveolar process is diagnosed by the observation that moving the displaced tooth causes the neighbouring teeth to move.

7.34 First aid for severe dental pain

Kyösti Oikarinen

General principles

- A GP can give first aid independent of the cause of the dental pain. Treatment possibilities include systemic analgesics and antibiotics, local treatment or a combination of these.
- A GP can treat pain and inflammation after extraction or operation when dental consultation is not possible. All other cases should be referred to a dentist as soon as possible.

Dental pain

- Pain is provoked by a current of air or by thermat (cold) or physical (sweet) irritation.
- Caries is the most typical cause of dental pain. The second most common cause is exposure of dentinal tubules in the root surface due to apical recession of the gingiva caused, for example, by heavy tooth brushing.
- After filling the tooth can be painful, with the pain resembling that caused by caries or exposure of dentinal tubules.

Treatment

- Patient counselling. Tooth pastes that relieve the symptoms after exposure of dentinal tubules and that can be applied to sensitive root surfaces are available in pharmacies.
- A dentist can varnish exposed dentinal tubules with fluoride or calcium hydroxide paste.
- The treatment of carious or advanced abrasions in the root are treated with conventional fillings.
- The pain after filling a tooth subsides in a few days. During that time the tooth is sensitive, and the patient should avoid cold and sweet food and drinks.

Pulpitis

- Pulpitis is mostly caused by caries that has advanced to the dental pulp but can also be caused by, for example, dental trauma.
- Pulpitis causes acute, severe and pulsating dental pain that is provoked by hot and relieved by cold irritation. Initially the pain localizes to one tooth, but may later become more diffuse.

Treatment

- Non-steroidal analgesics are often ineffective. Centrally acting analgesics are usually the drugs of choice. Sometimes a combination of peripherally and centrally acting analgesics is most effective.
- Local anaesthesia relieves the pain immediately.
- Infiltrative local anaesthesia is possible in all upper teeth and anterior lower jaw. **Technique**: 1 ml of anaesthetic solution (e.g. Ultracain-Suprarenin® 5 µg/ml) is injected submucosally on the bone and periosteum. Lower jaw molar teeth require block anaesthesia, which is usually given by a dentist. The anaesthetics used by dentists include prilocaine + felypressin or articaine + adrenaline 5 µg/l.
- Pulpectomy and root canal treatment are performed by a dentist. The first aid treatment in the dental chair is opening of the pulpal cavum through the crown. Sometimes grinding of the occlusal contact relieves the symptoms.

Periostitis

- Caused by an untreated pulpitis that develops into perapical osteitis. Pus moves into the buccal soft tissues through the periosteum. This causes palpable and tender swelling in the vestibulum, sometimes also seen extraorally.
- Severe pain is caused by distraction of the periosteum.

Treatment

- Incision and drainage of the abscess, usually in the sulcus, can be performed with a sharp knife.
- Systemic antibiotics, primarily penicillin (erythromycin in case of penicillin allergy)
- A widespread dental abscess often needs hospitalization, especially if the patient has systemic symptoms (weakness, fever, difficulties in swallowing etc.).

Pericoronitis

- Pericoronitis is caused by bacterial inflammation in the soft tissue around the crown of an unerupted tooth, usually the lower third molar.
- The symptoms are fever, swelling, pain, odour and limitation of mouth opening.

Treatment

- Systemic antibiotics, primarily penicillin. Erythromycin in case of penicillin allergy.
- Extraction of the upper third molar if it is the cause of mechanical irritation
- The lower pericoronitic third molar should be extracted after the symptoms/infection have subsided if it causes pain or recurring infections.
- Extraction of the tooth involved is performed after acute infection has been cured.

Bruxism/grinding of the teeth

- Bruxism can cause dental pain resembling that caused by pulpitis.
- The symptoms can involve one or several teeth simultaneously and are a result from unusually strong masticatory stress.

Treatment

- An occlusal splint made by a dentists is worn at nights on the teeth to prevent unphysiological night-time grinding of the teeth
- Occlusal adjustment by selective grinding of the teeth performed by a dentist.

Severe pain after tooth extraction, dry socket

- Pain is most common after extraction of lower molar teeth, especially wisdom teeth and results from a disturbance in the clotting of the extraction socket.
- This dry alveolitis is characterized by pain that intensifies markedly on the third or fourth postextraction day and by lack of response to peripherally acting analgesics.

Treatment

- Tamponation with a solution containing anaesthetics and analgesics, for example Chlumsky ointment that contains camphor, phenol and ethanol.
- The tampon is changed daily because the drugs have a short duration of action.
- A systemic antibiotic is needed only if the patient has general symptoms.
- Normal postextraction pain can usually be managed with peripherally acting anti-inflammatory drugs. Centrally acting analgesics can be used when necessary either alone or combined with peripherally acting drugs.

7.36 Emergency treatment of a gingival abscess

Jukka Ainamo

- Abscesses may occur either on the buccal or lingual side of the row of teeth. An abscess in the gingival region can be caused by:
  - an acute inflammation in the dental pulp (see pulpitis and its complications 7.34).
  - an inflammation in a deep periodontal pocket.
- A general practitioner may initiate antibiotic therapy.
- A dentist should then scrape the infected tissue and bacterial plaque away.

Periodontal inflammation: periodontitis

- In periodontitis bacterial deposits grow down along the root surface and at the same time destroy the root attachment permanently. Abscesses can develop in the periodontal pocket and may subsequently empty spontaneously through fistulae.
- When a chronic deep gingival pocket (abscess) turns into an acute state, antibiotics can be used in order to alleviate the condition. Abscesses from deep gingival pockets seem to respond particularly well to orally administered metronidazole (400 mg twice a day). The antibiotic does not, however, eliminate permanently the cause of the inflammation, the hard and soft bacterial deposits. The anaerobic bacterial flora can re-establish itself on the root surface of the deep pocket.
- When the acute inflammation has subsided, a dentist performs thorough curettage and root planing, preferably under local anaesthesia. The root surface must be rendered totally clean with regard to both dental calculus and soft bacterial coverings. Finally, the patient should take particularly good care of his or her oral hygiene in order to avoid relapse.

Gastroenterology

Evidence Based Medicine Guidelines. Edited by the Duodecim Editorial Team
 ISBN: 0-470-01184-X

8.1 Involuntary weight loss

Rauli Leino

Basic rules

- Investigate a patient with significant involuntary weight loss (at least 5% of body weight = 3.5 kg in a 70-kg patient in 6 months) and follow-up the patient if the initial investigations do not resolve the cause.
- Identify diabetes or hyperthyroidism at the first consultation on the basis of symptoms and laboratory test results.
- Identify peptic ulcer and coeliac disease.
- Identify anorexia nervosa as the cause of weight loss in a young woman.
- Perform adequate investigations to detect lung or gastrointestinal cancer in elderly patients, and haematological malignancy in patients of all ages.
- Examine dentures and assess the ability to eat in an old patient before more invasive tests.
- Recognize depression as a cause of weight loss.

Diagnostic clues

- See Table 8.1.

The most common causes of involuntary weight loss

- Cancer (pancreas, liver, lungs, ovary, prostate, lymphoma, leukaemia)
- Gastrointestinal disease (other than cancer)
- Psychiatric disease (anorexia nervosa, depression)
- Moderate or severe dementia
- Heart failure (after general oedema has been treated)
- Pulmonary causes (other than cancer)
- Dietary causes (including alcohol)
- Endocrine diseases
- The cause is not found in 25% of the patients.

Table 8.1 Diagnostic clues in the assessment of involuntary weight loss

Clinical picture	Disease
History	
Abdominal pain	Peptic ulcer, infection, tumour, coeliac disease
Vomiting	Peptic ulcer, obstruction
Dysphagia	Gastrointestinal malignancy or ulcer
Diarrhoea	Inflammatory bowel disease, coeliac disease
Constipation	Anorexia, tumour
Faecal colour	Black: melena; pale (and floating); malabsorption
Smoking	Lung cancer, peptic ulcer, COPD
Alcohol use	Cirrhosis of the liver
Fear of gaining weight, desire to be underweight, distorted body image, sports activities	Anorexia nervosa
Use of psychotropic drugs, death of a close relative, other personal loss, stress, psychosocial situation, financial problems, poor appetite	Depression
Problems with memory	Dementia
Cough, dyspnoea	Tumour, infections, heart failure
Fever, perspiration, fatigue	Infections, hyperthyroidism
Menses	If normal the weight loss is rarely significant
Bone pains	Metastases, myeloma
Haematuria	Tumour of the urinary tract
Physical signs	
Skin temperature and colour	
• Warm skin	Hyperthyroidism
• Pigmentation	Addison's disease
• Jaundice	Cancer of the pancreas, liver diseases
• Petechiae, ecchymoses	Thrombocytopenia, cirrhosis, cancer
• Carotenaemia	Anorexia
Dental prosthesis, toothlessness	Undernourishment
Palpation of the abdomen	Conditions causing hepatomegaly or abdominal masses
Palpation of lymph nodes	Lymphoma
Touch per rectum, type of faeces	Rectal tumour
Pelvic examination	Tumours

Investigation strategy

- In about 50% of the patients the main symptom suggests a specific disease.

1. Objective assessment of weight loss
    - Check earlier weight recordings in the patient's medical record, ask about clothes that have become too spacious, and about the observations of the next of kin.
    - In about 50% of the patients the weight loss cannot be verified.
2. A chest x-ray is the most useful examination. It should always be taken at the initial phase.
    - Lung cancer
    - Infections

- Enlarged lymph nodes (lymphoma, sarcoidosis)

3. Laboratory examinations
    - Blood count, ESR
    - Fasting blood glucose
    - Serum ALT, alkaline phosphatase
    - Serum sodium, potassium, calcium, albumin
    - HIV serology if there are risk factors
    - Serum TSH
    - Urine test and culture (haematuria in particular should be investigated thoroughly)
    - Faecal occult blood test.
4. The patient's history may suggest anorexia nervosa in an adolescent girl or young woman (34.10).
    - Further tests are not necessary.
5. The symptoms suggest a gastrointestinal aetiology or the above-mentioned investigations have not revealed the cause of weight loss.
    - Perform upper gastrointestinal examination (gastroscopy) first, and then lower gastrointestinal investigations (colo-noscopy or sigmoidoscopy together with colongraphy) unless lower gastrointestinal symptoms indicate the opposite order.
    - If endoscopies have not revealed the cause, consider the imaging examinations of the abdomen.
    - In a very elderly patient in poor general condition consider the potential benefit of the investigations (i.e. of diagnosing cancer) in the selection of treatment and whether the treatment helps the patient.
6. The history and above-mentioned investigations do not reveal the cause of weight loss.
    - If a specific cause is to be found it is usually by combining the information from the history, clinical examination, laboratory and imaging examinations, and endoscopy.
    - If the initial investigations do not reveal the cause, a follow-up of 1–2 months is a better option than ordering more non-targeted investigations.

Indications for specialist consultation

- If anorexia nervosa is suspected and the general condition is good, refer the patient to an outpatient clinic of adolescence psychiatry.
- Refer the patient for gastrointestinal endoscopy and imaging if they cannot be performed locally.
- The patient has symptoms or signs suggesting an organic disease that has not been diagnosed by initial examinations in primary care.
- A depressive patient should be referred according to local conventions.

8.2 Nausea and vomiting

Editors

Basic rules

- Identify conditions needing urgent treatment: myocardial infarction, hypoglycaemia, pancreatitis, intestinal obstruction, appendicitis, meningitis and other bacterial infections, acute glaucoma, acute cerebrovascular disorders, and intoxications.
- In cases of prolonged or paroxysmal nausea obtain a careful history and perform the clinical examination and initial investigations in outpatient care.

Diagnostic approach in nausea and vomiting

Duration and severity of the symptoms

- Do you have only the feeling of nausea or do you actually vomit?
- Are the symptoms associated with meals?
- Content of the vomit
- Preceding illnesses, use of medication and alcohol
- Pregnancy?
- Nausea and vomiting of acute onset is typical of gastroenteritis, labyrinthic vertigo and somatic causes that should be readily identified.
- Prolonged symptoms often suggest a metabolic cause, a chronic disease or psychogenic origin.
- In children and in the elderly nausea and vomiting may be the presenting symptom of many bacterial infections (otitis media, pneumonia, urinary tract infection).

Essentials of the clinical examination

- Fever, systemic symptoms, dehydration, involuntary weight loss, jaundice
- Palpation of the abdomen: tenderness, palpable masses
- Auscultation of the abdomen: high-pitched bowel sounds (obstruction)
- Size of the liver
- Auscultation of the heart and the lungs
- Neurological examination (meningism, nystagmus, optic fundi, unilateral symptoms)

Diagnostic clues

- See Table 8.2.

Table 8.2 Nausea and vomiting–diagnostic clues

Symptom or sign	Most probable diagnoses	Consider in differential diagnosis
Headache	Migraine	Cerebrovascular disorders, meningitis, encephalitis
Rotatory vertigo	Vestibular neuronitis, Ménière's disease	TIA/intracerebral bleeding
Fever	(Severe) infection	Meningitis
Diarrhoea	Gastroenteritis	
Abdominal pain	Peptic ulcer Gastritis	Pancreatitis Myocardial infarction
Chest pain	Myocardial infarction	Oesophagitis
Neurological symptoms or signs	Cerebrovascular disorder	
Large dose of digoxin Recent onset of new medication	Nausea and vomiting caused by a drug	

Clues from the history suggesting the aetiology

- Sudden vomiting without preceding nausea is typical of increased intracranial pressure.
- Dehydration and weight loss suggest an organic disease.
- Morning nausea and vomiting are typical of early pregnancy, alcoholic gastritis, biliary reflux gastritis following ventricle resection, and uraemia.
- Vomiting after a meal suggests pyloric obstruction (gastric or duodenal ulcer, carcinoma).
- Voluminous, bile-stained vomiting suggests proximal intestinal obstruction.
- Haematemesis suggests bleeding ulcer, acute gastric mucosal damage, Mallory-Weiss ulceration, or oesophageal varices.
- Faecal vomitus is caused by distal intestinal obstruction.
- History of travelling is a clue to eventual infectious aetiology. The symptoms of acute hepatitis include food aversion and nausea. Nausea and vomiting may be the cardinal symptoms of giardiasis.
- Lactose intolerance may present as nausea and vomiting without intestinal symptoms particularly in young persons.
- The patient's medication may be cause (digoxin in toxic concentrations, nitrofurantoin, sulphasalazine, imidazoles, erythromycin, tetracycline, metformin).
- If the general condition remains unaffected the symptoms may be of psychogenic origin.

Investigations

- Consider first whether hospitalization is indicated (8.9).
- If the patient is not referred to hospital the following tests are indicated according to the history and clinical signs:
  - CRP, blood glucose, urine amylase (dipstick test), ECG, and urine test, particularly in the elderly
- In prolonged symptoms (in addition to the former)
  - Blood count, serum creatinine, potassium, sodium, ALT, alkaline phosphatase, ESR, serum digoxin

Further investigations

- Plain radiograph of the abdomen if intestinal obstruction is suspected (vomiting, pain, bowel sounds)

Prolonged symptoms

- Gastroscopy
- Abdominal ultrasonography
- Neurological examination
- Psychiatric assessment (eating disorders)

Drug therapy of nausea and vomiting

Migraine, labyrinthic, intestinal, or cerebrovascular vomiting

- Metoclopramide
  - Dosage
    - P.o. 10–20 mg × 3
    - As a suppository 20 mg × 1–3
    - I.m. or i.v. 10–20 mg × 1–3
  - Extrapyramidal symptoms may occur as adverse effects.
- Prochlorperazine (especially vestibular nausea and vertigo)
  - Dosage
    - P.o. 5–10 mg × 3, in migraine 25 mg × 1
    - As a suppository 5 mg × 1 or 25 mg × 1
    - I.m. 12.5–25 mg
  - The adverse effects include extrapyramidal symptoms that can be treated with biperiden 2.5–5 (–10) mg i.m. or slowly i.v. In mild cases also perorally 2 mg 1/2–1 tablets 1–4 times daily, maximum 9 tablets/day.

Vomiting caused by chemotherapeutic drugs

- See 16.2.

Motion sickness

- See 8.3.
- Scopolamin
  - 1 depot patch 5–6 hours before the start of the journey. The effect lasts 72 hours.
- Antihistamines
  - Cyclizine 50 mg tablets

Hyperemesis gravidarum

- Rest is the most important treatment
- Meclozine
  - 25 mg × 2 p.o.
  - Suppository 50 mg

Vomiting and pain associated with colic (biliary or ureteral)

- Analgesics i.v., i.m., suppositories, or p.o.
  - Indometacin 50 mg slowly i.v.
  - Diclofenac 75 mg during 15 min–2 hours i.v.
  - Several anti-inflammatory drugs are available as suppositories

Vomiting associated with increased intracranial pressure

- Dexamethason
  - p.o. 0.5–3 mg × 3

Nausea and vomiting associated with opioid medication

- Haloperidol
  - Initially 0.5 mg × 2 or 2 mg in the evening. Metoclopramide can be added if necessary (B) [1 2].
  - Substituting morphine by oxycodone may help.

References

1. Hirayama T, Ishii F, Yago K, Ogata H. Evaluation of the effective drugs for the prevention of nausea and vomiting induced by morphine used for postoperative pain: a quantitative systematic review. Yakugaku Zasshi. Journal of the Pharmaceutical Society of Japan 2001, 121(2), 179–185.
2. The Database of Abstracts of Reviews of Effectiveness (University of York), Database no.: DARE-20013485. In: The Cochrane Library, Issue 3, 2002. Oxford: Update Software.

8.3 Motion sickness

Hannu Laaksonen

Basic rules

- Mild symptoms need no other treatment than advice to the patient.
- Occasional symptoms and symptoms in children under 10 years of age can be treated with antihistamines (cyclizine).
- Severe symptoms and symptoms in persons above 10 years of age can be treated with a scopolamine patch.
- The medication is most efficient if started before the journey.

Pathogenesis and epidemiology

- Motion sickness is caused by motion, either of the body or just the visual field. Irritation of the semicircular canals is the pathogenetic mechanism.
- About a third of the population is susceptible to motion sickness. Children under 2 years are rarely affected, but children aged 2–12 years suffer from motion sickness most frequently. Women are more often affected than men, particularly during menses and pregnancy.

Symptoms

- Paleness and cool, sweating skin
- Yawning, increased salivation, sighing
- Nausea that is temporarily relieved by vomiting
- Increased respiratory frequency, belching, flatulence, and constipation or diarrhoea.
- Other variable symptoms include: headache, confusion, a cold feeling on face and limbs, agitation, loss of appetite, a feeling of weakness, a pressing sensation on the chest, feeling hot.

Prevention

- Avoidance of alcohol before and during travel. Alcohol is not a medication for motion sickness.
- Light meals and sufficient fluid intake during travel. On short trips the intake of food should be avoided.
- Staying in the middle section of vehicles such as boats, ships, or aeroplanes. In the car the best place is on the front seat with a view ahead. In a boat it is best to stay on deck with sight directed far to the horizon.
- Having the neck bent forwards is the worst posture. For example, children susceptible to motion sickness should not read while travelling in a car. Supporting the head on the head-support is recommended.
- Lying is the best position, preferably with the eyes closed.
- Strong odours may predispose to motion sickness. Fresh air and good ventilation should be ensured.
- Warm clothing may prevent motion sickness.
- Psychological factors may play a role. Do not intimidate persons with the risk of motion sickness. Passengers should have something to occupy themselves with rather than merely wait to become motion sick.

Drug treatment

1. **Scopolamine** as a depot patch is the most efficient drug.
   - Place the patch behind the ear on dry, clean, hairless skin 5–6 hours before travel.
   - The duration of action is 72 hours. If a shorter action is needed the patch can be removed earlier (even during the journey): the blood concentration of the drug decreases slowly as the drug absorbed by the skin is slowly released into the circulation.

- If a longer action is needed the patch is removed after 3 days, and a new patch placed behind the other ear.
- Wash hands after handling the patch because the drug may dilate the pupils if transferred to the eyes on the hands. The site where the patch was worn should also be washed thoroughly.
- Contraindications for use include glaucoma and hypersensitivity to scopolamine. Adverse effects are minimal if the drug is used properly: dryness of the mouth, somnolence, and impairment of near vision.
- Scopolamine is not recommended for children below 10 years of age or for pregnant women. Alcohol should not be used during treatment.

2. **Antihistamines** are the most commonly used drugs
   - **Cyclizine** probably causes the least drowsiness. The drug is also suitable for children.
   - Promethazine hydrochloride is the most effective but also causes the most drowsiness. The drug can be taken in the evening if motion sickness is associated with insomnia.
   - Meclozine can be used during pregnancy if treatment is really indicated. Suppositories are also available.
3. **Metoclopramide**, thiethylperazine, and prochlorperazine are as efficient as mild antihistamines and do not cause much fatigue. Most are available as suppositories, too. They can be recommended for occasional motion sickness for patients also using these drugs for other purposes.

Principles of drug treatment

- All drugs are most effective if taken before travel.
- Conditioning for motion occurs after 2–3 days at sea, and the need for drugs decreases.
- Tolerance for drugs often develops; avoid regular routine medication if there are no clear indications.
- For the vomiting patient suppositories are most efficient.
- The drowsiness due to medication may affect driving ability, although probably less than severe motion sickness itself.
- Alcohol and drugs acting on the CNS increase the drowsiness caused by drugs used for motion sickness.

8.4 Dysphagia

Jouko Isolauri

Basic rule

- Identify patients with dysphagia and refer them to appropriate investigations.

Definition

- Dysphagia can be defined as the feeling of food remaining in the oesophagus after swallowing.

Epidemiology

- Dysphagia is uncommon in comparison with other dyspeptic symptoms.
- The patients usually seek help after the symptoms have lasted for weeks or months, even years. Rapid exacerbation of the dysphagia prompts an earlier consultation.

The most common causes of dysphagia

Benign causes

- Oesophagitis
- Strictures caused by oesophageal reflux disease
- Oesophageal diverticula
- Congenital oesophageal rings
- Corrosion injuries of the oesophagus
- Motility disorders of the oesophagus (achalasia, diffuse spasm)
  - The most common cause for oesophageal dilatation is achlasia (impaired dilatation of the lower oesophageal sphincter, and motility disorder of the middle segment of the oesophagus).
- Systemic diseases imparing oesophageal motility (scleroderma)

Malignant causes

- Oesophageal carcinoma (incidence 40 cases/million/year)
- Carcinoma of the cardia (30 cases/million/year)
- Risk factors for esophageal squamous cell carcinoma include smoking and consumption of alcohol. Adenocarcinoma often affects patients with Barrett's esophagus.

Diagnostic approach

History

- Has the patient had oesophageal symptoms in the past?
- Is there a history of a corrosion injury (drugs or accidental ingestion of a corrosive chemical)?
- Are the symptoms increasing in severity?
- Does the patient have systemic symptoms?

Acute dysphagia

- Severe pain and shock may suggest **oesophageal perforation,** which is a life-threatening condition (mortality 20–50%).
- Dysphagia associated with symptoms of infection may be caused by **pharyngeal abscess** (38.20), pharyngitis, viral oesophagitis, or candida oesophagitis. Consider also

epiglottitis (31.16) if the patients has fever and poor general condition.

- If a **foreign body or piece of food** has been stuck in the oesophagus the cause for sticking should be determined.
- **Cerebrovascular disorders** may cause dysphagia, which is associated with other neurological symptoms, such as diplopia, salivation, and pareses.

Dysphagia that has lasted for weeks or months

- Dysphagia that develops slowly during weeks or months in an elderly patient suggests a **tumour**. In younger patients achalasia should be suspected. Weight loss is typical of both diseases.
- Short, severe pain associated with the passage of a piece of food suggests a developing **stricture** of the oesophagus (tumour or benign stricture).

Chronic dysphagia that has lasted for years

- Intermittent dysphagia lasting for more than a year suggests a **motility disorder** of the oesophagus.
- Intermittent symptoms that are not related to the consistence of the swallowed food may indicate a **psychogenic problem** (see also anorexia 34.10).

Investigations

- The basic investigations include clinical examination, local lymph nodes, palpation of the neck, chest x-ray ECG, blood count, and ESR.
- In the next phase **all patients should have gastroscopy** with biopsies for histological examination.
  - Usually the macroscopic findings already differentiate between a benign lesion (oesophagitis, stricture, diverticulum) and cancer. The findings are verified by histological examination.
  - Dilatation of the oesophagus suggests achalasia. Other motility disorders cannot be diagnosed reliably by gastroscopy.
- If the diagnosis is not evident after gastroscopy the investigations should proceed with double contrast examination or manometry of the oesophagus or both in order to detect a motility disorder, diffuse oesophageal spasm, achalasia, diverticula, or hiatus hernia.

Indications for radiological examination of the oesophagus and ventricle

- After oesophageal dilatation has been diagnosed, the degree of the dilatation can only be determined by radiological examination. In achalasia the degree of dilatation is a prognostic indicator of treatment outcome.
- Stricture caused by carcinoma that cannot be passed with gastroscopy. Tumours affecting a segment longer than 10 cm are usually inoperable.
- Radiological examination is more accurate than gastroscopy in the determination of the size and location of oesophageal diverticula before a planned operation.

Manometry

- Manometry is indicated in the diagnosis of motility disorders. Manometry should be performed if gastroscopy is normal in a patient with dysphagia.

24-hour monitoring of oesophageal pH

- If a patient has oesophageal stricture of unknown origin (negative history for reflux symptoms or corrosion injury) the contribution of reflux can be determined by pH monitoring after endoscopic dilatation of the stricture.

Treatment (stricture, carcinoma, motility disorders, diverticula)

Oesophageal stricture

- Endoscopic dilatation is the treatment of choice.
- If the stricture is caused by reflux disease the acid reflux is prevented pharmacologically or surgically.
- In most cases repeated dilatations are needed.

Carcinoma of the oesophagus

- The oesophagus is resected and substituted by the stomach, which is pulled to the chest cavity in case the tumour does not adhere to adjacent structures (trachea, aorta, mediastinum) and there are no metastases.
- In other cases the treatment is palliative and aims at keeping the oesophagus patent for eating. The palliative measures include laser vaporization, ethanol injections, intraoesophageal stents, and irradiation.

Disorders of oesophageal motility

- Endoscopic balloon dilatation of the lower oesophageal sphincter is the treatment of choice for achalasia.
- Heller myotomy of the distal muscular layer is indicated if dilatation does not alleviate the symptoms B [1 2].
- Diffuse oesophageal spasm is treated with calcium channel blockers that relax the muscular layer of the oesophagus.

Oesophageal diverticula

- If the diverticulum is symptomatic (the patient has dysphagia or regurgitation) surgical resection is indicated.

References

1. Spiess AE, Kahrilas PJ. Treating achlasia from whalebone to laparoscope. JAMA 1998;280:638–642.
2. The Database of Abstracts of Reviews of Effectiveness (University of York), Database no.: DARE-989009. In: The Cochrane Library, Issue 2, 2000. Oxford: Update Software.

8.5 Haematemesis

Martti Matikainen

Goals

Primary

- To prevent hypovolaemic shock
- To find the cause and to stop the bleeding

Secondary

- To prevent recurrent bleeding
- To repair the primary cause for bleedings (ulcer disease, etc.)

Epidemiology

- More than 5% of surgical emergency patients have acute gastrointestinal bleeding, and 80% of them have upper gastrointestinal bleeding.

History

- The patient's history can yield good clues of the underlying cause, but it seldom has any effect on the acute management of the bleeding patient.
- Important factors in the patient's history are
  - use of analgesics and non-steroidal anti-inflammatory drugs (NSAIDs) (gastric erosions)
  - previous ulcer history
  - liver cirrhosis (variceal bleeding).

Clinical findings

- The severity of the bleeding is estimated by clinical examination.
- The signs on **severe bleeding** are
  - sudden onset
  - signs of hypovolaemic shock or preshock, as paleness and dizziness in upright position.
- Patient in a hypovolaemic shock is pale and coldsweating, the pulse is rapid and thin and the blood pressure low. When the blood pressure is measured one must keep in mind that even moderately low values can be serious if the patient has hypertension.
- Rectal examination is mandatory in every patient with haematemesis. Melaena (dark, tarry faeces) tells that the patient has had the bleeding already for some hours. Normal faeces does not rule out bleeding in case of doubt. In extremely severe upper gastrointestinal bleeding the faeces can be bloody, **haematochezia**.
- Signs of chronic liver disease are
  - large or hard liver on palpation
  - spider naevi, palmar erythema
  - gynaecomastia
  - jaundice.
- Mucosal abnormalities
  - Teleangiectasias associated with the Rendu–Osler–Weber syndrome

Primary investigations

- If the patient has signs of shock, the treatment must be started immediately and the patient referred to hospital.
- In case of slower bleeding and if the diagnosis of bleeding is uncertain, the haematocrit value can be useful. It is typical that the patient has a very low haematocrit value without shock, if the bleeding has been slow (days). On the other hand, quite heavy acute bleeding can cause only a slight decrease in the haematocrit value because of haemoconcentration.

First aid

- If there is any doubt about significant bleeding, an i.v. infusion is started.
- If the patient has a shock, two i.v. cannulas are recommended.
- Blood volume substitution is mandatory. Use balanced electrolyte solutions.
- All patients with acute gastrointestinal bleeding should be referred to a surgical unit, because operative treatment may be necessary. If the bleeding is profuse, it is a good policy to inform the receiving unit in advance.

Management in the hospital emergency unit

- I.v. infusion is continued.
- Haematocrit, blood typing, and cross-check are the most important primary blood tests.
- Coagulation tests (thromboplastin time, platelets) and transaminases are also useful.
- Gastroscopy should be performed for the bleeding patient as soon as possible.
  - In practice gastroscopy is often performed during the duty hours. If the patient is admitted at nighttime, it can be performed on the next morning if the bleeding is in control. In case of continuing bleeding gastroscopy should be performed immediately.
- Shock patients should be managed in an **intensive care unit.**

Aetiology and the treatment of haematemesis

Oesophageal varices

- The most common cause for oesophageal bleeding are oesophageal varices. The bleeding is usually massive and there is "blood all over". Sudden bleeding often also stops rapidly, but starts easily again. Mortality is considerable.

- Variceal bleeding is suspected, if the haematemesis is bright and the patient has signs of liver cirrhosis and elevated portal pressure, such as ascites, gynaecomastia, spider naevi, jaundice and large veins on the abdominal wall.
- Treatment
  - Haemodynamics is maintained with sufficient infusions of volume expanders and with packed red cells.
  - Platelets and frozen plasma are given when necessary.
  - Proper oxygenation is sustained.
  - As a first aid somatostatin analogues are given B [1 2 3 4 5].
  - If the bleeding continues a Linton or Sengstake–Blakemoore tube is introduced. The gastric balloon is filled and put on traction. This is usually sufficient to stop the bleeding. The right place of the balloon should always be checked by radiography. **The variceal origin of the bleeding must be confirmed by gastroscopy before any balloon tamponades.**
  - Endoscopic sclerotherapy in acute bleeding is quite a demanding procedure. It is repeated at one to three week intervals until the varices have disappeared.
  - As a long-term treatment beta-blockers and nitrates may lower mortality.
  - The most important prognostic factor in variceal bleeding is the severity of the liver disease.

Mallory–Weiss tear

- Forceful vomiting can cause a tear on the prolapsing gastric mucosa. This so-called Mallory–Weiss tear can bleed considerably, but the bleeding usually stops spontaneously. The tear is located at the gastro-oesophageal junction.
- The history of Mallory–Weiss tear is quite typical: forceful vomiting with normal gastric content is followed by haematemesis. Treatment with acid inhibiting agents is not necessary.

Peptic ulcer disease

- Peptic ulcer disease is the most important single cause for upper gastrointestinal bleeding. Gastric and duodenal ulcer cause about one third of these bleedings.
- Treatment
  - If the ulcer is bleeding during endoscopy (Forrest 1a or 1b) or a "visible vessel" (Forrest 2a) is seen, the ulcer is treated during the investigation (adrenaline injection, electrocoagulation, heater probe or fibrin glue).
  - When the ulcer is treated endoscopically a control endoscopy should always be performed within the next 24 hours. Repeated endoscopic treatment after short observation period (<24 hours) reduces re-bleedings significantly.
  - If the endoscopic treatment is unsuccessful after several attempts (bleeding continues or the patient still has signs of shock after infusion of five units of packed red cells) surgery is indicated.
  - Acid inhibiting agents have not been shown to have any effect in the treatment of an acute bleeding peptic ulcer. However, they have a crucial role in the treatment of the ulcer disease and in the prevention of rebleeding A [6 7].
- Follow-up treatment
  - During acute endoscopy a helicobacter test should be performed. If it is positive, eradication regimen can be started immediately after the bleeding has stopped and recurrences can be avoided.

Bleeding gastric erosion

- Anti-inflammatory drugs (NSAIDs) cause an increasing number of gastric bleedings, particularly in the elderly. These drugs cause mucosal erosions that may also bleed.
- The treatment is usually endoscopic according the same principles as in the peptic ulcer bleeding. To prevent recurrent bleeding, the need for further use of ASA and NSAIDs should be evaluated. Also prophylactic treatment with proton pump inhibitors should be considered.

References

1. Gøtzsche PC. Somatostatin analogues for acute bleeding oesophageal varices. Cochrane Database Syst Rev. 2004;(2): CD000193.
2. Imperiale TF, Birgisson S. Somatostatin or octreotide compared with H2 antagonists and placebo in the management of acute nonvariceal upper gastrointestinal hemorrhage. Ann Intern Med 1997;127:1062–1071.
3. The Database of Abstracts of Reviews of Effectiveness (University of York), Database no.: DARE-988099. In: The Cochrane Library, Issue 4, 1999. Oxford: Update Software.
4. Imperiale TF, Teran JC, McCullough AJ. A meta-analysis of somatostatin versus vasopressin in the management of acute oesophageal variceal haemorrhage. Gastroenterology 1995;109:1289–1294.
5. The Database of Abstracts of Reviews of Effectiveness (University of York), Database no.: DARE-952897. In: The Cochrane Library, Issue 4, 1999. Oxford: Update Software.
6. Bustamante M, Stollman N. The efficacy of proton-pump inhibitors in acute ulcer bleeding: a qualitative review. Journal of Clinical Gastroenterology 2000, 30(1), 7–13.
7. The Database of Abstracts of Reviews of Effectiveness (University of York), Database no.: DARE-20000229. In: The Cochrane Library, Issue 2, 2002. Oxford: Update Software.

8.6 Faecal incontinence

Kari-Matti Hiltunen

Basic rules

- Faecal incontinence associated with acute gastroenteritis does not indicate proctological investigations unless it becomes prolonged or recurrent.

- Inquire actively about faecal incontinence in patients with anorectal problems, as incontinence is not often reported spontaneously.

Epidemiology

- The prevalence of the condition is 4/1000 according to the results of a British study. The symptom is most common in the elderly but a considerable proportion of the patients are of working age.

Aetiology

- Acute infectious diarrhoea
- Faecal impaction (overflow incontinence)
- Over-consumption of laxatives (common in the elderly)
- Injuries of the anal sphincter
    - Operations: anal fistula, dilatation of the anus
    - Delivery
    - Pelvic fractures and other direct injuries
- Rectal prolapse
- Anorectal tumours
- Congenital malformations
- Neurological diseases: sequelae of cerebral infarction, multiple sclerosis, tetraplegia, intervertebral disk herniation, dementia
- Proctitis, colitis
- Idiopathic (neurogenic)

Investigations

- Ask about the duration and frequency of the symptom, consistency of leaking faeces (hard? diarrhoea?), surgery on the lower abdomen and the back, and, particularly, neurological diseases and drugs used by the patient (over-consumption of laxatives).
- Proctological examination is the basis of diagnosis: inspection, proctoscopy, and recto-sigmoidoscopy. These examinations are always indicated, with the exception of transient infectious diarrhoea.
- Urinary incontinence developing together with faecal incontinence suggests spinal cord disease.
- Inspection
    - A widely open anus indicates injury of the anal sphincter
    - Ask the patient to push as in defecation and observe the motion of the perineum. If the perineum is lowered to the level of the ischial tuberosities a neurogenic disorder is likely
    - Identify eventual rectal prolapse, and vaginal or uterine prolapse in female patients
- Touch per rectum
    - Determine the tone of the anal sphincter, both at rest and during contraction
- Proctoscopy and rectoscopy or sigmoidoscopy
    - Identify tumours and inflammation

Treatment

Conditions suitable for treatment by the general practitioner

- Acute infectious diarrhoea
- Overflow incontinence
- Incontinence caused by medication
- Any patient with mild or moderate incontinence that is not caused by a tumour and who has been sufficiently investigated as regards neurological or other systemic disease, is eligible for a therapeutic trial.

Medication

- If the patient has altering consistency of the stools and only loose stools cause incontinence, bulk laxatives may be effective.
- In the beginning, overflow incontinence often requires enemas.
- Weakness of the internal anal sphincter is treated with loperamide. The initial dose is 2 mg, and the dose can be increased up to 16 mg/day.
- About 15% of patients become continent after medication C [1].

Physiotherapy

- Mild faecal incontinence can be treated by exercises of the pelvic floor muscles C [2] similar to those recommended for urinary stress incontinence.

Indications for specialist consultation

- Total incontinence or daily soiling of the underwear, unless the cause is definitely untreatable (severe dementia or neurological disease).
- The surgical treatment options include repair of a ruptured anal sphincter, plastic corrections of pelvic floor muscles and the perineum, and substitution of the anal sphincter D [3]. In some cases a stoma is made. This allows to keep the bowel empty when sphincter function cannot be restored.

References

1. Cheetham M, Brazzelli M, Norton C, Glazener CMA. Drug treatment for faecal incontinence in adults. Cochrane Database Syst Rev. 2004;(2):CD002116.
2. Norton C, Hosker G, Brazzelli M. Biofeedback and/or sphincter exercises for the treatment of faecal incontinence in adults. Cochrane Database Syst Rev. 2004;(2):CD002111.
3. Bachoo P, Brazzelli M, Grant A. Surgery for faecal incontinence in adults. Cochrane Database Syst Rev. 2004;(2): CD001757.

8.7 Obstipation in the adult

Editors

Basic rules

- Rule out acute intestinal occlusion (total obstipation, pain, vomiting, visible peristalsis, swelling of the abdomen).
- Refer patients with suspected organic disease for further investigations (pain, bloody stools, change in bowel habits, systemic symptoms, chronic obstipation in a young person).
- Identify overflow diarrhoea as a symptom of obstipation.
- Identify drugs as a cause of obstipation.
- Start prophylactic medication for obstipation in patients who receive strong opioids for pain.
- Give written instructions (48.91)

Definition

- Decreased frequency and difficulty of defecation. Normally defecation occurs at 8–72 hour intervals.

Epidemiology

- Obstipation occurs in 1–6% of healthy adults.
- Up to 80% of immobilized elderly people have obstipation.

Aetiology

- Lifestyle
  - Lack of exercise
  - Diet low in fibre
  - Insufficient fluid intake
  - Neglecting the natural feeling of need to defecate (army, school)
- Drugs
  - Opioids
  - Verapamil and, to a lesser extent, other calcium antagonists
  - Anticholinergic drugs (neuroleptics, antidepressants, drugs for Parkinson's disease)
  - Stimulating laxatives in long-term use
  - Sucralfate, antacids
  - Diuretics
  - Iron preparations
- Organic causes
  - Tumours
  - Anal fissure
  - Bowel stenosis
  - Hypothyroidism
  - Several other endocrine disorders (hypo- and hyperparathyroidism, Addison's disease, panhypopituitarism)
  - Diabetic neuropathy
  - Aganglionosis (Hirschsprung's disease)
  - Neurological diseases (Parkinson's disease, cerebrovascular disease, spinal cord injury, multiple sclerosis)
- Psychogenic causes
  - Anorexia nervosa
  - Depression

GAS

History

- The definition of the patient's problem is most important.
- Find out all drugs used by the patient.

Symptoms suggesting habitual obstipation

- No other changes in bowel habits or general symptoms
- A long history of obstipation

Symptoms suggesting organic disease

- Increasing abdominal pain
- Pain associated with defecation
- Change in bowel habits
- Melaena or anal haemorrhage
- General symptoms (weight loss, fatigue)

Investigations

- Abdomen: inspection (scars), palpation
- Touch per rectum, proctoscopy: haemorrhoids, fissures, faecal prop
- General physical examination as necessary
- If the symptoms suggest an organic disease the following investigations may be helpful:
  - Plain abdominal x-ray if intestinal obstruction or paralytic ileus is suspected
  - Sigmoidoscopy or rectoscopy
  - Colonography
  - Colonography, rectal biopsies, and anorectal manometry are indicated if Hirschsprung's disease is suspected (in young people with obstipation from childhood).

Treatment

- Treatment is indicated only if obstipation causes symptoms.

Temporary obstipation

- Stimulating laxatives can be used temporarily.
- A mini-clysma relieves severe obstipation.

Chronic obstipation

- Correction of diet, adding fibre B [1 2] and fluids. Give written instructions.
  - Fibre is effective also during pregnancy B [3]

- Increasing exercise
- Regular defecation (e.g. every morning after breakfast)
- Stimulating laxatives are discontinued (senna, danthron, bisacodyl)
- Obstipation-inducing drugs are discontinued or their doses are reduced.
- Laxatives for increasing the volume of the stools B [1 2]
  - Bulk laxatives
  - Lactulose
  - Magnesium milk
- Sodium picosulfate can also be used.
- A mini-clysma relieves severe obstipation. If necessary, a large-volume water clysma can be used, but it involves a small risk of perforation.

Special cases

- A bowel-cleansing solution, e.g. Colonsteril®, is effective for otherwise therapy-resistant obstipation. If the patient cannot drink sufficiently the drug can be given through a naso-gastric tube.
- A small amount of senna may improve the effectiveness of a bulk laxative in bedridden patients.
- Neurogenic obstipation
  - Obstipation caused by low-level injury should NOT be treated with bulk laxatives but with regular mini-clysma at 4–6 day intervals or by finger evacuation.
  - Obstipation caused by a higher injury can be treated by bowel training, finger evacuation or bulk laxatives.

References

1. Tramonte SM, Brand MB, Mulrow CD, Arnato MG, O'Keefe ME, Ramirez G. Treatment of chronic constipation in adults: a systematic review. J Gen Int Med 1997;12:15–24.
2. The Database of Abstracts of Reviews of Effectiveness (University of York), Database no.: DARE-970266. In: The Cochrane Library, Issue 4, 1999. Oxford: Update Software.
3. Jewell DJ, Young G. Interventions for treating constipation in pregnancy. Cochrane Database Syst Rev. 2004;(2):CD001142.

8.8 Abdominal pain and swelling–the irritable bowel

Simo Tarpila

Basic rules

- Lactose intolerance should be detected or ruled out before other investigations.
- Coeliac disease should be diagnosed.
- Diseases causing obstruction or delayed emptying of the stomach or bowel should be diagnosed: tumours, chronic inflammatory diseases, pseudo-obstruction, diverticula (bacterial overgrowth).
- The symptom is classified as functional (the irritable bowel, aerophagia) after the forementioned diseases have been ruled out with acceptable certainty (see diagnostic approach below).

Epidemiology

- Abdominal swelling occurs in 20–40% of the population. The patient usually contacts a doctor only after the symptoms have lasted for a long time.

Etiology

- Development of gas, bowel contractions, or increase of pressure in any part of the gastrointestinal tract is experienced as pain, swelling or both.
- The patients often have a low pain threshold for stretching or a decreased ability to cope with stress.
- The reasons for collecting of gas in the different parts of the gastrointestinal tract vary.

Stretching of the stomach

- Aerophagia
  - May be subconscious or associated with rapid swallowing of food.
  - May be related to excessive use of chewing gum.
  - Aerophagia is often related to psychological factors.
  - Belching is the most common symptom.
- Antroduodenal motility disorder
  - Slow emptying of the stomach or duodenogastric reflux, or both.
  - The symptoms consist of belching and early filling of the stomach at meals.
  - If the patient has epigastric pain or vomiting it is important to perform gastroscopy to exclude peptic ulcer disease causing pyloric obstruction.

Swelling of the small bowel

- Lactose intolerance
- Food intolerance (see colonic swelling below)
- Small bowel diverticula
  - Most commonly occur in the duodenum
  - The diverticula contain anaerobic bacterial flora of the colon that causes gas formation and pain due to bacterial metabolism.
  - The patients tolerate poorly a diet rich in fibre.

Colonic swelling

- Nutritional factors
  - Consumption of beans, peas, cabbage, bananas

- Inabsorbable carbohydrates (saccharides or some fruit and vegetables, fructose, sorbitol, carbohydrates of wheat and dark bread) or proteins.
- Motility disorder with increased gas formation
    - Accelerated small bowel passage time increases the amount of fermentable food in the colon, thus increasing gas formation.
- Pain threshold for stretching is low.
- Psychosocial factors are often involved. The psychologic symptoms may be associated with
    - panic disorder
    - depression
    - anxiety
    - general somatization tendency.

Clinical picture of the irritable bowel syndrome

- Diffuse abdominal pain, sometimes cramps
- Left epigastric pain (flexura lienalis syndrome)
- Right epigastric pain (flexura hepatica syndrome)
- Variable consistency of faeces
- Abdominal swelling and pain, often relieved by defecation
- Long history of symptoms
- Frequent consultations and periods of treatment in the hospital

Examination of the patient

- A good history is the key to diagnosis
    - Typical symptoms of the irritable bowel syndrome (see above)
    - The association between food and symptoms (lactose intolerance, intolerance to other foods)
- Palpation of the abdomen and touch per rectum
- Blood count, AST, alkaline phosphatase
- Lactose ingestion test
- Occult blood in the faeces
- Transglutaminase or endomysium antibodies in order to detect coeliac disease.
- Abdominal ultrasonography (gallstone disease)
    - increased ALT or alkaline phosphatase
    - right epigastric symptoms
- Gastroscopy (in order to detect peptic ulcer or coeliac disease)
    - Epigastric symptoms
    - Symptoms of stomach retention
    - Symptoms of malabsorption
- Sigmoidoscopy and colongraphy or colonoscopy (in order to detect tumors, polyps, diverticulosis and spastic colon)
    - Positive occult blood in the faeces
    - The patient is aged over 50 years.
- Small bowel passage (reveals small bowel diverticula and the rare pseudo-obstruction, determines passage time)
    - Performed on selected patients if the symptoms continue and are severe, and results of other investigations are negative.
- Psychological factors should always be considered as psychiatric disorders, such as anxiety, panic disorder and depression, are common in patients with functional abdominal problems.

GAS

Treatment

- It is essential to establish a positive relationship with the patient. The symptoms and exacerbating factors are discussed with the patient. Explaining the pathophysiology of the symptoms is often beneficial.
- Often the patient is afraid of cancer. A thorough examination is the best way of controlling fear. If the symptoms are diagnosed functional after the examination, this fact should be presented to the patient as a positive result by telling that the diagnosis is now clear–not by stating that nothing was found in the investigations.
- The patient should understand that his way of reacting to foods and life situation is characteristic to him, and that symptoms may recur.
- The diagnosis of functional abdominal problems is usually reliable and the diagnosis should be retained if the symptoms do not change.
- Some patients have an underlying psychiatric disorder most commonly depression. Treating this may help to cure the symptoms Ⓐ [1 2].

Diet therapy

- There is no standard diet, but the patient should avoid foods that cause symptoms.
- Poorly absorbable carbohydrates, such as fructose, xylitol, and sorbitol, may be the reason for diarrhoea.
- Sometimes carbohydrate starch (cereals, potatoes, maize) is not absorbed totally, causing symptoms in the colon.

Drug therapy

- In controlled studies no drug therapy has been conclusively effective against symptoms of irritable bowel. Symptomatic treatment is occasionally necessary.
- If the patient has obstipation, a diet rich in fibre may be of benefit. Wheat bran 10–30 g/day with a sufficient amount of water, or bulk laxatives (particularly roughly ground flaxseed) gradually combined in the diet may help. The treatment trial should last at least 2–3 months.
- Dimeticone may help in flatulence by reducing surface tension.
- Anticholinergic medication may be tried for convulsions, and loperamide Ⓑ [3 4] for paroxysmal diarrhoea. Both should be taken only when needed.
- For nightly abdominal cramps a small dose of amitriptyline combined with chlordiazepoxide may be beneficial.

Follow-up

- Long-term, supporting doctor-patient relationship is often essential for successful treatment.
- A follow-up appointment (history and physical examination) annually may be beneficial.
- Factors that exacerbate the symptoms (foods, psychological factors) should be discussed thoroughly with the patient, and the persistent and variable nature of the symptoms should be explained.

References

1. Jackson JL, O'Malley PG, Tomkins G, Balden E, Santoro J, Kroenke K. Treatment of functional gastrointestinal disorders with antidepressant medications: a meta-analysis. Am J Med 2000;108:65–72.
2. The Database of Abstracts of Reviews of Effectiveness (University of York), Database no.: DARE-20000291. In: The Cochrane Library, Issue 3, 2001. Oxford: Update Software.
3. Jailwala J, Imperiale TF, Kroenke K. Pharmacological treatment of the irritable bowel syndrome: a systematic review of randomized controlled trials. Annals of Internal Medicine 2000;133:136–147.
4. The Database of Abstracts of Reviews of Effectiveness (University of York), Database no.: DARE-20008660. In: The Cochrane Library, Issue 3, 2001. Oxford: Update Software.

8.9 Acute abdomen in the adult

Antero Palmu

Basic rules

- Deciding on the urgency of treatment is more important than making an exact diagnosis.
- The first thing to do is to decide whether the patient needs referral to a hospital, an urgent operation, or whether there is time for further investigations.

Condition demanding urgent treatment

- Rupture of an abdominal aortic aneurysm
- Peritonitis
  - The patient should not be examined thoroughly, if an urgent operation is needed, and the cause for the condition is determined in the operation. A delay results in complications and increased mortality.
- Intestinal obstruction
  - Abdominal pain associated with suspected obstruction that becomes continuous may be a sign of strangulation, which must be operated immediately.
- Abdominal catastrophes
  - Worsening general condition, decreased diuresis, and acute confusion suggest an abdominal catastrophe. For example in pancreatitis these indirect clues are more important than local symptoms that may be misleadingly vague.
- Dehydration and loss of electrolytes
  - Acute abdomen may quickly result in dehydration and loss of electrolytes.

Aetiology of acute abdomen

- Surgical causes, see Table 8.9.1
- Gynecological causes, see Table 8.9.2
- Other causes, see Table 8.9.3.

Investigations

History

- Is this a new acute problem in a patient or an exacerbation of a prolonged abdominal discomfort?
  - Acute onset may indicate perforation or colic.

Table 8.9.1 Surgical causes for acute abdomen (diagnostic clues)

Cause	Diagnostic clue
Appendicitis	Common. Results of laboratory examinations characteristic of inflammation are often normal.
Intestinal obstruction	Hernias, surgical scars, periodical symptoms (risk for strangulation!)
Perforated peptic ulcer	Acute onset, peritonism. Often the first symptom of peptic ulcer disease
Acute cholecystitis	Localized symptoms; clinical manifestations of an infection. Often the first symptom of gallstone disease.
Acute pancreatitis	History of alcohol consumption. Consider gallstones as possible aetiology. Urine and serum amylase may be normal in severe cases.
Mesenterial thrombosis	May be difficult to diagnose on the basis of clinical manifestations. The patient often has cardiovascular problems.
Diverticulitis of the colon	The most common site is the sigmoid colon.
Volvulus	Sigma is the most common site. Symptoms of intestinal obstruction (risk for perforation!). Volvulus of the caecum develops more slowly.
Testis torsion	The testis is tender on palpation. Often pain and tenderness in lower abdomen.

Table 8.9.2 Gynaecological causes for acute abdomen (diagnostic clues)

Cause	Diagnostic clues/examples
Ectopic pregnancy	Pain; referred pain in shoulder. Urine pregnancy test may be normal, sensitive serum test is usually positive.
Ovarial disease	Infection; ruptured cyst; torsion of a cyst
Myoma	Torsion; necrosis; bleeding into the abdominal cavity, infection

Table 8.9.3 Non-surgical causes for acute abdomen (examples)

Cause	Example
Metabolic disorders	♦ Diabetic ketoacidosis ♦ Porphyria ♦ Hypertriglyseridaemia ♦ Haemochromatosis (24.65)
Infectious causes	♦ Gastroenteritis ♦ Diverticulitis (8.82) ♦ Hepatitis ♦ Perihepatitis ♦ Mononucleosis ♦ Herpes zoster ♦ Pyelonephritis ♦ Epididymitis, orchitis ♦ Sepsis
Referred pain	♦ Myocardial infarction ♦ Pericarditis ♦ Pleuritis ♦ Pulmonary infarction ♦ Heart failure (hepatic stasis) ♦ Renal calculi
Immunological disorder	♦ Angioneurotic oedema ♦ Polyarteritis nodosa ♦ Henoch–Schönlein purpura ♦ Hypersensitivity reaction

- The location of referred pain suggests the extent of the pathological process
  - Pancreatic pain is felt in the epigastrium; retroperitoneal irritation resulting from the affection of the entire pancreas causes referred pain in the back.
- Food intolerance and the association of pain with meals may help in the diagnosis
  - Postprandial pain is typical of gastric ulcer but may be caused by other diseases of the upper gastrointestinal tract.
- Vomiting suggests obstruction
  - Vomiting of food suggests pyloric stenosis.
  - Vomiting of bile suggests obstruction of the proximal small bowel.
  - Vomiting of faeces suggests of distal ileal or colonic obstruction.
  - Proximal intestinal obstruction causes heavy and abundant vomiting. Distal obstruction results in mild vomiting.
  - Reflectory vomiting may be associated with severe pain.
- Obstipation is often chronic. A change in bowel habits is an important symptom and suggests organic disease.
- Always ask about diarrhoea, blood or mucus in the stools, and pain during defecation.

Type of pain and palpation findings

- The pain in **acute appendicitis** is at first diffuse, shifting and often located mainly in the upper abdomen. It feels deep and dull around the umbilicus, and nausea or vomiting are often present. As the inflammation penetrates the serosa the pain becomes parietal (superficial, severe, and localized) and lateralizes in the right lower quadrant. Muscular guarding (defence) develops simultaneously.
- If the appendix is perforated, a generalized peritonitis develops and the tension and rigidity of the abdominal wall increases.
- Wave-like, rhythmically changing and paroxysmally disappearing pain is typical of diseases of the bowel as well as of biliary obstruction and ureteral calculi. If the pain becomes continuous strangulation should be suspected.
- Extremely rapid onset of pain is typical of ulcer perforation. The abdominal wall becomes rigid in an instant.

Physical examination

- General examination
  - Heart and lungs
  - Blood pressure
  - General neurological examination
- Inspection of the abdomen
  - Flat or swollen?
  - Surgical scars
  - Hernias (visible or palpable)
- Palpation of the abdomen
  - Pain and the location of maximal pain
  - Abdominal wall (soft, or hard suggesting peritoneal irritation?)
  - Palpable masses
  - Sites of hernias
  - Ascites
- Palpation of the genitals
  - Hernias
  - Pain or swelling of the testes
- Touch per rectum
  - Tumour, bleeding
  - Prostate
  - Is there faeces in the rectum? The colour of the faeces.
- Auscultation of the abdomen
  - A very useful examination
  - Tense bowel sound (obstruction), absent sounds (adynamic ileus), splashing sounds (obstruction)

Laboratory examinations

- Of minor importance in patients with acute abdomen
- Blood count, CRP B [1 2], dipstick test for urine, urine amylase and ALAT and ALP if cholecystitis is suspected

Imaging

- Plain abdominal radiograph
  - Air in the abdominal cavity (perforation), dilatated bowel segments (obstruction), fluid levels (ileus).
- Sonography
  - Acute cholecystitis, abscesses, aortic aneurysm, gynecological disease, fluid in the abdominal cavity
  - Sonography (also called "sonopalpation") performed by the primary care doctor on duty is useful.
- Chest x-ray
  - Look for pleural effusion, pericarditis, or heart failure.
- ECG
  - Always indicated if a cardiac cause is suspected.

Emergency treatment

- During the initial investigations the degree of metabolic derangement should be assessed and fluid therapy should be started before transport to a hospital, unless the distance is very short.
- Start measuring urine output.
- Insert a nasogastric tube if the patient vomits repeatedly.
- Wide-spectrum antibiotics should be started simultaneously with induction of anaesthesia when peritonitis and other infections are present.
- The most serious disorders of fluid and electrolyte balance should be quickly corrected before an operation, without delaying the operation. Isotonic physiological saline is best.

References

1. Hallan S, Asberg A. The accuracy of C-reactive protein in diagnosing acute appendicitis. Scand J Clin Lab Invest 1997;57:373–380.
2. The Database of Abstracts of Reviews of Effectiveness (University of York), Database no.: DARE-971078. In: The Cochrane Library, Issue 4, 1999. Oxford: Update Software.

8.10 Syndroma pelvis spastica

Kari-Matti Hiltunen

Definition

- A syndrome with pain deep in the rectal area

Types of pain

- The pain may be paroxysmal and even arouse the patient at night. The duration of an attack varies from a couple of minutes to a couple of hours. Such episodic pain is also called proctalgia fugax.
- Another type of pain is precipitated by prolonged sitting. This more continuous pain is called coccygodynia.
- The third group of pain is continuous neuralgia-type pain in the anus (idiopathic proctalgia). It most commonly occurs in elderly women without any pathological findings.

Aetiology

- A spasm of the levator muscle is considered the cause of the pain. The site of the pain reflects the localization of the spastic portion of the muscle.
- Psychogenic factors often play a role.

Investigation and treatment

- Examine the patient carefully and convince him or her of the benign nature of the symptom. Many patients can cope with their symptoms after they have been properly informed.
- NSAIDs and spasmolytes may be effective but equally often they fail to produce an effect.
- Of physical treatment modalities, galvanic current with an intra-anal probe (high-voltage therapy) can be tried. The treatment causes contraction of the levator muscle. The intensity of the current is adjusted so as not to cause unpleasant pain. The treatment must be repeated every two days, about 10 times altogether. 50–80% of the patients may obtain a benefit.

8.20 Organizing endoscopy in primary care

Ilkka Kunnamo

Need for investigations

- Gastroscopy: a minimum of 200 investigations/10 000 inhabitants/year
- Fibreoptic sigmoidoscopy or colonoscopy: a minimum of 100 investigations/10 000 inhabitants/year.
- The proportion of investigations of the colon should be increased (diagnosis of adenomas and colon carcinomas).

Educational requirements

- Gastroscopy: tens of examinations performed under the supervision of a gastroenterologist.

- Fibreoptic sigmoidoscopy: 5–10 investigations under the supervision of a physician who masters the examination
- Other assistant personnel: at least one day in an endoscopy unit.

Personnel requirements

- The doctor needs 30 minutes for gastroscopy or sigmoidoscopy and a full hour for colonoscopy.
- 1–2 assistants are required.
- Preparations before the examination and washing of the instruments after it takes almost an hour. A washing machine shortens the time somewhat.

Cooperation

- Primary care endoscopy services should be organized in cooperation with a specialized unit.
  - Training of primary care endoscopists
  - Delegation of patient follow-up to primary care
  - The biopsy specimens should be examined in the same laboratory as those from the specialized unit.

Recommendations

Fibreoptic sigmoidoscopy

- Fibreoptic sigmoidoscopy services in primary care should be based on a population of at least 10 000.
- Because the investigation is always elective (and requires cleansing of the bowel) the instrument can be transported from one health centre to another. In many centres sigmoidoscopes are being replaced with colonoscopes. Colonoscopy is a more demanding procedure than either sigmoidoscopy or gastroscopy and should be concentrated in the hands of fewer physicians.

Gastroscopy

- Gastroscopy services in primary care can be considered for a population of at least 10 000–15 000 if there is enough personnel, if there are preferably two interested physicians who want to learn gastroscopy, the services are needed in the area, and the services can be organized in good cooperation with a specialized unit.
- Because some examinations are performed on acutely ill patients, transportation of the instrument from one health centre to another is not always feasible.

What should be considered before starting primary care endoscopy

Benefits

- Improved diagnostics as symptomatic patients can be examined quickly
- Travelling times and costs are less in scarcely populated areas.
- The continuity of care improves.
- The use of specialized services decreases, but the costs of organizing endoscopy in primary care should be considered.
- The resources of the specialized unit can be reserved for other services.
- Examination of patients with anal haemorrhage by fibreoptic sigmoidoscopy helps to detect curable colorectal cancers and precancerous lesions. Rigid rectoscopy should be replaced with fibreoptic sigmoidoscopy.
- There is no firm evidence of improvement in the prognosis of gastric cancer with free endoscopy, but this is to be expected.

Problems

- Endoscopy services require time and resources that might be better used for more essential primary care services.
- Maintaining competence requires a large number of yearly examinations per doctor (at least 100, preferably 200).

The consultative role of the primary care endoscopist?

1. Examinations (sigmoidoscopy) are performed only on those patients the doctor is seeing him/herself. The responsibility for further treatment lies clearly on the doctor performing the examination.
2. Examinations are performed as a consultation for other physicians. The demands on the accuracy of the diagnosis are then higher. Concentrating the examinations in the hands of a few doctors ensures a sufficient number of investigations annually.

- If endoscopy is introduced to a primary care unit, the doctors performing the examinations will in practice act as consultants.

8.21 Gastroscopy

Ilkka Kunnamo

Indications for gastroscopy

Gastroscopy as a diagnostic investigation

- Dyspepsia in a patient over 50 years of age
- Dyspepsia in a patient below 50 years of age if vomiting, weight loss, anaemia or dysphagia are associated or if the symptoms continue or recur after a 2–4-week treatment trial.
- In patients aged under 50 years screening for helicobacter with a urea breath test or antibody test and treatment

of helicobacter-positive patients before gastroscopy is an efficient and safe treatment alternative

- In patients with functional dyspepsia eradication of helicobacter has little effect on the symptoms of dyspepsia A [1]; however, the benefit of cured peptic ulcer disease, which is associated with helicobacter infection, is achieved.

- Helicobacter-positive patients with symptoms of dyspepsia and increased risk of ulcer (those using NSAIDs and smokers)
- Continuous symptoms suggesting reflux disease
- Pain or difficulty in swallowing
- Chest pain of unknown aetiology
- Recurrent vomiting and early filling of the stomach (pyloric stenosis)
- Abnormal or unclear finding on abdominal radiography
- Acute upper gastrointestinal bleeding; the examination must be performed within 24 hours
  - Vomiting of blood (with the exception of a small amount of bright blood following heavy vomiting probably originating from a Mallory-Weiss tear)
  - Melena (peptic ulcer bleeding)
- Iron deficiency anaemia or suspicion of chronic bleeding
- Suspicion of coeliac disease
- Severe epigastric pain also at night (suspicion of peptic ulcer)
- Dyspepsia in a patient on NSAIDs and peroral steroids
- Involuntary weight loss (suspicion of peptic ulcer or cancer)
- Suspected coeliac disease (e.g. antibodies for gliadin, reticulin, endomysium or transglutaminase)
- Control of ventricle ulcer healing
- Follow-up of Barrett's esophagus
- Positive test for faecal occult blood (after the colon has been examined and no reason for the bleeding has been found)

As a follow-up examination

- Follow-up of Barrett's oesophagus
- Follow-up of the healing of an oesophageal ventricle or stoma ulcer
- Follow-up of the healing of severe oesophagitis
- Follow-up of adenomatous polyp or carcinoid of the ventricle
- Follow-up of dysplasic changes in the ventricle
- For ensuring the efficacy of gluten-free diet in coeliac disease

Gastroscopic procedures

- Polypectomy
- Treatment of bleeding and prevention of re-bleeding
- Sclerotherapy or ligations for varicose veins
- Dilatation of strictures
- Ablation of oesophageal tumour
- Stenting
- Percutaneous endoscopic gastrostomy

Gastroscopy is usually not indicated

- Unnecessary use of gastroscopy should be avoided. The following conditions do not fulfil the criteria
  - Mild symptoms suggesting gastro-oesophageal reflux that responds to changes in life style or mild medication
  - Dyspepsia in a patient under 50 years of age that cures during a 2–4-week treatment trial unless the patient has alarming symptoms and does not use NSAIDs.
  - Symptoms of dyspepsia when the patient has already undergone gastroscopy with normal findings
  - Symptoms suggesting lactose intolerance before a trial with milk-free diet
  - Symptoms suggesting irritable bowel syndrome, such as abdominal pain, distention, alternating diarrhoea and constipation
  - Active gastroenteritis

Gastroscopy is the first investigation in dyspepsia

- The biopsy findings are helpful in determining the diagnosis: gastritis, helicobacter infection, atrophy, malignant ulcer, coeliac disease and giardiasis can be diagnosed or ruled out.
- Superficial pathology such as haemorrhagic gastritis, mild oesophagitis and telangiactasias can be seen.
- An active peptic ulcer can also be identified in a deformed bulbus.
- Postgastrectomy problems can be investigated reliably.
- The patient is not exposed to radiation

Preparation for the investigation and care after it

- The patient must not take food after 8 o'clock on the preceding evening, or for a minimum of 6 hours before the examination.
- Sucralfate, antacides (which adsorb on the gastric mucosa) and drugs that delay gastric emptying should be stopped (1-) 2 days before the investigation. Other drugs can the taken as usual.
- After the investigation the patient should eat cool, soft food. If a local anaesthetic has been used the patient should not drink or eat during the first 1–2 hours after the examination (risk of aspiration).

Significant gastroscopic findings

- Gastroscopic and histological findings with clinical significance are listed in Table 8.21.1.

Gastroscopic findings of uncertain clinical significance

- For gastroscopical findings with uncertain clinical significance, see Table 8.21.2

Table 8.21.1 Gastroscopy findings and histological changes with proven clinical significance

Finding	Clinical significance
Oesophagus	
Erosive striae	Oesophagitis
Strictures, ulcers	Complicated oesophagitis; biopsies
Barrett's oesophagus (histological verification)	An area of intestinal metaplasia that may require follow-up by gastroscopy because of increased risk of cancer; biopsies
Ventricle	
Retention	Slowered emptying of the ventricle
Ulcer	Large size, undefined borders, nodular base suggest malignancy; always biopsies
Tumour	Submucotic tumours are often benign if less than 3 cm in size; polyp should be removed, with the exception of hamartomatous polyps of the corpus.
Bleeding lesion, angioectasia	Can often be coagulated endoscopically
Severe dysplasia	Risk of cancer
Severe atrophy	Risk of cancer; patients with symptoms should be readily followed up by repeated gastroscopy
Duodenum	
Ulcer	No risk of cancer
Erosive or deformed bulbus	Suggests the risk of duodenal ulcer
Histological bulbitis	Suggests the risk of duodenal ulcer
Loss of circular folds	Suggests villus atrophy
Mosaic-like appearance of the mucous membrane	Suggests villus atrophy
Histological villus atrophy	Coeliac disease very probable
Histological giardiasis	Treatment is almost always necessary

Contraindications to and complications of gastroscopy

- Uncompensated heart failure and severe pulmonary disease are contraindications to gastroscopy.
- Recent myocardial infarction is a relative contraindication, although endoscopy seldom causes ischaemia in haemodynamically stable patient
- Pregnancy is not a contraindication.

Reference

1. Moayyedi P, Soo S, Deeks J, Delaney B, Harris A, Innes M, Oakes R, Wilson S, Roalfe A, Bennett C, Forman D. Eradication of Helicobacter pylori for non-ulcer dyspepsia. Cochrane Database Syst Rev. 2004;(2):CD002096.

Table 8.21.2 Gastroscopy findings and histological changes in a dyspepsia patient with uncertain clinical significance

Finding	Possible clinical significance
Oesophagus	
Gastric heterotopia in the upper third	Innocent congenital anomaly
Redness, reddish patches, ill-defined striae	Unspecific for oesophagitis
Hiatus hernia	Not always associated with the symptoms
Histological oesophagitis without erosion	May be a normal finding in the distal end; sensitivity and specificity are poor.
Ventricle	
Bile reflux	No clear correlation with the symptoms
Redness, erosions	No correlation with gastritis or symptoms
Prepyloric deformed folds (+ erosions)	Correlation with symptoms unclear
Histological gastritis and helicobacter infection	No correlation with the symptoms
Intestinal metaplasia	Associated with atrophy, does not require follow-up
Duodenum	
Redness and swelling	No correlation with histological duodenitis

8.22 Sigmoidoscopy and colonoscopy

Ilkka Kunnamo

- See also article on organizing endoscopy in primary care 8.20.

Principles

- Fiberosigmoidoscopy should replace rectoscopy with a stiff instrument whenever sigmoidoscopy is available. Fiberosigmoidoscopy should be available in primary care. Even colonoscopy can be carried out in primacy care.
- Adequate cleansing of the bowel is a prerequisite for successful examination.
- Sigmoidoscopy must always be complemented by proctoscopy and touch per rectum in order to detect abnormalities of the anal canal.
- Sigmoidoscopy is often sufficient in the investigation of bloody or prolonged diarrhoea or fresh blood from the anus if the cause of the bleeding becomes evident in the investigation. Microscopic colitis can almost always be diagnosed from the sigma.
- Sigmoidoscopy must be complemented by colongraphy, or colonoscopy should be performed as the initial investigation

if the patient has iron deficiency anaemia or occult blood in the faeces. **Thorough investigation of these patients is the key to an early diagnosis of colon cancer and precancerous adenomas.**

- If an adenoma is detected in sigmoidoscopy, colonoscopy must always be performed.

Indications for sigmoidoscopy

- Anal haemorrhage (8.50)
  - Sigmoidoscopy (+colongraphy) should be performed on patients over 50 years of age.
  - Proctoscopy is sufficient for younger patients if an anal fissure (8.63) or typical haemorrhoids (8.62) are detected and the symptoms are consistent with these findings.
- Iron deficiency anaemia of unknown origin (sigmoidoscopy + colongraphy or colonoscopy as the first examination)
- Occult blood in faeces, and the patient has no epigastric symptoms indicating gastroscopy as the first examination.
- Chronic diarrhoea: suspicion of inflammatory bowel disease (proctitis, ulcerative colitis or Crohn's disease) according to the patient's symptoms.
  - If the patient has diarrhoea or bloody diarrhoea after a course of antibiotics, rectoscopy as an on duty examination (even without bowel emptying), or a Clostridium difficile test or both is sufficient to make the diagnosis of Clostridium difficile colitis.
  - Even if a patient with diarrhoea has a normal appearing colonic mucosa, a biopsy must always be performed in order to diagnose colitis.
- A change in bowel habits in a person above 50 years of age, particularly if the patient has abdominal pain.
- Ill defined, novel and worsening lower abdominal symptoms (innocent irritable bowel symptoms commence already at a young age and are periodical).

Cases where sigmoidoscopy is not the first examination

- Melena (black, tar-like faeces). The most common cause is upper gastrointestinal bleeding, and gastroscopy should be performed first.
- If the patient has symptoms suggesting lactose intolerance, a diet without milk products should be tried first.

Preparing the patient for sigmoidoscopy

- The patient is advised to:
- Avoid berries and vegetables with seeds (tomatoes, whortleberries, cucumber) and linseed for one week preceding the examination.
- Drink only water or mineral water from the evening before the examination. No other food during that time.
- Start drinking the polyethylene glycol lavage fluid on the morning of the examination. 3–4 litres of fluid should be taken over 3–4 h. During the first hour bowel movement becomes more frequent and a diarrhoea develops. When the fluid coming out is clear or almost clear, it is time to start with the examination.
- Sodium phosphate enema is a good alternative to polyethylene glycol lavage (A) [1 2].

Techniques of fiberosigmoidoscopy

1. The patient lies on his left side with hips and knees slightly flexed.
2. Touch per rectum is performed first to detect lesions near the anus. If something is felt by finger, a proctoscopy should be performed first. Eventual biopsies from the rectum are taken after the sigmoidoscopy.
3. The tip of the instrument is lubricated with lidocaine gel before insertion into the ampulla.
4. The lumen is made visible by infusing air into the bowel. The instrument can be advanced only after the lumen has become visible, and visual control must be maintained always when the instrument is passed on. Advancing the instrument blindly may result in the tip passing into a diverticulum and perforating the bowel. The instrument is passed on to its maximal range without delay, and the bowel is inspected during retraction of the instrument. If a lesion is seen during insertion its position (cm from the anus) should be recorded.
5. If the lumen disappears and cannot be found when bending the instrument and infusing more air the instrument should be returned a few centimeters until the lumen is again visible. If the insertion of the instrument does not succeed the patient should change to supine position with the hips and knees flexed and heels on the examination table. The change of position may straighten the bends of the bowel.
6. After the instrument has been inserted into its maximal range (or a bend in the bowel prevents advancing it despite repeated attempts) the inspection is started by slowly pulling the instrument back while bending its tip to see the entire mucosa.
7. Biopsies should be taken from macroscopically suspect sites (usually at least 2 biopsies from one site, even more from an adenoma). If the mucosa looks normal to the experienced eye, histology rarely detects anything abnormal. Routine biopsies need not be taken **unless the patient has diarrhoea**. A small polyp can be totally removed with the biopsy forceps. Several biopsies should be taken from larger tumours. If the mucosa looks inflamed (unglossy, bleeding, membranotic) biopsies should be taken both from the abnormal mucosa as well as from normal-appearing mucosa surrounding it. Report the distance from the anus, or otherwise describe the place where the biopsies were taken, on the biopsy containers. **If the examination is performed as follow-up of an inflammatory bowel disease always take biopsies even if the bowel looks normal.**

Findings of clinical importance

- Polyps (adenomas) and tumours
- Ulcerations

- Membranes that cannot be rinsed away or the removal of which causes bleeding.
- Petecchiae or bleeding on light touch of the instrument
- Unglossy appearance of the mucosa, lack of normal vascular pattern
- Pipelike bowel without haustration
- Telangiectasias (angiodysplasias)
- Diverticula
- Haemorrhoids
- Histological inflammation, dysplasia or adenoma

References

1. Hsu CW, Imperiale TF. Meta-analysis and cost comparison of polyethylene glycol lavage versus sodium phosphate for colonoscopy preparation. Gastroint Endosc 1998;48: 276–282.
2. The Database of Abstracts of Reviews of Effectiveness (University of York), Database no.: DARE-981598. In: The Cochrane Library, Issue 2, 2000. Oxford: Update Software.

8.30 Heartburn; reflux oesophagitis

Juhani Lehtola

Basic rules

- Exclude life-threatening diseases, such as cardiovascular diseases, severe oesophagitis, complicated peptic ulcer disease and tumours of the oesophagus and stomach, in cases where heartburn is associated with other sudden or serious symptoms such as chest pain, abdominal pain, or haematemesis.
- Treat other patients with heartburn symptomatically, and perform further investigations if the pain becomes prolonged.

Definition

- Heartburn is a burning sensation behind the sternum. It is not frank pain. Cold or hot drinks, citrus juice, and alcohol often exacerbate heartburn, antacids typically alleviate it.
- In reflux oesophagitis the patient becomes susceptible to the associated complications and may suffer from deterioration in quality of life.

Epidemiology

- According to an American study, 7% of healthy hospital personnel had heartburn daily and 14% weekly.
- During pregnancy heartburn is even more common (25–80%).
- Heartburn and symptoms of gastro-oesophageal reflux increase with age.
- Only a minority of the patients seek medical help.

Aetiology

- Heartburn is usually caused by gastro-oesophageal reflux. The symptom can be associated with
  - gastro-oesophageal reflux disease (with or without oesophagitis)
  - motility disorders of the oesophagus (achalasia, diffuse spasms, nutcracker oesophagus)
  - peptic ulcer disease
  - disorders of gastric emptying
  - irritable bowel syndrome
  - tumours of the oesophagus and stomach
  - hiatus hernia
- Reflux without anatomical abnormalities is common. A hiatus hernia is usually not associated with reflux symptoms.
- Transient lower oesophageal sphincter relaxation (TLESR) is the most important aetiopathogenetic factor. The resting pressure of the lower sphincter may be normal or low, and the level of acid secretion may be normal on average. Oesophageal acid clearance and gastric emptying may also be pathogenetic factors.

Complications

- Reflux oesophagitis is usually a mild disease without serious complications.
- Chronic, untreated inflammation may result in the substitution of squamous epithelium by metaplastic columnar epithelium (Barrett's epithelium). It can be detected in 8–20% of patients with oesophagitis, and it is associated with increased risk for adenocarcinoma.
- Chronic, ulcerating oesophagitis may cause strictures and dysphagia. Oesophagitis is the cause in 7% of all gastrointestinal bleedings. The bleeding is nearly always gradual and results in anaemia.
- Reflux disease without obvious oesophagitis probably does not lead to permanent oesophageal injuries.
- Reflux disease may be associated with aspiration and recurrent respiratory infections, particularly in infants and the elderly.
- Tooth enamel defects have been suggested to be associated with reflux disease.

History and clinical examination

Symptoms suggesting reflux disease

- Heartburn is the main symptom; 75% of patients with reflux disease have it. However, the sensitivity of the symptom is poor.
- The symptom is associated with meals: large, fat-containing meals, chocolate, coffee, strong beverages, and sour juices

exacerbate the symptoms. Milk and antacids often alleviate the symptoms.

- Bending, lifting, tight clothes, and lying down aggravate the symptoms.
- Heartburn is associated with other oesophageal symptoms: chest pain, dysphagia, belching, and sour regurgitation.
- Patients with reflux disease often have other functional gastrointestinal symptoms such as constipation, abdominal distention, and flatulence.
- The elderly may have nocturnal attacks of coughing because of aspiration.
- Alarming symptoms indicating immediate endoscopy include
  - haematemesis
  - haemorrhage
  - anaemia
  - dysphagia
  - feeling that food gets stuck
  - chest pain.

Symptoms suggesting a condition other than reflux disease

- Abdominal pain and epigastric tenderness suggest a peptic ulcer or other organic disease of the upper abdomen.
- Exertional chest pain is often cardiogenic. Occasionally both oesophageal and cardiac symptoms may be aggravated by the same factors. Nitrates also alleviate oesophageal pain. Reflux disease may exacerbate the symptoms of ischaemic heart disease.
- Dysphagia is associated with oesophageal stricture, tumour or primary motility disorders.

Trial of drug therapy before gastroscopy

- A diagnostic drug trial with proton pump inhibitors can be carried out in patients under 50 years of age with typical but not alarming symptoms of reflux disease. Unnecessary endoscopies can be avoided with this strategy. Mild symptoms can be treated initially with the mildest drug: antacids, H_2-blocker (A) [1].
- Perform initial investigations if the symptoms last for more than 3 weeks or recur repeatedly after drug treatment. If the cause of the symptoms has been elucidated and the symptoms recur after treatment, the same treatment can be repeated.

Initial investigations

- Should be performed on all patients who have had daily or frequently recurring symptoms for more than 3 weeks.
  - Gastroscopy
  - Blood count
- Reflux oesophagitis can be diagnosed reliably by gastroscopy with biopsies. The significance of histologically verified oesophagitis without macroscopic findings is controversial.
- Gastroscopy detects or rules out other causes of heartburn, such as a peptic ulcer and tumours of the oesophagus and stomach.

Endoscopic grading of reflux disease

- The selection and duration of drug therapy depend on the severity of oesophagitis (see Table 8.30).

Further investigations

- If oesophagitis is not detected endoscopically and the patient has recurrent severe symptoms, noncardiac chest pain or symptoms of aspiration, try to confirm the presence of reflux disease or motility disorder.
  - Continuous ambulatory monitoring of oesophageal pH reveals increased total reflux time (pH $<$ 4 for more than 5% of the time), and long periods of reflux ($>$5 min).
  - Lower oesophageal sphincter pressure should be measured before an operation or when motility disturbance, such as achalasia, is suspected.
  - A contrast radiograph of the oesophagus is indicated if a motility disorder is suspected. Normal radiology does not rule out a mild motility disorder.
- Cardiac causes should be considered if the patient has (exertional) chest pain.
  - Chest x-ray
  - ECG
  - Ergometer test

Treatment of gastro-oesophageal reflux disease

- Main goal is to alleviate reflux symptoms.
- Most patients also need long-term maintenance treatment.

Goals for therapy

- Abolishment of symptoms

Table 8.30 Assessment of oesophagitis (Los Angeles Classification System)

Grade[1)]	Endoscopic finding[2)]
A	One or more mucosal breaks no longer than 5 mm, none of which extends across the tops of the mucosal folds
B	One or more mucosal breaks more than 5 mm long, none of which extends across the tops of two mucosal folds
C	Mucosal breaks that extend across the tops of two or more mucosal folds, but which involve less than 75% of the oesophageal circumference
D	Mucosal breaks that involve at least 75% of the oesophageal circumference

1. Grades C and D = Severe oesophagitis. The complications of oesophagitis, such as strictures, ulcers and Barret's metaplasia are graded separately.
2. Mucosal break is a clearly distinct reddish or fibrin-covered area.

- Endoscopical recovery
- Prevention of relapse
- Prevention of complications

Lifestyle changes and antacid therapy

- Lifestyle changes and antacids are often unsatisfactory.
  - Elevation of the head of the bed (a water mattress is unsuitable)
  - Reduction of body weight
  - Avoidance of evening meals
  - Frequent, small meals
  - Avoidance of irritating foods (citrus fruit, strong beverages, tomatoes, coffee)
  - Stopping smoking
  - Avoidance of certain drugs (nitrates, calcium antagonists, anticholinergics, theophylline preparations)
  - Alginate or antacids when needed

Drug therapy

- Drug therapy is similar in non-endoscoped, endoscopy-negative and mild oesophagitis.
- For grades of severity of oesophagitis see LA classification above.
- Curing symptoms and oesophagitis
  - Mild oesophagitis (grade A and B)
    - Proton-pump inhibitor for 4–6 weeks **A** [1]
      - Esomeprazole 40 mg × 1
      - Omeprazole 20 mg × 1 **B** [2]
      - Lansoprazole 30 mg × 1 **A** [3 4]
      - Pantoprazole 40 mg × 1
      - Rabeprazole 20 mg × 1
    - H_2-blocker as a normal dose twice a day (ranitidine, nizatidine 150 mg × 2, famotidine 20 mg × 2) for 12 weeks
    - Cisapride should no longer be used because of the risk of arrhythmias.
  - Severe symptoms of grade C or D oesophagitis **A** [1]
    - Esomeprazole 40 mg × 1 for 8–12 weeks
    - Omeprazole 20–40 mg × 1–2 for 8–12 weeks **B** [2]
    - Lansoprazole 30 mg × 1–2 for 8–12 weeks **A** [3 4]
    - Pantoprazole 40 mg × 1–2 for 8–12 weeks
    - Rabeprazole 20 mg × 1–2 for 8–12 weeks
- Prevention of recurrence (oesophagitis or symptoms recur in 60–80% of the patients within one year.)
  - No oesophagitis or mild oesophagitis
    - Proton-pump inhibitor **C** [5 6 7 8] once a day. The smallest dose is often sufficient.
    - Cisapride is not recommended.
    - Esomeprazole 20 mg is effective also when used on demand as symptoms recur.
  - Moderate or severe oesophagitis
    - Proton-pump inhibitor **C** [5 6 7 8] once a day as a normal dose or low therapeutic dose.
      - Omeprazole 10–20 mg × 1
      - Lansoprazole 15–30 mg × 1
      - Pantoprazole 20–40 mg × 1
      - Esomeprazole 20 mg × 1

Long-term treatment

- Symptoms of reflux disease recur in 80% of the patients within one year of the cessation of antisecretory therapy.
  - At present, the aim is to use the mildest therapy that keeps the patient free of symptoms.
- Long-term maintenance therapy with proton pump inhibitors is effective and safe.
- **Surgery** (Nissen fundoplication) is required in about 10% of cases. The indications are the following:
  - Oesophagitis does not respond to drug therapy or recurs frequently.
  - Complications of oesophagitis: strictures, Barrett's epithelium and continuous oesophagitis, haemorrhage, severe symptoms of aspiration.

Follow-up

- Mild oesophagitis need not be followed up endoscopically if the symptoms are alleviated.
- The healing of severe or moderate oesophagitis must be confirmed endoscopically. Endoscopy is also indicated if the symptoms change.
- In Barrett's oesophagus follow-up endoscopy is indicated at 2-year intervals, irrespective of whether active oesophagitis has healed. Patients with Barrett's oesophagus carry an increased risk for adenocarcinoma.
- If no oesophagitis is detected in endoscopy, the reflux disease should be treated in the same way as reflux oesophagitis. Repeated endoscopy or follow-up is unnecessary if the symptoms subside.

Primary motility disorders of the oesophagus

- See also 8.4.
- The goal of treatment is to alleviate symptoms and prevent complications, particularly pulmonary complications of achalasia.

Treatment of motility disorders

- Drug therapy can be tried as initial treatment for diffuse oesophageal spasms. The results vary.
  - Short-acting glyceryl nitrate before meals or
  - Isosorbide mononitrate before meals.
- If the symptoms do not respond to nitrates, try calcium channel blockers such as nifedipine or diltiazem. Note that calcium antagonists may increase reflux symptoms.
- The treatment of choice for achalasia is pneumatic dilatation. If this fails myotomy (Heller operation) is recommended.

References

1. van Pinxteren B, Numans ME, Bonis PA, Lau J. Short-term treatment with proton pump inhibitors, H2-receptor antagonists and prokinetics for gastro-oesophageal reflux disease-like symptoms and endoscopy negative reflux disease. Cochrane Database Syst Rev. 2004;(2):CD002095.
2. Vroomen PC, de Krom MC, Wilmink JT, Kester AD, Knottnerus JA. Lack of effectiveness of bed rest for sciatica. N Engl J Med 1999;340(6):418–23.
3. Manzionna G, Page F, Bianchi Porro G. Efficacy of lansoprazole in the short- and long-term treatment of gastro-oesophageal reflux disease: a systematic overview. Clin Drug Invest 1997;14:450–456.
4. The Database of Abstracts of Reviews of Effectiveness (University of York), Database no.: DARE-980160. In: The Cochrane Library, Issue 4, 1999. Oxford: Update Software.
5. Garg PP, Kerlikowske K, Subak L, Grady D. Hormone replacement therapy and the risk of epithelial ovarian carcinoma: a meta-analysis. Obstetrics and Gynecology 1998;92:472–479.
6. The Database of Abstracts of Reviews of Effectiveness (University of York), Database no.: DARE-981528. In: The Cochrane Library, Issue 1, 2001. Oxford: Update Software.
7. Lacey JV, Mink PJ, Lubin JH, Sherman ME, Troisi R, Hartge P, Schatzkin A, Schairer C. Menopausal hormone replacement therapy and risk of ovarian cancer. JAMA 2002;288:334–341.
8. Anderson GI, Judd HI, Kaunitz AM, Barad DH, Beresford SAA, Pettinger M, Liu J, McNeeley SG, Lopez AM. Effect of estrogen plus progestin on gynecologic cancers and associated diagnostic procedures. JAMA 2003;290:1739–1748.

8.31 Dyspepsia

Pekka Pikkarainen

Basic rules

- Gastroscopy is the primary investigation for a dyspeptic patient.
- A therapeutic trial before further investigations is indicated in patients below 50 years of age who do not use NSAIDs (A) [1 2 3].
- Upper abdominal ultrasonography is not useful as a primary investigation.
- The policy of determination of antibodies against Helicobacter pylori or performing urea breath test followed by eradication in test-positive patients depends on the availability and cost of gastroscopy (A) [1 2 3].

Epidemiology

- Dyspepsia is a common symptom. Dyspeptic symptoms occur in 20–40% of the population, at an equal frequency in women and men. Dyspeptic symptoms in the past 6 months are reported more often in people aged 20–40 years than in older people, with the exception of heartburn, which is less common in the younger age group.
- Dyspepsia is the main complaint in 3% of all encounters in primary care. According to interviews, only a quarter of dyspeptic people consult a doctor. The probability of consultation is
    - not dependent on the severity of symptoms
    - more common in the lower social classes and the elderly
    - dependent on how concerned the patient is about the symptoms.

Causes of dyspepsia

- According to endoscopic studies the following causes can be identified (B) [4 5]:
    - Peptic ulcer 18%
    - Oesophagitis 15%
    - Duodenitis 8%
    - Gastric cancer 2%
    - Functional dyspepsia 57%
- **Functional dyspepsia** can be defined as pain or discomfort centred in upper abdomen without an organic cause explaining the symptoms. If heartburn and acid regurgitation are the main symptoms **gastro-oesophageal reflux disease** is usually diagnosed. Helicobacter gastritis is not associated with symptoms.

Diagnostics

Symptoms and signs suggesting organic disease and requiring further investigations

- Age above 50 years
- Symptoms
    - Severe
    - Long-lasting symptoms that have not been investigated before
    - Pain radiating in the back
    - Melaena, haematochezia
    - Repeated vomiting
    - Feeling of food getting stuck in the oesophagus, dysphagia
    - Objectively verified weight loss (8.1)
- Anaemia
- Heavy smoking
- Excess consumption of alcohol
- Use of NSAIDs
- Heredity
    - Peptic ulcer disease
    - Gastric cancer
    - Coeliac disease
- Severe cancerophobia

Findings suggesting functional dyspepsia that allow the use of a therapeutic trial before further investigations

- Age below 50 years
- Symptoms
  - Short-lived
  - Mild
  - No weight loss
  - Normal colour of the faeces
- Results of the basic laboratory tests are normal

Types and symptoms of functional dyspepsia

- Dysmotility-like dyspepsia
  - Feeling of non-painful sensation (discomfort) in the upper abdomen
  - Abdominal fullness and early satiety
  - Nausea
  - Variable food intolerance
  - Temporary symptoms suggesting irritable bowel syndrome may coexist
- Ulcer-like dyspepsia
  - Pain centred in upper abdomen
- Symptoms suggesting aerophagia
  - Repeated belching without relief of symptoms
  - Abdominal swelling, nausea
  - The symptoms occur at the same time of the day (after the meal)
  - The symptoms are exacerbated by stress.

Diagnostic strategy

- Musculoskeletal pain can be differentiated from gastrointestinal pain by clinical examination. Epigastric tenderness is as common in peptic ulcer disease as in functional dyspepsia.
- If the patient has symptoms suggesting an organic disease the following laboratory tests can be performed: blood count, serum ALT, serum alkaline phosphatase. The chronological order of further examinations is as follows.

1. Test of Helicobacter pylori and treatment of positive patients or upper gastrointestinal endoscopy and biopsies verifying:
   - Gastro-oesophageal reflux disease
   - Strictures
   - Peptic ulcer disease and gastric mucosal erosions
   - Tumours
   - Coeliac disease
   - Giardiasis (diagnosed from duodenal biopsies)
2. Lactose provocation test
   - Lactose intolerance
3. 24-hour pH monitoring of the oesophagus
   - Indicated if a therapeutic trial of proton-pump inhibitors does not bring adequate long-term relief, and oesophageal reflux disease is suspected.
4. Upper abdominal ultrasonography
   - Gallstone disease
   - Pancreatic tumours
   - Most gallstones are asymptomatic. Dyspeptic symptoms are as frequent in patients with gallstones as in patients without them. Therefore, gallstones detected in dyspeptic patients should not be considered the cause of the dyspepsia **C** [6]. Belt-like epigastric pain lasting several hours is typical of gallstones. Upper abdominal ultrasonography should be performed only after gastroscopy, lactose provocation test, and therapeutic trials for functional dyspepsia have been performed and their results have been negative.
5. Others: computed tomography, ERCP, colonoscopy, etc.

Antibodies against Helicobacter pylori or urea breath test

- Gastritis caused by chronic Helicobacter infection is common and does not cause symptoms.
- Helicobacter test can be used when patients under 50 years of age are selected for gastroscopy. The patients with a positive test result can be treated with antibiotics with no further examination **A** [1 2 3]. A negative result means that the patient probably does not have an ulcer unless they have used NSAIDs.
- If gastroscopy is performed in any event there is no indication for a non-invasive Helicobacter test because the detection of Helicobacter from biopsies is reliable.

Therapeutic trials before definite diagnosis

- A therapeutic trial of 4–8 weeks with proton pump inhibitors can be performed on a patient below 50 years of age before further investigations **A** [1 2 3].
- A therapeutic trial is also indicated first if the patient has been previously examined for similar symptoms and the results have been negative.

Treatment of functional dyspepsia

- The aim of treatment is to make the patient understand the functional nature of the symptoms and their tendency to recur.
- The visceral threshold for pain may be lowered, but the pain is real, not imaginary. A good doctor–patient relationship is essential and prevents a vicious circle of multiple investigations.
- When ordering diagnostic tests in patients below 50 years of age it is wise to anticipate that their results will probably be normal. Such an approach may help to avoid unnecessary repeated investigations.
- Follow-up examination has shown that the symptoms of functional dyspepsia decrease for a few months after endoscopy but recur thereafter.
- Very few patients develop an organic disease during follow-up.
- For the treatment of dyspepsia, reflux oesophagitis and peptic ulcer disease see 8.32.

Further investigations after a therapeutic trial

- If the patient's symptom is not relieved in 2 weeks or if there are symptoms after a 4–8 week therapeutic trial the patient should be referred for endoscopy.
- The sensitivity and specificity of double-contrast gastric radiography is inferior to endoscopy in the diagnosis of oesophagitis, peptic ulcer disease and early gastric carcinoma.

Upper abdominal ultrasonography in the assessment of dyspepsia

- Upper abdominal ultrasonography is of less importance in the assessment of dyspepsia unless the symptoms suggest
  - gallstone disease (bouts of severe steady epigastric pain lasting for hours, abnormal results of liver function tests)
  - chronic pancreatitis (history of alcohol abuse)
  - cancer of the pancreas.

Organic causes of dyspepsia

Reflux oesophagitis

- See 8.30.
- If the patient has erosive oesophagitis the treatment should last 1–3 months. Control endoscopy after treatment is usually not needed. The risk of recurrence is considerable after the treatment is discontinued.
- If the patient has severe reflux symptoms but no oesophagitis endoscopically 24-hour ambulatory pH monitoring is useful in making the diagnostics and selecting treatment.

Peptic ulcer

- A **gastric ulcer** can be malignant (in about 5% of cases) and should always be biopsied. Healing must be confirmed by endoscopy. NSAID use is a risk factor. Helicobacter pylori must be eradicated.
- A **duodenal ulcer** is hardly ever malignant. Healing of the ulcer need not be confirmed by endoscopy. Helicobacter pylori must be eradicated in all patients, including those who have had an ulcer in the past but who have remained symptom-free with acid-suppressing drugs.

Gallstone disease

- See 9.24.
- Dyspeptic symptoms are as common in people with gallstones as in those without them.
- Only a typical gallstone colic–epigastric or right-sided severe pain radiating in the back–can be considered as a specific symptom of gallstone disease. In such cases upper abdominal ultrasonography is the primary investigation.

Chronic pancreatitis

- See 9.31.
- A rare cause of abdominal pain, usually associated with chronic alcohol consumption.
- Ultrasonography is often diagnostic in severe pancreatitis. Mild forms can be diagnosed by secretin stimulation test and endoscopic retrograde pancreatography (ERP) or magnetic resonance cholangiopancreatography (MRCP).
- The determination of faecal elastase is useful in the diagnosis of moderate or severe pancreatic insufficiency.

Coeliac disease

- See 8.84.
- Mild coeliac disease causes vague dyspeptic symptoms.
- Duodenal biopsies taken during gastroscopy are essential in the diagnosis.

Lactose intolerance

- See 8.83.
- In dysmotility-type dyspepsia lactose intolerance should be ruled out by a lactose provocation test, with observation of symptoms caused by the test.
- Hypolactasia can also be established with genotyping.
- Another diagnostic approach is to observe the symptoms during a 2 week elimination of lactose from the diet.

Gastric cancer

- Gastric cancer may cause symptoms at the initial stage. The risk of cancer increases with age. Therefore, in elderly patients gastroscopy must be performed more readily.
- The treatment consists of surgical resection. Adjuvant chemotherapy is probably not beneficial (B) [7 8].

References

1. Delaney BC, Moayyedi P, Forman D. Initial management strategies for dyspepsia. Cochrane Database Syst Rev. 2004;(2): CD001961.
2. Ofman JJ, Rabeneck L. The effectiveness of endoscopy in the management of dyspepsia: a qualitative systematic review. Am J Med 1999;106:335–346.
3. The Database of Abstracts of Reviews of Effectiveness (University of York), Database no.: DARE-990745. In: The Cochrane Library, Issue 4, 2000. Oxford: Update Software.
4. Colin-Jones DC. Practical approaches to the management of dyspepsia. The Medicine Group, Langhorne, Pennsylvania 1989.
5. Heikkinen M, Pikkarainen P, Takala J, Räsänen H, Julkunen R. Etiology of dyspepsia: Four hundred unselected consecutive patients in general practice. Scand J Gastroenterol 1995;30: 519–523.
6. Heikkinen M, Pikkarainen P, Takala J, Räsänen H, Julkunen R. Etiology of dyspepsia: Four hundred unselected consecutive patients in general practice. Scand J Gastroenterol 1995;30:519–523.
7. Agboola O. Adjuvant treatment in gastric cancer. Cancer treatment Reviews 1994;20:217–240.

8. The Database of Abstracts of Reviews of Effectiveness (University of York), Database no.: DARE-940336. In: The Cochrane Library, Issue 4, 1999. Oxford: Update Software.

8.32 Treatment of dyspepsia, peptic ulcer and helicobacter infection

Pekka Pikkarainen

Basic rules

- Mild dyspeptic symptoms can be treated on the basis of the clinical picture.
- If heartburn or acid regurgitation are the main symptom, the patient has gastro-oesophageal reflux oesophagitis (8.30).
- Determination of Helicobacter pylori antibodies or breath urea test and the treatment of positive cases is an efficient and safe approach to the management of patients below 50 years of age without alarming symptoms.
  - In patients with functional dyspepsia, the effect of Helicobacter pylori eradication on the symptoms is limited (A) [1]; however, the associated peptic ulcer will be cured.
- If dyspeptic symptoms are severe (8.31) or occur for the first time at the age of 50 year or above, treatment should not be started before gastroscopy.
- Helicobacter pylori must always be eradicated in a patient with a gastric or duodenal ulcer.

Definition of dyspepsia

- Dyspepsia (8.31) is defined as pain or discomfort centred in the upper abdomen with the source of pain located in the upper gastrointestinal tract.
- Dyspepsia can be caused by a peptic ulcer, gastric cancer or (in most cases) by a functional disorder.

Therapeutic trial for heartburn or retrosternal pain

- If the symptoms are present daily and have lasted for more than 4 weeks, gastroscopy should be performed.
- Depending on the frequency and severity of symptoms
  - Liquid-form or chewable antacids, sucralfate, or alginate on demand
  - Proton pump inhibitor once daily or H_2-blocker twice daily
  - Proton pump inhibitor 1–2 times a day
- Advice on lifestyle modifications
  - For treatment of reflux, see 8.30.

Therapeutic trial for ulcer-like dyspepsia

- The pain awakens the patient at night and is relieved by meals.
- The patient is below 50 years of age.
- The duration of the pain should not exceed 2–4 weeks. If the pain lasts longer or recurs, gastroscopy should be performed.
- Helicobacter test and eradication (A) [1]
- Proton pump inhibitor once a day
- H_2-blocker after supper or for the night as one dose

Therapeutic trial for other types of dyspepsia

- The placebo effect is considerable.
  - Antacids can be tried.
- Spastic symptoms
  - Anticholinergic drugs
- Abdominal swelling, feeling of satiety
  - Metoclopramide 10 mg × 3 before meals
- Dyspepsia symptoms can also be treated with the helicobacter eradication regimen (A) [1]

Treatment of peptic ulcer (both gastric and duodenal ulcer)

- Eradication of Helicobacter pylori (see below) is always indicated if an infection has been detected by rapid urea test or biopsy.
- Smoking and NSAID use should be stopped (paracetamol is allowed).
- If the rapid test for Helicobacter is negative (and before the results of biopsies are available)
  - A proton pump inhibitor (A) [2 3 4 5 6 7] (esomeprazole 40 mg × 1, omeprazole 20 mg × 1 (A) [8 9 10 11], lansoprazole 30 mg × 1 (A) [12 13], pantoprazole 40 mg × 1 or rabeprazole 20 mg × 1).
- If a peptic ulcer has not been cured in 8 weeks, a proton pump inhibitor once a day in the morning for 8 weeks is the most effective further treatment.

Helicobacter infection

Epidemiology

- In most patients the infection is symptomless; however, in 10–20% it results over the years in the development of a gastric or duodenal ulcer and increases the risk of stomach cancer by 2–6 fold.

Diagnosis

- In previously untreated patients the following tests are recommended before gastroscopy: IgG class antibody determination or ^{13}C urea breath test. Faecal antigen determination is also an option.
- The sensitivity and specificity of qualitative whole blood serology are not always satisfactory.
- When the tests are taken in connection with endoscopy, biopsy and urease test are the best methods.
- At present screening of the symptom-free population is not considered justified.

Treatment of helicobacter pylori infection

- **Duodenal or gastric ulcer in a patient with** Helicobacter **infection is always an indication for eradication of the microbe** A [14 15 16 17 18 19].
- Helicobacter eradication can be carried out without gastroscopy in helicobacter-positive dyspepsia patients who are below 50 years of age and do not have severe symptoms (8.31).
- Nowadays, eradication is recommended also in cases of persistent functional dyspepsia after thorough investigation, although controlled studies have shown that this therapy alleviates the symptoms of dyspepsia only in a small minority of patients A [1].
- A rapid urease test for Helicobacter pylori should be performed during gastroscopy. If the test is positive, eradication can be started immediately.
- **See Table 8.32 for treatment recommendation** A [20 21 22 23].
  - Metronidazole is not included in the first-line recommendation because resistence of H. pylori to metronidazole is common (clarithromycin is recommended as first-line drug if metronidazole resistance is above 30%) B [24 25].
  - Resistence to amoxicillin has not been detected. Proton pump inhibitors A [20 21 22 23] and ranitidine bismuth citrate A [26 27 28] are probably as effective.

Table 8.32 Recommended eradication treatment for Helicobacter pylori

Primary treatment	Repeated treatment after one unsuccessful treatment
• Proton pump inhibitor, normal dose[1)] + clarithromycin 500 mg + amoxicillin 1 g, all drugs twice daily for 7 days OR Ranitidine bismuth citrate 400 mg + clarithromycin 500 mg + amoxicillin 1 g, all drugs twice daily for 7 days	Ranitidine bismuth citrate 400 mg × 2 + metronidazole 400 mg × 3 + tetracycline 500 mg × 4 for 7 days

- Omeprazole 20 mg, esomeprazole 40 mg, lansoprazole 30 mg, pantoprazole 40 mg, rabeprazole 20 mg or esomeprazole 20 mg

- The duration of the treatment is 7 days. In active peptic ulcer disease the proton pump inhibitor can be continued for 2–4 weeks. Esomeprazole 40 mg × 2, lansoprazole 30 mg × 2, pantoprazole 40 mg × 2 or rabeprazole 20 mg × 2 can be used instead of omeprazole.
- A combination of only two drugs is less effective and should not be used.
- Preceding treatment with a H_2-blocker or proton pump inhibitor is not a contraindication for eradication treatment.
- Repeated treatment must be based on the detection of persistent infection, not only on symptoms (or serology) that remains positive for a long time after eradication.
- Consult a gastroenterologist if eradication fails even with a second-line drug regimen.
- Eradication is successful in 85–90% of adult patients C [29 30] and in at least 75% of children B [31 32 33] given triple therapy.
- **It is essential to motivate the patient to continue the medication despite mild adverse effects.** In practice adverse effects rarely prevent completing the course of treatment, with the exception of allergic reactions (most often caused by amoxicillin). The most common adverse effects include
  - abdominal symptoms and diarrhoea
  - taste of metal (metronidazole) or dark colour of faeces (bismuth).
- H. pylori develops resistance to metronidazole and clarithromycin, but not to amoxicillin.
- **The success of the eradication must be verified in duodenal ulcer disease by a urea breath test** or fecal antigen test one month after cessation of the treatment (sampling can be performed in ambulatory care or even at home).
- **The healing of a gastric ulcer must always be confirmed endoscopically** because the ulcer may be caused by carcinoma. During endoscopy biopsies should be taken to verify the success of the eradication.

References

1. Moayyedi P, Soo S, Deeks J, Delaney B, Harris A, Innes M, Oakes R, Wilson S, Roalfe A, Bennett C, Forman D. Eradication of Helicobacter pylori for non-ulcer dyspepsia. Cochrane Database Syst Rev. 2004;(2):CD002096.
2. Poynard T, Lemaire M, Agostini H. Meta-analysis of randomised clinical trials comparing lansoprazole with ranitidine or famotidine in the treatment of acute duodenal ulcer. Eur J Gastroenterol Hepatol 1995;7:661–665.
3. The Database of Abstracts of Reviews of Effectiveness (University of York), Database no.: DARE-952659. In: The Cochrane Library, Issue 4, 1999. Oxford: Update Software.
4. Eriksson S, Langstrom G, Rikner L, Carlsson R, Naesdal J. Omeprazole and H_2-receptor antagonists in the acute treatment of duodenal ulcer, gastric ulcer and reflux oesophagitis. Eur J Gastroenterol Hepatol 1995;7:467–475.
5. The Database of Abstracts of Reviews of Effectiveness (University of York), Database no.: DARE-951295. In: The Cochrane Library, Issue 4, 1999. Oxford: Update Software.

6. Langtry HD, Wilde MI. Omeprazole: a review of its use in helicobacter pylori infection, gastro-oesophageal reflux disease and peptic ulcers induced by NSAIDs. Drugs 1998;56:447–486.
7. The Database of Abstracts of Reviews of Effectiveness (University of York), Database no.: DARE-981678. In: The Cochrane Library, Issue 3, 2000. Oxford: Update Software.
8. Meta-analyses of cisapride, omeprazole and ranitidine in the treatment of gastrooesophageal reflux disease: implications for treating patient subgroups. Clin Drug Invest 1998;16:9–18.
9. The Database of Abstracts of Reviews of Effectiveness (University of York), Database no.: DARE-981284. In: The Cochrane Library, Issue 2, 2000. Oxford: Update Software.
10. Tunis SR, Sheinhait IA, Schmid CH, Bishop DJ, Ross SD. Lansoprazole compared with histamine-2-receptor antagonists in healing gastric ulcers: a meta-analysis. Clin Therap 1997;19:743–757.
11. The Database of Abstracts of Reviews of Effectiveness (University of York), Database no.: DARE-971237. In: The Cochrane Library, Issue 2, 2000. Oxford: Update Software.
12. Moore RA. Helicobacter pylori and peptic ulcer: a systematic review of effectiveness and an overview of the economic benefits of implementing what is known to be effective. Oxford: Pain Relief Research Unit VII 1995;37.
13. The Database of Abstracts of Reviews of Effectiveness (University of York), Database no.: DARE-950348. In: The Cochrane Library, Issue 4, 1999. Oxford: Update Software.
14. Laine L, Hopkins RJ, Girardi LS. Has the impact of Helicobacter pylori therapy on ulcer recurrence in the United States been overstated: a meta-analysis of rigorously designed trials. Am J Gastroenterol 1998;93:1409–1415.
15. The Database of Abstracts of Reviews of Effectiveness (University of York), Database no.: DARE-981610. In: The Cochrane Library, Issue 2, 2000. Oxford: Update Software.
16. Hopkins RJ, Girardi LS, Turney EA. Relationship between Helicobacter pylori eradication and reduced duodenal and gastric ulcer recurrence: a review. Gastroenterology 1996;110: 1244–1252.
17. The Database of Abstracts of Reviews of Effectiveness (University of York), Database no.: DARE-960755. In: The Cochrane Library, Issue 4, 1999. Oxford: Update Software.
18. Penston JG, McColl KE. Eradication of Helicobacter pylori: an objective assessment of current therapies. Br J Clin Pharmacol 1997;43:223–243.
19. The Database of Abstracts of Reviews of Effectiveness (University of York), Database no.: DARE-970424. In: The Cochrane Library, Issue 4, 1999. Oxford: Update Software.
20. Evaluation of treatment regiments to cure Helicobacter pylori infection: a meta-analysis. Aliment Pharmacol Ther 1999;13:857–864.
21. The Database of Abstracts of Reviews of Effectiveness (University of York), Database no.: DARE-991562. In: The Cochrane Library, Issue 2, 2001. Oxford: Update Software.
22. Houben MH, Van de Beek D, Hensen EF, De Craen AJ, Rauws EA, Tytgat GN. A systematic review of Helicobacter pylori eradication therapy: the impact of antimicrobial resistance on eradication rates. Aliment Pharmacol Ther 1999;13:1047–1055.
23. The Database of Abstracts of Reviews of Effectiveness (University of York), Database no.: DARE-991702. In: The Cochrane Library, Issue 1, 2001. Oxford: Update Software.
24. Vondracek TG. Ranitidine bismuth substrate in the treatment of Helicobacter pylori infection and duodenal ulcer. Ann Pharmacother 1998;32:672–679.
25. The Database of Abstracts of Reviews of Effectiveness (University of York), Database no.: DARE-981113. In: The Cochrane Library, Issue 2, 2000. Oxford: Update Software.
26. Pipkin GA, Williamson R, Wood JR. Review article: one week clarithromycin triple therapy regimens for eradication of Helicobacter pylori. Aliment Pharmacol Ther 1998;12:823–37.
27. Xia HX, Talley NJ, Keane CT, O'Morain CA. Recurrence of Helicobacter pylori infection after successful eradication: nature and possible causes. Dig Dis Sci 1997;42:1821–1834.
28. The Database of Abstracts of Reviews of Effectiveness (University of York), Database no.: DARE-971219. In: The Cochrane Library, Issue 4, 1999. Oxford: Update Software.
29. Oderda G, Rapa A, Bona G. A systematic review of Helicobacter pylori eradication treatment schedules in children. Aliment Pharmacol Ther 2000, 14(Supplement 3), 59–66.
30. The Database of Abstracts of Reviews of Effectiveness (University of York), Database no.: DARE-20002174. In: The Cochrane Library, Issue 3, 2002. Oxford: Update Software.
31. Gottrand F, Kalach N, Spyckerelle C, Guimber D, Mougenot JF, Tounian P, Lenaerts C, Roquelaure B, Lachaux A, Morali A, Dupont C, Maurage C, Husson MO, Barthélemy P. Omeprazole combined with amoxicillin and clarithromycin in the eradication of Helicobacter pylori in children with gastritis: A prospective randomized double-blind trial. J Pediatr 2001;139:664–668.

8.33 Safe use of non-steroidal anti-inflammatory drugs (NSAIDs)

Arja Helin-Salmivaara

NSAID-induced peptic ulcer disease

- Approximately 25% of long-term users of NSAIDs develop a chronic gastric or duodenal ulcer. Gastric ulcer is approximately twice as common as duodenal ulcer.
- Risk factors for a NSAID-induced ulcer include
  - age over 65 years
  - a history of previous ulcer
  - concurrent corticosteroid, anticoagulant or SSRI treatment
  - concurrent use of more than one NSAIDs
  - large daily dose of an NSAID
  - treatment duration of 1-3 months.
- NSAID-induced ulcer is often asymptomatic, and it may first present as bleed or perforation. Less than half of the patients have abdominal symptoms indicative of an ulcer before complications develop.

- Of the patients with life-threatening ulcer related complications approximately 60% have a history of NSAID use. Among ulcer related deaths the corresponding figure is as high as 80%.
- The NSAID used by a patient with peptic ulcer should be withdrawn or replaced by a safer drug (e.g. paracetamol).
- Both Helicobacter pylori (HP) infection and NSAID use seem to increase the risk of peptic ulcer independently. HP eradication is always indicated in a patient with NSAID-associated ulcer with HP positive gastritis. Screening for, and eradication of, HP infection before starting NSAID treatment is recommended, particularly in high-risk patients.
- NSAIDs can also harm the small intestine and cause colitis as well as aggravate reflux oesophagitis.

Preventive treatment of NSAID-induced peptic ulcers

- Misoprostol is a synthetic analogue of prostaglandin E1, and it effectively prevents gastroduodenal ulceration and associated complications among NSAID users (A) [1 2 3]. The recommended prophylactic dose is 200 µg 2–3 times daily. The combination of misoprostol and an NSAID (diclofenac) is a good choice for some patients, although gastrointestinal adverse effects (mainly diarrhoea) may restrict its use.
- Proton pump inhibitors (e.g. omeprazole 20 mg o.d.) are slightly more effective than misoprostol in the prevention of erosions and particularly ulcers associated with NSAIDs, and have fewer adverse effects.

Renal effects and blood pressure

- Acute renal failure may develop rapidly after commencing NSAID treatment in patients with risk factors, such as advanced age, diabetes, heart failure, dehydration, infection and use of other drugs. The disorder is reversible upon discontinuation of the medication.
- The possibility of analgesic nephropathy, usually associated with products containing phenacetin, has been known for a long time. Long-term use of NSAIDs can apparently also cause a chronic form of analgesic nephropathy, but the incidence of the disease is not known. Furthermore, the effect of NSAIDs on the progression of chronic kidney disease has not been established.
- NSAIDs can cause hyperkalaemia, fluid retention and hyponatraemia.
- NSAID treatment may reduce the efficacy of diuretics and other antihypertensive agents.

Asthma and allergies

- NSAIDs cause bronchospam in 5–10% of the patients with astma. Patients whose asthma symptoms include rhinitis and nasal polyps are particularly prone to this kind of hypersensitivity.
- The bronchospasm is a class effect of NSAIDs. All NSAIDs are contraindicated for patients who have ever developed a serious asthma attack after taking an NSAID.

Micturition disturbances

- Tolfenamic acid causes dysuria in some patients, which resolves rapidly after the medication is stopped.
- Long-term use of tiaprofenic acid has been reported as having caused severe cystitis in some patients.

Selective and specific inhibitors of COX-2

- The gastrointestinal effects of moderately selective COX-2 inhibitors (meloxicam, nabumetone, nimesulide, etodolac) are dose dependent. According to epidemiological studies they appear to be somewhat safer for the gastrointestinal tract than the non-selective NSAIDs.
- During the use of selective COX-2 inhibitors, i.e. coxibs, (celecoxib (B) [4], parecoxib which is suitable for postoperative pain relief and the recently licensed etoricoxib) the incidence of endoscopically verified gastroduodenal ulcers is similar to that observed with placebo. Furthermore, coxibs do not affect blood clotting. With the use of coxibs the incidence of symptomatic and complicated ulcers is halved, as compared with non-selective NSAIDs. The safety of coxibs may be lost in patients who require concurrent low-dose acetylsalicylic acid for thrombosis prophylaxis. Rofecoxib was withdrawn in October 2004 because of increased risk for cardiovascular events in long-term (>18 months) use.
- Coxibs may cause fluid retention to the same degree as non-selective NSAIDs. Coxibs should be administered with caution to patients with renal impairment.

Prescribing NSAIDs

- When prescribing always consider whether an analgesic other than NSAID would be suitable.
  - An NSAID is usually the best choice for inflammatory rheumatic disease, pain caused by acute injury or acute back pain. On the other hand, for pain in osteoarthritis, paracetamol or an opioid may be more effective and safe.
  - A NSAID should hardly ever be prescribed for chronic back pain.
- An increase in the dose of any NSAID significantly increases the risk of adverse effects. The differences between the various drugs are partly attributable to the fact that some drugs are generally prescribed in smaller doses than others. NSAIDs that are administered as injections or as suppositories are not safer than those used orally; however, products that are absorbed through the skin have been found to cause no other systemic adverse effects than attacks of asthma, which are extremely rare.
- The adverse effect profiles of different NSAIDs vary. Of the older drugs, particularly ibuprofen seems relatively safe regarding gastrointestinal toxicity, while piroxicam seems to carry the highest risk. Diclofenac affects liver function more often than the other drugs.

- Assess the risks involving the gastrointestinal tract and kidneys, particularly in patients aged 65 or more.
- Consider other risk factors and the possibility of drug interactions.
- Choose a COX-2 selective drug for patients at high risk for gastrointestinal adverse effects, or use protective medication. The cost-effectiveness of COX-2 selective NSAIDs is poor, unless their use is limited to high-risk patients.
- Select a suitable preparation for the patient's symptoms, regarding the timing of its action and required dose.
- Slow-release preparations may be suitable as a short course for acute pain, but rapidly acting preparations may enable more precise and safe dosing in long-term use.
- Check the indications for the medication at regular intervals: is the drug used to treat pain or inflammation?
- Ensure that the patient is informed of possible adverse effects and the appropriate measures to be taken should they occur.

References

1. Rostom A, Dube C, Wells G, Tugwell P, Welch V, Jolicoeur E, McGowan J. Prevention of NSAID-induced gastroduodenal ulcers. Cochrane Database Syst Rev. 2004;(2):CD002296.
2. Koch M, Dezi A, Ferrario F, Capurso L. Prevention of nonsteroidal anti-inflammatory drug-induced gastrointestinal mucosal: a meta-analysis of randomised controlled trials. Arch Intern Med 1996;156:2321–2332.
3. The Database of Abstracts of Reviews of Effectiveness (University of York), Database no.: DARE-968492. In: The Cochrane Library, Issue 4, 1999. Oxford: Update Software.
4. Simon LS, Weaver AL, Graham DY, Kivitz AJ, Lipsky PE, Hubbard RC, Isakson PC, Verburg KM, Yu SS, Zhao WW, Geis GS. Anti-inflammatory and upper gastrointestinal effects of celecoxib in rheumatoid arthritis. A randomized controlled trial. JAMA 1999;282:1921–1928.

8.40 Orientation on diarrhoea in adult patients

Tapio Pitkänen

Aims

- Identify patients with diarrhoea needing emergency surgical intervention.
  - Acute appendicitis
  - Intestinal obstruction
- Identify and treat patients who are suffering from a curable infection (8.41) (8.42).
  - Infections caused by bacteria
  - Colitis caused by Clostridium difficile
  - Simultaneous diarrhoea and malaria or bacterial meningitis
- Identify patients who have an infection with no known effective therapy, and those who are suffering from secondary diarrhoea, not from an infectious disease.
- Laboratory resources should be used with discretion for both the patient's benefit and for restricting communicable diseases that are significant from a public health viewpoint.
- A swift and systematic approach is good when there is solid evidence of a food-borne epidemic.
- The possibility of HIV infection should be remembered when diarrhoea has continued for more than two months.

GAS

Signs pointing to infectious diarrhoea

- Clearly abrupt onset of diarrhoea
- Fever, vomiting, aches in the limbs
- An intense sense of sickness in bacterial gastroenteritis
- Bowel sounds are strong and rapid

Important history

- Has the patient recently been on antibiotics?
- Has the patient or someone in the family been travelling; country, town, hotel?
- Does anyone in the family work in food production or delivery business?
- Is anyone else ill in the neighbourhood?
- Does the family have children in a daycare centre?

Incubation period and aetiology

- See Table 8.40

Types of diarrhoea

- In food poisoning, watery diarrhoea and vomiting; botulism is an exception
- Watery diarrhoea, no fever, no severe abdominal pain
- Dysentery (bloody faeces, fever, often abdominal pain)
- Typhoid syndrome; headache, high fever, sense of sickness, abdominal pain, nausea and relative bradycardia, i.e. pulse

Table 8.40 Incubation period and aetiology of infectious diarrhoea

Incubation period	Aetiology
1–2 days	Food poisoning
1–5 days	Virus
3–10 days	Bacteria
10–20 days	Salmonella typhi
♦ range 4–50 days	♦ severely ill patient

rate under 100 per minute when fever is over 39°C (100.2°F).

- Typhoid fever is almost always associated with typhoid syndrome. Typhoid fever may be fatal.
- Typhoid syndrome occurs in every tenth hospitalized salmonella "alia" patient and may be fatal.

Clinical findings

- General condition
- State of dehydration
  - Tongue
  - Eye sockets
  - Skin of the abdomen in children
- Auscultation of bowel sounds, palpation of the abdomen, and where relevant continue with tests for acute appendicitis
- Pulse of the severely ill patient
  - Slow pulse and high fever point to typhoid syndrome
  - Hypotension may be associated with toxic shock syndrome

Differential diagnosis

- An urgent surgical condition must be excluded or referred
  - Diarrhoea together with acute appendicitis
  - Recently perforated appendix
  - Intestinal obstruction in an elderly patient
  - Invagination in children
  - Cholecystitis

Examinations

- If the patient has fever or the general condition is impaired, it is relevant to assay serum C-reactive protein and serum sodium and potassium to check the serum electrolyte balance. High CRP indicates a bacterial cause for the diarrhoea.

Faecal examinations

- Faecal culture is not needed for every diarrhoea patient. Salmonella, Shigella, Campylobacter and Yersinia should be investigated
  - if the disease is not over within two weeks
  - if the patient is a professional food handler (even those with mild symptoms)
  - if diarrhoea is accompanied by arthritis or arthralgia.
- Recent use of antibiotics may indicate Clostridium difficile (8.42).
  - A negative Clostridium difficile toxin test does not exclude pseudomembranous colitis, nor diarrhoea caused by antibiotics. Rectoscopy is recommended, but may show normal appearance of mucosa in mild infections.
- An incubation period of over seven days or prolonged diarrhoea warrants parasitological examination of faeces for protozoan and other parasites.
  - Salmonella, Shigella, Campylobacter and Yersinia, faecal culture
  - Faecal parasitology
  - Tests for viral pathogens in faeces only for children in hospital
- Two faecal specimens on the same day seldom differ in results; however, faecal cultivation tests taken on successive days result in 16–20% more diagnoses in Campylobacter and Salmonella infections. Prolonged, persistent diarrhoea may be diagnosed from faecal culture that is repeated three times or by parasitological investigations that are repeated even more often.
- Faecal parasitological examination is not necessary before the patient returns complaining of prolonged diarrhoea, unless parasite infection is likely. Good parasitological examination of faeces is based on the formalin ether concentration method, which gives 10–15 times more diagnoses compared with a faecal swab on an objective slide.
- A patient suffering from prolonged diarrhoea for over two months and from loss of weight, should be requested to make a self-estimation of whether HIV infection could be possible. The patient's opinion decides whether HIV test is performed. Further discussion is necessary only if there is a history of previous venereal disease or hepatitis B or if Candidiosis of the oesophagus or the mouth is diagnosed.

Diarrhoea caused by hepatitis A virus

- Hepatitis A infection is not associated with jaundice in four out of five patients under the age of two years.
- A single serum test for hepatitis A IgM becomes diagnostic about ten days from the beginning of the illness.

Cholera

- In endemic areas cholera is a common cause of diarrhoea. In non-endemic areas a history of travelling in endemic areas or consumptions of certain foods (smuggled and poorly boiled oysters) may suggest this aetiology.

Diarrhoea due to poliovirus

- Loose stools or diarrhoea may be a symptom of polio infection.

Examinations when an epidemic is suspected

- See 8.43
- It is wise to wait for the diagnosis of the index case(s). A telephone call is often necessary to speed up the results from the laboratory. In connection with a new epidemic, the most common mistake is to collect specimens only from those who are symptomatic. A reasonable number of asymptomatic persons who have been in contact with

the symptomatic ones should be included when food-borne infection is the case.
- A water-borne or large epidemic indicates selective sampling according to the resources of the laboratory. In addition, follow-up requires cooperation between the local laboratory and clinical personnel.

Serological examinations

- If the patient's diarrhoea is complicated by abdominal pain, arthritis, arthralgia or carditis, serological tests for Yersinia, Salmonella and Campylobacter might be useful.
- Among patients with diarrhoea only those who are severely ill may benefit from diagnosis by means of a paired serum test in cases where the culture of faecal specimens remains negative.
- Hepatitis A IgM test is indicated in a jaundiced patient with diarrhoea.

8.41 Clinical features and treatment of diarrhoea in adults according to aetiology

Tapio Pitkänen

Principles

- The recognized specific causative agent and the clinical features of the patient both affect the treatment decisions.
  - There are usually no reactive complications associated with viral and parasitic gastroenteritis, nor with cholera, which is associated with rice-water diarrhoea caused by the cholera toxin.
  - Reactive complications such as arthritis, carditis, urticaria, erythema nodosum, conjunctivitis and Reiter's syndrome are associated with Salmonella, Campylobacter, Yersinia enterocolitica and Shigella.
- In addition to oral rehydration fluid, specific antibiotic treatment should be considered
  - for symptomatic, and especially severely ill patients, at the time of diagnostic results
  - for both symptomatic and asymptomatic pregnant women with Campylobacter infection
  - for all Shigella and Yersinia enterocolitica patients.
  - With quinolone antibiotics the treatment of adult Salmonella patients has become more active compared with the pre-quinolone period. However, in a meta-analysis antibiotics did not shorten the duration of diarrhoea or fever in previously healthy adults. The studies did not include immunocompromised hosts, or neonates. Many studies had also excluded severely ill patients. Ciprofloxacin has been used in children only in serious cases, because on the basis of animal studies the drug is feared to accumulate in the cartilages. In addition, quinolones are not recommended during pregnancy and lactation.

Treatment of a diarrhoeal patient without a specific diagnosis

- **Oral rehydration solution (ORS) -type treatment** is the key to success. Dehydration is combated by water that contains salt and sugar in measured proportions. A common mistake is to drink only sweet beverages, which may result in osmotic diarrhoea.
  - Advice to adults: "A cup of tea without milk should have 2 teaspoons of sugar; drink with salted biscuits. In addition, water or mineral water may be consumed until the feeling of thirst disappears. Not more than one third of the fluids may be sweet beverages, which are not absolutely necessary."
  - There is no evidence that fasting will benefit adults; even less so for children. Small meals should be eaten as long as the diarrhoea continues.
- Treatment with **antibiotics** may shorten a travellers' feverish diarrhoea. Norfloxacin (400 mg) or ciprofloxacin (500 mg) may be used twice a day for three days as a short treatment when the treatment starts within 24 hours of the beginning of fever and diarrhoea as long as the causative agent is not known. Some unwanted problems may arise:
  - Increased bacterial resistance to quinolones
  - The possibility that the patient becomes a carrier in case of salmonella infection.
- A diarrhoeal disease after a visit to a place where Giardia lamblia is endemic may be treated as **giardiasis** (1.60). Faecal specimens should be examined only if the treatment is not successful. Metronidazole has an antabus side effect.

Indications for hospital referral

- Severe abdominal pain, clear tenderness on abdominal palpation; remember surgical conditions in the differential diagnosis of diarrhoea.
- Severe dehydration demanding intravenous fluid therapy; especially elderly patients.
- Carditis and pancreatitis.
- Arthritis with severe symptoms; often diarrhoea has preceded arthritis by 2–4 weeks.
- Typhoid syndrome. Typhoid fever causing domestic typhoid syndrome is rare, but in 5–10% of other salmonella infections treated in hospital there is typhoid syndrome.
  - High fever starting with headache, sense of sickness, abdominal pain, nausea, relative bradycardia (pulse under 100 per minute) when fever is higher than 39°C (100.2°F), as well as diarrhoea or constipation. The list has the main features of typhoid syndrome.

  - Typhoid syndrome occurs in 1–2% hospital-treated patients with Campylobacter enteritis and mixed infections caused by intestinal bacterial pathogens.
  - Searching for typhoid syndrome helps to estimate the need for hospital referral. The more criteria are fulfilled the more certainly hospital referral is needed.
- Guillain-Barré, syndrome after Campylobacter enteritis.

Sick leave, follow-up faecal specimens and treatment of carriers

- Sick leave of one week is necessary for a person suffering from diarrhoea and working as a food-handler. Extension of sick leave should be considered for those who continue to have diarrhoea or those who have been diagnosed to excrete Salmonella or Shigella. After three negative faecal specimens a carrier of Salmonella or Shigella may start again as a food-handler. In the case of Campylobacter it is enough that the person is asymptomatic, although many patients with fever and diarrhoea need sick leave of one week to recover.
- A new salmonella patient, even without symptoms, may need sick leave until hygiene matters have been discussed and possible food-handler's restrictions issued. A surgeon in hospital may start work after a course of antibiotics, but a food-handler should produce negative faecal specimens if the causative agent has been Salmonella or Shigella.
- Carriers of Salmonella, Shigella and EHEC-bacteria should be kept from food-handlers' work. Long-term carriers are becoming rarer because adults can be treated with ciprofloxacin, 750 mg twice per day for 15 days.
- Communicable diarrhoeal diseases of public health importance are Salmonella, Shigella, EHEC-infection and cholera. These should be notified to health officials.
- Children who are carriers of Salmonella should be treated with ciprofloxacin only where there are vital indications. Follow-up faecal specimens should be taken weekly until three consecutive negative results have been obtained. After four positive results it is reasonable to extend the interval up to 2–4 weeks in order to save resources and to reduce the stress.
- A child who is a carrier of Salmonella, Shigella or EHEC-bacteria should not attend day care.
- Faecal specimens for follow-up should be taken in general only from those who have not recovered, those who are working as food-handlers and those who have had Salmonella, Shigella or cholera.

Advice for personal hygiene

- There is no evidence that disinfecting the toilet bowl at the patient's home would prevent the spread of the bacteria. Washing hands after defecation is important as well as before starting to prepare a meal. Hands should be washed with soap and dried with disposable paper napkins.
- Health care personnel who are asymptomatic carriers of intestinal pathogens may remain undiagnosed because of a faulty gall bladder that hides the pathogen. When the problem has been recognized the carriers may continue in specified duties and should be asked to use a separate toilet facility. A gall-bladder operation may be necessary to eliminate the carrier state. If antibiotics are started several days after the onset of a diarrhoeal disease caused by Salmonella, they tend to prolong Salmonella detection in stools.

Enterotoxigenic Escherichia coli (ETEC)

- Enterotoxigenic Escherichia coli is the most common cause of travellers' diarrhoea. The disease is usually self-limiting and the patient recovers rapidly.
- Standard laboratory faecal culture of Salmonella, Shigella, Yersinia enterocolitica and Campylobacter do not reveal ETEC, which thus remains undiagnosed.
- Short treatment with norfloxacin, 400 mg twice per day for three days, when treatment has been started within 12 hours of the onset of the disease, may give some advantage: approximately one day less diarrhoea, relapse less often and subjective recovery more often than with placebo. For problems of short treatment, see treatment without a specific diagnosis (above).

Enterohaemorrhagic Escherichia coli (EHEC)

- Diarrhoea is the main symptom; sometimes blood-stained stools. The kidneys may become damaged, necessitating dialysis.
- EHEC bacteria have been detected in the stools of cattle, and the bacteria have been isolated from beef.
- No antibiotic treatment C [1].
- EHEC cases should be notified to health officials.

Salmonella alia

- Salmonella "alia" here means any other Salmonella but Salmonella typhi. At the time of diagnosis any moderately ill patient with Salmonella alia or one who has been excreting Salmonella alia for one month or longer may be treated with ciprofloxacin, 750 mg twice per day, or norfloxacin, 400 mg twice per day for 15 days. Treatment of a carrier will be appropriate if culture is accompanied by sensitivity tests. A faulty gall bladder or schistosomiasis may explain prolonged excretion.

Salmonella typhi

- Typhoid fever should be treated in hospital on the basis of mere suspicion as soon as a blood culture test has been taken. Treatment consists of ciprofloxacin, 750 mg twice per day, norfloxacin, 400 mg × 2, chloramphenicol, 500 mg 3–4 times per day, or trimethoprim-sulpha, 160/800 mg twice per day for 10–15 days.

- Relapses occur in about 5% of patients. Extension of chloramphenicol or trimethoprim-sulpha courses has not decreased the number of relapses. Quinolones abolish symptoms sooner than the traditional antibiotics.

Shigella

- According to the WHO specialists' consensus only Shigella dysenteriae infection should be treated by antibiotics, whereas they have no effect on the disease caused by Shigella flexneri.
- Norfloxacin 400 mg twice per day, or ciprofloxacin 500 mg twice per day for 5–10 days is more effective than traditional ampicin or trimethoprim-sulpha for 7 days, and often the sensitivity test is more favourable for quinolones. Even a single dose of norfloxacin (800 mg) has been as effective as trimethoprim-sulpha 160/800 mg twice per day for 5 days. Asymptomatic patients should also be treated. Mesillinam can be used for children.

Campylobacter

- Campylobacter enteritis is usually self-limiting and the patient often recovers without intervention. The patients feel much more sick than in cases of travellers' diarrhoea caused by enterotoxigenic Escherichia coli.
- Campylobacter may spread from one person to another.
- A patient who is symptomatic at the time of diagnosis should receive a five-day course of antibiotic. The first choice is erythromycin 500 mg × 4, and other macrolides may be effective. The second line antibiotic is doxycycline, and for children, clindamycin. Fluoroquinolones are not widely used because of the many resistant strains of Campylobacter.
- Pregnant patients should be treated with erythromycin.
- In cases of prolonged fever, complications or immunosuppression the antibiotic course should be doubled; from five days to 10 days or even more.
- Campylobacter enteritis is the second most common infection, after respiratory infections, to precede the Guillain-Barré, syndrome by several days or even week.

Yersinia enterocolitica

- Both symptomatic and asymptomatic patients should be treated with fluoroquinolones for 7–10 days: norfloxacin, 400 mg twice per day, or ciprofloxacin, 500 mg twice per day. Tetracycline, 500 mg 3 times per day for 10 days is another choice. Treatment has not been shown to prevent reactive arthritis. Children can be treated with trimethoprim-sulpha. For adults the dose is 160/800 mg twice per day for 10 days.

Clostridium difficile

- See 8.42.
- Clostridium difficile may cause pseudomembranous enterocolitis or prolonged diarrhoea during an antibiotic course (especially cefuroxim axetil orally, other cephalosporins, clindamycin and other broad-spectrum antibiotics).
- It is common that antibiotic treatment in hospital causes prolonged diarrhoea in the discharged patient at home.
- A typical picture in rectoscopy is a patchy creamy covering and watery faeces.
- In patients with moderate symptoms it is worth trying ordinary ORS-type therapy before possible specific antibiotic treatment of Clostridium difficile.
- Mild cases of prolonged, but not feverish, Clostridium difficile diarrhoea may be treated at home with metronidazole 400 mg 3 times per day for two weeks, but cases with fever and the severely ill should be referred to hospital to be treated with metronidazole as mentioned above or with vancomycin orally, 125–250 mg 3 times per day for two weeks. An increase in the use of vancomycin has spread hospital epidemics caused by vancomycin-resistant Enterococci (VRE).

Diarrhoea caused by viruses

- Diarrhoeas caused by viruses such as norovirus (calicivirus), rotavirus or adenovirus are treated symptomatically with ORS-type therapy because there is no specific treatment.

Giardia lamblia

- See 1.60.
- Giardia lamblia should always be treated. The best medication is tinidazole (a 2000 mg single dose), but also metronidazole is suitable as a single dose of 2400 mg, or 250–400 mg 3 times per day for seven days (A) [2]. Warn about the possible antabus effect. Relapses occur.

Entamoeba histolytica

- If faecal Entamoeba histolytica has not been typed for pathogenicity, both symptomatic and asymptomatic patients should be treated with metronidazole, 400 mg 2–3 times per day for 10 days. Relapses and amoebic liver or other abscesses indicate specialist consultation, or the patient should be referred to a clinic of infectious diseases.

Cryptosporidium

- Effective and specific treatment is not known. Consult a specialist in infectious diseases.

Candida albicans or spp

- Occasionally candidosis may appear in the intestines of healthy persons. Treatment is a single dose of fluconazole (150 mg), or 50 mg once daily for 7–14 days. Both the dose and the course should be doubled for immunosuppressed patients.
- Previously healthy persons should be asked if they have recently received broad-spectrum antibiotics. Oesophageal

and oral candidosis should lead to consideration of the HIV test or a differential count of leucocytes to exclude haematological cancer. However, candidosis of the vagina is such a common finding after any antibiotic that treatment with a single dose of fluconazole (150 mg) is enough without further examination. Pregnancy is considered a contraindication to fluconazole.

Pneumocystis carinii

- May cause diarrhoea although the common symptoms are in the lungs. Pneumocystis carinii is associated with immunosuppression and AIDS. The infection is often treated in hospital with trimethoprim-sulpha, 15–20 mg per kg per day, divided in three doses, or with pentamidine, 4 mg per kg per day as a slow i.v. infusion. The latter has been given as an aerosol once per day with less severe side effects. Both antibiotics have been used to prevent Pneumocystis carinii infection.

Cholera

- Rice-based ORS in patients with cholera is effective in reducing stool output **A** [3]

References

1. Wong CS, Jelacic S, Habeeb RL, Watkins SL, Tarr PI. The risk of the hemolytic –uremic syndrome after antibiotic treatment of Escherichia coli O157:H7 infections. N Engl J Med 2000;342:1930–1936.
2. Zaat JOM, Mank ThG, Assendelft WJJ. Drugs for treating giardiasis. Cochrane Database Syst Rev. 2004;(2):CD000217.
3. Fontaine O, Gore SM, Pierce NF. Rice-based oral rehydration solution for treating diarrhoea. Cochrane Database Syst Rev. 2004;(2):CD001264.

8.42 Antibiotic diarrhoea

Editors

Basic rule

- Remember the possibility of Clostridium difficile infection and treat symptomatic patients.

Aetiology

Clostridium difficile

- Toxigenic Clostridium difficile causes a majority of all cases of diarrhoea following antibiotic treatment in adults. In children it is less common.
- Most antibiotics may cause C. difficile colonization, but the risk varies according to the antibiotic. Compared with penicillin V or G, the risk is 8-fold with ampicillin, 12-fold with quinolones and clindamycin, and up to 34-fold with cephalosporins.

Haemorrhagic colitis

- Treatment with penicillin antibiotics may cause haemorrhagic colitis.

Clinical manifestations and diagnosis

- Watery, quite often bloody, profuse diarrhoea begins 4–9 days after the start of antimicrobic therapy, sometimes only after the antibiotic course has ended.
- Fever is common in Clostridium colitis, but rare in haemorrhagic colitis.
- In severe pseudomembranotic Clostridium colitis rectoscopy or sigmoidoscopy reveal typical yellowish grey membranes. Haemorrhagic colitis often affects the ascending colon.
- ESR and serum CRP are increased according to the severity of the disease.
- Detection of Clostridium toxin in the faeces with ELISA method and Clostridium difficile culture are of equal value as diagnostic methods. The result of the former is available earlier.
- Latex agglutination test for the toxin is not accurate enough (gives false positive results).
- After treatment asymptomatic patients do not need control tests.

Treatment

Mild diarrhoea, no fever

- Stopping the antibiotic is often all that is needed.
- If the diarrhoea is prolonged perform the C. difficile toxin test or culture. The treatment is chosen according to the test result.

Abdominal pain, profuse diarrhoea, bloody diarrhoea or fever

- A clinical suspicion is a sufficient basis for starting the therapy, at least in patients with severe symptoms or fever. If possible, the toxin test or culture is performed before starting the treatment.
  - Metronidazole 400 mg × 3 × 10 p.o. is the drug of choice **B** [1 2 3 4].
  - In severe disease necessitating hospitalization vancomycin 125 mg × 4 p.o. can be used (not effective when administered intravenously).
- Fluid replacement is given according to the severity of diarrhoea and the patient's general condition.
- The diarrhoea relapses in one out of five patients. The treatment is a new course of metronidazole, or vancomycin for the second relapse.

Prevention

- Avoid unnecessary use of antibiotics.
- Clostridium difficile spreads through direct contact on hospital wards. Wash hands and use gloves when treating a symptomatic patient. Patients with diarrhoea should be transferred from a room with uninfected patients.

References

1. Zimmerman MJ, Bak A, Sutherland LR. Review article: treatment of clostridium difficile infection. Alim Pharmacol Therapeutics 1997;11:1003–1012.
2. The Database of Abstracts of Reviews of Effectiveness (University of York), Database no.: DARE-980109. In: The Cochrane Library, Issue 4, 1999. Oxford: Update Software.
3. Teasley DG, Gerding DN, Olson MM, Peterson LR, Gebhard RL, Schwartz MJ, Lee JT Jr. Prospective randomised trial of metronidazole versus vancomycin for Clostridium-difficile-associated diarrhoea and colitis. Lancet 1983:1043–1046.
4. Wenisch C, Parschalk B, Hasenhundl M, Hirschl AM, Graninger W. Comparison of vancomycin, teicoplanin, metronidazole, and fusidic acid for the treatment of Clostridium difficile-associated diarrhea. Clinical Infectious Diseases 1996;22:813–818.

8.43 Food poisoning

Tapio Pitkänen

Principles

- Treatment of patients is symptomatic, with the exception of botulism. Consider therapy again when the cause of food poisoning is known.
- The aim is to stop an epidemic and to disclose the cause.
    - Stool specimens should be taken from the index case(s), and from persons with and without symptoms around and in connection with the index case. In the case of a large epidemic the faecal specimens should be examined for Salmonella, Shigella, Campylobacter and Yersinia as well as viral agents.
    - A suspected water-borne epidemic or an epidemic involving a large group of people indicates screening of faecal specimens. The target groups and the number of sampled persons should be decided with the laboratory or environmental authorities.
    - A specimen of the suspected food item should be taken.

Definition

- Food poisoning is caused by bacteria, bacterial toxin(s), or viruses. Symptoms appear abruptly soon after eating contaminated food, generally within 24 hours. In cases involving Salmonella and Campylobacter the incubation period may be longer.

Aetiology

- The most common causes of food poisoning are:
    - Bacteria: Staphylococcus aureus, Clostridium perfringens, Bacillus cereus, Salmonella and Campylobacter
    - Viruses: rotavirus, SRSV (small round structured viruses), adenovirus, astrovirus, calicivirus. SRSV affects all age groups; other viruses mainly paediatric age groups.
    - Other agents and unknown causes
- Food poisoning from abroad is often caused by some of the Salmonella types.
- Botulism
    - Very rare but severe poisoning caused by the soil bacterium Clostridium botulinum
    - Typically caused by home-made preservatives
    - Symptom that include tiredness, dizziness and dryness of the mouth begin within 12–36 hours of ingesting the toxin. At the same time or within 3 days neurological symptoms develop: visual symptoms, difficulty in swallowing, muscle weakness.
    - Symptoms affecting the GI tract are absent
    - Differential diagnosis includes Guillain–Barré syndrome, polio, encephalitis and myasthenia gravis
    - Although the disease is rare, it is important to know and identify as early treatment (antitoxin, assisted respiration) may save the patient's life.
- For symptoms of the most common types of food poisoning caused by bacteria, see Table 8.43.

History

- Exact time of the onset of symptoms.
- Description of the symptoms: diarrhoea, vomiting, fever, sense of sickness, aches.
- Travel history: staying abroad within recent weeks.
- History of meals within 24 hours.
    - Foods consumed; who prepared them?
    - Eating places?
    - Who else and how many have eaten the same food?
    - How many are sick?
    - Which food item does the patient suspect?
- Does the patient belong to a group at risk of spreading Salmonella at work?
    - Professionals in the food industry
    - Nursing personnel
    - School children
    - Children attending day care
- Severity of food poisoning in relation to age (newborns and the elderly are vulnerable) and to the patient's chronic diseases.

Table 8.43 Symptoms of food poisonings caused by common bacteria

	Staphylococcus aureus	Clostridium perfringens	Bacillus cereus	Salmonella
Onset	abrupt	abrupt	abrupt	often abrupt
Incubation time	3–4 (1–6) h	10–12 (–20) h	8–16 h	6–72 h
Vomiting	almost always	seldom	seldom	often
Diarrhoea	heavy	heavy	heavy	common
Abdominal pain	moderate	severe	severe	moderate
Fever	not regularly	not common	not common	common
Sense of illness	severe, abrupt	mild	mild	common
Pain in joints	no	no	no	may occur
Symptoms last	5–12 h	6–24 h	6–24 h	a few days

Treatment

- Sufficient amounts of fluid, at least one third similar to oral rehydration fluid (8.41).
- Rest; if necessary sick leave for 1–2 days.
- Symptomatic treatment of persistent diarrhoea in addition to fluid therapy.
- If Salmonella or Campylobacter is suspected, consider antibiotics for thc newborn, elderly and chronically ill patients.
  - Advice about toilet hygiene: After defecation and always before touching foodstuffs the hands should be washed with warm water and soap. Hands should be dried with disposable paper napkins, which are used for as long as diarrhoea or the presence of a possible causative agent continues
  - The patient must avoid preparing meals for other persons
  - Those who belong to possible risk groups should be taken off work in kitchens, schools and day-care centres for the time being
- No antibiotic before stool specimen.

To clear up the cause of an epidemic

- When there is a group of sick persons the head of local primary care services or the officer in charge of communicable diseases should evaluate of the situation. The public health inspector should take faecal specimens. When suspicion of food poisoning arises outside office hours, it is wise to contact immediately any medical officer in charge.
- If the infection is suspected to have originated in a public eating place, a take-away or a grocery, the medical officer in charge contacts the place. If the patient/client makes the first contact, it often happens that the suspected food has been "eaten up or thrown away".
- The history of the patients may often give a clue as regards a particular microbe or foodstuff. Common infectious vehicles are foodstuffs that contain animal protein and are served cold:
  - poorly heated or frozen meat or fish
  - cut cold meat, chicken
  - oysters
  - bean sprouts, salads, sauces and frozen berries
  - eggs and mayonnaise
  - milk products, confectionery
  - holiday-imported meat, meat products and cheese
- These and raw materials for the meals should be sampled for bacteriological and/or virological examinations.
- In addition to foodstuffs the inspection should include food-handlers and utensils.
  - Hands: wounds, cutaneous eruptions; specimens of infections
  - Possible symptoms: **food-handlers with symptoms should be taken off work if spreading of infection is likely**.
  - Utensils: knives, cutting boards, towels, food machinery etc.
- Faecal specimens should be taken from at least a few persons who are suffering from diarrhoea.

8.44 Prolonged diarrhoea in the adult

Markku Ellonen

- For acute diarrhoea see article 8.40.

Basic rules

- Identify infection diarrhoeas that can be specifically treated (Giardia, Clostridium difficile).
- Perform primary investigations for early diagnosis of common malabsorption disorders (coeliac disease, lactose intolerance) and inflammatory bowel diseases (IBD: ulcerative colitis, Crohn's disease).
- Exclude malignancy.
- The most common disorder is functional diarrhoea (irritable bowel syndrome, (IBS)), which is a diagnosis by exclusion. The patients need follow-up because in organic diarrhoeas

there are not always abnormal clinical signs or laboratory findings at the initial stage. Benign microscopic colitis resembles IBS.

- Identify overflow diarrhoea caused by obstipation in the elderly.

Criteria for prolonged diarrhoea

- More than 3 defecations daily
- Duration of diarrhoea exceeds 3–4 weeks.
- Even minor changes in bowel function may suggest the onset of disease.

Aetiology

- Drugs
  - Laxatives, antibiotics, cholinergics, magnesium-containing antacids, iron, quinidine, cholestyramine
  - Antibiotics may cause Clostridium difficile colitis that can be a serious disease in the elderly.
  - Yeast colonization caused by antibiotics is of unknown significance; usually the condition is cured without medication.
- Malignancy
  - Cancer of the colon and other gastrointestinal malignancies (particularly lymphoma).
- Systemic diseases
  - Hyperthyroidism, AIDS, diabetic autonomic neuropathy, uraemia, pancreatic insufficiency, malabsorption of various causes.
- Inflammatory bowel diseases
  - Ulcerative colitis and Crohn's disease (8.80).
- Microscopic colitis: collagen colitis and lymphocytic colitis
- Infections
  - Bacteria or parasites only seldom cause prolonged diarrhoea. Clostridium and Camphylobacter are the most common causes, sometimes also EHEC, Yersinia.
  - Diarrhoea associated with giardiasis (1.60) typically begins after travel abroad. Negative faecal tests are unreliable, and a trial of single-dose medication may be the best option. The treatment of amoebiasis should last longer.
- Ischaemic colitis: the patients often have a severe generalized vasculitis.
- Dietary factors
  - Lactose malabsorption (8.83) is common. It is often an incidental finding, not the cause of the diarrhoea. Hypolactasia may be secondary to coeliac disease or occur in the convalescent phase of severe gastroenteritis.
  - Poor absorption of xylitol, sorbitol, or fructose may cause diarrhoea.
  - Coeliac disease (8.84) is caused by gluten in wheat, rye, and barley.
  - Adult-onset food allergies are a rare cause of diarrhoea. Fresh root allergy may cause symptoms in the oral cavity and upper gastrointestinal tract.
  - The existence and significance of yeast allergy is controversial.
- Irritable bowel syndrome (IBS) can be set as the diagnosis after all other diseases have been excluded.

Assessment of a patient with prolonged diarrhoea

History

- Onset and duration of diarrhoea
  - Infectious colitis starts acutely with fever and general symptoms.
  - Inflammatory bowel disease starts insidiously unless triggered by an infection.
  - Prolonged diarrhoea with long asymptomatic periods suggests a functional disorder.
- Diarrhoea starting after travelling abroad requires more comprehensive microbiological investigations.
- Consider the patient's medication and earlier bowel surgery as the aetiology of the diarrhoea.

Therapeutic trial

- Lactose malabsorption may be a misleading and insignificant finding that prevents correct diagnosis. Avoidance of lactose should alleviate the symptoms within two weeks. In many patients lactose intolerance is associated with irritable bowel syndrome, which makes the interpretation of therapeutic trials difficult.

Laboratory investigations

- The primary investigations include blood count, ESR, CRP, faecal occult blood × 3, faecal bacterial culture and clostridium toxin or culture, and, if indicated, parasites.
- Elimination–provocation test can be used as an alternative to lactose tolerance test.
- Problems with interpretation of the result may arise from individual differences in lactose tolerance in patients with hypolactasia. In unclear cases a gene test is useful.
- For further examinations, colonoscopy (or sigmoidoscopy complemented with barium enema).

Diagnostic clues

Age

- In young and middle-aged patients prolonged diarrhoea is often functional (8.8), caused by malabsorption, or a result of food allergies that have been present from childhood. Bloating, pains, flatulence and mucorrhea together with diarrhoea of varying severity are consistent with the irritable bowel syndrome.

- Inflammatory bowel diseases also occur in young people. In Crohn's disease ESR and CRP are often elevated.
- In the elderly systemic diseases and malignancies should be considered.

Occult or visible blood in the stools

- If blood is detected in the stools consider ulcerative colitis, Crohn's disease, ischaemic colitis, and malignancy. Investigate the patient without prior therapeutic trials. Diverticles can be considered the cause of bleeding if no other cause is found.
- Mucus in the stools is not a serious sign, but bloody mucus or visible blood is. Mucus alone may be present in the irritable bowel syndrome.

Fever and elevated infection parameters

- Fever and elevated CRP and ESR are often present in the early stages of infectious diarrhoea and in Crohn's disease.
- In ulcerative colitis these findings are seen only in the most severe forms.

Small volume of stools and frequent defecation

- Suggestive of distal colitis or proctitis.
- (Bloody) mucus is often present on the surface of the stools.
- The primary investigations include sigmoidoscopy and biopsy.
    - Ulcerative colitis at an early stage may be difficult to differentiate from infectious colitis, but histology is often helpful.
    - Biopsy is mandatory, even if endoscopy findings are normal; microscopic colitis is detected only by histological examination.

Large volume of stools, weight loss and anaemia

- Suggestive of proximal bowel disease or malabsorption (coeliac disease).
- Stools floating in water most often indicate fermentation and trapped air in the stools rather than fatty diarrhoea.
- Pain around the umbilicus and in the right lower quadrant suggests proximal bowel disease.
- Prolonged watery diarrhoea with a varying course may also be caused by collagen colitis (8.80) or lymphocytic colitis; in these conditions there are no general symptoms or weight loss.
- Further investigations should be performed to detect lactose intolerance (8.83), coeliac disease (8.84), ulcerative colitis, Crohn's disease (8.80), and pancreatic insufficiency (9.32).

Serious symptoms and signs requiring investigations and follow-up without therapeutic trials

- Repeatedly visible blood in the stools.
- Weight loss, fever or malaise (remember HIV infection!).
- Acute onset and continuous worsening.
- Diarrhoea that also occurs at night.
- Onset of diarrhoea in old age.
- Abnormal results of laboratory tests (haemoglobin, ESR, CRP, liver function tests, faecal occult blood).
    - Laboratory test results are normal in functional disorders, lactose malabsorption and microscopic colitis.

Indications for specialist consultation

- Suspicion of coeliac disease if small bowel biopsy (gastroscopy) is not available in primary care.
- Ulcerative colitis and Crohn's disease.
- Severe symptoms and obscure diagnosis.
- See 8.83

8.50 Examining a patient with rectal bleeding

Matti V. Kairaluoma

- Causes of bleeding (8.51)

Definition

- Rectal bleeding is defined as fresh or clotted blood in the faeces or in association with defecation.
- The colour of the faeces may be otherwise normal, in contrast to melena, which is defined as black, tar-like stools or the maroon stool often seen with caecal bleeding.

Basic rules

- Identify the site and cause of the bleeding, most importantly separating bleeding from the anal canal versus the proximal colon. The former can often be handled locally, whereas the latter requires a more global approach.
- Identify patients with a tumour, inflammatory bowel disease, or other condition requiring specific treatment.
- Identify patients with haemorrhoids, anal fissure, excoriation of anal skin, or other condition that can be treated symptomatically.

History

Type of rectal bleeding

- Does the bleeding occur only in association with defecation or also at other times?
- Is the blood fresh (bright red), clotted or old (maroon)?

- Is the bleeding seen
  - during cleansing (external or prolapsed haemorrhoids, anal fissure or excoriation)
  - dripping in the water (internal haemorrhoids)
  - on the surface of the stools (tumour)?
- What is the colour and consistency of the stools? Most importantly are the stools liquid or solid?
- Are there other symptoms associated with the bleeding?
  - anal pain (fissure)
  - abdominal pain or tenesmus (tumour, inflammation of the bowel)?
- Ask about the duration, frequency, and eventual exacerbation of the symptoms
- Are the bowel movements normal?
- Are there other symptoms (abdominal or systemic symptoms, weight loss)?

Medical history

- Ingestion of aspirin, ibuprofen, warfarin or other antiplatelet drugs.
- Earlier investigations or surgery?
- Colorectal cancer in the family? Here it is important to inquire as to the health history of each family member rather than simply ask the global question... Has anyone had..? (8.70)
- History of cirrhosis, other liver disease, diabetes (haemochromatosis), foreign travel.
- Sexual history (best obtained patiently and with some sensitivity).

History of symptoms

- Ask about the duration, frequency and eventual exacerbation of the symptoms.
- Are the bowel movements normal? Has there been a change in bowel habits?
- Are there other symptoms (abdominal or systemic symptoms, **weight loss**)?

Physical examination

- Palpation and auscultation of the abdomen (tenderness distension, ecchymoses, palpable mass, width, tenderness and contour of the liver edge).
- Inspection by spreading the anal margins: fissure, sentinel fold, rhagades, fistular orifices.
- Diagnose eventual mucosal or rectal prolapse by spreading the anal margins and asking the patient to push as if he were defecating. This is better accomplished either by having the patient stand for a moment if the anal canal is very flaccid, or by having the patient sit for a time on the toilet as if to defecate and then bend forward so the anus can be visualized in this position. Lastly rectal prolapse can be visualized during dynamic proctography, a type of barium enema with moving pictures taken during defecation on a comode.
- Digital rectal examination (DRE): tonus and strength of the anal sphincter, fissure (pain!), anal crypts, ampullar mucosa, prostate, cervix, rectovaginal septum, coccyx, sacrum, colour of the stools.

Further investigations

- Always identify the origin of rectal bleeding.
- If an evident fissure is diagnosed in a young patient (under 50 years) it is sufficient to treat it and follow up. In other cases at least a sigmoidoscopy should be performed, even if it seems that the bleeding is only caused by haemorrhoids.
- In all patients over 50 years of age, colonoscopy is recommended to rule out malignancies.
- What tools exist for the identification of the source of rectal bleeding?
  - **Ears**
  - **Eyes**
  - **Finger** (digital rectal examination)
  - **Anoscope** – the best instrument for evaluating the anal canal. Hard to use if the patient has anal pain.
  - **Rigid 25-cm proctosigmoidoscope**. Obsolete as a cancer screening tool but the best instrument for evaluating the distal colo-rectum in emergency settings or in un-prepared patients. The best first test in the evaluation of diarrhoea with or without bleeding – to see, to biopsy and to culture.
  - **60-cm flexible sigmoidoscope**. This has replaced the proctoscope as a cancer screening tool and for the elective evaluation of bleeding and diarrhoea. A valuable primary care tool
  - **Colonoscope.** The gold standard. The most definitive instrument for the evaluation of the entire colon as well as a therapeutic tool. Almost impossible to use in unprepared patients.
  - **Barium enema.** This has no place in the emergency evaluation of rectal bleeding. It is still a good cancer screening tool but of no value in the evaluation of diarrhoea.
  - **Labelled red cell scanning**. The best second test for massive rectal bleeding (after rigid proctosigmoidoscopy), though the results are often crude, only separating right from left colon.
  - **Mesenteric angiography.** The most precise test to localize bleeding from the intestine in the actively bleeding patient.

8.51 Diseases causing rectal bleeding

Matti V. Kairaluoma

Anal fissure

- See 8.63.
- Common in young and middle-aged persons whose anal sphincter tonus is high.

- Pain and smarting on defecation is the initial symptom. As the fissure becomes chronic the pain often lasts from one to two hours after defecation.
- Bright blood is occasionally seen on the toilet paper after cleansing.
- The fissure is usually situated dorsally on the skin of the anal canal. Aberrant (non-midline) location of the fissure, multiple almost asymptomatic fissures, and a macerated anus may suggest Crohn's disease. Other causes of fissure include anal neoplasm, leukaemia, lymphoma, sexually transmitted disease, tuberculosis.

Investigations

- If a young person has findings that are consistent with the symptoms, careful and gentle external examination of the anus, spreading the buttocks is often a sufficient investigation.

Treatment

- See 8.63.

Haemorrhoids

- See 8.62.
- Haemorrhoids are defined as cushions on the anal sphincters that contain blood vessels and connective tissue. They are a normal structure of the anal canal.
- Strain causes congestion that dilates the haemorrhoids, resulting over time in prolapse outside the anal canal.
- A congested haemorrhoid may bleed during defecation if there is a mucosal tear. The bleeding is associated with strain on defecation, and the blood is bright red, dripping or jetting, and it discolours the toilet water. Prolapsed (grade 3–4) haemorrhoids may bleed from friction even at other times.
- Other symptoms associated with haemorrhoids include perianal irritation and itch resulting from mucous leakage related to prolapse. Only incarcerated or thrombosed haemorrhoids cause pain. Haemorrhoids may also cause soiling because of incomplete closing of the anal canal due to tissue oedema.

Investigations

- Haemorrhoids can be diagnosed by proctoscopy; however, at least sigmoidoscopy should be performed on all patients who have had rectal bleeding. Endoscopy should also be performed for patients without rectal bleeding if their history and symptoms are not very typical. If the patient is above 50 years of age then colonoscopy or barium enema are usually indicated to rule out cancer, even if haemorrhoids are obviously present.

Treatment

- See 8.62.

Bleeding from diverticula

- Bleeding from diverticula is one of the most common causes of rectal haemorrhage in elderly patients. The diagnosis is based on the exclusion of other causes of bleeding. The site of bleeding is only rarely seen.
- The bleeding originates from an artery at the fringe of the diverticulum, or an arterio-venous malformation can be profuse, causes bloody diarrhoea, and may sometimes lead to shock.

Bleeding from angiodysplasia

- Angiodysplasias are submucosal AV malformations occurring predominantly in the aged. Their origin is unknown. The bleeding may be profuse or slow and may cause anaemia and require transfusions or surgery.

Treatment

- Resuscitate
- Localize
- Correct coagulopathy
- With these therapies alone bleeding will stop in about 80–90% of patients.
- Further non-surgical therapies include intravenous or arterial pitressin, embolization, endoscopic coagulation and finally surgical resection.

Inflammatory bowel diseases

- See 8.80.
- In inflammatory bowel diseases the bleeding and/or diarrhoea are usually associated with exacerbations of the disease. An earlier diagnosed disease or earlier intestinal bowel symptoms are the most important clues from the history.
- The diagnosis is obtained in sigmoidoscopy most often. In less acute situations by colonoscopy and in more urgent situations by radiolabelled white cell scanning. The treatment consists of medication, and if necessary, correction of the general condition with transfusions and parenteral nutrition. Fulminant colitis not responding to other treatments should be treated surgically.

Rectal bleeding associated with a tumour

- Suspect a tumour always when a person aged over 50 years has blood on or mixed in the faeces or in younger patients if there is involuntary weight loss, a positive family history or abdominal findings on physical examination.
- Ribbon-like faeces, abdominal pain, palpable tumour, weight loss, and symptoms of intestinal obstruction are alarming signs.
- Fibreoptic sigmoidoscopy with double contrast colonography and colonoscopy alone are the investigations of choice when a colorectal tumour is suspected.

Ischaemic colitis

- Ischaemic colitis is a poorly characterized disease that is a cause of bloody diarrhoea in the elderly.
- The elderly patient typically often has a history of a cardiovascular disease.
- The attack starts with abdominal pain followed by bloody diarrhoea. Bloody diarrhoea, and palpable tenderness in the region of the affected part of the bowel are observed. The bleeding is rarely so heavy that it requires a transfusion. The risk of ischaemic colitis is highest in the first few postoperative days after the repair of an abdominal aortic aneurysm.
- Can be diagnosed with colonoscopy. The differential diagnosis should include pseudomembranous colitis and infectious enteritides, especially in younger patients.

Treatment

- Resuscitation
- Localization
- Optimize mesenteric blood flow –this often means cessation of digitalis and other medications that might cause mesenteric spasm.
- Close monitoring for signs of transmural ischaemia or necrosis, which require emergency surgery.
- Angiography is often of little value.
- Endoscopy and radiolabelled white cell scanning are the most accurate means of making the diagnosis.

8.52 Melena

Editors

Basic rule

- Identify the cause of bleeding in all cases at least by gastroscopy and, if necessary, by colonoscopy or sigmoidoscopy and colonography. The exceptions are the following:
  - The cause of bleeding is evident on the basis of earlier investigations.
  - The general condition of a terminally ill patient is so poor that no active treatment is planned.

Definition

- Black, tar-like stools indicate the mixing of blood with the contents of the bowel. If fresh blood or clots are visible in the faeces, see the article on rectal bleeding (haemorrhagia ex ano) 8.51.

Table 8.52 Causes for gastrointestinal bleeding

Cause	%
Oesophageal varices	10
Oesophageal tear or ulceration	9
Ventricle ulcer or gastric erosions	15
Cancer of the stomach	2
Benign tumour	1
Duodenal ulcer	18
More distal cause	15
Unknown	25

Epidemiology

Causes of gastrointestinal bleeding

- See Table 8.52.

Urgency of investigations and treatment

- If the patient has symptoms resulting from low haemoglobin concentration or hypovolaemia (collapse, dizziness, vertigo, exacerbation of heart failure) the bleeding has been profuse, and the patient should be referred immediately. Correction of hypovolaemia with Ringer's solution is often indicated during transportation (not if the patient has heart failure).
- A haemoglobin concentration under 80 g/l is usually an indication for red cell transfusion.
- If the patient is asymptomatic, and the haemoglobin concentration is above 100 g/l the patient can be referred the following morning after a telephone consultation. However, follow-up in a hospital should be arranged immediately if there is any doubt.
- The first investigation is always gastroscopy. Gastroscopy may be available in primary care or at an outpatient clinic, and the optimal place for the examination should be determined by assessing the risk of continuous bleeding. If it is probable that the bleeding will continue the patient should be referred to a hospital where endoscopic treatment or surgery can be performed.
- Sigmoidoscopy and colonography can be performed at an outpatient clinic.

8.60 Anal pain

Kari-Matti Hiltunen

Basic rules

- Identify patients that can be examined and treated in primary care.

- Identify patients with conditions (anal abscess or incarcerated haemorrhoids) that need investigation and treatment in a hospital.

Epidemiology

- Anal pain is a common symptom. It is usually caused by a benign condition, most commonly anal fissure.
- A tumour is a rare cause of anal pain.
- Patients often try self-medication with topical over-the-counter ointments. Patients often delay seeking medical care for anal problems.

Causes of anal pain

- Common causes and sources of anal pain are listed in Table 8.60.
- Rare causes include
  - Crohn's disease
  - Anal cancer
  - Rectal cancer
  - Other anorectal malignancies
  - Rectal prolapse
  - Anal mucosal prolapse
  - Anal fistula
  - Leukaemia
  - Suppurative hidradenitis
- The cause of anal pain can usually be treated in primary care.

Table 8.60 Common types and sources of anal pain

Symptoms and signs	Probable source
Pain associated with bleeding or weight loss	Rule out cancer, colitis
Pain of recent onset, constant or increasing, with or without fever	Abscess
Sudden onset of pain	Thrombosed haemorrhoid
Chronic short or intermittent pain associated with defaecation	Fissure
Tenesmus or cramping associated with bleeding or diarrhoea	Proctitis, colitis
Deep, aching intermittent pain, not associated with defaecation	Levator spasm
Chronic itching, no associated symptoms	Pruritus ani
Itching, diarrhoea	Proctitis
Itching, mucosal prolapse	Haemorrhoids
Bleeding	Haemorrhoids, cancer, colitis
Palpable mass	Prolapsed haemorrhoids, sentinel pile associated with fissure, tumour, condylomata, abscess, foreign body

- Carefully taken history and clinical examination are usually sufficient for diagnosis. Further investigations mainly aim at the exclusion of precancerous and cancerous conditions and inflammatory bowel diseases.
- The major problems with the evaluation of anal pain are:
  - The sensitivity of the area; physically and psychologically. Patients are therefore very sensitive about being examined.
  - The anatomy of the area is complex and creates difficulties with diagnosis and therapy.
  - There are multiple causes of anal pain, some potentially life threatening.

History and clinical examination

- It is important to ask about other symptoms that can give a clue to the diagnosis. The patient usually complains of haemorrhoids irrespective of the actual cause of the symptoms. Other common proctological symptoms include bleeding, itch, discharge, incontinence, and mucosal prolapse.
- The proctological examination consists of local examination and palpation of the abdomen and inguinal lymph nodes. The anus can most easily be examined when the patient is lying on his left side with the hips and knees flexed. Good focal and general light is necessary.
- Proceed slowly with the examination so that the patient can overcome his anxiety and relax; the doctor thus obtains more information. Explain to the patient the course of the examination, as he/she cannot see what happens behind his/her back.

Inspection

- Reassure the patient that you will do your utmost to perform the examination gently. The patient should be relaxed, preferably in a prone jack-knife position, but alternatively in the left lateral decubitus position.
- Palpate the perineum for the presence of a hidden abscess in patients who complain of pain.
- If the inspection is difficult because of large buttocks elevate the right buttock to make the anus visible.

The following conditions can be diagnosed at inspection

- Incarcerated haemorrhoids
- Perianal haematoma
- Pruritus ani
- Anal fistula
- Anal fissure
- Prolapsed haemorrhoids
- Rectal prolapse
- Anal malignancies
- Anal condylomas

Digital rectal examination (DRE)

- DRE can usually be performed, with the exception of very painful conditions such as incarcerated haemorrhoids fissure or perianal abscess.

Structures that can be examined by DRE

- Rectal mucosa
- Anal canal
- Internal and external sphincter
- Levator muscle (the so-called anorectal ring)
- Anovaginal septum
- Sacrum and pre-sacral space
- Sites of pain
- Palpable masses – cervix, prostate
- Finally, the material visible on the glove should be examined, particularly for the presence of blood.

The following conditions can be diagnosed at DRE

- Anal stenosis
- Anal fissure
- Rectal tumours
- Tumours of the anal canal
- In syndroma pelvis spastica (also known as anismus, non-relaxing puborectalis levator syndrome) the levator muscle may be tender on palpation, and moving the puborectalis in the posterior midline between the anus and the coccyx will be painful.
- Anal stenosis may result from Crohn's disease or anal (postoperative) scars.

Anoscopy

- Anoscopy is part of adequate proctological practice. It cannot be replaced by rectoscopy.
- No emptying of the rectum is necessary.
- The most common finding on proctoscopy is haemorrhoids, but conditions of the anal canal and distal rectum can also be distinguished.

Conditions that can be diagnosed by proctoscopy

- Haemorrhoids
- Anal fissure
- Anal stenosis
- Polyps of the anal canal
- Hypertrophic anal papillae

Further investigations

- The above-mentioned investigations do not require any preparation.
- Fibreoptic sigmoidoscopy, and colonoscopy can be performed only after emptying the bowel.
- All examinations can be performed in primary care but both the procedures and interpretation of the findings require experience.
- Rectoscopy can be easily performed in primary care. Its value lies in the diagnosis of rectal adenomas and polyps. Proctitis can also be diagnosed. The first 15–18 cm of the rectum can nearly always be inspected, but sharp bending of the bowel at the rectosigmoid border, often made sharper by hysterectomy, or spasm, may prevent passing the instrument further.
- In fibreoptic sigmoidoscopy the descending colon and rectum can be visualized, and the examination is definitely better than rigid endoscopy for cancer screening.

GAS

General remarks on treatment

- Proctological diseases often require some (surgical) procedure. Medical treatment is rarely sufficient, with the exception of nitroglycerin ointment for anal fissure B [1 2 3].
- Ointments for haemorrhoids alleviate symptoms, as might bulk fibre laxatives.
- Do not prescribe ointments for haemorrhoids before careful proctological assessment and exclusion of malignant disease.
- The treatment of levator spasm must begin with the simplest therapies and progress slowly to the more complex. In this case, begin with bulk laxatives and warm baths. Muscle relaxants might be tried next, warning the patient of their side effects. If there is still no improvement, referral to a specialized centre where such things as electrogalvanic stimulation, biofeedback and epidural blocks might be employed is needed

Guidelines for specific diseases

- Haemorrhoids (8.62)
- Anal fissure (8.63)
- Pruritus ani (8.61)
- Syndroma pelvis spastica (8.10)
- Anal abscess (8.64)

Follow-up

- Verify the outcome of treatment and encourage the patient to contact medical services again if the symptoms recur.
- Repeat the examinations when necessary.

References

1. Chase D, Milne R. Glyceryl trinitrate for chronic anal fissures. Southampton: Wessex Institute for Health Research and Development. Wessex Institute for Health Research and Development. DEC Report No. 96. 1999.
2. The Health Technology Assessment Database, Database no.: HTA-998495. In: The Cochrane Library, Issue 1, 2001. Oxford: Update Software.

3. Lund NJ, Scholefield JH. A randomised, prospective, double-blind placebo-controlled trial of glyceryl trinitrate in treatment of anal fissure. Lancet 1997;349:11–14.

8.61 Pruritus ani

Kari-Matti Hiltunen

Basic rules

- Exclude rectal causes that need treatment (proctoscopy is often indicated)
- Do not confuse superficial skin excoriations with anal fissure.
- Remember pinworms as a cause for anal itch (1.55).
- For the majority (60%) of patients, no specific cause for anal itch can be established. Washing habits, haemorrhoids (that keep perianal skin moist), and local reactions to topical drugs may be the cause of perianal dermatitis.

Symptoms

- While itch is the main symptom, many patients also complain of poignant pain.
- The area of affected perianal skin may be considerable.

Treatment

- Pruritic skin needs air, and anal hygiene is mandatory (showering or washing after defecation followed by gentle drying).
- Zinc ointment can be used topically. For severe itch, 1% hydrocortisone cream or fungisidic preparations (in combination with hydrocortisone) can be used as topical treatment. Avoid sensitizing combinations of topical drugs.
- In persistent cases a skin biopsy from the affected skin may be indicated.

8.62 Haemorrhoids

Matti V. Kairaluoma, Kari-Matti Hiltunen

Principles

- Haemorrhoids refer to the enlargement and prolapse of haemorrhoidal tissue ("anal cushions").
- Symptoms associated with haemorrhoids are common and usually self-limited, but they tend to recur.
- It is important to take a detailed history and ensure that the presenting complaints is in fact caused by haemorrhoids.
- A general practitioner can examine and treat over 90% of patients with haemorrhoids.
- Surgery is usually reserved only for patients with persistently prolapsed (grade IV) haemorrhoids.

Symptoms

- Rectal bleeding is the most common complaint (haematochezia). Ask the patient about the type of bleeding (visible on toilet paper, soiling the pants, dripping after defecation). Blood mixed in faeces is suggestive of a tumour.
- Other symptoms include uncomfortable feeling, itching or problems with personal hygiene. Pain is more likely to be caused by perianal haematoma, thrombosed haemorrhoids, or anal fissure.

Diagnosis

- **Visual inspection**
  - Observe for external skin tags, anal fissure, tumours
- **Digital rectal examination**
  - Note the resting tone, force of contraction and presence of tumours
- **Proctoscopy**
  - Without bowel preparation during the appointment. The grade of the haemorrhoids may be assessed by asking the patient to strain with the proctoscope in situ. With the patient straining withdraw the proctoscope, and any haemorrhoids will prolapse through the anal orifice with the scope.
- **Sigmoidoscopy/colonoscopy**
  - Before any treatment is instigated, sigmoidoscopy must be carried out in all patients; patients over 50 years of age are also recommended to undergo colonoscopy to exclude carcinoma and adenoma. For melaena see 8.50.

Differential diagnosis

- Anal fissure (8.63)
  - Painful; situated dorsally; may be palpated on digital rectal examination (lidocaine gel necessary for the examination).
- Perianal abscess (8.64)
  - Incision preferably under general anaesthesia.
- Perianal fistula
  - Surgery often indicated.
- Mucosal prolapse

- Prolapse of the rectal mucous membrane outside the anal canal. Diagnostics are the same as for haemorrhoids. Radial mucosal folds are apparent on visual inspection.

Grading

- Grade I: Congested haemorrhoidal tissue.
- Grade II: Protrude up to the anal orifice with straining, but reduce spontaneously into the anal canal.
- Grade III: Protrude outside the anal canal, and require manual reduction.
- Grade IV: Remain prolapsed outside the anal orifice.

Treatment

- No symptoms: no specific treatment
- Minor symptoms: local treatment
  - Personal hygiene is most important.
  - Local creams
  - Constipation should be treated in all patients (bulk laxatives) C [1].
- Bleeding haemorrhoids:
  - Rubber band ligation A [2]
- Prolapsed haemorrhoids:
  - Surgery
- A summary of treatment strategies is presented in Table 8.62.

Rubber band ligation

- Can be performed by general practitioner.
- Use a banding instrument with suction (not forceps).
- A headlamp may be used as the light source.
- The suction cup of the instrument is inserted through a proctoscope at least 3 cm into the rectum (approx. 1 cm above the dentate line) on the haemorrhoid or over a site proximal to the haemorrhoid if it is located lower. A ligature closer to the anal orifice is painful and should be avoided.
- After the cup has been positioned in the right place, turn the suction on, and suction the mucosal fold containing the hemorrhoid tissue into the cup. Trigger the ligation band. Turn the suction off and detach the suction catheter from the instrument. Withdraw the instrument gently together with the proctoscope.
- Reinsert the proctoscope to check the correct positioning of the rubber band (a "blueberry" can be seen if the procedure was successful).
- Up to three haemorrhoids can be ligated at the same occasion.
- The ligated haemorrhoids or mucosal folds will fall out within a week, and any haemorrhoids below the ligature will atrophy as their venous connection have been severed.
- The procedure can be repeated 3–4 times within an interval of one month if residual hemorrhoids exist.
- Complications are rare, but may include bleeding and infection of the adjacent rectal tissue.

Table 8.62 Treatment strategies

Grade	Management	Alternatives
Asymptomatic haemorrhoids	No treatment	
Symptomatic grade I-II	Rubber band ligation	Creams, dietary fibre
Symptomatic grade III	Rubber band ligation × 3–4	Sitz baths, dietary fibre, surgical excision
Symptomatic grade IV	Surgical excision	
Bleeding haemorrhoids or patients with hepatic cirrhosis or coagulopathies	Rubber band ligation	Sclerotherapy, (surgical treatment)

Strangulated haemorrhoids

- Strangulated haemorrhoids (acute haemorrhoidal crisis) require hospital treatment. The onset is abrupt with severe pain. Accompanying mucosal prolapse will contribute towards mucous discharge and bleeding.
- The diagnosis is apparent on inspection.
- Conservative treatment is effective, but will take several days of hospital treatment. Urgent haemorrhoidectomy is preferable.

Perianal haematoma ("thrombosed haemorrhoids")

- Perianal haematoma occurs when a venous plexus, or subcutaneous haematoma, becomes thrombosed and acutely painful and forms a hard, dark red blister.
- Treatment: Infiltrate a small area of the skin with 1% lidocaine and make an incision with a narrow-tipped scalpel. Evacuate the clot by gently pressing with fingers or by curettage. Any bleeding can be controlled by compression.
- After the procedure, the patient should be advised to wash the area 1–3 times daily.

Rectal prolapse

- Rectal prolapse refers to the prolapse of the entire rectal muscular wall outside the anal orifice. The prolapse is accompanied by pain, mucous discharge and bleeding.
- The condition is most common in individuals aged 60–70 years. The majority of the patients are women.
- A total rectal prolapse will not reduce spontaneously in adults, but requires surgery. The patient must be referred to the care of a specialist team. A prolapse of the rectal mucosa alone can usually be treated with repeated rubber band ligations.

References

1. Perez-MM, Gomez CA, Leon CT, Pajares J, Mate JJ. Effect of fiber supplements on internal bleeding hemorrhoids. Hepato-gastroenterology 1996;43:1504–1507.
2. MacRae HM, Macleod RS. 1995. Comparison of hemorrhoidal treatment modalities: a meta-analysis. Diseases of the Colon & Rectum 1995;38:687–694.

8.63 Anal fissure

Kari-Matti Hiltunen

Basic rules

- Conservative treatment should be preferred in newly diagnosed cases. Nitroglycerin cremor should always be tried.
- A chronic fissure often needs surgery.
- Remember inflammatory bowel diseases and cancer in the differential diagnosis.

Aetiology

- A fissure is often caused by obstipation and ischaemia, which results in a mechanical tear caused by defecation.
- A fissure may also be caused by frequent cleaning during a diarrhoeal disease.

Location

- A fissure is usually located dorsally in the midline of the anal canal (>80%). The second most common site is the anterior midline (>10%).
- Suspect Crohn's disease if a fissure is not located in the midline.

Symptoms

- The main symptom is anal pain that intensifies during defecation.
- Small amounts of bright blood may be seen in the toilet paper.

Treatment

- Spontaneous recovery occurs in 60–80%. If the symptoms have not been present for longer than a month spontaneous recovery should be expected. Local anaesthetic gel before and after defecation may alleviate pain. Toilet hygiene should be good. Warm sitz baths (40°C) twice daily for 15–20 min may relax sphincter spasm and alleviate pain.
- Nitrate gel (0.2%) daily on the anal skin has been shown to be significantly better than placebo (B) [1 2 3]. If a ready-made preparation is not available, one of the following recipes can be used, applying the preparation 3 times a day for 8 weeks:
    - Glyceryl trinitrate 150 mg + Vaselin alb. 40 g, or
    - Percutol® (glyceryl trinitrate 2% ointment) 5 g + Vaselin alb. 30 g, or
    - Diltiazem 0.8 g mixed with emollient (oil in water emulsion) 40 g. (Doesn't cause headache like glyceryl nitrate does.)
- Obstipation is managed with bulk laxatives.

Chronic fissure

- If a fissure persists for more than 2 months the condition should be classified chronic. The fibres of the internal sphincter muscle are visible at the bottom of the fissure. A "sentinel fold" is often seen in the anus, and there is a hypertrophic anal papilla at the dentate line in the anal canal.
- Conservative treatment with nitrate gel should be tried as 50% heal with this therapy. Botulin toxin injections have also been successful.
- In surgical therapy, internal sphincterectomy is performed under local or general anaesthesia. Manual anal sphincter dilatation is no longer recommended (A) [4]. Internal sphincterectomy in local anaesthesia can be performed in ambulatory care. The fissure itself does not need to be treated.
- A disturbingly large sentinel fold and hypertrophic anal papilla can be excised.

References

1. Chase D, Milne R. Glyceryl trinitrate for chronic anal fissures. Southampton: Wessex Institute for Health Research and Development. Wessex Institute for Health Research and Development. DEC Report No. 96. 1999.
2. The Health Technology Assessment Database, Database no.: HTA-998495. In: The Cochrane Library, Issue 1, 2001. Oxford: Update Software.
3. Lund NJ, Scholefield JH. A randomised, prospective, double-blind placebo-controlled trial of glyceryl trinitrate in treatment of anal fissure. Lancet 1997;349:11–14.
4. Nelson R. Operative procedures for fissure in ano. Cochrane Database Syst Rev. 2004;(2):CD002199.

8.64 Anal abscess

Kari-Matti Hiltunen

Basic rules

- Anal abscesses are treated surgically.
- Follow-up the patient to detect anal fistula.

Symptoms

- An anal abscess causes severe acute pain, and often (but not always) fever.
- Difficulties in voiding can be associated with a deep abscess.

Investigations

- Inspection of the anus usually reveals the diagnosis: a tender mass is observed near the anus.
- Touch per rectum may be impossible because of the pain. Perineal palpation may reveal a painful mass in these patients.

Treatment

- Antibiotics alone are not effective. The abscess requires incision and drainage.
- General anaesthesia is necessary for clinical examination and sufficiently wide incision.
- The patient must be followed up after incision of the abscess, because an anal fistula requiring surgical treatment develops in about 30–40% of the patients.

8.70 Colorectal cancer

Jukka-Pekka Mecklin

Classification and prognosis of colorectal cancer

- Dukes' classification is used widely. The classification is based on examination of the whole surgical preparate, detection of metastases during the operation, and complementary investigations.
- The prognosis and the probability of recurrence can be roughly determined on the basis of the Dukes' class and the grade of differentiation (poor, intermediate, high) of the tumour. Molecular detection of micrometastases may become an additional tool in the near future.
- See Table 8.70.

Risk of recurrence

- See 8.71.
- A Dukes' A tumour, if correctly staged, does not recur.
- A well-differentiated Dukes' B tumour rarely recurs; a poorly differentiated tumour recurs more often.

Table 8.70 Dukes' classification and prognosis of colorectal cancer

Dukes' class	Staging	Proportion of all patients	5-year survival rate
A	Confined to the mucosa	20–25%	>90%
B	Invading the muscular layer	40–45%	60–70%
C	Lymph node metastases	15–20%	35–45%
D	Distant metastases or residual tumour	20–30%	0–5%
All (in the best patient series)			50–60%

- A well-differentiated Dukes' C carcinoma with metastases in lymph nodes adjacent to the tumour (Dukes' C1) may be cured permanently.
- A poorly differentiated Dukes' C tumour with metastases near the margins of the resected mesentery (Dukes' C2) nearly always recurs.
- A Dukes' D carcinoma can be cured permanently only in cases where a solitary liver metastasis can be removed surgically. The prognosis of these patients is identical to the average prognosis of all patients with colorectal cancer.

Radiotherapy and antineoplastic drugs

- Adjuvant antineoplastic drugs improve the prognosis in Dukes' C tumours (A) [1 2 3 4 5 6].
- Radiotherapy and cytostatic drugs may decrease the size of solitary metastases temporarily (partial response) but the life expectancy of the patients is probably not increased (with the exception of hepatic artery infusion of floxuridine which may slightly improve survival (A) [7 8]).
- According to some studies the rate of local recurrence of rectal cancer has decreased with preoperative or postoperative radiotherapy, but there are also observations to the contrary.

Heredity

- See 8.73.
- 1–5% of all patients with colorectal cancer belong to families where colorectal cancer is inherited dominantly.
- Young age and/or colorectal cancer in the family may suggest hereditary cancer.
- The genetic basis of familial colorectal cancer has recently been identified (see 8.73), and relatives of the cancer patient can be investigated with a blood sample.
- **To identify persons who carry a high risk of cancer the family history should be requested from all patients with colorectal cancer (i.e. have the parents, sisters, or brothers had cancer).**

References

1. Dube S, Heyen F, Jenicek M. Adjuvant chemotherapy in colorectal carcinoma: results of a meta-analysis. Dis Colon Rectum 1997;40:35–41.
2. The Database of Abstracts of Reviews of Effectiveness (University of York), Database no.: DARE-970196. In: The Cochrane Library, Issue 4, 1999. Oxford: Update Software.
3. Figueredo A, Germond C, Maroun J, Browman G, Walker-Dilks C, Wong S. Adjuvant therapy for stage II colon cancer after complete resection. Cancer Prevention and Control 1997;1:379–392.
4. Figueredo A, Fine S, Maroun J, Walker-Dilks C, Wong S. Adjuvant therapy for stage III colon cancer after complete resection. Cancer Prevention and Control 1997;1:304–319.
5. The Database of Abstracts of Reviews of Effectiveness (University of York), Database no.: DARE-984000. In: The Cochrane Library, Issue 4, 2000. Oxford: Update Software.
6. The Database of Abstracts of Reviews of Effectiveness (University of York), Database no.: DARE-984002. In: The Cochrane Library, Issue 4, 2000. Oxford: Update Software.
7. Harmantas A, Rotstein LE, Langer B. Regional versus systemic chemotherapy in the treatment of colorectal cancer metastatic to the liver: is there a survival difference? Meta-analysis of published literature. Cancer 1996;78:1639–1645.
8. The Database of Abstracts of Reviews of Effectiveness (University of York), Database no.: DARE-961716. In: The Cochrane Library, Issue 4, 1999. Oxford: Update Software.

8.71 Prevention and screening of colorectal cancer

Editors

Detection and follow-up of adenomas

- Screening is justified on the basis of the assumption that removing adenomatous polyps from symptomless individuals reduces the incidence of and mortality from colorectal cancer
- The prevalence of adenomas in unselected autopsy series is as high as 30%.

Symptomatic patients

- If a polyp is detected the whole colon should be examined and all polyps removed.
- If colonography suggests a polyp not exceeding 5 mm in diameter in a patient above 75 years of age there is no absolute indication for colonoscopy and polyp removal.
- Suspicion of a polyp in a young patient or a polyp exceeding 5 mm in diameter is always an indication for colonoscopy.

Asymptomatic persons

- The use of colonoscopy for screening of asymptomatic individuals is indicated only in cases with marked familial susceptibility to cancer, or if an adenoma has earlier been removed endoscopically.
- Follow-up after the initial investigations is not indicated in persons with a single small tubular adenoma in the rectum, or in patients above 75 years of age.
- Individuals with a history of one large adenoma or several adenomas of any type should undergo screening colonoscopy at 3–5-year intervals.

Preventive measures

- Although diet is considered to be a major environmental cause of colorectal cancer there is insufficient evidence to recommend dietary changes for prevention. On the other hand, the diet suggested for prevention, with a reduced content of fat and energy along with an increased content of fruit and vegetable fibre, is in accordance with recommendations for the treatment and prevention of other diseases.

Population-based screening

- The results of large trials involving screening for faecal occult blood indicate a reduction in mortality from colorectal cancer (A) [1], but such screening results in colonoscopy being performed on a large proportion of the screened population. The cost-effectiveness of screening is controversial. Only about 50% of those invited can be expected to attend screening (B) [2 3].

Screening family members of cancer patients

- Always obtain a thorough family history from a patient with colorectal cancer. If there are cases of colorectal cancer or other adenocarcinomas (e.g. of the breast, uterus or ovaries) in the family consider the possibility of familial cancer and screening of the relatives (C) [4 5].

Examining a symptomatic patient

- Patients with colorectal cancer often present with non-specific gastrointestinal problems. Because both the sensitivity and specificity of faecal occult blood are rather poor, a negative result does not exclude colorectal cancer in a symptomatic patient.

References

1. Towler BP, Irwig L, Glasziou P, Weller D, Kewenter J. Screening for colorectal cancer using the faecal occult blood test, Hemoccult. Cochrane Database Syst Rev. 2004;(2):CD001216.

2. Vernon SW. Participation in colorectal cancer screening: a review. J Nat Canc Instit 1997;89:1406–1422.
3. The Database of Abstracts of Reviews of Effectiveness (University of York), Database no.: DARE-971223. In: The Cochrane Library, Issue 4, 1999. Oxford: Update Software.
4. Brewer DA, Fung CL, Chapuis PH, Bokey EL. Should relatives of patients with colorectal cancer be screened? A critical review of the literature. Diseases of Colon and Rectum 1994;37:1328–1338.
5. The Database of Abstracts of Reviews of Effectiveness (University of York), Database no.: DARE-954069. In: The Cochrane Library, Issue 1, 2001. Oxford: Update Software.

8.72 Postoperative follow-up of colorectal cancer

Jukka-Pekka Mecklin

Basic rules

- The aim of postoperative follow-up (A) [1 2 3 4 5] is to detect solitary liver (C) [6 7] or pulmonary metastases that are suitable for surgical resection. This implies that follow-up is indicated (A) [1 2 3 4 5] in patients whose age and general condition would allow liver or lung surgery.
- Locally recurring tumours (the most common form of recurrence) are usually not suitable for reoperation. Instead, the primary operation should be radical: besides hemicholectomy, a locally invasive left loop tumour can be treated with pancreatic and gastric resection, splenectomy, and left-sided nephrectomy.
- It is important to look for new tumours in patients who have had colorectal cancer (8.73).

Follow-up investigations

- History and symptoms.
- Clinical examination. Do not forget touch per rectum and palpation of the perineum.
- Serum carcinoembryonic antigen (CEA) concentration should be determined at every follow-up examination.
- The remaining colon should be examined 1–2 times during the follow-up period.
- The anastomosis should be examined with fibreoptic endoscopy after anterior resection.
- After the first five years of follow-up, endoscopy of the remaining bowel is performed on patients under 65 years of age until the age of 70 years in order to detect eventual new tumours.

Table 8.72 Post-operative follow-up of colorectal cancer

Time	Place	Investigations (in addition to clinical examination, which is always performed
4–6 weeks	Hospital	Blood count (BC) C-reactive protein (CRP); is post-operative healing proceeding well?
3 months	Primary care (PC)	BC, carcinoembryonic antigen (CEA)
6 months	PC	BC, CEA
9 months	PC	BC, CEA
12 months	Hospital	BC, CEA, ultrasonography, colonoscopy
15 months	PC	BC, CEA
18 months	PC	BC, CEA
21 months	PC	BC, CEA
24 months	Hospital	BC, CEA, ultrasonography
30 months	PC	BC, CEA
36 months	PC	BC, CEA
42 months	PC	BC, CEA
48 months	Hospital	BC, CEA, ultrasonography
60 months	Hospital	BC, CEA, colonoscopy. Need for further follow-up?

Postoperative follow-up in primary care

- Because 60% of patients with colorectal cancer are aged above 70 years, and they often have many diseases, follow-up of the patient (not of the cancer!) is the best option for many of them.
- In this form of follow-up the patient visits his or her personal doctor. No special investigations are necessary in addition to clinical examination.

Follow-up scheme

- See Table 8.72

References

1. Jeffery GM, Hickey BE, Hider P. Follow-up strategies for patients treated for non-metastatic colorectal cancer. Cochrane Database Syst Rev. 2004;(2):CD002200.
2. Richard CS, McLeod RS. Follow-up of patients after resection for colorectal cancer: a position paper of the Canadian society of surgical oncology and the Canadian society of colon and rectal surgeons. Can J Surg 1997;40:90–100.
3. The Database of Abstracts of Reviews of Effectiveness (University of York), Database no.: DARE-970594. In: The Cochrane Library, Issue 4, 1999. Oxford: Update Software.
4. Bruinvels DJ, Stiggelbout AM, Kievit J, Vanhouwelingen HC, Habbema JDF, van de Velde CJH. Follow-up of patients with colorectal cancer: a meta-analysis. Ann Surg 1994;219:174–182.

5. The Database of Abstracts of Reviews of Effectiveness (University of York), Database no.: DARE-940048. In: The Cochrane Library, Issue 4, 1999. Oxford: Update Software.
6. Beard SM, Holmes M, Majeed A, Price C. Hepatic resection as a treatment for liver metastases in colorectal cancer. Guidance Note for Purchasers. Sheffield: University of Sheffield, Trent Institute for Health Services Research. Guidance Notes for P. 1999. 1–67.
7. The Database of Abstracts of Reviews of Effectiveness (University of York), Database no.: DARE-20008029. In: The Cochrane Library, Issue 1, 2001. Oxford: Update Software.

8.73 Long-term follow-up of patients at risk of colorectal cancer

Jukka-Pekka Mecklin

Risk groups

- Patients with colorectal cancer
- Patients with adenomas
- Patients with dominantly inherited predisposition to colorectal cancer
  - Hereditary non-polyposis colorectal cancer (HNPCC)
  - Hereditary colonic adenomatosis
- Patients with ulcerative colitis
- **Remember to ask about family history in all cases of colorectal cancer.**

Method of follow-up

- Colonoscopy

Recommended frequency of screening

Patients with colorectal cancer or adenoma (age below 70 years)

- At 2–3-year intervals in patients with
  - HNPCC and an adenoma
  - multiple colorectal cancers
  - multiple adenomas
- At 3–5-year intervals in patients with
  - colorectal cancer
  - one large adenoma
  - an adenoma with moderate or severe dysplasia
  - a villous or tubulovillous adenoma.
- At 5–10-year intervals in patients with
  - 1–2 tubular adenomas less than 1 cm in diameter.
  - According to present opinion, follow-up after a single tubular adenoma that is <5 mm in diameter is not necessary.
- Long-term follow-up is carried out on patients above 70 years of age only if there are special indications.

Ulcerative colitis

- Colonoscopy is performed at 2–3-year intervals among patients who have had ulcerative colitis for more than 8 years.
- Precancerous dysplasia is sought from random biopsies. Detecting dysplasia from the histological specimens requires experience. If dysplasia is detected and confirmed, prophylactic colectomy is performed.
- The diagnosis of carcinoma associated with colitis is difficult. The tumour usually does not grow in an exophytic or circular manner, instead it can be a benign-looking stricture or a poorly demarcated plaque.

Hereditary colonic adenomatosis and hereditary non-polyposis colorectal cancer (HNPCC)

- Both conditions are carcinoma syndromes that are inherited dominantly. Persons with the genetic trait usually become affected before their 40th birthday if prophylactic colectomy (in adenomatosis at the age of 20–25 years) or prophylactic adenoma removal (in HNPCC at screening colonoscopies at 3-year intervals) is not performed.
- In some countries there are national registers of these syndromes, where all affected families are noted. Screening of persons at risk in these families is the responsibility of those maintaining the registers.
- If cancer is found in a HNPCC patient, colectomy and ileosigmoidostomy are performed (30–35 cm of the colon is left).

8.80 Chronic inflammatory bowel disease

Pekka Pikkarainen

Basic rules

- Identify chronic inflammatory bowel disease in patients with recurring abdominal pain, weight loss or recurrent or prolonged (bloody) diarrhoea.

- Identify patients with fulminant colitis requiring hospitalization.
- Arrange long-term follow-up for patients with colitis because of the risk for malignancy (8.73).

Epidemiology

- The yearly incidence of ulcerative colitis is eight new cases per 100 000 inhabitants, and its prevalence is about 200/100 000.
- The prevalence of Crohn's disease is on average one third to one half of the prevalence of ulcerative colitis.

Symptoms and signs

- See Table 8.80.
- If colitis is caused by Crohn's disease the most common symptom is diarrhoea. Terminal ileitis manifests as abdominal pain, fever, elevated ESR and decreased serum albumin.
- Signs of severe colitis include defecation frequency >6/day, tachycardia, fever, elevated ESR and CRP, and decreased serum albumin.

Investigations

- Sigmoidoscopy or colonoscopy are the methods of choice. Ulcerative colitis is nearly always detected, but some patients with Crohn's disease have normal colonic mucosa. Biopsies must always be taken even if the mucosa looks normal.
    - In the acute phase of the disease differentiating between infectious colitis and ulcerative colitis is not always possible, but the histology is often suggestive.
    - Granulomas that ascertain the diagnosis of Crohn's disease are often found in mucosa that appears normal.
- If sigmoidoscopy is not available in primary care, a biopsy taken at rigid rectoscopy often reveals inflammation (and helps to differentiate the disease from infectious colitis).
- In all patients except those with mild colitis confined to the rectum (as assessed by sigmoidoscopy), the extent of the disease should be determined either by colonoscopy or leukocyte scintigraphy.
- If Crohn's disease is suspected, double-contrast passage radiography or CT/MRI-enterography is often diagnostic.

Table 8.80 Differential diagnosis of ulcerative colitis and Crohn's disease

Symptom	Ulcerative colitis	Crohn's disease
Abdominal pain	+	+++
Diarrhoea	+++	++
Bloody diarrhoea	+++	+
Proctitis	+++	+
Perianal fistula	-	+
High ESR	+	+++
Tender mass	-	++

Differential diagnosis

- Infectious colitis (faecal bacterial culture, mucosal biopsy)
- Clostridium difficile colitis and other diarrhoeas caused by antibiotics (preceding antibiotic regimen) (8.42).
- Ischaemic colitis (in patients above 50 year of age with abdominal pain followed by bloody diarrhoea).
- Colitis following radiation therapy (even years after the therapy)
- Periappendicular abscess (often detected by palpation)
- Tumours
- Diverticulitis (diverticula detected by low colonography or CT enterography using soluble contrast material or in endoscopy, no mucosal changes, symptoms confined to the left colon)

GAS

Treatment

Drug therapy

- In proctitis and distal colitis the drug of choice is **sulphasalazine, mesalazine or olsalazine** in 2 or 3 daily doses A [1 2 3].
- Supportive drug therapies include enemas and suppositories
    - 5-ASA enema is the first choice B [4 5]
    - Prednisolone enema
    - Hydrocortisone foam
    - Budesonide enema
    - Sulphasalazine or mesalazine suppositories for proctitis.
- Systemic steroids can be given for a short period if the symptoms are not controlled by other therapies B [6 7]. Corticosteroids do not significantly reduce the risk of relapses in Crohn's disease C [8].
- Sulphasalazine, olsalazine or mesalazine are used continuously for a long period to prevent recurrences A [1 2 3]. In distal colitis the drugs can be stopped after a few years if there are no inflammatory changes in biopsy samples. Also azathioprine is effective in maintaining remission A [9].
- A primary care physician can start the therapy after the primary investigations (endoscopy and biopsy) have been performed. Colonoscopy or leukocyte scintigraphy are recommended if they are easily available. These examinations will yield negative results within a few weeks from the start of effective initial therapy. A specialist should be consulted about the treatment plan.
- A mild recurring episode of colitis can be treated by a primary care physician
    - If the symptoms are mild start sulphasalazine 3–4 g daily, mesalazine 800–1000 mg 3 or 4 times daily, or olsalazine 500 mg 3 or 4 times daily A [1 2 3]. The dose can be increased in a graded fashion during one week.
- If the patient has even moderate symptoms (bloody diarrhoea) prednisolone 30–40 mg daily for 1–2 weeks should be given, then tapering the dose during 4–8 weeks.
- In severe cases metronidazole, ciprofloxacin and immunosuppressive drugs (azathioprin A [10], cyclosporin, rarely methotrexate) are also used. The patients should be treated and followed up by a specialist.

- Stopping smoking helps to prevent recurrences of Crohn's disease after surgery.

Reasons for consulting a specialist

- The symptoms of a recurrent episode are not alleviated within 1–2 weeks.
- Corticosteroids cannot be stopped within 2 months.
- Pregnancy, even if the patient is asymptomatic
- Extraintestinal symptoms (liver, skin, joints, low back, eyes)

Extraintestinal manifestations

- Joints: peripheral arthritis, ankylosing spondylitis
- Skin and mucosa: erythema nodosum, aphtous stomatitis, pyoderma gangrenosum
- Eyes: episcleritis, iritis, uveitis
- Liver: fatty liver, chronic hepatitis, sclerosing cholangitis, pericholangitis, cholangiocarcinoma
- Others: autoimmune haemolytic anaemia, venous thrombosis

Follow-up

- The activity of a symptomatic disease is followed up with colonoscopy as required.
- Because of the risk for malignancy, colonoscopy should be performed on patients who have had ulcerative colitis for 8 years, and thereafter the examination should be repeated at 1–3 years intervals to detect dysplasia (C) [11 12]. Surgery is indicated if high-grade dysplasia is detected.
- To ensure adequate follow-up the patients should be included in a local register.
- The risk of malignancy in colitis caused by Crohn's disease is similar to that of ulcerative colitis.
- Ask the patient about intestinal, articular, spine, and ocular symptoms at follow-up visits.
- The ordinary laboratory tests include ESR, serum CRP, blood count, ALT, alkaline phosphatase, albumin.
- Reversible oligospermia is a possible side effect of sulphasalazine.

Microscopic colitis

- In ca. 10% of patients suffering from chronic diarrhoea, inflammatory changes can be found in histological biopsies taken from an (in endoscopy) otherwise healthy-looking colon.
  - Collagenous colitis: a thickened collagen layer under the epithelium.
  - Lymphocytic colitis: an increased lymphocyte-dominant cell population within the epithelium
  - The changes are usually most prominent in the beginning and middle parts of the large intestine, but they also appear in the distal part of the intestine, so sigmoidoscopy is sufficient for making the diagnosis.
- The aetiology of microscopic colitis is unknown.
- The patients are usually over 50 years of age, more often women than men.
- The symptoms include continuous or recurring watery diarrhoea with abdominal pain, flatulence and abdominal distention.
- The patients often (in collagenous colitis up to 40%) have some chronic inflammatory or autoimmune disease (rheumatoid arthritis, other connective tissue disease, thyroid disorder, coeliac disease or diabetes).
  - Coeliac disease should always be excluded with antibody determination (gliadin, endomysium and transglutaminase, gastroscopy if necessary)
- The prognosis is good: the disease can be asymptomatic for years or cure spontaneously. No association with an increased risk for malignancy has been observed and colonoscopy follow-up is not necessary.
- Drug therapy is symptomatic and often there is no need for long-lasting maintenance therapy.
  - Loperamide if necessary.
  - Sulphasalazine and 5-ASA alleviate the symptoms in some patients.
  - Budesonide capsules help (B) [13], but the symptoms often recur.
  - Prednisolone in large doses should be given only temporarily for severe symptoms.

References

1. Sutherland L, MacDonald JK. Oral 5-aminosalicylic acid for induction of remission in ulcerative colitis. Cochrane Database Syst Rev. 2004;(2):CD000543.
2. Messori A, Brignola C, Trallori G, Rampazzo R, Bardazzi G, Belloli C, d'Albasio G, De Simone G, Martini N. Effectiveness of 5-aminosalisylic acid for maintaining remission in patients with Crohn's disease: a meta-analysis. Am J Gastroenterol 1994;89:692–698.
3. The Database of Abstracts of Reviews of Effectiveness (University of York), Database no.: DARE-953513. In: The Cochrane Library, Issue 4, 1999. Oxford: Update Software.
4. Marshall JK, Irvine EJ. Rectal corticosteroids versus alternative treatments in ulcerative colitis: a meta-analysis. Gut 1997;40:775–781.
5. The Database of Abstracts of Reviews of Effectiveness (University of York), Database no.: DARE-970863. In: The Cochrane Library, Issue 4, 1999. Oxford: Update Software.
6. Kornbluth A, Marion JF, Salomon P, Janowitz HD. How effective is current medical therapy for severe ulcerative and Crohn colitis: an analytic review of selected trials. J Clin Gastroenterol 1995;20:280–284.
7. The Database of Abstracts of Reviews of Effectiveness (University of York), Database no.: DARE-951799. In: The Cochrane Library, Issue 4, 1999. Oxford: Update Software.
8. Steinhart AH, Ewe K, Griffiths AM, Modigliani R, Thomsen OO. Corticosteroids for maintenance of remission in Crohn's disease. Cochrane Database Syst Rev. 2004;(2):CD000301.
9. Pearson DC, May GR, Fick G, Sutherland LR. Azathioprine for maintenance of remission in Crohn's disease. Cochrane Database Syst Rev. 2004;(2):CD000067.

10. Sandborn W, Sutherland L, Pearson D, May G, Modigliani R, Prantera C. Azathioprine or 6-mercaptopurine for induction of remission in Crohn's disease. Cochrane Database Syst Rev. 2004;(2):CD000545.
11. Griffiths AM, Sherman PM. Colonoscopic surveillance for cancer in ulcerative colitis: a critical review. J of Pediatric Gastroenterology and Nutrition 1997;24:202–210.
12. The Database of Abstracts of Reviews of Effectiveness (University of York), Database no.: DARE-978168. In: The Cochrane Library, Issue 1, 2000. Oxford: Update Software.
13. Chande N, McDonald JWD, MacDonald JK. Interventions for treating collagenous colitis. Cochrane Database Syst Rev. 2004;(2):CD003575.

8.81 Intestinal obstruction, paralytic ileus, and pseudo-obstruction

Editors

Basic rules

- Identify and treat acute mechanical intestinal obstruction immediately. The treatment of strangulation is particularly urgent (see also acute abdomen 8.9).
- In paralytic ileus start conservative treatment as soon as possible.
- Treat pseudo-obstruction of the colon by removing air or with neostigmin.

Aetiology

Mechanical obstruction

- Adhesions resulting from abdominal surgery
- Tumour of the gastrointestinal tract (particularly colorectal cancer)
- Invagination
- Strangulated hernia
- Strangulation (rotation of the intestine stops local circulation)

Paralytic ileus

- Surgery
- Severe systemic disease (e.g. infection)
- Intractable constipation in the elderly may have characteristics of both mechanical obstruction and paralytic ileus.

Colonic pseudo-obstruction (Ogilvie's syndrome)

- Marked dilatation and air filling (megacolon) may be associated with any disease affecting the general condition, surgery, or medication suppressing intestinal motility.

Symptoms and signs

Mechanical obstruction

- Abdominal pain is colicky, and at first paroxysmal.
- In strangulation the pain becomes continuous, and the general condition of the patient deteriorates subsequently.
- Vomiting is an early symptom in proximal obstruction, and a late symptom in colonic obstruction.
- Abdominal distension is marked in colonic obstruction.
- In the colic phase, bowel sounds are frequent and high-pitched.
- In the later ileus phase, bowel sounds become quiet.

Paralytic ileus

- Bowel movements cease (no defecation or passing of air).
- The abdomen becomes distended.
- Bowel sounds are absent.
- Splashing may sometimes be heard when the abdomen is pushed from the side while the patient is lying supine.
- There is no pain or the pain is mild and diffuse, not colicky.

Colonic pseudo-obstruction

- The abdomen distends and there are no bowel movements.
- The whole length of the colon is distended in plain abdominal x-ray.

Investigations

- Auscultate the bowel and palpate the abdomen repeatedly (observe tenderness and splashing).
- Plain x-ray of the abdomen should always be carried out with the patient in an upright position or lying on one side if the patient's general condition is poor.
  - Air-filled, distended bowel loops or fluid levels confirm the diagnosis and give a clue to the level of the obstruction.
  - A large amount of impacted faeces can often be seen in the x-ray.
  - Always look for free air in the abdominal cavity (under the diaphragm in an upright x-ray). Detecting free air is an indication for immediate surgical consultation.
- Carry out infection tests (CRP) in paralytic ileus if the cause is not evident. Remember abdominal infections (pancreatitis, cholecystitis).

Treatment

Choosing the place of treatment

- If intestinal obstruction or ileus is suspected the patient should be evaluated in a hospital, with the exception of constipation that can be relieved at an outpatient clinic.

- Patients with good general condition with paralytic ileus or mild mechanical obstruction can be treated at a community hospital if the aetiology is known (old adhesions, constipation).
- A patient with painful obstruction should be referred to a surgical unit. It is particularly important to recognize strangulation, which can cause perforation of the necrotic bowel.

Fluid therapy

- Both mechanical and paralytic ileus is associated with fluid retention in the bowel, dehydration, and salt loss.
  - Infuse isotonic saline; initially 2000–4000 ml, and thereafter guided by peripheral circulation, urine output, signs of dehydration, and serum sodium and potassium levels.

Relieving the bowel

- Do not give fluid or food perorally before the obstruction has become resolved or bowel motility has resumed and bowel sounds are present in paralytic ileus.
- Nasogastric suction is useful in proximal obstruction but not necessarily in paralytic ileus if the patient is not vomiting.
- Empty the bowel and remove air with a rectal tube if the abdomen is distended.
- The treatment of colonic pseudo-obstruction consists of decompressing the colon with a rectal tube, or if necessary, by suction with a colonoscope (or sigmoidoscope).
- 2 mg of neostigmine intravenously is effective **B** [1] but precautions should be taken to treat bradycardia (keep atropin available).
- Surgery is contraindicated in pseudo-obstruction.

Treating the underlying cause

- Infection, for example, should be treated in paralytic ileus.

Reference

1. Ponec RJ, Saunders MD, Kimmey MB. Neostigmine for the treatment of acute colonic pseudo-obstruction. N Engl J Med 1999;341:137–41.

8.82 Diverticulitis and diverticulosis

Editors

Basic rules

- Before starting conservative treatment of diverticulitis make sure that the patient does not have a bowel obstruction or perforation necessitating surgery.
- Do not diagnose prolonged or recurring lower abdominal symptoms as diverticulosis before examining the patient thoroughly (knowing that the patient has diverticula must not prevent from investigating the cause of abdominal symptoms) **C** [1]

Symptoms and signs

Diverticulitis

- Pain and tenderness on palpation, usually in left lower quadrant or the abdomen
- Mild fever (usually below 38.5°C)
- ESR and serum CRP are often increased. If CRP exceeds 100 mg/l the patient should be hospitalized.
- The diagnosis should be verified (by detecting diverticula) with
  - distal colongraphy with water-soluble contrast medium in the acute phase, or
  - ordinary colongraphy or sigmoidoscopy one month after the acute episode.

Diverticulosis

- Usually asymptomatic
- Symptoms may resemble those of irritable bowel syndrome.
- Bleeding from a diverticulum may be the cause of blood in the faeces.
- The diagnosis is based on colongraphy or sigmoidoscopy showing diverticular orifices.

Treatment of diverticulosis

- Obstipation should be treated.
- Diet rich in fibre is probably beneficial in the prevention and treatment of diverticulosis irrespective of whether the patient has constipation **C** [2 3].

Treatment of diverticulitis

- If peritoneal irritation is detected the patient should be hospitalized and intravenous fluids should be given. Surgical treatment is indicated if the disease advances to a perforation.

Parenteral treatment

- Is indicated if there is peritoneal irritation or serum CRP is markedly increased.
- Second generation cephalosporins (e.g. cefuroxim 1.5 g × 3 i.v.) in combination with an imidazole compound (e.g. metronidazol 400 mg × 3) is the drug of choice.

Peroral treatment

- Can be used in mild cases.

- Cephalosporin (cephalexin, cephadroxil) 500 mg × 3 or doxycyclin 150 mg × 1 in combination with metronidazol 400 mg × 3 for 10 days.

Recurrent diverticulitis

- Young or middle-aged patients should be treated surgically (resection of the affected part of the colon).

References

1. Schnyder P, Moss AA, Thoeni RF, Margulis ARA. Double-blind study of radiologic accuracy in diverticulitis, diverticulosis, and carcinoma of the sigmoid colon. Journal of Clinical Gastroenterology 1979;1:55–66.
2. Brodribb AJ. Treatment of symptomatic diverticular disease with a high-fibre diet. Lancet 1977;1:664–666.
3. Taylor I, Duthie HL. Bran tablets and diverticular disease. BMJ 1976;1:988–990.

8.83 Lactose intolerance

Editors

Basic rules

- Identify lactose intolerance as the cause of flatulence and diarrhoea before performing more extensive investigations.
- Make the diagnosis if the lactose ingestion test shows a pathological result and the patient has typical symptoms during the test. The diagnosis may also be based on a gene test.
- Avoid over-diagnosis of lactose intolerance in children below 5 years of age. Perform a lactose ingestion test in children only when there are clear indications. (The test frequently yields false positive results.)

Definition and aetiology

- Hypolactasia is defined as lactase deficiency inherited as an autosomal recessive trait.
- Lactose intolerance is defined as symptomatic hypolactasia.
- Secondary hypolactasia may be a result of coeliac disease or chronic infection of the bowel (e.g. giardiasis).
- Hypolactasia is not always the only cause of the patient's abdominal symptoms, and it does not cause anaemia or malabsorption of nutrients.
- The symptoms are the result of lactose absorbing water in the intestine by osmosis, which speeds intestinal transport. Lactose is then metabolized by colonic bacteria producing gas.

Epidemiology

- Hypolactasia occurs in 17% of Northern European inhabitants. It is more common in the Mediterranean area and much more common in many tropical countries. About half of the patients have weekly symptoms. It is very uncommon for lactose as an ingredient of tablets to cause symptoms.
- In children hypolactasia rarely develops before the age of 5 years. At the age of 7 the prevalence is 2–3%.

Symptoms

- Flatulence and meteorism
- Ill-defined abdominal pain
- Diarrhoea
- The symptoms start 1–2 hours after a lactose-containing meal.

Diagnostics

Lactose provocation test

- Fifty grams of lactose dissolved in 400 ml of water is ingested. The blood glucose (or galactose) level is determined at 20, 40 and 60 minutes.
- The test result is positive if the increase in blood glucose does not exceed 1.1 mmol/l, and the patient has typical symptoms during the test or within 3 hours after the test. The result should not be interpreted as positive if no symptoms appear.
- In diabetics the rise in blood glucose may be above 1.1 mmol/l even if the patient has hypolactasia. The occurrence of symptoms often indicates hypolactasia in such cases. The lactose-ethanol test also suits diabetic patients. In the test the serum galactose concentration is determined once 40 minutes after the ingestion of lactose and ethanol (ethanol at a dose of 0.15 g/kg prevents the metabolism of galactose).
- In children false positive results (a lack of increase in blood glucose concentration) occur as frequently as in 30% of the individuals tested.

Gene test

- A gene test, which can be performed from a blood sample, gives accurate information on the lactase activity of an adult person.

Treatment

- Decrease the amount of lactose in the food (2–3 g of lactose per day does not result in symptoms in the majority of patients with hypolactasia); cf. coeliac disease where an absolutely gluten-free diet is mandatory.
- After diagnosis the patient should avoid all milk products for 2–3 weeks. Thereafter the ingestion of milk products can be increased according to tolerance.

- Sour milk products contain relatively small amounts of lactose.
- Products containing hydrolyzed lactose contain less than 1% lactose (ordinary dairy products contain about 4.8%).
- Lactase capsules may be effective.
- Ripened cheese does not contain lactose.
- Patients with severe symptoms should remember that bread and other bakery products, sausages, butter, margarine and milk chocolate contain lactose. Mashed potatoes may also contain lactose.
- Patients on a strict lactose-free diet should ensure adequate calcium intake, with cheese or calcium preparations.
- Ask the patient to consult again if the symptoms do not disappear completely with a lactose-free diet. Usually the cause is non-compliance with the diet, but the patient may also have coeliac disease or some other form of malabsorption.

8.84 Coeliac disease

Pekka Collin

Basic rules

- Bear in mind the variable manifestations of coeliac disease: lassitude, gastrointestinal symptoms (often mild), deficiency of nutrients, associated conditions.
- Antibody testing can be used for initial screening.
- Confirm the diagnosis by small bowel biopsy (gastroscopy).
- Make sure that effective treatment is implemented
- Encourage the patient to adhere to a gluten-free diet.

Definition

- In coeliac disease, cereal gluten causes small bowel damage, villous atrophy and crypt hyperplasia in genetically susceptible persons. The damage is reversed with a gluten-free diet, but reoccurs if the patient resumes a normal diet.
- Coeliac disease can also manifest as a skin disease, dermatitis herpetiformis (13.70), in which itching, blistering rash erupts especially in the area of elbows, knees and buttocks. Small bowel mucosal damage is present also in dermatitis herpetiformis, but it is often milder than in coeliac disease. IgA deposits found by immunofluorescence in skin biopsies taken from uninvolved skin are diagnostic.

Symptoms

- Common symptoms include lassitude, loose stools, upper abdominal swelling, weight loss, and, in children, retarded growth or puberty. A history of self-experienced intolerance towards products containing wheat flour is rare in coeliac disease.
- The symptoms are often mild and may have been present for years. Frank steatorrhoea is rare.
- The most common biochemical sign of malabsorption is anaemia, which may be caused by iron deficiency (hypochromic, microcytic), folic acid deficiency (macrocytic) or both. Vitamin B_{12} deficiency is less common.
- Calcium malabsorption and osteoporosis may also occur.
- Atypical but not uncommon symptoms include enamel defects in permanent teeth, ulcers on oral mucous membrane (aphthae), and various joint symptoms.
- The diagnosis may be reached on the basis of neurological symptoms (ataxia, polyneuropathy, memory disturbance), infertility or recurring spontaneous abortions.
- Lactose intolerance may be a sign of coeliac disease, especially when the symptoms are not alleviated by lactose-free diet.
- Silent coeliac disease is found accidentally either as the result of a routine biopsy in connection with gastroscopy or by directing antibody screening especially at risk groups.

Risk groups

- First-degree relatives of coeliac disease patients.
- In patients with IgA deficiency the risk of coeliac disease is approximately 10 times higher than in the normal population.
- Patients with autoimmune diseases. Coeliac disease may concur with type 1 diabetes, hypothyroidism, Sjögren's syndrome or Down's syndrome and may be silent. Coeliac disease may sometimes be the reason for elevated liver enzymes and liver disease.

Prevalence

- According to screening studies the actual prevalence of coeliac disease may be up to 1 in 100 inhabitants B [1 2 3].
- 60–75% of coeliac disease patients are women; dermatitis herpetiformis is equally common in men and women.
- The disease is most often diagnosed in adults and in children over 10 years of age; coeliac disease in small children has become rarer. However, the disease can be found at any age after the consumption of cereals has begun.
- Dermatitis herpetiformis occurs in 1 in 4 patients with coeliac disease.

Diagnosis

- Coeliac disease should be suspected on the basis of symptoms and the presence of related antibodies.
  - IgA class antibodies against endomysium and transglutaminase are positive in 80–95% of untreated coeliac disease and dermatitis herpetiformis patients. The accuracy of these tests is about 95%.

- False-positive results are obtained particularly for gliadin antibodies; the specificity of endomysium and transglutaminase antibodies is 90–98%.
- It should be noted that IgA class antibodies do not reveal the coeliac disease patient with selective IgA deficiency.

♦ The diagnosis should always be based on small bowel (or skin) biopsy.
- The biopsy is taken during gastroscopy as distally in the small bowel as possible; however, a special capsule has been developed for this purpose and is used mainly in small children (Crosby or Watson capsule).
- Treatment should never be started without confirmation by biopsy, as reaching a diagnosis later on is often difficult.
- In dermatitis herpetiformis, the biopsy is taken from uninvolved skin.
- In borderline cases, when the interpretation of the small bowel specimen is difficult or villous atrophy is mild, the inflammatory cells of the small bowel can be examined with a more sensitive immunohistochemical method (diagnostic test for latent coeliac disease).
- In the latent phase, an inflammation is often detected in the small bowel. In particular, the density of intraepithelial gamma-delta cells is increased. The finding is not, however, pathognomonic and correct interpretation calls for experience.

Principles of diagnostics

♦ If a suspicion of the disease is strong, a small bowel biopsy (skin biopsy in dermatitis herpetiformis) should always be taken; antibody screening can be used to verify the diagnosis.

♦ In mild and atypical symptoms, antibody screening can be used as the initial method and small bowel biopsy may be reserved for antibody-positive patients. IgA class antibodies to gliadin, endomysium (reticulin) and transglutaminase can be used in screening. Patients with selective IgA deficiency remain negative for these tests; in these cases IgG class gliadin antibodies or serum total IgA can be used. A small bowel biopsy should be readily taken from patients with symptomatic IgA deficiency. IgG class antibodies to gliadin are elevated in most of these patients provided they have coeliac disease.

♦ IgA class antibodies (and serum total IgA) can be used to screen asymptomatic first-degree family members and risk groups (patients with autoimmune diseases) (D). Endomysium and reticulin antibodies are well suited for this purpose as false-positive results are rare. The sensitivity and specificity of IgA transglutaminase antibody test are approximately as high as those of endomysium antibodies. This test will probably replace gliadin antibody screening.

♦ The diagnosis of coeliac disease should always be based on a biopsy specimen taken while the patient is on gluten-containing diet. Small bowel biopsy is recommended also in dermatitis herpetiformis even though skin biopsy is diagnostic.

♦ If the biopsy finding is not obvious or the patient has antibodies but the biopsy finding is normal, testing for genetical susceptibility can be considered. Most coeliac disease patients are found to have the HLA DR3-DQ2 or DR4-DQ8 haplotypes; their absence speaks strongly against coeliac disease or latent, developing disease. These genotypes are common in the population and therefore the genetic test can only be used to rule out and not to diagnose coeliac disease.

Treatment

♦ Treatment consists of permanently gluten-free diet with avoidance of wheat, rye and barley and all products that contain these cereals; the diet is lifelong and should be as strict as possible. In borderline cases and latent cases, more studies are needed to evaluate the benefits of dietary treatment.

♦ Instructions given by a dietician are mandatory first after diagnosis and also later on, if considered necessary.

♦ According to recent studies, most coeliac disease and dermatitis herpetiformis patients can eat a moderate amount of oats (50 g/day) (B) [4 5 6]; however, oats-containing products must not be gluten-contaminated. The patient should consult his doctor on the use of oats.

♦ The initial treatment of dermatitis herpetiformis includes dapsone.

♦ During treatment the symptoms usually disappear within a few weeks or months. Skin symptoms alleviate more slowly: despite adherence to gluten-free diet dapsone therapy is often required for 1–2 years.

♦ Starch products made of wheat may contain small residues of gluten. Evidence suggests that coeliac disease can be managed successfully with these products, however, the most sensitive patients may get symptoms.

Outcome of treatment

♦ On gluten-free diet, the mucosal morphology and clinical symptoms improve. The malignant development is very rare in long-term treated patients and bone mineral density recovers by diet. The diet can improve the quality of life, and depression, poor wellbeing and gastrointestinal complaints can be alleviated. The life expectancy of well-treated coeliac patients does not differ from that in the population.

Follow-up

♦ A decrease in antibody levels indicates that the diet is gluten-free. Repeat the biopsy from the small bowel about one year after the diagnosis in order to ascertain the healing of the small bowel mucosa. Thereafter, regular biopsies are not necessary, unless symptoms reoccur.

♦ In dermatitis herpetiformis, a small bowel biopsy is not necessary in most cases as the disappearance of the rash is a good measure of the success of the treatment. In this disease, IgA deposits are found in the skin long after the correct diet has been started; skin biopsy is thus not used for monitoring treatment.

- Adherence to diet may theoretically be weaker if the patients are not followed up regularly. This is why a yearly control visit for examination of general condition is recommended. Blood count and antibody titres can be monitored in this connection.

Treatment failure

- First check the diet. The use of gluten may be intentional, or products that have been thought to be gluten-free may be contaminated with gluten. The patient may also start to use naturally gluten-free products. It should be kept in mind that also these products may be gluten contaminated.
- In treatment-resistant cases, verify the diagnosis. This requires specialist level examinations.
  - All symptoms are not necessarily caused by coeliac disease; the patient may suffer from some other disease or from e.g. irritable bowel syndrome.
  - Check readily thyroid gland function; up to 10% of coeliac disease patients may have hyper- or hypothyroidism.
- Coeliac disease may be associated with an increased risk of malignant lymphoma. This should be noted particularly in cases of treatment-resistant disease, especially if the patient is elderly and the disease has been diagnosed within 5 years. Lymphoma suspicion requires specialist care.
- Immunosuppressive treatment (corticosteroids) is nowadays seldom needed. This treatment is given by specialists.

Where to diagnose and treat coeliac disease

- Suspicion: primary health care
- Diagnostic examinations are performed in a unit with the capacity to take biopsy samples (also in primary health care where gastroscopy can be performed). A dermatologist sets the diagnosis of dermatitis herpetiformis.
- Patients showing borderline findings in the small bowel biopsy should be referred to a specialist unit for evaluation.
- Treatment should be started in a unit where dietary counselling is available. Dermatitis herpetiformis is managed by dermatologists. When the rash can be kept in check simply by a gluten-free diet, the patient can be followed up in primary health care.
- Children with coeliac disease are diagnosed and treated in specialist units.
- Complications are examined and treated in specialist units.

Complications

- Malignant lymphoma
  - Usually associated with untreated coeliac disease and is nowadays much more rare than, for example, 20 years ago.
  - Sometimes lymphoma is seen as the first manifestation of coeliac disease.
  - The possibility of lymphoma should be kept in mind if the patient does not improve on the diet or if a previously asymptomatic patient begins to have symptoms.
  - Treatment-resistant severe coeliac disease may indicate malignant development.
- Osteoporosis may be seen in patients failing to take a strict gluten-free diet.

References

1. McMillan SA, Watson RPG, McCrum EE, Evans AE. Factors associated with serum antibodies to reticulin, endomysium, and gliadin in an adult population. Gut 1996;39:43–7.
2. Johnston SD, Watson RGP, McMillan SA, Sloan J, Love AHG: Prevalence of coeliac disease in Northern Ireland. Lancet 1997;350:1370.
3. Kolho K-L, Färkkilä MA, Savilahti E: Undiagnosed coeliac disease is common in Finnish adults. Scand J Gastroenterol 1998;33:1280–1283.
4. Janatuinen EK, Pikkarainen PH, Kemppainen TA, Kosma V-M, Järvinen RMK, Uusitupa MIJ, ym. A comparison of diets with and without oats in adults with celiac disease. N Engl J Med 1995;333:1033–7.
5. Hardman CM, Garioch JJ, Leonard JN, Thomas HJW, Walker MM, Lortan JE, Lister A, Fry L: Absence of toxicity of oats in patients with dermatitis herpetiformis. New England J Med 1997;337:1884–7.
6. Reunala T, Collin P, Holm K, Pikkarainen P, Miettinen A, Vuolteenaho N, Mäki M: Tolerance to oats in dermatitis herpetiformis. Gut 1998;43:490–3.

8.85 Hernias

Editors

Inguinal and femoral hernias

Types

- An indirect (lateral) inguinal hernia descends in the inguinal canal towards the scrotum or labia. An indirect hernia tends to grow and cause symptoms.
- A direct (medial) hernia bulges at the bottom of the inguinal canal. In general it occurs in elderly men and rarely causes complications.
- A femoral hernia penetrates under the inguinal ligament in the femoral canal. The risk of incarceration is high.
- A hernia is considered incarcerated if it is painful on palpation and the patient is unable to reposition it as before.

Clinical examination

- Examine the patient in standing and supine positions.
- In male patients the examining finger should be passed into the inguinal canal from the scrotum while the patient coughs; bulging of the hernia is felt.
- Bulging of a femoral hernia can be felt in the femoral canal when the examining finger is in the inguinal canal.

Indications for surgery

- An adult patient with an incarcerated hernia should be referred for an operation immediately. Reposition of the hernia should not be tried because an attempt may result in complications.
- An incarcerated hernia in an infant can be repositioned as the risk of intestinal necrosis is small and the procedure is usually easy. A specialist should be consulted the following day at the latest. The best time for surgery is 2–3 days after repositioning.
- A scrotal hernia in a man should always be treated surgically. The hernia is always indirect and it can grow and become incarcerated.
- If a hernia does not reach the scrotum in a man or if the patient is a woman it is not always possible to classify the hernia as direct or indirect on the basis of the clinical presentation.
    - Symptomatic hernias should always be treated surgically unless a concomitant disease increases the operative risk.
    - If a hernia does not reach the scrotum and causes no or minimal symptoms, follow-up is warranted. A male patient should be seen again after 6 months in order to check if the hernia has descended into the scrotum. If it has not, the patient should be asked to return if the hernia becomes symptomatic. A female patient with minimal symptoms does not need a follow-up visit unless the symptoms worsen.
- A femoral hernia carries a high risk of incarceration, and the patient should always undergo operation.
- In the operation a mesh is implanted in the abdominal wall Ⓐ [1].
- A laparoscopic procedure has the benefit of more rapid recovery Ⓑ [2 3 4], but the complication rate may be slightly increased.

Abdominal hernias

Types

- **Umbilical hernias** usually occur in infants and children.
- **Ventral hernias** develop in operative scars.

Indications for surgery

- An umbilical hernia in an infant nearly always heals spontaneously or with an adhesive bandage. The patient should be referred for surgical consultation if
    - the diameter of the canal in the abdominal wall is more than 1.5 cm (the doctor's little finger can easily be passed through the canal).
    - the patient has symptoms of incarceration
    - the hernia persists to the age of 4 years.
- An umbilical hernia in an adult carries the risk of incarceration and operation should be performed early. Minor, symptomless bulging in the umbilical region does not, however, require surgery.
- A ventral hernia is often large. In very elderly patients and in patients in a poor general condition an operation should be avoided because of the high risk of complications.
- In the operation a mesh is implanted in the abdominal wall.

Hernias of the diaphragm

- A hernia of the diaphragm is often detected in gastroscopy or contrast examination of the ventricle performed because of dyspeptic symptoms.

Types

- **A sliding hernia** is common and usually an incidental finding without clinical significance.
- In a **paraoesophageal hernia** the gastric fundus ascends above the diaphragm on the left side of the oesophagus and may cause symptoms.
- **Hernias of Morgagni and Bochdalek** are congenital hernias of the diaphragm. Morgagni's hernia causes symptoms (abdominal pain and occasionally haematemesis as a result of incarceration) in middle-aged patients. Bochdalek's hernia may be associated with respiratory distress in the newborn.

Diagnostics

- Contrast examination of the ventricle or gastroscopy. Sometimes a hernia of the diaphragm is visible in a chest x-ray as a supradiaphragmatic opacity.

Indications for surgery

- A sliding hernia should be treated surgically if the patient has reflux symptoms that do not respond to conservative treatment or if the symptoms recur frequently. The operation is Nissen's fundoplication.
- Paraoesophageal, Morgagni's and Bochdalek's hernias should nearly always be treated surgically.

Other hernias

- Obturator hernia, Spigel's hernia and some internal hernias are rare causes of abdominal pain and occasionally also of intestinal obstruction.

References

1. Scott NW, McCormack K, Graham P, Go PMNYH, Ross SJ, Grant AM on behalf of the EU Hernia Trialists Collaboration. Open Mesh versus Non-Mesh for Groin Hernia repair. Cochrane Database Syst Rev. 2004;(2):CD002197.
2. McCormack K, Scott NW, Go PMNYH, Ross S, Grant AM on behalf of the EU Hernia Trialists Collaboration. Laparoscopic techniques versus open techniques for inguinal hernia repair. Cochrane Database Syst Rev. 2004;(2):CD001785.
3. Cheek CM, Black NA, Devlin HB, Kingsnorth AN, Taylor RS, Watkin DF. Groin hernia surgery: a systematic review. Annals of the Royal College of Surgeons of England 1998;80(suppl 1):S1–S80.
4. The Database of Abstracts of Reviews of Effectiveness (University of York), Database no.: DARE-981408. In: The Cochrane Library, Issue 2, 2001. Oxford: Update Software.

8.86 Postoperative gastric problems

Pekka Pikkarainen

Basic rules

- Treat common postoperative problems (dyspeptic symptoms, heartburn, vomiting) conservatively during the first few months. The symptoms usually become alleviated with time. Elective ulcer operations are rarely performed today.
- Consider a control gastroscopy if the intensity of the symptoms increases after a quiet period (recurring peptic ulcer; increased risk of carcinoma after an operation).
- Detect and treat nutritional problems (anaemia, calcium deficiency, steatorrhoea).
  - Avoid reactive hypoglycaemia (23.10) in gastrectomized patients.

Dumping

- Nausea and epigastric fullness, feeling hot, perspiration, elevated blood pressure, regurgitation and vomiting, palpitation, and dyspnoea
- Symptoms of dumping commence immediately after the operation in many patients undergoing gastric resection. The symptoms are probably caused by rapid gastric emptying. Early dumping, with symptoms 10–20 min after a meal, is more common than late dumping, with symptoms 90–120 min after a meal.

Treatment of dumping

Diet

- The patient should eat slowly and only small amounts at a time.
- Drink between and not at meals.
- Avoid strongly spiced foods because of their hyperosmolality.
- Consume few carbohydrates, but plenty of protein.

Drug therapy

- Response to drug therapy is usually poor.
- Anticholinergic drugs or guar gum can be tried.

Surgical treatment

- Consider surgery if
  - afferent loop syndrome lasts for more than 12 months
  - the patient loses weight, and does not respond to conservative treatment.

Nutritional disturbances

- Megaloblastic anaemia (malabsorption of vitamin B_{12}) (15.24)
- Iron deficiency anaemia (gastrointestinal bleeding) (15.21)
- Calcium deficiency (change in diet, malabsorption)
- Steatorrhoea

Other problems

Postoperative recurrent ulcer

- Screening and eradication of Helicobacter pylori if necessary.
- Occurs in 1% of patients after resection of the stomach and in 10% of patients after vagotomy.
- Symptoms are vague or absent. Remember screening for anaemia!
- Ask about use of non-steroidal anti-inflammatory drugs and aspirin.
- If the patient has recurrent ulcers after operation consider hypergastrinaemia or hypercalcaemia: assay serum gastrin and serum calcium.
- Primary therapy is conservative, following normal principles of ulcer treatment. Reoperation is indicated in therapy-resistant cases.

Alkaline reflux oesophagitis

- Acid suppression is of little benefit.

Carcinoma of the gastric stump

- Risk of carcinoma is increased if more than 20 years have passed since the operation.

Hepatology and Pancreatic Diseases

Evidence Based Medicine Guidelines. Edited by the Duodecim Editorial Team
 ISBN: 0-470-01184-X

9.10 The icteric patient

Pekka Pikkarainen

Basic rules

- Identify patients with obstructive jaundice that can be treated surgically or endoscopically. Upper abdominal ultrasonography should be performed on all acutely icteric patients preferably within 24 hours from onset.
- Diagnose haemolysis (15.25) and Gilbert's syndrome (9.11) (bilirubin is unconjugated).
- Find out whether jaundice due to hepatic cell damage is associated with acute or chronic liver disease.
- Differentiate true icterus from hypercarotinaemia in patients who eat a lot of carrots.

Definition

- Jaundice is observed in the skin or sclerae, or serum bilirubin is >20 μmol/l.

Pathophysiological classification of jaundice

Haemolysis or Gilbert's syndrome

- The bilirubin is **unconjugated** (total bilirubin is increased, conjugated bilirubin is not).

Parenchymal jaundice

- The concentration of conjugated bilirubin is increased.
- Acute jaundice
  - Acute viral hepatitis
  - Drug-induced hepatitis or by herbal products
  - Right-sided heart failure
  - Postoperative jaundice
  - Sepsis
  - Intravenous nutrition
- Chronic jaundice
  - Alcoholic hepatitis
  - Cirrhosis of the liver
  - Autoimmune hepatitis
  - Chronic viral hepatitis (HBV, HCV)
  - Hepatoma
  - Intrahepatic cholangiocarcinoma
  - Liver metastases

Obstructive jaundice

- Common bile duct stone
- Cholecystitis
- Carcinoma of the pancreas
- Cholangiocarcinoma of the extrahepatic bile ducts
- Acute or chronic pancreatitis
- Spasm of sphincter of Oddi
- Postoperative stricture of the biliary ducts

Icterus due to hypercarotinaemia

- There is no icterus on the sclerae.
- Liver function tests are normal; usually a history and normal physical findings are sufficient for making the diagnosis.

The patient's history

- Duration of the jaundice
- Itch (suggestive of obstruction or intrahepatic cholestasis)
- Abdominal pain (common in obstruction but may also occur in alcoholic hepatitis)
- Cholecystectomy
- Loss of appetite (viral hepatitis)
- Loss of weight (malignancies)
- Travel abroad, contact with an icteric patient, transfusions
- Drugs
- Consumption of alcohol; ask the patient's family or friends, too.

Findings

- Tenderness (cholecystitis)
- Liver size (enlarged liver – alcoholic fatty liver, hepatitis, tumour)
- Consistency of the liver
- Signs of portal hypertension: spider naevi, palmar erythema, gynaecomastia, splenomegaly, ascites
- Palpable, untender gallbladder (carcinoma of the pancreas)
- Injection scars

Upper abdomen ultrasonography

- An acutely jaundiced patient should be referred to hospital for the following morning. If obstructive icterus lasts for more than three weeks a permanent liver damage results. The obstruction should be relieved before that.
- Ultrasonography can differentiate obstructive jaundice from parenchymal jaundice: the intrahepatic bile ducts are usually dilated in obstructive jaundice (they may be normal during the first few days). Gallbladder stones, cholecystitis, and hepatic metastases can be visualized.

Laboratory investigations

- Blood count, serum CRP, bilirubin, conjugated bilirubin, ALT, AST, alkaline phosphatase, GGT, serum or urine amylase, serum albumin, prothrombin time, HAV-IgM antibodies, HBsAg, HCV antibodies.

- Interpretation
  - Increased bilirubin and normal liver enzymes: the diagnosis is Gilbert's syndrome (9.11) if conjugated bilirubin is normal and there are no signs of haemolysis (normal reticulocyte count, lactate dehydrogenase and haptoglobin)
  - Alkaline phosphatase > 1000 U/l suggests obstructive jaundice.
  - Increased E-MCV, increased GGT/alkaline phosphatase ratio, increased AST/ALT ratio suggest alcoholic liver disease.
  - Decreased serum albumin or increased prothrombin time suggest parenchymal disease.

Other investigations

- **Endoscopic retrograde cholangiography (ERCP)** is the best investigation for finding out the location and type of obstruction. If needed, the obstruction can be alleviated by extraction of stone or by stenting the malignant stricture.
- MRI cholangiography is the method for screening the cause of obstruction before ERCP if the pretest probability of gallstones is low or moderate.
- Doppler ultrasonography (changes or obstruction of flow in the portal vein and hepatic veins), CT or MRI are performed in special cases (haemochromatosis, tumours)
- **Liver biopsy** is the best method to investigate the aetiology, severity and prognosis of chronic liver disease (liver enzyme concentrations increased >6 months).

9.11 Gilbert's syndrome

Markku Ellonen

Basic rule

- This common disorder presenting as asymptomatic jaundice should be identified and unnecessary examinations and referrals avoided.

Epidemiology

- The prevalence in White and Asian populations is estimated to be 3–7%.

Aetiology and findings

- Gilbert's syndrome is an autosomally inherited disorder of bilirubin metabolism characterized by an increase of serum unconjugated bilirubin and intermittent jaundice.
- The disorder is caused by defective conjugation and decreased clearance of bilirubin in the liver.
- The condition is benign.
- Jaundice is usually first observed at the age of 20–30 years in association with fasting (B) [1] or alcohol consumption.

Diagnosis

- Clinical jaundice or increased serum bilirubin concentration (usually below 50 μmol/l). Level of conjugated bilirubin is normal and that of unconjugated bilirubin is increased.
- The typical patient is a young man, who is fit and well. Other liver function tests (ALT, GGT) are normal.
- No haemolysis is detected (serum haptoglobin and blood reticulocytes are normal).
- No liver biopsy or ultrasonography is necessary. The diagnosis can be made in primary health care.

Treatment

- There is no need for treatment, advice on living habits or follow-up.

Reference

1. Felsher BF. Effect of changes in dietary components on the serum bilirubin in Gilbert's syndrome. Am J Clin Nutr 1976;29:705–709.

9.12 Assessing a patient with an abnormal liver function test result

Pekka Pikkarainen

Basic rules

- Identify patients with hepatic or biliary disease requiring specific treatment (chronic viral hepatitis, autoimmune hepatitis, haemochromatosis, Wilson's disease, biliary obstruction).
- Follow up patients with slightly abnormal results and refer them for liver biopsy if the liver function test results remain abnormal for more than 6 months or deteriorate during follow-up.
- AST and ALT are sensitive indicators of liver damage. Alkaline phosphatase is increased in cholestasis but also in bone diseases.

Causes of increased AST or ALT concentrations

- Toxic hepatocellular injury (alcohol, anabolic steroids, drugs, herbal products)
- Obesity and diabetes (fatty liver and steatohepatitis)
- Heart failure (liver congestion)
- Biliary obstruction
- Acute and chronic viral hepatitis
- Hepatic tumours
- AST is also increased in myocardial injury

Slight increase (<3 x upper limit of reference value), no symptoms

- Initial investigations
  - ALT, alkaline phosphatase, GGT, bilirubin
  - Thromboplastin time, albumin
  - Upper abdominal ultrasonography is also recommended.
- If transaminase levels remain increased the following should be assayed after follow-up of 4–12 weeks:
  - HBsAg, HCV antibodies, IgG, IgM, IgA, smooth muscle antibodies, mitochondrial antibodies, serum iron, serum transferrin, serum ferritin
- **Alcoholic liver disease** is suggested by
  - daily alcohol consumption of >40 g in women, >60 g in men
  - AST/ALT ratio > 1.5, increased MCV, increased GGT
  - normalization of enzyme levels after 2 weeks of abstinence. MCV and GGT are normalized more slowly.
  - If the values are increased for more than 3 months or if there are signs of impaired liver function, such as decreased levels of coagulation factors (abnormal thromboplastin time) or albumin, liver biopsy can be performed to assess the severity of the condition. The biopsy result does not influence the treatment of definite alcoholic liver disease but may help to rule out other chronic liver diseases.
- If hepatic injury caused by a drug is suspected the drug should be discontinued. The use of certain drugs (e.g. statins) can be continued if liver function tests are monitored at 1–3-months intervals.
- **Fatty liver** is suggested by
  - marked obesity (BMI > 30)
  - NIDDM
  - bright echogenic liver in ultrasonography.
- Liver biopsy is indicated if the transaminase levels remain increased for more than 6 months (aiming at differential diagnosis between fatty liver and steatohepatitis which has a more severe prognosis).
- **Biliary obstruction** is suggested by
  - epigastric colic
  - increased serum alkaline phosphatase
  - increased serum amylase
  - Upper abdominal ultrasonography reveals gallstones, biliary tract obstruction (dilated biliary ducts), hepatic and pancreatic tumours, and complicated pancreatitis.

Remember rare (but often treatable) liver diseases

- Chronic autoimmune hepatitis (ALT usually higher than AST, high serum IgG, positive antinuclear antibodies and smooth muscle antibodies)
- Chronic viral hepatitis (HBsAg, HCV antibodies)
- Haemochromatosis (serum iron, transferrin, transferrin saturation > 60%, ferritin) (24.65)
- Wilson's disease (low ceruloplasmin concentration)

ALT markedly increased (>3 x upper limit of reference value)

- If there are no symptoms, repeat the tests after 1–2 weeks, and perform tests to determine the aetiology at the same time (see above).
- If the patient has symptoms, such as fatigue, itch, jaundice or anorexia, refer him or her to a hospital.
- For investigations of jaundice see 9.10, and for increased serum alkaline phosphatase see 9.13.

9.13 Alkaline phosphatase (ALP)

Kerttu Irjala

Site of origin

- Serum alkaline phosphatase can originate from different tissues:
  - Liver, biliary tract, intestine
  - Bones
  - Placenta

Conditions where ALP concentrations are increased

- Serum ALP concentration increases physiologically during pregnancy and skeletal growth (check the reference values from your laboratory)
- Biliary tract obstruction
- Primary biliary cirrhosis
- Liver metastases
- Acute and chronic parenchymal diseases of the liver
- Intestinal disease is only rarely the cause of increased ALP.
- Bone diseases (osteomalacia, osteitis deformans, rickets, metastases)

- Slightly increased serum concentrations of skeletal ALP may be detected in hyperparathyroidism and sarcoidosis as well as during the healing of fractures.

Assessment of a patient with an increased serum ALP concentration

- Because the origin of an increased serum ALP concentration is usually either the liver or the bones, other investigations are often helpful.
  - In liver diseases serum glutamyl transferase activity parallels that of ALP or is even more increased.
    - If glutamyl transferase activity is normal an elevated concentration of ALP does not originate from the liver.
    - Drugs rarely cause an increase in ALP concentration. In such cases glutamyl transferase (and ALT) are more sensitive indicators of liver affection.
  - In the diagnosis of bone diseases it is helpful to assay serum calcium, phosphorus, PTH, and 25-OH-cholecalciferol (if deficiency of vitamin D is suspected).
  - In practice, ALP isoenzyme analyses to determine the tissue of origin of the increased concentration are needed only rarely.

Reference values

- The upper reference limit for adults is 105 U/l using the analysis method recommended by the International Federation of Clinical Chemistry and Laboratory Medicine (IFCC).
- An increase in serum ALP concentration of more than 30% may be of clinical importance even if concentration is within reference limits.
- See the reference values of your own laboratory.

9.20 Viral hepatitis

Maija Lappalainen, Martti Färkkilä

Basic rules of hepatitis prevention

- Food and water hygiene is the best prophylaxis against hepatitis A and E.
- Proper precautions in risk occupations and sexual relationships prevent hepatitis B infections. Use of i.v. drugs is the most important single risk factor for hepatitis C.
- Prophylaxis against hepatitis A by vaccination or gammaglobulin is indicated before travelling to high-risk countries.
- Hepatitis B vaccination is indicated in high-risk occupations and for risk groups
- (N.B.: Vaccination recommendations in this article are based on Finnish guidelines.)

Basic rules of diagnosis

- If acute viral hepatitis is suspected, the following tests should be performed: IgM antibodies against hepatitis A, HBsAg, IgM antibodies against hepatitis B core antigen and hepatitis C antibodies.
- If a mild hepatitis is associated with symptoms of mononucleosis (fever, lymphadenopathy, splenomegaly, upper respiratory symptoms) the following additional tests are indicated: mononucleosis rapid test or EBV antibodies, cytomegalovirus antibodies.

Hepatitis A

Incubation period

- 15–50 days

Route of infection

- Usually faeco-oral

Clinical picture

- Acute onset
- Poor appetite and nausea are the initial symptoms.
- Fever
- Jaundice

Laboratory tests

- Serum ALT and AST are increased, and smooth muscle antibodies are detected.
- A specific diagnosis can be made by determining serum IgM antibodies against HAV.
- Total (IgA and IgM) antibodies can be determined to assess the need for prophylaxis. (The presence of IgG antibodies is a sign of an earlier infection that protects against the disease.)
- See Figure 9.20.1

Prophylaxis

- Avoid susceptible foods (especially mussels and shellfish) when travelling in high-risk countries.
- For short trips (less than 1 to 2 months), 2 ml of gammaglobulin i.m. for an adult or 0.02–0.04 ml/kg for a child prevents the disease (80% protection).
- Those who stay a long time or travel frequently to a high-risk country should be vaccinated.
  - For adolescents aged 15 or over and for adults, two doses (Havrix® 1440 ELISA-U/ml) of vaccine are given at months 0 and 6–12.
  - For children aged 1–15 years half the adult dosage is given at months 0, 1, and 6–12.

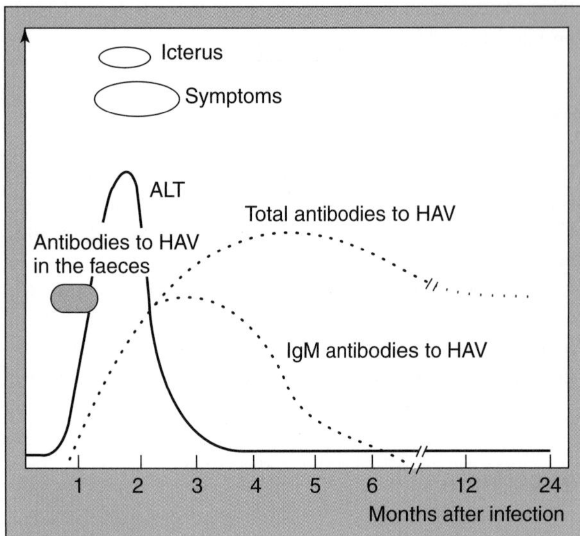

Figure 9.20.1 Typical course of hepatitis A virus infection.

- Epaxal® vaccine is given the same doses for adults and children over 2 years of age.

♦ Hepatitis A + B combination vaccine
- Given in three doses at months 0, 1, and 6.
- A separate vaccine is available for children below 16 years of age.

♦ Hepatitis A prophylaxis is always recommended for tourists travelling to the African and Asian coasts of the Mediterranean. In the Baltic countries, Russia and former Eastern European countries prophylaxis is recommended if the intended stay exceeds 1 month or repeated trips will be made.

Contagiousness

♦ After one week from the onset of jaundice virus particles are no longer excreted in the faeces.
♦ There are no permanent carriers of the virus.

Course of the disease and follow-up

♦ The disease is self-limiting, and no specific therapy is known.
♦ Serum ALT concentrations should be monitored weekly until they start to decline.

Indication for hospital referral

♦ Acute fulminant hepatitis (rapidly progressive jaundice, cerebral symptoms)

Hepatitis B

Incubation period

♦ 1–6 months

Route of infection

♦ Parenteral (syringes for illegal drugs, blood products)
♦ Sexual intercourse
♦ Perinatal transmission

Clinical picture

♦ The onset of the disease is slower than in hepatitis A.
♦ Joint symptoms occur in 10–20%.
♦ Skin symptoms
♦ Liver transaminase concentrations rise more slowly than in hepatitis A.

Laboratory diagnosis

♦ Increased serum ALT and AST
♦ A specific diagnosis is made by determining serum HBsAg and IgM antibodies against hepatitis B core antigen.
♦ For assessment of infectivity HBeAg should be determined. (If the result is positive, the disease is easily transmitted because the virus is continuously replicating.)
♦ See Table 9.20 and Figure 9.20.2

Prophylaxis

♦ Avoidance of high-risk behaviour (unprotected intercourse with potential virus carriers, use of unclean injection needles).
♦ Avoidance of blood contact in occupations that involve contact with human blood.

Vaccination

♦ Target groups
- Neonates of mothers and fathers positive for HBsAg **B** [2 3]
- Persons who have been exposed to HBsAg-positive blood through needlestick injury, wounds, mucous membrane or damaged skin
- Users of intravenous illegal drugs and their sexual partners and family members
- Sexual partners of HBsAg carriers and patients with an acute HBV infection
- People moving to work in hyperendemic areas
- People with a bleeding disorder (if the blood products are potentially infectious)
- family members of carriers and patients with an acute HBV infection
- people with high-risk sexual behaviour

♦ Vaccination is also recommended for
- personnel in outpatient departments for drug addicts **A** [1]
- personnel in oral and maxillofacial surgery **A** [1]
- personnel having risk of getting exposed to HBV

♦ Administration of the vaccine
- Hepatitis B vaccine (e.g. H-B-Vax®) 1.0 ml i.m. (0.5 ml for children).

Table 9.20 Interpretation of hepatitis B serology

	HBsAg	HBsAb	HBc-IgG	HBc-IgM	HBeAg	HBeAb
Non-infected	−	−	−			
Vaccinated	−	+	−			
Natural immunity	−	+[1]	+			+
Acute infection						
• early	+[2]	−	−	−	+/−	
• late	+	−	+	+++	+	
Carrier						
• infective	+	−	+	+/−	+	−
• less infective	+	−	+	−	−	+

1. Negative in about 10–15% of infected persons. HBcAg is the only marker of infection in such cases.
2. The first test to become positive (before clinical symptoms)

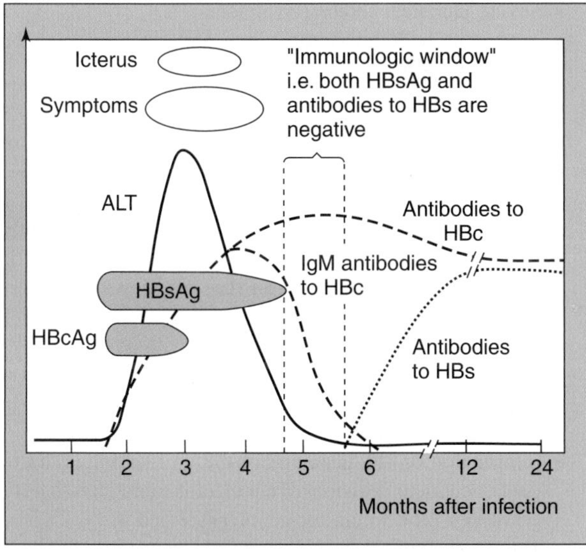

Figure 9.20.2 Typical course of hepatitis B virus infection.

- The dose is repeated at 1 and 6 months. No boosters are necessary after the initial series of successful vaccinations.
- About 10% of the vaccinated persons do not obtain sufficient immunity. If the risk of exposure to the virus is high and long-lasting, the presence of immunity should be confirmed serologically about 2 months after the third dose. If there is no antibody response, the risk of exposure should be decreased by e.g. job arrangements.

Immune prophylaxis after exposure to the virus

- Hepatitis B immunoglobulin (Aunativ® 0.5 ml i.m.) is given to neonates of HBsAg positive mothers (+HBV vaccinations) **B** [1,2].

Action after exposure to infectious blood

- Clean blood from the wound, clean the skin with alcohol and water, and rinse mucous membranes with ample water.
- Determine HBsAg and HBc antibodies from the suspected source of infection if the carrier status is not already known.
- Determine HBs and HBc antibodies from the exposed person.
- Give 5 ml of hepatitis B immunoglobulin and a vaccination. If the exposure is verified, continue with vaccinations at 1 and 6 months.

Infectivity

- Most patients with HBV infection recover; however, about 5–10% remain carriers of the virus (if the infection occurs in adults).
- The determination of HBeAg is helpful in the assessment of infectivity.

Course of the disease and follow-up

- Most cases are self-limiting.
- In the active stage of the disease serum ALT concentrations are monitored weekly until they start to decline.
- HBsAg is determined 3 months after disease onset.

Chronic stage of the disease

- Interferon alpha for 4–6 months cures about 40% of patients (HBeAg disappears from the blood) **A** [3,4]. The drug is effective in both adults and children **B** [5,6]. Drug addicts should be abstinent for one year before the treatment can be considered.
- The risk of hepatoma is increased in chronic carriers of hepatitis B.

Indications for specialist consultation

- Acute fulminant hepatitis
  - Rapidly progressive jaundice, cerebral symptoms
- Chronic active hepatitis
  - Serum ALT is increased or HBsAg is positive for more than 3 months after disease onset.

Hepatitis C

- The most common type of hepatitis in most countries.
- Most cases of non-A-non-B hepatitis after transfusion have been caused by hepatitis C. There are about 500 million carriers of hepatitis C.

Incubation period

- 20–120 days

Route of infection

- Parenteral as in hepatitis B but the infectivity is much lower. Intravenous drug use, tattooing and unprotected sexual intercourse with a hepatitis C-positive person are sources of exposure. Infectivity via sexual intercourse, however, is pretty low and safe sex is not absolutely necessary in settled relationships.
- Hepatitis C was a common cause of transfusion hepatitis during the period when hepatitis C was not screened from blood products.
- There are cases of hepatitis C who have not received transfusions and who do not belong to any risk group.

Clinical picture

- The clinical presentation is usually mild. Only about 25% of infected individuals develop jaundice, compared with 50% of those infected with hepatitis B. The disease is often asymptomatic.
- Extrahepatic manifestations such as essential cryoglobulinaemia, glomerulonephritis, autoimmune thyroiditis, Sjögren's syndrome, and porphyria cutanea tarda have been reported in patients with chronic hepatitis C.

Laboratory diagnosis

- Often the only manifestation of non-A-non-B hepatitis is fluctuating levels of hepatic transaminases, with normal or periodically normal results. Serum ALT and AST concentrations rarely exceed 800 U/l.
- A specific diagnosis is obtained by determining serum hepatitis C antibodies and RNA (HCV RNA).
  - Antibodies can be detected only after 4–6 months from exposure, and after 2–4 months from the onset of symptoms.
  - HCV RNA is usually positive from the onset of symptoms.

Infectivity

- 50–70 (–90)% of patients develop chronic hepatitis.
- The majority of patients with positive antibodies are carriers of the virus and may spread the infection.

Course of the disease and follow-up

- The acute phase is milder than in hepatitis B but the disease becomes chronic in 70–80% of patients.
- Transaminase assays are not helpful in the acute phase because they tend to fluctuate.
- The average times from primary infection to liver disease are: chronic hepatitis 13 years, active hepatitis 18 years, cirrhosis 21 years, and hepatoma 28 years. Some patients (20–30%) develop cirrhosis of the liver as soon as 5–7.5 years after disease onset.

Indications for specialist consultation and treatment

- Acute fulminant hepatitis
  - Severe jaundice, cerebral symptoms
  - Treatment with interferon alpha and ribavirin may be considered **A** [7 8 9].
- Chronic hepatitis
  - Increased serum ALT 6 months after the onset of symptoms; normal ALT does not, however, rule out chronic hepatitis.
  - A patient with a positive HCV-PCR-test and permanently elevated ALT most probably has a mild chronic hepatitis and treatment decisions can be made without liver biopsy in genotypes 2 and 3.
  - Liver biopsy is indicated in a patient with positive HCV-PCR-test and normal ALT, and with genotypes 1 and 4 before considering therapy, signs of chronic hepatitis in the biopsy are an indication for treatment.
  - Information on the genotype of the virus is important to guide treatment decisions. Treatment is more effective for genotypes 2 or 3 than for genotypes 1 and 4.
  - Treatment with a combination of interferon alpha or pegylated inferferon alpha **A** [10 11] and ribavirin **B** [12 13] **A** [14] is used for 48 weeks for genotypes 1 and 4, and for 24 weeks for genotypes 2 and 3.
  - When treating genotypes 1 or 4, if there is no response at 12 weeks (HCV-PCR still positive), the treatment is discontinued.
  - Liver transplantation is indicated if the expected survival is about 6 months.

Delta agent (hepatitis D)

- Occurs as a superinfection with hepatitis B caused by a satellite virus that can only infect a person with hepatitis B. Both viruses can be acquired at the same exposure.
- Usually occurs in intravenous drug addicts and in HBV carriers.

- The course of the disease can be fulminant.
- A specific diagnosis can be made by determining serum antibodies against HDV and HDV antigen.
- Treatment with interferon alpha has been tried B [15 16].

Hepatitis E

- A disease resembling hepatitis A that occurs mainly in developing countries.
- A specific diagnosis can be made by determining serum IgG and IgM antibodies against HEV.
- Hepatitis E should be suspected in patients who have recently visited a developing country.
- During pregnancy hepatitis E may be fulminant and result in 20% maternal mortality.
- Treatment and follow-up are carried out as in hepatitis A.

Other viral hepatites

- Some cases of viral hepatitis still remain without an aetiological diagnosis. There may still be unknown hepatitis viruses.
- Hepatitis occurs in both Epstein-Barr and cytomegalovirus infections in 90% of such patients. The disease is usually mild, and only about 5% of the patients become icteric.

Treatment of hepatitis

Acute hepatitis

- Itching can be treated by antihistamines or cholestyramine (4 g/day).
- All drugs that are metabolized in the liver should be avoided.
- The diet should contain plenty of energy and carbohydrates.
- The severity is assessed by determining serum albumin and thromboplastin time (TT normotest and pro-thrombin time; INR is not suitable). The disease is mild if TT is over 0.40 and serum albumin above 30 g/l.

Consultation and indications for treatment

Acute fulminant hepatitis (A, B or C)

- Intense icterus, cerebral symptoms, progressing liver damage.
- Intensive care is indicated. Liver transplantation may be lifesaving.

Chronic hepatitis B

- Consultation is indicated in chronic hepatitis B. A remission (no HBeAg in the blood) can be induced in about 30% of patients with chronic hepatitis B with interferon alpha A [3 4]. Peroral lamivudine is an alternative to interferon. Patients who have used i.v. drugs are required to have abstained for over a year before treatment is initiated.

Chronic hepatitis C

- Consultation is indicated in chronic hepatitis C if serum ALT remains elevated and there are no contraindications to antiviral therapy (decompensated cirrhosis, severe liver dysfunction, cytopenia, immunosuppressive state, HIV positivity, drug or alcohol abuse, severe depression, autoimmune disease, severe generalized disease, pregnancy).
- If liver biopsy reveals obvious hepatic changes and increased fibrosis, the treatment of hepatitis C is started in most cases with a combination of interferon alpha or pegylated interferon and ribavirin. The duration of treatment is determined on the basis of the viral genotype B [17 18 19 20 21 22 23 24]. The teratogenic effect of ribavirin calls for reliable birth control for 6 months after treatment. The same applies to partners of male patients receiving the treatment.
- About half of the patients become virus-free with combination therapy.
- Liver transplantation can be performed when life expectancy is about 6 months.

Other viral hepatites

- In part of hepatites the causative virus remains unidentified, and it is possible that hepatitis viruses other than those described above exist.
- Mononucleosis caused by both the Ebstein-Barr virus and the Cytomegalovirus cause hepatitis in up to 90% of the patients. The clinical manifestations are usually mild, and only about 5% develop icterus.

Working ability

- In the acute phase sickness leave is prescribed according to normal principles: work is allowed as soon as the patient's general condition allows.
- Chronic carrier state should not prevent the person from working.

References

1. Andre FE, Zuckerman AJ. Review: protective efficacy of hepatitis B vaccines in neonates. J Med Virol 1994;44: 144–151.
2. The Database of Abstracts of Reviews of Effectiveness (University of York), Database no.: DARE-940807. In: The Cochrane Library, Issue 4, 1999. Oxford: Update Software.
3. Malaguarnera M, Restuccia S, Receputo G, Giugno I, Pistone G, Trovato BA. The efficacy of interferon alfa in chronic hepatitis B - a review and meta-analysis. Current Ther Res Clin Exp 1996;57:646–662.
4. The Database of Abstracts of Reviews of Effectiveness (University of York), Database no.: DARE-961665. In: The Cochrane Library, Issue 4, 1999. Oxford: Update Software.

5. Torre D, Tambini R. Interferon-alpha therapy for chronic hepatitis B in children: a meta-analysis. Clin Infect Dis 1996;23:131–137.
6. The Database of Abstracts of Reviews of Effectiveness (University of York), Database no.: DARE-961259. In: The Cochrane Library, Issue 4, 1999. Oxford: Update Software.
7. Myers RP, Regimbeau C, Thevenot T, Leroy V, Mathurin P, Opolon P, Zarski JP, Poynard T. Interferon for acute hepatitis C. Cochrane Database Syst Rev. 2004;(2):CD000369.
8. Camma C, Almasio P, Craxi A. Interferon as treatment for acute hepatitis C: a meta-analysis. Dig Dis Sci 1996;41:1248–1255.
9. The Database of Abstracts of Reviews of Effectiveness (University of York), Database no.: DARE-961165. In: The Cochrane Library, Issue 4, 1999. Oxford: Update Software.
10. Zeuzem S, Feinman SV, Rasenack J et al. Peginterferon alfa-2a in patients with chronic hepatitis C. N Engl J Med 2000;343:1666–1672.
11. Heathcote J, Shiffman ML, Cooksley GE et al. Peginterferon alfa-2a in patients with chronic hepatitis C and cirrhosis. N Engl J Med 2000;343:1673–1680.
12. Antiviral therapy for chronic hepatitis C. Bloomington, MN: Institute for Clinical Systems Improvement (ICSI). 2002. Institute for Clinical Systems Improvement (ICSI). (www.icsi.org/index.asp).
13. Health Technology Assessment Database: HTA-20030535. The Cochrane Library, Issue 1, 2004. Chichester, UK: John Wiley & Sons, Ltd.
14. Kjaergard LL, Krogsgaard K, Gluud C. Ribavirin with or without alpha interferon for chronic hepatitis C. Cochrane Database Syst Rev. 2004;(2):CD002234.
15. Malaguarnera M, Restuccia S, Pistone G, Ruello P. Giugno I, Trovato BA. A meta-analysis of interferon-alpha treatment of hepatitis D virus infection. Pharmacotherapy 1996;16: 609–614.
16. The Database of Abstracts of Reviews of Effectiveness (University of York), Database no.: DARE-961376. In: The Cochrane Library, Issue 4, 1999. Oxford: Update Software.
17. Camma C, Giunta M, Linea C, Pagliaro L. The effect of interferon on the liver in chronic hepatitis C: a quantitative evaluation histology by meta-analysis. J Hepatol 1997;26:1187–1199.
18. The Database of Abstracts of Reviews of Effectiveness (University of York), Database no.: DARE-970845. In: The Cochrane Library, Issue 4, 1999. Oxford: Update Software.
19. Niederau C, Heintges T, Haussinger D. Treatment of chronic hepatitis C with alpha-interferon: an analysis of the literature. Hepato-Gastroenterology 1996;43:1544–1556.
20. The Database of Abstracts of Reviews of Effectiveness (University of York), Database no.: DARE-970102. In: The Cochrane Library, Issue 4, 1999. Oxford: Update Software.
21. Carithers RL, Emerson SS. Therapy of hepatitis C: meta-analysis of interferon alfa-2b trials. Hepatology 1997;26 (suppl 1):S83–S88.
22. The Database of Abstracts of Reviews of Effectiveness (University of York), Database no.: DARE-971157. In: The Cochrane Library, Issue 3, 2000. Oxford: Update Software.
23. Camma C, Giunta M, Pinzello G, Morabito A, Verderio A, Pagliaro L. Chronic hepatitis C and interferon alpha: conventional and cumulative meta-analyses of randomized controlled trials. American Journal of Gastroenterology 1999;94:581–595.
24. The Database of Abstracts of Reviews of Effectiveness (University of York), Database no.: DARE-990690. In: The Cochrane Library, Issue 2, 2001. Oxford: Update Software.

9.21 Chronic hepatitis

Pekka Pikkarainen

Aetiology and classification

- Complication of acute hepatitis B or C.
- Associated with inflammatory bowel disease
  - Ulcerative colitis
  - Crohn's disease
- Sometimes associated with chronic pancreatitis
- Often the aetiology remains unknown.
- Chronic hepatitis is classified according to aetiology, histological stage (severity) and disease activity (grade).
- The most common types of chronic hepatitis are chronic autoimmune hepatitis and chronic hepatitis C.
- **Specific** causes of hepatitis that should be considered in differential diagnosis include
  - Wilson's disease
  - Alfa-1-antitrypsin deficiency
  - Medicines, herbal remedies

Autoimmune hepatitis

- 70% of all patients with chronic autoimmune hepatitis are women. Half of the patients become affected before their 30th birthday.

Symptoms and signs

- Fatigue, loss of appetite, weight loss, aversion for fatty foods and alcohol
- The most common initial finding is increase in liver transaminase concentrations.
- A third of the patients have acute hepatitis at presentation.
- Jaundice is observed in 30%.
- Women have amenorrhoea, men have gynaecomastia.
- Hepato- and splenomegaly
- Spider naevi
- Chronic diarrhoea, skin lesions, joint symptoms, ulcerative colitis, pleuritis, or pericarditis are sometimes associated with the disease.

Mild forms of the disease

- "Chronic persistent hepatitis"
- Often asymptomatic; the increase in liver transaminases is detected incidentally.

Laboratory findings

- Serum alanine aminotransferase (ALT) is markedly increased (often 10 times above reference values).
- Serum alkaline phosphatase (ALP) and serum bilirubin are increased to a lesser extent.
- Serum IgG is elevated most in hypergammaglobulinaemia.
- Antibodies against smooth muscle are detected in 40–60% of the patients
- Antinuclear antibodies are detected in 50–80% of the patients.
- Serology for viral hepatitis is negative (HBs Ag, HB-IgM antibodies, HCV antibodies, HCV-RNA)

Mild forms of the disease

- Serum transaminases are slightly or moderately increased.
- Serum ALP, albumin and gammaglobulin concentrations are usually normal, serum IgG is slightly increased.
- The diagnosis is based on liver biopsy, which should not be done before 6 months have elapsed since an episode of acute hepatitis.

Diagnosis

- The above mentioned laboratory findings in a young woman suggest autoimmune hepatitis.
- The diagnosis is confirmed by liver biopsy, which is not always diagnostic. However, liver biopsy is the only method for assessing the activity of the disease. During follow-up liver biopsy should be repeated every 2–3 years if the serum transaminases remain elevated.
- The differential diagnostic alternatives include viral hepatitis, drug-induced hepatitis, Wilson's disease and alpha-1-antitrypsin deficiency.

Treatment and prognosis

Severe autoimmune hepatitis

- The initial therapy consists of prednisolone 20–60 mg daily as long as the aminotransferase concentrations have become normal or close to normal, thereafter prednisolone 5–15 mg daily + azathioprine 1 mg/kg daily for 2–3 years, and thereafter only azathioprine 2 mg/kg daily up to 4–5 years.
- 80–90% of treated patients are alive after 10 years compared with the 5-year survival rate of 50% in patients without treatment.
- Liver transplantation can be performed.

Mild forms of the disease

- The disease may regress spontaneously, and the prognosis is good without drug therapy.

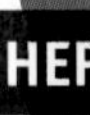

9.22 Cirrhosis of the liver

Pekka Pikkarainen

Definition

- In cirrhosis the liver cells are replaced by connective tissue. The decrease in functioning liver parenchyma, portal hypertension, and activity of the underlying liver disease determine the severity and prognosis of cirrhosis.

Aetiology

- Alcoholic hepatitis
  - Susceptibility to cirrhosis cannot be predicted. Women are more susceptible than men.
  - Alcoholic hepatitis is often cured if the patient stops drinking.
- Chronic immunological liver diseases
  - Chronic autoimmune hepatitis (9.21)
  - Primary biliary cirrhosis (9.23)
  - Sclerosing cholangitis (9.25)
- Chronic viral hepatitis
  - Hepatitis B
  - Hepatitis C
- Metabolic diseases
  - Diabetes and metabolic syndrome (steatohepatitis)
  - Haemochromatosis (24.65)
  - Alpha-1-antitrypsin deficiency
  - Wilson's disease

Diagnosis

- At an early stage cirrhosis is often asymptomatic.
- Fatigue, itching, jaundice, and abdominal swelling are late symptoms or are associated with the underlying disease.
- In alcoholic cirrhosis alcoholic hepatitis can be considered as an intermediate phase.
- The development of alcoholic cirrhosis is preceded almost always by continuous consumption of alcohol for more than 10 years (at least 60 g daily in men, 40 g daily in women).
- The type and severity of alcoholic liver disease can be diagnosed reliably and other diseases ruled out only by liver biopsy.

- Fatty liver is reversible. Heavy fatty transformation, steatonecrosis, and perivenular sclerosis precede progression to cirrhosis.

Findings suggesting cirrhosis

- Small, palpable liver
- Palpable spleen
- Spider naevi on the upper trunk and face
- Palmar erythema
- Gynaecomastia and atrophy of the testes
- Dilated abdominal surface veins
- Ascites
- Jaundice

Laboratory investigations

- The basic investigations when liver disease is suspected include
  - ESR, basic hematology, ALT, alkaline phosphatase, GGT, bilirubin, prothrombin time, albumin, prealbumin, potassium, natrium and creatinine.
- Investigations to determine the aetiology include
  - HBsAg, HCV antibodies, smooth muscle antibodies, mitochondrial antibodies, antinuclear antibodies, serum IgG, IgA, IgM, serum iron, transferrin, ferritin, alpha-1-antitrypsin, ceruloplasmin.
- Indicators of poor prognosis include
  - serum bilirubin above 300 μmol/l
  - serum albumin below 20 g/l
  - INR above 2.

Upper abdominal ultrasonography

- A "bright" liver indicates fatty transformation or cirrhosis, but is an unspecific finding.
- Spleen enlargement, dilated vessels of the portal system, and visible collaterals suggest portal hypertension.
- Even a small amount of ascites can be detected easily.

Liver biopsy

- The only reliable method to diagnose cirrhosis (with regenerative nodules and connective tissue septa).
- The result may be false negative, if the needle avoids the connective tissue.
- Liver biopsy can be performed if the coagulation factors are at an acceptable level (INR < 1.3, platelets > 60).
- Ultrasonographic guidance improves safety.

Treatment of cirrhosis and its complications

- Abstinence improves prognosis in alcoholic cirrhosis. If a patient who stops drinking has not had variceal bleeding, jaundice or ascites, cirrhosis does not affect his/her prognosis. A diet rich in energy and protein is needed, because cirrhosis is often associated with malnutrition. Due to catabolism, the patient may even be advised to eat before going to bed.
- No antifibrotic medication is available, but the treatment of the underlying liver disease may halt the progression of cirrhosis.

Portal hypertension

- If the patient has had a variceal bleeding, a recurrence can be prevented by
  - ablating the varices by rubber band ligation **A** [1 2 3] or by sclerotherapy
  - by lowering portal pressure with propranolol **A** [4 5] (the heart rate is titrated 25% lower than before medication with a beta-blocker) and with isosorbide-5-mononitrate **B** [6] (meta-analysis **B** [7 8]).
  - shunt surgery or transjugular intrahepatic portosystemic shunt (TIPS) if the aforementioned methods fail **B** [9 10].
- If the patient has not had variceal bleeding, the first bleeding can be prevented by using propranolol **A** [4 5] and isosorbide-5-mononitrate.

Ascites

- Salt restriction (1–3 g of sodium daily)
- Water restriction, if the patient has hyponatraemia (serum sodium below 120 mEq/l)
- Spironolactone 50–400 (–600) mg daily
- If necessary, spironolactone can be combined with a loop diuretic (e.g. frusemide 20–80 mg daily, bumetadine 1–2 mg daily).
- Excessively rapid weight loss should be avoided (>0.5 kg daily if there is no peripheral swelling).
- Prostaglandin inhibitors (anti-inflammatory drugs) may impair renal function.
- In therapy-resistant ascites even a large paracentesis (4–6 litres) is safe if 6–8 g of albumin is infused intravenously for every removed litre of ascites. The ascites puncture is performed with a needle for percutaneous cystostomy.
- Complications include renal insufficiency, hyponatraemia (control Na, K, diuresis, body weight).
- If the ascites does not respond to therapy consult a surgeon or a radiologist: shunt, TIPS.

Hepatic encephalopathy

- Initially protein restriction 40 g daily is recommended, but as the symptoms alleviate the protein content of the diet is returned to normal.
- Lactulose should be given 15–30 ml 2–3 times daily aiming at 2–3 loose stools per day. It can also be used prophylactically. Lactitol can be used instead of lactulose.
- Consider liver transplantation in end-stage cirrhosis.
  - In alcohol cirrhosis liver transplantation is rarely indicated, and there must be evidence of abstinence.

References

1. Laine L, Cook D. Endoscopic ligation compared with sclerotherapy for treatment of esophageal variceal bleeding: a meta-analysis. Ann Int Med 1995;123:280–287.
2. Heresbach D, Jacquelinet C, Nouel O, Chaperon J, Bretagne JF, Gosselin M. Sclerotherapie versus ligature au cours de l'hemorragie par rupture de varices oesophagiennes: meta-analyse directe des essais randomises. Gastroenterologie Clinique et Biologique 1995;19:914–920.
3. The Database of Abstracts of Reviews of Effectiveness (University of York), Database no.: DARE-960289. In: The Cochrane Library, Issue 4, 1999. Oxford: Update Software.
4. Bernard B, Lebrec D, Mathurin P, Opolon P, Poynard T. Beta-adrenergic antagonists in the prevention of gastrointestinal rebleeding in patients with cirrhosis: a meta-analysis. Hepatology 1997;25:63–70.
5. The Database of Abstracts of Reviews of Effectiveness (University of York), Database no.: DARE-970162. In: The Cochrane Library, Issue 4, 1999. Oxford: Update Software.
6. Angelico M, Carli L, Piat C, Gentile S, Rinaldi V, Bologna E, Capocaccia L. Isosorbide-5-mononitrate versus propranolol in the prevention of first bleeding in cirrhosis. Gastroenterology 1993;104:1460–1465.
7. Bernard B, Lebrec D, Mathurin P, Opolon P, Poynard T. Propranolol and sclerotherapy in the prevention of gastrointestinal rebleeding in patients with cirrhosis: a meta-analysis. J Hepatol 1997;26:312–324.
8. The Database of Abstracts of Reviews of Effectiveness (University of York), Database no.: DARE-970301. In: The Cochrane Library, Issue 4, 1999. Oxford: Update Software.
9. Papatheodoridis GV, Goulis J, Leandro G, Patch D, Burroughs AK. Transjugular intrahepatic portosystemic shunt compared with endoscopic treatment of variceal rebleeding: a meta-analysis. Hepatology 1999;30:612–622.
10. The Database of Abstracts of Reviews of Effectiveness (University of York), Database no.: DARE-991730. In: The Cochrane Library, Issue 1, 2001. Oxford: Update Software.

9.23 Primary biliary cirrhosis

Editors

Definition

- An autoimmune disease with unknown aetiology characterized by inflammation of small bile ducts.

Epidemiology

- Annual incidence is 6–11 per million.
- 90% of the patients are women.
- The age of onset is (20–) 40–60 (–70) years.

Symptoms and signs

- Often asymptomatic in the initial stage.
- Generalized itch, initially only in the evening, is usually the presenting symptom.
- The itch may appear during the use of oestrogens or drugs causing cholestasis, and sometimes in association with pregnancy.
- Jaundice is the presenting symptom in 10% of the patients.
- Hepatomegaly is detected in 50% of the patients on presentation.
- Splenomegaly, xanthelasmas, or cirrhosis of the liver is detected in some patients already on presentation.

HEP

Laboratory findings

- Serum alkaline phosphatase is often markedly elevated.
- Serum transaminases are moderately increased.
- Mitochondial antibodies are detected in 95% of the patients.
- Serum IgM is increased in 80% of the patients.
- ESR is usually increased.
- Serum bilirubin and cholesterol are increased.

Diagnosis

- If a middle-aged woman is affected with itch, jaundice or hepatomegaly, or if serum alkaline phosphatase is increased, the following tests should be taken: GGT (increased if the increase in serum alkaline phosphatase results from a liver disease), serum IgM and mitochondrial antibodies.
- If mitochondial antibodies are positive, the diagnosis should be confirmed by liver biopsy.

Therapy

- No medication has been definitely shown to slow the progression of the disease. Ursodeoxycholic acid has been used, but it confers only a marginal benefit C [1 2 3 4 5 6 7 8 9].
- The itch can be treated by cholestyramine or cholestipol, which are also beneficial in the concomitant hypercholesterolaemia.
- Calcium and vitamin D should be taken in sufficient amounts to prevent bone affection.
- Liver transplantation B [10 11]

Prognosis

- The course of the disease is difficult to predict. Elevated serum bilirubin concentration is a sign of poor prognosis.
- After the patient has become symptomatic, life-expectancy is 5–10 years.

References

1. Gluud C, Christensen E. Ursodeoxycholic acid for primary biliary cirrhosis. Cochrane Database Syst Rev. 2004;(2): CD000551.

2. Goulis J, Leandro G, Burroughs AK. Randomised controlled trials of ursodeoxycholic-acid therapy for primary biliary cirrhosis: a meta-analysis. The Lancet 1999;354:1053–1060.
3. The Database of Abstracts of Reviews of Effectiveness (University of York), Database no.: DARE-999683. In: The Cochrane Library, Issue 2, 2001. Oxford: Update Software.
4. Eriksson LS, Olsson R, Glauman H, Prytz H et al. Ursodeoxycholic acid treatment in patients with primary biliary cirrhosis. A Swedish multicentre, double-blind, randomised controlled study. Scand J Gastroenterol 1977;32:179–186.
5. Lindor KD, Dickson ER, Baldus WP et al. Ursodeoxycholic acid in the treatment of primary biliary cirrhosis. Gastroenterology 1994;106:1284–1290.
6. Heathcote EJ, Cauch Dudek K, Walker V et al. The Canadian multicenter double-blind randomised controlled trial of ursodeoxycholic acid in primary biliary cirrhosis. Hepatology 1994;19:1149–1156.
7. Combes B, Carithers RL Jr, Maddrey WC et al. A randomised, double-blind, placebo-controlled trial of ursodeoxycholic acid in primary biliary cirrhosis. Hepatology 1995;22:759–766.
8. Vuoristo M, Färkkilä M, Karvonen AL, Leino R, Lehtola J, Makinen J, Mattila J, Friman C, Seppälä K, Tuominen J et al. A placebo-controlled trial of primary biliary cirrhosis treatment with colchicine and ursodeoxycholic acid. Gastroenterology 1995;108:1470–1478.
9. Gonzalez-Koch A, Brahm J, Antezana C, Smok G, Cumsille MA. The combination of ursodeoxycholic acid and methotrexate for primary biliary cirrhosis is not better than ursodeoxycholic acid alone. J Hepatol 1997;27:143–9.
10. Bravata DM, Olkin I, Barnato AE, Keeffe EB, Owens DK. Health-related quality of life after liver transplantation: a meta-analysis. Liver Transplantation and Surgery 1999;5:318–331.
11. The Database of Abstracts of Reviews of Effectiveness (University of York), Database no.: DARE-994128. In: The Cochrane Library, Issue 1, 2001. Oxford: Update Software.

9.24 Cholelithiasis

Ilmo Kellokumpu

Basic rules

- Identify patients whose pain is caused by gallstones and offer appropriate surgery.
- Complications are rare in asymptomatic gallstones, and surgery is not usually recommended.
- Acute cholecystitis and other complications of cholelithiasis (obstructive jaundice, suppurative cholangitis, empyema or gangrene of the gall bladder, enterobiliary fistula, gallstone ileus) should be treated as soon as possible after the onset of the symptoms.
- Patients with cholelithiasis often have other illnesses (e.g. peptic ulcer, gastro-oesophageal reflux disease, lactose intolerance, coeliac disease, functional dyspepsia, irritable bowel syndrome, pancreatitis or even cancer). Any symptoms suggestive of the above illnesses usually warrant endoscopic, laboratory or imaging studies before surgery.

Risk factors

- Age
- Female sex
- Hereditary disposition
- Obesity
- Past deliveries
- Diabetes
- Diseases of the ileum
- Total parenteral nutrition

Clinical manifestation

- Two-thirds of patients with gallstones are asymptomatic.
  - The pain often radiates into the shoulders or back. An attack is often accompanied by nausea and vomiting.
    - Biliary pain lasting more than 12 hours with accompanying fever or jaundice is indicative of acute cholecystitis or cholangitis.

Diagnosis

- Ultrasonography is the investigation of choice for the diagnosis of both uncomplicated and complicated cases. It detects stones in the gall bladder with over 90% sensitivity, but its sensitivity in detecting common bile duct stones is only 25%.
- Special investigations
  - ERCP (endoscopic retrograde cholangiopancreatography) may be used both for the diagnosis and extraction of common bile duct stones.
  - Increased serum concentrations of ALT, alkaline phosphatase and bilirubin, associated with an attack of pain, are indicative of common bile duct stones. However, about 40–60% of ERCP investigations, carried out on elevated liver function tests alone, turn out to be normal.
  - For the diagnosis of cholecystitis, and for the assessment of its severity, serum CRP and liver function tests (ALT, alkaline phosphatase, bilirubin) should be determined, in addition to clinical examination. Serum amylase concentration and an ultrasonography of the upper abdomen are used to exclude pancreatitis.

Complications

- Acute cholecystitis: biliary pain lasting more than 12 hours, fever and increased CRP.
- Acute cholangitis: high fever, pain and jaundice
- Acute pancreatitis: severe pain, increased serum (and urine) amylase, increased liver function tests, history
- Jaundice
- Carcinoma of the gall bladder

- Gallstone ileus (a large gallstone passes into the duodenum through a cholecystoduodenal fistula and obstructs the bowel). The clinical picture is typical of intestinal obstruction. Plain abdominal x-ray may show air in the bile ducts.

Indications and urgency of treatment

- **Asymptomatic gallstones** need not be treated (with the exception of a totally calcified "porcelain" gall bladder which is associated with a markedly increased risk of cancer, immunosuppressive medication).
- Patients with repeated episodes of **biliary pain** should be operated on within a few months, those with severe symptoms even more urgently. Pain-triggering foods should be avoided while waiting for the operation. NSAIDs or spasmolytics are given to alleviate the colicky pain.
- **Acute cholecystitis** should be treated surgically within 2–7 days from the onset of the symptoms. Elderly patients and those in poor general health should also be referred for surgical evaluation. Intravenous fluids and analgesics are given for initial treatment. An antibiotic such as cefuroxime 1.5 g t.d.s., should be administered (the causative agent is usually E. coli).
- Patients with **acute biliary pancreatitis** must be immediately referred to hospital. Intravenous fluids and analgesics are given for initial treatment. MRCP (magnetic resonance cholangiopancreatography) (or ERCP) is carried out to verify the presence of common bile duct stones. If an impacted stone or cholangitis is detected during the urgent (within 48 hours) ERCP, a sphincterotomy and removal of the stone is carried out. Cholecystectomy is carried out within a month to prevent the recurrence of pancreatitis.
- A jaundiced patient must be referred to hospital for investigations and treatment within the next 24 hours.
- Carcinoma of the gall bladder is often an incidental finding during cholecystectomy. It is also occasionally diagnosed in patients with jaundice or other severe biliary symptoms. Individual decisions need to be made regarding further investigations and surgery.

Current treatment trends and choice of methods

- The complications of cholelithiasis should be treated with surgery within a few days of the onset of symptoms.
- Even very old patients and patients in poor general health can be treated with both conventional operative measures and with less invasive newer methods (radiological and endoscopic methods).
- Laparoscopic cholecystectomy is used increasingly for the removal of the gall bladder and common bile duct stones **B** [1,2]. The benefits of this approach include shorter hospitalisation time and sick leave. A laparoscopic cholecystectomy must sometimes be converted to open surgery half way through the procedure **B** [1,2].
- Common bile duct stones can be removed with ERCP. In some cases it is possible to leave the gall bladder in situ in the elderly and in patients in poor general health. However, up to half of the patients will continue to experience attacks of pain, which will eventually lead to cholecystectomy in over a third of the patients.
- Residual or recurrent stones after cholecystectomy can often be removed with ERCP.
- Asymptomatic gallstones are not removed surgically, as the operative risk (although minimal) exceeds the expected benefit.
- Gallstone dissolution and other experimental methods have not become routine practice as yet **A** [3,4].

Abdominal pain after cholecystectomy

- Abdominal pain after cholecystectomy may be caused by residual or recurring stones in the biliary tract, biliary strictures or spasms. Increased concentrations of serum ALT or alkaline phosphatase may suggest these conditions.
- The symptoms may have other than biliary aetiology, e.g. diseases of the stomach or colon (see the aforementioned list). Specialist investigations (endoscopy, imaging, laboratory investigations) should be carried out if necessary or the patient may need specialist consultation (always if laboratory tests are abnormal).

References

1. Shea JA, Healey MJ, Berlin JA, Clarke JR, Malet PF, Staroscik RN, Schwartz JS, Williams SV. Mortality and complications associated with laparoscopic cholecystectomy: a meta-analysis. Ann Surg 1996;224:609–620.
2. The Database of Abstracts of Reviews of Effectiveness (University of York), Database no.: DARE-961865. In: The Cochrane Library, Issue 4, 1999. Oxford: Update Software.
3. May GR, Sutherland LR, Shaffer EA. Efficacy of bile acid therapy for gallstone dissolution: a meta-analysis of randomized trials. Alimentary Pharmacology and Therapeutics 1993;7: 139–148.
4. Tudyka J, Wechsler JG, Kratzer W, Maier C, Mason R, Kuhn K, Adler G. Gallstone recurrence after successful dissolution therapy. Digestive Diseases And Sciences 1996;41:235–41.

9.25 Sclerosing cholangitis

Editors

Definition

- Sclerosing cholangitis is a chronic, fibrotizing and constrictive inflammation of the biliary ducts that progresses slowly and leads to cholestatic liver damage and cirrhosis.

Epidemiology

- Prevalence 5–10/100 000
- More common in men than in women
- Age at onset is 25–45 years.

Aetiology

- 70% of the cases are associated with ulcerative colitis. Respectively, 5% of patients with ulcerative colitis in turn are affected with sclerosing cholangitis.
- Coeliac disease, sarcoidosis, rheumatoid arthritis
- HLA associations and circulating antibodies suggest an autoimmune aetiology.

Symptoms, signs and diagnosis

- Most patients are asymptomatic at the time of diagnosis; abnormal liver function tests (alkaline phosphatase) are detected incidentally.
- Cholangitis with fever, weight loss and jaundice are symptoms of a late phase.
- The diagnosis is based on endoscopic retrograde cholangiography (ERCP).
- Colonoscopy to detect silent colitis is indicated in all patients.

Complications

- Strictures of the biliary tract
- Increased risk for gallstones
- Cholangiocarcinoma develops in 10% of the patients.
- Cirrhosis develops at the end stage of the disease.

Treatment

- There is no evidence on the effect of any treatment.
- Ursodeoxycholic acid and methotrexate have been tried.
- Biliary strictures can be dilatated endoscopically.
- Liver transplantation

9.30 Acute pancreatitis

Pauli Puolakkainen

Basic rules

- Suspect acute pancreatitis in any patient with epigastric pain and impaired general condition in association with history of alcohol consumption.
- Identify acute pancreatitis at an early stage on the basis of the clinical presentation and determination of urine amylase or trypsinogen-2-status (dipstick test).
- Refer to central hospital all patients with acute pancreatitis who have
  - impaired general condition, or
  - clearly elevated serum CRP concentration.

History

- Excessive consumption of alcohol is the cause in the majority of cases in Finland.
- Ask about biliary diseases and earlier episodes of pancreatitis.

Physical examination

- The general condition is most important.
- Shock, respiratory distress, anuria and mental confusion may indicate severe pancreatitis.
- Record epigastric tenderness and palpable masses.
- Examine the skin of the flanks and navel for haematomas.
- Observe symptoms and clinical findings of peritonitis or intestinal paralysis.

Laboratory examinations

- Urine trypsinogen-2 dipstick test is the best method for screening.
- Urine amylase above 2000 U/l (serum amylase > 300 IU/l) suggests pancreatitis, and a concentration above 6000 U/l (serum amylase > 900 IU/l) is considered diagnostic. Amylase (also dipstick) determinations are suitable for primary diagnosis, bearing in mind that the amylase test is unspecific, and that the amylase concentration does not correlate with the severity of pancreatitis.
- Serum CRP is a good test in the assessment of the severity of pancreatitis. A clearly elevated concentration above 100 mg/l suggests severe pancreatitis.
- Marked elevations (3×) of ALT or AST suggest gallstone pancreatitis C [1 2]

Radiological investigations

- Plain x-rays of the abdomen may be useful in differential diagnosis (perforated peptic ulcer, intestinal obstruction).
- The usefulness of ultrasonography is decreased by intestinal air that prevents reliable visualization of the pancreas. Furthermore, ultrasonography is not suitable for the assessment of severity.
- Contrast-enhanced computed tomography is the most accurate imaging method for diagnosing and assessing the severity of pancreatitis. MRI study is also a promising but more rarely available imaging method.
- If the pancreatitis is caused by a wedged gallstone in the papilla, an emergency endoscopic papillotomy accelerates healing and improves prognosis.

Treatment of mild pancreatitis

- Even mild pancreatitis should be followed up in a hospital because of the risk of complications.
- Sufficient early fluid resuscitation is the basis of conservative treatment. Even mild pancreatitis causes dehydration, and the minimum requirement for fluids during the first 24 hours is 5 l. Fluid resuscitation is continued according to the clinical condition and urine output. Glucose-saline solutions are the most suitable.
- Adequate analgesia and follow-up are an essential part of the treatment.
- Antibiotics **A** [3], other medications, with the possible exception of antisecretory agents **B** [4 5], and nasogastric suction are of no benefit according to the results of controlled studies. A nasogastric tube can be used if the patient vomits profusely because of intestinal paralysis.
- The outcome of conservative treatment is almost invariably good.
- Serum CRP, blood glucose, blood count, serum calcium, sodium, and potassium should be determined daily. Serum or urine amylase concentrations do not correlate with the severity of pancreatitis.
- The patient should be maintained on intravenous fluids as long as he has symptoms.

Interventions for gallstone pancreatitis

- Urgent (during the first day) sphincterotomy and removal of gallstones from the common bile duct on ERCP improves the prognosis in severe pancreatitis, if there are signs of biliary obstruction or cholangitis.

Necrotizing pancreatitis

- The treatment of necrotizing pancreatitis should be concentrated to units of specialized care with the best experience and intensive care readiness because of the risk of complications and high mortality.
- The symptoms of severe pancreatitis include peritonitis shock, respiratory distress, anuria, and mental confusion.
- An increased serum CRP concentration (above 100 mg/l) is the most accurate indicator of severe pancreatitis, along with an impaired general condition and findings in contrast enhanced computed tomography.
- The treatment of necrotizing pancreatitis has been changed in favour of conservative approach including aggressive fluid resuscitation (in the initial stage up to 10 l/day) and conservative measures maintaining cardiovascular and respiratory function (in intensive care). However, surgery may still be indicated. The primary indication for surgery is the infection of pancreatic necrosis.
- If pancreatitis is caused by a gallstone wedged in the papilla of Vater, emergency papillotomy speeds recovery and improves prognosis.
- Prophylactic antibiotics are indicated in severe pancreatitis **B** [6 7 8 9].

References

1. Tenner S, Dubner H, Steinberg W. Predicting gallstone pancreatitis with laboratory parameters: a meta-analysis. Am J Gastroenterol 1994;89:1863–1866.
2. The Database of Abstracts of Reviews of Effectiveness (University of York), Database no.: DARE-940874. In: The Cochrane Library, Issue 4, 1999. Oxford: Update Software.
3. Bassi C, Larvin M, Villatoro E. Antibiotic therapy for prophylaxis against infection of pancreatic necrosis in acute pancreatitis. Cochrane Database Syst Rev 2003(4):CD002941.
4. Andriulli A, Leandro G, Vlemente R, Festa V, Caruso N, Annese V, Lezzi G, Lichino E, Bruno F, Perri F. Meta-analysis of somatostatin, octreotide and gabexate mesilate in the therapy of acute pancreatitis. Alim Pharmacol Therap 1998;12:237–245.
5. The Database of Abstracts of Reviews of Effectiveness (University of York), Database no.: DARE-980804. In: The Cochrane Library, Issue 2, 2000. Oxford: Update Software.
6. Kramer KM, Levy H. Prophylactic antibiotics for severa acute pancreatitis: the beginning of an era. Pharmacotherapy 1999;19:592–602.
7. The Database of Abstracts of Reviews of Effectiveness (University of York), Database no.: DARE-991015. In: The Cochrane Library, Issue 1, 2001. Oxford: Update Software.
8. Golub R, Siddiqi F, Pohl D. Role of antibiotics in acute pancreatitis: a meta-analysis. Journal of Gastrointestinal Surgery 1998:2; 496–503.
9. The Database of Abstracts of Reviews of Effectiveness (University of York), Database no.: DARE-2000. In: The Cochrane Library, Issue 1, 2002. Oxford: Update Software.

9.31 Recurrent or chronic pancreatitis

Editors

Basic rules

- Consider chronic pancreatitis as the cause of recurrent abdominal pain, weight loss and diarrhoea.
- Detect diabetes at an early stage in patients with chronic pancreatitis. Be careful not to induce hypoglycaemia in patients on insulin.
- Recurrent severe pain and complications are indications for surgical treatment.

Aetiology

- Alcohol in over 75% of cases

  - With few exceptions the patient is a heavy drinker who has consumed 150–175 g of pure alcohol daily over 10–15 years before disease onset
- Gallstone disease
- Metabolic disorders (hypertriglyceridaemia, hyperparathyroidism)
- Hereditary chronic pancreatitis (hereditary pancreatic calcification)
- Autoimmune pancreatitis is associated with primary sclerosing cholangitis, primary biliary cirrhosis, and Sjögren's syndrome.

Symptoms

- Abdominal pain that radiates to the back with possibly associated nausea and vomiting.
- Within approx. 8 years 50% of the patients develop endocrine and exocrine pancreatic insufficiency manifested as steatorrhoea, weight loss and diabetes. (9.32)

Diagnosis

Laboratory examinations in primary care

- Urine amylase, urine trypsinogen-2 and blood leukocyte count are often increased during attacks of pain.
- Serum concentrations of alkaline phosphatase, ALT and bilirubin are increased in biliary obstruction.
- Fasting blood glucose should be determined for early detection of diabetes.
- For tests of exocrine pancreatic function see 9.32

Conservative treatment

- Treatment of diabetes
  - Small doses of insulin are often needed (hypoglycaemia tends to develop easily)
- An attack of acute pancreatitis
  - Should be treated conservatively.
  - Fluid resuscitation and analgesics are usually indicated.
  - The patients often recover quickly.
- The patient must stop the use of alcohol.
- Small meals are of benefit in cases of pain and steatorrhoea. The diet should be low in fat with no fibre. Enzyme substitution is indicated if 24-hour faecal fat is >15 g. The effect of enzyme substitution on pain is not proven D [1 2]

Indications for specialist consultation

- Differential diagnosis
- Recurrent bouts of severe pain
- Suspected complications (pancreatic pseudocyst or abscess)
  - The symptoms include vomiting and weight loss (gastric retention), icterus and cholangitis, fistulas into adjacent organs, and oesophageal bleeding (portal hypertension)

References

1. Brown A, Hughes M, Tenner S. Banks PA. Does pancreatic enzyme supplementation reduce pain in patients with chronic pancreatitis: a meta-analysis. Am J Gastroenterol 1997;92:2032–2035.
2. The Database of Abstracts of Reviews of Effectiveness (University of York), Database no.: DARE-971420. In: The Cochrane Library, Issue 4, 1999. Oxford: Update Software.

9.32 Pancreatic insufficiency

Editors

Basic rules

- Consider pancreatic exocrine dysfunction as a cause of chronic diarrhoea.
- Abstinence and diet are the treatments of choice. In advanced cases pancreatic enzyme substitution is required.
- Determine fasting blood glucose regularly to detect diabetes caused by endocrine insufficiency.

Aetiology

Primary causes

- Chronic pancreatitis (9.31) is the most common cause.
- Carcinoma of the pancreas (9.33)
- Extensive resection of the pancreas
- Pancreatic trauma
- Hereditary diseases
  - Hereditary pancreatitis
  - Cystic fibrosis (31.23)
- Undernutrition

Secondary causes

- Gastrinoma (Zollinger–Ellison syndrome)
- Gastric operation (Billroth I, vagotomy and pyloroplasty)

Clinical features

- Diarrhoea
- Weight loss
- Postprandial abdominal pain
- Voluminous foul-smelling stools

Laboratory investigations

- Serum cholesterol concentration is typically low.

- Serum albumin is decreased.
- Hypocalcaemia (real)
- Blood glucose is elevated in 50% of the patients.
- Serum alkaline phosphatase is elevated if the patient has biliary obstruction or deficiency of vitamin D.
- Pancreatic function tests (serum trypsin and pancreatic amylase concentrations are low, secretin-stimulated pancreatic bicarbonate secretion is low).
- Faecal elastase I determination is useful in the diagnosis of moderate or severe pancreatic dysfunction.
- Investigations for pancreatic dysfunction should be performed if the cause of diarrhoea and malabsorption is not evident on the basis of the patient's history (alcoholic pancreatitis, pancreatic carcinoma).

Treatment of pancreatic exocrine dysfunction

Diet

- Total abstinence
- Frequent, small meals
- Only 20–25% of total energy should come from dietary fats.
- The diet should not contain a lot of fibre because fibres inhibit pancreatic enzymes.
- High intake of carbohydrates

Pancreatic enzymes

- Pancreatic enzymes should be given if the patient has
  - abdominal pain D [1,2]
  - low body weight
  - steatorrhoea.
- Treatment
  - Lipase should be given sufficiently (30 000 units) at meals.
  - Lipase is inactivated at low pH.
- H_2-blockers, proton-pump inhibitors, or coated enzyme preparations should be used as adjuvant therapy.
- Sodium bicarbonate

Medium chain triglyceride oil

- Should be considered if adequate nutritional state cannot be maintained with diet and pancreatic enzyme preparations.

Vitamins

- Deficiency of vitamin D may develop. Deficiencies of vitamins A, E, and K are rare.

Secondary diabetes associated with pancreatic diseases

- Insulin and glucagon deficiencies are typical.
- Ketosis is rare.
- Periods of hypoglycaemia (23.10) are common.
- Vascular complications are rare.
- The daily requirement of insulin is usually 20–30 units. Even a small dose should be divided in two because of the risk of hypoglycaemia.

HEP

References

1. Brown A, Hughes M, Tenner S. Banks PA. Does pancreatic enzyme supplementation reduce pain in patients with chronic pancreatitis: a meta-analysis. Am J Gastroenterol 1997;92:2032–2035.
2. The Database of Abstracts of Reviews of Effectiveness (University of York), Database no.: DARE-971420. In: The Cochrane Library, Issue 4, 1999. Oxford: Update Software.

9.33 Carcinoma of the pancreas

Editors

Basic rules

- Suspect carcinoma of the pancreas in a patient with
  - continuous dyspeptic symptoms with weight loss
  - painless icterus (a late symptom)
- Consider the possibility of carcinoma of the pancreas in patients with recent-onset diabetes or acute pancreatitis.

Epidemiology

- Adenocarcinoma of the pancreas is among the ten most common cancers.
- Endocrine tumours of the pancreatic isles (insulinoma, gastrinoma, vipoma, glucagonoma, somatostatinoma, carcinoid tumour) are very rare.

Symptoms and occurrence

- Weight loss 90%
- Dyspeptic symptoms 80%
- Jaundice 55%
- Epigastric pain radiating to the back 30%
- Recent-onset diabetes 30%
- Loss of appetite 20%
- Malaise 15%
- Symptoms caused by endocrine activity of the tumour

Diagnostics

- Routine laboratory examinations are not helpful in early diagnosis.

- The sensitivity and specificity of CA 19-9 is about 80%, and this test can be used to investigate a suspicion of cancer in patients without jaundice.
- Ultrasonography and computed tomography (+ guided biopsy) are the basic examinations.
- ERCP or endoscopic ultrasonography can be performed as further investigations.

Treatment

- Pancreaticoduodenal resection (Whipple's operation) can be performed if the tumour has not spread to adjacent tissues.
- Radiotherapy for tumours that have spread to adjacent tissues provides palliative relief to about 50% of the patients but does not improve long-term prognosis.
- Palliative surgery (occasionally).
- Some patients may benefit from chemotherapy C [1 2].
- In addition to analgesics, coeliac plexus block can be used for severe pain B [3 4].

Prognosis

- In adenocarcinoma the 5-year age- and gender-adjusted survival rate is below 10%.
- The prognosis of periampullar carcinoma is better (because diagnosis is made earlier).

References

1. Kollmannsberger C, Peters HD, Fink U. Chemotherapy in advanced pancreatic adenocarcinoma. Cancer Treatment Reviews 1998;24:133–156.
2. The Database of Abstracts of Reviews of Effectiveness (University of York), Database no.: DARE-981512. In: The Cochrane Library, Issue 1, 2001. Oxford: Update Software.
3. Eisenberg R, Carr DB, Chalmers TC. Neurolytic coeliac plexus block for treatment of cancer pain: a meta-analysis. Anesth Analg 1995;80:290–295.
4. The Database of Abstracts of Reviews of Effectiveness (University of York), Database no.: DARE-950978. In: The Cochrane Library, Issue 4, 1999. Oxford: Update Software.

Nephrology

Evidence Based Medicine Guidelines. Edited by the Duodecim Editorial Team
 ISBN: 0-470-01184-X

10.1 Polyuria

Leo Niskanen

Introduction

- Establish whether the patient has true polyuria with excessive amounts of dilute urine, or does he/she have increased urinary frequency with the amount and concentration of the urine excreted being normal.

Definition

- Polyuria is a condition characterized by excessive excretion of urine in a 24 hour period. The definitions vary but >2 l in 24 hours is probable and >3 l is definite polyuria (a more accurate method is calculating the amount in relation to bodyweight, i.e. >30 ml/kg/24 hrs)
- Polyuria can be further divided into two categories:
  - Water diuresis (low urine osmolality, i.e. <300 mosm/kg H_2O)
  - Osmotic diuresis (usually high urine osmolality).

Aetiology

- The most common cause of **osmotic diuresis** is glycosuria induced by diabetes mellitus. More rare aetiological factors include increased urea following parenteral or enteral feeding, administration of mannitol or following a contrast medium investigation (transient).
- **Water diuresis** can be further classified as:
  - Primary polydipsia (plasma sodium and serum osmolality normal or low)
  - Diabetes insipidus (plasma sodium and serum osmolality normal or high)
    - Pituitary: inadequate ADH (antidiuretic hormone) secretion
    - Gestational
    - Nephrogenic: inadequate effect of ADH
- Primary polydipsia
  - Excessive fluid intake will lead to the accumulation of fluid in the body, to lowered plasma osmolality and to the prevention of ADH secretion. This will result in large amounts of dilute urine. A healthy individual is able to consume up to 20 litres of fluid in 24 hours without adverse effects. However, if ADH secretion is impaired either for physiological reasons (e.g. nausea) or through medication, water intoxication may ensue.
  - Primary polydipsia is further divided into psychogenic and dipsogenic subtypes. In psychogenic polydipsia the consumption of large amounts of water is either due to the perceived health benefits gained or compulsive desire to drink (schizophrenia; note that ADH secretion may be abnormal in schizophrenia). In dipsogenic polydipsia the patient has a dysfunction of the thirst centre which becomes stimulated even though plasma osmolality remains normal. The cause may originate from medication, a central nervous system illness or be unknown.
- Aetiology of diabetes insipidus
  - **Pituitary**: idiopathic, hereditary, head injury, autoimmune, brain tumour, infection, pituitary surgery, compression by an aneurysm
  - **Nephrogenic**: medication (particularly lithium), hypokalaemia and hypercalcaemia (24.21) (easily reversible), toxins (ethanol, ethylene glycol), pyelonephritis and many tubulo-interstitial renal diseases, congenital forms
  - **Gestational**: in some cases a history of previous, undiagnosed mild diabetes insipidus of pituitary origin. The placenta degrades endogenic ADH, but not synthetic desmopressin. Will reverse after delivery.

Diagnosis and treatment

1. History is important. Try to distinguish between polyuria and increased urinary frequency.
   - The duration of the problem?
   - Does the amount of urine vary from day to day?
   - At what time of the day is the problem worst? Particularly nocturnal micturition, i.e. nocturia, is an early sign of polyuria.
   - How many episodes of micturition during the day and night?
   - Does reducing fluid intake affect the amount of urine?
   - Problems with continence?
   - Pain or discomfort during micturition?
   - Aggravating factors?
   - Colour of the urine?
   - Nocturnal enuresis?
   - Medication (diuretics in particular)?
   - History of urinary tract infections?
   - Lifestyle; fluid intake per 24 hours? Coffee, alcohol, added salt at table?
2. Basic investigations.
   - Serum creatinine
   - Plasma potassium and sodium
   - Serum total or ionized calcium
   - Plasma glucose (diabetes mellitus)
   - Urinalysis: no abnormal findings in polyuria caused by water diuresis
   - Protein in urine –renal disease?
   - Blood in urine –bladder tumour, renal stone or infection?
   - Bacterial culture of the urine to exclude infection
   - In men, PSA (remember to palpate the prostate)
   - Possibly plasma ADH

3. If history and basic investigations are still suggestive of polyuria:
   - Following overnight fluid deprivation (if possible) measure plasma sodium, and both plasma and early morning urine osmolality, as well as plasma ADH
     - If plasma osmolality (plasma sodium) is normal and early morning urine osmolality > 800 mosm/kg H_2O, renal concentration of urine is normal and the patient has no significant problems of water metabolism.
     - Low plasma osmolality (sodium) in a polyuric patient is suggestive of primary polydipsia. Basic investigations are, however, often normal.
     - If plasma osmolality > 295 mosm/kg H_2O and urine osmolality <300 mosm/kg H_2O, diabetes insipidus can usually be diagnosed. In partial diabetes insipidus it is not possible to make differential diagnosis based on basic investigations.
4. Further investigations and initiation of treatment is carried out by a specialist team (endocrinology or nephrology). Further investigations may include:
   - Differential diagnosis; is the condition of pituitary or nephrogenic origin? Plasma ADH is low in pituitary causes, high in nephrogenic causes (interpretation requires ensuring the stimulus is sufficient, i.e. increased plasma osmolality). Response to desmopressin (urine not concentrated in nephrogenic causes).
   - To diagnose partial lack of ADH secretion, enhanced water deprivation test can be carried out with hypertonic saline infusion.
   - In pituitary diabetes insipidus, MRI of the head
   - Diagnosis and treatment of renal disease (nephrology)
   - Treatment is aimed at the causative factor. Lack of ADH is treated with synthetic arginine vasopressin.

10.2 Elevated serum creatinine

Jukka Mustonen

Reference values and interpretation

- In women less than 95 μmol/l
- In men less than 105 μmol/l
- The production of creatinine correlates with muscle mass. A creatinine concentration of 135 μmol/l in a muscular man does not necessarily indicate renal insufficiency. However, a creatinine concentration of 200–300 μmol/l in a slim woman may indicate significant renal failure.
- The reference values for children vary with age.
- When about half of the kidney function has been lost, serum creatinine rises above normal values and continues to rise steadily as the kidney damage progresses.
- In severe renal insufficiency, the extrarenal creatinine clearance and tubular secretion of creatinine lead to serum creatinine no longer being a linear and reliable indicator of renal insufficiency.

Causes of elevated serum creatinine

URO

- The cause can be acute or chronic renal insufficiency or a chronic condition becoming acute.
- The aetiology of both acute and chronic conditions can be either prerenal (hypovolemia, cardiac failure), renal (kidney disease) or postrenal (urinary tract obstruction).

Indications for measuring serum creatinine

- Suspicion of urinary tract disease at the renal level (pyelonephritis, epidemic nephropathy).
- Basic evaluation of a hypertensive patient
- To find out if the kidneys are affected by a systemic disease, such as SLE.
- Suspicion of organ complications related to an underlying disease, such as diabetes
- A severely ill patient with an undetermined diagnosis

How to act when an elevated serum creatinine level is observed incidentally or as a result of screening

1. Check if the patient's creatinine has been measured previously, and find out his/her medication and possible diseases.
2. Find out if the patient takes drugs that affect kidney function
   - Analgesics, except paracetamol
   - Antimicrobial drugs: penicillin and cephalosporin derivatives, aminoglycosides, vancomycin, trimethoprim, amphotericin B
   - Antituberculous drugs: rifampicin, isoniazid
   - Antirheumatic drugs: aurothiomalate, penicillamine
   - Angiotensin converting enzyme inhibitors, angiotensin receptor blockers
   - Lithium
   - Allopurinol
   - Cytotoxic drugs
   - Cyclosporin (A) [1 2]

Investigations

- Clinical examination
  - Blood pressure
  - Heart auscultation
  - Peripheral pulses
  - Palpation of abdomen
  - Palpation of prostate
  - Skin colour

- Primary laboratory investigations
  - Blood picture, ESR (systemic diseases, myeloma) (15.46)
  - Electrolytes (Na, K, Ca, Pi)
  - Blood glucose
  - Dipstick tests of urine
  - Protein in urine, see 10.3.
  - Blood in urine, see 11.5.
  - Infection in urine, see 10.10.
  - Glucose in urine, the patient may have diabetes.
- Imaging
  - Ultrasonography of the kidneys is a primary imaging study.
    - Size and structure of the kidneys?
    - Hydronephrosis?
- Hospital investigations
  - The need for investigations performed in hospital is assessed based on the findings from primary investigations. Hospital investigations include:
    - Examination of renal circulation (Doppler ultrasonography, renal angiography)
    - Other imaging of urinary tracts (CT scan, MRI)
    - Kidney biopsy
    - Outruling of multiple myeloma (protein fractions of serum and urine, bone marrow examination)

Follow-up

- The frequency of follow-up visits depends on the underlying disease.
- In chronic renal failure, the serum creatinine should be measured with an interval of a few months, at least twice a year.

Acute renal failure

- If acute renal failure is suspected, refer to hospital as an emergency.
- The most common causes
  - Bleeding, severe dehydration
    - A hypotensive patient in poor general health
  - Shock
    - Cardiogenic circulatory shock
    - Septic shock
  - Acute kidney damage
    - Nephrotoxin: cooling agents consumed by alcoholics, nephrotoxic drugs
    - Rhabdomyolysis (10.41)
    - Nephritis; acute glomerulonephritis (10.31), acute pyelonephritis (10.10)
    - Epidemic nephropathy (1.43)
    - Occlusion of a renal artery or vein
  - Obstruction of urinary tract
  - Prostatic hypertrophy
  - Tumour in the region of bladder or pelvis

References

1. Vercauteren SB, Bosmans JL, Elseviers MM, Verpooten GA, De Broe ME. A meta-analysis and morphological review of cyclosporine-induced nephrotoxicity in auto-immune diseases. Kidney International 1998;54:536–545.
2. The Database of Abstracts of Reviews of Effectiveness (University of York), Database no.: DARE-981271. In: The Cochrane Library, Issue 2, 2000. Oxford: Update Software.

10.3 Proteinuria

Ilpo Ala-Houhala

Principles

- Unnecessary, routinely performed urinalyses should be avoided. There is no need to screen for proteinuria at health check-ups, as it is unlikely that a symptomless, remediable disease will be revealed.
- Mild, harmless postural proteinuria can be identified without further investigations.
- The magnitude of proteinuria is assessed by measuring daily urinary excretion of protein.
- If the excretion of protein exceeds in about 5% further investigations and follow-up are usually indicated.
- It should be remembered that absence of proteinuria does not exclude severe renal disease.
- If proteinuria is detected in a pregnant woman, the possibility of pre-eclampsia should always be considered (see 26.1).

Normal urinary excretion of protein

- In the healthy adult, no more than 150 mg protein/24 h is excreted in the urine. This is mostly albumin, but other serum proteins, e.g. immunoglobulins, are also excreted.
- In the diabetic, microalbuminuria (excretion of more than 20 μg/min of albumin, i.e. about 30 mg/24 h) indicates incipient diabetic nephropathy.

Evaluation of proteinuria with a Waldenström's test strip

- The test strip is the most commonly used semi-quantitative method for assessing proteinuria. Its sensitivity for protein is > 0.15 g/l. The method is unsuitable for the detection of urinary light chains (myeloma).
- False positive test strip results may be caused by
  - contamination
  - very alkaline urine.

- False negative results are most commonly caused by considerably diluted urine.

Transient and periodic proteinuria

- May be functional or postural. Albumin is usually the predominating fraction; the total excretion is less than 1 g/24 h.
- Common causes of functional proteinuria include fever, inflammatory disease and physical exertion.
- Organic diseases causing functional proteinuria include
  - severe congestive heart failure
  - hypertension
  - extensive skin lesions (e.g. burns)
  - high blood concentrations of protein (parenteral administration of albumin or plasma).
- Postural proteinuria is seen in 5% of all young men. For confirmation of the diagnosis, urine is collected after rest and after being upright (immediately after waking and in the afternoon). A negative result after rest and a positive after being upright confirm the diagnosis. Follow-up and further investigations are not needed, provided urinary protein excretion during the day does not exceed 1 g/24 h.
- If the patient also has haematuria, some other disease than functional proteinuria must be suspected.

Persistent proteinuria

- Suggests renal damage even in a symptom-free patient, who does not have haematuria or renal insufficiency.
- Causes of persistent albuminuria include:
  - glomerulonephritis
  - diabetic nephropathy
  - amyloidosis
  - nephrosclerosis (associated with hypertension or atherosclerosis)
  - certain drugs, for example penicillamine and gold preparations
  - various types of interstitial nephritis, such as chronic pyelonephritis
  - reflux nephropathy
  - structural anomalies
  - renal tissue loss caused by various disease
  - toxic renal damage (heavy metals, aminoglycosides, amphotericin B)
  - eclampsia or pre-eclampsia in pregnancy.
- Excretion of low molecular weight proteins in the urine may be detected in
  - hereditary tubular diseases
  - Fanconi's syndrome
  - tubular acidosis
  - chronic hypokalaemia
  - rejection of a kidney graft
  - Wilson's disease
  - interstitial viral nephritides
- A finding of heavy proteinuria (15–20 g/24 h) should raise suspicion of excessive quantities of some extra protein in the blood. Usually, the diagnosis has already been suggested by the clinical symptoms. Such disorders include:
  - lysozymuria in leukaemia
  - excretion of amylase in pancreatitis
  - excretion of myoglobin in extensive muscle injuries (rhabdomyolysis causes brown urine)
  - excretion of haemoglobin after haemolysis
  - excretion of monoclonal immunoglobulin light or heavy chains in gammopathies, such as multiple myeloma, Waldenström's macroglobulinaemia and AL amyloidosis.

Proteinuria detected incidentally – primary investigations

A weakly positive result in the strip test

- The initial diagnostic work-up does not require a visit to the doctor, but can be done on the basis of the medical records.
  1. Possible results of previous urinalyses are checked.
  2. The possibility that the patient is suffering from a disorder associated with kidney disease is considered:
     - diabetes
     - hypertension (blood pressure should be measured unless recently recorded)
     - a chronic inflammatory disease (e.g. rheumatoid arthritis)
     - urinary tract infection (mild proteinuria is normal during inflammation and does not require re-examination).
  3. Further investigations (see the following paragraph) are performed only if the patient has previously had proteinuria or if there is reason to suspect renal disease.

If the result of the strip test is clearly positive or if further investigations are indicated (according to paragraph 3 above)

1. A new urinary sample is collected in the morning and analysed with the test strip. If two new samples give a negative result, the patient probably has harmless postural proteinuria and no further work-up is needed. However, even mild accompanying haematuria calls for additional investigations.
2. If there is protein in the new morning urine sample, the patient should visit the physician. A more detailed history should be taken and further investigations performed.
   - The history
     - Has there been proteinuria before?
     - Are there urinary tract symptoms (dysuria, pollakiuria, lower abdominal pain, colicky back pain)?

- Is there a recent history of fever, sore throat, inflammatory disease, or physical stress?
- Does the history reveal heart or kidney disease, diabetes, rheumatic disease or structural anomalies of the urinary tract?

• Physical examination
  - The blood pressure should be measured.
  - The presence of oedema should be recorded (congestive heart failure, nephrotic syndrome).
  - Auscultation of the heart should be performed.
  - The lower abdomen should be palpated and the back patted for tenderness.

• Laboratory investigations
  - Serum creatinine
  - A 24-hour urine collection and measurement of protein excretion
  - The urine sediment (haematuria? casts?) and bacterial culture
  - A blood count, ESR

Indications for follow-up and further investigations

♦ If the results of the laboratory test are normal and the urinary protein excretion is less than 0.3 g/ 24 h, no further work-up is needed.

♦ If 24-hour urinary protein excretion exceeds 0.3 g but is less than 1.5 g and the serum creatinine level is normal:
  - If proteinuria occurs in association with fever or physical exertion, the 24-hour urinary protein excretion is reassessed a few days after the exercise or 1–3 weeks after cure of the infection. Epidemic nephropathy should not be forgotten (1.43).
  - In the case of a young and otherwise healthy patient whose proteinuria does not exceed 1.5 g/24 h, postural proteinuria is sought by repeating the orthostatic test: the nocturnal urinary excretion of protein is assessed separately (the patient empties his urinary bladder in the evening before going asleep, in the morning immediately after getting out of bed, and in the afternoon after being upright during the day). If the quantity of protein in the urine is much smaller at night than in the daytime, the patient probably has harmless postural proteinuria.
  - If proteinuria is not postural but urinary protein excretion does not exceed 1.5 g/24 h, quality of the urinary protein is examined: urinary albumin-, alpha-1 microglobulin excretion and/or urinary protein electrophoresis is performed.
  - If proteinuria is accompanied by haematuria, further investigations are indicated. See haematuria 11.5.
  - If the patient is hypertensive, a renal cause should be excluded by appropriate investigations.
  - Congestive heart failure or poorly controlled hypertension should be treated. If proteinuria is not relieved, further investigations are indicated.
  - If the urine contains immunoglobulin light chains or if there is low molecular weight (tubular) proteinuria (increased alpha-1 microglobulin excretion), the patient should be admitted for the exclusion of systemic disease.
  - If there is mainly albuminuria and the quantity is less than 1.5 g/24 h, a follow-up visit at 6-month intervals is sufficient (blood pressure, urinary protein/24 h, serum creatinine). If proteinuria is persistent or increases, the patient should be admitted for the consideration of a kidney biopsy.

♦ If urinary protein excretion exceeds 1.5 g/24 h or renal function is impaired:
  - The patient is admitted for a further diagnostic work-up: Doppler ultrasonography of the kidneys, kidney biopsy. The possibility of a systemic disease causing proteinuria is considered. If the patient is elderly and in a poor state of health, consider whether the patient would really benefit from an aetiological diagnosis.
  - A specialist is consulted concerning the treatment of the underlying disorder (diabetic nephropathy, amyloidosis).

10.4 Sampling and investigating urine

Editors

Basic rules

♦ Urine examination is not necessary in uncomplicated cystitis in women (D).

♦ A phased investigation strategy is recommended.

♦ A dipstick test is the primary investigation in acute urinary symptoms and in cases where a disease of the urinary tract must be ruled out.

♦ Urine bacterial culture is indicated in patients with symptoms of a urinary tract infection but with a negative dipstick test.

♦ Both a bacterial culture and an antibiotic sensitivity test are indicated in other cases of urinary tract infection.

Components of the test request

1. Dipstick test
2. Urine sediment
3. Urine bacterial culture and antibiotic sensitivity test
4. Special culture and antibiotic sensitivity test

Selection and phased strategy of urine tests

- A phased investigation strategy is recommended: abnormal results of the dipstick test are followed by further tests according to a fixed scheme in the laboratory.
  - If phased microscopy is performed, the urine sediment is examined only in cases where the dipstick test shows blood or albumin but leukocytes and nitrites are negative.
  - In phased bacterial culture the culture is performed only in cases where the dipstick test for leukocytes or nitrites is positive.
- In some cases bacterial culture or microscopy of the urine sediment should be requested directly (e.g. in patients with a strong suspicion of renal disease or a transplanted kidney)

Suspicion of acute urinary tract disease (infection, haematuria, abdominal pain)

- Usually a dipstick test and, if necessary, a bacterial culture is performed. Because a negative dipstick test is rather common in urinary tract infection, bacterial culture should usually be performed in cases with symptoms suggesting a urinary tract infection but with a negative dipstick test.
- In acute cystitis in women neither dipstick test nor bacterial culture is necessary D.
- Both a bacterial culture and an antibiotic sensitivity test are indicated in other patients with urinary tract infection (in order to monitor antibiotic resistance in the area).
- In ambiguous cases (a diluted sample with insufficient retention time in the bladder before sampling) a new morning urine sample may be indicated.

Timing and transportation of the urine specimen

- The dipstick test and bacterial culture should be performed as soon as possible (within 30 minutes of sampling) but they can be performed as much as 24 hours later if the sample has been stored at +4°C (refrigerator, ice or cold container).
- Microscopy should be performed at the latest 4 hours after sampling.
- Samples other than morning urine are usually sufficient unless the urine is strongly diluted. The recommended retention time in the bladder before sampling is 4–6 hours.
- Samples for cytological examination should be from fresh urine (with a retention of time of 2–3 hours before sampling). If the specimen cannot be transported to the laboratory within 2 hours it should be centrifuged and the sediment should be fixed with 50% alcohol.
- A bladder puncture specimen (0.1–5 ml) should be injected directly to an aerobic blood culture bottle and placed in a warm incubator.

Method of sampling

- The ureter meatus is cleaned with water, **not with a disinfectant**.
- The sampling container should be sterile.
- A midstream urine sample is best in adults. For girls, a midstream sample can be obtained by placing the container in the anterior part of the pot.
- A urine bag used for sampling from infants should be changed and the washing repeated once an hour. Bladder puncture (31.61) is always indicated if a urinary tract infection cannot be confirmed or ruled out easily in infants and small children.
- A catheter sample should be taken after the first few ml have been passed from the catheter.
- A sample from an indwelling catheter should be taken by puncturing the cleaned catheter pipe from the side after the catheter has been closed for 4 hours (if the condition of the patient allows) and the urine initially retained in the catheter has been passed. A catheter often causes microscopic haematuria.

Quick interpretation

- Adequately performed dipstick tests are more sensitive in detecting pyuria and haematuria than a counting chamber or microscopy of the sediment. The sensitivity of the dipstick tests corresponds to about 3 cells or 1–2 erythrocytes in a high-power field (hpf). The dipstick test also detects dissociated cells.
- The reference values in urine sediment microscopy (× 400) are as follows:
  - First morning urine sample in women: less than 3–4 granulocytes/hpf, 1–2 epithelial cells/hpf, 1–2 erythrocytes/hpf; in men: 1–2 granulocytes/hpf, and 1–2 erythrocytes/hpf.
  - No casts should be present.
- Positive test for nitrites
  - Usually indicates a large number of bacteria in the bladder and confirms infection.
  - A negative test result does not rule out infection. (The sensitivity for infection is 40%. In infections caused by Staphylococcus saprophyticus and some enterococci the nitrite test is always negative.)
- Bacteriuria associated with pyuria is a certain sign of infection.
- Recurrent significant pyuria (>5 leukocytes/hpf) with a negative bacterial culture should raise the suspicion of chlamydial infection or tuberculosis.

Bacterial culture

- The most common causes of urinary tract infection include
  - E. coli 70–80%
  - Staphylococcus saprophyticus 5–10% (as high as 40% in young women)

URO

Table 10.4 Clinically significant counts of uropathogens and yeasts

Clinical situation or sample type	Significant bacterial count (microbes/ml)
Asymptomatic bacteriuria	• 10^5
Catheter sample from a female patient	• 10^4
Catheter sample from a male patient	• 10^3
Symptomatic patient with suspected urinary tract infection and a midstream urine sample	• 10^3
Bladder puncture sample	• 10^2
Bladder puncture sample, enrichment	No lower limit

- Klebsiella 3–9%
- Proteus mirabilis 2–5%
- Enterococci 2–4%

- For clinically significant counts of uropathogens and yeasts, see Table 10.4.
- The combination of a bacterial growth of 100 000/ml and one bacterial species is an almost certain sign of an infection.
- A sample with strong bacterial growth should be verified before treatment if
    - the patient is asymptomatic and the microscopy is normal
    - the sample contains 3 or more species of bacteria.
- If the sample contains 10 000–100 000 bacteria/ml, only 1 bacterial species is detected, and the patient has symptoms, an infection is probable.
- Staphylococcus saprophyticus, even in small numbers, indicates infection.

10.10 Treatment of urinary tract infection

Risto Ikäheimo

Aims

- Treat according to the level of the infection.
- Identify patients with obstructed urinary flow and treat the cause of obstruction.
- In children (31.60) and male patients the underlying cause must be identified already after the first UTI.
- Monitor recovery in risk patients (pregnant women, children, patients with pyelonephritis).
- Avoid unnecessary check-ups in patients who have had an acute uncomplicated lower UTI if the patient becomes asymptomatic.
- Healthy women with uncomplicated symptomatic cystitis can even be treated on the basis of history alone without laboratory diagnostics if the infection is unquestionable.
- Avoid unnecessary sampling in patients who do not have any symptoms of symptoms of UTI (asymptomatic bacteriuria should not be searched for, asymptomatic infections are treated only in risk patients).

Types of infection

- Chronic covert bacteriuria
- Acute uncomplicated UTI
- Acute pyelonephritis
- Recurrent UTI
- Complicated UTI
- Special groups: children, pregnant or breastfeeding women, the elderly, diabetics, men with prostatitis, and men in general

Asymptomatic bacteriuria

- Occurs in less than 0.5% of men, 1–4% of girls, 5–10% of women
- Screening is indicated only in the following risk groups:
    - fever of unknown origin or other symptoms in a child aged below 6 years
    - pregnancy A [1]
    - (immunodeficiency)
- Screening and treatment are not necessary for women with diabetes B [2].
- Treat risk-group patients as in acute UTI.
- In the elderly, covert bacteriuria does not usually warrant treatment.
- Further evaluation (referral) is necessary in children. Urinary tract anomalies are found in 20–50%.

Urethral syndrome

- Dysuria, increased urinary frequency, difficulty in urination but no bacteriuria.
- If pyuria or mild bacteriuria occurs, the patient has cystitis.
- If a patient has pyuria but no bacteriuria, specimens for examinations for chlamydia should be taken, particularly from young patients.
- Oestrogen therapy may be helpful for postmenopausal women.
- If no infection is found, gynaecological evaluation is performed or the patient is referred to a urologist (cystoscopy and/or urethral dilation may be helpful; interstitial cystitis).
- In some patients, oxybutynin or tolterodine may be helpful.

Acute UTI in outpatients

- In acute uncomplicated UTI of an adult woman urine specimen is not required if the clinical picture is perfectly clear.

Table 10.10.1 Clinically significant concentrations of uropathogens

Clinical condition or method of sampling	Significant concentration (microbes/ml)
Midstream specimen, patient with symptoms or bladder time < 4 h [1)]	• 10^3
Midstream specimen, bladder time > 4 h	• 10^{4-5}
In men specimen obtained by catheterisation	• 10^3
In women specimen obtained by catheterisation	• 10^4
Covert bacteriuria	• 10^5
Suprapupic puncture specimen	All growth

1. Even small concentrations of uropathogens may be significant. Usually one uropathogen is identified, in some cases two and only exceptionally three or more. If the sample shows more bacteria strains than what has been set as the standard, the results is 'mixed bacterial flora'. In this case the possible pathogen cannot be identified, and a new specimen is necessary for diagnosis of UTI.

Table 10.10.2 Antimicrobial therapy in acute urinary infection for outpatients

Drug	Dosage	Observe
1. Trimethoprim	♦ 160 mg × 2 × 5 or ♦ 300 mg × 1 × 5	
Nitrofurantoin	75 mg × 2 × 5	Not in renal failure
Pivmecillinam	200 mg × 3 × 5	
2. Norfloxacin	400 mg × 2 × 3	
Ofloxacin	200 mg × 1 × 3	
Cefalexin	500 mg × 2 × 5	
Cefadroxil	500 mg × 1 × 5	
Fosfomycin	3 g × 1 × 1 as a single dose	
3. Ciprofloxacin	♦ 250 mg × 2 ×7 ♦ (500 mg × 2 in severe infections)	Pseudomonas infections and other multiresistant bacteria

- In all other cases of UTI, bacterial culture should be used to support diagnosis and treatment decisions (see Table 10.10.1) even if the results are not available when therapy is started. See 10.4.

Lower UTI

- Duration of treatment is 3–5 days; short treatment is enough if symptoms have not lasted for long **B** [3]. Single-dose treatment is not recommended during pregnancy **C** [4].
- In choosing a first-line antibiotic (Table 10.10.2), consider resistance in the geographical area concerned–particularly for trimethoprim!
- The primary empirical starting drug should be varied; do not use only 1–2 drugs.
- Diabetes or urinary tract anomalies: duration of treatment 5–7 days, choice of medication as above.

Acute pyelonephritis (urosepsis)

- The patient usually has fever. In the elderly the only symptom may be the deterioration of general condition (CRP determination is useful, in pyelonephritis requiring parenteral therapy it is usually > 50 mg/l).
- Duration of treatment should be 10–14 days.
- Begin by giving cefuroxim i.v. 750–1500 mg × 3. Continue with a first-generation cephalosporin or fluoroquinolone p.o when the patient no longer has fever.
- Another option is fluoroquinolone p.o. (when hospitalization is not needed and the patient is able to take oral medication).

Renal insufficiency

- I.v. cephalosporins (reduction of dose)
- Cephalexin, cefadroxil, amoxicillin, pivmecillinam
- Remember to reduce the dose in cases of severe insufficiency.
- Nitrofurantoin is not suitable in renal insufficiency.

Pregnancy

- Duration of treatment is 5 days **C** [5], monitor recovery.
    - Pivmecillinam 200 mg × 3 (repeated mecillinam courses should be avoided during pregnancy because pivmecillinam lowers serum carnitine levels)
    - Nitrofurantoin 75 mg × 2
    - First-generation cephalosporins (e.g. cefadroxil 500 mg × 2 or cephalexin 500 mg × 3)

UTI in male

- Palpate the prostate gland, determine the volume of residual urine (42.4), examine serum prostate-specific antigen and creatinine.

Monitoring is necessary

- in patients who remain symptomatic after completion of medication
- always in cases of upper UTI
- in risk-group patients (pregnancy) 3–7 days after completion of medication

Check-ups are not necessary

- in cases of uncomplicated lower UTI (of an adult woman)

Self-management

- An alternative to prophylactic medication in cases of recurrent infection with burning sensations on urination, which are common in young women, particularly after intercourse.
- The patient should take trimethoprim 300 mg, sulphatrimethoprim (2 high-dose tablets) or nitrofurantoin 75 mg × 2 for two days immediately after the first symptoms have appeared. If this medication is not sufficient to control the infection, a longer course (3–5 days) should be prescribed.

URO

Acute UTI in an inpatient

- Causative bacteria include also Klebsiella, Proteus, Pseudomonas, enterococci.
- Treat with narrow-spectrum antibiotics, e.g., nitrofurantoin.
- Avoid sulphonamides, tetracyclines, possibly also trimethoprim.

Recurrent UTI

- The same strain: 1–3 weeks since the previous infection (relapse)
- New strain: 1–2 months since the previous infection (reinfection)
- Urodynamic disturbance is seldom the cause; 3–6% of patients need surgery.
- In cases of frequent recurrence, perform ultrasonography, a residual urine test, cystoscopy.
- General protective measures (not evidence-based)
  - Abundant diuresis (more than 2 litres of non-caloric fluids per day)
  - Frequent emptying of the bladder (at 3-hour intervals during the day, and after intercourse)
  - Good hygiene
  - Postcoital medication if necessary: 160 mg of trimethoprim
  - Avoiding exposure to cold
- A patient may start a 3-day medication after dysuria appears (trimethoprim, quinolone, nitrofurantoin). A midstream urine specimen should be taken after one week.
- Patients with a tendency to frequent recurrence should be given a prophylactic medication either daily or on 3 days/week for a period of 3, 6 or 12 months.
- Indications for long-term prophylaxis (3–6 months, rarely longer):
  - Renal damage or urinary tract anomaly
  - Intermittent catheterization (patients with indwelling catheter do **not** benefit)
  - Pregnancy
  - Quality of life aspects in special cases (fear of recurrence, social stigma at work)
- Medication: trimethoprim 100 mg × 1, nitrofurantoin 75 mg × 1, norfloxacin 200 mg × 1 or methenamine hippurate 1 g × 2 C [6]. Beta-lactam antibiotics are used for prophylaxis only in exceptional cases.

Chronic pyelonephritis

- Diagnosis by imaging (scar deformities + history)
- Rare; risk factors include reflux in children, infection, analgesics.
- Bacteriuria is present in only some patients.
- Symptomatic infection treated on the basis of results of sensitivity determinations. Chronic pyelonephritis alone is not an indication for continuous prophylactic medication or repeated urine samples in asymptomatic patients.
- A midstream urine specimen should be checked at 3–4-month intervals.

References

1. Smaill F. Antibiotic vs no treatment for asymptomatic bacteriuria in pregnancy. In: Neilson JP, Crowther CA, Hodnett ED, Hofmeyr GJ (eds.) Pregnancy and Childbirth Module of The Cochrane Database of Systematic Reviews, (updated 02 December 1997). Available in The Cochrane Library (database on disk and CDROM). The Cochrane Collaboration; Issue 1. Oxford: Update Software; 1998. Updated quarterly.
2. Harding GKM, Zhanel GG, Nicolle LE, Cheang M, for the Manitoba Diabetes Urinary Tract Infection Study Group. N Engl J Med 2002;347:1576–1583.
3. Leibovici L, Wysenbeek AJ. Single-dose antibiotic treatment for symptomatic urinary tract infections in women: a meta-analysis of randomized trials. Quarterly Journal of Medicine 1991;285:43–57.
4. Villar J, Lydon-Rochelle MT, Gulmezoglu AM. Duration of treatment for asymptomatic bacteriuria during pregnancy. In: Neilson JP, Crowther CA, Hodnett ED, Hofmeyr GJ (eds.) Pregnancy and Childbirth Module of The Cochrane Database of Systematic Reviews, (updated 02 December 1997). Available in The Cochrane Library (database on disk and CDROM). The Cochrane Collaboration; Issue 1. Oxford: Update Software; 1998. Updated quarterly.
5. Vazquez JC, Villar J. Treatments for symptomatic urinary tract infections during pregnancy. Cochrane Database Syst Rev. 2004;(2):CD002256.
6. Lee B, Bhuta T, Craig J, Simpson J. Methenamine hippurate for preventing urinary tract infections. Cochrane Database Syst Rev. 2004;(2):CD003265.

10.20 Acute renal failure

Eero Honkanen

Definition

- In acute renal failure glomerular filtration decreases during hours or days leading to a disturbance of acid-base and fluid-sodium balance, and accumulation of end products of nitrogen metabolism. Because of this the serum creatinine increases by 50–100 μmol/l/day.
- A rate of urine flow less than 30 ml/h (less than 400 ml/24 h) is characteristic of acute renal failure. Failure to concentrate the urine without reduced urine volumes is a considerably less common condition.

Principles

- Acute renal failure should be recognized when the rate of urine flow decreases or ceases even before there is a significant increase in the serum creatinine concentration. Urine flow should be monitored in all severely ill patients.

- Pre- and postrenal causes are distinguished by a review of the medical history and by clinical examination.
  - Hypovolaemia is the most common cause of oliguria and is correctable with fluid administration. Ileus, in which litres of fluid are sequestered in the intestine, is a common condition calling for fluid repletion.
  - Acute cessation of urine production without hypovolaemia is often caused by obstruction of the urinary tract.
- If no pre- or postrenal cause is detected, a renal cause should be considered.
- Administration of diuretics is usually not recommended before hypovolaemia has been ruled out, initial diagnostic procedures have been performed and the results of urinalysis and serum sodium and potassium measurements are available.

Diagnostic hints

- In urethral obstruction with cessation of urine production, palpation and percussion usually reveal a distended urinary bladder. Prostatic hypertrophy or malignancy should be considered. Remember to examine the prostate by touch per rectum.
- In anuria caused by hypovolaemia, blood pressure is usually low, the limbs are cool and filling of peripheral veins is poor. High blood pressure may suggest intrinsic renal disease or occlusion of the renal artery (dissection of the aorta!).
- Macroscopic haematuria colours the urine dark. Rhabdomyolysis (10.41) is suggested by the combination of dark urine, a strip test positive for blood, and absence of erythrocytes in the sediment. This diagnosis should be borne in mind when treating alcoholics and patients who have not been fully conscious ("found in a poor general state of health").
- Fever suggests infection (e.g. pyelonephritis, nephropathia epidemica).
- Involvement of drugs or toxic agents should always be considered if the obvious cause of renal failure is not hypovolaemia or urinary tract obstruction. Use of nephrotoxic drugs may be associated with non-oliguric acute renal failure. Causes of acute interstitial nephritis or acute tubular injury include:
  - non-steroidal anti-inflammatory drugs (NSAID)
  - many antibiotics (e.g. penicillins, cephalosporins, aminoglycosides, sulphonamides, rifampicin!)
  - diuretics
  - radiocontrast agents (intravenously administered)
  - ethylene glycol
  - organic solvents
  - mushroom poisoning (Cortinarius sp.)
- In the elderly, vascular procedures (angioplasty, surgery) may cause a cholesterol embolism.
  - This is marked by decreasing renal function and symptoms of systemic embolization (livedo reticularis, distal cyanosis)

Laboratory investigations

- A **urine sample** is analysed promptly (a sample of catheter urine should be collected, see below).
  - Protein, blood and casts in the urine suggest renal disease.
  - Dark urine, a strip test showing blood, and absence of erythrocytes in the sediment suggest myoglobinuria or rhabdomyolysis.
- **Serum electrolytes and creatinine** (and indices of the acid-base balance, whenever available) should be determined as soon as possible. Serum CK and myoglobin should be investigated in case rhabdomyolysis is suspected.
  - Hyperkalaemia is the most serious complication of acute renal failure, and it is worsened by acidosis.
- Ultrasonography of the urinary system may reveal
  - hydronephrosis caused by postrenal urinary tract obstruction
  - oedematous kidneys associated with acute parenchymal disease or
  - shrunken kidneys if there is underlying chronic renal failure.
- ECG (hyperkalaemia!) and chest x-ray (congestion/oedema?)
- A renal biopsy is mostly needed in a case of suspected acute glomerulonephritis (profuse proteinuria, haematuria, red cell casts).

Treatment

- Prophylactic treatment should be remembered in contrast media examinations
  - Risk groups (decreased renal function especially in the elderly and in diabetic patients).
  - Adequate fluid therapy: infusion of 0.45% or 0.9% NaCl 1ml/kg/hour, 12 hours before and after the examination.
  - Acetylcysteine may be of benefit.
  - Contrast mediums used in magnetic resonance imaging are not nephrotoxic.
- Nephrotoxic drugs, such as ACE inhibitors and non-steroidal anti-inflammatory drugs should be avoided when renal function begins to fail acutely.
- There is no need to catheterize a patient who is able to urinate.
- In a case of suspected postrenal obstruction, an indwelling urinary catheter should be inserted (or a percutaneous cystostomy performed promptly if palpation reveals a distended urinary bladder or if catheterization is unsuccessful). In this way, obstruction of the urethra is diagnosed and treated.
- Hourly measurement of urine flow should be started.
- In a case of anuria the catheter must be removed (risk of infection).
- If the patient has cool extremities, a systolic blood pressure below 90 mmHg, and no audible rales on pulmonary auscultation, an infusion with isotonic (0.9%) sodium chloride 15 ml/kg/h should be started. The infusion is continued until symptoms of hypovolaemia are relieved and production of urine increases.

- Observe for and take care of possible hyperkalaemia 24.11 and acidosis (see 10.21).
- The patient should be observed and care should be taken not to cause pulmonary oedema by too vigorous fluid replacement.
  - Colloid solutions C [1] or albumin B [2] are not recommended.
  - Patients with acute renal failure should as a rule be treated at hospital.
  - The patient can be transported to the hospital when infusion of fluid has been started and the patient's general condition permits transportation.
- There is no convincing evidence of the usefulness of drugs in the treatment of acute renal failure.
- Increasing doses of intravenous furosemide (2–10 mg/kg i.v.) may be tested. In case urinary output increases, constant infusion (10–40 mg/h) may be started.
- Consider prompt initiation of renal replacement therapies (dialysis, continuous filtration) in case there is:
  - severe overhydration
  - hyperkalaemia (K > 6.5 mmol/l)
  - metabolic acidosis
  - persisting oligouria (>12 hours), or marked retention of uraemic toxins (assessed by serum urea, creatinine).

References

1. Alderson P, Schierhout G, Roberts I, Bunn F. Colloids versus crystalloids for fluid resuscitation in critically ill patients. Cochrane Database Syst Rev. 2004;(2):CD000567.
2. The Albumin Reviewers (Alderson P, Bunn F, Lefebvre C, Li Wan Po A, Li L, Roberts I, Schierhout G). Human albumin solution for resuscitation and volume expansion in critically ill patients. Cochrane Database Syst Rev. 2004;(2):CD001208.

10.21 Treatment of chronic renal failure

Jukka Mustonen

- In clinical practice, serum creatinine serves as an index of renal function.

Therapeutic approaches to slow the progression of renal disease

- Treatment of hypertension
- Prevention of hyperparathyroidism
  - Diet
  - Drugs
- Treatment of hyperlipidaemia  [1,2]
- Avoidance of toxic agents
- Infections are treated actively
- Smoking is avoided
- Control of the electrolyte balance
- Glycaemic control in diabetic subjects

Treatment of hypertension

- It is important to treat hypertension in order to slow the progression of renal disease.
- The aim is normotension (130/80 mmHg).
- Most of the common antihypertensive drugs can be used (diuretics, beta-blockers, calcium channel blockers, ACE inhibitors, angiotensin receptor blockers).
- Thiazide diuretics are often ineffective if serum creatinine is above 200 μmol/l. Loop diuretics are then recommended. Potassium-sparing diuretics may cause hyperkalaemia. Therefore they should be used with caution and combination with ACE inhibitors or angiotensin receptor blockers should be avoided.
- ACE inhibitors and angiotensin receptor blockers are generally suitable as primary drugs. They can be combined with diuretics and the other above-mentioned drugs. ACE inhibitors reduce proteinuria A [3,4,5,6] and slow down progression of renal failure A [7,8,9,10].
- If the patient has only one kidney, bilateral renal artery stenosis (often occurs in association with peripheral obliterative atherosclerosis!) or congestive heart failure, meticulous use of ACE inhibitors and angiotensin receptor blockers is recommended.
- Prior to treatment with ACE inhibitors or angiotensin receptor blockers, serum creatinine, serum potassium and serum sodium should be measured and the tests should be repeated 2–4 weeks after starting treatment. In the beginning of the therapy a mild elevation in creatinine (<20% of baseline) is sometimes detected. This does not prevent from continuing therapy; however, careful monitoring is necessary.
- Starting doses of ACE inhibitors:
  - Captopril 12.5 mg × 1
  - Enalapril 5–10 mg × 1
  - Lisinopril 5–10 mg × 1
  - Perindopril 2–4 mg × 1
  - Ramipril 2.5 mg × 1
  - Quinapril 5–10 mg × 1
  - Cilazapril 1 mg × 1

Prevention of hyperparathyroidism

- Renal failure is usually associated with a low serum calcium level, a high serum phosphate level (phosphate retention) and secondary hyperparathyroidism.

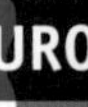

Dietary treatment

- Implies restriction of the intake of protein (A) [11] [12] [13] [14] [15] and phosphate.
- The acceptable upper limit of protein intake is usually (0.6–0.8 g/kg body weight/24 h).
- In practice, the use of milk products should be reduced. This should be started when renal insufficiency is mild (serum creatinine 150 μmol/l).
- Treatment is initiated at a specialist clinic.

Drug treatment

- Calcium carbonate binds phosphate in the food, inhibits the absorption of phosphate and increases the intake of calcium. Calcium carbonate is best started when the serum phosphate concentration exceeds the upper normal level or the serum calcium value falls below the lower normal level.
    - The dose is 0.5–1.0 g of calcium with meals.
- Calcium acetate binds phosphate slightly more effectively than calcium carbonate.
- Drugs that interfere with acid production in the stomach tend to reduce the effect of calcium carbonate.
- If hypocalcaemia persists and the serum phosphate concentration is normal, vitamin D analogues may be used. The aim is to control hyperparathyroidism. This requires careful monitoring because of the risk of hypercalcaemia.
    - The initial dose is alphacalcidol 0.25–0.50 μg/24 h
- Sevelamer is phosphate binder which is calcium-free. The use is so far scarce.

Monitoring of dietary and drug treatment

- The following variables should be monitored: Serum calcium (ionized calcium is preferred, total serum calcium is not as reliable), serum phosphate, serum protein, serum creatinine, serum urea nitrogen, the acid-base balance.
- The treatment aims at keeping the ionized serum calcium concentration between 1.15 and 1.30 mmol/l, the total serum calcium between 2.20 and 2.50 mmol/l and the serum phosphate between 0.8 and 1.5 mmol/l.
- Ca × Pi product must not exceed 5.5 $(\text{mmol/l})^2$ because this level involves the risk of soft tissue calcification.

Disturbances in electrolyte and fluid balance

- The recommended intake of fluid is 2–3 litres/24 h.
- The intake of sodium usually has to be restricted to 3–5 g/24 h. If necessary, a loop diuretic may be given.
- The intake of potassium is restricted, if necessary. Occasionally an ion exchange resin (polystyrene sulphonate) is used.
- The risk of hyperkalaemia associated with the use of ACE inhibitors, angiotensin receptor blockers, potassium-sparing diuretics or non-steroidal anti-inflammatory drugs and especially with various combinations of these preparations, should always be remembered.
- Oedemas are managed by restricting sodium intake and by loop diuretics.

Treatment of acidosis

- Acidosis should be corrected if the serum bicarbonate concentration is lower than 18 mmol/l, or at the latest when it falls below 15 mmol/l.
- Applicable drugs include calcium carbonate 2–6 g/24h, sometimes also sodium bicarbonate 1–6 g/24 h.
- The aim is to maintain the standard bicarbonate concentration >20 mmol/l and base excess <5.

Treatment of hyperlipidaemia

- Polyunsaturated fats should be preferred in the diet.
- Hyperlipidaemia may speed up the progression of renal failure. The mechanism remains unknown; possibly acceleration of glomerulosclerosis occurs in hyperlipidaemia.
- Statins (C) [1] [2] and fibrates may be used. In renal failure the dose of fluvastatin or atorvastatin does not need to be reduced; however, the dose of other statins and fibrates must be lowered.

Treatment of anaemia

- Decreased production of erythropoietin in the kidneys is the main cause of renal anaemia. Anaemia may be corrected by exogenous erythropoietin (A) [16]. Erythropoietin may be given to patients receiving dialysis treatment or to patients with a milder degree of renal insufficiency. It should be administered intravenously or subcutaneously. The dose needed varies widely as well as the frequency of administration (from one time every second week to three times a week).
- It is important to ensure the supply of iron, which is given either orally or intravenously.
- The iron concentration is monitored by measuring serum ferritin (target 200–600 μmol/l) and transferrin saturation (target >20%).
- With exogenous erythropoietin, the haemoglobin level is usually elevated to 110–130 g/l.
- Knowledge of the serum erythropoietin level is not needed when treatment decisions are made.

Avoidance of toxic agents

- The aim is to avoid all exogenous agents with potential renal toxicity.

- First of all, nephrotoxic drugs should be avoided and the dose of drugs should be adjusted according to renal function.
- In practice, the most important nephrotoxic agents include
  - aminoglycosides
  - non-steroidal anti-inflammatory drugs
  - gold preparations
  - hydralazine
  - ACE inhibitors and angiotensin receptor blockers (see above)
  - x-ray contrast mediums (the patient should be adequately hydrated prior to radiological investigations, diabetic patients require extra precautions).

Management of infections

- Infection often aggravates chronic renal failure. The cause may be the infection itself, dehydration or hypertension, or the adverse effects of drugs (NSAIDs and antibiotics).
  - The patient should be referred to hospital readily.

Smoking

- Cardiovascular diseases are the most common causes of death in patients with chronic renal failure. Therefore these patients should avoid smoking. Apparently smoking also speeds the progression of chronic renal disease.

Follow-up

- In stable, slowly progressing renal failure the patients can be followed up at an outpatient unit at 6–12-month intervals. It is often feasible to arrange intermediate controls at a health centre or local hospital for a patient who is otherwise followed up at a university hospital.
- On control visits the following symptoms and findings should be noted: tiredness, nausea, loss of appetite, weight loss, dyspnoea, itching, muscle cramps, hypertension, oedemas and the condition of the skin.

Treatments initiated in hospital

- Erythropoietin, parenteral iron
- Vitamin D, sevelamer
- Pharmacotherapy for hyperlipidaemia
- Dietary counselling

References

1. Massy ZA, Ma JZ, Louis TA, Kasiske BL. Lipid lowering therapy in patients with renal disease. Kidney International 1995;48:188–198.
2. The Database of Abstracts of Reviews of Effectiveness (University of York), Database no.: DARE-951884. In: The Cochrane Library, Issue 4, 1999. Oxford: Update Software.
3. Gansevoort RT, Sluiter WJ, Hemmelder MH, deZeeuw D, Dejong PE. Antiproteinuric effects of blood-pressure lowering agents: a meta-analysis of comparative trials. Nephrology, Dialysis, Transplantation 1995;10:1963–1974.
4. The Database of Abstracts of Reviews of Effectiveness (University of York), Database no.: DARE-960061. In: The Cochrane Library, Issue 4, 1999. Oxford: Update Software.
5. Weidmann P, Scneider M, Bohlen L. Therapeutic efficacy of different antihypertensive drugs in human diabetic nephropathy: an updated meta-analysis. Nephrol Dial Transpl 1995;10(suppl 9):pp. 39–45.
6. The Database of Abstracts of Reviews of Effectiveness (University of York), Database no.: DARE-960106. In: The Cochrane Library, Issue 4, 1999. Oxford: Update Software.
7. Kshirsagar AV, Joy MS, Hogan SL, Falk RJ, Colindres RE. Effect of ACE inhibitors in diabetic and nondiabetic chronic renal disease: a systematic overview of randomized placebo-controlled trials. American Journal of Kidney Diseases 2000:35; 695–707.
8. The Database of Abstracts of Reviews of Effectiveness (University of York), Database no.: DARE-20000916. In: The Cochrane Library, Issue 1, 2002. Oxford: Update Software.
9. Giatras I, Lau J, Levey AS. Effect of angiotensin-converting enzyme inhibitors on the progression of non-diabetic renal disease: a meta-analysis of randomized trials. Ann Intern Med 1997;127:337–345.
10. The Database of Abstracts of Reviews of Effectiveness (University of York), Database no.: DARE-978302. In: The Cochrane Library, Issue 4, 1999. Oxford: Update Software.
11. Fouque D, Wang P, Laville M, Boissel JP. Low-protein diets in renal failure. The Cochrane Database of Systematic Reviews, Cochrane Library number: CD001892. In: The Cochrane Library, Issue 2, 2002. Oxford: Update Software. Updated frequently.
12. Pedrini M, Levey A, Lau J, Chalmers T, Wang P. The effect of dietary protein restriction on the progression of diabetic and nondiabetic renal diseases: a meta-analysis. Ann Intern Med 1996;124:627–632.
13. The Database of Abstracts of Reviews of Effectiveness (University of York), Database no.: DARE-968176. In: The Cochrane Library, Issue 4, 1999. Oxford: Update Software.
14. Kasiske BL, Lakatua JD, Ma JZ, Louis TA. A meta-analysis of the effects of dietary protein restriction on the rate of decline in renal function. Am J Kidney Dis 1998;31:954–961.
15. The Database of Abstracts of Reviews of Effectiveness (University of York), Database no.: DARE-981020. In: The Cochrane Library, Issue 2, 2000. Oxford: Update Software.
16. Cody J, Daly C, Campbell M, Donaldson C, Grant A, Khan I, Pennington S, Vale L, Wallace S, MacLeod A. Recombinant human erythropoietin for chronic renal failure anaemia in pre-dialysis patients. Cochrane Database Syst Rev. 2004;(2):CD003266.

10.22 Kidney transplantation

Jukka Mustonen

Organization

- The most common indications include diabetic nephropathy, chronic glomerulonephritis, cystic renal diseases, nephrosclerosis, and amyloidosis.
- Most transplantations are cadaveric, where the donor's diagnosis is cerebral death, the cause usually being intracerebral haemorrhage or skull trauma.
- The proportion of related donors and child donors is small.

Immunosuppressive medication

- Should be used as long as there is a functioning graft.
- Usually a combination of three, sometimes two drugs C [1 2]
- Immunosuppressive medication increases the susceptibility to infections (1.71) and cancer (skin and thyroid cancer).

Corticosteroids

- The maintenance dose should usually be very small, for example methylprednisolone 4 mg every other morning. In stressful situations (surgery, severe infections, traumas), the dose should be increased. The adverse affects of high-dose corticosteroids are described in 24.43.

Cyclosporin

- The dose is adjusted according to blood cyclosporin levels. The adverse effects usually depend on the dose. The most common adverse effects are nephrotoxicity (elevated serum creatinine), hypertension, tremor, cephalalgia, nausea, gingival hypertrophy and hypertrichosis. Careful monitoring of renal function is mandatory if the patient concurrently uses non-steroidal anti-inflammatory drugs, ACE inhibitors and angiotensin receptor blockers. Aminoglycosides and amphotericin B should not be combined with cyclosporin. Other interactions are described in 21.66.

Mycophenolate mofetil

- 1–2 g/day in two doses.
- Prevents acute rejection possibly better than azathioprine.
- Adverse effects include GI disturbance, diarrhoea and increased risk for cytomegalovirus infections.

Azathioprine

- The dose is usually 75–150 mg/day. Side effects (anaemia, leucopenia, thrombocytopenia, liver toxicity) may necessitate dose reduction.

Tacrolimus

- The dosage is regulated according to blood concentrations.
- The adverse effects are similar to those of cyclosporin; both may cause nephrotoxicity. Cyclosporin causes more hypertension and tacrolimus more diabetes.

Clinical examination at follow-up

- Initially, weekly visits at the outpatient clinic. Later on, intervals may be prolonged to 3–4 months.
- The general condition, skin, hairiness, blood pressure, pulse and cardiac status, oral and dental status, body weight.
- Palpation and auscultation of the graft (arterial bruits?)

Laboratory investigations during follow-up

- Blood haemoglobin, leucocyte and platelet counts
- Renal function and electrolytes: Serum creatinine, serum urea nitrogen, serum sodium, potassium, calcium and inorganic phosphate.
- Liver function: Serum alanine transaminase, serum alkaline phosphatase
- Blood cyclosporin level
- Blood glucose, serum cholesterol, HDL cholesterol, triglycerides
- Urine: protein, blood, glucose, leucocytes, bacteria

Radiological investigations at follow-up

- Chest x-ray annually
- Ultrasonography of the graft if required
- Ultrasonography of the native kidneys at intervals of about 2 years (for possible development of acquired polycystic degeneration and malignant transformation)
- Doppler ultrasonography or angiography (when renal artery stenosis is suspected) of the graft, if required.

When should acute rejection be suspected?

- Poor state of health, fever
- Reduced production of urine
- Palpatory tenderness and swelling of the graft, hypertension
- Increase in serum creatinine, proteinuria

How to act when acute rejection is suspected

- The patient should be transferred quickly to a university hospital or a central hospital.

URO

- The diagnosis is confirmed by a biopsy of the graft.
- The treatment consists of an increase in the dose of corticosteroids, for example methylprednisolone 3 mg/kg/24 h.
- Another indication for referral to hospital is inability of the patient to take the immunosuppressive medication, for example because of vomiting.

Cost-effectiveness of kidney transplantation

- Renal replacement is very cost-effective. In a Finnish study replacement paid for itself before the end of the second year.
- According to a US study the average costs of a kidney transplantation operation correspond to the costs of 2.7 years of dialysis.
- Calcium channel blockers given in the peri-operative period may reduce the incidence of acute tubular necrosis in kidney transplant recipients (C) [3].
- Interleukin 2 receptor antagonists for prophylaxis against acute rejection in kidney transplant recipients are as effective as other antibody therapies and with significantly fewer side effects (A) [4].

References

1. Kunz R, Neumayer HH. Maintenance therapy with triple versus double immunosuppressive regimens in renal transplantation. Transplantation 1997;63:386–392.
2. The Database of Abstracts of Reviews of Effectiveness (University of York), Database no.: DARE-973216. In: The Cochrane Library, Issue 2, 2000. Oxford: Update Software.
3. Shilliday IR, Sherif M. Calcium channel blockers for preventing acute tubular necrosis in kidney transplant recipients. The Cochrane Database of Systematic Reviews, Cochrane Library Number: CD003421. In: Cochrane Library, Issue 1, 2004. Chichester, UK: John Wiley & Sons, Ltd.
4. Webster AC, Playford EG, Higgins G, Chapman JR, Craig J. Interleukin 2 receptor antagonists for kidney transplant recipients. The Cochrane Database of Systematic Reviews, Cochrane Library Number: CD003897. In: Cochrane Library, Issue 1, 2004. Chichester, UK: John Wiley & Sons, Ltd.

10.30 Nephrotic syndrome

Eero Honkanen

Aim

- Nephrotic syndrome should be recognized as a relatively rare cause of oedema.
- Familiarize yourself with its treatment which is symptomatic.

Definition

- Nephrotic syndrome is caused by increased glomerular capillary wall permeability. In nephrotic syndrome proteins are lost in the urine >3–3.5 g/day and serum albumin concentration is <30 g/l.
- This will lead to decreased colloid osmotic pressure and, in most cases, to oedema.
- The clinical picture also includes hyperlipidaemia and abnormal blood clotting, predisposing the patient to thrombosis.

Aetiology

- Chronic glomerulonephritis (10.31)
- Diabetic nephropathy
- Renal amyloidosis
- Drugs: non-steroidal anti-inflammatory drugs, gold
- Multiple myeloma

Signs and symptoms

- Symptoms emerge at the latest when the serum albumin concentration falls below 25 g/l due to excess proteinuria.
- The most important symptom is oedema of the lower limbs, which is caused by accumulation of fluid in the tissues as the serum protein concentration decreases and the capacity of the body to excrete sodium is reduced.
- The extent of oedema correlates fairly poorly with the blood albumin concentration.

Diagnosis

- The diagnosis is based on the clinical picture and on the results of laboratory investigations (see definition).
- To establish the aetiology, a renal biopsy is usually required. Therefore, the patient should be admitted to hospital for investigations.

Treatment

- Treatment of the underlying disease
  - Certain types of glomerulonephritis may be treated with immunosuppressive medication (glucocorticoids, cytotoxic drugs, ciclosporin) (B) [1].
- Reduction of proteinuria
  - Both ACE inhibitors and angiotensin-II receptor antagonists reduce proteinuria.
  - Their use (in some cases their combinations) is recommended at least in the treatment of proteinuria associated with diabetes or glomerulonephritis.

- Optimal treatment of hypertension
  - Aim = 125/75 mmHg.
- Reduction of oedema
  - Restricted salt intake (aim <3 g of NaCl/day)
  - A diuretic
    - Furosemide 20–80 mg two to four times daily orally. In severe oedema, treatment may be instigated with intravenous administration (the corresponding doses are 10–40 mg).
    - The dose of furosemide is increased according to response.
    - A thiazide diuretic enhances the effect of furosemide. The dose of hydrochlorothiazide is 25–50 mg/day (higher in renal failure).
    - Avoid excessive weight loss; 0.5–1 kg/day is appropriate.
  - An infusion of intravenous furosemide and albumin has been used in oedema resistant to other therapy, but its use remains controversial.
  - Ultrafiltration may be required to remove excess fluid.

Complications

- Hypercoagulability; risk of venous thrombosis of the lower limbs, pulmonary embolism and renal vein thrombosis.
  - Aspirin should be given routinely.
  - Prophylactic anticoagulation is usually not administered. However, it should be instigated in patients with a history of a thromboembolic event and continued whilst the patient remains nephrotic.
- Susceptibility to infections. The loss of IgG in the urine predisposes the patient to infections.
  - Pneumococcal vaccine is recommended.
- Gradual muscle wasting as a consequence of hypoproteinaemia
  - The diet should include high quality protein, approximately 1 g/kg/day.
  - Energy intake should be 35 kcal/kg/day.
- Atherosclerotic changes as a consequence of hyperlipidaemia
  - Statins are usually indicated.
- Altered calcium metabolism
  - Calcium supplementation and vitamin D are recommended
- Altered protein binding of drugs.

Reference

1. Hodson EM, Knight JF, Willis NS, Craig JC. Corticosteroid therapy for nephrotic syndrome in children. Cochrane Database Syst Rev. 2004;(2):CD001533.

10.31 Glomerulonephritis

Jukka Mustonen

URO

Aims

- Acute glomerulonephritis should be suspected when the patient presents with oedema, hypertension or macroscopic haematuria in association with or shortly after an infectious disease.
- Classical acute (poststreptococcal) glomerulonephritis is nowadays much more rare than rapidly progressing acute glomerulonephritis.
- Rapidly progressing glomerulonephritis must be recognized to be treated early enough.
- Chronic glomerulonephritis should be suspected when the patient presents with haematuria, proteinuria (usually both), hypertension, or an elevated serum creatinine concentration.
- In all patients with glomerulonephritis, blood pressure should be monitored and effectively controlled.

Acute glomerulonephritis

Aetiology

- A complication of a streptococcal infection (tonsillitis, erysipelas)
- Infections caused by other bacteria or by viruses
  - Endocarditis
  - "Shunt nephritis"
  - Septicaemia
  - Pneumococcal pneumonia
  - Other bacterial infections
  - Hepatitis B, infectious mononucleosis

Symptoms

- The onset of symptoms usually occurs 1–3 weeks after the primary infection.
- Oedema, especially facial
- General symptoms: headache, fever, abdominal pain, nausea and vomiting
- Always proteinuria, usually haematuria, sometimes oliguria or anuria
- Hypertension
- Symptoms of congestive heart failure

Laboratory findings

- Haematuria, proteinuria and casts in the urinary sediment
- Raised serum creatinine
- For the final diagnosis, histological examination of a kidney biopsy is required.

Treatment

- Supportive measures: control of fluid balance and blood pressure
- Identification and eradication of the infectious focus

Prognosis

- Children who fall ill during an epidemic will usually recover without permanent renal damage.
- Adults and children who fall ill sporadically may develop a rapidly progressing or chronic glomerulonephritis.

Rapidly progressing acute glomerulonephritis

Aetiology

- May complicate glomerulonephritis caused by infectious agents or systemic disease or be associated with primary glomerular disease.
- It is often associated with vasculitis (Wegener's granulomatosis).

The clinical picture

- In the course of a few weeks or months, a progressing glomerular injury develops, which leads to severe renal insufficiency and often anuria.
- The aetiology determines the clinical picture.

Diagnosis

- Based on renal biopsy. The finding is usually crescent glomerulonephritis.
- C-ANC antibodies are suggestive of vasculitis.

Treatment

- Results of conservative treatment are usually unsatisfactory.
- Pulse steroid treatment may stop the progression of the disease. The treatment should be started without delay at the hospital.
- Cyclophosphamide is used in vasculitic syndromes.
- Dialysis if necessary
- Kidney transplantation

Chronic glomerulonephritis

Aetiology

- Usually diagnosed incidentally (haematuria and proteinuria)
- A sequela of acute glomerulonephritis
- A preceding infection is often not identified
- Systemic diseases
  - SLE (21.41)
  - Vasculitic syndromes (21.44)
  - Henoch-Schönlein purpura (32.53)

Symptoms

- Vary from an incidentally detected abnormal result of urinalysis to chronic renal failure and nephrotic syndrome.
- Late manifestations include hypertension and other findings characteristic of chronic renal failure.

Diagnosis

- Based on renal biopsy
- The most common ones are IgA nephropathy (10.32), minimal change nephropathy, focal segmental glomerulosclerosis, and membranous glomerulonephritis.

Treatment

- Corticosteroids and other immunosuppressive agents **B** [1 2 3 4], particularly when there is a systemic disease or nephrotic syndrome (10.30).
- See treatment of chronic renal failure 10.21.
- IgA nephropathy, see 10.32.

References

1. Hogan SL, Muller KE, Jennette JC, Falk RJ. A review of therapeutic studies of idiopathic glomerulopathy. Am J Kid Dis 1995;25:862–875.
2. The Database of Abstracts of Reviews of Effectiveness (University of York), Database no.: DARE-951607. In: The Cochrane Library, Issue 4, 1999. Oxford: Update Software.
3. Imperiale TF, Goldfarb S, Berns JS. Are cytotoxic agents beneficial in idiopathic membranous nephropathy? A meta-analysis of the controlled trials. J Am Soc Nephrology 1995;5:1553–1558.
4. The Database of Abstracts of Reviews of Effectiveness (University of York), Database no.: DARE-951187. In: The Cochrane Library, Issue 4, 1999. Oxford: Update Software.

10.32 IgA nephropathy

Jukka Mustonen

Epidemiology

- The most common of the chronic glomerulonephritides

Symptoms and signs

- Usually the patient has both microscopic haematuria and proteinuria.

- Recurrent macroscopic haematuria, particularly in association with respiratory tract infections.
- Manifests rarely as acute glomerulonephritis or nephrotic syndrome.
- Hypertension is seen in 30% of all patients at diagnosis. At follow-up, hypertension is recorded in at least 50% .
- Renal insufficiency is rare at diagnosis.
- Serum IgA concentration is elevated in 50% of all patients.
- May present as glomerulonephritis only or as part of the Henoch-Schönlein syndrome.

Diagnosis

- Suspicion of IgA nephropathy should arise if a person has asymptomatic microscopic haematuria and proteinuria, often associated with high blood pressure.
- Recurrent episodes of macroscopic haematuria in a young patient should raise suspicion of IgA nephropathy.
- The diagnosis is based on renal biopsy, where IgA deposits are seen by immunofluorescence.

Prognosis

- Chronic renal failure may occur (in 10–20%).
- A poor prognosis is indicated by the following factors: absence of macroscopic haematuria, massive proteinuria, raised creatinine level at diagnosis, overt hypertension and histologically demonstrable severe glomerular and tubular damage indicate.

Treatment and follow-up

- No specific therapy is available.
- Treatment of hypertension is important, even if the rise in blood pressure is minor. Combination drug therapy is often necessary. Normotension is targeted.
- Corticosteroids and other immunosuppressive medication are given in selected cases B [1 2 3].
- Treatment of chronic renal failure may be necessary (10.21).
- Follow-up usually occurs in outpatient health care; blood pressure, serum creatinine, basic urine tests (albumin and erythrocytes) and urinary protein (24-hour urine sample) are measured at least once a year.

References

1. Pozzi C, Bolasco P, Fogazzi G, Andrutti S, Altieri P, Ponticelli C, Locatelli F. Corticosteroids in IgA nephropathy: a randomised controlled trial. Lancet 1999;353:883–887.
2. Schena FC, Montenegro M, Scivittaro V. Meta-analysis of randomised controlled trials in patients with primary IgA nephropathy. Nephrol Dial Transplant 1990;suppl 1:47–52.
3. Samuels JA, Strippoli GFM, Craig JC, Schena FP, Molony DA. Immunosuppressive agents for treating IgA nephropathy. Cochrane Database Syst Rev 2003(4):CD003965.

10.40 Renal cysts

Jukka Mustonen

UR

Solitary cysts

- Solitary renal cysts are associated with ageing and do not usually have clinical significance when detected as incidental findings on ultrasonography (in as many as 50% of patients above 50 years of age). The sonographic criteria of a benign cyst are
    - no internal echoes
    - acoustic enhancement behind the cyst
    - sharply defined, imperceptible wall
    - round or oval shape.
- If all these criteria are met, further evaluation or follow-up is not required.
- A solitary cyst may also be malignant. Malignant cysts can usually be differentiated from benign cysts by ultrasonography (see above). Additional investigations include computed tomography or needle biopsy performed by a radiologist.

Renal polycystic disease

- Infantile form
    - Is inherited as an autosomal recessive trait.
    - Prevalence 1:40 000
    - Enlarged kidneys are usually discovered straight after birth.
    - Diagnosis by ultrasonography
- Adult form
    - Is inherited as an autosomal dominant trait.
    - Prevalence 1:1500
    - Symptoms appear after 20 years of age.
    - Abdominal pain and haematuria are the most common initial symptoms.
    - Diagnosis by ultrasonography
    - About 50% of the patients are hypertensive.
    - Renal insufficiency develops slowly.
    - In advanced disease the cystic kidneys may be palpable. The liver may also contain cysts.
    - Cerebral artery aneurysms are present in 5% of the patients. Also valvular heart disease and colon diverticulosis are present more often than normally.
    - Conservative treatment
        - Urinary tract infections are treated and prevented by prophylactic medication.
        - High blood pressure is treated effectively.
        - Renal insufficiency is treated (10.21).
    - Dialysis and renal transplantation.

10.41 Rhabdomyolysis

Heikki Saha

Aims

- Suspect rhabdomyolysis in patients with typical history (particularly those found unconscious or those who have suffered a crush injury), symptoms and clinical findings.
- When suspicion arises diagnosis is easy to verify (serum creatine kinase, CK).

Definition

- Rhabdomyolysis refers to an injury of striated muscle. It may result in acute renal failure unless treatment is instigated early enough.

Aetiology

- The most common causative factor is lying unconscious on a hard surface either as a result of intoxication (alcohol or medication), or due to an illness. The long lasting pressure will cause muscle damage.
- Crush injury, excessive muscle strain (running, body building etc.) and convulsions
- Alcohol and illegal drugs (heroin, cocaine)
- Medication (statins)
- Hyperthermia (malignant hyperthermia, neuroleptic malignant syndrome)
- Metabolic disorders (hyperosmolar coma, ketoacidosis, hypokalaemia, hypophosphataemia)
- Infections (pneumococcus, salmonella, legionella, influenza, cytomegalovirus)
- Myopathy (congenital muscle enzyme deficiency, alcohol)

When to suspect?

- A typical history involves a patient
  - who has been lying unconscious on a hard surface due to excess alcohol, medication or another reason, or
  - with excessive muscle strain over the preceding hours or days.
- Signs and symptoms:
  - The affected area (limbs, buttocks, back) is painful, swollen or tender to touch.
  - The patient may be unconscious, confused, dehydrated or febrile.
  - Paresis or sensory disturbance may be present in the limbs (increased compartment pressure).
  - Urine may be dark (myoglobin), or the patient may be oliguric or anuric.
- Urine strip test may be positive to haematuria (due to myoglobin), even when no red cells are seen in the sediment.

Diagnosis

- If rhabdomyolysis is suspected, measure serum creatine kinase (CK).
- CK activity is often > 10 000–100 000 U/l.
- In clinical practice, the measurement of other muscle enzymes is not needed.
- Other typical laboratory findings include:
  - hypocalcaemia (calcium deposited in muscle tissue)
  - hyperkalaemia
  - hyperphosphataemia (renal failure and release from cells)
  - urine Hb positive in approximately 50% of patients
  - increased serum creatinine as renal failure develops.
- Differential diagnosis: Local symptoms may resemble those of deep venous thrombosis.

Treatment

- The patient is usually admitted to hospital.
- In primary care the first aid consists of the correction of hypovolaemia and dehydration.
  - Start with physiological saline
    - 1000 ml during the first hour
    - followed by 400–500 ml/h
  - The aim is to prevent the development of acute renal failure, caused by myoglobin which is being released from the muscles.
- In the hospital the follow-up treatment consists of the following:
  - Correction of dehydration to maintain diuresis. Forced alkaline diuresis should be used to prevent renal failure; aim to keep urine pH at 7.5.
    - Initially 1000 ml of 0.9% NaCl over 1 hour
    - Followed by 0.3% NaCl with 5% Glucose 400 ml/hr
    - Urine is alkalinized with a side infusion of 1.4% NaHCO3 administered 50–100 ml/h or 7.5% NaHCO3 administered 10–20 ml/h.
    - Diuresis may be encouraged with 20–40 mg of intravenous furosemide.
  - Dialysis is indicated in renal failure if the patient is anuric and diuresis is not induced with rehydration.
    - Dialysis will have no effect on the renal state, but will keep the patient alive until renal function spontaneously returns. This may take several days, even weeks.

- Fasciotomy is indicated if increased compartment pressure threatens to cause muscle necrosis or nerve damage.
- Correction of symptomatic hypocalcaemia must be carried out cautiously, because hypercalcaemia often develops during recovery. Asymptomatic hypocalcaemia requires no treatment.

Prognosis

- ♦ Prognosis is good even in cases where renal failure has developed, since the failure is reversible.
  - If compartment syndrome is not treated early enough, residual nerve and muscle damage may persist.

Urology

Evidence Based Medicine Guidelines. Edited by the Duodecim Editorial Team
 ISBN: 0-470-01184-X

11.2 Poor urine flow

Teuvo Tammela

Aetiology

- Men above 60 years of age usually have an enlarged prostate (hyperplasia (11.12) or carcinoma (11.13)).
- Anatomical or functional urethral stricture
- Detrusor sphincter dyssynergia in a neurogenic bladder associated with, for example, spinal cord disease or injury.
- Poorly contracting detrusor muscle
- In women, prolapse of the uterus or urethral mucous membrane

Investigations

- Digital rectal examination (DRE) of the prostate.
- Palpation and percussion of the bladder to detect retention (11.3).
- Measurement of residual urine volume: ultrasonography (42.4) (or single catheterization) after voiding.
- Difficulties with catheterization may suggest urethral stricture.
- Serum prostatic antigen (PSA) in men (11.12)
- Symptom questionnaire.
- In hospital, urine flow measurement is the primary investigation.

11.3 Urinary retention

Teuvo Tammela

Basic rules

- Acute symptomatic urinary retention must be treated immediately at the first encounter (at the clinic).
- Considerable retention (above 1000 ml) should be treated by cystostomy, indwelling catheter, or repeated catheterization.
- Consider the patient's medication as a potential cause of retention (anticholinergic and sympathomimetic drugs!).

Symptoms and signs

- Lower abdominal pain (often absent in slowly developing retention)
- Overflow incontinence or increased urinary frequency
- Enlarged palpable bladder
- Enlarged bladder by percussion (often a more sensitive examination than palpation)

Aetiology

- Benign prostatic hyperplasia (BPH) (age, DRE)
- Postoperative retention
- Urethral stricture
- Urethral mucosal prolapse or uterine prolapse in women
- Neurogenic causes (spinal cord injury, intervertebral disc herniation, multiple sclerosis, diabetes, neuropathy caused by alcohol or toxic substances)
- Functional causes (pain, tension, exposure to cold)
- Drugs (sympathomimetics, anticholinergic drugs, tricyclic antidepressants)

Treatment

- Before commencing treatment, ultrasonography should be performed first to assess the volume of retention if it is not definitely large and the examination can be performed without delay (42.4).
- Perform **single catheterization** if
  - the retention is not large
  - in postoperative retention more than 6 hours have elapsed since last voiding and the patient is unable to void despite encouragement and analgesics.
- **Suprapubic cystostomy** (11.32) is recommended as the first procedure if
  - the retention is large (above 1000 ml according to ultrasonography or the bladder reaches the navel)
  - the patient has a complicated urethral stricture
  - a large prostate has caused difficulties in catheterization earlier.
- The cystostomy catheter can be removed when voiding is repeatedly successful and the residual urine is less than 200 ml.
- A large retention without anatomical catheterization problems can be treated with an **indwelling silicone catheter** (11.31). Aim at removing the catheter within 3 days.
- The whole volume can be emptied at one time. In the final phase of emptying, the urine may be bloody because of small tears on the bladder mucosa caused by over-distension.
- **Medical treatment**
  - In postoperative retention a short course of alpha-blockers or the cholinergic drug like carbachol, 2 mg × 3, is useful.
  - For retention caused by BPH use alpha-blockers (tamsulosin hydrochloride or alfuzosin) (11.12). The treatment requires careful follow-up of symptoms and residual urine volume.
- For indications for surgical treatment see 11.12.

Further investigations

- In most cases of BPH-related retention the episode is the first occurrence of retention and therefore warrants follow-up.

- A cleanly voided urine specimen should be taken from all patients.
- No other investigations are necessary if the patient had his first retention and there is a predisposing factor, e.g. alcohol, exposure to cold, postoperative state, or bed rest associated with an acute illness.
- Retention without an evident cause and recurrent retention are indications for the following laboratory examinations: serum creatinine, blood glucose, and, in men, serum prostate-specific antigen (PSA). If an increase of serum creatinine concentration during retention was due to obstruction it normalizes rapidly. Note! Retention and catheterization raise PSA, and a value obtained at this point is not reliable. If the value is elevated, it should be controlled after 3–4 weeks.
- Specialist consultation is indicated in recurrent urinary retention.

11.4 Urinary incontinence in women

Juha Mäkinen

Basic rule

- Differentiate between the two main types of incontinence: stress incontinence and urge incontinence.

Types of incontinence

1. Loss of urine on exertion (**stress incontinence**) is the problem in 3/4 of adult incontinent patients.
2. **Urge incontinence** is due to bladder dysfunction where the need to void is so sudden that loss of urine occurs before the patient makes it to the toilet. It occurs typically in elderly women after the menopause, but also in young women.
3. A combination of the two types is called **mixed incontinence**.
4. Other types such as **overflow** occurs after surgery, **reflux** incontinence rarely occur in women.
5. In institutionalized patients, incontinence often is caused by cerebral ischaemia or dementia.

Epidemiology

- The prevalence in adult women (of 25 to 55 years of age) is about 20%. Every second patient conceals her problem.
  - The prevalence is 15% in women of 35, and 28% in women of 55.
- After retirement, about 50% of women and men suffer from urinary incontinence.

Aetiology

- In **stress incontinence** the pelvic floor may be weakened because of excessive body weight (>20% overweight), pregnancy, deliveries, and heavy work. Stress incontinence may also be caused by connective tissue weakness, asthma, or muscle-relaxant drug such as prazozine.
- **Urge incontinence** is a consequence of chronic bladder irritation. It can be related to
  - sequelae of urinary tract infections
  - past surgery for incontinence
  - oestrogen deficiency after menopause
  - diabetes or multiple sclerosis
  - use of medicines, such as neuroleptics and diuretics.

URO

Investigations

- Exclude urinary tract infection by urine culture.
- A questionnaire differentiates fairly well between stress incontinence and urge incontinence.
- Exclude tumours by examination (and endoscopy if required).

Indications for specialized investigations (ultrasonography, radiography, urodynamics)

- Annoying symptoms, especially if dominated by urge incontinence.
- Recurrence of symptoms after surgery.

Conservative treatment

- Postmenopausal women with minimal symptoms should try local oestrogen therapy (a vaginal suppository or tablet once or twice a week) **B** [1 2 3 4]. Local oestrogen is more effective than systemic oestrogen for either type of incontinence.
- Patients with mild stress incontinence
  - Weight reduction
  - Exercises for strengthening the muscles of pelvic floor **A** [5 6 7]
- Patients with mild urge incontinence
  - Bladder schooling (normalizing the micturition interval) **B** [8 9 10]
  - Anticholinergic medication **A** [11] has been used
    - The starting dose of oxybutynin is small (2.5–3 mg), the dose should be raised individually to the maximum of 5 mg × 3/day. The new slow release tablet (10 mg) taken once daily causes less side effects.
    - Tolterodine is as effective as oxybutynin in urge incontinence, but may have fewer anticholinergic side effects (dryness of the mouth and visual disturbances). The dose is 2 mg × 2 from the start.

- Trospium chloride is the newest drug for urge incontinence. The dose is 20 mg × 1–2/day. The effect is at least equal to the other drugs but it may have even fewer side effects.

- Electrical stimulation is worth trying in both types of incontinence (in stress incontinence the muscles of the pelvic floor are stimulated, in urge incontinence the overactivity of bladder muscles is decreased) D [12 13].
- A questionnaire assessing the seriousness of the problem helps in determining the urgency of investigations and treatment.

Surgical therapy

- Stress incontinence may be treated surgically according to the judgment of an urogynaecologist.
  - Burch colposuspension was the Golden standard up to the end of 1990s. It can also be performed endoscopically quite easily either using a mesh or stitches.
  - The most frequently used method nowadays is TVT, which is rather simple and can even be performed under local anaesthesia. The results are at least as good as with the Burch method. Even newer procedure TOT seems to replace TVT.
- In urge incontinence, surgery usually is not effective. In extreme cases an operation aimed at enlarging the bladder may be indicated by a specialist.
- The treatment for mixed incontinence is selected according to the dominant type of incontinence.

Aids

- Aids: bandages, diapers, urinals, and plastic bed sheets prevent leaking. Vaginal bullets and cones A [14] and vaginal tampons help to find the muscles in pelvic floor muscle training and prevent incontinence in short-lasting physical strain. A specialized nurse is responsible for supplying the aids and educating the patient.

References

1. Fantl JA, Cardozo L, McClish DK. Estrogen therapy in the management of urinary incontinence in postmenopausal women: a meta-analysis: first report of the Hormones and Urogenital Therapy Committee. Obst Gynecol 1994;83:12–18.
2. The Database of Abstracts of Reviews of Effectiveness (University of York), Database no.: DARE-953435. In: The Cochrane Library, Issue 4, 1999. Oxford: Update Software.
3. Zullo MA, Oliva C, Fanconi G, Paparella P, Mancuso S. Efficia della terapia oestogenica sull'incontinentia urinaria: studio meta-analitico. Minerva Ginecologica 1998;50:199–205.
4. The Database of Abstracts of Reviews of Effectiveness (University of York), Database no.: DARE-983808. In: The Cochrane Library, Issue 2, 2000. Oxford: Update Software.
5. Hay-Smith EJC, Bø K, Berghmans LCM, Hendriks HJM, de Bie RA, van Waalwijk van Doorn ESC. Pelvic floor muscle training for urinary incontinence in women. Cochrane Database Syst Rev. 2004;(2):CD001407.
6. Berghmans LC, Hendriks HJ, Bo K, Hay-Smith EJ, de Bie RA, van Waalwijk van Doorn ES. Conservative treatment of stress urinary incontinence in women: a systematic review of randomized clinical trials. British Journal of Urology 1998;82:181–191.
7. The Database of Abstracts of Reviews of Effectiveness (University of York), Database no.: DARE-981413. In: The Cochrane Library, Issue 3, 2000. Oxford: Update Software.
8. Wallace SA, Roe B, Williams K, Palmer M. Bladder training for urinary incontinence in adults. Cochrane Database Syst Rev. 2004;(2):CD001308.
9. Berghmans LC, Hendriks HJ, De Bie RA, Van Doorn E, Bo K, Van Kerrebroeck PH. Conservative treatment of urge urinary incontinence in women: a systematic review of randomized clinical trials. BJU International 2000;85:254–263.
10. The Database of Abstracts of Reviews of Effectiveness (University of York), Database no.: DARE-20000524. In: The Cochrane Library, Issue 3, 2001. Oxford: Update Software.
11. Hay-Smith J, Herbison P, Ellis G, Moore K. Anticholinergic drugs versus placebo for overactive bladder syndrome in adults. Cochrane Database Syst Rev. 2004;(2):CD003781.
12. Bo K. Effect of electrical stimulation on stress and urge urinary incontinence: clinical outcome and practical recommendations based on randomized controlled trials. Acta Obst Gyn Scand 1998;77(suppl 168):3–11.
13. The Database of Abstracts of Reviews of Effectiveness (University of York), Database no.: DARE-981604. In: The Cochrane Library, Issue 2, 2000. Oxford: Update Software.
14. Herbison P, Plevnik S, Mantle J. Weighted vaginal cones for urinary incontinence. Cochrane Database Syst Rev. 2004;(2):CD002114.

11.5 Haematuria

Erna Pettersson

Aims

- Exclude urinary tract infection and blood contamination (menstruation, sexual trauma, etc.).
- Further investigations should be carried out in all patients with confirmed haematuria that is not explained by the above causes C [1 2].

Macroscopic haematuria

- Less than 0.5 ml of blood in 500 ml of urine causes macroscopic haematuria. Depending on the urine pH the colour of urine may vary from bright red to almost black. Usually the patient is correct when he/she has noticed the urine to be "bloody".

- Red coloured urine may also be caused by
  - certain foods (beetroot)
  - medication (nitrofurantoin, rifampicin)
  - acute porphyria.

Microscopic haematuria

- More than three erythrocytes/high power field in sediment analysis.
- More than five erythrocytes/0.9 mm^3 in counting chamber.

Investigations of patients with haematuria

- It should be noted that there is not necessarily a correlation between the degree of haematuria and the severity of the underlying disease. Thus, scant haematuria should be investigated as thoroughly as more significant haematuria.
- If a dipstick test is positive for blood, the finding must be confirmed with a fresh urine sample after a couple of days. The urine must also be examined microscopically. Confirmed haematuria is always an indication for further investigations.
- Exclude urinary tract infection and contamination
- All patients
  - Thorough clinical investigation
  - Urinanalysis: proteinuria, erythrocyte morphology, casts, leucocytes
    - If the erythrocyte morphology (acanthocytes or red-cell casts) in microscopic haematuria is suggestive of glomerular aetiology, and the patient has no proteinuria or renal impairment (creatinine normal), no further investigations are needed. However, the patient should be monitored with occasional checks (first follow-up at 6 months and annually thereafter) for the possible development of proteinuria or renal impairment.
  - Blood tests (see below)
  - Ultrasound examination of the kidneys and urinary tract
    - All patients if glomerular haematuria has not been verified with urinalysis or blood tests.
  - Cytology (daytime sample) for patients over 40 years of age.
- Cystoscopy
  - In patients over 50 years of age; in younger patients only if haematuria has been macroscopic or the patient has risk factors for bladder cancer (smoking, occupational exposure, history of cyclophosphamide treatment).
  - Suspicious cells in cytology
  - Increased serum prostate specific antigen (PSA)
  - Ultrasound examination suggestive of bladder pathology
- Other investigations for selected patients
  - Computed tomography (investigation of choice for suspected urinary calculi or tumour of the upper urinary tract)
  - Urography
  - Angiography
  - Pyelography
  - Renal biopsy

Medical history

- In what circumstances was haematuria noted (fever, physical activity etc.)?
- Are there any other symptoms or signs (increased urinary frequency, dysuria, lower abdominal or flank pain)?
- Is haematuria seen at the initiation of, throughout or at the end of voiding? Blood at the initiation suggests a urethral pathology, continuous haematuria a renal or ureteral problem and blood at the end a bladder pathology.
- Are there any hereditary diseases or a tendency for urinary calculus formation?
- Travel abroad (exclude infectious diseases, such as schistosomiasis, malaria etc.)
- Medication: use of nonsteroidal anti-inflammatory drugs (NSAIDs) or treatment with cytotoxic agents (cyclophosphamide)? These drugs may cause interstitial nephritis (NSAIDs), interstitial cystitis or uroepithelial cancer (cytotoxic agents).

Clinical investigation

- Look for petechiae, bruising or enlarged lymph nodes.
- Check blood pressure.
- Abdominal palpation (the size and contour of the liver, spleen, kidneys).
- Palpation of the prostate via the rectum.
- Laboratory tests should include coagulation analysis, tests for prostatic disease, IgA nephropathy and tests for systemic disease and renal function (blood counts, ESR, CRP, creatinine, PSA, possibly IgA).

Urinalysis

- Dipstick tests for blood are sensitive and reliable. False-positive results may be seen in
  - haemoglobinuria
  - myoglobinuria.
- Reducing agents such as ascorbic acid or gentisic acid (a metabolite of acetyl salicylic acid) reduce and even inhibit the staining reaction.
- A positive dipstick test must be confirmed by analysing the urine sediment.
  - A semiquantitative sediment analysis or quantitative counting chamber may be used. The semiquantitative sediment analysis is reliable in validated conditions.
  - The analysis is carried out on a fresh urine sample, voided before ingesting any fluid (an early morning sample). After the urine is centrifuged the sediment is analysed under a microscope using a 400 × magnification.

- The analysis offers much more information if the sediment is stained or analysed under a phase-contrast microscope. These methods enable observation on the shape of the erythrocytes, which in turn helps to localise the source of bleeding. Symmetric, round and normal appearing red blood cells (RBCs) are seen as a consequence of bleeding in the lower urinary tract, whereas dysmorphic RBCs (acanthocytes) are seen in association with parenchymal renal disease ("glomerular bleeding").

- ♦ Culturing midstream urine and analysing urine sediment may not only confirm haematuria, but reveal an infection or the presence of leucocytes, casts or abnormal cells. Abnormal cells are suggestive of a urinary tract malignancy. However, urinary cytology must always be included in the investigations.
- ♦ Sterile pyuria is typical not only of genitourinary tuberculosis, but is also seen in association with calculi and tumours. Concurrent proteinuria is usually suggestive of a renal parenchymal disease.
- ♦ Cellular, granular, fatty or waxy casts in the sediment analysis are suggestive of a renal parenchymal disease.

Subsequent investigations

- ♦ Ultrasound of the kidneys and, if necessary, urography.
- ♦ Cytology of the urine
- ♦ Cystoscopy
- ♦ The importance of these investigations depends partly on the age of the patient. In children urography must be done only after careful consideration and cystoscopy is seldom necessary.
- ♦ Ultrasound investigation of the kidneys is safe and, particularly in pregnancy, the only recommended investigation. Sometimes additional investigations are needed, such as urography with tomography studies, computed tomography, angiography and antegrade or retrograde pyelography.
- ♦ Urinary cytology: a random daytime sample is better than an early morning sample, but bladder wash cytology is the best. Generally three separate samples should be analysed for the highest diagnostic yield. Up to 80–90% of transitional cell bladder carcinomas may be diagnosed with urinary cytology.
- ♦ If the patient also has pyuria the urine should be cultured for tuberculosis.
- ♦ Cystoscopy is performed at the outpatient clinic under local anaesthesia.

Additional investigations and follow-up

- ♦ Possible additional investigations depend on the primary findings. The more investigations carried out the more likely it is that the underlying cause will be found. Urological investigations will reveal a cause in up to 80% of the cases.
- ♦ A renal biopsy will reveal a renal parenchymal disease. Renal biopsy should be considered particularly if the patient has simultaneous proteinuria, pathological casts or dysmorphic erythrocytes suggestive of a glomerular haematuria. With this approach the patient may be saved from unnecessary antibiotic therapies, repeated radiographic investigations or cystoscopies.
- ♦ Some causes of haematuria are listed in Table 11.5 according to severity (serious causes indicate findings that necessitate major medical intervention or threaten the life of the patient).
- ♦ Haematuria in a young patient is usually caused by urinary tract infection, calculi or parenchymal renal disease, particularly IgA nephropathy, whereas malignancy must be considered in patients over the age of 40 years. Therefore, haematuria must always be taken seriously.
- ♦ The cause of haematuria is not always revealed despite meticulous investigations. It may be necessary to follow up these patients, for example once a year, with a check-up of blood pressure and routine blood tests and urinalyses.

Table 11.5 Causes of haematuria according to severity

Serious	Moderate	Minor
♦ Renal carcinoma ♦ Uroepithelial cancer ♦ Ureteral stones ♦ Prostate cancer ♦ Hydronephrosis ♦ Tuberculosis ♦ Polycystic kidney disease ♦ Parenchymal renal disease	♦ Kidney stones ♦ Urinary tract infection ♦ Interstitial cystitis ♦ Bladder stones	♦ Asymptomatic prostatic hyperplasia

References

1. Buntinx F, Wauters H. The diagnostic value of macroscopic haematuria diagnosing urological cancers: a meta-analysis. Family Practice 1997;14:63–68.
2. The Database of Abstracts of Reviews of Effectiveness (University of York), Database no.: DARE-970347. In: The Cochrane Library, Issue 4, 1999. Oxford: Update Software.

11.6 Urinary bladder tamponade (blood clots in the bladder)

Teuvo Tammela

First aid

- ♦ Infuse physiological saline to ensure adequate circulating blood volume.
- ♦ Perform catheterization with an open-ended Ch 16–20 catheter; preferably a PVC catheter (which does not collapse

with suction). The bladder should be flushed repeatedly with isotonic saline to remove clots. If a three-way catheter is available, start continuous lavage and refer the patient to hospital, preferably to a urological ward.
- Bleeding after transurethral resection of the prostate may stop with gentle pulling of a catheter balloon filled with 50–80 ml of saline. It is important to **hold the penis in an upward direction** to avoid urethral trauma.
- Tranexamic acid (1 g × 3) may be of benefit.
- The patient must usually be hospitalized (the bleeding may continue)
- During transportation the catheter should be in place in the bladder.

11.7 Haematospermia

Editors

Aetiology

- Usually no cause is found.
- Urethral trauma, e.g. in association with sexual activity.
- Prostatovesiculitis.
- A tumour is a rare cause of haematospermia.

Investigations

- A urine test with microscopy should always be performed to detect haematuria. For investigations into haematuria see article 11.5.
- Palpation of the prostate (touch per rectum) to detect a tumour.
- Repeated haematospermia is an indication for further investigations (serum prostate-specific antigen, cystoscopy), particularly in men above 50 years of age.

Treatment

- The symptoms usually need no other treatment than reassuring the patient.

11.10 Acute prostatitis

Teuvo Tammela

Symptoms

- Increased urinary frequency, burning sensation in lower abdomen = symptoms of urinary tract infection.
- Voiding difficulties, painful voiding.
- The patient often has fever and feels ill.

Differential diagnosis

- Sexually transmitted diseases (chlamydia, gonorrhoea)
  - Take samples for culture or PCR test.
- Chronic bacterial prostatitis (11.11).

URO

Clinical and laboratory findings

- Tenderness in the lower abdomen.
- Very tender prostate on palpation.
- A large amount of leucocytes, mucus and bacteria in the urine specimen = findings consistent with UTI.

Treatment

- Peroral fluoroquinolone or trimethoprim-sulphamethoxazole in normal (UTI) doses is usually sufficient. Of the fluoroquinolones, ciprofloxacin and norfloxacin yield the highest concentrations. The duration of treatment is at least 4 weeks.
- If the patient has fever and severe symptoms the initial treatment should consist of intravenous cefuroxime in a hospital for one week, followed by oral medication for 3 weeks.
- Massage of the prostate is **contraindicated**.
- Suprapubic cystostomy may occasionally be necessary to secure the emptying of the bladder no catheterisation.

11.11 Chronic prostatitis

Teuvo Tammela

- See also Spastic pelvis syndrome 8.10

Basic rules

- Inform the patient thoroughly.
- Avoid unnecessary antibiotics.
- In frequently recurring prostatitis search for bacterial aetiology by fractionated urine sampling.

Aetiology

- Usually (in 70% of the cases) the patient has sterile prostatodynia. The condition tends to recur several times a year.
- The disease may be caused by bacteria residing in the prostatic ducts.

Symptoms

- The symptoms are similar to those of acute prostatitis but milder and recurring
  - Increased urinary frequency
  - Voiding difficulties and pain
  - Burning sensation in the lower abdomen, scrotum, perineum, glans, or inner thighs.
- Feeling of incomplete emptying of the bladder
- Feeling of pressure in the perineum, anus or anterior to the anus
- Sitting may cause difficulty, or the patient feels as if he were sitting on a pillow
- Bloody semen, painful ejaculation
- Decreased libido, erectile dysfunction

Clinical and laboratory findings

- Tenderness of the prostate. However, lack of tenderness does not exclude chronic prostatitis
- Normal urine test results

Fractionated urine sampling

- Should be performed only if frequently occurring acute symptoms result in repeated courses of antibiotics.
  - Sample of initial stream urine
  - Prostate massage
  - A sample of urine voided after massage of the prostate, which is examined under microscope and cultured.
- If the sample taken after massage contains bacteria and more than 10 leucocytes/field, and the first samples is clean or shows a much smaller number of bacteria, the findings suggest chronic bacterial prostatitis.
- A sample for chlamydia should be taken if there is pyuria without bacterial growth.

Treatment

- Warm clothing
- Warm sitz baths C [1]
- NSAIDs
- alpha-blockers
- 5-alpha-reductase inhibitors
- Massage of the prostate sometimes alleviates the symptoms
- Continuity of the doctor–patient relationship; reassurance of the benign nature of the condition and treatment of eventual depression
- Antibiotics are not indicated for prostatodynia
- Take a fractionated urine sample in frequently recurring cases. If bacteria are detected, treat with a 1–2-month course of fluoroquinolones (starting with e.g. norfloxacin 400 mg × 2, lowering the dose later on) or trimethoprim-sulfamethoxazole.
- If the patient has pyuria without bacterial growth try the same regimen as above; however, if this is not beneficial, do not give repeated courses of antibiotics.

Reference

1. McNaughton Collins M, Mac Donald R, Wilt T. Interventions for chronic abacterial prostatitis. Cochrane Database Syst Rev. 2004;(2):CD002080.

11.12 Benign prostatic hyperplasia

Teuvo Tammela

Aims

- The diagnosis of benign prostatic hyperplasia is based on symptoms and basic investigations. Other causes of voiding disturbances (prostate cancer in particular) are excluded.
- Conditions requiring surgical management are recognized.
- Follow-up alone or drug therapy are good options in patients with relatively mild symptoms and no complications of urinary tract stricture.

Symptoms

- Storage symptoms
  - Extraordinary voiding frequency
  - Nocturia
  - Urinary urgency
  - Urge incontinence
- Voiding symptoms
  - Difficulty in the initiation of voiding
  - Poor urine flow
  - Need to strain while voiding
  - Discontinued voiding
  - Feeling of inadequate bladder emptying
  - Urinary retention

Primary investigations

- Symptom questionnaire
  - A commonly used questionnaire is IPSS
  - The questionnaire is useful in the assessment of severity symptoms when decisions are made between follow-up, drug treatment and surgery.
- Writing down details associated with voiding
- DRE (digital rectal examination)
- Urinalysis
- Serum creatinine
- Serum prostate-specific antigen (PSA)
- Residual urine volume is determined by ultrasonography (42.4) (or if ultrasonography is not available by catheterization). Ultrasonography is useful in the determination of prostatic size (calculated with the same equation as residual urine volume (42.4)), shape, and eventual hydronephrosis.

Table 11.12 Differential diagnosis on benign prostatic hyperplasia

Condition or disease	History or finding
Prostate cancer	Finding in DRE, elevated serum PSA concentration
Urinary bladder cancer	Haematuria, abnormal cytological finding
Bladder calculi	Haematuria, ultrasonography finding
Urethral stricture	Box-shaped flow curve
Stricture of the bladder neck	Earlier invasive treatment
Bladder neck dyssynergia	Small prostate gland, disturbing symptoms associated with voiding
Prostatitis	Tender prostate gland
Overactive bladder	Urgency with possible urge incontinence

- Differential diagnosis, see Table 11.12.

Indications for specialist consultation

Indications for diagnostic investigations by the urologist

- The patient is below 50 years of age.
- DRE is suspicious (nodules)
- Serum PSA is above 10 mg/ml (above 3 mg/ml in patients below 65 years of age)
  - If the serum total PSA concentration is in the range of 3–10 mg/ml, measuring free/total PSA ratio is recommended. If this value is under 0.15, the probability of prostatic cancer is increased and a urologist should be consulted.
  - DRE before determination of serum PSA level does not influence the result.
- Rapidly developing symptoms
- Haematuria (cystoscopy)
- Diabetics who may have neuropathy
- History of pelvic surgery or irradiation
- Neurological disease or injury affecting the function of the urinary bladder
- Necessary medication affecting the function of the urinary bladder
- Lower abdominal pain as the main symptom
- Discrepancy between symptoms and findings
- The investigations performed by the urologist usually include:
  - urine flow measurement
  - transrectal ultrasonography,
- and if necessary also
  - cystometry and pressure-flow examination (recommended before deciding on surgery if the peak flow is >10 ml/s and also when there is a discrepancy between symptoms and findings or the patient has undergone surgery of the lower urinary tract)
  - urethrocystography
  - urography
  - prostatic biopsies
  - cystoscopy.

Surgical treatment is indicated in the following cases:

- Urinary retention, overflow incontinence or repeatedly more than 300 ml of residual urine
- Severe symptoms
- Dilatation of the upper urinary tract
- Impairment of renal function
- Recurrent macroscopic haematuria
- Urinary tract infections
- Bladder calculi
- Severe or moderate symptoms in a patient who wants rapid relief or if satisfactory results have not been obtained with other treatments.

URO

Conservative treatment

Follow-up

- As the symptoms of BPH vary greatly and the course of the disease in an individual cannot be fully predicted, follow-up is a suitable approach in patients with mild symptoms. Also in moderate symptoms, follow-up can be the initial approach if the symptoms do not essentially affect the quality of life and complications have not developed.
- Follow-up includes explaining to the patient the nature of the disease and carrying out basic investigations annually or when symptoms have changed. Opportunistic follow-up during other encounters in primary care is one method of screening.

Drug treatment

- Although the effectiveness of drug treatment is not as good as that of surgery it is often sufficient for reducing or alleviating the symptoms.
- When deciding on the treatment, cost-effectiveness should also be evaluated, i.e. when would invasive therapy, which usually gives complete cure, cost less and be more convenient for the patient than drug therapy continuing for years (for example, to avoid one invasive treatment, 20 men have to be treated with finasteride for 4 years). Transurethral resection is more cost-effective than drug treatment.
- Patients on drug treatment should be followed up regularly at 6–12-month intervals to detect complications resulting from urethral obstruction.
- The size of the prostate and total serum PSA determine the selection of the therapy C [1 2]. If the prostate is not markedly enlarged on palpation or in ultrasonography (<40 g) and PSA is <1.5 mg/ml the first choice is an alpha$_1$-blocker (e.g. tamsulosin or alfuzosin). If the prostate is markedly enlarged or PSA is > 1.5 mg/ml either 5-alpha-reductase inhibitor (finasteride, dutasteride) A [3 4] or an alpha$_1$-blocker can be used.
- A combination of 5-alpha-reductase inhibitor and alpha$_1$-blocker alleviates symptoms more effectively than either drug alone B [5].

Alpha-blockers

- Tamsulosin, alfuzosin, doxazosin, terazosin and prazosin.
- $Alpha_1$-blockers decrease symptoms, increase peak urinary flow and reduce the volume of residual urine significantly more than placebo.
- The effect of $alpha_1$-blockers is seen rapidly and it has been shown to continue for several years.
- The patients should be followed up initially at 1–3-month intervals.
- The side effects include dizziness, postural hypotension, and retrograde ejaculation. With selective tamsulosine and alfuzosin the risk of hypotension is lower.

5-alpha-reductase inhibitors

- The dose of finasteride is 5 mg × 1 and that of dutasteride is 0.5 mg × 1.
- The symptoms are alleviated, the urine flow is increased, and the obstruction is decreased A [3 4].
- The effect is at its best in patients with large prostates C [1 2].
- The effect starts slowly, sometimes as late as 6 months after the onset of treatment. If no effect is observed in 6 months the indications for surgery should be reconsidered.
- The drug decreases prostatic size but the prostate returns to its original size a few months after discontinuation of treatment.
- Impotence may occur as an adverse effect.

Surgical and other invasive treatments

- Transurethral resection of the prostate (TURP)
  - The only treatment for complicated prostatic hyperplasia and the best documented treatment for uncomplicated disease.
  - Results very seldom in erectile dysfunction (though in most cases already before operation), almost always retrograde ejaculation.
- Transurethral incision of the prostate (TUIP)
  - Suitable for patients with prostates <30 ml and no prominent median lobe.
- Open prostatectomy
  - Rarely used nowadays (prostate >100 ml)
- Thermotherapy (microwave treatment)
  - Alleviates irritative symptoms
  - Long-term results are not available.
- Stent or spiral
  - Can be used in selected cases in patients with a poor general condition.

Catheter

- Percutaneous cystostomy is indicated in patients with urinary retention waiting for surgery.
- In selected cases repeated catheterization can be used (preferably by the patient himself).
- A silicon catheter with the balloon filled with hypertonic (5%) saline or glyserol can be used, but percutaneous cystostomy is preferred.

Treatment after TURP

- Urine bacterial culture should be taken routinely 4–6 weeks after the operation to detect bacteriuria, and always if a urinary tract infection is suspected (pyuria and haematuria may occur as long as 3 months after the operation).
- If bacterial growth is detected, antibiotics are indicated.
- Stress incontinence may be alleviated within 1 year: exercises of pelvic floor muscles may help.
- Antimuscarinic drugs (oxybutynin, tolterodine, trospium chloride) can be used for the treatment of urge incontinence and nocturia.

References

1. Boyle P, Gould AL, Roehrborn CG. Prostate volume predicts outcome of treatment of benign prostatic hyperplasia with finasteride: meta-analysis of randomised trials. Urology 1996;48:398–405.
2. The Database of Abstracts of Reviews of Effectiveness (University of York), Database no.: DARE-961572. In: The Cochrane Library, Issue 4, 1999. Oxford: Update Software.
3. Wilde MI, Goa KL. Finasteride: an update of its use in the management of symptomatic benign prostatic hyperplasia. Drugs 1999;57:557–581.
4. The Database of Abstracts of Reviews of Effectiveness (University of York), Database no.: DARE-990978. In: The Cochrane Library, Issue 4, 2000. Oxford: Update Software.
5. McConnell JD, Roehrborn CG, Bautista OM, Andriole GL Jr, Dixon CM, Kusek JW, Lepor H, McVary KT, Nyberg LM Jr, Clarke HS, Crawford ED, Diokno A, Foley JP, Foster HE, Jacobs SC, Kaplan SA, Kreder KJ, Lieber MM, Lucia MS, Miller GJ, Menon M, Milam DF, Ramsdell JW, Schenkman NS, Slawin KM, Smith JA; Medical Therapy of Prostatic Symptoms (MTOPS) Research Group. The long-term effect of doxazosin, finasteride, and combination therapy on the clinical progression of benign prostatic hyperplasia. N Engl J Med 2003;349(25):2387–98.

11.13 Prostate cancer

Editors

Basic rules

- Palpation and prostate-specific antigen (PSA) determination are used to exclude prostate cancer in patients suffering from prostate hyperplasia or with urinary tract infection.

- Identify metastatic prostate cancer as a possible cause of skeletal pain.

Epidemiology and risk factors

- The most common malignant neoplasm in men.
- The presence of androgens is necessary for the development of the cancer.
- Known risk factors include high intake of dietary fat, obesity and smoking.
- Only 5% of the patients are under 60 years of age at diagnosis.
- Asymptomatic prostate cancer is a common finding at post-mortem examination (in 30% of those over 50 years, in 70–80% of those over 80 years).
- The natural course of the disease is difficult to predict. In about 80% of the patients in whom the disease is confined within the prostatic capsule the disease does not progress during a follow-up of 10 years.

Symptoms

- The symptoms resemble those of bening prostatic hyperplasia. The symptoms may include
  - increased urinary frequency
  - poor urinary flow
  - urinary retention
  - urinary tract infection
  - sensation of inadequate bladder emptying
  - haematuria (rare symptom of prostate cancer)
  - symptoms caused by metastases (skeletal pain, particularly in the ribs and spine).

Diagnosis

- Screening tests are not indicated, as there is no evidence of their effect on life expectancy or morbidity C [1 2 3 4]. Patients whose disease will progress and who thus would benefit from early treatment cannot be identified with present methods.
- Rectal palpation of the prostate and serum PSA determination are indicated in men over 50 years of age who have symptoms (see above) suggesting prostatic disease C [1 2 3 4].
  - Prostate cancer is found in about 30% of the patients with a palpable nodule.
- PSA is a useful test in assessing the spread of the disease.
  - The upper limit of the reference range is 3 μg/l.
  - In benign prostatic hyperplasia, a concentration as high as 10 μg/l can be considered "normal".
  - A concentration above 20 μg/l often indicates prostate cancer, and a concentration above 50 μg/l indicates metastatic cancer.
- Refer the patient to a urologist if
  - **a nodule is felt on rectal examination or serum PSA is above 10 μg/l**
  - **the patient is below the age of 65 and has serum PSA above 3 μg/l.**
  - **total PSA is in the range 3–10 μg/l, and free/total PSA ratio is less than 15%**
- The diagnosis is verified by a histological examination of a needle biopsy obtained during transrectal sonographic examination C [1 2 3 4].
- Radioisotope scanning is the method of choice for detecting skeletal metastases. If serum PSA is below 10 μg/l, the probability of bone metastases is very low (below 1%). Bone radioisotope scan should be carried out if a patient with recently diagnosed prostate cancer has skeletal pain, his PSA is over 10 μg/l or serum alkaline phosphatase is elevated. During follow-up, an isotope scan should be performed if skeletal pain emerges or alkaline phosphatase becomes elevated.
- At diagnosis, about 20% of the cancers are localised, 40% have spread outside the prostatic capsule and 40% have sent metastases.

Treatment

- A **localised prostate cancer** (intracapsular cancer) can be treated with four alternative methods C [1 2 3 4]:
  - Active follow-up ("watchful wait") is suitable for elderly patients who do not want surgery or radiotherapy, or wish to avoid the associated adverse effects. Target group: T1 - 2N0M0, Gr 1, Gleason 2–4, age >70 years, little/no symptoms.
  - Radical prostatectomy is suitable for patients in good health, generally <70 years, who want the tumour removed. Target group: T1b-2N0M0, Gr 1–3, Gleason 2–9. A Scandinavian study, which compared patients assigned to either radical prostatectomy or watchful waiting, showed that erectile dysfunction (80% vs. 45%) and urinary leakage (49% vs. 21%) were more common after radical prostatectomy, whereas symptoms of urinary obstruction (28% vs. 44%) were less common C [5].
  - Radiotherapy (about 30 treatment sessions) is equally effective as radical prostatectomy. Target group: T1–3, Gr 1–3, Gleason 4–9. Adverse effects include irritation of the bladder and rectum. Internal radiation therapy (brachytherapy) where radioactive particles or needles (palladium, iodide^{125}) are inserted into the tissue under ultrasound guidance has increased during recent years.
  - Bicalutamide. Target group: T1-T3NXM0, Gr 1–3, Gleason 2–9.
- Treatment of an **advanced cancer** is hormonal.
  - 80% respond to therapy.
  - Within 5 years the tumour becomes unresponsive to hormonal therapy in almost 80% of the patients.
  - Orchiectomy is effective and can be carried out even on very old patients under local anaesthesia. The adverse effects include impotence and hot flushes.
  - LHRH analogues are an alternative to orchiectomy. The medicine is administered subcutaneously, usually with an

interval of three months. The efficacy and adverse effects are similar to orchiectomy.
- Oestrogen therapy (intramuscular injections of polyestradiol phosphate) is another alternative to orchiectomy. This treatment has become less popular because of cardiovascular complications (thrombosis) and other adverse effects (gynaecomastia, hot flushes, fluid retention, depression).
- Antiandrogens (cyproterone acetate, bicalutamide, flutamide, nilutamide) can be used as primary or add-on therapy for selected patients Ⓐ [6 7].

♦ The **second-line** treatment of an **advanced cancer** after the tumour no longer responds to hormonal therapy may include estramustine, certain cytotoxic agents or radiotherapy. The aim is to improve the quality rather than the duration of life.

♦ Palliative treatments
- Electroresection of the prostate alleviates urinary retention.
- Radiotherapy is effective against skeletal pain.
- A small dose of radiation on the breasts prevents gynaecomastia associated with anti-androgen and oestrogen treatment.
- Clodronate is effective in hypercalcaemia (and possibly also in skeletal pain in some patients).
- The effect of cytotoxic agents is limited (only 2–19% of the patients respond).

Prognosis

♦ 5-year life expectancy is 65%.

♦ Life expectancy in metastatic cancer is on average 2–3 years.

Follow-up

♦ Follow-up visits at 3-month intervals during the first year, at 6 month intervals during years 2–3, and annually from year 4 onward are recommended.

♦ In addition to regular follow-up, the patient needs to know where or who to contact if necessary.

♦ The follow-up of an **incidental localised cancer** (detected for example during transurethral resection of the prostate) can be carried out by PSA determinations and rectal palpation with 6–12 month intervals. Doubling of the PSA concentration is considered a sign of disease spread and an indication for referral to a urologist.

♦ Patients treated with **radical prostatectomy or radiotherapy** are initially followed up at the initial place of treatment, and subsequently referred to the care of a urologist or oncologist. The follow-up of an elderly patient may be carried out by his general practitioner.

♦ Patients receiving **hormonal therapy** have their first follow-up visit at the initial place of treatment. If the patient responds to the treatment his care may be undertaken by his general practitioner.

♦ If the **disease advances despite hormonal therapy**, the patient is monitored more frequently. The continuity of the doctor–patient relationship and the early recognition of symptoms and complications affecting the quality of life are important.

Investigations during the follow-up of advanced prostate cancer

♦ Ask about the patient's symptoms and problems (pain, voiding problems, impotence, depression).
- Skeletal pain is an indication for urological or oncological consultation.
- Local tumour growth may cause voiding problems. Refer the patient to a urologist.

♦ Measure serum PSA if the patient wishes to know whether the disease is progressing, before the symptoms become evident. A rise in serum PSA level precedes the symptoms by about one year.
- Doubling of the PSA concentration is an indication of the advancement of the disease and requires urological consultation.
- PSA determinations are not indicated in metastatic cancer unless the effect of a change in therapy needs to be monitored.

♦ In addition to the above investigations, the following tests may be carried out: haemoglobin, creatinine, alkaline phosphatase, midstream urine and residual urine.

♦ Chest x-rays are not indicated in routine follow-up, neither are other imaging investigations.

References

1. Selly S, Donovan J, Faulkner A, Coast J, Gillatt D. Diagnosis, management and screening of early localised prostate cancer. Health Technology Assessment 1997;1:1–96.
2. The Database of Abstracts of Reviews of Effectiveness (University of York), Database no.: DARE-988277. In: The Cochrane Library, Issue 4, 1999. Oxford: Update Software.
3. Coley CM, Barry MJ, Fleming C, Mulley AG. Early detection of prostate cancer part 1: prior probability and effectiveness. Ann Intern Med 1997;126:394–406.
4. The Database of Abstracts of Reviews of Effectiveness (University of York), Database no.: DARE-978080. In: The Cochrane Library, Issue 4, 1999. Oxford: Update Software.
5. Stanford JL, Feng Z, Hamilton AS, Gilliland FD, Stephenson RA, Eley JW, Albertsen PC, Harlan LC, Potosky AL. Urinary and sexual function after radical prostatectomy for clinically localized prostate cancer. The Prostate Cancer Outcomes Study. JAMA 2000;283:354–360.
6. Bertagna C, De Gery A, Hucher M, Francois JP, Zanirato J. Efficacy of the combination of nilutamide plus orchidectomy in patients with metastatic prostatic cancer. A meta-analysis of seven double-blind randomized double blind trials (1056 patients). Br J Urol 1994;73:396–401.
7. The Database of Abstracts of Reviews of Effectiveness (University of York), Database no.: DARE-940104. In: The Cochrane Library, Issue 4, 1999. Oxford: Update Software.

11.20 Balanitis, balanoposthitis, and paraphimosis in the adult

Pekka Autio

Basic rules

- The aetiology is determined critically (avoid overdiagnosing candidiasis)
- Most often the treatment is symptomatic, and sometimes directed to the cause.
- Paraphimosis must be treated without delay to avoid the risk of necrosis of the glans.
- Consider circumcision in severe cases.

Definitions

- Balanitis can be defined widely to include all inflammatory dermatoses in the glans. In this article the following classification is used:
- Balanitis means inflammation of the epithelium of the glans.
- Balanoposthitis means inflammation of the glans and the inner surface of the foreskin.
- Paraphimosis ("Spanish collar") (Figure 11.20.1) occurs when a tight foreskin is retracted and the resulting stasis causes marked swelling of the distal foreskin.

Aetiology

- Balanitis can be caused by
  - Irritants, neglecting hygiene, tight foreskin, irritation by smegma
  - Seborrhoeic dermatitis; check scalp, the skin behind the ears, and skin folds

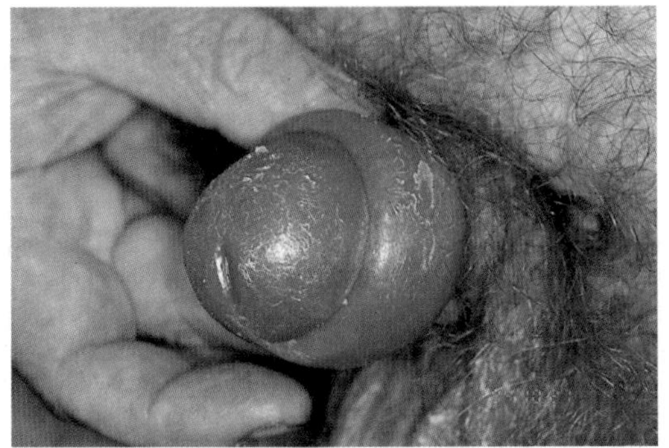

Figure 11.20.1 Balanoposthitis ("Spanish collar") is a manifestation of seborrhoeic eczema, and not caused by bacteria or fungi. If the swollen foreskin is very tight, the circulation of the glans is compromised. Reposition and class II corticosteroids improved the condition in one week. Photo © R. Suhonen.

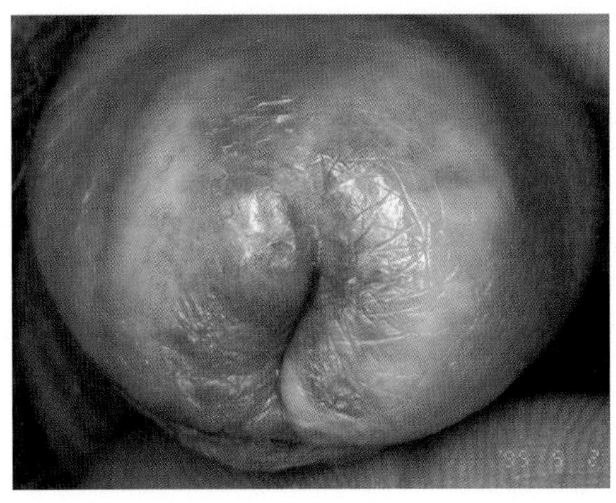

Figure 11.20.2 Balanitis xerotica obliterans, male Lichen sclerosus et atrophicus affects the glans and prepuce. Effective therapy is needed to prevent the stricture of the urethral meatus and phimosis. This disease carries a certain risk of development of malignancy if not treated and followed properly. Photo © R. Suhonen.

  - Candida; a positive culture result does not yet prove causality. Candidiasis is overdiagnosed.
  - Contact allergy
    - Latex and additives used in rubber manufacture
    - constituents of skin care products (used by the patient and his partner)
  - Balanitis xerotica obliterans (BXO, lichen sclerosus et atrophicus) (Figure 11.20.2).
  - Balanitis circinata are there other signs of Reiter's disease?
  - Balanitis plasmacellularis Zoon (rare)
- In the same location as balanitis may also occur
  - Lichen (ruber) planus–it is more common in the glans than is generally believed.
  - Psoriasis–check other typical locations of psoriasis
  - Erythema fixum (particularly caused by tetracyclines)
  - Erythroplasia Queyrat (a variant of Bowen's disease in the glans), which is a carcinoma in situ.

Investigations

- Bacterial culture (bacteria, candida) should be taken only if there is a clear suspicion of infection. Interpret the result critically.
- Patch tests (in cases of suspected allergy): refer to a dermatologist.
- Biopsy (if malignancy is suspected e.g. in BXO): refer to a urologist or a dermatologist.

Treatment

- Relevant treatment against specific aetiology (bacteria, candida)
- Potassium permanganate (1:10 000) is nearly always beneficial.
- Corticosteroid creams (class I–II) for eczema

- Refer BXO to a specialist (dermatologist or urologist)
- Treat phimosis by circumcision. If the foreskin of an adult man cannot be retracted in the sulcus of the glans after the balanitis has cured a circumcision is indicated.
- Paraphimosis should be treated by immediate reposition. Use lidocaine gel and squeeze the tip of the glans long enough to reduce swelling so that the foreskin can be liberated. If reposition is not successful, an incision of the foreskin should be made.

11.21 Peyronie's disease (Induratio penis plastica)

Editors

Symptoms and signs

- A fibrotic induration of corpus cavernosum
- The aetiology of is unknown; however, 15% of the patients have Dypyutren contracture of the palms.
- The skin is normal and freely mobile at the site of induration.
- The penis is curved in the direction of the induration during erection.
- In differential diagnosis consider the spread of prostatic carcinoma into the penis (palpate the prostate).

Treatment

- No therapy is indicated unless intercourse becomes difficult. Explain the condition to the patient.
- Refer to a urologist if the penis is painful or markedly curved.

11.22 Testis pain

Editors

- Swelling of the scrotum, see article 11.23.

Basic rules

- Diagnose and treat testis torsion immediately (always suspect torsion in children and young adults who are not yet sexually active).
- Treat epididymitis with antibiotics.
- Diagnose varicocele as a cause of prolonged or recurrent testis pain.

Testis torsion

- Pain, which is often felt initially in the lower abdomen and only later in the scrotum, and unilateral swelling of the scrotum start suddenly.
- The testicle rises in the upper part of the scrotum and lies there horizontally. The cremaster reflex is absent.
- Torsion of appendix testis and epididymitis may resemble testis torsion. The differential diagnosis can often be made only in an operation.
- Testis torsion should be treated with an urgent operation to avoid permanent damage to the testis.

Epididymitis

- Swelling and tenderness are located in the epididymis, but the testis itself may also be tender.
- The causative agents include bacteria causing urinary tract infections, and in sexually active patients also chlamydiae and sometimes gonococci. In older men retention problems may be a predisposing factor.
- Epididymitis occurs also before the sexually active age.
- In children epididymitis is apparently caused by the passage of sterile or infected urine to the deferent duct. In recurrences, ultrasonography of the urinary tracts is a worthwhile examination for excluding e.g., ectopic ureter. Attention should also be paid to enuresis and difficulties in voiding.
- In all age groups manipulation of the urethra, such as prolonged indwelling catheterization and urological interventions, predispose to epididymitis.
- Investigations
  - Urine test and culture
  - Chlamydial and gonococcal culture or PCR
- The treatment consists of trimethoprim-sulphamethoxazole or cephalosporin derivative (in children), doxycycline 150 mg × 1 × 10–14 (in adolescents) or cephalosporin derivative or fluoroquinolone (in the elderly).
- A suspensor to support the scrotum, cool bandages, and NSAIDs relieve pain.

Orchitis

- The swelling is located in the testis itself.
- Orchitis is very uncommon in countries where mumps has disappeared as a result of vaccinations, but may sometimes be associated with epididymitis (epididymo-orchitis).
- The differential diagnosis of orchitis and testicular torsion is difficult (refer to hospital urgently if there is the slightest doubt).
- Investigations
  - Parotitis serology (paired serum samples) from the unvaccinated
- Treatment
  - Pain relief (see above)

Varicocele

- In a young man the symptoms are visible varicose veins, pain (rarely) and decreased fertility.
- For details see article 11.23.

11.23 Enlarged scrotum or palpable mass in scrotum

Editors

Basic rules

- An enlarged testicle should be considered a tumour unless this is ruled out. Always refer the patient to a specialist.
- If the swelling can be located **outside the testicle**
  - identify a hydrocele without special investigations
  - identify a spermatocele without special investigations, and verify that the condition is innocent by sufficient follow-up.
  - detect a hernia and refer the patient for surgery
  - detect a varicocele (which may cause infertility)

Hydrocele

- A hydrocele is a collection of fluid inside the tunica vaginalis surrounding the testicle and appendix testis.
- Easily differentiated from a solid tumour by transilluminating the scrotum in a dark room with a sharp light. The light easily traverses a hydrocele, but not a testicular tumour.
- A hydrocele can be freely deformed unlike a solid tumour.
- The diagnosis can be verified by ultrasonography.
- A small hydrocele need not be treated. A large hydrocele can be treated surgically or with sclerotherapy. Needle aspiration is not beneficial as the fluid collection recurs.

Spermatocele

- A spermatocele is a round, soft mass above the testicle clearly separated from it.
- A spermatocele transilluminates fairly well.
- Aspiration of the contents may be diagnostic. A spermatocele contains fluid that may be grey because of semen.
- An annoyingly large spermatocele can be treated surgically.

Varicocele

- Usually left-sided
- Dilatated veins can be seen as worm-like swellings in the base of the scrotum when the patient is standing. The Valsalva manouvre may be helpful in doubtful cases. In the supine position dilated veins disappear.
- Particularly in young men varicocele causes a feeling of weight in the testes, see article on testis pain (11.22).
- In a middle-aged or elderly patient a rapidly appearing left-sided varicocele may indicate renal vein thrombosis (which can be caused by renal carcinoma). Right-sided varicocele may indicate obstruction of the inferior vena cava.
- Treatment is indicated if the varicocele causes symptoms or infertility (D) [1]. The testicular vein can be ligated surgically, laparoscopically, or by a radiological procedure.

Inguinal hernia

- Visible as a swelling at the orifice of the inguinal canal. Reposition by pressing with fingers is usually easy. Read more about hernias (8.85)

Testicular cancer

- An enlarged, solid testicle or a nodule in the testis is the typical finding.
- The prognosis is rather good with the combination of surgery, irradiation and chemotherapy.

Reference

1. Evers JLH, Collins JA, Vandekerckhove P. Surgery or embolisation for varicocele in subfertile men. Cochrane Database Syst Rev. 2004;(2):CD000479.

11.30 Choosing a method for bladder emptying

Teuvo Tammela

- Repeated catheterization is the preferred method (11.31).
- If this is not feasible (the patient has an obstruction, urinary output/hour must be monitored, catheterization cannot be performed at home in long-term care, or the patient has considerable retention >1000 ml) suprapubic cystostomy (11.32) is preferred.
- If the need for catheterization is temporary, the capacity of the bladder is small, or there are operative scars in the

lower abdomen (risk of bowel perforation at insertion in cystostomy) a thin silicone or PVC catheter should be used.

- If ultrasonography is available immediately before percutaneous cystostomy the absence of bowel between the bladder and the abdominal wall can be confirmed relatively reliably.

- If the urine is bloody a Ch 16 PVC catheter can be used (11.6).
- A permanent indwelling catheter should not be inserted without a medical cause in an incontinent patient in long-term care.

11.31 Catheterization of the urinary bladder

Teuvo Tammela

Catheters

- The number of the catheter gives its circumference in millimetres. The diameter of the catheter is roughly the circumference divided by 3.
- Silicone and PVC are the most suitable materials for long-term catheterization as they cause the least tissue irritation.

Catheterization

- Wash the urethral orifice with an antiseptic solution (e.g. 0.01% chlorhexidine).
- Inject 20 ml gel into the urethra of men (and somewhat less for women). Use preferably a gel containing a local anaesthetic.
- Both gel injection and insertion of the catheter should be performed gently and slowly.
- In men the penis should be straightened to an angle of 90 degrees to the body in order to facilitate catheter insertion.
- Fill the balloon only after making sure that both the tip of the catheter and the balloon are in the bladder: the urine flows freely, or if the bladder is empty, saline solution injected into the catheter flows in easily.
- If the catheter cannot be inserted with gentle handling try a Thieman catheter. Do not attempt repeatedly but perform a cystostomy (11.32). If the patient has an enlarged prostate, changing to a bigger catheter is often helpful.

Repeated catheterization

- The most physiological means of emptying the bladder.
- Teach the patient in the hospital (and provide written instructions).
- Catheterization should be repeated frequently enough so that the bladder is not filled above 500 ml.
- If the patient is totally unable to void spontaneously, the recommended frequency is 4 times a day. If the treated residual is large, fewer catheterizations may suffice.
- The best catheter type is one that has been covered with a hydrophilic lubricant and that can be moistened and lubricated by water. Additional lubrication with gel is thus not needed.
- In self-catheterization it is sufficient for the patient to wash hands well before the procedure. In hospital aseptic techniques should be used.
- Antimicrobial medication is not recommended, even if it would prevent the development of bacteriuria in cases of single catheterization or in patients using an indwelling catheter temporarily. Only symptomatic infections are treated. Routine urine specimens are not collected as most patients undergoing repeated catheterization have bacteriuria that has no clinical significance.

Long-term catheterization

- A silicone catheter (size 12–14) is preferable. A PVC catheter (with a larger internal diameter) is most practical if the urine is bloody and flushing of the bladder is necessary.
- In long-term catheterization the balloon should be filled with 5% saline or glycerol solution.
- The catheter must not be pulled downwards by gravity (use a thigh bag).
- Prophylactic antibiotics are not indicated for a patient with an indwelling catheter. Symptomatic UTIs should be treated. Before starting medication take a sample by puncturing the catheter aseptically.

11.32 Suprapubic cystostomy

Teuvo Tammela

Inserting the catheter

1. Check that the procedure is indicated.
2. The bladder should be filled with at least 300 ml of urine (urinary retention or a minimum of 4 hours since last voiding). If ultrasonography is easily available, determining the location and volume of the bladder before the procedure is always recommended (42.4). Use ultrasonography also to ensure that there is no bowel between the bladder and abdominal wall.
3. Clean the skin with, e.g., 0.01% chlorhexidine solution.
4. Infiltrate 1% lidocaine in the skin fold just above the symphysis (approximately the width of two fingers) or just proximal to it with a long thin needle (e.g. a lumbar puncture needle). Aspiration of urine confirms the location

of the bladder and its depth. Do not inject the aspirated urine into the tissues of the abdominal wall while drawing the needle back. It is important to inject the anaesthetic also to the bladder wall.

5. Make a small skin incision with a lancet, insert the cystostomy needle perpendicular to the skin into the bladder, and insert the catheter.
6. Withdraw the needle and ensure that the catheter is not withdrawn. Remove the needle.
7. Fix the catheter either by inflating the balloon or by sutures.
8. The patient can try to void with the catheter in place (after it has been closed). If voiding is repeatedly successful and the residual volume is less than 200 ml, a catheter inserted because of urinary retention can be removed.

11.40 Impotence

Outi Hovatta

Basic rules

- Impotence is often of organic origin. However, problems in self confidence and couple relationship are always associated with it. They have to be taken into account when treating these men.
- Primary impotence of a young man has to be examined by a specialist. A general practitioner can well treat older men with impotence that has developed gradually.

Aetiology

- Vascular factors (about 20%)
  - Atherosclerosis, heavy smoking, venous leakage
- Endocrine causes (about 10%)
  - Testosterone deficiency
    - Elderly men often have testosterone deficiency that can be treated using testosterone or dihydrotestosterone. This is often related to overweight, which induces high sex hormone-binding globulin and low free testosterone levels.
    - Small testes and infertility are associated with Klinefelter's syndrome.
  - Hyperprolactinaemia, disorders in thyroid function
- Neurological causes (about 20%)
  - Diabetic neuropathy, alcohol neuropathy, autonomic neuropathy, multiple sclerosis, spinal cord injury, pelvic traumas, operations in the pelvic area etc.
- Alcohol over-use (about 20%)
  - Erections improve in 50% after abstaining from alcohol
- Drugs (10%)
  - Among pharmaceutical agents used for arterial hypertension, calcium channel blockers and ACE inhibitors are less harmful than the others, but they may also have effects. Untreated hypertension, on the other hand, is also associated with erectile dysfunction.
  - Digoxin, thiazide diuretics, spironolactone
  - Anticholinergic substances
  - Many psychopharmaceutical agents; benzodiazepines, sulpiride
  - Opioids
  - Antiandrogenic drugs; cimetidine, ranitidine, cyproterone acetate
- Severe systemic diseases
- Psychological causes (about 20%)

Investigations in erectile dysfunction

History

- Did the symptoms begin suddenly, or little by little?
- How severe is the symptom? Does it occur continuously? Is erection sufficient for penetration in one out of five attempts, or less or more frequently?
- Are there morning erections (circulation probably sufficient)?
- Factors connected to certain situations, difficulties in couple relationship
- Drugs, alcohol consumption, smoking
- If erectile dysfunction began gradually and progressed slowly, the cause is often organic.
- If erectile dysfunction is connected with a certain partner, if there are morning erections, and masturbation is successful, the cause is probably psychological.

Clinical signs

- Blood pressure, peripheral arterial pulses
- Thyroid
- Tendon reflexes
- Prostate
- Signs of hypogonadism; size and consistency of the testes, pubic and axillary hair, growth of the beard, gynaecomastia etc.

Laboratory tests

- Specialist investigations on erection are seldom needed.
  - Devices for these investigations are expensive
  - One method is to place a band around the penis for the night; the band breaks during erection.
- Prostaglandin injection test; see later
- Blood tests are chosen according to the situation; haemoglobin, sedimentation rate, C-reactive protein, blood glucose, liver function tests, serum total cholesterol, HDL-cholesterol, triglycerides, thyroid-stimulating hormone, creatinine, testosterone, prolactin, prostate-specific antigen.

Investigation strategy in general practice

1. Possible underlying diseases are diagnosed and treated. Medication is checked, and changed when suspected of influencing erectile dysfunction. Diabetes and hypertension are treated to as a good balance as possible. A recommendation is given to stop smoking and alcohol consumption for at least a test period. A new appointment is given, for 2–3 months later.
2. If dysfunction has not improved (or when the patient would like to try the medication immediately, without the follow-up period) the following tests are carried out:
   - Serum testosterone (in all cases. Note that a man with diabetes can also have hypogonadism)
   - Serum prolactin, especially if sexual desire is also low
   - Other above-mentioned blood tests according to suspected aetiology.
3. Young men (below 40–50 years of age) without any systemic diseases are sent to a urologist after the first investigations (the cause may be operatively treatable, as in venous leakage). A general practitioner may treat older men.

Treatment of impotence

- If a man with erectile dysfunction has low serum testosterone, a normal prostate, normal serum levels of prostate-specific antigen and serum lipids, **testosterone** treatment can be started. It has been shown to be effective in erectile dysfunction caused by hypogonadism in a placebo-controlled study .
  - Testosterone enantate (Primoteston depot®) or a combination of testosterone esters (Sustanon "250"®), 1 amp. i.m. every 3rd week
  - Testosterone undecanoate (Panteston®), 40 mg × 3–5, taken together with a meal
  - Testosterone transdermal patch (Atmos®), 2 patches per day
  - Follow-up
    - The size of the prostate (ultrasound scan) and assay of serum prostate-specific antigen once a year
    - If erectile dysfunction has not improved within a few weeks, therapy is stopped, and other causes and treatments are sought.
- **Sildenafil** (Viagra®) is efficient for impotence of various aetiologies.
  - The initial dose is 50 mg, and it is taken 1 hour before intercourse (A) [1 2 3 4 5 6 7]. In the elderly and in severe renal insufficiency or hepatic insufficiency the initial dose is 25 mg. Exceeding a dose of 100 mg brings no further benefit.
  - Maximum frequency is one dose daily.
  - Sexual stimulation is necessary.
  - The hypotensive effect of nitrates is potentiated by sildenafil. **Its use is contraindicated in patients on nitrates.**
  - Other contraindications include severe cardiovascular disease, severe hepatic insufficiency, very low blood pressure, recent cerebral infarction or myocardial infarction or hereditary degenerative retinal disease.
  - The most common adverse effects include headache, flushing, dyspepsia, nasal stuffiness and transient visual disturbances.
  - The drug is not intended for women.
- **Vardenafil** (Levitra®) has a similar effect as sildenafil.
  - The drug is taken 25–60 minutes before intercourse.
  - The average dose is 10 mg, and the maximum dose is 20 mg. In the elderly and in patients with liver or kidney insufficiency the dose is 5 mg.
- **Tadalafil** (Cialis®) has a similar effect as sildenafil, but a longer duration of action.
  - The tablet can be taken 0.5–12 hours before intercourse.
  - If 10 mg is not enough, the dose can be raised to 20 mg. With liver or kidney insufficiency the maximum dose is 10 mg.
- **Apomorphine** (Uprima®) acts centrally and is effective in impotence of various aetiologies.
  - One tablet is taken 20 minutes before planned sexual activity.
  - The recommended starting dose is 2 mg. The dose can be raised to 3 mg for obtaining the desired clinical effect.
  - The minimum interval before the next dose is 8 hours.
- **Intracavernous prostaglandin injections** are the choice if the serum testosterone concentration is normal, and sildenafil has proved not to be effective (C) [8 9]. Several drugs and combinations of drugs have been studied, and **alprostadil** (Caverject®) has been shown to be effective in impotence due to many causes .
  - A test is first carried out in the clinic to see if the injection is effective, and to find the appropriate dose. If the injection proves effective the technique is taught to the patient and maybe his partner. A written patient's guide including the injection technique and what to do if a prolonged erection (4–6 hours) occurs, is given.
  - Injection technique:
    - The starting dose in young men with neurogenic impotence is 0.25 ml (5 µg), in older men 0.5–1.0 ml (10–20 µg). If necessary, the dose can be increased to 2 ml (40 µg).
    - The solution is injected into the penile erectile tissue (the proximal third). The needle is directed from above, somewhat laterally. The urethra can hence be avoided.
    - An injection pen can be used if the use of an ordinary needle is difficult.
  - Side effects
    - Pain in the penis, in every second man, seldom severe
    - Prolonged erection (4–6 hours) in 5%
    - Prolonged erection over 6 h (requiring treatment) in 1%
  - Treatment of prolonged erection

- Physical activity, for example, walking up and down stairs
- Cool showers
- Blood (100–200 ml) can be aspirated from the penis by using a needle and syringe
- An alpha-adrenergic drug (such as Effortil®, 0.5 mg, or noradrenaline, 0.02–0.04 mg) can be injected into the erectile tissue, repeatedly if necessary. Referral to a hospital urology unit if there are any difficulties in treatment.

- **Yohimbine** is a peroral drug with controversial treatment results. In a meta-analysis (A) [10 11 12] it was more effective than placebo in a group of patients, but in a recent placebo-controlled randomized study, no effect could be seen.
- **Intraurethral alprostadil** (Muse®) (B) [13 14 15]. The alprostadil gel is injected into the urethra using an applicator, and the penis is massaged gently for about 10 min. Intraurethral alprostadil is a good option in psychogenic, neurogenic or mild vascular impotence.
- A **vacuum pump** is an option for men who do not want to use drugs (C) [8 9]. An erection of some kind can be obtained in up to 90% of users. Being mechanical devices, they are not easily accepted by all men. Side effects are numbness and pain in the penis, sometimes bruises (contraindicated in men with problems of bleeding or anticoagulant treatment). There is little literature regarding the treatment results .
- **Vascular surgery** has been used for selected groups of patients. It has proved effective in young men with traumatic vascular lesions. In men with general atherosclerosis the benefit is only temporary . The results from venous surgery are still controversial .
- **Penile prostheses** are used by urologists as the last option, when all other treatments have been ineffective (C) [8 9].

References

1. Langtry HD, Markham A. Sildenafil: a review of its use in erectile dysfunction. Drugs 1999;57:967–989.
2. The Database of Abstracts of Reviews of Effectiveness (University of York), Database no.: DARE-991320. In: The Cochrane Library, Issue 1, 2001. Oxford: Update Software.
3. Burts A, Clark W, Gold L, Simpson S. Sildenafil: an oral drug for the treatment of male erectile dysfunction. Birmingham: University of Birmingham, Department of Public Health and Epidemiology. 12. 1998. 1–94.
4. The Database of Abstracts of Reviews of Effectiveness (University of York), Database no.: DARE-999267. In: The Cochrane Library, Issue 2, 2001. Oxford: Update Software.
5. Goldstein I, Lue TF, Padma-Nathan H, Rosen RC, Steers WD, Wicker PA. Oral sildenafil in the treatment of erectile dysfunction. N Engl J Med 1998;338:1393–404.
6. Morales A, Gingell C, Collins M, Wicker PA, Osterloh IH. Clinical safety of oral sildenafil citrate (ViagraTM) in the treatment of erectile dysfunction. Int J Impot Res 1998;10:69–74.
7. Mitka M. Viagra leads as rivals are moving up. JAMA 1998;280:119–220.
8. Montague DK, Barada JH, Belker AM, Levine LA, Nadig PW, Roehrborn CG, Sharlip ID, Bennett AH. Treatment of erectile impotence with drugs and prostheses (sildenafil not included). J Urol 1996;156:2007–2011.
9. The Database of Abstracts of Reviews of Effectiveness (University of York), Database no.: DARE-961894. In: The Cochrane Library, Issue 4, 1999. Oxford: Update Software.
10. Ernst E, Pittler MH. Yohimbine for erectile dysfunction: a systematic review and meta-analysis of randomized clinical trials. Journal of Urology 1998;159:433–436.
11. The Database of Abstracts of Reviews of Effectiveness (University of York), Database no.: DARE-980212. In: The Cochrane Library, Issue 4, 2000. Oxford: Update Software.
12. Carey MP, Johnson BT. Effectiveness of yohimbine in the treatment of erectile disorder: four meta-analytic integrations. Arch Sex Behav 1996;25:341–60.
13. Hellstrom WJ et al. A double-blind, placebo-controlled evaluation of the erectile response to transurethral alprostadil. Urology 1996;48:851–6.
14. Spivac AP et al. Long-term safety profile of transurethral alprostadil for the treatment of erectile dysfunction. J Urol 1997;157:792.
15. Padma-Nathan H et al. Treatment of men with erectile dysfunction with transurethral alprostadil. N Engl J Med 1997;336:1–7.

URO

11.41 Urinary calculi

Pekka Hellström

Basic rules

- An acute attack is treated with intravenous NSAIDs at the first place of treatment.
- The diagnosis is confirmed with urography, or increasingly with spiral CT; the vitality of the kidneys is verified by follow-up.
- The stone is removed and analysed.
- Laboratory investigations to find out the aetiology of urinary calculi are always indicated to prevent recurrences.

Types of stones and their aetiology

Calcium stones

- 75–85% of all urinary calculi
- Occur mostly in men above 20 years of age
- A hereditary predisposition is often evident
- Aetiology
  - Idiopathic hypercalciuria 25–30%
  - Hypocitraturia 20–25%
  - Hyperuricosuria 10%
  - Primary hyperparathyroidism 5%
  - Hyperoxaluria (diet, after bowel resection) 15–30%

Urate stones

- 5–8% of all urinary calculi
- More common in men
- Aetiology
  - Gout in 50%
  - Hereditary in 50% (often triggered by dehydration), urine pH <5.5 may rouse suspicion.

Stones associated with urinary tract infection

- Often composed of magnesium ammonium phosphate
- 10–15% of all urinary calculi
- More common in women
  - Formed as a result of urinary tract infection (Proteus, staphylococci, E. coli).

Cystine stones

- An inherited metabolic defect
- About 1% of all urinary calculi

Symptoms and signs

- Intense, colicky pain radiates from the costal arch obliquely to the lower abdomen, groins, and testes.
- Nausea and vomiting is common.
- Microscopic, or rarely macroscopic, haematuria in 90%
- Earlier episodes are often recognized from the history, and there are cases in the family. Tendency for recurrences is 50% in 10 years.
- Tenderness of the kidneys on percussion is often observed.
- The patient has difficulty in keeping still (in contrast to, e.g. perforated peptic ulcer, where the patient prefers to lie still).
- 90% of the stones are radio-opaque (urate stones are invisible, and cystine stones may be poorly visible).

Differential diagnosis

- Colon-related pain
- Appendicitis
- Attack of biliary cholic, dyspepsia
- Aortic aneurysm
- Gynaecological conditions
- Renal infarction

First aid for an attack

- Intravenous (B) [1 2] prostaglandin inhibitor (A) [3 4] (rapid relief) or i.m. (slower onset of action), e.g.
  - diclofenac 75 mg i.m. or a slow i.v. infusion (>30 min), or
  - ketoprofen 50–100 mg i.m. or 100–200 mg as a slow i.v. infusion (>30 min)
  - indomethacin 50 mg i.v. slowly (>5 min)

Investigation strategy

- See Figure 11.41.1
- Spiral CT is used increasingly in specialist hospitals as an on-call investigation.
- If the stone can be analysed at the beginning, the investigations can be directed according to the suspected aetiology.
- After the first attack the following tests are indicated: serum calcium, urate, creatinine, and urine bacterial culture.
- If repeated attacks occur at intervals less than 2 years the following tests should also be performed: 24-hour urine creatinine, calcium (24.21), and citrate. Routine investigation of oxalate, urate (21.50) and magnesium is not recommended.

Treatment

- The patient should be treated in a facility where urography is available (42.2).
  - If the diameter of the stone is under 5 mm, the patient does not have hydronephrosis, and serum creatinine is normal, only follow-up is needed.

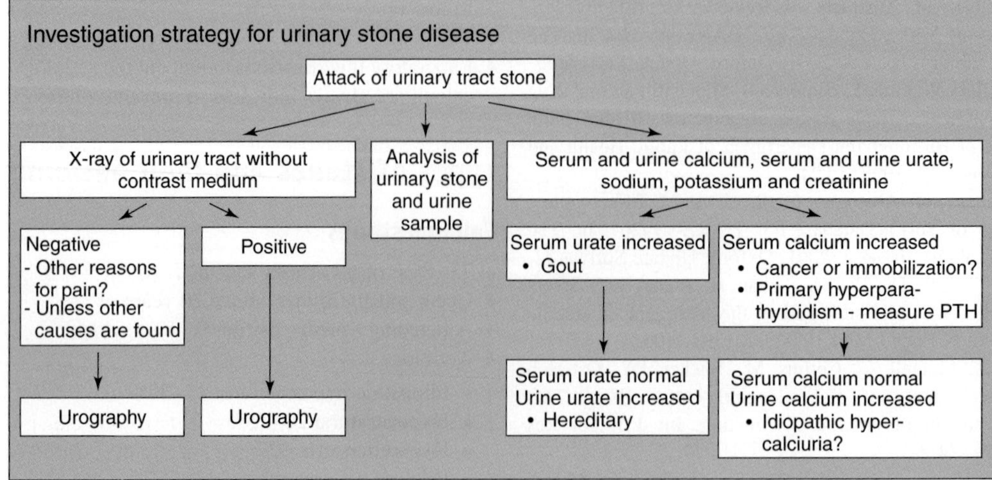

Figure 11.41.1

- A urologist should be consulted if the above-mentioned investigations are not locally available, the diameter of the stone exceeds 5 mm, or the patient has a urinary tract infection, has only one kidney, is pregnant, or has a recurrence.

Conservative treatment

- All patients are advised to drink 6–8 glasses of water every day.
- If the patient has hypercalcaemia (and hypercalciuria) its aetiology should be determined. For investigations see article 24.21.
- The precipitation of oxalate should be prevented by diet. The patient should:
  - Drink plenty of water
  - Avoid oxalate-containing foods such as dried fruit, gooseberry, nettle, asparagus, parsley, beans, spinach, nuts, rhubarb, chocolate, cocoa, and tea.
- Idiopathic hypercalciuria has been treated with a diet low in calcium, but a diet with restricted intake of animal protein and salt, but normal intake of calcium, may be more effective (C) [5]. If necessary, with a thiazide diuretic 50 mg × 1 and potassium supplementation (remember the possibility of gout). 24-hour urine calcium should be determined 3 and 6 months after onset of treatment.
- If serum urate is increased, a specific diagnosis of gout should be aimed for (clinical picture, analysis of synovial fluid in patients with joint symptoms (21.11)). The condition is treated with fluids, diet (21.51), and allopurinol.
- If the patient has only an elevated serum urate (but no symptomatic gout) the stones may be composed of either calcium or urate. The treatment of choice is
  - diet, or
  - alkalinization of urine (if diet fails), or
  - allopurinol in severe cases.
- If an infection is detected in the urine test, it should be treated according to the antibiogram. Follow-up urine tests are always indicated, as is (usually) prophylactic medication (10.10).

Control examinations

- If a stone suitable for conservative treatment has been detected the passage of the stone is ascertained with plain radiographs or renography after 1 (–3) months. If the stone persists, the follow-up is continued (plain x-rays, ultrasonography to rule out hydronephrosis, serum creatinine) until the stone has been passed and the patient is asymptomatic. If the stone has not been passed by 6 months it should be removed surgically.

Indications for shock-wave lithoripsy and endoscopic stone removal

- The diameter of the stone exceeds 4–5 mm.
- A smaller stone is not passed spontaneously and causes recurrent pain. The passing of a small asymptomatic stone can be followed up for 6 months if hydronephrosis does not develop.

References

1. Tramer MR, Williams JE, Carroll D, Wiffen PJ, Moore RA, McQuay HJ. Comparing analgesic efficacy of non-steroidal anti-inflammatory drugs given by different routes in acute and chronic pain: a qualitative systematic review. Acta Anaesth Scand 1998;42:71–79.
2. The Database of Abstracts of Reviews of Effectiveness (University of York), Database no.: DARE-980293. In: The Cochrane Library, Issue 2, 2000. Oxford: Update Software.
3. Labrecque M, Dostaler LP, Rouselle R, Nguyen T, Poirier S. Efficacy of nonsteroidal anti-inflammatory drugs in the treatment of acute renal colic: a meta-analysis. Arch Intern Med 1994;154:1381–1387.
4. The Database of Abstracts of Reviews of Effectiveness (University of York), Database no.: DARE-948041. In: The Cochrane Library, Issue 4, 1999. Oxford: Update Software.
5. Borghi L, Schianchi T, Meschi Tiziana, Guerra A, Allegri F, Maggiore U, Novarini A. Comparison of two diets for the prevention of recurrent stones in idiopathic hypercalciuria. N Engl J Med 2002;346:77–84.

11.43 Cancers of the urinary system and testes

Olavi Lukkarinen

- For cancer of the prostate see article 11.13.

Renal carcinoma (hypernephroma)

Epidemiology

- The incidence is about 1/10 000/year.
- Smoking and overweight are the only known risk factors.
- Patients with hereditary von Hippel–Lindau disease carry a high risk of renal carcinoma (up to 30%).

Symptoms and signs

- The symptoms include haematuria (37%) (C) [1 2], pain, weight loss, fever, fatigue, hypersedimentation, anaemia (but 3–5% of the patients have erythrocytosis because of erythropoietin secretion), rapidly developing varicocele, and a palpable mass.
- Ultrasonography is the most important diagnostic examination, complemented by guided biopsy if necessary. Small tumours are not visible in urography. Computed tomography is useful in assessing the extent of the disease.

- Renal carcinoma often infiltrates the surroundings. Metastases occur in lymph nodes, the skeleton, lungs, and subcutaneously.

Treatment

- Extrafascial nephrectomy is the routine treatment for localized disease. A more radical operation, adjuvant irradiation or antineoplastic drugs are of no proven benefit. Even a carcinoma that has infiltrated the inferior vena cava should be operated on. Solitary metastases (e.g. in the lungs) can be removed surgically.
- Treatments for metastases include surgery, irradiation (bone pain, symptomatic metastases), antineoplastic drugs (vinblastine), immunomodulators (IFN A [3], IL-2), and follow-up. Response to treatment is modest.

Follow-up

- Follow-up is aimed at detection of solitary, treatable metastases.
- Follow-up examinations are usually carried out at the treatment unit at 3–6 months intervals until 2 years have elapsed.
- If no relapse is detected, further follow-up can be carried out in primary care at intervals of 6 months to 1 year for up to 5 years.
- The follow-up examinations include ESR, blood count, ALT, alkaline phosphatase, serum creatinine, urine test. A chest x-ray should be taken yearly. CT scan, bone scan etc. are performed if necessary.

Bladder cancer

Epidemiology

- The incidence is about 1.5/10 000/year.
- Smoking and certain chemicals are risk factors.
- More than 90% of the cancers originate from transitional type epithelium.

Symptoms and signs

- The symptoms include haematuria in 85%, and bladder irritation in 30% of the cases.
  - More than 5 erythrocytes per microscopic field in the urine sediment indicate cytological examination of the urine, cystoscopy, and renal ultrasonography. For haematuria see 11.5.
- The spread of bladder cancer depends on the stage of differentiation and the depth of invasion. The most common sites of metastases are pelvic lymph nodes, lungs, and bones.

Treatment

- The treatment options include electroresection and coagulation, bladder resection, bladder removal, irradiation, and intravesical treatments (epirubicin, mitomycin C or BCG A [4] [5] [6] 5–6 times at one-week intervals, then once a month for one year).
- The selection of treatment is determined by the grade, TNM classification B [7] [8], and age. In the case of metastases antineoplastic drugs can be tried (about 30% of the patients respond).
- On average 70% of the tumours recur but local recurrences can usually be treated effectively. After 5 years the risk of recurrence declines to under 5%.

Follow-up

- Follow-up should be carried out in a urology unit and consists of cystoscopy, urine cytology, and if necessary, imaging.
- Cystoscopy is performed at 3-month intervals for the first year, at 6-month intervals for the next two years, and yearly after that.
- If the tumour has not recurred within 5 years, further follow-up with urine tests, including cytology, performed in primary care, may suffice.

Cancer of the testis

Epidemiology

- The incidence is about 10/million/year.
- Seminomas are the most common type in men aged 30–35 years, whereas non-seminomas are the most common type in men aged 25–29 years.
- There are many histological types of tumour. About 90% are germ cell tumours, and of these about 50% are seminomas, and 50% other tumours (e.g. embryonal carcinomas, teratomas, teratocarcinomas, placental tumours).

Symptoms and signs

- The symptoms include enlargement of the testis (which should always be investigated), a lump, a change in consistency, vague pain, and prolonged epididymitis.
- Ultrasonography usually reveals an enlarged, non-homogeneous tumour within the testis.
- Computed tomography is used to detect possible retroperitoneal lymph node metastases.

Treatment

- The treatment always begins with an operation, followed by irradiation for seminomas.
- Antineoplastic drugs are used if the tumour has metastasized widely. Over 90% of patients even with widespread tumours, are cured.
- 60–70% of metastasized non-seminomas can be cured with antineoplastic drugs.
- Fertility is preserved in about 65% of irradiated patients. Semen can be frozen before treatment.

Follow-up

- Follow-up should be carried out in a specialized unit.
- Patients with seminomas treated by surgery only are controlled for 5 years at 4-month intervals, and patients with seminomas treated with antineoplastic drugs are controlled

for 3 years at 3-month intervals, and thereafter at 6-month intervals up to 5 years.
- Patients with non-seminomas are controlled once a month for the first year, at 3-month intervals for the next year, and at 6-month intervals thereafter for a total of 5 years.
- Follow-up consists of assay of biochemical markers (AFP, HCG, if the concentrations were increased before the operation), a chest x-ray at 2–3-month intervals, and computed tomography at 2–6-month intervals.
- Further follow-up with longer intervals should be continued for a long time, as the tumour may recur even more than 10 years after the primary operation. Recurrent tumours usually respond favourably to treatment.

References

1. Buntinx F, Wauters H. The diagnostic value of macroscopic haematuria diagnosing urological cancers: a meta-analysis. Family Practice 1997;14:63–68.
2. The Database of Abstracts of Reviews of Effectiveness (University of York), Database no.: DARE-970347. In: The Cochrane Library, Issue 4, 1999. Oxford: Update Software.
3. Coppin C, Porzsolt F, Kumpf J, Coldman A, Wilt T. Immunotherapy for advanced renal cell cancer. Cochrane Database Syst Rev. 2004;(2):CD001425.
4. Shelley MD, Court JB, Kynaston H, Wilt TJ, Fish RG, Mason M. Intravesical Bacillus Calmette-Guerin in Ta and T1 Bladder Cancer. Cochrane Database Syst Rev. 2004;(2):CD001986.
5. Huncharek M, Geschwind JF, Witherspoon B, McGarry R, Adcock D. Intravesical chemotherapy prophylaxis in primary superficial bladder cancer: a meta-analysis of 3703 patients from 11 randomized trials. Journal of Clinical Epidemiology 2000:53; 676–680.
6. The Database of Abstracts of Reviews of Effectiveness (University of York), Database no.: DARE-20001523. In: The Cochrane Library, Issue 1, 2002. Oxford: Update Software.
7. Pawinski A, Sylvester R, Kurth K, Bouffioux C, van der Meijden A, Parmar MK, Bijnens L. A combined analysis of European organisation for research and treatment of cancer, and medical research council randomized clinical trials for the prophylactic treatment of stage TaT1 bladder cancer. J Urol 1996;156:1934–1941.
8. The Database of Abstracts of Reviews of Effectiveness (University of York), Database no.: DARE-973046. In: The Cochrane Library, Issue 4, 1999. Oxford: Update Software.

11.45 Hypogonadism in the aging male

Sakari Rannikko

Introduction

- Hormone replacement therapy is effective in lessening the symptoms of hypogonadism in the aging male.
- Treatment warrants a careful consideration of benefits and possible risks as well as close monitoring.
- So far, the significance and safety of hormone replacement therapy in the activation of latent prostate cancer or its precursor (PIN, prostatic intraepithelial neoplasia) is not known.
- Medicalization of the normal aging process may also be considered a concern.

URO

Hormone activity in the aging male

- Some aging males suffer from symptoms associated with hormonal decline.
- Symptoms of ADAM (androgen decline in the ageing male):
  - deterioration of physical, emotional and sexual functions.
- As the population becomes older, the number of aging males will also increase; in 2010, 14% of men will be over 65 years of age.

Signs and symptoms of ADAM

- Symptoms resemble those seen during the female climacteric (hot flushes, sweating, depression, tiredness, sleep disturbances).
- Several symptoms are attributable to dysfunction of organs targeted by testosterone (erectile dysfunction, reduced muscular strength).
- Slowing down of physiological responses.
- Many of the symptoms are not only connected with the reduced amounts of testosterone but other factors also play a part:
  - loss of muscle tissue (growth hormone?)
  - osteopenia (oestrogens?)
  - truncal obesity (leptin?)
  - atherosclerosis (oestrogens?)
  - decreased libido (oestrogens?)
  - erectile dysfunction
  - impaired memory and learning
  - emotional fatigue
  - sleep disturbances (melatonin?)

Investigations

- When replacement therapy is considered the risk of prostate cancer must be evaluated:
  - symptoms, family history, palpation of the prostate
  - PSA, serum testosterone, LH, haematocrit (increased risk of thrombosis if above 52%), lipids
  - Other causes of hypogonadism, see (24.61).

Replacement therapy

- Before deciding to instigate treatment, the benefits and possible risks should be carefully considered.
- Before treatment is instigated, both the physician and the patient must be fully aware of the associated risks.

- The patient must commit himself to long-term monitoring, which may last for several years.
- Hormone replacement therapy may be prescribed, if
  - the patient presents with typical signs and symptoms of ADAM and
  - serum testosterone level is low (mean−2 SD)
    - Testosterone < 11 nmol/l
    - Free testosterone < 0.255 nmol/l.

Treatment choices

- Transdermal preparations are the best treatment choice for maintaining the normal circadian pattern of testosterone concentrations, and are therefore recommended.
- Testosterone patches
- Testosterone gel
- Testosterone capsule
  - Testosterone undecanoate is absorbed via the lymph pathways and therefore exerts no extra strain on the liver
- Testosterone injection–testosterone propionate - isocaproate -undecanoate

Contraindications

- Absolute:
  - Suspicion of prostate cancer
  - Benign prostatic hyperplasia with severe symptoms
  - Suspicion of malignant breast tumour
  - High haematocrit (>52%)
- Relative:
  - Severe sleep apnea
  - Hepatic dysfunction
  - High blood lipid values and coronary heart disease.

Follow-up

- The first follow-up visit should be at 3 months. The intervals between subsequent visits can gradually be lengthened. The visits should, however, be at least annual.
- Monitor the development of symptoms (ADAM and micturition), palpate the prostate.
- Measure PSA. Suspect prostate cancer
  - if increased >1.5 ug / l or
  - the rate of increase >0.75 μg / l / year
- Blood count (haematocrit >52%)
- Testosterone levels will normalize during replacement therapy and there is, therefore, no need to measure the levels during treatment.

Sexually Transmitted Diseases

Evidence Based Medicine Guidelines. Edited by the Duodecim Editorial Team
 ISBN: 0-470-01184-X

12.1 Chlamydial urethritis and cervicitis

Timo Reunala

Aims

- To diagnose the disease and treat the patient in time to avoid the serious complications of prolonged or recurrent infection (pelvic inflammatory disease, infertility, ectopic pregnancy)
- To examine and treat the person who is the source of the infection and any other persons who might have been subsequently infected, in order to prevent the spread of the chlamydial infection

Epidemiology

- Young adults with many sexual contacts are especially at risk, and the use of oral contraceptives increases the likelihood of contracting the disease.
- Asymptomatic infections promote the spread of the disease. The time from infection to diagnosis is on average four weeks but may be up to many months.
- By the time of diagnosis, a quarter of patients have already had a new sexual relationship, which presents a challenge for tracing the infection.
- On the basis of extensive material, men are most commonly (60%) infected by a temporary sexual partner and women by a permanent partner. Prostitutes and foreigners do not constitute a significant source of infection in most countries.

Early symptoms

- The "incubation period" from chlamydial infection to the emergence of symptoms is one to three weeks, i.e. longer than in gonorrhoea. About a quarter of men and most women experience no particular early symptoms from chlamydial infection, and many of them become asymptomatic carriers of chlamydial disease.
- In men, urethritis is marked by scant, watery (later mucous) discharge from the urethra. Other symptoms include an aching pain and dysuria. In women, there is dysuria, pollakisuria and mild leucorrhoea. Cervicitis is a relatively common finding. It is manifested as mucopurulent discharge and oedema or bleeding tendency of the orifice of the uterus.

Late symptoms and complications

- In women, prolonged chlamydial infection often results in **endometritis** and **salpingitis**. These conditions are not always associated with severe symptoms; the patient may have just slight fever or mild lower abdominal pain. Endometritis may also cause irregular uterine bleeding. **Pelvic inflammatory disease (PID)** is an important late complication of chlamydial infection; it generally requires inpatient treatment. Perihepatitis is a rare complication of chlamydial infection.
- Late complications of extensive and, especially, recurrent chlamydial infection also include tubal damage which in turn causes **infertility** and **ectopic pregnancies**.
- In men, chlamydial infection is an important cause of **epididymitis**, whereas the etiological significance of chlamydia in prostatitis is considered small.
- Chlamydial infection can trigger the development of **reactive arthritis** (uroarthritis, Reiter's disease) in both men and women.

Diagnostics

- **Clinical symptoms and signs**. Chlamydial infection can be suspected but never diagnosed on the basis of symptoms alone. A burning sensation and mucous discharge from the urethra are common symptoms in men after unprotected sexual intercourse with a temporary partner. Although Gram or methylene blue stains of plain smear specimens are usually rich in white blood cells, chlamydia is found to be the cause of the infection in only half the patients. A reliable diagnosis of chlamydial infection in both men and women can therefore be reached only by appropriate microbiological sampling.
- **Laboratory diagnostics** has undergone a profound change in recent years. Conventional chlamydial culture has been relegated to a minor role, and immunological staining methods of poor sensitivity have been abandoned. New gene amplification methods have replaced previous techniques, and first-void urine samples have acquired an established position in chlamydial diagnostics in both men and women.
- **Gene amplification methods**, such as polymerase chain reaction (PCR) and ligase chain reaction (LCR), are based on multiplication of chlamydial nucleic acids with specific probes. The main assets of the methods are their high sensitivity and the fact that they, unlike culture methods, yield a positive result also when there are no living chlamydia in the sample. Compared with traditional culture methods, gene amplification methods reveal 5–7% more cases of chlamydial infection, and false positives are practically nonexistent. The price of these tests has come down to an acceptable level. Today chlamydia and gonorrhoea can be analysed on the same sample if required.
- **First void urine samples** are used for chlamydial diagnostics in both men and women. Samples are taken when at least five to seven days have passed since the potential time of acquirement of infection. The patient has to refrain from voiding for 2 h before urine sampling. The sample (10 ml) is sent to a laboratory in the normal way. If needed, the sample may be kept refrigerated for one or two days.

- As an alternative to first-void urine, women may give urethral and cervical swab samples that are then analysed by the same gene amplification methods. Even samples from the cornea of the eye can be examined by gene amplification techniques.
- Gene amplification is a rapid method, with results being available within as little as 24 h. In practice, large laboratories analyse samples two or three times a week.
- First-void urine samples are well suited for home screening of risk groups or sexual partners.
- **Chlamydial culture** has been rendered secondary in importance for several reasons. It has a sensitivity of 80% but a specificity of close to 100% . The sample for chlamydial culture is obtained with a special swab from the urethra or cervix. It should be transported to the laboratory without delay, and the result becomes available after two or three days. In chronic infections, the test is often negative because of low numbers of bacteria. Unlike gonorrhoea, chlamydial infections are not associated with resistance problems.
- **Serology**. Chlamydial serology may be useful in chronic infections. High IgG antibody titres are often present in pelvic infections and also in other complications. An isolated positive test indicates that the patient has a history of chlamydial infection.

Treatment of chlamydial infection

- Chlamydia trachomatis is sensitive to macrolides and tetracyclines. Clindamycin is also relatively effective against this species, fluoroquinolones less so. The common cephalosporins and penicillin have poor efficacy.
- **Azithromycin 1 g as a single dose** is the treatment of choice for chlamydial infection. Other alternatives are tetracycline 500 mg × 3/day or doxycycline 100 mg × 2/day for 7–10 days. Patients who are pregnant should receive erythromycin 500 mg × 4/day for seven days B [1]. Some 10% of patients get mild gastric side effects from azithromycin and tetracyclines. Azithromycin therapy has the benefit of 100% compliance; it is more expensive than the common tetracyclines, however. Controlled studies have shown similar therapeutic outcomes for these drugs, with 95–97% of patients being cured.
- Chlamydial infections of the throat, anus or eyes are treated with azithromycin for three to five days. For mild complications, patients are given tetracycline or doxycycline for two to three weeks, for reactive arthritis triggered by chlamydial infection even longer. In pelvic infections, combinations of antibiotics are used, as other bacteria, such as anaerobes, may be involved.
- The permanent sexual partner of the index patient should be tested before any treatment since the partner is not necessarily infected. The suitability of the antibiotic for the partner should also be ascertained, as well as ensuring that the female partner to be treated is not pregnant. Furthermore, the partner may have transmitted the infection to other persons; an issue that can only be clarified by having the partner visit the physician or clinic.

Post-treatment follow-up and tracing the contacts of the patient

- A follow-up visit should only take place after three to four weeks because the presence of gene traces may produce a false positive result in an earlier re-test.
- Every physician treating patients with chlamydial infections is required to trace the sexual contacts of their patients B [2]. The physician should enquire the index patient whether the person who is the source of the infection and any persons potentially infected have been tested for chlamydia and received treatment as needed. If desired, the attending physician may delegate the screening of sexual partners to a physician responsible for communicable diseases.

DER

Screening for asymptomatic infections

- It has been shown that targeted screening for chlamydial infections is effective in preventing pelvic inflammatory disease (PID) and ectopic pregnancies.
- Screening for chlamydial infection is cost-effective if the prevalence of chlamydial infection exceeds 3% in the population screened. Systematic screening for chlamydial infection has been considered relevant among family planning clinic customers and in general those young women who see their physician to renew their contraceptive pill prescription, especially if there is a history of temporary sexual partners.
- Tracing the contacts of the patient is the most effective way of combating the disease. Partner screening normally yields 20–30% positive cases. The practice of taking first-void urine samples from the partner at home has increased the number of detected infections by 50% compared with the usual practice of partner notification. Many young people are unaware that chlamydial infection is often asymptomatic, which reduces and delays testing for chlamydia.
- Recent seroepidemiological studies have indicated an association between a history of chlamydial infection and the development of cervical carcinoma. The exact causal relationship remains to be determined, however. Therefore, no seroepidemiological screening programmes have been undertaken as yet.

References

1. Brocklehurst P, Rooney G. Interventions for treating genital chlamydia trachomatis infection in pregnancy. Cochrane Database Syst Rev. 2004;(2):CD000054.
2. Mathews C, Coetzee N, Zwarenstein M, Lombard C, Guttmacher S, Oxman A, Schmid G. Strategies for partner notification for sexually transmitted diseases. Cochrane Database Syst Rev. 2004;(2):CD002843.
3. Oxman AD, Scott EA, Sellors JW, Clarke JH, Millson ME, Rasooly I, Frank JW, Naus M, Goldblatt D. Partner notification for sexually transmitted diseases: an overview of the evidence. Can J Publ Health 1994;85(suppl 1):41–47.

4. The Database of Abstracts of Reviews of Effectiveness (University of York), Database no.: DARE-945071. In: The Cochrane Library, Issue 4, 1999. Oxford: Update Software.
5. Turrentine MA, Newton ER. Amoxicillin or erythromycin for the treatment of antenatal chlamydial infection: a meta-analysis. Obst Gynecol 1995;86:1021–1025.
6. The Database of Abstracts of Reviews of Effectiveness (University of York), Database no.: DARE-960039. In: The Cochrane Library, Issue 4, 1999. Oxford: Update Software.

12.2 Gonorrhoea

Timo Reunala

Aetiology

- Caused by Neisseria gonorrhoeae (gonococcus), which is a gram-negative diplococcus.
- Transmitted almost exclusively by sexual intercourse and multiplies in the columnar epithelium of the mucous membranes.

Epidemiology

- The incidence of gonorrhoea varies considerably between countries, as does resistance to drugs.
- Pharyngeal gonorrhoea and ophthalmia neonatorum are nowadays rare in developed countries, as is concurrent chlamydial infection in a gonorrhoea patient.

Incubation time and symptoms

- Men, 2–5 days after exposure.
- Women, 1–2 weeks after exposure.
- Symptoms are commonly mild or totally absent. Distinct symptoms occur in about 60% of men and 30% of women.
- In men the symptoms are urethritis and a yellowish urethral discharge; women have vaginal discharge, pain on urinating and lower abdominal pain.

Complications

- In women the most serious complication is pelvic inflammatory disease (PID), in men gonorrhoea may sometimes cause epididymitis.
- Pustular dermatitis and arthritis are rare complications of untreated gonorrhoea.
- Proctitis and proctocolitis may be acquired in anal intercourse.

Laboratory investigations

- A smear of pus on a glass slide (methylene blue or Gram staining) containing leucocytes with intracellular diplococci is a suggestive finding.
- Culture is the basic method for diagnosis and for determining antibiotic resistance.
- The sample is obtained with a dacron swab from the urethra and cervix and, when necessary, also from the pharynx and the rectum. Store at +4°C, if storage is necessary.
- Cultured in a special medium. A negative result is obtained within a few days. A final positive result and ciprofloxacin sensitivity of the gonococcus are available 1–3 days later.
- Gonococcal nucleic acid amplification test
  - This sensitive test that is performed by special laboratories replaces culture. Its use is increasing.
  - First void urine sample or a sample taken with a swab is examined by nucleic acid amplification (A) [1 2]. The result is available on the same day.
  - The same sample can be used to test for both gonorrhoea and chlamydial infection.
  - Determination of antibiotic resistance is not possible with this method.

Treatment

- The susceptibility of Neisseria gonorrrhoeae to antibiotics varies greatly in the world. Resistance to quinolones is increasing, particularly in South-East Asia where up to 20% of strains are resistant.
- Culture is necessary when antibiotic resistance is suspected.

Uncomplicated acute infection

- Ciprofloxacin 500 mg × 1 is the basic treatment.
- For resistant strains use ceftriaxone 250 mg × 1 i.m. or spectinomycin 2 g × 1 i.m.
- During pregnancy and breastfeeding treat with spectinomycin 2 g × 1 i.m. (C) [3].

Complicated infection

- Ciprofloxacin 500 mg × 2 for 5–7 days orally

Post-treatment follow-up

- A control sample is important for verifying cure.
- A culture sample is taken one week after treatment and a sample for nucleic acid amplification test is taken three weeks after treatment.
- The outcome of treatment is controlled at least twice if the strain is resistant to ciprofloxacin, and special attention is paid on identifying partners.
- See also 12.1.

References

1. Koumans EH, Johnson RE, Knapp JS, St Louis ME. Laboratory testing for neisseria gonorrhoeae by recently introduced nonculture tests: a performance review with clinical and public health considerations. Clinical Infectious Diseases 1998;27:1171–1180.
2. The Database of Abstracts of Reviews of Effectiveness (University of York), Database no.: DARE-982037. In: The Cochrane Library, Issue 3, 2000. Oxford: Update Software.
3. Brocklehurst P. Antibiotics for gonorrhoea in pregnancy. Cochrane Database Syst Rev. 2004;(2):CD000098.

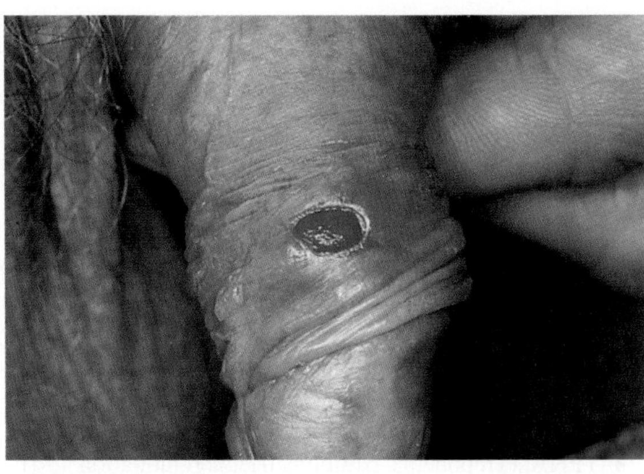

Figure 12.3.1 Lues primaria presenting as an ulcer at the site of inoculum. This foreskin ulcer was relatively painless; it has sharp borders, and it is clean, without debris. If pressed, syphilitic spirochetes can be seen in microscopy using the dark field technique. In this case serological tests for syphilis were positive, but they may be negative in other cases. In suspected cases the tests should be repeated later. The possibility of other venereal diseases should also be remembered (gonorrhoea, chlamydia, HIV). Photo © R. Suhonen.

12.3 Syphilis

Timo Reunala

Aims

- Suspected syphilis should be verified with the appropriate clinical and serological tests and the patient should be treated with the most efficient antibiotics.
- Syphilis is a dangerous infectious disease that should be prevented and treated effectively.

Aetiology and transmission

- The pathogen is the spirochete Treponema pallidum.
- Easily transmitted by sexual intercourse and also from the mother to the foetus
- Contagiousness is highest (30–60%) in the primary and secondary phases. After 2 years, the patient ceases to spread the disease.

Clinical picture

- Asymptomatic incubation period lasts for 3–4 weeks after which two thirds of the patients (not all!) have visible symptoms.
  - Primary symptoms (local infection)
    - An ulcer, the "primary lesion", with a clean, hard base (Figure 12.3.1) appears in the genital region, sometimes also in anus or the oral region.
    - There is local lymphadenopathy without tenderness.
  - Secondary stage 6–8 weeks after exposure (general infection).
    - General symptoms include indisposition, fever and enlarged lymph nodes.
    - Roseola eczema resembles widely spread viral eczema or drug eruption.
      - * Syphilids, i.e. formations of papules are found in the hands and feet or spread all over the body. May be large, cauliflower-like formations (condylomata latum) around the anus or necrotic in patients with a poor immune response (e.g. HIV).
    - Alopecia syphilitica, typical "moth-eaten" spotty baldness in some patients.
  - Late symptoms occur in about one third of untreated patients in 10–30 years. The most important are neurological (atypical psychosis, paralytic dementia) and vascular symptoms (aortic aneurysm, valvular regurgitation).

Differential diagnosis

- Primary syphilis
  - Genital herpes. Incubation time is short in primary infection, lesions occur in groups and they are painful. Lymphadenopathy is less pronounced, however, the nodes are tender.
  - Ulcus molle (soft chancre)
  - Infected coital or other traumas.
    - Secondary syphilis
  - Roseola may resemble pityriasis rosea, drug eruption, measles (rubeola), German measles (rubella) or scarlet fever (scarlatina).
  - Syphilids may resemble papular lichen ruber planus, psoriasis, scabies or infectious eczema of the feet (e.g. tinea). Condyloma latum may resemble condyloma acuminata.

Diagnosis

1. History of exposure (unprotected sex) and/or clinical picture.
2. Plain specimen. A dark field microscope may reveal spirochetes in lesion discharge and confirm the diagnosis.
3. Serology
   - The cardiolipin test becomes positive 3–4 weeks after infection. It is the primary test for screening. High titres (>16) are almost always specific. A low titre is in many cases a false positive result (pregnancy, connective tissue disease, infection) or a serological scar of an earlier treated infection or latent syphilis.
   - TPHA (Treponema pallidum haemagglutination test) is the test of choice for verifying syphilis. The result becomes positive slightly later than that of the cardiolipin test, but it is specific (almost 100%) and suitable for following up response to treatment.
   - FTA-abs (fluorescence test) is a specific syphilis test used in special cases (neurosyphilis, suspicion of neonatal syphilis) as it detects also IgM antibodies.
   - Gene amplification methods are already being used for screening.

Treatment

- Procaine penicillin 1.2 million IU × 1 i.m. for 10 days (primary and secondary syfilis, in latent syphilis treatment is received for three weeks), in neurosyphilis i.v. penicillin.
- For patients allergic to penicillin the alternatives are doxicycline (200mg/day for 15 days) or ceftriaxone injection (1 g/day).

Follow-up and identification of partners

- After antibiotic therapy the cardiolipin and TPHA tests are performed at 3 and 6 months and one year. In primary stage infection the tests become negative in most cases, in other recent infections the titre falls by at least two dilutions when the treatment has been successful.
- All sexual partners who have been exposed to infection should be screened with the cardiolipin test. If the result is negative, the test should be repeated after 3 months.

12.4 Human papillomavirus (HPV) infection (Condyloma)

Jorma Paavonen

Basic rules

- Visible condylomata should be treated.
- Precancerous changes caused by HPV should be treated.

Epidemiology

- Transmitted mainly in sexual contact; causative agent is human papillomavirus (HPV).
- Time of transmission is impossible to determine (from 1 to 8 months, may be latent for a long time).
- The infection may present with classical cauliflower-like warts, condyloma acuminatum, but in most cases it presents as flat subclinical lesions that are detected in women by Pap smear.
- Common in conditions involving immunosuppression (HIV, medication).

Symptoms

- The HPV-infection may be completely symptomless and the condylomata are often detected accidentally.
- Intense pruritus and ulcerations may occur occasionally in the regions of vulva, anus, and prepuce.
- Urethral warts may cause burning on urination and haematuria.
- Some of the symptoms may be caused by other concurrent infections (Candida, herpes, Chlamydia).

Diagnosis

- Classical exophytic warts are usually readily diagnosed by the naked eye (Figure 12.4.1). It is advisable to examine also the anus (Figure 12.4.2) (proctoscopy) and distal urethra (e.g. with a small nose speculum).
- Flat HPV-infection in women is usually detected by PAP smear (koilocytic atypia). A patient with repeated abnormal findings on PAP smear (class II or ASCUS) should be referred to colposcopy.

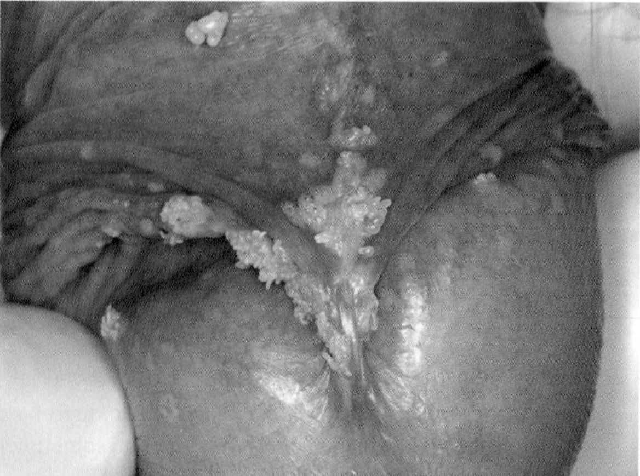

Figure 12.4.1 Condyloma acuminatum (genital warts) is a common viral infection of predominantly genital mucous membranes. The therapeutic alternatives are podophyllotoxin, various cauterization methods, cryotherapy and most recently imiquimod. Especially in female patients the condition may prove to be highly resistant to treatment. Photo © R. Suhonen.

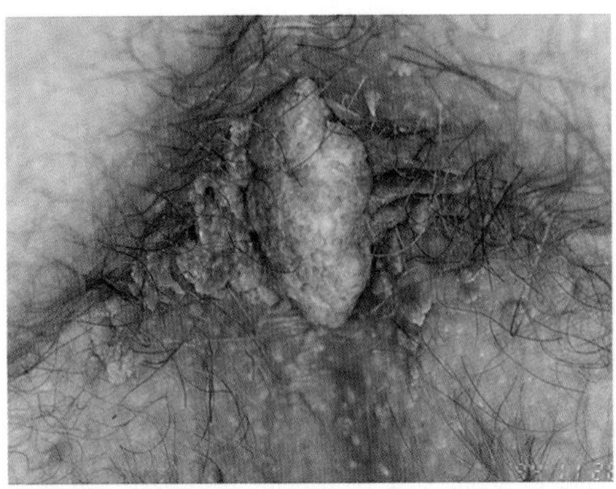

Figure 12.4.2 Condylomata accuminata are less common in the anal region than in the genital area. In male patients the possibility of homosexual behaviour should be considered, with the possibility of an increased risk of HIV infection. Photo © R. Suhonen.

- Acetic acid application (3–5%) makes flat lesions visible as pale plaques (acetowhitening) in both sexes, but the finding is unspecific and difficult to interpret without a colposcope. Histological confirmation is needed for the diagnosis. The latter is not recommended as a clinical routine because the majority of healthy adults bear the virus without having a disease.
- Biopsy is recommended, if there are
  - naevus like lesions, especially if pigmented
  - treatment-resistant warts
  - chronic symptoms (intensive itching, ulcerations).
  - repeated mild abnormalities on Pap smears (class II or ASCUS)

Differential diagnosis

- Acetowhitening reactions may be seen in cases of unspecific infectious lesions and scar formation.
- About 30–40% of young men have papulae around the glans; these are not associated with HPV (Figure 12.4.3).

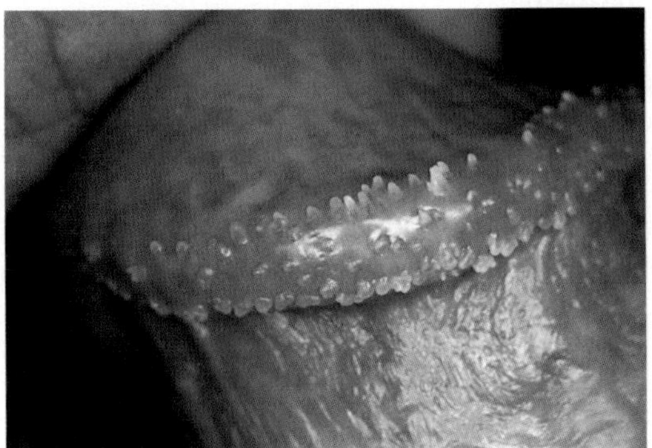

Figure 12.4.3 Penile pearly papules are harmless, but often confused with condylomata acuminata and consequently quite often a target of therapeutic trials with podophyllotoxin or other "therapies". Photo © R. Suhonen.

- Candida (itching, fissures), herpes (tender ulceration)
- Several skin diseases (e.g., lichen sclerosus et atrophicus, lichen planus, psoriasis, allergic eczema).

Management of condylomata

- Pap smear is indicated for women
- Remember other sexually transmitted diseases!

DER

Treatment alternatives

- **Podophyllotoxin**
  - May be self-applied by the patient on visible warts twice daily on 3 consecutive days. The course may be repeated at 1 week intervals.
  - Best for small solitary condylomata.
  - Not during pregnancy and not in the vagina or on the vaginal part of cervix.
- **Imiquimod cream**
  - New immune response modifier
  - Applied on intact skin every other day (3 times per week), to be washed away in the morning (6–10 hours later)
  - Treatment is continued until the warts have disappeared, not longer than 16 weeks.
- **Excisional removal**
  - Scissors, conchotome, or similar (local anaesthesia, e.g., with lidocaine/prilocaine cream)
  - Suited for solitary large-sized warts
- **Cryotherapy**
  - Best for external warts
- **Electrocoagulation**
  - Controlling the depth of the tissue damage is difficult
- **Laser vaporization**
  - Best method for wide or recurrent lesions irrespective of the location
  - Especially suitable for warts in the urethral orifice, in the vagina or in the anus

Treatment of subclinical HPV-infections

- Treatment is determined by the colposcopy (vulvoscopy/ peniscopy) and histological findings.
- Cervical lesions are treated according to their extent and severity by removal either with an electric loop or with laser (conization).
- Vaginal lesions can be treated with laser (CO_2) in association with colposcopy.
- The problematic flat HPV-lesions in the vulva or in the perineal or anal regions (itching, burning, ulcerations) may also be treated with CO_2-laser using a colposcope.

Treatment results

- Recurrence is common after all treatments.

- Screening and treatment of symptomless men does not affect the healing of mucosal lesions in their female partners.
- There are controversial results concerning the effect of condom use on the transmission of HPV or on the healing process.

12.5 Genital herpes

Eija Hiltunen-Back

Basic rules

- The clinical picture of genital herpes is often typical and easy to diagnose. Problems arise when the manifestations are atypical, such as intermittent itching in the genital area, fissures and erythema. In order to provide adequate care and prevent the patient from spreading the disease it is essential to recognize these as symptoms of herpes.

Aetiology

- In most cases genital herpes is a chronic sexually transmitted infection caused by the Herpes simplex virus 2 (HSV-2). However, around 20% of the infections are nowadays caused by HSV-1. After infection the virus always remains latent in the body.

Epidemiology

- The virus is particularly contagious in the symptomatic phase; however, asymptomatic virus shedding is also known to occur. Partners who are unaware of carrying the virus transmit the virus in about half of the cases. In females the risk of infection is greater than in males.
- HSV-1 recurs less frequently and less severely than HSV-2.
- Genital herpes lesions increase the risk of HIV infection.

Symptoms

Primary herpes

- The symptoms appear 4–14 days after infection.
- General symptoms include
  - fever
  - headache
  - myalgia.
- Genital symptoms include
  - vesiculae
  - stinging pain
  - dysuria
  - inguinal lymphadenopathy
  - ulcerating cervicitis.
- The lesions are bilateral.
- The symptoms persist for 2–3 weeks.
- Primary herpes infection may also be asymptomatic.
- Virus secretion continues for about two weeks.
- During pregnancy the risk of foetal infection is 50% in primary herpes, but less than 5% in recurrent herpes.

Recurrent herpes

- Occurs in about 80% of patients who have had primary herpes (HSV-2).
- Lesions are unilateral.
- Lesions and symptoms are usually limited to the genitals: in females to the external genitals, and less frequently the cervix.
- General symptoms are rare.
- The frequency of recurrences varies individually.
- The infection may recur after physical or mental stress, in females frequently during menstrual period.
- The duration of symptoms is about 7 days.

Diagnosis

- Herpes simplex virus can be isolated from the lesion either by viral culture or by antigen detection methods. Culture sample must be taken to the laboratory within 24 hours while samples for antigen detection tolerate transportation and storage better.
- The sample is taken from the lesion with a cotton swab by rubbing.
- Antibody tests detect HSV-1 and HSV-2 seropositivity, i.e. carrier status, but not the location of the infection.
- PCR is especially well applicable for the diagnosis of neonatal herpes from the spinal fluid.

Treatment

- **In primary herpes** oral medication shortens viral secretion from 12 to 9 days. Mere clinical suspicion is a cause for starting medication: acyclovir 200 mg × 5, valaciclovir 500 mg × 2 or famciclovir 250 mg × 3, all three drugs for 5–10 days.
- Indications for intravenous administration are
  - severe clinical manifestations
  - meningeal irritation causing a headache
  - neonatal herpes.
- **In recurring herpes** oral acyclovir 200 mg × 5 × 5 days or valaciclovir 500 mg × 2 × 5 days ameliorates the symptoms and shortens the duration of the symptomatic phase.
- Locally applied acyclovir ointment is not as efficient in recurring genital herpes simplex as it is in labial herpes.

- Short-term prophylaxis can be used in a targeted manner, for example, during holidays.
- In frequent and difficult recurrence long-term prophylactic medication can be employed (6 months–): acyclovir 400 × 2, valaciclovir 500 mg × 1 or famciclovir 250 mg × 2.
- Prophylactic medication can reduce viral secretion considerably. Transmission is, however, still possible.
- At present there is no drug for eradication of the virus from neural sensory ganglions.
- To identify early symptoms and thus reduce the risk of transmission, the patient needs information on the natural course of the infection and infectivity.
- The need for medical care varies with the patient's life situations.

12.6 Rare venereal diseases: chancres

Timo Reunala

Ulcus molle (soft chancre, chancroid)

Aetiology

- Haemophilus ducreyi

Epidemiology

- A rare disease in Scandinavian countries, but in the tropics, such as in Africa, it is the most common venereal disease in some regions. In males the disease is ten times as frequent as in females. The disease is usually contracted from prostitutes.
- Incubation period 4–7 days

Symptoms

- One or more tender and painful genital ulcerations with a purulent exudate and surrounded by an erythematous halo. Ulcerations are generally shallow, but may persist for months or years without healing.
- Frequently acute unilateral inguinal adenitis with fused inguinal nodes (bubo) which may spontaneously rupture. A general infection does not develop.
- Of the typical ulcerations some may be mixed syphilis and chancroid (mixed chancre).

Diagnosis

- Gram's stain of lesion specimens frequently reveals strands of small gram-negative rods but only rarely in lymph node samples.
- Culture is not used routinely in low-incidence areas. In high-incidence areas a M-PCR technique is used. Its sensitivity in revealing H. ducreyi is 95%.
- Differential diagnoses are syphilis and herpes. A rare type of **transient** chancroid may be confused with lymphogranuloma venereum. Ulcus molle increases the risk of HIV infection.
- The possibility of concomitant lymphogranuloma venereum or granuloma inguinale and ulcus molle must be kept in mind.
- All patients should have a serologic test for syphilis at the initial examination and one month after all lesions have healed.

DER

Treatment

- Ciprofloxacin 500 mg × 2 × 3–5 days per os
- Ceftriaxone 250 mg × 1 i.m.
- Erythromycin 500 mg × 3 × 5 days per os.
- Roxithromycin 300 mg × 1 × 7 days or longer per os.
- Azithromycin 1 g single dose per os.

Lymphogranuloma venereum (LGV)

Aetiology

- Chlamydia trachmomatis serotype L1, L2 or L3
- The disease is most frequently spread by venereal contact, but the portal of entry may also sometimes be the eye.

Epidemiology

- The disease is global in distribution, but rare. In the tropics there are several endemic areas.

Clinical picture

- The primary lesion, a small papule, usually appearing 3–30 days after the infective contact, is not always noticed (e.g. located in the rectum).
- Suppurating fused inguinal lymph nodes (inguinal bubo), and sometimes genital ulcerations are found about two weeks after the primary lesion. The location of the primary lesion determines which nodes will be involved.
- The infection may be complicated by rashes, arthritis, conjunctivitis and meningoencephalitis.
- The incubation period prior to chronic lymphadenitis can be several months.
- The clinical picture may be accompanied by urethritis, proctocolitis and at a later stage by chronic and constricting fistulas and contracting scars. Rectal strictures are common in females and in male homosexuals. Elephantiasis of the labia and clitoris or of the penis and scrotum may occur. Hypergammaglobulinaemia is frequently observed in chronic cases. The diagnosis is supported by elevated chlamydial antibody concentrations.

Treatment

- Tetracycline 2 g × 1 × 2–4 weeks per os or 4 g × 1 × 2 weeks per os.
- Doxycycline 200 mg × 1 × 2–4 weeks per os.

- Erythromycin 2 g × 1 × 2–4 weeks per os.
- The clinically cured patient may remain infective and continue to spread the disease.

Granuloma inguinale (fourth venereal disease, granuloma venereum, donovanosis)

Aetiology

- The aetiologic agent is the pleomorphic rod Donovania granulomatis occurring intracellularly, singly or in clusters. (It has antigenic similarity with Klebsiella.)
- Microscopy reveals so-called Donovan bodies in mononuclear cells.

Epidemiology

- In India, Africa and the West Indian islands quite common, frequently endemic.

Symptoms

- Onset is insidious and without prodromal symptoms.
- In males it usually produces at first a vesicle, papule or nodule, and within a few days an ulceration with a beefy-red granular base on the glans, praeputium and rectum and frequently also urethritis.
- 14–90 days later a package of fused inguinal lymph nodes becomes unilaterally evident.
- The possibility of concomitant syphilis, lymphogranuloma venereum and ulcus molle must be kept in mind.
- Secondary elephantoid enlargement of the vulva and clitoris or of the penis and scrotum may occur.
- Without treatment the disease progresses to a chronic, granulomatous and tissue-destructing infection. Ulcerations may become extensive and invade the whole pudendal region, lower abdomen, thighs and buttocks.

Diagnosis

- Diagnosis of granuloma inguinale should be based on the demonstration of Donovan bodies in the pathognomonic cells in spreads or biopsies (e.g. Giemsa stain).

Treatment

- Tetracycline 500 mg × 4, 3–4 weeks per os.
- Chloramphenicol, ampicillin and fluorocinolones are also effective.

Dermatology

Evidence Based Medicine Guidelines. Edited by the Duodecim Editorial Team
 ISBN: 0-470-01184-X

13.1 One-glance diagnosis of dermatoses

Editors

Basic rules

- One in six patients visiting a GP have dermatosis.
- Eczematous dermatitis, urticaria, dermatophytosis and onychomycosis are the most common dermatoses.
- Diagnosis is often possible at one glance.

Diagnostic hints

Dermatitis of the eyelids

- Atopic dermatitis is the most usual diagnosis; seborrhoeic dermatitis is also possible but allergic contact dermatitis is rare.

Stubborn dandruff of the scalp in infants

- The diagnosis is the seborrhoeic form of infantile (atopic) dermatitis, very rarely true seborrhoeic dermatitis. Food allergy is associated with this condition as often as with the nummular form of infantile (atopic) dermatitis.

Dandruff of the scalp in adults

- In northern countries every third person has seborrhoea. In Central Europe the percentage is lower, and even lower in Mediterranean areas. Seborrhoea usually means dandruff, most often on the temples. Atopic dermatitis of the scalp of a young adult closely resembles seborrhoeic dermatitis. Exact diagnosis is not necessary because the treatment is the same.
- In psoriasis, the lesions are well demarcated and the scales are coarse.
- Lichen simplex of the neck (Neurodermatitis nuchae) is a sign of atopy.
- Dermatophytosis is possible but rare. When a dermatophyte occupies the hair shaft, the hair will break off close to the scalp surface. Mycological culture should be performed in suspected cases.

Urticaria

- Diagnosis is more difficult than expected. The weal and flare lesions should disappear or at least migrate in 24 hours.
- If the weal persists for longer than 24 hours, the correct diagnosis is not usual urticaria and further investigations are indicated.

Dermatitis of the sole of the foot

- In children, scaling and fissuring dermatitis of the plantar surfaces of the forefeet is known as juvenile plantar dermatosis and is seen especially in atopic dermatitis. Dermatophytosis of the feet is very rare in children below 15 years of age. Tinea of the feet is usually located under and between the lateral toes. Allergic contact dermatitis (shoe dermatitis) is rare. "Moccasin foot" means dry, scaly dermatosis of the whole plantar surface of the feet, extending to the dorsal surfaces of the toes. It is caused by Trichophyton rubrum or other dermatophytes. Remember mycological culture! If the moccasin foot is unilateral, tinea is even more probable.
- Two main types of plantar warts exist: common warts that are raised from the skin surface and flat mosaic warts. Mosaic warts are only 2–3 mm in diameter and usually occur in groups.
- Dermatitis of the sole may also be caused by sweating feet and occlusive boots (Figure 13.1.1).

Dermatitis of the palms

- Symmetric dermatitis on the palmar surfaces of the hands in a young person is atopic dermatitis.
- The aetiology of palmar dermatitis in adults usually remains unknown. It is called chronic hand dermatitis, or sometimes infectious hand dermatitis. Delayed contact hypersensitivity is sometimes encountered (Figure 13.1.2).
- Chronic hand dermatitis in a dairy farmer may be due to immediate or delayed allergy to cow dander.
- Severe chronic (infectious) hand dermatitis may be a sign of excessive alcohol consumption. Smoking is another aggravating factor.
- Unilateral palmar dermatitis is often tinea. Remember mycological culture.
- Nummular eczema may appear also in hands (Figure 13.1.3).

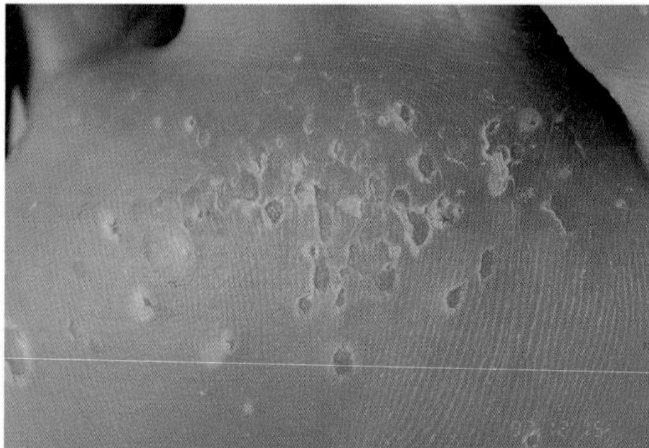

Figure 13.1.1 Pitted keratolysis on the sole. Sweating feet and occlusive boots may lead to bacterial overgrowth in plantar skin. The "punched out" depressions of the skin can be healed also by using aluminium chloride-containing antiperspirants and by eliminating occlusion. The main differential diagnosis is plantar mycosis caused by T. rubrum. Photo © R. Suhonen.

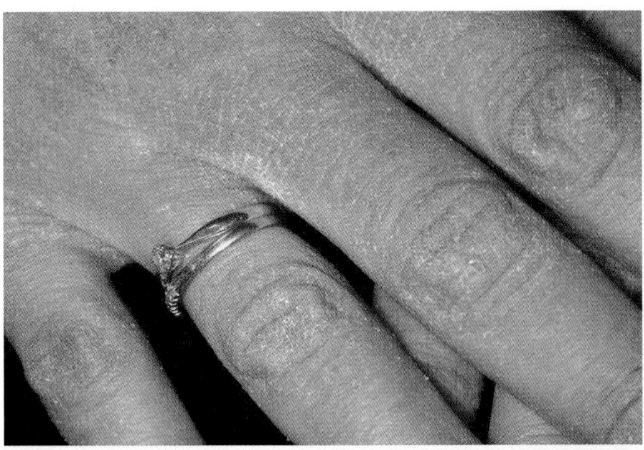

Figure 13.1.2 Toxic dermatitis on the dorsal aspect of the fingers—a typical phenomenon in atopic ladies who do household work involving exposure to water. Protection of the hands against irritants is recommended, and topical corticosteroids and emollients are usually beneficial. The possibility of a contact allergy should be investigated by patch testing. Photo © R. Suhonen.

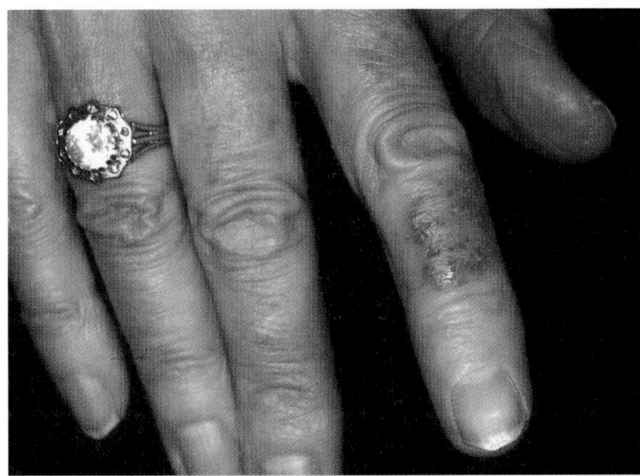

Figure 13.1.3 Nummular (discoid) dermatitis affects mainly the skin of the body and extremities. A solitary patch in a finger is a common feature of nummular dermatitis. The cause of this common, severely pruritic eruption is unknown. Photo © R. Suhonen.

Patchy hyperkeratosis of the palms and/or soles

- In middle-aged patients the condition is usually inherited and connected with climacterium, also in males!
- Psoriasis and contact allergy to chromate and cobalt are the most common differential diagnoses.

Anogenital dermatosis

- Seborrhoeic dermatitis (intertrigo) and inguinal tinea are the most common complaints in the anogenital area. Psoriasis and Candida intertrigo due to obesity and/or diabetes are the next most frequent causes.

Balanitis

- Often seborrhoeic balanitis. You can also find seborrhoeic dermatitis in other places, e.g. the scalp and face.
- Circinate balanitis is a sign of Reiter's disease. It may be hidden by another inflammation.
- Psoriasis and lichen planus appear as well-demarcated, chronic, slightly infiltrated patches.

Perianal dermatitis

- Nearly always seborrhoeic dermatitis
- Scratching leads to lichen simplex (neurodermatitis).
- Flexural psoriasis closely resembles seborrhoeic dermatitis.

Itching dermatitis of the lower leg

- Is usually circumscribed lichen simplex ("neurodermatitis") or nummular eczema.
- A thick reddish-blue patch may also be chronic hypertrophic lichen planus.

Fingertip dermatitis

- Scaling and fissuring chronic dermatitis of the finger tips.
- Seen in middle-aged and elderly women. Aetiology unknown.
- Also myxoid cyst (Figure 13.1.4) and glomus tumour (Figure 13.1.5) may appear in finger.

Angular cheilitis

- In children plump cheeks and a deep labial sulcus form a furrow in which Candida and staphylococci thrive.

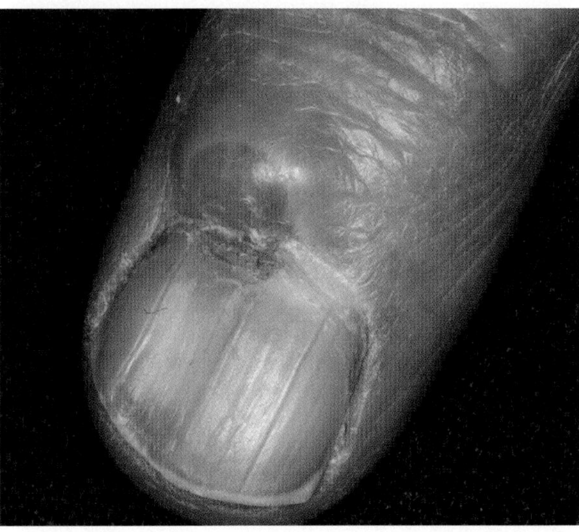

Figure 13.1.4 A myxoid cyst at the level of the proximal nail fold may cause a longitudinal depression on the nail plate. The nail can return to its normal shape only if the cyst is removed. Skilful surgery is most effective, but puncture, opening of the cyst with subsequent exposure to solid silver nitrate, or liquid nitrogen cryotherapy can also be tried. Recurrence is not uncommon with any method of therapy. Photo © R. Suhonen.

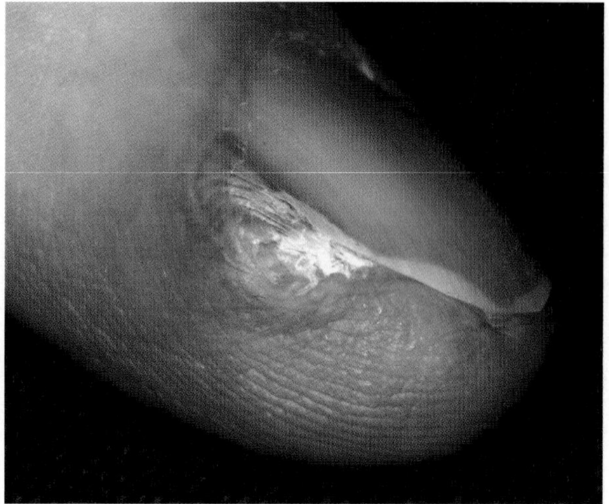

Figure 13.1.5 Glomus tumour is a quite rare, extremely tender, benign tumour. Most often the patient is a middle-aged woman who has a painful lesion under a fingernail. The treatment is by surgery. Damage of the matrix must be avoided in order to prevent nail damage. Photo © R. Suhonen.

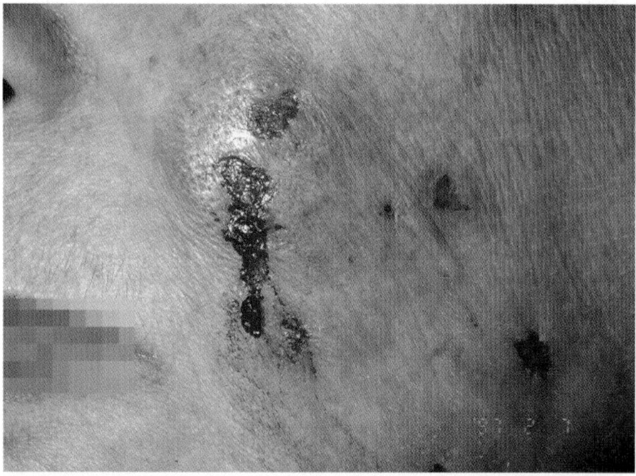

Figure 13.1.6 Self-induced - most commonly with a nail - skin lesions may cause problems with differential diagnosis. Pruritic skin diseases may cause similar secondary skin changes. Still more difficult is to achieve the patient's acceptance to the theory of the psychogenicity of the problem. Photo © R. Suhonen.

- Elderly patients are usually edentulous.
- Diabetes and immunodeficiency are also predisposing factors.

Dry cheilitis

- A sign of atopy, especially in children. Breathing through the mouth and food allergies aggravate the inflammation.

Other dermatose

- Dermatosis may also be self-inflicted (Figure 13.1.6) or caused by e.g. music instrument (Figure 13.1.7).

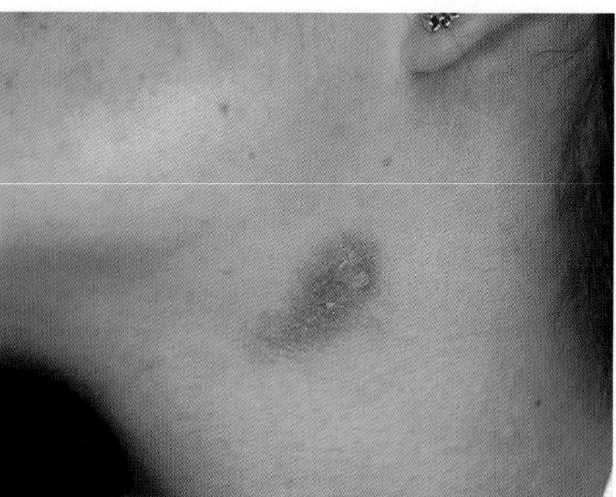

Figure 13.1.7 Fiddler's neck. Repeated, long-standing pressure and friction from the body of a violin provokes a reddish-brown patch on the neck. There is no cure if the contact is not eliminated. Photo © R. Suhonen.

13.2 Itch

Pekka Autio

Basic rules

- Identify causes of itch for which specific treatments are available (scabies, eczemas, dermatitis herpetiformis).
- If no dermatological cause can be found search for systemic diseases that cause itching (e.g. liver diseases, Hodgkin's disease, uraemia).

Localized itch

- The cause is often a local condition (eczema, neurodermatitis, topical drug reaction, insect bite), sometimes psychogenic.

Generalized itch

- Skin diseases: urticaria, widespread eczemas; systemic drug reactions, liver diseases, Hodgkin's disease, chronic scabies.

Diagnostic clues by the site of the itch

Scalp

- Seborrhoeic dermatitis
- Atopic dermatitis
- Psoriasis (itch is common)

- Irritation or allergy (hairdresser's chemicals)
- Head lice

Face

- Atopic dermatitis
- Seborrhoeic dermatitis
- Allergic dermatitis (cosmetics, nail polish)
- Impetigo (children)
- Herpes simplex (often painful)

Trunk

- Atopic dermatitis
- Seborrhoeic dermatitis (13.15)
- Allergic dermatitis (13.13)
- Urticaria (13.74)
- Pityriasis rosea (13.72)
- Insect stings and bites (13.42)
- Ringworm

Genital region

- Atopic dermatitis
- Seborrhoeic dermatitis (13.15)
- Ringworm (men) (13.50)
- Pubic lice (13.41)
- Scabies (13.40)
- Psychological causes

Anal region

- Seborrhoeic dermatitis (13.15)
- Non-specific dermatitis
- Allergic dermatitis (haemorrhoid ointments) (13.13)
- Haemorrhoids
- Anal fissure (painful)
- Secondary candidiasis (occasionally) (13.50)
- Psychological causes
- Pinworms (rare)

Extremities

- Atopic dermatitis
- Irritant dermatitis (13.14)
- Allergic dermatitis
- Stasis dermatitis (leg)
- Scabies (13.40)
- Insect bites
- Neurodermatitis
- Dermatitis herpetiformis
- Gianotti-Crosti syndrome (Figure 13.2.1)

Widespread itch with a visible cause

- Atopic dermatitis
- "Dry skin" (in the winter season in old people)
- Urticarias (13.74)
- Lichen planus (13.73)
- Psoriasis (13.71)

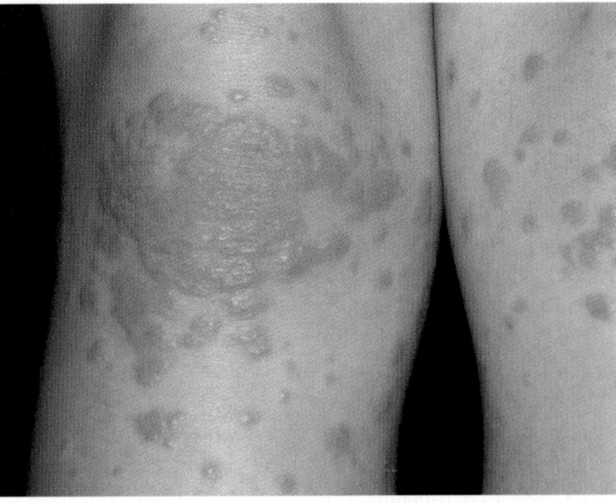

Figure 13.2.1 Gianotti-Crosti acropapulosis is a transient (weeks-months) eruption often of viral origin. The disease affects children. Possible pruritus can be treated with low potency corticoids. The papules are met in the face and extremities, seldom on the trunk. Photo © R. Suhonen.

- Widespread extrinsic allergic reactions (13.13)
- Endogenous allergic reactions (13.13)

Generalized itch without visible skin pathology

- Infrequent compared with itching skin diseases
- Dermographism (make a scratch!)
- Uraemia
- Liver diseases
- Hepatic cholestasis of pregnancy
- Hodgkin's disease
- Polycythaemia vera
- Diseases of the thyroid gland
- Psychogenic itch (?)

Investigations

Itch and a dermatological disease

- If the cause is a dermatological condition look for specific aetiology (allergies, infections, scabies).
- Symptomatic treatment is often the best you can do (atopic dermatitis, other non-specific eczemas, lichen planus).
- Many skin diseases are cured spontaneously.

Generalized itch without clinical skin pathology

- Thorough clinical examination (jaundice, lymph node enlargement)
- History of concomitant/past diseases and medications
- Blood count, ESR, creatinine, ALT, alkaline phosphatase, bilirubin (total and conjugated)
- Chest x-ray
- Consultation by a dermatologist, a specialist in internal medicine, or psychiatrist as required

Treatment of itch

- Treat a dermatological disease according to aetiology.
- Dry skin is often associated with itch. Moisturizers are indicated, especially in the winter season for elderly patients.
- Ask about the patient's washing habits. Often the use of soap or washing liquids can be restricted. A moisturizing cream should be applied to moist skin after washing.
- Hydroxyzine for the night is a good symptomatic treatment. The so-called non-sedating antihistamines are effective against urticaria, but for other causes of itch their effect is comparable to placebo.
- Light therapy (SUP/UVB/PUVA) is effective for many causes of itch: atopic dermatitis, seborrhoeic dermatitis, psoriasis, lichen planus, urticarias, uraemic itch).
- Treatment of itch in a terminal patient: see also 13.13.

Indications for specialist referral

- If no sufficient explanation is found for the itch or the response to treatment is poor. A patient with annoying itch without visible cause will eventually be examined by a specialist.

13.3 Hair loss

Eero Lehmuskallio

Alopecia areata

- Patchy hair loss (Figure 13.3.1).
- Small patches recover spontaneously over several months.
- The prognosis of widespread hair loss is poor, particularly if the eyelashes, eyebrows, and beard are also affected.
- The cause may also be discoid lupus erythematosus (Figure 13.3.2).

Treatment

- Treatment is not decisive as regards prognosis but it may increase hair growth to some extent.
- Topical corticosteroid liniments
- PUVA treatment usually brings only temporary improvement.
- Steroid injections in the affected scalp, given by a dermatologist, may be partly effective.
- Wigs
- Experimental treatments carried out by dermatologists include sensitisation treatments based on contact allergy.

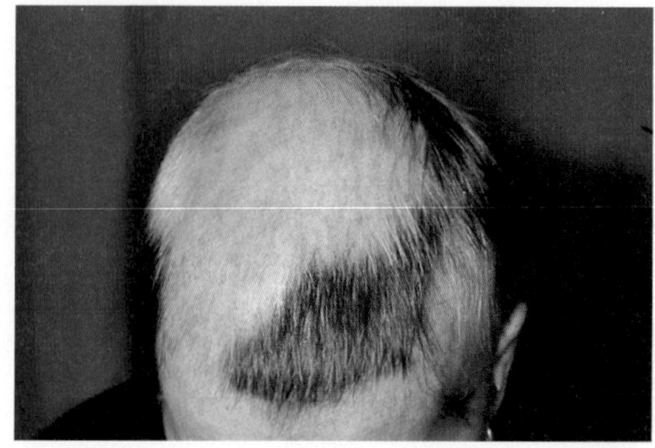

Figure 13.3.1 Alopecia areata is probably an autoimmune phenomenon, where bald areas of variable size appear in any hair-growing area of the body. Limited cases have a good tendency for spontaneous healing; in more extensive cases, e.g. alopecia totalis or alopecia universalis, the prognosis is less favourable. Therapeutic trials have had variable success. Photo © R. Suhonen.

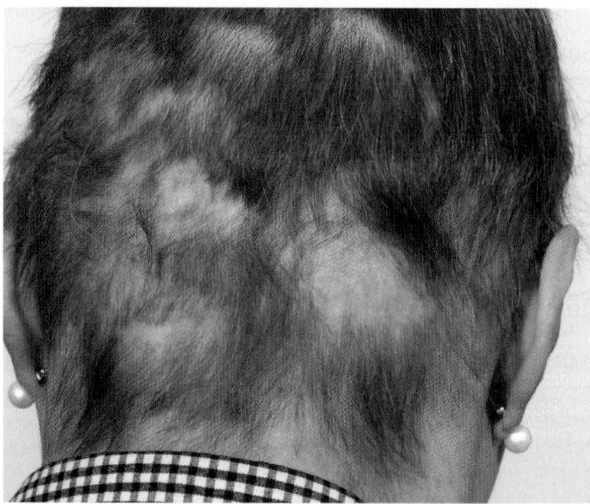

Figure 13.3.2 Discoid lupus erythematosus is one of the most common diseases causing cicatrical alopecia. The hair is lost permanently in the affected scalp area. Photo © R. Suhonen.

Male-type baldness

- Usually affects elderly men but may occur in young men in some families.
- There is no convincing evidence of the effect of minoxidil. If the drug works effectively its effect is lost when its use is discontinued.
- Minoxidil is also used for alopecia androgenica in women.
- Peroral treatment with 1 mg/day finasteride has a similar effect as topical minoxidil on premature male-type baldness.
- Before commencing the treatment the patient should be informed that the treatment with minoxidil or finasteride must be continued throughout life to be effective and that it is expensive. Discontinuation of the treatment results in all effects being lost in 3–12 months. Re-instituted treatment does not restore the condition that was obtained before discontinuation.

- Hair transplantation and other plastic surgical techniques may result in an acceptable outcome.

13.5 Diagnostic tests in dermatology

Editors

Skin prick tests

- Skin prick tests (SPT) and scratch tests are needed for finding allergens and aggravating factors in atopic dermatitis in children and sometimes also in adults. Standard inhalation and food allergen series are used most often.

Indications

- In children, SPTs are indicated in widespread dermatitis and also in patients with rapidly exacerbating dermatitis. Dermatitis in the eyelids or on the perioral or perianal areas is also an indication for skin testing, especially when the patient also has gastrointestinal disturbances, rhinitis or asthma.
- In adults, widespread dermatitis
- SPT results may give hints for detecting clinically significant allergies.
- Indications for SPTs also include contact urticaria, protein contact dermatitis and suspicion of immediate-type allergy to local anaesthetics. Natural rubber latex, animals and flours are typical causes of immunological contact urticaria and protein contact dermatitis.
- Antihistamines should be discontinued before the tests as follows: Astemizole 6 weeks; other antihistamines 2–4 days prior to testing. A small amount of a systemic corticosteroid (e.g. prednisolone 20 mg or less per day in adults) does not influence the result.

Patch tests

- The standard series of patch tests (PT) usually includes 20–30 chemicals. It covers 70–80% of all contact allergies. Other test series are available for plastics, glues, acrylic resins, chemicals used in hairdressing, toothbrushes, etc. Chemicals brought by the patient him/herself can also be used.
- Finn Chamber® or Scanpor®-system (Epitest Ltd, Tuusula, Finland) is used in most countries and is the gold standard. The allergens are usually mixed with white petroleum jelly or water. Other methods such as the gel-based TRUE™ test (Pharmacia, Uppsala, Sweden) and various chambers may also be used. The tests are usually fixed on the upper back skin for 48 hours. Sometimes 24 or 72-hour exposure times are used.
- The results are read 3–5 days after application. Reactions to topical corticosteroids may be delayed by up to 9–10 days. A test becoming positive later than on day 10 is usually a sign of active sensitization.
- Antihistamines do not interfere with patch testing but systemic corticosteroids may weaken the reactions.
- Photopatch tests are done when photoallergic or phototoxic reactions are suspected. The tests are applied in the same way as the ordinary PTs but with double sets of patches. After 24-hour occlusion, the test strips are removed and one test series is irradiated with UVA, 5–20 J/cm^2. The results are read 2–5 days after the application. The test is used for normal contact allergies and photoallergies of either toxic or allergic origin.

DER

Phototests

- Suspected photosensitivity is the main indication for phototesting. Phototests are done separately with UVB and UVA or preferably by using several wavelengths of UVB and UVA. UV-induced urticaria is seen as soon as 10–30 minutes after the irradiation, eczema in 1–3 days.
- In polymorphous light eruption the same skin site is irradiated on 3–5 consecutive days, and the test is followed up for 5–7 days.

Special tests in urticaria

Dermographism

- Scratch the skin of the back firmly with the blunt end of a pen and wait for 15–20 minutes. Mild redness that disappears in a few minutes is the normal reaction. 5% of people react with a weal. If the diameter of the weal does not exceed the width of the pen end the patient usually does not have dermographism. In symptomatic dermographism, the weal is wider than the stroke, and pseudopodia can also be seen. Systemic or local antihistamine abolishes the reaction, but systemic or topical steroids do not.

Test for cold urticaria

- The test can be performed either with ice cubes or with cold (7°C) water. Ice cubes wrapped in plastic bags are fixed on the arm skin for periods varying from 1 to 10 minutes. The weals appear when the skin is warming up. The test with cold water is somewhat more reliable. In cold urticaria restricted to certain areas, the test may be negative on the arm but positive on the symptomatic area.

Test for heat urticaria

- A test tube with 42°C water is placed on the arm skin for 5–10 minutes. Alternatively, the arm may be immersed in warm (42°C) water for 5–10 minutes. In positive cases, weals appear during the warming up period.

Cholinergic urticaria

- An exercise during which the patient's sweat produces tiny weals on the trunk.

Challenge tests

Single open application test

- In contact urticaria and protein contact dermatitis, the suspected agent is spread and gently rubbed onto a 5 × 5 to 10 × 10 cm area, preferably on previously affected skin. The result is read in 15–30 minutes, possibly also after 24 hours.

Repeated open application test, ROAT

- A small amount of the suspected material is spread twice daily for 7 days onto the antecubital fossa. In positive cases, dermatitis will usually appear in 2–4 days.

Usage test

- The suspected product is used as normally for 1 month. The response is checked weekly.

Peroral challenge test

- In drug hypersensitivity, atopic dermatitis and sometimes also in urticaria suspected drugs/foods are given perorally in a double blind manner. The first dose should be so small that no serious consequences can be expected.

Subcutaneous challenge

- Subcutaneous challenge is especially utilized in diagnosing allergy to local anaesthetics: for example, 0.5–1 ml of 1% lidocaine is injected subcutaneously in the arm. The result is followed up for 1 hour, sometimes for 24 hours.

Who performs the tests?

- In dermatological indications, skin prick, patch, photo- and photopatch tests are done in dermatological units.
- Special tests for urticaria (dermographism, cold, heat and cholinergic urticaria tests) are carried out by the GP.
- Specialists usually do challenge tests.

13.6 Indications for and techniques of skin biopsy

Markku Helle

Basic rules

- Make a clear working diagnosis and ask the right questions
- Inform the pathologist adequately (duration of the disease, site of the lesions, site of biopsy)
- Ensure the technical quality of the biopsy specimen.
- Take the biopsy from a suitable site.

Indications for skin biopsy

Tumours

- Send all tumours to a pathologist, with the exception of typical seborrhoeic verrucosis and atheromas (with a content of sebaceous mass). If the benign nature of a skin lesion is not evident, a biopsy is preferable to follow-up alone.
- Children very seldom have malignant skin tumours. Refer children with unidentified skin tumours to a specialized unit.

Other skin diseases

- Differential diagnosis of bullous skin diseases; immunohistochemical analysis is also usually necessary (immunofluorescence examination). Formalin fixation is not allowed in these cases –refer the patient to a specialized unit.
- Skin infiltrates resembling tumours.
- Some genodermatoses (e.g. ichthyoses; rare diseases that should be treated by specialists).

Clinical diagnosis can be supported by skin biopsy in the following cases:

- Psoriasis (often histology is not very specific)
- Lichen ruber planus (biopsy findings are distinctive)
- Lupus erythematosus (a specimen from sun-exposed skin for immunofluorescence is often also indicated)
- Granulomatous diseases (granuloma annulare, necrobiosis lipoidica, sarcoidosis, lupus vulgaris)

Techniques of performing skin biopsy

- An ordinary skin biopsy should be taken with a scalpel (no. 15) to include the complete depth of the skin to the subcutaneous adipose tissue. Choose the site of the biopsy so that underlying structures do not prevent a sufficiently deep incision. Incise in the direction of skin folds in order to minimize scar formation. A specimen measuring 0.5 × 1.5 cm is recommended. The thickness is determined by the site.
- In the case of a plaque-like, homogeneous lesion a 3–4 mm punch may be more convenient. Take a specimen down to the subcutaneous fat. The wound usually needs no sutures. Cover the wound with a hydrophilic colloid dressing (e.g. Duoderm® or Comfeel®) to promote healing. Leave the dressing in place until the wound is closed.
- Do not squeeze or tear the biopsy specimen. Use small surgical forceps, a hook or a needle.

Site of skin biopsy

- Take the biopsy from a newly but fully developed lesion (a biopsy sample from a fresh lesion is important particularly in bullous diseases).
- If the whole lesion cannot be excised it is recommended to take the biopsy from the outer part of pathological lesion, extending radially to the centre of the lesion. Inform the pathologist about the location of the lesion and the site of the biopsy in the lesion.
- Take small blisters unbroken into the biopsy specimen (do not try to do this with a punch because the roof of the blister may be detached and the diagnosis will be impossible!).
- Try to remove small tumours completely.
- If the pathological diagnosis and the clinical presentation are in disagreement take a new biopsy or refer the patient to a specialist. The pathological diagnosis is not the whole truth, so you should yourself take responsibility for diagnosis and treatment.

13.10 Hand dermatitis

Pekka Autio

Basic rules

- Hand dermatitis is not contagious or dangerous but it may interrupt sleep and seriously affect the patient's occupation.
- The treatment of hand dermatitis is easy to start: a tube of a corticosteroid cream. If initial treatment is not successful the patient must be examined. Early investigations and a treatment plan may save the patient from the worst –chronic hand dermatitis.
- Before prescribing corticosteroids determine whether the patient has dermatitis or another skin disease. Corticosteroid treatment does no harm in psoriasis, lichen planus, or palmoplantar pustulosis, but tinea, scabies, and syphilis need specific treatment.

Identifying causes that need specific treatment

- Tinea is rare in the hand. It is improbable if there is no tinea in the feet, or in men, in the inguinal creases.
- Scabies should be diagnosed by detecting furrows made by female mites. They can usually be found with a stereomicroscope in the palms, wrist folds, or between the fingers.
- Syphilis is common in many countries. Palmar lesions in secondary syphilis may look innocent. The same maculae can be found on the soles of the feet. Condylomata lata, which is not a viral disease but a sign of secondary syphilis, can often be found in the region of genital organs.

Investigating hand dermatitis

Aims

- The aim of treatment is to eliminate the cause of visible and itching dermatitis that interferes with work and hobbies. Hence the underlying cause must be identified.
- The examination should be started by looking at the soles of the feet and between the toes. Foot tinea may be associated with an id-reaction in the hands, that does not involve fungi but is best treated by first treating tinea of the feet.

History

- Do bananas or avocados cause itching of the palate? The patient may be allergic to natural rubber latex.
- Did the patient get a rash after the application of Nobecutan® on the skin after surgery? The patient may have thiuram allergy which also prevents the use of most rubber gloves.
- Is the patient a gardener, and does the eczema reside in fingers I–III? The cause may be tulips or alstroemeria.
- Is there diffuse eczema here and there on a woman's neck and face? Eczema around in the nail folds may be caused by toluenesulphonamide formaldehyde-containing nail varnish.
- Has your patient been on sick leave because of the eczema? Did the eczema improve during sick leave and how rapidly? If there is no improvement after one week and if there is eczema also on the soles, the eczema is not likely to be work-related.
- The cause of irritant dermatitis is often evident. The patient is often atopic, and even mild detergents remove the protective lipid layer of the skin of the hands. A young mother may have recently come from the maternity hospital. In fear of bacteria she may "boil" her hands in soapy water. Staphylococci prefer such injured hands with dermatitis (Figure 13.10.1).

Skin tests

- Epicutaneous tests are the basic investigative method in hand dermatitis. The causative agent is often difficult to identify without tests because the symptoms may appear several days after exposure. Epicutaneous tests cannot and need not always be performed as the first step. Treatment can be started with topical corticosteroids, and the patient can be tested later. Testing in the acute phase may cause difficulties in interpretation and exacerbate the eczema. Epicutaneous tests should be performed by a qualified dermatologist.
- Prick tests may reveal IgE-mediated allergy to natural rubber latex, to animal dander (e.g. cows) or to animal proteins (butchers), but the allergies may also be of the delayed type.

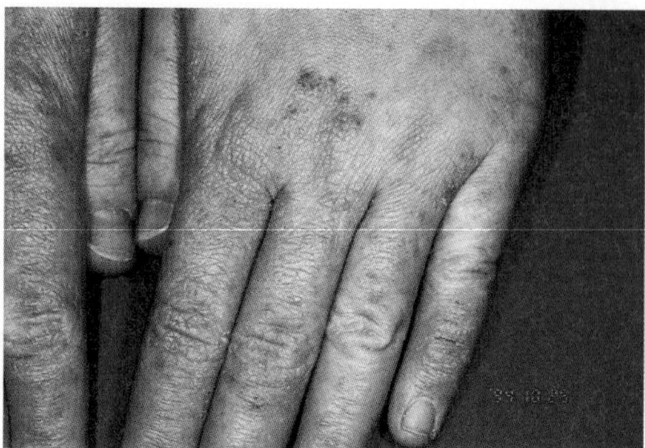

Figure 13.10.1 A typical irritant dermatitis on the dorsal aspect of the hands. The photograph could also be an example of adult atopic hand dermatitis. The patients are usually atopic (females), who handle water and detergents. Photo © R. Suhonen.

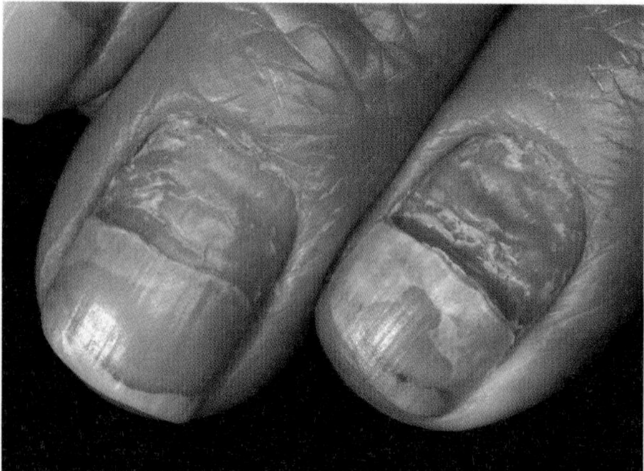

Figure 13.10.2 An episode of heavy paronychial dermatitis some months earlier led to temporary arrest in nail growth with transverse grooves in the affected nail plates. If these symptoms are seen synchronously in all nails, the possibility of systemic disease should be considered (Beau's lines). Photo © R. Suhonen.

Chronic eczema

- Chronic eczema is a diagnosis of exclusion. This "diagnosis" is made after careful and targeted disease history and well-planned testing have not identified the cause of the eczema.
- Eczema in the nail fold can disturb nail growth (Figure 13.10.2). Staphylococci may also enter, as well as Candida in the chronic stage. All this can lead to Beau's lines (Figure 13.10.3).

Treatment

Topical treatment

- The initial treatment is symptomatic.
- A corticosteroid cream or an ointment is usually all that is needed.

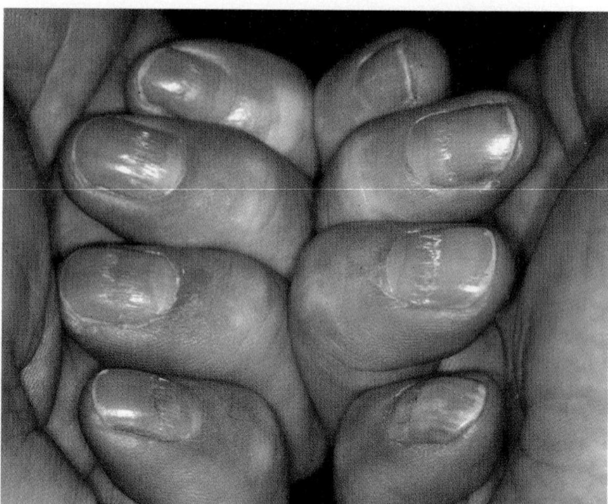

Figure 13.10.3 Transverse grooves in the nail plate are often due to repeated worsening periods of chronic hand dermatitis also affecting the nail fold region. The symptom usually affects only one or a few nails. If a single transverse groove is found in all nails, it is due to a systemic health problem (febrile disease, malnutrition, trauma etc.): Beau's lines. Photo © R. Suhonen.

  - The cream becomes a lotion if a wet compress is applied on it for the night.
  - If an emollient is preferred apply it on moist skin.
  - Cream works best for dry eczema if it is covered by a fat-based ointment.
- The recommended potency of a topical corticosteroid depends on the type of eczema, the age of the patient, and the location of the eczema (palm or dorsum of the hand).
  - Mild steroid cream for children and the aged.
  - Steroid cream of intermediate potency for working-aged persons.
  - Persistent, vesiculating eczema of the palms may need potent steroids.
  - The milder steroids may be used twice daily; the most potent steroids only for the night.
- If a potent corticosteroid is not alternated with a base cream the efficacy is decreased, and the skin becomes atrophic.
- The effectiveness of a combination of a topical antibiotic and a corticosteroid has not been well documented, and the antibiotic may cause contact allergy.
- A persistent plaque of eczema in the middle of the palm can often be treated by applying potent or very corticosteroid scalp liniment on the palm and covering it with a hydrocolloid dressing that is left in place for several days. The treatment can be repeated a couple of times.
- In addition to corticosteroid preparation prescribe plenty of emollients. The choice of cream versus fatty ointment is mainly a matter of taste. Patients tend to prefer lighter creams even lotions. A fatty emulsion (oily cream, unguentum, lipogel), however, is preferred for dry scaling eczema. Applying emollient before dirty work makes hand washing easier. Preparations marketed as "barrier creams" may do more harm than good (Figure 13.10.4).

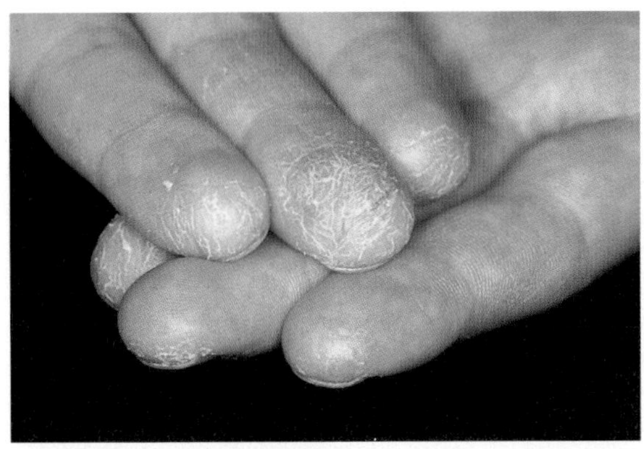

Figure 13.10.4 Finger tip dermatitis is common in housewives with atopic background and constant exposure to water and detergents. This clinical picture is quite resistant to therapy, which should combine potent topical corticosteroid to regular use of emollients and protection of the skin against irritants. Photo © R. Suhonen.

Antibiotics

- If the hand eczema is clearly infected or if the patient has lymphangitis and enlarged lymph nodes an oral antibiotic is indicated: cephalexin or cefadroxil 500 mg × 2–3 for 7–10 days are good choices. Treat the eczema concomitantly.
- Tetracyclines (1 g/day) often improve vesiculating infectious eczema of the palm. The treatment should be continued for 1–2 months, and in responding but recurring cases for 6 months or longer. Remember restrictions in use associated with young age, pregnancy, and lactation.

Peroral corticosteroids

- May be considered as a short course in the acute phase of a case of fulminant eczema (30 tablets of 5 mg prednisolone, starting with 30 mg/day).

Light therapy

- Sunlight alleviates hand eczema during the summer. During the winter it can be replaced with UVB or selective UV-phototherapy (= SUP = UVA + UVB irradiation).
- Ultraviolet light may be more effective when the whole body is treated.
- Other treatments must usually be combined with light therapy, but skin creams or ointments should not be applied just before it.

Protective gloves

- If the patient can do with cotton gloves the problem is often solved. However, protection against water and chemicals is usually needed, and the problem is that the hands get wet with perspiration in the gloves. Sometimes frequent change of combined cotton–plastic/rubber gloves may help.
- In vesicular endogenous eczema of the palms occlusion by a protective glove may worsen the situation.
- When composite resins are handled the allergens may penetrate ordinary protective gloves in minutes.

Sick-leave

- Try to treat the eczema first with the patient continuing with his work. Adjustments should be made at the workplace to minimize exposure to irritant agents and physical conditions. The skin should tolerate normal life.
- If re-education is considered necessary the new occupation must be chosen so that eventual hand eczema does not prevent working.

Prognosis

- If a patient has hand eczema before the age of 10 he will also have it in adulthood.
- Allergy to nickel (junk jewellery) may make the hand eczema chronic.
- Smoking, excessive consumption of alcohol, and hand eczema are often associated, with occupational exposure also playing a role.

13.11 Inguinal dermatitis

Pekka Autio

Basic rules

- Treat symptomatically but minimize risks, or treat curatively if the cause is identified.
- Do not treat before making a diagnosis.
- If a dermatophyte infection is suspected treatment can be started empirically while waiting for the results of fungal culture, which should always be carried out. Native microscopy is a quick adjunct to diagnosis.
- Avoid over-diagnosis of Candida infections.

Diagnostics

Children (infants)

- Nappy rash is the most common condition. Round erosions (craters) may be present in severe nappy rash. Erythema and papules are the usual presentation.
- Detecting Candida albicans on the skin does not prove its causative role. In real candidiasis there are usually satellite lesions around a larger (severely affected) lesion.
- Atopic dermatitis is usually not seen in the nappy area (the urea/carbamide in the urine cures the eczema)
- During the first months of life seborrhoeic eczema may be fulminant in the nappy area.
- "Dermatophytosis" in the inguinal region of children is nearly always a false diagnosis (take a sample for culture!).

Adults

- **Inguinal ringworm** is common in men but rare in women. If ringworm occurs in the inguinal region it can also almost invariably be found between the toes –always examine the feet. Ringworm usually presents with an active margin, occasional folliculitis, and even pustules. Take a sample for fungal culture, as even experienced clinicians make false clinical diagnoses.
- **Eczema** (seborrhoicum) is common in the inguinal region. Examine other typical sites for seborrhoeic eczema. Seborrhoeic eczema may have an elevated margin and it may resemble ringworm.
- **Psoriasis** often affects the inguinal folds. It presents with marked, often moist erythema. Examine the navel, armpits, buttock furrow, knees, elbows, nails, and scalp.
- **Erythrasma** of the inguinal region is uncommon. It usually looks inactive and it does not have an elevated margin. No fungi are detected in culture.
- **Candida infection** in the inguinal folds of an adult person usually indicates diabetes. Fasting blood glucose is a more important examination than culture for Candida.
- **Tinea incognito** is an iatrogenic condition where ringworm has been treated with corticosteroids. The clinical presentation consists of striae and atrophy. The condition is caused by omnipotent clinicians who "do not need fungal cultures".
- Itching of hairy skin may indicate **pubic lice** (Phthiriasis pubis). Use a magnifying lense (or stereomicroscope) to detect the eggs, sometimes even the lice. Examine also the eyelashes for eggs.
- Papules in the penis and scrotum are typical of **scabies**. Examine the wrists and interdigital folds of the fingers.

Treatment

Children

- Nappy rash (32.40) should be treated by avoiding the irritating effect of urine and faeces. Frequent nappy changes, avoidance of skin contact by occlusive plastics, using protective ointments (containing zinc), and removing nappies whenever possible are the basis of treatment. The ulcerative form may be therapy-resistant.
- Combination preparations (containing antimycotics and corticosteroids) are the most suitable for candida infections, but do not use corticosteroids for extended periods, and watch for possible adverse effects.
- The treatment of choice for eczema is mild hydrocortisone (0.5–1%). Restrict use to limited periods, follow the clinical response and observe safety precautions.

Adults

- Inguinal ringworm is almost invariably cured with topical antimycotics. Do not forget to treat the ringworm at other sites (e.g. between the toes).
- Eczema can be treated with mild or intermediate potency corticosteroids. Stronger corticosteroids should not be used, and even the use of moderately potent steroids should be restricted to very limited periods. A poor response to treatment suggests false diagnosis.
- Psoriasis is relatively easy to treat in the inguinal region. The same treatment applies as for eczema. Calcipotriol can also be used (sic!).
- Erythrasma is a bacterial disease that can be treated with imidazole preparations for 2–3 weeks.
- Candida is a significant pathogen only in diabetics. It can be treated with topical antimycotics.
- Permethrin or malathion shampoos are effective against pubic lice.
- Scabies: treat the whole family with malathion or permethrin.

Indications for specialist referral

- Difficulties in diagnosis and treatment.

13.12 Leg dermatitis

Jaakko Karvonen

Basic rules

- Identify and treat common skin diseases on legs according to the diagnosis.
- Consider the possibility of contact allergy.
- Avoid unnecessary antibiotic and antiseptic ointments, because patients with leg dermatitis (and particularly those with leg ulcers) are often allergic to topical drugs.

Common types of leg dermatitis

Nummular eczema

- Occurs typically on the legs and on the arms as round or ovoid patches or plaques.
- It is most common in the winter.
- Do not confuse with dermatophytosis (which is rare in the legs).
- Mild corticosteroids are usually not sufficient. Nummular eczema requires potent corticosteroids (e.g. betamethasone valerate).

Static eczema (eczema venosum hypostaticum)

- Signs of venous insufficiency are usually obvious.
- Typically occurs as pigmented dermatitis (Figure 13.12.1) surrounding leg ulcers.
- Remember that these patients are often allergic to topical drugs, especially topical antimicrobial agents.
- The underlying venous insufficiency should be treated surgically before venous ulcers develop.

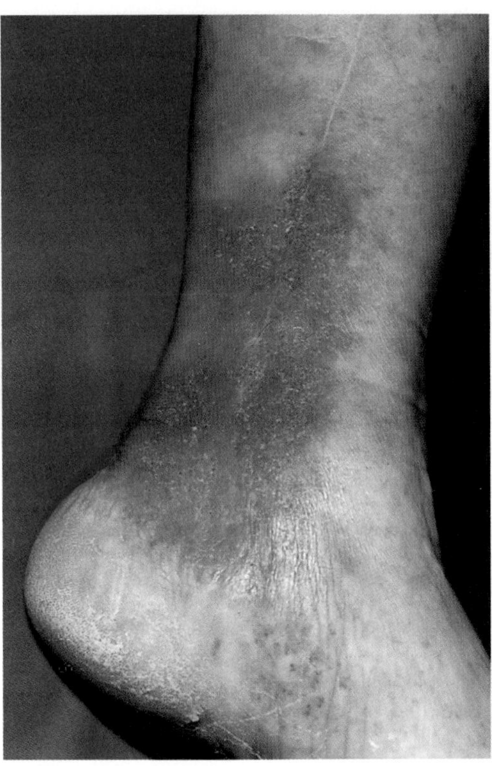

Figure 13.12.1 Stasis dermatitis (Eczema staticum) is common in venous insufficiency. Although topical corticoids are necessary in therapy, more important is a regular use of supporting bandages or stockings which are chosen individually. Cooperation of a GP, a dermatologist and a vascular surgeon leads to best results. Contact allergies to many therapeutic agents are not uncommon. Photo © R. Suhonen.

- Compression stockings or intermittent compression devices should be used if there is leg oedema.

Contact dermatitis (eczema allergicum)

- Allergic contact dermatitis of the leg is usually caused by topical drugs. Erythema may become widespread around the original eczema, and occur on other skin areas that have been in contact with hands contaminated by the sensitizing drug (13.13). The patient has often observed that the ointment does not feel good. Ulcerated skin is particularly prone to the development of contact allergy.
- Rubber boots sometimes cause allergic leg eczema.

Neurodermatitis (lichen simplex chronicus)

- Neurodermatitis may appear without evident cause, but often it is a complication of preceding itching eczema, e.g. atopic eczema.
- The ankle and leg are typical sites for chronic neurodermatitis.
- The condition may last for years or even a lifetime because of the vicious circle of itching and scratching.
- Potent steroid ointments are required for treatment.
- Occulsion therapy can also be used:
  - Apply potent corticosteroid scalp liniment and cover the site with a hydrocolloid dressing.
  - Change the occlusion dressing 2–3 times at 2–4-day intervals.
- The condition often recurs despite adequate treatment.
- Prurigo nodularis is the most chronic and therapy-resistant form of neurodermatitis.

Psoriasis

- See Article 13.71.
- The same principles of treatment apply as on other skin areas.

Lichen planus

- Lichen planus (13.73) typically occurs on the wrists, ankles, and legs.
- Chronic hypertrophic lichen planus almost invariably occurs on the leg and greatly resembles chronic neurodermatitis.

Erysipelas

- Rapid onset, high fever, and well-demarcated, tender erythema and oedema of one leg are typical of erysipelas (13.20) and make the diagnosis easy.
- Effective, preferably intravenous antibiotics should be started immediately.

Other skin diseases on legs

- **Nodular diseases of the leg** include a variety of diseases such as erythema nodosum (13.75), erythema induratum, polyarteritis nodosa, nodular vasculitis, and superficial thrombophlebitis. The diagnosis is often difficult to make and requires biopsies. The diagnostic examinations are often best performed at dermatological outpatient departments.
- **Necrobiosis lipoidica** (Figure 13.12.2) is often associated with diabetes. The lesion is yellowish, centrally atrophic, even ulcerating, and most pronounced on the margins.

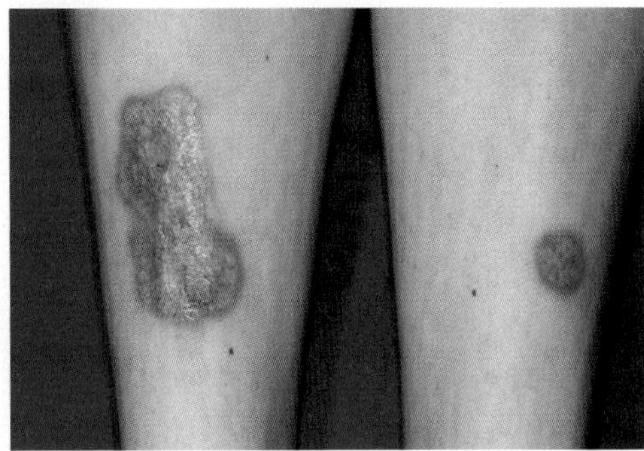

Figure 13.12.2 Necrobiosis lipoidica is most common in patients with insulin-dependent diabetes mellitus. Therapy may be problematic. In cases with ulceration, skin grafting may be considered. Photo © R. Suhonen.

- Erythema migrans on the leg may be a sign of Lyme disease (1.29).

Indications for specialist referral

- Need for epicutaneous tests in suspected contact allergy.
- Suspected rare nodular diseases of the leg.

13.13 Allergic dermatitis

Editors

Aetiology

- **Delayed cell-mediated immunity**
  - Usually results from an exposure lasting for weeks or months
  - The most common causative agents are nickel, rubbers and glues, chrome and cobalt, perfumes, and other compounds used in skin care products (Figures 13.13.1 and 13.13.2).
- **Immediate allergic reaction**
  - Less frequent than the former. The causative agents include latex, bovine hair and dandruff, and vegetables.

Symptoms

- The symptoms initially occur at the site of contact but they may spread to other areas.
- The symptoms recur within 1–2 days from the onset of a new exposure and cease gradually after the exposure has stopped.

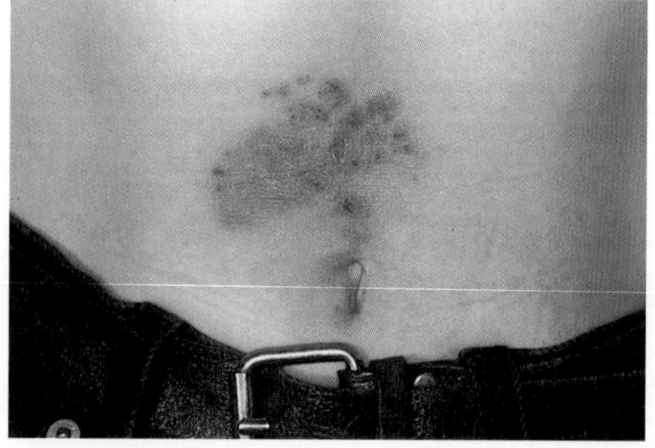

Figure 13.13.1 A belt buckle sensitized this boy to nickel. The allergy is usually life-long, but the symptoms disappear by avoiding nickel contact. Symptomatic therapy against dermatitis is only palliative. Photo © R. Suhonen.

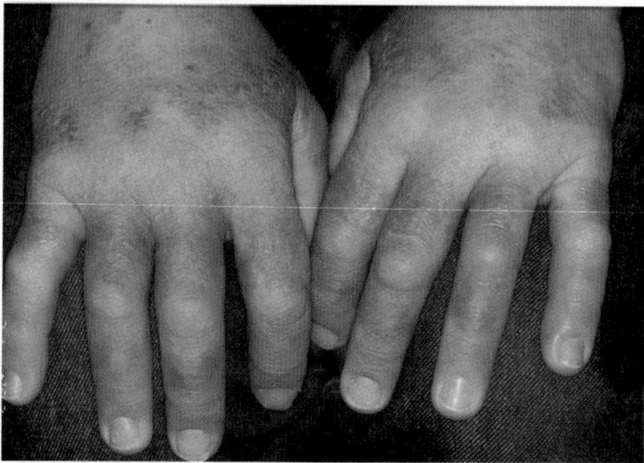

Figure 13.13.2 A violent dermatitis in the hands caused by contact allergy to epoxy resin, confirmed by patch testing. The sensitivity led to a change of profession. Very minimal exposure to the causative agent may provoke symptoms in a sensitized individual. Photo © R. Suhonen.

Diagnostics

- Allergic dermatitis should be suspected on the basis of the location. Typical sites for allergic eczema include
  - face and neck (cosmetics)
  - armpits (clothes, deodorants)
  - wrists and hands (metals, leather, tools, chemicals)
  - waist (latex, metals)
  - buttocks (haemorrhoid ointments and suppositories)
  - thighs and legs (socks, rubber boots, topical treatments for leg ulcers)
  - feet (metals, gum, leather, dyes, contact glue, chromium, antimycotics)
- Verifying the diagnosis: see article 13.5.

Treatment

- Treatment should always be directed at eliminating the sensitizing agent.
- Topical corticosteroid preparations

13.14 Toxic eczema

Eero Lehmuskallio

Aetiology

- A chemical (rarely physical) irritant can injure the skin and cause an inflammatory reaction if the exposure is strong enough and continues long enough.
- Persons with atopic, dry skin are most susceptible.

- The most common causative agents
  - Detergents and water (cleaners, housewives)
  - Substances with a high pH
  - Lipid solvents
- Diaper dermatitis is also a form of toxic eczema.

Symptoms

- Usually a hand eczema starting between the fingers and on the back of the hand, spreading later to the palm.

Diagnosis

- History reveals exposure to typical irritating factors, and the positive effect of avoiding exposure (e.g. during holidays).
- Contact allergy can often be excluded with epicutaneous tests
  - The tests should be performed if avoiding exposure does not control the eczema.
- Diagnosing atopic eczema does not rule out the possibility of toxic eczema in the same person.

Treatment

- The irritating factor should be avoided.
- Protective gloves (of plastic rather than of rubber) should be used.
- Moisturizing emollients should be used regularly to protect the skin.
- Corticosteroid creams are usually effective.

13.15 Seborrhoeic dermatitis

Eero Lehmuskallio

Epidemiology

- Usually occurs in adults (aged 18–40 years) in areas rich in sebaceous glands.
- Men are more commonly affected than women.

Symptoms and signs

Sites of predilection

- Affected skin areas in order of frequency
  - Scalp
  - Face; eyebrows, nasolabial creases, sideboard (sideburn) areas
  - Ears and ear canals
  - Mid-upper parts of the chest and back ("perspiration creases")
  - Buttock crease, inguinal area, genitals, and armpits
  - Only rarely becomes generalized.

Clinical picture

- Greasy or dry scaling of the scalp, sometimes a "cradle cap"
- Mildly scaling eczematous patches on the face at typical locations, often with itch and stinging
- Itch and inflammation of the ear canal
- Blepharitis
- Well-demarcated eczematous patches on mid-upper trunk.
- Intertrigo

Aetiology and pathophysiology

- Increased layer of sebum on the skin, quality of the sebum, and the immunological response of the patient favour the growth of Pityrosporum yeast.
- Degradation of the sebum irritates the skin and causes eczema.

Diagnosis

- Based on the typical clinical presentation and location of the eczema.
- In psoriasis (13.71) the scales are thicker, and the sites of predilection are different (elbows, knees). Psoriasis often has a familial occurrence.

Treatment

- The treatment does not cure the disease permanently. Therefore it must be repeated when the symptoms recur, or even prophylactically **B** [1].

Removing the thick scales and decreasing the amount of sebum

- The scales can be softened with a cream containing salicylic acid and sulphur (but not vaseline) or by wetting and washing.
- Seborrhoeic skin should be washed more often than usual.

Decreasing fungal growth

- Washing the scalp with ketoconazole shampoo **B** [1]
- Topical treatment with creams containing imidazole derivatives
- Antimycotic on skin creases (rarely necessary)
- Sometimes ultraviolet light therapy

Symptomatic topical treatment

- Corticosteroid liniments for the scalp (from mild to potent) B [2]
- Corticosteroid creams for other parts of the body (from mild to potent)
- Moisturizing emollients after washing
- Ketoconazole shampoo and corticosteroid liniments must often be combined in therapy-resistant cases.

References

1. Peter RU, Richarz-Barthauer U. Successful treatment and prophylaxis of scalp seborrhoeic dermatitis and dandruff with 2% ketokonazole shampoo: results of a multicentre double-blind, placebo-controlled trial. Br J Dermatol 1995;132:441–5.
2. Hersle K, Mobacken H, Nordin P. Mometasone furoate solution 0.1% compared with ketoconazole shampoo 2% for seborrheic dermatitis of the scalp. Current Ther Res Clin Exp 1996;57:516–22.

13.16 Nummular eczema

Editors

Aetiology

- The aetiology is unknown.
- The disease is often called infectious eczema although no infectious aetiology has been verified (Figure 13.16.1).
- Stress may be a causative factor.

Clinical presentation

- Well-demarcated, itching plaques
- Often recurs at varying intervals.
- Patients with atopic or seborrhoeic eczema may have lesions that can be classified as nummular eczema.
- Occurs in all age groups.

Diagnostics

- Diagnosis is based on the clinical presentation.
- Fungal culture from single lesions may be indicated.
- Bacterial culture from discharging lesions is useless. Staphylococcus aureus is usually detected, but its clinical significance is controversial.
- Biopsy is of no value.

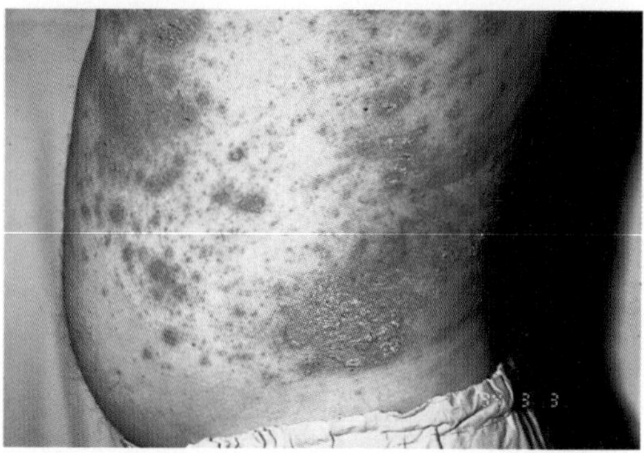

Figure 13.16.1 This might be called "nummular" or "infectious" eczema. Antibiotics, topical corticosteroids, possibly combined with UV-therapy are helpful. The disease tends to be more therapy-resistant in smokers. It is unusual to find relevant contact allergy in a patient with this dermatosis. Photo © R. Suhonen.

Differential diagnosis

- Fungal infection (ringworm)
  - Occurs most often in the calves.
  - Examine the feet and the nails.
  - Ask about contacts with pets and farm animals.
- Psoriasis
  - Look for lesions at sites typical for psoriasis.
  - Psoriatic nail dystrophy?
  - Psoriasis in the family?
  - Nummular eczema may be impossible to differentiate from psoriasis. In these cases treatment is directed against nummular eczema, and not specifically against psoriasis.
- Superficial basiloma
  - A solitary plaque that has remained silent for a long time (even years).

Treatment

- Some patients respond to a mild corticosteroid preparation, others do not respond even to very potent preparations (Figure 13.16.2).
- In the wet phase (Figure 13.16.3) apply cream on the skin and cover it with wet compresses (water, saline, or sometimes silver nitrate 0.01–0.1%).
- Potassium permanganate
  - Total body bath (dilution 1:25 000) is sometimes necessary. (The solution will stain the bath.)
- SUP or UVB light therapy
- Response to treatment is variable.

Indications for specialist consultation

- If the eczema responds poorly to treatment there may be a need to check the diagnosis and investigate secondary allergies (to preparations used in the treatment), and a need for effective combination therapies.

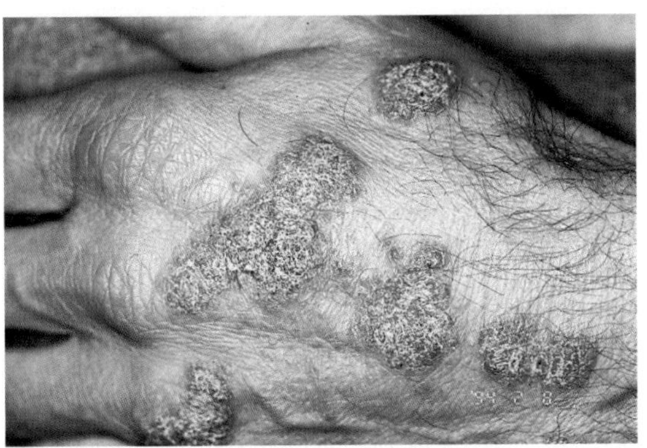

Figure 13.16.2 Crusted, exceptionally florid nummular dermatitis on the back of the hand. Some patients have an atopic background, but mostly no cause initiating this itchy dermatosis is found. The response to therapy varies; sometimes combined therapy with corticoids, different UV sources and emollients is needed. There is some evidence that nummular dermatitis is more therapy-resistant in smokers. Photo © R. Suhonen.

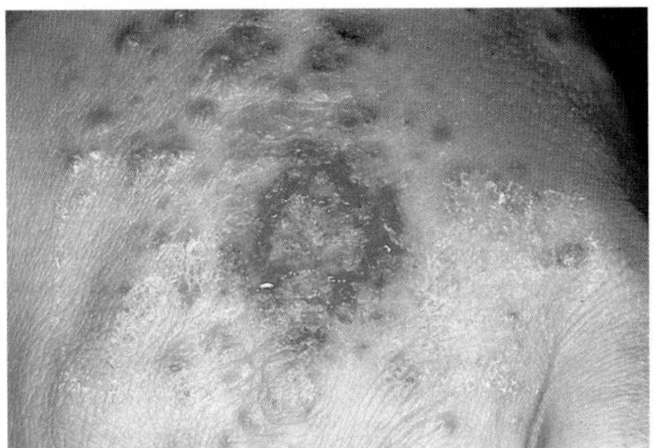

Figure 13.16.3 Nummular eczema may be weeping in the acute phase, as here on the back of the hand. The descriptive character of the diagnosis gives the correct impression of a disease with unknown aetiology. The itching may be quite problematic. Topical corticosteroids are usually beneficial. Photo © R. Suhonen.

13.18 Herpesvirus skin infections

Editors

General notions

- Infections caused by viruses of the Herpesviridae family are the most common viral infections in man.
- Following the primary infection, all herpesviruses can cause a latent infection, which may become reactivated later on.

Human herpesviruses

- This group includes eight herpesviruses:
  - Herpes simplex viruses 1 and 2
  - varicella zoster virus
  - Epstein–Barr virus (causes a febrile disease with mild symptoms in children and mononucleosis in young adults (1.42))
  - cytomegalovirus
  - human herpesviruses types 6–8 (HHV-6–8).
    - HHV-6 causes exanthema subitum in children (31.54).
    - Clinical symptoms caused by type 7 are not yet known.
    - In the majority of Kaposi's sarcoma patients the appearance of HHV-8 antibodies precedes the development of the disease.

HSV1 and HSV2 infections

- Both HSV-1 and HSV-2 are transmitted in direct contact, HSV-1 mainly by other than sexual contact.
- Many HSV-1 infections are subclinical.
- In 1–3-year-olds the primary infection is often a symptomatic stomatitis, with widespread vesicles in the mouth and pharynx. Associated symptoms include fever, pain, nausea, and enlarged lymph nodes (32.20).
- HSV-1 recurs mainly on the lips. Recrudescence may be triggered by external factors (e.g. UV light), hormonal variation or psychological stress.
- Immunodeficiency predisposes to herpesvirus infections.
- In HSV infections affecting the skin, the vesicles usually occur in dense groups (Figure 13.18.1).
- On the skin of the fingers, HSV may cause a painful herpetic abscess.
- Herpes infection around the eye can easily cause keratitis and thus requires consultation with an ophthalmologist (Figure 13.18.2).
- In atopic persons HSV infection may cause widely spread eczema, particularly in the face and head (eczema herpeticum) (Figure 13.18.3)

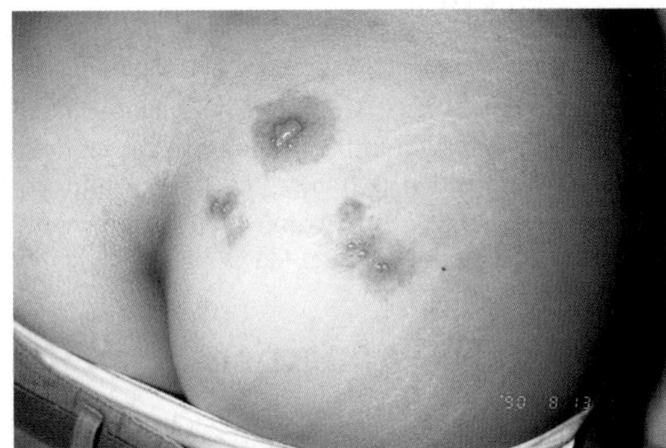

Figure 13.18.1 Recurrent HSV infection is not uncommon in the sacral region. During the recurrence simultaneous pain is possible in the lumbar-genital area. If recurrences are frequent, oral antivirals should be considered—even as continuous prophylactic therapy. Photo © R. Suhonen.

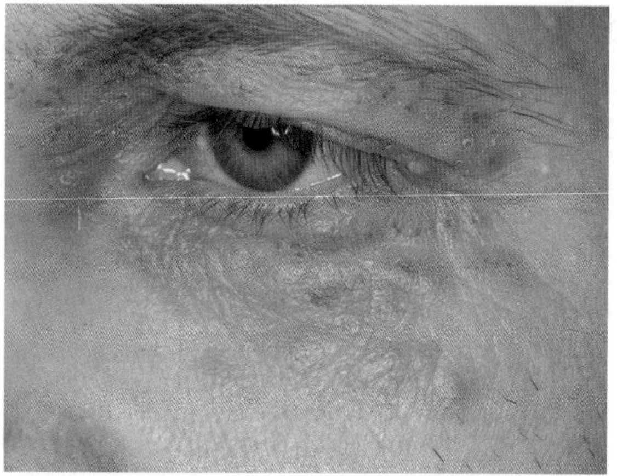

Figure 13.18.2 The recurrent HSV infection is spreading rapidly—eczema herpeticum. Normally immediate therapy by oral acyclovir (or analogues) will stop the progression. In case there are any ocular symptoms an immediate ophthalmologic consultation is indicated. Photo © R. Suhonen.

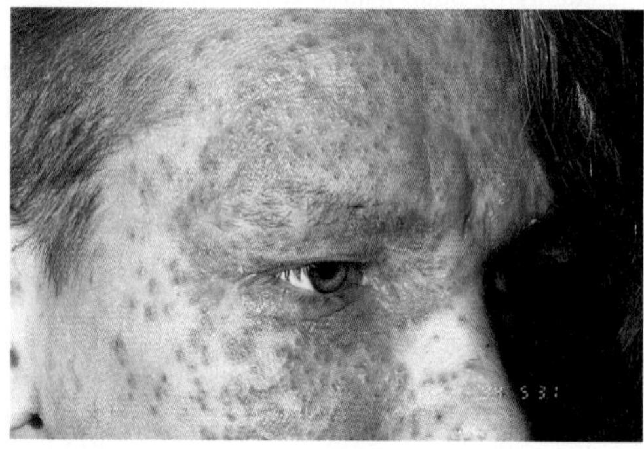

Figure 13.18.3 Recurrence of HSV (or a primary infection) may spread rapidly on the face: eczema herpeticum, i.e. Eruption varicelliformis Kaposi. This eruption must be treated immediately with oral acyclovir or its analogues. This patient with redness in the eyes must be referred to an ophthalmologist immediately (risk of herpes keratitis). Photo © R. Suhonen.

Primary genital herpes

- See article 12.5.
- May be caused by both HSV-1 and HSV-2, and sometimes recurs as a skin infection in the pelvic or sacral regions.
- Neonatal HSV infection is transmitted to the child in the birth canal and causes a serious infection with a mortality of 65% . Incubation time is 2–26 days.

Diagnostics of HSV infections

- Usually based on the clinical picture.
- Virus detection with fluorescent antibody (FA) test is a rapid method.
- Viral culture may succeed if the sample is taken within 3 days from the appearance of vesicles.
- Serology is useful only in primary infections.

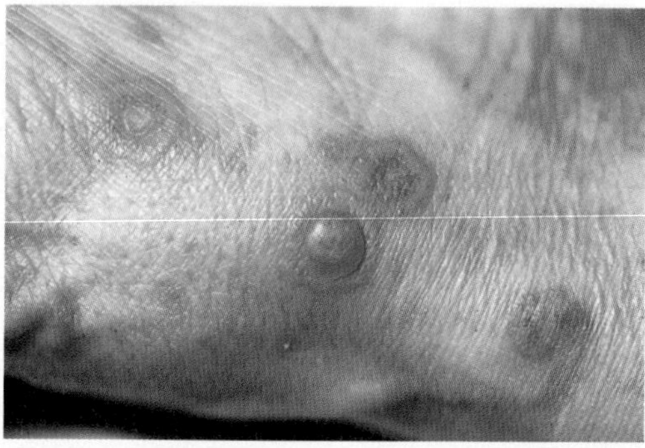

Figure 13.18.4 Erythema multiforme is worthy of its name, with wide variation in expression of the lesions. In this case the clinical picture is typical: target lesions with central bulla formation. Mostly the background of the symptoms remains obscure, but recurrent HSV infection may precede the lesions—or is even found in the multiforme lesions. Photo © R. Suhonen.

Treatment of HSV infections

- Antiviral drugs acyclovic, valacyclovir or famcyclovir can be used for therapy. These drugs prevent viral replication but are not harmful to human cells.
- The therapeutic efficacy of topical forms (cream/ointment) is low (acyclovir, pencyclovir); however, these products reduce pain and burning and are useful in mild recurrent infection (e.g. male genital infections).
- In severe cases the drugs are administered orally: acyclovir 200 mg × 5, valacyclovir 500 mg × 2 or famcyclovir 125 mg × 2 for 5 days.
- Prophylactic therapy should be considered only if the infection recurs 1–2 times a month. For prophylaxis the doses are acyclovir 400 mg × 2 or valacyclovir 250 mg × 2 or 500 mg × 1.

Erythema multiforme

- Recrudescent herpes is one of the most common causes of erythema multiforme. Other causes include e.g. drug eruptions (14.3) and various viral infections.
- The favourite sites of this eczema are the extensor surfaces and it typically appears 1–2 weeks after herpes infection (Figure 13.18.4).
- Oral steroid may alleviate symptoms.

13.20 Erysipelas

Jaakko Karvonen

Basic rules

- Diagnose erysipelas quickly and start antibiotics immediately, preferably parenterally.

♦ Check the skin of the legs if the patient has a high fever without other obvious cause.
♦ Examine the interdigital folds of the toes to detect fungal infection and treat it.

Aetiology

♦ Erysipelas is caused by group A beta-haemolytic streptococci. Usually the skin has to be disrupted for the bacteria to invade it.

Symptoms

♦ High fever of sudden onset (fever may sometimes be absent, particularly in facial erysipelas) (Figure 13.20.1).
♦ Headache and vomiting are common.
♦ A well-demarcated erythema, increased skin temperature, and swelling on the lower leg (Figure 13.20.2), rarely on other skin areas (upper extremities, head).
♦ A delay in treatment may cause bullous or ulcerating skin affection. The bullae may contain blood.

Diagnosis

♦ The clinical picture is often typical. Leukocytosis, high ESR and CRP values are usually observed.
♦ Differential diagnostic problems may be caused by
  • erythema nodosum (often raised nodules) (13.75)
  • deep vein thrombosis
  • early herpes zoster on the face (1.41)
  • severe local allergic reaction, e.g. to local treatments for a leg ulcer
  • erysipelothrix in the hands (1.22)
  • in diabetics Charcot's foot (23.44) (arthropathy most commonly in the ankle, CRP normal)

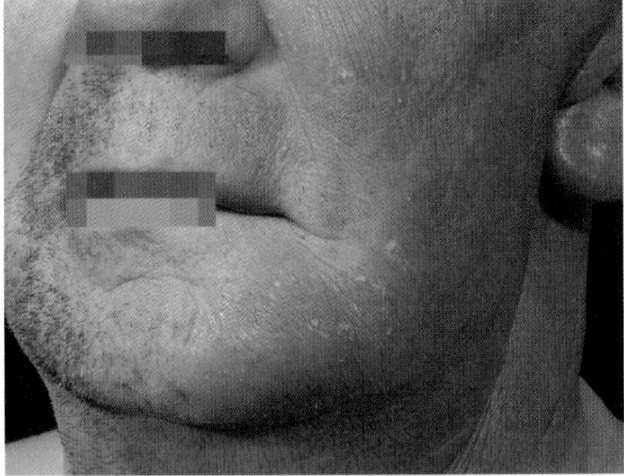

Figure 13.20.1 Sudden rise in body temperature, often malaise and red swelling are typical signs of erysipelas. In the face it may either be in the midline (origin in nose) or unilateral (origin in ear region), but the spread is not limited to the midline like in HZ. Parenteral penicillin is the drug of choice for this life-threatening, almost invariably streptococcal infection. Photo © R. Suhonen.

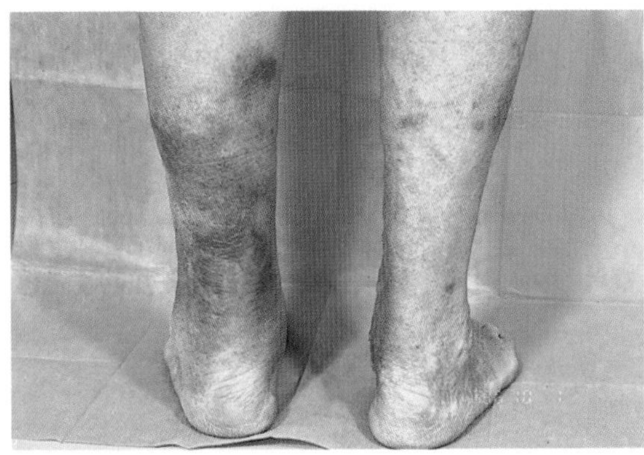

Figure 13.20.2 Erysipelas, an acute, febrile, serious infection commonly affects leg. The infection is almost always caused by group A pyogenic streptococci. Fever may arise very rapidly to a high level, the patient may be confused, the leg is swollen, red, often haemorrhagic/purpuric and bullous lesions may develop. The therapy of choice is intravenous penicillin G. There is a tendency for recurrence. Check toe clefts for tinea and other possible dermatoses. Photo © R. Suhonen.

Treatment

♦ Bed rest, often hospitalization as an emergency
♦ Antibiotics should be started parenterally. Penicillin is the drug of choice, e.g. penicillin G 2 million units × 4 i.v. (procain penicillin 1.2–1.5 million units × 1 i.m. in ambulatory care). After the fever has subsided peroral penicillin (3–4 million units/day) is sufficient.
♦ If the skin ulcerates, or fever lasts for several days despite penicillin medication, a staphyloccal superinfection may be present. First or second-generation cephalosporins or cloxacillin is then the drug of choice.
♦ Patients allergic to penicillin can be treated with clindamycin 350–450 mg × 4 i.v. for 3–5 days, thereafter perorally. If severe (anaphylactic) allergy is not suspected also cephalosporins can be used.
♦ The antibiotics should be continued long enough, at least 3 weeks even in uncomplicated cases and for 6–8 weeks in recurrences. Patients with erysipelas in a leg with swelling caused by poor circulation or with an ulcer also need a long course of antibiotics.
♦ Wet compresses are used in bullous or ulcerating cases. If the skin is intact no local treatment is necessary but even in these cases a wet compress may decrease swelling and bring relief to the patient.
♦ The source of infection, usually interdigital fungal infection, should be identified and treated.

Recurrent erysipelas

♦ In recurring erysipelas (three times within a few years) consider first long-lasting (6–24 months) or even lifelong penicillin prophylaxis. The regimens that can be used are long-acting benzyl penicillin 1.2–1.5 million units i.m. at 3–4 week intervals, or more often if necessary, or peroral penicillin V 1–2 million units/day. Persons allergic to penicillin can usually take first-generation cephalosporins.

13.21 Necrotising fasciitis and gas gangrene

Janne Laine, Janne Mikkola

Aims

- Make a clinical diagnosis quickly.
- Infected tissue must be surgically debrided.
- Follow-up care in a high dependency unit.

Epidemiology

Necrotising fasciitis

- Certain serotypes of group A streptococci (particularly T1M1) may cause invasive infections, the initial clinical picture of which may resemble erysipelas.
- Necrotising fasciitis caused by mixed pathogens (Bacteroides, E.coli, Enterococcus faecalis, etc) often starts from a wound or the genital region (Fournier's gangrene).
  - Nearly half of the patients have no predisposing factors.
  - One patient in three has a history of alcohol abuse.
  - Predisposing factors include rheumatoid arthritis, renal insufficiency, diabetes, puerperium, the neonatal period, immunodeficiency and chickenpox.

Gas gangrene

- Gas gangrene is caused by common clostridia species found in the soil and the intestinal flora.
- May be traumatic or spontaneous, non-traumatic.
- in the latter case, predisposing factors include gastrointestinal surgery, diverticulitis, malignancy or immunodeficiency

Signs and symptoms

- Toxic shock syndrome (fever, diarrhoea, rash, and low blood pressure) (1.70) which is not to be mistaken for febrile gastroenteritis.
- The portal of entry of necrotising fasciitis is usually a site of minor trauma or an infected postoperative wound
  - Symptoms include a rapid onset of swelling, redness and very severe pain.
  - The skin may blister and discolour to a purplish red. The skin manifestations may be misleadingly slight. The subcutaneous tissue becomes gangrenous.
- In gas gangrene, the necrotic wound becomes swollen with palpable crepitus.
- The swelling spreads quickly (within hours), in suspected cases repeated clinical assessment is important.
- In gas gangrene bacterial staining of a tissue sample may show large gram-positive rods. A sample should be sent for an anaerobic culture (tissue swabs transported in Stuart's transport medium or other suitable anaerobic tube).

Treatment

- The treatment of necrotising fasciitis and gas gangrene is urgent surgical debridement. All infected tissue and the overlying skin must be removed.
- Prescribe a broad-spectrum intravenous antibiotic (e.g. imipenem 1 g t.d.s.) (Staph. aureus, Clostridium perfringens and various mixed infections may cause a similar clinical picture). When streptococcal aetiology has been confirmed, prescribe benzylpenicillin 2 million IU intravenously every four hours.
- Hyperbaric oxygen, in combination with surgical debridement and antibiotics, may be beneficial in the treatment of necrotising fascitis caused by mixed pathogens. However, transportation to a hyperbaric oxygen therapy site must not delay radical surgery by more than one hour.

Prevention

- When treating deep contaminated and ragged wounds all devitalized tissue must be debrided.

13.22 Impetigo and other pyoderma

Pekka Autio

Aims

- Impetigo should always be treated because it spreads easily in the family, daycare centre and school.
- Bacterial cultures and antibiograms should be used to determine antibiotic susceptibilities.
- Remember the possibility of post-infectious glomerulonephritis in streptococcal impetigo.

Clinical features

- Children are most commonly affected.

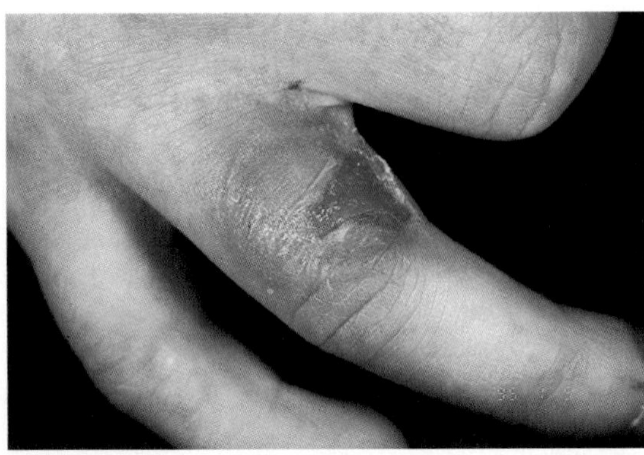

Figure 13.22.1 Staphylococcus aureus infection on the side of a finger. Bulla formation is typical of certain strains of staphylococci. Photo © R. Suhonen.

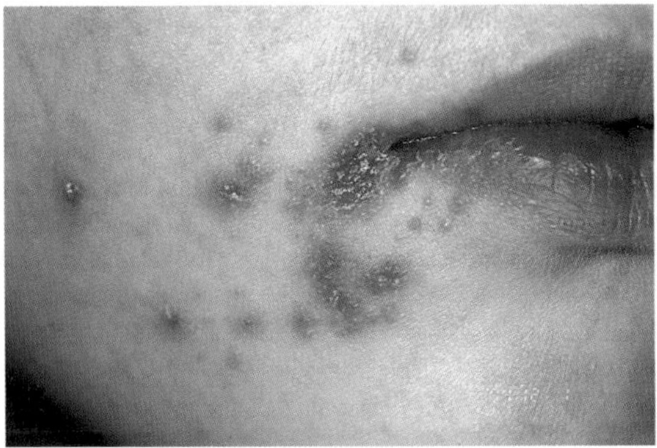

Figure 13.22.2 The angular region of the lips is a common site for impetigo contagiosa as well as for atopic dermatitis. In young persons, both diseases are typical at this location, often causing a mixed disease, as here. The eradication of bacterial infection (here S. aureus with follicular "satellites") as well as therapy and prevention of dermatitis are needed. Photo © R. Suhonen.

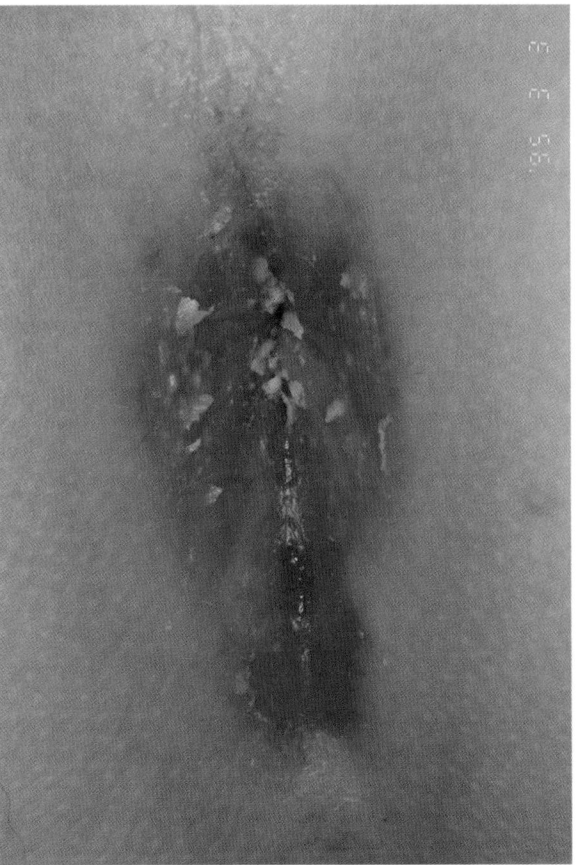

Figure 13.22.3 Perianal streptococcal dermatitis is a relatively common disease. The clinical picture is fairly typical, with bright red skin around the anus. Bacterial culture confirms the clinical diagnosis. Oral antibiotics are needed for cure. The main confusing diagnosis is candidal infection. If both group A pyogenic streptococcus and Candida albicans are found simultaneously, the latter is probably saprophytic; treat the streptococcus. Photo © R. Suhonen.

- Streptococcal infection typically makes crusts or small ulcerations; staphylococcal infection tends to make blisters (Figure 13.22.1).
- "Pemphigus neonatorum" in infants is actually impetigo. The infection is caused by S. aureus phage type II.
- The crusts usually appear in the surroundings of the nostrils, on the chin, and generally on the face (Figure 13.22.2).
- Thick crusts are characteristic.

Differential diagnosis

- Primary herpes simplex infection may resemble impetigo.
- Ringworm (Tinea corporis)
- If impetigo tends to recur in the scalp and neck consider the possibility of head lice.

Causative agents

- Group A beta-haemolytic streptococci (Figure 13.22.3)
- Staphylococcus aureus
- Eczema may predispose the skin to impetigo.
- The infection usually spreads by autoinoculation.
- Recurrences are caused by bacteria remaining in the nostrils.

Treatment

- Treatment is started on the basis of the clinical presentation.
- If the disease is confined to a small area the treatment consists of soaking the crusts so that they are detached, and applying an antibiotic ointment (sodium fusidate **B** [1 2] or a combination of neomycin and bacitracin e.g.).
- If the disease is more widespread (>6 cm^2) use a systemic antibiotic (first generation cephalosporin, e.g. cephalexin or cefadroxil 50 mg/kg daily for 7–10 days **B** [3] or amoxicillin-clavulanic acid. Patients with cephalosporin allergy can be treated with clindamycin.
- Macrolides are no longer recommended **D**.
- If the patient has eczema a topical preparation containing a corticosteroid and an antimicrobial agent should be used

together with systemic antibiotics until the skin is intact. Do not forget further treatment of the eczema.

- The most common reasons for poor response to treatment:
  - The diagnosis is incorrect. The patient has scabies, lice, or ringworm.
  - The crusts have not been soaked and removed. The bacteria can survive under crusts.
  - The underlying eczema has not been treated.
  - The nostrils serve as reservoir for bacteria (apply neomycin-bacitracin ointment into the nostrils. Mupirocin should not be used for this disease as its use should be limited to the eradication of methicillin-resistant Staphylococcus aureus) (D).

References

1. White DG, Collins PO, Rowsell RB. Topical antibiotics in the treatment of superficial skin infections in general practice—a comparison of mupirocin with sodium fusidate. Journal of Infection 1989;18:221–9.
2. Morley PA, Munot LD. A comparison of sodium fusidate ointment and mupirocin ointment in superficial skin sepsis. Current Medical Research and Opinion 1988;11:142–8.
3. Demidovich CW, Wittler RR, Ruff ME, Bass JW, Browning WC. Impetigo. Current etiology and comparison of penicillin, erythromycin, and cephalexin therapies. Am J Dis Child 1990;144:1313–5.

13.23 Skin abscess and folliculitis

Jaakko Karvonen

Basic rule

- Uncomplicated superficial abscesses should be treated by incision and drainage without antibiotics.

Aetiology and terminology

- The causative agent is usually **Staphylococcus aureus**.
- If the infection affects only the hair follicle the condition is called folliculitis (Figure 13.23.1)
- If the infection spreads into the surrounding skin and subcutaneous tissue the condition is called furunculosis.
- Sycosis barbae is deep folliculitis in the beard region.

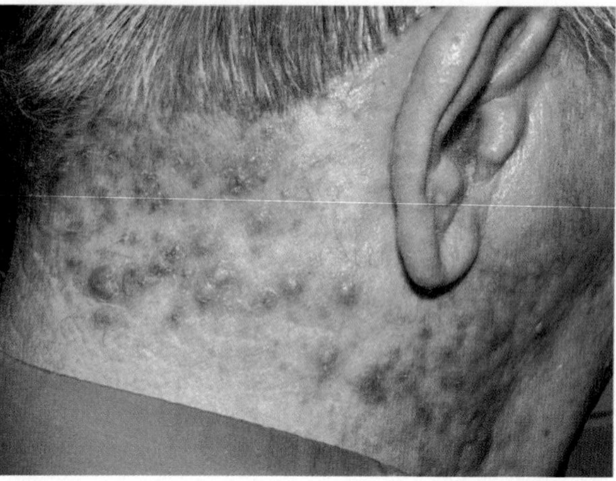

Figure 13.23.1 Staphylococcal folliculitis is relatively common in the hairy neck area. In spite of combined topical and oral antibacterial medication recurrences are common. Photo © R. Suhonen.

Treatment

- Topical antiseptic preparations (e.g. chlorhexidine) are usually sufficient in superficial folliculitis. Antibiotic creams (e.g. neomycin) can be used temporarily. On hairy skin mild folliculitis is a physiological phenomenon that need not always be treated.
- Deep or widely spread folliculitis is an indication for systemic antibiotics effective against staphylococci.
- Sycosis barbae is always an indication for systemic antibiotics.
- Surgical incision and drainage (Figure 13.23.2) without antibiotics is the treatment of choice for a superficial abscess (B) [1 2 3]. Antibiotic treatment is indicated, if
  - the patient has fever or general symptoms
  - the abscess is large and tissue damage extensive
  - the abscess is located in the nasal region
  - concomitant diseases make the patient susceptible to infections (diabetes, immune deficiency, artificial joint, use of corticosteroids).

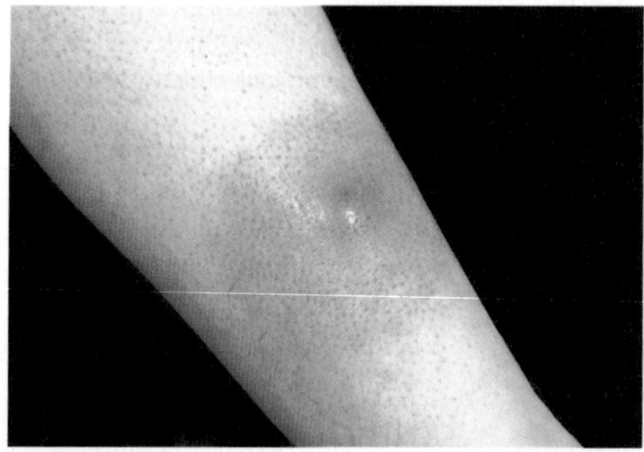

Figure 13.23.2 Staphylococcus aureus was the causative agent of this carbuncle. Oral antibiotic therapy and subsequent surgical drainage of the boil should be performed without delay. Photo © R. Suhonen.

- The drug of choice is first generation cephalosporine (500 mg × 3, children 50 mg/kg/day). Alternatively, amoxicillin-clavulanic acid or cloxacillines can be used.
- In case of recurrent abscess, hygiene is improved, antibacterial lotions or creams are used, and in severe cases (more than 3 recurrences in 6 months), clindamycin 150 mg × 1 is given as preventive medication for three months.

References

1. Llera JL, Levy RC. Treatment of cutaneous abscess: a double-blind clinical study. Annals of Emergency Medicine 1985;14:15–9.
2. Macfie J, Harvey J. The treatment of acute superficial abscesses: a prospective clinical trial. Br J Surg 1977;64:264–6.
3. Stewart MP, Laing MR, Krukowski ZH. Treatment of acute abscesses by incision, curettage and primary suture without antibiotics: a controlled clinical trial. Br J Surg 1985;72:66–7.

13.30 Warts (verruca vulgaris)

Pekka Autio

Aims

- Conservative treatment or spontaneous recovery yields the best cosmetic result. Because a wart is an epidermal viral tumour its treatment should not destroy the dermis. Avoid operations leading to scar formation.

General

- Warts caused by Papilloma viruses are common in all age groups. Details on their epidemiology are poorly known.
- There is no evidence to suggest measures to avoid Papilloma virus infections. Do not impose restrictions on your patient. An innocent viral disease is less of a burden than efforts to avoid it.
- Warts are not precancerous lesions (with the exception of genital warts).

Diagnosis

- Elevated (filiform) warts occur on the face.
- On the extremities the warts are only slightly elevated and their surface is often broken by fissures (Figures 13.30.1 and 13.30.3).
- In the nail cuticula, and particularly in the soles and heels, the warts present as flat mosaic. In the soles they compress the deeper structures and are painful. A clavus often develops around a plantar wart. The diagnosis of a wart is clinically confirmed by point haemorrhages caused by cutting the wart horizontally with a scalpel or paring it.
- Young persons may have flat warts (Verruca plana) affecting the dorsa of the hands and the face.
- Surgical excision in order to obtain a biopsy is necessary only if the diagnosis is not clear. A traumatically haemorrhagic plantar wart may be difficult to differentiate from a melanoma.

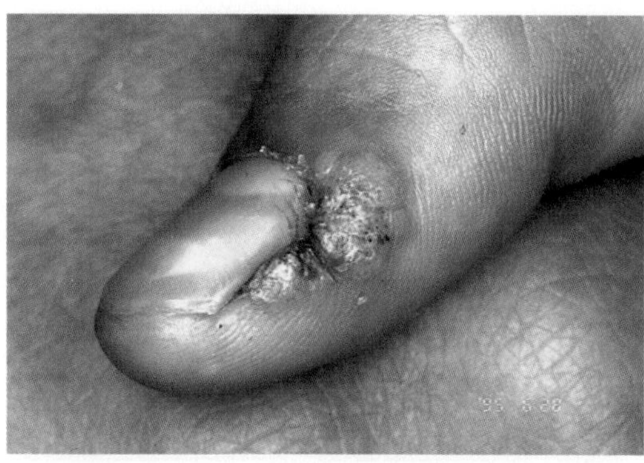

Figure 13.30.1 Characteristic common warts in the lateral nail fold of a schoolboy. A single treatment session of cryotherapy yielded an excellent result. Photo © R. Suhonen.

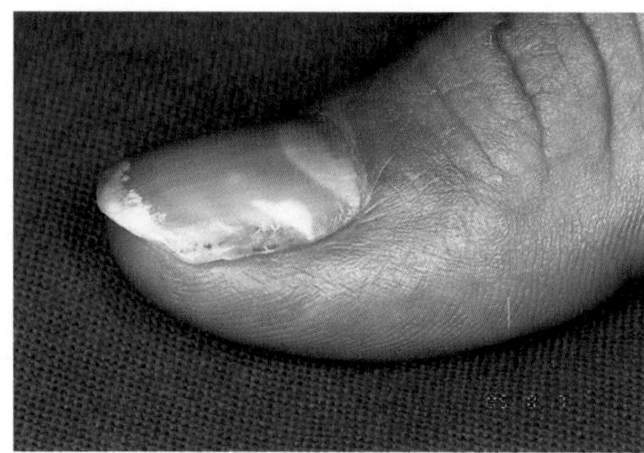

Figure 13.30.2 The same nail as in Figure 13.30.1. The white band in the nail plate, a temporary keratinization disturbance caused by the cryotherapy, will travel distally with the growing nail and disappear. A minor deformity of the nail is seen distally, caused by the pressure from the wart. New nail growth is normal. The cryotherapy did not harm the morphology of the nail fold. Photo © R. Suhonen.

Prevention

- There is no evidence on the effect of preventive measures. Do not burden the patient with unnecessary "advice".

Conservative treatment

- Over-the-counter preparations and 40% salicylic acid  [1] tapes are the first choice.

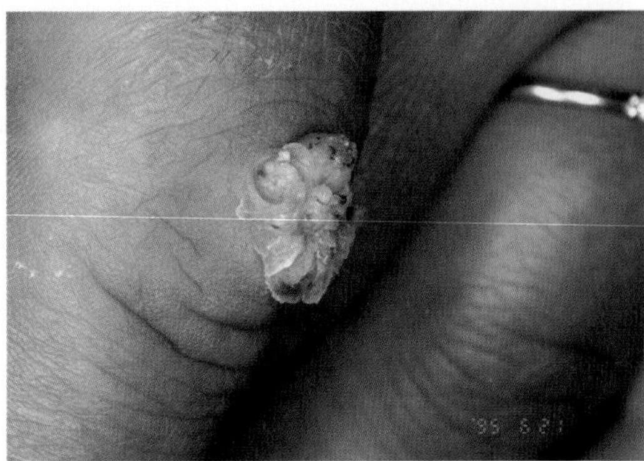

Figure 13.30.3 A cauliflower-resembling common wart at the PIP joint of a finger. A single treatment session with liquid nitrogen spray was successful. Photo © R. Suhonen.

- Paring of the wart after soaking it or without soaking is essential before the drug is applied.
- After the medicine has dried on the wart it can be covered with a hydrocolloid patch.
- The response to treatment is slow. Do not book a control visit in less than 2 months' time.
- The pain caused by plantar warts is relieved soon after treatment has made the warts thinner.
- For flat warts, waiting is best; aggressive treatment efforts may spread the warts. Topical tretinoin cream can be used according to the tolerance of the skin.
- Imiquimod has been suggested to be effective against common warts .

Mechanical removal, electrocauterization, and cryotherapy

- Facial warts can be removed with a curette even without local anaesthesia, with a good cosmetic outcome. The operation causes less bleeding if electrocauterization of the wart (without anaesthesia) is performed first.
- The use of a local anaesthetic bears the risk of cauterizing too deeply, resulting in a scar.
- Common warts of the extremities can be electrocauterized without anaesthesia and wiped away (Figure 13.30.3).
- Plantar warts on the soles need prolonged treatment (Figure 13.30.4). If the patient is not prepared to have them treated conservatively and active treatment is wanted the doctor can curette the warts after local anaesthesia and cauterize the base with care. However, there is a risk of scars, even keloids. Surgical excision is not recommended because keloids may develop and the warts often recur in the operative scar.
- Freezing with liquid nitrogen yields good results (Figure 13.30.2). Effective freezing of the sole is painful and may require local anaesthesia. However, the pain is less than that associated with laser treatment, and freezing is much less expensive.
- Carbon dioxide laser treatment is expensive, and the results are not dramatically better than with other treatment modalities. Its use is best justified in the treatment of therapy-resistant plantar warts.

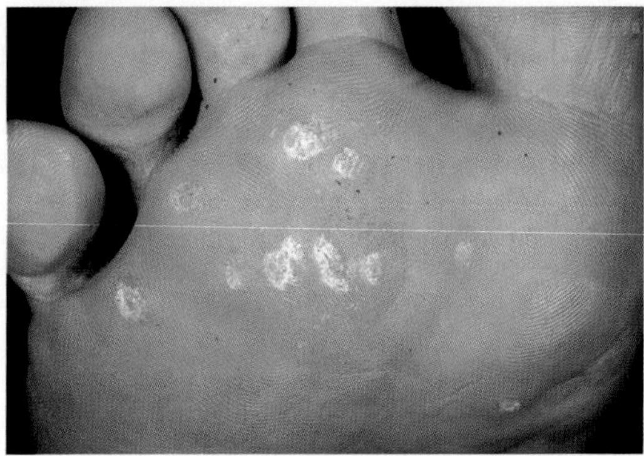

Figure 13.30.4 The plantar wart is a real challenge to medicine. The wide selection of therapeutic approaches is symbolic of the difficulty of eradicating this simple viral disease. A plantar wart is often painful when walking. It is best to start any therapy with paring of the hyperkeratotic layers. Keratolytics combined with regular filing may help, cryosurgery or laser are painful. The best help to the patient and doctor alike is the spontaneous healing tendency of viral warts. Photo © R. Suhonen.

Indications for specialist consultation

- The indications for specialist consultation are not purely medical, and the tolerance of the patient and doctor play a role.

Reference

1. Gibbs S, Harvey I, Sterling JC, Stark R. Local treatments for cutaneous warts. Cochrane Database Syst Rev. 2004;(2):CD001781.

13.31 Molluscum contagiosum

Pekka Autio

Basic rule

- Lesions disappear spontaneously without treatment. If a cooperating child has just a few papules, healing can be speeded by mechanical means.

Epidemiology

- Molluscum contagiosum is common in children, particularly in those with atopic dry skin (Figure 13.31.1). Apparently the development of specific immunity prevents recurrence.

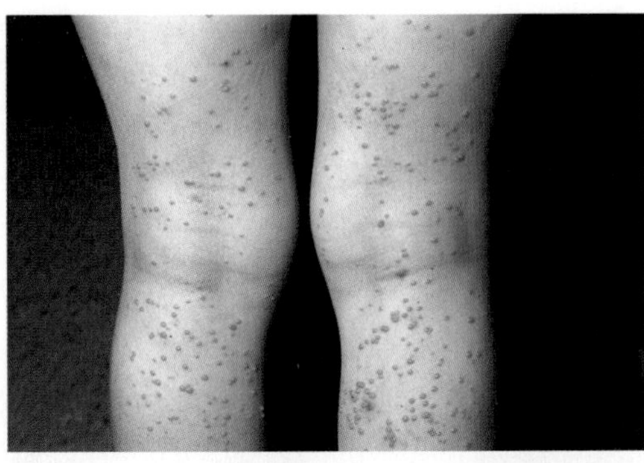

Figure 13.31.1 Mollusca contagiosa are small viral tumours most common in children. Atopic persons are especially prone to suffer. Good spontaneous tendency for cure allows to wait for quite a long time before starting therapy. There is no specific therapy. Older children may allow cautious freezing with liquid nitrogen (spray technique, no frozen halo, no aesthetic risks). Other methods (forceps, needle, curette) for abolishing individual molluscae are used commonly. Use of a topical analgesic (e.g. prilocain) may improve patient compliance. Photo © R. Suhonen.

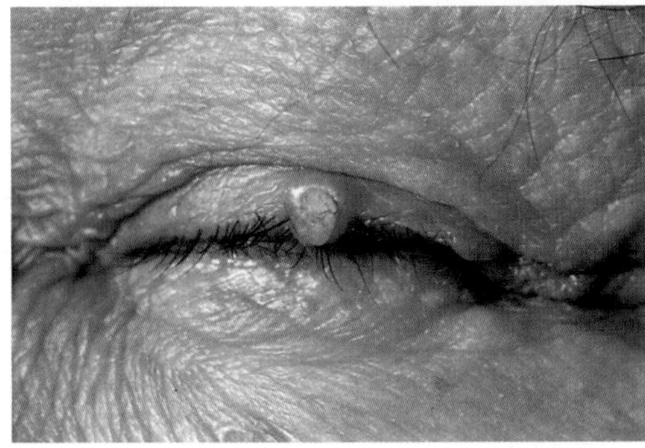

Figure 13.31.2 The tumour at the margin of the upper eyelid is molluscum contagiosum. The patient is an elderly female on cytostatic medication. Molluscum contagiosum in adult patients should lead to the consideration of the possibility of an immunologic disturbance. However, AIDS cannot be diagnosed on the presence of molluscum contagiosum alone! The majority of adult patients with molluscae are otherwise healthy. Photo © R. Suhonen.

- There is no reason for limiting contacts with other children because of an innocent common virus, and the child can attend daycare or school normally.
- Papules sometimes occur in adults. Numerous papules may be a sign of immunodeficiency, e.g. HIV infection.

Diagnostics

- Typical lesions presenting as small papules (of a few mm) with dimpling in the centre cause no problems as regards differential diagnosis, particularly when they are numerous (Figure 13.31.2).
- In a very early stage the typical features may be lacking, and a single papule may be difficult to identify. In an adult patient it may resemble an early basal cell carcinoma or sebaceous gland hyperplasia.

Treatment

- Active treatment of the first few papules may stop the spread of the disease. The simplest treatment is to break the papule with special forceps, a needle, or curette. In a child local lidocaine/prilocaine cream for 20–30 min before the procedure ensures adequate anaesthesia (B) [1]. Its application on of large areas of the skin is not recommended.
- Cryotherapy with liquid nitrogen is effective but not totally painless.
- If mechanical treatment of a child patient cannot be performed without struggling it is better to wait for spontaneous healing.
- In adults curettage without anaesthesia is an adequate treatment. Remember the possibility of HIV infection.
- General anaesthesia is not indicated for the treatment of lesions. Treating atopic eczema coexisting with molluscum contagiosum lesions with corticosteroids and emollients does not appear to compromise the healing of lesions, and it helps the patient.

Complications

- If all lesions become irritated and eczema develops around them the probable cause is the onset of an immune response and not a bacterial infection.
- If pyoderma develops it should be treated with antibiotics. In practice, true pyoderma are seen rather rarely.

Indications for specialist consultation

- There is no real indication for specialist consultation. The general practitioner can treat all lesions.

Reference

1. de Waard van der Spek FB, Oranje AP, Lillieborg S, Hop WC, Stolz E. Treatment of molluscum contagiosum using a lidocaine/prilocaine cream (EMLA) for analgesia. J Am Acad Dermatol 1990;23:685–8.

13.40 Scabies

Pekka Autio

Basic rules

- Treatment given "just in case" may cause problems. Aim at diagnosis.

- Scabies is easily transmitted: it is important to treat all members of the same household, not only those with symptoms.
- Clothes and bed clothes must be washed and either heated or frozen.

Epidemiology

- Scabies is not a sexually transmitted disease, but sharing a bed is a common source of infection.
- Scabies may be transmitted in a short contact, even at physical examination.

Symptoms

- Itch, especially in the evening and during the night, is most intensive in the buttocks, wrists and folds between the fingers.
- The symptoms commence a few weeks after inoculation. In reinfections the latent period is shorter.
- Avoid attempts at determining the time of inoculation in individual patients.

Diagnosis

- Annoying itch
- Varying papules, vesicles, and signs of scratching on the skin (Figure 13.40.1). The face is not affected in adults (with the exception of patients with mental retardation or immunosuppression who have rare generalized scabies).
- Intraepidermal burrows made by female scabies mites are seen nearly always in the wrist folds, between fingers (Figures 13.40.2 and 13.40.3), and in children also in the palms and soles. The mite can be easily extracted from its burrow, using a stereomicroscope, to be identified under an ordinary microscope.

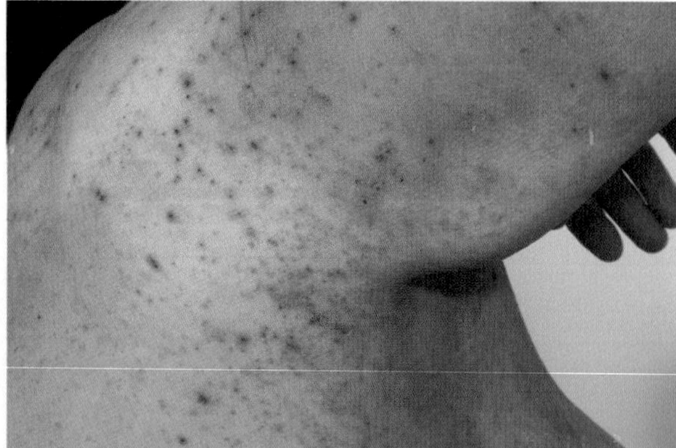

Figure 13.40.1 Old lady with itchy dermatosis for six months: examine the hands and wrists properly. The scratch marks come from scabies mites unless otherwise proven. Verify the diagnosis with 100% accuracy; long-lasting scabies in an old-age home has transmitted the disease to multiple contacts—it is better to be sure of the diagnosis. Photo © R. Suhonen.

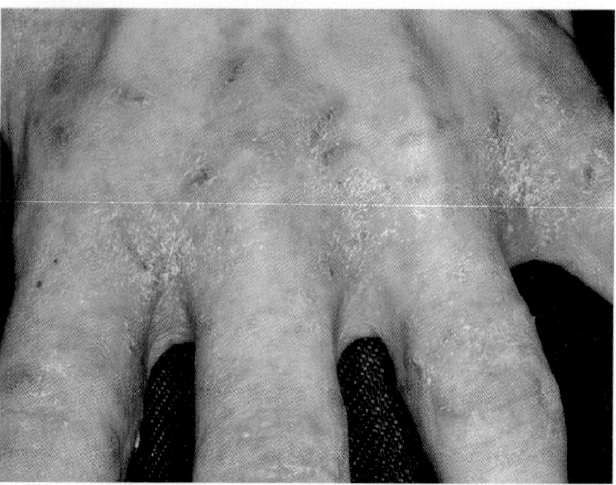

Figure 13.40.2 Secondarily infected, eczematous scabietic infestation in the finger webs. The easiest and most reliable way to confirm the diagnosis is to pick a single scabies mite on the object glass for microscopy. Stereoscopic microscopy is valuable help in this procedure. Photo © R. Suhonen.

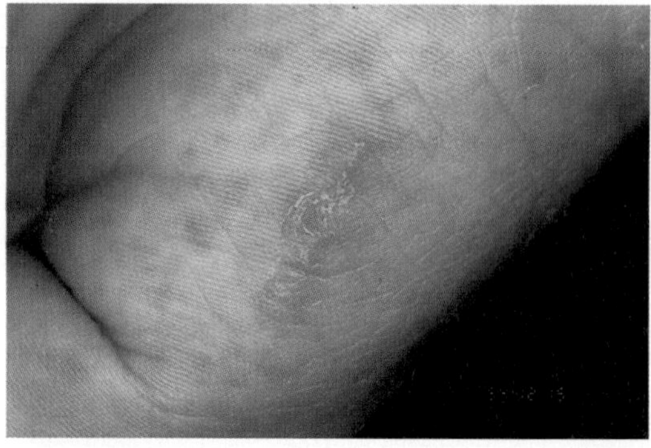

Figure 13.40.3 Scabies on the side of the hand. The female Sarcoptes scabiei mite can be seen as a darker spot at the end of its tunnel. Picking the mite on the object glass and looking at it with the laboratory microscope is quite convincing to the patient and very helpful should there arise problems later in therapy. Photo © R. Suhonen.

- Itching, erythematous papules in male genitalia suggest scabies.
- Do not forget to look at the wrists and between the fingers of the mother of a child with suspected scabies.

Differential diagnosis

- Vesicles may resemble those occurring in eczema.
- Folliculitis may resemble scabies. The typical localisation of the lesions and the occurrence of symptoms in other persons living in the same household suggest scabies.

Treatment

- Permethrin cream is a safe treatment for scabies 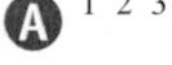 [1 2 3]
  - The cream is applied all over the skin from toes to apex, including the folds between the fingers and genitals.

The drug should be washed away after 8–15 hours. The hands should not be washed during treatment, or the drug must be applied again after washing. During treatment clothes that have touched the skin and bed clothes are washed.
- The package contains detailed instructions on how to destroy the mites in clothes with cold and hot. The manufacturer also recommends treating clothes once with permethrin. One course of treatment may suffice, but the response can be ensured by giving a new course of treatment after one week, mainly because the treatment of many family members simultaneously often results in failure to complete the treatment.

- After treatment the patient may have itching papules for longer than one month. The condition need not be treated unless mites are discovered. The itch and secondary dermatitis can be treated with mild corticosteroids and chlorhexidin cream, and more potent corticosteroids can be applied on solitary papules.
- Not uncommonly a false diagnosis or two coexistent diseases is the reason for a poor response to treatment. In problematic cases it is often revealed that only symptomatic family members have been treated.
- A dermatologist should be consulted in therapy-resistant cases.

References

1. Walker GJA, Johnstone PW. Interventions for treating scabies. Cochrane Database Syst Rev. 2004;(2):CD000320.
2. Brown S, 2002 J, Bady W. Treatment of ectoparasitic infections: review of the English-language literature, 1982–1992. Clin Infect Dis 1995;20(suppl 1):pp. 104–109.
3. The Database of Abstracts of Reviews of Effectiveness (University of York), Database no.: DARE-950852. In: The Cochrane Library, Issue 4, 1999. Oxford: Update Software.

13.41 Head lice and pubic lice

Pekka Autio

Symptoms

- Itching and red papules in the scalp and pubic hair.
- Secondary pyodermia often develops in the scalp, and the lymph nodes in the nuchal region become enlarged.
- Pubic lice make red bite marks that cause severe itch in the genital area.
- In children pubic lice from the parents may reside in the eyelashes, and there may be vague bluish maculae on the trunk (“maculae coerulae”).

Diagnosis

- Nits (louse eggs) are visible in the hair and pubic hair. Nits can remain in hair for months, which is why only nits found less than 6 mm from the scalp are a definite sign of living parasites (hair grows approximately 1 mm in a month). Nits are best found with a louse comb.
- Pubic louse nits also typically occur in the hair of the anterior thorax and eyelashes.
- Do not mix the “hair cast” phenomenon (a ring of dandruff that glides along the hair) with nits. A nit does not glide but is strongly attached to the hair.
- In children the diagnosis of pubic lice can be based on maculae coerulae and nits in the eyelashes.

Treatment

- Application of permethrin shampoo (A) [1 2 3 4] according to the instructions in the package.
- If this is not effective, malathion shampoo or solution can be used.
- Nits should be combed away with a louse comb (distance between tooths 0.2–0.3 mm) from the very root of the hair. Other combs and brushes are washed with the above-mentioned shampoos.
- In daycare centres and schools the whole community should be alerted to the problem.

References

1. Vander Stichele RH, Dezeure EM, Bogaert MG. Systematic review of clinical efficacy of topical treatments for head lice. BMJ 1995;311:604–608.
2. Dodd CS. Interventions for treating headlice. Cochrane Database Syst Rev. 2004;(2):CD001165.
3. Vander Stichele RH, Dezeure EM, Bogaert MG. Systematic review of clinical efficacy of topical treatment of head lice. BMJ 1995;311:604–608.
4. The Database of Abstracts of Reviews of Effectiveness (University of York), Database no.: DARE-952233. In: The Cochrane Library, Issue 4, 1999. Oxford: Update Software.

13.42 Insect bites and stings

Editors

Complications caused by bites and stings

- Hymenoptera stings may cause an anaphylactic reaction.
- Ticks spread borreliosis and tick-borne encephalitis.
- Mosquitoes spread malaria, tularemia, and arbovirus diseases (Alphavirus, Flavivirus and Bunyavirus genera) with potentially dangerous consequences (serous encephalitis).

Diptera (mosquitoes and flies)

Mosquitoes

- Mosquito sting causes a rapidly developing urticaria-like papule that almost always disappears spontaneously but that may also result in a long-lasting, itching papule in sensitized persons. In the autumn mosquitoes may cause large papules, even vesicles, in the Mediterranean region.

Black fly (Simuliidae) (Buffalo gnat)

- Black flies may also bite under clothing. Many develop a reaction of papules that may last to up to a few weeks. Some people become allergic to black flies and may get a local oedematous reaction.

Biting midge (Culicoides)

- The biting midge is smaller that the black fly and may be found in large swarms. They penetrate through mosquito nets also to city houses and may sting under the bed linen.

Deer louse fly (ked) Lipoptena cervi

- May cause isolated papules on the scalp, especially in the neck that last for up to months.
- Causes problems late in the summer.
- Common in Eastern Europe.
- Insect repellents are not efficient.

Horsefly (gady) (Tabanidae)

- A horsefly bite often causes a large swollen papule with a watery spot in the middle.

Hymenoptera

- Hymenopterous insects cause the most dangerous allergic reactions.
- Sometimes the anaphylactic reaction leads to death.
- A wasp, (honey)bee or bumblebee sting causes severe pain and swelling at the site of the sting immediately.
- Sensitization to hymenoptera venom causes many anaphylactic reactions annually.

Lice (Anoplura)

- Head lice epidemics may occur in schools or day care centres.
- Body lice affect homeless persons.
- Body lice are found in the seams of clothes.
- Regular washing of the clothes in a washing machine is sufficient to sterilize the clothes.

Bedbugs (Cimicidae)

- Occurs in old, dirty buildings.
- Sucks blood at nights causing lumps on the skin.

Fleas

- Fleas carried by birds, squirrels (fur farmers) and rats also bite humans. Fleas carried by man, dog and cat are very rare or extinct.
- Symptoms occur most frequently in the spring when people are out in the nature (cleaning bird nests, visiting summer houses for the first time, etc).
- Fleas cause solid, intensely itching papule with a biting mark in the middle, usually in groups of a few bites (Figure 13.42.1). Apparently, fleas often cause a papular urticaria that children sometimes have in the summer (strophulus).
- The patient usually has no idea of the cause of the rash.

Larvae

- The larvae of some moths (Lepidoptera) may cause both toxic and allergic reactions.

Ticks

- The Ixodes ricinus tick spreads borreliosis (1.29), Kumlinge tick-borne encephalitis virus and Uukuniemi virus.
- The best protection is to wear long boots and trousers when walking in the nature (ticks are found in the grass not in trees).
- Bird (chicken farmers), dog and cat ticks often cause groups of a few itching papules on the extremities and the trunk in areas covered by clothing. A biting mark is seen in the middle of the papule.

Spiders

- The bite of the European garden spider (Araneus diadematus) may be painful.
- The bite of a big bird spider is not dangerous.

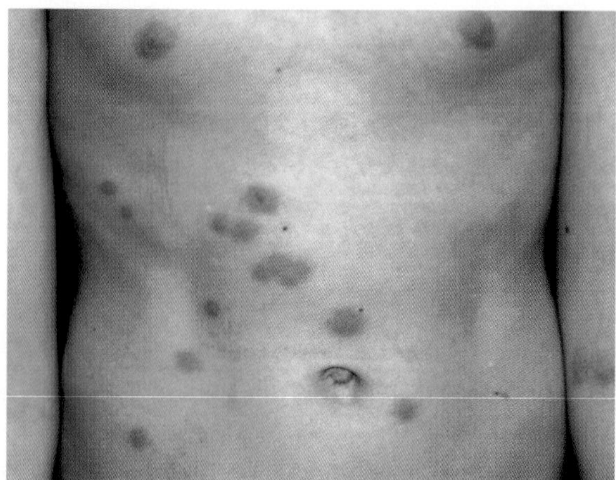

Figure 13.42.1 Insect bite reaction, typically grouped in 2-5 red, itchy papules. Bird fleas or Cheyletiella from dogs or cats are common causes of this clinical picture. The symptoms appear only in those persons specifically sensitized to the causative parasite. Only symptomatic therapy is needed, but the source of the parasite (dog, cat) should be desinfected. Photo © R. Suhonen.

Therapy for reactions caused by insect bites

Hymenoptera bites

- After a bee has stung, the sting and the attached venom pouch remain in the skin. The sting is removed as quickly as possible, preferably within two seconds. Whether one squeezes the venom pouch or not is not as significant as muscles attached to the pouch will continue to pump the venom after the bee has detached itself. The sting of a wasp and a bumblebee is removed from the skin when the insect detaches itself.
- Cold compress is a good first aid for hymenoptera stings. Persons who have been stung several times should be observed for an hour in case systemic symptoms develop.
- **Severe anaphylactic reactions**: The patient must avoid exposure and carry and adrenaline injection at all times (Epipen®). If the patient has taken the adrenaline injection, 50 mg of predniso(lo)ne is given. For first aid, see 14.1. Consult a dermatologist or an allergologist always when your patient reports of swelling associated with the sting that is not limited to the site of the sting, of dyspnoea or collapse. Desensitization therapy may need to be considered; however, it is not a routine solution. The therapy has its risks, it is not known how long the therapy should continue, it does not abolish other therapies and is costly.

Other stings and bites

- In mild local reactions hydrocortisone cream is sufficient. Sometimes secondary bacterial infection requires treatment. Oedema that blocks the eye does not necessitate automatically oral steroids or other special therapy.
- An antihistamine tablet taken preferably before exposure may diminish symptoms. In double-blind studies, cetirizine has been shown to alleviate symptoms.
- Severe reactions require a steroid course of a few days, e.g. prednisolone 30 mg/day.

13.50 Dermatomycoses

Editors

Basic rules

- Before starting treatment make sure that the patient has dermatomycosis and not another skin disease resembling it. Take a specimen for fungal culture; however, in typical tinea found only between the toes this is not necessary.
- Remember the adverse effects of fungicidal drugs and the interactions of azole drugs with other drugs.

Infectiousness

- Exposure to fungi is common. Infections are much more uncommon.
- Genetic factors play a role in the infectiousness of nail and foot mycoses.
- Mycoses of animals (e.g. cows, guinea pigs, cats) spread easily to humans and cause ringworm on the extremities, trunk, and face.

DER

Obtaining a specimen for fungal culture

- Clean the skin with an alcohol-ether solution and scratch scales from the margin of the lesion into a dry tube and send the specimen to the laboratory by ordinary mail. Hair can also be taken or slices can be cut from a nail as specimens and scales can be scratched from the nail matrix.
- The laboratory performs native microscopy with potassium hydroxide and a fungal culture.
- There is a delay of 2–6 weeks before the results of the culture are available.
- If the result is negative and mycosis is strongly suspected, take a new sample.

Antimycotic spectra of the drugs

General properties

- Modern drugs have shortened the treatments and improved the results. However, a permanent cure (= clinical cure after follow-up of 1–2 years) is obtained in less than half of the patients.
- Ringworm should usually be treated with topical drugs (A) [1], whereas most cases of onychomycosis require systemic medication.

Indications

- Terbinafine (cream and tablets) are effective only against dermatophytes.
- Nystatin and natamycin are effective only against yeasts.
- Topical azoles (clotrimazole, econazole, miconazole, thioconazole, ketoconazole), amorolfine (cream and nail varnish), and systemic ketokonazole, itraconazole, and fluconazole are effective against both dermatophytes and yeasts. There are no significant differences in the efficacy of the topical drugs.

Adverse effects and interactions

- The risk of interactions with terbinafine is apparently small. A typical but rare side effect is impairment or even complete loss of the sense of taste for 1–2 months. Some cases of drug exanthema have also been described. They may vary from mild symptomless or itching exanthemata to serious blister-forming erythema multiforme that may last for more than a month.

- Ketoconazole may affect liver function in some patients, and its use should be restricted to short periods.
- Itraconazole and ketoconazole C [2] [3] may lengthen the effects of triazolam and midazolam considerably. They may increase the concentration of terfenadine (risk of arrhythmias), digoxin, warfarin as well as that of the calcium-blockers felodipine, and isradipine. An increase in the blood levels of calcium antagonists may result in leg oedema. Interaction with calcium antagonists has also been described with fluconazole.

Ringworm (Tinea)

- Cutaneous ringworm usually has an elevated, erythematous, scaling margin that spreads as a ring and causes itching.
- The rings are often multiple but incomplete.
- Particularly in inguinal and scalp ringworm there may be solitary folliculitic pustules, or even larger pustules.
- An insidious "moccasin" form, ringworm of the sole (Figure 13.50.3) may remain undetected. It is often accompanied by onychomycosis.
- Scalp ringworm may spread aggressively.

Foot ringworm (Tinea pedis)

Clinical presentation

- "Athlete's foot" is the typical presentation (Figure 13.50.1).
  - Most commonly occurs between the 4th and 5th toes.
  - The skin is erythematous, macerating, or even ulcerating, and there may be vesicles at the margins of the lesion.
  - There is a severe itch.
  - A secondary bacterial infection may occur.
  - Fungal vesicles on the hands and soles may be associated with the acute phase.
  - Despite its aggressiveness the disease is easily cured by topical treatments.
- Dry type or moccasine ringworm (Figure 13.50.2)
  - Often there are no subjective symptoms (Figure 13.50.3).

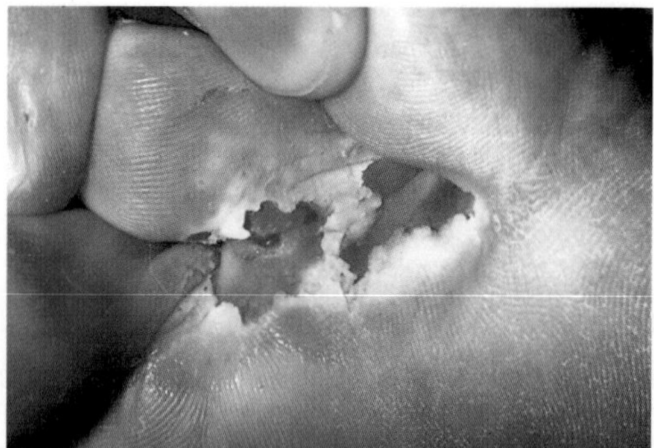

Figure 13.50.1 Athlete's foot is the combination of fungal and bacterial infection. The digital clefts and soles are macerated, often with bullous lesions. Wet compresses and antibacterials are necessary at first and are followed by antifungal therapy. Photo © R. Suhonen.

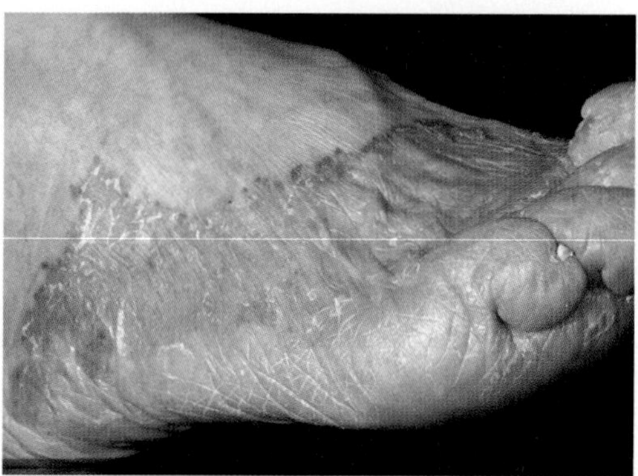

Figure 13.50.2 Plantar tinea often spreads to the lateral border of the foot—sometimes even as high as in the photograph. The causative agent is T. rubrum. Such a widespread plantar tinea indicates the possibility of a specific immunological defect in the antifungal defence mechanism, and oral antifungal medication is recommended. Photo © R. Suhonen.

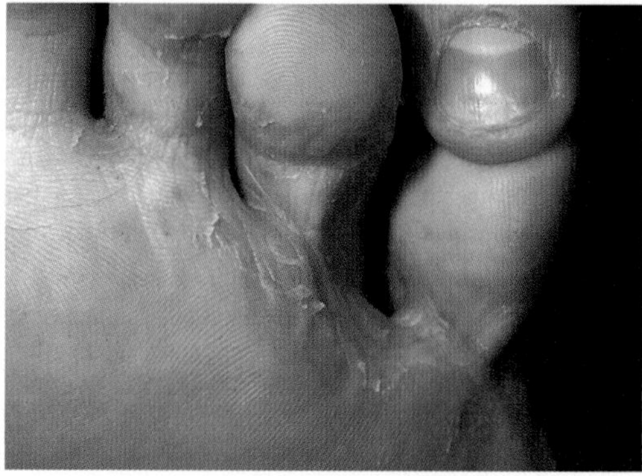

Figure 13.50.3 A quiescent, typical interdigital tinea is mildly scaling, with itchy episodes, and may even show blistering. A topical antifungal therapy is normally curative. Photo © R. Suhonen.

  - The skin is slightly hyperkeratotic, often mildly erythematous, scaling.
  - Unilateral affection is common, as well as partial (distal) affection of the forefoot. The scaling margin of the lesion is clearly visible (Figure 13.50.4).
  - A similar lesion may be visible on the palms, often unilateral (Figure 13.50.5).
  - Onychomycosis often coexists with this type of infection.
  - Topical treatments are relatively ineffective.

Aetiological agents

- The causative agent is nearly always Trichophyton rubrum, sometimes T. mentagrophytes, and very rarely Epidermophyton floccosum.
- Candida may also be isolated from macerated skin between the toes but this does not imply a pathogenic role.

Treatment

- Ringworm between the toes is most effectively treated with terbinafine emulsion for two weeks applied as a thin layer in

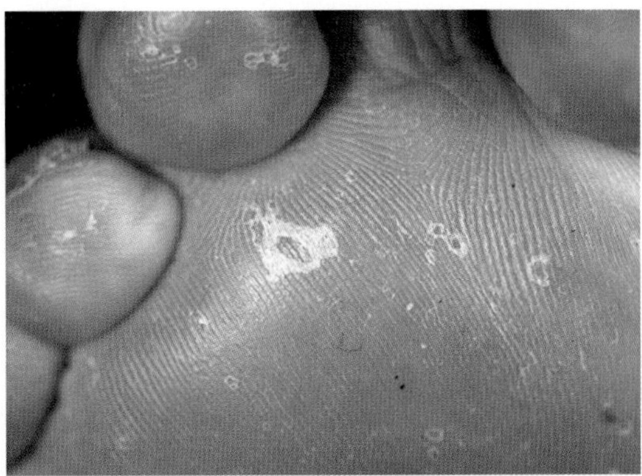

Figure 13.50.4 Circular, tiny, often unilateral scales on plantar skin are diagnostic for "dry-type tinea", probably resulting from genetically determined predisposition to this silent dermatophyte (T. rubrum) infection. Plantar tinea is more common than believed. The next step is onychomycosis, which brings the patient to seek help. It is beneficial to recognize the infection already on the skin and save the patient from longer therapy of nail infection. Oral fungicidal therapy is preferred to guarantee long-term cure. Photo © R. Suhonen.

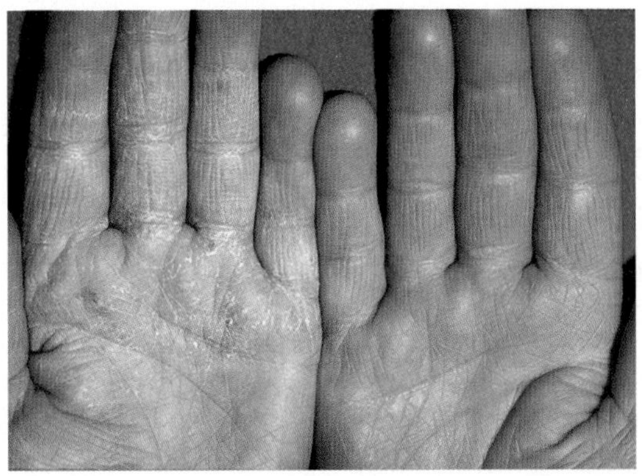

Figure 13.50.5 Fungal infection is uncommon in the hands. Fine scaling with an advancing border and only slight itching is the normal finding. In most cases only one hand is affected ("one hand—two feet-syndrome"). Oral antifungals are needed for permanent cure. The nails are also often affected which determines the duration of the therapy. Photo © R. Suhonen.

the evening B [4]. The duration of treatment is one month with azole derivatives.

- Foot hygiene: Normal daily washing, careful drying, and change of socks. The shoes need not be changed or disinfected.
- Moccasin ringworm of the sole is difficult to treat and usually requires systemic medication: terbinafine 250 mg × 1 for 2–4 weeks or itraconazole, 100 mg × 1 for 4 weeks.

Onychomycosis

Clinical picture

- Occurs most commonly in the toenails, often in just one or a few nails.

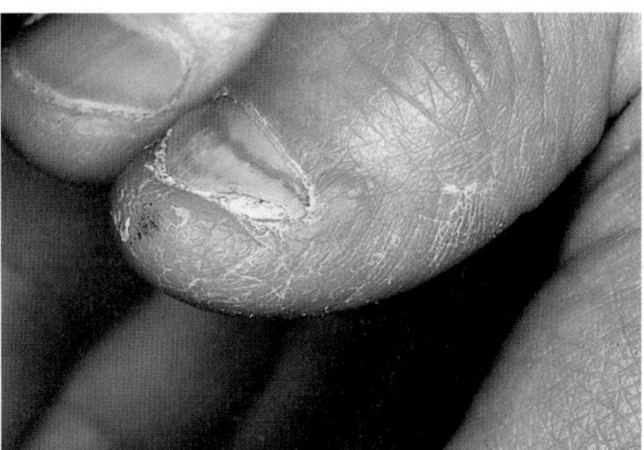

Figure 13.50.6 Trichophyton rubrum—dermatophyte has invaded both the skin and nail of the thumb. This situation is almost always preceded by an infection of the soles of the feet and toenails. Photo © R. Suhonen.

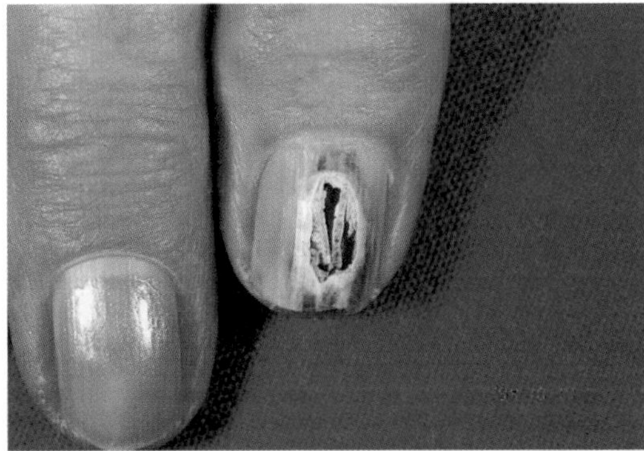

Figure 13.50.7 A green colour of the nail is usually a sign of infection caused by Pseudomonas aeruginosa, as here. The "window" into the hollow onycholytic space has been filed by the patient. Photo © R. Suhonen.

- Fingernails are infrequently affected (Figures 13.50.6 and 13.50.7).
- Onychomycosis is rare in children. Predisposition for the disease may be hereditary.
- 'Twenty nail dystrophy' (Figure 13.50.8).
- Onychomycosis usually begins under the nail, spreads linearly towards the base of the nail, makes the nail thick, and produces keratin under the nail. The disease may totally destroy the nail, but never permanently, as successful treatment restores the normal appearance of the nail (Figure 13.50.9).
- Moccasin ringworm of the sole often coexists.

Treatment

- The diagnosis should be verified by culture, because the treatment is neither risk-free nor cheap.
- Topical treatment (amorolfin nail varnish) is effective only against very distal onychomycosis and onychomycosis in children. The treatment should be continued according to the instructions in the package until the nail is totally normal (about 6 months for fingernails, 12 months for toenails).

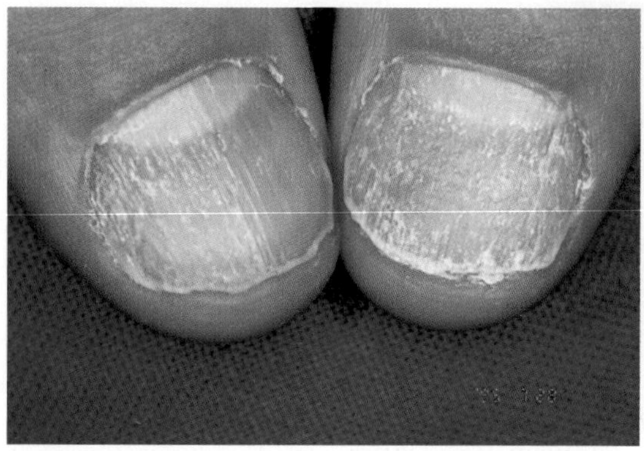

Figure 13.50.8 Trachyonychia may be secondary to alopecia areata, lichen planus, psoriasis; however, it may often affect all 20 nails ("twenty nail dystrophy") without any evident concomitant skin disease. Usually the affection is seen more easily in fingernails. There is no "best therapy", but oral biotin may be tried. Photo © R. Suhonen.

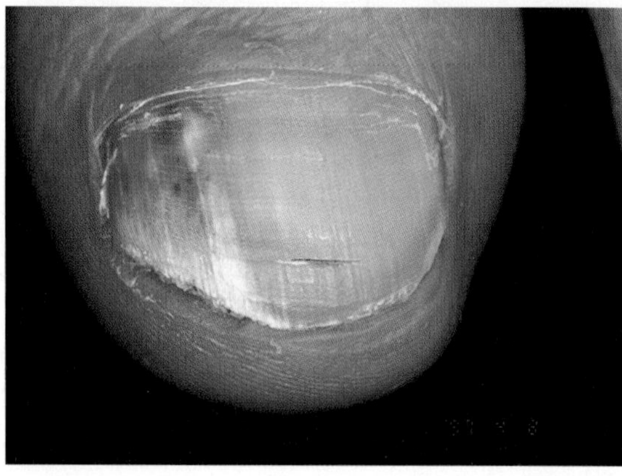

Figure 13.50.9 The most common location for onychomycosis is the big toenail. The infection starts distally at the nail bed, spreading proximally and, with time, affects the nail plate as well. However, the fungus will not destroy the germinative matrix—the fungal nail deformity is reversible with effective therapy. Photo © R. Suhonen.

- Urea ointment therapy of deformed nails administered by a chiropodist improves the treatment results.
- The most efficient therapy for onychomycosis is terbinafine at 250 mg × 1 for 3 months for toenails and 1 month for the treatment of fingernails **B** [5].
- Itraconazole is best administered as pulse therapy: 200 mg × 2 at meals for one week each month for a total of 3 months. Remember interactions!
- With terbinafine toenail culture remains negative for more than a year in 70–80% of the patients, with itraconazole pulse therapy in 40–50%.
- The efficacy of fluconazole has not been firmly established.
- There is no contraindication for a combination of local and systemic treatments.
- Urea ointment therapy
  - Urea 40.0, Crea alba 5.0, Adeps lanae 20.0, Vaselin album 25.0, Silica gel type H 10.0.
  - Another formula: Urea 40.0, miconazole cream ad 100.0
  - The ointment is spread on the nail and an occlusive bandage is placed on top for less than 7–10 days. Protect the surrounding skin from the ointment, for example, by cutting a finger off from a rubber glove and making in it a hole the size of the nail. The ointment listed first is easier to spread under the bandage.
- The success rate in onychomycosis of the big toe in older age groups is slightly above 50%. Consider the indications for treatment before starting the medication.

Inguinal ringworm (Tinea cruris)

Clinical picture

- A unilateral, itching, well-demarcated ring or several concentric rings with erythematous margins are observed (Figure 13.50.10), at least at the initial phase. Mycotic folliculitis or even small abscesses may be detected in the lesion and in the surroundings.

Treatment

- Terbinafine cream in the evening for a couple of weeks **A** [1].
- Ketoconazole **A** [1] or amorolfin cream in the evening for 3–4 weeks.
- Other azole creams **A** [1] should be applied twice daily for 4 weeks.
- In mycotic folliculitis or furuncles the treatment should be prolonged or systemic medication should be used: itraconazole, 100 mg × 1 or terbinafine 250 mg × 1 for two weeks.
- For dermatoses of the inguinal region see also article 13.11.

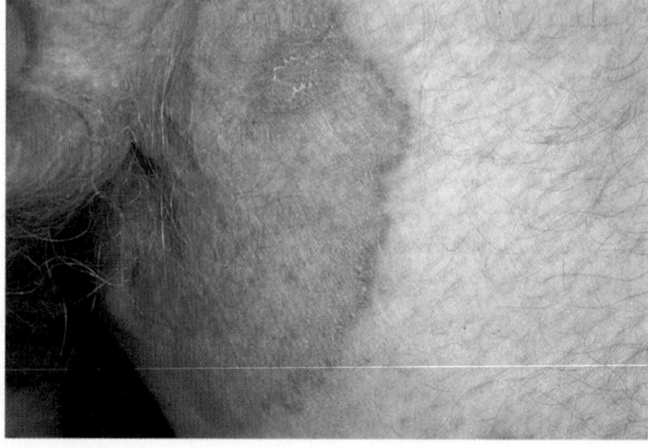

Figure 13.50.10 Fungal infection of the inguinal region, Tinea cruris, is typically most active at the advancing border. This clinical feature, together with positive mycology helps to make a definite diagnosis. This form of dermatophyte infection is common in men, but quite rare in women. In most cases simultaneous tinea is found also in the feet. Topical therapy is nearly always sufficient for eradicating the fungus from the groin. Photo © R. Suhonen.

Ringworm on the trunk (Tinea corporis)

Diagnosis

- Easily confused with nummular eczema. The diagnosis cannot be reliably made on clinical grounds.
- Fungal culture and a history of animal contacts (guinea pig, cat, dog, cattle) helps to confirm the diagnosis.
- The species of fungus found in the culture helps to detect the source of infection.

Treatment

- Similar to inguinal ringworm (see above) A [1].
- In widespread disease systemic medication may be indicated.

Wrestler's ringworm

Aetiology and diagnosis

- The causative agent is Tricophyton tonsurans.
- The disease easily spreads in wrestlers and spreads from the trunk to the scalp.
- Fungal culture should always be carried out. Use protective gloves when taking the sample.

Treatment

- Systemic medication in all cases
  - Itraconazole (100 mg/day) for patients weighing less than 40 kg, and 200 mg/day for those weighing more than 40 kg for two weeks in trunk infections, and for 4 weeks in scalp infections
  - Terbinafine at 62.5 mg/day for patients weighing less than 20 kg, 125 mg/day for patients weighing 20–40 kg, and 250 mg/day for patients weighing more than 40 kg for 4 weeks.
- Wrestling and contact training should be interrupted for at least 2 weeks after the onset of systemic medication.
- Asymptomatic family members and training companions as well as asymptomatic family members of the training companions should be treated with ketoconazole shampoo once a day for one week. A couple of teaspoons of the shampoo is spread on moist skin and left there for 3–5 minutes.
- The wrestling mats and washrooms should be washed with sodium hypochlorite once a week during the treatment course.

Scalp ringworm (Tinea capitis)

Aetiology and diagnosis

- Uncommon in Western countries.
- The diagnosis should always be based on a positive culture result.
- The causative agent is usually Microsporon canis (from cats), T. mentagrophytes (from several kinds of pet), or T. violaceum (in children from developing countries).

Clinical picture

- There are short, broken stumps of hair in a scaling, erythematous, rough, bald plaque.
- In a rapidly progressive, pus-forming infection ("kerion") a rapid start of treatment is necessary to prevent permanent hair loss.
- Take scaling skin or broken hair stumps with forceps. If there is pus it should also be sampled. In cases of kerion the treatment should start immediately after the specimen for fungal culture has been taken.

Treatment

- Terbinafine for 1 month at a dose of 250 mg/day B [6]. Itraconazole has been used at a dose of 100 mg/day for one month, or as pulse therapy with 200 mg × 2 for one week, repeated 2–3 times. An oral solution (4 mg/kg) is available for children. Consult a dermatologist C [2 3].
- The duration of treatment can be longer if necessary. See Wrestler's ringworm for children's doses.

Candida infections

- Candida infections are commonly over-diagnosed. The diseases falsely labelled as candidiasis include lichen planus and "stomatodynia" in the mouth, atopic eczema in the angles of the mouth in children, and seborrhoeic eczema in skin folds. "Candidial balanitis" is often seborrhoeic eczema, and "candidial intertrigo" between the fingers is toxic eczema.
- The most common aetiological agent of true candidiasis is Candida albicans.
- Isolating Candida albicans from a culture specimen does not prove that it is the pathogenic agent, because Candida is a normal human saprophyte.
- Candidiasis in the angles of the mouth, under the breasts, and in the inguinal folds in the elderly is often macerated, and ulcerating in the bottom of the fold, and with small satellite lesions at the margins.
- Predisposing factors include diabetes, long-term antibiotic treatments, immunosuppression (particularly HIV infection), polyendocrinopathies, and dental prostheses.

Oral candidiasis

Clinical picture

- Typical white exudates on the buccal mucosa in infants.
- More infrequent in adults than expected, and difficult to diagnose. Both exudative and atrophic forms of the disease exist.

Treatment

- See article 31.30.

DER

Cheilitis angularis Monilia

Clinical picture

- Occurs with concomitant oral candidiasis or even alone (see 7.11).
- Wearing a low dental prosthesis deepens the skin fold in the angle of the mouth, keeps it moist, and predisposes the subject to candidiasis.

Treatment

- Azole ointment; sometimes a combination ointment to treat secondary eczema and bacterial infection.
- The disease tends to recur, and the treatment must be repeated.

Candida intertrigo

Clinical picture

- Avoid over-diagnosis: often the cause is seborrhoeic eczema (particularly in the anal region) or psoriasis of the infolds.
- Occurs under the breasts, in the navel, in the inguinal folds, between the buttocks, and between fingers.
- Is more aggressive than ringworm, but less pronounced at the margins of the lesions, more evenly erythematous, and often moist. There are satellite lesions near the margins.

Treatment

- Normal washing, preferably with acid lotions.
- Miconazole-hydrocortisone (A) [1] combination ointment is recommended initially.
- Usually there is no need for peroral antifungal medication (fluconazole, itraconazole). In recurrent infections consider fluconazole resistance, which easily develops in yeasts.
- Two weeks of treatment is sufficient.
- Frequently recurring candidiasis is an indication for the determination of blood glucose, and consider the possibility of immunodeficiency.

Paronychia Monilia

Clinical picture

- Identify eczemas, psoriasis, periungual warts, and tumours.
- The infection is often mixed: Candida albicans + S. aureus.
- Working with moist hands (e.g. in cleaners and kitchen personnel) predisposes the subject to the disease.
- In chronic paronychia a recurrent horizontal growth disturbance results in a wavy appearance.
- An acute disease does not damage the nail permanently, as is the case with chronic paronychia.

Treatment

- At the acute phase it is often best to treat the bacterial infection with systemic antibiotics.
- Liquid-form azole medication is used against the candida infection.
- Refer a patient with chronic paronychia to a dermatologist.
- Keeping the hands dry is the best prophylaxis.

Candida balanitis

- Most cases of "candidial balanitis" are falsely diagnosed seborrhoeic eczema.
- Over-diagnosis of candidiasis causes unnecessary concern; female partners have vaginal yeast without symptoms–they need not be treated.
- Culturing candida yields so many false positive results that it is not recommended in balanitis.

Clinical picture

- The symptoms of candidial balanitis include itch, erythematous erosions, and easily breaking pustules on the glans and inner preputium.
- A white exudate may be visible occasionally (check the patient's sanitary habits before diagnosing candidiasis!).

Treatment

- Although seborrhoeic eczema and candidial balanitis are often confused, this does not cause severe problems with the treatment: both can be treated with miconazole-hydrocortisone cream. A couple of weeks of treatment is usually effective for both.
- Potassium permanganate bath (1:10 000) daily for 15 min can also be used initially (be careful not to stain clothes and vessels!).
- A mild silver nitrate solution in the form of a compress (0.01–0.1%) may alleviate symptoms of infection on mucosal surfaces.

References

1. Crawford F, Hart R, Bell-Syer S, Torgerson D, Young P, Russell I. Topical treatments for fungal infections of the skin and nails of the foot. Cochrane Database Syst Rev. 2004;(2):CD001434.
2. Abdel-Rahman SM, Nahata MC. Treatment of tinea capitis. Ann Pharmacother 1997;31:338–348.
3. The Database of Abstracts of Reviews of Effectiveness (University of York), Database no.: DARE-970404. In: The Cochrane Library, Issue 4, 1999. Oxford: Update Software.
4. Bell-Syer SEM, Hart R, Crawford F, Torgerson DJ, Tyrrell W, Russell I. Oral treatments for fungal infections of the skin of the foot. Cochrane Database Syst Rev. 2004;(2):CD003584.
5. Glyn E, Evans V, Sigurgeirsson B for the LION study group. Double-blind, randomised study of continuous terbinafine compared with intermittent itraconazole in treatment of toenail onychomycosis. BMJ 1999;318:1031–1035.

6. Fuller LC, Smith CH, Cerio R et al., A randomized comparison of 4 weeks of terbinafinen vs. 8 weeks of griseofulvin for the treatment of tinea capitis. Br J Dermatol 2001;144: 321–327.

13.51 Pityriasis versicolor

Pekka Autio

Aetiology

- The rash is caused by exceptionally abundant growth of Pityrosporum ovale (Malassezia furfur). The reason why this lipophilic fungus grows in large numbers in some patients is not known.

Symptoms

- Irregular, mildly scaling maculae are seen on the trunk, neck and proximal parts of the limbs (Figure 13.51.1).
- The colour varies from pale to brown, even "dirty" grey. On light skin the maculae are brown, on tanned skin they are more light-coloured than the surrounding skin.

Investigations

- The clinical appearance is diagnostic.
- Pityrosporum also grows on normal skin. Therefore fungal culture is of no benefit.
- In microscopy of a scraped sample (methyl blue staining) the appearance of Pityrosporum is typical.

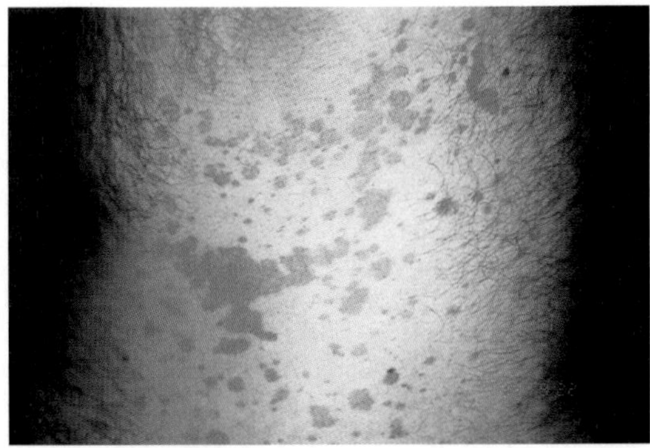

Figure 13.51.1 Pityriasis versicolor mostly affects the skin of the upper thorax; less often the proximal extremities. It is caused by a commensal lipophilic yeast, Pityrosporum ovale (Malassezia furfur). This yeast is hosted by virtually all people. Do not call this a contagious disease! The most effective therapy is ketoconazole, either as a topical shampoo or an oral single dose of 400 mg preferably with an acidic drink. A single dose of ketoconazole is not a risk as regards hepatic welfare. Photo © R. Suhonen.

Treatment

- Ketokonazole shampoo is applied on the skin for 10 minutes on a few evenings, followed by a shower. Later, a single night's treatment every month controls the disease.
- Ketokonazole tablets (400 mg = 2 tablets) as a single dose with a small amount of food.
- About 2 hours later the patient should exercise intensely enough to cause perspiration as this increases the concentration of the drug on the skin. A shower should not be taken during the next 10 hours. The treatment can be repeated when the disease recurs (on average after 8 months).
- Pityriasis versicolor is not a contagious disease. Treatment does not mean eradication but control of the colonisation of an innocent saprophyte fungus.

DEF

13.60 Acne

Jorma Lauharanta

Classification of acne

- Comedonic acne (A. comedonicus) (Figure 13.60.1)
  - Plenty of open or obstructed comedos, but scant inflammatory changes
- Common acne (A. vulgaris) or pustular acne
  - Pustules and comedos
- Cystic acne (A. cystica) (Figure 13.60.2)
  - Cystic foci of infection that result in scars
- Acne conglobata
  - Multilobular inflammatory cysts containing volatile pus
  - Therapy resistant, scar forming
- Acne fulminans
  - An uncommon variant of acne in young men characterized by systemic symptoms (fever, arthralgia, skeletal foci of inflammation)
  - Systemic corticosteroids, not antibiotics, are the drugs of choice.
  - Refer patients with suspected acne fulminans to a dermatologist without delay. The painful disease is not well known, and is often left untreated for a long time.

Treatment

Local treatment

- Local treatment is usually sufficient for comedonic acne and mild common acne.

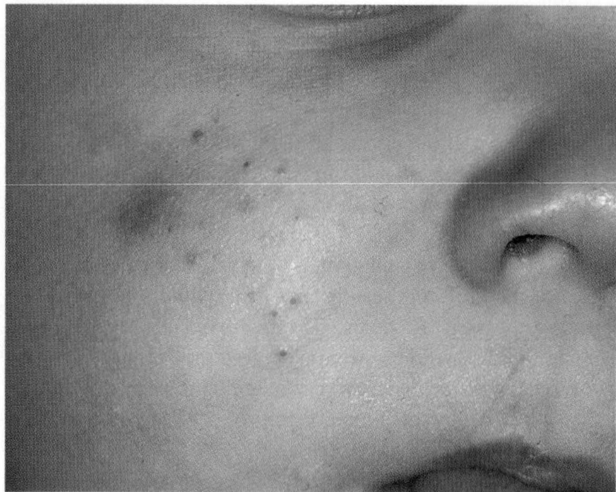

Figure 13.60.1 Even a small child may have acne. This baby acne with comedones is best treated with topical tretinoin or adapalene. Photo © R. Suhonen.

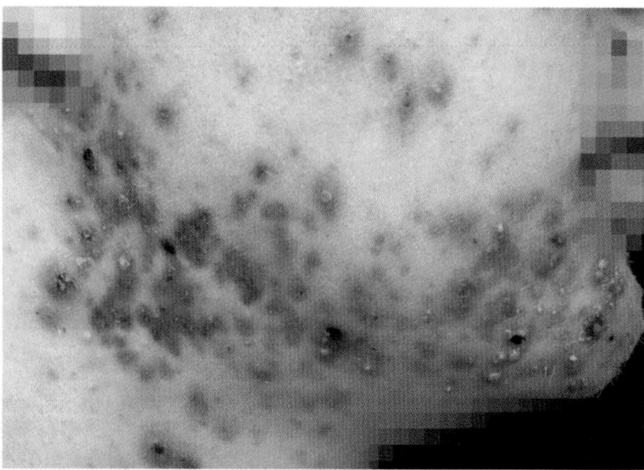

Figure 13.60.2 This case of acne of the cystic and indurate type in a teenager boy was completely and permanently cured with oral isotretinoin. Other treatment modalities (antibiotics, various topical remedies) may at best give a temporary relief of acne with this degree of severity. Photo © R. Suhonen.

- Wash the skin with soap or antibacterial detergents
- Comedonic acne can be treated with
  - Retinoic acid cream or solution
  - Adapalen gel
  - Benzoyl peroxide (3–10%)
  - All above drugs can be irritating at first. Use a low concentration of the active drug initially, and advise the patient to wash the drug away after a few hours. The tolerance of the skin increases with time.
- Common acne can be treated with
  - Local antibiotics (e.g clindamycin solution)
  - Ultraviolet light therapy (as a course of 15 treatments added to other treatment) for widespread disease
- Consider systemic treatment if the effect of local treatment is unsatisfactory 2–3 months from the onset of treatment.

Systemic treatment

- Antibiotics
  - Tetracycline B [1] and erythromycin are equally effective. The usual dose is 250–500 mg/day for a few months. Six months' treatment with tetracycline or erythromycin 1 g/day is more effective than a shorter treatment with a smaller dose. Do not use tetracyclines in children below 12 years of age.
  - Local treatment and light therapy can be used simultaneously with systemic treatment.
  - Local treatment is not sufficient in cystic acne and conglobate acne. Use systemic antibiotics or consider referral to a dermatologist. Pus-containing cysts can be drained by incising them with a large-calibre injection needle or narrow-tipped scalpel.
- Hormonal treatment for women
  - Cyproterone acetate (an anti-androgen) + oestrogen for 6 months reduces the excretion of sebaceous glands and alleviates acne.

Acne scars

- Consider treatment of scars by skin abrasion or laser therapy D [2 3 4 5] only after the activity of the disease has totally subsided.
- Scars can be treated either by a dermatologist or a plastic surgeon.

Indications for specialist consultation

- Severe forms of acne (A. cystica, conglobata, fulminans)
- If ordinary treatment fails, the dermatologist can consider isotretinoin. However, it has considerable teratogenicity.

References

1. Garner SE, Eady EA, Popescu C, Newton J, Li Wan Po A. Minocycline for acne vulgaris: efficacy and safety. Cochrane Database Syst Rev. 2004;(2):CD002086.
2. Jordan R, Cummins C, Burls A. Laser resurfacing of the skin for improvement of facial acne scarring. West Midlands: Department of Public Health and Epidemiolog. West Midlands Development and Evaluation Service. 11. 1998. 1–51.
3. The Database of Abstracts of Reviews of Effectiveness (University of York), Database no.: DARE-999269. In: The Cochrane Library, Issue 2, 2001. Oxford: Update Software.
4. Jordan R, Cummins C, Burls A. Laser resurfacing of the skin for the improvement of facial acne scarring. Birmingham: Department of Public Health and Epidemiology, University of Birmingham. West Midlands Development and Evaluation Service, Department of Public Health and Epidemiology (DPHE). DPHE Report No. 11. 1998. pp51.
5. The Health Technology Assessment Database, Database no.: HTA-998502. In: The Cochrane Library, Issue 1, 2001. Oxford: Update Software.

13.61 Rosacea

Editors

Aims

- Identify the disease.
- Avoid corticosteroid creams.

Clinical picture

- Rosacea is a chronic skin disease with paroxysmal exacerbations. It is most common in women aged 30–50 years.
- The etiology is not known.
- The typical clinical presentation includes acne-like pustules, dilated blood vessels (telangiectasia), and redness of the skin (Figure 13.61.1).
- The typical site is the central area of the face (Figure 13.61.2).
- There are no comedos.
- Exacerbating factors include hot drinks, strong spices, sun light and sauna baths. Reaction to these factors varies among individuals.

Differential diagnosis

- Acne (13.60) occurs in younger patients and is associated with comedos.
- Perioral dermatitis (13.62) is situated around the mouth and lacks telangiactasia.
- The skin affection in SLE may be difficult to differentiate from rosacea. The lack of systemic symptoms aids in diagnostics.

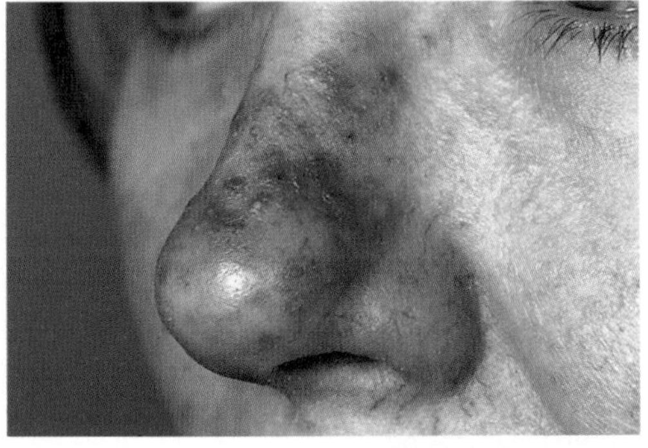

Figure 13.61.1 Rosacea is a disease of the sebaceous glands affecting mainly the skin of the nose and cheeks. Telangiectases, diffuse redness, and small pustules are the main clinical features. It is good to remember that possible ocular problems (e.g. keratitis) are often one of the symptoms of rosacea. Oral tetracyclines are the mainstay in rosacea therapy, although in many cases topical metronidazole may be effective. Photo © R. Suhonen.

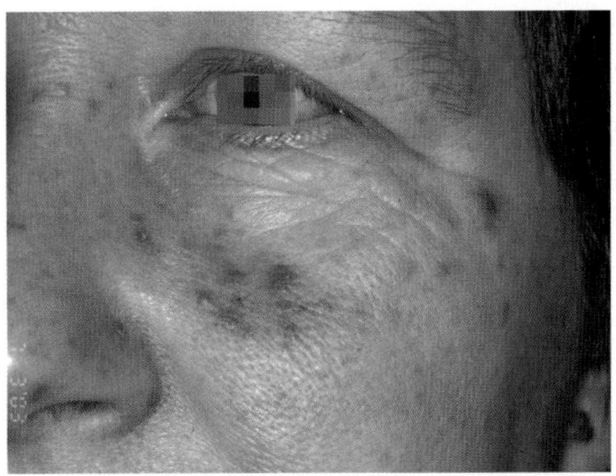

Figure 13.61.2 Rosacea affects both men and women in their middle ages. Usually the telangiectases, small pustules, and in some cases also papules, are most numerous on the central facial area. Sometimes also extrafacial skin areas are affected (e.g. pubic region), and it is also good to keep in mind that rosacea may affect eyes (e.g. keratitis). Oral tetracyclines and topical metronidazole are beneficial in most cases. Photo © R. Suhonen.

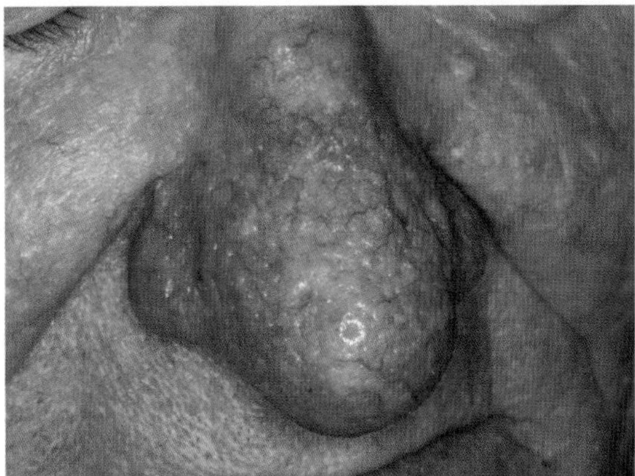

Figure 13.61.3 Rhinophyma is an uncommon hypertrophic growth of nasal sebaceous glands with increased vascularity. It affects mainly men. The nose can be re-shaped by surgery, electrocautery or carbon dioxide laser. Photo © R. Suhonen.

Treatment

- Metronidazole ointment (1%) is the drug of choice **B** [1]. It can be used as long as necessary.
- Azelaic acid **B** [1] and possibly permethrin ointment are also effective.
- A local ointment with 1–3% sulphur can also be used.
- Corticosteroids must absolutely be avoided.
- Persons whose rosacea aggravates in the spring may benefit from sun-protective creams.
- Tetracycline as a course lasting 1–2 months is usually effective **B** [1]. The dose is smaller than in the treatment of acne. After an initial daily dose of 750–1000 mg the dose can be decreased to 250 mg daily.
- Sebaceous gland hyperplasia in the nose (rhinophyma) (Figure 13.61.3) sometimes necessitates surgical treatment. Isotretinoin often controls hyperplasia effectively.

Reference

1. van Zuuren EJ, Graber MA, Hollis S, Chaudhry M, Gupta AK. Interventions for rosacea. The Cochrane Database of Systematic Reviews, Cochrane Library Number: CD003262. In: Cochrane Library, Issue 1, 2004. Chichester, UK: John Wiley & Sons, Ltd.

13.62 Perioral dermatitis

Pekka Autio

Aetiology

- The aetiology is unknown.
- Cosmetics and local corticosteroids on the face have been suspected as causative agents (the disease almost invariably affects women).

Clinical features

- Small erythematous papules and single small pustules, but no comedones or scars (Figure 13.62.1).
- Occurs in young or middle-aged women in the surroundings of the nose and mouth; sometimes also around the eyes (periocular dermatitis), which can become worse especially with corticoid creams.

Investigations

- No diagnostic tests are available.

Treatment

- Tetracycline, 500 mg/day, is usually effective within 2–3 weeks **B** [1 2]. The treatment is continued for 1–2 months.

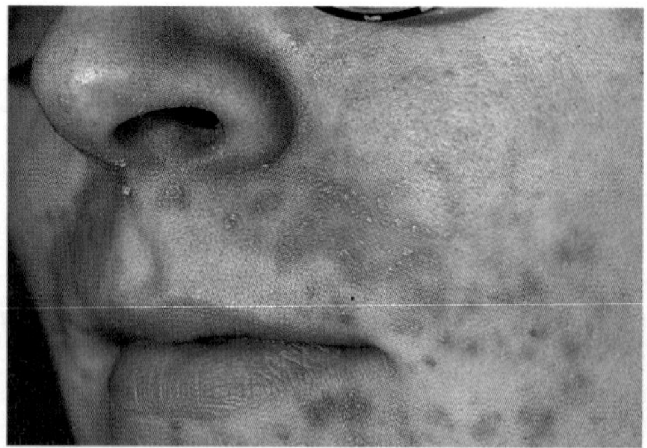

Figure 13.62.1 Perioral dermatiti—red spots around the mouth, which spare a zone of 5–10 mm immediately outside the lip margin, is a typical skin disorder in women. The symptoms are common also around the nose and eyes. Oral tetracycline is the drug of choice. Photo © R. Suhonen.

- Topical treatment alone is usually less effective. A metronidazole cream can be tried.
- After a treatment lasting 2 months the lesions often do not recur until after a few years.

References

1. Weber K, Thurmayr R, Meisinger A. A topical erythromycin preparation and oral tetracycline for the treatment of perioral dermatitis: A placebo-controlled trial. J Dermatol Treat 1993;4:57–59.
2. Veien NK, Munkvad JM, Nielsen AO, Niordson AM, Stahl D, Thormann J. Topical metronidazole in the treatment of perioral dermatitis. J Am Acad Dermatol 1991;24:258–60.

13.70 Chronic bullous diseases (dermatitis herpetiformis, pemphigoid)

Pekka Autio

Aim

- Dermatitis herpetiformis and pemphigoid should be diagnosed.

Organization of treatment

- Chronic bullous diseases are rare. Diagnosis requires special investigations (immunohistochemistry), and treatment (dapsone, peroral corticosteroids, cytotoxic drugs) may cause complications, which is why these diseases should be treated by a specialist.

Dermatitis herpetiformis

Diagnosis

- Typical vesicles on erythematous skin, and scratches on the elbows and knees (Figure 13.70.1), sacrum, and scalp.
- Ordinary histopathology is usually non-specific, but immunohistopathology is useful.
- The existence of gliadin, reticulin, endomysium or transglutaminase antibodies may suggest the coexistence of coeliac disease (abdominal symptoms!).
- Gastroscopy and small bowel biopsy are indicated before starting diet therapy.
- Remember to ask about other cases in the family.

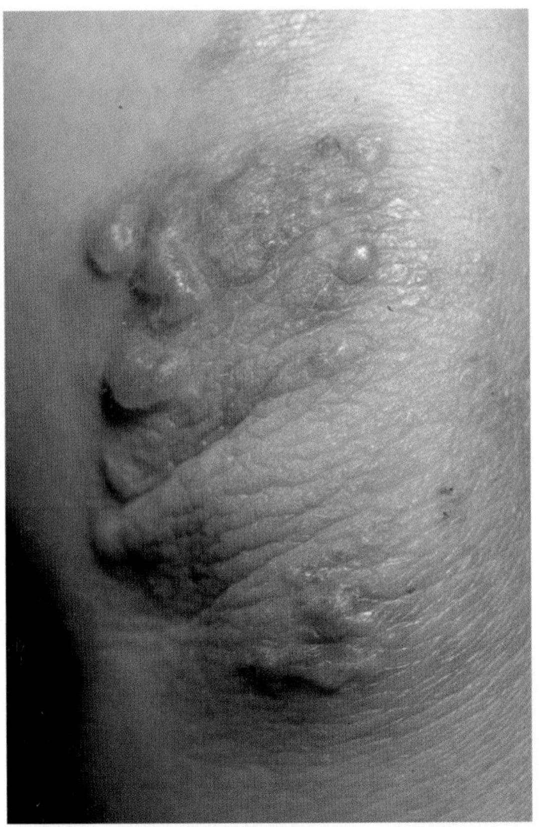

Figure 13.70.1 Dermatitis herpetiformis forms itchy vesicles on the elbows, knees and the sacral region, sometimes also on other skin areas. The patients have almost invariably atrophy of duodenal villi. Dapson heals the skin lesions rapidly, but the patients should be advised to follow a gluten-free diet. Photo © R. Suhonen.

Treatment

- A gluten-free diet has a favourable effect on the skin symptoms in cases of dermatitis herpetiformis even if the patient does not have coeliac disease. Adequate diet councelling is essential.
- The use of dapsone (which is effective against the skin symptoms) bears a risk of haemolysis. Repeated laboratory examinations and clinical follow-up are absolutely necessary.
- Local corticosteroids may alleviate the skin symptoms.

Indications for specialist consultation

- A specialist should always be consulted on the diagnosis, treatment, and follow-up of dermatitis herpetiformis.

Pemphigoid

Definition

- An autoimmune disease of the elderly presenting with vesicles or large bullae. Skin basal membrane antibodies are present.

Symptoms

- Pemphigoid affects elderly people (>60 years of age)
- Large thick-walled, translucent, and itching vesicles or bullae develop on erythematous skin of the trunk and proximal parts of the extremities.
- Mucosal surfaces are usually unaffected.
- The general condition of the patient is unaffected.

Diagnosis

- A biopsy should be taken from a fresh (small) vesicle or from an erythematous skin lesion. If a vesicle is biopsied the complete base of the vesicle should be included in the specimen.
- The epithelium under an older vesicle has often already regenerated, and interpretation of the histology is difficult. Immunohistology is diagnostic.
- Basal membrane antibodies may be detectable in the serum (an auxiliary examination that should not delay the onset of treatment!).

Differential diagnosis

- Pemphigus (vulgaris, foliaceus, erythematosus, vegetans)
  - The age distribution is wider.
  - Very rare in comparison with pemphigoid.
  - Immunohistology is diagnostic.
  - More difficult to treat than pemphigoid. Pemphigus vulgaris may be life threatening.
  - Epidermolysis bullosa
  - A rare genodermatosis
  - Porphyrias
  - P. cutanea tarda presents with vesicles on the dorsa of the hands
  - Rare
  - Dermatitis herpetiformis
  - Sometimes presents as a widespread disease that is difficult to identify.

Treatment

- Systemic corticosteroids
  - The dose is individual. The initial dose is relatively large (40–60 mg/day of prednisolone **C** [1]).
  - Continuous medication is seldom needed.
- Sometimes corticosteroid treatment must be combined with dapsone or cytostatics.
- Local treatment with very potent corticosteroids may suffice in limited disease **B** [2].

Indications for specialist consultation

- Confirmation of the diagnosis and differential diagnosis (immunohistology) are tasks of a specialist. The patient should be referred without delay.

References

1. Morel P, Guillaume JC. Treatment of bullous pemphigoid with prednisolone only: 0.75 mg/kg/day versus 1.25 mg/kg/day.

A multicenter randomized study. Ann Dermatol Venereol 1984;111:925–928.
2. Khumalo N, Kirtschig G, Middleton P, Hollis S, Wojnarowska F, Murrell D. Interventions for bullous pemphigoid. Cochrane Database Syst Rev. 2004;(2):CD002292.

13.71 Psoriasis

Erna Snellman

Definition and prevalence

- Psoriasis is a chronic disease of the skin, characterized by well-defined plaques bearing adherent, silvery scales.
- The prevalence of psoriasis in Scandinavia and Western Europe is approximately 2%. It is rare below 5 years of age (Figure 13.71.1). There are two peaks of onset: between 16 and 22 years of age in Type I psoriasis and between 57 and 60 years of age in Type II psoriasis. The genetic background of these two types differ.
- Genetic predisposition to psoriasis follows a multifactorial pattern. As many as seven susceptibility genes (locus) have been identified. The most significant locus (PSORS1) lies within chromosome 6p21.3. Only about 10% of the susceptibility gene carriers will develop the disease (low penetrance).
- Psoriasis is characterized by an abnormal regulation of the interaction between T cells and keratinocytes. T cell cytokine secretion profile resembles that of Th-1.
- External factors (infections, streptococcal in particular, skin injuries, certain drugs) often trigger the onset of psoriasis. Stress, smoking and excessive alcohol consumption may also be connected with the onset of psoriasis.

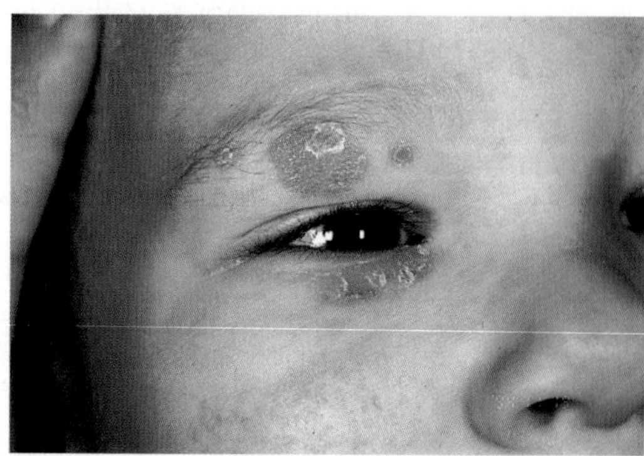

Figure 13.71.1 Psoriasis is uncommon in young children. Characteristic patches, covered with silvery scales are present here on the eyelids, which further complicates the therapy. I this case emollients were mostly used and two years later the patches had disappeared. Photo © R. Suhonen.

Clinical features

- Characteristic cutaneous lesions facilitate diagnosis.
  - The plaques are sharply demarcated, slightly elevated and covered with silvery scales (Figure 13.71.2)).
  - Gentle scraping of the scales reveals minute capillary bleeding points (Auspitz sign).
  - The elbows, knees, legs, lower back and scalp (Figure 13.71.3) and glans penis (Figure 13.71.4) are the sites of predilection.
- Involvement of the nails is common.
  - Pitting
  - Separation of the distal nail plate from the nail bed (onycholysis), yellowish flecks beneath the nail plate ("oily macules") and subungual hyperkeratosis (Figure 13.71.5).
  - Acrodermatitis continua of Hallopeau is a painful, localized pustular form of psoriasis which often leads to nail deformity (Figure 13.71.6).

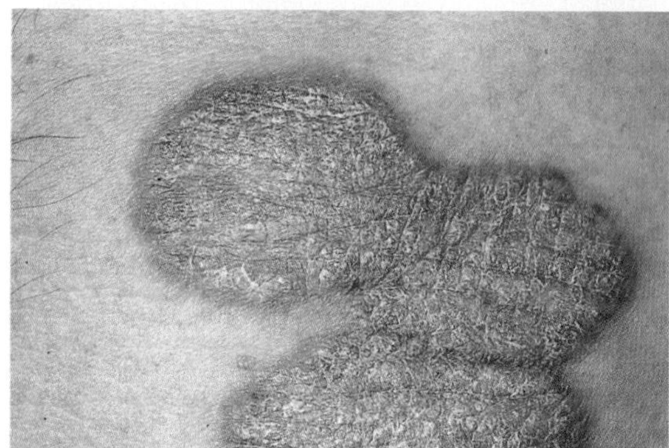

Figure 13.71.2 Psoriatic plaques generally have distinct margins and they appear red and scaly. In this case the scaling is less prominent and of smaller particle size than usual. Photo © R. Suhonen.

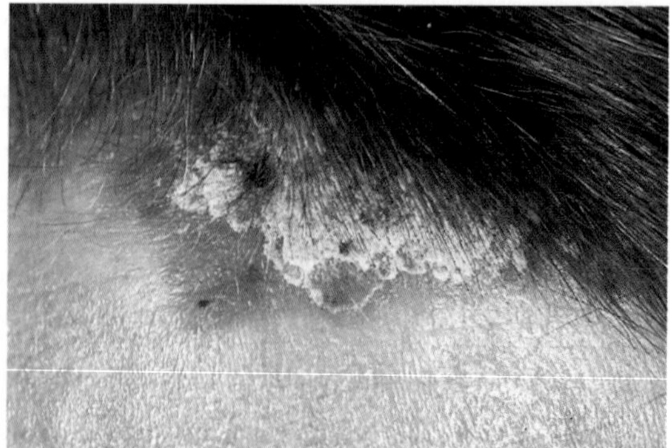

Figure 13.71.3 Psoriatic lesions on scalp skin are common near the hair margins. Here the silvery scales are exceptionally widely visible, even outside the hair margin. Often, as here, the red background is wider than the scaling. Differential diagnosis between psoriasis and seborrhoeic dermatitis is often difficult, even impossible, if only the scalp is affected. Photo © R. Suhonen.

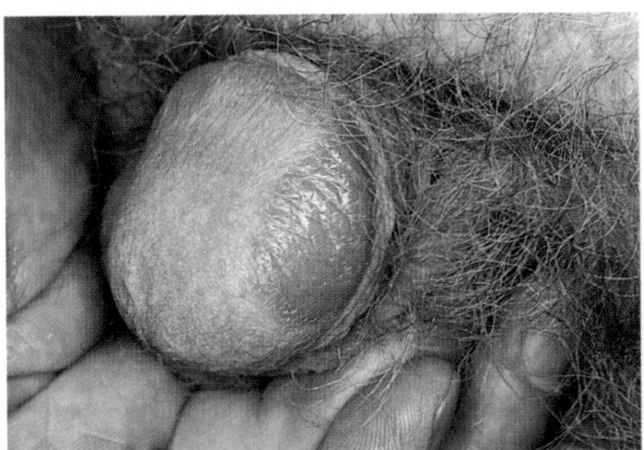

Figure 13.71.4 Glans penis is not an uncommon site for a psoriatic plaque. The best diagnostic method for this location is the careful study of other skin sites—psoriasis is seldom unifocal. Photo © R. Suhonen.

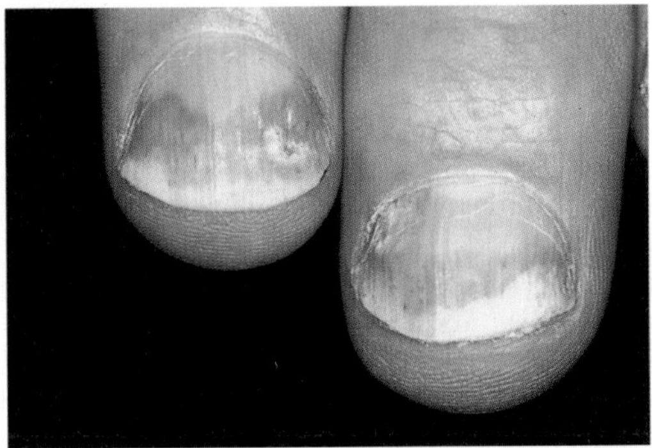

Figure 13.71.5 Psoriatic nails with all the common features: all the nails are affected, there is distal onycholysis and subungual hyperkeratosis, the nail surfaces are irregular with pronounced pitting and "oil spots" are seen under the nail plates. Mycology specimens test negative in psoriatic nails. Photo © R. Suhonen.

Common manifestations of psoriasis

- The most common type is plaque psoriasis, which is a stationary form of the disease with the lesions often covered with thick silvery scales.
- Guttate psoriasis is often triggered by tonsillitis. It is widely distributed throughout the body.
- Flexural psoriasis is localised within the main skin folds (genitocrural area, navel, axillae, submammary region).
- Erythrodermic psoriasis is generalized form of the disease and is the most refractory to treatment. It may also appear in a pustular form (pustular psoriasis).
- Psoriasis may also affect joints in 5–10% of cases.

Differential diagnosis

- Diagnosis is based on the clinical picture.
- A biopsy may exclude some other skin diseases resembling psoriasis, but it rarely is pathognomic.
- A family history of psoriasis may be helpful: up to 50% of patients report an affected relative.

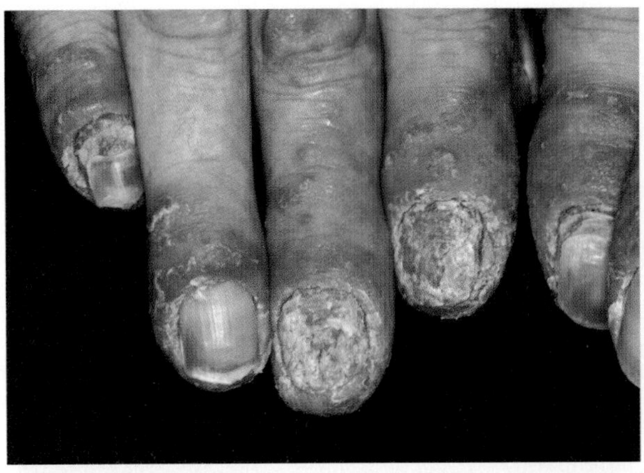

Figure 13.71.6 Acrodermatitis continua is a severe form of psoriasis affecting the distal fingers and toes. Redness, swelling, pustules and gross nail deformity are characteristic features. Often the best control of symptoms is achieved by oral methotrexate. Photo © R. Suhonen.

Scalp

- In **seborrhoeic dermatitis** (13.15) the flakes are thinner, "greasier" and the condition responds better to treatment. It is often difficult to differentiate seborrhoeic dermatitis from psoriasis unless other skin areas offer additional information.
- **Fungal infection** of the scalp (13.50) is uncommon in the Western populations. It mostly affects children. This diagnosis can be excluded by microscopy and negative culture for fungi.
- **Neurodermatitis** of the neck (lichen simplex nuchae) is characterised by an isolated, itchy plaque covered with thin scales.

Flexures

- **Seborrhoeic dermatitis** may resemble flexural psoriasis. Examine other skin areas. It is not always necessary to differentiate between these two conditions, as the treatment is the same.
- **Fungal infection** (tinea) (13.50) may resemble psoriasis; however, it usually heals in the centre and expands peripherally. KOH (potassium hydroxide) and fungal culture is diagnostic.
- **Candidiasis** is not often seen in the young or middle aged patients. It presents as a moist area of erythema and maceration with outlying "satellite eruptions".
- **Erythrasma** is a macular brown area with few symptoms, most often found in the armpit or groin. It is caused by an overgrowth of diphtheroids of the normal skin flora. These areas fluoresce coral pink under long-wave ultraviolet radiation (Wood's light)

Hands, feet

- **Hyperkeratotic eczema** of the palms and **palmoplantar pustulosis** may be difficult to differentiate from psoriasis (Figure 13.71.7). Examine the entire skin.

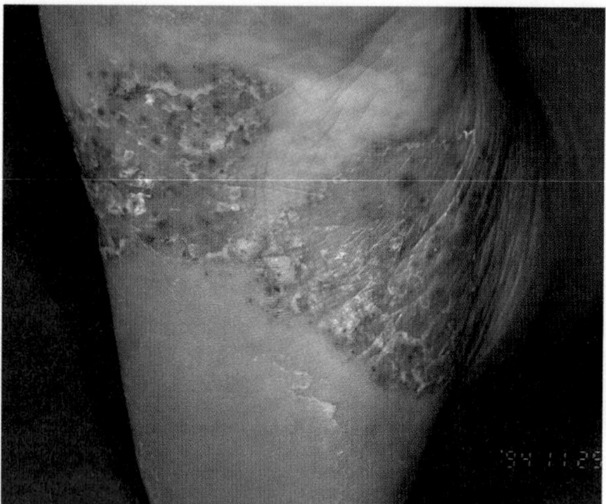

Figure 13.71.7 Pustulosis (palmo-) plantaris is one of the most therapy-resistant skin diseases. The cause is unknown and its relationship to psoriasis unclear. Potent topical corticosteroids, calcipotriol, oral tetracyclines, acitretin or even cyclosporin are therapeutic alternatives. Smokers are at an increased risk of this disease. Photo © R. Suhonen.

- **Fungal infection** (13.50) can easily be diagnosed with microscopic examination and culture.

Treatment

- The choice of treatment depends on the psoriasis subtype and the extent, severity and site of the lesions and, importantly, on the patient's preferences. In addition to the age of the patient, the availability, feasibility and cost of the treatment as well as response to earlier treatment also have an influence on the choice.
- Any comorbidities (e.g. hepatic disease, hypertension, alcohol abuse, HIV), or a possible pregnancy of the patient, must also be taken into account.
- It is not necessary to treat psoriasis if it has no effect on the patient's quality of life (minor psoriasis on the elbows or knees).

Topical treatment

- The main form of treatment available for a general practitioner is the use of various ointments and creams.
- Topical treatment may also enhance the effect of other treatment forms.
- The active treatment of mild to moderate plaque psoriasis may consist of vitamin D derivatives (calcipotriol and calcitriol) or a retinoid derivative (tazarotene). These are suitable for long-term use. Topical corticosteroids are also suitable, but their use should be intermittent.
- **Emollients** may be used as a general treatment in non-acute phases of the disease. They can also be used to soften and remove the scale from the scalp (plenty of emollient rubbed into the scalp in the evening and washed out in the morning). The scalp must not be scratched to remove the scale since this may worsen the symptoms (Köbner phenomenon). An emollient base with 5% salicylic acid enhances the exfoliating effect.
- **Topical corticosteroid** Ⓐ [1] ointments are usually more effective than creams. On the face and flexures only mild to moderately potent topical corticosteroids should be used. On the other body areas treatment results will only be achieved with potent to very potent ointments. Topical corticosteroids can well be used on the scalp too. The duration of a course of a corticosteroid ointment may vary from one week up to four weeks, depending on the age of the patient, the area to be treated and the potency of the preparation. The treatment should then be stopped. Then an emollient can be used or another suitable treatment regime. Corticosteroids are not suitable for the treatment of large skin areas. The treatment of psoriasis in children is usually prescribed only after consulting a dermatologist. Systemic corticosteroids must not be used for the treatment of psoriasis, as disease progression to an extensive form of pustular psoriasis is possible.
- Preparations of **coal tar** are suitable for the treatment of extensive guttate psoriasis or as follow-up treatment of other treatment forms. At present, coal tar preparations are not much used due to their smell and mess.
- **Dithranol** (anthralin) is used as a "short contact" regimen. 1–3% dithranol formula is applied and left on for 20–30 min. The preparation is washed off after the application time. The preparation may permanently stain the wash basins. Dithranol is also suitable for the treatment of scalp psoriasis.
- **Calcipotriol** (calcipotriene) is a vitamin D analogue. It is available as an ointment or cream as well as scalp solution. Its efficacy is similar to that of a potent topical corticosteroid. The maximum weekly dose is 100 g of 50 μg/g ointment, cream or solution.
- **The combination of calcipotriol with a potent topical corticosteroid** is more effective than either component alone Ⓐ [1]. The combination formula is suitable as an initial treatment of plaque psoriasis in adults. Once daily dosing is sufficient, which may improve compliance. The treatment may last for up to four weeks. The patient must be observed for corticosteroid-induced signs of skin atrophy (thinning of the skin, papery skin, dilated capillaries, bruising). Follow-up treatment may be carried out for example with calcipotriol alone.
- **Calcitriol** Ⓐ [2 3] is an active form of vitamin D, and it is available as an ointment. Its efficacy is similar to that of a potent topical corticosteroid. The treated area must be not more than 35% of total body surface area. The maximum dose is 30 g of the ointment (3 μg/g) daily or 210 g weekly. It can also be applied lightly to sensitive skin areas, such as the face and flexures. The ointment should be applied twice daily. It has also been used together with a topical corticosteroid.
- **Tazarotene** is a topically applied retinoid used as a gel once daily Ⓑ [4]. Its efficacy is similar to that of a potent topical corticosteroid. Irritation is seen in some patients.

The addition of a potent topical corticosteroid to tazarotene therapy increases the treatment success.

Phototherapy

- Phototherapy may be used for extensive psoriasis (>20% of the body surface) Ⓐ [5 6 7]. Phototherapy should only be prescribed with firm criteria. The prescribing physician must be well versed in the prescribed form of phototherapy and the doses necessary for the patient's particular skin type.
- Indications, suitable doses and frequency of exposure to phototherapies and concomitant treatment require the experience of a dermatologist. PUVA (ultraviolet A radiation with a psoralen) and retinoids may only be prescribed by dermatologists.
- Various combination regimens (e.g. retinoids) are recommended to reduce the cumulative UV dose and with the intention to reduce the long-term adverse effects of phototherapy.
- Climatotherapy (heliotherapy). Skin must tolerate exposure to the sun (i.e. the skin must be able to tan and it may not burn easily). Sunbathing is started with small UV doses. The time to sunbathe is dependent on the skin phototype and degree of tanning. Furthermore, the geographical location, time of day, season, weather, altitude and other factors like pollution have a major influence on the time needed for sunbathing. Therefore, no single predetermined time schedule can be given. As regards plaque psoriasis, a three-week course is usually necessary for a good result. Contraindications include alcoholism and severe mental health problems. Photosensitising medications (e.g. amiodarone, piroxicam and doxycycline) are also a contraindication, as is poor general health. Heliotherapy is an effective but relatively expensive treatment modality due to the lost working days.
- Ultraviolet B (UVB) radiation is particularly beneficial in guttate psoriasis. UVB treatments are divided into the conventional broad-band (TL12) UVB therapy (wavelength 385–400 nm) and the narrow-band (TL01) UVB therapy (wavelength 309–313 nm). The latter (TL01) is now regarded in most clinics as the treatment of choice in the field of phototherapy.
- The efficacy of narrow-band UVB therapy is at least comparable to that of PUVA. The long-term adverse effects of narrow-band UVB are not yet known.
- The efficacy of UVB therapy may be enhanced with the addition of a systemic retinoid (ReUVB)and various topical agents compatible with phototherapy which may reduce the cumulative UV dose received by the patient.
- PUVA therapy is an effective but also highly demanding form of phototherapy. The photosensitising effects of different psoralens vary ten-fold. During RePUVA therapy the patient receives a concomitant systemic retinoid (acitretin). The PUVA therapies have fallen out of favour due to increased risk of skin cancer associated with tablet-PUVA therapy. Despite the associated risks, PUVA may still be the best choice for some patients in problematic cases.

Systemic treatment

- Acitretin, methotrexate Ⓒ, hydroxyurea Ⓒ, ciclosporin Ⓐ and sulfasalazine Ⓑ [8] may be prescribed by a dermatologist to patients with severe psoriasis. The administration of these modalities requires special experience and regular follow-up. In a recent study, methotrexate and ciclosporin proved to be equally effective for moderate to severe plaque type psoriasis in a randomized controlled trial.
- Biologicals, such as alefacept, efalizumab, etanercept and infliximab, have recently been introduced for the treatment of severe psoriasis. Alefacept and efalizumab inhibit T-cell activation. TNF-alpha antagonists infliximab and etanercept are also effective in psoriatic arthritis. A special risk associated with TNF-alpha antagonists is an activation of latent infections (e.g. tuberculosis).

Referral to specialist

- Children suffering from psoriasis and adults requiring combination treatment regimens, or suffering from psoriasis (regardless of the extent) that does not respond to usual treatment modalities, should be referred to a dermatologist.
- An experienced dermatologist can be more helpful in the diagnosis of problematic psoriasis than sending off a skin biopsy.
- If excessive corticosteroid use is suspected the patient should be referred to a dermatologist.

References

1. Mason J, Mason AR, Cork MJ. Topical preparations for the treatment of psoriasis: a systematic review. Br J Dermatol 2002;146:351–64.
2. Ashcroft DM, Li Wan Po A, Williams HC, Griffith CE. Systematic review of comparatative efficacy and tolerability of calcipotriol in treating chronic plaque psoriasis. BMJ 2000;320:963–967.
3. The Database of Abstracts of Reviews of Effectiveness (University of York), Database no.: DARE-20008265. In: The Cochrane Library, Issue 3, 2001. Oxford: Update Software.
4. Weinstein GD, Krueger GG, Lowe JL et al. Tazarotene gel, a new retinoid, for topical therapy of psoriasis: Vehicle-controlled study of safety, efficacy and duration of therapeutic effect. J Am Acad Dermatol 1997;37:85–92.
5. Griffiths CEM, Clark CM, Chalmers RJG, Li Wan Po A, Williams HC. A systematic review of treatments for severe psoriasis. Health Technol Assess 2000;4(40).
6. Spuls PI, Witkamp L, Bossuyt PM, Bos JD. A systematic review of five systemic treatments for severe psoriasis. Br J Dermatol 1997;137:943–949.
7. The Database of Abstracts of Reviews of Effectiveness (University of York), Database no.: DARE-980690. In: The Cochrane Library, Issue 1, 2000. Oxford: Update Software.
8. Griffiths CEM, Clark CM, Chalmers RJG, Li Wan Po A, Williams HC. A systematic review of treatments for severe psoriasis. Health Technol Assess 2000;4(40).

13.72 Pityriasis rosea

Eero Lehmuskallio

Aetiology

- Pityriasis rosea is a self-limited skin disease. It may be caused by some virus.

Symptoms

- Initially a primary lesion ("herald patch") appears on the trunk. The lesion is oval, rose-coloured, and up to 3 cm in diameter (Figure 13.72.1). Later slight circular scaling develops around the lesion.
- After a few days several smaller (0.5–3cm) patches develop, most commonly on the chest. Their long axis aligns the ribs.
- Some patients have slight itching.
- The disease is not contagious. It is most common in the spring and autumn.

Differential diagnosis

- Patients with guttate psoriasis (13.71) often have a family history of psoriasis, and scaling is more marked.
- Pityriasis versicolor is more slender and the lesions develop more slowly. The colour of the lesions is usually not rose and there is no herald patch.
- Secondary syphilis is very rare. If the patient is sexually active and the history is suggestive, the cardiolipin test (or corresponding test) may be indicated.

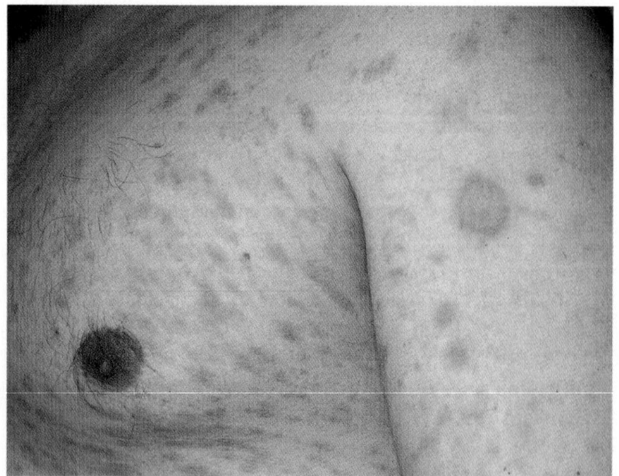

Figure 13.72.1 Pityriasis rosea is a common, often pruritic exanthema, lasting a few weeks, maximally two months. The "primary medallion" seen in the upper arm, appeared a couple of weeks before the spread of the eruption. Typical mild "collar scaling" is seen best in this primary patch. The longer axis of the ellipsoid lesions on the chest follows the direction of the ribs. Photo © R. Suhonen.

Treatment

- The disease is self-limited, and the lesions usually disappear in 6–8 weeks. The lesions do not recur.
- The patient should be reassured that the prognosis is good and the lesions are harmless. Usually no other treatment is needed.
- Itching can be treated with mild corticosteroid lotions or oral antihistamines.

13.73 Lichen planus

Pekka Autio

Aetiology

- The aetiology is unknown.

Clinical features

- Bluish-red, flat, glistening, polygonal papules (Figure 13.73.1) with a pale mesh-like surface (Wickham striae).
- Some of the papules may have bullae (L. bullosus).
- On the legs the lesions may become hypertrophic (L. hypertrophicus).
- On the mouth mucosa a pale mesh-like surface is typical. It may ulcerate.
- The **Koebner phenomenon**: Scratches on the skin become affected with papules.
- Typical sites include the volar fold of the wrist, flexor surfaces of the arms, and the ankle (Figure 13.73.2). Common sites also include the proximal palms, soles, lower

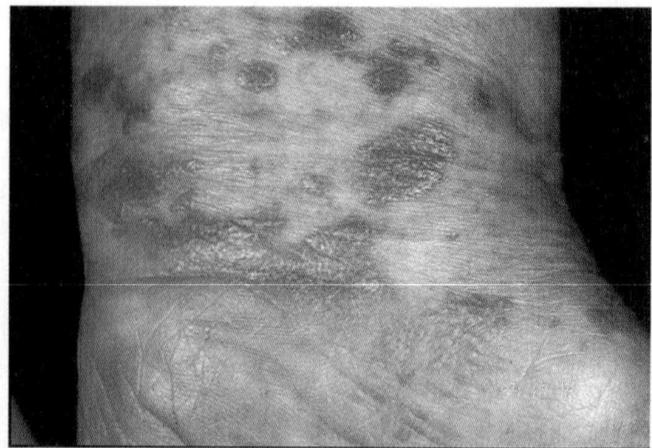

Figure 13.73.1 Lichen planus in one of the most typical locations—the ventral side of the wrist. Potent topical corticoids for limited period are mostly efficient. Recurrence is not unusual—it may affect up to 50% of the patients. Photo © R. Suhonen.

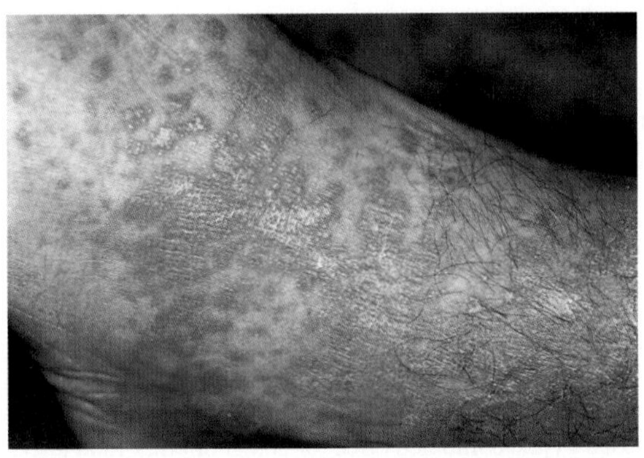

Figure 13.73.2 Prominent lichen planus in the ankle region. A lilac red colour, woven in a whitish Wickham stria-network, is a typical clinical feature. A controlled use of (very) potent corticosteroid ointments of a few weeks' duration often proves beneficial. Photo © R. Suhonen.

lip and glans penis. Papules are often distributed on the trunk, especially in the sacral area.

- The lesions are almost invariably itchy.

Diagnostics

- The clinical presentation is usually sufficient for diagnosis.
- Skin biopsy is diagnostic.

Treatment

- An alternative to all modes of treatment is to wait for spontaneous recovery. There is no predictable time-course for spontaneous healing. Imagine yourself in the position of the patient when making treatment decisions.
- Potent corticosteroid preparations C [1 2] often clear the lesions in a couple of weeks.
- Do not use potent steroids without controlling for the outcome!
- Lichen planus on the oral mucosa is difficult to treat. Corticosteroids, retinoids, cyclosporin C [1 2], or sometimes cryotherapy may be of benefit C [3 4 5 6]. The possible irritating or sensitizing effect of amalgam fillings may be worth consideration.
- Do not treat pigmented remnants of lichen papules. They return to normal colour spontaneously with time.
- If widespread, active lichen planus is not cured by local treatments a dermatologist may consider acitretin C [1 2], griseofulvin C [1 2], cyclosporin, or PUVA C [3 4 5 6].
- The disease recurs in at least 50% of the patients–often after a few years.

References

1. Cribier B, Frances C, Chosidow O. Treatment of lichen planus: an evidence-based medicine analysis of efficacy. Archives of Dermatology 1998;134:1521–30.
2. The Database of Abstracts of Reviews of Effectiveness (University of York), Database no.: DARE-990129. In: The Cochrane Library, Issue 1, 2002. Oxford: Update Software.
3. Chan ES-Y, Thornhill M, Zakrzewska J. Interventions for treating oral lichen planus. The Cochrane Database of Systematic Reviews, Cochrane Library number: CD001168. In: The Cochrane Library, Issue 2, 2002. Oxford: Update Software.
4. Buajeeb W, Kraivaphan P, Pobrurksa C. Efficacy of topical retinoic acid compared with topical fluocinolone acetonide in the treatment of oral lichen planus. Oral Surg Oral Med Oral Pathol Oral Radiol Endod 1997;83:21–5.
5. Harpenau LA, Plemons JM, Rees TD. Effectiveness of a low dose of cyclosporin in the management of patients with oral erosive lichen planus. Oral Surg Oral Med Oral Pathol Oral Radiol Endod 1995;80:161–7.
6. Lundquist G, Forsgren H, Gajecki M, Emtestam L. Photochemotherapy of oral lichen planus. A controlled study. Oral Surg Oral Med Oral Pathol Oral Radiol Endod 1995;79: 554–8.

13.74 Hives (urticaria)

Editors

Aims

- The diagnosis is clinical–avoid unnecessary investigations.
- Identify different forms of urticaria and find out precipitating factors.
- Treat the patient's symptoms effectively.

Symptoms and signs

- The skin lesions are often pink or pale hives. There may be erythema in the surrounding skin (Figure 13.74.1).
- There may be considerable itching. Signs of scratching are rare.
- The size of the lesions varies from 1 mm to large confluent hives.
- The hives often cover large areas of the skin.
- Single lesions disappear within 24 hours.
- One patient in three has Quincke's oedema.

Differential diagnosis

Signs suggesting a disease other than urticaria

- The lesions leave a sign, e.g. mild ecchymosis or purpura.
- A single lesion remains in place for more than 24 hours.
    - For example, the following diseases should be considered in such cases: exanthemas, erythema multiforme, erythema nodosum, erythema fixum, and urticarial vasculitis.

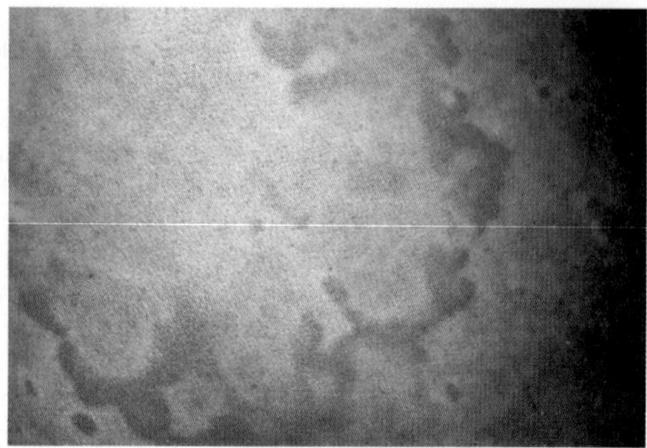

Figure 13.74.1 A red urticaria wheal (hives). In acute forms of urticaria the aetiology often can be found or at least suspected. In chronic urticaria (lasting for more than 1 month) a specific cause seldom is found, although there is no general agreement on this matter. Antihistamine drugs are the therapy of choice. Photo © R. Suhonen.

Diseases that should be considered in the differential diagnosis

- Angioneurotic oedema (Quincke's oedema): oedema in the lips, eyelids, hands, etc. The duration of the lesions is 1–3 days. The disease occurs alone or concomitantly with urticaria.
- Strophulus or papular urticaria. The duration of the lesions is several days, even a few weeks. Antihistamines do not help.
- Urticarial vasculitis. The duration of the hives is 1–3 days. Antihistamines do not help.

Acute urticaria (duration <3 months)

- Most acute urticarias are associated with infections, although the aetiological connection remains unproven. The drugs used for the infection are often blamed although they are usually not the causative factor.
- If urticaria commences during a course of medication reconsider the need for the drug. (Is the disease requiring medication already cured? Was the course given for a vague indication such as a prolonged cough?) Change the drug if further treatment is indicated.
- Provocation tests are needed to prove a drug as the cause of urticaria. Drug provocation tests are performed in a hospital only when the patient has recovered completely.
- In urticaria caused by penicillin, a RAST test is often positive. The positive reaction usually disappears within one year from the reaction.

Treatment

- An antihistamine or a combination of antihistamine-vasoconstrictor perorally in normal doses as long as the urticaria continues.
- Adrenalin (1:1000) 0.5 mg subcutaneously for oedema of the mouth, pharynx or airways, or for severe systemic symptoms.
- In exceptionally severe urticaria a single 40–60 mg dose of prednisolone can be given perorally.
- Sick leave may be indicated in some patients.
- Hospitalization is rarely necessary, but a few hours' follow-up is sometimes indicated.

Recurrent acute urticaria

- Recurrent urticarias occur at intervals of years or months during infections or irrespective of them. Finding the cause is exceptional, and investigations are usually unrewarding.
- Acute attacks of urticaria and anaphylaxis may sometimes be caused by the combined effect of cereal or other food allergy and exercise. They may also be caused by the combined effect of infection and exercise (particularly when associated with hangover).
- Urticaria may also be caused by contact with, for example, animal saliva, latex or semen.

Investigations

- No investigations are necessary in acute urticaria.
- In recurrent acute urticaria the patient can be referred to a specialist.

Chronic urticaria (duration >3 months)

- Chronic urticaria is sometimes associated with infections, allegies, drugs or other diseases
  - Identify infection foci, allergies etc. depending on the case
  - Remove/manage the causing factor
- Idiopathic chronic urticaria
  - The symptoms are often daily.
  - No clear cause is found
  - Any antihistamine can be used as treatment.
- Autoimmune urticaria
  - Symptoms occur daily, as in idiopathic urticaria
  - The symptoms are severe and the patient responds poorly to antihistamines
  - Hives persisting longer than 24 hours occur, resembling urticarial vasculitis
  - Intradermal test with the patient's own serum is positive
  - Immunoglobulin therapy is often efficient
  - Refer to a specialist
- Dermatographism (urticaria factitia)
  - A (viral) infection is often a triggering factor.
  - The duration of the disease is usually < 1 year in young people, 2–4 years in middle-aged people.
  - Any antihistamine that causes less drowsiness can be prescribed.
- Local cold urticaria
  - When cooled skin is rewarmed redness and swelling appears locally. The phenomenon usually lasts for some years.
  - The diagnosis is made by placing a piece of ice on a skin area where the symptoms usually occur.

- Treatment: warm clothing. UVB light therapy (about 30 times) is usually helpful. Doxepin 10 (–25) mg × 1–3 is moderately effective.

♦ Perspiration urticaria
  - In young adults severely itching hives 1–2 in diameter are triggered by perspiration (and excitement).
  - The duration of the symptom is < 2 hours at a time.
  - The diagnosis is made with "a staircase test": any exercise resulting in perspiration.
  - Treatment: UVB light therapy, avoiding perspiration.

♦ In Quincke's oedema (most commonly caused by ACE inhibitors or angiotensin receptor blockers, sometimes also by other drugs) antihistamines do not help. In most cases the cause remains unidentified. If the swelling is severe and annoying 30–60 mg of prednisone or prednisolone can be given perorally to an adult. If necessary, 0.5 mg of adrenalin (1:1000) should also be given. The patient can also be managed at home if symptoms subside.

13.75 Erythema nodosum

Editors

Aims

♦ Identify erythema nodosum.
♦ Exclude the possible underlying causes, such as streptococcal infection, sarcoidosis, and yersiniosis.

Epidemiology

♦ More common (3–5 times) in women than in men.
♦ Racial and geographical differences (in the prevalence of the underlying causes) influence the incidence rates.
♦ Young adults are most commonly affected.
♦ Most cases occur in the winter and spring.

Aetiology

♦ Infectious diseases
  - Streptococcal tonsillitis (7–14 days before the nodules appear)
  - Chlamydia pneumoniae infection
  - Yersiniosis, salmonellosis
  - Primary infection of tuberculosis

♦ Sarcoidosis
♦ Drug reaction
  - Sulphonamides

♦ Hormonal causes
  - Contraceptive pills, hormonal treatment

♦ Rare causes
  - Inflammatory bowel diseases
  - Malignancies (e.g. Hodgkin's disease)

♦ Often the aetiology remains unknown.

Symptoms and signs

♦ Solitary red, tender, elevated nodules on the anterior aspect of the legs; rarely in other parts of the body.
♦ Fatigue, fever, and arthralgia, rarely arthritis, may occur.
♦ High ESR.

DER

Investigations

♦ The investigations aim at detecting an underlying disease that can be treated specifically.
♦ Ask also about symptoms in family members.

Basic investigations

♦ Throat streptococcal culture
♦ Chest radiograph (sarcoidosis, tuberculosis)
♦ ESR, CRP
♦ Blood count, urine test (other infections)

According to individual judgment

♦ Antistreptolysin (a change in the titre or a high titre may suggest streptococcal infection)
♦ Yersinia antibodies
♦ Chlamydia pneumoniae antibodies if the patient has respiratory symptoms

Treatment

♦ Rest
♦ Treatment of the underlying disease
♦ NSAIDs, cooling compresses

13.76 Solar keratosis

Pekka Autio

Aim

♦ Treat solar keratosis to avoid the risk of development of carcinoma and aesthetic harm.

Definition

♦ Solar keratosis is a degenerative disorder of epidermal cell growth. It is a precancerous lesion that can develop into an

epidermoid carcinoma that does not (yet) infiltrate through the basal membrane.
- Solar keratosis can be treated without affecting the dermis (i.e. without causing a scar).

Epidemiology

- Common among those with fair skin. Occurs in old age on sun-exposed areas of the skin.
- The face, bald scalp, upper corners of the ear lobes, and dorsum of the hand are sites of predilection.

Diagnostics

- An erythematous, asymptomatic, well-demarcated small plaque is the first manifestation (Figure 13.76.1).
- The plaque grows up to a diameter of a few centimetres, scales, and may develop thick hyperkeratosis, even a cornu cutaneum.
- In most cases there are multiple lesions.
- Take a biopsy or refer the patient to a dermatologist.

Treatment and prophylaxis

- Before treatment exclude an epidermoid carcinoma (13.77).
- Cryotherapy with liquid nitrogen is effective, cheap, and the aesthetic outcome is good.
- Simple excision of small lesions is adequate but the cosmetic result is not as good as with cryotherapy.
- Imiquimod and photodynamic therapy are emerging treatment options.
- Tretinoin cream (0.05%) can be used for the treatment and prophylaxis of very thin lesions B [1]. The cream can be used for long periods, even continuously.
- Assess healing after 2–3 months.
- Sunscreen preparations slow the development of new lesions B [2].

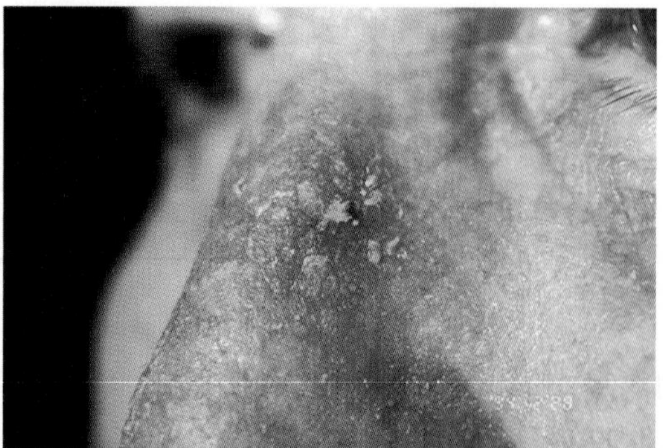

Figure 13.76.1 Actinic/solar keratosis is a premalignant, sun-provoked lesion. Over the years it may progress into epidermoid carcinoma. Often the best therapy is cryosurgery, which—using the appropriate technique—eliminates the epidermal disorder without unacceptable aesthetic adverse effects. Bowen's disease and epidermoid carcinoma are diagnostic alternatives. Photo © R. Suhonen.

Prognosis

- In following years new lesions will probably appear.
- If left untreated for years solar keratosis may develop into an epidermoid carcinoma.

Indications for specialist consultation

- Cryotherapy with liquid nitrogen is usually performed by a dermatologist.
- A dermatologist is the best diagnostician as the diagnosis (a stereomicroscope is useful).

References

1. Marks R, Lever L. Studies on the effects of topical retinoic acid on photoageing. Br J Dermatol 1990; 122 Suppl 35:93–5.
2. Thompson SC, Jolley D, Marks R. Reduction of solar keratoses by regular sunscreen use. N Engl J Med 1993;329:1147–51.

13.77 Skin cancer

Editors

Basic rules

- The most important indication for excision of a naevus is suspicion of malignancy. Other indications include aesthetic considerations or the location of the naevus in an area exposed to friction. If naevi are excised for cosmetic reasons always estimate the eventual consequences of a scar and the tendency of the patient to develop keloids.
- A general practitioner can excise any naevus under local anaesthesia. Very large lesions and strong suspicion of melanoma should be referred to a specialist.

Naevi, melanoma

- The incidence of melanoma is increasing. Suspect a melanoma if a naevus starts to grow, change its colour, develop satellites, bleed, or discharge. A melanoma cannot be ruled out on clinical grounds, and it may develop on previously intact skin.

1. "Ordinary looking" naevus

- The need for excision depends on the history given by the patient concerning changes, and aesthetic considerations or annoying location. Requests for the removal of solitary naevi should generally be granted even if the doctor considers the lesion benign.

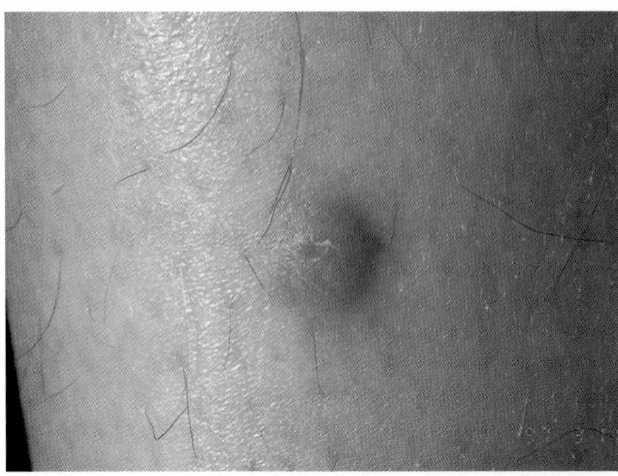

Figure 13.77.1 Dermatofibroma is one of the most common tumours on the legs in adulthood. A hard, smooth, regular nodule, often with diffuse hyperpigmentation around the outer border, are typical features. Cryosurgery, excision or no therapy at all are the therapeutic alternatives. Photo © R. Suhonen.

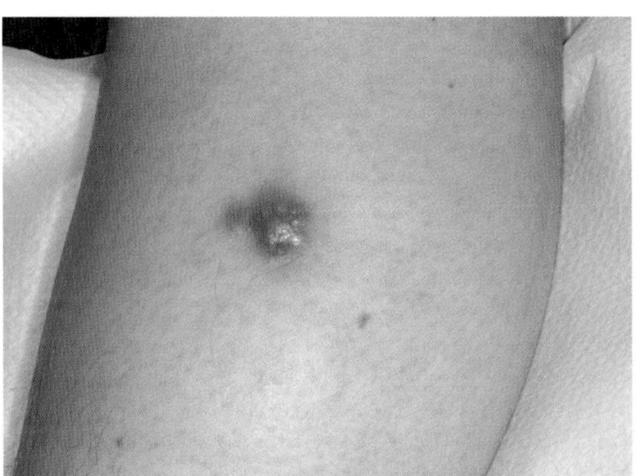

Figure 13.77.2 An unusually large, reddish, multilocular dermatofibroma on the leg. The diffuse pigmentation around the outer margins is characteristic for this benign and common skin tumour. Photo © R. Suhonen.

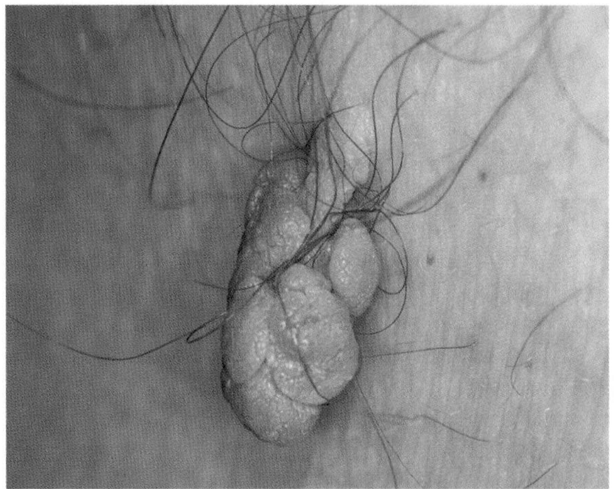

Figure 13.77.3 Fibroma molle, a soft fibroma is a benign skin tumour. If it becomes twisted it may lose its blood supply, which eventually leads to pain and necrosis. Soft fibroma can easily be treated by electrocautery, excision or cryosurgery. Photo © R. Suhonen.

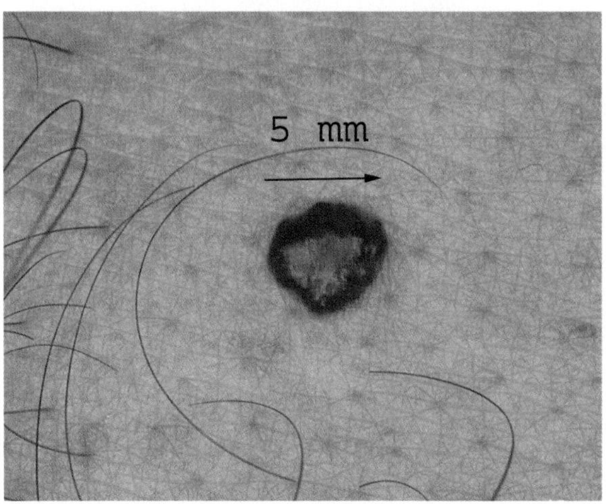

Figure 13.77.4 Cherry angioma, also called senile angioma. The common lesions are usually of 1–5 mm in diameter. They are harmless, but can be treated, e.g. with liquid nitrogen cryotherapy, if necessary for cosmetic reasons. Photo © R. Suhonen.

- The naevus is removed totally, but the margin of intact skin can be small.
- Benign lesions that may concern the patient include dermatofibroma (Figures 13.77.1 and 13.77.2), fibroma molle (Figure 13.77.3), and cherry angioma (Figure 13.77.4).
- The general practitioner often sees patients who require the removal of a large number of naevi either one at a time or at the same consultation. Usually a reassuring conversation and the removal of a few large naevi calms the patient, unless the patient suffers from conversion, in which case the same problems occur again later.

2. "Slightly suspect" naevus

- For example, a naevus that looks benign but that has grown or changed colour (darker) or has bled or discharged according to the patient C [1,2].
- Such a naevus should always be removed, and the excision margin is determined by the appearance and location of the naevus.
- Granuloma pyogenicum is a benign growth that usually develops at the site of disrupted skin (Figure 13.77.5).
- The following lesions may be difficult to differentiate from melanoma:
  - 'blue naevus' (Figure 13.77.6)
  - lentigo (Figure 13.77.7)
  - naevus spilus (Figure 13.77.8)
  - Spitz naevus (Figure 13.77.9)

3. Strong suspicion of a melanoma

- Refer the patient to a plastic surgeon, surgeon, or a specialist in otorhinolaryngology or ophthalmology if a naevus has

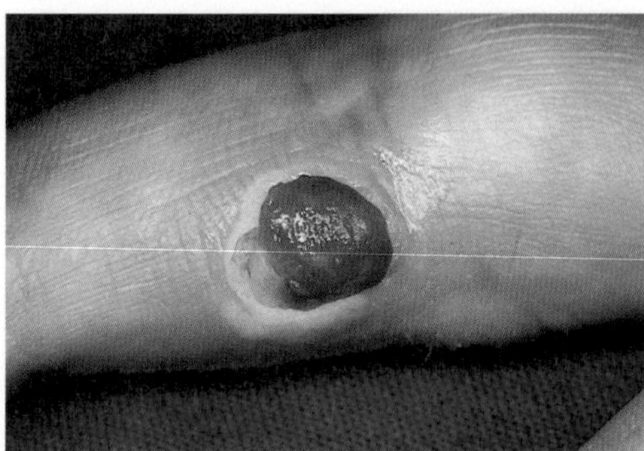

Figure 13.77.5 Pyogenic granuloma (Telangiectatic g.) is not uncommon in the fingers. The lesion may be initiated by a minor trauma. The benign, easily bleeding tumour may be treated by curettage and/or liquid nitrogen cryosurgery, electrodesiccation or laser. Photo © R. Suhonen.

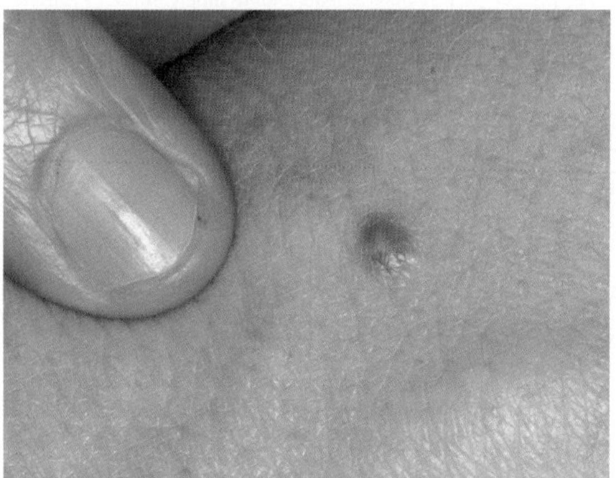

Figure 13.77.6 Blue naevus, naevus coeruleus, is a benign skin tumour, which may mimic malignant melanoma. It is best excised with small margins for histopathology. Photo © R. Suhonen.

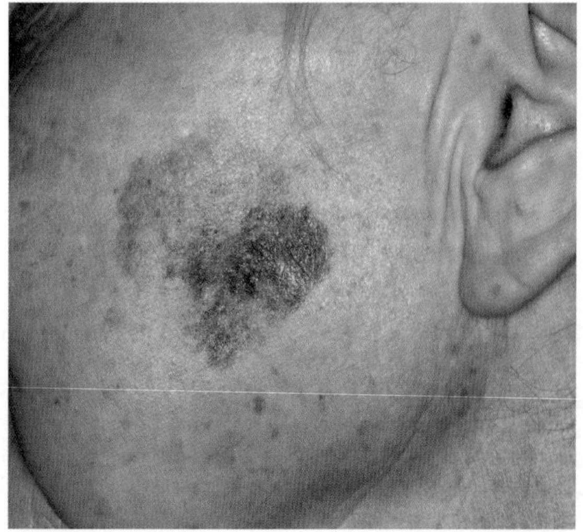

Figure 13.77.7 The unevenly pigmented lesion of an elderly lady proved to be lentigo maligna, in situ—malignant melanoma. One year earlier several biopsies showed a benign lentigo. The lesion was excised. Photo © R. Suhonen.

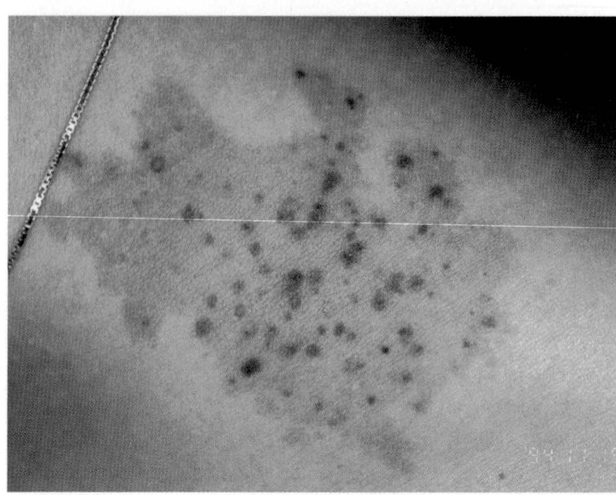

Figure 13.77.8 Naevus spilus is characterized by a brownish macular patch including small scattered darker spots. There is very little tendency towards malignant transformation and consequently excision of the lesion is not routinely recommended. Photo © R. Suhonen.

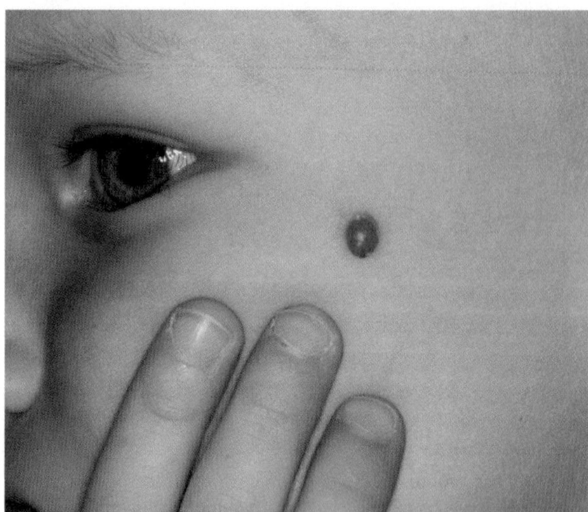

Figure 13.77.9 Spitz naevus, spindle cell naevus, is a benign skin tumour of childhood. Erroneously it has earlier been called "juvenile melanoma", which should now be avoided to avoid therapeutic and prognostic confusion. The colour may vary from dark pigmented to pink red. Excision with small margins for histopathologic study is the preferable therapy. Photo © R. Suhonen.

- markedly grown and changed its colour (Figure 13.77.10)
- become exceptionally large (Figure 13.77.11)
- developed satellites
- appeared on the site of a melanoma that has been excised before.

♦ Make sure that the patient has been reserved an appointment and that the naevus was removed.

Treatment and follow-up of a melanoma

♦ In cases of melanoma the patient should be referred for further surgical treatment, and the referring physician should make sure that the patient is treated without delay.

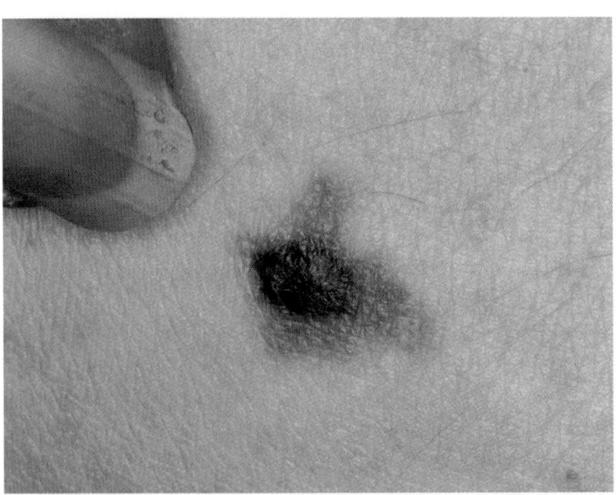

Figure 13.77.10 A small black area in previously harmless naevus is a strong indication for excisional biopsy. The tumour proved to be a malignant melanoma. Photo © R. Suhonen.

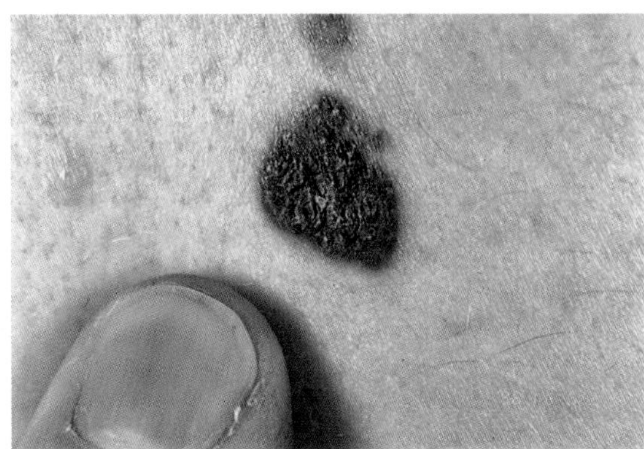

Figure 13.77.12 This pigmented lesion on the skin of the back of a middle-aged male was excised with 2-mm margins for histopathological study. It proved to be malignant melanoma. Some weeks earlier a punch biopsy specimen had shown only benign features. Any pigment lesion with irregularity in colour and shape should be excised totally for microscopic study. Photo © R. Suhonen.

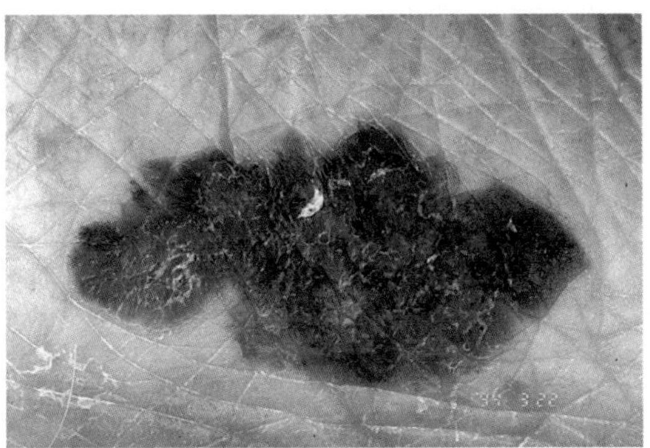

Figure 13.77.11 Malignant melanoma (MM) on the lateral side of the right foot. Irregular border, variation in colour hue and intensity are typical features of this highly malignant tumour. Excision and free grafting were performed. Photo © R. Suhonen.

- A larger excision of the skin and subcutaneous tissue is performed around the tumour. The extent of the excision is determined by the location, thickness (Breslow classification) and depth of infiltration (Clark classification) of the tumour.
- Very superficial melanomas (Clark I–II, Breslow < 1 mm) should be excised with a 1 cm margin of intact tissue (Figure 13.77.12). Deeper melanomas should be removed with a 2–5 cm margin. The site of excision is reconstructed with a pedicle flap or free graft. Prophylactic evacuation of lymph nodes is performed in some cases of melanoma.

Follow-up of a melanoma

- Patients with a melanoma are followed-up every 3 months until 2 years have passed from the diagnosis. Thereafter, follow-up is continued every 6 months for 5 years. The unit responsible for follow-up (hospital or primary care) can be decided on locally. It is important that the same doctor always sees the patient.
- If the patient has numerous naevi or the syndrome of hereditary dysplastic naevi, follow-up of a melanoma should take place in a dermatological unit. High-quality photographs facilitate follow-up. These patients should be followed up throughout their life.
- At follow-up visits the general condition and symptoms are investigated, and the site of excision and local lymph nodes are palpated. Satellites of melanoma are usually felt as subcutaneous nodules and they are visible under the skin as dark spots.
- A melanoma first metastasizes into regional lymph nodes which should be followed-up carefully by palpation. If the clinical examination suggests the spread of a melanoma, a chest x-ray, blood count, liver function tests, and liver ultrasonography should be performed.
- If a melanoma has infiltrated the regional lymph nodes they are removed surgically. A metastasized melanoma is treated by an oncologist. Cytostatics and interferon have been moderately effective in the treatment of metastasized melanoma.

Basiloma (basalioma, carcinoma basocellulare, basal cell carcinoma, BCC)

- Basiloma or basal cell carcinoma is the most common malignant tumour in man. It is typically located in the face of an elderly person (Figures 13.77.13 and 13.77.14).
- A typical basiloma is a glittering tumour with elevated margins. Often ulceration develops in the centre. A so-called morphoid basiloma is difficult to recognize and its borders are difficult to determine.
- A superficial basiloma usually occurs on the trunk (Figure 13.77.15). Differentiation from psoriasis or eczema may sometimes be difficult.

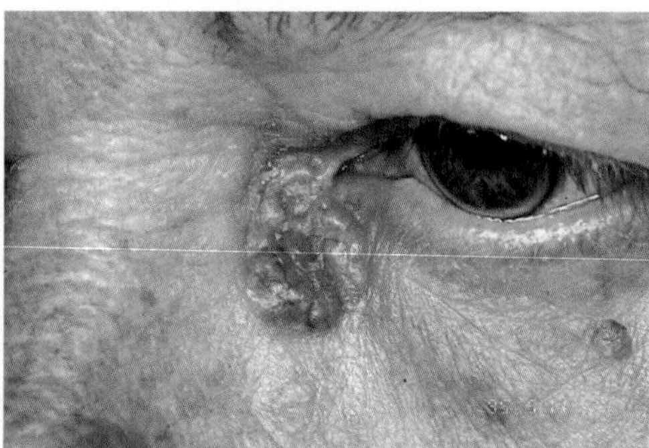

Figure 13.77.13 Basal cell carcinoma in the inner canthus is a real challenge to therapy. The size of the basalioma in this location is a regrettable sign of neglect of the health care system. There is obvious difficulty in operating with safe margins. Recurrence in cartilaginous structures may be an ocular catastrophe. There is no place for cryosurgery in this location. Photo © R. Suhonen.

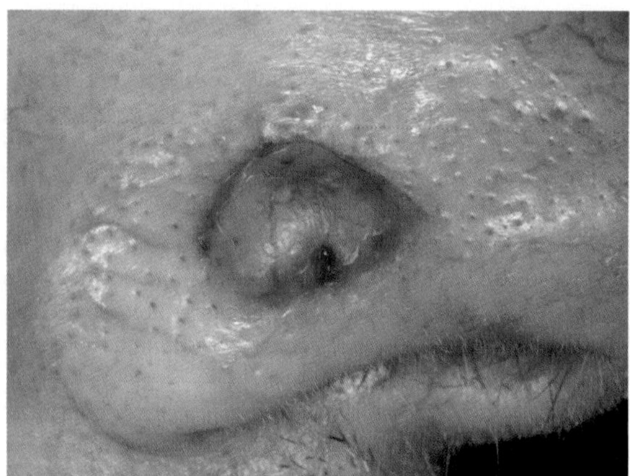

Figure 13.77.14 The side part of the nose is a typical site for basalioma. In this nodular BCC typical telangiectases are seen. Both cure and good aesthetic outcome are important in this location. The choice of proper treatment method should be carefully considered. Photo © R. Suhonen.

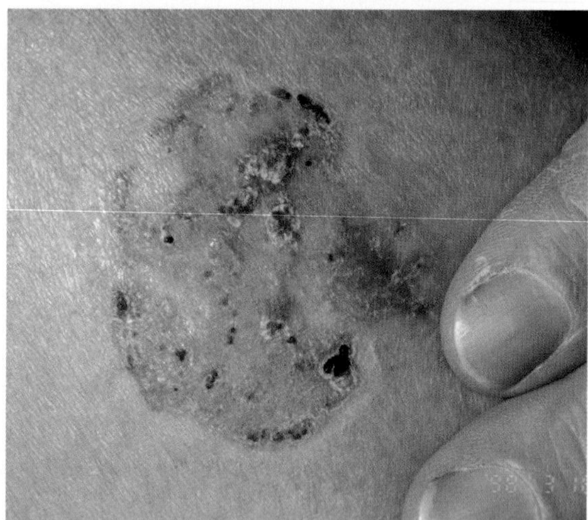

Figure 13.77.15 The superficial type of basalioma is most common on the trunk, where it may resemble inflammatory dermatosis. The lesion is typically reddish, sharply demarcated, often with a faint "necklace of pearls". If biopsied, take a sufficiently large sample; false negative specimens are not uncommon in superficial BCCs. Photo © R. Suhonen.

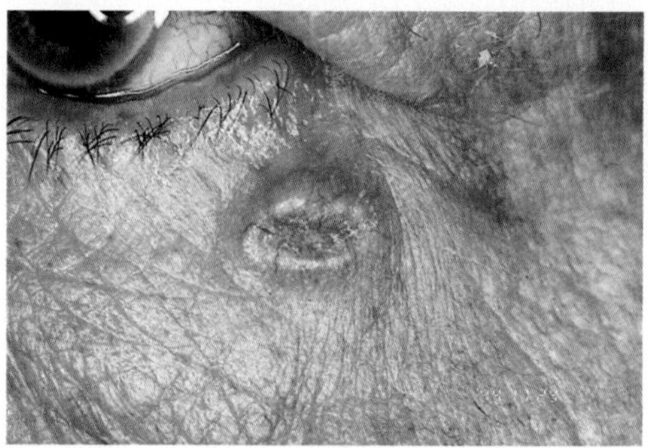

Figure 13.77.16 Basal cell carcinoma in the eyelid is a good target for cryosurgery (medial canthus excluded). Cryosurgery is at least as curative as plain surgery and the aesthetic result is mostly good to excellent. Cryosurgery is a low-cost dermatologic office procedure. Photo © R. Suhonen.

Treatment and follow-up

- The general practitioner can excise C [3 4 5] a small, typical basiloma if he/she is familiar with the operative techniques in the area. Patients with a suspected basiloma on the eyelids or in the vicinity of the nostrils or ear canal should be referred to a specialist.
- The treatment of choice is surgery. The tumour is excised under local anaesthesia with a 5-mm margin of intact tissue, and reconstruction is performed if necessary by pedicle flap or free graft. A patient with basiloma should be followed-up for 5 years after surgery. Shorter follow-up may suffice for a solitary, small basiloma.
- A superficial basiloma, and some common basilomas, particularly in the elderly, can be treated with liquid nitrogen cryotherapy in a unit familiar with the technique (Figure 13.77.16).
- A basiloma metastasizes rarely. Because local spread is common special care should be taken in the treatment and follow-up of basilomas near the eyelids, nostrils, or ear canal.
- Small basilomas in non-risk areas can be excised by the general practitioner who is also responsible for follow-up.
- Consider referring a young patient with basiloma to a dermatologist. Basiloma may be a manifestation of some rare inherited diseases (Figure 13.77.17).

Epidermoid carcinoma (c. epidermoides, c. spinocellulare, c. squamocellulare, spinalioma)

- Epidermoid carcinoma is rare compared with basiloma. It most commonly occurs on the face and hands. The usual form is an ulcerating prominence or scaling plaque.

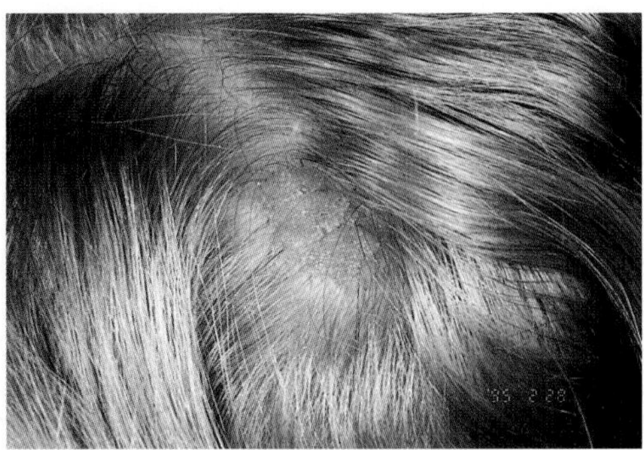

Figure 13.77.17 Sebaceous naevus on the scalp. This principally benign, congenital hamartoma has a malignant tendency in adults. Basal cell carcinomas are especially prone to develop among sebaceous naevi. Photo © R. Suhonen.

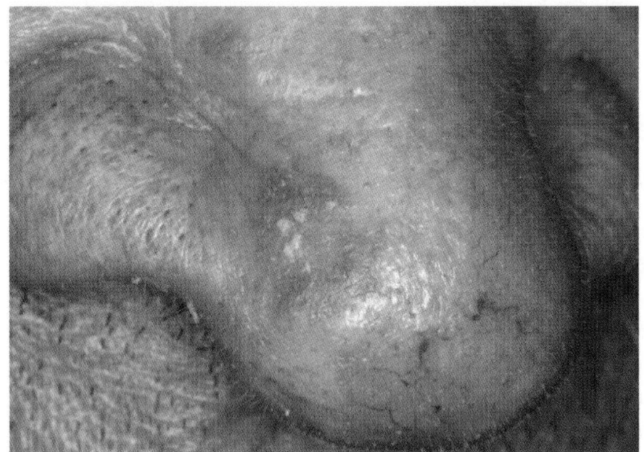

Figure 13.77.18 Solar keratosis is the result of life-long sun exposure. Skin changes with reddish, rough skin surface, often multiple, and which are non-responding to topical corticoids, are usually solar (actinic) keratosis. In the case shown here the treatment method of choice is cryosurgery with liquid nitrogen. In more widespread cases a good alternative is photodynamic therapy. Photo © R. Suhonen.

- An epidermoid carcinoma should be treated by surgical excision with a margin of 1–2 cm, and by subsequent reconstruction. A developing epidermoid carcinoma on sun-exposed skin can be treated by liquid nitrogen cryocoagulation by an experienced specialist. Distinguish from solar, actinic or senile keratosis (Figure 13.77.18) (13.76).
- Keratoacanthoma is a rapidly growing benign tumour (Figure 13.77.19).
- Bowen's disease is a superficial, "incipient" (in situ) carcinoma (Figure 13.77.20). It can be removed either surgically or by liquid nitrogen cryotherapy. The operation is usually performed by a surgeon, plastic surgeon, otologist, ophthalmologist, or dermatologist specialized in cryotherapy.
- A patient with epidermoid carcinoma should be followed-up at 6-month intervals for at least 5 years after treatment.

Lip carcinoma

- Lip carcinoma (epidermoid carcinoma of the lip) is usually situated in the lower lip. It presents first as an erosion or ulceration that can be preceded by leukoplakia.

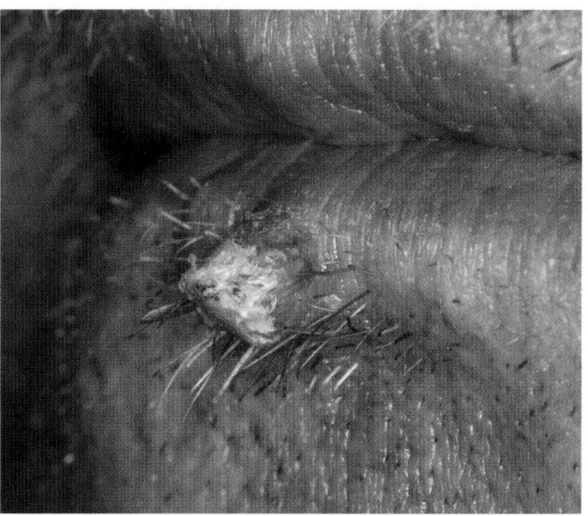

Figure 13.77.19 Keratoacanthoma in the lower lip. Keratoacanthoma is a rapidly growing benign tumour. Differential diagnosis with squamous cell carcinoma may be difficult. Rapid growth, and central heavy keratinous growth surrounded by an epithelial rim are characteristics favouring the diagnosis of keratoacanthoma. Photo © R. Suhonen.

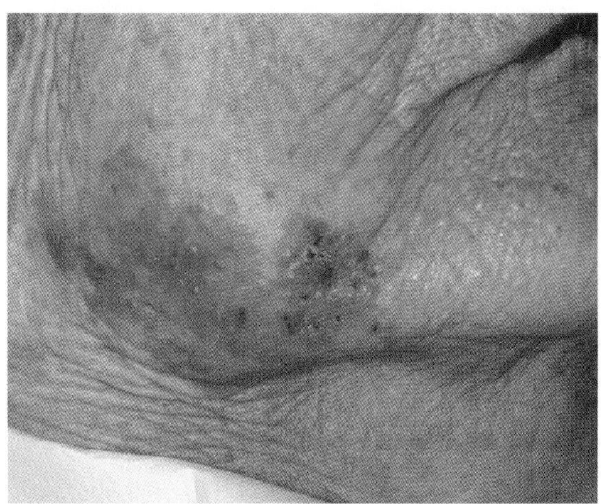

Figure 13.77.20 Bowen's disease, an intraepidermal epidermoid carcinoma, should be treated before it changes into an invasive carcinoma. Today, in an extensive case like this, the treatment of choice would probably be photodynamic therapy (PDT). Photo © R. Suhonen.

- A lip carcinoma is treated surgically by excising the lip at the site of the tumour, with a margin and by performing reconstruction.
- A lip carcinoma easily metastasizes in the lymph nodes under the skin, which should be palpated at follow-up examinations.

Prevention of skin cancer

- There is little evidence of interventions to prevent skin cancer. Sunscreens may be effective in the prevention of solar keratoses C [6] [7]

DER

References

1. Whited JD, Grichnik JM. Differential diagnosis of mole and melanoma. JAMA 1998;279:696–701.
2. The Database of Abstracts of Reviews of Effectiveness (University of York), Database no.: DARE-988293. In: The Cochrane Library, Issue 4, 1999. Oxford: Update Software.
3. Thissen MR, Neumann MH, Schouten LJ. A systematic review of treatment modalities for primary basal cell carcinomas. Archives of Dermatology 1999;135:1177–1183.
4. The Database of Abstracts of Reviews of Effectiveness (University of York), Database no.: DARE-992074. In: The Cochrane Library, Issue 1, 2001. Oxford: Update Software.
5. Bath FJ, Bong J, Perkins W, Williams HC. Interventions for basal cell carcinoma of the skin. Cochrane Database Syst Rev. 2004;(2):CD003412.
6. Prevention of skin cancer: a review of available strategies. University of Bristol Health Care Evaluation Unit 1995;31.
7. The Database of Abstracts of Reviews of Effectiveness (University of York), Database no.: DARE-950349. In: The Cochrane Library, Issue 4, 1999. Oxford: Update Software.

13.79 Keloid

Pekka Autio

Aims

- Prevent the formation of keloids (a previous keloid means risk for new keloids)
- Treat keloids that cause aesthetic or mechanical problems or symptoms. A newly formed keloid is easier to treat than an old one.

Definition

- A keloid is a pathological, tumour-like scar formation in a surgical wound, burn, earring holes or as a consequence of acne on the trunk that spreads beyond the original injury and does not regress spontaneously.

Diagnosis

- A typical case is easy to recognise. A keloid is at first a rubber-like, red, later dark red, solid, often tender, smooth growth of connective tissue covered by thin skin.
- The size can vary from a very small one to the size of an orange.
- A benign hypertrophic scar becomes soft and smaller within 6 months, whereas a keloid does not.
- Some cases occur familiarly.

Typical features

- Excessive scar formation is detected within 3–4 weeks from the injury. The growth may continue for months or years.
- Young women (from puberty to the age of 30) are at the greatest risk.
- Wound infection and tension increase the risk for keloid formation.
- The predilection sites include earlobes (holes!), upper trunk (particularly over the sternum), shoulders, chin, neck, and lower limbs. The palms, soles, and facial skin are less frequent sites.

Indications for treatment

- Aesthetic harm
- Restriction of skin motion, tenderness, or severe itch

Treatment

- A combination of liquid nitrogen cryotherapy and corticosteroid injection has yielded promising results C [1]. The keloid is frozen thoroughly with liquid nitrogen spray. After 5 minutes the swollen keloid is infiltrated with e.g. methylprednisolone 40 mg/ml (small syringe, thin needle). The treatment is repeated 1–2 times at 6 weeks intervals. The treatment is usually performed by a dermatologist.
- Pressure therapy may also be successful, but the treatment is laborious and takes a long time.
- In severe cases a plastic surgeon should be consulted. Simple excision usually provokes a new keloid.

Reference

1. Layton AM, Yip J, Cunliffe WJ. A comparison of intralesional triamcinolone and cryosurgery in the treatment of acne keloids. British Journal of Dermatology 1994;130:498–501.

13.80 Ingrowing toenail: avulsion of the nail edge and phenolization

Editors

Basic rule

- If bathing the toe and using spacious shoes does not result in healing the best treatment is the cutting and simple avulsion of the nail edge combined with phenolization. The method is more effective A [1] and less traumatic than surgical excision.

Techniques

- The 4 digital nerves are blocked with 1% lidocain.
- Cut a 3–5 mm slice from the lateral edge of the nail with scissors. Continue the incision through the proximal nail margin. Detach the slice from the nailbed and extract it, e.g. with forceps. The whole proximal "root" of the slice should be removed.
- Dry the resulting hole and insert a thin cotton wool bud dipped in 80% phenol into it. Replace a new bud 2–3 times and move (rotate) the buds for about a total of 45 s. Take care to prevent the phenol from spreading onto the surrounding skin. Clean the area and remove excessive phenol with a cotton wool bud dipped in saline or by injecting saline into the wound with a syringe (without a needle).
- Cover the toe with dressings.
- Instruct the patient to start showering the toe on the next day for 10–15 min twice a day as long as there is discharge from the wound.
- Acute infection around the nail edge is not a contraindication for the procedure.

Treatment of paronychia

- The excision and phenolization of an ingrowing nail is often sufficient (see above).
- A symptomatic abscess should be incised and bathed in $KMnO_4$ (dilution: 0.5 g in 5 l of water), which is an effective antiseptic. A first-generation cephalosporin or cloxacillin is indicated in severe infection.
- Avoid repeated wetting of the hands while working. For toxic eczema a corticosteroid cream, or a combination of a corticosteroid and an antifungal agent is beneficial (particularly in the fingers).
- Advise the patient to use spacious shoes and dry socks.

Reference

1. Rounding C, Bloomfield S. Surgical treatments for ingrowing toenails. Cochrane Database Syst Rev. 2004;(2):CD001541.

13.81 Protecting the skin from freezing, sun, and drying

Editors

Protecting the skin from freezing

- Avoid soap and cleansing products.
- Avoid shaving lotions and foam.
- Cold protection creams, including the most greasy ones, may **increase the risk of freezing** because they lower skin temperature.
- The outer layer of clothing should be wind-proof, the inner layer should be air-containing and voluminous.
- Avoid perspiration by decreasing clothing during exercise: several thin layers of clothing are better than one thick layer.
- Avoid exposing the head and neck to airflow.
- Thermal insulation for the feet can be improved by spacious shoes, a detachable inner sole in a rubber boot, a plastic bag between two layers of socks, and the prophylactic application of talc on perspiring feet.

DER

Protecting the skin from the sun

- According to the results of epidemiological studies, UVB radiation in particular predisposes the skin to the development of basiloma, epidermoid carcinoma, and solar keratosis.
  - UVB is the most important single risk factor for epidermoid carcinoma, and the risk of basiloma is directly proportional to the cumulative dose of UVB radiation.
  - Recurrent sunburn rather than a high cumulative light exposure is considered a risk factor for melanoma.
- Reflection from sand, water, and especially snow increase the amount of ultraviolet radiation. Adequate skin protection is mandatory in conditions where there is a lot of reflected light.
- Adequate clothing and avoidance of light exposure especially around noon help to protect from the sun.
- Sunscreen creams with a protection factor of 15 or more are also beneficial **B** [1 2] but they do not substitute for adequate clothing.

Protecting the skin from drying

- Protective cream should always be used when the skin feels dry and rough, or there are fissures.
- Recurrent wetting and particularly the use of soaps predispose the skin to drying. Hands should be washed only once a day, and patients with contact allergy should use protective gloves.
- Protection is most important in patients with atopy and contact dermatitis. Atopic persons should use creams on wider skin areas than just those that feel dry. Two or three different barrier creams should be used alternatingly in 2–3-week periods to avoid tachyphylaxis.
- Keratolytic ointments (e.g. salicylic acid or carbamide preparations) are needed for soles with fissures.

References

1. Thompson SC, Jolley D, Marks R. Reduction of solar keratoses by regular sunscreen use. N Engl J Med 1993;329:1147–51.

2. Naylor MF, Boyd A, Smith DW, Cameron GS, Hubbard D, Neldner KH. High sun protection factor sunscreens in the suppression of actinic neoplasia. Archives of Dermatology 1995;131:170–5.

13.82 Drugs and light sensitivity

Pirkko Paakkari

Definition

- Light eruption may be a toxic or an allergic reaction (Figure 13.82.1).
  - Phototoxic reactions are more common than allergic ones and usually occur already during the first course of the drug if exposure to light is sufficient.
  - Photoallergic reactions usually appear after repeated or long-term use of the drug.

Symptoms and signs of light sensitivity

- **In a photoallergic reaction** after exposure to sun or solarium light the skin may react with an erythematous, blistery, exudative or urticaria-like rash with severe itching often associated.
- **A toxic reaction** looks like a sunburn, is strictly demarcated to the sun-exposed area, and there is minimal or no itching.
- When the rash is in a light-exposed area, the patient should be asked about his/her medication, including natural remedies, skin creams and other cosmetic products. Even sunscreens may contain substances that cause photosensitivity.
- Plants containing psoralens may cause toxic reactions. Examples of such plants are the family Heracleum (e.g. giant hogweed or cow parsnip), rues (e.g. Ruta graveolens and Dictamus albus). Also celery can sensitize to light.

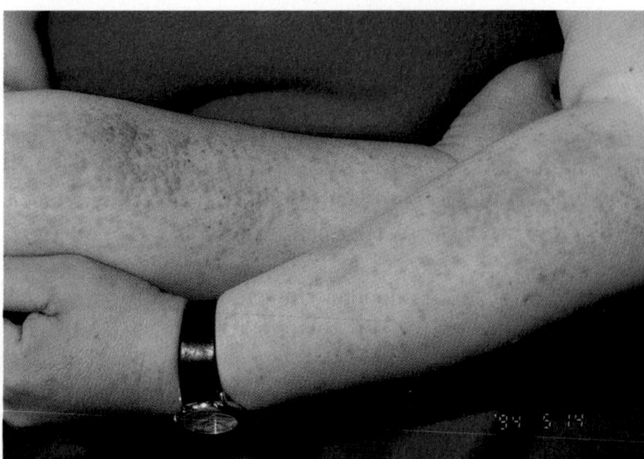

Figure 13.82.1 Chronic polymorphous light eruption (CPLE) is a common disease of unknown origin. The sun-exposed areas react on the evening of the first sunny days of spring-summer. Itching is the main symptom. Protection of the skin with clothes is the best prophylaxis. Topical UV protecting preparations are of limited benefit. Photo © R. Suhonen.

Medicines that can cause light sensitization

Antimicrobic drugs

- Tetracyclines, doxycycline
- Isoniazid
- Quinolones, e.g.: norfloxacin, ofloxacin, ciprofloxacin, levofloxacin, moxifloxacin, sparfloxacin
- Sulphonamides, trimethoprim-sulphamethoxazole

Neuroleptics and antidepressants

- Chlorpromazine (more than other neuroleptics)
- Promazine, levomepromazine
- Perphenazine
- Fluphenazine

Cardiovascular drugs

- Thiazide diuretics
- Furosemide
- Quinidine
- Amiodarone

NSAIDs

- Piroxicam
- Tenoxicam

Dermatological drugs

- Isotretinoin
- Acitretin

Local treatment

- Tar products
- Benzoyl peroxide
- Tretinoine
- NSAID-containing gels
- Chlortetracycline
- Antihistamines

Herbal products

- St. John's Wort

Other drugs

- Tricyclic antidepressants, sulphonylureas used for diabetes, neurological drugs: amantadine, phenytoin, carbamazepine, and cytotoxic drugs: fluorouracil, methotrexate, vinblastine also cause sensitization to light.

13.83 Prevention and treatment of pressure sores

Editors

Phases of pressure sore development

- The first sign of a developing pressure sore is hyperaemia. The following steps are detachment of epidermis, blisters and crust, a clean ulcer, and eventually an infected ulcer (Figure 13.83.1).

Classification of pressure sores

- Pressure sores are classified into four grades according to the extent of tissue injury:
  - Non-blanching erythema on intact skin
  - Skin defect limited to the epidermis or dermis
  - Injury penetrating the whole dermis into subcutaneous tissue, demarcating in the underlying fascia.
  - Skin defect with tissue destruction or necrosis, penetrating into muscle, bone, or connective tissue.

Initial assessment

- Determine the grade and size of the sore (measurement).
- Record fistulas, cavities, discharge, necrosis, granulation tissue, and epithelialization.

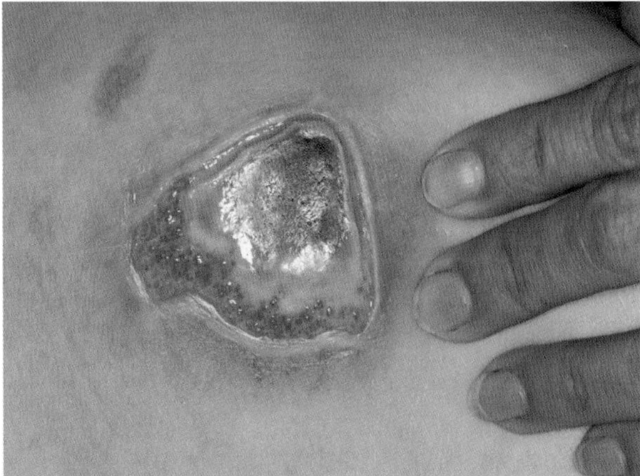

Figure 13.83.1 Prevention is the best therapy for pressure ulcers. Necrosis may extend deep into the tissues and demand reconstructive surgery. Pressure ulcer preventive mattresses are the best health care investment. Photo © R. Suhonen.

- Assess the underlying diseases, nutritional state, degree of pain, and mental status of the patient.
  - Diabetes, impaired peripheral circulation, connective tissue disease, immune deficiencies, psychosis, and depression are risk factors for delayed or unsuccessful healing.
  - Assay of serum albumin is useful in the assessment of the nutritional state.

Prevention

DER

- The patient's position is changed frequently (at intervals of less than 2 hours if personnel resources allow). Note hyperaemia of the skin every time the position is changed.
  - The sacral area is the most vulnerable. Lying on the side in a position resulting in pressure directly on the trochanter should also be avoided.
  - Avoid excessive elevation of the patient's head and upper body for long periods.
- A decompression mattress should be used for patients who are at a high risk of pressure sores, particularly if there already is one (A) [1]. Decompression mattresses can be classified as static and dynamic.
- A static decompression mattress (where the air or water does not move from one compartment to another) is sufficient for patients who can change their position themselves and when the weight of the patient does not collapse the mattress against the hard base. A light water bed is the best static bed, approaching the efficiency of dynamic beds.
  - Check the adequacy of the mattress by putting your hand under the patient and estimating the thickness of the mattress at a place where the pressure is greatest (the thickness should be at least 2–3 cm).
  - Sheepskin or elbow and heel pads (not rings that merely transfer the pressure from one place to another) and pillows can be used as augments.
- A dynamic mattress (in which the air or water is pumped from one compartment to another) is indicated for patients who cannot change position themself, whose weight collapses a static mattress, or whose sores do not show signs of healing.
- A low-air-loss or air-fluidized mattress (A) [1] is indicated in cases of large grade 3 or 4 sores.
- Optimal hydration and cleaning of the skin
  - No soap for frail skin. Use emulsions, moisturizing cream, or soft lotion for skin folds instead.
  - Wash normal skin with gentle soap or acid washing emulsions.
  - Dry the skin by patting and use talc. Massage gently.
  - An indwelling urinary catheter is recommended for incontinent patients.

Treatment

- Hyperaemia or superficial skin detachment
  - Minimize pressure

- Adhesive hydrocolloid dressings (e.g. Duoderm®)
- Avoid friction
- Air baths

♦ Blister or scab

- Do not break a blister.
- If the tissue under a scab is painless and non-infected, and there is no fluctuation or discharge from the sore or erythema of the surrounding skin, leave the scab intact and cover it with clean dressings. In particular, scabs on the heels should be treated in this way.
- Minimize pressure

♦ Clean ulcer

- Minimize pressure
- Clean the surface of the ulcer with an antiseptic preparation (e.g. 10% povidone iodine). Note, however, that there is little evidence of the effectiveness of cleansing D [2 3].
- Apply 1% silver nitrate solution D [2 3].
- Cover the ulcer with a greasy dressing or a hydrocolloid dressing (e.g. Duoderm®)
- Consider surgical treatment (skin transplantation)

♦ Necrotic ulcer

- Remove necrotic tissue at the onset of treatment and at every change of dressings.
  - Mechanical debridement with a scalpel is the quickest method. It is recommended if there is a lot of necrotic tissue, or if an infection (cellulitis, sepsis) is imminent.
  - Alternate dry and moist dressings (not on a granulating surface)
  - Use enzymatic debridement if the patient does not tolerate mechanical debridement, and the ulcer is non-infected. For infected ulcers enzymatic debridement is too slow.

♦ Infected ulcer

- Wash with water, preferably by showering.
- Apply hydrogen peroxide to an ulcer that smells on change of dressings; wash it away.
- 0.1% silver nitrate compresses should be kept moist by adding silver nitrate solution when needed.
- Use cleaning topical treatments (absorbing gel or adsorbing dressings that can be covered by plastic film or a saline compress).
- Use a systemic antibiotic if there is infection in adjacent tissues (erysipelas!)

♦ Providing adequate nutrition C [4]

- Maintaining a positive nitrogen balance requires 30–35 kcal/kg/day, and 1.25–1.5 g protein/kg/day.

References

1. Cullum N, Deeks J, Sheldon TA, Song F, Fletcher AW. Beds, mattresses and cushions for pressure sore prevention and treatment. Cochrane Database Syst Rev. 2004;(2):CD001735.
2. Margolis DJ, Lewis VL. A literature assessment of the use of miscellaneous topical agents, growth factors, and skin equivalents for the treatment of pressure ulcers.
3. The Database of Abstracts of Reviews of Effectiveness (University of York), Database no.: DARE-950955. In: The Cochrane Library, Issue 4, 1999. Oxford: Update Software.
4. Langer G, Schloemer G, Knerr A, Kuss O, Behrens J. Nutritional interventions for preventing and treating pressure ulcers. Cochrane Database Syst Rev 2003(4):CD003216.

Allergology

Evidence Based Medicine Guidelines. Edited by the Duodecim Editorial Team
 ISBN: 0-470-01184-X

14.1 Anaphylaxis

Editors

Aims

- Adrenaline should be given as soon as possible in reactions suspected to be anaphylactic.
  - In severe reactions intravenous adrenaline is used. In mild reactions intravenous administration may cause more harm than benefit.
- All patients who have experienced an anaphylactic reaction are given preloaded adrenaline syringes.
- Immediate readiness to treat anaphylactic reactions (adrenaline available) should be available in locations where vaccinations, allergy tests or radiographic examinations with contrast medium are carried out.

Aetiology

- In theory, any food (or other agent) can trigger anaphylaxis.
- Drugs and vaccines
  - Antibiotics and analgetics
  - ACTH, insulin
- Insect stings
  - Wasp, bee, mosquito
- Foods
  - Nuts (tree nuts and peanuts), fish, shellfish, celery, kiwi, egg, milk
- Radiographic contrast media, blood products, allergenic products used in examinations and treatment
- Natural rubber (latex) (14.5)
  - Gloves, catheters, condoms, balloons
- Physical exercise, shaking, cold
- The patient is often atopic

Clinical features

- The more rapidly the symptoms start and progress, the more severe is the reaction.
- First symptoms
  - Erythema, burning of the skin, stinging
  - Tachycardia
  - A feeling of thickness in the pharynx and chest, coughing
  - Possibly nausea and vomiting
- Secondary symptoms
  - Swelling of the skin (especially the eyelids and lips)
  - Urticaria
  - Laryngeal oedema, hoarseness, wheezing, bouts of coughing
  - Abdominal pain, nausea, vomiting, diarrhoea
  - Hypotension, sweating, paleness
  - In severe cases laryngeal spasm, shock, respiratory and cardiac arrest

Differential diagnosis

- Acute asthma attack
  - No skin symptoms
  - Blood pressure normal or elevated
  - Can develop over several days.
- Fainting
  - No skin or respiratory symptoms
  - Bradycardia
- Hereditary angioneurotic oedema (HANE) (14.10)
  - No urticaria
  - Adrenaline does not help!

Management

- Stop the administration of the causative agent immediately.

1. Adrenaline

- Intramuscular adrenaline 1:1000 (1 mg/ml) 0.5 ml or 0.1 ml/10 kg up to 0.5 ml for children, administered deep into the thigh or to the upper arm, see Table 14.1.
- Adrenaline injection can be repeated after 5 (–15) minutes.
- Adrenaline 1:10 000 (0.1 mg/ml) 1–3 ml intravenously can be given slowly (in 5–10 minutes) to an adult patient in profound shock, and for children 0.1–0.5 ml.

2. Supportive treatment

- The patient should lie flat with the legs raised.
- Make sure that the patient is breathing. Oxygen should be administered if it is available.

3. Intravenous corticosteroids

- For an adult methylprednisolone 80–125 mg, and for children 2 mg/kg intravenously. Alternatively, hydrocortisone 250–500 (–1000) mg for adults and for children 10 mg/kg intravenously. The total dose for a child must not exceed the dose for adults.
- Predniso(lo)ne orally for 3–5 days as additional treatment, 30–50 mg for the first day.

Table 14.1 Administration of adrenaline in anaphylaxis

Weight of the patient	Adrenaline dose (1:1 000 = 1 mg/ml)
5 kg	0.05 ml
10 kg	0.1 ml
15 kg	0.15 ml
20 kg	0.2 ml
50 kg	0.5 ml
80 kg	0.8 ml

4. Intravenous fluid therapy

- Intravenous Ringer's solution or physiological NaCl solution should be started immediately. For an adult 500–1000 ml should be given during the first hour. For children 10–20 ml/kg over 30 minutes.

5. Beta2-sympathomimetics

- Corticosteroid and adrenaline are effective for asthma symptoms. Use also the inhaled drug that the patient normally takes for asthma attacks.
- In severe bronchial obstruction that does not respond to other drugs, administer e.g. salbutamol 5–10 mg by nebulizer.

6. Antihistamines

- Orally, e.g. hydroxyzine
  - for adults 25–50 mg
  - for children a solution containing 2 mg/ml
    - below 1 year 2.5 ml
    - 1–5 years 5 ml
    - 6–10 years 10 ml
- Intramuscularly e.g. promethazine 25–50 mg may be administered alternatively.

7. Follow-up

- Refer the patient to hospital for follow-up. Usually the patient recovers quickly, but there is always a possibility of recurrence.

Long-term management

- Patients should carry a preloaded adrenaline syringe for self-treatment of anaphylaxis. This is a disposable intramuscular adrenaline injection, and the patient and family members should be taught how to use it.
- In wasp and bee allergy specific immunotherapy is given by the allergologist.
- The patient should not try out foods that might cause allergy at home.

14.2 Investigation of atopy

Minna Kaila

Choice and timing of investigations

- Medical history is the best investigation of allergy.
- Treat the patient, not the test results.
- **Skin prick tests** are the basic method for all ages.
- **Total IgE level** in blood is insensitive and usually of little benefit. A normal level does not exclude allergy but a high level suggests atopic tendency. However, it does not reveal the allergen.
- Tendency for atopy can be screened by testing **IgE antibodies towards common inhalation** antigens. A positive result indicates hypersensitivity and may warrant investigations for specific allergens.
- Food hypersensitivity should not be screened.
- Allergy = proof of immunological sensitization + clinical symptoms

Rhinitis

- In clearly seasonal rhinitis (induced by airborn pollens) allergological investigations are not mandatory.
- In persistent rhinitis it might be beneficial to test for and then eliminate a special allergen.
- IgE-mediated sensitization must be verified when specific immunotherapy is considered.

Asthma

- Taking a history of allergies is essential. Skin tests of relevant inhaled allergens are sufficient in most cases.
- Exaggerated elimination of allergens is seldom beneficial. For example, duvet and pillow down has been shown to be quite safe.
- Instructions on how to avoid allergens are given individually based on the verified sensitization or allergies.

Eczema

- Extensive atopic eczema, eczema around mouth or eyes or anal fold, especially if the patient also has gastrointestinal or airway symptoms suggest allergy in children. Extensive testing (e.g. skin prick tests) should be avoided (Figures 14.2.1 and 14.2.2).
- So-called "winter-foot" symptom (Figure 14.2.3) is not usually associated with allergy.
- Extensive atopic eczema in an adult indicates investigations.
- Healing of eczema during the summer speaks strongly against food allergy.

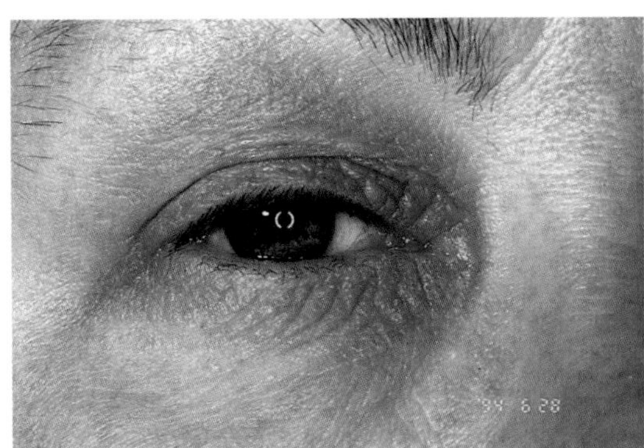

Figure 14.2.1 Atopic dermatitis in the eyelid region. The clinical picture does not allow the evaluation of the possible role of airborne allergies (e.g. dander of cats or dogs). Topical corticoids of low potency, emollients and elimination of possible allergens are necessary for cure. Photo © R. Suhonen.

ALL

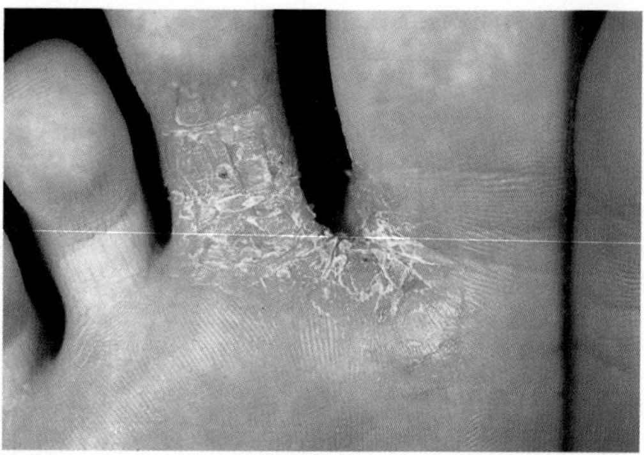

Figure 14.2.2 Skin eruption between the toes is most often caused by a dermatophyte. In this case, however, the young patient has atopic dermatitis affecting the first interdigital space where fungal infection regularly is situated as a rule in the most lateral toewebs. Photo © R. Suhonen.

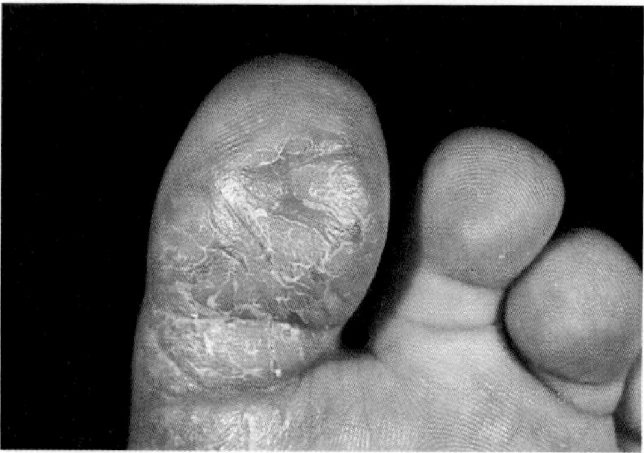

Figure 14.2.3 "Atopic winter foot", juvenile plantar dermatosis (JPD), is common in young boys. The skin of the contact surface of feet (and fingers) may be irritated, scaling, often also fissuring and painful. Views on whether this is a form of contact allergy vary greatly. JPD regularly heals spontaneously in some years, which does not suggest contact allergy. Topical corticosteroids and emollients help when waiting for the eventual spontaneous cure. Photo © R. Suhonen.

- Investigations for food allergy: see 14.6.
- Indications of skin prick tests in dermatological diseases and withdrawal of antihistamine drugs: see 13.5.

Skin prick testing

- Assesses immediate (IgE mediated) allergy
- Follow the instructions of test material producer.

Basic series of skin prick tests

- Include, for example:
  - Birch (Betula sp.)
  - Timothy (Phleum pratense)
  - Fescue (Festuca pratensis)
  - Mugwort (Artemisia vulgaris)
  - Cladosporium herbarum mould
  - Dog
  - Cat
  - Horse
  - House mite (D. pteronyssimus)
  - Natural rubber (latex)

Interpretation of skin prick test

- Histamine solution is used as a positive control and the basic solution of allergenic extraction is used as a negative control.
- A positive reaction is indicated by an itching wheal or papule surrounded by erythema. The reaction usually reaches its peak after 15 minutes of pricking.
- The lower limit for a positive result is a wheal of 3 mm in diameter. The diameter (the average of the biggest and smallest diameter (D+d)/2) should be written down. The size of the reaction wheal must be at least half of the size of the wheal caused by histamine in order to be significant.
- At the same time the negative control must be truly negative, i.e. no papule.
- The clinician treating the patient is the one who decides the true clinical value of the test result.
- Especially the clinical significance of sensitization to foods should be evaluated critically against the symptoms.
- Some people have a tendency to dermographism: in these cases injecting the skin always causes a small papule. Do not confuse this reaction with allergy.

14.3 Hypersensitivity to drugs

Kristiina Alanko

Basic rules

- Skin reaction are the most frequent manifestations of drug hypersensitivity, but many other organs such as lungs, kidneys, liver and bone marrow can also be involved. Fever and other general symptoms are present in the most severe skin reactions.
- Drug eruptions have non-specific clinical features. Similar clinical eruptions may be caused by other sources, e.g. various infections. If the reaction has been falsely attributed to a drug, later use of the drug is prevented unnecessarily by the fear of a new reaction.
- An allergic reaction can always be reproduced. It occurs every time the patient uses the drug and the new reaction is often stronger.
- The reaction may need an external factor, such as light energy, to occur.
- It is often impossible to identify the responsible agent on the basis of clinical appearance alone (13.1). One drug can cause several types of eruptions, and conversely, morphologically similar eruptions can be induced by quite different drugs.
- Exanthematous eruptions and urticaria are the most common types of drug eruptions. Rarer manifestations

include erythema multiforme, Stevens-Johnson syndrome, toxic epidermal necrolysis (Lyell's syndrome), eczematous reactions, erythrodermia, i.e. exfoliative dermatitis, lichenoid reactions, lupus erythematosus-type reactions, erythema nodosum and photoallergic or phototoxic reactions.

- In summary, drugs can cause almost any kind of eruptions and the clinical picture may include different morphological features of typical skin reaction types.
- Topical skin application results in delayed-type allergy which is manifested clinically as contact dermatitis. In a person previously topically sensitized, e.g. from neomycin or gentamycin cream, an eczematous eruption, a so-called systemic contact dermatitis may occur after systemic administration of the same or related drug.

Causative drugs

- The most common causes are antibiotics (sulphonamides and penicillins in particular), non-steroidal anti-inflammatory drugs (NSAIDs) and drugs acting on the central nervous system (usually phenytoin and carbamazepine) (Figure 14.3.1).
- Sulphonamides and trimethoprim have caused most cases of severe drug reactions (Stevens-Johnson and Lyell's syndromes).
- Serum sickness-type reactions are caused particularly by penicillins, acetylsalicylic acid (ASA), streptomycin and sulphonamides.
- Penicillins usually cross-react with each other. In estimated 10% of cases, cephalosporins cross-react with penicillins.

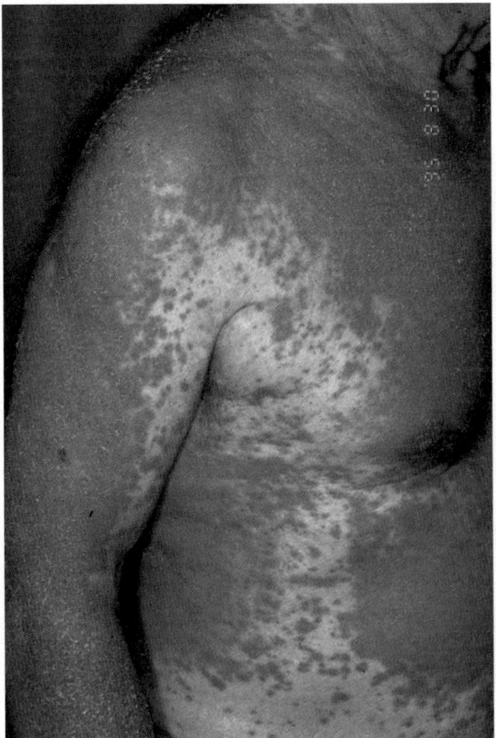

Figure 14.3.1 Carbamazepine is an important drug, but its use may lead to allergic exanthema. In spite of the often florid clinical picture the condition improves rapidly with oral corticosteroids - if the causative drug is replaced. Photo © R. Suhonen.

Exanthematous eruptions

- The most common type of drug eruption, often called rash (Figure 14.3.2).
- Almost any drug can cause exanthematous eruptions. Most frequently they are caused by antibiotics (especially penicillins and sulphonamides) and anticonvulsive agents, phenytoin, carbamazepine, oxcarbazepine and lamotrigine.
- The clinical symptoms vary greatly. The rash is formed of erythematous macules or maculopapules which may coalesce and form large red oedematous areas.
- Usually arises quite symmetrically on both sides of the body.
- Exanthematous eruptions may also be triggered by infections caused by several viruses and other microbes.
- E.g. poxes, such as measles, rubella and scarlet fever, are exanthematous eruptions.
- Together with acute mononucleosis, ampicillins cause an exanthematous eruption, the exact mechanism of which is unknown.

Immediate reactions

- Type I immediate allergic reactions are IgE antibody-mediated. Most cases of immediate-type drug reactions are, however, pseudoallergic, i.e. transmittors are released without an immunological mechanism. Drugs can e.g. release histamine directly from mast cells without a preliminary immunological reaction. The clinical symptoms are similar, but the distinction has significance in diagnostics.
- Pseudoallergic reactions may not be reproduced like the true allergic reactions.
- Drug-induced pseudoallergic reactions may be caused, e.g. by NSAIDs, codeine, opiates, hydralazine, quinine and radiographic contrast media. Anaphylactoid reactions caused

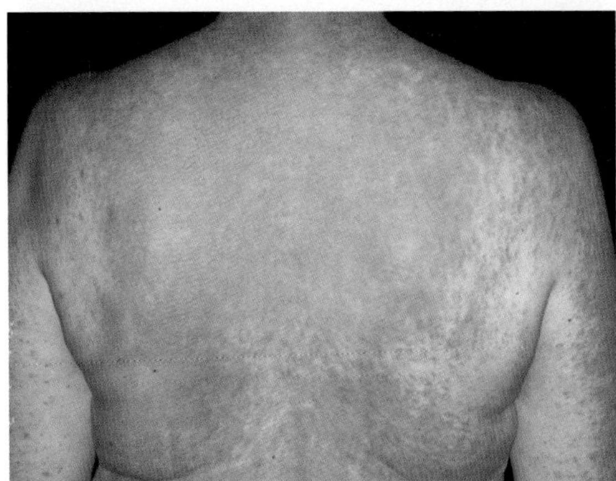

Figure 14.3.2 An allergic reaction to oral medication manifests itself commonly as exanthema. The appearance of the skin eruption does not allow conclusions about the specific causative agent. Photo © R. Suhonen.

by muscle relaxants and other anaesthetic agents as well as angioedemas caused by ACE inhibitors are examples of these pseudoallergic reactions.

- During surgery, an immediate-type allergic reaction can also be caused by natural rubber latex in surgical gloves or by chlorhexidine in skin disinfectants.
- An immediate-type reaction in connection with local anaesthesia can be induced even by vasovagal collapse.

Urticaria

- The most common causes are penicillins and related antibiotics (both allergic and pseudoallergic reactions) as well as ASA and related substances (pseudoallergic reactions).
- Urticaria can be caused by several other factors (e.g. viral infections) and by different pathological mechanisms.
- Characterized by mildly elevated wheals which are erythematous or pale and often itchy. They appear, disappear and change place within only a few hours.

Angioedema

- Angioedema is a deeper skin inflammation. It may appear together with urticaria or separately. Predilection areas are the lips, eyelids and fingers. In severe cases laryngeal mucosa is involved (i.e. anaphylactic reactions).

Vasculitis

- Purpura and skin lesions may be caused by vasculitis leucocytoclastica (Figure 14.3.3).

Anaphylactic shock

- See 14.1.

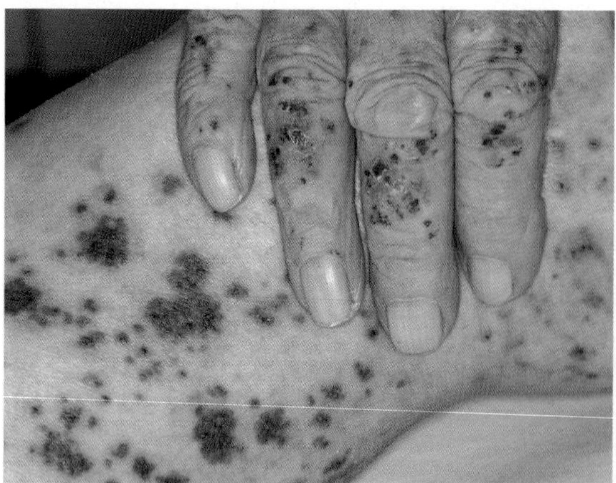

Figure 14.3.3 Vasculitis leucocytoclastica (v. allergica) is a small-vessel vasculitis, with purpura and superficial necrosis of the skin. Most lesions are in the lower extremities; in the case shown here the fingers are also affected. An infection or drugs may cause the symptoms, but in most cases no explanation is found. Photo © R. Suhonen.

Fixed drug eruption

- The only skin reaction which is solely provoked by drug hypersensitivity.
- Most common causative agents are sulphonamides, trimethoprim, tetracyclines, carbamazepine and in the past also barbiturates. Phenazone salicylate-containing antipyretic analgesics are a frequent cause of fixed drug eruptions. These products have been taken from the market in some countries.
- A round, sharply marginated, usually intensely red patch which may develop into a blister (Figure 14.3.4)
- One or several patches on various sites of the body, also on mucous membranes.
- The patch is usually followed by a dark brown pigmentation which may persist for months.
- Reappears at the same sites when the causative drug is readministered.
- If the use of the drug continues, the patches spread to new sites.

Diagnosis

- Based on patient history and clinical picture.
- In most cases no other methods are available.

Patient history

- Is the eruption really drug-induced? An exanthematous eruption or urticaria suspected to be caused by an analgesic or antibiotic is often caused by the underlying infection itself.

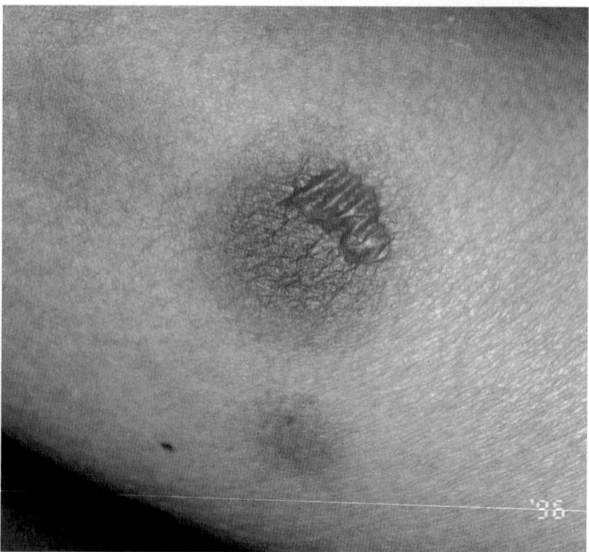

Figure 14.3.4 Fixed drug eruption (Erythema fixum) may be bullous and after healing leaves a darkish hue in the skin. The lesion may be solitary or multifocal. Here the causative agent is the most common one: phenazone salicylate. The pruritic lesion recurs without exception on every exposure to the drug, a few hours after intake. Photo © R. Suhonen.

- Which among the drugs used by the patient could be the causative one? Drugs taken only occasionally are easily forgotten. Inquire also about them.
- The clinical picture of the eruption? Only few drugs, e.g. ASA and penicillins, are commonly associated with a specific type of skin reaction (urticaria).
- Does the reaction reappear? Often the cause is revealed by a spontaneous reappearance of the reaction after spontaneous readministration of the drug.
- Timing? If there has been no previous exposure, the allergic reaction may appear after a latent period of several days or even two weeks of the therapy. On readministration, the reaction appears more rapidly, usually within 24 hours, and is often more severe.
- Elimination? Withdrawal of the suspected drug helps to identify the cause. The eruption is usually cured when use of the causative drug is discontinued.

Drug challenge test

- A peroral provocation test is the most reliable diagnostic method.
- Performed after the reaction has healed completely, at the earliest after 1–2 months.
- The suspected drug is given orally at a test dose significantly lower than the therapeutic dose and chosen individually. If no reaction occurs, the test can be repeated with a larger dose until the normal therapeutic dose. The aim is to bring about the reappearance of the reaction in a mild form.
- The test should be performed in controlled circumstances, preferably in a hospital under the care of a specialist, since the challenge test always includes the hazard of an unexpectedly strong reaction.
- The test should be started in the morning, and the flare-up of the reaction, pulse rate, blood pressure and other clinical symptoms should be followed up at 1-hour intervals until the evening. The recommended total follow-up time is 24 hours, but in most cases the symptoms appear within a few hours.
- Because drug challenge tests are time-consuming, expensive and possibly dangerous, the indications should be considered thoroughly. The challenge is worthwhile if the patient really needs the drug in the future or if the patient has several suspected drug allergies and, for example, finding a suitable antibiotic is difficult.
- Absolute contraindications include anaphylactic reactions, severe life-threatening skin reactions, haematological dysfunctions and lupus erythematosus -type (SLE) systemic reactions.

Other investigations

- Available only in rare cases.
- Routine laboratory examinations are of no help in purely skin reactions.
- Immediate allergy is usually investigated by skin prick tests and specific serum IgE antibody assays (RAST). However, most immediate drug reactions are pseudoallergic and cannot be investigated by the above methods. It is also uncertain whether a pseudoallergic reaction can be reproduced by a challenge test.
- In IgE-mediated drug allergy, skin prick tests and IgE antibody assays are generally available only for penicillins (penicilloyl G and penicilloyl V), as well as some large molecular weight drugs e.g. ACTH and insulins.
- Skin prick tests with drugs should be performed only at expert dermatology/allergology units because of the hazard of anaphylactic reactions. Penicillin skin prick tests are somewhat more reliable than blood assays. Skin prick tests are also sometimes used to study immediate-type reactions to local anaesthetics and agents used in general anaesthesia. Allergy is rarely confirmed, as most reactions are pseudoallergic.
- Intracutaneous (intradermal) tests are also used occasionally for studying both immediate and delayed allergy type reactions.
- Patch tests are not routinely used to study reactions caused by systemic drugs. Patch testing is the method for detecting delayed, cell-mediated allergy (e.g. contact dermatitis).

ALL

Treatment

- First of all, the patient must stop taking the suspected drugs (preferably all drugs in use).
- Stopping the use of the drug is usually sufficient therapy for mild exanthematous eruptions. If necessary, corticosteroid cream or peroral steroids can be used.
- Urticaria reactions are treated by oral antihistamines. Do not hesitate to prescribe large doses. If necessary, peroral corticosteroids are used.
- Anaphylactic reactions, see 14.1.
- Prolonged and severe reactions with general symptoms are treated by peroral corticosteroids. Consider referral to a specialist.
- The most severe reactions in which the skin is detached require therapy at an intensive care unit.

Further use of drugs

- If the reaction is verified (typical clinical picture, recurrences, challenge test positive), the patient must not use the drug again.
- Uncertain cases are decided individually, taking into consideration the type and severity of the reaction.
- A patient may report a history of drug allergy, but the symptoms have been headache, diarrhoea or other gastrointestinal complaint. In these cases the drug can be used.
- If the suspected reaction has been exanthematous eruption, the drug can be tried again with caution. The use of the tried drug must be stopped immediately if any skin symptoms or fever appear.
- Drug eruptions involve many false diagnoses, and in these cases forbidding the use of the suspected drug is unnecessary. On the other hand, a hazard in recurring

reactions is a more severe reaction. Urticaria may develop into anaphylaxis and exanthematous eruption into a serum sickness or pseudolymphoma-type reaction.

- If the reaction has been of immediate type, giving the same drug again is not safe. If serum IgE antibody tests are available (penicillins, up to 1–6 months after the reaction) they should be performed. A positive result confirms the diagnosis. If the test is negative, skin prick tests or a challenge with the drug can be considered. If the suspicion of allergy is strong, consider skin prick tests instead of a drug challenge in penicillin allergy.
- After severe haematological or pulmonary reactions the suspected drug should not be used.

Annotations and reporting

- A note of the allergy must be written in a clearly visible place in the patient records, including the date and a detailed description of the reaction.
- The patient should write a note of the drug allergy for his/her own use.
- Depending on the local policy, the reaction must be reported to the authorities. Only verified allergies and severe reactions are reported.

14.4 Food additives and hypersensitivity

Kirsti Kiviranta

- Food industry uses chemical additives in order to improve processing, taste, flavour, colour and texture, or the shelf life of foods. They are natural on near-natural products. The use of additives is regulated by law. All the additives known to induce adverse reactions must be listed on the ingredients label, as names or E-code numbers. Many alcoholic drinks contain sulphites, but these are not listed.
- The use of synthetic azo dyes in foods was banned in some European countries due to evidence of their harmful effects. Renewed permission for their use was granted 1996, according to EC directives. Some azo dyes are also used in drugs.

Epidemiology

- Hypersensitivity to food additives is not common. In a European study the estimated prevalence was 0.01–0.23%. There is no difference between atopic or non-atopic persons.

Symptoms

- Immediate within minutes, or late reactions after several hours
- Urticaria
- Flush
- Oedema of the mouth and throat
- Rhinitis, asthma
- Nausea
- Anaphylactic shock, see 14.1
- Worsening of atopic eczema
- Allergic purpura

Examinations

- The mechanism of these adverse reactions is not known. If there is an immunological IgE-mediated mechanism skin prick tests are positive, as in occasional cases of sulphite-allergic patients.
- The history of the symptoms and probable connection with recently ingested foods is important.
- The diagnosis is confirmed in hospital with a double blind challenge test. If this is not possible the patient must avoid the suspected additives by reading the ingredient labels.

Additives that most commonly cause hypersensitivity symptoms and their use in food

- **Benzoic acid and benzoates** (E210–219): lingonberries, jam, spice puree, stock cubes containing fish, meat or vegetable mixtures, preserved and spiced fish, mushrooms and cucumbers, smoked fish, soft drinks, soft-centred sweets and chocolates.
- **Sulphitic acid and sulphites** (E220–228): wines and beers, dried fruit, mushrooms and vegetables, industrially peeled potatoes, preservatives, jams, juices, soft drinks, horseradish paste, mustard sauce, vinegar. Sulphites evaporate on boiling.
- **Glutamic acid and L-glutamates** (E620–625): aroma salt in Chinese restaurant food, sausages, preserved meat, spice mixtures.
- **Tartrazine and other azo dyes**: sweet, soft drinks, pastry. There is cross-reactivity between azo dyes and hypersensitivity to aspirin and other non-steroidal anti-inflammatory drugs. Patients allergic to aspirin can usually take paracetamol; however, they should avoid hot or cold drinkable remedies containing analgesics, as these often contain azo dyes. Carmine (cochineal, E120), which is used in alcoholic beverages, can trigger an anaphylactic reaction or other symptoms of allergy with an IgE-mediated mechanism revealed by skin prict tests or RAST.
- Patients who are hypersensitive to food additives ought to avoid them in their diet. They should not use preservatives, soft drinks, sweets and prepared foods, and they must cook using pure foodstuffs.

14.5 Latex allergy

Kristiina Turjanmaa

Aim

- Suspect latex allergy in a patient or a member of health care personnel who gets symptoms from rubber gloves, condoms, balloons, babies' dummies or instruments containing rubber.

Aetiology and epidemiology

- Latex allergy is an immediate (type I) reaction to proteins of the rubber tree. Delayed (type IV) reaction to chemicals added to natural rubber latex is called rubber allergy.
- About 0.1% of population and 3–10% of health care personnel suffer from latex allergy.

Factors triggering an allergic reaction

- Surgical, examination or household gloves
- Catheters
- Radiographic balloons (e.g. in barium enema)
- Manometry balloons (e.g. in the investigation of the oesophagus)
- Cofferdam of the dentist
- Rubber parts of blood pressure meter and stethoscope tubing that can contaminate the hands by which the allergens can be carried to the face.
- Balloons and rubber toys
- Babies' dummies
- Condoms
- Rubber bands
- Intubation tubes
- Anaesthesia masks

Symptoms

- Local or generalized urticaria, itching
- Hand eczema
- Conjunctivitis
- Rhinitis
- Asthma
- Anaphylactic reaction

Risk groups

- Usually persons who are atopic or suffer from hand eczema
- Repeatedly (especially as a child) operated patients (e.g. spina bifida patients)
- Health care personnel, especially physicians and operating room nurses, dentists and nurses
- Persons using household gloves
- Young children suffering from food allergies
- The most severe reactions are usually caused by direct contact of natural rubber latex with mucous membranes during an operation, delivery and different investigations. Skin contact is also dangerous in case of eczema.
- Every patient scheduled to undergo surgery should be asked about symptoms from gloves, condoms and balloons.

Cross-reactions with bananas and other fruit

- Cross-reactions to fruit and vegetables (banana, avocado, kiwi, raw potato) have been observed to occur in persons allergic to natural rubber latex. Inquire about possible symptoms from patients.

Diagnosis

- Based on skin prick tests.
- RAST is not as specific and sensitive.
- Challenge tests (skin, lung) are performed at a specialist clinic.

Treatment and prophylaxis

- Products containing natural rubber latex should be avoided.
  - All staff members working in the same area should use low allergenic gloves because natural rubber allergens spread into the air by contaminated glove powder.
  - Allergic staff members can use low allergenic surgical and examination gloves if they do not suffer from any symptoms, otherwise gloves without natural rubber or vinyl gloves should be used.
- Health care personnel must use gloves without natural rubber latex when they treat patients with latex allergy.

14.6 Food hypersensitivity and allergy

Minna Kaila

- Food hypersensitivity includes both food allergy and food intolerance.
- In food allergy, the symptoms are related to an immunological mechanism. A skin-prick test or tests for specific IgE antibodies in the serum may be used in the determination of an immunological mechanism.
- Most infants suffering from food allergy to nutritionally important foods (milk, cereals) recover at pre-school age.

- School-aged children may develop allergy to vegetables or fruit.

Epidemiology

- Up to half of the parents of children younger than 2 years of age associate some of the child's symptoms with food, however, most suspicions of allergy dissolve with time.
- In a survey of school children, 24% reported to be or to have been allergic to food at some point.

Prevention

- To prevent allergies, the risk groups should be identified reliably, and an efficient preventative measure should be available.
- There is some evidence that an avoidance diet during lactation could delay the onset of atopic eczema; however, this applies only to high-risk families.
- Maternal avoidance of food allergens during pregnancy (third trimester) does not prevent atopic manifestations in the infant C [1].
- The existing studies have been carried out in children at high risk of atopy, while the general population has not been studied.
- Exclusive breast feeding for at least 4–6 months is recommended.
- Partially hydrolysed formulas are effective when breast-feeding is not available for high-risk infants (at least one first-degree relative with correctly diagnosed allergy) A [2 3 4]. These products may not be marketed in all countries.

Causes of food allergy

- In principle any food can cause allergy. There is no allergy-safe diet.
- If a baby does not eat a particular food substance, he cannot become sensitised to it. He also cannot develop tolerance to it.
- See 14.8.

Cow's milk and cereal allergies are nutritionally most significant

- Mainly seen in young children
- Rarely after pre-school age
- Symptoms caused by these foods usually appear in infancy soon after the food has been introduced to the child's diet.
- See 14.7.

Allergens related to birch pollen allergy

- Allergens associated with birch pollen allergy include the following
    - Root vegetables: potato, carrot, celery, parsnip
    - Fruit and other vegetables: apple, pear, peach, kiwi fruit, plum, mango, tomato, sweet pepper
    - Spices: mustard, caraway, turmeric, ginger, cinnamon
    - Others: walnut, almond
- In most cases preparation of vegetables (cutting, freezing and especially cooking) removes the allergenicity, the majority of persons allergic to birch pollen can eat cooked vegetables.
- After pre-school age, the avoidance of allergens should be based on symptoms, not test results. Due to cross-reactions, the number of false-positive results is high in skin-prick and RAST testing, and they are therefore not recommended.

Other allergens

- Peanuts, soya, fish, shellfish, eggs, wheat, barley, oats, rye, buckwheat, banana, avocado
- Linseeds, sesame seeds and poppy seeds
- Mushrooms, especially shiitake
- Causes of intolerance (no allergy mechanism)
    - Strawberry, citrus fruit, chocolate, tomato
- Alcoholic drinks
    - Cereal allergens, aniseed, colouring agents, metabisulphite, benzoic acid

Anaphylactic reaction

- May, in theory, occur with any food.
- In infants with milk and egg allergy
- Possible allergens both in children and adults: fish, shellfish, peanuts, soya, celery, kiwi fruit, linseeds and sesame seeds

Symptoms of food allergy

- Typically several symptoms are manifested: stomach pain, diarrhoea, cutaneous eruptions etc.
- In 50–80% of infants admitted to hospital with atopic eczema, i.e. with severe eczema, a food allergy is found to aggravate the symptoms (14.2).
- Atopic eczema can also be exacerbated by air-borne allergens: birch pollen in the spring, grass pollen suspended in water and contact with pets (eczema in areas exposed to air is suggestive).
- Eczema can also occur in contact areas (touching a dog, peeling potatoes).
- Of gastrointestinal symptoms, the most obvious one is contact allergy around the mouth and lips which appears almost immediately after ingestion and is easy to connect with the food (tomatoes, citrus fruit and apples in those allergic to birch pollen).
- Other symptoms that appear soon after ingestion of the food (loose stools, vomiting) are also rather easy to connect with the allergen, especially if the association occurs repeatedly.
- Delayed gastrointestinal reactions, or worsening of the atopic eczema, are very difficult to associate with a particular food.
- The frequency of bowel motions varies greatly between individuals. For example, in infancy defecation 10 times a day or once a week may be normal (provided that the child is well and developing normally).

- All changes in the diet can cause temporary changes in bowel function, as can courses of antibiotics.

Other symptoms

- Food hypersensitivity may also be linked to exacerbation of asthma.
- There is no evidence supporting an association between food (hypersensitivity) and migraine, arthritis, cystitis or nephritis.

Diagnosis of food hypersensitivity

- See also 14.7, 14.8.
- As a basic rule, skin or blood testing of older children for food hypersensitivity should be avoided unless there is a strong suspicion.
- The diagnosis should be based on elimination and reintroduction trials. For the nutritionally important foods (milk and wheat in young children) a more formal elimination–challenge test should be carried out.
    - The suspected food(s) are eliminated from the diet totally (for 1–2 weeks).
    - The onset/disappearance of symptoms is recorded in a symptom diary.
    - Reduction or disappearance of symptoms supports food allergy, but is not diagnostic. The food needs to be reintroduced (challenge).
    - A small amount of the food is reintroduced to the diet and as long as the child remains asymptomatic the amount is increased gradually to the normal (age-adjusted) amount consumed daily.
    - Symptoms usually reappear within a week (symptom diary) after, consuming large enough amounts.
- History reveals immediate reactions. Foods that are nutritionally less important need not be tested but can be eliminated from the diet and reintroduced at a later stage.
- Suspicion of anaphylactic reactions caused by food: careful analysis of the causative factor. NEVER instruct the patient to reintroduce the suspected food at home.
- A result from a skin-prick test may be considered fairly reliable in indicating true food allergy only in infants.
- The presence of specific IgE antibodies is not enough for a diagnosis. IgA and IgG antibodies are detected in everyone and are not useful in diagnostics.
- Patch or epicutaneous test. Its suitability for the diagnosis of food allergy requires extensive further research (14.7). So far such testing has only been studied in selected patients in specialist settings.

Follow-up

- Specific items of food that are not nutritionally important may be eliminated when the association between the symptoms and food is clear. Formal tests are not necessarily needed (elimination reintroduction can be carried out at home whilst keeping a symptom diary).
- Indications for referral to specialist care
    - An infant with widespread eczema or worsening symptoms
    - An infant with difficult or perplexing symptoms, and the parents are convinced of food allergy.
    - Failure to thrive.
    - Diet limited by the parents to dangerously few foods.
    - An older child needs to be referred if the diet threatens to become too limited.
- In primary care
    - The growth of a child on an elimination diet is monitored by growth charts.
    - Vaccinations are given according to the normal programme. Allergy to eggs does not prevent vaccination unless the child has had an anaphylactic reaction to eggs.
    - The family is encouraged to expand and rationalise the diet towards a normal diet.
    - The childs diet should be re-evaluated at 5 years of age at the latest: is the avoidance of certain foods based on an eliminationchallenge test? Should a specialist re-evaluate the situation?
    - All elimination diets at school-age should be based on an elimination–reintroduction, not skin or blood tests.

ALL

References

1. Kramer MS, Kakuma R. Maternal dietary antigen avoidance during pregnancy and/or lactation for preventing or treating atopic disease in the child. Cochrane Database Syst Rev. 2004;(2):CD000133.
2. Baumgartner M, Brown CA, Exl BM, Secretin MC, van't Hof M, Haschke F. Controlled trials investigating the use of one partially hydrolyzed whey formula for dietary prevention of atopic manifestations until 60 months of age: an overview using meta-analytical techniques. Nutr Res 1998;18:1425–1442.
3. The Database of Abstracts of Reviews of Effectiveness (University of York), Database no.: DARE-980427. In: The Cochrane Library, Issue 2, 2000. Oxford: Update Software.
4. Osborn DA, Sinn J. Formulas containing hydrolysed protein for prevention of allergy and food intolerance in infants. Cochrane Database Syst Rev 2003(4):CD003664.

14.7 Cow's milk allergy

Minna Kaila

Aims

- To recognize cow's milk allergy leading to symptoms of persisting dermatitis, diarrhoea, and/or growth failure in an infant.

- Diagnosis by clinical elimination and challenge test.
- Securing adequate nutrition and normal growth during the elimination diet.
- Rechallenge to demonstrate achieved tolerance.
- Discontinuation of the elimination diet on negative (re)challenge and tolerance.

Epidemiology

- About 3% of children show symptoms of allergy to cow's milk, usually soon after the introduction of regular use of cow's milk protein-containing foods.
- Cow's milk allergy occurs in infants and small children.
- Cow's milk allergy may appear during exclusive breast feeding.

Symptoms

- Cow's milk allergy refers to allergic inflammation associated with cow's milk proteins, with symptoms in the skin, gut and/or the respiratory system.
- Symptoms are classified according to the affected organ or time of appearance.
  - Immediate symptoms that appear after ingestion (urticaria, spitting out or vomiting, exanthema around the mouth, rhinitis, cough and diarrhoea).
  - Reactions within a day after consumption or later (loose stools, diarrhoea, obstipation, chronic atopic exzema, impaired growth and, more rarely, chronic respiratory symptoms). The symptoms may appear over a time of several days; however, in the majority they begin within a week.
- Anaphylactic reaction/anaphylaxia occurs seldom (rapid onset).
- Symptoms may include in addition restlessness, abdominal pain, irritability.
- In most cases the child has a combination of several symptoms.
- The underlying abnormal immunological mechanism is IgE-mediated in most cases.
- Lactose intolerance (hypolactasia) is not cow's milk allergy.

Diagnosis

- Diagnostic criteria
  - Symptoms suggesting cow's milk allergy appear on a cow's milk protein-containing diet (in breast-fed children mother's diet may be the cause).
  - Symptoms remit on (diagnostic) elimination of these products from the diet (symptom diary).
  - Symptoms reappear on (diagnostic) clinical challenge with cow's milk protein-containing foods (same symptoms with same time delay, symptom diary).
  - Symptoms remit again on (therapeutic) elimination.
    - Any home reintroductions with positive results should be confirmed.
    - A symptom diary helps in evaluating changes in symptoms.
  - Infections and hypolactasia are excluded.
    - Infection is a rare cause of prolonged diarrhoea; however, they may aggravate skin symptoms.
    - Repeated courses of antimicrobial drugs may sustain a recurring/continuous diarrhoea.
    - Hypolactasia is rare in preschool children, while cow's milk allergy typically first becomes symptomatic within the first year of life.
- Laboratory tests play a secondary role in the diagnostic work-up.
  - Skin prick test is too sensitive and simultaneously not specific enough.
  - Patch tests cannot be used for diagnostics.
  - Measuring serum specific IgE (RAST) is similarly problematic.
- Laboratory testing can be helpful in designing the elimination diet in infants when multiple food allergy is suspected.

Clinical challenge (diagnostic and repeated)

- In most cases, do not challenge if anaphylaxis has been the symptom.
- Should preferably be begun under the supervision of a physician; a symptom diary should be kept for a week before and a week after commencement of the challenge.
- Protocols vary, but the basic principle is to start with a small dose and gradually raise the dose to the amount consumed by a child of that age (unless symptoms occur).
- Examples:
  - Place a drop of cow's milk on the lip, observe possible reaction.
  - After 5 minutes, if the child has no symptoms, give a small amount of milk with a spoon. Observe for possible symptoms for 20–30 minutes.
  - If the child continues to be symptomless, give increasing portions at 20–30 minute intervals (e.g. 10 ml–25ml–50ml–100ml).
  - On appearance of unambiguous symptoms (write down), the challenge is discontinued, and the diagnosis of cow's milk allergy can be made. When in doubt, consider readministration of the latest dose.
  - If the patient remains asymptomatic during the follow-up in the office, the challenge is continued at home + a symptom diary.
  - Arrange for a control visit one week later if challenge is continued at home. The diagnosis is made by a physician: no cow milk allergy or cow milk allergy.

Treatment of cow's milk allergy

- The present view is that all cow's milk proteins should be eliminated from the diet. The level of elimination should be individualized: when symptoms appear after greater amounts, extremely strict elimination is not mandatory.

- If possible, a dietician should help in implementing the diet.
- Give written instructions, the family may need courses for cooking special foods.
- Special formulas (breast milk substitutes) are necessary up to the age of 2 years.
- Special formulas: soy formulas, whey hydrolysate, casein hydrolysate, amino acid-based formulas (price rises in this order)
  - Under the age of 6 months use primarily a more degraded product (whey or casein hydrolysate).
  - In older children, use soy formula.
  - Synthetic amino acid-based formulas are reserved for infants with documented multiple food allergy (particularly if they have a growth disturbance). These formulas should always be replaced by hydrolysate or soy formula as the child grows. Only less than one in ten cow's milk allergic infant needs an amino acid based formula.
  - Older children are given calcium supplementation (500 mg of calcium carbonate/day), and intake of sufficient amounts of protein and energy substituents is ensured. This approach may be considered in children older than 1 year of age.

Follow-up

- Infants and those with severe symptoms should be readily referred to a paediatrician for diagnosis and initial treatment.
- Follow-up treatment and challenge tests can be performed in primary care when the parents manage the diet.
- Growth is monitored using a growth chart and sufficient nutrition is secured.
- Therapeutic cow's milk elimination diet is not lifelong; repeated challenges are therefore necessary.
- Most rechallenges can be carried out at the home of the child by the parents.

Prognosis

- The majority of children recover in early childhood.
- Strong atopic tendency: a considerable percentage of the children becomes sensitized to inhalation allergens and develops asthma.

14.8 How to investigate symptoms associated with foods?

Minna Kaila

Aims

- Long-lasting elimination diets should only be started with good reasons. The evidence on the beneficial effects of long-lasting elimination diets in the treatment of e.g. atopic eczema is very limited.
- Elimination diets started in infancy or preschool age should be discontinued in time (before school starts).

Main questions on history when investigating food allergy

- Family (particularly first-degree family: allergies, asthma, skin diseases, gastrointestinal diseases)
- Early history (pregnancy + delivery, position in sibling series)
- Breastfeeding (accurate history of exclusive breastfeeding, total duration + first administration of formula + starting additional foods)
- The mother's possible diet during breastfeeding
- Age at the onset of skin rash and locations of rash
- Foods that have caused symptoms in the child (+ what symptoms + how soon after consuming the food)
- Foods suspected by parents
- Itching
- GI symptoms (be particularly careful in assessing whether these are real symptoms or just normal variation)
  - Spitting up, loose stools/diarrhoea, malodorous/strange coloured stools, constipation, and abdominal pain
- Courses of antibiotics (effect on abdominal symptoms)
- Present diet, foods that may already have been eliminated + justification for elimination
- Growth (height, weight, head circumference)
- Skin care (emollients, use of cortisone)
- Respiratory symptoms
- Smoking (also outdoors, in the car, at grandparents' house)
- Metabolic disease, coeliac disease or lactose intolerance
- Pets (also grandparents), form of daycare

Infant (1 year)

- History
  - Are the symptoms so severe that they call for further investigation, or just part of normal infancy?
  - Family (Do parents or siblings have allergies? Food allergies?)
  - Environment: Pets, smoking
  - Onset of symptoms: Accurate description, what were the symptoms and what happened then?
  - Foods that parents suspect to cause allergy
  - The child's present diet
  - The child's symptoms during breastfeeding (association with foods)
  - In what order have foods been introduced to the diet? Are the symptoms and order correlated?
  - As symptoms usually begin within a few weeks from the introduction of a new foodstuff, the first foods to be eliminated are the 1–5 latest ones.
  - Main basic foods cannot be eliminated in primary care: the child needs to be referred to a specialist (14.7).

- Adhering to a diet is laborious, and parents need good instructions. Find out what information is available to patients (by nutritionists/organizations).
- Symptom diary is useful.
- An analysis of confounding factors is particularly important.

♦ Removing the foods that have been last introduced to the diet and then monitoring the symptoms (without otherwise changing the diet) can be tried. If this is helpful, then new foods can be tried out one at a time.
♦ Foods are introduced one at a time and tried for one week each. This helps to identify possible causes for symptoms.
♦ During this assessment period it is important that new foods are not added randomly.
♦ Special diets that have had no effect on the symptoms are stopped.

Older child

♦ Food-induced symptoms are more unlikely.
♦ For cross-reactions in birch pollen allergy, see 14.6.
♦ Skin rash that is alleviated in the summer is most likely not food allergy.

14.9 Allergen-specific immunotherapy

Erkka Valovirta

Basic rules

♦ The effect of allergen-specific immunotherapy is good in periodic allergic rhinitis and in allergy to Hymenoptera venoms.
♦ Allergen-specific immunotherapy is also used in allergic asthma as a part of anti-inflammatory treatment.

General

♦ Allergen-specific immunotherapy is the causal treatment of IgE-mediated
- allergic rhinitis and conjunctivitis
- allergic asthma and
- allergy to wasp and bee venoms (i.e. Hymenoptera).

♦ During allergen-specific immunotherapy allergic inflammation in target organs diminishes.
♦ In allergy to Hymenoptera venoms allergen-specific immunotherapy decreases the number of life-threatening reactions.
♦ The treatment is usually continued for 3 (–5) years.
♦ The treatment has an effect in 80–90% of the patients and the effect lasts several years (for 10 years according to the latest studies) after it has been stopped.
♦ The decision to start the treatment is made by a specialist, preferably a specialist in allergology.

Preconditions to be met before starting allergen-specific immunotherapy

♦ The patient has confirmed IgE-mediated allergy (allergic rhinoconjuctivitis) that causes symptoms.
♦ Elimination and avoidance of allergens and drug treatment have not removed the symptoms.
♦ Allergic disease is at an early stage. (The risk of pollen-allergic children developing asthma diminishes when allergen-specific immunotherapy is started sufficiently early.)
♦ There are no contraindications to the treatment.
♦ Trained personnel are available to give and follow up the treatment.
♦ The patient has been informed about the duration of the treatment, the restrictions and possible side effects caused by it and wishes to have the treatment. This improves compliance.

Indications

♦ Allergy to hymenoptera venoms
♦ Allergic rhinoconjuctivitis caused by
- pollens
- house dust mite
- animals/pets (in special cases)

♦ Asthma (A) [1 2 3]
- pollens
- house dust mite
- animals/pets (in special cases)

♦ Allergy to moulds (not indicated for symptoms associated with water-damaged houses as these are usually irritation symptoms).
♦ Occupational allergies
- animals

♦ The effect is good in pollen, animal and house dust mite allergies. In allergy to hymenoptera venoms allergen-specific immunotherapy is the only effective causative treatment. Asthma in itself is hardly ever treated solely with allergen-specific immunotherapy.

Contraindications

♦ Other immunological or malignant disease
♦ Severe heart and respiratory illnesses
♦ Continuous oral corticosteroid medication (over 10 mg of prednisolone or corresponding steroid per day)
♦ Age under 5 years
♦ Pregnancy and breastfeeding

Practical aspects

- The treatment is administered around the year by giving subcutaneous injections of aluminium hydroxide-bound depot allergen extracts.
- During the updosing phase the injection dose is increased every 1–2 weeks. After the updosing phase the treatment can be given in a health care centre in cooperation with the centre where it was first started.
- In the maintenance phase the injections are usually given every 6 (4–8) weeks.
- The maintenance dose is individual (the largest dose the patient can tolerate), but no more than recommended by the manufacturer of the allergen extract (the side-effects increase, but the effect does not).
- The next dosage is dictated by the possible reaction from the previous injection and the symptoms the patient has at that time.
- During the pollen season the dose of allergen extract depends on the patient's symptoms. Detailed directions can be obtained from the manufacturers of the allergen extracts.

Precautions

- Emergency equipment for the treatment of anaphylactic reactions must be available.
- A qualified nurse should give the injections and a medical doctor should always be present at the centre.
- The patient is interviewed about possible reactions after the previous visit before giving the injection.
- The patient should be followed up for at least 30 minutes supervision after the injection.
- Patients below 15 years of age must be accompanied.
- Intensive physical exercise and alcohol must be avoided after the injection.

Treatment-related reactions

- Various injection reactions are a natural part of the treatment: local redness and swelling.
- The dosage of the extract is estimated every time on the basis of the swelling reaction (a clear lump which can be felt and measured with the finger, not a possible prick lump on the skin!).
- Generalized reactions (urticaria, asthma, fatigue, generalized allergic reaction) might occur.
- The patient is given medication for the reactions:
  - antihistamine
  - corticosteroid cream
  - a bronchodilatator
  - possibly self injected adrenaline

Treatment follow-up

- The doctor who first started the treatment should evaluate the efficacy at least annually.
- This evaluation is based on the allergic symptoms and the use of other medication.
- So-called VAS evaluation (visual analogue scale) is a new method for evaluating efficacy. The patient gives his estimate of the effect yearly by using the VAS. The evaluation is based on changes in symptoms and use of medication during the treatment.

References

1. Abramson MJ, Puy RM, Weiner JM. Allergen immunotherapy for asthma. Cochrane Database Syst Rev. 2004;(2):CD001186.
2. Malling HJ. Immunotherapy as an effective tool in allergy treatment. Allergy 1998;53:461–472.
3. The Database of Abstracts of Reviews of Effectiveness (University of York), Database no.: DARE-981030. In: The Cochrane Library, Issue 2, 2000. Oxford: Update Software.

ALL

14.10 Hereditary angioedema (HAE) and ACE inhibitor-induced angioedema

Hanna Jarva, Seppo Meri

Aims

- Consider the possibility of hereditary angioedema (HAE) in the differential diagnosis of anaphylactic reaction if the patient has, or has had
  - episodes of mucocutaneous oedema
  - bouts of abdominal pain
  - bouts of headache
  - a family history of HAE.
- Remember that angioedema is a possible adverse effect of ACE inhibitors.

HAE

Definition

- Hereditary angioedema (HAE) is a rare illness transmitted as an autosomal dominant trait. It causes angioedema as a result of a deficiency or dysfunction of the C1-inhibitor (C1-INH) of the complement system.
- Used to be called HANE (hereditary angioneurotic oedema).

Symptoms

- The patient typically presents with episodes of mucocutaneous oedema lasting for 1–5 days. The oedema may be accompanied by erythematous rash, whereas urticaria, pruritus and pain are not typical manifestations.
- Oedema of the intestines causes attacks of abdominal pain which may be the only symptom. Vomiting and diarrhoea may occur.
- If surgery is carried out for the abdominal pain, the operative findings will include oedematous intestines and copious amounts of ascites.
- Laryngeal oedema may occur in up to 50% of the patients, and it might be the first sign of the illness. Laryngeal oedema may be life-threatening.
- Urinary retention
- Headache
- Attacks may be triggered by trauma, injury to the skin, mental or physical stress, menstruation, ovulation or pharyngitis. ACE inhibitors and oestrogen may also trigger an attack (progestogen-only contraceptive pills may be used). Dental procedures and surgery around the head may induce laryngeal oedema. Often no triggering factors can be identified.
- Symptoms may manifest themselves in childhood, youth or adulthood. Symptoms emerging in late adulthood or old age are suggestive of acquired angioedema (AAE) or angioedema associated with ACE inhibitors.

Diagnosis

- **History.** Has the patient had similar episodes in the past? Is there a family history of similar symptoms? A third of the patients are the first ones in their family to be afflicted. A negative family history does therefore not exclude the possibility of HAE.
- **Laboratory investigations**. C1-inhibitor concentration, biochemical C1-inhibitor function as well as C3 and C4. The measurement of C1-inhibitor concentration alone is not sufficient for the diagnosis or exclusion of the condition.
- In Type I HAE (about 85% of HAE patients) the antigen levels and biochemical function of C1-INH as well as the concentration of C4 are decreased. The concentration of C3 is normal.
- In Type II HAE (about 15% of HAE patients) the antigen levels of C1-INH are normal or higher than normal, but the biochemical function is markedly decreased. The concentration of C4 is decreased, but the concentration of C3 is normal.
- Type III HAE has recently been described. It occurs only in women and the C1-INH measurements are normal.
- In acquired C1-inhibitor deficiency (acquired angioedema, AAE), the symptoms generally first appear in midlife or later. Some patients suffer from B-cell lymphoma, cancer or an autoimmune disease, while others only have C1-INH antibodies. C1-INH and C4 concentrations are decreased. In contrast to HAE, the concentration of C1q is decreased.
- Since the condition is so rare a specialist referral is warranted after the initial investigations.

Differential diagnosis: Anaphylaxis or HAE?

- It is not possible to distinguish between the cutaneous oedema caused by an anaphylactic reaction and one caused by HAE.
- Urticaria is often seen in an anaphylactic reaction but not in HAE.
- During the attack, or 1–2 days before it, some HAE patients develop pink, delicate non-itching ring-shaped patches.
- Anaphylactic reaction is a systemic reaction, whereas in HAE the life-threatening symptoms are caused by pharyngeal and laryngeal oedema: hoarse voice is the first symptom, after which the patient is unable to speak and may suffocate.

Treatment of an attack

- Mild oedema; limb oedema in particular: tranexamic acid 1.5 g t.d.s.
- Severe oedema; around the head and neck in particular, or severe abdominal pain:
  - C1 esterase inhibitor concentrate (Cetor® 500 IU, CLB, Netherlands) 1000–2000 units as an infusion.
  - If C1 esterase inhibitor is not available fresh frozen plasma may be administered (4–6 units, according to response).
  - Methyl prednisolone (40–)80 mg intravenously because some patients are also atopic.
  - The patient should be admitted to a hospital, and the staff should prepare for possible tracheal intubation.

Prophylaxis

- If the patient has recurring, severe attacks with laryngeal oedema, prophylactic medication should be commenced with anabolic steroids (stanozolol or danazol). Stanozolol is not available in all countries, and the use of danazol for this indication may be unlicensed. The starting dose of danazol is 400 mg per day, and the dose is subsequently decreased down to 50–200 mg per day, based on the response. Danazol is not suitable for children or pregnant women.
- Tranexamic acid (0.5–1 g t.d.s.) is another alternative for prophylactic use.
- Short-term preventive measures should be instigated before dental or other surgical procedures. Tranexamic acid may be administered for 2 days prior to the procedure (dose as above) or danazol for 5 days prior to the procedure (dose is 600 mg per day). The prophylactic medication should then continue for 3 days after the procedure.

Angioedema caused by ACE inhibitor medication

- Angioedema is a possible adverse effect of ACE inhibitors. With the increased use of ACE inhibitors the incidence of this adverse effect has also increased. Angiotensin-II receptor blockers can cause a similar reaction.

- Tissue oedema occurs most often in the face, pharynx and larynx. The aetiological mechanism is based on the ACE inhibitor-mediated accumulation of bradykinin in the body; C1-INH is also a potent regulator of the bradykinin system.
- Pharyngeal oedema is managed with adrenalin and intravenous corticosteroids (for dosage see 14.1).
- In life-threatening situations C1 esterase inhibitor concentrate (Cetor® 500 IU, CLB, Netherlands) may also be administered (1000 units as an infusion).

Haematology

Evidence Based Medicine Guidelines. Edited by the Duodecim Editorial Team
 ISBN: 0-470-01184-X

15.1 Bone marrow examination

Juhani Vilpo

Basic rules

- Bone marrow examination is an easy and inexpensive outpatient examination. It is necessary for confirmation or exclusion of haematological malignancies.
- It is very advisable to examine the blood film simultaneously. Bone marrow iron stain has been a golden standard in iron deficiency diagnostics. Bone marrow trephine biopsy is necessary in "dry tap" situations and helpful in several others.

Purpose

- Bone marrow aspiration has a central role in examination of diseases of the blood. It may be the only way in which correct diagnosis is made. In addition, many actual blood diseases can be excluded by a normal finding. Sometimes bone marrow examination has a prognostic value. It may also be used to follow the response to treatment, for instance, during chemotherapy of leukaemia.
- The diagnosis of several diseases is solely or essentially based on bone marrow examination. These include megaloblastic anaemias (15.24), leukaemias (15.45), myelodysplastic syndromes (15.48), multiple myeloma (15.46), Waldenström's macroglobulinaemia (15.47), bone marrow metastases and some storage diseases.
- Examination of a bone marrow aspiration sample also completes the picture in several other diseases, such as aplastic anaemia, agranulocytosis, idiopathic thrombocytopenic purpura and hypersplenism.

Specific conditions (aspiration)

- Undefined anaemia
- Undefined thrombocytopenia
- Leucocytopenia, leucocytosis
- Undefined lymphadenopathy, splenomegaly, hepatomegaly
- Fever of unknown origin
- (Suspected) bone marrow involvement of
  - haematological malignancy
  - metastatic malignancy.
- Follow-up of chemotherapy
- Lymphoma staging
- Local bone pain
- Metabolic diseases of the bone

Specific conditions (trephine)

Necessary

- No bone marrow aspirated
  - Dry tap
  - Blood tap
- Myelofibrosis
- Bone marrow necrosis
- Metabolic diseases of the bone

Useful

- Aplastic anaemia
- Search for bone marrow metastases
- Lymphoma staging
- Granulomas
  - Tuberculosis
  - Sarcoidosis

Puncture

- The usual sites of aspiration biopsy in adults are the sternum and the iliac crest.
- Trephine samples are usually taken from the posterior iliac crest.
- In young children, from birth to 1-(2) years, the medial aspect at the border between the middle and upper third of the tibia is a good site. In older children the posterior iliac crest is the site of choice. This site can also be used for children younger than 2 years.

Interpretation

- Good collaboration between the clinician and the examiner is a prerequisite of successful bone marrow examination.
- The examiner should be provided with information about
  - clinical background (also medication)
  - size of the spleen and liver, icterus
  - lymph node status
  - current blood picture: haemoglobin, haematocrit, MCV, mean cell haemoglobin (MCH), leucocyte count and differential, platelet count. In anaemia reticulocyte count is also useful.
- Fruitful collaboration requires that the examiner is active and clear as regards reporting the results and conclusions. An immediate contact is sometimes necessary if the findings demand an urgent response. Hence the examiner must be provided with the name and phone number (fax, e-mail) of the clinician in charge.

15.2 Blood films

Juhani Vilpo

- For absolute normal reference ranges of different cell types in adults, see 15.4.

Basic rules

- The concept of blood film is not definite or unambiguous. Local practice determines the content and use of blood films.
  - **Differential white cell count** is usually automated and only abnormal findings are checked manually by a laboratory technician. Sometimes a differential white cell count also includes a description of red cell morphology and an estimate of the number of platelets.

Table 15.2 Diseases where blood film examination may be helpful or even diagnostic although the numerical blood picture (haemoglobin, WBC, platelets and sometimes white cell differential) may be normal

Condition	Findings
Compensated haemolysis	Spherocytosis, polychromasia, red cell agglutination
Hereditary spherocytosis	Spherocytes, polychromasia
Hereditary elliptocytosis	Elliptocytes (ovalocytes)
Thalassaemia	Hypochromasia, target cells
Sickle-cell disease	Sickle cells
Myelofibrosis, bone marrow infiltrates	Teardrop cells, leucoerythroblastic picture
Asplenia (after splenectomy, spleen infiltrates, atrophy)	Howell-Jolly bodies, acanthocytes, target cells
Lead poisoning	Punctate basophilia
Early deficiency of vitamin B_{12} or folate	Hypersegmentated neutrophils
Myeloma, macroglobulinaemia	Rouleaux formation
DIC and mechanical haemolysis	Fragmented red cells (schistocytes)
Severe infections	Neutrophilia, harsh ("toxic") granulation of neutrophils
Infectious mononucleosis	Transformed (reactive) lymphocytes
Some storage diseases	Vacuolated lymphocytes
Hereditary anomalies involving leucocytes and platelets	Specific morphological changes in affected cells (e.g. giant platelets in Bernard–Soulier syndrome)
Agranulocytosis	Neutropenia
Allergic conditions	Eosinophilia
Chronic lymphocytic leukaemia	Relative lymphocytosis, smashed lymphocytes
Hairy cell leukaemia	Hairy cells
Acute leukaemias (in the early stage)	Blasts

  - **Blood morphology** is a complete examination of the blood film by a medical specialist. This usually requires a referral with a clinical problem.

Indications

- Blood morphology examination is always indicated in the assessment of the following conditions, unless the cause is otherwise apparent:
  - leucocytopenia
  - leucocytosis
  - polycythaemia
  - thrombocytosis
  - thrombocytopenia
  - other than iron deficiency anaemia.
- Differential white cell count and blood morphology are rarely suited for follow-up; WBC or a more specific parameter (for example reticulocytes in haemolysis) is preferred.
- Table 15.2 lists some diseases in which blood haemoglobin concentration and both leucocyte count and thrombocyte count may be normal and blood morphology may lead to the correct diagnosis.

15.3 Elevated ESR (hypersedimentation)

Editors

Reference values

- Men
  - age < 50 years < 15 mm/h
  - age > 50 years < 20 mm/h
- Women
  - age < 50 years < 20 mm/h
  - age > 50 years < 30 mm/h
- The significance of a slightly elevated ESR is difficult to assess, particularly in the elderly. The threshold for starting investigations can be set considerably higher if the patient is asymptomatic or if the ESR has not increased during follow-up (see below).

Factors affecting the ESR

- Marked effect
  - Acute phase reactants (particularly fibrinogen)
  - Increased concentration of immunoglobulins

- Decreased concentration of albumin
- Pregnancy (see below)

♦ Small effect

- Anaemia, irrespective of its cause
- High serum cholesterol
- The ESR is usually low in polycythaemia (even in diseases that usually raise the ESR).

Hypersedimentation is nearly always associated with the following diseases

♦ A normal ESR usually rules out these diseases. Conditions in which the ESR is a better indicator of disease activity than serum CRP are indicated with an asterix (*).

- Septicaemia (with symptoms for more than 2 days)
- Deep abscesses, osteomyelitis
- Polymyalgia rheumatica and temporal arteritis
- Symptomatic subacute thyroiditis
- Myeloma and other paraproteinaemias (*)
- Widespread lymphoma (*)
- Nephrotic syndrome (*)

Hypersedimentation is often associated with the following diseases

♦ Pyelonephritis
♦ Bacterial pneumonia (the ESR may also be elevated in viral pneumonia)
♦ Active rheumatoid arthritis and ankylosing spondylitis
♦ Systemic connective tissue diseases (*)
♦ Tuberculosis
♦ Crohn's disease
♦ Ulcerative colitis (*)
♦ Marked hyperlipidaemia (*)
♦ Fibrotizing alveolitis (e.g. farmer's lung)
♦ Sarcoidosis (*)
♦ Chronic hepatitis (*)
♦ Cirrhosis of the liver (*)
♦ Metastasized cancer (*)
♦ Renal carcinoma (hypernephroma) (*)
♦ Cholesterol embolism (*) (5.61)
♦ The level of the ESR is dependent on the activity of the disease. In many situations the CRP concentration decreases with disease activity but the ESR remains high because of hypergammaglobulinaemia.

The ESR is often normal in the following diseases

♦ Most cancers, particularly those of the gastrointestinal tract
♦ Osteoarthrosis
♦ Viral infections

Assessment of a patient with hypersedimentation

♦ **Symptomatic** patients should be investigated to diagnose the underlying disease. The nature of the symptoms determines the urgency of the investigations.
♦ In **asymptomatic** patients or patients with **minimal symptoms,** find out whether the ESR has steadily increased from a normal value, and what is the direction of change. If the ESR is markedly elevated (more than 20 mm/h above the upper reference value) further investigations should be planned as follows.

History

♦ Always ask about

- Fever
- Impaired general condition
- Local symptoms (pain, tenderness)
- Joint symptoms (particularly morning stiffness) and myalgias; also earlier episodes
- Bowel habits, consistency of the stools
- Cough, sputum
- History of tuberculosis

Investigations

♦ General physical examination, particularly lymph nodes, palpation of the thyroid gland, skin, lungs, abdomen, joints, teeth
♦ If the history of the patient does not suggest any particular diagnosis, perform the following examinations:

- Complete blood count (automated differential count is sufficient)
- Urinalysis and bacterial culture
- Serum CRP
- Serum ALT, alkaline phosphatase
- Serum creatinine
- Serum protein electrophoresis (differentiation between polyclonal and monoclonal increase in the gammaglobulin concentration)
- Serum rheumatoid factor (if the patient has joint symptoms)
- Chest, sinus etc. x-rays according to the clinical findings
- Fine needle biopsies

Indications for hospital investigations in hypersedimentation of unknown origin

♦ If the general condition of the patient is markedly affected the investigations should be started immediately.
♦ Asymptomatic young or middle-aged patients should be referred after the aforementioned investigations if the ESR does not decrease. A very high ESR (>80 mm/h) is an indication for more urgent investigations.

- In the elderly the general situation of the patient determines the scope of the investigations. Sometimes no investigations are necessary after serious diseases and treatable conditions have been excluded.

15.4 Leucocytosis

Juhani Vilpo

Basic rules

- Leucocytosis refers to an elevation of the total number of white cells in blood. This can be caused by a rise in the amount of one or more leucocyte types:
  - Neutrophilia
  - Lymphocytosis
  - Monocytosis
  - Eosinophilia
  - Basophilia.
- The division of leucocytoses (especially neutrophilias) according to their aetiology is directly useful in clinical diagnostics.
  - Infections and inflammations
  - Medication-related (corticosteroids, granulocyte growth factors, others)
  - Stress-related (physical, emotional)
  - Leukaemias (rare in comparison to the previous-mentioned)

Aims

- A severe infection as a cause of leucocytosis should be urgently recognized and therapy initiated.
- Leucopenia or a normal leucocyte count, on the other hand, does not necessarily exclude a severe infection.
- Leucocytosis of unknown origin may be associated with rheumatic diseases, other chronic inflammations or haematological malignancies. The cause of leucocytosis can usually be revealed with a small number of investigations.

Reference intervals

- See Table 15.4.

Approach

- If the clinical picture explains the occurrence and extent of leucocytosis, no specific investigations are required.
- If the underlying disease is unknown, the leucocyte differential count helps in orientation.

Neutrophilia ($>7.5 \times 10^9$/l) is the most common form of leucocytosis

- Neutrophilia occurs most frequently with **infections**; the neutrophil count is related to the severity of infection as

Table 15.4 Reference ranges (mean ± 2 SD or 95%) for white cell parameters

Patients	Leucocytes ($\times 10^9$/l)	Differential (%)	Absolute number ($\times 10^9$/l)
Adults	3.4–8.2		
Neutrophils		40–75	(1.5)–2.0–7.5
Lymphocytes		20–50	1.5–4.0
– B lymphocytes		10–20	0.2–0.6
– T helper (CD4)		30–45	0.4–1.5
– T suppressor (CD8)		15–30	0.2–1.0
– CD4/CD8 = 1.2–2.8 (average 1.6)			
Monocytes		2–10	0.2–0.8
Eosinophils		1–6	0.04–0.4
Basophils		<1	0.01–0.1
Children			
Newborn	9.0–38.0		
1–2 weeks	5.0–21.0		
3–4 weeks	5.0–19.5		
1 month–1 year	6.0–17.5		
2–6 years	5.0–14.0		
7–12 years	4.5–13.0		
>12 years	4.5–13.0		

Leucocyte count may be increased during pregnancy (up to 15–20 $\times 10^9$/l), physical activity, psychological stress, and after meals. The leucocyte count is lower in the morning than in the afternoon. The upper reference limit of the leucocyte count for adults is such that 5–10% of healthy persons may have values slightly greater than 8.2 $\times 10^9$/l.

well as to the microbiological aetiology. Pyogenic cocci (staphylococcus, streptococcus, pneumococcus, gonococcus and meningococcus) and bacilli (E. coli, Proteus and Pseudomonas) are common causes of neutrophilia. The leucocyte count is usually 15–30 × 10^9/l, but sometimes even 50–80 × 10^9/l. Immature neutrophils (bands, metamyelocytes) and "toxic" granulation are characteristic in the acute phase.
- Neutrophilia is also relatively common in non-pyogenic infections. These include rheumatic fever, scarlet fever, diphtheria (1.25), polio, typhoid fever, cholera, and shingles (1.41). The leucocyte count is usually 12–18 × 10^9/l.
- Sometimes neutrophil leucocytosis with immature granulocytes is so marked that it is called a leukaemoid reaction.
- Other causes of neutrophil leucocytosis include:
  - bleeding
  - trauma
  - cardiac diseases (infarction, atrial fibrillation)
  - drugs (e.g. corticosteroids), poisonings
  - metabolic diseases (renal insufficiency, diabetic coma, gout attack, eclampsia)
  - blood diseases: myeloid leukaemias (15.40), polycythaemia vera (15.41), myelofibrosis (15.42)
  - rheumatoid arthritis, vasculitis
  - blood transfusion

Eosinophilia is relatively common

- See 15.6

Lymphocytosis (>4.0 x 10^9/l) is also relatively common

- Marked lymphocytosis is seen in chronic lymphocytic leukaemia (15.43), infectious mononucleosis and in pertussis.
- Milder lymphocytosis is common in various infections.

Monocytosis (>0.8 x 10^9/l) is uncommon

- It can be associated with various infections (typhoid fever, brucellosis, tuberculosis, subacute endocarditis, malaria (2.30)), rheumatoid arthritis and other connective tissue diseases, Hodgkin's disease and monocytic leukaemias.

Basophilia is rare

- It is sometimes seen in the accelerated phase of chronic myeloid leukaemia (CML) (15.40).

Investigations

- Bone marrow examination (15.1) is necessary if the aetiology of leucocytosis remains unknown, especially if the white cell differential count or the clinical picture indicates the possibility of a haematological malignancy.
- Chronic benign leucocytosis with immature neutrophils shall be distinguished from CML by genetic analyses (15.40)
- If the symptoms and findings are unremarkable, follow-up of 1–2 weeks and a new leucocyte count may be the method of choice. A significant proportion of underlying conditions (infections) are harmless and temporary. Treatment is directed against the cause of leucocytosis.

15.5 Leucocytopenia

Juhani Vilpo

Aims

- Neutropenia is suspected on the basis of acute or chronic weakness and fatigue associated with infections of the skin or mucous membranes.
- Hospitalization is advisable if the patient has fever or if the leucocyte count is less than 0.5 × 10^9/l.

Basic rules

- In leucopenia, the leucocyte count is below the reference range, i.e. less than 3.4 × 10^9/l (when the reference range is set to 3.4–8.2 × 10^9/l). However, the leucocyte count of healthy persons may permanently be 3.0–4.0 × 10^9/l or even less than that. The reason for this can be a deficiency of circulating neutrophils in spite of normal storage pools (i.e. "peripheral neutropenia"). The reference values for children vary with age.
- Leucopenia may indicate
  - neutropenia (neutrophil count less than 1.5–2.0 × 10^9/l)
  - lymphopenia (lymphocyte count less than 1.5 × 10^9/l)
  - a combination of both.
- If AIDS is excluded, leucopenia is nearly always a result of **mild neutropenia**.
- In **severe leucopenias** both neutrophils and lymphocytes are decreased.
- **Lymphopenia** is seldom associated with specific conditions with the exception of rare inherited and acquired immune deficiency syndromes. A deficiency of helper T cells (CD4) is used as an indicator of disease stage in HIV infection (1.45).
- Neutropenia is associated with an **increased risk of bacterial infection**. In particular, a continuously declining neutrophil count calls for special attention.
  - Owing to a rich bone marrow storage pool, a neutrophil count of 1.5–2.0 × 10^9/l does not indicate an increased risk.
  - A moderate infection risk exists if the neutrophil count is 0.5–1.0 × 10^9/l
  - Severe bacterial infections are frequent if the neutrophil count is less than 0.5 × 10^9/l.

- Septic infections are common when the neutrophil count is less than 0.1×10^9/l.

Kinetics

- There are two kinetic groups of leucopenia–mostly caused by neutropenia.
  - Increased consumption
    - e.g. at the focus of pyogenic infections.
  - Decreased production in the bone marrow
    - e.g. in aplastic anaemia when the production of all cells has decreased or ceased, or owing to large bone marrow infiltrations of a metastatic tumour.
  - Both can occur simultaneously. The kinetic nature of leucopenia is not known in all cases.

Aetiology

- Infections
  - Bacterial (typhoid, paratyphoid, brucellosis)
  - Viral (influenza, measles, rubella, infectious hepatitis, viral pneumonia)
  - Rickettsial
  - Protozoal (malaria)
  - Severe infections, such as miliary tuberculosis and infections in the elderly and in patients having decreased resistance
- Leukaemia (also aleukaemic)
- Drugs
  - Causing selective neutropenia
  - Causing aplastic anaemia
- Aplastic anaemia
- Hypersplenism
- Idiopathic neutropenia
  - Acute or chronic
- Bone marrow infiltrates
  - Cancer metastases
  - Lymphomas
  - Myelofibrosis (15.42)
  - Multiple myeloma (15.46)
- Megaloblastic anaemia (15.24)
- Connective tissue diseases
  - SLE
  - Sjögren's syndrome
- Severe iron deficiency anaemia
- Other causes
  - Toxic chemicals
  - Ionizing irradiation
  - Other

Clinical manifestations of neutropenia

- Local and generalized clinical manifestations are related to infections.
- Mild and symptomless neutropenia may be associated with many diseases.
- The clinical picture may be broadly classified as acute or chronic.

Neutropenia with symptoms

- May often be associated with
  - acute leukaemia
  - many drugs
  - aplastic anaemia
  - hypersplenism
  - severe idiopathic neutropenias (rare)

Acute neutropenia

- Clinical manifestations
  - sudden fever, chilliness, sweating
  - headache
  - muscle ache
  - tiredness
- There may be a 1–2-day prodromal phase characterized by weakness.
- Local infections are most frequent in the skin and mucous membranes, especially in the oral cavity.
  - The throat first becomes reddish and swollen.
  - Within 1–2 days necrotic areas become demarcated. Gangrenous ulceration is covered with a yellow-grey-greenish membrane.

Chronic neutropenia

- The clinical picture is less dramatic with milder symptoms (tiredness, weakness).
- Infections are mostly located in the skin and mucous membranes. Infections tend to be chronic and they do not respond well to antibiotics. Necrosis and ulceration are common. Owing to the shortage of granulocytes, pus formation is scarce.
- Wound healing is slow.

Examinations

- Neutropenia is established by total and differential white cell counts or a neutrophil count.
- Careful history (drugs, chemicals, previous infections, family) and clinical examination are necessary and helpful.
- Bone marrow examination (15.1) usually reveals the kinetic type (decreased production or increased peripheral consumption) of neutropenia and often also gives information about the underlying cause.
- **Spleen size** determination (palpation, ultrasound) is helpful. Splenomegaly (>10–12 cm) may indicate an underlying disease or it may be associated with hypersplenism.
- **Abscesses** may be imaged using a gamma camera and **radioactively labelled granulocytes**.
- Determining circulating anti-neutrophil antibodies is a too complicated investigation to be used in primary care.

Treatment

- **Hospitalization is advisable for rapid diagnosis and treatment, if a patient with neutropenia has fever or if the neutrophil count is less than 0.5 × 10^9/l.** This is justified because neutropenia is commonly associated with fatal bacterial infections. These require rapid and accurate microbiological diagnostics and effective antibiotic treatment combined with supportive measures.
- In severe neutropenia, **haematopoietic growth factors** (G-CSF and GM-CSF) effectively increase the neutrophil count if there are progenitors in the bone marrow. These parenteral drugs are most commonly used in chemotherapy-induced neutropenia (A) [1] and in severe chronic neutropenia.
  - The effect starts within the first 24 h and should be clearly seen after a few days.
  - **In severe chronic neutropenias** the maintenance dose is tailored individually. After discontinuing therapy, the neutrophil count decreases by 50% within 1–2 days and returns to baseline in 1–7 days.
  - **During chemotherapy** a temporary increase in neutrophil count is seen in 1–2 days. To achieve a long-term therapeutic response, therapy is continued until the lowest count has been passed and the normal count has been achieved. In some cases therapy has to be continued for up to 14 days.
  - Treatment is expensive; however, carefully targeted and implemented therapy is indicated in certain cases. The treatment strategy is planned by an experienced specialist (haematologist, oncologist, a specialist in internal medicine or a paediatrician).

Reference

1. Clark OAC, Lyman G, Castro AA, Clark LGO, Djulbegovic B. Colony stimulating factors for chemotherapy induced febrile neutropenia. Cochrane Database Syst Rev. 2004;(2): CD003039.

15.6 Eosinophilia

Juhani Vilpo

Basic rules

- Eosinophils normally account for 1–6% of peripheral blood (3.4–8.2 × 10^9/l) leucocytes. The reference range in absolute numbers is 0.04–0.4 × 10^9/l.
- In practice, an eosinophil count of >0.4 × 10^9/l can be regarded as eosinophilia. In infants (below 1 year) the upper limit is higher and >1.0 × 10^9/l means eosinophilia.
- Consider the following:
  - Could the eosinophilia be a sign of some underlying disease, which needs medical attention (based on history and status)?
  - Can the eosinophilia itself pose a threat to the patient (eosinophils can cause tissue damage by secreting proinflammatory cytokines)?
- There is diurnal variation in the blood eosinophil count. It has an inverse relationship with blood glucocorticoid levels. The blood eosinophil count is highest in the evening and lowest in the morning. Eosinophil levels are slightly higher during menstruation. Physical strain temporarily increases the blood eosinophil count, but psychological stress and beta-blockers may decrease it.

Underlying diseases

- The list of factors causing eosinophilia is almost endless. The issue is further complicated by the fact that eosinophilia seems to appear randomly, that is, its absence does not rule out a suspected cause.

Most important causes of eosinophilia (>0.4 x 10^9/l)

- Allergy
  - Asthma, allergic rhinitis, drug eruptions, urticaria, etc.
- Parasitic infections
  - Ascariasis infection (1.54), trichinosis (1.53), echinococcosis (1.51), human toxoplasmosis (1.62) and tropical parasites, e.g. schistosomiasis (2.33).
- Drugs
  - Penicillin, streptomycin and chlorpromazine when associated with icterus alone
  - Gold (21.62)
  - Antibiotics, e.g. ofloxacin and nitrofurantoin
  - Tryptophan-use is associated with eosinophilia-myalgia syndrome (probably caused by the impurity present in tryptophan that is used as a natural remedy).
- Skin diseases
  - Eczema, pemphigus, psoriasis, dermatitis herpetiformis, prurigo, etc.
- Lung involvement (infiltrates in radiography and blood eosinophilia) (6.42)
  - Löffler's syndrome (mild, often resolves in 4 weeks)
  - Prolonged form of the disease (no asthma symptoms, fluctuating course, duration 2–6 months)
  - Pulmonary eosinophilia + asthma
  - Tropical eosinophilia
  - Churg–Strauss syndrome
  - Nitrofurantoin lung
- Infections

- In many bacterial infections eosinophilopenia is common in the acute phase, but eosinophilia may be seen when neutrophilia starts to decrease.

♦ Malignant haematological diseases

- Chronic myelocytic leukaemia, polycythaemia vera, Hodgkin's disease (as many as 10% of the patients), sometimes also in multiple myeloma. Eosinophilic leukaemia is extremely rare.

♦ Carcinomas

- Especially in metastatic or necrotic carcinomas and following radiotherapy (in about 30%)

♦ Eosinophilic fasciitis

- A rare connective tissue disease that resembles scleroderma.
- Often begins after hard physical strain.
- The skin of both upper and lower extremities swells and becomes hard as in scleroderma. The disease often progresses rapidly.
- Laboratory tests show elevated ESR in addition to eosinophilia.
- Biopsy of affected skin or fascia is diagnostic.
- Treated with high doses of corticosteroids

♦ Familial eosinophilia

- Very rare

Clinical approach

♦ The assessment of eosinophilia requires a multifaceted approach. Eosinophil values obtained from automated white blood cell differential counting are used in follow-up.

- When the eosinophil count is $0.4–0.5 \times 10^9$/l, and the patient is symptomless, the clinical situation and the eosinophil (morning) count is checked at 1–2-month intervals.
- When eosinophilia is more pronounced, thorough investigations are warranted (unless the probable cause is known and the basic disease is already treated). The patient's condition determines the need for further investigations.

♦ Some patients are considered to suffer from hypereosinophilic syndrome (HES). The following criteria have been suggested:

- Eosinophil count $> 1.5 \times 10^9$/l for more than 6 months
- Signs of end-organ involvement
- Absence of an identifiable cause.

♦ The higher the eosinophil count the more likely is end-organ involvement. The occurrence increases when the count exceeds $5–10 \times 10^9$/l. Examination of symptomatic patients (respiratory and cardiac symptoms and involvement) is the responsibility of a specialist. Some patients may need

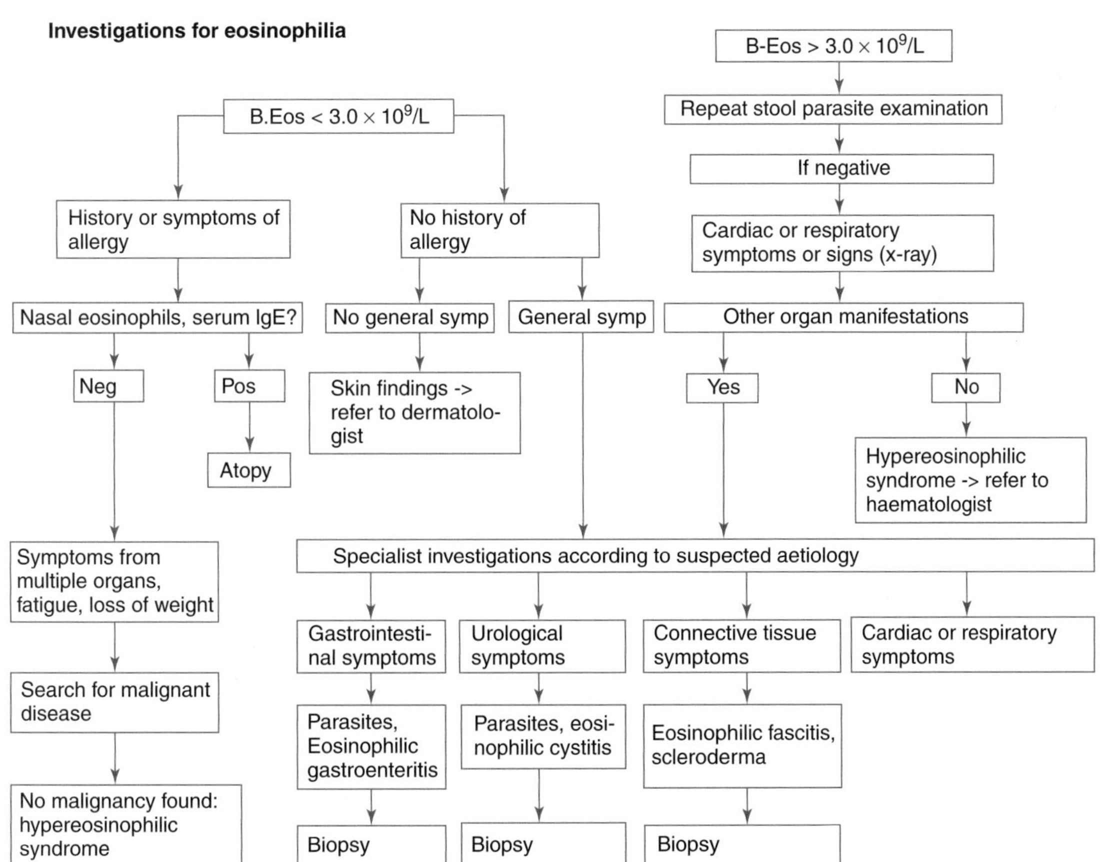

Figure 15.6.1 The aetiology of eosinophilia is variable. A logical empirical investigation strategy should be followed.

antihistamines to alleviate symptoms and possibly also glucocorticoids or even cytotoxic agents to prevent end-organ manifestations.

Diagnostic strategy

1. Faecal parasites
2. If parasites are not found, continue examinations as shown in the algorithm (Figure 15.6.1). In investigation of atopy skin prick tests are indicated (13.5).

15.7 Erythrocytosis

Juhani Vilpo

Aims

- Distinguish primary polycythaemia (polycythaemia vera, PV) from secondary and relative erythrocytosis (elevated haemoglobin, normal red cell mass).

Basic rules

- Erythrocytosis refers to an elevation of the total number of red cells in blood. In practical terms it can be defined by measuring one of the following:
    - Blood haemoglobin concentration
    - Packed cell volume or haematocrit
    - Erythrocyte concentration.
- Erythrocytosis means:
    - In women; haemoglobin > 155 g/l, haematocrit > 0.46, or erythrocytes $> 5.2 \times 10^{12}$/l.
    - In men; haemoglobin > 167 g/l, haematocrit > 0.50, or erythrocytes $> 5.7 \times 10^{12}$/l.
- Erythrocytosis may be **relative** (normal red cell mass) or **absolute** (elevated red cell mass). Absolute erythrocytosis may be **primary** (PV) or **secondary**.
- PV (15.41) is a chronic myeloproliferative disease. It is a true "poly"cythaemia because usually leucocyte and platelet concentrations are also increased.

Causes

True polycythaemias

- PV
- Secondary polycythaemias
    - Hypoxia-induced
        - High-altitude erythrocytosis
        - Congenital heart disease
        - Chronic pulmonary disease
        - Others (acquired heart disease, rigid thorax, marked obesity, heavy smoking)
    - Other causes (secondary to aberrant erythropoiesis)
        - Renal diseases
        - Some neoplastic diseases
- Familial erythrocytosis
- Abnormal haemoglobins (such as Hb Helsinki, Hb Linköping)
- Medications (doping), erythropoietin, androgens

Relative erythrocytoses

- Dehydration
- Decreased plasma volume
- Pseudopolycythaemia or stress polycythaemia (common among heavy smokers and obese persons)

Clinical approach

- The general practitioner evaluates the need for special investigations.
    - Severe heart and lung diseases are often associated with polycythaemia and no special investigations are necessary.
    - PV patients often have splenomegaly (>10–12 cm), thrombocytosis and leucocytosis as well as general symptoms (tiredness, itching, nausea). Bleeding and thrombotic complications are common.
- Differential diagnosis may be difficult if a PV patient does not have pancytosis or splenomegaly. Identification of

Table 15.7 Differential diagnostic studies of erythrocytosis

Analyte	Polycythaemia vera	Secondary polycythaemia	Relative erythrocytosis
Red cell mass	Increased	Increased	Normal
Leucocytosis	Usually	No	No
Thrombocytosis	Usually	No	No
Splenomegaly	Often	No	No
Oxygen, partial pressure, arterial	Normal	Decreased or normal	Normal
Leucocyte alkaline phosphatase stain	Increased	Normal	Normal
Serum erythropoietin	Decreased	Increased or normal	Normal
Spontaneous growth in stem cell culture	Usually	No	No

secondary polycythaemia may be difficult if the underlying disease remains obscure. True polycythaemia can be ascertained only by red cell mass determination, available only in the outpatient clinics of larger hospitals.

- Table 15.7 lists the central differential diagnostic investigations.

Treatment

- Treatment of PV (15.41).
- In secondary polycythaemia, treatment is directed against the underlying disease. Venesections (400–500 ml at a time) are seldom necessary. They are used to prevent central nervous system complications associated with blood hyperviscosity.
- In relative erythrocytosis, the cause is eliminated. Dehydration is corrected. Obesity and chain-smoking are treated by counselling etc.

15.8 Macrocytosis (increased MCV)

Juhani Vilpo

Aims

- Mean (red) cell volume or MCV denotes average red cell volume in femtolitres. Traditionally it has been calculated on the basis of haematocrit and red cell count; MCV = haematocrit/red cell count, where the latter has been estimated by chamber counting. Owing to the relatively low number of cells counted, the reproducibility of this parameter has been poor. Hence, MCV should not be based on chamber counting of red cells.
- Nowadays MCV is determined directly in haematological analysers using either light scatter or impedance (Coulter method). Although very precise, the result is not necessarily accurate. This is why the reference intervals for different laboratories may be slightly different.
- In most laboratories the MCV value is reported automatically together with haemoglobin values, although the clinician may not necessarily have asked for it. It is therefore quite common to find values higher than the upper limit of the reference value (98 fl).

Causes of increased MCV (macrocytosis)

- The causes of macrocytosis (MCV > 100 fl) can be divided into two groups:
  - Normoblastic erythropoiesis
    - Reticulocytosis (bleeding, haemolysis)
    - Liver disease
    - Severe hypothyroidism
    - Severe hypopituitarism
    - High consumption of alcohol
  - Megaloblastic erythropoiesis or dyserythropoiesis (15.24)
    - Hypovitaminosis (folate or B_{12})
    - Myelodysplastic syndrome (15.48)
    - Malignant blood disease
    - Defective DNA synthesis (Mostly drug-induced. Rarely inherited.)

Artefacts in determination

- Abundant red cell rouleaux formation or agglutination
- Severe hyperglycaemia
- Marked leucocytosis

Clinical approach

- If a patient has anaemia, haematological investigations are carried out as usual (15.24), (15.20).
- If the haemoglobin level is normal, the situation can be evaluated practically as follows:
  - Alcoholism and alcohol abuse are the most common causes of macrocytosis. If past history and the clinical impression make ethanol a likely cause, no other investigations are required. The situation is explained to the patient and counselling started. If there is hope of improvement, MCV can be followed. Its normalization takes several months. Gamma glutamyltransferase (GGT) returns to the reference range earlier, if abstinence is successful.
  - If alcoholism is not evident, additional investigations are carried out: blood reticulocyte count, serum GGT, serum vitamin B_{12} and red cell folate. Hypothyroidism should be excluded by thyroid function tests. Blood and bone marrow microscopy are not usually helpful as first-line investigations. Macrocytosis often remains unexplained (idiopathic). Among men the respective figure may be about 10% and among women as much as 40%.

15.9 Thrombocytosis

Juhani Vilpo

Aims

- Differential diagnosis between
  - secondary (reactive) thrombocytosis and
  - thrombocytosis associated with chronic myeloproliferative disorders (particularly essential thrombocythaemia, but also polycythaemia vera, chronic myelogenous leukaemia and myelofibrosis), i.e. clonal thrombocytosis.

Basic rules

- The reference range of the blood platelet count is broad ($150-360 \times 10^9/l$). On the other hand, there is little intra-individual variation between days.
- Thrombocytosis (platelet count $> 360 \times 10^9/l$) can be classified into three categories:
  - Physiological
  - Reactive or secondary
  - Primary, i.e., clonal (essential thrombocythaemia and thrombocytosis associated with other chronic myeloproliferative disorders).
- Of these, only clonal thrombocytosis causes symptoms and complications. These are not met in reactive thrombocytoses even if the platelet counts may be markedly increased. The primary disease in itself may of course pose a risk of thrombosis or bleeding.

Causes of thrombocytosis

- Clonal thrombocytoses, i.e., those associated with malignant haematological diseases (follow-up or treatment needed)
  - Myeloproliferative disorders (essential thrombocythaemia (15.49), polycythaemia vera (15.41), chronic myeloic leukaemia (15.40), myelofibrosis with myeloid metaplasia (15.42))
- Secondary, i.e., reactive (attention is paid to finding and treating the primary disease)
  - Transient
    - Acute haemorrhage
    - Over-compensation (recovery phase of thrombocytopenia, especially in connection with bone marrow suppression)
    - Acute infection or inflammation
    - Marked physical strain, childbirth, adrenaline
  - Chronic
    - Iron deficiency anaemia (15.21)
    - Haemolytic anaemia (15.25)
    - Asplenia (e.g., following splenectomy)
    - Cancer
    - Chronic infection or inflammation
    - Reactions to medications (vincristine, retinoid acid, cytokines, growth factors)

Clinical approach

- Distinction between different forms of secondary thrombocytosis versus chronic myeloproliferative disorders (particularly essential thrombocythaemia, but also polycythaemia vera, chronic myelogenous leukaemia and myelofibrosis) is most important. Sometimes, however, differential diagnosis may be difficult. Helpful examinations are listed in Table 15.9.

Table 15.9 Differential diagnosis of thrombocytosis: clinical picture and laboratory investigations

Findings	Clonal thrombocytosis*	Reactive thrombocytosis
Primary disease	No	Often apparent or easily found
Ischaemia in cerebral circulation, fingers or toes	Frequently (in untreated disease)	No
Thrombosis in arteries or veins	Increased risk	No
Bleeding	Increased risk	No
Splenomegaly	Ca. 40% of patients	No
Blood smear	Giant platelets	Platelet morphology normal
Bone marrow	Abnormal megakaryocytes	Megakaryocytes normal

*Clonal thrombocytosis includes essential thrombocytosis and other myeloproliferative diseases.

Treatment

- In secondary thrombocytosis, treatment is directed against the underlying disease.
- In myeloproliferative disorders, thrombocytosis is associated with an increased risk of thrombosis and bleeding. The risk increases considerably with age as well as with other simultaneous risk factors, which is why diagnosis and treatment of myeloproliferative disorders is worthwhile. Consultation with a specialist (specialist in internal medicine, haematologist) is necessary in unclear cases and when deciding the course of treatment.

15.10 Thrombocytopenia

Juhani Vilpo

Clinical approach

- Remember the possibility of so-called pseudothrombocytopenia.
- Stop drugs possibly causing thrombocytopenia unless vitally indicated.
- If the thrombocytopenic patient has symptoms of bleeding, immediate hospitalization is advisable.

Basic rules

- The pathophysiological mechanism of thrombocytopenia (blood platelet count $< 150 \times 10^9/l$, in late pregnancy $< 120 \times 10^9/l$) may be

- decreased production in the bone marrow
- increased peripheral consumption
- increased sequestration in the spleen.

♦ Artificially low platelet counts are occasionally obtained when counted from EDTA-anticoagulated blood (pseudothrombocytopenia). When thrombocytopenia ($<100 \times 10^9$/l) is detected in a patient for the first time, the same blood sample should be checked manually for the presence of thrombocyte aggregates.

♦ Thrombocytopenia is only a symptom, the cause of which should be clarified. Typical manifestations of thrombocytopenia are **skin bruising and petechiae and mucous membrane bleeding**. In particular, **gum and nasal bleeding** is common. Bleeding may also take place in the **gastrointestinal and urinary tracts**. **Menorrhagia** is also common.

♦ A tendency towards bleeding is uncommon if the platelet count is $50-100 \times 10^9$/l. Platelet concentrations of $10-50 \times 10^9$/l are frequently associated with spontaneous bleeding and haemorrhages are often severe with platelet counts of $<10 \times 10^9$/l.

Causes of thrombocytopenia

Decreased production

♦ Inborn causes
  - Pancytopenias and thrombocytopenias
  - Bone marrow infiltrates
  - Rubella
  - Maternal use of thiazide diuretics during pregnancy

♦ Acquired causes
  - Aplastic anaemia
  - Bone marrow infiltrates (carcinoma, leukaemia, myelofibrosis, myelodysplasia, tuberculosis)
  - Ionizing radiation, other causes of myelosuppression
  - Drugs (trimethoprim-sulfamethoxazole, gold, thiazide diuretics, alcohol, oestrogens, interferons)
  - Deficiency of vitamins and other essential trace elements or nutrients (B_{12}, folate, iron)
  - Viral infections (in Henoch–Schönlein purpura, the thrombocyte count is normal)
  - Uraemia
  - Heavy drinking
  - Pregnancy

Increased consumption

♦ Inborn causes
  - Non-immunological (haemolytic disease of the newborn, prematurity, maternal pre-eclampsia, renal vein thrombosis, infections)
  - Immunological (drug-induced, isoimmune neonatal thrombocytopenia, maternal idiopathic thrombocytopenia purpura (ITP))

♦ Acquired causes
  - Non-immunological (infections, disseminated intravascular coagulation, thrombotic thrombocytopenic purpura, haemolytic-uraemic syndrome, drug-induced overconsumption of platelets)
  - Immunological (drug-induced, in connection with anaphylaxis, following blood transfusion, chronic and acute ITP (32.2))

Platelet sequestration

♦ Hypersplenism and hypothermia

Loss of platelets

♦ Haemorrhage and haemoperfusion

HAE

Clinical approach

Symptomless patient, platelet count $100-150 \times 10^9$/l

♦ The general practitioner can safely follow the situation, initially at intervals of a few months. If no underlying disease becomes evident and thrombocytopenia remains stable, no further follow-up is required. All drugs causing thrombocytopenia should be avoided if possible.

♦ Many drugs cause thrombocytopenia relatively frequently C [1 2]. These include heparin, quinidine, chloroquine, gold, salicylates, sulphonamides, thiazides, allopurinol, phenytoin, carbamazepine and trimethoprim. NSAIDs (especially acetosalicylic acid) and some other medicines (clopidrogel) frequently impair platelet function and bring about a bleeding tendency. This tendency is disproportionately strong among thrombocytopenic patients. Paracetamol appears not to impair platelet function.

Symptomless patient, platelet count $< 100 \times 10^9$/l

♦ Thrombocytopenia-causing drugs should be stopped. Basic investigations are performed: haemoglobin, leucocyte count and differential, platelet count and bone marrow examination.

♦ If the situation does not improve, referral to a specialist in internal medicine or haematology is advisable.

♦ If there are no obvious reasons for thrombocytopenia, platelet antibody assessment should be carried out early.

♦ Sometimes it is necessary to measure platelet life-span with radioactively labelled platelets. This investigation gives information about the kinetic nature (poor platelet production or decreased survival) of thrombocytopenia.

♦ Pseudothrombocytopenia: thrombocytes are aggregated in an EDTA tube.

If a thrombocytopenia patient has symptoms of bleeding

♦ He/she needs specialist care

♦ It is important to detect the possible cause. Remember that the list of drugs possibly causing thrombocytopenia is very long. All these drugs should be avoided.

ITP

- Treatment is planned by a specialist in internal medicine, a paediatrician or haematologist.
- In adults, predniso(lo)ne continues to be the first-line therapy. The starting dose is 1–2 mg/kg/day. Response to treatment is often achieved in 1–4 weeks. At least a partial response is observed in 70–90% of cases, but a good one (i.e. platelet count > 100 × 10^9/l) in only 30–50% of the patients. After a maximal response is observed, the drug is slowly (over weeks) tapered to the smallest dose resulting in an acceptable clinical situation, say a platelet count > 50 × 10^9/l, with no symptoms of bleeding. Among paediatric haematologists the use of corticosteroids in ITP has been more controversial, because spontaneous remissions are very frequent (32.2).
- Intravenous gammaglobulin infusions may induce a response faster than corticosteroids. Non-responders are treated with immunosuppressants or splenectomy.
- Fibrinolysis inhibitors may be used to reduce excessive mucous membrane haemorrhages, such as nasal, gastrointestinal and urinary tract bleeding and menorrhagia. Platelet transfusions are effective if no platelet antibodies are present. Massive bleeding is compensated with red cells, fresh-frozen plasma and platelet concentrates.

References

1. George JN, Raskob GE, Rizvi Shah S, Rizvi MA, Hamilton SA, Osborne S, Vondracek T. Drug-induced thrombocytopenia: a systematic review of published case reports. Annals of Internal Medicine 1998;129:886–890.
2. The Database of Abstracts of Reviews of Effectiveness (University of York), Database no.: DARE-989740. In: The Cochrane Library, Issue 3, 2000. Oxford: Update Software.

15.20 Assessment of anaemia in adults

Juhani Vilpo

Principles

- The physician should answer three questions:
  - What is the type of anaemia (according to automated MCV determination)?
    - microcytic (MCV < 80 fl)
    - normocytic (MCV 80–100 fl)
    - macrocytic (MCV > 100 fl)
  - What is the mechanism (decreased production or increased destruction of red cells)?
  - What is the diagnosis: the pathophysiology and underlying cause of the anaemia?

Basic rules

- The WHO criteria for anaemia are as follows:
  - children; blood haemoglobin <110 g/l
  - women; blood haemoglobin <120 g/l, during pregnancy <110 g/l
  - men; blood haemoglobin <130 g/l
  - However, even lower haemoglobin levels may be normal. For instance, a 2.5–97.5% reference interval of 117–155 g/l for women was recently confirmed in Finland.
- The prevalence of anaemia ranges from 0.7 to 6.9%. It is more common in women and often a "side diagnosis". Haemoglobin determination is often a routine examination.
- In many patient series, iron deficiency is found to be the most common mechanism of anaemia (about 50% of patients in ambulatory care).
- **Anaemia is not a final diagnosis, but a symptom. The reason for this symptom, i.e. the underlying cause, must be determined.**
- The lowering of a patient's haemoglobin value by more than 20 g/l from his/her normal level can similarly be regarded as a symptom, even if the haemoglobin value is still within reference range.

Mechanisms of anaemia

- Anaemia may result from increased destruction of red cells (haemorrhage or haemolysis), poor production of red cells in the bone marrow or both.

Diagnostic assessment

- When blood haemoglobin is determined, the MCV is usually also measured.
- If haemoglobin is determined because of suspected anaemia, it is advisable to determine **ESR, leucocytes, MCV and reticulocyte count** at the same time.

Classification according to MCV count

- **Microcytic anaemias** (MCV < 80 fl)
  - iron deficiency
  - secondary anaemias (in a minority of cases)
  - thalassaemias.
- **Normocytic anaemias** (MCV 80–100 fl)
  - secondary anaemias (most cases)
  - haemolytic anaemia (most cases)
  - acute haemorrhage
  - aplastic anaemia or bone marrow infiltration.
- **Macrocytic anaemias** (MCV > 100 fl)
  - vitamin B_{12} deficiency
  - folate deficiency

- blood loss (> 2 days previously through haemolysis or bleeding; marked reticulocytosis)
- liver disease
- heavy alcohol consumption
- others (myelodysplasia, haematologic malignancy, hypothyroidism)
- macrocytosis without anaemia, see 15.8.

Diagnosis

- If the anaemia is microcytic, no underlying disease can be found and ESR is not elevated, iron deficiency anaemia (15.21) is most probable. The prevalence of thalassaemia syndromes must however be taken into account.
- **Reticulocytosis** is a strong indicator of bleeding or haemolysis (15.25) and **reticulocytopenia** indicates impaired erythrocyte production.
- **Macrocytosis** associated with anaemia is mostly caused by megaloblastic anaemia (15.24).
- **Normocytic anaemia** is usually associated with a chronic disease, i.e. secondary by nature (15.23).
- **Bone marrow examination** is an essential part of the assessment of anaemia, and it should be performed in most unclear cases where iron deficiency is not the probable cause (15.21).
- Determination of serum soluble transferrin receptor (TfR) level is useful in the diagnosis of iron deficiency anaemia (in iron deficiency the concentration is above 2.3 mg/l).

15.21 Iron deficiency anaemia

Juhani Vilpo

Aims

- Exclusion of secondary anaemias
- Demonstration of the likely mechanism of iron deficiency before treatment.

Basic rules

- The majority of cases of microcytic anaemia (MCV <80 fl) are caused by iron deficiency. However, ca. 10% of these have secondary anaemia, and on the other hand, ca. 30% of cases of iron deficiency anaemia have MCV > 80 fl (depending on the patient population).
- If the patient has microcytic anaemia (MCV <80 fl) and secondary anaemia appears to be excluded, iron deficiency anaemia is likely. Secondary anaemias are unlikely if there is no relevant chronic disease and past history, clinical status, erythrocyte sedimentation rate, CRP or leucocytosis do not indicate the presence of an underlying disease. If the cause of iron deficiency is certain or evident, the situation is sufficiently well characterised and iron therapy may be initiated. Among some ethnic groups and especially in known families thalassaemias may be the primary causes of microcytic anaemia.
- If the situation is not clear enough, the category of anaemia is ascertained with certain laboratory investigations. The cause of iron deficiency should be uncovered.
- Sometimes it is impossible in practice to demonstrate the cause of iron deficiency. In such cases adequate iron therapy is initiated and a good response and its permanence are ascertained.
- Starting iron therapy as a trial with a diagnostic goal may also be a good option.

Causes

- Chronic haemorrhage
- Defective nutrition
- Malabsorption (most commonly caused by coeliac disease)

Diagnostics

- Iron deficiency without any other apparent causes (growth spurt, pregnancy, gynaecological haemorrhage, intestinal haemorrhage) is detected with serum ferritin: S/P-Ferritin <30 μg/l is a sign of iron deficiency.
- Iron deficiency in association with a chronic disease is determined with a serum soluble transferrin receptor assay (TfR). TfR > 2.3 mg/l is a strong indicator of iron deficiency. The assay is not reliable in all situations, e.g. pregnancy, acute haemorrhage, haemolysis, sickle cell anaemia, thalassaemia and polycythaemia. In these cases determine serum ferritin, transferrin iron saturation percentage (based on iron and transferrin values; fP-TS <15% indicates iron deficiency) or both.
- With the development of biochemical assays, bone marrow examination has lost its role as a central investigation. In unclear cases and when suspecting an actual haematological disease, bone marrow examination is still indicated.

Determining the cause of iron deficiency

- Iron deficiency anaemia is only a symptom. The underlying pathogenic mechanisms must be uncovered.
- In fertile women the most likely cause is **excessive menstrual bleeding**. If the history of menstrual bleeding does not indicate excessive blood loss, gastrointestinal haemorrhage should be sought by means of two or three successive faecal blood tests (see below).
- **Haemorrhages**, especially gastrointestinal ones (gastric ulcer, intestinal tumours, also haemorrhoids) are common (8.52). **If menstrual bleeding does not explain the iron deficiency, gastrointestinal causes must be carefully checked.** The patient's age and past history together with current symptoms determine the order of investigations.

- Blood in the faeces has previously been determined with faecal human haemoglobin tests (e.g. Hemolex®) and guaiac-based tests (e.g. Fecatwin Sensitive®). These are now being replaced by a single test (e.g. Actim®) which detects human haemoglobin in the faeces.
- It is advisable to investigate the colon in all patients over 50 years of age (sigmoidoscopy (8.22), colonoscopy or double-contrast barium enema). Gastroscopy is the first examination if the patient has (had) melena (8.52) or there are symptoms compatible with a gastric ulcer. A faecal blood test is not a prerequisite for gastrointestinal investigations, because a negative result does not exclude a gastrointestinal tumour as a cause of iron deficiency anaemia.
- With younger patients the examinations begin with gastroscopy, especially if there are gastric symptoms. If the symptoms point to a disease at the distal end of the gastrointestinal tract or if gastroscopy does not explain the anaemia, the colon should be examined (at least by sigmoidoscopy).

♦ **Nutritional causes** and **malabsorption** are rarer causes.

- Coeliac disease (8.84) is diagnosed in gastroscopy.

Treatment

♦ It is most important to prevent excess iron (blood) losses and to guarantee the sufficient iron content of the diet.

♦ Iron substitution is usually given orally. Daily amounts of 100–200 mg, given in 2–4 doses are sufficient.

- In moderate to severe iron deficiency anaemia there is a reticulocyte response usually seen 5–10 days after starting therapy.
- Normalization of haemoglobin and MCV values is expected in 2–4 months.

♦ **Iron substitution should be maintained for 2–3 months after full response in order to fill body iron stores.**

♦ Patients who do not respond normally to iron therapy should be referred to a specialist.

15.22 Anaemia of pregnancy

Juhani Vilpo

Aims

♦ To make a distinction between physiological haemodilution and true anaemia.

Basic rules

♦ Normal decrease of blood haemoglobin to level ≥110 g/l (first trimester) or ≥100 g/l (later on in the pregnancy): no interventions necessary.

♦ Haemoglobin decreasing to level <95–100 g/l and MCV < 84 fl: iron deficiency likely, begin iron therapy as a trial.

♦ Continuously declining haemoglobin (Hb < 100 g/l) or Hb 90–95 g/l: further investigations necessary.

Starting points

♦ The WHO criterion for anaemia of pregnancy is a haemoglobin level < 110 g/l.

♦ Physiological haemodilution begins at weeks 8–12 of pregnancy and usually increases towards the end of pregnancy: haemoglobin levels < 110 g/l are observed in 10–20% of women with normal pregnancy. The physiological explanation is that the relative increase of plasma volume (up to 50%) is larger than that of the red cell mass (up to 25%).

Causes of anaemia

♦ In addition to the physiological decrease of haemoglobin values, **iron deficiency** is common in pregnancy. During the second trimester increased amounts of iron are required to expand the mother's red cell mass and during the last trimester for the growing foetus. The role of routine iron therapy is unclear. Prophylaxis after week 20 of pregnancy is recommended at least in some Nordic countries (60–100 mg/day).

♦ The need for **folate** is also increased during pregnancy and folate deficiency is a possible cause of anaemia. Some specialists recommend folate substitution (0.3–0.4 mg/day) during pregnancy (A) [1].

♦ Other causes are less common.

Diagnosis

♦ Iron therapy as a trial (at least for 4–6 weeks), if blood haemoglobin < 95 g/l and mean cell volume (MCV) < 84 fl: 60–100 mg/day. The target Hb level is 100–120 g/l.

♦ Normocytic anaemia (no primary disease), if blood haemoglobin < 95–100 g/l: ESR, CRP, haemoglobin, MCV, reticulocytes and ferritin. In inflammatory conditions the ferritin level may be unreliable. The level of soluble transferrin receptor may be useful (a normal value indicates secondary anaemia), but pregnancy in itself may increase the value.

♦ Macrocytic anaemia (MCV > 100 fl): fE-folate and serum vitamin B_{12}.

♦ Unclear cases: also bone marrow examination.

Reference

1. Mahomed K. Folate supplementation in pregnancy. Cochrane Database Syst Rev. 2004;(2):CD000183.

15.23 Secondary anaemia

Juhani Vilpo

Aims

- To exclude "specific" anaemias (iron deficiency, vitamin deficiency, haemolysis, acute haemorrhage, myelodysplastic syndrome and malignant haematological diseases). This can be done with basic investigations of anaemia (15.20).
- Assess whether the severity of the anaemia can be explained by the severity of the primary disease.
- Avoid unnecessary iron therapy in secondary anaemia, but aim at finding those patients who would benefit from iron, i.e. who have combined anaemia.

Basic rules

- A heterogeneous group. Most often these are divided into (a) anaemia associated with a chronic disease and (b) anaemias associated with certain "organ-diseases" (chronic renal and hepatic diseases and certain endocrinopathies). This division is primarily clinical, because for the time being, the aetiopathogenesis is in most cases unclear.
- Pathogenesis: inhibition of erythropoiesis by cytokines and other mediators of inflammation. Usually appears 1–2 months after onset of the primary disease.
- Common in some patient groups (e.g. in severe rheumatoid arthritis and renal insufficiency (10.21)).
- Is not caused by a deficiency of vitamins or mineral elements.
- Differentiation from other anaemias may be difficult.

Underlying diseases

- Anaemia associated with a chronic disease
  - Chronic infections
  - Other chronic inflammatory diseases (autoimmune disease, severe traumas and burns)
  - Malignomas (without infiltrates to bone marrow)
  - Others (alcoholic liver disease, congestive heart failure, thromboflebitis, ischaemic heart disease, idiopathic)
- "Organ-specific" causes
  - Chronic renal failure (10.21)
  - Cirrhosis and other liver diseases
  - Endocrinopathies (hypothyroidism, hyperthyroidism, adrenal failure, androgen deficiency, hypopituitarism, hyperparathyroidism, anorexia nervosa)

Diagnostic assessment

- Ascertain the underlying disease. Include erythrocyte sedimentation rate, CRP and blood white cell count determinations in the routine laboratory examination of anaemia (the others are: haemoglobin, MCV and reticulocyte count).
- Consider whether the underlying disease can explain the degree of anaemia. In moderate and mild diseases the haemoglobin concentration is usually 100–110 g/l and in more severe diseases it may be 80–90 g/l or even lower.
- If the haemoglobin level is disproportionately low, search for specific causes of anaemia.
- Exclude increased red cell loss (bleeding or haemolysis, reticulocyte count increased).
- Exclude iron deficiency (P-TfR > 2.3 mg/l) and megaloblastic anaemia (MCV > 100 fl).
- Bone marrow examination is useful in all obscure cases.
- An iron therapy trial is a practical approach if iron deficiency is combined with the secondary anaemia. Iron stores are restored in 2–3 months and the true level of secondary anaemia is revealed.
- Serum transferrin-receptor/ferritin ratio is a very promising parameter to reveal "functional" iron deficiency.

HAE

Treatment

- Treat the underlying disease.
- Certain groups of renal or cancer patients are treated with recombinant human erythropoietin (always consult a specialist). The use of erythropoietin is spreading to other secondary anaemias.
- Red cell transfusions are restricted to patients who absolutely require them.
- It is important to explain the nature of secondary anaemia to the patient.

15.24 Megaloblastic anaemia

Juhani Vilpo

Aims

- Detect megaloblastic anaemia on the basis of increased MCV in the blood count.
- In many countries (e.g. Nordic ones), pernicious anaemia is the leading cause of megaloblastic anaemia. In some populations folate deficiency may be more prevalent.
- Pernicious anaemia is characterised by:
  - vitamin B_{12} deficiency
  - atrophic gastritis
  - a good response to vitamin B_{12} therapy.
- Distinguish from pernicious anaemia other conditions that require some other type of treatment.

Symptoms

- In milder cases the symptoms are related to the severity of anaemia.
- In more advanced cases of pernicious anaemia there is also:
  - weight loss
  - glossitis
  - mild icterus
  - neurological symptoms associated with vitamin B_{12} deficiency (paraesthesiae, muscle weakness, and psychological symptoms such as dementia and impaired memory).

Causes of megaloblastic anaemia

Vitamin B_{12} deficiency

- The aetiology in about 90% of the cases.
- Often caused by a gastric disease, i.e. an intrinsic factor deficiency + atrophic gastritis (pernicious anaemia), gastrectomy, rarely gastric cancer.
- Rarely a disease of the terminal ileum (Crohn's disease, resection, inborn vitamin B_{12} malabsorption).
- Diphyllobothrium latum infection and other parasites.
- Dietary deficiency.

Folate deficiency

- Dietary deficiency (frequent in alcoholics)
- Increased requirements (pregnancy, prematurity, haemolysis, cancer).
- Malabsorption (coeliac disease).
- Increased loss (some skin and liver diseases, dialysis).

Drugs

- Folic acid antagonists: methotrexate, trimethoprim
- Purine analogues (antineoplastic and antiviral drugs and immunosuppressives): acyclovir, azathioprine, mercaptopurine, thioguanine
- Pyrimidine analogues (antineoplastic and antiretroviral drugs): azacytidine, fluorouracil, cytarabine, stavudine, zidovudine
- Ribonucleotide reductase inhibitors (antineoplastic drugs): hydroxyurea
- Antiepileptics: phenytoin, phenobarbital, primidone
- Other drugs that interfere with folate metabolism: oral contraceptives, glutethimide, cycloserine
- Drugs that interfere with vitamin B_{12} metabolism: para-aminosalicylic acid, metformin, phenformin, colchicine, neomycin
- Others: isoniazid, mefenamic acid, nitrofurantoin, pentamidine, phenacetin, pyrimethamine, triamterene

Diagnostic assessment

- Can mostly be performed in primary care.
  - Past history concerning nutrition and the gastrointestinal tract is important.
  - Investigate serum vitamin B_{12} level and fasting serum and red cell folate. Bone marrow examination may be helpful but is not absolutely necessary in this phase.
  - In hypovitaminosis, investigate the cause. If vitamin B_{12} and folate levels are normal, perform bone marrow examination.

Additional investigations

- **Vitamin B_{12} deficiency alone** (vitamin B_{12} < 170 pmol/l, fasting serum folate > 4.5 nmol/l, erythrocyte folate may be at the low reference range). Note, these reference ranges have been determined for the author's laboratory! Use pertinent reference intervals.
  - If there are no other obvious reasons for vitamin B_{12} deficiency, perform gastroscopy and biopsies to reveal atrophic gastritis.
  - Faecal parasites should be investigated twice.
  - If the pathogenesis of vitamin B_{12} deficiency remains obscure, refer to a specialist for malabsorption studies. These include
    - vitamin B_{12} absorption test (Schilling I without intrinsic factor and Schilling II with intrinsic factor. These give indirect information about the function of the stomach and terminal ileum)
    - serum pepsinogen I (low in atrophic gastritis)
    - serum gastrin (high in atrophic gastritis)
    - endoscopies with biopsies.
- **Folate deficiency alone** (serum vitamin B_{12} level > 170 pmol/l, fasting serum folate < 4.5 nmol/l and erythrocyte folate < 280 nmol/l. Use your own reference ranges!).
  - If diet has been folate-deficient, give nutritional counselling. Tablet substitution is advisable at the beginning.
  - If diet has been adequate, refer to a specialist (in internal medicine; gastroenterologist).
- **All values normal (serum vitamin B_{12}, fasting serum folate and erythrocyte folate concentration)**
  - Check drug use and, if possible, drop drugs known to cause megaloblastic anaemia. Check haemoglobin and MCV values after 1–2 months.
- **Combined deficiency of folate and vitamin B_{12}**
  - Follow instructions given above. These are assessed separately.

Treatment

- In megaloblastic anaemia the patients are well adapted to very low haemoglobin values (even 40–60 g/l). **Avoid red cell or blood transfusions.** If vitally required for oxygenation, transfuse slowly in order to minimize the possibility of overloading or inducing a hyperkinetic state (for example, one unit per 2–4 hours). Samples for vitamin determinations should be taken before transfusion.
- **Vitamin B_{12} substitution** in pernicious anaemia is started with intramuscular injections of 1 mg hydroxycobalamin at

1–2-day intervals for 1–2 weeks. Thereafter the dosing is 1 mg (at least 100 µg) per month, but 1 mg every 3 months is also sufficient. Either hydroxy- or cyanocobalamin may be used.

- **In neuropathy** the initial treatment is more intensive: 1 mg hydroxycobalamin is given intramuscularly every other week up to 6 months. **Folate substitution is contraindicated** (improves the blood picture, but may make neuropathies worse).
- Ascertain the efficacy of the remedy. A significant increase in reticulocyte count should be observable 5–7 days after initiation of therapy. A good response predicts a favourable outcome. MCV and haemoglobin concentration are checked after 1 and 4 months. Thereafter, routine blood controls in pernicious anaemia are not necessary.
- If vitamin B_{12} therapy does not correct the haemoglobin concentration, the reason may be simultaneous iron deficiency (MCV becomes smaller but the anaemia persists). Determine the ferritin and transferrin receptor concentrations. Start iron therapy when required.
- If still unresponsive, refer the patient to a specialist in internal medicine or to a haematologist.

♦ Oral therapy (2 mg/day) appears to be as efficient as parenteral therapy (B) [1 2].

♦ **Folate deficiency** is mostly caused by a deficient diet. Nutritional counselling is given. Oral substitution is mostly sufficient (1 mg/day), even in malabsorption, when the doses are higher (5–10 mg/day).

References

1. Kuzminski A, Del Giacco E, Allen R, Stabler S, Lindenbaum J. Effective treatment of cobalamin deficiency with oral cobalamin. Blood 1998;92:1191–8.
2. Elia M.Oral or parenteral therapy for B12 deficiency. Lancet 1998;352:1721–2.

15.25 Haemolytic anaemia

Juhani Vilpo

Aims

♦ Remember blood reticulocyte count as an indicator of haemolysis.

♦ Comprises of ca. 200 subtypes. The aetiopathogenesis should nevertheless be determined.

Epidemiology

♦ Haemolytic anaemias are rare in Nordic countries (less than 5% of anaemias) but common, for example in the Mediterranean area. In the Nordic countries, the most prevalent is autoimmune haemolytic anaemia: approximately one new case per year per 75 000 persons.

Basic rules

♦ In haemolysis the life span of red cells is shortened from the norm of 120 days to as short as a few minutes.

♦ Red cells are destroyed either extravascularly (in the reticuloendothelial system, particularly in the spleen), intravascularly (in the blood stream) or already as precursors in the bone marrow.

♦ The consequences of haemolysis are:

- compensatory enhancement of bone marrow erythropoiesis resulting in blood reticulocytosis
- increase of haemoglobin catabolic products
- increased plasma free haemoglobin concentration in intravascular haemolysis, and sometimes even haemoglobinuria and haemosiderinuria.

Causes of haemolytic anaemia

♦ Increased destruction of red cells may be caused by:

- damage or defects in red cells themselves (hereditary haemolytic anaemias and paroxysmal nocturnal haemoglobinuria or PNH)
- external causes (acquired haemolytic conditions)

♦ Specific haemolytic anaemias are listed in Table 15.25.

Diagnostic assessment

♦ The goals are

- to ascertain the presence of haemolysis
- to uncover the specific diagnosis, i.e. the aetiopathogenesis of the haemolytic conditions

♦ Haemolysis is seen as reticulocytosis in basic anaemia laboratory tests (haemoglobin, haematocrit, CRP, MCV, reticulocyte count, ESR and leucocyte count). Marked haemolysis also increases the MCV value. A normal reticulocyte count practically excludes the possibility of significant haemolysis.

♦ In unclear cases study also:

- Lactate dehydrogenase
  - Sensitive but non-specific indicator of haemolysis
- Haptoglobin
  - Is decreased in haemolysis but also in liver diseases. It is increased in inflammatory states and this may mask the decrease caused by haemolysis.
- Bilirubin
  - The concentration of conjugated bilirubin increases in haemolysis.

Table 15.25 Causes of haemolytic anaemias

Pathological red cells	External causes
Membrane defects	**Immunohaemolytic anaemias**
♦ Hereditary spherocytosis ♦ Hereditary elliptocytosis	♦ Autoimmune haemolytic anaemia ♦ Cold haemagglutination ♦ Transfusion reaction ♦ Mother-child immunization ♦ Drug-induced haemolysis
Enzymopathies **Haemoglobinopathies** **Thalassaemias** **PNH**	**Fragmentation haemolysis** ♦ Artificial surfaces (prosthetic valves, other prostheses, haemoperfusion) ♦ Vasculitis ♦ March haemoglobinuria ♦ DIC (disseminated intravascular coagulation) ♦ TTP (thrombotic thrombocytopenic purpura) ♦ HUS (haemolytic uraemic syndrome)
	Other external causes ♦ Infections, toxins, burns, hypersplenism

- A specific diagnosis is approached early on. Family history is crucial in hereditary forms of haemolytic anaemia. There are also other informative laboratory investigations useful for a general practitioner.
  - A direct antiglobulin test (Coombs' test; a positive test result points to autoimmune haemolytic anaemia or AIHA)
  - Blood smear and, if necessary, bone marrow examination
  - Urine haemosiderin examination (positive in intravascular haemolysis when the kidney threshold has been exceeded).
- More specific investigations are available in specialised clinics. However, the general practitioner can fairly easily exclude the possibility of significant haemolysis as a cause of anaemia. **Reticulocyte count determination is always a basic investigation of anaemia.**

Treatment

- Treatment depends on the specific condition and is mostly carried out in collaboration with a specialist in internal medicine or a haematologist.
- Remember drugs as a possible cause or an enhancer of haemolysis.

15.30 Easy bruising, petechiae and ecchymoses

Juhani Vilpo

Aims

- Conclude from the clinical picture and history whether a patient has a normal or an increased tendency to bruise or have petechiae.
- Purpura is most commonly caused by a tendency to bleed or by vasculitis. Make a distinction between these two.
- Remember the possibility of physical abuse as a cause of "spontaneous" bruising, especially in children.

Terminology

- **Purpura** is a group of disorders characterized by intradermal or submucosal haemorrhages that are purplish or brownish red in colour. Haematomas are petechiae or ecchymoses.
- **Petechiae** are well-defined small (1–3 mm), intradermal or submucous spots caused by haemorrhage. They are not elevated from the skin. They do not disappear when pressed, for example, with a glass. Note the difference to haemangiomas and telangiectases.
- An **ecchymosis** is a small haemorrhagic spot, larger than a petechia, in the skin or mucous membrane, forming a non-elevated, rounded or irregular, blue or purplish patch.

Basic rules

- Everybody has occasional bruising after minor trauma or even without a noticed trauma at all. There is large inter-individual variation in sensitivity. Solitary bruises, even without a noticed trauma, are usually harmless and do not necessarily require further laboratory investigations.
- Petechiae are most common at sites where venous pressure is highest, for example, in the legs as well as distally in association with tight socks or bandages. Heat, e.g. a sauna, may increase capillary leakage and induce petechiae.

The following are typical of "non-pathological" bruising and do not require additional investigation

- A bruise is formed at the site of trauma.
- A single bruise (<3 cm) anywhere on the body. No other symptoms. Unnoticed bruises are common, especially on the limbs.
- Elderly people may have bruises on the arms and on the back of their hands. These are caused by excessive movement of the skin resulting in capillary breaks.

Petechiae do not require additional investigation if

- The patient has cardiac or vein insufficiency and petechiae are located in the legs and deteriorate during oedema (walk, hot weather, sauna).

Petechiae and bruises require additional investigation if

- The patient also has other symptoms of unknown origin, such as fever, tiredness etc.
- They are formed spontaneously in various sites of the body, even if the patient has no other symptoms.
- In these cases it should be clarified whether or not the patient has purpura.

Causes of purpura

- Purpura is common in diseases affecting blood vessels and platelets (thrombocytopenia or -pathy), but is uncommon in coagulopathies.

Autoimmune diseases

- Allergic purpuras
  - Henoch–Schönlein purpura is frequently associated with arthralgia and gastrointestinal symptoms (32.53).
  - Other similar purpuras.
- Idiopathic thrombocytopenic purpura or ITP (15.10), (32.2)
- Drug-induced vascular purpuras (iodides, atropine, quinine, procaine penicillin, aminophenazone, aspirin, chloral hydrate, other sedatives, sulphonamides, coumarin derivatives)
- Purpura fulminans

Infections

- Bacterial (meningococcaemia and other septicaemias, typhoid fever, scarlet fever, diphtheria, tuberculosis, endocarditis)
- Viral (influenza, measles, others)
- Rickettsial
- Parasitic (malaria, toxoplasmosis)

Structural malformations

- Hereditary haemorrhagic telangiectasia or Osler's disease
- Hereditary connective tissue diseases (Ehlers–Danlos disease, osteogenesis imperfecta, pseudoxanthoma elasticum)
- Acquired connective tissue diseases (scurvy, corticosteroid-induced purpura, Cushing's disease, senile purpura, purpura associated with cachexia)

Miscellaneous

- Autoerythrocyte sensitization and related syndromes
- Paraproteinaemias
- Purpura simplex and related disorders (orthostatic and mechanical purpura, factitious purpura)
- Purpura associated with skin diseases
- Others (blood-borne tumour emboli, Kaposi's sarcoma, snake bites, haemochromatosis, amyloidosis)

Clinical pictures of various forms of purpura

Allergic purpura

- Appearance
  - Variable
  - Small bruises, urticaria, bullae, sometimes small ulcers.
- Sites
  - Symmetrical, proximal in limbs, legs and buttocks.
- Other findings
  - Itching, also joint and abdominal symptoms, no general tendency to bleed.

Purpura fulminans

- Appearance
  - Large, symmetrical bruises. Skin infarctions with sharp borders. Petechiae unusual.
- Sites
  - Often symmetrical, in distal parts of the limbs and in the genitals.
- Other findings
  - Distal gangrene in the limbs (fingers and toes). Fever, tiredness, general tendency to bleed and coagulopathy.

Scurvy

- Appearance
  - Petechiae common around hair follicles. Bruises, large subcutaneous haematomas.
- Sites
  - Often symmetrical. Like a saddle in the thighs and buttocks.
- Other findings
  - Tiredness, pains in the limbs, periosteal haemorrhages in children, general tendency to bleed.

Autosensitization to red cells

- Appearance
  - Solitary, often large dark red bruises on a reddish and swollen base.
- Sites
  - In limbs, proximally, in thighs, lower legs and abdomen. Occasionally on the back.
- Other findings
  - Prodromal symptoms, lesions often painful

- Nausea, vomiting, and general symptoms
- Hysteric and neurotic symptoms
- Menorrhagia, haematuria, nasal bleeding
- Skin test positive.

Thrombocytopenic purpura

- Appearance
  - Purple/red and dark petechiae
  - Superficial bruises of variable size and form.
- Sites
  - Everywhere. Preferentially at sites of venous compression and high venous pressure.
- Other findings
  - Generalised tendency to bleed in mucous membranes.

Clinical approach

- If it is likely or evident that there is increased susceptibility as regards bruises and petechiae, the approach can be as follows.
- Children. It should be considered whether the clinical picture is compatible with
  - Henoch–Schönlein purpura (32.53)
  - Idiopathic thrombocytopenic purpura (ITP) (32.2)
  - Infection which is commonly associated with purpura; remember the possibility of meningococcaemia if the patient is in poor condition and feverish.
  - Physical abuse
  - For orientation, some laboratory investigations are helpful
    - Haemoglobin, white cell count and platelet count
    - Urinalysis (microscopic haematuria?)
    - C-reactive protein (bacterial infection?).
- Adults. Firstly, the use of non-steroidal anti-inflammatory analgesics (NSAIDs) and oral anticoagulants should be investigated.
  - If an otherwise symptomless patient has used NSAIDs, easy bruising is probably a result of these drugs. The medication should be stopped or replaced with paracetamol or a cyclooxygenase-2 inhibitor and the clinical situation checked after one month. If purpura is still present, further investigations are indicated. If purpura is massive or sudden, it is advisable to initiate the above-mentioned laboratory investigations, even if the patient is using NSAIDs.
  - If the patient is using oral anticoagulants and has bruising but is otherwise symptomless, then INR measurement helps in orientation. If the value is within the therapeutic range, the possible role of oral anticoagulants in bruising is explained to the patient. The patient is counselled to contact the physician if the bruising tendency increases or if general symptoms appear. The clinician has to judge whether the patient requires immediate laboratory investigations or hospitalization. Despite a "therapeutic" prothrombin time, this is always the situation if a severe defect in haemostasis is imminent.
- The medication is checked in order to reveal drugs possibly causing thrombocytopenia or platelet dysfunction. Drugs used during the last month before purpura are of the most interest. The antihaemostatic effect of NSAIDs lasts about one week.
- Infections as a cause of purpura must be checked (remember the possibility of a septic infection if the patient is in poor condition or feverish).
- If there are no simple explanations for purpura, such as drugs or an infection, the next question to be answered is: does the patient have an increased tendency to bleed (most likely one affecting platelet function, usually thrombocytopenia), or does purpura have a vascular aetiology (allergic, skin disease)?
  - The primary laboratory investigations are the same as for children (see above). The cause of thrombocytopenia (platelet count $< 100 \times 10^9$/l) should be clarified (see thrombocytopenia, 15.10 and ITP, 15.10 and 32.2. It should be remembered that purpura is seldom associated with moderate thrombocytopenia (platelet count 50–100 $\times 10^9$/l) unless there are other aggravating factors.
  - If thrombocytopenia is excluded (platelet count $> 100 \times 10^9$/l) as a cause of purpura, platelet function is assessed, preferably with a PFA device or alternatively as bleeding time. Normal bleeding time indicates a vascular aetiology rather than platelet dysfunction. If Henoch–Schönlein purpura is unlikely, the accurate diagnosis of vascular diseases often requires skin biopsy and immunohistochemistry (skin biopsy, see 13.6).
  - If platelet function is impaired, the patient should be referred to specialist care (unless the condition can be explained by e.g. medication).

15.31 Assessment and treatment of a patient with bleeding diathesis

Editors

Basic rules

- Consider the possibility of a clotting disorder if the patient has
  - exceptionally profuse bleeding after surgical procedures or trauma
  - spontaneous purpura, large ecchymoses, haematomas, haemarthrosis, or menorrhagia. For example, continuous bleeding overnight after dental extraction is abnormal.
- Identify the cause of bleeding as soon as possible and arrange further treatment
  - Disseminated intravascular coagulation

- Acute leukaemia
- Overdose of warfarin (can be treated in primary care if the bleeding is controlled)

Causes of bleeding diathesis

- Hereditary bleeding disorders
  - Haemophilia A (deficiency of factor VIII)
  - Haemophilia B (deficiency of factor IX)
  - von Willebrand's disease
- Acquired bleeding disorders associated with an underlying disease
  - Liver disease: decrease of plasma concentrations of the "hepatic factors" (prothrombin, F VII, F IX, F X)
  - Renal disease, uraemia: platelet dysfunction, thrombocytopenia, disorders of clotting and fibrinolysis
  - Bleeding disorder associated with an infection
  - Haematological disease: leukaemia, thrombocytopenia, polycythaemia
  - Disseminated intravascular coagulation
  - Malignancies
  - Autoimmune diseases
  - Vascular bleeding disorders: Osler's disease (hereditary haemorrhagic telangiectasia)
- Bleeding disorders associated with drugs
  - Therapeutic action: warfarin, heparin
  - Adverse effect: aspirin, NSAIDs, drugs causing thrombocytopenia (15.10)
- Examples of bleeding disorders that may result from a bleeding diathesis but that in most cases have a local origin
  - Epistaxis
  - Menorrhagia
  - Gastrointestinal bleeding
  - Suggillation (37.21)

Diagnosis

- Look for signs of bleeding on the skin and mucous membranes.
- Inspect the appearance and range of movement of the joints.
- Jaundice, enlarged lymph nodes, tenderness on bones, or enlarged liver or spleen may indicate an underlying disease causing the tendency to bleed.
- **Typical symptoms of bleeding diathesis caused by vascular disorders, thrombocytopenia or platelet dysfunction include**
  - bleeding in the skin (petecchiae, purpura, bruising)
  - mucous membrane bleeding (gingival bleeding, epistaxis, menorrhagia).
  - The bleeding starts immediately after trauma, can be stopped by compression and does not recur after having stopped once.
- **Typical signs of a clotting disorder include**
  - deep haematomas
  - bleeding into joints
  - haematuria
  - retroperitoneal bleeding.
- Traumatic bleeding often has a delayed start, and stops normally but recurs after 2–3 days. Bleeding from a wound cannot be permanently stopped by compression.

Investigations

- If a generalized bleeding diathesis is suspected, discontinue all aspirin preparations and perform the following tests:
  - Platelet count
  - Bleeding time, using a sensitive method (not Duke's method)
  - Thromboplastin time
    - measures the extrinsic clotting factors (factors VII and X and prothrombin)
    - Note that the accurate measuring range of tests used in the monitoring of anticoagulant treatment (e.g. Thrombotest® (TT-TT)) is in the "therapeutic" range. If clotting factor levels near the normal range are assessed, other tests (such as TT-SPA or TT-NT) should be carried out.
  - Activated partial thromboplastin time (APTT)
    - A general measure of the function of the intrinsic clotting mechanism (fibrinogen, prothrombin, factors VI, VIII, IX, X, XI and XII); does not measure factors VII and XIII.
    - Can be determined from a sample that has been cooled to +4°C for transportation if the patient's situation allows the delay.
- If the patient has thrombocytopenia, prolonged bleeding time or abnormal thromboplastin time, he/she can be referred for further investigations without the determination of APTT.

Further investigations

- See 15.10 for **isolated thrombocytopenia.**
- If the platelet count, APTT and thromboplastin time are normal but the **bleeding time** is prolonged, suspect von Willebrand's disease or platelet dysfunction. Further investigations should include assessment of factor VIII and platelet function.
- If the platelet count and bleeding time are normal the cause of the bleeding diathesis is probably deficiency of clotting factors.
  - **Normal APTT and thromboplastin time**: the patient probably does not have a severe clotting disorder. Normal results do not rule out a mild clotting factor deficiency or deficiency of factor XIII. Further investigations are indicated if bleeding diathesis is evident. If the diathesis is mild, follow-up without further investigations is sufficient.
  - **Prolonged APTT, normal thromboplastin time**: the patient has haemophilia A or B, deficiency of factor XII (which is not associated with a bleeding diathesis) or a

HAE

severe form of von Willebrand's disease. For hereditary thrombophilias see 15.32.

- **Normal APTT, decreased thromboplastin time**: the patient has a disorder of the extrinsic clotting mechanism (prothrombin, factor VII or X). Prolonged thromboplastin time (high INR) is common in liver diseases and deficiency of vitamin K (and naturally in patients on warfarin therapy).
- **Prolonged APTT, decreased thromboplastin time**: multiple defects, circulating anticoagulants or a disorder at the end of the clotting pathway (factors X, V, prothrombin, fibrinogen).

Treatment

- Profuse bleeding that cannot be controlled is always an indication for immediate referral to a hospital. Intravenous fluids, monitoring of the blood pressure, and preparations for transfusion are essential as first aid.
- Immediate referral is also indicated if leukaemia, a severe infection or DIC is suspected.
- In bleeding associated with liver or renal disease investigations and treatment can be performed locally if sufficient resources are available.
  - If the patient has a decreased thromboplastin time and mild bleeding caused by liver disease, give 1–3 drops (20 mg/ml) or one 10 mg tablet of vitamin K. If rapid onset of action is required give 10–20 mg of vitamin K as a slow intravenous injection or infusion. The therapeutic action starts within 6–12 hours. Dangerous bleeding should be treated with frozen plasma (10–15 ml/kg).
  - An overdose of warfarin is treated with 1–2 mg of vitamin K perorally, intramuscularly, or intravenously. If a larger dose of vitamin K is used, anticoagulation is difficult to manage during the next few weeks. Dangerous bleeding should be treated with frozen plasma (10–15 ml/kg) or Prothromplex T®.

15.32 Haemophilia and von Willebrand's disease

Editors

Basic rules

- A general practitioner should know all haemophiliacs in the population he/she is caring for.
- Organisation of treatment in cases of bleeding should be planned in advance and the clotting factor concentrate should be readily available.

Principles

- Aspirin should not be given to patients with disorders of haemostasis. The analgesic drug of choice is paracetamol or a combination of paracetamol and codeine. Mefenamic acid, tolfenamic acid, and diflunisal are allowed. Dextropropoxyphene or tramadol can be used for severe pain.
- Drug treatment is necessary for bleeding in the joints, muscles, the face, neck, mouth, tongue and eyes, a severe blow on the head or a severe headache, severe bleeding anywhere, severe pain or swelling anywhere, wounds requiring sutures, large trauma, dental extractions and surgery.
- Minor soft tissue bleeding can be treated with immobilisation, bandaging, cold compression and eventually analgesics.
- **When a haemophiliac patient suspects bleeding take him/her seriously even if there are no visible signs!**
- In cases of bleeding, the coagulation system must be transiently normalized by infusing a clotting factor concentrate. Use frozen plasma only if there is no specific clotting factor concentrate available for the patient's disease.
- Do not perform diagnostic arthrocentesis. If arthrocentesis is indicated because of pain it should be performed under the protection of clotting factor concentrate. Further doses are indicated after arthrocentesis.
- If the diagnosis of bleeding is difficult, ultrasonography should be performed. X-rays are rarely useful.
- Determine haemoglobin concentration if the bleeding is profuse. Other laboratory tests are not indicated because of bleeding. Anaemia is corrected with red cell concentrate if necessary.
- If the bleeding continues despite drug treatment suspect production of antibodies and consult a specialist.
- Orthopaedic surgery, other elective surgery, dental surgery, and treatment of patients with clotting factor antibodies should be carried out in specialized centres.
- Patients receiving blood products should be protected against hepatitis B by vaccination.

Haemophilia A and B

- Haemophilia A is an X-linked hereditary deficiency of factor VIII and haemophilia B is a deficiency of factor IX. Men are affected by the disease, carriers (women) rarely have symptoms.
- The annual incidence of haemophilia is about 1/million.
- The activated partial thromboplastin time (APTT) is prolonged, and the bleeding time is normal. Further investigations should include determination of specific clotting factors.

Treatment of bleeding

- Patients with **haemophilia A** should be treated with Amofil®, which is free from risk of hepatitis and HIV.
- In cases of minor bleeding a single dose of a clotting factor concentrate (10–15 units/kg) is used.
- For other bleeding in muscles or joints the dose is 25–40 units/kg. The treatment must often be continued for 2–4 days, with doses of 10 units/kg at 8–12-hour intervals.

- For bleeding in the head, neck, and abdominal and chest cavities the initial dose is 40–50 units/kg. Further treatment is always indicated, and the dose is adjusted according to the plasma level of factor VIII.
- Patients with **haemophilia B** should be treated with Bemofil®, which is free from risk of hepatitis and HIV. The dose is about 30% higher than the dose of factor VIII. In further treatment the interval between doses is 12 hours.

Von Willebrand's disease

- The disease is caused by a decreased concentration (type 1), structural abnormality (type 2), or severe deficiency (type 3) of the von Willebrand's factor (vWF). Types 1 and 2 are inherited autosomally dominantly, type 3 (which is very rare) is inherited autosomally recessively.
- The disease occurs in both men and women (unlike the haemophilias).
- The symptoms are caused by functional abnormalities of the platelets (bruising, mucosal bleeding, prolonged epistaxis or menstrual bleeding).
- The incidence is about 2/10 000. More than 90% of the cases are mild (type 1), and the disease often remains undiagnosed.
- Prolonged bleeding time but normal APTT is suggestive of the disease. Prolonged APTT suggests a severe form of the disease.

Treatment

- Mucosal bleeding (epistaxis, excessive menstrual bleeding) can usually be treated with tranexamic acid at normal doses.
- Mild bleeding and minor surgery in patients with type 1 disease can be handled with desmopressin, administered either as an infusion (0.3 μg/kg), subcutaneously, or intranasally (300 μg for adults, 150 μg for children). The dose can be repeated after 12–24 hours if necessary. The patient can also administer the nasal spray himself/herself.
- Bleeding in patients with type 2 or 3 disease and other types of bleeding in type 1 disease should be treated with Haemate® (or Cryo-AHG®). The initial dose is the same as in haemophilia A. The interval between doses is 12 hours.

15.39 Tumours of haematopoietic and lymphoid tissues: general guidelines

Juhani Vilpo

Aims

- Recognize the signs and symptoms
- Be familiar with diagnosis and treatment outlines
- Bone marrow examination to exclude malignant blood diseases (not effective for lymphoma)
- Familiarize yourself with the appropriate local care pathways, and refer the patient accordingly for further investigations and treatment.

Definition

- Tumours of haematopoietic and lymphoid tissues.
- Includes the following: leukaemias, lymphomas (non-Hodgkin's lymphoma), Hodgkin's disease, myeloma and myelodysplastic syndromes.
- Contains a total of approximately one hundred disease types, see the WHO Classification of Tumours of Haematopoietic and Lymphoid Tissues (Table 15.39).

Table 15.39 Summary of the WHO Classification of Tumours of Haematopoietic and Lymphoid Tissues

Category	Number of tumour types
Chronic myeloproliferative diseases	7
Myelodysplastic/myeloproliferative Diseases	4
Myelodysplastic syndromes	6
Acute myeloid leukaemias (AML):	
♦ AML with recurrent cytogenetic abnormalities	4
♦ AML with multilineage myelodysplasia	2
♦ AML myelodysplastic syndromes, therapy related	3
♦ AML not otherwise categorized	12
Acute leukaemia of ambiguous lineage	1
B-cell neoplasms	
♦ Precursor B-cell lymphoblastic lymphoma/leukaemia	2
♦ Mature B-cell neoplasms	17
♦ B-cell proliferations of uncertain malignant potential	2
T-cell and NK-cell neoplasms	
♦ Precursor T-cell lymphoblastic lymphoma/leukaemia	3
♦ Mature T-cell and NK-cell neoplasms	14
♦ T-cell proliferations of uncertain malignant potential	1
Hodgkin lymphoma	6
Histiocytic and dendritic-cell neoplasms	
♦ Macrophage/histiocytic neoplasm	1
♦ Dendritic cell neoplasms	7
♦ Mastocytosis	6

Signs and symptoms

- Leukaemias prevent the normal formation of blood cells in bone marrow. This will lead to cytopenias with corresponding signs and symptoms: leucopenia and neutropenia (infection), thrombocytopenia (proneness to bruising, bleeding), anaemia (insufficient oxygen delivery to tissues).
- Signs and symptoms of lymphomas are non-specific and vary according to the organ infiltrated by the tumour, the pressure exerted by the tumour and the degree of disturbed functioning of the damaged organ. The patient may also present with general symptoms (also seen in leukaemias), such as fever, sweating, weight loss etc.
- Lymphadenopathy, hepatomegaly, splenomegaly and localized tumours may be seen in lymphomas, and also in leukaemias (depending on the subtype).

Diagnosis, subtyping, staging

- Basic diagnosis:
  - Conventional morphology from MGG stained bone marrow and blood smears (malignant blood diseases).
  - For lymphomas, histological examination of the tumour.
- Subtyping:
  - Immunologic and enzymatic phenotyping of malignant cells (special stains).
  - Karyotyping and molecular genetics to confirm chromosomal and gene changes.
- Staging:
  - Malignant blood diseases are, in theory, already widespread at diagnosis.
  - In Hodgkin's disease and non-Hodgkin's lymphomas, prognosis and the choice of treatment is dependent on the extent of the tumour mass. Staging is carried out with the use of a CT scan and bone marrow biopsy.

Guidelines to determine the urgency of diagnosis and treatment (new presentation or a change in the condition of a patient with confirmed diagnosis)

- Immediate admission to hospital (according to local guidelines to a hospital with appropriate facilities):
  - Maintenance of vital functions requires immediate measures (treatment of infections, arresting bleeding, blood transfusion to ensure oxygen supply to tissues). In these cases, the diagnosis of the specific subtype is irrelevant.
- Hospital admission within 24 hours:
  - Complications involving organs (for example, severe renal insufficiency in myeloma)
  - Pathological fractures
  - Thromboses, haemorrhage
  - Suspected cases of acute leukaemia in a child (clinical picture, blasts in the blood, cytopenia).
- Hospital admission within a few days:
  - Suspected cases of acute leukaemia in an adult (clinical picture, blasts in the blood, cytopenia)
  - "Impending situations" (severe cytopenia, infections, haemorrhage, worsening anaemia, other)
  - Complicated cases.
- Specialist appointment within a few weeks (the patient may initially be managed by a primary care physician):
  - Monitoring of blood picture in a relatively asymptomatic patient (chronic leukaemia, polycythaemia vera, essential thrombocythaemia)
  - Follow-up of a patient with monoclonal gammopathy (monoclonal gammopathy of unknown significance, i.e. MGUS, myeloma)
  - Follow-up of an enlarged lymph node (more than 2 cm).

Treatment

- Treatment modalities are very varied, they change rapidly and require specialist expertise (destruction of malignant cells and supportive treatment). The treatment is increasingly subtype specific, and targets are set taking the patient's age into consideration.
  - Destruction of malignant cells: chemotherapy, radiotherapy, biological therapy (stem cell transplantation in some cases)
  - Supportive treatment: antibiotics for an immunosuppressed patient, blood transfusions (cell therapy), growth factors, general care of a cancer patient.
- Treatment is carried out by a haematologist, oncologist, consultant physician or paediatric oncologist, as dictated by local policies.
- The increasing tendency is for the follow-up appointments and monitoring to be carried out by primary care physicians, in co-operation with the treating specialist centre.

15.40 Chronic myelogenous leukaemia (CML)

Juhani Vilpo

Basic rules

- Recognize the rare CML among the common neutrophilia.

- A sufficient and necessary finding upon diagnosis is the demonstration of Philadelphia chromosome or corresponding genetic abnormality (BCR/ABL) in a specialized laboratory.

Pathology

- CML is a slowly progressing haematopoietic stem cell disorder characterised by a considerable increase in the number of leucocytes with accumulation of all forms of mature and immature granulocytes in the blood and bone marrow. Often, megakaryocyte (in bone marrow) and platelet (in blood) numbers are also increased.

Epidemiology

- One new case/100 000/year
- CML accounts for 20% of all leukaemias
- The are no sex differences in the incidence of CML.
- The majority of patients are 30–60 years old, the incidence peak being around the age of 45 years.
- Occurs rarely in children.

Aetiology

- Remains unknown in individual patients.
- Ionizing irradiation and apparently also benzene increase the risk.

Diagnostic criteria

- Philadelphia chromosome or corresponding genetic abnormality (BCR/ABL).

Differential diagnostics

- Other leucocytoses (infections, tissue necrosis, neoplasias, other myeloproliferative diseases).

Clinical picture and laboratory findings

- Steadily increasing leucocytosis
- Anaemia
- Splenomegaly (often)
- Symptoms and signs associated with hypermetabolism, such as night sweats, mild fever, malaise and weight loss.
- The disease has three phases: asymptomatic phase, chronic phase and metamorphosis, which can be further divided into accelerated phase and acute transformation, **blast crisis**. Sometimes the disease is first detected only in the blast crisis stage.

Laboratory findings

- Correspond to the phase of the disease.
- Leucocytosis and immature gralunocytes are detected, often also thrombocytosis.
- Blast crisis: blasts > 30% in blood and bone marrow.

Basic investigations

- Blood picture
- Bone marrow examination
- Abdominal ultrasonography (spleen size?)
- Blood urate (hyperuricaemia and even gout are common)
- Lactate dehydrogenase (changes reflect disease activity or myeloid mass)
- Serum creatinine
- The specific diagnosis is always confirmed with karyotyping and a DNA test.

HAE

Complications

- Bleeding
- Thrombosis and infarctions resulting from leucostasis
- "Giant splenomegaly"
- Blast crisis is a natural phase in the course of the disease.

Course of the disease and prognosis

- If left untreated, the course of the disease is usually quite typical, although the duration of the phases may vary: asymptomatic phase, chronic phase and metamorphosis.
- Median survival is 4–5 years. Old cytotoxic drugs have had little effect on survival even though they have prolonged the symptom-free phase.
- New therapy forms will bring about changes but the end results are not quite known yet.

Treatment and follow-up

- The course of treatment is planned by a haematologist.
- Therapy options include allogeneic stem cell transplantation (patients younger than 30–50 years and a proper donor available), imatinib (a tyrosine kinase inhibitor) and interferon (A) [1 2].
- Cytostatics (hydroxyurea possibly combined with cytarabine) are used to reduce large tumour masses. This may be the only therapy option for elderly patients.
  - When leucostasis, i.e. high leucocyte count that slows down circulation (in the brain, lungs, and heart) becomes life-threatening, leucopheresis is used.
  - Splenectomy requires special indications.

References

1. Chronic Myeloid Leukemia Trialists' Collaborative Group. Interferon alfa versus chemotherapy for chronic myeloid leukemia: a meta-analysis of seven randomized trials. Journal of the National Cancer Institute 1997;89:1616–1620.

2. The Database of Abstracts of Reviews of Effectiveness (University of York), Database no.: DARE-971375. In: The Cochrane Library, Issue 1, 2000. Oxford: Update Software.

15.41 Polycythaemia vera (PV)

Juhani Vilpo, Petri Oivanen

Basic rules

- The major goal of the treatment is to prevent thrombotic complications and haemorrhages.
- This is best achieved by maintaining moderately low haemoglobin values (haemoglobin < 145 g/l and haematocrit < 0.45).
- Allopurinol is used to prevent gout symptoms and hyperuricaemic kidney lesions if urate levels are at the upper end of the normal range.
- A low dose of aspirin (100 mg/day) is given to reduce the risk of distal ischaemia and transcient ischaemic attacks. This dose has also been shown to reduce the risk of thrombosis (in cerebral and coronary circulation) in unselected PV patient material (B) [1].

Pathology

- PV is a chronic and progressive haematological malignancy. The growth of all myeloid cell lineages (erythrocytes, granulocytes and megakaryocytes) is increased in the hypercellular bone marrow. Increased erythropoiesis and high haemoglobin levels are usually the most prominent features.

Epidemiology

- Approximately 2 new cases/100 000/year.
- Most common among middle-aged and elderly people. Most patients are 40–70 years old. PV often begins around the age of 50 years.

Aetiology

- Unknown

Criteria for diagnosis

- WHO classification (the diagnosis of polycythaemia vera requires A1 + A2 plus one other A criterion, or A1 + A2 and two B criteria):
  - A1: Elevated eryhtrocyte mass (>25% above the reference value) or Hb > 185 g/l (men), >165 g/l (women)
  - A2: When possible causes of secondary polycythaemia have been excluded
    - Hereditary erythrocytosis
    - Causes of excessive erythropoietin (EPO) production: hypoxia (aB-O_2 ≤ 92%); high oxygen affinity of haemoglobin; mutation of EPO receptor; autonomic production of EPO by the tumour
  - A3: Splenomegaly
  - A4: Some other clonal anomaly than Ph+ (Philadelphia)
  - A5: Spontaneous colony growth in stem cell culture
  - B1: Blood platelet count > 400×10^9/l
  - B2: Blood leucocyte count > 12×10^9/l
  - B3: Bone marrow examination: increased cellularity and increased proliferation of both the erythrocyte and megakaryocyte cell lines.
  - B4: Decreased serum EPO level

Diagnosis

- In normal clinical situations, the diagnosis can be made without performing all possible investigations. For example, venesections must sometimes be started immediately, and red cell mass measurement cannot be performed. Furthermore, there are polycythaemia vera cases where the above-mentioned criteria are not strictly applicable. When making the diagnosis a haematologist should be consulted in order to place a clinically sufficiently accurate diagnosis and determine the course of treatment.
- See also Table in 15.7.

Differential diagnostics

- Secondary erythrocytoses
  - Often associated with cardiopulmonary diseases
  - High O_2 affinity haemoglobins (Hb Helsinki, Hb Linköping)
  - Anabolic steroids, erythropoietin (keep in mind the increased incidence of doping)
- Relative erythrocytoses (red cell mass normal)
  - "Stress" polycythaemia
  - Dehydration
- Other myeloproliferative conditions

Clinical picture

- Tile-red skin
- Congestive mucous membranes
- Splenomegaly (>10–12 cm on ultrasonography) in approximately 75% of cases at diagnosis
- Hyperviscosity symptoms
  - Headache, dizziness
  - Numbness of the fingertips and erythromelalgia

- Itching
- Gastrointestinal symptoms, often haemorrhages
- Arthralgias
- Neurological symptoms

Laboratory findings

- Erythrocytosis (erythrocyte count often 8–9 × 10^{12}/l). Also high haemoglobin and haematocrit unless iron deficiency is apparent.
- Hypercellular bone marrow
- See also diagnostic criteria (above).

Disease progression and prognosis

- Progression is usually very slow and even. Median survival is around 10 years, which is as long as that of the age-matched general population.
- Thrombosis and bleeding are the major fatal complications.
- Vascular catastrophes can be avoided in the majority of cases. The disease often progresses naturally to myelofibrosis and may sometimes end finally as acute leukaemia.

Complications

- Thromboses, haemorrhages

Treatment and follow-up

- The major goal is to avoid vascular complications by maintaining normal blood viscosity and moderate platelet levels (haematocrit < 0.45, haemoglobin < 145 g/l). This can be achieved by venesections which decrease thrombophilia and bleeding tendencies. The course of treatment is planned according to a haematologist's evaluation and may largely be carried out in primary care.
- Therapy is started with venesections of 400–500 ml initially every other week. The equipment used and duration of venesection follow the principles of blood donation. If haemoglobin is >200 g/l, 400 ml can be taken daily up to the maximum of 1500–2000 ml.
- If the annual number of venesections exceeds 6–12, myelosuppressive treatment or interferon is added to the regimen. In younger patients this treatment should be postponed for as long as possible.

Myelosuppressive treatment

- Given in primary care in collaboration with an experienced specialist.
- Drugs of choice are interferon, hydroxyurea or ^{32}P (elderly patients).
  - With hydroxyurea response in leucocytes is seen in one week; therapy requires intense follow-up in the beginning. Treatment is often long-lasting. Haemoglobin reduction starts to be seen in about one month.
  - ^{32}P (i.v. or p.o.) as a single dose. Effect begins in about 2 weeks (first in leucocytes, then in platelets and lastly in red cell counts) and lasts <2 years.
  - Interferon is a good option, if the patient can tolerate it.
  - Busulphan sometimes controls spleen size satisfactorily.
  - Anagrelide is useful in the control of thrombocytosis refractory to hydroxyurea.

Symptomatic treatment

- Antihistamines for itching, and H_2 receptors blockers (cimetidine) for abdominal symptoms and also itching. A response to itching has also been reached with interferon alpha (is suitable if cytoreductive therapy is also needed), psoralen photochemotherapy, cholestyramine, iron (watch out for "burst" of erythropoiesis in microcytosis) and paroxetine (worth a try when cytoreductive therapy is not needed).
- Allopurinol is used to prevent symptoms of gout and kidney damage, especially if serum urate is elevated.
- Aspirin (50 mg/day) is used to prevent thrombotic complications if the patient already has distal ischaemia, TIA symptoms or risk factors (atherosclerosis, hypertension, smoking).
- There is little experience of using new platelet aggregation inhibiting medicines in polycythaemia vera.

Follow-up

- According to the therapy
  - Hydroxyurea treatment: initially every 1–3 weeks, later every 1–2 months.
  - ^{32}P: first control after 1 month, thereafter every 2–4 months. In stable disease, every 4–12 months.
  - Interferon: in the same way as in hydroxyurea treatment.

Reference

1. Landolfi R, Marchioli R, Kutti J, Gisslinger H, Tognoni G, Patrono C, Barbui T,. Efficacy and safety of low-dose aspirin in polycythemia vera. N Engl J Med 2004;350(2):114–24.

15.42 Myelofibrosis (MF)

Juhani Vilpo

Basic rules

- Therapy is mostly supportive and palliative.
- It is important to explain the nature of the disease and the cause of anaemia to the patient.
- Cytostatic therapy is given in marked leuco- and thrombocytosis.

HAE

Pathology

- MF is a progressive haematological malignancy. The prominent feature is pathological proliferation of bone marrow myeloid cells, particularly megakaryocytes. This is associated with a gradual replacement of haematopoietic marrow by fibrotic tissue.
- Has over 30 synonyms, e.g. chronic idiopathic myelofibrosis, agnogenic myelogenous metaplasia, myelofibrosis and myelogenous metaplasia.

Epidemiology

- Estimated incidence is <1 case/100 000/year.
- The peak incidence is between the ages of 40–70 years. It is rarely seen in young adults and very rarely in children.
- There is no sex difference.

Aetiology

- In individual patients aetiology remains unknown.
- Benzene increases the risk, as does ionizing radiation.
- The advanced or myelofibrotic stage of polycythaemia vera resembles idiopathic myelofibrosis.

Diagnostic criteria

- Splenomegaly (on ultrasonography > 10–12 cm)
- Anaemia and leuko-erythroblastic blood picture
- Dry tap in bone marrow aspiration
- Bone marrow trephine biopsy (collagen and reticulin staining) confirms the diagnosis.

Differential diagnostics

- Other splenomegalies
  - Chronic myeloid leukaemia, polycythaemia vera, essential thrombocytosis
  - Lymphomas
  - Other causes
- Other causes of leuko-erythroblastic blood picture
  - Bone marrow metastases
  - Multiple myeloma
  - Lymphomas
  - Storage diseases
  - Acute myelofibrosis (resembles acute leukaemia)
- Secondary myelofibrosis
  - Bone marrow metastases
  - Tuberculosis
  - Lymphomas and leukaemias

Clinical picture

- Progression usually very slow
- Earliest findings:
  - anaemia
  - splenomegaly.
- Later symptoms:
  - weight loss
  - poor condition
  - tiredness
  - haemorrhages
  - gout, hyperuricaemia
  - bone pains
  - leg cramps.

Laboratory findings

- Blood picture
  - Anaemia
  - Leuko-erythroblastic picture
  - Teardrop cells
- Bone marrow
  - Dry tap on aspiration
  - Typical histology in trephine biopsy
- Other
  - Often increased blood lactate dehydrogenase and bilirubin levels
  - Sometimes folate deficiency

Basic investigations

- Blood picture (numerical and blood film examination)
- Abdominal ultrasonography (spleen size?)
- Bone marrow trephine biopsy with reticulin and collagen stains
- Other: blood urate, lactate dehydrogenase, folate and creatinine

Disease progression and prognosis

- Often very slow progression (progresses from the profibrotic to the fibrotic stage of bone marrow)
  - Median survival 5–7 years
  - Some patients live >20 years
- In more severe forms
  - Anaemia requiring red cell transfusions (and iron chelation therapy)
  - Increasing splenomegaly
  - Cardiac insufficiency
  - Haemorrhages, infections
  - In ca. 25% of cases the disease progresses to acute leukaemia

Complications

- Haemorrhages, spleen infarctions and (seldom) spleen rupture

Treatment and follow-up

- Treatment is supportive and palliative.
  - Anaemia is treated in symptomatic cases by red cell transfusions. Remember also trivial causes of anaemia, such as iron deficiency.
  - Myelosuppressive therapy for massive splenomegaly and for leuco- and thrombocytosis. Results are usually temporary.
  - Sometimes splenectomy relieves symptoms and prolongs transfusion intervals.
- The overall treatment strategy is planned by a haematologist, but the general practitioner may have a major role in supportive care and in follow-up.

15.43 Chronic lymphocytic leukaemia (CLL)

Juhani Vilpo

Basic rules

- Usually diagnosed incidentally (lymphocytosis) during investigations for some other disease.
- Immunocytopenias (AIHA and ITP) are detected on the basis of anaemia and bruising tendency.
- Antiviral drugs should be readily used in herpes zoster (acyclovir, penciclovir or valaciclovir).
- Avoid living vaccines.
- Explain the chronic course of the disease to the patient.
- When the disease is progressing rapidly (doubling time of lymphocytes in blood < 6 months) and the mortality risk is high, radical cytostatics (fludarabine ± cyclophosphamide) combined with stem cell transplantation may be tried.

Pathology

- CLL is a haematological malignancy, where mature-looking lymphocytes slowly accumulate in bone marrow, blood and lymphatic tissues.
- According to current classification, CLL is a B-cell disease.

Epidemiology

- CLL is the most prevalent form of leukaemia in Western countries accounting for about 30% of all leukaemias.
- 90% of the patients are older than 50 years. CLL has not been found in children.
- CLL is twice as common in males compared with females.

Aetiology

- The aetiology is unknown. In contrast to other leukaemias, ionizing radiation and viral infections have not been linked to leukaemogenesis in CLL.

Diagnosis

1. Absolute chronic lymphocytosis ($>5\times10^9$/l)
2. Bone marrow: hyper- or normocellular, >30% of cells are small, mature lymphocytes.
   - If the patient is symptomless, urgent diagnosis is not necessary. Bone marrow examination is sufficient for the diagnosis of CLL.

Differential diagnostics

- Other mature-cell lymphoid leukaemias: histology (lymph-node biopsy, bone marrow trephine) may be helpful.
- Reactive lymphocytoses.

Laboratory investigations and clinical picture

- Slowly increasing lymphocytosis.
- Approximately 50% of the patients have hypogammaglobulinaemia, and about 5% have a serum M component.
- During disease progression, lymph nodes, spleen and liver become enlarged. The symptoms of advanced disease include fever, night sweats, tiredness and weight loss.
- The clinical problems result from anaemia, aggravation of other cytopenias, infections or lymphocyte infiltrates in other organs.

Basic investigations

- The completion of investigations can be delayed to a later, symptomatic stage, if the basic diagnosis is otherwise ascertained. All investigations must be completed before therapy is initiated.
  - Chest x-ray (mediastinum, pulmonary hilum, lung parenchyma)
  - Abdominal ultrasonography (spleen and liver size and parenchyma), lymph nodes
  - Serum protein electrophoresis (M component?), serum immunoglobulins (IgG, IgA, IgM and possibly IgG subclasses)
  - Direct antiglobulin test (Coombs' test)
  - Serum creatinine and urate concentrations

Special investigations

- In a disease that is progressing rapidly or otherwise requires treatment, the investigations aim at evaluating the mortality risk of the patient:

- Flow cytometric immunophenotyping (including antigens CD38 and ZAP-70)
- Analysis of chromosome changes
- Assessment of the mutation status of the immunoglobulin genes with gene sequencing (based on this investigation, the patients may be divided into two groups according to their prognosis; in the more favourable group the median life expectancy is double compared with the less favourable group).

Disease progression and prognosis

- Very slow in half of the patients.
- Median survival is in the range of 5–10 years.
- May transform to a more aggressive form associated with immature cell morphology (approximately 5–10%)
  - prolymphocytic leukaemia
  - Richter's syndrome (immunoblastic lymphoma)
  - a condition resembling acute lymphoid leukaemia.
- Staging according to Binet's or Rai's classification determines when and whether or not therapy is initiated and gives more accurate prognostic information.

Complications

- AIHA (autoimmune haemolytic anaemia) in 5–10%
- ITP (immunological thrombocytopenia) in 1% or more
- Infections associated with severe hypogammaglobulinaemia but also from other causes. Recurrent bacterial infections may be a severe problem.
- Usually harmless virus infections may be severe or even fatal (herpes zoster and even generalized herpes simplex infections). Avoid routine administration of living vaccines.

Follow-up and chemotherapy

- Symptomless patients do not benefit from chemotherapy. These patients may have high lymphocyte counts, for example $100–150\times10^9$/l.

Follow-up

- After diagnosis, every 2–4 months. If progression is slow, then every 6–12 months.
- Investigations:
  - Laboratory investigations: haemoglobin levels < 100 g/l and platelet counts < 100×10^9/l indicate bone marrow insufficiency and they are taken into account in clinical staging.
  - Infections
  - Lymph nodes
  - Size of the spleen
  - If a total response to treatment has been achieved, the residual disease of the bone marrow is followed-up with the help of flow cytometry (and sometimes with PCR).
- Chemotherapy and special investigations are planned by a specialist, but a local general practitioner may collaborate by performing the intermittent follow-up checks.

Indications of chemotherapy

- General symptoms
- Rapid progression
- Anaemia caused by bone marrow infiltrates (haemoglobin < 100 g/l) or thrombocytopenia (<100×10^9/l)
- Disturbingly large lymph nodes or spleen
- Symptoms or cytopenias usually appear when the leukocyte count exceeds 100×10^9/l.

Implementation of therapy

- In milder forms the usual starting combination is chlorambucil-prednisolone, preferentially given as intermittent courses.
- In hypersplenism the therapy is splenectomy or splenic irradiation.
- In chlorambucil-resistant cases the specialist usually prescribes fludarabine (± cyclophosphamide), chlorodeoxyadenosine, high-dose chlorambucil or a regimen of cytotoxic drugs (COP, CHOP). Also monoclonal antibodies (rituximab, alemtuzumab) that destroy leukaemic cells are used in special cases.
- In immunocytopenias (AIHA, ITP) corticosteroids are preferred.
- Intravenous immunoglobulin therapy may be beneficial for some individual patients suffering from frequent bacterial infections.
- Radical cytostatics and stem cell transplantation may be considered for younger patients and in rapidly progressing or otherwise high-mortality diseases.

15.44 Lymphomas

Lasse Teerenhovi

Basic rules

- Adults with an enlarged lymph node (>2 cm) that does not decrease in size during a follow-up of one month should be referred to a specialist to obtain a biopsy.
- If a patient has prolonged symptoms after treatment of lymphoma, thorough investigations are indicated to rule out recurrence.
- Consider the possibility of late adverse effects of treatment (early menopause, hypothyroidism, cardiac disease, certain infections and secondary malignancies).

Definition

- Hodgkin's disease and non-Hodgkin's lymphoma represent a heterogeneous group, as far as their clinical picture and prognosis are concerned, of diseases of the lymphoreticular system. Non-Hodgkin's lymphoma is further divided into indolent (slow-growing) lymphomas (i.e. follicular, lymphocytic, marginal zone and mantle zone lymphoma) and aggressive (fast-growing) lymphomas (i.e. large B-cell, Burkitt's and lymphoblastic lymphoma as well as most T-cell lymphomas).

Epidemiology

- The annual incidence of Hodgkin's disease is about 2/100 000 in the Nordic countries. The age distribution of Hodgkin's disease is bimodal: i.e. the first peak occurs at the age of 30 years and the second at the age of 50 years.
- The annual incidence of non-Hodgkin's lymphoma is about 19/100 000 in the Nordic countries. The mean age at onset is about 60 years.
- The incidence of non-Hodgkin's lymphomas is increasing in all Western countries, particularly in the Nordic countries. The reason for the increase is not known. The incidence of Hodgkin's disease, however, has slightly declined in recent decades.

Signs and symptoms

Hodgkin's disease

- Most patients have no symptoms, or the symptoms are associated with the pressure caused by the tumour mass, such as a cough in hilar tumours and retrosternal feeling of heaviness, or superior vena cava syndrome, in mediastinal tumours.
- A minority of patients have systemic symptoms: fever, night sweats and unexplained weight loss (known as the B symptoms), severe pruritus or pain in the affected glands after alcohol consumption. The latter symptom only occurs in Hodgkin's disease.
- The disease usually starts in the supraclavicular lymph nodes and spreads through the lymphatic system to the axillae or mediastinum, or both, and further to the retroperitoneal lymph nodes.
- The disease may infiltrate from lymph nodes to other organs (for example from mediastinal lymph nodes to the pericardium, from hilar lymph nodes to the lung tissue or from para-aortic lymph nodes to the spinal cord).
- A mediastinal tumour in a young adult is often Hodgkin's disease.
- A typical lymph node in Hodgkin's disease is hard, rubbery and multilobular.
- Haematogenic spread to the bone marrow or liver is a late manifestation of the disease that follows the spread of the disease to the spleen from lower mediastinal or para-aortic lymph nodes.

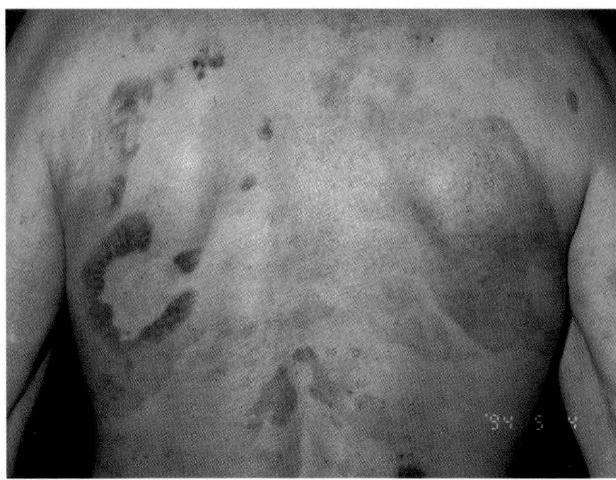

Figure 15.44.1 Mycosis fungoides (T-cell lymphoma of the skin) has a variable clinical picture. In this case the skin at the back shows palpable plaques. The patient also had facial tumour lesions. A dermatologist or oncologist should be consulted. Photo © R. Suhonen.

Non-Hodgkin's lymphoma

- Symptoms are non-specific and dependent on the organs infiltrated by the tumour mass. Many patients are totally asymptomatic when lymphoma is diagnosed.
- About 25% of patients with non-Hodgkin's lymphoma have at least one of the aforementioned B symptoms. The more advanced the disease the more common the symptoms. The prevalence of symptoms is also dependent on the histology of the lymphoma; patients with an aggressive non-Hodgkin's lymphoma are most likely to manifest B symptoms.
- In about 50% of the patients, only in the lymph node areas are affected at the diagnosis. On the other hand, almost 20% of the patients have lymphoma tissue only in extranodal organs. These organs include the stomach, skin, bone, brain, thyroid gland and intestine (Figure 15.44.1).
- Although diagnosis cannot be made on the basis of the clinical presentation alone, non-Hodgkin's lymphoma should be suspected in the following cases:
  - Lymphadenopathy involving several lymph node areas in an elderly patient is often indicative of an indolent non-Hodgkin's lymphoma, usually follicular lymphoma.
  - Lymphocytosis in an elderly patient is often indicative of an indolent non-Hodgkin's lymphoma.
  - Prolonged tonsillitis not responding to antibiotics may indicate lymphoma.
  - A fast-growing local lymphadenopathy is often caused by an aggressive non-Hodgkin's lymphoma.

Diagnosis and determination of tumour spread

- The diagnosis of Hodgkin's disease and non-Hodgkin's lymphoma is always based on a thorough histopathological examination. A surgical biopsy is necessary. If a patient has a palpable lymph node more than 2 cm in diameter that does not decrease in size during a follow-up of one month, or a similar lymphadenopathy is observed in a chest x-ray, he/she should be referred to a specialist to obtain a biopsy.

- Laboratory investigations are not particularly helpful in diagnosis, with the exception of significant lymphocytosis seen in some indolent lymphomas. The World Health Organization classification of hematological malignancies should be used as a guideline of pathological diagnosis.
- Determination of tumour dehydrogenase (LDH) pathologically to more than one extranodal the poorer the prognosis.
  - The spread of Hodgkin's disease is determined by clinical examination, computed tomography and bone marrow biopsy.
  - The same methods are used to determine the spread of non-Hodgkin's lymphoma.
  - In both types of lymphoma the extent of the disease is expressed using the Ann Arbor Staging System (I-IV A-B).
  - In Hodgkin's disease, the prognosis is better the lower the Ann Arbor stage. The presence of B symptoms worsens the prognosis.
  - In non-Hodgkin's lymphoma, prognosis can also be evaluated by the International Prognostic NHL Index (IPI). Points, which indicate poor prognosis, are allocated for the following factors:
    - Age $\geq$ 60 years
    - Ann Arbor Stage > II
    - WHO performance status > 1 (incapable of work because of symptoms)
    - Serum lactate dehydrogenase (LDH) pathologically high
    - The disease has spread to more than one extranodal organ.
  - The higher the score the poorer the prognosis.

Treatment and prognosis

Hodgkin's disease

- Local and asymptomatic (Ann Arbor I–IIA) Hodgkin's disease is treated by combination chemotherapy, i.e. the ABVD regime (Adriamycin/doxorubicin, bleomycin, vincristine and dacarbazine). The duration of treatment varies from two to six months, depending on the response. The ABVD therapy is followed by radiotherapy to the involved area.
- The treatment of widespread disease, or disease with B symptoms, consists of combination chemotherapy (ABVD or BEACOPP, i.e. bleomycin, etoposide, Adriamycin, cyclophosphamide, Oncovin [vincristine], procarbazine and prednisolone) of six to eight months' duration. If considered appropriate, any residual tumours are then treated with radiotherapy. Radiotherapy will lead to a slightly improved tumour control but has not been shown to affect the long-term outcome B [1 2 3 4].
- The ten year mortality from Hodgkin's disease is only about 20% in patients under 60 years of age at diagnosis, whereas the corresponding figure for those aged 60 or more is 40–50%.

Non-Hodgkin's lymphomas

- Indolent lymphomas remain local in 10–20% of patients (Ann Arbor stage I or II). A proportion of these patients can be cured. Radiotherapy to the affected sites is the treatment of choice.
- Asymptomatic patients with a more widespread disease can first be monitored without treatment, but if the patient develops symptoms or the disease spreads further, oral cytostatics (e.g. chlorambucil) are indicated. The fewer IPI points the patient has the better the life expectancy. On average, life expectancy is 6–9 years; no patient will be totally cured. However, in patients with mantle zone lymphoma the average life expectancy is only about three and a half years. This subtype is therefore treated in the same way as an aggressive lymphoma.
- The lower the IPI score the better the prognosis of aggressive lymphomas. The main treatment modality is combination chemotherapy, which aims at complete treatment response. If complete response is not achieved, the patient will die of the disease. The higher the IPI score the less likely it is that the patient has a complete response to chemotherapy. The intensity and duration of chemotherapy is determined according to the patient's personal IPI score.
- Local lymphoma, stage I-II, (IPI score 0–1) is treated with three cycles of the CHOP regimen (i.e. cyclophosphamide, doxorubicin, vincristine, prednisolone) followed by radiotherapy to the affected site.
  - The treatment of a more widespread disease with worse prognosis consists of combination chemotherapy of 4–6 months' duration (e.g. CHOP, M-BACOD (methotrexate, bleomycin, doxorubicin, cyclophosphamide, vincristine, dexamethasone, leucovorin), new experimental regimens). If considered appropriate, chemotherapy may be followed by radiotherapy to the major tumour sites. The adding of rituximab, an anti-CD 20 antibody, to combination chemotherapy improves the prognosis of patients with diffuse, large B-cell lymphomas.
- Of the patients with none of the above factors indicating poor prognosis, about 80% under 60 years of age can be cured; however, if all the factors are present only 30–40% will be cured.

Follow-up

- The risk of recurrence of Hodgkin's disease is greatest during the first 5 years of disease onset.
- Aggressive lymphomas usually do not recur if 3 years has elapsed from the initial treatment.
- Indolent lymphomas may recur at any time during the remainder of the patient's life.
- At the initial stage the aim of follow-up is to detect recurrence as early as possible. While the risk of recurrence

remains high follow-up visits should be carried out every 3 months. A thorough history should be taken during the visits, and palpation of lymph nodes is essential. Any symptom that has continued for several weeks, and/or has become worse, warrants thorough investigation to rule out the possibility of a recurrence. Imaging the focus of the symptoms (computed tomography or magnetic resonance imaging) is the primary examination.

- An increased ESR may indicate the recurrence of Hodgkin's disease and an increased serum LDH the recurrence in cases of non-Hodgkin's lymphoma. Other laboratory tests are of little value in the detection of recurrence.
- After the risk of recurrence has decreased, follow-up is aimed at detection of late sequelae of treatment and the disease.

Radiotherapy

- Follow-up is dependent on the area irradiated.
  - Thyroid gland—risk of hypothyroidism
  - Ovaries—risk of early menopause
  - Heart—risk of pericarditis, insufficiency, valvular disorders, early coronary heart disease
  - All areas—increased risk of secondary malignancies >10 years after initial treatment
    - Cessation of smoking
    - Removal of naevi from irradiated skin areas

Chemotherapy

- Follow-up is dependent of the combination of chemotherapy used:
  - Alkylating drugs—risk of secondary leukaemia after 3–6 years
  - Alkylating drugs—risk of early menopause, infertility
  - Anthracyclines—risk of heart failure

Splenectomy

- Risk of septic infection
  - Vaccination against pneumococci, haemophilus and meningococci

References

1. Sprecht L, Gray RG, Clarke MJ, Peto R. Influence of more extensive radiotherapy and adjuvant chemotherapy on long-term outcome in early-stage Hodgkin's disease: a meta-analysis of 23 randomized trials involving 3,888 patients. Journal of Clinical Oncology 1998;16:830–843.
2. The Database of Abstracts of Reviews of Effectiveness (University of York), Database no.: DARE-980477. In: The Cochrane Library, Issue 1, 2000. Oxford: Update Software.
3. Loeffler M, Brosteanu O, Hasenclever D et al. Meta-analysis of chemotherapy versus combined modality treatment trials in Hodgkin's disease. Journal of Clinical Oncology 1998;16:818–829.
4. The Database of Abstracts of Reviews of Effectiveness (University of York), Database no.: DARE-980476. In: The Cochrane Library, Issue 1, 2000. Oxford: Update Software.

15.45 Acute leukaemia in adults

Juhani Vilpo

Basic rules

- Suspect acute leukaemia in patients with anaemia, granulocytopenia, thrombocytopenia and associated systemic symptoms such as infection and bleeding, particularly mucosal bleeding.
- Remember that blasts are not found in the peripheral blood in about 10% of leukaemia patients. The diagnosis of leukaemia can only be made on the basis of bone marrow examination.

HAE

Definition

- Acute leukaemia is a haematological disease where blast cells accumulate in the bone marrow and in most cases also in the peripheral blood. In some cases the proportion of mature (but pathological) cells is remarkable.
- Leukaemic cells also invade other organs.

Epidemiology

- The annual incidence is about 3–4/100 000.
- The incidence is about 2/100 000 up to the age of 40–50 years. Thereafter the incidence increases up to 15–20 cases/100 000 by the age of 75.
- Men are slightly more frequently affected than women (the incidence is highest in young boys and elderly men).
- About 80% of the patients have acute myeloid leukaemia (AML), and 20% have acute lymphatic leukaemia (ALL).

Aetiology

- The aetiology remains unknown in most individual patients.
- Well-known risk factors include ionizing radiation, organic solvents (particularly benzene) and some cytotoxic drugs.
- Secondary leukaemias following the treatment of other cancers are becoming more common and comprise about 10% of all leukaemias.
- The above-mentioned factors increase the risk of AML much more than the risk of ALL.

Diagnostic criteria

- The main criterion for acute leukaemia: blasts > 20% of bone marrow population (new WHO recommendation for classification) or > 30% (old FAB classification).

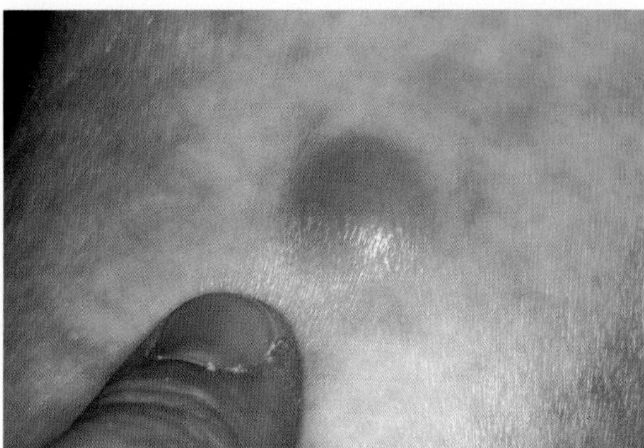

Figure 15.45.1 Skin tumours may be a feature of leukaemias. The nature of the tumour is defined on the basis of a skin biopsy. Photo © R. Suhonen.

- According to the new WHO classification, AML (including its subtypes) is still considered as its own group of diseases. ALL on the other hand is grouped here together with lymphomas as "precursor B- and T-cell neoplasms". ALL is discussed in this guideline and lymphomas separately in (15.44).
- The accurate diagnosis is currently based on traditional morphology (blood picture, aspiration and trephine samples from the marrow and biopsy from the lymphoma), and also cytochemistry, immunophenotyping, chromosome and molecular biological studies (15.39).
- Preliminary investigations (bone marrow examination, biopsy) can be carried out in primary care but in order to coordinate the diagnosis, a haematologist should be consulted already at an early stage to plan the course of diagnosis and treatment.
- AML subtyping (WHO classification)
  - AML with a standard chromosomal change (4 subtypes)
  - AML with myelodysplasia of several cell lines (2 subtypes)
  - Previous type, but therapy-related (3 subtypes)
  - AML, unclassified (12 subtypes, according to the dominating cell type and degree of maturity)
- ALL subtyping
  - B-cell diseases
  - T-cell diseases

Differential diagnosis

- AML: myelodysplastic syndromes
- ALL: lymphoblastic lymphomas (in these the prominent tumour is outside the bone marrow)

Clinical picture and laboratory findings

- The growing leukaemic cell population affects normal haematopoiesis.
- Anaemia, neutropenia, thrombocytopenia, and associated systemic symptoms such as infection and bleeding, particularly mucosal bleeding.
- Abnormal cells in the peripheral blood (blasts) are the most common laboratory finding. Most patients have leucocytosis. About 10% of the patients have no blasts in the differential count. **The diagnosis of leukaemia can only be made on the basis of bone marrow examination.**
- Other laboratory tests yield non-specific results.

Primary investigations

- Blood count and differential, and bone marrow examination
- The primary investigations (including bone marrow aspiration) must be completed in a few days in patients with suspected acute leukaemia. Diagnosis and treatment are performed according to the division between specialist and primary care.

Natural course of the disease and prognosis

- If untreated the disease is fulminant and results in death in a few weeks in most cases.
- In some patients the disease progresses slowly and life expectancy without treatment is about 1–2 years.

AML

- Remission is obtained in 50–80% of the patients. The prognosis is worsened by age: remission is obtained in 55–80% of patients below age 60, but in only 33–76% of patients above age 60. The median duration of remission is about one year and the median life expectancy of patients with AML is about 2 years.
- About 20–40% of patients with AML are cured by chemotherapy.

ALL

- The mean age of the patients is younger than in AML.
- Remission is obtained in 70–90% of the patients, and the median duration of remission is 18–24 months. Long-term remission is obtained in about 20–40% of the patients.
- The prognosis is significantly better in patients treated by allogeneic bone marrow transplantation.

Complications

- Infections
- Bleeding
- Neuroleukaemia
- Complications of chemotherapy

Treatment and follow-up

- Most patients are treated with intensive combined chemotherapy. The therapy is tailored individually according to the risk of mortality related to each case. The goals of the therapy are:

- to rapidly restore normal haematopoiesis (induction therapy)
- to prevent the formation of resistent leukaemia cell populations (induction therapy)
- to eliminate pockets that are not reached by antineoplastic drugs (e.g. radiation therapy of central nervous system)
- to prevent the formation of multiple drug resistance (consolidation therapy following remission).

- The central drugs in the treatment of AML are cytarabine and anthracyclines. In ALL the combinations almost without exception include vinca alkaloid and predniso(lo)ne.
- Allogeneic stem cell transplantation is attempted in patients below 40–50 years of age, particularly if the prognosis of the particular disease type is poor. Autologous stem cell transplantation is also used as adjunct treatment C [1 2] although this treatment modality is not yet fully established.
- Central nervous system prophylaxis is an established treatment in ALL.
- The treatment is carried out in specialized centres. Less intensive treatment may be indicated in the very aged and in patients who are otherwise unsuitable for intensive chemotherapy.
- Supportive treatment of acute leukaemia is demanding. The most important components are blood products and treatment of infections.
- Palliative treatment in patients with acute leukaemia can be performed by the general practitioner in cooperation with a haematologist. A hospital bed is often needed even for palliative care.

References

1. Johnson PW, Simnett SJ, Sweetenham JW, Morgan GJ, Stewart LA. Bone marrow and peripheral blood stem cell transplantation for malignancy. Health Technology Assessment 1998;2:1–188.
2. The Database of Abstracts of Reviews of Effectiveness (University of York), Database no.: DARE-989011. In: The Cochrane Library, Issue 3, 2000. Oxford: Update Software.

15.46 Multiple myeloma (MM)

Juhani Vilpo, Petri Oivanen

Aim

- To recognize symptoms that require early intervention.

Pathology

- MM is a clonal bone marrow proliferation of mature B cells (plasma cells) characterized by a monoclonal immunoglobulin fraction (M component) in the serum or sometimes only in urine protein electrophoresis.
- Benign disease forms (MGUS or monoclonal gammopathy with unknown significance and benign paraproteinaemia) are about 100 times more common than myeloma.

Epidemiology

- Approximately 3–4 new cases/100 000/year.
- Diagnosis is usually made at the age of 50–70 years; rarely before the age of 40 years.
- No sex differences.

Aetiology

- In individual patients aetiology remains unknown.
- Ionizing radiation slightly increases the risk.

Diagnosis

- The main diagnostic difficulty is to make a distinction between early cases of MM and "benign" paraproteinaemias, especially MGUS.

Criteria for diagnosis of multiple myeloma (WHO classification)

- A. The diagnosis of multiple myeloma requires one main criterion and at least one additional criterion OR three additional criteria, which include C1 and C2. In addition, the disease has to be symptomatic and progressive.
- B. Main criteria
  - Bone marrow plasmacytosis (>30%)
  - Plasmacytoma in biopsy
  - M component
    - Serum/plasma: IgG > 35 g/l, IgA > 20 g/l
    - Urine: > 1 g/24 h
- C. Additional criteria
  - Bone marrow plasmacytosis (10–30%)
  - M component (smaller than in point B)
  - Osteolytic lesions
  - Decrease of polyclonal immunoglobulins in serum
    - IgG < 6 g/l
    - IgA < 1 g/l
    - IgM < 0.5 g/l

Differential diagnostics

- MGUS (plasma cells in bone marrow < 10%; IgG < 35 g/l or IgA < 20 g/l, no osteolytic foci, no symptoms)
- Waldenström's macroglobulinaemia (15.47)
- Lymphomas with an M component in some cases
- Other rare diseases where there is an M component

Clinical picture

- Often:
  - Osteolytic lesions and bone pains
  - Mild anaemia, hypercalcaemia, hyperuricaemia
  - Renal insufficiency.
- Rarely:
  - Hyperviscosity syndrome (IgA myeloma).

Typical laboratory findings

- Increased erythrocyte sedimentation rate (not in light-chain myeloma)
- M component in serum and/or urine
- Decreased haemoglobin level, often also leuco- and thrombocytopenia
- Malignant plasma cell infiltrates in the bone marrow
- Osteolytic lesion in bone x-ray
- Often increased serum urate and calcium but diminished albumin concentration

Basic examinations

- Blood picture, serum calcium, potassium, natrium and creatinine and ESR
- Bone marrow examination
- Serum and urine protein electrophoresis (M component can be found exclusively in urine in 10–20% of MM patients)

Additional investigations when MM is likely

- X-ray (skull, thorax/ribs, vertebrae, scapulae, pelvis and long bones of the extremities)
- Serum/plasma total protein, albumin, potassium, sodium, calcium, ionised calcium, creatinine, urate and immunoglobulins (IgG, IgA, IgM)
- Identification of M component heavy and light chains by immunofixation or by other means
- Magnetic resonance imaging is more sensitive than radiography, but is seldom indicated in basic diagnosis.

Complications requiring attention preferably within 24 hours (particularly in new patients)

- Sepsis or pneumonia (intravenous broad-spectrum antibiotics)
- Renal insufficiency (dialysis or haemofiltration)
- Hyperviscosity (plasmapheresis)
- Hypercalcaemia (fluid replacement, bisphosphonates, steroids)
- Spinal cord compression (surgical decompression, radiotherapy?)
- Pathological fractures (pain medication, stabilization)
- Vertebral compression (orthopaedic treatment)

Disease progression and prognosis

- With traditional therapies, median life expectancy at diagnosis is about 3.5–4 years and somewhat longer with more intensive treatments. Marked individual variation exists.
- Myeloma cells become gradually resistant to chemotherapy.
- Myeloma cell infiltrates occupy the bone marrow causing anaemia, thrombocytopenia and leucopenia.
- Infections, haemorrhages and renal insufficiency are frequent complications.

Follow-up and treatment

- If the patient is symptomless, no chemotherapy is usually given, as it does not improve the patient's wellbeing or prolong life.
- Symptomatic patients are treated actively.

In follow-up, attention is paid to

- The amount of M component (serum and/or urine)
- The blood picture (reflects the degree of bone marrow infiltrates)
- General condition and symptoms, infections and (bone) pains
- Osteolytic lesions (x-ray)
- Renal function and hypercalcaemia.

Chemotherapy

- According to instructions given by a haematologist or a specialist in internal medicine who is familiar with the treatment of haematological diseases: the aim is intensive therapy and two successive autologous stem cell transplantations (patients under 70 years).
- VAD (vincristine, adriamycin and dexamethasone) or similar combinations when stem cell transplantation is considered or a rapid response is needed.
- MP therapy (a combination of melphalan and prednisolone) especially for patients over 70 years of age and also for younger patients if stem cell transplantation is not considered.
- Refractory cases
  - VAD (vincristine, adriamycin and dexamethasone)
  - MOCCA (vincristine, cyclophosphamide, lomustine, melphalan and methylprednisolon), high-dose melphalan or other cytostatics
  - Thalidomide
  - Dexamethasone
- Interferon may be tried B [1] [2] especially for maintaining an otherwise reached good response.

Supportive therapy includes

- Maintenance of fluid and electrolyte balance (to prevent renal failure)

- Treatment of hypercalcaemia
- Treatment of infections
- Maintenance of mobility in order to prevent osteoporosis and pathological fractures
- If necessary, treatment of anaemia and thrombocytopenia.

Stem cell transplantation

- Autologous stem cell transplantation is used increasingly and is often the first-line treatment for patients over 70 years of age C [3] [4].
- Allogeneic stem cell transplantation is also used increasingly, but is still possible only for few patients.

References

1. Trippoli S, Becagli P, Messori A, Trendi E. Maintenance treatment with interferon in multiple myeloma: a survival meta-analysis. Clin Drug Invest 1997;14:392–399.
2. The Database of Abstracts of Reviews of Effectiveness (University of York), Database no.: DARE-971500. In: The Cochrane Library, Issue 4, 1999. Oxford: Update Software.
3. Johnson PW, Simnett SJ, Sweetenham JW, Morgan GJ, Stewart LA. Bone marrow and peripheral blood stem cell transplantation for malignancy. Health Technology Assessment 1998;2:1–188.
4. The Database of Abstracts of Reviews of Effectiveness (University of York), Database no.: DARE-989011. In: The Cochrane Library, Issue 3, 2000. Oxford: Update Software.

15.47 Waldenström's macroglobulinaemia (WM)

Juhani Vilpo, Petri Oivanen

Basic rules

- Remember Waldenström's macroglobulinaemia as a rare cause of a high ESR.

Definition

- Clonal proliferation of relatively mature B lymphocytes (differentiation at the lymphocyte–plasma cell level) with an M component (an immunoglobulin fraction in protein electrophoresis) consisting of IgM.

Epidemiology

- Far less frequent than myeloma (ca. 15% of cases of multiple myeloma)
- Usually occurs in persons aged 50–70 years.
- Both sexes are equally affected.

Aetiology

- Unknown

Diagnostic criteria

- Lymphocyte–plasma cell infiltrates in the bone marrow and a serum M-component consisting of IgM

Differential diagnosis

- Other conditions with M component (WM accounts for ca. 15–20% of these conditions):
    - IgM-MGUS (monoclonal IgM-gammopathy of undetermined significance, drawing the line between IgM-MGUS and WM is difficult). These patients have approximately a 46-fold risk of developing WM.
    - B-lymphoplasmocytic neoplasms (IgM myeloma which is extremely rare, and extramedullary plasmocytoma)
    - B-lymphocytic neoplasms (chronic lymphatic leukaemia, diffuse lymphoma)
    - Benign conditions (e.g., cold agglutination syndrome)

Clinical picture and laboratory findings

- Symptoms caused by cytopenias and immunodeficiency
    - Weakness
    - Bleeding (thrombocytopenia and -pathy)
    - Infections
- Extramedullary tumour infiltrates
    - Splenomegaly (15%)
    - Hepatomegaly (20%)
    - Lymphadenopathy and other neoplasms (15%)
- Hyperviscosity symptoms (15%; usually serum IgM > 40 g/l)
    - Cerebral ischaemia (retinal changes are typical)
    - Dyspnoea
    - Neurological symptoms
- Laboratory findings
    - High ESR
    - M component in serum protein electrophoresis which in immunofixation is typed as IgM
    - Increased serum viscosity can be detected in 50% of the patients (is worth monitoring only in symptomatic patients, who usually have IgM > 40 g/l)
    - Often anaemia or thrombocytopenia
- Osteolytic lesions are very rare (point towards IgM multiple myeloma).

Primary investigations

- Blood count and bone marrow aspiration

HAE

- Serum protein electrophoresis (immunofixation should be performed if an M component is detected)
- Serum IgG, IgA and IgM
- Serum creatinine and serum urate
- Chest x-ray and upper abdominal ultrasonography

Course of the disease and prognosis

- Variable
- WM is a long-lasting disease and its progression may be very slow.

Complications

- Hyperviscosity syndrome
- Cryoglobulinaemia
- Chronic cold agglutination disease
- Haemorrhages and infections

Treatment and follow-up

- Hyperviscosity syndrome can be treated with plasmapheresis.
- No suitable studies are available as regards chemotherapy. The following regimen has often been used:
  - Chlorambucil (initial dose 6–10 mg/day, maintenance dose 2–6 mg/day) or cyclophosphamide (haematologists often try to avoid alkylating agents in the treatment of patients between 55–65 years of age because of the potential leukaemogenic effect)
  - Prednisolone is usually added.
  - Fludarabine, cladribine
  - Monoclonal antibodies (rituximab)
  - Thalidomide (limited experience).
- The follow-up interval is 4–12 months; during chemotherapy 2–3 months.

15.48 Myelodysplastic syndromes (MDS)

Juhani Vilpo

Definition

- A heterogenic group of stem cell diseases.
- The disease manifests clinically as cytopenias (anaemia, neutropenia, thrombocytopenia) or dysfunction of blood cells.

Epidemiology

- The incidence is ca. 1.5–2 × that of acute leukaemia. The incidence grows steadily in higher age groups; under 50 years ca. 0.5/100 000, over 80 years ca. 90/100 000.
- The mean age at diagnosis is ca. 70 years. The disease is rare in children and adolescents.

Aetiology

- The aetiology is unknown.
- Ionizing radiation, cytostatics (previous antineoplastic medication), benzene and certain other chemicals increase the risk.
- Genetic factors probably have a role in the aetiopathogenesis of myelodysplasia.

Diagnostic criteria

- The current classification, with 8 subtypes is from WHO (2001) (15.39). The classification requires several specialist investigations and can be difficult to apply. The basic starting-point is bone marrow examination, which can provide classification for some of the subtypes. Attention is paid to the following:
  - Cytopenias of blood
  - Cell morphology, where e.g. pathological lobulation of nuclei (e.g. pseudo-Pelger-Huët anomaly and overlobulation), neutrophil hypogranularity and micromegakaryocytes point to dysplasia.
  - Number of bone marrow blasts (class boundaries 5%, 10% and 19%)
  - Presence of pathological ringed sideroblasts.

Differential diagnosis

- Acute myeloid leukaemia, chronic myeloproliferative diseases, chronic myelomonocytic leukaemia
- Megaloblastic anaemias and toxic bone marrow disorders (e.g. ethanol)

Clinical picture and laboratory findings

- A heterogenous group
- Some patients are asymptomatic; the diagnosis is suggested by incidental findings in a blood count (cytopenias).
- Symptoms resulting from cytopenias or impaired blood cell function:
  - Anaemia
  - Infections
  - Bleeding.
- Laboratory findings:
  - Cytopenias
  - Macrocytosis in some patients
  - Structural anomalies in neutrophils
  - Dysplastic features in bone marrow

- Dysfunction of neutrophils and platelets detectable by special tests
- Many patients have chromosomal aberrations in the bone marrow.

Primary investigations

- Peripheral blood smear
- Bone marrow examination (with iron staining to detect pathological ringed sideroblasts)
- The WHO classification requires in most cases chromosome and molecular biology examinations in addition to bone marrow examination (15.39). Because the treatment and prognosis are determined by the MDS subtype, a consultation with a haematologist is in order in the first months.

Clinical course and prognosis

- The clinical course and prognosis vary greatly. The prognosis is estimated according to the MDS subtype and clinical features. In the unfavourable class the median life expectancy is less than one month and over 24 months in the most favourable.

Complications

- Anaemia
- Infections
- Bleeding
- Acute leukaemia

Treatment and prognosis

- There is no specific or curative treatment for most patients. Allogeneic stem cell transplantation can be considered in young patients and in cases where the expected disease progression is rapid. Follow-up with active supportive therapy is usually the best option.
  - Treatment of infections (antibiotics)
  - Control of bleeding (platelet transfusions)
  - Red cell transfusions (the transfusion threshold is decided individually; usually a haemoglobin concentration of 70 g/l necessitates transfusions).
- Chemotherapy is usually palliative, but in some cases the goal is long-lasting remission, which can be attained with intensive chemotherapy and, if necessary, stem cell transplantation.
- Some patients have responded to various other treatments (erythropoietin, growth factors G-CSF and GM-CSF, vitamin A, retinoids, glucocorticoids, haemearginate, pyridoxal phosphate, apoptosis-inhibitors, antiangiogenics, tumour necrosis factor alpha inhibitors (anti-TNFs)).
- The treatment is planned by a specialist.
- The follow-up interval is 1–6–12 months according to the patient's condition.

15.49 Essential thrombocythaemia (ET)

Juhani Vilpo

Pathology

- ET is a chronic myeloproliferative haematological malignancy characterized by accelerated platelet production and gradually worsening thrombocythaemia.

Epidemiology

- ET is less common than chronic myeloid leukaemia or polycythaemia vera.
- The estimated incidence is $<$ 1 case/100 000/year.

Aetiology

- Unknown.

Criteria for diagnosis (WHO recommendations)

- Positive criteria
  - Long-lasting thrombocythaemia (months): blood platelet count $\geq 600 \times 10^9$/l
  - Bone marrow sample: increased amount of megakaryocytes, abnormal morphology
- Conditions that need to be excluded
  - Polycythaemia vera (15.41)
  - Chronic myelogenous leukaemia (15.40)
  - Myelofibrosis (chronic, idiopathic) (15.42)
  - Myelodysplastic syndromes (15.48)
  - Reactive thrombocytoses (15.9)

Differential diagnosis

- Secondary thrombocytosis (see Table 15.49).
  - Rheumatoid arthritis and other connective tissue diseases
  - Infections, inflammations
  - Malignant tumours
  - Tissue damage
  - Haemorrhage and iron deficiency
- Other myeloproliferative disorders (polycythaemia vera, myelofibrosis, chronic myelogenous leukaemia)

Clinical picture

- ET is detected incidentally in routine blood examination in symptomless patients.

Table 15.49 Differential diagnosis of thrombocytosis: clinical picture and laboratory investigations

Clinical picture and laboratory findings	Reactive thrombocytosis	Essential thrombocytosis
Thrombosis/bleeding	Rare	Frequent
Course	Temporary	Permanent, deteriorating
Splenomegaly	No	60–80%
Platelet count ($\times 10^9$/l)	Usually < 1000	Usually > 1000
Platelet morphology and function	Normal	Often pathological
Leucocyte count	Mostly normal	Increased (in ca. 90%)
Leucocyte alkaline phosphatase staining	Normal	Often increased
Bone marrow	Often normal	Megakaryocytes: increased number and pathological morphology
Spontaneous growth in stem cell culture	No	In most cases

- Ischaemic symptoms in cerebral circulation and in fingers and toes (known as erythromelalgia; in over 15% of patients)
- Thrombosis (in 10–15%)
- Haemorrhages, particularly in mucous membranes, easy bruising (in less than 10%)

Laboratory findings

- See also Table 15.49.
- Blood platelet count permanently > 600×10^9/l.
- Bone marrow morphology is often typical.
- Splenomegaly in advanced cases
- Spontaneous colony formation in stem cell culture (often)

Disease progression and prognosis

- Chronic
  - Median survival approximately 5 years
  - Increasing use of thrombocyte count reveals milder cases more often.

Complications

- Haemorrhages
- Thrombosis
- Leukaemic transformation (rare)

Treatment and follow-up

- There is a shortage of reliable clinical information concerning the treatment of ET. It is therefore advisable to consult a haematologist when making the diagnosis.
- Patients below 60 years without risk factors of thrombosis are not treated, if the blood platelet count is below 1500×10^9/l.
- A trial of antiplatelet aspirin prophylaxis (100 mg/day) is indicated in patients with arterial hypertension, atherosclerosis or ischaemic symptoms, and in smokers. Symptoms resolve within hours and the Aspirin effect lasts for 2–3 days.
  - A high risk for thrombosis or haemorrhage: previous thrombosis or haemorrhage, age over 60 years or thrombocyte count > 1500×10^9/l are other risk factors for thrombosis.
- Cytoreductive therapy
  - Hydroxyurea: fast (effect starts within a few days) and short-lasting effect. Only slightly leukaemogenic.
  - Busulphan: effect starts more slowly and lasts longer.
  - ^{32}P: most appropriate for elderly people.
  - Anagrelide
  - Thrombapheresis and ASA are given as emergency treatment, if there are severe cerebral symptoms or danger of necrosis.
- Treatment strategy is planned in cooperation with a specialist in internal medicine or haematology.
- Follow-up at the beginning every 2–4 months and in the stable phase every 6–12 months.

15.60 Indications for and techniques of red cell transfusion

Editors

Basic rule

- Clinically significant (symptomatic) acute or chronic anaemia should be corrected by transfusion if there is no specific treatable cause or if the clinical condition requires rapid correction of the anaemia.

Indications for red cell transfusion

- Red cell transfusion can be performed in primary care in the following cases:
  - **After acute bleeding (e.g. epistaxis or wound) if the blood loss is between 20 and 40% of total blood volume.**
    - Physiological saline can always be used as first aid in acute anaemia.
    - The general condition of the patient and underlying diseases should always be taken into account when deciding on the need for red cell transfusion. The

haemoglobin concentration is just one of the criteria. In patients with ischaemic heart disease even a small decrease in the haemoglobin may increase the risk of myocardial infarction.
  - If the patient has lost more than 50% of his/her blood volume, plasma constituents must be administered in addition to volume correction and red cell transfusion. Refer the patient to a specialized hospital.
  - If bleeding continues (in the gastrointestinal tract) the patient should be referred to a hospital where transfusions can be performed and the bleeding stopped endoscopically (8.52).
  - Peroral iron substitution (100 mg $Fe^{++} \times 2$) should be started at once and continued for at least 2 months.
- **Chronic therapy-resistant (normovolaemic) anaemia** (15.23)
  - The main target is to maintain the patient's usual physical exercise capacity.
  - Transfusions are not routinely recommended for patients with malignant disease or severe systemic disease unless the transfusions can be expected to improve the patient's condition or independence.
  - The transfusion threshold must be individually determined for each patient. Most patients have annoying symptoms of anaemia if the haemoglobin concentration is below 70 g/l. Transfusion of 2–4 units of red cells is usually performed. If the patient has cardiac or pulmonary symptoms the threshold haemoglobin value (determined by the symptoms) is higher. In some patients the haemoglobin concentration must be kept above 120 g/l, with the drawback that spontaneous red cell production may decrease and the interval between transfusions may be shortened.

Selection of the red cell concentrate in special cases

- **Red cell concentrate without leucocytes**: correction of anaemia in patients who must avoid HLA immunisation or cytomegalovirus infection.
  - Aplastic anaemia or leukaemia
  - Before and after organ transplantation
  - Patients with suspected haematological disease
  - Paroxysmal nocturnal haemoglobinuria (PNH)
  - Pregnancy
  - Patients who have had a febrile reaction from leucocytes in a red cell concentrate B [1,2].
- PNH; washed red cells (complement has been removed)
- Deficiency of IgA; washed red cells (IgA has been removed)
- Deficiency of IgA and anti-IgA antibodies; red cells from a donor with IgA deficiency or five times washed red cells
- Immunodeficiency associated with, for example, cytostatic drugs or immunosuppression; irradiated red cells (to prevent graft versus host reaction)
- Typed red cells if the patient has clinically significant antibodies
- The red cell unit should be warmed (+37°C) before transfusion if the patient has cold agglutinins.

Techniques of red cell transfusion

1. **Take a blood sample for blood group and compatibility test**
   - Check the identity of the patient.
   - With the exception of emergencies, blood samples for blood group determination and compatibility tests should be taken at different times by different persons.
   - The samples should be stored in a refrigerator as whole blood. They remain analysable for five days.
2. **Check the blood unit**
   - The blood group on the bag label corresponds to the blood group recorded in the patient's notes (see below).
   - Red cells from donors with other than identical (but compatible) blood groups can be used much more freely than whole blood products (15.7). The rules on acceptable incompatibility should be clear in advance.
   - Check the compatibility test: the numbers on the bag and on the tube should match (the compatibility test has been performed using the correct unit) and the compatibility test should have been recorded as performed.
3. Check the patient's **identity**.
4. Check vital functions (**blood pressure, pulse, temperature**) before the transfusion.
5. **Infusion**
   - The infusion needle should be sufficiently thick (e.g. a green Viggo® needle).
   - One unit (about 320 ml) is infused over 1–2 hours in a normovolaemic patient. Two units can be infused one after another; thereafter a break of a few hours is recommended, at least in elderly patients.
   - If the patient has heart failure and oedema or pulmonary congestion 20 mg of furosemide should be administered intravenously during the transfusion of each unit.
   - Monitor the patient carefully, particularly during the first 15 minutes of the transfusion. For actions to be taken if a transfusion reaction occurs see 15.61.

References

1. Gibis B, Baladi JF. Leukoreduction: the techniques used, their effectiveness and costs. Canadian Coordinating Office of Health Technology Assessment 1998;6E:1–79.
2. The Database of Abstracts of Reviews of Effectiveness (University of York), Database no.: DARE-988596. In: The Cochrane Library, Issue 4, 1999. Oxford: Update Software.

15.61 Transfusion reactions

Editors

Actions to be taken when a transfusion reaction is suspected

- Stop the administration of blood products immediately.
- Treat the reaction with supportive measures.
- Consult a specialist in a national/regional transfusion centre.
- As a precaution for assessing transfusion reactions the compatibility blood samples should be stored in the laboratory and a piece of the tubing of every transfusion bag should be stored at the ward for about five days after the transfusion.

The most common transfusion reactions

- See Table 15.61.
- **Fever** is treated symptomatically. Fever caused by a transfusion usually subsides rapidly (in 8–10 hours at the latest).
- **Urticaria** occurs in 1–2% of patients receiving a transfusion. The causative agent is probably a substance in the transfused blood to which the patient is allergic. Antihistamines can be used for symptomatic treatment. Serological investigations are not indicated.
- Fever, restlessness, a feeling of pressure in the chest, and particularly low back pain are signs of an **immediate haemolytic reaction**. The urine turns reddish brown. The patient is often hypotensive. Treatment consists of fluid therapy (maintenance of adequate diuresis), and intravenous corticosteroids.
- Rapid development of anaemia, and sometimes fever, nausea, and jaundice are signs of a **delayed haemolytic reaction.** The laboratory results include a high serum concentration of unconjugated bilirubin, a positive direct Coombs' test result, and an increased serum concentration of lactate dehydrogenase. The condition is rarely serious.
- **Anaphylaxis** caused by IgA antibodies is a rare but very dangerous transfusion reaction.

Table 15.61 The most common transfusion reactions

Reaction	Incidence / 1 million of population annually	Aetiology
Fever	About 100	Leucocyte antibodies
Urticaria	About 100	Unknown
Delayed haemolytic reaction	5–10	Erythrocyte antibodies
Immediate haemolytic reaction	0.4–1	Erythrocyte antibodies

Oncology

Evidence Based Medicine Guidelines. Edited by the Duodecim Editorial Team
© 2005 John Wiley & Sons, Ltd ISBN: 0-470-01184-X

16.1 Adverse effects of radiotherapy

Risto Johansson

- Radiotherapy is a local treatment modality and therefore the side effects are almost invariably local. Systemic adverse effects are seen after half- or total-body radiotherapy or in radiation accidents.

Skin and mucosal lesions

- **Skin reactions** comprise redness and dry or moist epithelitis. These often appear already during the radiotherapy. A mild reaction will heal by itself within two to four weeks.
- Severe reactions are treated like burn wounds.
- Late symptoms include thinning of skin and even telangiectasia; no specific treatment is needed. The function of sweat glands is impaired, and the skin feels thin and dry.
- **Loss of hair** from the irradiated area occurs three to six weeks after the start of therapy. Generally the hair will regrow, albeit sometimes in different colour or more curled.
- Depending on the site of irradiation, mucosal irritation manifests as **stomatitis, oesophagitis, intestinal irritation or diarrhoea**.
- Irritation of the mouth and oesophagus is treated with sucralfate, topical antifungal agents and, if required, lidocaine gel before a meal. Very warm, coarse and spicy foods must be avoided.
- Diseases of the teeth and mouth should be treated before radiotherapy to the jaw area. After radiotherapy special attention should be paid on oral and dental hygiene and regular check ups and treatment are necessary **C** [1 2]. Gingival and dental operations should be avoided; if needed urgently, these should be performed at specialist dental units. The mouth feels dry if the salivary glands are irradiated. Treatment consists of artificial saliva and dietary councelling.
- The treatment of **diarrhoea** is symptomatic, ensuring sufficient hydration. Late effects may include intestinal stenoses up to several years afterwards. Persistent diarrhoea calls for faecal culture; treatment is based on the result of the culture.
- **Irritation of the urinary bladder** manifests as frequent micturition, sometimes as pain. Infections have to be excluded and treated. Treatment consists of analgesics according to the severity of symptoms. Warm sitz baths are used as local therapy.
- Irradiation of the eye region causes **conjunctivitis**. Treatment consists of locally administered eye drops.
- **Cataract** is a late effect from irradiation of the eye; treatment consists of cataract surgery.

Other organ damage

- **Radiation pneumonitis** appears two to six months after irradiation hitting the lungs. The symptoms comprise dry, nonproductive cough and mild fever. Chest x-rays may show shadowing in the irradiated area. Radiation pneumonitis is treated with antitussives, sometimes even with codeine tablets. An antibiotic and prednisolone at 10–25 mg three times daily may be administered for two to four weeks.
- Parts of renal tissue are usually spared in a way that the damage does not cause clinical symptoms. Local reactions include atrophy and fibrosis as well as occlusion of small vessels.
- Radiotherapy to the heart area may cause fibrosis, increased cardiac morbidity and, in the worst case, constrictive pericarditis as late sequelae.
- The hormone and gamete production of the reproductive system is damaged by a fairly low dose of irradiation.
- The spinal cord tolerates about 45 Gy in 5 weeks. Higher doses involve the risk of insidious, progressing paraparesis that begins within months of the treatment and that may be difficult to distinguish from symptoms caused by a tumour.

Haematological adverse effects

- **Leuco- and thrombocytopenia**, sometimes anaemia, are encountered after extensive radiotherapy, such as half- or total-body radiotherapy. These are self-limiting and subside within a few weeks. In rare cases, blood cell transfusions, growth factors or even bone marrow transplantation may be required. A moderate decrease in blood count after normal radiotherapy does not require treatment; however, severe neutro- or thrombopenia is managed in an oncology unit.

General symptoms

- Radiotherapy of the head can cause oedema and elevation of **intracranial pressure**. The treatment is dexamethasone 3–9 mg three times daily tapered off gradually after the end of radiotherapy.
- **Nausea** may result from total-body, half-body, intestinal or head irradiation. Treatment consists of metoclopramide and, in central nervous system irritation, corticosteroids. Administration of serotonin-3 receptor antagonists is worth trying if other drugs are not effective **B** [3 4].
- The occurrence of **fatigue and mental symptoms** is variable. The treatment is symptomatic. Appropriate mental support should be arranged.
- In total-body radiotherapy and radiation accidents the first symptoms appear within minutes or hours after high doses of radiation. These include nausea, fatigue, loss of muscle strength, and confusion. A person who is initially asymptomatic may develop the gastrointestinal syndrome within a few days (nausea, diarrhoea, mucosal damage of the intestine, bleeding). If left untreated the syndrome can progress to fatal paralytic ileus. Even a lower dose of irradiation causes leuco- and thrombopenia within a few weeks, which can also be fatal if not treated.
- Radiotherapy of children may cause **disturbances of bone and cartilage growth** as well as impairment of mental development.

References

1. Kowanko I, Long L, Hodgkinson B, Evans D. The effectiveness of strategies for preventing and treating chemotherapy and radiation induced oral mucositis. Adelaide: The Joanna Briggs Institute for Evidence-Based Nursing and Midwifery. A systematic review. 1998. 1–84.
2. The Database of Abstracts of Reviews of Effectiveness (University of York), Database no.: DARE-999776. In: The Cochrane Library, Issue 2, 2001. Oxford: Update Software.
3. Tramer MR, Reynolds DJ, Stoner NS, Moore RA, McQuay HJ. Efficacy of 5-HT3 receptor antagonists in radiotherapy-induced nausea and vomiting: a quantitative systematic review. European Journal of Cancer 1998;34:1836–1844.
4. The Database of Abstracts of Reviews of Effectiveness (University of York), Database no.: DARE-990019. In: The Cochrane Library, Issue 2, 2001. Oxford: Update Software.

16.2 Adverse effects of antineoplastic drugs

Risto Johansson

Nausea and vomiting

- Different antineoplastic drugs and their combinations cause a varying degree of nausea. Some drugs do not affect the patient more than placebo, while the most problematic drugs, such as cisplatin, doxorubicin and dacarbazine, cause nausea in almost all patients.
- Acute nausea or vomiting begins already during drug infusion or within 2–6 hours after the infusion. With mildly emetogenic drugs metoclopramide 20 mg is effective, with more emetogenic ones serotonin 5-HT3-receptor antagonists (ondansetron 8 mg, tropisetron 5 mg, or granisetron 3 mg B [1 2]) are given i.v. 30–60 minutes before infusion of the antineoplastic drug to prevent vomiting A [3 4]. Concomitant administration of corticoids (dexamethasone 10 mg i.v.) increases the efficacy of the treatment.
- Metoclopramide 10–30 mg three times daily is effective in prolonged and delayed vomiting (2–6 days after infusion of the antineoplastic drug), concomitantly with corticoids, if necessary. An oral 5-HT3-receptor antagonist may be used if other treatments fail.
- Anxiolytic drugs prevent anticipatory nausea (the mere fear of treatment, e.g. smell or sight of hospital, may be enough to initiate nausea), e.g. lorazepam 1–5 mg p.o., or even i.m. injection of benzodiazepine a few hours before admission to the hospital.

Blood cytopenias

- Potent antineoplastic treatments cause leucopenia, thrombocytopenia and even anaemia. These typically appear within 1–3 weeks.
- Neutropenia (15.5) is associated with increased risk of infections. Treatment with **colony stimulating factors** (G-CSF or GM-CSF) decreases the risk. The effect is best if the treatment is initiated within 24–48 hours after the antineoplastic infusion, when the blood count still is normal. In a prolonged neuropenia, colony-stimulating factor may be given even later on. Initially, the white cell count decreases further, but within 6–14 days of treatment the values start improving. Severe blood cytopenias are treated in a special care unit, with bone marrow or stem cell transfusion, if necessary.
- **Thrombocytopenia** is sometimes treated with thrombocyte transfusion, but most often a spontaneous remission can be expected. Factors stimulating thrombopoiesis are under investigation.
- **Anaemia** is treated with red cell transfusions, a prolonged anaemia with erythropoietin.

Hair loss

- Hair loss is a common adverse effect of most antineoplastic drugs. Choosing another antineoplastic drug can sometimes prevent it. The use of a special cooling cap during the infusion of cytostatics may inhibit or decrease alopecia.
- Hair is lost 3–5 weeks after the first antineoplastic infusion and it usually grows back, after cessation of the treatment, sometimes already during it.

Organ-specific effects

- Anthracyclines (doxorubicin and epirubicin) cause myocardial damage, which may manifest even months after the treatment. The condition is rare if the cumulative dose is kept low. Sometimes the damage becomes apparent first months or years after the administration of the drug.
- Bleomycin, busulphan, mitomycin and methotrexate may damage the lungs. Differentiating this condition from changes caused by the cancer, such as lymphangitis carcinomatosa, and from infections is often difficult.
- Cisplatin and high doses of methotrexate may damage the kidneys.
- Many antineoplastic drugs cause immediate tissue damage if they escape the vein. The damage may progress chronically and requires extensive surgical removal of the damaged tissue. Pain during infusion (if not caused by drug outside the vein) can be alleviated by slowing the infusion rate or with an irrigating solution. Fluorouracil can cause innocent discoloration of the veins even when administered properly intravenously.
- Cisplatin, vincristine and taxanes cause peripheral neuropathy, which appears as numbness and muscular weakness in the extremities.

- Cyclophosphamide and iphosphamide cause irritation in the urinary bladder. This may be prevented with uromitexan (mesna).
- Many drugs cause mucosal damage, liver dysfunction, electrolyte disturbances, functional cardiac symptoms, and allergic reactions.

References

1. Perez EA. Review of the preclinical pharmacology and comparative efficacy 5-hydroxytryptamine-3-receptor antagonists for chemotherapy-induced emesis. J Clin Oncol 1995;13:1036–1043.
2. The Database of Abstracts of Reviews of Effectiveness (University of York), Database no.: DARE-950862. In: The Cochrane Library, Issue 4, 1999. Oxford: Update Software.
3. Jantunen IT, Kataja VV, Muhonen TT. An overview of randomised studies comparing 5-HT3 receptor antagonists versus conventional anti-emetics in the prophylaxis of acute chemotherapy-induced vomiting. Eur J Cancer 1997;33:66–74.
4. The Database of Abstracts of Reviews of Effectiveness (University of York), Database no.: DARE-970313. In: The Cochrane Library, Issue 4, 1999. Oxford: Update Software.

16.10 Pharmacological treatment of cancer pain

Eija Kalso

Basic rules

- Therapies that are effective against the cancer itself, such as antineoplastic agents, radiotherapy and surgery, often also relieve pain efficiently. If these treatments are not sufficient alone or if they cannot be used, pain is managed with medications or regional anaesthesia.
- Pain medication is increased stepwise D [1] [2] (Figure 16.10.1).
  - Treatment is started with NSAIDs or paracetamol, unless these are contraindicated.
  - An opioid is added when the pain becomes more severe.
- The principles of pain management are
  - effectiveness
  - feasibility
  - continuous pain relief at a stable dose by using a sustained-release drug

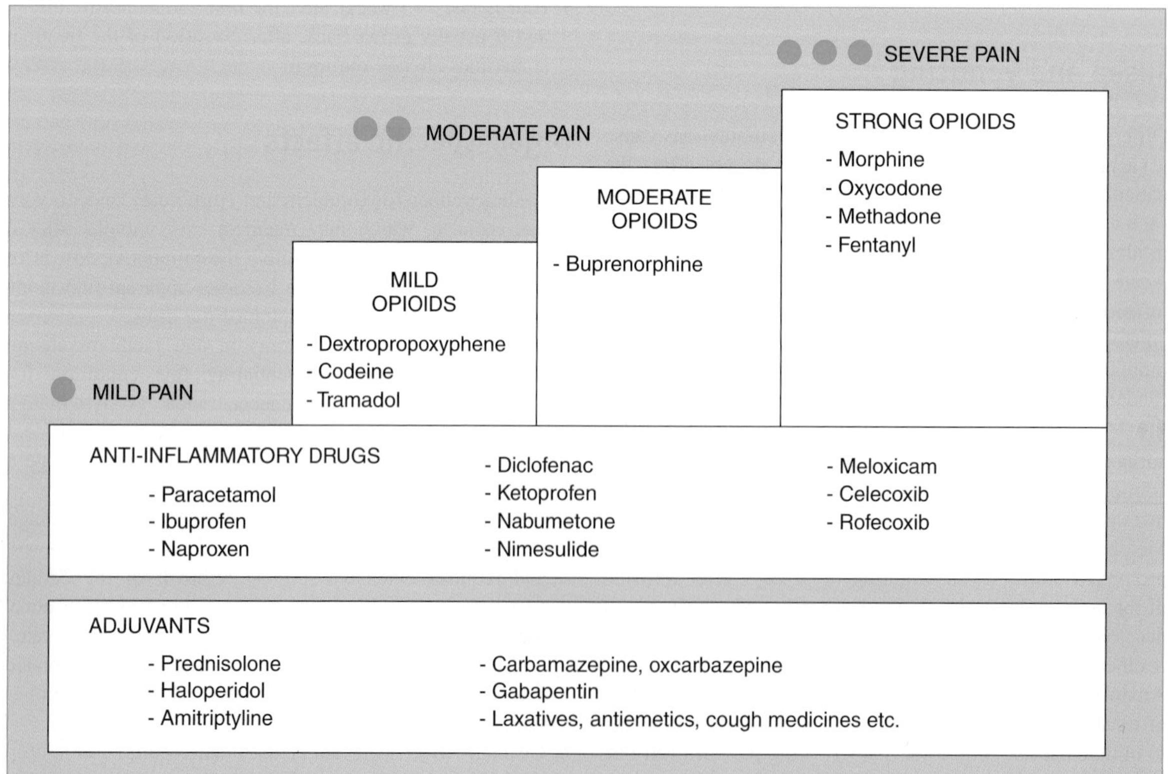

Figure 16.10.1 WHO's Pain Relief Ladder

- management of pain peaks with a rapid-acting drug
- minimization of adverse effects by changing the opioid or route of administration or by managing them with suitable drugs.
- regular follow-up of the therapy:
  - does the patient use the prescribed drugs?
  - if not, why (misconceptions, adverse effects?)
  - is pain relieved with the prescribed dose?
  - measurement of pain

NSAIDs

- The efficacy of different NSAIDs in the management of cancer pain has not been compared. In the range of recommended doses, a clear dose-response has been shown for various NSAIDs (better pain relief with higher doses).
- Adverse effects to be considered include hypersensitivity and effects on gastric mucosa, thrombocytes and renal circulation **C** [3].
  - During treatment with some cytostatics (e.g. methotrexate) only paracetamol is safe to use.
  - Gastric irritation can be alleviated with sucralfate, H_2 antagonists, proton pump inhibitors (omeprazole, lansoprazole and pantoprazole), and with a prostaglandin E_1 analogue (misoprostole).
  - Selective COX-2 inhibitors cause less GI damage and do not prevent thrombocyte aggregation. As to renal function, they have no advantage over other NSAIDs.
- Different NSAIDs should not be administered simultaneously. If the drug is not efficient alone, an opioid should be combined with it.
- An NSAID should be continued with the opioid if it has been beneficial as these two drugs with different modes of action usually give better pain relief when they are combined.

Opioids

- Severity of pain determines which opioid should be used. Opioids can be classified into three groups on the basis of their efficacy and ceiling effect:
  - Weak opioids
    - Dextropropoxyphene, codeine (only in combination products) and tramadol
  - Medium-strength opioids
    - Buprenorphine
  - Strong opioids
    - Methadone
    - Morphine
    - Oxycodone
    - Fentanyl (as a transdermal patch)
- Interindividual differences in adverse effects and efficacy may be significant. If an adequate dose of one opioid is not effective, change to another.
- If your patient is in severe pain, start with a rapid-acting oxycodone or morphine solution or with normal release oxycodone tablets. When the right dose has been found, the patient can change to a sustained-release tablet.
- If your patient has breakthrough pain, prescribe morphine or normal release oxycodone solution or oxycodone tablets in addition to sustained-release tablets.
- Opioids very rarely cause psychological dependence in cancer patients.
- Because of neuroadaptation (physiological dependence) sudden discontinuation of opioid medication leads to withdrawal symptoms (this is not psychological dependence). Therefore, **opioids should not be discontinued abruptly**.
- If the pain is opioid-sensitive (alleviated with opioids), the effect will not wear off even if the patient uses the drug for several years.

HAE

Constant pain relief and treatment of pain peaks

- Morphine **A** [4] and oxycodone are available as sustained-release tablets that are administered twice daily. The effect of sustained-release preparations begins within one to two hours.
- Breakthrough pain requires rapid relief, which is achieved with morphine or oxycodone solution or normal release oxycodone tablets. The additional dose for breakthrough pain is one sixth of the normal daily dose of the corresponding preparation.

Avoid intramuscular injections!

- Oral opioids are a more simple and humane option compared with intramuscular injections; a terminal-phase patient has little muscle tissue left, injections are painful and have to be repeated at 2–4-h intervals. A patient in poor condition has trouble learning to pull a small amount of the drug into the syringe and to inject it.
- Oral administration of a liquid opioid is as effective as i.m. administration, as long as the dose is sufficient.

Subcutaneous infusion when oral administration is unsuccessful

- If the patient cannot take oral medication because of a GI obstruction or severe nausea, constant pain relief can be achieved with subcutaneous infusion. Both morphine (1/3 of the daily oral dose) and oxycodone (1/2 of the daily oral dose) can be given as a subcutaneous infusion.
- An antiemetic can be administered concomitantly with the opioid infusion (haloperidol 2–5 mg/day).
- Transdermal fentanyl **A** [4] is an alternative to subcutaneous infusion. The patch is changed every 72 hours. The dose of transdermal fentanyl can be calculated from the daily oral dose of morphine (Table 16.10).

Table 16.10 Dose of transdermal fentanyl

Oral dose of morphine (mg/24h)	Dose of transdermal fentanyl (μg/h)
<135	25
135–224	50
225–314	75
315–404	100

Problematic pains

- Opioids as such do not always provide adequate pain relief. Pain caused by nerve damage or fractures may be problematic.
- A cancer patient may have a purely **neuropathic pain**, e.g. polyneuropathy caused by antineoplastic agents. This pain is managed as neuropathic pain in general: with **antidepressants** (amitriptyline 25–75 mg daily) or **antiepileptic drugs** (carbamazepine 400–800 mg D [5 6], oxcarbazepine 300–600 mg daily or gabapentin 900–3200 mg daily).
- The tumour may compress or infiltrate nerve tissue. Management often requires large doses of opioids or regional anaesthesia (consult an anaesthesiologist).
- In severe pain spinal drug delivery may be considered (opioid, local anaesthetic agent, alpha-2-adrenergic agonist such as clonidine, NMDA antagonist such as ketamine), freezing of sensory nerves, and neurosurgical procedures
- The role of psychosocial factors should not be underestimated in the management of terminal phase cancer pain.

Examples of oral opioids

Codeine

- Ibuprofen 200 mg + codeine 30 mg A [7 8]
- Paracetamol 500 mg + codeine 30 mg B [9 10]
- Approximately 10% of caucasians are "slow metabolizers" who do not metabolise codeine to morphine and the drug has no effect.

Dextropropoxyphene

- 65 mg × 3–4, (sustained-release) 150 mg × 2
- Dangerous with alcohol. Cardiotoxic.

Tramadol

- Nausea is the most common adverse effect. Tramadol inhibits serotonin and noradrenaline re-uptake. Its weak opioid effect is transmitted mainly by metabolites. Metabolism is affected by drugs that inhibit the CYP 2D6 isoenzyme.

Buprenorphine

- Maximum daily dose is approximately 4.2 mg.
- Buprenorphine is a partial opioid agonist. In high doses it's analgesic efficacy may decrease as well as that of other opioids. Dizziness and nausea are the most common adverse effects.

Strong opioids

- Strong opioids do not have maximum doses. If pain is alleviated by opioids, more relief is expected if the dose is increased. Therefore, only starting doses are given for strong opioids. The starting dose is determined by the intensity of pain and the patient's condition. Elderly persons are usually more susceptible than younger patients.

Methadone

- Orally administered methadone has a good bioavailability. It may be more effective than other opioids in the management of neuropathic pain.
- Pharmacokinetics of methadone is complicated. Only to be administrated by experienced personnel.

Morphine

- Morphine is the basic opioid. With oral administration its bioavailability is poor and variable. The parenteral dose is usually 1/4–1/3 of the oral dose. In renal failure, the dose must be reduced. Morphine is a potent releaser of histamine.

Oxycodone

- The bioavailability of oxycodone with oral administration is good. The parenteral dose is usually 1/2–2/3 of the oral dose. Adverse effects are the same as those of morphine. Some patients have less nausea and nightmares compared with morphine.

Fentanyl

- Fentanyl is a very potent opioid. Treatment with transdermal patches is suited only in patients whose pain is well managed. Fentanyl is not suited when the dose is first being titrated or when the severity of pain varies greatly during the day.
- Pain relief begin within 12 hours after the first patch has been placed. When the patient changes from sustained-release morphine or oxycodone tablets to a fentanyl patch, the last tablet is given when the first patch is placed.
- Fentanyl patch is indicated in patients who cannot take pain medication orally. If several patches are required to manage the pain, consider changing the mode of administration (s.c. infusion).
- Fentanyl does not release histamine at all.
- For choice of fentanyl patch, see Table 16.10.
- The patch is changed every 72 hours.

Equipotent oral daily doses for the starting phase

- Morphine 60 mg
- Oxycodone 40 mg
- Fentanyl 25 μg/hour (transdermal patch)
- These doses are suggestive. Titration must be carried out individually. When the patient changes from one strong opioid to another after having used it even for a week, the dose relationships may vary unexpectedly.

The most common adverse effects of opioids and their management

- Sedation (usually alleviated after the starting phase)
- Nausea (usually alleviated soon)
    - Management: haloperidol 0.5–1 mg × 3. If nausea is severe and/or persists, try changing the opioid and, in complicated cases, the mode of administration
- Constipation (unavoidable and persistent)
    - Management: laxatives, e.g. sodium picosulphate and lactulose
- Pruritus (usually a direct opioid receptor effect; morphine releases histamine, which may be the cause of pruritus)
- Sweating
- Accommodation disturbance (difficult to read!)
- Nightmares (both at night and/or during the day)
    - Management: change the opioid or start haloperidol
- Muscle cramps (particularly with high doses of morphine)
    - Management: change the opioid, try benzodiazepines
- Respiratory depression is usually not a problem if the dose is related to the amount of pain. If the pain is suddenly alleviated by, for example, regional anaesthesia, respiratory depression may occur.
    - Management: oxygen. Urge the patient to breathe. In emergency situations give naloxone intravenously e.g. 0.4 mg.
- Palliative treatment, see also 16.11.

Prescriptions of opioid solutions (examples)

- Morphine solution (4 mg/ml); the solution may be more potent, e.g. 10 mg/ml)
    - Morphine hydrochloride 4 mg
    - Methyl paraoxybenzoate 1 mg
    - Aqua menth. piperit. ad 1 ml
    - M.D. 500 ml S.
    - 5 ml × 6 daily for severe pain.
- Oxycodone solution (3 mg/ml); equals morphine solution 4 mg/ml
    - Oxycodone hydrochlorid 3 mg
    - Aqua menth. piperit. c. conservans ad 1 ml
    - M.D. 500 ml S
    - 5 ml × 6 /day orally for severe pain.

References

1. Jadad AR, Browman GP. The WHO analgesic ladder for cancer pain management: stepping up the quality of its evaluation. JAMA 1995;274:1870–1873.
2. The Database of Abstracts of Reviews of Effectiveness (University of York), Database no.: DARE-968010. In: The Cochrane Library, Issue 4, 1999. Oxford: Update Software.
3. Perez Gutthann SP, Garcia Rodriquez LAG, Raiford DS, Duque Oliart AD, Ris Romeu JR. Nonsteroidal anti-inflammatory drugs and the risk of hospitalisation for acute renal failure. Arch Intern Med 1996; 156: 2433–9.
4. Wiffen PJ, Edwards JE, Barden J, McQuay HJM. Oral morphine for cancer pain. Cochrane Database Syst Rev 2003(4):CD003868.
5. McQuay H, Carroll D, Jadad AR, Wiffen P, Moore A. Anticonvulsant drugs for management of pain: a systematic review. BMJ 1995;311:1047–1052.
6. The Database of Abstracts of Reviews of Effectiveness (University of York), Database no.: DARE-953055. In: The Cochrane Library, Issue 4, 1999. Oxford: Update Software.
7. Li Wan Po A, Zhang WY. Analgesic efficacy of ibuprofen alone and in combination with codeine or caffeine in post-surgical pain: a meta-analysis. Eur J Clin Pharmacol 1998;53:303–311.
8. The Database of Abstracts of Reviews of Effectiveness (University of York), Database no.: DARE-980366. In: The Cochrane Library, Issue 4, 1999. Oxford: Update Software.
9. de Craen AJM, di Giulio G, Lampe-Schoenmaechers AJEM, Kessels AGH, Kleijnen J. Analgesic efficacy and safety of paracetamol-codeine combinations versus paracetamol alone: a systematic review. BMJ 1996;313:321–325.
10. The Database of Abstracts of Reviews of Effectiveness (University of York), Database no.: DARE-968384. In: The Cochrane Library, Issue 4, 1999. Oxford: Update Software.

16.11 Palliative treatment of cancer

Rita Janes

Aims

- The duration of palliative treatment for cancer ranges from months and years to a few days. Treatment of the cancer with antineoplastic drugs or radiotherapy may alleviate the symptoms of a patient in a better condition efficiently, while care and alleviation of pain (16.10) are central in the treatment of a dying patient. At each stage of the disease the aim is to find therapies with beneficial effects outweighing the adverse effects. The treatment alternatives given in this article should be considered from this perspective.
- Discuss treatment alternatives with the patient. Explain the probable aetiology of the symptoms, engage family members in the treatment, and consult with specialists.

Respiratory symptoms

Cough: causes and treatment alternatives

- Heart failure, asthma, COPD: treatment according to the disease.

- Infection: antibiotics, antipyretics.
- Lung metastases, tumour-induced irritation of the pharynx and airways
  - Prednisone 40–60 mg × 1 or dexamethasone 6–9 mg × 1 with dose tapering according to response
  - Antitussive medication, see below.
  - Radiotherapy
- Pleural effusion
  - Pleural aspiration (not more than 1500 ml at a time), drainage +/− sclerotherapy
  - Prednisone 40–60 mg × 1 or dexamethasone 6–9 mg × 1 with dose tapering according to response
  - Antitussive medication, see below.
- Haemoptysis
  - Tranexamic acid 1000–1500 mg × 3
  - Prednisone 40–60 mg × 1 or dexamethasone 6–9 mg × 1 with dose tapering according to response
  - Radiotherapy
- Drug- (bleomycin, methotrexate) or radiotherapy-induced pneumonitis. Radiation pneumonitis may appear (1–) 3 months after radiation of the lungs. It is seen as an opacity with the shape of the irradiation field on the chest x-ray. Fever may be present and CRP may be elevated.
  - Rest
  - Prednisone 40–60 mg × 1 or dexamethasone 6–9 mg × 1 with dose tapering according to response
  - Antitussives (see below), antibiotics if infection co-exists.
  - If you suspect drug-induced pneumonitis, contact the centre giving the cytostatic therapy.
- Pulmonary aspiration (pharyngeal palsy, obstructing tumour)
  - Pharyngeal palsy: eating sitting up with chin pointed downwards
  - Fluid is made thicker (e.g. Thick and Easy)
  - Radiation of the obstructive tumour, laser therapy or bypassing using a stent
  - Gastrostoma
- Productive cough/mucus secretion
  - Infection: antibiotics
  - Pain prevents the patient from coughing productively, coughing is difficult when the patient is lying down
    - Management of pain
    - Position therapy
    - Breathing into a bottle
  - Humidification of the air
  - Mucolytes (e.g. bromhexine 8 mg × 3)
  - If the patient is too weak to cough
    - Antitussives, see below
    - Aspiration of mucus from the airways is seldom necessary and it is unpleasant for a conscious patient.
    - Anticholinergics, e.g. glycopyrrolate 0.2 mg × 1–6 s.c. or 0.6–1.2 mg daily continuous s.c./i.v. infusion decreases mucus production in the airways but also dries the mouth.
- Antitussive medication
  - Opioids, e.g.
    - codeine 30–60 mg × 3–4
    - paracetamol 500 mg + codeine 30 mg 1–2 × 3–4
    - ibuprofein 200 mg + codeine 30 mg 1–2 × 3–4
    - morphine solution with a starting dose of 12–20 mg × 1–6
    - long-acting morphine with a starting dose of 10–30 mg × 2

Dyspnoea; causes and treatment alternatives

- Heart failure, asthma, COPD: treatment depends on the disease
- Pulmonary embolism: anticoagulant therapy
- Pneumonia: antibiotics, antipyretics
- Anaemia: red cell transfusion; in some cases erythropoietin may be indicated
- Fever: antipyretics.
- Partial pulmectomy, lung fibrosis: symptomatic therapy
- Drug- (bleomycin, methotrexate) or radiotherapy-induced pneumonitis, see under cough above.
- Tumour-induced causes of dyspnoea in the neck and thorax
  - Compression of the trachea, bronchi or the vena cava superior, atelectasis, lung metastases, lymphangitis carcinomatosa:
    - dexamethasone 3–10 mg × 1–3 with dose tapering according to response
    - radiotherapy
    - consider laser therapy or a stent
  - Pleural effusion
    - Pleural aspiration (not more than 1500 ml at a time), drainage +/− sclerotherapy
    - Prednisone 40–60 mg × 1 or dexamethasone 6–9 mg × 1 with dose tapering according to response
  - Pericardial tamponade
    - Aspiration
- Ascites, enlarged liver or large abdominal tumour:
  - Ascites puncture, diuretics
  - Elevation of the upper body, half-sitting position
  - Prednisone 40–60 mg × 1 or dexamethasone 6–9 mg × 1 with dose tapering according to response
- Anxiety, hyperventilation
  - Calming down, safe environment, a benzodiazepin
- Non-pharmacological management of dyspnoea
  - A patient with dyspnoea is often very restless. Anxiety may aggravate dyspnoea. Explain to the patient the course of the disease and teach how to act during acute attacks.
  - Consider whether you should discuss the fear of suffocation. Patients with a lung tumour or metastases may fear suffocation also when there is no risk of severe dyspnoea: "In these situations, some of my patients have been afraid of suffocating..." Suffocation caused by cancer is very rare (tracheal obstruction or bleeding caused by a tumour in the head and neck region).
  - If dyspnoea continues to be severe despite treatment, you can agree with the patient and his/her family to keep the level of consciousness so low that the patient need

not suffer from the feeling of suffocation; instructions on medication are given below
- Plan of action for attacks of dyspnoea
  - Pre-planned drugs readily available, e.g. in the pocket, on the night table
  - (Half-) sitting resting position, calm breathing, window open, etc.
  - How to call for help: wristband alarm, bell, phone (telephone number must be written down clearly and readily at hand!)
- Physiotherapy, relaxation exercises
- Physical strain depending on functional capacity
- Oxygen, if hypoxaemia is present and its correction is beneficial

♦ Pharmacotherapy for dyspnoea
- If obstruction is associated (see also section on the treatment of asthma)
  - Inhaled bronchodilatator
  - Teophylline mixture may bring subjective relief.
- Prednisone 20–80 mg × 1 or dexamethasone 3–10 mg × 1–3 with dose tapering according to response
- Opioids are effective in the treatment of dyspnoea (A) [1].
  - Starting dose with a morphine solution 12–20 mg × 1–6
  - Starting dose with a long-acting morphine 10–30 mg × 2
  - Dose is increased by 20–30% (up to 50%)
- Benzodiazepines
  - Diazepam (5–)10–20 mg at night, 5–10 mg × 1–3 p.o./p.r.
  - Lorazepam 0.5–2 mg × 1–3 p.o., i.m., i.v. or 2–4 mg/day s.c./i.v. infusion
- If necessary, start antidepressive medication.
- Give the patient (written) instructions on medication for acute attacks of dyspnoea: the patient should always have 1–2 doses of morphine solution and 1–2 doses of benzodiazepine available.
- If sedation is required
  - Continue the symptomatic medication
  - Titrate effective morphine medication
  - Add a benzodiazepine, e.g. diazepam (2.5)–5–10 mg p.o./p.r. i.v. once every hour until the patient is calm; plan continuous medication on the basis of the dose needed to calm the patient.
  - Haloperidol often enhances sedation, e.g. haloperidol 2.5 mg i.m. once every hour until the patient is calm; plan continuous medication on the basis of the dose needed to calm the patient
- Agree upon emergency medication if an emergency, e.g. tracheal bleeding/compression, is to be expected:
  - The patient must not be left alone, everyone must stay calm
  - For example, diazepam 5–20 mg i.v. or 10–20 mg per rectum +/– morphine 10–20 mg i.v./i.m. (the dose is determined by the patient's earlier medication).
  - If necessary, repeat the dose until the patient becomes/is unconscious.

Dry mouth and stomatitis

♦ See also article on dry mouth 7.10.

Dentist

♦ Helps with oral hygiene and with dental repairs. Gives instructions on the use of fluorine.

Oral hygiene

♦ Soft toothbrush

♦ No strong mouth rinses or toothpastes

♦ Well-fitted prostheses that are cleaned twice daily and not worn at nights.

♦ Frequent mouth rinsing and gargling
- Water
- Saline solution (1 tsp of salt in 2 dl of water)
- Salt-sodium bicarbonate solution (1 tsp of salt + 1 tsp of sodium bicarbonate in 2 dl of water)
- Chlorhexidine diluted

HAE

Eating

♦ Lukewarm, mildly spiced soft foods.

♦ Nothing very cold or hot.

Treatment of candida and herpes infections

♦ Candida is the most common cause of infection.

♦ Local therapy:
- Miconazole gel 2% 2.5 ml × 4
- Natamycin drops 25 mg/ml 1 ml × 4
- Nystatin drops 100000 IU/ml 1 ml × 4
- Amfotericin B tablet 1 × 4 (difficult if dry mouth)

♦ In severe candida stomatitis give fluconazole systemically

♦ Herpes infection:
- Valaciclovir 500 mg × 2 for 5 days

Treatment of pain

♦ Local therapy:
- Lidocaine mouth rinse 5 mg/ml 15 ml for gargling + 15 ml swallowed × 1–8 (note allergy and danger of aspiration)
- Lidocaine mixture (20 mg/ml) 5–10 ml first gargled and then swallowed slowly × 1–6 (note allergy and danger of aspiration)
- Sucralfate first gargled and then swallowed 200 mg/ml 5 ml × 4–6 (if this induces vomiting, the patient should not swallow the dose) may reduce the need for analgesics.
- Systemic pain medication (16.10). In severe stomatitis caused by chemotherapy, radiotherapy or tumour infiltration, strong opioids are often required.

Anorexia

♦ This section deals with causes of anorexia, some of which can be treated. It is quite common for a patient approaching the end of life to lose interest in eating and drinking. Knowing that the loss of appetite is a common problem in the course of advanced cancer may help the patient and family members to give up a compulsory search for suitable foods.

- There is no clear evidence of the correlation of fluid status and the feeling of thirst C [2 3].
- Causes of anorexia
  - Medication, such as antineoplastic agents, interferon, analgesics.
  - Oral Candida infection (common); sore or dry mouth; see article on the treatment of a stomatitis and dry mouth (7.10).
  - Nausea and vomiting, see section on the treatment of nausea.
  - Early feeling of satiety, which may be caused by
    - Constipation (see section below on management)
    - Abdominal tumour or large liver (corticosteroids may reduce swelling: prednisone 20–40 mg × 1 or dexamethasone 3–6 mg × 1)
    - Ascites (puncture, diuretics)
    - Half-sitting position, small portions, metoclopramide 10–20 mg × 3–4 given 20 minutes before a meal and at night.
  - Metabolic causes, e.g. hypercalcaemia, uraemia, see 10.21, 24.21
  - Pulmonary aspiration (pharyngeal palsy, obstructing tumour) (see above cough)
  - Pain (pain medication)
  - Depression: comforting, medication
  - Unpleasant surroundings for eating
- Cold food (ice cream etc.)
- Small portions on small plates. Pleasantly set meals at short intervals when the patient wishes. A smell-free place for eating.
- Shared meals by the table dressed up instead of eating in the bed wearing nightwear.
- An aperitif may improve the patient's appetite; any alcoholic drink is suitable (NB antabus interaction with metronidazole)
  - A recipe for egg-nog: 1 raw egg, 0.5–1 dl of cream, 2 teaspoonfuls of sugar, 1 tablespoonful of orange juice, 10–15 ml of cognac.
- Medication may improve the patient's appetite
  - Corticosteroids: dexamethasone 3–6 mg × 1 or prednisone 10–20 mg × 1
  - Megestrol acetate 160 mg × 2 up to 800 mg/day
  - Medroxyprogesterone acetate 100 mg × 3 –500 mg × 2.

Nausea and vomiting; causes and treatment alternatives

- Chemotherapy
  - Acute chemotherapy-induced emesis: antiemetic medication is given at the hospital
  - Delayed chemotherapy-induced emesis:
    - metoclopramide 10–30 mg × 3–4 p.o, p.r. ± dexamethasone 3–4.5 mg × 1–2 for 2–4 days
  - Other drugs, for example, opioids (nausea caused by opioids seldom lasts more than a week), digoxin (concentration), NSAIDs
    - Stop unnecessary drugs, change the drug, and check dosage.
  - Irradiation of the abdomen or large pelvic field
    - Metoclopramide 10–20 mg × 3–4 p.o., p.r.
- Constipation is a common and curable cause of nausea; see below and separate article for treatment (24.21).
- Increased intracranial pressure: brain tumour, brain metastases:
  - dexamethasone 3–10 mg × 1–3 with dose tapering according to response, radiotherapy, surgery.
- Enlarged liver, ascites: steroids, ascites puncture, diuretics.
- Uraemia, liver failure: symptomatic treatment.
- Oesophagitis, gastritis (8.32), remember the possibility of candida stomatitis and oesophagitis.
- Anxiety, fear, depression
  - Appropriate treatment of nausea, psychological support and anxiolytic and/or antidepressive medication, when necessary.
- Cough resulting in vomiting: see section on treatment of cough above.
- Symptomatic medication at suggestive doses
  - Metoclopramide 10 mg 1–2 × 3–4 p.o./p.r./i.v./i.m., 20–50 mg/day as a continuous s.c./i.v. infusion
  - Haloperidol 1–2 mg at night, 0.5–2 mg × 1–3 p.o., 2.5–5 mg × 1–3 i.m., 5–10 mg daily s.c./i.v. infusion
  - Lorazepam 0.5–2 mg × 1–3 p.o., i.m., i.v., 2–4 mg/day as a s.c./i.v. infusion
  - Dexamethasone 3–9 mg × 1 p.o., 5–10 mg × 1–2 i.m., i.v., prednisone 20–60 mg1
  - Prochlorperazine 5–20 mg × 1–3 p.o., 25 mg × 1–3 p.r.
  - Levomepromazine 2.5–12.5 mg at night
  - Cyclizine 25–50 mg × 1–3, hydroxyzine 20 mg at night
  - Above drugs in combinations.

Constipation

- Constipation is a very common symptom in a patient with advanced cancer. It is associated with the disease itself, changes in diet, reduction of exercise, drugs, lack of privacy in the hospital or a combination of these factors. Rule out intestinal obstruction (vomiting, cramp-like pain, visible peristaltic activity, swelling of the stomach), see below section on intestinal obstruction and acute abdomen.
- In the beginning of treatment, auscultate abdominal sounds, palpate the stomach and confirm/exclude blockage of the rectum by touch per rectum.
- Causes:
  - Cancer: obstruction, peritoneal carcinosis, ascites, spinal cord compression

- Drugs: opioids, anticholinergics (e.g. neuroleptics, antidepressants), vinka-alkaloids, 5-HT3 antagonists.
- Changes in nutrition, dehydration: recommend ample amounts of fluids, juices and, if possible, fibre
- Reduction in physical activity: encourage physical activity (and treat pain that prevents it)
- Painful anal fissure, irritated haemorrhoids: treat
- Hypercalcaemia (24.21)
- Lack of privacy in the hospital: ensure sufficient privacy

- ♦ Constipation is a private complaint: ask actively about it and inform the patient.
- ♦ Start prophylactic medication for constipation when opioids are initiated!
- ♦ Medication is given preferably orally. Suppositories are used when necessary or bowel movement is induced by giving an enema.
    - Bulk laxatives require ample amounts of fluids and are not suitable for a patient in poor condition.
    - Osmotic laxatives (e.g. lactulose 20–30 ml × 1–2(–4)) are used alone or with stimulant laxatives
    - Stimulant laxatives (senna, sodium picosulphate, docusate, bisacodyl) alone or combined with osmotic laxatives.
    - Prokinetic agents: metoclopramide 10–20 mg × 3–4
    - Some centres have used octreotide in treatment-resistant cases 25–100 μg × 1–3 s.c. also for other conditions than the carcinoid syndrome.

Diarrhoea

- ♦ Treatment-related causes:
    - Diarrhoea in a cancer patient is most often caused by cytotoxic agents, e.g. 5-fluorouracil, irinotecan, topotecan
    - Irradiation of the pelvic region
    - Postoperative causes: resection of the intestine or pancreas, blind-loop syndrome
    - Antibiotics: Clostridium difficile
- ♦ Cancer-related causes:
    - Carcinoid syndrome: causative and symptomatic treatment, including octreotide.
    - Pancreas cancer: osmotic diarrhoea, pancreatic enzyme substitution, consultation with a therapeutic dietitian
    - Constipation may cause “overflow” diarrhoea.
    - Some nutrients may aggravate diarrhoea: spicy, greasy, fibre-rich foods, dairy products
- ♦ Consultation with a therapeutic dietitian may be useful, particularly after surgery and in pancreatic cancer.
- ♦ Parenteral fluid therapy is indicated when the overall situation is such that benefit is to be expected.
- ♦ Treat symptomatically by giving
    - Charcoal tablets
    - Loperamide 4 mg starting dose, and 2 mg after each diarrhoeic voiding up to 16 mg/day.
    - Morphine solution 12–20 mg × 1–6 or oxycodone solution 10–15 mg 1 × 6
    - Long-acting morphine 10–30 mg × 2 or oxycodone 20 mg × 2
    - Morphine or oxycodone; starting doses 4–10 mg × 4–6 s.c.

Intestinal obstruction

- ♦ If the patient’s condition allows surgical intervention consult a surgeon.
- ♦ Inoperable obstruction:
    - Discontinuation of food intake, intravenous hydration and nasogastric suction are indicated only in preparation for an operation.
    - When the obstruction is located proximally in the gastrointestinal tract vomiting occurs rapidly after food or drug ingestion; in a distal obstruction oral medication may be successful.
    - The need for parenteral fluid therapy or nutrition must be considered individually. When the intestine is permanently obstructed the cancer is usually so advanced that parenteral therapy is not beneficial.
    - Nausea, vomiting, colic pain
        - Haloperidol 5–15 mg daily s.c./i.v. infusion or 1–2 mg × 3 p.o.
        - Morphine 30–60 mg/day s.c. /i.v. infusion, 10–30 mg × 2 p.o., starting doses
        - Glycopyrrolate 0.6–1.2 mg/day continuous s.c./i.v. infusion, 0.2 mg × 1–6 s.c.
        - Dexamethasone 6–20 mg × 1 may reduce swelling around the tumour
        - Chlorpromazine 10–25 mg × 3 daily p.o.; may cause sedation.
        - Some centres have used octreotide in treatment resistant cases at 25–100 μg × 1–3 s.c. C [4].
- ♦ If your patient vomits continuously despite medication, discuss the pros and cons of the nasogastric tube with him/her.

Hiccups

- ♦ Causes:
    - Irritation of the phrenic nerve or the diaphragm (tumour, distention of the ventricle, enlarged liver, diaphragmatic hernia, ascites, ulcer, gastritis, oesophagitis)
    - Brain tumour
    - Uraemia.
- ♦ Non-pharmacological treatments, e.g.: the patient should try sitting up, breathing into a paper bag, drinking two glasses of water or swallowing two tsps of sugar.
- ♦ Metoclopramide 10–20 mg × 3–4 daily p.o./p.r. or parenterally.
- ♦ Haloperidol 0.5–2 mg × 1–3 daily p.o., or 2.5–5 mg i.m. × 1–3, 5–10 mg/day s.c./i.v. infusion
- ♦ Chlorpromazine 25–50 mg × 1–3 daily p.o (may cause sedation).
- ♦ Baclofen 5–20 mg × 2–3 p.o.
- ♦ If the cause is a brain tumour, antiepileptic medication may be effective.

HAE

Ulcerations caused by skin metastases or ulcerating tumours

Treatment

- Radiotherapy
- If the skin is exudative, shower × 2–often, cover with a moist dressing, e.g. physiological saline bandages.
- Foul smell, infection
  - Showering and antiseptic bandage
  - Absorbing activated charcoal bandages reduce smell.
  - Consider systemic antibiotics that are effective against anaerobes
  - Bad smell in the room can be reduced, for example, by lemon slices or a scented (tar)candle.
- Treatment-resistant focal ulcer: consult a (plastic) surgeon.

Itching; causes and treatment alternatives

- Skin diseases: treatment of the basic disease.
- Allergic reactions: stopping or changing medication, treatment of allergic reaction.
- Morphine is a rare but possible cause of itching: try changing to oxycodone or fentanyl.
- Uraemia: (symptomatic) treatment of uraemia
- Itching caused by skin metastases; radiation therapy; see section above for treatment of skin ulcers
- Polycythaemia vera: causative treatment, low-dose ASA, note bleeding complications.
- Cancer-induced cholestasis
  - In extrahepatic cholestasis bile acids can be drained, in some cases radiotherapy may be an option
  - Prednisone 20–80 mg × 1 or dexamethasone 3–10 mg × 1–2 with dose tapering according to response
  - Good skin care, see below
  - Symptomatic medication, with sedation as the main benefit. In some cases night-time dosing is sufficient
    - Antihistamines (especially sedative ones) such as hydroxyzine 10–25 mg × 1–3.
    - Haloperidol 0.5–2 mg × 1–3 p.o., 2.5–5 mg ×1–3, or 5–10 mg/day s.c./i.v. infusion
    - Benzodiazepines
      - Lorazepam 0.5–2 mg × 1–3, 2–4 mg/day s.c./i.v. infusion
      - Diazepam 5–10 mg p.o./p.r. at night, 5–10 mg × 1–3 p.o./p.r., 5–10 mg/day i.v. infusion
    - Chlorpromazine 25–50 mg × 1–3 p.o., NB: sedative effect
    - Opioids, e.g. long-acting morphine 10–30 mg × 2, oxycodone 20 mg × 2, starting doses
    - Cholestyramine binds bile acids, suggested dose is 4 g × 4 daily p.o.; rarely applicable in practice for a cancer patient.
- Skin care: the most common cause of pruritus in cancer patients is dryness of the skin. Skin care is a central form of treating itching regardless of its aetiology.
  - Dryness aggravates pruritus. The greasier the ointment, the longer the effect. Less greasy creams may feel more pleasant: apply more often. Soap should be avoided, and an emulsion cream is applied to the skin before a bath/shower or oil is added to the bath water. Dry the skin patting lightly.
  - Cooling menthol ointments can be used as skin cream.
  - Menthol-alcohol solutions are available at pharmacies.
  - Heat, anxiety, boredom and lack of activity make pruritus worse.
  - Cotton gloves for the night, short nails to prevent scratching, light cotton clothing.

Palliative radiotherapy

- Indications
  - Bone pain that does not respond to pain medication (including opioids): at least partial palliation is achieved in about two thirds of patients and total relief on pain in about half. The onset of pain relief varies from a few days to four weeks and palliation lasts on average 3–6 months; most patients benefit from repeated treatment.
  - Prevention of fractures of the weight-bearing bones. If the risk of fracture is already present (more than half of the cortex is destroyed or there is a larger than 2–3 cm lytic metastasis in the diaphysis), consult a surgeon first.
  - Treatment of spinal cord compression; NB: if the patient is developing paraparesis, tetraparesis, or the cauda equina syndrome, i.e. he/she has progressive neurological symptoms, radiotherapy (or surgical therapy) should be given as an emergency treatment. The neurological status of the patient at the time the therapy is started determines the outcome. Start the patient on steroids: see instructions below.
  - Managing pressure symptoms: e.g. brain metastases, brain tumour, nerve compression
  - Haemorrhage: haemoptysis, haematuria
  - Treatment of skin metastases
  - Reducing obstructions (bronchus, vena cava superior, ureter)
- If pressure symptoms occur in the beginning of the treatment, or if they are to be expected during therapy, start the patient on a steroid, e.g. dexamethasone 3–10 mg × 1–3 p.o. or parenterally (some centres use doses up to 100 mg per day in medulla compression (A) [5 6]).
- The aim of palliative radiotherapy is to relieve symptoms quickly with as few adverse effects as possible.
- On the average, palliative radiotherapy is administered in 1–10 fractions; at times, longer courses of radiotherapy are needed.

References

1. Jennings AL, Davies AN, Higgins JPT, Broadley K. Opioids for the palliation of breathlessness in terminal illness. Cochrane Database Syst Rev. 2004;(2):CD002066.

2. Viola RA, Wells GA, Peterson J. The effects of fluid status and fluid therapy on the dying: a systematic review. Journal of Palliative Care 1997;13:41–52.
3. The Database of Abstracts of Reviews of Effectiveness (University of York), Database no.: DARE-985105. In: The Cochrane Library, Issue 1, 2000. Oxford: Update Software.
4. Feuer DJ, Broadley KE. Corticosteroids for the resolution of malignant bowel obstruction in advanced gynaecological and gastrointestinal cancer. Cochrane Database Syst Rev. 2004;(2):CD001219.
5. Loblaw DA, Laperriere NJ. Emergency treatment of malignant extradural spinal cord compression: an evidence-based guideline. J Clin Oncol 1998;16:1613–1624.
6. The Database of Abstracts of Reviews of Effectiveness (University of York), Database no.: DARE-980717. In: The Cochrane Library, Issue 2, 2000. Oxford: Update Software.

16.20 Public health policy on screening for cancer

Matti Hakama

Prerequisites

- Before a screening programme is run as a public health policy there should be evidence that
  - the programme will be effective, i.e. result in a reduction in mortality, or that the quality of life of the target population will be improved
  - the adverse effects of the programme will be acceptable compared to the benefit, i.e. effectiveness
  - the cost of the programme will be acceptable compared to the cost of health services in the target population.
- Three screening programmes for cervix, breast and colorectal cancer are based on class A evidence and could be run as a public health policy. The evidence deals only with the effect on mortality. There is only a limited amount of evidence on benefits to quality of life and on adverse effects. There is no scientific evidence on the comparative weighing of benefits, harms and costs.

Screening for cervical cancer

- The evidence is based on large routine screening programmes world-wide. The effects have been substantial and the evidence is sufficient even in the absence of randomized screening trials.

Recommendation

- Screening with a Pap test can achieve an 80% reduction in mortality from cervical cancer in the target population of women aged from 25 to 60 years.
- A sufficient screening interval is 5 years.
- The younger the women screened the smaller the marginal effect and the larger the number of women diagnosed and treated with preinvasive lesions, that would not have progressed to invasive cancer even in the absence of screening. At high ages attendance and the quality of the smear fall and the effect is reduced.

Screening for breast cancer

- The evidence is based on randomized screening trials in several countries.

Recommendation

- Screening with mammography can achieve a 30% reduction in mortality from breast cancer in the target population of women aged from 50 to 70 years **A** [1 2 3 4]. The effectiveness of screening as public health policy may be somewhat less than that achieved in randomized trials.
- A sufficient screening interval is 2 years.
- The evidence of effectiveness for women younger than 50 years is limited **C** [5 6 7]. Shorter intervals may be needed between screening rounds for the screening to be effective.

Screening for colorectal cancer

- The evidence is based on randomized screening trials but screening was never carried out as an organized screening programme (where e.g. low adherence may be a problem **B** [8 9]).
- Screening with an occult blood test can result in reduction in mortality **A** [10], but there is no good evidence to support recommendations on ages and intervals of screening.

Screening for lung cancer

- According to randomized screening trials in several populations (comparing intensive screening with less intensive screening, but not screening with an unscreened control group), screening for lung cancer with cytology and/or radiology will not result in reduction in mortality from lung cancer **A** [11]. No randomized screening trials are available with spiral CT or biomarkers and mortality as an end point. Therefore, screening for lung cancer is not recommended as a public health policy.

Screening for cancers of other primary sites

- There are screening tests proposed for several cancer sites. None of them has been tested regarding their effect on mortality. Therefore, at the present state of knowledge, they cannot be recommended as a public health policy.

References

1. Olsen O, Gøtzsche PC. Screening for breast cancer with mammography. Cochrane Database Syst Rev. 2004;(2):CD001877.

HAE

2. Kerlikowske K. Efficacy of screening mammography. JAMA 1995;273:149–154.
3. The Database of Abstracts of Reviews of Effectiveness (University of York), Database no.: DARE-950297. In: The Cochrane Library, Issue 4, 1999. Oxford: Update Software.
4. IARC Handbook, Volume 7: Breast Cancer Screening.
5. Smart CR, Hendrick RE, Rutledge JH, Smith RA. Benefit of mammography screening in women ages 40 to 49 years: current evidence from randomized controlled trials. Cancer 1995;75:1619–1626.
6. The Database of Abstracts of Reviews of Effectiveness (University of York), Database no.: DARE-952088. In: The Cochrane Library, Issue 4, 1999. Oxford: Update Software.
7. Vernon SW. Participation in colorectal cancer screening: a review. J Nat Canc Instit 1997;89:1406–1422.
8. The Database of Abstracts of Reviews of Effectiveness (University of York), Database no.: DARE-971223. In: The Cochrane Library, Issue 4, 1999. Oxford: Update Software.
9. Towler BP, Irwig L, Glasziou P, Weller D, Kewenter J. Screening for colorectal cancer using the faecal occult blood test, Hemoccult. Cochrane Database Syst Rev. 2004;(2):CD001216.
10. Manser RL, Irving LB, Stone C, Byrnes G, Abramson M, Campbell D. Screening for lung cancer. Cochrane Database Syst Rev. 2004;(2):CD001991.

16.21 Problems of long-term survivors of childhood cancer

Anne Mäkipernaa

Basic rules

- Survivors of childhood cancer may suffer from different physical and psychological problems in later life. In addition to the disease itself and its treatment, many hereditary and environmental factors play a role in the development of problems in adult life.
- Whilst the child is still growing, the follow-up should be carried out by a specialized hospital. An individual follow-up instruction should be planned thereafter according to the type of cancer and the treatment received.

Bones and soft tissues

- Radiotherapy in a growing child may cause soft tissue hypoplasia or slow down skeletal development. Bone mineral density will be reduced, particularly in survivors of acute lymphoblastic leukaemia (ALL). They are also at a higher risk of fractures and osteonecrosis. The risk is increased by low levels of oestrogen, the female gender and, in particular, cranial radiotherapy. Appropriate hormone and calcium replacement therapy should be considered. Survivors of childhood cancer should be advised to refrain from smoking and to pay particular attention to their physical well being.

Central nervous system

- Cranial irradiation and large doses of intrathecal or intravenous cytotoxic drugs may cause problems with learning, perception, and memory, particularly when given in early childhood.

Heart

- Patients treated with anthracyclines (doxorubicin, daunorubicin) or thoracic irradiation have an increased risk of late cardiac effects. The risk is increased by high cumulative doses of anthracyclines, the female gender and treatment in early childhood.
- Cardiomyopathy, chronic pericarditis and occlusion of the coronary arteries are all possible and may not manifest themselves until several years after the treatment.
- Echocardiography and an exercise test are therefore recommended as follow-up tests for all patients who have received these forms of treatment.

Metabolic syndrome

- Survivors of childhood cancer tend to be overweight and have a high body mass index (BMI). Cranial irradiation is likely to pose an extra risk factor.
- An abnormal lipid profile will predispose the patients to early atherosclerotic changes. These changes are most marked in patients with a history of cranial irradiation and who suffer from growth hormone deficiency. On the other hand, similar findings have been encountered in patients with no growth hormone deficiency.
- Hypertriglyceridaemia and reduced HDL-cholesterol concentration have been noted in association with reduced glucose tolerance, hyperinsulinaemia and truncal obesity, particularly after stem cell transplantation, but also in other cancer patients.

Lungs

- Lung irradiation, and some cytostatics, especially bleomycin, may cause fibrosis. Usually lung problems are mild and mostly restrictive (the mobility of the chest is restricted by the disease and its treatment).

Urinary tract

- Cisplatin may cause renal damage (both glomerular and tubular injury). Usually the renal impairment does not progress after the end of the treatment.

Endocrine system

- Cranial irradiation may decrease the secretion of growth hormone.

- Thyroid irradiation and scattered irradiation may cause hypothyroidism, which may be almost asymptomatic for a long time.
- Irradiation of the lower abdomen may damage the ovaries and prevent the growth of the uterus, and miscarriages are therefore possible. The prepubertal ovary, however, is quite resistant to cytotoxic treatment. When high dose cytotoxic therapy (including alkylating agents) is associated with stem cell transplantation and combined with irradiation the patient is at risk of ovarian damage. Appropriate hormone replacement therapy may be needed.
- The testes are easily harmed by irradiation. Furthermore, many cytotoxic drugs may affect semen production, and testosterone replacement therapy may be needed.
- Recent advances in the treatment of infertility have offered significant help in overcoming these problems. Moreover, the methods to preserve the fertility of a cancer patient have improved.

Teratogenicity

- The offspring of survivors of childhood cancer do not have a significantly increased risk of cancer, with the exception of certain hereditary cancer syndromes (retinoblastoma, Li-Fraumeni).
- There is no strong evidence of a higher incidence of congenital abnormalities among the offspring of survivors of childhood cancer compared with the offspring of the rest of the population.

Secondary malignancies

- People who have survived cancer are at an increased risk of developing other cancers or leukaemia. Depending on the study, the cumulative risk after 20 years varies between 3% and 10% and is 5–20 times the risk seen in the general population.
- Both malignant and benign tumours may develop in body areas that have received irradiation, e.g. breast cancer, skin cancer or tumours of the thyroid gland, brain, bone or soft tissue.
- Both breast and thyroid cancer often develop relatively soon after irradiation. However, secondary cancers usually manifest themselves more than 10 years after the treatment.
- Leukaemia resulting from treatment with cytotoxic drugs usually develops a few years after the treatment.

Psychosocial problems

- Psychosocial coping after childhood cancer is usually considered to be fairly good among the survivors. However, appropriate support should be offered, particularly if physical effects emerging in later life cause morbidity.

Anaesthesiology

Evidence Based Medicine Guidelines. Edited by the Duodecim Editorial Team
 ISBN: 0-470-01184-X

17.1 Resuscitation

Maaret Castrén

Course of resuscitation when the patient has been seen or heard to loose consciousness

♦ Any acute attack characterized by **loss of consciousness, lifelessness, convulsions, loss of muscular tone** and possibly a **bluish-grey skin colour** call for the following measures:

- Confirm whether the patient can be waken up (shake and ask loudly)
- Confirm whether the patient breathes:
  - Open the airways by lifting the lower jaw with one hand and by tilting the patient's head with the other while pressing on the forehead.
  - Is the chest rising?
  - Is there a flow of air from the mouth or nostrils?
- If the patient does not breathe or the breathing is abnormal
  - Confirm whether the patient is breathing and clean the patient's mouth and throat as necessary (a denture that sits well in place is not removed).
  - Start mouth-to-mouth **resuscitation by blowing two even breaths** and confirm that the patient's chest is rising. The amount of air in one breath should be 700–1000 ml when extra oxygen is not available.
  - If you use mask ventilation for oxygenation, remember extra oxygen and oxygen reserve bag. Press the fingers of one hand together with the ventilating bag between them. This amount of air (400–600 ml) is sufficient.
- Check for signs of circulation (watch, listen, feel for 10 s).
  - Breathing, moving, clearing the throat and swallowing are signs of circulation as is a palpable carotid pulse.
  - Do not use more than 10 seconds at the most.
- If no signs of circulation, **begin cardiopulmonary resuscitation (CPR).**
  - If a defibrillator is not available, try giving a punch with your fist (a hard punch in the middle of the chest). A punch is useful only during the first 30 seconds of cardiac arrest.
  - Before intubation the ratio of 15 cardiac compressions to two breaths is used in all cases (also when there are two rescuers).
  - Compression frequency is 100/minute for patients of all ages.
  - Do not compress the heart when air is being blown in.
- **Defibrillation** is vital and must be performed at once.
- CPR is started immediately. When a defibrillator is available, note the patient's heart rhythm and defibrillate immediately if the rhythm can be converted (VF, pulseless VT). A semi-automated defibrillator analyses the rhythm automatically and functions accordingly. Remember to place the apical electrode sufficiently laterally in midaxillary line 10 cm down from the axilla.
- If necessary, defibrillation should be repeated twice immediately. If the device is monophasic use 200 J, 200 J and 400 J. If the device is biphasic use the joules recommended by the manufacturer. When a manual devise is used, monitoring electrodes are attached to the patient after the first three shocks.
- The patient should be **intubated** as soon as it is feasible without delaying defibrillation. An attempt to intubate may not take more than 30 sec.
- If intubation is unsuccessful, ventilate with a mask and try again. After intubation blow 12 times/min and continue compressions at 100 times/min without pauses.
- Open an **infusion line**. Use the neck or arm veins (see section on infusion).
- If VF or VT continues, give 1 mg of adrenaline.
- Continue CPR for one minute.
- Resuscitation may be discontinued only for analysing the rhythm and for defibrillation.
- If VF/VT persist, consider antiarrhythmic medication (see below: resuscitation drugs), repeat defibrillation as instructed above.
- Repeat: if VF/VT persists, give 1 mg of adrenaline (at one minute intervals) and continue resuscitation. Consider antiarrhythmic medication.
- If the patient has recurring VT, i.e. has a momentary sinus rhythm, an antiarrhythmic drug is always preferred to adrenaline.
- If the patient has a rhythm that cannot be converted by defibrillation (asystole/pulseless electrical activity (PEA)), 1 mg of adrenaline is the drug of choice. Continue CPR and repeat adrenalin every 3 minutes.
- Electrodes for monitoring the rhythm are placed at an early phase.
- Remember that the cause of cardiac arrest may be reversible: hypoxia, hypovolaemia, hypo- or hyperkalaemia, hypothermia (18.43), tension pneumothorax, cardiac tamponation, intoxication, pulmonary embolism.
- Aim to treat the cause, as obtaining sinus rhythm is otherwise very difficult.
- If hypovolemia, give i.v. fluids readily (Ringer's solution, 0.9% NaCl, or if necessary, hydroxyethyl starch) 1000–1500 ml.
- Remember that a massive pulmonary embolism is managed by rapid thrombolytic therapy. Use plasminogen activators, reteplase (10 mg i.v.) or alteplase (50 mg i.v.).
- Drain pneumothorax with needle thoracocentesis.
- In the above cases the original rhythm of the cardiac arrest is usually PEA, i.e. a pulseless rhythm where ventricular complexes are visible in the ECG.
- Continue resuscitation until circulation is restored or 30 minutes have elapsed from cardiac arrest, i.e. the

situation is hopeless and resuscitation can be stopped as useless.

Resuscitation procedure when cardiac arrest is noticed immediately and a defibrillator is available

- Analyse the rhythm with the defibrillator.
  - Defibrillate immediately if the arrhythmia responds to defibrillation (VF/VT).
  - Continue defibrillation, if necessary, up to 6 times before other procedures (200 J + 200 J + 360 J + 360 J + 360 J + 360 J (monophasic) or 150 J (biphasic) × 6).
  - If VT persists, give antiarrhythmic medication and basic life support for one minute.
  - Continue as described above in point 6.

Resuscitation is not started in following cases of cardiac arrest

1. The patient has secondary signs of death (livor, rigidity).
2. The patient has been found lifeless and the initial rhythm is asystole.
3. The patient has not been resuscitated in any way for 15 minutes and the initial rhythm is asystole.
4. The patient has traumas and the initial rhythm is asystole.
5. The patient carries a document forbidding resuscitation.
6. The patient is end-stage.

Resuscitation is discontinued as unsuccessful (hypothermia excluded)

- Resuscitation has been continued for 30 minutes since the beginning of lifelessness and emergency call, and normal rhythm has not been restored once during resuscitation.

Defibrillation

- Defibrillation is the primary procedure in cardiac arrest.
- In a medical facility defibrillation should be performed within 3 minutes of noticing lifelessness and elsewhere within 5 minutes.
- The first person present should perform defibrillation. In over 90% of the cases in a medical facility a nurse is the first person present and should thus perform the procedure.
- During every minute that passes from the onset of VT to the beginning of defibrillation 7–10% of the patients are lost. Waiting for a doctor to arrive thus worsens the prognosis.
- The rhythm of a lifeless patient is initially confirmed using the defibrillator electrodes when the device is semiautomatic or with paddles if the device is monophasic.
- Conducting paste or saline pads should be put on the paddles for enhancing the procedure already before first defibrillation. The paddles should be pressed against the patient's chest with a steady force that should be kept constant until defibrillation has been performed.
- A semiautomatic defibrillator, which gives advice, is attached with glue electrodes. Its program recognizes the rhythm. A semiautomatic defibrillator is the primary device for facilities where defibrillations are not performed routinely and resuscitation is not routine. Only intensive care units and emergency rooms and operating theatres should use a manual defibrillator.
- With a manual device, the personnel must interpret the rhythm, decide whether defibrillation is necessary and choose the energy to be used.
- Studies suggest that a biphasic waveform is more efficient than a monophasic one.

Resuscitation drugs and infusion

- Establish an i.v. line at the neck or the arm. Use an intraosseal needle if opening a venous line is difficult.
- Adrenaline is given in 1 mg doses at 1–3-min intervals, concentration 1:1 000, 1 mg/ml in a 5-ml ampule.
- If an i.v. line is not established, remember to use an intraosseal needle. If an infusion cannot be started, give 2–3 mg of adrenaline via the intubation tube. Its absorption from the lungs is, however, very uncertain. It is preferable to give the drug with a suction catheter deep into the bronchus and then give 10–20 ml of Ringer solution via the suction catheter. Ventilate a few times.
- If VT persists or recurs, antiarrhythmic medication is given after three defibrillation shocks and adrenaline administration. Drug administration must never delay other resuscitation procedures. No antiarrhythmic drug has been found to improve the final prognosis. The following three drugs can be used:
  - According to new international recommendations, **amiodarone** is the primary antiarrhythmic drug. Initial dose is 300 mg i.v., i.e. 6 ml into the vein with 200 ml of Ringer's solution given immediately thereafter into the same vein. The next doses are 150 mg, i.e. 3 ml.
    - Prepare to treat hypotension efficiently when normal rhythm is restored.
  - Lidocaine can be used for recurring VT when a pulsing rhythm has been achieved momentarily or in prolonged VT after the 9th defibrillation attempt.
    - Do not use together with amiodarone.
    - Starting dose of lidocaine is 1.5 mg/kg i.v. and thereafter 0.75 mg/kg (e.g. a patient weighing 70 kg: initially 100 mg and thereafter 75 mg).
    - Do not give more than 3 mg/kg during the first two hours.
  - Beta-blockers can be used in the management of prolonged or recurring VT.
    - For example, metoprolol is given up to the maximal dose of 10 mg as i.v. boluses of 4 mg + 3 mg + 3 mg.

TRA

Other resuscitation drugs

- Atropine is used when the initial rhythm cannot be defibrillated, i.e. the patient is asystolic or has PEA. It is given as a single dose of 3 mg i.v.
- Magnesium at a dose of 8 mmol is used for prolonged VT if hypomagnesaemia is suspected, e.g. because the patient is on potassium-wasting diuretics.
- Bicarbonate is not a routine drug in resuscitation. It may be given as a 7.5% solution (0.5–1 mmol/kg) if the patient is known to have acidosis, intoxication caused by tricyclic antidepressants or if the patient has been drowned.

Further treatment after successful resuscitation

- Normoventilation with the patient's pulse oximetry reading (oxygen saturation) >95%.
- For fluid therapy give Ringer's solution as a very slow infusion. More ample i.v. infusion is indicated only if hypovolaemia is suspected.
- In an adult patient systolic blood pressure should be at least 120 mmHg. Use dopamine, if necessary (concentration 1 mg/ml; dose 2–12 µg/kg/min).
- Register ECG. A 13-lead ECG (also V4R) registered 20 minutes after restoration of rhythm is the recording of choice.
  - If signs of infarction are present, give thrombolytics (plasminogen activator).
- Give sedatives so that the patient tolerates having an intubation tube and remains calm.
  - Begin with morphine 5–10 mg i.v., additional doses 5 mg.
  - If necessary, give also diazepam 2.5–5 mg i.v.
- Do not attempt to warm up the patient: mild cooling is beneficial. Keep the patient's head straight to avoid compression of the neck veins.
- Monitor the rhythm continuously. Keep the patient coupled to the defibrillator.
- Alert the receiving hospital. A doctor should accompany transportation. Monitoring and treatment are continued without interruption also during transportation.

17.2 Endotracheal intubation

Eija Kalso

- Tracheal puncture, see 6.60.

Equipment

- Laryngoscope, lamp operation confirmed
- Endotracheal tubes
  - For adult men: size 8–9 (inner diameter 8–9 mm)
  - For adult women: size 7
  - A one size smaller tube in reserve
  - Children's tubes
- Introducer
- Ribbon for fastening the tube
- Syringe for filling the cuff
- Stethoscope
- Laryngeal tube

Intubation

- The patient's head must be supported with a 3–5-cm thick pillow or some other elevation.
- The intubator holds the patient's head tilted backwards and inserts the laryngoscope with his left hand through the patients right mouth angle. In this way, the patient's tongue will stay on the left side of the groove of the laryngoscope when the head of the laryngoscope is inserted into the pocket between the epiglottis and the tongue.
- An assistant may try to improve visibility by pulling from the patient's right mouth angle and pressing on the cricoid cartilage so that the larynx is better visualized.
- The vocal cords usually come into sight without problems when the intubator lifts the laryngoscope in the direction of the handle.
- It is important to maintain visual control throughout the intubation; this will ensure that the endotracheal tube is passed between the vocal cords and that it is placed to a suitable depth (the distance between the upper edge of the cuff and the level of the vocal cords should be about 2 cm).
- If the vocal cords are not visualized within 30–60 s, the patient must be ventilated for a while with 100% oxygen, i.e. with a mask that has a bag attached to the bellows. The assistant is asked to connect an introducer to the endotracheal tube for the next intubation attempt. The introducer bends the distal tip of the tube upwards, facilitating the passage of the tube under (behind) the epiglottis even in the absence of visual control.

Avoiding oesophageal intubation

- To avoid oesophageal intubation when working outside the operating theatre or other well-equipped emergency facility, the following instructions should be adhered to:
  - Always try to intubate under visual control.
  - If you are unable to see the vocal cords or the arytenoid cartilage, use an introducer.
  - Auscultate the trachea, both lungs and the upper abdomen. Monitor also the movements of the chest.
  - If you have intubated without visual control, if the respiratory sounds are not symmetric and vesicular, or if you are otherwise unsure about the position of the

endotracheal tube, you should repeat the laryngoscopy and push the endotracheal tube against the hard palate so that you can see it between the arytenoid cartilages.

- If a capnometer is available, attach it to the endotracheal tube and make sure that the gas coming out contains carbon dioxide, which confirms the correct position of the tube. (Due to low cardiac output the $ETCO_2$ can be low)
- If you are still unsure about the placement of the endotracheal tube, remove the tube, ventilate the patient with 100% oxygen through a mask, and re-intubate as necessary.
- If the patient is to remain intubated, ensure the correct depth of the tube (tip 3 cm above the tracheal bifurcation) by chest radiography.

17.3 Prehospital emergency care

Timo Jama

I Basic rules

- Initially evaluate the patient's level of consciousness on a scale awake / arousable / unarousable. The level of consciousness should be further specified at a later stage using the Glasgow Coma Scale (GCS) (see Table 17.3.1), but only after the patient's airway and breathing have been secured and circulation evaluated.

A. Airway

- Identify and correct possible airway obstruction:
  - Chin lift/jaw thrust
  - Remove any foreign bodies.
  - Insert an oropharyngeal airway and, if necessary, intubate.

Table 17.3.1 Glasgow Coma Scale

Criteria		Score
Eyes open	Spontaneously	4
	To speech	3
	To pain	2
	None	1
Best motor response	Obeys commands	6
	Localizes/avoids pain	5
	Withdraws from pain	4
	Flexion	3
	Extension	2
	None	1
Best verbal response	Orientated	5
	Confused	4
	Inappropriate words	3
	Incomprehensible sounds	2
	None	1
		Total 3-15

B. Breathing

- Identify and treat respiratory failure (oxygenation and ventilation).
- Be aware of the most common conditions causing respiratory distress (failure) and treat accordingly:
  - Pulmonary oedema
  - Exacerbation of asthma and COPD
  - Pneumonia
  - Pulmonary embolism
  - Hyperventilation
  - Tension pneumothorax.
- Administer oxygen to all high risk patients.

C. Circulation

- Identify and treat circulatory failure.
- Arrest external bleeding by compression.
- Iv-access to all high risk patients.
- Treat life-threatening arrhythmias (ventricular fibrillation, ventricular tachycardia) before transportation.

D. Other

- Specify the level of consciousness accurately, i.e. GCS.
- Prevent further trauma (skeletal support, vacuum mattress).
- Minimize heat loss (electric or regular blanket, warm fluids).
- Start pain relief as necessary with i.v. opiates (alfentanil, fentanyl, oxycodone, morphine).
- Choose whether to 'load and go' or 'stay and play'.

E. Abstain from treatment when the patient has no chance of recovery

- Lifeless (= no breath or heart sounds and unresponsive) trauma patients, when the initial rhythm is asystole or PEA (pulseless electrical activity).
- Normothermic lifeless adult (unwitnessed collapse), when the initial rhythm is asystole.
- At least 15 minutes since cardiac arrest with no attempts at resuscitation.
- Secondary signs of death evident.
- Lifeless trauma patient with cranial crush injury or outflow of brain substance.

II When to intubate at the scene?

- Cardiac and/or respiratory arrest (when respiratory arrest is associated with heroin overdose treat by mask ventilation and i.v. naloxone).
- Low level of consciousness (GCS < 9) without readily treatable cause (hypoglycaemia, hypoxia, hypercapnia, bradyarrhythmia or tachyarrhythmia, hypotension, heroin or benzodiazepine overdose).

- Airway management, oxygenation and/or ventilation not successful or otherwise adequate by other means (oropharyngeal airway, oxygen therapy, CPAP, "Ambu-bag" and mask ventilation). Prevention of aspiration.
- Anticipated airway obstruction (inhalation burn, trauma to the facial or neck region, uncontrolled bleeding or allergic pharyngeal swelling).

III When to stabilize haemodynamics before transportation?

- Systolic blood pressure (BP) < 90 mmHg or > 220 mmHg, and the patient has cerebral manifestations.
- Diastolic BP > 140 mmHg.
- Heart rate < 40 or > 120/min.
- Even more readily in the presence of chest pain, dyspnoea, pulmonary oedema or altered level of consciousness.
- Remember disturbed autoregulation of cerebral circulation in patients with cerebral trauma, infarction or bleeding. A high blood pressure is usually compensatory because cerebral perfusion pressure is dependent on systemic blood pressure; blood pressure should not be lowered aggressively during the acute phase (recommended upper limits: subarachnoid haemorrhage 160/100, intracranial bleed 180/100, cerebral infarction 220/_) The safest medication for blood pressure reduction is labetalol in boluses of 10–20 mg i.v.; nifedipine may even be harmful!

IV When is transfer to hospital urgent?

- **Load and go**: The patient will benefit from rapid transportation to the final point of care.
  - Sharp trauma (shooting, stabbing) in the trunk or neck region.
  - Blunt trauma, if suspicion of continuing bleeding into a body cavity.
  - Other uncontrolled bleeding and/or signs of shock.
  - Clinical suspicion of massive pulmonary embolism.
  - Clinical suspicion of acute stroke (thrombolysis may be considered at the hospital).
- **Stay and play**: The patient's condition should be stabilized at the scene before transportation.
  - Resuscitation (17.1)
  - Respiratory distress and facilities are available for symptomatic treatment (asthma, COPD, pulmonary oedema).
  - Bradyarrhythmia (atropine, external pacemaker) or tachyarrhythmia (cardioversion, antiarrhythmics).
  - Acute myocardial infarction, if thrombolytic therapy can be administered.
  - Lowered level of consciousness, when the underlying cause is treatable (hypoglycaemia, hypoxia, hypotension, hypercapnia, bradyarrhythmia or tachyarrhythmia, certain intoxications) and adequate treatment facilities are available.
  - The patient meets the criteria for intubation (see Section II).
  - Needle thoracocentesis for tension pneumothorax (Figure 17.3.1).
  - Mechanical ventilation should not be instigated in a patient with pneumothorax without a chest drain in situ (risk of tension pneumothorax).
  - A patient with a cranial/cerebral trauma will benefit from early anaesthesia/ intubation and controlled ($etCO_2$) ventilation.

V Recommendation for the equipment of a basic and advanced life support (ALS) ambulance

- See Table 17.3.2.
- The physician responsible for prehospital emergency care will decide on the regional requirements and the level of equipment needed for ambulances.

VI Emergency care of the most common patient groups

- Establish venous access in all patients. Administer oxygen, monitor the patient's vital signs and continually observe the cardiac monitor, pulse oximetry as well as the patient's level of consciousness.

Resuscitation

- See 17.1.
- In ventricular fibrillation and ventricular tachycardia defibrillation is vital and must be carried out without delay.

Chest pain and myocardial infarction

- 13-lead ECG is essential. If it is not available, only administer basic therapy and transport the patient to the nearest care facility.
- Basic therapy (all patients): patient at rest, supplemental oxygen 8 l/min, ASA 250 mg p.o (cave: allergy for aspirin, asthma patients and active GI-bleeding) and isosorbide dinitrate (ISDN) spray until pain is reduced, i.v.-line, EKG-monitoring"
- **Treatment of unstable angina pectoris**. If ST depression and/or T wave inversion is evident on a 13-lead (V4R!) ECG, consider beta-blockade (e.g. metoprolol 2.5 mg i.v. until heart rate down to 60-70/min), nitrate infusion (starting dose 20 μg/min, the dose is increased by 10 μg/min at a time, targeting a systolic BP reduction of about 15% in normotensive and 25% in hypertensive patients, diastolic BP must remain >60), opiates (morphine 4–6 mg i.v., until pain-free) and enoxaparin 40 mg i.v.
- **Acute myocardial infarction**
  - Thrombolytic therapy, if not contraindicated.
  - If immediate defibrillation (and preferably external pacing) facilities are not available, thrombolytic therapy should not be administered outside the hospital.

Table 17.3.2 Equipment recommendation for a basic and advanced life support (ALS) ambulance.

Equipment	Basic	ALS	Medication	Basic	ALS
Automated external defibrillator (AED) with a monitor screen	X	X	adenosine		X
13-lead ECG + telemetry		X	adrenaline 1 mg/ml	X	X
External pacemaker		X	adrenaline 0.1 mg/ml		X
Sphygmomanometer	X	X	racemic adrenaline		X
Stethoscope	X	X	alfentanil, fentanyl		X
Cannulas and other equipment for fluid therapy	X	X	aspirin	X	X
Syringe or infusion pump		X	atropine		X
Intraosseal needle		X	diazepam, rectal	X	X
Intubation kit	X	X	diazepam i.v.		X
Set of oropharyngeal airways	X	X	dopamine		X
Set of laryngeal masks		X	flumazenil		X
Nebulizer		X	glucagon		X
Peak flow meter		X	10% glucose	X	X
Pulse oximeter	X	X	glyseryl trinitrate		X
Ventilator		X	oxygen	X	X
Ambu-bag + set of masks	X	X	enoxaparin [1)]		X
Capnometer with grafic display		X	hydroxyethyl starch	X	X
CPAP equipment		X	ipratropium bromide		X
Blood glucose meter	X	X	isosorbide dinitrate	X	X
Thermometer	X	X	activated charcoal	X	X
Set of cervical collars	X	X	lidocaine, i.v.		X
Set of vacuum mattresses and splints	X	X	metoclopramide/droperidol		X
Suction device	X	X	metoprolol		X
Alcohol breathalyzer	X	X	methylprednisolone		X
Stretchers	X	X	morphine/oxycodone		X
			naloxone		X
			reteplace or tenecteplace[1)]		X
			Ringer's solution	X	X
			salbutamol		X

[1)] If the crew has been trained to administer thrombolysis and have the facility to transmit 13-lead ECG readings telemetrically.

Arrhythmias

- The patient is haemodynamically unstable if his/her BP < 90 and he/she complains of chest pain and/or has respiratory distress/pulmonary oedema and/or lowered level of consciousness.
- **A. Bradyarrhythmias** (heart rate <40/min)
  - External pacing in Mobitz type II and total heart block irrespective of haemodynamic state, at least by using the "on demand" function (the condition usually worsens during transportation). In distal block, atropine is usually of no benefit.
  - In other bradyarrhythmias (trifascicular block, SSS, sinus arrest/block, Mobitz type I), external pacing is usually applied only if the patient is haemodynamically unstable or has a recent history of syncope.
  - In other cases, atropine 0.5 mg i.v., up to 2 mg, may be beneficial.
  - If external pacing is ineffective, consider dopamine (5–15 μg/kg/min) and/or adrenaline infusion (0.02–0.2 μg/kg/min), both titrated according to response.
- **B. Tachyarrhythmias** (heart rate > 120/min)
- Electrical cardioversion is indicated if the patient is haemodynamically unstable.
  - If the patient is unresponsive and no carotid pulses can be felt (see Resuscitation), administer a non-synchronized direct current shock of 200 J.
  - A synchronized direct current shock is indicated if the rate is fast (whether broad or narrow complex, heart rate usually more than 150/min) and the patient's condition is unstable. Start with 50–100 J. In atrial fibrillation start with 200 J, increasing up to 360 J (monophasic defibrillator). Sedation is usually required (e.g. propofol 30–50 mg in boluses or diazepam 5–10 mg + alfentanil 0.5–1 mg i.v.). Be prepared for a brief respiratory arrest.
- If the patient is haemodynamically stable, medical therapy is usually sufficient.
  - Supraventricular tachycardia (narrow-complex, regular): adenosine 6+(12 +18 if needed) mg i.v. (as a rapid bolus into the antecubital or jugular vein, flushed with 20 ml of Ringer's solution/NaCl 0.9%) or verapamil 5+(5 if needed) mg i.v.
  - Broad-complex, regular tachycardia in a cardiac patient is usually ventricular tachycardia. If the patient remains stable treat with lidocaine (50–100 mg)/ beta-blocker (e.g. metoprolol 5–10 mg) / amiodarone 150–300 mg i.v., otherwise cardioversion. In rare cases, SVT + aberrant accessory conduction pathway.

- Recent-onset atrial fibrillation does not usually require treatment outside the hospital, unless the patient is haemodynamically unstable. Beta-blockers can be used to slow down the conduction.
- In WPW syndrome, cardioversion is the safest alternative (avoid digoxin, verapamil, beta-blockers).
- Atrial flutter can be slowed with beta-blockers or verapamil.

Respiratory distress

- You must be able to differentiate between the most common conditions that cause respiratory distress and tension pneumothorax as well as foreign bodies in the airways.
- Note whether the patient is able to speak in sentences/only use single words/unable to speak, record the respiratory rate, I/E ratio, breath sounds, SpO_2, skin colour and the possible use of accessory muscles.

Emergency treatment at the scene

- **Exacerbation of asthma and COPD**
  - The underlying disease is usually known. A half-sitting or forward-leaning position will help.
  - Inhaled bronchodilators (e.g. salbutamol 5 mg + ipratropium bromide 0.5 mg × 1–2), theophylline 5 mg/kg i.v., methylprednisolone 125 mg i.v. and adrenaline inhaled/i.v. in a severe attack.
  - A COPD patient also requires supplemental oxygen in hypoxia, use a Venturi mask with adequate flow; a conscious patient does not stop breathing while receiving supplemental oxygen, the SpO_2 target is about 90% or the patient's own earlier level. If the level of consciousness deteriorates and/or the respiratory rate drops, reduce inspired oxygen fraction. A high carbon dioxide concentration does not kill the patient, but inadequate oxygenation will!
- Pulmonary oedema
  - Consider aetiology, i.e. cardiogenic or non-cardiogenic (sepsis/pneumonia, intoxication, hepatic failure, pre-eclampsia, airway obstruction).
  - Start CPAP at 1 cm H_2O/10 kg and a nitrate infusion with 20 µg/min (if cardiogenic aetiology and the patient is peripherally cold and systolic BP > 100). In the presence of underlying ischaemia, administer beta-blockers with caution (metoprolol in 1 mg i.v. boluses), morphine 4–6 mg i.v. and, in associated bronchial obstruction, theophylline 200 mg as a slow i.v. injection over 5 minutes.
- Pulmonary embolism
  - Oxygen and transportation to the nearest diagnostic unit (spiral TT, lung scan).
  - If haemodynamically unstable, dopamine infusion 5–10 µg/kg/min.
  - Favourable case reports have been obtained with early thrombolytic treatment in resuscitation situations: reteplase as a 20 U bolus.
- Pneumonia
  - The patient is usually febrile with gradually worsening respiratory distress, unilateral rales on pulmonary auscultation.
  - Oxygen therapy usually improves oxygenation; if not sufficient: CPAP is needed.
  - If haemodynamically compromised start dopamine infusion at 5–10 µg/kg/min.
- Foreign body in the airways
  - Usually evident from the history: preceding meal, paediatric patients.
  - Heimlich manoeuvre.
  - Unconscious patient: laryngoscopy and removal of the foreign body under visual control.
  - If not helpful, intubation and manipulation of the foreign body into another main bronchus.
- Pneumothorax
  - Spontaneous pneumothorax is common: acute respiratory distress, sudden sharp or general chest pain and unilateral quiet breath sounds. If breathing is not too laboured and oxygenation remains good, give oxygen and send the patient to hospital.
  - Remember the possibility of tension pneumothorax, particularly in trauma patients. The signs and symptoms include: severe respiratory distress and increased respiratory effort, tracheal deviation towards the contralateral side, tympany on percussion and decreased/absent ipsilateral breath sounds, distended neck veins and, finally, circulatory collapse.
- Treatment of tension pneumothorax (Figure 17.3.1)
  - Immediate needle thoracocentesis and, if possible, insertion of a chest drain before transportation (at least if mechanical ventilation is indicated).

Lowered level of consciousness and seizures

- Recognize the most common, readily treatable conditions that cause disturbances of conscious level, i.e. hypoglycaemia (i.v. glucose), a low blood pressure and/or too fast/slow heart rate (see Haemodynamic therapy), hypoxia (oxygenation), hypercapnia (ventilation), intoxication (heroine, benzodiazepines; antidotes).
- If the cause is not easily treatable: see Section II.
- Remember that hypothermia may explain the lowered level of consciousness (the so-called urban hypothermia may develop even whilst the patient remains at home).
- Seizures can usually be treated with i.v. diazepam/lorazepam, remember the post-ictal phase (consider hypoglycaemia as a possible cause for seizures). If diazepam at a dose of up to 20–30 mg i.v., or lorazepam up to 8 mg i.v, is not effective, give a loading dose of fosphenytoin. If seizures continue the patient should be intubated under anaesthesia (requires the presence of an anaesthetist or emergency medicine physician).

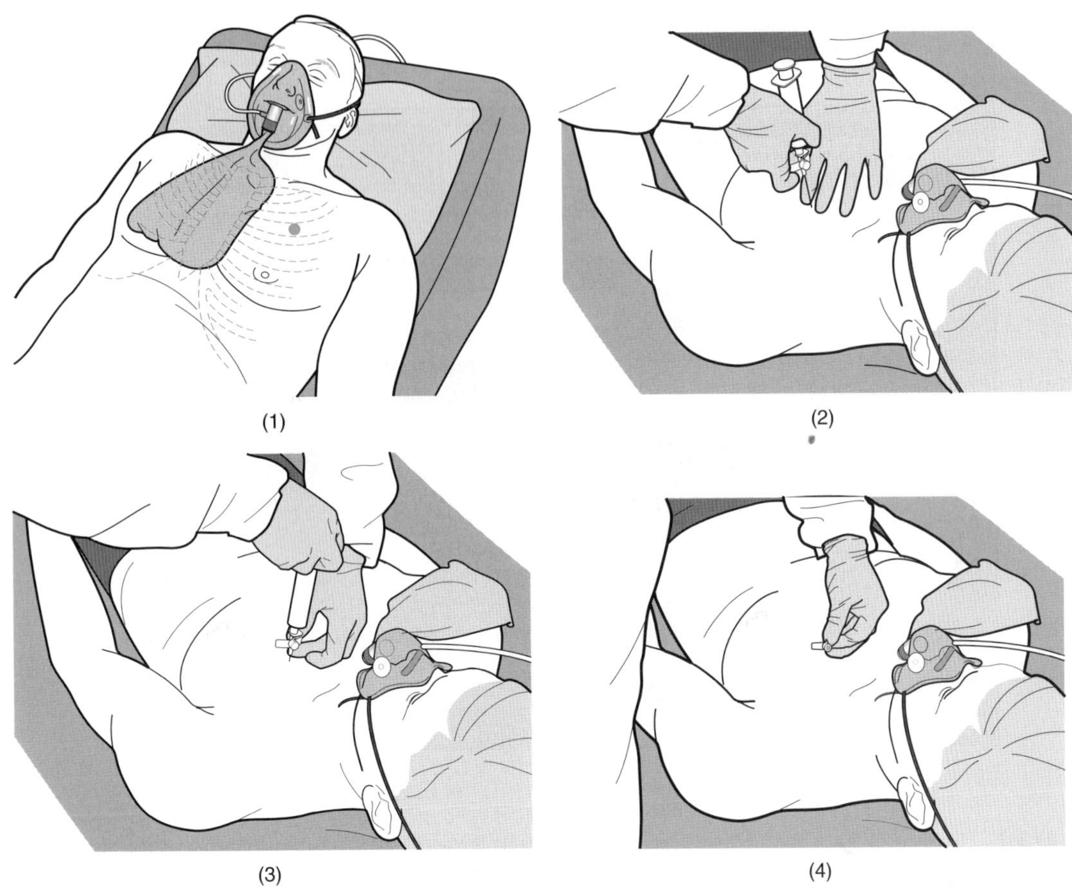

Figure 17.3.1 1) The puncture site is the second intercostal space (between ribs 2 and 3) in the midclavicular line, on the side of the suspected tension pneumothorax. Clean the skin with disinfectant, use local anaesthetic if necessary. 2) A large calibre cannula (preferably with a diameter of at least 2 mm), with the drip chamber removed, is joined with a 10 ml syringe. The cannula is inserted through the skin at a straight angle, following the upper border of the 3rd rib. 3) After piercing the skin, pull back on the plunger of the syringe to create a slight negative pressure and continue inserting the cannula for its entire length. 4) Remove the syringe and mandrin and air will flow out at a high pressure. Leave the cannula inside and connect it with a three-way stopcock with which you can regulate the air flow. Remove the cannula only after inserting a chest drain.

Intoxication

- See 17.20
- Emergency treatment should be targeted at respiratory and circulatory support as described above. Do not hesitate to intubate if needed.
- Give activated charcoal (orally if conscious, and by nasogastric tube when the level of consciousness is impaired, intubate first!) if less than 2 hours have elapsed from the ingestion, if the substance is highly toxic, if the substance is known to depress intestinal functioning (opiates, tricyclic antidepressants) or when sustained release medications have been ingested.
- Antidotes for emergency treatment (administered according to response):
  - naloxone 0.08–0.2 mg i.v. (opiates, heroine), see also 17.21
  - flumazenil 0.1–0.2 mg i.v. (benzodiazepines)
  - glucagon 5–10 mg i.v. (0.1 mg/kg) + infusion 3–5 mg/h (beta-blockers)
  - calcium chloride 1 g/5 min i.v., the dose can be repeated at 10–20 min intervals or given as an infusion 3–4 g/h (calcium-channel blockers)
  - hydroxycobalamin 5 g/30 min i.v. (cyanide, combustion gases).
- In cases of carbon monoxide poisoning, ending exposure and administering 100% oxygen are the vital components of treatment (use an oxygen mask with an oxygen reservoir. Note: a conventional oxygen mask only delivers about 35–40% FiO_2) (17.24). Consider hyperbaric oxygen therapy (HBOT) if the patient remains symptomatic despite oxygen therapy of 4–6 hours duration. HBOT is always indicated in serious cases (impaired conscious level, circulatory failure).

Trauma patients

- For transportation tactics see Section "When is transfer to hospital urgent"?

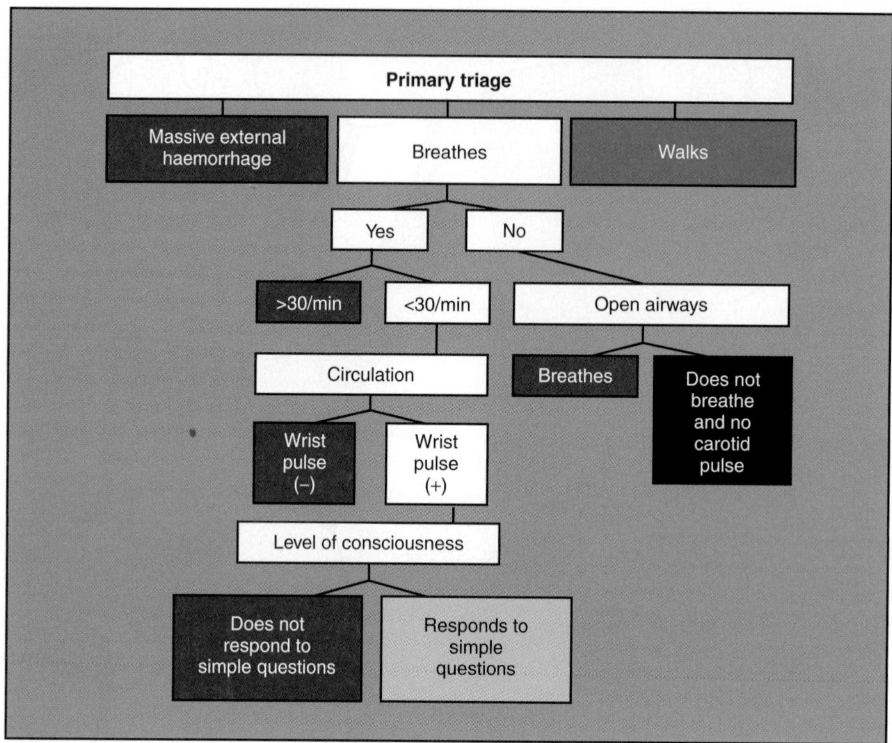

Figure 17.3.2

Table 17.3.3 Instructions for secondary triage, which takes place at the scene after emergency treatment and, if necessary, whilst waiting for transportation. (Note: A patient may move from red to yellow if, for example, an airway obstruction has been treated by intubation.).

Priority class	Trauma or finding
I	Airway obstruction (e.g. severe facial trauma)
	Chest trauma with respiratory distress
	Unconscious patient with airway problems even in the recovery position; patients who lose consciousness during treatment (epidural bleed)
	Inhalation injury and facial burns
	Skin burns 20–75%
	Massive external bleeding
	Hypovolaemic shock
	Multiple trauma patients (mere suspicion is not enough)
	Extensive open fractures
	Eviscerations (prolapses or internal organs)
II	Chest trauma without respiratory problems
	Abdominal and/or urinary tract trauma
	Unconscious patients (except Class I priority group patients)
	Large bone fractures and open fractures other than those in Class I
	Unstable pelvic fracture
	Patients with chest pain
III	Injury to spine or spinal cord or suspicion of such trauma
	Cranial/cerebral traumas (GCS 14–15/15 = speaking contact or bleeding from the ear in a conscious patient)
	Simple fractures and bruises
	Burns other than those of Class I
	Slight facial trauma (jaw/nose fractures etc.)
	Eye injuries
	Usually all walking patients
IV	Open brain injury with herniated brain tissue
	Burns > 75% of total body area
	Situations leading to cardiac arrest (-> DNR)
	Other dying patients

- A patient with a high-energy trauma usually needs two (or more) large calibre venous cannulas (diameter 1.7–2.0 mm). Take blood samples during cannulation.
- In a patient who is bleeding into a body cavity systolic blood pressure of around 80 mmHg is probably sufficient, but in cranial/cerebral trauma blood pressure should be kept higher (120 mmHg).
- Fluid therapy: crystalloid/colloid 1:1 until the target blood pressure is reached, a patient with cranial/cerebral trauma probably benefits from hypertonic saline.
- Give burn patients Ringer's solution or NaCl 0.9% at the rate of 1000 ml/h.
- Intubation criteria, see Section II.
- Remember the possibility of tension pneumothorax in a trauma patient. Treatment consists of immediate needle thoracocentesis.
- A patient with chest trauma requiring mechanical ventilation will need a chest drain before transportation.
- Consider all unconscious patients, those thrown out of a car and those with trauma to the head/neck region to have cervical spine injuries until proven otherwise.

Multiple-casualty incident

- Multiple-casualty incident refers to an incident with two or more injured persons.
- Major incident refers to an incident the management of which will considerably increase the normal workload of health care providers.
- A Major Incident Plan is to be drawn up by local authorities to ensure the provision of medical assistance to casualties (medical staff and other stand-by groups, number of ambulances available, potential to increase the normal operation of hospitals and health centres).
- The Regional Medical Officer will decide when to dispatch a medical or stand-by group to the site of the incident, unless written instructions are in force giving the Dispatch Centre the right to dispatch such a group without a formal request.
- In order to gain experience medical and other stand-by groups should also be used for the routine management of accidents.
- On the way to the scene of the incident, verify the type of accident, estimated number of casualties and the amount of ambulance equipment already summoned to the scene. If necessary, make a request for further assistance via the Dispatch Centre (ambulances and crew members, medical staff or other stand-by groups from neighbouring regions) and if a true major incident has occurred alert local hospitals accordingly.
- At the incident scene, report to the rescue leader (the chief fire officer) and take responsibility for the medical operations.

Triage during a major accident

1. Primary triage

- Primary triage is carried out by the first medical team at the scene.
- In primary triage, patients are quickly assessed and divided into four treatment categories (Figure 17.3.2) according to urgency of treatment. The assessment should not take more than 20 seconds/patient; the two patient interventions allowed during the assessment include turning an unconscious patient into a recovery position and arresting massive external bleeding.
- The patients are colour or number coded according to their relative priority for treatment:
  - I red (critical)
  - II yellow (urgent)
  - III green (minor injuries, able to walk)
  - IV black (dead = not breathing, unresponsive, absent carotid pulse).
- In a major incident, a place is to be designated where the casualties are moved after primary triage (for emergency treatment).
- Emergency treatment is initiated for patients in the red (I) group according to available resources.
- Walking patients (green group III) are assembled in a separate area (a bus or other feasible alternative, if available).

2. Secondary triage

- Table 17.3.3
- After emergency treatment, the patients are re-triaged at the scene according to their injury.
- Triage is repeated again as the patients arrive at hospital.
- After emergency treatment, a patient may be allocated to a different group, e.g. an unconscious patient with airway obstruction moves from red to yellow after airway has been secured (intubation).

17.10 Blood gas analysis and acid-base balance

Timo Jama

Blood specimen

- Capillary blood or preferably arterial blood is used.
- The blood specimen should be examined as soon as possible after sampling (freeze the sample if this is not possible, <10 min).
- Venous blood can be safely used for pH evaluation.

Measurements

- Partial pressure of oxygen (pO_2) (not from capillary blood)
- pH
- Partial pressure of carbon dioxide (pCO_2)

TRA

- Base balance (base excess (BE) (metabolic alkalosis), base deficit (BD) (metabolic acidosis))
- BE is used to describe both conditions: the + and the −sign indicate whether the condition is alkalosis (+) or acidosis (−).
- Instead of BE, a standard bicarbonate (SBC) value can also be used.

Reference values

- Arterial blood
  - pO_2 average > 11 kPa (with lower values in advancing age)
  - pH 7.35–7.45
  - pCO_2 4.5–6.0 kPa
  - BE 0 ± 2.5 mmol/l
  - Standard bicarbonate (SBC) 22–26 mmol/l
- Capillary blood
  - pO_2 varies and has no clinical significance
  - pH 7.35–7.45
  - pCO_2 4.5–6.0 kPa
  - BE 0 ± 2.5 mmol/l
  - SBC 22–26 mmol/l

Severity of hypoxaemia and hypercapnia

- See Table 17.10.1.
- aB-pO_2 < 7.3 (−7.9) kPa in a patient with chronic obstructive pulmonary disease is an indication for continuous oxygen therapy when additional criteria are met.
- aB-pO_2 < 8 kPa, pCO_2 > 6.7 kPa indicates acute respiratory insufficiency.
- When pCO_2 rises acutely to >10–12 kPa carbon dioxide narcosis results.

Table 17.10.1 Severity of hypoxaemia and hypercapnia

Severity	Hypoxaemia aB-pO_2 (kPa)	Hypercapnia aB-pCO_2 (kPa)
Mild	8–11	6.1–6.6
Moderate	6–7.9	6.7–8
Severe	<6	>8

Disturbances of the acid–base balance

- See Table 17.10.2.
- Causes of metabolic acidosis (BE < −2.5)
  - Ketoacidosis (diabetic, alcohol-induced)
  - Renal failure or tubular pathology (renal tubular acidosis)
  - Shock, insufficient oxygen supply to the tissues
  - Lactic acidosis
  - Severe diarrhoea
  - Intoxication (ammonium chloride, methanol, salicylates, ethylene glycol)
- Causes of metabolic alkalosis (BE > +2.5)
  - Vomiting
  - Overdose of bicarbonate
  - Insidious hypovolaemia
  - Thiazide diuretics/furosemide
- Causes of respiratory acidosis
  - Acute or chronic ventilatory insufficiency (6.5)
- Causes of respiratory alkalosis
  - Hyperventilation (6.4)
  - Insensitivity of the respiratory centre to changes in pCO_2 as a result of a trauma or a disease process.
  - Psychogenic causes (panic disorder)
  - Hypoxaemia

Table 17.10.2 Disturbances of the cid-base balance.

Disturbance		Blood pH	Blood pCO_2	Blood BE	Urine pH
Metabolic acidosis	Uncompensated	decreases	normal	decreases	decreases
	Fully compensated	normal	decreases	decreases	
Metabolic alkalosis	Uncompensated	increases	normal	increases	
	Fully compensated	normal	increases	increases	increases
Respiratory acidosis	Uncompensated	decreases	increases	normal	decreases
	Fully compensated	normal	increases	increases	
Respiratory alkalosis	Uncompensated	increases	decreases	normal	
	Fully compensated	normal	decreases	decreases	decreases

17.11 Pulse oximetry

Timo Jama

Principles

- Hypoxaemia is common, difficult to detect and deleterious. An experienced clinician can detect hypoxaemia on the basis of cyanosis only when blood oxygen saturation is 80% or less.

- Pulse oximetry is an easy-to-use and effective method for detecting hypoxaemia when the device recognizes a good pulse wave B [1 2].
- Pulse oximetry should be used routinely for monitoring oxygen saturation, however, it tells nothing about ventilation.

Method of operation

- The measurement of blood oxygen saturation is based on the fact that two different wavelengths of light are absorbed unequally in reduced haemoglobin and oxyhaemoglobin.
- Only net absorption during a pulse wave is measured. This minimizes the influence of tissues and venous or capillary blood on the result.
- The device is usually calibrated at 75–99% SaO_2 values with an error marginal of approx. 2%.

Clinical use

- Detection of hypoxaemia associated with
  - anaesthesia
  - cardiorespiratory insufficiency
  - (severe) pulmonary embolism
  - sleep apnoea syndrome
- Controlling oxygen therapy

Interpretation

- A decrease in oxygen saturation to below 90% (a shift to the steeply sloping part of the oxyhaemoglobin dissociation curve) is an indication of a significant reduction in oxygen partial pressure. Higher saturation values do not mirror reliably the partial pressure of oxygen.
- Fever, acidosis and high concentration of CO_2 in arterial blood move the oxyhaemoglobin dissociation curve to the right resulting in increased dissociation of oxygen from haemoglobin, i.e. oxygenation of the tissues becomes more efficient.

Interventions in hypoxaemia

- See Table 17.11.

Table 17.11 Actions to be taken in hypoxaemia

Oxyhaemoglobin saturation (%)	Actions
90–95	Determine oxygen saturation regularly, particularly at night. If the result is unexpected, rule out sources of error. Find out the reason for the hypoxia.
80–90	As above + administer oxygen as long as the saturation exceeds 90%.
<80	As above + start continuous monitoring of oxygen saturation. Consider assisted ventilation.

Sources of error

Decreased peripheral circulation

- The most important source of error B [1 2]
- Causes
  - Cold weather or low body temperature
  - Hypotension, vasoconstriction
- Peripheral circulation can be improved by
  - warming
  - massage
  - local vasodilating therapy (e.g. a small amount of nitroglycerin ointment)
  - removing tight clothing or blood pressure torniquette.
- Error caused by movement: tremor, waving of the hands and vibration of the ambulance.

Venous pulsation

- Heart failure
- Tricuspidal insufficiency

Dyshaemoglobinaemias

- Carboxyhaemoglobin (carbon monoxide poisoning) B [1 2]
  - A misleadingly high saturation is recorded (the instrument interprets carboxyhaemoglobin as oxyhaemoglobin)
- Methaemoglobinaemia
  - The reading is about 85% irrespective of true oxygen saturation.

Problems with illumination

- The probe is placed incorrectly
  - Light must not leak into the probe
- Xenon and infrared lights
- Bright daylight, fluorescence-inducing light

Obstacles to absorption

- Nail polish, skin pigmentation, etc.

Advantages compared with blood gas analysis

- Continuous monitoring
- Easy-to-use and reliable instrument
- Fewer sources of error
- Pain and nervousness during artery sampling cause hyperventilation, which increases oxygen saturation values. Blood gas analysis may lead to an overestimation of oxygenation.

Restrictions

- Pulse oximetry does not give information on acid-base balance.

TRA

- Pulse oximetry does not detect hypoventilation (increased partial pressure of carbon dioxide) in a patient breathing air with increased concentration of oxygen. In a patient breathing normal air hypoventilation usually reduces oxygen saturation. Pulse oximetry does not thus replace clinical monitoring of respiration e.g. after anaesthesia.
- In a critically ill patient the method is unfortunately often unreliable because of peripheral vasoconstriction (the device does not recognize the pulse wave).

References

1. Meta-analysis of arterial oxygen saturation monitoring by pulse oximetry in adults. Heart and Lung 1998;27:387–408.
2. The Database of Abstracts of Reviews of Effectiveness (University of York), Database no.: DARE-982122. In: The Cochrane Library, Issue 2, 2000. Oxford: Update Software.

17.20 Treatment of poisoning

Ari Alaspää

Principles

- Drug (17.21) or some other poisoning is the most common cause of unconsciousness in a previously healthy (especially young) person, if asymmetry is not observed on neurological examination.
- The treatment is classified in the following manner:
  - Immediate action (Figure 17.20.1)
  - Prevention of absorption of orally taken drugs
  - Other specific therapy (antidotes and dialysis)
  - Follow-up treatment (finding out the cause of poisoning, psychiatric treatment).
- Risk assessment in based on the amount of drug taken and the time that has elapsed since. The patient may be momentarily misleadingly fit.
- The history of the ingested amount of drug is often erroneous.
- In most cases the poisoning results from a mixture of alcohol and several drugs, and the typical symptoms (Table 17.20.1) may be absent.

Examination of the intoxicated patient

- After immediate action
- More precise determination of the level of consciousness: Glasgow coma score (Table 17.20.2).
- Exclusion of other causes (e.g. use the MIDAS memory rule for an unconscious patient: Meningitis, Intoxication, Diabetes, Anoxia, Subdural haematoma)
- Breathing
  - Oxygen saturation
  - Frequency
  - Audible breathing sounds
- Circulation
  - Blood pressure
  - Pulse
  - ECG readily
- Other basic examination
  - Basic blood tests, blood glucose in disturbances of consciousness, blood count, CRP, serum sodium and potassium, creatinine, astrup, blood alcohol.
  - Qualitative drug screening from urine in unclear and serious cases.
  - Forensic samples (blood + contents of the stomach)

Prevention of absorption

- The most effective mode of therapy.
- The effect is reduced rapidly with time; however, individual responses vary greatly and the effect also depends on the substance.

Medicinal charcoal

- The most recommended therapy, also out-of-hospital.
- The recommended dose for adults is 50 g, for children 1 g/kg (5 ml of Carbomix solution). Can be mixed with e.g. ice cream. The relative effect becomes weaker if the charcoal:drug dose relationship is less than 10:1 (e.g. 50 g:5 g of drug) => increase the dose. Repeat by giving 20–50 g every 2–4 hours.
- Administered as a drink to a conscious patient who is able to talk. In other patients the airways must be secured first.
- Not effective against alcohols, metals (Fe, Pb, As, Li) cyanide, solvents.
- Charcoal is contraindicated if the patient has ingested corrosive substances (hampers endoscopy).

Gastric lavage

- Gastric lavage is clearly less useful than medicinal charcoal, and it involves more complications. It delays the administration of charcoal considerably.
- Consider gastric lavage in cases where medicinal charcoal does not absorb the toxic substance and/or the intoxication is life threatening.
- An unconscious patient must be intubated before gastric lavage.
- Procedure:
  - The patient should be kept preferably on his/her left side, head lower than the body.
  - A large calibre nasogastric tube (diameter 1 cm) is installed (not forcefully) to a depth that has been measured beforehand (nose-ear lobe-processus xiphoideus). The location of the tube must be verified (gastric content flows from the tube) before lavage.
  - In an adult patient, 200 ml of body temperature fluid is poured down at a time.

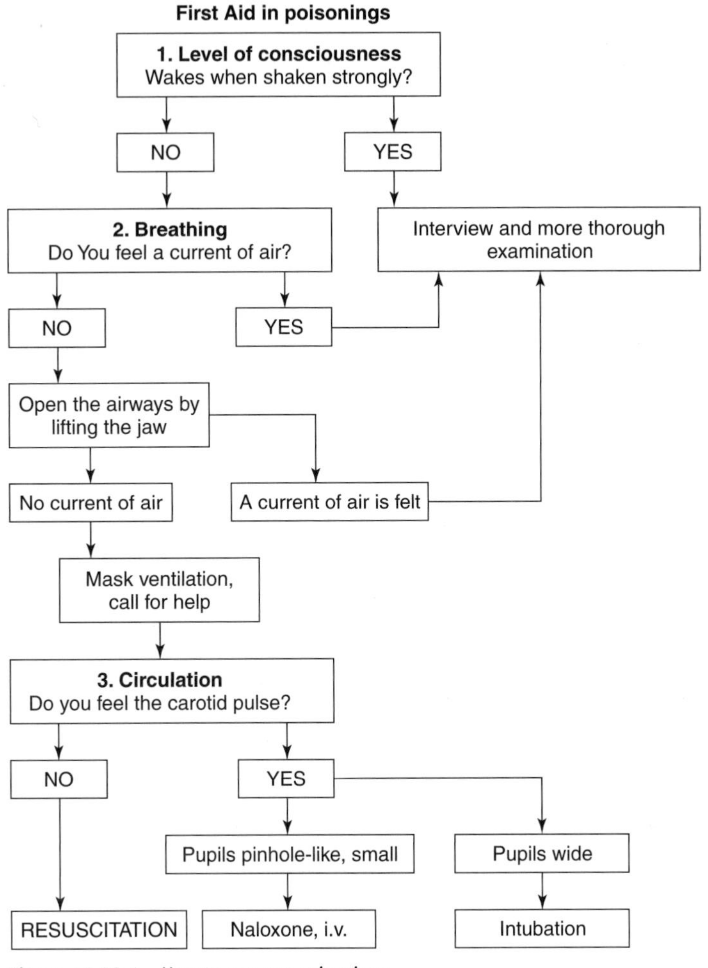

Figure 17.20.1 How to manage poisonings.

- Lavage is continued until the fluid that comes back from the tubing no longer contains any drug.
- After lavage, medicinal charcoal is given.

♦ Contraindications

- The patient has ingested corrosive acid or base
- Ingestion of solvents => only if airways have been secured (fully conscious/intubated).

Intestinal lavage

♦ Little evidence of effect

♦ Consider if

- the intoxication is life threatening and/or
- the drug has been ingested a long time ago and/or
- the drug is a depot formulation.

♦ Intubate before the procedure if the criteria are met (see section on airways).

♦ Performance

- Charcoal is given first (if it is assumed to adsorb the drug)
- Polyethylene glycol solution, e.g. Colonsteril®/Clean-Prep® is given to an adult at 1–2 l/hour orally or via a nasogastric tube until charcoal is detected in the stool.
- Do not forget to give medicinal charcoal repeatedly.
- Nausea is managed with metoclopramide 10 mg i.v.

Induced emesis

♦ Not as efficient. The use of emetics is not recommended because of uncertain and slow response.

Position therapy

♦ Placing the patient immediately in a recumbent position on the left side may delay absorption.

Other specific treatment

♦ Antidotes, see specific intoxications

♦ Elimination therapies (haemodialysis, haemoperfusion)

- Rarely used
- Determine the place of treatment, usually available only in larger hospitals
- Possible only with a few substances
  - Amphetamine

Table 17.20.1 Syndromes caused by poisonings.

Syndrome	Causes	Pulse/BP	Consciousness	Pupils	Peripheral temperature	Other
Adrenergic	Amphetamine, cocaine, teophylline, sympathomimetics (asthma drugs)	++/++	Agitation, psychosis	Dilated	Lowered, sweating	Myocardial infarction, cerebral haemorrhage, arrhythmia
Anticholinergic	Tricyclic antidepressants, neuroleptics, antihistamines	++/++	Agitation, confusion	Dilated	Elevated, dry, reddish	Mucous membranes, skin dryness, urine retention, fever
Cholinergic	Organic phosphates, cholinergic (MS, Alzheimer) drugs, funghi	—	Agitation, confusion unconsciousness	Constricted	Sweating	Secretion of saliva, secretion from the bronchi +, muscle strength -, asthma, convulsions, urine incontinence
Opioids	Heroin, euphorizing analgesics	No effect	Alcohol intoxication, unconsciousness	Very constricted		Respiratory failure
Sedative	Alcohol, benzodiazepines	No effect or lowers	Alcohol intoxication, confusion, unconsciousness			
Serotonergic	Antidepressants, moclobemide, selegiline, triptane, tramadol, dextrometorphane, amphetamine, cocaine		Agitation, confusion, unconsciousness			Fever, myoclonus, tremor, diarrhoea, muscle rigidity

- Asetylsalicylic acid
- Epilepsy medications (phenytoin, carbamazepine, sodium valproate)
- Lithium
- Theophylline
- Substitute alcohols (methanol and ethylene glycol)

• Decision is based on the severity of the symptoms and/or concentration of the toxic substance.

Symptomatic therapy

♦ The most common form of treatment!

Airways

♦ Intubate if the patient's level of consciousness is less than 8 with the Glasgow coma score (Table 17.20.2).

♦ Intubation is called for in the following conditions
  • Loss of pharyngeal reflex (irritation caused by the tracheal tube is tolerated)
  • Audible breathing sounds (rasping/snoring)
  • Respiratory/haemodynamic failure

♦ Exception
  • The level of consciousness is expected to rise quickly (e.g. hypoglycaemia).

Table 17.20.2 Glasgow coma score

Criteria		Score
Best eye response	Eyes open spontaneously	4
	Eye opening to verbal command	3
	Eye opening to pain	2
	No eye opening	1
Best motor response	Obeys commands	6
	Localizing pain	5
	Withdrawal from pain	4
	Flexion to pain	3
	Extension to pain	2
	No motor response	1
Best verbal response	Orientated	5
	Confused	4
	Inappropriate words	3
	Incomprehensible sounds	2
	No verbal response	1
		Total 3–15

  • The use of an antidote may be safer than intubation if the medical staff is not experienced in intubation.

♦ If intubation cannot be performed, place the patient on his/her left side, insert a tracheal tube, establish an i.v. line and arrange for transfer of the patient to further treatment with accompanying staff.

- An unconscious or drowsy patient should be positioned on his/her side because of the risk of vomiting and aspiration.

Respiration

- When pulse oximetry (17.11) functions well, it reveals disturbances in oxygenation sensitively.
  - Limitations: does not reveal false haemoglobins (carbon monoxide, cyan- and methaemoglobin) or insufficient ventilation during oxygen administration.
- Observation of breathing
  - Use of auxiliary muscles, breathing movements, ability to speak
  - Breathing becomes more difficult in oxygen saturation disturbances, aspiration and metabolic acidosis.

Circulation

- Clinical assessment: fullness of neck veins, oedemas, peripheral temperature, blood pressure, pulse.
- Hypotension is the most common problem. Often hypovolaemia is the underlying cause (unconscious/found patients). A direct effect of the ingested drug is a more rare cause.
- Treat hypotension with fluids: 500 ml of physiological saline or Ringer's solution/20 min. The dose can be repeated if the patient's condition does not worsen clearly. If fluids are not sufficient, start dopamine infusion > 5 μg/kg/min.
- Arrhythmias are managed if
  - haemodynamics fails (low BP)
  - the patient has ventricular tachycardia.
- Treatment options include electric cardioversion under sedation or administration of short-acting drugs (lidocaine 1.5–3 mg/kg i.v.).
- In torsade des pointes ventricular tachycardia, give magnesium sulphate 1–2 g i.v. or use external pacing.
- In slow arrhythmias give atropine 0.01 mg/kg i.v. If not response is seen, prepare for external pacing or try dopamine/isoprenal infusions.

Convulsions

- Sign of severe intoxication; may also be caused by severe haemodynamic failure (shock/arrhythmia).
- Hypoglycaemia should always be excluded first and treated accordingly.
- Convulsions caused by tricyclic antidepressants call for alkalinization (sodium bicarbonate 75 mg/ml, 1 ml/kg).
- Alcohol or drug withdrawal symptoms must always be remembered as a cause of convulsions.
- Treatment
  - Adults: diazepam at 5 mg doses i.v. up to 30 mg. For children, the dose is 0.2 mg/kg.
  - More long-acting lorazepam at 2 mg doses i.v. up to 8 mg
  - If no response => general anaesthesia + intubation: e.g. propofol 1–2 mg i.v. and infusion 4–12 mg/kg i.v.
  - If avoiding intubation is important, a diazepam infusion can be tried.

Aspiration pneumonia

- In justified suspicion 2 million units of G penicillin × 6 i.v. or cefuroxime 1.5 g × 3 i.v. may be started.

Rhabdomyolysis

- See 10.41.
- Risk is high if the patient has been found unconscious, has had convulsions or has signs of pressure necrosis in the skin or obvious muscle tenderness.
- Urine is dark or red in colour and dipstick test shows blood (cross-reaction with myoglobin).
- Serum creatine kinase (CK) and/or myoglobin reveal the degree of severity.
- Treat with ample fluids and alkalized diuresis (sodium bicarbonate infusion).

TRA

Choosing the location of treatment

- In most cases the patient needs only follow-up and symptomatic treatment.
- Some patients may require acute invasive procedures.
- Some treatments are available in local hospitals (most antidotes) and some only in specialist hospitals (e.g. dialysis).
- Determination of the blood concentration is useful in poisoning caused, for example, by alcohols, digoxin, lithium, paracetamol and theophylline. Therefore laboratory determination must be available in severe poisonings (17.21).

17.21 Drug poisoning

Ari Alaspää

Benzodiazepines

- The most common group of drugs that cause poisonings
- Symptoms:
  - Sedative syndrome
  - Hypotension may occur; it is mainly mild and associated with multiple drug and/or alcohol intoxications.
  - Respiratory depression possible; however, in most cases it is caused by a blocked airway in an unconscious person.
- Preparations used as sleep medication are more dangerous than the less sedative ones (e.g. oxazepam).
- For example, the lethal dose of diazepam is around 1 g.
- The toxicity of benzodiazepines is increased by other drugs that lower the level of consciousness and by alcohol =>

blood alcohol concentration must be measured with a breath alcometer.

- Treatment
  - Symptomatic
  - The antidote is flumazenil. Dosage: 0.25 mg i.v. repeated up to 2 g. Effective also in zopiclone, zalepton and zolpidem poisonings.
    - Continue with an infusion at the dose of 0.1–0.4 mg/h
    - Multiple drug/alcohol poisonings involve potentially lethal reactions (convulsions, etc), which is why the antidote should be used only in exceptional cases.

Antidepressants

- Tricyclic antidepressants are clearly most dangerous.
- Serotonin syndrome is a possible adverse effect of all antidepressants, particularly SSRI drugs.

Tricyclic antidepressants

- Doses exceeding 1 g are dangerous.
- Cause anticholinergic syndrome, see Table 17.20.1, and at the same time delay gastric emptying => the effect of medicinal charcoal lasts longer (recommended when less than 12 hours have elapsed from drug ingestion). However, severe symptoms have been reported several days after drug ingestion.
- Typical symptoms of severe intoxication
  - CNS symptoms: impaired consciousness, convulsions
  - Cardiac symptoms: conduction disturbances (AV conduction, branch blocks) and arrhythmias (both atrial and ventricular brady- and tachycardias)
  - Wide QRS complex, >0.12 sec, on ECG is a warning sign.
- Treatment
  - Monitoring of the heart rhythm is mandatory if the ingested dose is dangerous or not known.
  - Readiness for intensive care (special care unit), sufficient follow-up time.
  - Administration of charcoal and intestinal lavage are useful even in later stages of poisoning
  - If haemodynamics is instabile or the patient has convulsions
    - Alkalinization reduces cardiotoxicity: sodium bicarbonate 75 mg/ml, 1 ml/kg i.v. in 20 minutes.
    - Intubate readily to avoid respiratory acidosis.

Serotonin re-uptake inhibitors

- Usually cause mild intoxications.
  - CNS symptoms (agitation, restlessness, confusion, muscle rigidity, convulsions)
  - Symptoms of the autonomic nervous system (tachycardia, sweating, flushes, mydriasis)
  - Rhabdomyolysis is possible
- Serotonin syndrome may occur as a result of concomitant use of a serotonergic drug and other drugs.
  - Opioids (dextrometorphan, tramadol, pethidine)
  - MAO inhibitors (moclobemide, selegiline)
  - Stimulating drugs (amphetamine, cocaine, crack, ecstasy, etc).
  - Triptanes (sumatriptan, zolmitriptan, naratriptan)
  - Other drugs: buspirone, carbamazepine, lithium)
- Symptoms suggesting serotonin syndrome
  - Hyperthermia
  - Myoclonus (muscle jerks)
  - Irreversible symptoms develop eventually: convulsions, hyperthermia, increased intracranial pressure, death.
- Treatment
  - Usually symptomatic
  - If signs of serotonin syndrome are present => refer to intensive care. Before intensive care
    - cool down externally, give sufficient amounts of fluids and primarily haloperidol 5 mg or chlorpromazine 50 mg i.m.
    - treat convulsions; even general anaesthesia may be necessary.

Neuroleptics

- High-dose neuroleptics (levomepromazine, chlorpromazine, etc) have been considered more harmful than low-dose neuroleptics (e.g. haloperidol).
  - Cardiorespiratory depression is more severe.
- The elimination half-life of many neuroleptics is long and anticholinergic effect is common => sufficiently long follow-up and administration of charcoal are necessary even in the later stages of poisoning.
- Symptoms:
  - Anticholinergic syndrome
  - Frequently hypotension and tachycardia
  - Arrhythmias, particularly rapid ones (torsade des pointes ventricular tachycardia occurs particularly with thioridazine)
  - Extrapyramidal symptoms (particularly with low-dose neuroleptics)
  - Unconsciousness, convulsions, respiratory depression
- Treatment
  - Symptomatic
  - i.v. fluids are usually efficient in hypotension
  - Extrapyramidal symptoms: diazepam 5–10 mg i.v. or biperiden 2–5 mg i.m.

Opioids

- These drugs are abused, and oral preparations are also injected.
- Remember combination preparations (e.g. paracetamol + codeine) and treat all drug intoxications

- Typically an opioid syndrome that is aggravated by other sedative drugs or alcohol.
  - Altered level of consciousness
  - Pinhole pupils
  - Respiratory depression (bradypnoea and cyanosis)
- Atypical symptoms are caused by
  - tramadol (convulsions, nausea, seldom respiratory depression)
  - dextropropoxyphene (myocardial depression, conduction disturbances and asystole) already at low doses.
- Treatment
  - Be prepared to treat severe intoxications
  - These drugs slow gastric emptying => administration of medicinal charcoal is useful also later.
- The antidote naloxone
  - is administered if the patient has symptoms of opioid syndrome (for immediate actions, see Figure 17.20).
  - The dose is 0.4 mg iv./0.8 mg i.m. at a time (use lower doses with heroin (17.22) up to 10 mg i.v. If a response is obtained, start an infusion with 2/3 of the dose that waked the patient up given per hour (not in heroin intoxication).
  - The efficacy is less certain in buprenorphine, dextropropoxyphene and tramadol poisonings.

Other analgesics

- The most harmful substances are over-the-counter ASA and paracetamol!
- Because of the large amount of drug in the tablets the dose of medicinal charcoal often needs to be increased.

ASA (Acetyl salicylic acid)

- Doses exceeding 150 mg/kg are dangerous (in a person weighing 70 kg this equals 10 g = 20–40 tablets!)
- Symptoms
  - GI symptoms (nausea, vomiting, diarrhoea, abdominal pain)
  - CNS symptoms (tinnitus, convulsions, unconsciousness)
  - Hypoglycaemia, severe acidosis and hyperventilation.
- Treatment
  - Symptomatic
  - In severe cases alkalised diuresis, sometimes even dialysis.

Paracetamol (acetaminophen)

- Harmful doses >150 mg/kg, individual variation is great. Apparently alcoholics are more susceptible to liver damage, while children tolerate large doses better.
- Symptoms
  - GI symptoms (nausea, vomiting, abdominal pain)
  - Liver failure appears later.
- Administration of the antidote acetyl cysteine B [1] depends on the blood concentration and symptoms => refer to hospital readily.

Other non-steroidal anti-inflammatory drugs

- Usually cause mild poisonings
- Mainly GI symptoms
- Severe symptoms (convulsions, renal failure, coagulation disturbances) are rare.

Cardiac drugs

- Poisonings are rare when compared with the wide use of these drugs. However, they are invariably dangerous.
- Drugs affecting the pumping ability and electric activation of the heart cause the most severe poisonings while less severe poisonings are caused by drugs with only vasodilating activity.

Beta-blockers

- May cause very rapidly (in only 30 min) a poorly manageable circulatory shock.
- Fat-soluble, non-selective preparations are most deleterious, e.g. propranolol.
- Symptoms
  - Bradycardia and hypotension, which may be provoked rapidly by, for example, vomiting.
  - Convulsions
  - Pulmonary oedema of non-cardiac origin
  - Bronchus obstruction in asthmatic patients
  - Hypoglycaemia
- Treatment
  - Be always prepared to treat a severe intoxication.
  - Glucagon 3–5 mg i.v. is the antidote. Effect begins within 20 min.
  - May cause vomiting => an unconscious patient must be intubated.
  - Fluid administration in excess of 1000 ml is not beneficial
  - High inotropic doses (dopamine 20 µg/kg/min, readily also a high-dose adrenaline infusion at 0.1–1 (sic!) µg/kg/min
  - External pacing is rarely necessary if the above treatment modalities are available.

Calcium channel blockers

- Cause symptoms resembling beta-blocker poisoning, but with a slower effect.
- Ten times the daily dose taken at one time is already dangerous.
- Bradycardia, bronchus obstructions and hypoglycaemia are more rare than in beta-blocker poisonings
- Treatment
  - Calcium is the antidote; dose $CaCl_2$ 1 g × 4 i.v. in one hour or calcium glucobionate 3 g × 4 i.v. DO NOT give if the patient has concurrent digoxin poisoning. Establish venous access if $CaCl_2$ is administered (risk of tissue necrosis).
  - Otherwise managed like a beta-blocker poisoning. Glucagon may be tried if an inotropic infusion is not helpful.

TRA

- There is preliminary evidence on the effect of a 0.5 IU/kg/h insulin infusion.

Digoxin

- Most poisonings are accidents and result from the narrow therapeutic range.
- Predisposing factors
  - Renal insufficiency (age!)
  - Hypokalaemia, hypercalcaemia
  - Hypoxia and acidosis (poor tissue circulation is thus an independent risk factor!).
- Interactions with other drugs: e.g. itraconazole, quinidine, spironolactone and verapamil increase the blood concentration of digoxin.
- Symptoms are variable
  - Impaired general condition and confusion
  - CNS symptoms: disturbances of colour vision, headache, weakness, unconsciousness, convulsions
  - Various arrhythmias, particularly bradycardia and conduction disturbances but atrial or ventricular tachyarrhythmias are also possible.
- Treatment
  - Stable haemodynamics and no serious CNS symptoms => interruption of medication
  - Severe poisonings arrhythmias/serious CNS symptoms => follow-up in a hospital
  - Readiness to treat arrhythmias (atropine, lidocaine).
  - In more severe cases an antidote (Digibind®) can be given after the blood concentration of digoxin has been determined. This drug is expensive.

Antiepileptic drugs

- In particular the older drugs phenytoin, carbamazepine and sodium valproate cause similar symptoms
  - GI symptoms (abdominal pain, nausea, vomiting)
  - CNS symptoms: loss of consciousness, convulsions
  - Circulatory and respiratory depression is possible.

Chloroquine

- Doses of only a few grams cause rapidly developing circulatory and respiratory depression. In children, a single tablet may be life threatening.
- Medicinal charcoal must be given as soon as possible.

Reference

1. Brok J, Buckley N, Gluud C. Interventions for paracetamol (acetaminophen) overdoses. Cochrane Database Syst Rev. 2004;(2):CD003328.

17.22 Poisoning caused by inebriating substances (alcohols, drugs)

Ari Alaspää

Alcohols

- Not to be underestimated: cause as many deaths as all medicine poisonings together.
- Alcohol has interactions, particularly with sedative drugs, which is why a clinical assessment of drunkenness is difficult and correlates poorly with the alcohol concentration measured from blood.
- Methods of prevention of adsorption are in practice inefficient: medicinal charcoal is not effective and gastric lavage is useful only immediately after consumption.

Ethanol

- The lethal dose is 3 g/kg in children and ca. 6 g/kg in adults.
- The risk of trauma and cerebral haemorrhage increase manifold under the effect of ethanol.
- The elimination of ethanol varies individually.
- A blood alcohol concentration < 2.5 per mil alone does not explain unconsciousness in an adult.
- Criteria for follow-up at a care unit
  - Alcometer reading > 3 per mil (recent consumption may raise the level)
  - No verbal response
  - Alcometer reading correlates poorly with the patient's condition (other causes are suspected).
- If the above criteria are not met and clinical examination does not suggest any other reason for follow-up, the inebriated patient can usually be discharged from the care unit, IF
  - he/she is able to take care of himself OR
  - someone else takes care of him (police, accompanying person who can function adequately)
- Clinical follow-up
  - Monitor the development in the state of consciousness
  - Blood glucose, serum sodium and potassium, if available
  - CRP, if infection is suspected, and acid-base balance if the use of alcohol substitutes is suspected
  - Body temperature, particularly if the patient appears febrile or the trunk feels cold (suspicion of hypothermia)
  - If the patient's condition has not improved in 3–4 hours, the diagnosis must be re-evaluated.
  - If mixed intoxication is suspected, medicinal charcoal can be given early on.

- In severe inebriation, management in a special care unit is necessary
  - Child
  - Unconsciousness or coma
  - Circulatory or respiratory symptoms

Isopropanol poisoning

- Isopropanol is found in carburettor fluid and in antifreeze solutions.
- The inebriating effect is stronger and longer lasting than that of ethanol.
- Treatment and follow-up are as in ethanol poisoning.

Methanol poisoning

- Methanol is found in windscreen cleaner solutions, paint removers, etc
- Lethal dose varies individually, on average 30 ml (2 tablespoonfuls!)
- If ethanol has been consumed simultaneously, symptoms may appear after a delay of a few days when ethanol has first been eliminated from the system.
- Because the symptoms are unspecific, methanol poisoning should be kept actively in mind as a possible cause when the condition of an alcohol-abusing person suddenly deteriorates. In such cases, metabolic acidosis verifies the diagnosis.
- Symptoms
  - Inebriation, confusion, gastric/chest pain, vomiting, in many cases elevated serum amylase
  - Metabolic acidosis => dyspnoea, hyperventilation
  - Visual symptoms (white spots or "snow fall", blindness, wide pupils that do not react to light, papillary oedema)
  - CNS symptoms (convulsions, unconsciousness) and hypoglycaemia are also possible.
- Treatment
  - If the patient has hyperventilation/decreased consciousness, or the ingested amount of methanol is >0.4 ml/kg, give 20% ethanol orally (200 ml of ethanol + 800 ml juice) at a rate of 300 ml in the first hour, thereafter 100 ml at 2-hour intervals, if the patient responds when spoken to.
  - To an unconscious patient, give 10% ethanol intravenously (100 ml of ethanol + 900 ml of 5% glucose solution) with 5–10 ml/kg in one hour as the starting dose and thereafter 0.15–0.3 ml/kg/hour. Give the upper limit of the dose range to chronic alcoholics. Aim: to maintain blood alcohol concentration at 1 per mil.
  - Sodium bicarbonate infusion of 1 ml/kg in 15 minutes
  - Fomepizole is an alternative to ethanol: the dose is 10–20 mg/kg in 100 ml of NaCl in the first 30 minutes, thereafter 10 mg/kg at 12-hour intervals.
- Treatment should always be given in a hospital where haemodialysis can be carried out.

Ethylene glycol poisoning

- Found in, for example, antifreeze solutions.
- The lethal dose is 100–150 ml.
- Symptoms
  - As in methanol intoxication, with the following differences
    - Visual symptoms are absent
    - Renal symptoms: haematuria and proteinuria are possible
    - Hyperglycaemia may occur.
- Treatment
  - As in methanol intoxication.

Drugs

- Drug addicts usually need acute care for the following causes: overdose, withdrawal symptoms and trauma.
- Multiple addiction is usual.
  - Several drugs
  - Medications
  - Alcohol
- Users of intravenous drugs may have blood-transmitted diseases (80% have hepatitis C).
- The concentration and purity of drugs varies, combinations of different drugs are common.

Heroin

- The risk of dying from an overdose is approx. 1% /year for a regular user.
- Overdose usually results only from intravenous administration.
- Mixed intoxication, particularly with alcohol, worsens symptoms.
- Symptoms
  - Opioid syndrome, see above
  - Unconsciousness is always an emergency.
- Treatment
  - For immediate actions, see Figure 17.20.
  - If oxygenation cannot be corrected rapidly with efficient mask ventilation AND/OR respiratory rales are loud, the patient must be intubated.
  - Naloxone is the antidote. The dose is smaller than with other opioids (0.08 mg at a time at 15–30 s intervals until respiration returns to normal, maximum dose is 2 mg), thereafter the rate of dosing is slower until the patient wakes up. The necessary dose is usually 0.4–0.8 mg and the patient wakes up in 10 minutes on average.
  - If an i.v. line is not established quickly, equal efficacy is obtained with s.c. or i.m. administration with a single dose of 0.8 mg.
- A follow-up time of 2 hours is generally recommended.
  - Rare adverse effects, e.g. convulsions

  - Recurring of opioid syndrome (rare when only heroin is used)
  - Other causes, e.g. aspiration pneumonia.
- An adult patient can be left without monitoring safely IF
  - the intoxication is caused by heroin alone (alcometer test, history) AND
  - the patient refuses treatment AND
  - the patient is fully orientated AND
  - an additional dose of naloxone 0.4–0.8 mg i.m. has been given.

Stimulants (amphetamine, cocaine, crack, ecstasy, etc)

- Symptoms: adrenergic syndrome, see Table 17.20.1
- Cocaine causes more severe cardiac symptoms (arrhythmias, MI) and convulsions than other substances.
- Severe dehydration, electrolyte disturbances and hyperthermia are associated particularly with ecstasy.
- Risk of sudden death is increased by the following conditions
  - Arrhythmias/chest pain
  - Intense agitation that required forceful management
- Treatment
  - Sedation with benzodiazepines, e.g. diazepam 5–10 mg i.v. or lorazepam 2–4 mg i.v. Give a sufficiently large dose, as an agitated patient is at risk of sudden death.
  - Chest pain/spell of unconsciousness/feeling of arrhythmia =>ECG
  - Hypertensive crisis
    - Calm the patient
    - Labetalol 20–50 mg i.v., if necessary as an infusion 60–120 mg/hour; the use of beta-blocker alone is not recommended (the remaining alpha-effect may cause a hypertensive crisis).
  - In myocardial ischaemia, give nitrates, e.g. nitroglycerin infusion 20–200 μg/min or even thrombolytic therapy
  - Arrhythmias and hyperthermia: see symptomatic treatment
  - With ecstasy, sufficient fluid administration is important.

Gammahydroxybutyrate (GHB)

- Often used as a sedative after stimulant abuse.
- Symptoms
  - Sedative syndrome resembling alcohol intoxication
  - Mild bradycardia is a typical symptom.
  - Symptoms last for 2–8 hours.

PCP

- Hallucinogenic => hallucinations, catatony, psychosis
- Typical symptoms include nystagmus and hypoglycaemia.
- Symptomatic treatment, sedation with benzodiazepines if necessary

17.24 Carbon monoxide poisoning

Markku Ellonen

Aims

- Remember to suspect carbon monoxide poisoning always when your patient suffers from unexplained headache, fatigue (unconsciousness), nausea and vomiting. Because the symptoms of are so unspecific, exposure to carbon monoxide is an under-diagnosed problem.
- Hyperbaric oxygen therapy is beneficial in severe carbon monoxide poisoning causing unconsciousness (COHb > 40 %) C [1 2 3 4 5 6 7 8 9].
- Pulse oximetry does not distinguish between carboxyhaemoglobin (COHb) and oxyhaemoglobin (OHb) and thus gives false normal results for a severely anoxic patient.

General comments

- Carbon monoxide poisoning leading to death is in most cases suicide. Accidental poisonings are caused by petrol-driven motors running at idle in a closed space, by various heaters that use fuels or gas at a low-burning flame, and also by traditional wood-burning heaters.
- Persons with cardiac and respiratory diseases develop symptoms of anoxia already at a smaller exposure to carbon monoxide (COHb 10–20 %). In basically healthy persons, the first symptoms are disturbances of consciousness of varying severity.
- In addition to anoxia, carbon monoxide has other toxic effects causing organ damage comparable to that caused by cyanide.
- The severity of poisoning is dependent on the concentration of CO and on the exposure time.

Symptoms and findings

- Symptoms are nonspecific and the diagnosis is often delayed. Sometimes the poisoning is diagnosed as respiratory or GI infection.
- Neurological symptoms include headache, tiredness, nausea and vomiting. Unconsciousness of varying level occurs in the most severe cases.
- Unconscious patients often have red lips and cheeks.
- As a consequence of CO poisoning the patient may develop slowly reversible or even permanent unspecific neurological changes.

Diagnosis

- Difficult to reach, particularly in milder cases in which exposure is not revealed.
- Diagnosis is made easier if several persons fall sick at the same time.
- Measuring blood COHb concentration confirms clinical suspicion (In smokers COHb concentration is frequently 5%.)

Treatment

- A mild poisoning is alleviated in fresh air over several hours.
- Breathing pure oxygen (100%) reduces the half-life of COHb to a couple of hours. Oxygen therapy should be given for 4–6 hours.
- In severe poisonings, rapidly started hyperbaric oxygen therapy reduces neurological damage.
- European consensus statement issued in 1994 recommends hyperbaric oxygen therapy to patients who have been unconscious or who have severe neurological or cardiac symptoms. COHb level above 40% also requires hyperbaric oxygen even if the patient is asymptomatic. COHb concentration does not always correlate with the severity of the poisoning!
- The results from hyperbaric oxygen therapy in the management of milder CO poisonings are contradictory.

References

1. Medical Services Advisory Committee. Hyperbaric oxygen therapy. Canberra: Medical Services Advisory Committee (MSAC). 2001. 131. Medical Services Advisory Committee (MSAC). www.msac.gov.au.
2. Hailey D. Hyperbaric oxygen therapy—recent findings on evidence for its effectiveness. Update. Edmonton: Alberta Heritage Foundation for Medical Research (AHFMR). 2003. 25. Alberta Heritage Foundation for Medical Research (AHFMR). www.ahfmr.ab.ca.
3. McDonagh M, Carson S, Ash J. Hyperbaric oxygen therapy for brain injury, cerebral palsy, and stroke. Rockville: Agency for Healthcare Research and Quality (AHRQ). 2003. Agency for Healthcare Research and Quality (AHRQ). www.ahrq.gov.
4. Saunders P. Hyperbaric oxygen therapy in the management of carbon monoxide poisoning, osteoradionecrosis, burns, skin grafts and crush injury. Birmingham: West Midlands Health Technology Assessment Collaboration, University of Birmingham (Collaborative effort with Wessex Institute). 2000. 52. West Midlands Health Technology Assessment Collaboration (WMHTAC).
5. Health Technology Assessment Database: HTA-20020065. The Cochrane Library, Issue 1, 2004. Chichester, UK: John Wiley & Sons, Ltd.
6. Health Technology Assessment Database: HTA-20030475. The Cochrane Library, Issue 1, 2004. Chichester, UK: John Wiley & Sons, Ltd.
7. Health Technology Assessment Database: HTA-20031127. The Cochrane Library, Issue 1, 2004. Chichester, UK: John Wiley & Sons, Ltd.
8. Health Technology Assessment Database: HTA-20000924. The Cochrane Library, Issue 1, 2004. Chichester, UK: John Wiley & Sons, Ltd.
9. Juurlink DN, Stanbrook MB, McGuigan MA. Hyperbaric oxygen for carbon monoxide poisoning. Cochrane Database Syst Rev. 2004;(2):CD002041.

17.30 Preoperative assessment

Markku Ellonen

TRA

Principles

- When interpreted widely, preoperative assessment of the patient should be based on the benefits of surgery to the patient. The physician referring the patient for surgery should also take part in this assessment.
- Assessment of anaesthetic risk is only a minor part of the total preoperative assessment.
- The task of the treating (referring) physician is to
  - individually assess the appropriateness of the proposed surgery
  - anticipate possible difficulties during recovery
  - carry out the set preoperative investigations
  - inform the surgeon about the patient's comorbidities which might affect the outcome of surgery
  - optimally treat chronic diseases and monitor the treatment if surgery is postponed.

Assessment of anaesthetic risk

- The most used tool for patient classification is the Physical Status Classification by the American Society of Anesthesiologists (ASA).
  1. A normal healthy patient, aged less than 65 years or aged more than 12 months (more than 1 month in some cases).
  2. A patient aged more than 65 years or with mild systemic disease (e.g. uncomplicated, controlled hypertension).
  3. A patient with severe systemic disease that is not a threat to life (e.g. type 1 diabetes with hypertension).
  4. A patient with incapacitating systemic disease that is a constant threat to life (e.g. uncontrolled diabetes or unstable angina pectoris).
  5. A moribund patient who is not expected to survive for 24 hours without surgery.

Preparation for surgery

- The surgical team and the general practitioner should agree on the basic investigations that can be carried out in primary care. The aim is to minimise the postponement of the operation and shorten the number of preoperative inpatient days.

- Before suggesting surgery to the patient, the treating physician must consider the availability of the particular surgery and its hazards. Any anticipated problems during recovery must also be addressed.
- If the waiting list is long, the treating physician must monitor the patient's condition for changes that could increase the operative risk, i.e.
  - TIA or stroke
  - worsening angina pectoris, myocardial infarction or exacerbation of heart failure
  - uncontrolled diabetes or emergence of complications
  - worsening of COPD.
- Even acute viral upper respiratory tract infection is an indication to postpone elective surgery.

Preoperative laboratory investigations

- Traditional extensive preoperative screening has been streamlined without compromising patient safety (A) [1 2]. The majority of the basic investigations can be carried out by the general practitioner.
- The following suggestions are for day case surgery:
  - Local anaesthesia: no investigations needed
  - An otherwise healthy patient aged less than 50 years (ASA 1):
    - No routine investigations (A) [1 2]. (Consider Hb for women and ECG for men.)
  - An otherwise healthy patient over 50 (ASA 1)
    - Blood count, ECG; if more than 60 years:chest x-ray.
  - A patient with cardiovascular disease, lung disease, diabetes or nephropathy:
    - Blood count, electrolytes, ECG, chest x-ray, creatinine, blood glucose
  - A diabetic patient:
    - In addition to the above, blood glucose on the morning of the procedure
  - Patients on anticoagulant therapy:
    - INR (also on the morning of surgery).

Division of tasks between primary and specialist care

- The referring general practitioner should inform the surgical team about:
  - the diagnosis of the disease in question, its severity and urgency of operation
  - the co-operating capacity of the patient, especially during the recovery period
  - possible dementia and other factors affecting the decision to operate that may be missed in hospital investigations
  - other co-existing serious conditions, recent changes in the health status in particular, as well as the latest laboratory findings.
  - an anaesthetic questionnaire may be given to the patient (or completed with him/her) prior to day case surgery under general anaesthesia, in accordance with local practice.
- **A specialist in internal medicine** should prescribe the pre- and postoperative medication for patients with serious diseases.
- **An anaesthetist** will assess the risks associated with anaesthesia and is responsible for the medication during anaesthesia.
- **A surgeon** makes the final decision on whether to operate and decides on the eligibility of the patient for day case surgery, for which all the necessary information must be at his/her disposal.

The risks of co-existing common diseases on surgery

Coronary heart disease

- The most important single disease as regards operative risk. Preliminary estimation of exercise tolerance can be judged from the medical history. The patient's NYHA class (I–IV) should be estimated. The risk of cardiac complications is low in NYHA classes I–II. In practice this means that the patient is able to climb one flight of stairs, carrying a small shopping bag, without cardiac symptoms.
- Operative risk is increased significantly if
  - less than 6 weeks have passed since myocardial infarction, angioplasty or coronary artery by-pass graft
  - the patient has poor exercise tolerance or heart failure after myocardial infarction
  - the patient has severe or unstable (newly diagnosed!) angina pectoris.
  - Only urgent surgery is usually carried out in these patients.
- Operative risk is increased slightly if
  - 3 months have passed since myocardial infarction, and the patient has good exercise tolerance. Diabetes increases the risk.
  - the patient has stable angina pectoris with good exercise tolerance.
- Beta-blocker protection is important for patients with coronary heart disease undergoing surgery. If no contraindications exist a beta-blocker is administered to patients before and during surgery and for 2 weeks after surgery. This will considerably reduce the incidence of severe cardiac events.

Heart failure

- Decompensated heart failure will significantly increase the operative risk, and only urgent surgery should be undertaken.
- Compensated heart failure (with history of decompensation) increases the risk moderately.

Valvular heart disease

- Symptomatic aortic stenosis represents a high risk as regards non-cardiac surgery. The patient should be referred for cardiac surgery.
- Asymptomatic valvular disease does not prevent surgery. Prophylaxis against endocarditis is often indicated. (4.81)
- Mitral valve prosthesis is subject to thrombosis. Anticoagulation must not be stopped even temporarily unless the indications are vital (4.12). Anticoagulation is carried out with heparin during the operative phase.

Arrhythmias

- In most cases arrhythmia only requires intensified monitoring but is not a contraindication to surgery. Acute atrial fibrillation must be treated before surgery; it is a common perioperative arrhythmia.

Anticoagulation therapy

- See 5.44.
- The treating physician should make a decision regarding the importance of anticoagulation.
- Anticoagulation therapy of patients with valve prosthesis must usually not be discontinued unless absolutely indicated. (4.12)
- Anticoagulation may often be reduced (INR 1.5) for a few days (when a moderately long time has lapsed since pulmonary embolism) or it can be temporarily discontinued for a few days (chronic atrial fibrillation, TIA).

Hypertension

- Controlled hypertension without complications does not significantly increase operative risk. Medication should continue right up to surgery. Complicated hypertension is often associated with impaired renal function and type 2 diabetes.

Diabetes mellitus

- Diabetes is associated with increased risk of cardiovascular disease and, in some cases, multi-organ damage.
- Metformin should be stopped a few days before surgery.
- The prevention of perioperative hyperglycaemia is very important in order to prevent complications and infections from occurring.
- Recovery may be complicated by reduced renal function, proneness to infections and delayed wound healing.
- The routine investigations include:
  - blood glucose both on the day before surgery and on the morning of surgery, HbA1c and creatinine
  - ECG
  - chest x-ray, if considered necessary.

Obesity

- Pathological changes in almost all vital organs follow weight gain exceeding normal weight by more than 20% (BMI > 30).
- Overweight patients are at an increased risk of operative, or postoperative, morbidity and mortality.
- Morbidly obese patients (BMI > 35) are not suitable for day case surgery under general anaesthesia.
- Anaesthetic risks arise from breathing and circulation problems.
- The pulmonary function of obese patients is impaired due to the reduced movement of the diaphragm.
- If surgery is planned for an obese patient, particularly abdominal or thoracic surgery, the following investigations are always necessary:
  - chest x-ray
  - ECG
  - spirometry and often blood gas analysis.

Respiratory diseases

- Acute viral upper respiratory tract infection usually calls for the postponement of the operation, except for urgent surgery.
- Chronic pulmonary disease must be treated optimally. Pulmonary obstruction of COPD and asthma patients must not be worse than normal, nor should these patients have bacterial infections which require treatment. COPD is often associated with coronary heart disease.
- Stopping smoking 1–2 months before surgery is important.
- If FEV_1 is less than 50% of normal, upper abdominal surgery poses a greater risk than gynaecological or orthopaedic surgery.
- Spirometry is used to assess the risks of respiratory problems and is indicated for
  - patients with asthma or COPD as well as heavy smokers if upper abdominal surgery is planned.
  - As well as carrying out spirometry, other diseases which may affect the patient's eligibility for surgery should be taken into account.

Neurological diseases

- Recent stroke and TIA will usually result in elective surgery being postponed by 3 months.

Special problems with patients with cataracts

- Cataract is usually operated on under local anaesthesia.
- General anaesthesia is required for restless, non-cooperative patients and those with marked tremor.
- After operation the patient is allowed to mobilise immediately.
- Patients with cataracts often have many concomitant diseases. Exercise tolerance is not important. Acute or chronic cough for any reason can be problematic for cataract surgery. Patients with orthopnoea are unsuitable for cataract surgery. A thorough drug history should be obtained.

Patient selection for day case surgery

- Most decisions regarding the patient's fitness for surgery are made by the surgeon during a preoperative interview. A preoperative interview with an anaesthetist is not a routine practice. Not all patients are necessarily interviewed before the procedure. In this case the surgeon should ensure that the medical records contain all the necessary information for him/her to make a decision regarding the need for a preoperative interview and whether the patient is eligible for day case surgery.
- Referral should include:
  - a list of diseases which may increase the operative risk, and their severity
  - medication and its necessity (warfarin!)
  - selected laboratory and radiographic investigations
  - home circumstances
  - responsible adult to take the patient home and stay with the patient overnight
  - capacity of the patient's own primary care team to provide support
  - an anaesthetic questionnaire, depending on local practice.
- Day case surgery is not suited for:
  - abdominal surgery (except laparoscopic surgery)
  - unstable ASA 3 or ASA 4 (stable is often suitable)
  - morbid obesity (BMI > 35)
  - moderate obesity combined with a systemic disease
  - alcoholism and drug abuse
  - social problems, a patient who will not give consent for surgery or who does not understand instructions or has no support person at home.
  - MAO inhibitor medication must be discontinued 1–2 days before general anaesthesia.

References

1. Munro J, Booth A, Nicholl J. Routine preoperative testing: a systematic review of evidence. Health Technol Assess 1997;1:1–63.
2. The Database of Abstracts of Reviews of Effectiveness (University of York), Database no.: DARE-988286. In: The Cochrane Library, Issue 4, 1999. Oxford: Update Software.

17.40 Chronic pain

Martina Bachmann

Basic rules

- Patients with the most severe chronic pains are referred to a specialized pain clinic.
- Pain is documented on every visit by using the Visual Analogue Scale (VAS) for pain (0–10).
- Rehabilitation is arranged for patients with poor treatment response to help with adapting to and coping with the symptoms.

General

- Pain in considered chronic when it has continued for more than 6 months or has lasted longer than what is the normal healing time of tissues.
- The situation is often problematic when the pathological findings are minimal and the functional disturbance is large.
- Depression, suffering and anxiety are associated with chronic pain. The patient's psychosocial condition is taken into account in treatment and rehabilitation.
- The pathophysiology of the pain is assessed as carefully as possible and treatment is planned according to the aetiology of pain.
- By treating acute pain as well as possible, pain can be prevented from becoming chronic.

Types of chronic pain

Nociceptive pain

- Pain arising purely from tissue injury (nociperception = perception of tissue injury)
  - Ischaemic pain
  - Musculoskeletal pain
  - Infection pain
  - Degenerative pain in connective tissues
- The reason for the pain comes outside the nervous system.
- Nociceptive pain may also involve sensitization to touch in the corresponding skin area.
- Long-term pain in the extremities in particular, may activate the sympathetic nervous system, appearing as a change in the temperature and colour of the limb.
- Sympathetic nervous system is also activated in ischaemic cardiac pain, interstitial cystitis, and in functional abdominal pain (colon irritabile), although the pain is nociceptive.

Neuropathic pain

- The injury is located in the pain pathway of the nervous system.
- As a result of changes in the nervous system, the sense of touch functions abnormally, and earlier painless stimulus, e.g. touch, may cause intense pain (allodynia).
- Allodynia and sensation of touch occur also without stimulus. Pain is diagnosed as neuropathic when the neuroanatomical location of pain is explained by the injury (is logical) and the function of the sense of touch is altered.
- **Peripheral nerve injury**
  - Diabetic neuropathy (23.42)
  - Compression disorders (36.88)

- Sequelae of peripheral nerve injuries
- Compression of nerve root caused by intervertebral disk herniation (20.30)

♦ **Central nerve injury**
- Phantom pain
- Neuropathic pains caused by multiple sclerosis
- Unilateral pains following disturbances of cerebral circulation.

♦ **Both peripheral and central nerve injury** may be the underlying cause in postherpetic and phantom pain.

Chronic pain syndrome

♦ In chronic pain syndrome clear tissue or nerve injury is not found.
♦ The patients may have similar changes in the concentrations of CNS neurotransmitters that have been found in depressive patients (e.g. atypical facial pains).

Examining a patient with pain

♦ Thorough history: life situation, family, community factors at work etc.
♦ A visual analogue scale (VAS) is used to measure pain (scale 0–10, 0 = no pain at all, 10 = worst conceivable pain).
♦ The pain is measured and documented on each visit.
♦ Sensory changes and location of the pain observed by the patient should be documented in a pain drawing.
♦ Pay attention to skin temperature, vitality and sweating (the activity of sympathetic nervous system).
♦ Neuropathic pain
- Test the following senses in neurological examination: touch, sharp touch, heat, vibration, and cold, as well as the reaction to a normally painless stimulus, such a gentle stroking of the skin.
- Tests for motor function, reflexes and cranial nerves give an idea of the location of the injury. Testing helps to clarify the diagnosis and tailor the therapy.
- Normal result in electroneuromyography (ENMG) (36.16) does not exclude the possibility of peripheral neuropathy.

Treatment of chronic pain

♦ Treatment is tailored individually depending on the mechanisms of pain and the patient's characteristics by testing one method at a time and by combining treatments based on different mechanisms.
♦ In many cases the treatment is merely symptomatic; aetiological treatment should be given immediately (e.g. relieving a compressed nerve).
♦ Symptomatic treatment is the more effective the earlier it is begun.
♦ Understanding the psychodynamic origins of the pain.

Nociceptive pain

♦ Curative therapy prevents the pain from becoming chronic.
♦ Common analgesics (NSAIDs and, with special indications, opioids)
♦ Physiotherapy
♦ Stimulation therapies (TENS **C** [1], acupuncture)
♦ Local anaesthesias
♦ Pain management group
- Groups for pain patients lead by physiotherapists or outpatient care psychologists.

Neuropathic pain

♦ Stimulation therapies (TENS **C** [1], acupuncture)
♦ Tricyclic antidepressants (particularly amitriptyline, nortriptyline)
♦ Epilepsy medications (particularly carbamazepine, gabapentine)
♦ Pain management group

Chronic pain syndrome

♦ Tricyclic antidepressants
♦ Pain management group

TRA

Opioids in chronic pain

♦ Mainly used only when all other alternatives have been tried.
♦ If the diagnosis is clear, e.g. an elderly patient has spinal stenosis or osteoporotic pain, opioid therapy can be started sooner.
♦ The aetiology of the pain should be investigated as well as possible.
♦ Other indications
- The pain is clearly alleviated with an opioid and the patient's functional capacity improves.
- The patient does not have a tendency for drug abuse.

♦ Opioid therapy should preferably be started as the joint decision of two physicians. The implementation of the therapy should be the responsibility of only one doctor, with follow up at 1–3-month intervals.
♦ The administration is started with an oral preparation and the dose is raised gradually over 4–8 weeks. The drug should be taken regularly, not "as needed".
♦ The patient should be well informed of the principles of medication, and he/she may increase the dose only according the previously agreed scheme.
♦ Other methods of pain treatment are continued.
♦ Tramadol is effective in the treatment of diabetic polyneuropathy.
♦ Opioids are used only to treat pain. Specific medication is used to treat anxiety and depression.
♦ Opioid therapy for problem patients and those with chronic (but non malign) pain with strong opioids should be started in special pain management units.

Tricyclic antidepressants

♦ Analgetic effect is independent of depression.

- Lower doses are needed for pain alleviation than for reducing depression.
- There is most research data on amitriptyline, which exerts an analgetic effect already in 4–5 days.
- Drug of choice in neuropathic pain **A** [2 3 4 5]
- Start with small evening doses, starting dose 10–25 mg. The drug also improves the quality of sleep.
- The dose is raised by 10 mg every other day, until maximal pain relief is achieved or side effects (tiredness, dry mouth, constipation, voiding problems, orthostatic hypotension) prevent raising the dose.
- The benefit can be assessed when the dose has been constant for 2 weeks.
- If side effects are problematic and do not relieve when the therapy is continued, try the metabolite of amitriptyline nortriptyline or combine a cholinergic drug (distigmine) to therapy.

Other antidepressants

- Venlafaxine and mirtazapine have an effect profile similar to that of amitriptyline, but without as much its problematic anticholinergic side effects.
- The analgetic effect of serotonin reuptake inhibitors is milder than that of tricyclic drugs.

Anticonvulsive medications

- Used particularly for pain caused by nerve injury with electric shock-type elements.
- Main indications are trigeminal neuralgia, post-herpetic neuralgia, diabetic neuropathy and paroxysmal pains in MS.
- Carbamazepine is the most widely used drug, with trigeminal neuralgia as a special indication.
  - Starting dose is 100 mg × 2 and the dose is raised until the daily dose is 600–800 mg.
  - Side effects include tiredness, ataxia, dizziness, visual disturbances, nausea and dryness of the mouth.
  - During carbamazepine therapy, liver enzymes and blood count must be monitored.
- Alternatives to carbamazepine are clonazepam 0.5–2 mg × 3–4 (facial pain, muscle tension), oxcarbazepine 300–600 mg × 2 or sodium valproate 300–500 mg × 3 (effective particularly in migraine).
- Gabapentin at a dose of 300–400 mg × 3 is effective for diabetic neuropathy **B** [6] and post-herpetic neuralgia (to be started carefully, raising the dose gradually).

Topical drugs

- Capsaicin cream (0.025% and 0.075%) is used topically in diabetic neuropathy and in pain following nerve injury.
- The effect is seen only after weeks.
- Topical anaesthetic (EMLA) is used for post-herpetic pain

TENS therapy (transcutaneous electrical nerve stimulation)

- In musculosceletal pain (fibromyalgia, arthritis and arthrosis) the electrodes can be placed in the area of pain or close to it. Treatment targeted at trigger points reduces sensitivity to pressure and relaxes muscles.
- In post-herpetic neuralgia the electrodes are placed above or below the sick dermatome.
- In nerve injury pain the electrode is placed normally on the area of skin with a sense of touch. Areas without sense of touch do not contain sensory fibres and in the area of sensitized skin the stimulation would be intolerably strong. The electrodes can also be placed on the corresponding dermatome on the healthy side.
- The treatment is most effective in the beginning. In some patients the effect wears out in long-term therapy **C** [1].
- Cardiac pacemaker is a contraindication.

Acupuncture

- Most useful in mild nociceptive tension-type pains affecting the musculoskeletal system and in migraine.
- Acupuncture may trigger autonomic reactions such as nausea, bradycardia and tiredness.

Local anaesthetic injections

- Series of injections of local anaesthetics have traditionally been used in the management of chronic pain, but the evidence on their effect has remained scarce.
- The analgetic effect is longer than the pharmacological anaesthetic effect. Epidural and spinal anaesthesias are given only by hospital pain clinics.
- The injections are helpful because the analgesia normalizes the function and motor activity on the painful area (eg. resolves muscle spasms).

Trigger anaesthetics

- In myofascial pain trigger point pain may be present. Trigger pain radiates widely and also causes autonomic reflexes.
- The site of injection is located by palpating for a pain-sensitive point and by fixing it between two fingers. The injection is given aseptically (bupivacaine 0.125–0.25 % has the longest duration of action) at doses of 1–3 ml in the neck region, 4–8 ml in the shoulder, back and pelvic regions and 10 ml in the lumbar region.
- Corticosteroids can be added to the injections, e.g. 4 mg/10 ml of dexamethasone. After anaesthesia the muscle should be stretched first passively, later actively.

Arranging the management of chronic pain and cooperation between primary and specialist care

- The most serious cases of chronic pain are identified in primary care and are referred to a pain clinic. Ensure that the patient receives a holistic treatment for pain with adequate follow up.
- Major hospitals have pain clinics where specialists representing at least two different fields are in charge of the treatment. The clinics usually have a multidisciplinary team with an anaesthesiologist specialized in pain management, physiatrist, psychologist, psychiatrist, neurologist, orthopaedist and social worker
- The role of the psychologist is prominent when a patient tries to identify his/her own mechanisms of pain management.

References

1. Carroll D, Moore RA, McQuay HJ, Fairman F, Tramèr M, Leijon G. Transcutaneous electrical nerve stimulation (TENS) for chronic pain. Cochrane Database Syst Rev. 2004;(2):CD003222.
2. Kingery WS. A critical review of controlled clinical trials for peripheral neuropathic pain and complex regional pain syndromes. Pain 1997;73:123–139.
3. The Database of Abstracts of Reviews of Effectiveness (University of York), Database no.: DARE-980065. In: The Cochrane Library, Issue 4, 1999. Oxford: Update Software.
4. McQuay JH, Tramer M, Nye BA, Carroll D, Wiffen PJ, Moore RA. A systematic review of antidepressants in neuropathic pain. Pain 1996;68:217–227.
5. The Database of Abstracts of Reviews of Effectiveness (University of York), Database no.: DARE-978044. In: The Cochrane Library, Issue 4, 1999. Oxford: Update Software.
6. Wiffen P, McQuay H, Carroll D, Jadad A, Moore A. Anticonvulsant drugs for acute and chronic pain. Cochrane Database Syst Rev. 2004; (2): CD001133.

TRA

Traumatology and Plastic Surgery

Evidence Based Medicine Guidelines. Edited by the Duodecim Editorial Team
 ISBN: 0-470-01184-X

18.1 Facial injuries

Editors

Introduction

- In a first aid situation, secure the airways by removing any clotted blood, dentures and free fragments from the mouth, particularly if the patient has an impaired level of consciousness.
- If the injury extends to the oral cavity or pharynx, oedema of the throat may be extensive. Patency of the airways must be ensured at an early stage, see also 6.60.
- The management of facial fractures requires good clinical experience and should be left to the care of a specialist. Approximately half of all facial fractures are missed if x-rays alone are examined.

Urgency of treatment

- Within hours
  - Gunshot wounds
  - Comminuted fractures of the middle third of the face with associated eye injury
  - Concurrent fracture of the maxilla and mandible with anticipated compromise of the airways.
  - Multiple fracture of the mandible with compromised airways.
- Within 24 hours
  - Open fractures of the mandible
  - Fractures of the middle third of the face without eye involvement
- On the next working day
  - Undisplaced fracture of the zygomatic bone
  - Nasal fractures
- Stage the urgency of treatment only after the airways have been secured.
- Severe facial soft tissue injuries and burn injuries demand careful evaluation and treatment by a specialist.

Fracture types

Nasal fractures

- Nasal fracture see 38.43.

Lateral fractures of the face

- Loss of sensation on the malar eminence is suggestive of a dislocated fracture and warrants a referral for specialist care.
- Often missed due to swelling. Diagnosis is easier if the face is viewed from above with simultaneous palpation. X-rays: occipito-mental and AP projections.
- Reduction should be carried out at an early phase.
- If left untreated may result in diplopia and sensory loss over the cheek bone area (damage to the infraorbital nerve).

Orbital fractures

- Should be suspected if the eye has received a direct blow. Symptoms:
  - periorbital oedema and haematoma
  - subconjunctival haemorrhage
  - diplopia, especially when looking up
  - displacement of the pupil (downward).
- In a blow-out fracture, the impact directed towards the eye transmits pressure to the orbit which will break at the weakest point.
- Often missed in plain x-rays. Consider CT scanning.

Maxillary fractures

- Fractures of the maxilla require urgent attention since the mid-portion of the face may move backwards leading to airway obstruction.
- The patient is often unconscious; ensure patency of the airways.
- In severe head injury, check paranasal sinuses from skull x-rays. Any shadowing over a sinus may be suggestive of bleeding and a fracture of the maxilla.
- Examine AP, lateral and occipito-mental projections. A CT scan is always indicated in high impact trauma.
- For classification, see Table 18.1.

Mandibular fractures

- Often caused by physical violence. Swelling of the mouth and pharynx may block the airways.
- Diagnosed by palpating the lower jaw, also from inside the oral cavity. Examination is often hampered by the patient's intoxicated state.
- Examine teeth and dental occlusion, often the patient is aware of abnormal occlusion.
- Examine orthopantomographs, transaxial and oblique projections.

Table 18.1 Le Fort fractures

Le Fort Type 1	The dentulous area of the maxilla is detached from the midface at the level of the maxillary sinuses and the base of the nose. The nose and orbits are intact.
Le Fort Type 2	The fracture line passes through the maxillary sinuses, the orbits and the bridge of the nose. The midface is mobile.
Le Fort Type 3	The fracture line passes through the lateral orbital edges and the bridge of the nose. The midface is detached from the base of the skull.

18.2 Skull and brain injury

Editors

Basic rules

- Recognize any injury to the brain.
- Evaluate the extent of the skull injury according to the history of the events and the patient's clinical state, i.e. concussion (18.3), contusion (18.4) and intracranial bleeding or haematoma (18.5).
- Monitor the level of consciousness, and send patients requiring immediate attention to a hospital with appropriate facilities.
- Monitor and support vital functions during transport.

Diagnosis of brain injury

Level of consciousness

- Record the patient's initial level of consciousness and monitor any changes, initially on a scale: awake / arousable / responds to movement / responds to pain / unarousable.
- Specify the level of consciousness at a later stage using the Glasgow Coma Scale (GCS) (Table 18.2).

Pupils

- Increased intracranial pressure may dilate the pupil on the side of the injury. Check pupil size and reaction to light. A fixed dilated pupil requires urgent intervention.

Table 18.2 Glasgow Coma Scale

Criteria		Score
Eyes open	Spontaneously	4
	To speech	3
	To pain	2
	None	1
Best motor response	Obeys commands	6
	Localizes/avoids pain	5
	Withdraws from pain	4
	Flexion	3
	Extension	2
	None	1
Best verbal response	Orientated	5
	Confused	4
	Inappropriate words	3
	Incomprehensible sounds	2
	None	1
		Total: 3–15

Body temperature

- Brain injury may disturb the temperature regulation leading to increased body temperature. If necessary, cool the patient down.

Skull x-rays

- If the patient's level of consciousness is impaired, send him/her directly to a casualty department of a hospital.
- Skull x-rays are indicated if a skull injury is associated with:
  - a suspicion of a penetrative injury
  - intoxication or
- if the patient's condition is difficult to assess, for example due to epilepsy or psychiatric problems.

Linear skull fracture

- A linear skull fracture is a finding on a skull x-rays and is often an indication for closer clinical observation, but seldom a sign of brain injury.
- A fracture may indicate
  - an increased (100-fold) risk of haematoma (18.5)
  - a risk of infection in the posterior wall of the paranasal sinuses.
- In children, a skull fracture may sometimes increase in size. A repeat x-ray of a skull fracture is therefore indicated in children (under 2–3 years of age) at a later stage.

Fracture of the base of the skull

- Often caused by a fall.
- May be associated with concussion or more severe injury.

Fracture of the anterior cranial fossa

- The symptoms include bleeding and CSF leakage from the nose, eyelid haematoma, loss of smell because of a severed olfactory bulb (38.6) and sometimes symptoms associated with the optic nerve.
- A skull x-ray is usually not diagnostic; a CT scan is warranted.

Fracture of the middle cranial fossa

- The symptoms include bleeding and (later) CSF leakage from the auditory canal, and impairment or loss of hearing.
- Facial paresis (36.93) is possible either immediately or within a couple of days.

Fracture of posterior cranial fossa

- Rare
- Symptoms resemble those of the fracture of middle cranial fossa.

Treatment

- Conservative treatment for 1 week. Follow-up at the hospital outpatient clinic.

- The use of antibiotics is controversial. Many physicians prescribe penicillin due to the involvement of the paranasal sinuses; the patient is at risk of **meningitis**.
- **Haematomas** are more likely in patients with fractures.
- If **CSF leakage** continues for more than one week, the brain may have herniated through a tear in the dura. Surgery at a neurosurgical unit is required.

Depressed fracture

- Depressions equal to or more than the thickness of the bone should be treated surgically.
- **An open fracture** should be operated on within 24 hours.
  - If there is no brain injury, the case is not urgent. However, a transfer to the care of a neurosurgical team is indicated.
  - A CT scan is useful to show possible injury under the bone.
  - The risk of epilepsy is increased if the dura is torn.
  - **A closed depression fracture** is also usually an indication for treatment even if only for cosmetic reasons.

Indications for neurological consultation

- In addition to a skull fracture the patient
  - is confused or shows signs of reduced level of consciousness
  - has localized neurological signs or
  - is fitting.
- Confusion or neurological signs last for more than 12 hours.
- The patient remains unconscious after resuscitation.
- There is a suspicion of open skull fracture or a fracture of the base of the skull.
- Depression fracture
- The level of consciousness deteriorates or neurological symptoms emerge.

18.3 Brain concussion (commotio cerebri)

Editors

- For central nervous system injuries in children, see 32.75.

Aims

- Arrange observation for a patient with concussion at home, at an outpatient clinic or on a ward.
- Recognize any signs of intracranial haematoma during the observation, and in such case refer the patient immediately.
- Refer for further examinations any patient who has been observed as an outpatient over 1 week and who still has symptoms.

Symptoms of brain injury

- A change in the level of consciousness is the main symptom of a brain injury.
- The injury is mild if the patient is conscious when coming to see the doctor.
- In concussion, the unconsciousness lasts for less than 15–30 minutes.
- If unconsciousness lasts for more than 30 minutes, brain contusion (18.4) is probable.
- Progressive intracranial haematoma (18.5) is the third possible diagnosis.
- Any patient who has been unconscious after a trauma should be observed for the sake of differential diagnosis. At least two physical examinations with 2 hours interval are needed before making any decisions about further treatment.

Concussion (commotio cerebri)

- The history includes a trauma caused by a fall or other mild injury. The patient is conscious when examined. Alcohol often causes diagnostic problems.
- Symptoms: loss of consciousness, amnesia, headache, vomiting and repetition of same phrase or word.
- The clinical examination (36.1) must not reveal any local neurological findings. The examination should be repeated within two hours.
- Skull x-rays are not necessary but provide further information. Discovery of a skull fracture means a 100-fold increase in the risk of intracranial haematoma.
- The patient may be cared for at home after observation for 24 hours:
  - symptomatic medication
  - rest until the next morning
  - return to work after 1–3 days.
- Appointment for follow-up visit after 1 week.
- Do not follow up a symptomatic patient for more than 1 week as an outpatient.
- **Refer for hospital treatment**
  - patients with violent vomiting, to arrange fluid therapy
  - children, see also 32.75
  - the elderly (recovery is slow)
  - patients with multiple injury (who cannot manage independently)
  - heavily drunk patients
  - symptomless patients with a high-energy injury
  - patients with an exceptionally severe headache
  - patients with abnormal neurological status
  - patients with a fracture of the skull
  - patients with an unclear history
  - patients with differential diagnostic problems: subarachnoid haematoma, epilepsy.

- A CT scan is indicated for most of the patients mentioned above. Radiology may reveal a clinically evident concussion to be a brain contusion.
- Patients with concussion recover fully and become symptom-free.
- Problematic cases require neurological examinations in a hospital: CT scan, EEG, and neuro-otological, ophthalmological and psychological tests, if necessary.

18.4 Brain contusion

Editors

Aims

- Monitor the level of consciousness in a patient with brain contusion.
- A CT scan is performed on every unconscious patient as soon as possible.
- Identify additional injuries, such as cervical spine injuries and injuries causing severe bleeding which require urgent treatment, before transporting the patient to a care unit.

Diagnosis

- The diagnosis of brain contusion is clinical, radiological and neurophysiological. The seriousness of the injury correlates with the level of consciousness and the duration of unconsciousness. The patient's age is a significant factor regarding prognosis.
- Brain contusion is often the only injury; however, 10% have multiple injuries.
  - It is important to exclude cervical spine injuries immediately. Treat the patient as if he/she had a cervical spine injury until an x-ray has been taken.
- Determination of the level of consciousness (36.5) and simple basic neurological examination are of central importance in monitoring the patient.
- The CT scan shows the location of brain contusions, possible larger pooling of blood, and the condition of the brain ventricles, and reveals pressure elevation. In cases of unconsciousness the CT scan must be performed immediately.

Treatment of the acute phase

- The basic treatment of an unconscious patient takes place in the intensive care unit.
- The measurement of the intracranial pressure and prevention or treatment of increasing pressure are special procedures for brain contusion.
  - Controlled hyperventilation is the basis of treatment D [1 2 3]. If the patient is intubated, hyperventilation can be started during transportation.
  - Pressure can be controlled for a short time with mannitol or furosemide. Corticosteroids are probably of no benefit A [4], although this therapy may be theoretically justified.
- Repeated CT scans will give additional information on late haematomas and when resection of severe local brain contusion is considered.

Further treatment

- The phase of acutely increasing intracranial pressure is usually over in 4–5 days. After this, the unconscious patient with tracheotomy can be treated on a ward.
- Over the next 3–4 weeks of basic follow-up, the prognosis and further treatment lines are decided upon.
  - Mild contusion injuries do not prevent normal recovery and return to work.
  - When unconsciousness continues for a long time, the cognitive changes and, in particular, changes in personality require a rehabilitation programme and further attention with special follow-up.
  - The prognosis for neurological deficiency symptoms is basically good but physiotherapy should be continued.
  - The incidence of epilepsy is under 5% during the first year, but intracerebral haematoma increases the incidence to up to 30%. After 10 years half of the patients are free of attacks.

TRA

References

1. Roberts I, Schierhout G. Hyperventilation therapy for acute traumatic brain injury. Cochrane Database Syst Rev. 2004;(2): CD000566.
2. Geraci E, Geraci T. A look at recent hyperventilation studies: outcomes and recommendations for early use in the head-injured patient. J Neuroscience Nursing 1996;28:222–4.
3. The Database of Abstracts of Reviews of Effectiveness (University of York), Database no.: DARE-965420. In: The Cochrane Library, Issue 4, 1999. Oxford: Update Software.
4. Alderson P, Roberts I. Corticosteroids for acute traumatic brain injury. Cochrane Database Syst Rev. 2004;(2):CD000196.

18.5 Intracranial haematomas

Editors

Aims

- Suspect an intracranial haematoma when a patient with a head injury
  - is unconscious or the level of consciousness is decreased

- has neurological symptoms down one side of the body, primarily hemiparesis
- has increasing restlessness and cranial nerve symptoms or pupils of unequal size.

♦ The diagnosis must be made immediately – within two hours after the injury for an unconscious patient. If you suspect a haematoma to be the cause of unconsciousness and referral would cause a delay, consult a neurosurgeon directly.

First aid

♦ Ventilation (intubation)
♦ Circulation (infusion)
♦ Blood transfusions and emergency operations indicated by other injuries

Diagnosis

♦ A CT scan is always mandatory: a haematoma must not be treated in a facility without this imaging method.

Extradural haematoma

♦ Typical in children and young people. The mechanism of injury may be mild, and often the patient is conscious at first.
♦ Rapid blurring of consciousness, neurological symptoms down one side of the body, and dilatation of either pupil are signs of serious herniation. At this stage the patient needs immediate care and doesn't stand out transportation if it would take more than about 2 hours.
♦ Haematomas are removed by craniotomy. Dural arterial bleeding is the most common reason. In 80% of the cases the haematoma is situated in the temporal lobe.
♦ Recovery is rapid and complete, assuming there are no additional injuries and no delay in treatment.

Subdural haematoma

♦ In emergency situations you may encounter an acute haematoma leading to symptoms within 48 hours or a subacute haematoma with symptom onset later.

Acute subdural haematoma

♦ Often in association with brain contusion. The patient is not necessarily conscious at all, which makes it more difficult to recognize possible deterioration of the condition.
♦ The patients are often elderly or alcoholics.
♦ Atrophy increases the risk of bleeding.
♦ Rupture of the sagittal sinus is one aetiological possibility. An urgent CT scan of an unconscious patient is therefore essential. Haematoma is large, often crossing over to the other hemisphere.
♦ The result of an operation depends on when the surgery is performed. The degree of injury and the patient's age are important prognostic factors. Mortality is still high, approximately 50%.

Subacute subdural haematoma

♦ The course is similar to that of an extradural haematoma, but the symptoms develop more slowly. Symptoms of local compression dominate the clinical appearance.
♦ The patients are often alcoholics whose initial symptoms are masked by drunkenness, and recurrent injuries are possible. Subdural haematoma is often found to be the reason for death during detention.
♦ Recovery is good if the treatment is begun before bilateral symptoms of incarceration develop (unconsciousness and reaction to pain with simultaneous extension of the extremities).

Chronic subdural haematoma

♦ Symptoms appear only several months after the injury.
♦ Patients are often elderly who may present with symptoms like confusion, balancing problems or problems with memory. The patients are often on anticoagulant medication.
♦ The primary injury is usually a mild one (e.g. falling over) and often forgotten. The diagnosis is often acute because of rapidly developing symptoms (headache, hemiparesis or, in many cases, fluctuating, blurred consciousness) indicating elevated intracranial pressure. A subsequent fall may worsen the situation, as in acute subdural haematoma.
♦ If possible, treat urgently.
♦ A patient with blurred consciousness should be operated on immediately.
♦ Only a burr hole is required for rinsing and draining a liquefied chronic haematoma.
♦ Recovery is rapid and usually complete.
♦ The haematoma is bilateral in 10% of the cases; both sides can be operated on in the same session. Common symptoms of bilateral subdural haematoma are difficulty in walking, weakness of both lower extremities, and blurring of consciousness.
♦ Recurrence is possible after the first few weeks, and follow-up is therefore needed. Re-operation is indicated, and is quite safe when necessary.

Intracerebral haematoma

♦ Some of the problems in brain contusion are often caused by an intracerebral haematoma. Haematomas are of varying size and sometimes multiple. They should therefore be treated on a case basis.
♦ The symptoms depend on the mechanism of injury: falling over usually causes bleeding in the temporal lobe.
♦ A significant haematoma that causes pressure symptoms should be operated on. Contusioned brain tissue may also be removed during the operation.
♦ The diagnosis and especially the decision on treatment often require frequent CT scans, observation of intracranial pressure, and the availability of basic facilities of an intensive care unit.

18.6 Dislocation of the temporomandibular joint

Editors

Introduction

- Dislocation may occur almost spontaneously in some persons or in association with
  - trauma
  - yawning
  - a visit to a dentist.
- Reposition is usually easy if the mandible is intact.
- If the mandible is dislocated backwards the patient has a condylar fracture. In such case, consult an oral and maxillofacial surgeon directly.

Symptoms

- The patient cannot shut the mouth.
- The tip of the jaw deviates to the opposite side in unilateral dislocation.

Treatment

- The patient is placed in a sitting position.
- Press the mandible with your thumbs as deep as possible behind the last molars inside the mouth and support the mandible with the rest of the fingers from the outside. Press the jaw straight downwards until the muscles snap the joint back to its right position.
- If repositioning is unsuccessful, refer the patient to an oral and maxillofacial surgeon, preferably on the same day.
- If the dislocation recurs frequently consult an oral and maxillofacial surgeon.

18.10 Fractures of the spine

Editors

Introduction

- Always remember the possibility of cervical spine injury in an unconscious patient (cervical spine x-rays are more important than a skull x-ray).
- The patient must be moved on a stretcher with the injured part supported. If the patient is conscious, a muscle spasm will provide some protection to the injured site. Moving an unconscious patient requires particular care.

Fracture of the cervical spine

- All fractures should be considered unstable until proven otherwise.
- The likelihood of cervical spine fracture is very small, and cervical spine x-rays are usually not needed in patients who have no localized midline cervical tenderness, no focal neurological deficit, and who have no co-existing diseases that could interfere with the diagnosis.
- A painful neck in an elderly patient after a fall should always be considered as a possible fracture. Monitor the neurological status.

Diagnosis

- The interpretation of cervical spine x-rays requires experience.
  - Examine the lateral projection for displacement of the vertebrae. Ensure that all relevant vertebrae (C1–T1) are shown on the x-ray.
  - Check the outline of the odontoid process for intactness, both from the lateral and AP projections.
  - Using an AP projection, check that the arch of C1 is not abnormally wide (evident as a lateral displacement of the lateral masses from their expected alignment in relation to the outline of C2).
  - Cervical spine x-rays may be taken in flexion if the patient is conscious and the plain x-rays are normal and the patient has no neurological signs or symptoms.

Treatment

- Fracture of a cervical spine always requires hospitalization. A vacuum splint or cervical collar must be applied before the patient is moved.
- Unstable fractures and dislocations require skull traction (1 kg/vertebra, i.e. fracture of C3 will require 3 kg).

Fracture of the thoracic and lumbar spine

Compression fracture

- The most common is a compression fracture of the thoracic or lumbar spine that is caused by vertical force.
- The patient is often an elderly person who has fallen on his/her buttocks. The fracture is also seen in younger patients, for example after falling from a roof. In these cases the patient often presents with concomitant fracture of the calcaneus.
- If the height of a vertebral body is decreased anteriorly by more than 50% (compare with an adjacent vertebra), the fracture will often need surgical treatment; otherwise the fracture may be treated conservatively.

TRA

- Pain may persist for several years after the injury.
- An osteoporotic compression fracture in an elderly patient may be treated on a general hospital ward. The patient may be mobilized as pain allows.
- Intranasal calcitonin 200 units/day may be prescribed, and bisphosphonate treatment could be considered.

Fracture of a transverse process

- A sudden movement with rotational or flexional force, for example an epileptic fit, may cause a fracture of a transverse process in the lumbar spine.
- Pain and muscle tension will persist for 6 to 8 weeks. Analgesia and mobilization suffice for treatment.

18.11 Spinal cord injuries

Antti Dahlberg

Basic rules

- Consider the possibility of spinal cord injury in all trauma patients, and ensure that transport does not aggravate the injury (the spine must be stabilised).
- The treatment and rehabilitation of spinal cord injuries should be carried out by specialist units.
- The problems following spinal cord injury are often multifaceted, difficult to treat and permanent. The treatment therefore calls for expertise and individual planning.

Acute injury

- **Is the trauma mechanism such that the patient might suffer from spinal cord injury?** An unconscious patient with a high-energy injury must be considered to have a spinal cord injury until proven otherwise.
- Paraplegia or tetraplegia are obvious signs of spinal cord injury. Less severe signs of neurological deficit may also denote spinal cord involvement if the trauma mechanism is suggestive and, in particular, if the patient complains of local symptoms in the back or neck.
- The patient should be sent immediately to a hospital with sufficient facilities to treat spinal cord injuries. The care of spinal cord injuries should be centralised to specialist units.
- It is vital that no action is taken at the site of the accident and during transportation which may have the potential to worsen the spinal cord injury.
- When preparing the patient for transportation the following should be considered:
  - Monitoring vital functions is a priority. The breathing of an unconscious patient may be ineffective. The assistance of breathing in a patient with a cervical cord injury usually requires the maintenance of an open airway. Care must be taken not to compromise immobilisation. In field conditions the use of an intubating laryngeal mask (ILMA) is the most appropriate method. However, the recommended method to keep the airways open is the method best mastered by the rescue team.
  - The mean blood pressure should be kept sufficiently high due to injury to the nerve tissue. Sympathetic dysfunction associated with high level (above T6) injuries should be treated with catecholamines (remember the risk of vagal bradycardia). Possible volume depletion of a multitrauma patient, caused by blood loss, should be corrected with intravenous fluids.
  - Use of special boards is usually considered better than the hands of several assistants when transferring the patient, or when the patient needs to be cut free at the scene of an accident. However, if necessary, the patient may be transferred onto a spinal board supported by three or four assistants.
  - The immobilisation of the spine for transportation is of vital importance whenever spinal cord injury is suspected. The board should be smooth and even to prevent the early development of pressure sores during transportation. Urine retention should also be treated.
- The latest study results are conflicting regarding the use of **methylprednisolone** in the acute phase (B) [1]. However, methylprednisolone has been accepted as standard therapy in many countries and should be administered as soon as possible.
  - The initial dose is 30 mg/kg intravenously. If the treatment has been started within 3 hours of the accident the medication should be continued as an infusion (5.4 mg/kg/h) for 24 hours; if 3–8 hours have passed since the accident the infusion should be continued for 48 hours. Methylprednisolone should not be administered if more than 8 hours have passed since the accident.

Rehabilitation

Rehabilitation in the acute phase

- The care and rehabilitation of patients should be centralised and take place in specialised units.
- The life of an injured person has suddenly changed dramatically. Centralising the care and rehabilitation allows the staff to become highly skilled and experienced. The support of other spinal injury patients is also of the utmost importance.
- Rehabilitation in the acute phase includes:
  - **The promotion of functional independency**
  - Any functioning muscles should be strengthened.
  - Two thirds of all patients will be bound to a wheelchair for the rest of their lives.
  - Being in an upright position and standing up are usually practiced.
  - The patient will be provided with personal aids and equipment and instructed in their use (e.g. wheelchair, environmental control systems).

- Independence and coping will be tested during short home visits.

- **Medical care:**
  - The best possible medical care should be offered to treat the altered bodily functions (e.g. urinary bladder, bowels and sexual functioning).
  - Complications (e.g. pressure sores) should be prevented.
- **Psychiatric support:**
  - The family must be included in the management of the crisis which follows the sudden disability.
  - Peer support can be obtained from previously injured patients.
- The patient should be advised about relevant benefits and compensation payments. Necessary aids and equipment are to be fitted to the patient's home (special housing if needed). The patient is offered vocational rehabilitation.
- Almost all patients with spinal cord injury are discharged home after the acute phase of rehabilitation. With the aid of a personal care even those with severe injuries can cope with independent living.

Continued rehabilitation

- To maintain their physical functioning, patients with spinal cord injuries may need to attend inpatient rehabilitation services at regular intervals. The aim should be to maintain or improve functional independence, treat any musculoskeletal problems and improve the patient's physical condition. Respite care may be offered in order to enable the carer of a severely disabled patient to take a short break.
- The need and extent of community-based physiotherapy should be decided case by case.
  - Tetraplegic patients often require regular community physiotherapy either once or twice a week, or periodically. Community physiotherapy should include functional exercises, maintenance of joint movements, alleviation of spasticity, muscle care etc.
  - Paraplegic patients may require regular community physiotherapy to attain the afore-mentioned goals as well as to maintain musculoskeletal functioning.
  - Vocational rehabilitation and adaptation training are usually introduced during the first few years after the spinal cord injury. However, the need for such rehabilitation may also arise later on in life after other issues relating to the disability have stabilised themselves.
  - Aids and equipment significantly improve self-reliance and often enable independent living. The need for equipment is assessed during the initial rehabilitation phase. The patient's situation will change over the years and the assessment should be repeated at regular intervals.

Sequelae of spinal cord injury

- The long-term treatment of a spinal cord injury patient will be the responsibility of his/her general practitioner.
- Due to the unique nature of late complications the patient should be assessed at regular intervals at a specialised centre which collaborates closely with the patient's general practitioner.

Urinary tract problems

- Symptomatic urinary tract infections should be verified from a sample of cleanly voided urine and by bacterial culture. Urinary tract infection should always be considered as the cause of acute systemic symptoms and fever, even in the absence of typical symptoms. Some patients who require intermittent catheterisation have chronic bacteriuria.
- A patient with recurrent infections should be referred to a urologist. Symptomatic urinary tract infections should be treated with longer courses of antibiotics than usual. Prophylactic antibiotics should not be prescribed routinely.
- A urologist should examine all patients every 1–3 years with ultrasound examination of the kidneys and urinary tract, renography or urography if needed. Urodynamic examination is only performed in special indications.
- The method for bladder emptying must always be decided individually. Intermittent catheterisation is currently the primary therapy for neurogenic bladder dysfunction, and it has been shown to prevent dilatation and reflux in the upper urinary tract.

Skin problems

- Pressure sores can be prevented with adequate counselling and aids. Careful prevention is important.
- If there is a threat of a pressure sore developing, decompression of the skin should be accomplished immediately (bed rest if necessary, changing position, redirecting the pressure onto healthy skin areas).
- A plastic surgeon should be consulted even for small pressure sores that do not appear to be healing with conservative treatment. Months of bed rest may be avoided with timely plastic surgery.

Pain

- Musculoskeletal pains should be treated according to common guidelines. The neck and shoulder pains, and problems of the upper extremities, of a wheelchair-bound patient require special attention, as the patient's functional independence is at risk.
- The diagnosis of visceral pain can be difficult because of sensory deficit.
- Pain associated with spinal cord injury is often neuropathic and difficult to treat. However, neuropathic pain should be treated appropriately as the pain will have a considerable impact on the patient's quality of life. Early referral to a pain clinic may be warranted.

Spasticity

- A typical complication of spinal cord injury.
- Increased spasticity may originate from a cause caudal to the level of the spinal cord injury. Such a cause is often identifiable (e.g. infection, skin problems or other processes normally capable of causing pain). If spasticity is associated with systemic symptoms it can be a sign of a serious process, e.g. acute abdomen.
- The cause of increased spasticity must be treated promptly.
- Treatment of spasticity see 36.83.

Sexual function, fertility, family counselling

- Disorders of sexual function (particularly loss of sensation) may strongly impair the quality of life.
- Information and sexual counselling are an important part of the initial rehabilitation process. The need may also arise later on, as life situations change.
- Oral medication for erectile dysfunction is usually effective. Some patients prefer to use injections.
- In men with spinal cord injury, anejaculation and poor semen quality nearly always cause infertility. However, with modern treatment methods (vibratory stimulation, electroejaculation or testicular biopsy) semen can be collected from nearly every man with spinal cord injury.

Post-traumatic syringomyelia (PTS)

- PTS signifies cystic dilatation of the central canal of the spinal cord.
- PTS should always be suspected when a patient's neurological condition suddenly deteriorates several years after injury. Intensified pain may be the first clinical symptom. Other symptoms include a rise in the level of the sensory injury, increased spasticity, progressive muscle weakness and symptoms suggesting autonomic nervous system involvement.
- Diagnosis is confirmed by magnetic resonance imaging. The patient should be referred urgently to a neurosurgical unit for evaluation.

Other complications

- The following should also be kept in mind: altered bowel function, autonomic dysreflexia syndrome and the risk of osteoporosis.

Reference

1. Bracken MB. Steroids for acute spinal cord injury. Cochrane Database Syst Rev. 2004;(2):CD001046.

18.12 Fractures of the ribs and pelvis

Editors

Introduction

- Fractures involving the ribs and pelvis may only require conservative treatment or they may be more serious:
  - unstable rib fractures may be accompanied by breathing difficulties
  - a fractured pelvis may lead to severe blood loss.
- Recognize tension pneumothorax in a trauma patient, see 6.61.

Rib fractures

Diagnosis

- A diagnosis can be made clinically, i.e. the site of the fracture is tender both on direct palpation and when pressure is applied to the fractured rib from the back.
- Auscultate the lungs; if the finding is asymmetrical, suspect pneumothorax.
- A chest x-ray is not always necessary, but should be considered if haemothorax or pneumothorax need to be excluded and in cases where multiple rib fractures are suspected.

Treatment

- Fracture of one or two ribs can usually be treated at a fracture clinic, but the treatment of multiple rib fractures requires hospitalization.
- Injection of bupivacaine (2 ml under the lower rib edge) will give pain relief for about 24 hours, and can be repeated if necessary. If injecting the fractured rib does not offer pain relief, an intact rib on both sides of the fractured rib may also be injected.
- A rib fracture will be markedly painful for three days. The pain will then ease but persist for three weeks.
- The patient should be advised to return to the clinic if he/she experiences breathing difficulties.
- Adhesive strapping may sometimes be applied to one side of the chest wall (not encircling the entire chest wall) to alleviate pain caused by chest wall movement. Adhesive strapping is not usually required.
- In the elderly, sputum retention may lead to chest infection. This should be prevented by providing adequate pain relief. Pneumonia should be suspected on the emergence of signs of an infection.
- Flail chest should be strapped and the patient should lie on the unstable chest wall during transport.

Fractures of the pelvis

- Classification of pelvic fractures, see 18.12.

High energy injuries of the pelvis

- A complicated unstable fracture of the pelvis may lead to the loss of 1–3 litres of blood, and intravenous infusion should therefore be provided during transport.
- If the patient has an unstable fracture of the pelvis, the pelvis should be stabilized with a body drape to reduce bleeding.

Fracture of the pelvis in an elderly patient

- Fractures of the acetabular floor following a fall are common in elderly patients.
- An x-ray examination of the pelvis should include both an AP projection and a lateral view of the affected side.
- The acetabular floor must be carefully studied from the x-rays. Are any fissures or displacement evident?
- A patient with a fracture of the pubic ramus can ambulate and weight bear within the limits of the pain; the treatment can be carried out on a general hospital ward (injuries caused by a fall).
- Antithrombotic prophylaxis is usually initiated after 24 hours when the risk of bleeding has subsided.

Fracture of the coccyx

- After a fall or childbirth. A very painful fracture.
- Treatment consists of pain relief and the provision of a suitable seat.

Table 18.12 Fractures of the pelvis

Type of fracture	Prevalence	Treatment
Avulsion	In athletes: muscle contraction leads to avulsion of a bone fragment	Internal fixation often required, e.g. with screws
Single bone	Typically in an elderly person following an injury, e.g. fracture of the pubic ramus	Pain relief and early mobilization
Complicated: the pelvic ring fractured at several points	Compression injury in trauma patients	Usually surgical fixation, milder injuries treated conservatively
Acetabulum	Dislocation of the hip, e.g. in a car accident. Fracture of the acetabular floor in the elderly.	Dislocated hip needs immediate treatment, milder cases treated conservatively

18.20 Fractures of clavicula and scapula

Editors

Clavicula

- An arm sling is worn for 3–4 weeks. Ossification takes 6–8 weeks in adults.
- Surgery is necessary in
  - nerve, blood vessel or pleural injury
  - a lateral fracture extending to the articular surface
  - a lateral fracture combined with a rupture of the coracoclavicular ligament (the space between the coracoid and the clavicula is widened when compared with the intact side)
  - many middle third fractures, when the dislocation is more than the thickness of the clavicula or there is a shortening of more than 15 mm
  - non-ossified fracture which is over 6 months old and is still symptomatic.

TRA

Scapula

- An arm sling is worn for 2–4 weeks. Duration of sick leave depends on the recovery of the range of movement in the shoulder.
- Fractures of the scapular neck require CT examination and assessment of the need for operative treatment.

18.21 Dislocation of the shoulder

Editors

Basic rules

- Reduce a dislocated shoulder emergently.
- If you fail in reduction, refer the patient for surgical treatment.
- Always control a primary luxation with x-ray.

Aetiology

- Usually falling on an outstretched arm
- Sometimes a quick movement of the upper extremity
- Seizure attack (the luxation is often posterior, which is the case also with dislocation caused by an electric shock)

Findings

- An x-ray is necessary for excluding a fracture and an acromioclavicular dislocation. Out of hours, the reduction is sometimes performed without x-ray.
- It is often possible to exclude a fracture by means of accurate history (direct, forceful violence being a common aetiological factor) and careful examination. Do not forget the possibility of pathological fracture.
- Because of pain and worsening oedema, reduction should not be postponed to the next morning.
- Always check both before and after treatment
  - circulation of the upper extremity (palpate the pulse)
  - neurological status (check the sense of touch, range of motion of the upper extremity and spreading of the fingers).

Reduction

- The procedure is more likely to be successful if the patient can relax the shoulder. Tell the patient what you are doing, calm the patient and help him/her to relax the shoulder.
- You may use the methods of reduction in the following order:
  - Arm dangling
    - While supporting the arm, help the patient to lie down on the examination couch in prone position with his/her arm hanging over the edge. You can intensify the traction by binding a weight (for example a bag of sand) to the forearm. Encourage the patient to relax the shoulder. The shoulder is often reduced spontaneously, especially in recurrent dislocation, after 15–30 minutes.
  - Reduction while dangling
    - Sit down on a low seat. Calm and relax the patient, flex the patient's elbow 90° and support the forearm with your forearm. Pull the arm down by the elbow and rotate the upper arm cautiously inwards while you pull the upper part of the arm outwards with the other hand. If reduction fails give diazepam (5–10 mg i.v. or the same dose per rectum) and try again later.
  - Reduction by pulling upward
    - Can be used as an alternative to dangling and if the patient is not able to lie face downwards. The patient lies supine. Stand on a high seat (ca. 1 m) beside the patient (or place the patient on a mattress on the floor). Lift the relaxed upper arm straight upwards gently and for a long time, holding the wrist. Reduce with slow and calm rotational movements.
  - If the reduction is not successful or you suspect a fracture, refer the patient to a hospital (an ambulance may be necessary) for imaging and possible reduction under general anaesthesia.

Further treatment

- Successful reduction can be felt when the shoulder goes back to its socket with a snap. Pain is relieved instantly. Reduction is confirmed by cautious examination of the range of movement of the shoulder. The reduction can also be confirmed by ultrasound (symmetrical findings!) if this investigation is easily available.
- Check the circulation and neurological status in the arm and hand and make notes in the medical records. Reposition should be verified by x-ray.
- To reduce post-injury pain, the arm is supported with a sling and attached to the body in adducted and pronated position for about three weeks. The patient may, e.g., wash the face and eat, but external rotation is avoided for 6 weeks.

Recurrent dislocation

- Recurrent dislocations occur without significant injury and are easily reduced.
- No immobilization
- After a third dislocation operative treatment is considered.
- Postoperative immobilization with an arm-to-chest bandage for 3 weeks. For 6 weeks no abduction over 90° is allowed; after 2 weeks, anterior elevation exercises are commenced.
- Primary surgery may be preferable in the treatment of first traumatic anterior shoulder dislocation in young adults engaged in highly demanding physical activities, while non-surgical treatment remains the primary treatment option for other patient categories C [1].

Reference

1. Handoll HHG, Almaiyah MA, Rangan A. Surgical versus non-surgical treatment for acute anterior shoulder dislocation. The Cochrane Database of Systematic Reviews, Cochrane Library Number: CD004325. In: Cochrane Library, Issue 1, 2004. Chichester, UK: John Wiley & Sons, Ltd.

18.22 Dislocation of the acromioclavicular joint

Editors

Symptoms and findings

- Usually caused by falling on the shoulder

- Local tenderness and oedema around the acromioclavicular (AC) joint
- The dislocated head of the clavicula is felt as a prominence and can often be pressed downwards and sometimes also moved sideways.
- The dislocation is seen on an AP view of the x-ray when compared with the other side. Weighted x-rays in which the patient holds weight of approx. 7 kg in both hands may not improve diagnostics considerably.
    - Pay special attention to the possible rupture of the coracoclavicular (CC) ligament: is the gap between the clavicula and the coracoid widened?

Treatment

First-degree luxation

- The joint is painful and tender when palpated; no radiographic changes.
- Mobilization as much as the pain allows

Second-degree luxation

- Full rupture of the AC ligaments, with the CC ligaments intact
- The x-ray shows mild dislocation upwards, which is more prominent in weighted x-rays (displacement usually no more than 50% of the width of the clavicula).
- An arm sling is worn for one to three weeks and then the arm is mobilized.

Third-degree luxation

- The AC and CC ligaments are ruptured, and the joint is instable when palpated. The gap between the clavicula and the coracoid is widened on the x-ray.
- The conventional treatment is operative fixation for patients under 50 years of age, even if the evidence of efficacy is scarce C [1,2]. An arm sling is worn for three weeks, and the fixation material is removed in an out-patient clinic after 6 weeks.
- Conservative treatment for the elderly: mobilization as soon as the pain allows.

References

1. Phillips AM, Smart C, Groom AF. Acromioclavicular dislocation: conservative or surgical therapy. Clinical Orthopaedics and Related Research 1998;353:10–17.
2. The Database of Abstracts of Reviews of Effectiveness (University of York), Database no.: DARE-981504. In: The Cochrane Library, Issue 2, 2001. Oxford: Update Software.

18.23 Treatment of humeral and forearm fractures

Editors

- For wrist and metacarpal fractures, see 18.25.

Humeral fractures

- The basic aim is to mobilize the shoulder early in order to avoid stiffening of the joint.

Greater tubercle of the humerus

- If the dislocation is so minimal (up to 3 mm) that the detached part cannot be wedged under the acromion, immobilize the joint in a sling for a maximum of 2–3 weeks. Passive and active mobilization without load begins at once when pain is tolerable.
- In major dislocations surgery is needed.
- X-ray controls on weeks 1 and 2 after the injury are important.
- Sick leave: in light work about 4 weeks; in strenuous work up to 8 weeks.

Neck of the humerus

- Conservative treatment and cautious early mobilization (like in luxation) when the primary dislocation is minimal or when an acceptable position is achieved with reduction (dislocation less than 1 cm, angulation below 30–45 degrees). Note also patient's age.
    - Arm sling or collar-cuff sling is worn for 4–6 weeks to control pain and when moving around.
    - Mobilization immediately when pain is tolerable C [1] (no later than 3 weeks after); passive and pendulum exercises from the beginning.
    - Later physiotherapy is important.
- More severely dislocated fractures should be reduced and immobilized with an arm-to-chest bandage for 3–6 weeks. After immobilization, passive mobilization and pendulum exercises are begun.
- If the angle of dislocation exceeds 45 degrees consult an orthopaedist about the need for surgery.
- If the fracture is complicated by dislocation of the humeral head, surgery is the therapy of choice.
- Sick leave: 6–12 weeks depending on the recovery of the range of movement and the strenuousness of work.

Diaphysis and distal part of the humerus

- Reduction performed preferably in a sitting position

TRA

- Criteria of an acceptable position of the fracture:
  - Lateral displacement no more than two thirds of the bone diameter
  - Axial error no more than 10 degrees
- Immobilization with a U cast or orthosis and a collar–cuff sling for 6 weeks. Depending on the instability of the fracture, immobilization may be extended. Instead of a cast a Velcro tape orthosis may be used in this phase.
- From week 3 onward, cautious abduction exercises and passive exercises (pendulum) are allowed. At 6 weeks, active upper extremity mobilizing is started.
- Surgery (fixation with a plate and screws or with an intramedullary nail) is needed primarily in open fractures or if there is suspicion of radial nerve entrapment at the site of fracture. In a very unstable fracture with a short fracture line, operative treatment should be considered already in the primary stage or on week 6 if the fracture continues to be clearly unstable.

U cast

- Equipment
  - Tube gauze, padding, 3–4 rolls of cast, (width 20 cm for adults), one or two assistants
- Preparing the cast
  - Place the patient preferably in a sitting position or supine, with an assistant holding the upper extremity somewhat abducted.
  - Wrap tube gauze and padding first, do not use crepe paper.
  - Prepare an 8-layer thick cast plate extending from the greater tubercle down around the elbow up to the armpit. The plate is moistened and padding is placed on top. The still moist plate is fixed by wrapping the upper arm in an elastic bandage. Correction of humeral axis is made as needed.
- Use a collar–cuff sling with the elbow in a 90–100-degree flexion.
- X-ray control immediately after reduction and 1 week after it.
- Consult an orthopaedist if there is radial nerve injury in a closed fracture.
- The need for sick leave (3–4 months) depends essentially on casting time. Sick leave should also be reserved for molibization.

Fractures of the elbow region

Condylar fractures of the humerus

- A non-dislocated fracture is treated conservatively with an angular cast for 3 weeks.
- A dislocated fracture (>2 mm) is usually operated on. The aim is to stabilize the fracture and to mobilize the elbow from the start.
- In severe comminuted osteoporotic fractures of the elderly, primary mobilization may be considered disregarding the fracture, or a primary endoprosthesis may be indicated.

Capitulum of the radius

- Immediate mobilization without load if the fracture is not dislocated or the dislocation is less than 2 mm. Pronation–supination movement is important in mobilizing. Do not treat with a cast!
- In adults, the so-called chisel fracture (extending across the articular surface) requires operation and osteosynthesis when the displacement is more than 2 mm or the fracture is comminuted.
- Sick leave: 4–6 weeks
- Late symptoms may sometimes require an endoprosthesis.

Fracture of the olecranon

- If dislocation exceeds 2 mm an operation is necessary.
- Non-dislocated fracture (dislocation less than 2 mm) is treated with a 60–90-degree angular cast for 3 weeks.

Monteggia fracture

- Proximal ulnar diaphysial fracture and dislocation of the capitulum of the radius.
- The treatment is always ulnar osteosynthesis and closed reduction of the head of the radius, if necessary by surgery.

Fractures of the ulna and the radius

- A non-dislocated fracture can be treated with an angular cast for 6–8 weeks (B) [2 3], however, it is usually operated on.
- A larger angle is acceptable when the fracture is located near the distal epiphyseal line. Correct axial alignment is important.
- X-ray controls after 1 and 2 weeks are essential in conservative treatment.
- Distal ulnar fractures with minimal axial errors and dislocation less than 50% of the diameter of the diaphysis can be mobilized with a supportive bandage or a forearm cast for 6 weeks (B) [2 3].
- A dislocated fracture requires surgery (usually plate and screws or intramedullary nail). Cautious mobilization is started postoperatively as soon as the osteosynthesis is stable (pronation and supination exercises).
- Sick leave: 8–12 weeks

Angular cast

Equipment

- Tube gauze, padding, 3–4 rolls of cast

Preparation

- Use tube gauze and padding under the cast, crepe paper should not be used.
- Make a 6–8-layer thick cast extending from the distal metacarpals up to the upper arm.

- The cast is made of two pieces each extending over the elbow, or of one piece if the elbow is strengthened with a separate 4-layer thick dorsal part. The wet cast is fixed with an elastic bandage.
- The elbow is set in 90-degree flexion, and the wrist in 30-degree dorsal flexion. In injuries around the elbow, the wrist may be left free.

References

1. Handoll HHG, Gibson JNA, Madhok R. Interventions for treating proximal humeral fractures in adults. Cochrane Database Syst Rev. 2004;(2):CD000434.
2. Mackay D, Wood L, Rangan A. The treatment of isolated ulnar fractures in adults: a systematic review. Injury International Journal of the Care of the Injured 2000, 31(8), 565–70.
3. The Database of Abstracts of Reviews of Effectiveness (University of York), Database no.: DARE-20001826. In: The Cochrane Library, Issue 2, 2002. Oxford: Update Software.

18.24 Dislocation of the elbow joint

Editors

Introduction

- The forearm is usually dislocated backwards.
- The arm is deformed and there is loss of movement.

Reduction

- Reduction is usually successful conservatively without anaesthesia.
- The forearm is pulled so that one person holds the upper arm with both hands and the other holds the forearm with both hands (near the antecubital area and on the wrist).
- Pull first in the direction of the forearm and then by extending the elbow gently.
- At the end of traction bend the elbow with the hand holding the wrist as the other hand pushes the forearm from the elbow towards the wrist. The assistant keeps the upper arm fixed during traction.
- Crepitation felt in the elbow joint is a sign of possible fracture and the attempt of reduction is discontinued.

Further treatment

- Confirm by x-ray that there are no fractures and that the joint is in place.
- An angular splint (90 degrees see 18.23) is set for 2–3 weeks, after which the arm is mobilized actively.
    - Passive exercise therapy and particularly manipulation must be avoided.
- A stable joint can be mobilized from the beginning; however, full extension should be avoided.
- An instable joint requires assessment by an orthopaedic surgeon. A surgical repair of the ligaments is often performed.

18.25 Treatment of wrist and metacarpal fractures

Editors

TRA

Treatment of typical (Colles') fracture of the radius with a dorsal cast

Equipment

- Tube gauge, elastic bandage, and two rolls of cast.

Preparing the cast

- If reduction is needed inject local anaesthetic into the fracture line B [1].
- Set the tube gauge.
- Prepare a 6–8 layers thick cast slab and cut one corner for the thumb.
- Reduction is performed with a steady and lengthy pull by the second and third finger. The elbow is in flexion and the assisting person pulls back from the lower part of the upper arm during the procedure. Finally press the dislocated fragment into place with your thumb from the dorsal side. Simultaneously move the wrist to a 20-degree flexion and **ulnar deviation** and pronation D [2] which is the position for immobilization.
- The traction and the reposition grip are maintained and a wet dorsal cast is put in place by a third person without padding and leaving the fingers and the thumb free.
    - The cast should extend from the distal metacarpal bones up to the elbow.
    - The cast must secure the ulnar deviation by supporting the second metacarpal bone from the side.
- Criteria for the correct position
    - Articular surface must not be dorsally angulated (a volar angulation of 10–15 degrees is ideal).
    - There is no radial shortening when compared with the ulnar articular surface.
- Repeated attempts of reduction may worsen the end result. After two attempts one can accept a slightly incorrect result in the elderly.

- External fixation or open osteosynthesis should be considered (C) [3] and an orthopaedist consulted if the position is incorrect.
- At least as important as a good reduction is to perform clench-fist exercises from the beginning and to maintain the range of motion of the elbow and shoulder joints during the whole cast immobilization. Prevent the following chain: immobilization, oedema, pain, and reflex sympathetic dystrophy. When treating pain the most important thing is to make clench-fist exercises and to keep the arm elevated.
- There are several methods for treating radial fractures conservatively but the evidence is insufficient to determine which methods are the most effective (D) [2].

X-ray controls

1. Immediately after applying the cast
2. Control x-ray after 5–6 days is important because unsuccessful reduction is still possible to correct.
    - At this stage, 0 degrees of dorsal tilting and <2 mm displacement on the articular surface is acceptable.
    - If the dislocation has increased when compared with the first control x-ray but still acceptable, a further control x-ray should be taken after one week.
    - If you are unsure about the correct position you may take a control x-ray on the intact other wrist.
    - X-ray control is not necessary when the cast is taken off.
3. Always when the fracture is repositioned take a control x-ray after two weeks. If the position is unsatisfactory, consult an orthopaedic surgeon.

Immobilization time

- 4–6 weeks

Smith's fracture

- Fracture of the distal radius with a volar inclination of the distal fragment
- Often unstable requiring operative treatment
- Traction is first performed as in the reduction of the Colles' fracture.
- The wrist is left in a slightly dorsally flexed functional position and turned supinated and into ulnar deviation. Radial fragment is pressed in dorsal direction.
- Apply a dorsal cast (6–8 layers) extending from the upper arm down to the knuckles. The cast can be alternatively applied to the volar side extending from the elbow down to the base of the fingers. The wet cast is bound with an elastic bandage.
- Immobilize for 5 weeks.

Fractures of the scaphoid bone

Diagnosis

- Local tenderness in the anatomical snuffbox (fossa tabatière)
- The fracture is seen best in the navicular projection of a x-ray.
- Repeat the x-ray examination (or take a technetium bone scan or MRI) after 1–2 weeks if the fracture is not found primarily and there is still suspicion of a fracture.

Treatment

- Cast in nondislocated fractures. Dislocated (more than 1 mm) fractures and fractures over 2 weeks old are best operated on.
- Pseudoarthrosis that may develop as a postinjury complication is operated on at least in young patients.

Preparing the cast

- Equipment: tube gauge, padding, no crepe paper
- Place the tube gauge over the arm; use padding only on the forearm.
- Wrap the cast on the padding from the elbow down to the knuckles. Wrap the proximal phalanx of the thumb into the cast, with the distal phalanx remaining free. Place the wrist and the thumb in a functional position. The thumb must be able to touch the index finger allowing pen grip.

Immobilization

- The cast is worn for 8–12 weeks.
- Sick leave for 12–16 weeks
- Ossification is difficult to assess on an x-ray. Take control x-ray without cast.
- Fracture of the navicular tuberculum needs only a dorsal cast for 3–4 weeks.

Other carpal bones

- The dorsal avulsion fracture of the triquetral bone is the most common and is often missed in lateral x-rays.
- Treat with primary mobilization depending on the pain or apply a plaster splint with the hand in a functional position for 3 weeks.
- Other carpal bone fractures are rare and are often missed. Good x-ray which are compared with the unaffected side are essential. Note the possible dislocation of the semilunar bone!
- Intra-articular avulsion fractures are operated on.

Fractures of the metacarpal bones

Non-dislocated fracture of the metacarpal bones II–V

- Dorsal, thin-padded, 6-layer-thick plaster splint from mid-forearm to knuckles.
- Bind the cast with an elastic bandage; do not use crepe paper.

- Place the wrist in a functional position leaving the fingers free.
- Angulation < 10 degrees and dislocation not exceeding 50% of the diameter of the diaphysis are acceptable. Malrotation must be corrected.
- Remove the cast after 3 weeks.

Dislocated fractures of the metacarpal bones II–V

- Reduction requires the use of a local anaesthetic. Usually the angulation is dorsal, and reduction will be successful if the MP joints are flexed 90 degrees and pressure is applied on the PIP joints towards the metacarpals and the fracture site is simultaneously supported from the dorsal side.
- Apply dorsal cast from mid-forearm over PIP joints flexing the MP joints about 70 degrees and PIP joints < 30 degrees. An adjacent finger is bound into the cast to support the fractures and to prevent rotational error. To avoid pressure skin necrosis on the PIP joints and at the site of the injury, do not press with the reposition grip after the cast is in place. Place the wrist in a functional position (30 degrees dorsal flexion).
- An axial error of 10 degrees is acceptable. In the fractures of the fifth metacarpal neck, however, an axial error up to 30–45 degrees is acceptable and the hand may even be primarily mobilized without a cast, just binding the fractured finger to the adjacent finger for support.
- The cast may be removed after 3 weeks.

Non-dislocated fractures of the first MC bone

- Apply a dorsal U-shaped cast from mid-forearm to the IP joint of the thumb. Distal phalanx is left free. Place the thumb in an abducted functional position (the thumb must be able to touch the index finger). Place the wrist in a functional position.
- Remove the cast after 3 weeks.

Dislocated fractures of the first MC bone

- Treat after reduction as a nondislocated fracture, but add a volar support on the thumb to secure reduction and to keep the MC I joint abducted.
- Axial error of 20° is accepted.
- Remove the cast after 4 weeks.

Bennett's fracture (intra-articular fracture of the base of the first metacarpal bone)

- See Figure 18.25.1
- A dislocated Bennett's fracture is often treated operatively. If the position is good, conservative treatment may be applied.
- Place foam padding on the base of the first metacarpal bone (to prevent skin necrosis).

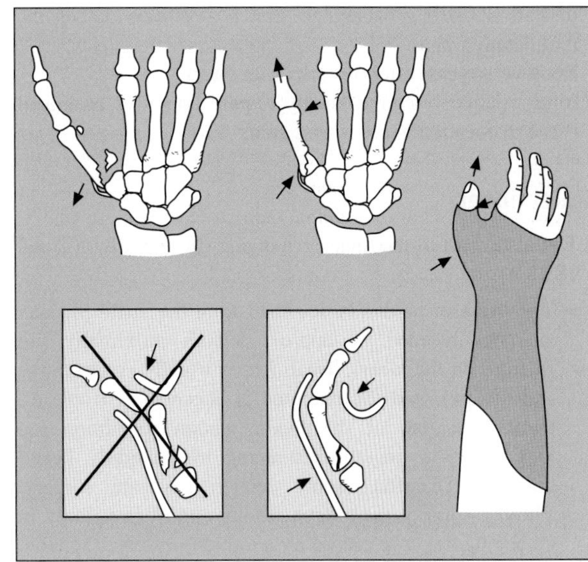

Figure 18.25.1 Conservative treatment of Bennett's fracture.

- Place a U-shaped cast from mid-forearm down to IP joint of the thumb. The cast is wrapped around the proximal phalanx of the thumb. Place the wrist in a functional position.
- Perform reduction while the cast is drying: the base of MC I bone is pressed inwards into a volar direction and the distal part of the MC I is simultaneously abducted with a grip on the metacarpal bone, not on the proximal phalanx.
- If the joint is dislocated and cannot be fully corrected by reduction, operation is indicated.
- X-ray controls are important (weeks 1 and 2) to ensure the maintenance of the correct position.
- You may remove the cast after 4 weeks.

Fractures of the fingers

A well-positioned fracture or dislocation

- Tie the injured finger to the adjacent finger with tape for 2–3 weeks.
- Full mobilization is allowed from the beginning.

Dislocated fracture

- Reduction requires the use of a local anaesthetic.
- Apply a volar cast or aluminium splint. The adjacent finger is also fixed to prevent rotation error. Place the basal joint in a 60–70-degree flexion and the wrist in a functional position. Remember the right axial direction (finger tips point in flexion to the tuberculum of navicular bone).
- It is important that the IP joints are always immobilized in full extension in all injuries where there is a suspicion that scar tissue may be formed distally of the basal joint during the healing process. In other case, the scar may draw the IP joints into a flexion contracture that cannot be stretched loose enough by the extensor muscles. The flexor muscles

instead are strong enough to stretch any scars during the mobilization phase.

- Remove the cast after 3 weeks (not later).
- Intra-articular fractures usually require operative treatment if the dislocation exceeds 1–2 mm.

Mallet finger

- The distal part of the finger is hanging (Figures 18.25.2 and 18.25.3)
  - The extensor tendon is detached from the distal phalanx and has receded by approx. 5 mm proximally (no fracture on the x-ray). Treatment is usually conservative (see below), and the outcome is acceptable. However, there is a risk of the flexor tendon remaining too long, and the fingertip remaining in a slightly flexed position. Therefore, some centres advocate surgery. Without surgery the trauma results almost invariably in a hanging fingertip caused by a too long extensor tendon.
  - If the x-ray shows a dorsal avulsion fracture of the distal finger, the DIP joint is immobilized in a hyperextended position (>20 degrees over the normal extension) so that the bone fragment becomes ossified as firmly as possible back to the avulsion site and so that the extensor tendon does not remain functionally too long. Use a padded two-fold hyperextension aluminium splint for 6 weeks. The splint must not be removed for any reason during the 5 week ossification period.
- If the detached fragment is large (over one-third of the distal phalanx) the joint often dislocates and an operation is needed. Bone avulsion as such does not require surgery.

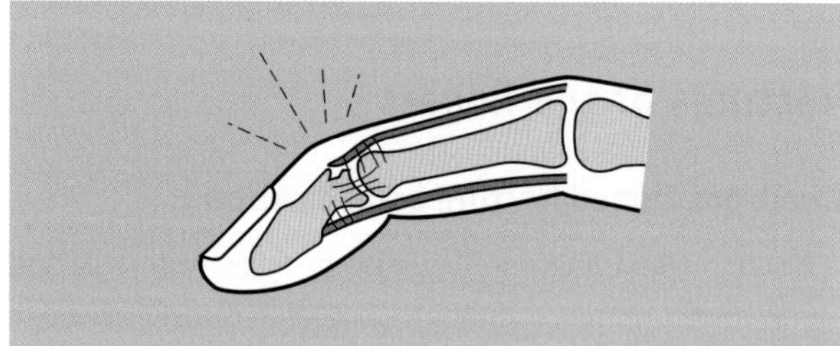

Figure 18.25.2 Mallet finger.

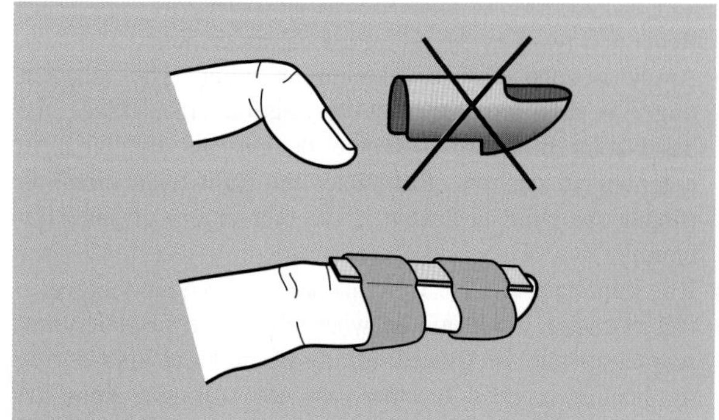

Figure 18.25.3 Extension splint.

References

1. Handoll HHG, Madhok R, Dodds C. Anaesthesia for treating distal radial fracture in adults. Cochrane Database Syst Rev. 2004;(2):CD003320.
2. Handoll HHG, Madhok R. Conservative interventions for treating distal radial fractures in adults. Cochrane Database Syst Rev. 2004;(2):CD000314.
3. Handoll HHG, Madhok R. Surgical interventions for treating distal radial fractures in adults. Cochrane Database Syst Rev. 2004;(2):CD003209.

18.26 Dislocation of the interphalangeal (IP) joint and injury of the first metacarpophalangeal (MCP) collateral ligament

Editors

Dislocation of the joint

Aetiology

- Usually caused by violent extension of a finger

Findings

- The digital joint is tender, in a forced position and deformed.
- An x-ray may be necessary to exclude a fracture, although in typical cases it is usually not needed.

Treatment

- Reduction is easier when the injury is recent. Do not wait until the next morning.
- Local anaesthesia is usually not needed. In special cases consider an interdigital nerve block or a small dose of diazepam to calm the patient.
- Calm the patient down by talking and help him/her to relax the muscles of the hand. The finger is pulled steadily but tightly in the distal direction, and the dislocated joint is simultaneously reduced. Function is checked, the position is re-examined, and possible fractures are found by x-ray.
- The finger is taped to the adjacent finger for two weeks, and on the third week mobilization is started.
- In an injury of the volar capsule of the PIP joint (avulsion), allow free flexion but limit extension to 30 degrees with a splint. If the mid-phalanx is dislocated (large avulsion fracture), fix with a K pin.

Buttonhole injury

- In the MP joint, and sometimes in the PIP and DIP joints, the dislocation may be of the buttonhole type: the head of the phalanx dislocates through the joint capsule or tendon and gets stuck.
- Reduction with traction is not possible. Refer the patient immediately for surgical treatment.

Injury of the ulnar MCP joint collateral ligament of the thumb

- Diagnosis is based on tenderness on the side of the MCP joint and instability of the joint (compare with the contralateral thumb). An abduction exceeding 30 degrees in the extended joint means total rupture. Local anaesthesia may be necessary for reliable investigation.
- Rupture of the ulnar ligament usually requires surgical treatment. More than 2 weeks' delay worsens the outcome.
- If an x-ray shows an avulsion fragment with dislocation less than 2 mm, the injury may be treated with a cast for four weeks.
- A collateral ligament injury on the radial side (rare) is treated with a splint worn for 4 weeks.

18.30 Femoral fractures

Editors

Introduction

- The incidence of osteoporotic fractures of the proximal femur are on the increase due to the aging of the population.
- Early mobilization and good management of co-existing illnesses are vital to avoid prolonged periods of hospitalization.

Fracture of the proximal femur

Findings

- Typically in an elderly patient, often following a low-energy injury (slipping, falling, falling out of bed).
- In a dislocated fracture, shortening and external rotation of the limb is usually evident.
- A non-dislocated fracture of the femoral neck may allow weight bearing, and therefore radiography with two projections is necessary.

Treatment

- Surgery without exception: osteosynthesis with a sliding hip screw or a gamma nail (DHS) C [1] (in intertrochanteric fractures), or hemiarthroplasty (in fractures of the femoral neck).
- Hemiarthroplasty is usually performed when the patient is over 70 years old and a fracture of the femoral neck is associated with dislocation.
- Before surgery the patient's mobility prior to the injury, medications and other co-existing illnesses must be evaluated. What caused the patient to fall? Was it due to an acute illness?
- The operation should be carried out as soon as possible, preferably within 24–48 hours of the injury.
- Antithrombotic A [2 3 4 5 6] and antibiotic prophylaxis should be started preoperatively (usually low-molecular-weight heparin, and cloxacillin or a first-generation cephalosporin).

Weight bearing after operation

- Osteosynthesis (screw-plate fixation, DHS) is carried out so as to allow weight bearing C [7] and is usually technically possible. Comminuted fractures of osteoporotic bone form an exception, and weight bearing is not allowed during the first stage.
- After hemiarthroplasty (Thompson, Austin Moore, etc.) full weight bearing is allowed immediately.
- Sometimes the fracture remains unstable even after fixation, and may demand 3–6 weeks of bed rest, after which the patient may mobilize with full weight bearing. Mobilization with partial weight bearing or non-weight bearing is usually not possible to achieve with an elderly patient. When mobilizing starts, crutches or a Zimmer frame, with or without wheels, is used for an appropriate length of time.

Restrictions to limb movements

- After osteosynthesis, no particular restriction is necessary in hip rotation.
- After hemiarthroplasty, in order to prevent the dislocation of the prosthesis, the following movements should be avoided for two months after surgery:
    - extensive internal rotation and flexion > 100° (in posterior approach)
    - external rotation and full extension (in anterior approach).

Physiotherapy and other postoperative treatment

- Active physiotherapy is essential; first sitting, then standing, followed by walking. Mobilization should start as soon as possible, preferably on the first postoperative day.
- Mechanical aids are of no particular benefit.
- Active medication for osteoporosis in the elderly has no short-term benefits.
- Provision of stimuli, empathy and a suitable analgesic, sometimes combined with a mild antidepressant, are usually beneficial.
- Padded trousers (external hip protectors) reduce the risk of femoral fracture. These are particularly useful for residents of a nursing home B [8 9].

Fracture of the shaft

Findings

- Usually as a result of a road traffic accident.
- The thigh is shortened and thickened.

Treatment

- The thigh should be splinted well during transport. Intravenous infusion is often warranted (may lose 2000 ml).
- Tibial traction whilst waiting for surgery, in a fracture of the femoral shaft 1:10 of the patient's weight.
- Intramedullary nail fixation is the usual choice of treatment.

Supracondylar fracture

- Often in an elderly patient with osteoporotic bones. Occurs in knee flexion or hyperextension.
- Treated with a screw-plate (or supracondylar intramedullary nail), mobilization of the knee and partial weight bearing for 3 months.

References

1. Parker MJ, Handoll HHG. Extramedullary fixation implants and external fixators for extracapsular hip fractures. Cochrane Database Syst Rev. 2004;(2):CD000339.
2. Handoll HHG, Farrar MJ, McBirnie J, Tytherleigh-Strong G, Awal KA, Milne AA, Gillespie WJ. Prophylaxis using heparin, low molecular weight heparin and physical methods against deep vein thrombosis (DVT) and pulmonary embolism (PE) in hip fracture surgery. Cochrane Database Syst Rev. 2002;(2):CD000305.
3. Efficacy and safety of low molecular weight heparin, unfractionated heparin and warfarin for thrombo-embolism prophylaxis in orthopaedic surgery: a meta-analysis of randomised clinical trials. Haemostasis 1997;27:75–84.
4. The Database of Abstracts of Reviews of Effectiveness (University of York), Database no.: DARE-973598. In: The Cochrane Library, Issue 4, 1999. Oxford: Update Software.
5. Howard AW, Aaron SD. Low molecular weight heparin decreases proximal and distal deep venous thrombosis following total knee arthroplasty: a meta-analysis of randomized trials. Thrombosis and Haemostasis 1998;79:902–906.
6. The Database of Abstracts of Reviews of Effectiveness (University of York), Database no.: DARE-983696. In: The Cochrane Library, Issue 2, 2000. Oxford: Update Software.
7. Handoll HHG, Parker MJ, Sherrington C. Mobilisation strategies after hip fracture surgery in adults. Cochrane Database Syst Rev. 2004;(2):CD001704.
8. Kannus P, 2001kari J, Niemi S, Pasanen M, Palvanen M, Järvinen M, Vuori I. Prevention of hip fractures in elderly people
with use of a hip protector. N Engl J Med 2000;343:1506–1513.
9. Lauritzen JB, Petersen MM, Lund B. Effect of external hip protectors on hip fractures. Lancet 1993;341:11–13.

18.31 Knee fractures

Editors

Fracture of the patella

Non-operative treatment

- In a fissure fracture with a smooth articular surface and with no separation of the fragments, immobilize the knee with a cylinder cast for 2 weeks. In a small fissure that does not cross through, an elastic bandage may be sufficient.
- A rule of thumb: if the patient can fully extend the knee, conservative treatment is usually successful.
- Limited weight bearing on the first days with crutches, full weight bearing later on.

Operative treatment

- Dislocated or comminuted fracture
- Consider always when the patient is completely unable to extend the knee.

Physiotherapy

- Quadriceps and hamstring muscles are exercised from the very beginning (first with isometric exercises).

Fracture of the tibial condyle

Non-operative treatment

- If the patient has haemarthron the blood is removed by aspiration. If the fracture is without dislocation and the knee is stable crutches are sufficient.
- Cylinder cast for 4 weeks or hinged orthosis for 6–12 weeks if
  - the dislocation (depression or lateral displacement) is less than 5 mm in a younger patient or less than 7 mm in an elderly patient
  - an elderly patient has an osteoporotic fracture even if the dislocation exceeds 7 mm
  - the fracture is stable.
- Weight bearing with limb weight continues for 6–12 weeks.

Operative treatment

- All other cases of tibial fracture

Physiotherapy

- Thigh muscle exercises
- If the patella is affected the exercises are not started from full flexion but only the last phase of extension is trained.

Fracture of the upper fibula

- Elastic bandage from the foot up to the knee
- Full weight bearing from the start
- Differential diagnosis: always examine the ankle for possible tenderness. If the fibular fracture is associated with a fracture of the ankle (with a rupture of the syndesmosis) as a result of twist injury, operative treatment is indicated. An isolated fibular fracture results from a direct blow.
- Recognize knee ligament injuries and injury of the peroneal nerve.

18.32 Dislocation of the patella

Risto Nikku

Mechanism of injury

- Valgus bend and external rotation of the lower leg while the knee is flexed causes the patella to dislocate over the lateral crest of femoral sulcus.

Symptoms and findings

- A typical patient is a teenager or a young adult with haemarthrosis of the knee.
- History (the patient him-/herself may have noticed the slipping of the patella; the injury leading to dislocation may be mild, whereas a higher energy injury is required for ligament damage)
- Difficulty in weight bearing
- Pain and palpable tenderness on the medial side of the patella, on the medial epicondyle of the femur and on the upper crest of the lateral condyle of the femur
- Sometimes the dislocation is visible.
- The patella can be displaced laterally more on the injured side compared with the intact side. This procedure is painful (the apprehension sign).
- X-ray (including the patellar axial projection) is necessary to find any bony fragments. Tilting and lateralization of the patella can be seen.

Treatment

Reduction

- The knee is extended and the patella is pressed in medial direction.

Evacuation of the haemarthrosis

- Major haemarthrosis is aspirated, which alleviates the pain. Presence of fat droplets suggests osteochondral fracture.

Indications for operative treatment

- Loose body on x-ray needing fixation
- In case of profuse haemarthrosis, arthroscopy and examination under anaesthesia should be considered.
- Operative treatment of recurrent dislocations is considered depending on the age of the patient and the frequency of dislocations. The key question is: Do you trust your knee?

Indications for conservative treatment

- Primary dislocation with only mild haemarthrosis
- Acute phase of recurrent dislocation. An operation is performed later if necessary.
- Quadriceps exercises are started and a patellar stabilizing orthosis is used when the oedema has diminished (2–3 days).
- Crutches may be needed for 1–2 weeks.

Recurrent dislocations of the patella

- The patient can usually reduce the patella by extending the knee, or the patella relocates spontaneously. Between recurrent episodes the knee may function without any problems.
- Try to find the structural or post-traumatic cause for the dislocation tendency.

Symptoms and findings

- Sensation of the knee giving way or being locked
- Pain around the patella and the inner side of the knee when going down the stairs and walking on rough terrain (often secondary chondromalacia)
- The patella may be displaced on the lateral condyle when the knee is flexed 20 degrees and the quadriceps muscle is relaxed. There is often unpleasant contraction of the quadriceps muscles if the patella is pushed to the side (apprehension sign).
- The patient often has valgus malposition and marked external rotation of the lower leg.
- On x-ray
  - a high-positioned patella (side view may reveal patella alta, i.e. the patellar ligament measured from the lower edge of the patella to the tuberositas tibiae is 20% longer than the patella itself)
  - patellar view may show tilting, lateralization and sequela of an avulsion fracture of the medial edge of the patella.

Treatment

- See above for the treatment of a dislocated patella.
- The extent of chondral damage seems to predict the results.

18.33 Knee injuries

Olli Korkala

Basic rule

- Diagnose and treat knee injuries early (short absence from work, minimal late sequelae).

History

- High or low energy injury?
- Past injuries?
- Was the injury caused by torsion?

Clinical examination

- Inspect and palpate the knee. Find out the site of tenderness.
- Can the patient bear weight on the knee? What is the range of motion?
- **Lachmann's test and drawer test** should be performed both forwards and backwards, and the range of movement compared with the other knee (injuries of the anterior and posterior cruciate ligaments).
- Test the medial and lateral collateral ligaments with the knee extended and in 30-degree flexion (**adduction-abduction test**).
- Determine the lateral shift tendency and tenderness of the patella, crepitation, and tenderness caused by friction of the patella against the femur when the patella is moved.
- **McMurray test:** The patient is lying supine. Palpate the posteromedial joint space and extend the knee gradually from extreme flexion in external rotation. A snap is felt and sometimes heard. Palpate the posterolateral joint space from the lateral side, and extend the knee in internal rotation.
- **Apley test:** The patient is lying prone with the tigh pressed against the surface. Perform the same rotation movements of the knee in a 90-degree flexion either while lifting from the foot (pain indicates a ligament injury) or while pressing the leg and the foot on the surface (pain and snapping in the joint space indicates meniscus injury).
- Perform a knee puncture if a hydrops is detected (Figure 18.33.1).
  - If the joint fluid is bloody, suspect ligament injury. Arthroscopy is usually indicated (except in some cases with dislocation of the patella). X-ray is indicated.
  - If the fluid contains both blood and fat droplets suspect fracture. X-ray is indicated.
  - If the fluid is clear the patient may have reactive effusion caused by trauma or synovitis.
  - If the fluid is turbid suspect bacterial infection (take bacterial culture, determine serum CRP).
- Plain x-rays should be taken in all but the mildest injuries.
- Arthrography doesn't anymore have much role in knee diagnostics, the investigation of a synovial cyst (Baker's cyst) maybe as a rare exception. Magnetic resonance imaging and arthroscopy have superior accuracy **A** [1 2 3 4].
- Fresh clear instability, deformity, haemarthrosis and locked knee (mechanical loss of extension) are indications for further investigations on emergency basis. Otherwise there is no hurry for specialist assessment but the situation may be followed up.

Treatment

- Mobilize mild injuries (no instability, hydrops, or locking) immediately. Use a supportive bandage, elevation, or an ice bag if necessary.
- In suspected internal injuries (possible instability, hydrops, or haemarthrosis, limitation of extension, or locking) x-rays and eventually arthroscopy (haemarthrosis) should be performed or the knee should be examined under anaesthesia. Primary (arthroscopic) surgery can be performed.

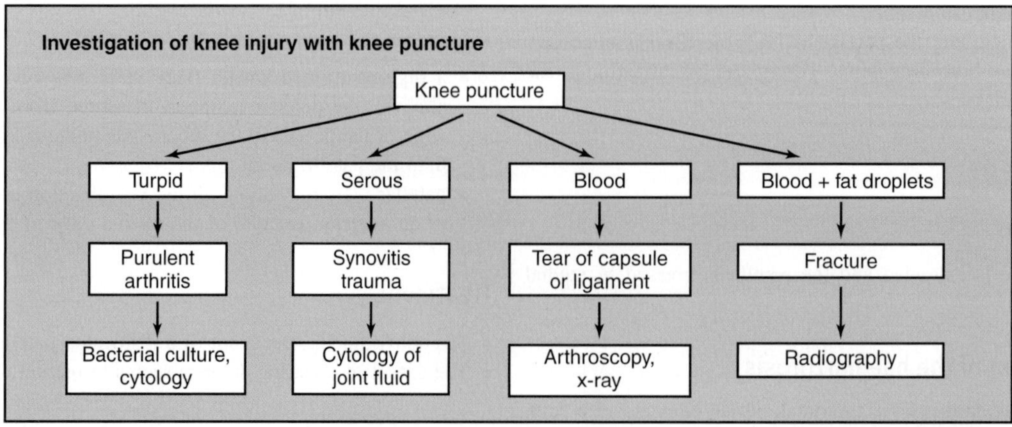

Figure 18.33.1

- If instability is evident (the drawer test is clearly positive, or instability is detected in the adduction-abduction test with the knee extended) eventual fracture or ligament injury should be corrected rapidly, usually by an operation.
- If acute dislocation of the patella has not been reduced spontaneously push the patella in place while extending the knee. Treatment is usually conservative at first if an osteochondral fracture is not detected. Consider surgery in recurrent dislocation of the patella (18.32).
- Minimize the time of cast immobilization and prefer dynamic knee supports (with a hinge). Such supports allow controlled mobilization, which enchances circulation and promotes healing.
- Arthroscopic surgery has shortened sick leaves in patients with menisceal tears. It is also probable that mini-invasive menisceal surgery improves late outcomes.
- Reparation of the anterior cruciate ligament (substituting the cruciate ligament by transplanted patellar tendon C [5 6] or hamstring tendon) at a later stage usually yields a good result and should be considered in young or working-aged patients.

References

1. Rappeport ED, Mehta S, Wieslander SB, Scwarz Lausten G, Thomsen HS. Magnetic imaging before arthroscopy in knee joint disorders. Acta radiologica 1996;37:602–609.
2. The Database of Abstracts of Reviews of Effectiveness (University of York), Database no.: DARE-961824. In: The Cochrane Library, Issue 4, 1999. Oxford: Update Software.
3. Mackenzie R, Palmer CR, Lomas DJ, DIxon AK. Magnetic resonance imaging of the knee: diagnostic performance statistics. Clin Radiol 1996;51:251–257.
4. The Database of Abstracts of Reviews of Effectiveness (University of York), Database no.: DARE-960778. In: The Cochrane Library, Issue 4, 1999. Oxford: Update Software.
5. Yunes M, Richmond JC, Engels EA, Pinczewski LA. Patellar versus hamstring tendons in anterior cruciate ligament reconstruction: a meta-analysis. Arthroscopy 2001, 17(3), 248–257.
6. The Database of Abstracts of Reviews of Effectiveness (University of York), Database no.: DARE-20010811. In: The Cochrane Library, Issue 3, 2002. Oxford: Update Software.

18.34 Fractures of the leg

Editors

Basic rules

- An isolated fracture of the fibula is treated with an elastic bandage if there is no ligament injury or rupture of the syndesmosis associated with the fracture (rupture of the syndesmosis is probable if the injury mechanism is torsion rather than direct impact and the ankle is tender).
- An isolated, well-positioned fracture of the tibia is treated with a lower extremity cast.
- Combined leg injury is reduced under spinal anaesthesia or treated surgically.

Fractures of the leg

- Most fractures of the leg heal well with conservative treatment.
- Operative treatment is necessary
  - when the fracture is dislocated (an acceptable position is not achieved by reduction)
  - there are large, soft tissue or vascular injuries that complicate the fracture and require surgery
  - there are multiple fractures.

Reduction

- Reduction should be performed as soon as possible. It often requires at least spinal anaesthesia. A slightly dislocated fracture can be reduced in an out-patient unit using analgesics or under "alcohol anaesthesia". Heel traction can used to help the reduction. Traction socks are available.
- Criteria for good reduction
  - No rotational error
  - Final angulation of the fractured parts 5 degrees or less
  - Lateral displacement no more than half the diameter of the diaphysis and shortening no more than 0.5–1 (–2) cm
  - The surfaces of the fracture should be in contact, and there should be no diastasis or slit caused by an edge in the bone.
- Casting: see 18.35.

Care after cast fixation

- The leg is kept raised for three days. When swelling has subsided, the patient is allowed to learn to move with crutches, and the cast is closed before discharging from the hospital. Toe and thigh muscle exercises are begun immediately.
- Control x-rays are taken on day 3 and thereafter on weeks 1–3, 6 (–8) and 10–12 after the injury, and later if necessary.
- Weight bearing with the weight of the leg is usually allowed immediately. The cast is changed to a light padded cast 6–8 weeks after the primary injury. When the fracture is clinically stable and there is no local tenderness a walking cast is fitted. Then the patient may walk with full weight bearing 2–4 weeks before the cast is finally removed. Walking cast may be made of fibreglass.
- If the primary dislocation is large, the healing process will probably be slow even if reduction is successful. If the fracture is still unstable after three months, bone transplantation is usually performed.

Primary operative treatment

- An AO plate or closed intramedullary rod techniques C [1 2] are used in the operation. With both techniques postoperative care is possible without a cast, and mobilization can be started immediately.

Prognosis

- With using conservative treatment the ossification takes an average of 20 weeks. After one year 98% of the fractures have ossified. After 24 weeks 55% of patients are able to walk without a stick, and after one year 95%.

Isolated fracture of the fibula

- Suspect a rupture of the syndesmosis of the ankle if the mechanism of injury in a proximal fibular fracture is torsion of the ankle or the ankle is tender on palpation and swollen. Syndesmosis rupture requires surgery.
- The fibula is not a weight-bearing bone, and fractures of the fibula caused by direct impact can be considered stable even when there is dislocation. Weight bearing on the injured side is permitted immediately. An elastic bandage extending from the toes to the knee prevents pain and swelling.
- Possible ligament injuries should be considered. A knee ligament injury or peroneal nerve injury can be associated with a proximal fibular fracture.

Isolated fracture of the tibia

- In isolated tibial fracture the position is usually good and the injury is treated with a lower extremity cast. The duration of immobilization is 8–12 weeks for adults, including 2–3 weeks with a walking cast. Sometimes a non-injured fibula causes a spring-like effect, angulating the fracture. In this case operative treatment is indicated because ossification might otherwise be delayed or a deformity may result.

References

1. Dervin GF. Skeletal fixation of grade IIIB tibial fractures: the potential of metaanalysis. Clin Orthop Related Research 1996; (332):10–15.
2. The Database of Abstracts of Reviews of Effectiveness (University of York), Database no.: DARE-961885. In: The Cochrane Library, Issue 4, 1999. Oxford: Update Software.

18.35 Casts in the treatment of lower extremity fractures

Matti Sävelä

Cylinder cast

Indications

- Patellar fractures; in vertical fractures, however, a hinged orthosis is often used
- Rarely other knee injuries (dynamic knee supports are becoming more common)

Equipment

- Tube gauze, padding, crepe paper, strips of foam, and 6–8 rolls of cast

Preparing the cast

- Place a stand under the ankle while an assistant supports the leg under the knee.
- Cover the extremity with tube gauge and pad the lower part of the ankle with a strip of foam.
- Padding and crepe paper are wrapped from the malleolar level up to the upper thigh and the cast is wrapped on the paper.
- An assistant supports the knee in a 10–15-degree flexion and changes the grip while supporting as the application proceeds to avoid dents. Make sure that the malleolar bones are free and that the ankle is free to move.
- The cast is moulded carefully around the knee and the thigh is supported from the sides to avoid later sliding of the cast.

Duration of cast treatment

- In patellar fracture, 5–6 weeks

Weight bearing

- Immediately, the pain allowing. Crutches may be used during the whole cast wearing period if necessary.

Long-leg cast

Indications

- Tibial fractures
- Rarely in knee fractures or ligament injuries where a hinge orthosis is most often used

Equipment

- Tube gauge, padding, crepe paper, 8–12 rolls of 15–20 cm wide cast

Preparing the cast

- Always have an assistant holding the leg and maintaining the ankle in a 90-degree dorsiflexion and the knee in a 20-degree flexion.
- The leg must be in the correct position before wrapping the padding and the crepe paper because later flexion of the ankle will make folds in the crepe paper. Such irregularities will press the skin inside the cast.
- To protect the skin, use tube gauge and put two layers of padding on it from the base of the toes to the upper thigh.

Pad the malleolar bones, the knee and the site of the injury especially well.

- Crepe paper is wrapped on the padding so tightly that the contours of the leg are visible.
- The cast is wrapped on the paper in five equally thick layers and is moulded, changing the supporting grip while proceeding. A splint formed of 4–5 layers of cast is placed on the sole from the base of the toes over the heel. This may be done at the end of the casting. Make sure that all toes are free to move. In the proximal end, the cast extends up to the greater trochanter and is supported on it. Round the edges by pulling the tube gauge over the cast.
- In acute injuries or after surgery, the cast including the paper is always split with a cast cutter and the leg is supported in an upright position. The cast is closed after 2–3 days (before the patient is discharged).
- If weight bearing is allowed, make the calf stronger and set a heel or a cast shoe.
- Isometric quadriceps exercises should be started without delay.
- Fibreglass cast can be used to strengthen the cast or as the only casting material if the trauma is not quite recent.

Immobilization time

- In a tibia fracture the first cast is worn for 5–6 weeks, followed by a walking cast for up to 3–4 months from the injury.

Weight bearing

- Weight bearing with limb weight is allowed from the beginning.
- Partial weight bearing enhances healing.
- Full weight bearing after 6 (–9) weeks if bone union is evident and the fracture is stabile.

Short cast boot

Indications

- Stable lateral malleolar fractures with dislocation less than 2 mm (bi- or trimalleolar fractures require surgery)
- After operative treatment of malleolar fractures
- After operative treatment of ankle ligament injuries; cast is not used in conservative treatment
- Mid-foot injuries

Equipment

- Tube gauge, padding, crepe paper, and 4–6 rolls of cast (width 15 cm for the ankle, 20 cm above the ankle)

Preparing the cast

- Place a stand under the knee, use tube gauge to protect the skin, and place the ankle in a 90-degree flexion.
- Wrap two layers of padding from the base of the toes up to upper calf and add crepe paper on the padding.
- The cast is wrapped on crepe paper leaving the toes free. The knee has to be free to bend. The cast should extend up to the level of the upper head of the fibula (to avoid peroneal nerve injury use enough padding, not a single dent is allowed). Round the edges by pulling the tube gauge over the cast. For making the sole, see instructions given for the long-leg cast.
- In acute injuries the cast is split with a cast cutter and closed after 2–3 days.
- If weight bearing is allowed make the calf stronger and set a heel or a cast shoe.

Immobilization time

- In lateral malleolar fracture, 6 weeks. On week 3 the cast is replaced by a walking cast.

Weight bearing

- Partial during the first 3 weeks, thereafter full weight bearing is allowed.

TRA

Patellar tendon bearing (PTB) cast

Indications

- As a primary treatment in stable fractures of the lower tibial shaft
- As a walking cast after a long boot cast

Preparing the cast

- Prepare like a short cast boot but include also patella and the patellar tendon in the cast to prevent rotation. The knee should bend 90–100 degrees. The part around the knee is made of a thick separate splint (5–6 layers), which is rounded with a sock. Do not use crepe paper in the patellar region.

18.36 Ankle fractures

Editors

Basic rules

- Identify the fracture type and plan treatment accordingly.
- Surgery is required always when
  - the fibula is fractured above the syndesmosis, which almost invariably results in a total rupture of the syndesmosis (exception: a fibula fracture caused by a direct blow)
  - the patient has a lateral malleolus fracture with a greater than 2 mm dislocation
  - the patient has a medial malleolus fracture that is even slightly dislocated

- the ankle is unstable
- the fracture of the posterior tibial triangle involves more than 1/4 of the joint surface.

- Active muscle exercises are begun while the cast is worn.
- A walking cast is worn before the cast is removed.
- After the cast has been removed, ensure that oedema is followed up and treated and that the patient is motivated to exercise.

Examining a suspected fracture

- See also article on sprain of the ankle 18.37.
- Find out the mechanism causing the trauma.
- Weight bearing: If the foot bears weight a fracture is unlikely, yet possible, as is a serious ligament trauma.
- Inspection: deformation, location of haematoma
- Palpation
    - Malleoli
    - Lower limb, also higher up (search for a proximal fibula fracture on the basis of pain on palpation)
    - Anterior and posterior tibiofibular and fibulocalcaneal ligaments (tenderness)
    - Stability: drawer sign, lateral stability, talar tilting by comparing with the healthy ankle.
- X-rays with anteroposterior and lateral projections are taken always when a fracture is suspected (no weight bearing, instability, tenderness on palpation suggesting fracture, age over 55 years)

Treatment according to fracture type (Weber classification)

- This classification is based on the location of the fibula fracture.

A. Fibula fracture below the syndesmosis

- Often a supination trauma
- Frequently a horizontal or avulsion-type fibula fracture (usually a benign trauma that seldom requires surgery)
- A possible medial malleolus fracture is vertical, found in the proximal part, with a large fragment.
- The posterior tibial triangle may have a fracture on the medial side (small fragment).
- Treatment
    - If dislocation is less than 2 mm, treat conservatively. Use a slit, padded walking cast boot. As the cast is drying, place your palm at the level of the calcaneal bone and push the medial malleolus towards the ankle from the lateral direction while the other hand opposes by holding from the medial side of lowest third of the leg. Control x-ray is recommended, particularly if there is a suspicion of even a small dislocation. The cast is worn for 4 weeks, with full weight bearing allowed from the beginning. See below for the follow up treatment of the immobilized extremity.
    - If the dislocation exceeds 2 mm or the ankle is unstable, surgery is required.

B. Fibula fracture at the level of the syndesmosis

- Most commonly a fracture of the lateral malleolus
- Often a supination–external rotation trauma
- Fibula fracture is often diagonal and vertical extending from the lower medial side to the upper lateral side.
- Some fractures include a syndesmosis rupture.
- The possible medial malleolus fracture is distal, and consists of a small fragment.
- The posterior triangle may have a lateral fracture.
- Treatment
    - If the fracture is completely undiscolated and the ankle is stable, treat conservatively: cast boot as in point A.
    - If the fracture contains even the slightest dislocation or the ankle is unstable, the patient should be referred to a hospital for evaluation of the need for surgery.

C. Fibula fracture above the syndesmosis

- Usually a pronation trauma
- Syndesmosis rupture is always present (exception, see above)
- The possible medial malleolus fracture is distal with small fragments.
- The posterior tibular angle may have a lateral fracture.
- Treatment
    - An operation is always required unless the patient has strong contraindications resulting from systemic diseases, vascular problems or chronic excema.

Treating the immobilized limb

- Padded, slit cast boot extending from below the knee to the base of the toes is worn for 1–2 weeks, thereafter the cast is closed and a control x-ray is taken.
- The patient excercises calf muscles while earing the cast and trains the rectus femoris muscle from the beginning of the treatment.
- The cast is changed after 3–4 weeks from trauma and a walking heel is added. Usually the patient is given permission for full weight bearing.
- The cast is removed after 6 weeks.
- Sick leave normally for 7–10 weeks.
- Pain and swelling may occur over one year from the trauma. If necessary, treat with a supportive bandage or compressive socks. Intermittent compression is also often beneficial. Keeping the leg elevated during the night is somewhat helpful.
- Weight bearing is necessary for healing even if pain is felt at first.
- Ankle exercises are performed at least three times a day, and each time the movements are repeated dozens of times.
- If a plate has been used for fixation, it should be removed from young patients within 6–12 months from the trauma.

A syndesmosis screw is removed after 8–12 weeks. Other screws are not removed unless they cause symptoms. See instructions on the removal of osteosynthetic material 18.39.

- A stable fixation with metal often allows treatment without a cast. In these cases, as in others, weight bearing is forbidden for 4 weeks.
- Some clinics use resorbable screws or rods for fixing fractures. In most cases a cast is worn. The advantage is that the fixation material does not need to be removed.

18.37 Sprain of the ankle

Olli Korkala

Aims

- Try to identify severe ligament injury and consider surgery for actively exercising patients under 30 years of age.
- Try to find malleolar fractures, which are immobilized or operated on.
- Mild injuries are mobilized early.

Mechanisms of injury

- The mechanism is nearly always inversion (supination).
- Eversion is far more rare than inversion and is usually associated with malleolar fractures (as are some inversion injuries).

History

- The history will suggest the grade of the injury. For example, torsion sustained in volleyball when landing after a jump often causes severe ligament injury, whereas an inversion injury while walking is rarely severe.

Clinical examination

- Ability to walk
  - Inability to bear weight or walk may indicate fracture and is usually an indication for x-ray. Ability to walk does not exclude severe ligament injury (or malleolar fracture).
- Tenderness
  - Maximal local tenderness around the anterior talofibular ligament (FTA) indicates FTA injury.
  - Tenderness around the fibulocalcaneal (FC) ligament indicates that the injury extends further back. (In practice injury nearly always begins from the anterior side extending back).
  - The FTP (posterior talofibular ligament) is rarely injured.
- Oedema (haematoma)
  - The degree of oedema does not correlate well with the degree of injury. However, absence of oedema indicates mild injury.
- Is the proximal fibula tender?
  - Proximal fracture of the fibula indicates rupture of a syndesmosis, which is an indication for operation.
  - Injury caused by a direct lateral blow to the fibula without a separate supination injury of the ankle makes an exception. The ankle is stable and without tenderness, and the treatment is conservative.

Indications for x-ray

- Patients with negative findings according to the Ottawa ankle rules are highly unlikely to have a fracture **A** [1 2]. X-rays are recommended if
  - The patient is not able to bear weight immediately after injury and is not able to take four steps in the consulting room.
  - Tenderness is observed on the malleolar bony structure of either the posterior edge or the tip.
  - Instability is observed in torsional tests (athletes and patients under 40 years old: see below further examinations).
  - Tenderness and oedema is observed on the medial side of the ankle.
  - A proximal fibular fracture is suspected.
- On the x-ray, attention is paid to widening of the ankle fork in addition to probable fractures.

Treatment

- In the first stage, using an ice pack and raising the leg often help to prevent extensive haematoma and pain.
- Partial ligament injury is treated conservatively with an elastic or adhesive bandage **B** [3 4 5 6] or semi-rigid ankle support **B** [7]. Several types of dynamic splints are also used **B** [8]. Full weight bearing is allowed at once, and antithrombosis exercises (ankle extension–flexion and periodical contractions of the calf muscle) are recommended from the start. Crutches are used if necessary. The bandage is worn for 1–3 weeks, depending on the symptoms.
- Severe ligament injury with clearly observed instability can be treated operatively by suturing the ligament and capsule **C** [9] if the patient is young (under 30–40 years old) and exercises actively. For older patients, an elastic bandage or orthosis is usually recommended. An actively exercising person can also be given an elastic bandage, and the corrective operation can be performed later if necessary. The tendency is to operate less frequently in the early stages because conservative treatment usually gives a good result **B** [3 4 5 6]. After an operation, immobilization with a cast or dynamic splint lasts 4 weeks and full weight bearing is allowed at once.

Recurrent ankle sprain

- Recurrent ankle sprain does not always require operative treatment; good results can be achieved with elastic supports

TRA

(ankle orthosis), boots with high ankles, and sometimes with exercises strengthening the peroneal muscles. However, operation should not be delayed unnecessarily because recurrent torsion injuries of the ankle prevent exercising and eventually cause talocrural arthrosis.
- The Evans' operation in which the lateral ligaments are reconstructed with the tendon of the short peroneal muscle (peroneus brevis) is used frequently. Another possibility is to perform a so-called anatomical reconstruction using periosteal tissue and suturing the remnants of the ligaments.

References

1. Markert RJ, Walley ME, Guttman TG, Mehta R. A pooled analysis of the Ottawa ankle rules used on adults in the ED. Am J Emerg Med 1998;16:564–567.
2. The Database of Abstracts of Reviews of Effectiveness (University of York), Database no.: DARE-981777. In: The Cochrane Library, Issue 2, 2000. Oxford: Update Software.
3. Ogilvie-Harris DJ, Gilbart M. Treatment modalities for soft tissue injuries of the ankle: a critical review. Clin J Sport Med 1995;5:175–186.
4. The Database of Abstracts of Reviews of Effectiveness (University of York), Database no.: DARE-951779. In: The Cochrane Library, Issue 4, 1999. Oxford: Update Software.
5. Pijnenburg AC, Van Dijk CN, Bossuyt PM, Marti RK. Treatment of ruptures of the lateral ankle ligaments: a meta-analysis. The Journal of Bone and Joint Surgery - American Volume 2000;82A:761–73.
6. The Database of Abstracts of Reviews of Effectiveness (University of York), Database no.: DARE-20001261. In: The Cochrane Library, Issue 1, 2002. Oxford: Update Software.
7. Kerkhoffs GMMJ, Struijs PAA, Marti RK, Assendelft WJJ, Blankevoort L, Dijk van CN. Different functional treatment strategies for acute lateral ankle ligament injuries in adults. Cochrane Database Syst Rev. 2004;(2):CD002938.
8. Kerkhoffs GMMJ, Rowe BH, Assendelft WJJ, Kelly K, Struijs PAA, van Dijk CN. Immobilisation and functional treatment for acute lateral ankle ligament injuries in adults. Cochrane Database Syst Rev. 2004;(2):CD003762.
9. Kerkhoffs GMMJ, Handoll HHG, de Bie R, Rowe BH, Struijs PAA. Surgical versus conservative treatment for acute injuries of the lateral ligament complex of the ankle in adults. Cochrane Database Syst Rev. 2004;(2):CD000380.

18.38 Treatment of foot fractures

Editors

Toes

- A shoe with an inflexible sole is worn for 1–4 weeks. Tape the fractured toe to the adjacent toe.
- Sick leave 1–4 weeks depending on the occupation
- Fracture of the proximal phalanx of the big toe requires correct reduction (operation if the dislocation exceeds 2 mm).

Metatarsal bones

- K-pin fixation should be considered if dislocation is severe or several bones are fractured. A dislocated fracture of the base of the fifth metatarsal bone is fixed with a screw. A cast is worn for 3 + 3 weeks (during the latter period a walking cast).
- In other fractures a walking cast for three weeks or an adhesive bandage support are sufficient. Walking is allowed at once depending on pain. The patient should use a shoe with an inflexible sole.

Fracture of a tarsometatarsal joint (Lisfranc's joint) combined with dislocation

- The diagnosis is easily missed.
- The basal joints of the metatarsal bones are dislocated dorsally and laterally, the first metatarsal bone often medially.
- Operative treatment

Talar-navicular dislocation (dislocation of the Chopart's joint)

- Reduction is usually easy, but may need fixation. Cast 3 + 3 weeks.
- A dislocated fracture of the navicular bone is operated on.

Talus

- Posterior complete dislocation of the corpus of the talus is reduced immediately because of the threat of skin necrosis. In other cases the treatment is selected according to the type of fracture and dislocation.
  - Conservative treatment if the fracture is non-dislocated: a cast for three weeks and a walking cast for five weeks
  - Screw fixation in a dislocated fracture

Calcaneus

- Anatomical reduction is usually neither possible nor necessary. The avulsion of the insertion of the achilles tendon is an exception and requires surgery. Severe deformations are treated by manipulation, if possible.
- Early mobilization and weight bearing as pain allows with supporting padded adhesive bandage. After 1–3 weeks a walking cast until the end of the sixth week. The pain is long-lasting (work disability 3–6 months).
- CT is often performed in order to choose the appropriate treatment approach.

18.39 Post-operative treatment of osteosynthesis and indications for the removal of the osteosynthetic material

Editors

Malleolar fracture of the ankle

Operation

- Malleolar bones are fixed with screws and lateral malleolar bone often also with a plate.
- If the syndesmosis is ruptured a syndesmosis screw is set through a hole in the lateral fixation plate.
- Casting time is 6 weeks.
  - Weight bearing with the weight of the extremity (10–15 kg) for 3–4 weeks after which the cast is changed
  - Half weight (30 kg) for 2 weeks
  - Full weight bearing for the last week

Removal of the syndesmosis screw

- The screw is removed 8 weeks after the operation. The screw can be removed in primary care following a strictly sterile technique. Under local anaesthesia a small cut is made in the scar after locating the screw by x-ray. The screw is driven off with hexagon-shaped screwdriver.
- If the wound of the operated ankle becomes infected (usually the lateral malleolus where the plate is fixed) antibiotic prophylaxis is necessary during ossification. All osteosynthetic material is removed from the infected side after ossification is complete.

Femoral and tibial intramedullary rod

- Is removed after 1 year at the earliest. In patients over 60 years of age the rod may be left in place, sometimes also in younger patients.
- The threat of re-fracture exists.
- Stressful exercises should be avoided (jumping, running) for 1 month after removal of the rod.

Femoral sliding screw (DHS)

- Remove from younger patients (under 50 years old) 1 year after ossification, usually in place 2 years from injury.
- The screw is left in place in older patients.

Ulnar and radial plates

- Usually removed after 8–12 months
- Threat of re-fracture is remarkable. Sometimes a proximal radial plate needs to be left in place if the radial nerve passing over the plate cannot be identified and released.
- Removed under anaesthesia and in blood vacuum.

AC-joint and lateral clavicular fracture

Operation

- Fixation with a screw, pins or "hook plate".
- A wrist-neck-sling is worn for 3 weeks. During the next 6 weeks abduction up to 90 degrees is allowed, and thereafter full mobilization.

Removal of screws and pins

- Screws and pins are removed after 5–6 weeks. Then patient may resume working. A hook plate is removed after 8–12 weeks.
- Screws and pins can also be removed in primary care under local anaesthesia.

Kirschner pins in fingers

- Pins inserted because of injury can be removed after 3–4 weeks. Pins used for arthrodesis can be removed after 3 months, if they are palpable.

18.40 Burn injuries

Editors

First aid

- Fight the fire with water or by suffocation and cool skin by immersing it in fairly cold water for 10–20 minutes if the burned area does not exceed 10% of the entire body surface area (corresponds to the surface of one arm). If the clothes catch fire, put the victim immediately in a lying position.
- Cover the burn with clean clothes or dressings.
- Protect the patient from hypothermia.
- Calm the patient.
- In children burns are most commonly caused by hot water, and the burned area is only a few per cent of the body surface. Treatment is sometimes more difficult because of the young age of the patient (1–3-year-olds).
- In injuries caused by flames (particularly in the face) remember the possibility of airway injury and prepare for intubation.
- Consider the possibility of carbon monoxide poisoning (17.24) (give normobaric or hyperbaric **C** [1 2] oxygen).

Table 18.40 Estimating the extent of burn (9% rule)

Injury	Adult%	1-year-old child%
Palm	1	1
Head	9	19
Upper limb	9	9.5
Upper body	36	32
Lower limb	18	15

Pulse oximetry gives a misleadingly high value in carbon monoxide poisoning.

- Corroding agents: rinse thoroughly with plenty of water.

Extent of burn injury (the 9% rule)

- See Table 18.40.

Estimating the depth of a burn injury

- Classification of burns into surface and deep injuries is important.

Surface injury (grades I–II)

- Sense of touch intact
- Capillary reaction: surface of the injured skin becomes pale under pressure and red again immediately after pressing.
- The wound surface is moist.
- If blisters develop in 4–16 hours from the incident the injury is usually grade I.
- Blisters develop in less than 2 hours from the injury: grade II.

Deep burns (grade III)

- Sense of touch impaired
- No capillary reaction (see above)
- The wound surface is dry
- The burn may deepen during up to 24 hours from the injury. Oedema and (blood vessel) thrombosis may worsen the injury. Do not underestimate the severity of a moderately deep burn immediately after injury.
- Injuries caused by flames are usually deep (grade III). A contact electric injury is always deep. Although the skin looks intact the muscle may be necrotic. An injury caused by an electric arc is comparable to that caused by flames.

Where to treat?

1. Mild burns: ambulatory care
    - Criteria: 10% or less of body surface area, with a maximum of 2% grade III (of which none on the face)
2. Moderate burns: hospitalization
    - Children with
        - II degree injuries exceeding 5% of the body surface area, even a smaller injury of the face, perineum (infection!), hands or soles
        - burns that are deeper than the moist grade II scalds.
        - **In slightest suspicion of a deep burn refer the child to a hospital.**
    - Adults with
        - grade II burns covering 10–30% of body surface area
        - electric burns
        - respiratory tract burns
        - other injuries associated
        - even a mild burn in an elderly patient
3. Severe injuries: Hospitalization in ICU or a specialized burns unit
    - Deep burns covering over 20% of body surface area

Treatment of mild injuries

- A burn is classified as a surface injury if the sense of touch, moistness and skin hair are intact.
- As first aid rinse with water for 10–20 minutes.
- Remove burned tissue, debris and dirt from the skin.
- Cover the burn with several layers of greasy mesh followed by sterile dressings at least 3–4 cm thick (gauze, cotton, wad) because the wound may secrete a 1-cm layer of fluid over the next 48 hours.
- The top layers of the moist dressing can be changed.
- On the third day from the injury the dressings are removed (if necessary by soaking), the depth of the injury is estimated and burst blisters and dead skin are evacuated.
- Tissue fluid must not come through the dressings.
- Antibiotic prophylaxis is not normally indicated.
- The dressings should be removed after 10 days. At that time they can in most cases be removed without force, revealing a clean, pink (thin, unpigmented) epithelium. Such skin can be showered with water and kept soft with mild creams or oils. Direct exposure to sunlight should be avoided. The pigmentation takes years to recover.
- In extensive and infected burns silver sulfadiazine cream can be used from the beginning.
- Give analgesics if necessary.
- Treat infection with 0.05% chlorhexidine or povidone iodine dressings.

First aid in severe burns

- Secure breathing (oxygen, intubation?)
- Circulation (arrythmias are common in burn injuries)
- Shock prevention: i.v. infusion (physiological saline) if the burn injury covers more than 15% of the body surface area in an adult and 5–10% in a child. Albumin is not recommended B [3].
- Calm the patient.

- Analgesics, if necessary: 5–10 mg morphine i.v. or s.c.
- Prevent hypothermia.
- Arrange for hospitalization. In severe cases inform the hospital in advance.
- If the injury of a child is more than 20% of the body surface and the transportation takes a long time, a physiological saline infusion should be started before transportation.
- Do not remove foreign material (e.g. asphalt) if it is tightly attached to the skin.

References

1. Tibbles PM, Perrotta PL. Treatment of carbon monoxide poisoning: a critical review of human outcome studies comparing normobaric with hyperbaric oxygen. Ann Emerg Med 1994;24:269–276.
2. The Database of Abstracts of Reviews of Effectiveness (University of York), Database no.: DARE-940524. In: The Cochrane Library, Issue 4, 1999. Oxford: Update Software.
3. The Albumin Reviewers (Alderson P, Bunn F, Lefebvre C, Li Wan Po A, Li L, Roberts I, Schierhout G). Human albumin solution for resuscitation and volume expansion in critically ill patients. Cochrane Database Syst Rev. 2004;(2):CD001208.

18.41 Electrical trauma

Editors

Basic rules

- In electric arc and contact injuries: surgical treatment
- Resuscitation must be continued for up to 4 hours in electric traumas that have caused asystole and respiratory arrest.
- After trauma, cardiac function is monitored for arrhythmia and infarction.
- Remember to rehydrate patients according to the extent of the burnt area.
- Renal insufficiency that may result from rhabdomyolysis (10.41) in electric trauma is prevented by enhanced diuresis and alkalization of urine. Fasciectomy decreases the pressure in muscle compartments.
- Late symptoms that may appear even years from the trauma include neurological defects and cataract. These should be identified.

Exposure to electricity

- The electrical power is determined by Ohm's law.
  - Electrical current I (in amperes, A) = voltage V (in volts, V) / resistance R (in ohms)
  - Resistance of the human body
    - dry skin, 100 000 ohm
    - moist skin, 1000 ohm
    - internal organs, 500 ohm
- A current over 2000 mA causes asystole, which returns spontaneously to normal rhythm. Respiratory arrest requires resuscitation, however.
- 100–2000 mA causes ventricular fibrillation and, as a late effect (1–3 h), myocardial infarction.
- 20–100 mA for over 1 minute may cause hypoxia in the brain and cardiac tissues.

Symptoms

Acute injuries

- Burn injury of the skin
- Deep injury causes oedema in the muscle compartments –rhabdomyolysis
- Asystole, arrhythmias, infarctions, sinus tachycardia
- Apnoea (hypoxia), coma (neuron damage)
- General vasoconstriction
- Lightning trauma may cause rupture of both tympanic membranes
- Internal organ perforation, necrosis
- Vertebral compression fractures due to contraction of paraspinal muscles

Delayed injuries (1 day–2 years)

- Nervous system
  - Neurological symptoms caused by demyelinization especially in the cervical and thoracic tract
  - Polyneuropathies
- Kidneys
  - Renal insufficiency caused by rhabdomyolysis
- Blood vessels
  - Delayed bleeding
- Eye
  - In head and neck tract electric trauma: cataract after 0–3 years

Care

- Remove the patient from the source of power: switch off and cut the conductors (work with gloves and insulated clothes).
- Resuscitation
  - Asystole: defibrillation
  - Shortness of breath: ventilation, intubation. Spontaneous breathing may return after 30 minutes.
  - Resuscitation must be continued for up to 4 hours. Rigid pupils may result from the effect of electrical power on the central nervous system. It does not always suggest a poor prognosis.
- Kidney function (rhabdomyolysis, see 10.41)
  - I.v. fluids quickly (hypotonic, e.g. 0.45% NaCl)

- Diuresis 100–400 ml per hour, 6–7 litres per 24 hours. In oliguria give mannitol if needed.
- Alkalize urine ($NaHCO_3$ drip until urine pH exceeds 7).
- Laboratory tests: serum creatine kinase, creatinine, sodium and potassium

♦ Manage arrhythmias

♦ Tachycardia, high blood pressure

- Beta-blockers

18.42 Frostbite injuries

Editors

Basic rules

♦ Thaw the frozen area quickly, but only if refreezing is not probable during transportation and the patient is not hypothermic.

♦ Unnecessary touching of the injured area should be avoided after thawing.

Clinical features

Frostbite injuries

♦ Stinging pain

♦ Numbness

♦ White blotch on the skin is the first sign of frostbite injury of the face.

♦ Pale, bluish or marble-like skin colour

♦ Severity cannot be estimated before thawing.

Immersion injuries

♦ Caused by cold water. The usual exposure time is several days or weeks.

♦ The injured extremity is insensitive and oedemic at the beginning of the warming process. Later, typical symptoms are redness and severe pain.

♦ The most serious immersion injuries cause ulcers and necrosis.

Care

♦ The main aim in emergency care is to avoid mechanical trauma.

♦ In the hospital, the first procedures are rectal temperature measurement and management of hypothermia before local injuries are treated. The extremities of a hypothermic patient must not be warmed.

♦ The best treatment is rapid thawing in warm water (40–42°C) for 15–30 minutes or until circulation returns to the injured area.

♦ When no thermometer is available, use your elbow to check the water temperature (must not burn).

♦ Refreezing is very harmful: avoid thawing at the scene of the accident if refreezing is likely during transportation.

♦ Prepare after thawing to manage intense pain.

♦ After thawing, the injured area is covered by soft sterile gauze pads.

♦ In post-thawing treatment, chlorhexidine or polyvidone fluids are used in daily bathing of the injured area.

♦ A swollen oedemic extremity is treated by cast in a functional position and by keeping the extremity raised.

♦ A dry gangrene is allowed to demarcate. Wet gangrene is removed quickly.

♦ Paraesthesias, sensitivity to cold, profuse sweating, joint pain, white fingers and causalgia may persist as post-injury symptoms for years.

18.43 Hypothermia

Editors

Basic rules

♦ A hypothermic patient with all the signs implicating death (no pulse, no breathing, dilated non-reactive pupils, muscle rigidity which resembles death rigidity) can sometimes be resuscitated.

♦ Resuscitation procedures (heart massage, artificial respiration) are avoided while the patient is unconscious and clearly hypothermic until he has been transported to a place where the ECG can be monitored.

- This procedure is followed especially if the patient has been found outside in the cold.
- Cold water cools the body quickly, and in icy water unconsciousness is possible in 15 minutes.

Pathophysiological changes in hypothermia

♦ See Table 18.43

♦ Sudden hypothermia develops if one falls into cold water. More slowly developing hypothermia (days or weeks) appears in persons who are lost outside or in elderly people living in poor housing conditions.

Table 18.43 Pathophysiology of hypothermia

Core temperature (°C)	Physiological abnormalities
35	Increased basal metabolic rate. Accelerated cardiovascular function. Polyuria
34	Impaired consciousness
30	Unconsciousness
27	Muscular rigidity
25	Spontaneous ventricular fibrillation
23	Cessation of breathing
19	Isoelectric ECG as in brain death
15	Asystole

Quick diagnosis

- If the patient has clothes on and the abdominal skin is cold when touching it with a hand of normal temperature, the patient is very likely hypothermic.
- If the patient is conscious, shivering and rectal temperature is over 33°C, the prognosis is good.
- Unconsciousness caused by cold is always life-threatening.
- A J-wave on the ECG is a diagnostic sign of hypothermia.

First aid

- Careless moving of the patient must be avoided because cold blood remaining in the extremities may cause ventricular fibrillation when it circulates to the heart.
- The patient is kept supine during transportation. When lifting the patient from water, avoid holding him under the armpits in an upright position.
- Ensure that airways remain open.
- Protect the patient from cold and wind, but avoid active heating. A warm pack can be placed on the chest if the patient is conscious.
- Wet clothes are not removed at the accident site. Vaporization is prevented by using blankets or plastic coverings. So-called space blankets are recommended for inclusion in first aid kits.
- Manual resuscitation is contraindicated if there are electric complexes on the ECG (may trigger ventricular fibrillation). If the patient has ventricular fibrillation or cardiac arrest, manual resuscitation and breathing assistance are started.
- Deeply hypothermic patient is best transported to a general hospital where the patient can be warmed up with a heart-lung machine.
- Defibrillation is (usually) not successful in patients with core temperatures below 28–30°C. If a severely hypothermic patient enters ventricular fibrillation, his temperature must be raised quickly to 30°C by immersing the patient in a warm (45°C) water pool, or by transporting him to a place where haemodialysis is possible.
- Slowly developing hypothermia is usually accompanied by hypoglycaemia.
- Low body temperature increases urine excretion and causes dehydration. If intravenous fluids are given, ensure that the fluid remains warm throughout the administration.

18.50 Indications for plastic surgery

Sirpa Asko-Seljavaara

- The following traumas, congenital abdomalities, diseases or conditions may be indications for plastic surgery:
  - skin cancer (13.77)
  - head and neck cancer (in cooperation with ENT and maxillofacial surgeons)
  - soft tissue sarcoma (20.91)
  - breast reconstruction (delayed or immediate reconstruction) (18.54)
  - leg ulcer (5.50)
  - ischaemic or diabetic ulcer of the foot (in cooperation with vascular surgeons)
  - pressure sore
  - lymph oedema (18.52)
  - facial paresis
  - trauma surgery
    - soft tissue injury of the face
    - replantation and other soft tissue defects of the hand (in cooperation with hand surgeons) (18.53)
    - complicated fracture of the leg (in cooperation with orthopaedic surgeons)
    - scar revisions (18.51)
    - burns
  - abnormalities of the face
    - cleft lip and palate
    - craniofacial surgery
  - aesthetic surgery
    - face lift, blepharoplasty, liposuction, rhinoplasty, body contouring, hair transplantation etc.

18.51 Injuries requiring plastic surgery

Sirpa Asko-Seljavaara

Facial injuries

- Laceration injuries of the face require primary plastic surgery. Debridement is carried out first, followed by meticulous closure.
- Skin and soft tissue injuries in the face, such as a dog bite, should be treated immediately by a plastic surgeon carrying out careful revision and immediate reconstruction.

TRA

- Shotgun injuries to the face should be treated primarily by a plastic surgeon together with a team comprising a neurosurgeon and a maxillofacial surgeon. Careful revision should be made. Reconstruction is carried out on emergency basis. In most cases free microvascular flaps are used. Shotgun injuries usually need multiple reconstructions.

Replantation

- See 18.53
- Hand and plastic surgeons cooperate in an emergency service to replant hands, fingers and other amputated parts of the body.
- The following parts of the body can be replanted (revascularized):
    - finger or fingers, hand, hand amputated at the wrist, upper extremity
    - lower extremity (indications have been extended because the replanted leg can be later lengthened).
    - ear, scalp, nose, lip
    - penis
- If any part of the body named above has been amputated, the patient is given first aid and a careful clinical examination is performed. The nearest hospital with readiness for replantation surgery is contacted by telephone as soon as possible. It is usually possible to assess already in the phone whether replantation is indicated.

Severe injuries of the lower extremity

- Compound fractures and other complicated injuries of the lower extremity are treated by plastic surgeons in co-operation with orthopaedic surgeons.
- Fasciotomy may be needed in the initial phase.
- After careful primary revision, the fracture is stabilized with external fixation. In special cases, a locking intramedullary nail or other internal osteosynthesis has been used.
- Soft tissue reconstruction and possible bone grafting are performed either immediately or a few days after the injury. Microsurgical tissue grafts are often required.

Scar revisions

- Scar corrections are common plastic surgery operations. General practitioners should not perform Z-plasties or other scar corrections.
- Most scars are corrected under local anaesthesia.
- A scar should not be corrected before 6 months have elapsed from the injury.
- If the scar hinders a joint to be extended, the mouth to be opened or an eye to be closed, scar revision and reconstruction should be carried out immediately.

Keloids

- For keloids see article 13.79.

18.52 Lymphoedema

Sirpa Asko-Seljavaara

Aetiology

- Chronic lymphoedema of an extremity is either caused by congenital hypoplasia of the lymphatic vessels or is acquired.
- Most lymphoedemas in the upper extremity are caused by breast cancer treatment. Most lymphoedemas in the lower extremity are due to treatment of cancer in the pelvis (e.g. ovarian or uterine carcinoma).

Conservative treatment

- Mild lymphoedemas are treated conservatively.
- The patient uses compression bandages or a compression garment (5.53), or receives pneumatic compression or manual lymph therapy (massage).
- Lymph therapy is beneficial in mild lymphoedema. The therapy should be given as courses of 10–15 treatments at 2–3-month intervals. It is given by physiotherapists and lymph therapists.
- The patient may have to consider changing her/his job if the condition is aggravated at work.

Surgical treatment

- If the patient has severe upper or lower extremity lymphoedema or lymphoedema of the penis or scrotum, the patient should be sent to a plastic surgeon for consultation.
- The surgical methods for treating lymphoedema include integumentectomy (removal of the skin and subcutatious tissue and free skin grafting). An attempt can also be made to improve lymph flow by transplanting lymph vessels into nearby veins using microsurgical methods (anastomoses) or by ultrasound liposuction.
- After surgery the patient must use a compression garment.
- After the treatment the sick leave is usually long.

18.53 Replantation of the extremity or part of the body

Sirpa Asko-Seljavaara

Basic rules

- At the scene of injury

- Stop the bleeding with pressure bandage. Lift the extremity up. Collect all the severed parts of the body to be taken with the patient. Remember the possibility of replantation. Indications, see below.

♦ In the emergency room
- Inspect the stump and the severed part visually and, if necessary, palpate carefully wearing sterile gloves. An x-ray may be taken.
- Cool the amputated part.
- The patient is transported quickly to the place where final operative treatment is available. Call the receiving facility when referring the patient.
- The patient's opinion about the utility of a replantation is also considered.

Indications of replantation

Absolute indications in all patients

- Thumb
- Amputation of two or more fingers
- Midpalm
- Wrist
- Distal forearm
- Other parts of the upper extremity sharply cut off
- Ear
- Scalp
- Nose
- Penis

Relative indications

- A single finger
- Proximal upper extremity (torn off)
- Tip of the fingers II–V
- Foot
- Leg
- (Thigh)

First aid

Stump

- Life threatening consequences of an accidental amputation must be treated first (the treatment of a haemorrhagic shock is always to be prioritized).
- Revisions and ligatures are avoided.
- A partly avulsed part that is still attached with a viable flap is not cut off.
- The stump will nearly always stop bleeding when it is bandaged tightly and held uplifted.

Avulsed part of the body

- Should be fetched immediately if left at the scene of injury.
- The part must not be prepared, or allowed to freeze or dry.
- The part is transported in a dry, clean, water tight bag, which is immersed to ice water (must not freeze).
- Consult the receiving hospital when you are referring the patient.

Post-operative treatment and late problems

- Physiotherapy is necessary for weeks to months after the replantation.
- A functionally good result is reached in about 70% of cases.
- Nearly all patients have cold intolerance in the replanted part.
- 20% have pain, which is less than the prevalence of phantom pain in an amputation stump.

18.54 Breast reconstruction

Sirpa Asko-Seljavaara

Indications for breast reconstruction

- Breast cancer is the most common carcinoma among females. In 40% of the cases the whole breast is removed (mastectomy). If the patient wishes, the breast can be reconstructed.
- The optimal time for reconstruction is 1–2 years after the mastectomy.
- Immediate reconstruction is indicated in certain types of breast cancers such as intraductal carcinoma in situ, multiple small carcinomas or in salvage mastectomy if the breast has been treated by lumpectomy and radiation therapy and the patient has had a small recurrence.

Methods of breast reconstruction

- Endoprosthesis under the pectoralis muscle
- Skin expansion and thereafter endoprosthesis
- Latissimus dorsi musculocutaneous reconstruction with or without endoprosthesis
- Microsurgical TRAM breast reconstruction (transverse abdominal muscle flap or DIEP flap = deep inferior epigastric perforator flap) is the best method when using the patient's own abdominal tissue. The flap is taken below the umbilicus symmetrically in the lower abdomen. Skin and subcutaneous tissue are harvested, as is a small piece of rectus abdominis muscle or only the perforating vessels (DIEP) from one side. TRAM breast reconstruction is a major plastic surgical operation. Immediate breast reconstruction is performed in cooperation by a general surgeon and a plastic surgeon following good oncological practice.

18.60 Subunguinal haematoma

Editors

Principles

- The haematoma is often pressurized and causes pain.
- Worth draining even several days after the injury

Drainage technique

- Hold the finger steadily pressing it against the table.
- Heat up the tip of a metal pin (for example an opened paper clip) until it is red hot and press it against the nail to make an opening for draining the blood. You may have to heat the pin up 2–3 times when perforating a thick nail.
- The nail does not need to be removed unless it is loose and gets stuck on objects, bothering the patient.

18.61 Muscle injuries

Editors

Basic rule

- The muscle should be immobilized immediately after the injury; however, active mobilization should begin soon (1–7 days from injury).

Diagnosis

- The severity of the injury may sometimes be underestimated because in most cases the patient is initially able to use the extremity almost normally.
- Muscle cramp causes a differential diagnostic problem when the patient is examined just after the injury has occurred.
- Muscle oedema (bleeding into the tissue) is best recognized in the thigh muscle by measuring the diameter of the thigh and comparing it to the healthy side.
- The loss of strength and function is correlated with the severity of the injury.
- Haematomas and irregular muscle consistency are revealed by ultrasound.
- Sharp laceration, blunt contusion, or rapid and strong stretching may cause a similar type of muscle injury.

Classification of muscle injuries

- Mild injuries (class I) do not cause a clear functional defect.
- Injuries that clearly hinder normal functioning belong to class II.
- Class III refers to a serious injury involving a total muscle rupture and loss of function.

Treatment

- **First aid**: elevation, compression, and ice packs.
- Early **immobilization** limits the size of the connective tissue scar. If immobilization lasts for more than one week, the settling of new muscle cells will be a problem; they will not settle parallel with old cells. The duration of immobilization is:
  - Class I injuries: 1–2 days
  - Class II (and III) injuries: up to 1 week
- **Mobilization** promotes parallelism of muscle cells, circulation, scar tissue resorption and stretching capacity.
- **Passive and active stretching** within the limits of pain can be started 1 week after injury, or in mild injuries 2–3 days after injury.
- NSAID, an elastic bandage, and ice pack on the injury if desired are recommended for 7–10 days.
- Muscle training and loading can be increased gradually. The antagonist muscle must also be trained to prevent inbalance in opposing muscle strengths.
- Activities involving intensive muscular efforts are allowed first when muscle strength and stretching are back to normal.
- **Surgical treatment** is rarely necessary; however, when it is indicated the best results are obtained when the operation is performed without delay.
  - A large haematoma can be aspirated or removed in an operation.
  - Sometimes a full rupture is repaired.
  - The symptomatic focus of myositis ossificans is operated on 6–12 months after the injury if necessary.

Complications

- A haematoma may encapsulate into a fibrotic pseudocapsule and sometimes form a fairly large haemorrhagic cyst.
- Myositis ossificans can be found by ultrasound or x-ray. Irregular shape and laminar bony structure are typical features.
- A rerupture of the muscle may occur if rigorous exercises are begun too early in a stage when the connective tissue scar formation and regeneration of the muscle are not complete.

18.62 Bite wounds

Editors

Basic rules

- Remember tetanus prophylaxis.
- Primary suturation is possible in mild, non-infected injuries, especially on the face.
- Antibiotic prophylaxis is recommended only in selected cases.

General

- Most bite injuries are caused by dogs, cats and humans, in this order.
- 5–20% of dog bites and 30–60% of cat bites become infected.
- Human bites are infected more often than dog bites and cause deep tissue complications of infection more often than other bites.
- Infective microbes usually originate from the biter's mouth, sometimes from the victim's skin or the environment.

Treatment of bite injuries

Immunization

- Tetanus (1.24) and, if needed, rabies immunization (1.46)

Suturation

- Infected bite injuries are not closed initially.
- Injuries with a probably low infection risk (superficial cat and dog bites) can be sutured or at least the edges of the wound can be secured together with tape.
- Bite injuries to the face are usually sutured for cosmetic reasons; bite injuries in the hands are left open to avoid infection.

Antibiotic prophylaxis in non-infected bite injuries

- Prophylaxis has not been shown with certainty to be effective in the prevention of infection.
- 3–5 days' prophylaxis may be needed in bite injuries that are under 8 hours old and involve a high risk of infection when
  - the bite is moderate or serious
  - the injury may reach a bone or a joint
  - the bite injuries are on the hands B [1]
  - the patient has an immune deficiency disease
  - the bite injury is near a joint endoprosthesis
  - the bite injury is near the genitals
  - the bite injury is caused by a cat or a human B [1].
- In lower risk bite injuries the primary prophylaxis is penicillin. The disadvantages of penicillin prophylaxis are its weak effect against Staphylococcus and only 50% effectivity against anaerobic microbes in the human mouth.
- In deep bite injuries and possibly in all human bites the best prophylaxis is amoxicillin-clavulanic acid.
- For those who are allergic to penicillin, good alternatives are tetracycline, cefalexin and cefuroxime.

Antibiotics used in infected bite injuries

- Usually peroral treatment with the medicines mentioned above continues for 5–10 days.
- Immobilization of the injured area and intravenous antibiotics are indicated when the victim has general symptoms or has an immunodeficiency disease.

Reference

1. Medeiros I, Saconato H. Antibiotic prophylaxis for mammalian bites. Cochrane Database Syst Rev. 2004;(2):CD001738.

TRA

18.63 Acute heat illnesses

Editors

Basic rules

- You should suspect heatstroke when physical activity is accompanied by hot skin, altered consciousness, hypotension, hyperventilation, nausea or diarrhoea.
- Measure the rectal temperature to distinguish between heatstroke and less severe heat illnesses (in heatstroke rectal temperature is over 39°C.) Axillary or ear temperature are not informative when examining a patient with a suspected heat illness.
- In heatstroke the first aid is cooling, which must be started without delay.

Predisposing factors

- Poor physical condition
- Hypovolaemia
- Physical activity in warm conditions
- Overweight
- Heart failure, diabetes, hyperthyroidism
- Medication (tricyclic antidepressants, phenothiazines, anticholinergics, antihistamines, diuretics, beta-blockers)
- Alcohol, psychostimulants
- Convalescence (common cold or gastroenteritis)
- Age (children and the elderly)
- Poor adaptation to heat (travelling)

Heatstroke

- The most severe type of illness caused by heat and may lead to death.
- Fitness events and working in hot conditions involve a risk of heart illness.

Symptoms

- In an acute heatstroke associated with physical stress, the consciousness is lost without prior symptoms or after short prodromal symptoms (disorientation, inappropriate behaviour).
- In a slowly developing heatstroke the prodromal symptoms such as poor appetite, weakness, nausea, diarrhoea and disorientation may appear in the course of a few days.

Findings

- Rectal temperature is usually 39°C or more (up to 45°C).
- Hypotension, tachycardia (over 100/minute)
- Skin is often dry in the slowly developing type and sweaty in the type associated with physical stress. Lack of sweating is often a symptom of a severe disturbance of temperature control.
- Signs of dehydration appear often.
- Laboratory findings
  - Hypernatraemia due to dehydration
  - Hypokalaemia is common in the first phase.
  - Hypoglycaemia sometimes appears after physical stress (drinking a lot of energy drinks containing short-chain carbohydrates may predispose to hypoglycaemia).
  - Renal failure occurs in the late phase, and hyperkalaemia and occasionally hypocalcaemia are found.
  - On the ECG, ST changes, T inversions and conduction abnormalities are seen (may sometimes simulate myocardial infarction).

Differential diagnosis

- Septicaemia, epileptic seizure, intracranial bleeding, ordinary syncope (normal body temperature)

Treatment

- Basic life support
- Side position
- Cooling as quickly as possible (starting on the scene)
  - The best method is to sprinkle, pour or spray water on the entire skin, and at the same time fan the patient with 2–3 fans or clothes.
  - Immersing in water is not recommended.
  - Ice packs are not beneficial.
- Oxygen
- Sufficient diuresis
- I.v. drip: isotonic NaCl, possible hypernatraemia should not to be worsened by infusing the wrong salts.
- Transportation to hospital (intensive care unit) after treatment to lower the body temperature has started. Continue treatment during transportation.

Laboratory tests

- Glucose (quick test)
- Serum potassium and sodium
- Blood count (leucocytosis is associated with dehydration)
- CRP (to differentiate from infection; should be analysed as early as possible)
- Acid-base balance
- Serum creatinine
- Serum creatinine kinase (isoenzymes as well), AST and lactate dehydrogenase
- Prothrombin time, activated partial thromboplastin time (aPTT)
- Lumbar puncture if there is any suspicion of central nervous system infection or subarachnoidal bleeding

Complications

- DIC (disseminated intravascular coagulation; the most common cause of death)

Prevention

- Adequate intake of fluids is ensured during physical strain
- Fluid resuscitation: 4 dl of water before strenuous physical activity, and 1–2 dl every 20 minutes during the activity (e.g. a marathon).

Sunstroke

- Caused by the heat stress directly on an uncovered head.
- Symptoms: headache, irritation, nausea, dizziness and other symptoms originating in the central nervous system.
- Treatment: taking shelter in a cool place, rest and drinking.

Heat oedema

- Hypertension and overweight predispose to oedema of the lower extremities.
- Treatment: rest, raising the legs and plenty to drink. Avoid diuretics if there is no pre-existing disease indicating their use.

Heat cramps

- Heat cramps occur most commonly in the calf muscles, especially when only water is used for rehydration during prolonged exercise.
- Treatment: oral energy drinks containing long-chain carbohydrates, 0.1% salted water (half a teaspoon of NaCl in 2 litres of water) or in severe cases i.v. infusion of isotonic saline.

Heat exhaustion

- Often a precursor to heatstroke. The main underlying factor is incorrect hydration. Three subtypes can be distinguished according to the nature of dehydration.

Hypertonic dehydration

- If fluid loss in not compensated, hypertonic dehydration will develop (hypernatraemia). It is usually caused by physical exercise and heat.
- Symptoms: tiredness, weakness, hyperventilation, disorientation, thirst and high temperature. (Remember serious bacterial infections in the differential diagnosis).
- Treatment: drinking water

Hypotonic dehydration (salt deficiency symptoms)

- If the patient is rehydrated with water alone, salt deficiency symptoms may develop slowly. The condition is rare.
- Symptoms: headache, weakness, nausea and GI symptoms. A feeling of thirst and elevated temperature is not as common as in hypertonic dehydration. Serum sodium is low, and in severe cases AST is elevated.
- Treatment: i.v. infusion of isotonic physiological saline

Isotonic dehydration

- Deficiency of both water and salts. Serum sodium is normal.
- Treatment: isotonic saline-glucose infusion or an oral glucose-salt solution. The oral solution should be hypotonic with regard to NaCl.

Other type of hyperthermia

- Hyperthermia can also be associated with the following conditions:
  - thyrotoxicosis (history!)
  - phaeochromocytoma
  - anaesthesia
  - cocaine/amphetamine overdose
  - malignant neuroleptic syndrome (35.14).

18.64 Stress fracture

Editors

Aims

- To identify a stress fracture by clinical examination. The findings may need to be confirmed by x-ray or by technetium bone scanning.
- To identify femoral neck stress fracture in military conscripts complaining of even mild groin, thigh or knee pain. The patient must stop all exercise immediately until stress fracture has been excluded.

Table 18.64 Sites of stress fractures in conscripts

Site	% of all stress fractures
Tibia	50–70
Metatarsals	20
Calcaneus	8
Femoral bone	5–10
Pelvic bones	4
Fibula	0.5

Risk groups

- 5–15% of military conscripts have stress fractures with most cases occurring at the beginning of the military training (see Table 18.64).
- Women athletes and military conscripts have a 2–10-fold risk compared with men; menstruation disturbances and pregnancy also predispose to stress fractures.
- Athletes and dancers who perform unusually strenuous walking or running exercises, especially on a hard surface
- Persons with leg length discrepancy

TRA

Symptoms

- At the beginning the pain occurs only during exercise, later local pain and aching are felt also at rest.
- Palpable local tenderness occurs at the exact site of fracture – sometimes a subperiostal nodule can be felt on palpation.

Radiological findings

- Changes become visible in plain x-rays 2 weeks to 3 months from the onset of symptoms. In long bones a narrow callus is seen at the site of the fracture (exactly where tenderness on palpation is present). In cancellous bone, sclerosis is usually seen first after 4 weeks.
- The fracture is seen on a bone scan within 3 days of the onset of symptoms. The sensitivity of the scan is almost 100%. The findings take several months to return to normal, sometimes up to 2 years.
- MRI is a sensitive and more specific examination than bone scan. It can be use for differential diagnosis, when necessary.
- In the pelvis, callus may be seen at the narrowest point of the pubic arch.
- Dense calcified line in a 90-degree angle to the trabecular structure of the bone may be seen at the inner edge of the femoral neck.
- Callus at the tibial or femoral shaft
- Horizontal calcified line in the medial condyle of the tibia near the epiphysis
- Dense spots and dense lateral horizontal line are seen in the posterior calcaneus.
- Callus of the second or third metatarsal bone, a dense line at the base of the first metatarsal bone horizontally to the shaft. Often an avulsion fracture is seen at the base of the fifth metatarsal bone.

Diagnosis

- Clinical diagnosis is usually sufficient: typical pain and palpable local tenderness. Stress fracture of the femoral neck is an exception to the rule: the diagnosis should be based on an x-ray as soon as the symptoms appear.

Clinical diagnosis and differential diagnosis

- X-ray is required during the healing process if the symptoms persist for 2–4 weeks despite avoiding exercise (to rule out bone tumours).
- If pain persists or the diagnosis is uncertain, x-ray may be repeated after 2–4 weeks or a technetium bone scan is performed (especially if a fracture of the femoral neck is suspected).
- Calcaneal stress fracture is painful when pressing on the sides, whereas pain in the plantar aponeurosis is experienced when palpating under the calcaneus.
- In medial tibial pain disorder the tenderness is located at the medial edge of the bone and bone scan shows a far-extending thickening.
- In bone tumours, radiographic finding (repeated imaging) is usually diagnostic in the end.

Treatment

- Avoidance of all strain and loading that causes pain is usually sufficient.
- Crutches may be used if the pain is severe.
- Do not give local steroid injections or massage.
- Metaphyseal fractures of the femoral neck or tibia do not usually require a cast.
- Healing usually takes 2–4 weeks, upper tibial fractures take 8–10 weeks, femoral shaft 1–4 months and femoral neck 3–4 months. Disappearance of pain is a sign of healing.
- Exercise is allowed when pain is no longer experienced in stress, palpation and when bending.
- Anti-inflammatory drugs are not recommended at the beginning of exercise.
- Fractures with a high risk of complications (consult an orthopaedist)
  - Femoral neck
  - Femoral supracondylar shaft
  - Patella
  - Anterior middle aspect of the tibia
  - Talus
  - Navicular bone
  - The base of the fifth metatarsal bone

Sports Medicine

Evidence Based Medicine Guidelines. Edited by the Duodecim Editorial Team
 ISBN: 0-470-01184-X

19.1 Physical activity in the prevention, treatment and rehabilitation of diseases

Katriina Kukkonen-Harjula, Ilkka Vuori

The fundamentals of physical exercise

- The physiological effects of physical activity are most marked in those parts of the body that are used during exercise, i.e. the muscles, joints, bones, energy metabolism, circulation, as well as hormonal and neural regulation.
- For the effects to persist, physical activity must be regular. The effects may persist when the duration and frequency of exercise is slightly reduced, particularly if the intensity remains the same.
- Physical activity is the best way of ensuring the maintenance of functional capacity. Physical activity is therefore especially important in the prevention of the detrimental effects of ageing and chronic illnesses.
- Excessive or otherwise incorrect exercise may cause functional disorders or sports injuries. The margin between suitable and excessive exercise, i.e. the therapeutic range of physical activity, may be narrow, particularly in those in poor health.
- The beneficial effects of endurance-type activity (aerobic exercise) to health and functional capacity have been studied the most. For endurance exercise to be beneficial, the intensity of the exercise in a healthy person needs to be at least 50%, preferably 60%, of the maximal aerobic power (maximal oxygen consumption, VO_2max). This means that the person's heart rate during exercise should be approximately 60–75% of his/her maximum heart rate. This type of exercise, for example brisk walking, is considered to be moderately intense. To improve cardiovascular fitness (energy metabolism and circulation), physical activity needs to include rhythmic movements of the large muscle groups which should be sustained for a considerable length of time (usually several tens of minutes). Walking, cross-country skiing, cycling and swimming are examples of endurance (stamina) building exercise. Less information is available regarding the health benefits of resistance training (weight training), which increases muscle strength.
- Physical activity plays a significant role in the prevention of coronary heart disease and other atherosclerotic diseases, hypertension, type 2 diabetes, osteoporosis and osteoporotic fractures, as well as some types of cancer (colon cancer and possibly also breast cancer). Exercise reduces the risk of all-cause mortality by approximately 10% and of cardiovascular diseases by 20%.

Exercise programmes

Cardiorespiratory (aerobic) fitness

- American College of Sports Medicine (ACSM), 1998
- Moderate intensity (50–85% of VO_2max, the effect is more significant if the minimum intensity is 60%) endurance training 3–5 times per week (see Table 19.1.1).

Health-related physical activity

- American College of Sports Medicine (ACSM) and Center for Disease Control and Prevention (CDC) (1995)
- Health-related physical activity refers to exercise that provides health benefits and does not cause significant health problems. The intensity of such physical activity should be moderate, brisk walking being a typical example. When the intensity is kept moderate, possible disadvantages of exercise (sports injuries and cardiac events associated with insidious coronary heart disease) are avoided, particularly in those not accustomed to exercise.
- **Recommendation**: Every adult should engage in moderate-intensity physical activity for at least 30 minutes on most, preferably all, days of the week. Moderate intensity is defined as 40–60% of maximal oxygen consumption (VO_2max). The 30-minute activity can also consist of shorter exercise bouts (minimum of 10 min) that are accumulated throughout the day (walking or cycling to work, shopping or running other errands etc.).

Prevention of coronary heart disease

- There is an inverse relationship between the occurrence of coronary heart disease and the amount of exercise taken, or aerobic fitness C [1].
- Physical activity can have a beneficial effect on the major risk factors of coronary heart disease (hypertension, dyslipidaemias, obesity, insulin resistance), on factors affecting

Table 19.1.1 ACSM exercise recommendation (1998)

Endurance training to improve and maintain cardiorespiratory fitness and to develop maintain body composition	Resistance training to improve and maintain muscular fitness and flexibility
• 3–5 times per week • (55–) 65–90% of HRmax • (40–) 50–85% of the VO_2 reserve (or HR reserve) • 20–60 minutes of continuous or intermittent (composed of bouts of at least 10 minutes accumulated throughout the day) exercise • Large muscle groups (rhythmic, aerobic)	• 8–10 exercises, 1 set, 2–3 times per week. Each exercise is repeated 8–12 times, older persons should repeat each exercise 10–15 times. • Flexibility (maintenance of the range of movement) at least 2–3 times/week

- VO_2 reserve = difference between maximal and resting oxygen consumption
- HRmax = maximal heart rate
- HR reserve = difference between maximal and resting heart rate

thrombosis formation, such as the function of the vascular endothelium, and possibly also on the electric stability of the heart. The most effective way of producing these effects is regular, frequent endurance training of moderate intensity. In practice, this means physical activity such as brisk walking for 30 to 60 minutes on most days.

Prevention and treatment of hypertension

- Persons who take regular exercise have lower resting blood pressure than those who exercise only a little. Endurance-type exercise lowers blood pressure on average by 4/3 mmHg **B** [2]. The effect is less significant on ambulatory blood pressure **C** [3]. Resistance training may also lower hypertension to the same degree as endurance training.
- The exercise recommendation of ACSM (1993) for mildly or moderately elevated blood pressure:
  - 40–70% of VO_2max, i.e. 55–80% of the maximal heart rate. The lower range of intensity is sufficient for the elderly.
  - 3 or 4 times weekly for at least 30 minutes at a time
  - Various endurance exercise modes are suitable. Resistance training (preferably circuit training) should not be the only form of exercise but should be combined with endurance training.
- Training at an intensity of about 50% of the VO_2max (moderate-intensity) is sufficient with regard to resting blood pressure reduction.
- There is little information regarding the effect of intermittent exercise, i.e. exercise bouts of less than 30 minutes duration, on the resting blood pressure. The reduction in blood pressure may be similar to that seen during exercise of longer duration.

Effect of physical activity on blood lipids

- Moderate-intensity endurance training may increase the serum concentration of HDL-cholesterol (approximately 5% from baseline) and decrease the concentration of LDL-cholesterol (5%) as well as triglycerides (4%) in healthy, sedentary individuals **B** [4].
- A high amount of moderate-intensity exercise over several months is needed in order to bring forth the beneficial effects on HDL-cholesterol concentration. In practice, this means brisk walking or similar exercise for 30–60 minutes almost daily.
- The effect of exercise on the LDL-cholesterol concentration is enhanced if the intake of saturated fats is reduced simultaneously. The above mentioned beneficial changes in the lipid profile may be further augmented with concurrent weight reduction (adipose tissue reduction). Larger serum lipid changes are seen with the combination of low fat diet and exercise.
- Information regarding the effect of resistance training on the blood lipoproteins varies, and HDL-cholesterol concentration does not always increase. The reason for this could be the lower energy consumption associated with moderate-intensity resistance training as compared with aerobic training.

Rehabilitation in coronary heart disease

- Cardiac rehabilitation programmes should consist of a multifaceted and multidisciplinary approach, exercise training being one of the facets. Cardiac rehabilitation may reduce both all-cause and cardiac mortality by around 20% **B** [5]. Cardiac rehabilitation with emphasis on exercise training does not differ markedly from conventional rehabilitation as regards all-cause mortality.
- Recommendation (American Heart Association, AHA, 1995)
  - Mainly endurance training
    - at an intensity of 50 (–60)–75% of symptom-limited VO_2max (or heart rate reserve, which is the difference between maximal and resting heart rate) for 30 minutes 3–4 times weekly (minimum); full benefit is obtained with 5–6 times/week; **and**
  - resistance training
    - at an intensity of 30–50% (up to 60–80%) of 1 RM (one repetition maximum), 12–15 repetitions, 1–3 sets twice weekly.

Other atherosclerotic diseases

Stroke

- Epidemiological research has shown that physical activity reduces the risk of stroke, and regular physical activity is one of the recommended methods of stroke prevention. Physical activity has an influence not only on atherosclerosis but also on other risk factors of stroke, such as hypertension, HDL-cholesterol, insulin resistance and blood coagulation factors. An exercise programme for the prevention of stroke is similar to the programme recommended for preventing coronary heart disease.
- In stroke rehabilitation, specific motor and physical exercises designed by professionals in neurology and physiotherapy are important in the correction of motor deficits.

Treatment and rehabilitation of obliterating peripheral arterial disease (intermittent claudication)

- Regular physical activity may protect against intermittent claudication.
- In lower limb atherosclerosis, physical exercise lengthens the painless walking distance **B** [6].
- In addition to smoking cessation, walking exercises up to the pain threshold several times a day form a central part of the treatment and of post-operative secondary prevention. Other types of exercise, such as resistance training, have not been shown to be clearly beneficial for symptom relief or for improvement of the functional capacity of the lower limbs.

Prevention and treatment of obesity

- Management of obesity always requires permanent changes to the diet. It is important to distinguish between the phases of weight loss and weight maintenance. The general aim of weight maintenance is to prevent weight gain, particularly after successful weight reduction. It may be best to increase the amount of physical activity, such as leisure-time exercise, when actual weight reduction ends.
- Exercise alone (usually endurance-type) without a change of diet only reduces weight by a few kilograms **A** [7 8]. Endurance training has a beneficial effect on body composition (amount of muscle tissue, i.e. fat-free mass (FFM), increases and that of fat tissue decreases), even if actual weight loss is limited. During a weight-reduction diet, resistance training preserves a few kilograms more of FFM compared with endurance training **A** [9].
- Exercise combined with a low-energy diet does not significantly improve weight reduction compared with diet alone; the additional weight loss is at the most only a few kilograms **B** [10 11 12 13].
- Exercise (increased physical activity) combined with a low-energy diet may improve weight maintenance after weight loss, compared with diet alone **C** [14 15 16]. In intervention studies, the effects of exercise on weight have been rather modest compared with epidemiological follow-up studies in which increased physical activity appears to reduce weight gain.
- In the prescribing of exercise the aim has usually been a weekly increase in energy expenditure of 4.2–8.4 MJ (1000–2000 kcal; Table 19.1.2), since adherence to a prescribed exercise programme is often difficult to achieve. To achieve successful weight maintenance, weekly energy expenditure of up to approximately 10.5–11.7 MJ (2500–2800 kcal) may be needed. This amount of energy consumption translates to 60–90 minutes of moderate-intensity physical activity daily (if the intensity is higher the duration may be decreased). However, even small amounts of daily physical activity (lifestyle activity) have been shown to have health benefits (regardless of whether the person loses weight or not) particularly on the risk factors of coronary heart disease.

Table 19.1.2 Total energy expenditure (kJ or kcal) of a person weighing 70 kg during one hour of different modes of exercise

Mode of exercise (and intensity)	kJ/h	kcal/h
Running (12 km/h)	3570	850
Cycling (20 km/h)	2690	640
Jogging (9 km/h)	2520	600
Swimming (50 m/min)	2310	550
Tennis	1760	420
Cycling (15 km/h)	1680	400
Brisk walking (6 km/h)	1390	330
Table tennis	1180	280
Volley ball	880	210
Dancing	880	210
Slow walking	800	190
Bowling	800	190

1. The above examples of energy expenditure are intended only as a guide. The most important factors affecting energy expenditure are the weight of the person, the intensity of the exercise and the performance technique. An overweight person, weighing more than 70 kg, consumes more energy than a person weighing 70 kg in sports that require the bearing of body weight, such as running or walking. The target energy expenditure of exercise for weight reduction should be at least an increase of 1.3 MJ (300 kcal) per day.

Prevention and treatment of type 2 diabetes

- A large amount of regular, moderate-intensity endurance training and ample lifestyle activity integrated into daily activities have a beneficial effect on the various components of the metabolic (insulin resistance) syndrome, such as obesity, hypertension, disturbance of lipid and glucose metabolism and insulin resistance. Similar effects might possibly also be achieved with resistance training. Increased physical activity reduces the risk of atherosclerotic artery diseases and type 2 diabetes.
- Frequent (at least 3 times a week) endurance exercise with at least moderate intensity increases insulin sensitivity, decreases plasma insulin concentration and enhances glucose tolerance. Endurance and resistance training may improve diabetic control (glycosylated haemoglobin) but only have a slight effect on weight reduction.
- This type of exercise may prevent the development of type 2 diabetes. The benefits of exercise are most prominent in persons with the highest risk of developing diabetes, for example, those with impaired glucose tolerance **B** [17 18].
- Physical activity reduces the risk of diabetic complications, such as coronary heart disease. On the other hand, the possibility or existence of any complications should be taken into account when prescribing exercise for people with type 2 diabetes. The risk of exercise-induced hypoglycaemia is negligible, unless the patient uses oral antidiabetic drugs.

Treatment of type 1 diabetes

- Regular, well-timed physical activity that has been adjusted according to insulin and nutrition intake can improve diabetic control. In addition, it has a beneficial effect on the risk factors of coronary heart disease and on life expectancy.
- Physical activity may, however, also impair diabetic control or cause hypoglycaemia. Hypoglycaemia can be prevented by consuming an extra amount of carbohydrates before exercise and by taking an additional 20–40 g per one hour of exercise. Hypoglycaemia may also be prevented by reducing the insulin dose before exercise, by avoiding physical activity during the peak action of insulin and by using an injection site that is not in an area where exercise (muscle work induces increased circulation) would fasten its absorption.
- If the patient's blood insulin level is low before exercise, glucose uptake by the muscles will not increase, but the liver will produce large amounts of glucose. This may lead to hyperglycaemia. Vigorous activity may also induce delayed hypoglycaemia.

- A patient whose diabetes is well controlled can take part in almost any type of physical activity. However, diabetic complications, such as neuropathies, atherosclerosis, retinopathy and poor recovery from infections, should be taken into account when planning an exercise programme.

Prevention of osteoporosis

- Peak bone mass increases in childhood and adolescence and it can be increased with regular exercise. The loss of bone mass becomes accelerated in menopausal women.
- Bone is strengthened when loading induces microscopic transient remodelling of its structure. The remodelling occurs only at the sites that are loaded.
- The mineral content of the bones is increased (or maintained) and the strength of the bone is improved by exercise that is varied, weight bearing and that requires at least moderate strength. The exercise should preferably include rapid, multidirectional movements, and controlled impacts. Examples of such exercise modes are aerobics, and other types of exercise which involve jumping, as well as rapid racket games, such as squash. The weaker the bones, the less loading is needed to influence their strength. For example, walking maintains the bone mineral content in the elderly.
- The loss of bone mass in postmenopausal women may be reduced by exercise. Aerobics as well as weight bearing and resistance training increase the bone density of the lumbar spine in postmenopausal women (A) [19]. Walking as such has an effect on the bone density of the femoral neck.
- Exercise also has a beneficial effect on the bone mass of premenopausal women.
- In men, exercise increases the bone mass at the femur, lumbar spine and calcaneus.
- Prevention of osteoporotic fractures
  - The aim is to maintain adequate bone mass and, in addition, to preserve gait and balance to prevent falls.
  - Versatile physical activity that maintains muscle control, moderate loading and strength as well as balance and agility, such as walking on uneven terrain, gymnastics, aerobics, dancing and racket games, is recommended within the limits set by the individual's physical condition and exercise skills.

Osteoarthritis of the lower limbs

- Normal daily activities probably provide sufficient loading for the joints. Prevention or reduction of excessive weight gain is probably beneficial in the prevention of osteoarthritis.
- Sudden overloading, incorrect joint loading during exercise, and various injuries predispose a person to osteoarthritis.
- Individually designed exercise programmes implemented under the supervision of a health care professional are beneficial in terms of overall fitness, joint problems and functional capacity. The programme should cover flexibility exercises, muscle strength training as well as endurance training.
- Exercise reduces the pain and functional disturbance in osteoarthritis of the knee (B) [20 21 22 23] and hip.

Rheumatoid arthritis

- Exercise (dynamic muscle work) improves muscle strength, joint flexibility and cardiovascular fitness in rheumatoid arthritis, but evidence on its long-term effect on functional capacity is still uncertain (B) [24]. Exercise does not have adverse effects on disease activity.

Prevention and rehabilitation of low back problems

- Regular exercise may prevent low back problems. So far, no consensus has been established on the contents of an optimal exercise programme. However, it is essential to regularly use the muscles of the back, trunk and lower extremities and to maintain the mobility of the back by moderate and varied physical activity. In the prevention of back problems the endurance of the muscles associated with the function of the back seems to be more important than their strength.
- Exercise is not particularly effective in the treatment of acute back problems, but in the rehabilitation of chronic back problems a quick return to normal physical activity has been shown to be more beneficial than passive bed rest (B) [25].

ORT

Asthma

- Endurance training improves the cardiovascular fitness of an asthmatic patient, but its long-term effects on lung function, overall health and quality of life require further studies (C) [26].
- In addition to traditional training programmes, interval exercises have been used as they may reduce exercise-induced asthma. Swimming (high air humidity) may cause less exercise-induced asthma than, for example, jogging.

COPD

- In COPD, physical exercise combined with conventional treatment improves functional capacity. Furthermore, exercise improves the quality of life, reduces dyspnoea and allows better mastery of the disease.

Mental health

- Physical activity may reduce anxiety. Both endurance and resistance training may improve mood and cognitive function in the elderly (C) [27 28].
- Physical exercise may reduce the symptoms of depression. It has not been established which mode of exercise is the most effective; however, it is important to prescribe exercise that the patient perceives as pleasant.

Sleep

- Physical activity can have both acute and long-term beneficial effects on sleep.
- Exercise can increase the duration of slow-wave sleep and total sleep time, and it is also related to a decrease in sleep onset latency and REM sleep.

Cessation of smoking

- Exercise may increase the success of smoking cessation as a part of the overall withdrawal therapy C [29 30].

Physical activity counselling by the physician

- Advising patients about physical activity forms a part of health education with the aim to introduce lifestyle changes. Physical activity counselling also includes patient education regarding his/her illness (does the illness set limitations to the amount of exercise; will exercise pose an increased risk?). Physical activity counselling is often combined with dietary advice. Physical activity promotion is a broader concept and is analogous with health promotion.
- According to international studies, physical activity counselling provided by a general practitioner or another health care professional in primary care is effective in producing short-term changes in physical activity, but adherence to the change is difficult A [31]. Advice should be individualised, and goals and monitoring should be agreed with the patient.
- Exercise carried out at home might be more successful than exercise in special sports facilities C [32]. This also emphasises the many possibilities of exercise incorporated into daily activities (lifestyle activity).
- Physical activity programmes have also been introduced at worksites, often integrated in activities to maintain and improve working capacity.

References

1. Foster C, Murphy M. Effects of physical activity on coronary heart disease. In: Primary prevention. Clinical Evidence 2002;7:91–123.
2. Halbert JA, Silagy CA, Finucane P, Withers RT, Hamdorf PA, Andrews GR. The effectiveness of exercise training in lowering blood pressure: a meta-analysis of randomised controlled trials of 4 weeks or longer. J Hypertens 1997;11:641–9.
3. Kelley G. Effects of aerobic exercise on ambulatory blood pressure: a meta-analysis. Sports Med Training Rehab 1996;7: 115–31.
4. Halbert JA, Silagy CA, Finucane P, Withers RT, Hamdorf PA. Exercise training and blood lipids in hyperlipidemic and normolipemic adults: A meta-analysis of randomized, controlled trials. Eur J Clin Nutr 1999;53:514–22.
5. Jolliffe JA, Rees K, Taylor RS, Thompson D, Oldridge N, Ebrahim S. Exercise-based rehabilitation for coronary heart disease (Cochrane Review). In: The Cochrane Library, Issue 1, 2001. Oxford: Update Software.
6. Leng Gc, Fowler B, Enrnst E. Exercise for intermittent claudication (Cochrane Review). In: The Cochrane Library, Issue 1, 2001. Oxford: Update Software.
7. Wing R. Physical activity in the treatment of the adulthood overweight and obesity: current evidence and research issues. Med Sci Sports Exerc 1999;31(11, suppl.):S547–52.
8. National Institutes of Health and National Heart, Lung, and Blood Institute. Clinical guidelines on the identification, evaluation, and treatment of overweight and obesity in adults. Evidence Report. Obes Res 1998;6(suppl. 2):51S–209S.
9. Garrow JS, Summerbell CD. Meta-analysis: effect of exercise, with or without dieting, on the body composition of overweight subjects. Eur J Clin Nutr 1995;49:1–10.
10. Wing R. Physical activity in the treatment of the adulthood overweight and obesity: current evidence and research issues. Med Sci Sports Exerc 1999;31(11, suppl.):S547–52.
11. National Institutes of Health and National Heart, Lung, and Blood Institute. Clinical guidelines on the identification, evaluation, and treatment of overweight and obesity in adults. Evidence Report. Obes Res 1998;6(suppl. 2):51S–209S.
12. Miller WC, Koceja DM, Hamilton EJ. A meta-analysis of the past 25 years of weight loss research using diet, exercise or diet plus exercise intervention. Int J Obes 1997;21:941–7.
13. Ballor DL, Keesey RE. A meta-analysis of the factors affecting exercise-induced changes in body mass, fat mass and fat-free mass in males and females. Int J Obes 1991;15:717–26.
14. Wing R. Physical activity in the treatment of the adulthood overweight and obesity: current evidence and research issues. Med Sci Sports Exerc 1999;31(11, suppl.):S547–52.
15. National Institutes of Health and National Heart, Lung, and Blood Institute. Clinical guidelines on the identification, evaluation, and treatment of overweight and obesity in adults. Evidence Report. Obes Res 1998;6(suppl. 2):51S–209S.
16. Fogelholm M, Kukkonen-Harjula K. Does physical activity prevent weight gain—a systematic review. Obes Rev 2000;1:95–111.
17. Tuomilehto J, Lindström J, Eriksson JG, Valle TT, Hämäläinen H, Ilanne-Parikka P, ym. Prevention of type 2 diabetes mellitus by changes in lifestyle among subjects with impaired glucose tolerance. N Engl J Med 2001;344:1343–50.
18. Knowler WC, Barrett-Connor E, Fowler SE, Hamman RF, Lachin JM, Walker EA, Nathan DM; Diabetes Prevention Program Research Group. Reduction in the incidence of type 2 diabetes with lifestyle intervention or metformin. N Engl J Med 2002;346:393–403.
19. Bonaiuti D, Shea B, Iovine R, Negrini S, Robinson V, Kemper HC, Wells G, Tugwell P, Cranney A. Exercise for preventing and treating osteoporosis in postmenopausal women. Cochrane Database Syst Rev. 2004;(2):CD000333.
20. McCarthy CJ, Oldham JA. The effectiveness of exercise in the treatment of osteoarthritic knees: a critical review. Physical Therapy Reviews 1999, 4(4), 241–250.
21. The Database of Abstracts of Reviews of Effectiveness (University of York), Database no.: DARE-20005145. In: The Cochrane Library, Issue 3, 2002. Oxford: Update Software.
22. Petrella RJ. Is exercise effective treatment for osteoarthritis of the knee? British Journal of Sports Medicine 2000, 34(5), 326–331.

23. The Database of Abstracts of Reviews of Effectiveness (University of York), Database no.: DARE-20002058. In: The Cochrane Library, Issue 2, 2002. Oxford: Update Software.
24. Van den Ende CMH, Vliet Vlieland TPM, Munneke M, Hazes JMW. Dynamic exercise therapy for rheumatoid arthritis (Cochrane Review). CD-Rom: The Cochrane Library, Issue 2, 2001. Oxford: Update Software.
25. Tulder MW van, Malmivaara A, Esmail R, Koes BW. Exercise therapy for low back pain (Cochrane review). CD Rom: The Cochrane Library, Issue 1, 2001. Oxford: Update Software.
26. Ram FSF, Robinson SM, Black PN. Physical training for asthma (Cochrane Review). In: The Cochrane Library, Issue 2, 2001. Oxford: Update Software.
27. Ethier JL, Salazar W, Landers DM, Petruzzello SJ, Han M, Nowell P. The influence of physical fitness and exercise upon cognitive functioning: a meta-analysis. Journal of Sport and Exercise Psychology 1997;19:249–77.
28. The Database of Abstracts of Reviews of Effectiveness (University of York), Database no.: DARE-988818. In: The Cochrane Library, Issue 1, 2001. Oxford: Update Software.
29. Ussher MH, West R, Taylor AH, McEwen A. Exercise interventions for smoking cessation (Cochrane Review). In: The Cochrane Library, Issue 1, 2001. Oxford: Update Software.
30. Marcus BH, Albrecht AE, King TE, Parisi AF, Pinto BM, Roberts M, ym. The efficacy of exercise as an aid for smoking cessation in women. A randomized controlled trial. Arch Intern Med 1999;159:1229–34.
31. Eakin EG, Glasgow RE, Riley KM. Review of primary care-based physical activity intervention studies: effectiveness and implications for practice and future research. J Family Pract 2000;49:158–68.
32. Hillsdon M, Thorogood M. A systematic review of physical activity promotion strategies. Br J Sports Med 1996;30:84–9.

19.2 Contraindications to physical exercise

Jouko Karjalainen

- Acute infection causing systemic symptoms
- Active myocarditis (4.82)
- Sustained ventricular tachycardia
- Refractory supraventricular tachyarrhythmia
- Decompensated heart failure or pathological cardiac dilatation
- Ischaemic heart disease (without permission from a specialized physician)
- Severe hypertension
- Cardiomyopathy
- Moderate or severe aortic valve stenosis (4.11)
- Conduction abnormalities
- Congenital long QT syndrome (4.1)
- Severe respiratory failure
- Pulmonary hypertension
- Deep venous thrombosis
- Recent embolism
- Dissecting aneurysm, annuloaortic ectasia, aortic root dilation in Marfan's syndrome
- Uncontrolled metabolic disorder (diabetes, thyrotoxicosis, hypothyroidism)

19.4 Diving medicine and hyperbaric oxygen therapy

Erik Eklund

ORT

Aims

- Identification of health risks associated with diving when assessing the fitness to dive
- Sufficient knowledge and readiness to treat diving-related medical conditions
- Persons with decompression sickness must be referred immediately to hyperbaric therapy.

Diving hazards

- Attacks of disease (somatic or psychiatric)
- Risk of misjudgment
  - Lack of knowledge
  - Panic reaction
  - Carelessness, negligence
- Equipment failure
- Risks of diving and their prevention, see Table 19.4.1.

Health check for divers

- Divers are usually required to bring along to the consultation a medical examination form approved by a national diving association or an internationally valid form where the obstacles to diving are noted.
- Professional and leisure divers have differing requirements for health check.
- Refer to a specialist in diving medicine all those requiring special consideration, see Table 19.4.2.
- Diver's medical examinations are recommended routinely for healthy persons
  - before diving is begun
  - every 5th year up to age of 40
  - every 3rd year up to age of 50
  - annually after age of 50.

Table 19.4.1 Risks of diving and their prevention

Risks	Causes	Prevention/treatment
Drowning	♦ Equipment failure ♦ Breathing gas runs out (mainly OC apparatus*) ♦ Breathing mixture unsuitable (mainly CC, SCC, ACOC apparatuses*) ♦ Unconsciousness ♦ Panic reaction	♦ Maintenance of equipment ♦ Diving plan, attention to diving time/depth ♦ Careful medical examination, observance ♦ Training, preventive medical examination
Barotrauma	♦ Deficient pressure balancing ♦ Panic reaction ♦ Pneumothorax ♦ Tension pneumothorax	♦ Knowledge ♦ Training, preventive medical examination ♦ Preventive medical examination ♦ Thoracocentesis at ambient pressure
Decompression sickness	♦ Decompression too rapid	♦ Adherence to diving table ♦ Hyperbaric chamber
Impossibility to get back	♦ Tension pneumothorax ♦ Entrapment ♦ Strong sea currents	♦ Thoracocentesis at ambient pressure ♦ Knowledge + equipment to secure breathing air* ♦ Observance
Injury	♦ Predatory or poisonous animals ♦ Waves, surges	♦ Knowledge, anticipation, observance
Hypothermia	♦ Diving without sufficient thermal protection, leading to hypothermia with impairment of reactions and judgement	♦ Appropriate equipment

*Different types of breathing apparatuses

- OC Open circuit with no rebreathing. Breathing mixture is discharged after inhalation.
- SCC: Semiclosed circuit with partial rebreathing. CO_2 is absorbed and used oxygen is replaced by an oxygen/inert gas mixture which guarantees a suitable oxygen partial pressure for the depth in question.
- CC: Closed circuit. Breathing mixture is rebreathed. CO_2 is absorbed and used oxygen is replaced by pure oxygen.
- ACOC: Alternating closed and open circuit. Breathing mixture is rebreathed until the oxygen partial pressure is above or near normal level and then discharged, and a new cycle starts with an inhalation of fresh mixture.

Barotraumas (damage caused by pressure changes)

- ♦ Water and tissues are practically not compressible contrary to a gas or a gaseous mixture: e.g. a air, however, is compressible. Volume of 10 litres (1 ata, depth 0 metres) becomes 5 litres at the depth of 10 metres, and only 1 litre at the depth of 90 metres. On descending, a failure in pressure adjustment may cause the following traumas:
  - Perforation of the tympanic membranes
  - Transudation or haemorrhage into the sinuses
- ♦ On ascending, the air volume increases respectively, causing symptoms and mechanical damage in air-filled body cavities.
  - Lungs: scars and emphysematous bullae can break and cause pneumothorax, leading to a worsening tension pneumothorax when the diver is ascending, which may require prompt thoracocentesis at actual depth.
  - Intestinal gases: hernias, gastrointestinal surgery

Decompression sickness

- ♦ When diving, inert gases (nitrogen, helium) in the breathing air are dissolved into tissue fluids as the surrounding pressure increases. If the ascent is rapid, the inert gas is not eliminated in time and its partial pressure takes up an increasing part of the available total pressure, affecting diffusive oxygen supply to tissues negatively.
- ♦ When the ambient external pressure decreases to less than the combined total pressure of the dissolved gas mixture (nitrogen, oxygen, carbon dioxide and water vapour) in the blood and extracellular and intracellular fluids, the excess gas is liberated as bubbles. These cause adverse haemodynamic effects, such as circulation obstruction by gas and fat emboli, activation of the coagulation system and diminished dissociative oxygen transport in the peripheral tissues. The elimination of nitrogen is a slow process, while a discrepancy between incoming and used oxygen in a short time leads to peripheral hypoxia.
- ♦ As a result of panic reaction, the diver may ascend too rapidly and predispose himself to both barotraumas and decompression sickness.

Symptoms

- ♦ Itching, pricking, spotty skin
- ♦ Unusually strong fatigue
- ♦ Arthralgia, particularly in large joints
- ♦ Dyspnoea
- ♦ CNS symptoms (paralysis, loss of sensation, disturbance of balance)

Table 19.4.2 Medical examination for divers

Diver's health check	Strong contraindications to diving	Possible obstacles, refer to a specialist in diving medicine	Other matters to consider
General condition		• Obesity, BMI > 30. Diving is possible when diving time and depth is restricted, e.g. diving to 8–10 metres (or deeper if nitrox breathing mixture is used)	• Diving is not recommended during pregnancy
Ear, nose, throat status	• Perforated tympanic membrane • Permanent disturbance of the vestibular organ • Ménière's disease	• Healed perforation of the tympanic membrane • Unilaterally congested nasal meatus • Deafness	• Perform the Valsalva test • Ears canals are cleaned thoroughly for full inspection
Visual acuity		• Impaired vision	
Mouth	• Loose denture (does not prevent diving if temporarily removed) • Cleft palate		• Poorly cleaned and cared teeth, air in fillings may cause pain when diving
Respiratory system	• Earlier spontaneous pneumothorax • Emphysema (grave or of bullous type) • Asthma (grave or poorly controlled)	• Tuberculosis scars • Symptomatic asthma • Chronic bronchitis • Other pulmonary failure • Sequela of pulmonary surgery	• Chest x-ray from all new divers. Flow-volume spirometry from those with pulmonary symptoms.
Circulatory system	• Coronary artery disease • Aortic valvular defects • Serious arrhythmias • Untreated hypertension and its complications	• Asymptomatic heart defects • Hypertension patients with good treatment balance. • Persons with pacemaker	• ECG from all new divers • Exercise ECG from over 40-year-old new divers
Haematological diseases	• Haemophilia • Polycythaemia	• Earlier severe haematological disease (e.g. leukaemia)	
GI/Kidneys and the urinary tracts	• Remarkable proteinuria, with unknown aetiology	• Peptic ulcer • Hernias	• Urine albumine
Nervous system; psyche	• Epilepsy • Serious head trauma within 3 months • Symptomatic psychiatric disorder • Emotional or cognitive immaturity • Learning difficulties that prevent understanding the theory of diving	• MS disease • History of convulsions • Suspicion of a mental health disturbance	
Endocrinological diseases	• Grave unstable diabetes mellitus, or severe diabetic complications	• All diabetics are referred to a specialist in diving medicine	• Urine glucose • Diabetics with a good treatment balance may be able to dive. Check ups at least annually, if not more often.
Drugs, narcotics	• Any severe illness requiring medication is considered a contraindication for diving without prior consultation with a specialist. • Addiction		• The diver should refrain from taking medications (e.g., antihistamines, analgesics) and from smoking or using alcohol or drugs immediately before diving.
Earlier case of decompression sickness		• Refer all to a specialist in diving medicine!	
Traumas	• Traumas that hamper swimming	• Arthritis, arthrodesis or amputation that does not prevent swimming	

ORT

- Symptoms may appear several hours after diving.
- The consequences of untreated decompression may include CNS damage and aseptic osteonecrosis, particularly on joint surfaces.

Prevention

- The divers should adhere to the ascending schedule, i.e. allow dissolved nitrogen to be eliminated by stopping at predetermined depths for a precalculated time.

Treatment

- Decompression sickness is managed with hyperbaric therapy, which diminishes bubble size (embolic effect is reduced) and increases the available partial pressure needed to supply oxygen to the tissues.
- Hyperbaric oxygen therapy is used to treat tissue hypoxia and to widen the "nitrogen window", which accelerates the elimination of nitrogen from tissues.
- Ample fluid therapy improves circulation and dilutes the partial pressure of the inert gas.
- Symptoms usually dissolve already within 20 minutes from the onset of therapy.

Hyperbaric oxygen therapy

- Mainly used to treat decompression sickness
- Scientific evidence on the effectiveness of hyperbaric oxygen therapy in the treatment of decompression sickness and gas embolism is available C [1 2 3 4 5 6 7 8 9].
- The treatment has also been used for acute acoustic trauma, severe carbon monoxide poisonings, osteoradionecrosis and osteomyelitis as well as to reduce sudden oedema of the brain and/or medulla resulting from severe contusion.
- A patient with disturbances of vital functions must be transferred to the managing unit as quickly as possible (with an ambulance, low-flying helicopter).

References

1. Medical Services Advisory Committee. Hyperbaric oxygen therapy. Canberra: Medical Services Advisory Committee (MSAC). 2001. 131. Medical Services Advisory Committee (MSAC). www.msac.gov.au.
2. Hailey D. Hyperbaric oxygen therapy - recent findings on evidence for its effectiveness. Update. Edmonton: Alberta Heritage Foundation for Medical Research (AHFMR). 2003. 25. Alberta Heritage Foundation for Medical Research (AHFMR). www.ahfmr.ab.ca.
3. McDonagh M, Carson S, Ash J. Hyperbaric oxygen therapy for brain injury, cerebral palsy, and stroke. Rockville: Agency for Healthcare Research and Quality (AHRQ). 2003. Agency for Healthcare Research and Quality (AHRQ). www.ahrq.gov.
4. Saunders P. Hyperbaric oxygen therapy in the management of carbon monoxide poisoning, osteoradionecrosis, burns, skin grafts and crush injury. Birmingham: West Midlands Health Technology Assessment Collaboration, University of Birmingham (Collaborative effort with Wessex Institute). 2000. 52. West Midlands Health Technology Assessment Collaboration (WMHTAC).
5. Health Technology Assessment Database: HTA-20020065. The Cochrane Library, Issue 1, 2004. Chichester, UK: John Wiley & Sons, Ltd.
6. Health Technology Assessment Database: HTA-20030475. The Cochrane Library, Issue 1, 2004. Chichester, UK: John Wiley & Sons, Ltd.
7. Health Technology Assessment Database: HTA-20031127. The Cochrane Library, Issue 1, 2004. Chichester, UK: John Wiley & Sons, Ltd.
8. Health Technology Assessment Database: HTA-20000924. The Cochrane Library, Issue 1, 2004. Chichester, UK: John Wiley & Sons, Ltd.
9. Juurlink DN, Stanbrook MB, McGuigan MA. Hyperbaric oxygen for carbon monoxide poisoning. Cochrane Database Syst Rev. 2004;(2):CD002041.

19.10 ECG in athletes

Editors

Typical abnormalities

- Sinus bradycardia as low as 30/min. A junctional rhythm that disappears during exercise may be observed.
- Prolonged PQ interval is common. Second-degree atrioventricular block that disappears during exercise may sometimes be observed.
- Voltage criteria for ventricular hypertrophy are often filled, particularly left, but also right ventricular hypertrophy. A narrow Q wave may be observed.
- Early repolarization is very common. It can be observed in leads V2–V4 as an elevation of 2 mm or more of the ST segment. The T wave is usually tall but its tail may be negative. The changes are corrected by exercise.
- A picture resembling partial right bundle-branch block (RBBB) is common.

Differential diagnosis

- The above-mentioned ECG changes may be difficult to differentiate from those caused by myocarditis, atrial septal defect, acute myocardial infarction, or hypertrophic cardiomyopathy.
- The diagnosis is easier if an earlier ECG is available for comparison.

19.11 Doping in sports

Markku Alén

National Antidoping Committees

- The National Antidoping Committees are responsible for doping control of athletes who participate in organized sports, especially in Olympic events. They continually update doping regulations that are based on the Anti-Doping Convention enacted by World Antidoping Agency (WADA) in co-operation with the International Olympic Committee (IOC) and various sports organizations.
- See internet: http://www.wada-ama.org

What is doping?

- Doping includes, for instance, the use of stimulants, beta2-agonists, euphorigenic analgesics, peptide hormones (e.g. growth hormone) or corresponding substance, erythropoietin, natural androgenic and anabolic hormones, their precursor steroids and synthetic derivatives, aromatase inhibitors, diuretics or blood transfusions or plasma expanders for the improvement of performance in sports.
- The manipulation of urine excretion, e.g. by means of probenecid or diuretics, or the physical manipulation of urine (e.g. exchange of urine) are also prohibited.
- The WADA list of doping agents mentions examples of the commonest prohibited active substances. In addition, it is stated that compounds related to those listed are also prohibited.
- The WADA lists of doping agents have been adopted as such into the rules of most sports organizations. Nevertheless, some international sports federations (for instance billiard, shooting, motorsports, modern pentathlon and soccer) have special provisions concerning the use of alcohol and beta-blockers. Therefore, physicians working for sports teams and organizations should also acquaint themselves with the rules applying to their specific sports event.
- Furthermore, restrictions have been placed on the use of local anaesthetics, corticosteroids, cannabis and certain antiasthmatic medications. For example, inhaled preparations containing formoterol, salbutamol, salmeterol and terbutaline may be used for asthma whereas other pharmaceutical forms and routes of administration of these substances are prohibited. However, the athlete must apply for an exemption from a specialist confirming a respiratory disease and its treatment.

Prescribing medicines to athletes

- To avoid mistakes, it would be safest for the athlete to use only medicines prescribed by a physician.
- Unscheduled (random) testing during the training season is primarily designed to detect the misuse of anabolic steroids and peptide hormones. During the training season the common cold and other upper respiratory diseases of athletes can, therefore, be treated according to the same principles as those of ordinary citizens (but this is not recommended because of the long elimination time after the use of some common preparations).
- Whenever a physician has to treat an athlete's illness by prescribing him/her a preparation containing prohibited stimulants or euphorigenic analgesics, the physician is at the same time obliged to forbid the athlete to compete until the drug and its metabolites have been totally cleared from the body and urine. The clearance time depends on the dose and substance used. For some preparates it may take only 4 days (e.g. ephedrine) and for some other even 7 days (e.g. selegiline).
- Even a healthy athlete undergoing doping tests is required to report all drugs (e.g. painkillers, antiallergic drugs, oral contraceptives, drugs for common cold) he/she has used during the past month.

Doping control

- Doping control concerns athletes who participate in organized sports, especially in Olympic events. If an athlete's urine test is positive, in other words, a prohibited substance is detected in the urine of the person tested, an expert group appointed by the Antidoping Committee will investigate whether doping has taken place.
- Apart from deliberate engagement in doping, a positive result on doping testing may be due to the use of a "wrong medicine" to treat an illness. Thus, an athlete should make every effort not to compete during an illness or when recuperating.
- An athlete who has used drugs for the purpose of improving his/her performance is guilty of doping irrespective of whether he/she was healthy or ill at the time. Refusal to have a doping test is also interpreted as doping.
- An athlete who has been found guilty of doping is punished in accordance with the rules of the international sports federation concerned.
- A physician, a trainer or a member of service personnel, who has been involved in doping can also be punished by excluding him/her from all sporting events for a defined time. This applies also to persons involved in smuggling, dealing and distribution of doping substances.

Physical Medicine and Orthopaedics

Evidence Based Medicine Guidelines. Edited by the Duodecim Editorial Team
 ISBN: 0-470-01184-X

20.1 Neck and shoulder pain

Eira Viikari-Juntura

Basic rules

- When treating neck and shoulder complaints, it may be difficult to arrive at a precise anatomical diagnosis.
- Based on history and clinical examination, neck injuries caused by trauma should be differentiated from neck pain associated with more serious illnesses. Nerve root compression and myelopathy should also be considered.
- Acute neck pain usually has a good prognosis and recovers spontaneously. Any factors which may aggravate the condition should be identified and alleviated.
- If the patient presents with localized non-specific neck pain it is safe to advise the continuation of normal activities within the limits set by the pain.
- In the treatment of chronic localized neck pain, active therapeutic exercise which improves muscular strength and endurance may be beneficial.

Incidence

- Neck pain is a common symptom. Two out of three people experience neck pain at some time in their life. Neck complaints constitute 3–4% of all visits to a general practitioner.
- Among the working age population, neck and shoulder complaints are a significant cause of incapacity to work.
- Many jobs involve a reduced need for muscular strength, while static work and psychosocial stresses have increased. The increased incidence of neck and shoulder complaints may be attributable to these changes.

Classification of neck pain

- Neck pain can be classified as follows:
  - Localized neck and shoulder pain
  - Radiating neck pain
  - Whiplash injury – related neck pain
  - Myelopathy (cord compression)
  - Other neck pain: pain associated with systemic illness and tumours, sequela of cervical spine fracture
- Depending on the symptom duration the first three groups may be further classified as being either acute (duration less than 12 weeks) or chronic (duration more than 12 weeks).

Examination of a patient with neck and shoulder pain

History

- Ask the patient about the incidents relating to symptom onset as well as about relevant background information, i.e.
  - injury or trauma
  - physical loads at work and leisure time
  - underlying illnesses (inflammatory rheumatic diseases, infections, tumours)
  - past treatment or procedures around the neck area
  - previous sick leave.
- Neck and shoulder symptoms
  - Where is the pain located (appropriate pain drawing may be useful)?
  - Does the pain or numbness radiate below the elbows or to the fingers?
  - How severe is the pain (on the scale from 0 to 10)?
  - Is the pain continuous?
  - Does anything aggravate the pain, for example head movements or coughing?
  - How much disability does the pain cause (special tools, or scale from 0 to 10)?
  - Are there sensory changes in the upper extremities?
  - Any muscle weakness?
  - Any problems with the lower extremities? Problems with walking and spasticity in myelopathy.
  - Any problems with the bladder or bowel? Reduced bladder control or incontinence are rare signs of advanced myelopathy.
  - Dizziness, tinnitus, headache, dysphagia and memory disturbances are suggestive of whiplash injury.
- Generalized signs and symptoms suggestive of a serious illness:
  - Malaise
  - Weight loss
  - Tiredness
  - Fever

Status

- Visual inspection (note atrophies, painful scoliosis, acute torticollis, dystonias, e.g. spasmodic torticollis)
- Mobility (restriction in movement and side-to-side differences, particularly in lateral flexion and rotation)
- Sensitivity especially to pain and touch (and vibration sense in suspected myeolopathy)
- Reflexes (biceps, brachioradialis, triceps and Babinski in suspected myeolopathy)
- Muscular strength
- Provocation and relief tests for radicular symptoms (neck compression test, axial manual traction, shoulder abduction)
- Muscle tenderness and tightness (reproducibility of palpation findings is poor as regards muscle tenderness and tightness. On the other hand, palpation may reveal unexpected findings, such as tumour or abscess).

Diagnostic tests

- There is no evidence to support the benefit of routine x-ray of the cervical spine, except in acute injury.
- X-rays are recommended if the history or findings are suggestive of a serious illness.

- If the neck pain persists for over three months, plain x-rays of the cervical spine are warranted. If the pain reoccurs at a later stage, new x-rays are not recommended, unless there are signs of severe illness.
- A specialist should be consulted if there is a need for imaging other than plain x-rays.
- ENMG studies (electroneuromyography, clinical neurophysiology) may be undertaken to demonstrate, or exclude, a lesion of neural origin.

Differential diagnosis

- Peripheral nerve entrapment of an upper extremity, see 20.20 (particularly carpal tunnel syndrome, see 20.61)
- Pain syndromes in the shoulder joint and rotator cuff
  - Rotator cuff tendinitis
  - Frozen shoulder
  - Reflex sympathetic dystrophy (the current official name is complex regional pain syndrome, CRPS)
- Angina pectoris, myocardial infarction
  - should be taken into consideration if the patient falls into a risk group and complains of pain radiating to the upper extremity on exertion.
- Others
  - Diaphragmatic irritation, e.g. biliary pain

When should a serious illness be suspected as the cause of neck pain?

- Unrelenting pain, which usually is unrelated to exercise, is suggestive of a serious illness as the cause of neck pain. The pain is often worse at rest and disturbs sleep.
- Systemic causes of neck pain are:
  - inflammatory joint disease, e.g. rheumatic arthritis, ankylosing spondylitis
  - primary malignancy or metastasis
  - inflammation (osteomyelitis, tuberculosis, sepsis).

Localized neck and shoulder pain

- Tension headache caused by tensed neck muscles, see 36.66.
- Neck pain that has persisted for less than 6 weeks is treated according to the history and clinical examination. There is no need to carry out laboratory tests or imaging, unless the history or findings give a reason to suspect a serious illness or an illness calling for specific treatment.
- Any aggravating factors at work, or during leisure time, should be addressed as early as possible. Such factors include any positions with sustained neck flexion, extension or rotation as well as working for long times with hands overhead and static postures.
- The importance of maintaining normal activity should be emphasized to the patient.
- **Analgesia**
  - Analgesics may be prescribed for a short time if pain relief can contribute towards maintaining physical activity.
  - Paracetamol is the drug of choice in milder neck pain. If the pain is more severe, a safe non-steroidal anti-inflammatory drug should be prescribed. If the pain is not managed with a non-steroidal anti-inflammatory drug alone, a mild to moderately potent opioid analgesic, such as codeine or tramadol, may be added to the treatment.
- **Skeletal muscle relaxants**
  - A skeletal muscle relaxant may be an alternative if non-steroidal anti-inflammatory drugs are unsuitable.
  - Nearly one-third of patients experience fatigue or vertigo as an adverse effect.
  - A combination of skeletal muscle relaxants and non-steroidal anti-inflammatory drugs is not recommended.
- **Physical activity and exercise therapy**
  - Light physical activity, such as walking, to maintain physical fitness is recommended.
  - Active exercise therapy to improve muscular strength and endurance may be beneficial in chronic localized neck pain C [1].
  - There is some evidence to support the beneficial effects of mobilization therapy in prolonged neck pain. Mobilization refers to the improvement of cervical spine mobility with the aid of exercises performed by the patient or techniques carried out by a therapist.
  - No evidence has been established on the efficacy of manipulation in the treatment of neck pain. Manipulation consists of a procedure of a few seconds duration with the aim to loosen a locked motion segment. The manipulation of the cervical spine is associated with a risk of serious complications, particularly when rotation techniques are employed.
- **Physical medicine**
  - Evidence on the efficacy of physical treatment modalities is inadequate B [2 3 4 5]. Evidence on the efficacy of massage as well as applying heat, cold or traction D [6 7] is insufficient.
  - Based on up to date study results acupuncture and laser treatments have no effect on neck pain.
- **Cervical collar**
  - There is no evidence that use of a cervical collar is beneficial in the treatment of neck pain.

A patient with radiating pain

- The majority of patients may be managed conservatively.
- A disc prolapse must be diagnosed (20.30). Typical signs and symptoms include neck pain of sudden onset which radiates to the fingers, or numbness of the fingers.
- A full neurological examination of the upper extremities should be carried out in the acute phase if the neck pain radiates. Subsequently the patient is frequently checked for sensory or reflex changes as well as for changes in muscle strength.
- The patient must be informed about the possibility of motor symptoms in the upper extremities or myelopathic symptoms. Should these occur the patient should seek medical advice.

- If the patient presents with marked or progressing muscle weakness or with excruciating pain, a referral should be made to an appropriate specialist.

Whiplash injury

Acute whiplash injury

- Whiplash injury is typically sustained in a car accident.
- The onset of pain ranges from a few hours to several days of the accident.
- The majority of patients recover within 3 months, but almost 10% still experience symptoms 12 months later.
- Active mobilization is the most effective treatment form in acute whiplash **C** [8, 9].
- Mobilization can be carried out as a home exercise programme.
- Cold treatment, or anti-inflammatory drugs, can be administered for pain in the acute stage.
- There is no evidence to support the use of a cervical collar.

Chronic whiplash injury

- Chronic whiplash presents a challenge since no specific treatment is available.
- There is evidence that help can be derived by adopting an active lifestyle.
- A multidisciplinary approach towards rehabilitation may alleviate pain and improve functional capacity.
- There is some evidence that radiofrequency denervation offers short-term relief for chronic cervical zygapophyseal joint pain which radiates to an upper extremity, when the pain was sustained in a car accident and confirmed by diagnostic local anaesthesia **C** [10, 11]. There is no evidence of long-term effects. Radiofrequency therapy is an invasive treatment modality which is not available freely in all countries.
- Botulinum toxin injections have also been used therapeutically, but so far evidence of their efficacy is insufficient.

References

1. Taimela S, Takala EP, Asklof T, Seppala K, Parviainen S. Active treatment of chronic neck pain: a prospective randomized intervention. Spine 2000;25:1021–7.
2. Binder A. Physical treatments in neck pain. Clinical evidence 2000;4:634–5.
3. van der Heijden GJ, Beurskens AJ, Koes BW, Assendelft WJ, de Vet HJ, Bouter LM. The efficacy of traction for back and neck pain: a systematic, blinded review of randomized clinical trial methods. Physical therapy 1995;75:93–104.
4. Kjellman GV, Skargren EI, Oberg BE. A critical analysis of randomised trials on neck pain and treatment efficacy. A review of the literature. Scand J Rehabil Med 1999;31:139–52.
5. White AR, Ernst E. A systematic review of randomized controlled trials of acupuncture for neck pain. Rheumatology (Oxford) 1999;38:143–147.
6. van der Heijden GJ, Beurskens AJ, Koes BW, Assendelft WJ, de Vet HJ, Bouter LM. The efficacy of traction for back and neck pain: a systematic, blinded review of randomized clinical trial methods. Physical therapy 1995;75:93–104.
7. The Database of Abstracts of Reviews of Effectiveness (University of York), Database no.: DARE-978020. In: The Cochrane Library, Issue 4, 1999. Oxford: Update Software.
8. Verhagen AP, Scholten-Peeters GGM, de Bie RA, Bierma-Zeinstra SMA. Conservative treatments for whiplash. Cochrane Database Syst Rev. 2004;(2):CD003338.
9. Binder A. Treatments for acute whiplash. Clinical Evidence 2000;4:636–7.
10. van Kleef M, Liem L, Lousberg R, Barendse G, Kessels F, Sluijter M. Radiofrequency lesion adjacent to the dorsal root ganglion for cervicobrachial pain: a prospective double blind randomized study. Neurosurgery 1996;38:1127–312.
11. Slappendel R, Crul BJ, Braak GJ, Geurts JW, Booij LH, Voerman VF, de Boo T. The efficacy of radiofrequency lesioning of the cervical spinal dorsal root ganglion in a double blinded randomized study: no difference between 40 degrees C and 67 degrees C treatments. Pain 1997;73:159–63.

20.2 Examination of the shoulder joint

Editors

- Examination of neck and shoulder pain, see 20.1.

A concise guide to the examination of the shoulder joint

- Inspection of the shoulder region: muscle atrophy (possible nerve or ligament injury)
- Active movements: abduction, flexion, rotations (pain, restrictions)
- "Painful arc" in 60° to 120° abduction (supraspinatus tendon, subacromial bursa)
- Passive movements if active movements are restricted or painful (possible causes: pain, adhesive capsulitis, muscular contractures, pareses)
- Resisted isometric 30° abduction (supraspinatus test)
- Resisted isometric external rotation (infraspinatus test)
- Resisted flexion of the supinated forearm (biceps test) (20.6)
- Palpation of the tendons
- Compression of the subachromial bursa
- Provocation test of the acromioclavicular joint (hyperabduction and cross arms test).

For differential diagnostic purposes

- Axial compression of the neck with the patient sitting (nerve root compression)

- Tests for "thoracic outlet syndrome" (20.60)
- Tests for epicondylitis
- Tests for carpal tunnel syndrome (20.61)
- Test for screening of neurological problems
  - Biceps, triceps (strength, reflexes)
  - Walking, Babinski

20.5 Disorders of the rotator cuff of the shoulder

Martti Vastamäki

Basic rules

- Rest, patient instruction and NSAIDs suffice for treatment in most cases of supraspinatus tendonitis.
- Prolonged cases of rotator cuff tendonitis are treated with steroid injections.
- Rupture of the rotator cuff should be identified. Major ruptures should be operated on within a few months of the trauma for a good result.

Prevalence

- The most common disorder affecting the rotator cuff of the shoulder is impingement syndrome in which the supraspinatus tendon is irritated (supraspinatus tendonitis).
- This disorder is very common in 40–50-year-olds.
- The majority of shoulder joint problems in working age persons affect the rotator cuff.
- When the shoulder becomes painful without a history of obvious trauma, the age of the patient is significant in the assessment of the disorder
  - In under 30-year-olds a chronic shoulder problem often arises from excess instability of the joint.
  - In the middle-aged, the cause is often impingement.
  - After the age of 50–55 years, the pain most often results from the rupture of the rotator cuff.

Supraspinatus tendonitis and impingement

- The most common shoulder disorder in 35–50-year-olds is supraspinatus tendonitis that is caused by irritation of the tissues of the shoulder joint, mainly the rotator cuff and the surrounding bursa.
- The tissues become inflammated and swollen and as a consequence the possibly already impinged joint becomes even more compressed and there is little space for the soft tissues between the bones and the ligaments, particularly when the arm is abducted.
- Abduction of the arm becomes difficult and night-time ache is disturbing.
- Supraspinatus tendonitis worsens with strain and a vicious circle may ensue with no response to any mode of therapy.

Treatment

- Initial management consists of rest and NSAID medication C [1 2 3].
- Cryotherapy is also often helpful, whereas warmth irritates, particularly in the early stages, as does exercise therapy. Therefore physiotherapy often aggravates the pain in the shoulder.
- In mild cases it is often sufficient that the patient is informed of the origin of the disorder. It is worthwhile to explain the mechanism with the help of an anatomic model and show how lifting the arm causes the irritated supraspinatus tendon to squeeze against the edge of the acromion.
- The patient is instructed to avoid pain-causing movements and is told that the condition usually resolves spontaneously within a few weeks or months.
- A corticosteroid-anaesthetic injection to the painful site under the acromion 1–3 times may give considerable relief C [1 2 3]. The pain may necessitate a long sick leave, particularly if the work requires holding the arms up.
- If no response is obtained within 6–12 months, surgery should be considered in the most severe cases.
- In prolonged conditions active movement C [4], e.g. swimming preferably crawl style, may also be beneficial.

Aetiology

- Supraspinatus tendonitis is a common strain disorder. Temporary strain, for example, thorough cleaning can cause a long-lasting pain in persons who do not normally strain their shoulders.
- The problem may also result from repeated, work-related strain.
- The cause of a chronic rupture is in many cases vascular insufficiency in the tendon and impingement of the tendon between the head of the humerus and the acromion and the coracoacromial ligament.
- For examination of the shoulder joint, see 20.2.

Injection technique in supraspinatus tendonitis

- For an injection use 1 ml of long-acting corticosteroid and 4 ml of local anaesthetic.
- The site of injection is in the middle of the lateral edge of the acromion. The posterior lateral border of the acromion is easily palpated and serves as a landmark for the injection site which is a couple of cm anteriorily. A thin 7–8 cm needle is most suitable. It is directed tangentially of the lower surface of the acromion to the subacromial bursa and to the insertion of the rotator cuff at tuberculum majus. This area is infiltrated largely, but do not aim to inject intra-articularly as the disorder affects extra-articular tissues. Mark the injection site by pressing with your nail and wash the skin well.

- A couple of minutes after the injection the patient may notice that abducting the arm is easier. Inform the patient the effect of the local anaesthetic lasts only for a couple of hours and that the effect of corticosteroid, if any, begins only after a few days.
- If necessary, the injection can be repeated after 2–4 weeks.

Calcifying tendonitis

- Sometimes the impingement involves calcium deposition in the tendon, and the disorder is called calcifying tendonitis.
- The calcium is usually deposited on the rotator cuff tendons, usually the supraspinatus tendon as a result of the function of specific cells. This accumulation of calcium is not a degenerative process as such. In the accumulation phase the calcium is hard and clearly visible on the x-ray. After months or a few years it becomes softer and is seen as a diffuse formation on the x-ray, whereafter it is resorbed spontaneously.
- Symptoms of calcifying tendonitis resemble those of impingement. In the resorption phase pain can be considerable. Puncture of the calcified area and suction of the calcium deposits through a thick needle may be indicated.
- A local cortisone injection is also helpful. If calcium is erupted suddenly in a joint or bursa, a severe pain called calcium arthritis or bursitis lasting for 2–3 days develops.
- The patient holds the affected arm tightly against the trunk and needs high doses of analgesics.
- Cryotherapy with an ice pack or a gel pack help best in acute calcifying tendonitis.
- Calcifying tendonitis is usually not treated surgically, unless there are other indications for an operation than removal of calcium deposits.

Acromioplasty

- May be considered for impingement if the symptoms have lasted for more than 6 months, conservative treatment is not effective and the patient is unable to work.
- If working ability is preserved, it is worthwhile to follow up the condition for up to a year, as the disorder has a high tendency for spontaneous recovery.
- In acromioplasty more space is created in the shoulder joint by removing bone and soft tissue.
- May be performed as open surgery or arthroscopically.
- After the procedure the arm is immobilized with an arm-to-chest bandage for one week.
- Pendulum exercises are begun on the first post-operative day, passive lifting of the arm to the front and side is begun after 1–2 weeks, and active exercises after 2–3 weeks.

Rupture of the rotator cuff

- Usually the sequel of a trauma: falling on the shoulder or outstretched hand.
- In over 45-year-olds shoulder dislocation often involves also rupture of the rotator cuff.
- The rupture is almost invariably in the area of the supraspinatus tendon and extends posteriorily to the area of the m. infraspinatus and, more rarely, anteriorily to the area of the subscapularis, or both directions.

Symptoms

- Symptoms include pain and restriction of movement and strength of the upper extremity. Abduction of the arm and external rotation lack strength.
- In a typical trauma-induced rupture of the rotator cuff the patient has experienced sudden pain and may have heard a cracking sound when falling, lifting a heavy load or receiving an impact on the shoulder region.
- The movements of the upper arm become restricted and lifting the arm above the shoulder level becomes impossible. The patient may continue work, but within 24 hours the pain becomes so intense that the patient seeks care.
- Night-time ache is disturbing. Light movement of the joint may alleviate pain.
- Pain may radiate as far as the fingertips and up towards the neck.

Diagnosis

- The active range of motion of the shoulder is found restricted on clinical examination. Often the patient is unable the raise the arm beyond the shoulder level, whereas the passive range of motion is usually normal.
- The patient tries to avoid this painful movement by lifting the arm with the help of the scapular movement and thus to avoid using the shoulder joint, i.e. the scapulohumeral rhythm is disturbed.
- Sometimes the range of motion of the joint may be normal, and the rupture is small, nevertheless painful.
- Measure the strength of the upper arm and compare it with the healthy arm; a rupture always causes weakness.
- Before surgery a rupture should always be verified with arthrography or echography.
- MRI can also be used, but it is a considerably more expensive investigation.

Treatment

- Initially conservative therapy, which is often sufficient in small tears.
- The most important treatment forms include physiotherapy for reducing pain and swelling, exercise, and corticosteroid injections.
- If pain, movement restriction and weakness still cause marked disability after 1–2 months of conservative therapy, surgery should be considered.
- A delay of 6 months leads to a poorer result.
- After surgery the patient wears an abduction splint, which is used to prevent the stretching of the corrected rotator cuff and re-rupture during immobilization.
- The patient should start passive mobilization at home 2–4 weeks from surgery while still wearing the splint.
- Mobilization is started after 4–6 weeks of immobilization at first by lifting the arm from a pillow.
- Final result is usually obtained 6 months from surgery.
- Surgery results in a completely healthy, painless, unrestricted normal-strength shoulder joint in only some patients.

Criteria for surgery

- Patients under 50 years of age
  - Sufficiently severe trauma, severe restriction, below the shoulder level, obvious weakness; operation as soon as possible, preferably within one month.
- 50–60-year-olds
  - First physiotherapy, analgesics, corticosteroid injection, rest if necessary, depending on the occupation; if the symptoms continue to be severe after 2–3 months, operation.
  - Sufficiently severe trauma, restricted movement and strength, pain, no signs of recovery after 1–2 months, operate after this follow up time.
- Over 60-year-olds
  - Impaired strength and range of motion, conservative treatment not helpful after 3–4 months.
  - Severe pain, no response to conservative therapy, operation after 6 months even if the range of motion and strength are good; the cause is usually a small and easily restored rupture.
- Over 70-year-olds
  - Operate only if the patient is active, the trauma is sufficiently severe and the patient does not have spinatus atrophy, or if the pain is severe and does not resolve with conservative therapy, strength and movements are poor and spinatus atrophy is severe; palliative surgery is also possible.

References

1. Green S, Buchbinder R, Glazier R, Forbes A. Interventions for shoulder pain. Cochrane Database Syst Rev. 2004;(2): CD001156.
2. Van der Heijden G, Van der Windt D, Kleijnen J, Koes B, Bouter L. Steroid injections for shoulder disorders: a systematic review of randomised clinical trials. Br J Gen Pract 1996;46:309–316.
3. The Database of Abstracts of Reviews of Effectiveness (University of York), Database no.: DARE-968205. In: The Cochrane Library, Issue 4, 1999. Oxford: Update Software.
4. Green S, Buchbinder R, Hetrick S. Physiotherapy interventions for shoulder pain. Cochrane Database Syst Rev 2003(1):CD004258.

20.6 Biceps muscle tendinitis and rupture

Editors

Symptoms

- Pain on the anterior aspect of the shoulder that is exaggerated by exercise.

Diagnosis

- Not very common as a single cause of shoulder pain.
- Tenderness on palpation of the biceps tendon at the sulcus in the anterior aspect of the humeral head.
- Resisted flexion of the elbow and resisted supination of the lower arm cause pain (the test is performed by fixing the upper arm against the patient's side with the elbow flexed 90 degrees and asking the patient to try to rotate the lower arm in both directions. Resist the rotation by a hand-in-hand grip as if shaking hands).
- Fluid around the biceps tendon can be detected easily by ultrasonography. In addition to biceps tendinitis, fluid in the tendon sheath may be present in a rupture of the rotator cuff. The diagnosis of biceps tendinitis is always clinical, not based on ultrasonography.
- If the tendon ruptures a part of the muscle protrudes to the lower end of the biceps. However, the flexion strength of the elbow joint remains intact.

Treatment

- Reduce physical strain.
- Inject a mixture of corticosteroid (e.g. methylprednisolone in depot form) and local anaesthetic near the tendon. Do not inject against a resistance.
- Results of operative treatment are poor.
- Prolonged treatment is often necessary.
- Muscle strength can be increased by physiotherapy.
- A tendon rupture is often left untreated as the limitations caused by it are minor. In special cases it may be corrected.

20.9 Winged scapula (Scapula alata)

Editors

Aetiology

- Paresis of the anterior serrate muscle due to lesion of the long thoracic nerve.
- The lesion can be caused by surgery (even the removal of a naevus on the neck), injury, neuritis or tumour.

Diagnosis

- Lifting the arm is not possible.
- Pushing forward with the arm causes winging of the scapula.
- Resisted flexion of the arms also causes winging.
- A chest x-ray should be taken and the chest and axillae should be palpated to find a possible nerve compressing tumour.
- The severity of a possible nerve injury is investigated by ENMG.

Treatment and prognosis

- If winging is considerable the scapula should be stabilized with a serratus support that prevents further stretching of the nerve.
- Muscle strengthening and range of motion preserving exercises
- Spontaneous recovery within a few monts up to one year.
- Even in chronic cases fixation of the scapula is rarely needed.

20.20 Tennis elbow

Olli Korkala

Basic rules

- Aim at relieving symptoms by rest and conservative treatment.
- Steroid injections are beneficial in the short term, but do not improve prognosis in the long term.

Aetiology

- Repetitive strain of the wrist and fingers that is considered to cause partial rupture or irritation of the tendon insertion.
- The patient is usually 30–40 years old.

Symptoms and signs

- The lateral (radial) epicondyle is tender on palpation, and the epicondyle is painful on strain of the extensor muscles.
- Pain at rest may occur.
- Resisted extension of the wrist starting from volar flexion causes typical pain at the lateral epicondyle. The chair-lifting test is often painful.
- In the differential diagnosis consider compression of the deep motor branch of the radial nerve (Frohse's syndrome) where the maximum tenderness is detected under the margin of the supinator muscle and where resisted supination is painful. ENMG is sometimes necessary in the differential diagnosis.
- Plain x-ray is indicated before eventual surgery to exclude a process in the bone. In prolonged symptoms a calcification may be visible at the tendon insertion.

Treatment

Acute phase

- Strain is avoided and the wrist is immobilized with an extension splint.
- A compressive (sticker) bandage on the arm near the elbow may relieve symptoms in the subacute phase (D) [1].
- Analgesics (paracetamol, NSAIDs (C) [2]) can be used in normal doses.

Prolonged symptoms

- A local corticosteroid injection is effective in prolonged symptoms (A) [3] [4] in the short term. About 90% of the cases are cured by conservative treatment.
  - Infiltrate about 0.5 ml of a depot corticosteroid suspension (e.g. methyl prednisolone) along the periost (the suspension can be diluted with 1% lidocain to obtain a total volume of 2–3 ml).
  - More than three injections are not recommended.
- Surgery may be indicated in prolonged cases if the symptom has lasted for at least six months.
- Before the decision to operate is made everything should be done to change the working conditions or eliminate irritation by sports activities.
- In practice the operation often aims at restoration of previous activity and working ability.
- The outcome of surgery is influenced by many factors. About four patients of five benefit, but symptoms that have lasted for years and treated with a number of corticosteroid injections tend to respond poorly.
- Postoperative immobilisation is usually not indicated. The sickness leave should last 2–4 weeks depending on the patient's work.

References

1. Struijs PAA, Smidt N, Arola H, Dijk van CN, Buchbinder R, Assendelft WJJ. Orthotic devices for the treatment of tennis elbow. Cochrane Database Syst Rev. 2004;(2):CD001821.
2. Green S, Buchbinder R, Barnsley L, Hall S, White M, Smidt N, Assendelft W. Non-steroidal anti-inflammatory drugs (NSAIDs) for treating lateral elbow pain in adults. Cochrane Database Syst Rev. 2004;(2):CD003686.
3. Assendelft W, Hay E, Adshead R, Bouter L. Corticosteroid injections for lateral epicondylitis: a systematic overview. Br J Gen Pract 1996;46:209–216.
4. The Database of Abstracts of Reviews of Effectiveness (University of York), Database no.: DARE-968185. In: The Cochrane Library, Issue 4, 1999. Oxford: Update Software.

20.21 Radial styloid tendovaginitis (De Quervain's disease)

Kaj Rekola

Definition and aetiology

- Constricting tendovaginitis of the common tendon sheath of the M. abductor pollicis longus and M. extensor pollicis brevis at the radial styloid process.
- The cause is mostly repetitive movements.

Symptoms

- Pain on movement of the wrist and thumb
- Gripping is painful.
- Grip is weak because of pain.

Clinical examination

- Pain provocation test. The affected tendons are stretched maximally by flexing the thumb and by deviating the wrist passively in the ulnar direction while simultaneously flexing it (Finkelstein's test). The test is positive if the typical symptoms are elicited in the styloid process region.
- Tenderness on palpation of the tendon sheath (may be fairly minor).
- At the acute phase some crepitation and oedema of the tendon sheath at the styloid process may be found.

Differential diagnosis

- Osteoarthritis of the carpometacarpal joint of the thumb.

Treatment

- Aims:
  - Treatment of tendovaginitis, prevention of adhesions and secondary prevention
- Rest (avoiding provocating activities, splint), steroid injection (if previous measures failed), ergonomics and surgery if needed (discision of the tendon sheath C [1])

Injection technique

- The affected tendons and the common tendon sheath are identified best at the radial styloid process if the patient resists abduction and extension of the thumb at the proximal phalanx of the thumb with the index finger of the other hand. A fine hypodermic needle is inserted tangentially to the tendon, slightly distally from the radial styloid process. The tip of the needle should be in the tendon sheath, not in the tendon. This can be checked by extending and abducting the thumb. If the needle follows the movement it is in the tendon.
- An injection consisting of 1 to 2 ml of 0.1 to 0.5% lidocaine with 0.5 ml of e.g. methyl prednisolone is injected into the tendon sheath. Do not inject against a resistance. A subcutaneous sausage-like bulge appears following the contours of the tendon sheath if the injection was placed correctly. The injection may be repeated, if necessary, after 4–6 weeks.

Reference

1. Harvey FJ, Harvey PM, Horsley MW. De Quervain's disease: surgical or nonsurgical treatment. J Hand Surg (|Am|). 1990 Jan;15(1):83–7.

20.22 Ganglion

Editors

Basic rules

- A ganglion is a gel-containing cystic structure attached to a joint or tendon sheath. As the amount of the gel-like contents increases the ganglion becomes painful.
- A ganglion is most often situated on the palmar side of the wrist, sometimes also on the dorsal side of the foot. Ganglions are also seen in flexor tendon sheaths in distal palm and the foot.
- The diagnosis is based on the gel-like contents at needle aspiration.

Treatment

- Treatment is necessary only if the ganglion causes pain or other inconvenience.
- Aspirate the fluid from the ganglion (viscous, glue-like, clear fluid is diagnostic).
- A corticosteroid preparation (triamcinolone, methylprednisolone in depot form) can be injected into the ganglion. An alternative method is to inject local anaesthetic and then crush the ganglion by pressuring strongly with the thumb.
- Aspiration and injection can be repeated if a symptomatic ganglion recurs.
- If repeated aspirations are unsuccessful and the ganglion causes symptoms, it can be removed surgically.
- About half of carpal ganglia resolve spontaneously, and active treatment may not improve cure rate in the long term C [1].

Reference

1. Dias J, Buch K. Palmar wrist ganglion: does intervention improve outcome? A prospective study of the natural history and patient-reported treatment outcomes. J Hand Surg [Br] 2003;28(2):172–6.

20.23 Lunatomalacia (Kienböck's disease)

Editors

Aetiology and epidemiology

- Young (20–35 years) male manual workers are most susceptible to this condition that usually occurs in the dominant hand.

ORT

- Hyperextension injuries, fractures or microfractures are probably the cause in some patients.
- A congenitally short ulna may predispose to this condition.

Symptoms

- Symptoms are periodical and often resolve over the years.
- There is pain in the wrist, occasionally also swelling dorsally. The maximal pain is felt over the lunatum.
- Dorsiflexion of the wrist is restricted and painful.
- Grip strength is decreased.

Diagnosis

- The diagnosis is based on x-rays: initially a reduction in the density of the bone is seen, later fragmentation and collapse. When initial symptoms appear, the x-rays may appear normal, but a bone scan or MRI is abnormal.

Treatment

- If symptoms are mild, avoidance of strain is recommended.
- Surgery is often needed; several methods are used but none of these is well established.

20.24 Dupuytren's contracture

Olli Korkala

Basic rules

- A newly diagnosed contracture is treated conservatively by extension exercises.
- Surgical treatment is indicated when flexion contracture is evident (the extension of MP joints is restricted by 20–30°).

Clinical picture

- The palmar aponeurosis is thickened and a progressive flexion contracture of the fingers develops.
  - The contracture typically affects the fifth and the fourth finger, less frequently the third finger, and rarely other fingers.
  - Thickening of the palmar fascia is the first clinical sign of the condition. A progressive flexion contracture develops in the course of years. Finally the finger may be contracted until it touches the palm.
  - Sometimes similar thickening is observed in the plantar fascia, usually together with Dupuytren's contracture in the hands.
- The cause is unknown. A family history is common. Diabetes predisposes to the condition.
- The condition is most common in men who have passed middle age, and it is usually bilateral.

Conservative treatment

- Active and passive extension exercises of the finger(s)

Surgical treatment

- A flexion contracture (exceeding 30° in the MP joint) is considered an indication for surgery. However, treatment is indicated only if the patient has functional impairment or is annoyed by the condition. Even the milder contracture of the PIP joint is an indication for surgery.
- The palmar fascia is excised surgically (fasciectomy, aponeurectomy). Partial excision or transsection (discision) of the aponeurosis usually results in a quick recurrence of the condition.
- Injury of a finger nerve is the most common surgical complication.
- The outcome of surgery is impaired if a contracture of the joint capsule has already developed. In severe contractures amputation of the finger may be the best option.
- Extension exercises of the fingers are important after surgery.

20.30 Low back pain

Antti Malmivaara

Basic rules

The patient expects an answer to the following questions

- What causes the back pain, and is this a serious disease?
- What is the natural course of the condition?
- What therapy would alleviate the symptoms?

For successful therapy

- Examine the patient carefully and take a good history.
- Treat pain adequately.
- Advise the patient to avoid bed rest.
- Advise to continue or resume ordinary activities as soon as possible.
- Convey the good prognosis to the patient.
- Follow the patient up and aim at restoring activity and ability to work.

Epidemiology

- Low back pain is a very common condition: nearly 80% of people experience a disabling low back pain at some point in their lives.
- Of all patients in general practice 4–6% of working age women and 5–7% of working age men present with low back pain as their main complaint.

Clinical examination

History

- Taking a history is the most important tool in the clinical examination of a back pain patient.
- Data obtained from the history can be classified as follows:
  - Earlier low back pain (onset of symptoms, visits at a doctor, earlier investigations, treatments and sick leaves)
  - Current low back pain (onset, nature and intensity of symptoms, pain radiating to the lower extremity, perceived disability in daily living, investigations, treatments and their effectiveness)
  - Other illnesses (operations, traumas, other musculoskeletal disorders, other diseases such as diabetes and arteriosclerosis in lower extremities, diseases of the urogenital system, allergies, current medication)
  - Social history (family, education, work and leisure time activities)
  - Lifestyle (physical exercise, smoking, drinking, diet)

Physical examination

- In the physical examination emphasis is placed on the assessment of signs of nerve root compression and functional status. The patient should undress to a sufficient degree. Assessment of signs of nerve root compression is indicated if the patient experiences pain radiating below the knee.

1. Inspection of the spine
   - Flattening of lordosis or scoliosis due to acute pain
2. Palpation of the vertebrae and the sciatic nerve
   - Unilateral tenderness of the buttocks and thighs is often associated with acute nerve root compression of the sciatic nerve.
3. The mobility of the lumbar spine gives an idea of the functional status of the back. Measuring mobility is useful in following up the condition.
   - **Adjusted Schober test:** The patients stands with his feet 15 cm apart. Three marks are drawn on his back: one in the midline between the spinae iliaca posterior superior, the second 10 cm above the first line and the third 5 cm below the first line, so that the latter two lines are 15 cm apart. The patient is asked to bend forward with his knees extended. The distance of the latter two lines should increase by 6–7 cm (the distance between the lines should be 21–22 cm in the flexed position).
   - **The sideways bending test**: A mark is drawn on the patient's thighs at the tips of both middle fingers when the patient is standing upright. After the patient bends maximally sideways (but not forward or backward), another line is drawn on the thigh on each side. The distance between the two lines should be about 20 cm in a symptomless person. Asymmetry is common in patients with low back pain.
   - In cases of prolonged pain, a physiotherapist's assessment of the muscular strength of the abdomen, back and lower extremities is useful.
4. Assessment of signs of nerve root compression
   - **Straight leg raising (SLR, Lasegue test)** is a rather sensitive test for verifying nerve root compression at S1 and L5 level **B** [1 2]
     - The test is positive when it causes pain radiating from the back to the lower limb. Back pain itself or tightness behind the knee are not a positive sign.
     - In nerve root compression passive dorsiflexion of the ankle increases the pain radiating to the limb.
     - Crossing pain: Intensified radiating pain when raising the contralateral limb is a specific sign of nerve root compression.
   - Muscular strength of the lower limbs
     - Extension strength of the ankle and the big toe (L5 root)
     - Walking on heels (L5 root) or on toes (S1 root)
   - Tendon reflexes
     - Patella (L4 root)
     - Achilles (S1 root)
   - Patients with lower limb symptoms are examined for sense of touch on the medial side of the knee (L4 root), medial (L5 root), dorsal (L5 root) and lateral (S1 root) sides of the foot.
   - Decreased muscle strength of both legs (paraparesis), enhanced or multiple tendon reflexes, and a positive Babinski's sign suggest a need for neurological or neurosurgical assessment. **Paraparesis is an indication for immediate referral.**
   - Rectal touch (tonus of the sphincter) and the sense of touch of the perineum should be examined when **cauda equina syndrome is suspected (immediate referral)**.
5. Other examinations according to the patient's history
   - Palpation of the arteries of lower limbs and Doppler stethoscope examination in patients over 50 years of age with intermittent claudication
   - Chest mobility and rotation and lateral movements of the spine become restricted early in the course of ankylosing spondylitis **C** [3 4].

Clinical classification

- Uncommon but serious causes of back pain should be recognized at an early stage. Also, signs of sciatic syndrome should be recognized.

ORT

- Back symptoms can be divided into three categories on the basis of the history and the findings in clinical examination:
  1. Possible serious or specific disease (tumour, infection, fracture, cauda equina syndrome, ankylosing spondylitis). Metastases can cause back pain, but also tumours of the internal organs may give referred back pain.
  2. Sciatic syndrome: Symptoms in the lower limbs suggesting nerve root dysfunction
  3. Non-specific back pain: Symptoms occurring mainly in the back without any suggestion of nerve root involvement or serious disease.
- The most common serious or specific causes for low back pain are presented in Table 20.30.1. Immediate or fast referral to a specialized unit is often warranted. Patients are explained the need for further investigations, but unnecessary guesses on the possible diseases behind the symptoms should be avoided. Normal findings in plain x-rays do not exclude a serious disease. Causal relation between x-ray findings and non-specific low back pain is weak C [5 6 7 8].

Serious or specific diseases

- Look for signs of a serious disease or conditions requiring specific treatment (see Table 20.30.1).
- Normal x-rays do not exclude the possibility of a serious disease. If there is a suspicion of a serious disease, the patient must be referred to a specialist for further examinations.

Sciatic syndrome

- The most common reason for an acute sciatic syndrome is intervertebral disc herniation. Usually the prognosis is good and surgery is not needed. About 50% of patients recover at least moderately well in 6 weeks and 90% within 90 days.

Conservative treatment

- Bed rest is not an effective treatment for intervertebral disc herniation and it should not be recommended as therapy B [9]. Severe pain may, of course, necessitate bed rest, and the psoas position often alleviates symptoms. The sciatica patient can continue his or her daily activities as far as the pain allows, avoiding positions that cause pain. NSAIDs or a combination of an NSAID and a weak opiate are recommended as analgesics. Dextropropoxyphen should be prescribed cautiously because of the potentially fatal interaction with alcohol. Buprenorphin may be considered for very severe pain.
- The is no evidence on the benefit of manipulation, stretching, or physical therapy, and they are not recommended.

Surgical treatment

- Absolute indications for surgery include cauda equina syndrome (urinary retention and anal incontinence, perineal numbness).
  - Refer immediately to a surgical unit where the patient can be operated on (as soon as possible, preferably within 6 hours from the onset of the symptoms).
  - Only about 2% of disc herniations lead to the cauda equina syndrome.
- Indications for early surgery include paresis of ankle extension or flexion and incapacitating pain
- If the patient has significant pain radiating to the lower limb and lasting for more than 6 weeks, further treatment

Table 20.30.1 The most common serious or specific causes for low back pain

Disease	Symptoms and signs, investigations
Cauda equina syndrome	Urinary retention, anal incontinence, perineal anaesthesia, sciatic symptoms. Emergency referral to a specialized unit with resources for emergency operation
Ruptured aortic aneurysm, acute aortic dissecation	Sudden, excruciating pain, age above 50 years, instable haemodynamics. Emergency referral to a specialized unit.
Malignant tumour	Age above 50 years, history of cancer, involuntary weight loss, symptoms do not decrease when lying in bed, duration of pain for over one month: Detailed clinical examination, blood count, ESR, x-rays. Referral to a specialized care unit. Paraparesis requires immediate referral.
Infectious spondylitis	Urinary tract or skin infection, immunosuppression, corticosteroid medication, abuse of intravenous drugs, AIDS. Examinations: blood count, ESR, CRP, urine specimen, radiology, Referral to a specialized unit.
Compression fracture	Age above 50 years, history of falling, peroral steroid medication: Examination: x-rays.
Spondylolisthesis	Adolescent (age (8–15 years). Examination: lateral x-ray of lumbar spine.
Spinal stenosis	Age above 50 years, neurogenic claudication. Examinations: blood count, ESR, x-ray. Further imaging (MRI or CT) in a specialized unit if necessary.
Ankylosing spondylitis	Age below 40 years at the onset of symptoms, pain is not alleviated by bed rest, morning stiffness, duration at least 3 months. Examinations: blood count, ESR, urine specimen, x-ray (including sacro-iliacal joints). Special investigations by a rheumatologist (HLA-B27, MRI of the sacro-iliacal joints, bone scanning).

options, including surgery, should be discussed with the patient B [10]. Before making the final decision to operate, a neuroradiological assessment must show that the patient has an intervertebral disc herniation at a location that matches with the symptoms B [11].

Non-specific low back pain

- Low back pain can be divided into three categories according to the duration of the disabling pain:
  - Acute low back pain (duration less than 6 weeks)
  - Subacute low back pain (duration from 6 to 12 weeks)
  - Chronic low back pain (duration more than 12 weeks)

Treatment of acute low back pain (duration less than 6 weeks)

- Recovery from acute low back pain usually takes some days or not more than some weeks. Recurrences are quite common but also then full recovery can be expected. Recurring, short episodes of back pain are treated like other short periods of pain.
- The treatment of short-term back problems that have lasted for less than 6 weeks should be based on history and clinical examination without laboratory tests or radiological imaging, unless there is reason to suspect a disease that is either serious or requires specific treatment.

Rest and activity

- The patient is informed about the benign nature of the condition and its good prognosis.
- The patient is encouraged to continue or resume ordinary daily activities as soon as possible B [12]. The patient can use his or her back in reasonable limits and continue light work.
- The patient is advised to avoid bed rest A [13 14 15].
- Light aerobic exercise that maintains the physical condition (e.g. walking) can be started in an early phase.
- There is no evidence for the benefit of specific strengthening or flexibility exercises for acute non-specific low back pain B [16]. However, improved fitness will promote general health.
- A short sick leave is often sufficient, and the aim is to return to work quickly.
- There is no reliable evidence on the effect of a supporting corset C [17].

Analgesics

- The effectiveness of NSAIDs in acute low back pain has been proved A [18 19].
- The risk of gastrointestinal adverse effects and NSAID allergies has to be considered when choosing the drug.
- The risk of an ulcer is increased with daily dose and age of the patient.
- The safest drug is paracetamol, which has an analgesic effect only B [20].
- There are differences between NSAIDs in the risk of ulcer. Ibuprofen is the safest of the commonly used NSAIDs. The new COX-2 selective NSAIDs are also quite safe.
- In severe pain the analgesic effect can be increased by adding a weak opiate to paracetamol or NSAIDs.
- Dextropropoxyphen should be used with caution because of its interaction with alcohol and the risk for fatal overdoses that have been reported. Tramadol has fewer side effects, but the duration of its effect is short and because of the risk of serious side effects it should not be used in combination with SSRI antidepressants. If necessary, stronger opiates like buprenorphin may be considered.

Muscle relaxants

- Muscle relaxants are more effective than placebo, but they are no more effective than NSAIDs, and the combination of muscle relaxants and NSAIDs brings no further benefit B [21].
- Muscle relaxants cause drowsiness or dizziness in almost one third of the patients.
- A muscle relaxant is, however, an alternative when NSAIDs are not suitable or cause side effects.

ORT

Physical activity and exercise therapy

- Light exercise that maintains fitness, such as walking, can be recommended.
- Active exercise therapy of the back is not beneficial in the early stages of acute disease.

Manipulation

- A certified manipulation therapist (a physician or physiotherapist with a manual therapy training, chiropractician, osteopath or naprapath) may treat a patient with acute low back pain of less than 6 weeks' duration if there is a delay in returning to ordinary activities.
- Manipulation may shorten the duration of pain in some patients, but it has not been shown to prevent the pain from relapsing or becoming chronic C [22 23 24]. In general, spinal manipulative therapy appears to provide no benefit over other standard treatments for patients with acute or chronic low-back pain B [25].
- Plain x-ray of the lumbar spine is recommended before manipulation, but the treatment can be performed without imaging, if there is no reason to assume that the patient has a contraindication.
- The contraindications of manipulation are:
  - Processes that weaken the vertebrae (advanced osteoporosis, tumour or infection)
  - Ankylosing spondylitis
  - Instability, spondylolisthesis
  - Advanced spondylarthrosis
  - Recent trauma
  - Bleeding diathesis
  - Suspicion of lumbar intervertebral disc herniation
  - Manipulation is not recommended for sciatic symptoms.

- Supportive corset
  - There is scant and uncertain evidence on the pain-alleviating effects of supportive corsets in short-term back pain (C) [17]. There is a moderate amount of evidence to show that supportive corsets do not help to prevent low back pain or the recurrence of pain.

Treatment of subacute low back pain (duration 6–12 weeks)

- If back pain becomes prolonged, the patient should be referred to further tests within 6 weeks of the onset of the pain in order to define the nature of the disease and possible need of surgical treatment, and when necessary, for planning a comprehensive rehabilitation plan.
- If there are no signs of a disease requiring surgery, the patient can also be treated by a multi-disciplinary team in primary health care or occupational health care.
  - Examine lumbosacral x-rays, take ESR (C) [3 4], blood count, urine sample and other laboratory tests if necessary.
  - Consult a physiatrist, orthopaedist or neurosurgeon to assess the diagnosis (special examinations), treatment, ability to work and function and the need for rehabilitation.
  - Patients with disc herniation often benefit from 6 weeks of conservative treatment before an orthopaedist or a neurosurgeon evaluates the need for surgery. The outcome of an operation is, however, best when it is performed within three months of the onset of symptoms.
  - The patient's illness behaviour, exhaustion and depression can be assessed in an interview and by pain drawings and questionnaires that the patient fills in him- or herself (e.g. depression inventory).
  - Waddell tests for assessing exaggerated illness behaviour can be used in clinical examination. These tests give suggestive information on exaggerated illness behaviour, but do not rule out serious disease.
  - Help the patient to analyse his situation by discussing problems linked with back pain.
- A primary care physiotherapist can make a physiotherapeutic assessment and educate the patient (ergonomy, relaxation, back school).
- Physicians should spend enough time with patients to provide them with answers to their questions, fear-reducing information, careful examination and a physiotherapist's advice on ergonomic use of the back, as well as information on how to exercise. Alternatively, health care centres could establish or refer patients to back clinics, where physicians and physiotherapists with special expertise on back pain could provide this mini-intervention.

Drug therapy

- Analgesics are used intermittently according to the intensity and nature of pain (A) [26 27].
- Paracetamol, NSAIDs or a combination of NSAIDs and a weak opiate can be used according to the intensity of pain.
- The adverse effects of NSAIDs must be considered especially in the elderly who are in the greatest risk for perforation or bleeding of peptic ulcer as a complication of NSAIDs.
- Antidepressants have so far not been shown to be better than placebo in the treatment of low back pain (C) [28 29], but amitriptylin is effective in chronic pain and fibromyalgia. In prolonged back pain antidepressants can be used as adjunctive therapy if the patient is depressive.
- Neuroleptics should not be prescribed for back pain.
- Benzodiazepines should be avoided.

The treatment of associated psychosocial problems

- Ensure continuity of care (a personal physician, other members of the primary care team).
- All persons involved in the treatment should support coping.
- The patient should be encouraged to find his own solutions.
- Alleviating associated problems can help the patient feel better, even if the treatment is not directed towards the back problem.

Psychological treatments

- Active psychotherapy using cognitive-behavioural methods combined with a visit to the work place has shown effectiveness in one study.
- Specific problems can be approached by psychotherapeutic methods with a behaviouristic approach. The effect of cognitive behaviouristic therapy has been shown in acute and chronic low back pain, when the assessment has been made immediately after the treatment.
- In studies with extended follow-up the effect of behaviouristic methods has not differed from that of other active treatments.
- The patient may learn to use different methods of coping with pain, stress and affective reactions (e.g. relaxation and reorganization).
- The patient may learn social skills, or a positive attitude, or understand his or her ways of action and their causes and consequences. The therapy often consists of group sessions.
- Psychotherapeutic treatment may alleviate fear, anxiety and depression.

Helping the patient to return to work

- In case of perceived ergonomic problems an occupational health nurse or physiotherapist should discuss these problems in detail and give appropriate advice to the patient, and if needed visit the patient's work place.
- The working conditions are assessed, with an aim to optimise the workload in cooperation with the occupational health professionals and the employer. Resumption of work may be facilitated by lightening the job temporarily.
- Sick leaves without clear indications are avoided in order to prevent chronicity.
- Ergonomic measures should balance the work demands and the worker's physical capacity.

Chronic back pain (duration over 12 weeks)

- The same recommendations are given as for subacute low back pain.
- A specialized unit for the treatment of pain may be consulted.
- The patient should participate in the treatment and rehabilitation decisions. The patient needs help in coping with the illness.
- Intensive (but not less intensive) multidisciplinary bio-psycho-social rehabilitation with a functional restoration approach improves pain and function A [30].
- However, exercise has not been shown to reduce the number of sick leaves or retirements among chronic low back pain patients. Rehabilitation and improving the capacity to work are described below.
- There is no evidence on the effect of a supportive corset, although patient compliance for corsets is good.
- There is no evidence for the benefits of trigger point or facet joint injections C [31 32].

Rehabilitation and promotion of working capacity

Definition

- Rehabilitation is defined as activities aiming at decreasing the disability caused by disease or trauma, improving the ability to function or work, and increasing the ability to cope.
- Rehabilitation also includes interventions on the physical and social environment.

Timing of rehabilitation

- Absence from work for 6 weeks or more predicts difficulties in returning to work. After a sick leave of 6 months about 50%, and after a sick leave of one year only about 10–20% of the patients return to work.
- Rehabilitation is an essential part of comprehensive therapy. Active rehabilitation is recommended if back pain lasts for 6 weeks or more, and it should be a part of the treatment chain from primary care to specialized care, with the aim of the patient returning to work and other daily activities.

Carrying out rehabilitation activities

- The individual needs and the patient's situation of life define the context of rehabilitation.
- The members and values of the rehabilitation team have a decisive influence on the results (the patient is part of the a team).
- Early rehabilitation can start with a rehabilitation assessment by a small primary health care team including the physician, physiotherapist and/or occupational health nurse.
- A back school may have some effect on the experience of pain, but there is no evidence of its effect on reducing the need for sick leaves B [33]. The efficacy of group education is not proven D [34 35].
- In studies comparing ambulatory and institutional rehabilitation no difference in effectiveness as measured by resuming work has been observed, but short-term effects on perceived disability are superior in institutional rehabilitation. In sparsely populated areas institutional rehabilitation is often the best solution. The opportunities for ambulatory rehabilitation should always be assessed as an alternative to institutional rehabilitation.

Measures promoting working capacity

- Promoting the working capacity of a patient with chronic back problems requires measures directed to the actual work. Actions that decrease the physical load of work aim at preventing work incapacity and at promoting the coping of disabled persons.
- It is important that the patient's co-workers are empathetic towards those having a disability caused by back pain.
- General practitioners and secondary care specialists should co-operate with the occupational health care units, which usually have the best possibilities to carry out the appropriate measures at the work places.

Patient educational material

- Giving patients correct information reduces anxiety and improves compliance. Information recommended by a British specialist group is listed in Table 20.30.2.

Table 20.30.2 Recommended patient education in back pain (Waddell et al, 1996)

Type of back pain	Patient information
Common, unspecific back pain –convey a positive message	No reason to worry, back pain is very common. No sign of a serious trauma or disease. Recovery usually takes days or weeks at the most. There will be no permanent harm. Recurrences are quite common, but even then tendency for recovery is good. Physical activity is beneficial. Too much rest is harmful. Pain does not mean that activity is harmful.
Sciatic pain –convey a cautiously positive message.	No reason for fear. In most cases conservative treatment suffices, however, recovery usually takes 1–2 months. Full recovery is to be expected. Recurrences are possible.
Possibly a serious disease –avoid conveying a negative message.	Further investigations are needed for making a diagnosis. Often the results of these investigations are normal. After the investigations a specialist will decide on the best possible therapy. Excessive physical strain should be avoided until the investigations have been completed.

ORT

References

1. Deyo RA, Rainville J, Kent DL. What can the history and physical examination tell us about low back pain? JAMA 1992;268:760–765.
2. Van den Hoogen HMM, Koes RW, van Eijk JTHM, Bouter LM. On the accuracy of history, physical examination and erythrocyte sedimentation rate in diagnosing low-back pain in general practice. A criteria-based review of the literature. Spine 1995;20:318–327.
3. On the accuracy of history, physical examination, and erythrocyte sedimentation rate in diagnosing low back pain in general practice. Spine 1995;20:318–327.
4. The Database of Abstracts of Reviews of Effectiveness (University of York), Database no.: DARE-978022. In: The Cochrane Library, Issue 4, 1999. Oxford: Update Software.
5. van Tulder MW, Assendelft WJ, Koes BW, Bouter LM. Spinal radiographic findings and nonspecific low back pain: a systematic review of observational studies. Spine 1997;22:427–434.
6. The Database of Abstracts of Reviews of Effectiveness (University of York), Database no.: DARE-970341. In: The Cochrane Library, Issue 4, 1999. Oxford: Update Software.
7. Kerry S, Hilton S, Patel S, Dundas D, Rink E, Lord J. Routine referral for radiography of patients presenting with low back pain: is patient's outcome influenced by GPs' referral for plain radiography? Health Technology Assessment. The national Coordinating Centre for Health Technology Assessment (NCCAHTA). 136665278. Vol. 4: No. 20. 2000. 110.
8. The Health Technology Assessment Database, Database no.: HTA-20000883. In: The Cochrane Library, Issue 1, 2001. Oxford: Update Software.
9. Vroomen PC, de Krom MC, Wilmink JT, Kester AD, Knottnerus JA. Lack of effectiveness of bed rest for sciatica. N Engl J Med 1999;340(6):418–23.
10. Gibson JNA, Grant IC, Waddell G. Surgery for lumbar disc prolapse. Cochrane Database Syst Rev. 2004;(2):CD001350.
11. Jensen MC, Brant-Zawadski MN, Obuchowski N, ym.: Magnetic resonance imaging of the lumbar spine in people without back pain. New Engl. J Med 331,2: 69 –73, 1994.
12. Hilde G, Hagen KB, Jamtvedt G, Winnem M. Advice to stay active as a single treatment for low-back pain and sciatica. Cochrane Database Syst Rev. 2004;(2):CD003632.
13. Waddell G, Feder G, Lewis M. Systematic reviews of bed rest and advice to stay active for acute low back pain. Br J Gen Pract 1997;47:647–652.
14. The Database of Abstracts of Reviews of Effectiveness (University of York), Database no.: DARE-978368. In: The Cochrane Library, Issue 4, 1999. Oxford: Update Software.
15. Malmivaara A, Hakkinen U, Aro T, Heinrichs ML, Koskenniemi L, Kuosma E, Lappi S, Paloheimo R, Servo C, Vaaranen V ym. The treatment of acute low back pain –bed rest, exercises, or ordinary activity? N Engl J Med 1995;332:351–355.
16. van Tulder MW, Malmivaara A, Esmail R, Koes BW. Exercise therapy for low-back pain. Cochrane Database Syst Rev. 2004;(2):CD000335.
17. van Tulder MW, Jellema P, van Poppel MNM, Nachemson AL, Bouter LM. Lumbar supports for prevention and treatment of low-back pain. Cochrane Database Syst Rev. 2004;(2):CD001823.
18. Tulder MW van, Koes BW, Bouter LM. Conservative treatment of acute and chronic nonspecific low back pain. A systematic review of randomized controlled trials of the most common interventions. Spine 1997;22:2128–2156.
19. van Tulder MW, Scholten RJPM, Koes BW, Deyo RA. Nonsteroidal anti-inflammatory drugs for low-back pain. Cochrane Database Syst Rev. 2004;(2):CD000396.
20. Laporte JR, Carne X, Vidal X, Moreno V, Juan J. Upper gastrointestinal bleeding in relation to previous use of analgesics and non-steroidal anti-inflammatory drugs. Catalan countries study on upper gastrointestinal bleeding. Lancet 1991;337:85–9.
21. Tulder MW van, Koes BW, Bouter LM. Conservative treatment of acute and chronic nonspecific low back pain. A systematic review of randomized controlled trials of the most common interventions. Spine 1997;22:2128–2156.
22. Koes BW, Assendelft WJ, van der Heijden GJ, Bouter LM. Spinal manipulation for low back pain: an updated systematic review of randomised clinical trials. Spine 1996;21:2860–2871.
23. The Database of Abstracts of Reviews of Effectiveness (University of York), Database no.: DARE-970192. In: The Cochrane Library, Issue 4, 1999. Oxford: Update Software.
24. Andersson GBJ, Lucente T, Davisw AM, Kappler RE, Lipton JA, Leurgans S. A comparison of osteopathic spinal manipulation with standard care for patients with low back pain. N Engl J Med 1999;341:1426–1431.
25. Assendelft WJJ, Morton SC, Yu Emily I, Suttorp MJ, Shekelle PG. Spinal manipulative therapy for low back pain. Cochrane Database Syst Rev. 2004;(1):CD000447.
26. van Tulder MW, Koes BW, Bouter LM. Conservative treatment of acute and chronic nonspecific low back pain: a systematic review of randomized controlled trials of the most common interventions. Spine 1997;22:2128–2156.
27. The Database of Abstracts of Reviews of Effectiveness (University of York), Database no.: DARE-971202. In: The Cochrane Library, Issue 4, 1999. Oxford: Update Software.
28. Turner JA, Denny MC. Antidepressants for chronic back pain. J Fram Pract 1993;37:545–553.
29. The Database of Abstracts of Reviews of Effectiveness (University of York), Database no.: DARE-940185. In: The Cochrane Library, Issue 4, 1999. Oxford: Update Software.
30. Guzmán J, Esmail R, Karjalainen K, Malmivaara A, Irvin E, Bombardier C. Multidisciplinary bio-psycho-social rehabilitation for chronic low-back pain. Cochrane Database Syst Rev. 2004;(2):CD000963.
31. Nelemans PJ, de Bie RA, de Vet HCW, Sturmans F. Injection therapy for subacute and chronic benign low-back pain. Cochrane Database Syst Rev. 2000;(2):CD001824.
32. Carette S, Leclaire R, Marcoux S, Morin F, Blaise GA, St.-Pierre A, Truchon R, Parent F, Lévesque J, Bergeron V, Montminy P, Blanchette C. Epidural corticosteroid injections for sciatica due to herniated nucleus pulposus. N Engl J Med 1997; 336:1634–1640.
33. van Tulder MW, Esmail R, Bombardier C, Koes BW. Back schools for non-specific low-back pain. Cochrane Database Syst Rev. 2004;(2):CD000261.
34. Cohen JE, Goel V, Frank JW, Bombardier C, Peloso P, Guillemin F. Group education interventions for people with low back pain: an overview of the literature. Spine 1994;19:1214–1222.

35. The Database of Abstracts of Reviews of Effectiveness (University of York), Database no.: DARE-940282. In: The Cochrane Library, Issue 4, 1999. Oxford: Update Software.

20.33 Lumbar spinal stenosis

Editors

Definition and epidemiology

- Lumbar spinal stenosis (LSS) is a condition in which the cauda equina is under compression in the lumbar spinal canal.
- LSS has two forms: central and lateral.
- The diagnostic criteria are fulfilled if
  - compression of the cauda equina and/or the nerve roots is verified by imaging (CT, MRI, and/or myelography).
  - the patient has one or both of the following symptoms: spinal claudication and/or chronic nerve root compression.
- Symptomatic LSS becomes more prevalent after the age of 50 years. The mean age of patients operated for LSS is approximately 60 years and that of patients operated for disc prolapse is about 40 years.
- The incidence of LSS in the general population is not known. Men are operated somewhat more often than women for LSS.
- The incidence and prevalence of LSS increase with ageing.
- LSS is also nowadays detected more often as the use of CT and MRI examinations increases.

Symptoms

- The patient typically reports that flexion of the spine relieves and extension worsens the symptoms.
- The symptom may be pain, numbness and/or weakness. It may be uni- or bilateral.
- **Spinal or neurogenic claudication** that appears when the patient walks, forcing him to stop; flexion of the spine, e.g. squatting or sitting, relieves the symptoms. Patients with claudication do not usually have symptoms when resting.
- **Chronic radicular compression** is usually continuous. Its severity varies depending on the position of the patient. It is more diffuse than dermatome pain in disc prolapse.
- **In mixed symptom** the patient has both disc prolapse and claudication type symptoms.
- **Cauda equina symptom** is rare, but it is important to remember to ask the patient about it.

Clinical findings

- A patient with LSS with spinal claudication is rather "well" when examined in the lying position. The examining physician should not let this mislead him/her.
- A patient with LSS with the disc prolapse symptom has pains when moving his back, and the Lasegue's sign may be positive.
- Extension test: the patient stands and extends his back for about 30–60 seconds. The examining physician can help by supporting him. If the patient has a remarkable stenosis, the condition will be provoked or aggravated.
- About half of the patients have sensory or reflex defects.
- Include touch per rectum in the clinical examination.

Diagnosis

- LSS is suspected on the basis of clinical history. A positive extension test supports the diagnosis of stenosis.
- LSS is verified by CT, MRI, and/or myelography.
- The diagnosis of LSS is set when history and clinical and radiological findings are in concordance.
- However, symptoms and radiological findings do not always correlate.

Differential diagnosis

- Intermittent claudication. If peripheral pulses are felt, arterial circulation of the lower extremities is undisturbed. Exception: If the arterial occlusion is in the pelvic region, peripheral pulses may be felt at rest.
  - The position of the back does not affect the symptom.
  - The symptom is relieved when standing, and the patient does not need to remain in flexion.
  - Bicycling provokes the symptom.
- Hip arthrosis
- Disc prolapse in the lumbar spine, especially in the elderly patients, simulates LSS.
- Referred pain from the region of the lumbar spine, the so-called pseudosciatica
- Neurological causes of lower extremity pain (e.g. polyneuropathy, spinal tumours, multiple sclerosis); Babinski sign and spasticity of the lower extremities

Treatment

- Evidence on the efficacy of surgical treatment is clear; however, that on conservative treatment is scarce.
- Randomized studies comparing surgical and conservative treatments are lacking.

Conservative treatment

- In long-term follow-up the condition of unoperated LSS patients is fairly good.
- It is usually worthwhile to start with conservative treatment.
- Indications for conservative treatment
  - The patient tolerates the symptoms sufficiently well.
  - The patient's capacity to function is adequate.
  - The patient can walk several hundred metres.
- If the symptoms are relieved by conservative treatment and the patient's capacity to function is adequate, the treatment

can be continued. Radiological finding alone is not an indication for surgical treatment.

- Pain medication
- A slightly flexing back support
- Stretching exercises of the flexor muscles
- Physiotherapy is aimed at reducing the pain and tightness of myofascial tissues of the lumbar back.
- The tightness of the muscles of the back, stomach, thighs and the loins is reduced with stretching exercises.
- Calcitonin
- Epidural anaesthetics

Surgical treatment

- Surgical management relieves the pain and lengthens the walking distance.
- Male gender and complete constriction in myelography predict a favourable outcome of the operation.
- The long-term result of surgical management is contradictory: the outcome remains good or deteriorates.
- Indications for surgery
  - Cauda equina syndrome is an indication for emergency surgery.
  - Progressive neurological deficit
  - Intolerable pain that is not alleviated with conservative management
  - Shortening walking distance (<200–300 m)
- Methods used in surgical treatment include total laminectomy C [1 2] and hemilaminectomy.
- Successful decompression shown on CT scan does not seem to correlate with the clinical outcome of surgery.

References

1. Niggemeyer O, Strauss JM, Schulitz KP. Comparison of surgical procedures for degenerative lumbar spinal stenosis: a meta-analysis of the literature from 1975 to 1995. Eur Spine J 1997;6:423–429.
2. The Database of Abstracts of Reviews of Effectiveness (University of York), Database no.: DARE-983339. In: The Cochrane Library, Issue 2, 2000. Oxford: Update Software.

20.34 Groin pain

Editors

Aims

- Septic infections warranting immediate treatment should be identified.
- A possible fracture of the femoral neck should be kept in mind (including a stress fracture) to avoid additional damage due to weight bearing prior to x-ray.

Young patients

- Stress-induced ligament lesion
- Acute synovitis of the hip joint (32.54)
  - Often after respiratory infection
  - Distinctly restricted internal rotation of the hip joint
- Stress fracture of the femoral neck or pubic bone in military conscripts
  - Due to extreme strain
- Acute osteoporosis of the femoral head
  - A rare condition that occurs mostly in middle aged or young males
  - After six weeks of pain and movement restriction periarticular osteoporosis and even changes in the joint surface will be seen in x-ray.
  - Resolves spontaneously in 2–12 months.
- Femoral head epiphysiolysis (32.61)
  - Teenage overweight boys
- Bone tumours (20.91)
  - Osteoid osteoma is the most frequent
  - Nocturnal pain
- Meralgia paraesthetica (20.63)
  - The pain is localised anteriorly in the thigh, includes paraesthesias and numbness
- Reactive arthritis, rheumatoid arthritis
  - Usually symptoms also in other joints
- Septic arthritis
  - Fever
- Painful lymph node in the groin
  - Erysipelas, tularaemia, genital or lower extremity infection
- Femoral hernia
  - Mostly a palpable lump
  - Abdominal symptoms
- Bursitis in the hip region
  - Resembles hip arthritis clinically but no fluid is found in the joint.
- Referred pain
  - In ureteric colic pain is referred into the side distinctly above the groin.
  - Referred prostate pain also is felt in lower abdomen.

Elderly patients

- In addition to the above
  - Hip osteoarthritis
    - The range of movements of the hip, especially internal rotation, is restricted.
    - X-ray show osteoarthritic changes.
  - Femoral neck fracture
    - An impacted fracture is possible despite ability to walk after the fall.

Testing

- X-rays are always necessary when pain arising from the hip joint or femur is suspected.
  - Indications for hip joint x-rays in children, see 32.54
- Except for suspicion of fracture, an x-ray is not necessary in off-hours but weight bearing is prohibited prior to ruling out fracture.
- Ultrasound reveals fluid in the hip joint and possible bursitis or ganglion.
- Bone scan is indicated in prolonged pain if the x-rays are normal (stress fracture of the femoral neck, tumour).

20.35 Buttock and hip pain

Kaj Rekola

Aim

- Nerve root syndromes, spinal stenosis, sacroiliitis, and malignant diseases should be identified.

Aetiology

- Children and adolescents
  - Synovitides, arthritides, traumas, congenital dislocation of the hip, epiphysiolysis of various origins
- Adults and the elderly
  - Disorders of intervertebral disks (even those of the lower thoracic spine), osteoarthrosis of the hip, trochanteric and other bursites, sacroiliitis, rheumatic diseases, aseptic bone necrosis, piriformis syndrome, and malignancies (lesser pelvis, prostate gland)

Diagnostic tips

- Spine-related pain
  - Buttock pain is common in acute back pain (20.30). The pain may increase during straight or oblique extension of the back.
- Arthritis or arthrosis of the hip
  - Restricted movement is a typical finding: limitations are first seen in inward rotation, thereafter in extension and finally in outward rotation and abduction.
  - Tenderness in the groin at the area of the hip joint
- Referred pain due to nerve root compression
  - Nerve root compression (sciatic syndrome) (20.30): Pain increases on forward flexion of the spine frequently radiating below the knee.
  - Spinal stenosis (20.33): Pain increases when walking; pain is felt also in the lower extremities.
- Piriformis syndrome
  - Pain can be provoked by lifting the ankle on the opposite knee and pulling the knee of the lifted foot towards the opposite shoulder (20.30).
  - Deep palpation of the buttock is painful.
- Sacroiliitis
  - May be the initial manifestation of ankylosing spondylitis (21.32) or reactive arthritis (21.31).
  - Typical symptoms include morning stiffness and stiffness after prolonged sitting.
  - ESR is occasionally elevated.
  - Pain in the ligament insertions may occur (enthesitis).
- Pubic bone stress fracture (18.64)
  - In military conscripts
- Strain induced pain in tendon insertions
- Claudication pain (spinal or vascular) (5.60)
  - When walking
- Trochanteric bursitis (20.36)
  - Maximal pain laterally to the hip joint, tenderness to palpation at the great trochanter
  - Pain is felt in extreme positions of the hip, and opposed movements cause pain.
- Tuber ischii bursitis
- Malignant diseases: lesser pelvis, prostate cancer (rectal touch!)

Testing

- Clinical diagnosis often suffices.
- Spinal x-rays are indicated, especially in persons under 20 years or over 45 years of age, in cases with prolonged or recurrent pain.
- Bone scan is the most sensitive test for sacroiliitis because of slowly developing radiological changes in this condition.
- Examination of the prostate is necessary; the piriform muscles can be palpated per rectum in conjunction with the examination.
- When vascular claudication is suspected the peripheral pulses should be examined and a blood pressure measurement at the ankles should be performed (doppler) (5.20).

20.36 Trochanteric bursitis

Editors

Basic rule

- Identify trochanteric bursitis as a cause of hip-thigh pain that can be easily treated by a steroid injection.
- The trochanter region contains 12–24 bursae at varying depths, which should be taken into account when injecting.

Symptoms

- Pain radiating both proximally and distally from the trochanteric area
- Pain on walking

Diagnosis

- The typical patient is a middle-aged or elderly woman. Overweight is a predisposing factor.
- Palpation of the greater trochanter indicates the site of tenderness.

Treatment

- The treatment of choice is an injection to the most painful site (use a 4–8 cm needle depending on the depth and the thickness of the thigh). Corticosteroid 1 ml + 4–5 ml 1% lidocaine. Insert the needle to bone contact, then lift the needle tip back about 5 mm. Inject half of the solution at the site of pain and the rest in different directions.
- The bursae may be located several cm from each other.
- If the first injection does not alleviate pain, the treatment can be repeated after a few weeks.

20.40 Painful knee

Editors

- The Table 20.40 includes the essential symptoms and findings indicating specific conditions and injuries.

20.41 Examination of knee instability

Editors

- Begin by examining the uninjured knee for further comparison.
- The range of movements of the injured knee is examined in a gentle manner to enable relaxation of thigh muscles. The tests for instability (Table 20.41) are performed by using gentle bending forces in the beginning.
- The most common injury leading to knee instability is rupture of the medial collateral ligament and anterior cruciate ligament (Item 1 in the table); the knee gives way in 30° flexion when it is forced into valgus.

Tests

Drawer test

- Usually performed with the patient lying supine with the knee in 90° flexion. The examiner moves the leg back and forth in the sagittal plane and compares the movement to the uninjured side.
- **Lachman's test**: The knee is held in 20° flexion and the tibia is moved back and forth in the sagittal plane in relation to the femur. This test gives a better picture of ligament integrity but may be difficult to perform in obese patients.

Pivot test

- The knee is held straight.

Table 20.40 The painfull knee – diagnostic clues

Symptoms, signs, typical cases	Condition
Pain on descending stairs or squatting; tenderness and crepitation at "grinding" the patella	Chondromalacia (20.42)
Tender and swollen tibial tuberosity; patient 10–15 years old	Osgood-Schlatter disease (32.63)
Tenderness at the lower margin of the knee and at the patellar tendon; sports including jumping	Jumper's knee (20.43)
Knee instability; injury or sequela of injury	Examination of knee instability (20.41) Knee injuries (18.33)
Locking, hydrops, giving way	Meniscal tear (20.44) Osteochondritis dissecans (20.47) Patellar dislocation tendency (33.1)
Swelling behind the knee	Baker's cyst (20.45)
Prepatellar swelling	Prepatellar bursitis (20.46)
Painful and/or swollen knee without injury, morning stiffness	Arthritis (21.2)
Pain on motion in middle-aged or older patient, periodic swelling, pain when starting motion or walking stairs	Osteoarthritis
Lateral pain on motion, tibial condyle is painful on lateral palpation	Insertion tendinitis of the iliotibial tract
Rotation movements of the hip joint are painful	Hip osteoarthritis (the pain radiates to the knee)

Table 20.41 Examination of the unstable knee

Instability	Test	Injury
Medial (valgus)	Knee in 30° flexion	Medial collateral, anterior cruciate
	Extended knee	Medial collateral, anterior cruciate, posterior cruciate, posterior capsule
Lateral (varus)	Knee in 30° flexion	Lateral collateral, anterior cruciate
	Extended knee	Lateral collateral, anterior cruciate, posterior cruciate, posterior capsule
Posterior	Drawer posteriorly	Posterior cruciate
Anterior	Drawer anteriorly	Anterior cruciate
Anteromedial	Drawer anteriorly in external rotation	Medial collateral, anterior cruciate
Hyperextension	Bending into hyperextension	Anterior cruciate, posterior cruciate, posterior capsule
Anterolateral	Pivot test (in internal rotation), lateral rotation	Anterior cruciate, lateral capsule, tractus iliotibialis, medial collateral
Posterolateral	Reversed pivot test (in external rotation)	Posterolateral capsule, posterior cruciate

- The leg is rotated internally from the ankle and the knee is simultaneously pushed into valgus.
- Keeping the internal rotation and valgus position the knee is flexed. At 40° to 45° a snapping sound indicates a positive test result as the lateral joint surfaces of the femur and the tibia snap into place pulled by the iliotibial tract.

The reversed pivot test

- Performed as above except for external rotation of the tibia.

Evaluation of test results and further action

- Evaluation of test results may be difficult.
- If the symptoms and signs indicate that arthroscopic or open surgery may be an option, a specialist with sufficient clinical experience and with facilities for magnetic resonance imaging and arthroscopy Ⓐ [1 2 3 4] should be consulted.

References

1. Rappeport ED, Mehta S, Wieslander SB, Scwarz Lausten G, Thomsen HS. Magnetic imaging before arthroscopy in knee joint disorders. Acta radiologica 1996;37:602–609.
2. The Database of Abstracts of Reviews of Effectiveness (University of York), Database no.: DARE-961824. In: The Cochrane Library, Issue 4, 1999. Oxford: Update Software.
3. Mackenzie R, Palmer CR, Lomas DJ, DIxon AK. Magnetic resonance imaging of the knee: diagnostic performance statistics. Clin Radiol 1996;51:251–257.
4. The Database of Abstracts of Reviews of Effectiveness (University of York), Database no.: DARE-960778. In: The Cochrane Library, Issue 4, 1999. Oxford: Update Software.

20.42 Patellar chondromalacia

Editors

Definition and epidemiology

- Chondromalacia commonly affects both genders after the age of 12 years and above. About 20% of the patients are less than 20 years old; 75% are under the age of 50.
- Chondromalacia is frequently associated with patellar instability and patellofemoral dysplasia as a histopathological finding.

Diagnosis

- Chondromalacia as such does not necessarily cause any symptoms; therefore, it should not be used solely as a clinical diagnosis.
- The clinical diagnosis is based on crepitation, pseudolocking, snapping, and/or pain on patellar "grinding". The medial and lateral margins of the patella may be tender. The finding can be verified by arthroscopy or MRI.

Causes

- The causes for patellar lateral dislocation tendency that results in reduced contact surface with the femur include valgus knees, increased Q-angle, condyle height imbalance, decreased sulcus angle, and muscular imbalance.
- Factors worsening the symptoms include squatting, walking stairs or on uneven terrain, bouncing associated with jumping, kneeling, and prolonged sitting with bent knees.

Treatment of the painful cartilage lesion

- The aim is to strengthen the medial quadriceps in particular and to stretch the tight Q and capsular system. Exercise therapy reduces pain Ⓒ [1].

The acute stage

- Rest for 1 to 3 weeks, pain medication

The exercise stage

- Straight leg lifting once per second with five repeats. The series is repeated three times a day for two weeks, thereafter five times a day. When this can be performed well, weights of 3–5 kg are attached to the ankle. The exercises are performed in a supine or sitting position. Dynamic exercises must never be started with a flexed knee. By palpating the quadriceps muscle the therapist should confirm that the patient is performing an isometric contraction, affecting the vastus medialis in particular. Progress can be monitored by measuring the muscle circumference.
- The patient should be advised that achieving pain relief might take several months. A specialist should be consulted not earlier than three months from the onset of symptoms. Patellar supports may be helpful, but may not press the patella against the femoral head.

Surgical treatment

- May be an option if active exercise does not relieve symptoms in six months.
- Lateral release or reinsertion of the tibial tubercle or both and anteromedialization or medial capsuloplasty is performed if patellar dislocation tendency is seen in the patellar projection of knee x-rays.

Reference

1. Heintjes E, Berger MY, Bierma-Zeinstra SMA, Bernsen RMD, Verhaar JAN, Koes BW. Exercise therapy for patellofemoral pain syndrome. Cochrane Database Syst Rev 2003(4):CD003472.

20.43 Jumper's knee

Editors

Definition

- A painful condition in the inferior or superior edge of the patella or in the distal insertion of the patellar ligament that occurs in athletes practicing sports requiring forceful jumping. The condition is the result of micro- or macroscopic ruptures resulting from repeated jumping.
- The symptoms may predict rupture of the patellar ligament.

Symptoms and signs

- Symptoms appear initially when jumping, later when running and walking, and in more advanced cases at rest.
- The inferior patellar edge and the adjacent patellar ligament are painful on palpation and when knee extension is resisted.
- X-rays may show a bony spur or a bone fragment in the inferior edge of the patella. Macroscopic ligament injuries are seen well by ultrasound.

Treatment

- Rest and NSAIDs in the beginning. Jumping on a hard surface with thin-soled sports shoes should be limited.
- A steroid/local anaesthetic injection into the attachment of the patellar ligament helps for pain, but repeated injections may cause degenerative changes in the ligament.
- Surgical treatment consists of removal of degenerated parts of the ligament and/or possible bone fragments.
- Jumping training may be resumed six weeks after surgery and full jumping after three months.

20.44 Meniscus tears

Editors

Mechanism of injury

- When the knee is flexed and the foot bears weight on the ground
  - A medial meniscus injury is caused by simultaneous abduction of the knee and internal rotation of the femur.
  - A lateral meniscus injury is caused by simultaneous adduction of the knee and external rotation of the femur.

Symptoms and signs

- Medial/lateral ratio: 6–8:1
- Knee pain appears at the time of injury, swelling appears within a couple of hours, and the knee may also lock immediately.
- Haemarthrosis is not associated with a meniscus tear if the meniscus has not detached from the joint capsule.
- Repeated locking and giving way of the knee
- Pain in the joint line, the patient feels snapping
- Pain on palpation of the joint line at the ruptured meniscus
- **Apley's test**: The patient lies prone with the knee in 90° flexion. By pressing the tibia vertically the meniscus is compressed between the articular surfaces which causes pain. Pulling the leg upwards relieves pressure on the meniscus but causes tension on the ligaments and possible pain. The purpose of the test is primarily to differentiate between meniscus and ligament injuries.
- **McMurray's test**: The knee is first flexed maximally and then extended while pressing the knee in the varus direction. The test is repeated by pressing the anterior, medial and

posterior aspects of the meniscus. If a snap is heard and the patient experiences pain at the same time, the test is considered positive.

- The diagnosis is confirmed by arthroscopy, magnetic resonance imaging (A) [1 2 3 4], or arthrography; arthrography is the least reliable method.

Treatment

- If meniscus injury is suspected, the patient should be referred to a specialist if surgical repair is an option (B) [5].
- Meniscus removal may cause secondary osteoarthritis (C) [6]; thus the meniscus should be preserved, if possible.
- Mild symptoms require only follow-up, exercise of the quadriceps muscle, and NSAIDs for pain relief.
- Partial arthroscopic excision of the injured meniscus (B) [5]
- Suturation of the ruptured meniscus either arthroscopically or during open surgery (especially in peripheral ruptures in younger persons)
- Postoperative treatment: It is essential to restore the strength of the quadriceps muscle. Crutches may be used for up to 14 days; by then full weight bearing should be achieved. Work disability lasts 3 to 4 weeks. Suturation of the meniscus requires a longer period of immobilization and sick leave.

References

1. Rappeport ED, Mehta S, Wieslander SB, Scwarz Lausten G, Thomsen HS. Magnetic imaging before arthroscopy in knee joint disorders. Acta radiologica 1996;37:602–609.
2. The Database of Abstracts of Reviews of Effectiveness (University of York), Database no.: DARE-961824. In: The Cochrane Library, Issue 4, 1999. Oxford: Update Software.
3. Mackenzie R, Palmer CR, Lomas DJ, DIxon AK. Magnetic resonance imaging of the knee: diagnostic performance statistics. Clin Radiol 1996;51:251–257.
4. The Database of Abstracts of Reviews of Effectiveness (University of York), Database no.: DARE-960778. In: The Cochrane Library, Issue 4, 1999. Oxford: Update Software.
5. Howell JR, Handoll HHG. Surgical treatment for meniscal injuries of the knee in adults. Cochrane Database Syst Rev. 2004;(2):CD001353.
6. Roos H, Lauren M, Adalberth et al. Knee osteoarthritis after meniscectomy. Prevalence and radiographic changes after twenty-one years compared with matched controls. Arthritis Rheum 1998;41:687–693.

20.45 Baker's cyst

Editors

Definition

- Synovial bulging in the back of the knee that can be congenital in children or in adults secondary to injury, arthritis, osteoarthritis or hydrops.

Treatment

- **In children**, the cyst may be followed up for a couple of years in case it does not interfere with the range of movement of the joint and does not cause pain. If a large cyst does not recede spontaneously, it can be removed surgically.
- **In adults**, the cyst can be drained with a syringe (avoiding puncture of vessels). Using the same needle methylprednisolone or triamcinolone can be injected into the drained cyst.

Rupture of Baker's cyst

- A ruptured Baker's cyst may cause swelling of the calf and pain resembling deep venous thrombosis.
- If the history of Baker's cyst is known and the patency of the popliteal vein can be confirmed with the doppler stethoscope or venous thrombosis can be excluded with the D-dimer test, venography is not necessary.
- Diagnostic ultrasound confirms the diagnosis.
- Ruptured Baker's cyst does not need treatment.

20.46 Bursitis (patella and elbow)

Editors

Aims

- Septic bursitis should be diagnosed and treated with antibiotics immediately.

Testing

- Septic bursitis should be suspected if the bursa region has rapidly become painful and red, or if the patient is feverish. Predisposing factors are often adjacent injuries, for example a skin lesion or an injury from direct pressure or friction (e.g. in a job requiring kneeling).
- If septic bursitis is suspected the bursa should be punctured and the sample should be cultured in a blood culture bottle (C) [1] (one aerobic culture bottle suffices) or, if a blood culture bottle is not available, a bacterial culture test tube can be used.
  - In septic bursitis the sample is often slightly bloody and reddish.
  - The cells in the bursa fluid are mostly granulocytes with a leucocyte count over 2000 × 10^6/l (C) but the absolute cell count is not reliable in distinguishing between septic and aseptic bursitis (in emerging septic bursitis very few cells may be found).
- Serum CRP concentration increases in septic bursitis usually within 12 hours of the first symptoms. ESR increases much

more slowly and is not useful for detecting a bacterial infection within the first 1–2 days.
- In practice, mere suspicion of bacterial bursitis is an indication for antibacterial therapy after a sample for bacterial culture has been taken.

Treatment

- **Septic bursitis**: an antibiotic against staphylococcus (a cephalosporin derivative, cloxacillin, etc.). Treatment should preferably be initiated parenterally (cefuroxime 750 mg i.v. or i. m. three times daily or ceftriaxone 1 g i.m. once daily for a couple of days). The injections can be administered at an outpatient clinic. The treatment is continued with cephalexin or cefadroxil 500 mg three times daily.
- **Aseptic bursitis**: The bursa should be injected with long-acting methylprednisolone or triamcinolone. The injection may be repeated after 2–4 weeks if the result of the first injection is not satisfactory.
- Trochanter bursitis, see 20.36.

Reference

1. Stell IM, Gransden WR. Simple tests for septic bursitis: comparative study. BMJ 1998;316:1877.

20.47 Osteochondritis dissecans in the knee

Editors

Definition

- Osteochondrosis is a condition where a fragment consisting of cartilage and underlying bone detaches from the joint surface (most often the medial femoral condyle). The condition is rare before the age of eight.

Symptoms and signs

- Slowly progressing pain
- A feeling of the knee giving way, swelling, lowered stress tolerance
- At later stages, as a consequence of the detached fragment, locking tendency develops.
- When the flexed and internally rotated knee is extended, pain is felt at the medial condyle in 30° flexion (Wilson's test).
- X-rays usually show the detached fragment well. Occasionally, a so called tunnel projection is needed. As the condition mostly is bilateral, both knees must be radiographed.
- MRI is the most accurate imaging method and also reveals early focuses of osteochondritis.

Treatment

- **In children and adolescents**, if no detachment has occurred, follow-up suffices; alternatively, a lower extremity cast for six weeks. The patient is not allowed to bear weight and must use crutches for walking.
- **In adults**, and always when fragment is detached, treatment consists of surgical removal of the fragment. In the elderly the fragment should be removed only if it interferes with moving.

20.50 Painful conditions of the ankle and foot in children and adults

Pentti Kallio

- The following disorders are usually detected easily on the basis of age, symptom location, and x-rays.

Köhler's disease

- Extremely rare aseptic necrosis of the navicular bone at the age of 5 to 7 years
- Symptoms include: pain, swelling proximally in the foot, and limping. Weight bearing worsens the symptoms.
- Diagnosis is based on x-rays; the navicular bone appears underdeveloped and fragmented. The x-rays should be compared with those of the other foot.
- Recovery is usually spontaneous. A cast can be applied for a short time to alleviate pain.

Freiberg's disease

- Aseptic necrosis of the head of the second metatarsal in children and young adults
- Symptoms include: pain and swelling at the metatarsal head; on palpation the head feels thickened. Limited motion of the MTP joint is evident.
- X-rays show a flattened and fragmented metatarsal head.
- Treatment: Shoes with thick soles, shoe inserts, or a transversal arch bar in the sole. A short cast treatment may be necessary, but surgical therapy is not usually warranted (removal of fragments, shaping of the head or removal) before conservative treatment has been tried for 1–2 years.

Sever's disease

- Pain in the achilles tendon insertion in children (7–11 years)
- The pain is worst after physical exercise.
- On palpation the sides of the heel bone are painful but not swollen.
- Radiology is not necessary if the symptoms and findings are typical.
- X-rays may show sclerosis and irregularities of the calcaneal apophysis, but this can be seen also in asymptomatic individuals.
- The pain disappears spontaneously in adolescence. In less severe cases, reducing load suffices. In mild cases the patient should avoid all jumping and running for 6 weeks.

Supernumerary navicular bone (os tibiale externum)

- A common accidental finding; a sesamoid bone in the posterior tibial tendon.
- May form a pseudarthrosis or may be attached to the navicular bone. The prominence may cause discomfort in association with flat feet, and cause compression in the shoe, particularly in skates and ski boots.
- Symptoms commence at pre-adolescence, and usually subside with skeletal maturity. Rarely symptoms persist in adulthood.
- Treatment includes temporary reduction of physical activity and well-fitting shoes or boots. In severe acute pain (recent partial tendon avulsion) below knee plaster cast for 4–6 weeks is indicated. Surgery is sometimes indicated.

Painful forefoot (Anterior metatarsalgia)

- Painful condition of the second and third metatarsal heads caused by collapse of the transversal arch, rheumatoid arthritis, or osteoarthritis of the metatarsophalangeal joints.
- Typically occurs in middle-aged and elderly individuals, especially in females used to wear shoes with high heels.
- The collapse of the transversal arch predisposes to hallux valgus, hammer toe and Morton's disease.
- The load can be reduced with a metatarsal bar. Severe and prolonged symptoms, particularly those caused by rheumatoid arthritis can be treated by removal of the metatarsal heads (Hybinette's procedure).

Stress fracture of metatarsal bones

- Caused by prolonged unusual stress, and is typical in military conscripts.
- The fracture cannot initially be seen in x-rays, but is revealed in MRI. A radiographic callus appears three weeks after the onset of the symptoms. Treatment consists of temporary reduction of stress on the affected foot.

Morton's disease

- A neuroma of the interdigital branch, most often between the third and fourth metatarsal heads
- The pain increases with a tight shoe and with manual sidewise compression of the forefoot.
- The condition is most frequent in middle-aged women.
- Treatment consists of wearing a shoe insert with a metatarsal pad to support the transversal arch. If the symptoms still persist, local steroid anaesthetic injections can be tried. The shoes should be sufficiently wide and have low heels. Surgical excision of the neuroma may be considered. Hypaesthesia of the interdigital area is an unavoidable adverse effect of surgery.

Hallux valgus

- See 20.53.

Flat foot (pes planovalgus)

- A painfree flexible flatfoot is a common physiological finding in a child. Most flatfeet will correct spontaneously with advancing age.
- The finding is benign and no treatment is needed.
- The effectiveness of orthoses or special shoes has not been proven.
- There is no evidence of the association of flat foot and other musculoskeletal problems such as growing pains in childhood or knee, hip or back problems in adulthood.
- A painful or rigid planovalgus is not physiological. It may be caused by arthritis, tarsal coalition, post-traumatic sequela or a tumour.

Obliterating arteriosclerosis

- A distal arterial obstruction may cause numbness of the sole or pain on walking.

20.51 Heel pain

Editors

Basic rule

- The causes of heel pain can generally be differentiated by the site of the pain and by clinical findings. X-rays may sometimes be useful.

Plantar fasciitis

- Most common painful condition, particularly in overweight persons and in those who walk much. Often caused by strain, sometimes by rheumatoid arthritis.
- On palpation, the pain is located centrally, anterior to the heel. The pain is felt most acutely after getting up from bed, sometimes after strain.
- Half of symptomatic patients have a bone spur on x-ray. This callus, which is formed in the plantar fascia enthesis, is also seen in 15% of asymptomatic persons.
- Treatment consists of a piece of plastic foam or a shoe insert with a U-shaped cut-out that relieves pressure in the painful area. The patient can make one him/herself or have one made by an orthotist. A silicone heel pad may be the best method. The load should be reduced and NSAID medication started.
- Corticosteroid/local anaesthetic injections C [1] can be administered into the painful area as needed at 3-week intervals. However, degeneration of the heel pad could occur as an adverse effect. The medication should be injected deep enough, not into the heel pad. The long-term benefits of injection treatment are uncertain.
- Dorsiflexion exercises are carried out twice daily to stretch the plantar fascia. Wearing an orthosis splint at nights has the same effect.
- The heel spurs seen on x-rays are a consequence, not the cause of the condition and do not require surgery. An operation should be considered when all other treatments have failed. With correct indications the results of surgery are good.
- A small minority of patients with plantar fasciitis have an underlying rheumatic disease in which case the condition is a manifestation of enthesopathy (Reiter's disease, ankylosing sponlylitis). History taking should include questions about morning stiffness, back and buttock pain, and tenderness in ligament insertions in the extremities; the joints and the ESR should be examined.

Nerve entrapment

- Diffuse radiating pain
- Provoked by the valgus position of the calcaneus bone
- Diagnosis by ENMG is difficult.

Heel pad pain

- The pain is located more posteriorly than the pain in plantar fasciitis.
- Treatment consists of temporary weight-relief, padding or heal cup.

Stress fracture of the calcaneus

- Occurs usually in military conscripts as a consequence of stress on the bone due to unusually strenuous running or walking.
- Occasionally it can be seen in pregnant women.
- The calcaneus is tender on lateral pressure.
- In about three weeks from the onset of symptoms a slightly sclerotic condensation can be seen on the x-rays.
- Treatment consists of temporary weight-relief.

Calcaneus apophysitis

- Common in adolescent boys (8–12 years)
- The painful spot is located at the insertion of the Achilles tendon where a lump often can be palpated. A x-ray is usually not needed.
- See 20.50.

Achilles tendon insertion pain in athletes

- Peritendinitis (20.52).
- Tendinosis
- Partial rupture (NB: no corticosteroid!)
- Retrocalcaneal bursitis
- Haglund's deformity

Other rare causes

- Cyst
- Osteoid osteoma and osteosarcoma
- Osteomyelitis
- Fracture of osteoporotic bone
- Talocalcaneal arthrosis (often secondary)

Reference

1. Crawford F, Thomson C. Interventions for treating plantar heel pain. Cochrane Database Syst Rev. 2004;(2):CD000416.

20.52 Achilles tendon peritendinitis and tendon rupture

Editors

Peritendinitis

Aetiology

- Achilles tendon peritendinitis is an overuse injury (running, jumping).

- The rupture of the Achilles tendon is a typical injury in 30–50-year-old men who are active in sports, particularly ball games (badminton, volley ball). The ruptured tendon almost invariably shows degenerative changes, although most patients have not had preceding symptoms.
- The use of fluoroquinolones increases the risk of Achilles tendon rupture, especially in over 60-year-olds and also when a steroid is used concomitantly C [1].

Symptoms and diagnosis

Peritendinitis

- Distinct tenderness on palpation around the Achilles tendon
- Movement pain when calf muscles are contracted and stretched

Tendon rupture

- Tendon rupture causes acute pain that soon eases off. The patient feels as if someone had kicked him/her from the back. Some ruptures may be painless.
- The patient is unable to stand on toes. Partial extension of the ankle may still be possible as the flexor tendons of the toes and peroneal tendons are functioning.
- A depression is felt at the site of the rupture. The longer the time from the rupture to the examination the less the depression is felt because of swelling and haematoma.
- The following tests can be used for diagnosis
  - In the **Thompson test** the patient lies prone with the ankle unsupported. Contraction of the calf muscles does not extend the ankle.
  - In the **Copeland test** the patient lies prone with his knee in 90-degree flexion. A blood pressure meter cuff is placed around the calf with a 100-mmHg pressure. Passive flexion of the ankle does not increase the pressure in the injured leg, whereas a rise of approximately 40 mmHg is observed in the healthy leg.
- Ultrasound is helpful in uncertain cases and when a long time has elapsed between the trauma and the investigation.

Treatment

Peritendinitis

- Rest and immobilization with a splint
- In case of **crepitating peritendinitis** low molecular weight heparin has been used (e.g. Fragmin®) 100 i.u./kg subcutaneously on three consecutive days D [2]. The patients should be advised about increased risk of haematomas. Haemorrhagic diathesis is a contraindication. Because heparin therapy requires several visits to the doctor and is associated with increased risk of haemorrhagic complications, it should be used only in competitive athletes who need to recover rapidly.
- NSAIDs are always recommended in distinct symptoms C [3 4]; however not in conjunction with heparin (paracetamol should be used instead).
- In **chronic peritendinitis** steroid injections D [2] can be administered in the peritendineum (never into the tendon itself because of increased risk of rupture). After steroid injections at least a 2-week rest is necessary before resuming heavy activities and the load must be increased gradually.
- Stretching the Achilles tendon and a heel raise are helpful.
- Surgical treatment is an option if the chronic peritendinitis does not react to conservative therapy.

Achilles tendon rupture

- Surgery is always warranted in the young, in athletes and in chronic ruptures. The rate of recurrence is only 1–2% for surgery and 10–15% for conservative treatment C [5 6]. After surgery up to 70% of the patients are able to resume sporting activities with the same level of intensity as before the injury.
- Conservative treatment is a good alternative for managing acute ruptures in elderly, less active patients C [5 6].

ORT

References

1. van der Linden PD, Sturkenboom MC, Herings RM, Leufkens HG, Stricker BH. Fluoroquinolones and risk of Achilles tendon disorders: case-control study. BMJ 2002;324:1306–7.
2. McLauchlan GJ, Handoll HHG. Interventions for treating acute and chronic Achilles tendinitis. Cochrane Database Syst Rev. 2004;(2):CD000232.
3. ALmekinders LC, Temple JD. Etiology, diagnosis, and treatment of tendonitis: an analysis of the literature. Medicine and Science in Sports and Exercise 1998;30:1183–1190.
4. The Database of Abstracts of Reviews of Effectiveness (University of York), Database no.: DARE-995382. In: The Cochrane Library, Issue 4, 2000. Oxford: Update Software.
5. Lo IK, Kirkley A, Nonweiler B, Kumbhare DA. Operative versus nonoperative treatment of acute Achilles tendon ruptures: a quantitative review. Clin J Sports Med 1997;7:207–211.
6. The Database of Abstracts of Reviews of Effectiveness (University of York), Database no.: DARE-970999. In: The Cochrane Library, Issue 4, 1999. Oxford: Update Software.

20.53 Hallux valgus

Markus Torkki

Basic rules

- Assess the biomechanical function and functional disturbance of the foot by clinical and radiological examinations.
- An observed functional disturbance is treated conservatively or surgically depending on the symptoms caused by the condition.

- The need and method of surgery is decided upon individually.
- Wearing well-fitting shoes prevents the development of hallux valgus.

Definition

- Hallux abductovalgus
  - Increased hallux valgus angle (between the first metatarsal bone and the proximal phalanx of the great toe). An angle below 16 degrees is considered normal.
  - The great toe is twisted inwards (valgus deformity).
- Medial exostosis of the distal end of the first metatarsal bone
- An increase in the intermetatarsal angle (IMA, the angle between the first and second metatarsal bones) is often associated with the above deformities. The normal angle is below 10 degrees.

Aetiology

- Disturbance of the biomechanical function of the foot exerts abnormal loading on the first metatarsal joint, leading to the formation of hallux valgus.
- Hereditary factors
- Footwear can contribute to the development of hallux valgus.
- Arthritis (rheumatoid)

Symptoms

- Functional defect
  - Functional disturbance of the foot (restricted supination on exertion) causes strain-related pain in the foot, ankle and leg.
  - Restriction of the range of movement or instability develops in the first MTP joint.
- Mechanical defect
  - Friction on the medial exostosis causes inflammation in the MTP joint (bursitis).
- Cosmetic harm (not sufficient for surgery)
- A functional disturbances often causes secondary changes: sores, local thickening of the plantar skin at the distal ends of the metatarsal bones II–IV.

Treatment

- Therapy is chosen on the basis of clinical and radiological examination.
- Fitting and spacious footwear with a good heel cup and sufficient rigidity, a buckle or laces for fastening and a heel less than 3 cm high are recommended.
- Functional foot orthoses can be tried in conservative therapy. They are prepared individually and are intended for correcting the biomechanical function of the foot.

Indications for surgery

- Surgery is indicated if the patient's problems are located in the region of the first metatarsal joint and are not resolved during follow up or by conservative therapy.
- The decision is never made on the basis of a plain x-ray alone.
- Cosmetic defect is not a sufficient indication.
- Angulation of first metatarsophalangeal joint > 20°
- Medial bursitis ("bunion")
- Pain on exercise

Surgical techniques

- More than 130 operation techniques have been described in the literature.
- Most operations are carried out under spinal anaesthesia in day surgery.
- The results of surgery are good or excellent in 80–90% of the patients if the indication is correct.
- In mild or moderate cases the most often used technique is the Chevron operation or distal transposition osteotomy of the first metatarsal bone.
- If the intermetatarsal angle is pathologically wide, proximal osteotomy or cuneiform osteotomy of the first metatarsal bone is necessary.
- If the first metatarsophalangeal joint is stiff, cheilectomy (removal of the dorsal exostosis of the first MT bone) or arthrodesis of the joint is performed.
- The Keller operation is used for elderly patients.

Further treatment

- The patient usually needs 3–6 weeks of sick leave.
- Further treatment depends on the performed operation. In osteotomy the great toe is supported in adduction with bandages or a special hallux support for 4–6 weeks. Exercises of the great toe are begun as soon as the stitches have been removed. On the first weeks the patient should bear weight on the lateral edge of the foot.
- Proper footwear is essential to prevent recurrences; orthopaedic shoes with a longitudinal arch support and sufficient space at the level of the transversal arch.
- If the longitudinal arch is clearly flattened and the patient has associated pain in the distal foot, a so-called metatarsal arch may be necessary.
- A special cushion, which is commercially available, can be kept between the first and second toes or the patient can use a supportive splint that turns the great toe (specialist stores for prosthesis or major shoe stores). When the MTP joint of the great toe is painful but a deformity has not yet developed, the splint should be worn for months at a time. The splint is sufficiently tight when it causes pain as it is put in place. After a bunion has developed a splint is hardly useful.

20.60 Thoracic outlet syndrome

Karl-August Lindgren

Symptoms

- Pain in the fingers, hand, antebrachium, and shoulder in the C7–Th1 dermatomes
- The pain can radiate to the chest.
- Working with the arms elevated to the level of the shoulders or higher provokes symptoms. Nocturnal pains after exertion are common.
- The symptom occurs more frequently in women compared with men. Static work that requires mainly the use of the upper extremities predisposes to symptoms. The syndrome is rare in persons over 50 years of age.

Diagnostic testing

- **Roos' test** (AER test): The upper arms are abducted and rotated outward and kept in this position for 1–3 minutes, at which point the fist is opened and closed. If the symptom is provoked, the test is positive.
- **Adson's test**: The patient turns her head to the side of the pain, inhales deeply, and holds her breath. Palpate for the possible disappearance of the radial pulse.
- With the head in different positions, auscultate the supraclavicular fossa for bruits indicating compression of the brachial artery.
- **Single provocations tests** are often positive also in asymptomatic patients. Therefore, the diagnosis should be based on several factors in the history and clinical status. The function of the entire superior thoracic aperture should be evaluated.
- **CRLF test** (cervical rotation lateral flexion test) is used to evaluate the function of the superior thoracic aperture. A positive test result suggests a function disorder.

Laboratory examinations and differential diagnostics

- Exclude the possibility of Pancoast tumour by thorax x-rays.
- X-rays of the cervical spine for detection of possible spondylosis or cervical rib
- Electroneuromyography is used primarily for excluding carpal tunnel syndrome.
- Imaging by using contrast medium is not a routine examination, unless there is reason to suspect venous thrombosis or serious arterial disease.

Treatment

- Conservative treatment is the primary option: it includes correcting a cyphotic posture, improving mobility of the upper neck and activating the scalenes for better mobility of the superior thoracic aperture. Conservative treatment should be long lasting, and instructions to the patient should be modified according to the achieved response.
- Surgery should be considered only if there are distinct neurological and vascular symptoms and signs (the connective tissue strand is removed, the scalenus anticus muscle is dissected or the first rib is resected).

20.61 Carpal tunnel syndrome (CTS)

Kaj Rekola

Aims

- Symptoms affecting the upper extremities, particularly nocturnal pains and numbness, should be identified as manifestations of carpal tunnel syndrome.
- Surgery (C) [1 2 3] before permanent paraesthesia and muscle dystrophy develop
- Nonspecific treatment (e.g. unnecessary physiotherapy) should be avoided.

Aetiology

- Increased pressure in the carpal tunnel can result from:
  - congenitally narrow tunnel
  - synovitis of the wrist and the tendon sheath (arthritis)
  - position of the wrist (ergonomics)
  - diseases of the nerve (diabetes, peripheral nerve diseases)
  - oedema (pregnancy, myxoedema)

Prevalence

- Two-thirds of affected persons are women 40–60-years of age.
- In 50% of the cases, the condition is bilateral.
- The syndrome is common in wrist fractures and during pregnancy.

Symptoms

- Symptoms of the upper extremity, particularly nocturnal pains and numbness, sense of swelling: shaking hands often gives relief (C) [1 2 3].
- The pain may be diffuse and is felt in the entire upper arms, not just the hand.
- Handling small objects, for example, buttoning may be difficult.
- Thenar muscles may become atrophied.

ORT

- Numbness symptoms
  - Pricking in the median nerve territory (digits I–III), most frequently in the middle finger. Pain in the hand awakens the patient early in the morning.
- The symptoms may continue for years without objective clinical findings.
- Untreated far progressed carpal tunnel syndrome may lead to permanent muscle atrophy and paraesthesia of the median nerve territory.

Diagnosis

- Nocturnal pain and numbness are important diagnostic clues. There may not necessarily be any positive clinical signs.
- **Phalen's test** (positive in 80% of the cases)
  - The wrists are kept in a maximally flexed position for one minute; if numbness or paraesthesias are provoked in the median nerve territory (usually the middle finger), the test is positive; there may be numbness and a sensation of tiredness also in the forearm.
  - An alternative (and complementary) approach is digital pressure for one minute over the carpal tunnel.
  - There is no numbness in an asymptomatic hand.
- **Tinel's sign** (positive in 45–60% of the cases) is obtained by tapping the medial nerve lightly with the fingertips or a reflex hammer, proximally to the carpal tunnel. In a positive test the patient experiences paraesthesias in the median nerve territory.
- Testing for skin sensitivity for touch (positive in approximately 80% of the cases) is the most sensitive test for nerve injury C [4 5].
  - The examiner strokes the patient's fingertips lightly with his/her own fingertips. The patient is asked if there are any differences compared with the ulnar nerve territory (the little finger, and lateral side of IV finger) and the contralateral hand. Two-point discrimination test is more objective.
- Atrophy of thenar muscles and weakness of palmar abduction of the thumb C [4 5] are signs of an advanced condition.

Differential diagnosis

- It is important to include the neck and the entire upper extremity in the examination.
  - Cervical radicular syndrome (C VI–VII) may cause similar symptoms.
  - One or several conditions may be present in addition to the CTS, e.g. a root compression syndrome or the so-called thoracic outlet syndrome (TOS).
  - Nerve compression of the proximal nerve may make the distal nerve more sensitive to pressure injury and vice versa (double crush effect). TOS-type symptoms may resolve after treatment of the carpal tunnel syndrome lesion.
- Differential diagnostics should also include other nerve compression syndromes of the upper extremity, shoulder pains, epicondylitis, vibration syndrome and polyneuropathy that may predispose to carpal tunnel syndrome.
- Occasionally, the median nerve may be entrapped at the cubital level (pronator teres syndrome) or at the forearm (anterior interosseal branch). These cases should be referred to a specialist.

Treatment

- Conservative treatment is possible in most cases.
- The symptoms often resolve if an underlying condition can be corrected, e.g. pregnancy is over or work load is relieved (diuretics, sick leave, ergonomics) C [6 7].
- If tendovaginitis of the finger flexors or carpal synovitis is suspected, a corticosteroid injection B [8] can be tried. The injection site is at the proximal volar transverse crease at the junction of the forearm and the palm, immediately ulnar of the palmaris longus tendon (Note: the tendon may occasionally be absent). The needle is directed at an angle of 45 degrees both distally and radially to a depth of 5–9 mm and 0.5–1 ml of a mixture containing steroid and local anaesthetic (methyl prednisolone and 0.5–1% lidocaine) is injected. Numbness or paraesthesias appearing in the median nerve territory are normal reactions, and will soon resolve. Do not inject against a resistance (a nerve or tendon).
- A functional splint (neutral position) can be used to avoid flexion of the wrist. Wearing a splint 24 hours a day may be more efficient than a splint at nights.

Referrals

Physiatrist, hand surgeon, or orthopaedist

- Clinical diagnostics – differential diagnostics
- Further examinations (ENMG)
  - Electroneuromyography should always be performed prior to deciding on surgery, especially if the clinical diagnosis is uncertain (differentiation from other, more rare, entrapment states).
- Assessment of the need for surgery
- Patients with suspected neuropathy should be referred to a neurologist.

Orthopaedist or hand surgeon

- Consultation necessary when the diagnosis is probable and conservative treatment has not helped.

Surgery

- Surgery is indicated if conservative treatment fails C [1 2 3]. In an ambulatory procedure, the carpal ligament is transected under local anaesthesia and after exsanguination. In advanced cases, recovery of sensory and motor deficits may take a year, or they are irreversible. Sick leave about 4 weeks; however, the scar may be painful for longer.
- The diagnosis should be re-evaluated if surgery does not resolve the symptoms.

References

1. Verdugo RJ, Salinas RS, Castillo J, Cea JG. Surgical versus non-surgical treatment for carpal tunnel syndrome. Cochrane Database Syst Rev. 2004;(2):CD001552.
2. Feuerstein M, Burrell LM, Miller VI, Lincoln A, Huang GD, Berger R. Clinical management of carpal tunnel syndrome: a 12-year review of outcomes. Am J Indust Med 1999;35:232–245.
3. The Database of Abstracts of Reviews of Effectiveness (University of York), Database no.: DARE-990383. In: The Cochrane Library, Issue 2, 2000. Oxford: Update Software.
4. D'Arcy CA, McGee S, Does this patient have carpal tunnel syndrome. JAMA 2000;283:3110–3117.
5. The Database of Abstracts of Reviews of Effectiveness (University of York), Database no.: DARE-20008316. In: The Cochrane Library, Issue 3, 2001. Oxford: Update Software.
6. Lincoln AE, Vernick JS, Ogaitis S, Smith GS, Mitchell CS, Agnew M. Interventions for the primary prevention of work-related carpal tunnel syndrome. Am Prev Med 2000, 18(4 Supplement S), 37–50.
7. The Database of Abstracts of Reviews of Effectiveness (University of York), Database no.: DARE-20001108. In: The Cochrane Library, Issue 3, 2002. Oxford: Update Software.
8. Marshall S, Tardif G, Ashworth N. Local corticosteroid injection for carpal tunnel syndrome. Cochrane Database Syst Rev. 2004;(2):CD001554.

20.62 Ulnar tunnel syndrome

Kaj Rekola

Definition and aetiology

- The (motor) end-branch of the ulnar nerve may be injured by compression in the so-called ulnar tunnel (Guyon's canal) at the site of pisiform bone. This causes pain and paresis of the ulnar-innervated muscles of the hand.
- Common causes are compression by a hand tool or curved bicycle handlebars, direct trauma, ganglion, muscle anomaly, or fracture.

Findings

- Weakness in the following test movements (and possibly muscular atrophy):
  - Scissors movement of the fingers
  - Adduction of the thumb
  - Abduction of the little finger
- Sensation is normal (the cutaneous branch of n. ulnaris deviates before the tunnel; diagnostic of the level of injury!).
- Tenderness and/or pain on compression of the ulnar tunnel.

Differential diagnostics

- More proximal nerve entrapments/lesions
  - Ulnar nerve lesion in the sulcus nervi olecrani or cubital tunnel
  - Thoracic outlet syndrome
  - Lesions of the brachial plexus and the nerve roots

Additional tests

- X-rays of the wrist
- Electroneuromyography

Treatment

- Occupation-related lesions
  - Watchful waiting for recovery after removing causative factors (regression of symptoms and signs, returning muscle strength)
  - Secondary prevention: ergonomics, tool design, cushioning (biker's padded gloves, padded handlebars)
  - Occasionally, trauma-related or occupational synovitis of the joint between triquetral and pisiform bones may cause compression of the ulnar nerve. Steroid can be injected into the joint via a fine needle.
  - Referral to a physiatrist or orthopaedist may be needed if the condition does not improve or further testing is needed.

20.63 Meralgia paraesthetica

Editors

Aetiology

- A fairly rarely occurring entrapment of the lateral femoral cutaneous nerve, located under the inguinal ligament, approximately 2 cm medially of the anterior superior iliac spine.
- May occasionally be caused by a more proximal lesion in the retroperitoneal space (L2 nerve root), due to a haemorrhage in patients on anticoagulants.

Diagnosis

- The patient is often overweight or pregnant.
- Symptoms include numbness, paraesthesias and pain in the anterior and lateral aspects of the thigh, which increases when standing.

- Hyperextension of the thigh with the knee flexed increases the pain.
- Compression of the entrapment site causes radiating pain into the thigh.
- Root compression is ruled out by using the straight leg rising test (Lasegue's test) and testing hip movements to rule out osteoarthritis-induced limitation.
- Electroneurophysiological tests may be used if the diagnosis remains uncertain.

Therapy

- Steroid/local anaesthetic injections into the entrapment site
- Stretching exercises of hip flexors
- Weight loss

20.72 Acupuncture

Seppo Junnila

Motto

- Acupuncture is needling but needling is not necessarily acupuncture.

Prior to treatment

- A correct diagnosis is needed, do not just implement the therapy the patient is asking for.
- Inform the patient about the limitations of acupuncture. It should not be the desperate last straw tried out but rather one of several options of medical therapies that fairly often alleviates symptoms and has negligible side effects.
- Using one needle once is not acupuncture. Three to four weekly sessions will often suffice, or, at least indicate if it is worth continuing.
- Reviewing your knowledge about anatomy to be sure what is beneath the surface improves diagnostics and safeguards against accidentally perforating organs.
- One third of the patients do not benefit from acupuncture; another third clearly get relief for their symptoms; the results achieved in the last third of the patients keep the reputation of acupuncture alive and makes acupuncture meaningful for the physician.
- Even a considerable experience in acupuncture does not help recognizing in advance whether the patients will get the best benefit of acupuncture.
- Do not try to treat hypochondriacs or paranoids, and do not suggest acupuncture to those who are seeking sick benefits instead of relief.
- Age or other ailments rarely are a specific contraindication for acupuncture; the indications should, however, be carefully considered if the patient has a heart valve prosthesis or receives immunosuppressants.
- Always use disposable needles. This is convenient and helps avoiding complications.
- Inform your patient in advance about the fact that the symptoms may worsen after the first three sessions – this helps avoid explanations afterwards.
- At least one patient in ten is tired after the session, some are even disoriented. Inform the patients in advance about this possibility and keep them under observation after the session.
- To avoid collapse the patient should lie down during the session; do not leave him/her alone, at least during the first few sessions – during the session you will have an excellent opportunity for complementary history taking.
- Acupuncture may temporarily enhance the effects of certain drugs. Especially diabetics and patients on antihypertensive medication should be monitored carefully after the therapy session.

Indications

- Acupuncture is especially indicated for treatment of pain; the best results are achieved in alleviation of musculoskeletal pain and dental pain B [1 2 3 4]. Acupuncture is useful in neck pain D [5 6] of muscular origin, soft tissue lesions in the shoulder region, and pain due to strain and sprain of back muscles, after conditions requiring surgical procedures are ruled out to avoid delay in appropriate surgical therapy.
- Pain related to osteoarthritis is also treatable (but evidence of efficacy is lacking D [7 8]): the osteoarthritic changes cannot of course be reversed but contracted muscles due to a changed gait pattern can be relaxed and the pain alleviated. Acupuncture has no effect in the treatment of rheumatoid arthritis C [9].
- Migraine and other recurrent or chronic, correctly diagnosed types of headache can be treated with acupuncture C [10]. There are always some patients for whom this is beneficial.
- Patients with sciatica and other prolonged back pain often get relief from acupuncture; again, keep in mind that some patients may need surgery. Even patients suffering from spinal stenosis may obtain relief while waiting for surgery or when surgery is not appropriate. In low back pain there is no clear evidence that acupuncture would be better than trigger point injection or transcutaneous nerve stimulation (TENS) C [11].
- Acupuncture as a complementary therapy in physiotherapy and rehabilitation is an interesting new approach. Training in acupuncture has been available for e.g. physiotherapists in some countries.
- Patients with symptoms of hemiplegia should be treated without delay; there is convincing evidence of the favourable vascular effects of acupuncture on circulation; in Sweden good, although conflicting results of faster recovery have been received after acupuncture.
- Treatment of neuralgia, neuropathies and phantom limb pain requires a more thorough understanding of the principles

of acupuncture and longer series of therapy sessions but results at times in a long-term and positive patient-physician relationship.

- Acupuncture has been tried as a treatment for tinnitus, but no evidence of its effect has been shown B [12 13]. Chronic eczemas, such as atopic eczemas, asthma and a vast spectrum of psychosomatic disorders may be indications for treatment for the experienced acupuncturist.
- Restless legs usually respond well to acupuncture. As is the case with restless legs, sleep disorders may sometimes, as a positive side effect, respond favourably to the treatment of other disorders.
- The treatment of drug addiction generally requires electroacupuncture; the results are, at least in the short term, surprisingly favourable. The effect of acupuncture on smoking cessation B [14] has not been shown; it can be regarded together with treatment for weight loss D [15 16] as a temporary fad. Acupuncture is used in many alcohol addiction clinics as an adjunct to detoxification. Acupuncture may also be useful in the treatment of postoperative or chemotherapy-related nausea C [17 18].
- The effect of acupuncture on animal reproduction and behavioural disorders has been favourable. Attempts have been made to treat menstrual disorders, unexplained sterility and depression but the results still remain mostly anecdotal.

Implementation

- Acupuncture should not be practised without consulting related textbooks.
- Traditional Chinese medicine is taught globally but for physicians with Western training it may be more convenient to participate in training specially designed for them. It may be advantageous to postpone learning about the oriental philosophy of man, disease, and therapy until one's own understanding of the possibilities of Western medicine has become clear.
- For starters one can learn to palpate the trigger- (tender) points in patients with musculoskeletal pain disorders. Needling of trigger-points alone is often perceived unpleasant; this does not result in as favourable long-term effects as does concomitant or exclusive use of classic acupuncture points.

Complications

- Most complications are caused by physicians who are unfamiliar with the correct techniques C [19 20 21 22]. Insufficient knowledge of anatomy, hurry, and inadequate preparation of the patient may have harmful consequences that could be avoided by using careful acupuncture techniques.
- Perforations of internal organs, such as pneumothorax, and complications from using non-sterile needles, e.g. hepatitis, are mostly caused by lay therapists.
- Haematomas may occur even using the most careful techniques, especially around the corner of the eye. Temporary worsening of pain, somnolence, euphoria etc., may also occur. Leaving a needle accidentally in place in the neck under a long hair is not a serious problem but may be an indication of too much hurry during the therapy session.

References

1. Ernst E, Pittler MH. The effectiveness of acupuncture in treating acute dental pain. A systematic review. British Dental Journal 1998;184:443–447.
2. The Database of Abstracts of Reviews of Effectiveness (University of York), Database no.: DARE-980926. In: The Cochrane Library, Issue 1, 2000. Oxford: Update Software.
3. Rosted P. The use of acupuncture in dentistry: a review of the scientific validity of published papers. Oral Diseases 1998;4:100–104.
4. The Database of Abstracts of Reviews of Effectiveness (University of York), Database no.: DARE-983869. In: The Cochrane Library, Issue 3, 2000. Oxford: Update Software.
5. White AR, Ernst E. A systematic review of randomized controlled trials on acupuncture for neck pain. Rheumatology 1999;83:143–147.
6. The Database of Abstracts of Reviews of Effectiveness (University of York), Database no.: DARE-991060. In: The Cochrane Library, Issue 2, 2001. Oxford: Update Software.
7. Ernst E. Acupuncture as a symptomatic treatment for osteoarthritis: a systematic review. Scand J Rheumatol 1997;26:444–447.
8. The Database of Abstracts of Reviews of Effectiveness (University of York), Database no.: DARE-980042. In: The Cochrane Library, Issue 4, 1999. Oxford: Update Software.
9. Casimiro L, Brosseau L, Milne S, Robinson V, Wells G, Tugwell P. Acupuncture and electroacupuncture for the treatment of RA. Cochrane Database Syst Rev. 2004;(2):CD003788.
10. Melchart D, Linde K, Fischer P, Berman B, White A, Vickers A, Allais G. Acupuncture for idiopathic headache. Cochrane Database Syst Rev. 2004;(2):CD001218.
11. van Tulder MW, Cherkin DC, Berman B, Lao L, Koes BW. Acupuncture for low-back pain. Cochrane Database Syst Rev. 2004;(2):CD001351.
12. Park J, White AR, Ernst E. Efficacy of acupuncture as a treatment for tinnitus: a systematic review. Archives of Otolaryngology Head and Neck Surgery 2000, 126(4), 489–492.
13. The Database of Abstracts of Reviews of Effectiveness (University of York), Database no.: DARE-2000863. In: The Cochrane Library, Issue 2, 2002. Oxford: Update Software.
14. White AR, Rampes H, Ernst E. Acupuncture in the treatment of nicotine addiction. Cochrane Database Syst Rev. 2002;(2):CD000009.
15. Ernst E. Acupuncture/acupressure for weight reduction. Wiener Klinische Wochenschrift 1997;109:60–62.
16. The Database of Abstracts of Reviews of Effectiveness (University of York), Database no.: DARE-978062. In: The Cochrane Library, Issue 4, 1999. Oxford: Update Software.
17. Acupuncture. Effective Health Care 2001; 7: 12.
18. The Database of Abstracts of Reviews of Effectiveness (University of York), Database no.: DARE-20018448. In: The Cochrane Library, Issue 2, 2002. Oxford: Update Software.
19. Ernst E, White A. Life-threatening adverse reactions after acupuncture? A systematic review. Pain 1997;71:123–126.

ORT

20. The Database of Abstracts of Reviews of Effectiveness (University of York), Database no.: DARE-979810. In: The Cochrane Library, Issue 4, 1999. Oxford: Update Software.
21. Norheim AJ. Adverse effects of acupuncture: a study of the literature for the years 1981–1994. Journal of Alternative and Complementary Medicine 1996;2:291–297.
22. The Database of Abstracts of Reviews of Effectiveness (University of York), Database no.: DARE-983104. In: The Cochrane Library, Issue 3, 2000. Oxford: Update Software.

20.75 Treatment of osteoarthritis

Hannu Väänänen

Basic rules

- The patient should be given instructions for self-management already in the early stages of the disease: the joint cartilage needs loading to function well.
- Paracetamol is the drug of choice for pain. Anti-inflammatory analgesics (NSAID) should be used sparingly and in courses to avoid their side effects. Topically applied preparations and glucosamine are useful options.
- If osteotomy is considered, it should be performed as soon as stress-induced pains appear constantly.
- A joint replacement implant should be considered before a loss of function or if intolerable pain cannot be controlled by other means (A) [1 2].
- Arthroscopic debridement or lavage in patients with osteoarthritis of the knee is not recommended as it does not improve function or reduce pain.

Aetiology

- Primary osteoarthritis develops in an anatomically perfectly normal joint. Its aetiology remains unknown, however, genetic factors play a role.
- The underlying factors in secondary osteoarthritis are diseases, traumas or disturbances in the development of the joint. In hip osteoarthritis clearly more than half of the cases are primary, whereas in knee osteoarthritis secondary cases dominate.
- Osteoarthritis of the ankle is always secondary and much more rare than either hip or knee arthrosis.
- The prevalence of osteoarthritis of the hip in persons aged 75 years or more has been estimated to be 20%. Knee arthrosis is 2–3 times more common in women, but in hip arthrosis there is no difference between the genders.
- Known risk factors of knee arthrosis are overweight, hard physical work and repeated heavy loading. In hip arthrosis the role of these factors is not as obvious.
- Traumas can cause arthrotic changes in any joint.

Symptoms of osteoarthrosis

- Initially pain during stress that increasingly limits the ability to move. Later pain at rest begins to disturb sleep.
- The range of motion of the joint gradually becomes restricted; in the hip the internal rotation and abduction are affected first, in the knee the extension.
- As the arthritis of the knee progresses, varus-valgus axis misalignment increases and aggravates the condition.

Principles of management

- In the early stages of the disease management consists of pharmaco- and physiotherapy.
- Surgical management is indicated early on if it helps to prevent the development of arthrosis. Mainly these procedures are used for treating later stages of the disease.

Pharmacotherapy

Analgesics

- Paracetamol is recommended for less severe pain (A) [3 4] because of few side effects. In the treatment of knee arthrosis its effect is comparable to that of naproxen and ibuprofen. Maximum dose is 3 g/day.
- If additional pain relief is needed, an NSAID can be combined with paracetamol. Slow-release preparations of these drugs should be used in courses of 7 to 21 days at a time. For hip (C) [5] and knee (C) [6] osteoarthritis different NSAIDs are probably equally effective (C) [5], and the choice of the drug should be based on tolerability and safety.
- To prevent renal side effects in long-term therapy, excessive dosage should be avoided and NSAIDs with a long half-life should be prescribed cautiously, although convincing evidence of harmful effects is not yet available.
- Topical NSAIDs administered as creams are more effective than placebo and have fever adverse effects than oral preparations (A) [7 8].
- Use of selective COX-2 inhibitors can be justifiably considered when the use of a non-selective NSAID involves an increased risk of gastrointestinal bleeding (8.33). Another option is to combine misoprostol with an NSAID.
- In severe arthrosis pain a centrally acting analgesic, such as tramadol, is sometimes needed.
- For side effects of anti-inflammatory analgesics, see 8.33.

Corticosteroids

- Intra-articular, long-acting glucocorticoid occasionally gives relief, particularly when symptoms of inflammation or intra-articular crystal deposition are present (21.10).
- In knee arthrosis the best response is obtained with short-term use.
- Short-term immobilization after a corticosteroid injection enhances the effect.

Hyaluronate

- The alleviating effect of hyaluronate in joint pain is apparently based on its anti-inflammatory and analgetic properties, but also on its direct effect on the cells of the joint capsule and cartilage.
- The primary target joint is the knee **A** [3 4], but hyaluronate is also used for arthrosis in other joints.
- It has been found the reduce the pain of knee arthrosis patients aged over 60 suffering from severe symptoms and to prolong their walking distance.

Glucosamine sulphate

- Peroral or intramuscular glucosamine is often effective and has few side effects **A** [9 10 11 12 13].

Physiotherapy

Physical activity

- The joint cartilage needs sufficient loading to function well.
- Long-term immobilization of the joint should be avoided as it causes deterioration of the cartilage and consequent new damage.
- Swimming and water gymnastics are suitable sports for maintaining overall fitness and joint function. Training in water is often possible even for patients with severe arthrosis.
- Out-of-pool training should be started with isometric exercises if pain is severe.

Overweight

- Weight loss is especially beneficial for patients with knee arthrosis, but is helpful also in other lower limb arthroses.
- Vicious circle of pain that prevents physical activity and results in weight gain should be avoided.
- Overweight complicates aftercare of knee and hip joint replacement surgery.

Orthotic devices

- Walking stick on the healthy side reduces the load of the joint by up to one third.
- Faulty positions of the knee or ankle and resulting loading problems can be managed with inserts worn in shoes.
- Acquisition of an orthotic device requires help from a podiatrist.
- Devices that lessen the impact on the heel (suitable footwear, shock-absorbing soles) are often a good addition to conservative therapy.

Environmental factors

- Environmental factors that affect the loading of the joints should be recognized: working conditions should be modified so that prolonged sitting or standing can be avoided.
- Multi-professional teamwork is often necessary (physiotherapists, occupational therapists).
- If working ability is threatened, a working age patient may need occupational rehabilitation. If necessary, refer the patient for evaluation.

Acupuncture

- There is no evidence for the effect of acupunture on osterarthrosis **D** [14 15].

Osteoarthritis of the hip

- Patient education **C** [16 17] should be started immediately after diagnosis.
- Instructions on physical activity are important for both treatment and prevention.
- The patient must be encouraged to maintain physical activity. Swimming, cycling and walking on soft terrain are good sports.
- Physiotherapy, articulation or traction may be effective in mild hip arthrosis
  - Abduction exercises are best performed when lying on the back, extension training when lying on the side.
  - If active stretching is not sufficient, contractures are treated with passive stretching of the flexor and adductor muscles with a pre-treatment regimen (warming with ultrasound and massage).
  - Technical devices may be necessary if the restriction of hip movement is considerable.
  - Stocking puller, raised toilet seat and bed legs, long picking forceps

ORT

Osteoarthritis of the knee

- Active self-management is efficient **B** [18 19 20 21]. Swimming, cross-country skiing or cycling are good sports.
- The aim of physiotherapy is to restore full range of movement. The following methods can be used
  - Thermal therapy (superficial thermal treatments, cold **C** [22]; ultrasound probably not effective **C** [23]) or transcutaneous electrical nerve stimulation **C** [24 25] for alleviating pain during treatment **C** [26].
- Active self-training of the knee is important **B** [27 28]. When the pain is severe, isometric training may be most suitable with resistance increased gradually.
- Physiotherapy is beneficial in the early stages of independent training for learning the right exercises **B** [18 19 20 21].
- Suitable devices and knee supports may help pain during physical activity.

Osteoarthritis of the ankle

- Primary osteoarthritis of the ankle is rare. Usually the condition is post-traumatic.
- Reduction of stress and shoe inserts that correct the alignment may be helpful.

- The range of movement may be restored with physiotherapy where gentle manual traction may be helpful.
- The patient should be taught exercises that improve the stability and coordination of the ankle.

Osteoarthritis of finger joints

- Warm water and paraffin baths are recommended.
- Strength training of finger muscles using a soft ball or silicone wax
- Resting splints in phases of pain exacerbation and especially in osteoarthritis of the metacarpophalangeal joint of the thumb
- Devices relieving stress on finger joints
- Fusion of distal interphalangeal joints or proximal interphalangeal joints of the index and little fingers may be indicated.

Surgical management

- Surgical management can be divided into three main types:
  - Osteotomy, which aims at correcting the mechanical properties of the joint
  - Joint immobilization, i.e. arthrodesis
  - Joint replacement where the joint is either fully or partially replaced with an artificial structure.
- In addition to correcting the mechanics of the joint, osteotomy often also prevents further arthrosis. Therefore the procedure should be carried out as soon as regular stress-induced pain has appeared.
- Arthrodesis and arthroplasty is not as urgent. However, one should resort to these procedures when the pain is no longer managed and the quality of life, ability to move and independent living cannot be maintained with conservative therapy.
- Joint prosthesis often improves considerably the patient's quality of life (A) [1 2].

References

1. Towheed TE, Hochberg MC. Health-related quality of life after total hip replacement. Arthritis Rheum 1996;26:483–491.
2. The Database of Abstracts of Reviews of Effectiveness (University of York), Database no.: DARE-961442. In: The Cochrane Library, Issue 4, 1999. Oxford: Update Software.
3. Towheed TE, Hochberg MC. A systematic review of randomised controlled trials of pharmacological therapy in osteoarthritis of the knee, with an emphasis on trial methodology. Semin Arthritis Rheum 1997;26:755–770.
4. The Database of Abstracts of Reviews of Effectiveness (University of York), Database no.: DARE-970656. In: The Cochrane Library, Issue 4, 1999. Oxford: Update Software.
5. Towheed T, Shea B, Wells G, Hochberg M. Analgesia and non-aspirin, non-steroidal anti-inflammatory drugs for osteoarthritis of the hip. Cochrane Database Syst Rev. 2004;(2):CD000517.
6. Watson MC, Brookes ST, Kirwan JR, Faulkner A. Non-aspirin, non-steroidal anti-inflammatory drugs for treating osteoarthritis of the knee. Cochrane Database Syst Rev. 2004;(2):CD000142.
7. Moore RA, Tramer MR, Carroll D, Wiffen PJ, McQuay HJ. Quantitative systematic review of topically applied non-steroidal anti-inflammatory drugs. BMJ 1998;316:333–338.
8. The Database of Abstracts of Reviews of Effectiveness (University of York), Database no.: DARE-988245. In: The Cochrane Library, Issue 4, 1999. Oxford: Update Software.
9. Towheed TE, Anastassiades TP, Shea B, Houpt J, Welch V, Hochberg MC. Glucosamine therapy for treating osteoarthritis. Cochrane Database Syst Rev. 2004;(2):CD002946.
10. Anonymous. Glucosamine and arthritis. Bandolier 1997;4:1–3.
11. The Database of Abstracts of Reviews of Effectiveness (University of York), Database no.: DARE-988123. In: The Cochrane Library, Issue 4, 1999. Oxford: Update Software.
12. Barclay TS, Tsourounis C, McCart GM. Glycosamine. Ann Pharmacother 1998;32:574–579.
13. The Database of Abstracts of Reviews of Effectiveness (University of York), Database no.: DARE-980948. In: The Cochrane Library, Issue 2, 2000. Oxford: Update Software.
14. Ernst E. Acupuncture as a symptomatic treatment for osteoarthritis: a systematic review. Scand J Rheumatol 1997;26:444–447.
15. The Database of Abstracts of Reviews of Effectiveness (University of York), Database no.: DARE-980042. In: The Cochrane Library, Issue 4, 1999. Oxford: Update Software.
16. Superio-Cabuslay E, Ward MMM, Lorig KR. Patient education interventions in osteoarthritis and rheumatoid arthritis: a meta-analytic comparison with nonsteroidal anti-inflammatory drug treatment. Arthritis Care & Research 1996;9:292–301.
17. The Database of Abstracts of Reviews of Effectiveness (University of York), Database no.: DARE-965403. In: The Cochrane Library, Issue 4, 1999. Oxford: Update Software.
18. Puett DW, Griffin MR. Published trials of nonmedicinal and noninvasive therapies for hip and knee osteoarthritis. Ann Intern Med 1994;121:133–140.
19. The Database of Abstracts of Reviews of Effectiveness (University of York), Database no.: DARE-948036. In: The Cochrane Library, Issue 4, 1999. Oxford: Update Software.
20. Van Baar ME, Assendelft WJJ, Dekker J, Oostendorp RAB, Bijlsma JW. Effectiveness of exercise therapy in patients with osteoarthritis of the hip or knee: a systematic review of randomized clinical trials. Arthritis and Rheumatism 1999;42:1361–1369.
21. The Database of Abstracts of Reviews of Effectiveness (University of York), Database no.: DARE-991430. In: The Cochrane Library, Issue 1, 2001. Oxford: Update Software.
22. Brosseau L, Yonge KA, Robinson V, Marchand S, Judd M, Wells G, Tugwell P. Thermotherapy for treatment of osteoarthritis. Cochrane Database Syst Rev 2003(4):CD004522.
23. Welch V, Brosseau L, Peterson J, Shea B, Tugwell P, Wells G. Therapeutic ultrasound for osteoarthritis of the knee. Cochrane Database Syst Rev. 2004;(2):CD003132.
24. Marks R, Ungar M, Ghasemmi M. Electrical muscle stimulation for osteoarthritis of the knee: biological basis and systematic review. New Zealand Journal of Physiotherapy 2000, 28(3), 6–20.
25. The Database of Abstracts of Reviews of Effectiveness (University of York), Database no.: DARE-20018129. In: The Cochrane Library, Issue 3, 2002. Oxford: Update Software.
26. Osiri M, Welch V, Brosseau L, Shea B, McGowan J, Tugwell P, Wells G. Transcutaneous electrical nerve stimulation for

knee osteoarthritis. Cochrane Database Syst Rev. 2004;(2): CD002823.
27. Petrella RJ. Is exercise effective treatment for osteoarthritis of the knee? British Journal of Sports Medicine 2000, 34(5), 326–331.
28. The Database of Abstracts of Reviews of Effectiveness (University of York), Database no.: DARE-20002058. In: The Cochrane Library, Issue 2, 2002. Oxford: Update Software.

20.76 Early recognition of complications after joint replacement

Editors

Recognition of an early infection

- Postoperative fever lasting more than one week should raise suspicion of a deep infection and the unit that performed the operation should be contacted.
- If infection is suspected, an attempt to aspirate fluid from the suspected area adjacent to the implant should be done using an absolutely sterile technique (keeping an alcohol-soaked compress on the puncture site for 5 minutes) to obtain a bacteriological specimen. If necessary, a surgical exploration should be made.
- If antibiotic medication is not started within two weeks of the implantation it is likely that the infection cannot be controlled without additional surgery.
- Patients with rheumatoid arthritis (RA) are at risk: infections occur 3–5 times more often than in patients with osteoarthritis.

Treatment and need of specialized care

- If the wound is infected but the patient does not have fever and CRP is not substantially elevated (max 40), a peroral antistaphylococcal antibiotic is started after taking the aspiration specimen. The wound should be cleaned by bathing (deep infection is not likely).
- Fever, a clearly elevated CRP or bacterial growth in the aspirated specimen is an indication for referral to specialized care.

Prevention of secondary infection of the implant

- RA patients and those receiving immunosuppressants (e.g. cancer patients) should be given antibiotic prophylaxis prior to a procedure that may cause bacteraemia.
- Purulent paronychia in RA patients should be treated with bathing in mild cases; in more severe cases peroral antibiotics are recommended.

Loosening of the implant

- An implant is considered loose when x-ray findings are associated with pain on loading.
- Patient-related causes of loosening
    - Overweight
    - Too much activity
- Infection is the cause of implant loosening in 10% of the cases and usually occurs within the first 3 years.
- Especially younger patients (<65 years) should be followedup radiologically (e.g. at one, four and eight years from the implantation); in case of loosening, even if associated with minimal symptoms, a revision should be made.
- In the elderly (>65 years), a revision is not necessarily made if the symptoms caused by the loosening are mild. However, the revision arthroplasty is easier to perform if the loosening has not caused damage to bony structures; therefore radiological follow-up may be indicated also in elderly patients.

Radiological findings associated with implant loosening

- Imaging should always be done in two projections; anteroposteriorly and sideways (not Lauenstein's projection). In the side projection the anteversion inclination will change and the other sides of the hip implant will be visible.
- Indications of loosening are:
    - A 2 mm or wider clear space between the cement and bone or between the implant and the cement
    - The whole cup/cement assembly has migrated compared with previous x-ray (the cup is likely to be loose)
    - Granulomatotic cavities indicating a foreign body reaction around the cement
    - Fracture of the cement is an indication of loosening of the stem.
    - A pronounced periostal reaction and thickening of the cortex on the lateral side of the diaphysis (the stem is compressing the cortex)
    - The entire stem/cement assembly has sunk lower in the bone marrow cavity.

Impression of the acetabular cup

- A complication of a haemiprosthesis
- Treated only if symptomatic
- Does not always require surgery because progression is variable and jamming of the trochanter against the rim of the acetabular cup may halt progression of the impression.

20.80 Restless legs, akathisia and muscle cramps

Hannu Lauerma

Definition

- Restless legs syndrome is a condition in which the patient experiences nocturnal, unpleasant sensations in the lower extremities alleviated by moving the legs. The condition may result in serious insomnia.
- Drugs that block the action of dopamine may cause akathisia (36.6).
- Muscle cramps are prolonged painful muscle contractions mainly in the lower extremities.

Predisposing factors

- Pregnancy, aging, scarcity of storage iron, uraemia, and family history of idiopathic symptoms may be the underlying causes of restless legs syndrome.
- Akathisia usually begins immediately after or within a few weeks of starting a predisposing medication.
- Electrolyte disorders (particularly hyponatraemia), dehydration, diuretics, leg oedema and denervation predispose to muscle cramps. Most patients suffering from muscle cramps do not have any known predisposing factor.

Tests

- Clinical examination of the lower extremities (oedema, varicose veins, eczema due to varicosis, patency of arteries, sense of touch).
- If restless legs syndrome is suspected, serum ferritin should be checked. If the concentration is in the lowest third of the reference range that is considered normal in investigation for anaemia, iron supplementation may be beneficial. If necessary, serum creatinine should be checked.
- In muscle cramps check serum sodium, potassium, blood glucose, haemoglobin, haematocrit, total red cell count, and differential count.

Treatment

- Instructions for improving sleep hygiene and iron supplementation are not always enough to calm restless legs. In mild cases a hypnotic or a low dose of benzodiazepine may be beneficial. Potent, short-acting benzodiazepines should be avoided. The best effect has been obtained with small evening doses of dopaminergic drugs (pramipexole 0.09–0.36 mg, ropinirole 0.25–1.5 mg or amantadine 100–300 mg) C [1 2 3 4 5]. The side effects of long-term therapy are not known. In severe cases opioids such as tramadol 50–100 mg in the evening have been used. Gabapentin may be useful in painful cases.
- If akathisia is suspected the dose is reduced or the drug is changed. If necessary a short course of propranolol 20 mg × 3, biperidine 1–2 mg × 3 or small doses of benzodiazepine may be used.
- Passive stretching of the cramped muscle can be used as a first-aid measure. For prophylaxis all triggering factors should be eliminated. In severe cases combinations including quinine sulphate B [6 7 8 9] and diazepam or meprobamate can be considered; the patients must be followed up during the first weeks of therapy to evaluate the efficacy and adverse effects.

References

1. Wetter TC, Stiasny K, Winkelmann J et al. A randomized controlled trial of pergolide in patients with restless legs syndrome. Neurology 1999;52:944–50.
2. Earley CJ, Yaffee JB, Allen RP. Randomized, double-blind, placebo controlled trial of pergolide in restless legs syndrome. Neurology 1998; 51:1599–602.
3. Montplaisir J, Nicolas A, Denesle R, Gomez-Mancilla B. Restless legs syndrome improved by pramipexole: a double-blind randomized trial. Neurology 1999;52:938–43.
4. Montplaisir J, Denesle R, Petit D. Pramipexole in the treatment of restless legs syndrome: a follow-up study. Eur J Neurol 2000;7 Suppl 1:27–31.
5. Evidente VG, Adler CH, Caviness JN et al. Amantadine is beneficial in restless legs syndrome. Mov Disord 2000; 15:324–7.
6. Man-Son-Hing M, Wells G. Meta-analysis of efficacy of quinine for treatment of nocturnal leg cramps in elderly people. Br Med J 1995;310:13–7.
7. The Database of Abstracts of Reviews of Effectiveness (University of York), Database no.: DARE-950302. In: The Cochrane Library, Issue 4, 1999. Oxford: Update Software.
8. Man-Son-Hing M, Wells G, Lau A. Quinine for nocturnal leg cramps: a meta-analysis including unpublished data. J Gen Intern Med 1998;13:600–606.
9. The Database of Abstracts of Reviews of Effectiveness (University of York), Database no.: DARE-981581. In: The Cochrane Library, Issue 2, 2000. Oxford: Update Software.

20.81 Muscle compartment syndromes

Editors

Aims

- Compartment syndrome should be suspected in leg injuries when the patient experiences atypical pain aggravated by extension of the distal joint.

Definition

- Ischaemic muscle pain caused by unproportionally large muscle volume constrained by a nonexpanding fascial compartment

Medial tibial syndrome (shin splint)

- Pain is felt medially in the leg at the medial edge of the tibia.
- Clinical signs include local tenderness and often a dense area at the medial edge of the tibia resembling a periosteal lump associated with tibial stress fractures.

Anterior tibial syndrome

- An acute tibial syndrome may be caused by extreme stress, crush injury or tibial fracture. Symptoms include:
  - Severe increasing pain anteriorly in the leg
  - Decreased strength of ankle and toe extensors
  - Numbness
  - Arterial pulses are usually not affected
- Chronic anterior tibial syndrome
  - Pain anteriorly and laterally in the leg
  - Diffuse tenderness at palpation of the anterior tibial compartment over a larger area than in the case of stress fracture

Treatment

- Acute anterior tibial syndrome should initially be treated with rest, cold packs, and furosemide 40 mg intravenously (or orally). The patient should be referred immediately to a hospital for possible emergency fasciotomy to prevent muscle necrosis.
- Chronic symptoms require rest, limited weight bearing, and NSAIDs. If the condition lasts several months, an extended fasciotomy should be considered.
- Possible foot misalignment should be corrected with orthotics. The patient should be advised to stretch the muscles.

20.90 Bone tumours

Olli Korkala

Diagnosis of primary bone tumours

- Radical surgery in the extremities often requires amputation. Nowadays sparing surgery with large endoprosthesis or allograftic bone is being used more frequently.
- The diagnosis of primary bone tumours is based on clinical suspicion and x-rays.
  - The abnormalities may be difficult to detect in x-rays, particularly in cases where the tumour is situated deep under soft tissues in the pelvis or spine.
- Bone scintigraphy is an important secondary examination.
- If malignancy cannot be ruled out, a bone biopsy should be taken in a specialized unit.
- Magnetic resonance imaging is valuable in the assessment of tumour invasion of the bone and soft tissues.

Osteosarcoma

- The most common primary malignant bone tumour occurs in children, adolescents, and young adults.
- The knee area is the site of predilection.
- X-ray findings are typical.
- Prognosis is improved by early diagnosis.
- The treatment consists of a combination of surgery and chemotherapy, and should be performed at specialized centres.

Benign bone tumours

- Exostosis (osteochondroma) and enchondroma (of the fingers) are the most common benign bone tumours.
- The diagnosis is usually evident on the basis of the native x-ray.
- Surgical treatment is often indicated.

Skeletal metastases

- The most common cancers seeding skeletal metastases are (oestrogen-receptor positive) breast cancer, lung cancer (particularly small cell lung cancer), prostatic, thyroid, and renal cancers.

Signs of good prognosis

- A highly specialized, slowly growing tumour
- A long period without metastases after primary treatment
- Sclerotic metastases initially
- Lytic metastases that become sclerotic during treatment
- A solitary bone metastasis
- Small total tumour load
- No metastases in vital organs
- Absence of hypercalcaemia
- Absence of leucoerythroblastoid anaemia

Sclerotic metastases

- Irradiation is effective in 80–90% of the patients.
- There is no risk of pathological fractures.

Lytic metastases

- There is a high risk of pathological fractures; particularly metastases in the femoral neck and diaphysis must be irradiated as soon as possible.

- Surgical stabilization should be considered even before a fracture has occurred!
- Metastases in the cervical spine are an indication for Schanz's collar before treatment is started; patients with metastases in the thoracal or lumbar spine should stay in bed at the initial stage. If threatening dislocations or neurological deficiencies develop surgery must be considered.

Treatment of pain

- Bisphosphonates are effective for skeletal pain and they also reduce skeletal events A [1 2 3].

Assessment of treatment outcome

- Relief of pain
- Recalcification of the metastases
- For the treatment of hypercalcaemia see article 24.21

References

1. Wong R, Wiffen PJ. Bisphosphonates for the relief of pain secondary to bone metastases. Cochrane Database Syst Rev. 2004;(2):CD002068.
2. Bloomfield DJ. Should bisphosphonate be part of the standard therapy of patients with multiple myeloma or bone metastases from other cancers: an evidence-based review. J Clin Oncol 1998;16:1218–1225.
3. The Database of Abstracts of Reviews of Effectiveness (University of York), Database no.: DARE-980479. In: The Cochrane Library, Issue 1, 2000. Oxford: Update Software.

20.91 Sarcomas

Risto Johansson

Basic rules

- In the early stages sarcomas cause very few symptoms. Bone sarcomas cause pain or locally increased skin temperature only at a late stage and when they are fairly large. Soft-tissue sarcomas are usually painless even in the late stage.
- Sarcomas spread mainly via the bloodstream, rarely to local lymph nodes. Sarcomas send metastases most typically to the lungs.
- Basic management consists of an appropriate combination of surgery, radiotherapy and chemotherapy.
- The treatment of both types of sarcomas should be given by highly specialized centres, starting with the diagnosis and biopsy taking. The histopathological diagnostics require special staining methods. Differentiating between benign and malignant sarcoma can be difficult.
- Metastases sent by soft-tissue sarcomas, e.g. solitary or few lung metastases should be removed by surgery.
- Of sarcoma patients who have received appropriate therapy, 50–80% are free of symptoms after 5 years.
- Amputation is rarely necessary. Experienced surgeons can perform radical surgery and yet spare the function of the limb by using prostheses or transplants.

Bone sarcomas

- E.g. osteosarcoma, chondrosarcoma, Ewing's sarcoma and malignant fibrous histiocytoma
- Pain, swelling, sometimes warmth or dysfunction of the adjacent joint arouse suspicion of bone sarcoma.
- In differential diagnosis most bone tumours are metastases sent by cancers elsewhere, myelomas or benign neoplasms.
- The diagnostics and treatment of all bone tumours belong to specialized hospitals with specific bone tumour teams.
- The outcome is good if appropriate treatment is administered from the very start.

Soft-tissue sarcomas

- E.g. fibrosarcoma, rhabdomyosarcoma, liposarcoma, leiomyosarcoma, synovial sarcoma, neurofibrosarcoma, malignant fibrous histiocytoma
- Soft-tissue sarcomas constitute about 1% of all malignancies.
- Half the tumours are in the limbs and half in the trunk, head or neck.
- A soft-tissue sarcoma is generally an asymptomatic lump that grows relatively slowly. Sarcoma should be suspected especially if the lump is under healthy skin, attached to the underlying tissue, hard and over 5 cm in diameter.
- If soft-tissue sarcoma is suspected, the patient should be referred without delay to a central hospital for surgical evaluation. University and specialized hospitals have multispeciality sarcoma teams who deal with urgent referrals.

Treatment

- Soft-tissue sarcomas are removed surgically with a wide margin (4–6 cm). In sarcomas of the limbs, it is preferable to remove the entire fascial compartment. Adjuvant radiotherapy is given after nonradical surgery or if surgery is not possible because of the location of the sarcoma.
- Chemotherapy is used in metastasized cases or to reduce the size of the tumour before surgery. Chemotherapy is an integral part of therapy in childhood sarcomas. Doxorubicin-based chemotherapy improves time to recurrence and recurrence-free survival in adult patients with soft tissue sarcoma A [1 2 3].
- The treatment of bone sarcomas depends on their histological structure. In low-grade malignant bone sarcomas radical surgery is usually sufficient. Surgery is the best alternative also in malignant fibrous histiocytoma and in chondrosarcomas. In high-grade malignant (Grade III–IV) osteo- and Ewing sarcomas treatment is started with aggressive chemotherapy. A few weeks later either radical surgery is performed or the patient receives radiotherapy, and

chemotherapy is continued with the same or a new drug combination for 6–9 months.

Follow-up

- Rehabilitation, prostheses and assistive devices are an essential part of further treatment. Many patients live long and recover well.
- Sarcomas are monitored at a cancer outpatient clinic at 3–6-month intervals for 5 years, then at 12-month intervals for up to 10 years. In follow-up the patient is examined for local recurrences and lung metastases as their early management often results in good long-term outcome.
- Treatment of bone sarcomas should be centralized to hospitals with special teams for managing bone tumours. The follow-up consists of thorough history, regular chest x-ray, bone scintigraphy, CT and, when necessary, MRI and biopsy.

References

1. Sarcoma Meta-analysis Collaboration (SMAC)* (see Acknowledgements Section for list of authors in SMAC). Adjuvant chemotherapy for localised resectable soft tissue sarcoma in adults. Cochrane Database Syst Rev. 2004;(2):CD001419.
2. Tieney JF, Mosseri V, Steward LA, Souhami RL, Parmar MK. Adjuvant chemotherapy for soft-tissue sarcoma: review and meta-analysis of the published results of randomised clinical trials. Br J Cancer Care 1995;72:467–475.
3. The Database of Abstracts of Reviews of Effectiveness (University of York), Database no.: DARE-968041. In: The Cochrane Library, Issue 4, 1999. Oxford: Update Software.

20.92 Fibromyalgia

Pekka Hannonen

Aims

- The diagnosis of fibromyalgia should be established to differentiate it from other disorders that can be treated more specifically, e.g. inflammatory rheumatic disorders, hypothyroidism, and menopausal symptoms.
- Factors that aggravate the symptoms should be explored.
- All patients should have an individually tailored treatment plan.
- Physical activity should be encouraged as it has been shown to reduce symptoms (A) [1].

American College of Rheumatology criteria for fibromyalgia

- A history of widespread pain
  - Pain in both sides of the trunk
  - Above and below the waist
- Pain on digital palpation in at least 11 of the following 18 tender points (each side is counted separately):
  - suboccipital muscle insertions
  - anterior aspects of the intertransverse spaces between C5 and C7
  - origins of supraspinatus muscle above the scapular spine
  - midpoint of upper border of m. trapezius
  - second costochondral junction
  - 2 cm distal to the lateral epicondyle
  - upper outer quadrants of the buttocks in the anterior fold of the muscle
  - posterior to the greater trochanter prominence
  - medial fat pad of the knee proximal to the joint line.

Additional symptoms and typical features

- Fatigue throughout the day
- Unrefreshing sleep (sleep arousals)
- Psychosomatic symptoms involving various organs (irritable bowel syndrome, frequent voiding, cardiac symptoms, gynaecological problems)
- Neurological symptoms (numbness, pricking, sense of tightness, headache)
- Mental disturbances (depression, anxiety; severe depression is rare)
- Cognitive problems (inability to concentrate, difficulty in learning new things)
- Subjective sensation of oedema
- 30–50% of the patients have joint hypermotility
- Tendency to blush (erythema fugax) that is limited to the upper body and, on the other hand, cold extremities are over-represented in these patients.
- Symptoms may fluctuate with changes in the weather and with the level of anxiety and stress.
- Fibromyalgia is not a separate disease entity but rather a combination of symptoms and findings that may develop by various mechanisms.

Treatment

- A continuous physician-patient relationship should be established.
- Exercising reduces symptoms (B) [2 3]. Aerobic capacity should be improved by physical exercise (walking, biking, cross-country skiing, or swimming) (B) [2 3] unless problems in the neck and shoulder region prevent training. A personal training programme should be established (C) [4].
- Sleep should be improved by eliminating disturbing factors (coffee, alcoholic beverages, noise, and stress).
- Small dose of amitriptyline from 10 to 25 (50) mg taken early at night has been shown to be effective in several randomized studies. The effect usually appears after one to two weeks (B) [5 6].

ORT

- Anti-inflammatory drugs (NSAID), analgesics, muscle relaxants and "modern" antidepressive drugs are not effective. Randomized studies regarding the effectiveness of paracetamol have not been conducted.
- A combination of paracetamol, carisoprodol, and caffeine was shown in a randomized study to be more effective than placebo C [7].
- In the most problematic cases best results are achieved using a comprehensive multidisciplinary rehabilitation programme D [8 9].

References

1. Busch A, Schachter CL, Peloso PM, Bombardier C. Exercise for treating fibromyalgia syndrome. Cochrane Database Syst Rev. 2004;(2):CD003786.
2. McCain GA, Bell DA, Mai FM, Halliday PD. A controlled study of the effects of a supervised cardiovascular fitness training program on the manifestations of primary fibromyalgia. Arthritis Rheum 1988;31:1135–1141.
3. Häkkinen A, Häkkinen K, Hannonen P, Alen M. Strength training induced adaptations in neuromuscular function of premenopausal women with fibromyalgia: comparison with healthy women. Ann Rheum Dis 2001; 60 (1):21–26.
4. Burckhardt CS, Mannerkorpi K, Hedenberg L, Bjelle A. A randomized controlled trial of education and physical training for women with fibromyalgia. J Rheumatol 1994;21: 714–720.
5. O'Malley PG, Balden E, Tomkins G, Santoro J, Kroenke K, Jackson JL. Treatment of fibromyalgia with antidepressants: a meta-analysis. Journal of General Internal Medicine 2000, 15(9), 659–666.
6. The Database of Abstracts of Reviews of Effectiveness (University of York), Database no.: DARE-20002036. In: The Cochrane Library, Issue 2, 2002. Oxford: Update Software.
7. Vaeroy H, Abrahamsen A, Foerre O, Kåss E. Treatment of fibromyalgia (fibrositis syndrome). A parallel double blind trial with carisoprodol, paracetamol and caffeine (Somadril comp) versus placebo. Clin Rheumatol 1989;8:245–250.
8. Karjalainen K, Malmivaara A, van Tulder M, Roine R, Jauhiainen M, Hurri H, Koes B. Multidisciplinary rehabilitation for fibromyalgia and musculoskeletal pain in working age adults. Cochrane Database Syst Rev. 2004;(2):CD001984.
9. Burckhardt CS, Mannerkorpi K, Hedenberg L, Bjelle A. A randomized controlled trial of education and physical training for women with fibromyalgia. J Rheumatol 1994;21: 714–20.

20.93 Tietze's syndrome

Editors

- **Symptoms**: Pain and occasionally swelling at one or several costochondral junctions. A typical location is the second costochondral junction at the sternal angle.
- Deep inhalation, coughing, bending or twisting the body aggravates pain.
- The costochondral junction is remarkably painful on palpation.
- **Differential diagnosis**: Ankylosing spondylitis or other spondylarthritic disorder causing inflammation in the sternoclavicular joint. In this case symptoms occur also elsewhere.
- **Treatment**: Steroid/local anaesthetic injections into the site of pain and physiotherapy to increase the motility of the ribs. The disorder is usually self-limiting.

20.94 Treatment of an amputated inferior limb

Editors

Postoperative days 1–3

- A pillow should not be placed under the residual limb (risk of contracture).
- The upper part of the body should not be elevated (risk of oedema in the residual limb).
- The patient should not sit for long periods.
- Lying prone is recommended.
- The scar should be protected from traumas during the healing process: even a small haematoma delays cure.

Day 4 to prosthetic fitting

- Exercise: initially extension and adduction exercises; five sets of exercises 3 to 5 times a day. Flexion contracture must be prevented.
  - Lying on the side, the residual limb is extended slowly and with maximal force as far back as possible.
  - Lying prone, push-ups while keeping the pelvis on the bed.
  - Standing, the residual limb is extended forcefully by stretching the hip flexors.
  - In all exercises the position is kept for 5 seconds.

Bandaging the residual limb

- The residual limb should be bandaged as needed up to 3 times a day as follows:
  - First the bandage is wrapped twice around the base of the residual limb.

- The bandage is then taken over the tip of the residual limb, pulling it tight and wrapping it twice around the tip.
- Finally, the part between the base and tip is bandaged by loosening the pressure proximally.

♦ Prior to binding, the tip of the residual limb should be massaged manually for 15 to 30 minutes until it softens.

Prosthesis training

♦ Use of the training prosthesis can begin two weeks after the operation if the wound has healed satisfactorily.

♦ When the bandaging has formed the residual limb, fitting of the permanent prosthesis can be started 6 to 8 weeks after the amputation.

♦ During the use of the prosthesis, swelling is controlled by massaging the residual limb manually and by tying it with a wide bandage for the night.

♦ Weight control is an important part of the treatment.

Later appearing residual limb pain

♦ Check first that the residual limb fits in the prosthesis.

Rheumatology

Evidence Based Medicine Guidelines. Edited by the Duodecim Editorial Team
 ISBN: 0-470-01184-X

21.1 Clinical examination of patients with joint inflammation in primary health care

Tapani Helve

- See sections on the painful knee 20.40, and painful conditions in the foot and ankle 20.50.

Aims

- Septic arthritis is a medical emergency. The diagnostic workup for other forms of monoarthritis should be performed within a week.
- Gout is diagnosed and treated specifically.
- Degenerative joint disease should be distinguished from inflammatory joint disease (21.3).
- The cause of a polyarthritis is established in a stepwise fashion during follow-up of the patient. Overuse of laboratory tests is not recommended.

Basic rules

- There are about 100 different potential causes of polyarthritis. Establishing the correct diagnosis may require follow-up for weeks or months.
- The therapy is directed against the pathophysiological process rather than against specific disease. Therefore, a specific diagnosis is not always necessary for starting treatment. The importance of early treatment for impending chronic joint inflammation cannot, however, be overemphasized.

Epidemiology

- See Table 21.1.1.

Diagnostic strategy

Clinical examination

1. The first step is to find out whether the symptoms originate from the joint itself or from adjacent tissues.
2. When the symptom has been localized to the joint, the next step is to evaluate clinically if there is joint inflammation (21.2). The aim of history taking is to differentiate between joint pain (arthralgia) and joint inflammation (arthritis), which is characterized by
   - pain on movement
   - ache
   - swelling
   - heat
   - stiffness.

Table 21.1.1 The epidemiology of inflammatory joint diseases (cases/10 000 adults; North-European figures)

Aetiology	Cases	Comments
Rheumatoid arthritis	5	
Unknown aetiology	8	Most often hydrops of the knee, often transient
Arthritis associated with HLA-B27-antigen	3	1 ankylosing spondylitis, 1 reactive uroarthritis and 1 enteroarthritis
Gout	5	
Psoriatic arthritis	1	
Systemic connective tissue disorder	1	
Others	2	(Septic and viral joint inflammations)

When the clinical criteria for joint inflammation are fulfilled the following procedures are recommended:

1. In acute monoarthritis, arthrocentesis is performed and the synovial fluid is analysed (21.11). If the patient is febrile or has a high serum CRP level, leucocytosis or hypersedimentation, arthrocentesis and cultures of the synovial fluid must be performed also in the case of polyarthritis. If the synovial fluid is purulent (leucocyte count exceeding 40 000 $\times$ 10^6/l), the patient should be admitted to hospital. A lower synovial fluid leucocyte count does not exclude bacterial arthritis; in such cases the decisions to start antimicrobial drug treatment (always parenterally at hospital) are based on the clinical picture and the serum CRP level. Synovial fluid is also necessary for the analysis of the presence of urate crystals to confirm the diagnosis of gout (21.3). It should also be obtained and this should be done as soon as possible because the fluid may quickly disappear.
2. The clinical picture and the synovial fluid findings are helpful for distinguishing degenerative joint disease from inflammatory joint disease (21.3). If the leucocyte count exceeds 2000 $\times$ 10^6/l, it indicates an inflammatory arthritis. A normal ESR supports the diagnosis of degenerative joint disease.
3. More specific investigations are performed according to Table 21.1.2, depending on the clinical picture. For diagnostic hints on the basis of clinical signs, see 21.3.

Investigations to be performed on a patient with joint inflammation

- See Table 21.1.2.

Indications for referral to hospital

1. Emergencies

Table 21.1.2 Investigations to be performed on a patient with symptoms of joint inflammation

	The clinical picture	Investigations
A	All patients with joint inflammation	♦ Microscopy of joint fluid (crystals) ♦ Serum urate, ESR
	Laboratory tests	♦ ESR, CRP, blood count, urinalysis ♦ Analysis of joint fluid whenever fluid can be extracted (cells, crystals, bacterial culture and Gram's stain if necessary)
	The history (for those marked [1)] see paragraph D below)	♦ Morning stiffness and its duration (more than 1 h?) ♦ Pain on motion, ache ♦ Low back pain during rest ♦ Preceding traumas ♦ Previous joint symptoms ♦ A positive family history for joint inflammation ♦ Signs of psoriasis (skin, nails) ♦ Preceding diarrhoea ♦ Eye inflammation[1)] ♦ Dysuria, purulent discharge from the urethra[1)] ♦ Sexual contacts[1)] ♦ Other infection symptoms (pharyngitis?) ♦ Raynaud's phenomenon ♦ Erythema on sun exposure ♦ Use of beer or diuretics, see B
B	Monoarthritis (gout, pseudogout, septic arthritis, reactive arthritis)	♦ Serum urate (normal serum urate does not exclude gout during acute attack) ♦ Joint fluid analysis; crystals, cells, bacterial culture and Gram's stain
C	Joint inflammation lasting for more than two weeks (rheumatoid arthritis?)	♦ Serum rheumatoid factor
D	Positive history for [1)] marked symptoms (see paragraph A) and acute arthritis in a young adult (infectious arthritis, reactive arthritis?)	♦ Anti-Yersinia, -Salmonella and -Campylobacter antibodies ♦ PCR for Chlamydia and gonococcus from urine ♦ Anti-Chlamydia antibodies (the titre may stay high for a long period after the infection. PCR-test is preferred because of superior sensitivity and specificity. ♦ Chest x-ray for sarcoidosis
E	A possible tick bite occurring in an area endemic for Lyme disease, or erythema migrans	♦ Anti-Borrelia burgdorferi antibodies (a negative result in early disease does not exclude Lyme disease)
	Pox-like exanthema	♦ Rubella? ♦ Alphavirus antibodies if the patient has itching rash in the summer or autumn. ♦ Parvovirus antibodies (31.53)
F	Preceding febrile pharyngitis (rheumatic fever?), a heart murmur, migratory polyarthritis, abnormal ECG (rheumatic fever?)	♦ Streptococcal pharyngeal culture ♦ ECG ♦ AST (analysed if rheumatic fever is suspected on clinical grounds, a negative result speaks against rheumatic fever) ♦ Chest x-ray
G	Erythema on sun exposure, Raynaud's phenomenon (SLE?)	♦ Anti-nuclear antibodies (not recommended if musculoskeletal symptoms are localized and there are no general symptoms)
H	Abnormal blood picture, severe pain at night (leukaemia)	♦ White cell differential and platelets ♦ X-ray of the joint(s) often needed

RHE

- **Febrile monoarthritis** because of the possibility of a bacterial infection. (Elderly people can be treated at the health centre ward if a sample of synovial fluid can be examined reliably.)
- Severe polyarthritis if the patient is febrile or in bad condition, especially if the indices of inflammation are high (CRP, ESR).
- Clinical suspicion of rheumatic fever (see Table 21.1.2, paragraph F).
- Clinical suspicion of cancer (abnormalities in the blood count, exceptionally severe nocturnal pain) either as an emergency (suspicion of leukaemia) or on the next working day.

2. Normal referral practice
   - **Suspicion of seropositive rheumatoid arthritis** as soon as a positive test for rheumatoid factor has been obtained.
   - **Mild but persistent seronegative inflammatory joint disease**: 1–2 months after the start of symptoms. Non-steroidal anti-inflammatory drugs and physiotherapy are started straight away and the course of the disease is followed.
3. The following conditions can be treated at the primary health care centre
   - All transient arthritides
   - Mild reactive arthritis the aetiology of which is certain (21.31). (In chlamydial arthritis the patient and the partner are given a course of tetracycline and in yersinia and salmonella arthritis the patients is given ciprofloxacin provided bacterial cultures are positive.)
   - Gout
   - Exertion-induced hydrops in the knee joint
   - Single joints can be treated with local corticosteroid injections provided bacterial infection has been excluded (culture negative, serum CRP value low in monoarthritis).

21.2 Diagnosis of joint inflammation in the adult

Ilkka Kunnamo

- See sections on chapters the painful knee 20.40, pain in the hands and wrists and pain in the ankles and feet 20.50.

Definition of arthritis

- A diagnosis of arthritis should always be based on clinical examination: without clinical signs no joint inflammation can be diagnosed. According to the ACR (American College of Rheumatology), arthritis is defined as follows: swelling and reduced mobility of the joint with associated heat, ache or pain on movement.

Examination of the joints

- The following scheme can be performed in less than ten minutes.
- **Skin temperature**: With the dorsum of your fingers, feel the temperature of symptomatic joints and compare it with that of the same joints on the other side. In the knees, ankles, elbows and wrists an asymmetric arthritis almost always causes a temperature difference. A "cold" hydrops in the knee is almost never caused by inflammation.
- **The fingers**: Flex all fingers, one after another, at the proximal interphalangeal and the distal interphalangeal joints while keeping the metacarpophalangeal joint straight. Normally, either the fingertips reach the palmar surface of the hands. There may be a flexion deficit even without visible swelling. Spindle-shaped, shiny swelling of the proximal interphalangeal joints is an almost certain sign of an inflammatory process.
- **The dorsum of the hands**: Swelling of the metacarpophalangeal joints is visible as filling up of the pits between the knuckles. Pain is elicited when the fingers are bent or when pressure is applied simultaneously from both the radial and the ulnar sides of the hands; there is a restriction of movement when the joints are flexed (normal flexion 90 degrees).
- Swelling of **the dorsum of the wrist** is often widespread, sometimes fluctuating. Dorsiflexion (normally at least 70 degrees) is first limited.
- Swelling of **the elbow joint** is visible below the olecranon on the dorsal side. Extension is the first movement to be limited.
- Rotation of **the shoulder joints** is tested.
- An asymmetric sausage-shaped thickening of **the toes** is seen on inspection by comparing the toes on both feet.
- Pain in **the metatarsophalangeal joints** is elicited by pressing the metatarsophalangeal region from both sides simultaneously.
- **The ankles**: Test the motility of the ankle joints (dorsiflexion, plantar flexion, inversion, eversion) and register possible differences between the right and left ankle. Swelling may be seen around the malleoli and, when viewed from behind, on both sides of the Achilles tendon.
- Inflammation of **the knee joint** is usually accompanied by hydrops. A massive hydrops causes suprapatellar swelling. A smaller hydrops is diagnosed by pressing the suprapatellar recess manually. A fluid wave on both sides of the patella is felt with the thumb and the index finger. The most sensitive way of diagnosing hydrops is the so-called bulge sign. Rotation of **the hip joints** is tested with the patient supine and the hip and knee in 90-degrees flexion. When the hip joints are inflamed, inward rotation is usually limited, asymmetric and painful. There is pain in the inguinal region, not on the lateral side of the hip (trochanteric bursitis!) nor in the buttock (sacroiliac joints). Detection of an extension deficit of the hip joint: With the patient supine the other hip joint is flexed maximally, whereby the lordosis of the lumbosacral spine is straightened. If there is an extension deficit of the opposite hip, that thigh is elevated, and the

angle between the thigh and the examination couch indicates the degree of extension deficit.

- **Sacroiliac joint** pain is elicited by pressing the pelvis firmly from one side and by simultaneously bending the crests of the ileal bone forwards in order to bring the anterior superior iliac spines closer: pain originating from the sacroiliac joint radiates towards the buttock. Alternatively, the pelvis can be pressed directly downwards towards the couch so that the iliac spines are brought further from each other. In the Gaenslen's test the patient lies supine near the edge of the couch, the other leg hanging right down with the hip joint hyperextended. In all these tests, the twisting of the sacroiliac joint causes pain in the buttock.
- When joint inflammation is suspected, **inspection of the skin and auscultation of the heart** should always be included in the clinical examination.

21.3 Disease-specific symptoms and signs in patients with inflammatory joint diseases

Tapani Helve

- This section gives a more detailed clinical description of the differential diagnosis of inflammatory joint diseases briefly presented in (21.1).

Osteoarthritis

- May resemble inflammatory arthritis, especially if there is an effusion of fluid in the knees or symptoms appear in the fingers.
- Characteristic symptoms are pain on exertion, followed by aching.
- Morning stiffness is absent or lasts for no more than 15 minutes, whereas morning stiffness in inflammatory diseases, particularly rheumatoid arthritis, lasts longer, often for more than two hours. Osteoarthritis is associated with stiffness at the initiation of movement.
- In the knee, an early symptom may be a small joint effusion caused by inappropriate joint loading. The overlying skin remains cool to the touch, or only slightly warm. No thickened synovium can be felt. In the synovial fluid, there is only a small number of leucocytes (usually less than 2000 $\times$ 10^6/l), with a predominance of mononuclear cells.
- Osteoarthritis in the fingers causes hard, bony thickening of the distal interphalangeal joints (Heberden's nodes) and a small flexion deficit (diastasis between finger tip and palm usually not more than 20 mm; see 21.2). The ESR and the CRP concentration are normal.

Rheumatoid arthritis

- The disease usually starts gradually with the first symptoms affecting the fingers, metatarsophalangeal joints or wrists, but any joint may be the first one to be affected. Fusiform synovitis of the proximal interphalangeal joint is characteristic of rheumatoid arthritis but may also be seen in other inflammatory joint diseases.
- The symptoms usually develop fairly slowly as the inflammation spreads. The disease may also have a palindromic onset with the symptoms lasting from a few hours to a few days at a time.
- The first symptoms may also be acute and fulminant. The inflammatory joint manifestation may be accompanied by tiredness, loss of appetite or fever.
- A symmetric onset is characteristic of rheumatoid arthritis.
- The inflamed joints are painful when moved, but pain at rest is not characteristic to rheumatoid arthritis.
- The more active the inflammation, the longer the morning stiffness lasts, i.e. feeling of slowness or difficulty moving the joints.
- The ESR and the CRP concentration are at least slightly elevated.
- Erosive osteoarthritis of the proximal and distal interphalangeal joints of the fingers may resemble chronic rheumatoid arthritis but can be distinguished by its localisation (it spares the wrists and metatarsophalangeal joints), absence of rheumatoid factor and the relatively low ESR.

Spondyloarthropathies

Reactive arthritis

- See 21.31.
- Is associated with the HLA-B27 antigen in 60–80% of cases. Predisposition for the disease is inherited. Family history may be positive.
- Usually presents as either mono- or oligoarthritis of the lower limbs with a relatively slow migratory or additive progress.
- In addition to arthritis, enthesopathy (tenderness at the site of muscular or fascial attachment to bone) and dactylitis are often seen.
- Some patients have ocular inflammations and urethritis (Reiter's syndrome).
- Rarely encountered in the elderly.
- A reactive monoarthritis causing severe symptoms and a marked increase in the ESR and CRP concentration may be difficult to distinguish from bacterial arthritis.

Psoriatic arthropathy

- Psoriatic arthropathy (21.30) is usually an asymmetric inflammatory joint disease (usually oligoarthritis). In the fingers, the distal interphalangeal joints are often involved.
- The sternoclavicular, sacroiliac and temporomandibular joints are often affected.

- The arthropathy is very often associated with psoriatic nail changes, and the psoriatic skin changes may sometimes be absent.
- Dactylitis of a finger or toe is often associated with psoriatic arthropathy.
- Family history may be positive.

Ankylosing spondylitis

- See 21.32.
- Associated with the HLA-B27 antigen in 95% of cases. Predisposition for the disease is inherited. Family history may be positive.
- About one third of the patients have peripheral arthritis, usually mono- or oligoarthritis, but there may be symmetric polyarthritis resembling rheumatoid arthritis.
- Characteristically, the back is stiff in the morning and after sitting down. Examination of the sacroiliac joints (21.1) may reveal sacroiliitis.
- Some patients have attacks of acute iritis.
- The patient may have enthesopathy.

Sarcoidosis

- Sarcoidosis may present as acute arthritis, which most often affects the ankles. The knees may also be affected.
- The ESR is usually increased.

Rheumatic fever

- See 21.31.
- Has become rare in industrialised countries.
- There is usually rapidly progressing migratory arthritis, but the joint complaints may be limited to pain.
- Carditis, which manifests as pancarditis, is an important prognostic factor.
- The ESR and CRP are usually markedly elevated.

Systemic lupus erythematosus (SLE)

- See 21.41.
- Joint symptoms are often more severe than the clinical investigation suggests.
- Usually there is symmetric polyarthritis/polyarthralgia.
- Joint symptoms are associated with general symptoms, various cutaneous manifestations and signs of other organ manifestations (headache in central nervous system involvement, proteinuria or haematuria in nephritis, thrombocytopenia, leucopenia, sometimes venous thromboses).
- The ESR is usually elevated but the CRP level may be normal.

Gout

- See 21.50.
- Usually starts at middle age and is more common among males.
- Starts from the first metatarsophalangeal joint in more than half of the cases.
- A trauma to the joint may elicit a gouty attack.
- The gouty attack usually begins at night and peaks within 24 hours. The signs of inflammation, i.e. pain, swelling and redness, are usually prominent.
- If the condition remains untreated, the attacks recur with increased frequency and gradually lead to chronic destructive polyarthritis.
- An acute gouty attack may be accompanied by fever, a moderately elevated ESR and CRP. The serum urate concentration is usually elevated.
- Often associated with the metabolic syndrome (truncal obesity).

Pyrophosphate arthropathy

- See 21.52.
- May clinically resemble gout or osteoarthritis.
- X-rays show calcification of the joint cartilage (chondrocalcinosis) and pyrophosphate crystals will be found in the synovial fluid.

Bacterial arthritis

- Usually a fulminant onset with septic fever. In elderly people and when prosthetic joints become infected, fever and other signs of inflammation may, however, be lacking.
- Acute monoarthritis should be regarded as a bacterial arthritis until proven otherwise. Oligoarthritis may also be bacterial in origin.
- CRP and ESR are usually markedly elevated, but leucocytosis may be absent.
- Crystal-induced arthritis may also be fulminant, resembling bacterial arthritis. (Remember to request an examination for crystals in the aspirate!)

Gonorrhoea

- See 12.2.
- The onset of gonococcal arthritis is usually more sudden than that of reactive arthritis.
- There is often mono- or oligoarthritis, which affects the joints of the upper limbs.
- The arthritis is often associated with tenosynovitis or periarthritis.
- Migrating joint symptoms and pustular skin lesions are characteristic of gonococcal arthritis.

Viral arthritis

- The viral arthritides usually manifest themselves either as mild poly- or oligoarthritis, have an acute onset and a benign and self-limited course.
- Joint inflammation is often particularly associated with rubella and arbovirus arthritis, which can be identified by the characteristic rashes. The rash in arbovirus arthritis is pruritic (1.44). Parvovirus B19 (31.53) is quite a frequent cause of arthritis or arthralgia in adults.

- In the viral arthritides, there is only a slight increase in the ESR and CRP concentration and there is usually (but not always) a predominance of mononuclear cells in synovial fluid.

Lyme disease

- A multi-faceted disease caused by the spirochete Borrelia burgdorferi, which is spread by tick bites (1.29).
- In the acute phase, a rash, called erythema migrans appears at the site of the tick bite. A considerable number of people with borrelia arthritis, however, have had no rash. At the start of the disease, there is usually fever, headache, myalgia and lymphadenopathy.
- Late manifestations of the disease include arthritis, neurological symptoms and carditis.
- Arthritis usually presents as recurrent mono- or oligoarthritis.
- For a favourable outcome early diagnosis is essential.

Hypertrophic osteoarthropathy

- A paraneoplastic phenomenon that includes synovitis and is accompanied by periostitis of the long bones of the limbs and digital clubbing.

Polymyalgia rheumatica

- See 21.45.
- Muscular tenderness around the shoulders and pelvic girdle.
- Synovitis of the wrists and knees is sometimes seen.
- Stiffness and difficulty moving the joints when getting up or after a rest.
- Note that rheumatoid arthritis in the elderly may start with shoulder pain resembling polymyalgia.

HIV infection

- Patients infected with HIV (1.45) often have reactive arthritis and arthralgia.

Trauma

- The patient may have forgotten an earlier joint trauma, which may make the diagnostic work-up more difficult.

21.4 Raynaud's phenomenon and acrocyanosis

Editors

Aims

- To be able to distinguish between harmless acrocyanosis and Raynaud's phenomenon.
- To be able to identify patients with connective tissue diseases among all those with Raynaud's phenomenon.
- To be able to identify cases caused by continuous vibration at work (5.62).

The clinical picture

Raynaud's phenomenon

- Intermittent ischaemic attacks of fingers or toes, marked by pallor and often accompanied by numbness and pain.
- At the end of the attack there is a reactive, often painful vasodilatation with intense redness of the skin.

Acrocyanosis

- Permanent (not intermittent), symmetric cyanosis and feeling of cold in the hands.
- Often sweating and clumsiness of the hands.
- Pressure with a finger causes a pale spot, which is slowly refilled from the margins.

Differential diagnosis

- Conditions that may cause cold, cyanotic or pale fingers and toes include
  - obliterative arteriosclerosis
  - vasculitides
  - cholesterol embolization (5.61)
  - endocarditis
  - polycythaemia vera
  - cryoglobulinaemia and hyperviscosity syndrome
  - myxoma.

Symptoms and signs of systemic disease

- Raynaud's phenomenon may be associated with a connective tissue disease, the course of which determines the prognosis of the patient.
- If no systemic disease can be found, Raynaud's phenomenon can be regarded as a benign condition.
- SLE (21.41) may be suspected if there is
  - a butterfly rash
  - photosensitivity
  - arthritis or arthralgia
  - nephritis, pleuritis or pericarditis.
- Scleroderma (21.40) may be suspected if there is
  - Swelling of the fingers (sausage fingers) followed by skin thickening and, later, shiny, atrophic skin and joint stiffness
  - skin tautness in the face
  - dysphagia
  - dyspnoea, and lung fibrosis on chest x-ray
  - arthritis.
- Polymyositis (36.85) or dermatomyositis may be suspected if there is

RHE

- proximal muscle weakness
- purple discolouration around the eyes, a rash on the neck or upper chest or on the extensor surfaces of the limbs
- arthritis.

♦ Mixed connective tissue disease (21.42) may be suspected if the clinical picture includes

- features of scleroderma, polymyositis and rheumatoid arthritis
- swelling of the fingers ("sausage fingers").

Laboratory investigations

♦ If the patient presents with mild Raynaud's phenomenon and does not have symptoms suggestive of any systemic connective tissue disease, no laboratory tests are needed.

♦ If there is severe Raynaud's phenomenon or if other clinical signs of a connective tissue disease are present, the following laboratory tests are recommended:

- A blood count
- The erythrocyte sedimentation rate (ESR)
- A test for anti-nuclear antibodies
- A test for rheumatoid factor
- Serum creatine kinase
- Urinalysis

Drug therapy

♦ Nifedipine as a slowly absorbable preparation (10–20 mg × 2) has been proved the most effective therapy. Intravenous iloprost is effective in patients with systemic sclerosis **B** [1].

♦ Prazosin is modestly effective for patients with Raynaud's phenomenon in scleroderma **C** [2].

♦ Some patients may benefit from nitroglycerin ointment applied to the fingers.

Indications for referral to a specialist

♦ Impending gangrene

♦ Symptoms, signs or laboratory test results indicating a connective tissue disease

♦ No benefit from drug therapy.

References

1. Pope J, Fenlon D, Thompson A, Shea B, Furst D, Wells G, Silman A. Iloprost and cisaprost for Raynaud's phenomenon in progressive systemic sclerosis. Cochrane Database Syst Rev. 2004;(2):CD000953.
2. Pope J, Fenlon D, Thompson A, Shea B, Furst D, Wells G, Silman A. Prazosin for Raynaud's phenomenon in progressive systemic sclerosis. Cochrane Database Syst Rev. 2004;(2):CD000956.

21.10 Local corticosteroid injections in soft tissues and joints

Ilkka Kunnamo

Basic rules

♦ Soft tissues, the glenohumeral joint, the subacromial bursa and the trochanteric bursa are treated with corticosteroids and an anaesthetic 1:1 or corticosteroids and 0.9% NaCl 1:1 (in the shoulder and trochanteric region 1:2–1:5). **Other joints and bursae are treated with corticosteroids only** and without an anaesthetic. An observed local effect of the anaesthetic soon after the injection serves as a diagnostic test.

♦ Intra-articular injections should be reserved for inflamed joints: swelling or hydrops and pain (see 21.2).

♦ **Triamcinolone**

- In the knee joint
- In other large joints (elbow, wrist) if there is obvious inflammation or if fluid can be aspirated.

♦ **Methylprednisolone**

- In smaller joints and soft tissues. Because of the risk of skin atrophy, intracutaneous or subcutaneous injection should be avoided.
- In the finger tendon sheaths.

♦ The needle should be as thin as possible (see Table 21.10) and care should be taken not to damage the joint cartilage.

♦ In weight-bearing joints (the knee and the ankle), more than three injections a year or injections more frequently than once monthly are not recommended. Smaller joints (other than weight-bearing joints) may be injected more frequently.

♦ Partial immobilization of the joint for 24 hours and avoiding vigorous exercise for a week after the injection improves the result of the treatment, at least at far as the large joints are concerned.

Table 21.10 Recommended needle size for injections into soft tissues and joins

Thickness	Site of injection
0.5 mm	Finger, toe, MTP joint, temporomandibular joint, tendon sheaths
0.6 mm	Wrist
0.7 mm	Talocrural and elbow joints, small knee hydrops without the need for aspiration
0.8 mm	Shoulder joint, superficial bursae, Baker's cyst
1.2 mm	Removal of major hydrops
2.0 mm	Rice body arthritis in the knee (local anaesthetic in injected first with a thin needle), emptying of haemarthrosis of the knee

Injection sites

Excellent result, injection recommended

- The metatarsophalangeal (MTP) joints of the feet
- The metacarpophalangeal (MCP) and proximal interphalangeal (PIP) joints of the fingers
- Hydrops in the knee (especially exertion-induced hydrops)
- Gout (especially a tender MTP joint of the big toe)
- Aseptic bursitis with fluid
- In the glenohumeral joint when movement is restricted, subacromial bursitis or inflammation of the supraspinatus tendon

Good result, injection useful

- Inflammation in the flexor tendons of the fingers
- The elbow, if there is recent swelling
- Lateral epicondylitis
- Insertion tendonitis and tendovaginitis
- Plantar fasciitis
- The temporomandibular joint
- Active polyarthritis (remember other types of treatment, not to many injections in weight bearing joints)

Poor result

- Osteoarthritis in the knee, no hydrops
- Ganglion carpi (20.22) (Emptying of the ganglion is, however, recommended before surgical treatment is considered.)

Injection contraindicated

- Acute monoarthritis when bacterial infection has not been excluded
- Infection or eczema at the site of the injection
- Unstable, weight-bearing joint

Effect of injection therapy

- The most long-acting local corticosteroid **triamcinolone** has proved more effective than methylprednisolone for the treatment of knee arthritis. Triamcinolone should be used for large joints with fluid accumulation, at least if the first injection with short-acting corticosteroids is unsuccessful. **Methylprednisolone** is a useful local corticosteroid preparation for many different purposes.
- For a shoulder joint with movement restriction a local corticosteroid injection has proved more effective than naproxen or physiotherapy.

Recommended quantity of injection fluid

- The knee joint: 1 ml
- Baker's cyst 0.5–1 ml
- The glenohumeral joint, the subacromial bursa: 1 ml of corticosteroids and 2–5 ml of local anaesthetic
- The ankle joint: 1 ml
- The wrist joint: 0.5 ml
- Soft tissues: 0.4–1 ml and the same quantity of local anaesthetic or 0.9% NaCl
- PIP, MCP and MTP joints, temporomandibular joints: 0.2–0.3 ml

Recommended needle size

- See Table 21.10.

Other injection therapies

- Osmic acid treatment of the knee joint should be considered if synovitis with fluid accumulation has not been relieved by repeated corticosteroid injections.
- Synovectomy should be considered after the above-mentioned types of treatment or as an alternative.
- The effect of intra-articular hyaluronate injections on osteoarthritic joints is uncertain.

21.11 Investigation of synovial fluid

Editors

Basic rules

- A bacterial culture of synovial fluid should always be obtained when there is a possibility of bacterial arthritis.

Table 21.11.1 Investigation of synovial fluid

Separate analyses	Total volume of the sample	
	Ample	Scant
♦ Sample on the glass slide for staining (and cell differential)	Gram-stain	Gram-stain and cell differential count, cell count in a chamber
♦ Sample for culture in an (aerobic) blood culture bottle	Can be used as such	Rinse the syringe with sodium chloride solution; use the instilled sodium chloride solution reaspirated from the joint
♦ Sample in heparin, fluoride oxalate or EDTA tubes (for the white cell count and differential)	Use as such	Not sufficient
♦ Sample for crystal analysis	In a clear tube as such	On a glass slide sealing the margins with nail polish

Table 21.11.2 Interpretation of synovial fluid findings

Diagnosis	Synovial leucocytes (× 10⁶/l)	Polymorphonuclear cells (%)	Comments
Bacterial arthritis	>40 000	>80	Synovial leucocytes may be low in early disease. Bacterial stains negative in every second patient.
Entero- or uroarthritis	>10 000	>60	Occasionally cell number remarkably high
Rheumatoid arthritis	>5000	(20-) 40–90	
Ankylosing spondylitis			
Borrelia arthritis	10 000–60 000	>50	
Gout			Strongly negatively birefringent crystals[1]
Pyrophosphate arthropathy	10 000–60 000	>50	Weakly positively birefringent crystals[1]
Viral arthritis	1000–20 000	5–90	Often mononuclear predominance
Osteoarthritis	200–2000	0–30	Very seldom polymorphonuclear predominance
Juvenile rheumatoid arthritis (early onset oligoarthritis)	1500–15 000	5–50	Seldom polymorphonuclear predominance
Juvenile rheumatoid arthritis (other)	5000–60 000	>50	Sometimes mononuclear predominance
Juvenile coxitis	1000–6000	10–80	Generally mononuclear predominance
Bacterial bursitis	>2000	>50	Cell number may be small in early disease.

1. Many other forms of crystals can also be found in synovial fluid (for example, persisting corticosteroid crystals after intra-articular injection). Therefore, microscopy requires experience in crystal analysis.

In addition, a gram staining should be performed when initiation of antimicrobial therapy is indicated on the basis of the clinical picture.

- On suspicion of gout, microscopy for crystal identification should always be performed.
- A total and differential white cell count should be performed when a joint inflammation has to be distinguished from other causes of fluid accumulation in the joint.

Samples

- See Table 21.11.1.

Interpretation of joint fluid analysis

- See Table 21.11.2.

21.20 Drug treatment of rheumatoid arthritis

Editors

Aims

- To prevent joint erosion.
- To reduce disability and the need for reconstructive rheumatic surgery.
- To improve quality of life and functional capacity.
- A curative effect is, however, achieved in only about 20% of patients. In most cases, the aim of the treatment is to slow down disease progression.

Basic rules

- Since it is not possible to predict the progress of the disease, standard disease-modifying antirheumatic drugs (DMARDs) should be prescribed to all patients after diagnosis. Early treatment aims at avoiding a delay during which joint destruction starts. For the commencement of therapy the classical diagnostic criteria for rheumatoid arthritis need not be fulfilled.
- The treatment should be active and aggressive. An effective medication is started on the assumption that the patient has a severe disease. If the treatment proves ineffective, the drug is substituted or another drug is added within 3 to 6 months.
- Confirmation of the diagnosis and initiation of antirheumatic drug therapy is best done by a specialist. Primary health care bears the responsibility for the safe continuation of the treatment (21.20.1) and for the identification of patients whose medication is inadequate.

Choice of DMARDs

- The primary drug is chosen on the basis of the clinical picture. However, it is not possible to tell from the start which drug will benefit the patient most.
- The two principal reasons for changing the therapy are treatment failure and adverse effects.

DMARDs in clinical practice

- Intramuscular gold (aurothiomalate) **A** [1]
- Peroral gold (auranofin) **A** [2]
- D-penicillamine **A** [3]
- Antimalarial drugs (chloroquine preparations) **B** [4]
- Sulfasalazine **A** [5]
- Azathioprine **C** [6]
- Methotrexate **A** [7]
- Podophyllotoxin
- Cyclophosphamide **B** [8]
- Chlorambucil
- Cyclosporin **B** [9]
- Leflunomide **A** [10] [11] [12]
- Tumour necrosis factor modulators **A** [13]

General principles for choosing an antirheumatic drug

- Chloroquine and oral gold have preserved their position as suitable drugs for the treatment of mild disease forms.
- If an antirheumatic drug proves effective, treatment should be continued for years. The dose may, however, be reduced if the disease remains well controlled.
- Prednisolone
  - Systemic corticosteroid therapy usually relieves the inflammatory symptoms of rheumatoid arthritis quickly. To minimize adverse effects the dose should be kept as low as possible.
  - There is some evidence of the anti-erosive effect of corticosteroids in the joints.

Table 21.20.1 Laboratory tests to ensure the safety of DMARDs

Drug	Laboratory tests
Aurothiomalate	
♦ Once every two weeks for two months,	Haemoglobin, white cell count, platelets, urine albumin
♦ thereafter before each injection and	Urine albumin
♦ before every third injection	Haemoglobin, white cell count, platelets
Auranofin	
♦ Once a month for 3 months, thereafter at 3 month intervals	Haemoglobin, white cell count, platelets, urine albumin
Penicillamine	
♦ Once every 2 weeks for 2 months, thereafter at 2–3 month intervals	Haemoglobin, white cell count, platelets, urine albumin
Sulfasalazine	
♦ Once every 2 weeks for 2 months, thereafter at 3 month intervals	Haemoglobin, white cell count, platelets, ALT
Azathioprine	
♦ Once every 2 weeks for 2 months, thereafter at 2–3 month intervals	Haemoglobin, white cell count, platelets, ALT
Methotrexate	
♦ Once every 2 weeks for 2 months, thereafter at 2–3-month intervals and	Haemoglobin, white cell count, platelets, ALT
♦ at 6 month intervals	Creatinine (creatinine clearance)
Podofyllotoxin	
♦ Once a month for 3 months, thereafter at 3 month intervals	Haemoglobin, white cell count, platelets, ALT
Cyclosporin	
♦ Once every 2 weeks for 2 months, thereafter at 2–3 month intervals	Creatinine, blood pressure
Cyclophosphamide	
♦ Once every 2-weeks for 2 months, thereafter at 1–3 month intervals	Haemoglobin, white cell count, platelets, ALT, urinanalysis
Chlorambucil	
♦ Once every 2 weeks for 2 months, thereafter at 1–3-month intervals	Haemoglobin, white cell count, platelets, ALT
Leflunomide	
♦ Once every 2 weeks for 6 months, thereafter at 2 month intervals	Haemoglobin, white cell count, platelets, ALT, blood pressure
Tumour necrosis factor modulators (infliximab, etanercept, anakinra)	
♦ Once every 2 weeks for 2 months, thereafter at 1–3 month intervals	Haemoglobin, white cell count, platelets

Table 21.20.2 The use of DMARDs during pregnancy and lactation. "Not usually" signifies that the drug can be considered if ensuring the safety of the pregnancy requires its use or if the drug has already been used during pregnancy

Drug	During pregnancy	During lactation
Aurothiomalate	No	Can be used
Auranofin	No	No
Chloroquine	Not usually	Not usually
Sulfasalazine	Can be used	Can be used
Penicillamine	No	No
Podofyllotoxin	No	No
Methotrexate	No	No
Azathioprine	Not usually	Not usually
Cyclosporin	Not usually	No
Cyclophos-phamide	No	No
Chlorambucil	No	No
Leflunomide	No (teratogenic, must be stopped some time before planned conception)	No
TNF-alpha modulators	No	No

- Small doses of corticosteroids (for example prednisolone 5–7.5 mg) are commonly used while waiting for the effect of slow-acting antirheumatic drugs.
- High-dose corticosteroids are often required for rheumatoid arthritis which causes systemic symptoms.
- Corticosteroid therapy of several years, duration will lead to a multitude of severe adverse effects.

The choice of drug in certain clinical presentations

♦ Active, polyarticular rheumatoid arthritis
  - If the disease process is particularly active, methotrexate is the drug of choice (A) [7]. In these cases combination therapy may also be initiated immediately, for example by combining sulfasalazine, methotrexate, hydroxychloroquine or a low-dose corticosteroid to the treatment (A) [1].

♦ Oligoarticular, seronegative rheumatoid arthritis
  - Sulfasalazine

♦ Palindromic rheumatism
  - Antimalarials, sulfasalazine, gold

♦ Systemic rheumatoid disease
  - Corticosteroids and cytotoxic drugs

♦ For medication during pregnancy, see Table 21.20.2.

Laboratory tests for ensuring the safety of the therapy

♦ See Table 21.20.1.

- The following test should be taken at follow-up visits: ESR, CRP, blood count, liver enzymes and urine sediment.
- When the drug dose is increased the tests are taken once with a shorter time interval, as when the drug was started.
- If blood white cell count is $<3.0 \times 10^9$/l differential count is needed.
  - If the blood count results are abnormal, medication is temporarily discontinued and the patient is referred to hospital (agranulocytosis) or the tests are repeated after 1–2 weeks.
- If urine album is positive, the medication is stopped for one week. If the repeat sample after one week remains positive, the urine is tested for protein.
- If the transaminase values increase to more than 80–100 U/l during methotrexate treatment, the dose should be reduced. If methotrexate is used concomitantly with leflunomide the liver enzyme values must be closely monitored.
- If transaminase values increase by more than 2–3 fold during leflunomide therapy, the patient needs close monitoring. If the increased values persist, the drug should be withdrawn and the introduction of cholestyramine considered.
- A marked rise in the transaminase values during azathioprine therapy is a contraindication for continuing the therapy.
- Cyclosporin may induce renal damage and close monitoring is indicated. If serum creatinine increases more than 30% from baseline (the mean of 2–3 initial measurements) the dose should be halved.

References

1. Clark P, Tugwell P, Bennet K, Bombardier C, Shea B, Wells G, Suarez-Almazor ME. Injectable gold for rheumatoid arthritis. Cochrane Database Syst Rev. 2004;(2):CD000520.
2. Suarez-Almazor ME, Spooner CH, Belseck E, Shea B. Auranofin versus placebo in rheumatoid arthritis. Cochrane Database Syst Rev. 2004;(2):CD002048.
3. Suarez-Almazor ME, Spooner C, Belseck E. Penicillamine for treating rheumatoid arthritis. Cochrane Database Syst Rev. 2004;(2):CD001460.
4. Suarez-Almazor ME, Belseck E, Shea B, Homik J, Wells G, Tugwell P. Antimalarials for treating rheumatoid arthritis. Cochrane Database Syst Rev. 2004;(2):CD000959.
5. Suarez-Almazor ME, Belseck E, Shea B, Wells G, Tugwell P. Sulfasalazine for treating rheumatoid arthritis. Cochrane Database Syst Rev. 2004;(2):CD000958.
6. Suarez-Almazor ME, Spooner C, Belseck E. Azathioprine for treating rheumatoid arthritis. Cochrane Database Syst Rev. 2004;(2):CD001461.
7. Suarez-Almazor ME, Belseck E, Shea B, Wells G, Tugwell P. Methotrexate for treating rheumatoid arthritis. Cochrane Database Syst Rev. 2004;(2):CD000957.
8. Suarez-Almazor ME, Belseck E, Shea B, Wells G, Tugwell P. Cyclophosphamide for treating rheumatoid arthritis. Cochrane Database Syst Rev. 2004;(2):CD001157.

9. Wells G, Haguenauer D, Shea B, Suarez-Almazor ME, Welch VA, Tugwell P. Cyclosporine for treating rheumatoid arthritis. Cochrane Database Syst Rev. 2004;(2):CD001083.
10. Hewitson PJ, DeBroe S, McBride A, Milne R. Leflunomide and rheumatoid arthritis: a systematic review of effectiveness, safety and cost implications. Journal of Clinical Pharmacy and Therapeutics 2000, 25(4), 295–302.
11. The Database of Abstracts of Reviews of Effectiveness (University of York), Database no.: DARE-20001983. In: The Cochrane Library, Issue 2, 2002. Oxford: Update Software.
12. Osiri M, Shea B, Robinson V, Suarez-Almazor M, Strand V, Tugwell P, Wells G. Leflunomide for treating rheumatoid arthritis. Cochrane Database Syst Rev. 2004;(2):CD002047.
13. Blumenauer B, Judd M, Cranney A, Burls A, Hochberg M, Tugwell P, Wells G. Infliximab for the treatment of rheumatoid arthritis. Cochrane Database Syst Rev. 2004;(2): CD003785.

21.21 Follow-up of a patient with rheumatoid arthritis

Editors

Basic rules

- Assess the activity of the disease and response to treatment; be prepared to reconsider the treatment plan if the need arises.
- Identify changes that are of importance for prognosis (erosions and a high serum CRP concentration as a sign of increased risk of amyloidosis).
- Monitor safety tests and side-effects of drugs.
- Assess and treat pain, tenderness and morning stiffness.
- Improve the patient's functional capacity (physiotherapy, orthoses, social support).

Inquire about the following from the patient

- Present problems and causes for concern (as a starting point for discussion)
- Duration of morning stiffness
- Activities of daily life or work that cause difficulties
- Joints with symptoms
- Adverse effects of drugs (especially gastrointestinal symptoms)
- Use of analgesics
- The experienced handicap caused by the disease: effect on social life, depression

Clinical examination

- Examine at least the symptomatic joints regularly (tenderness, swelling, and range of motion, recorded as numerical values), and whether or not symptoms are present check at least the following:
  - Is finger flexion restricted? If necessary, inject steroids into PIP or MCP joints or flexor tendon sheaths.
  - Is extension in the wrist or elbow joints restricted?
  - Can the upper arms be fully abducted (limitation of motion may develop subtly)?
- Systematic joint examination (21.2)
  - Annually for all patients
  - Before a change in medication and 2–6 months after it

Laboratory investigations for assessing disease activity

- ESR, CRP and haemoglobin concentration should be determined at least every 3 months.
- A persistently elevated CRP value may predict the development of amyloidosis, and may be a cause for changing medication.
- A low haemoglobin concentration associated with a high ESR is a sign of disease activity. Iron medication should not be given in most cases. Gastrointestinal haemorrhage (NSAIDs!) should be remembered as a cause of real iron deficiency anaemia.
- Rheumatoid factor is not a measure of disease activity, and it should not be assayed repeatedly.

Indications for x-rays

- Flexion-extension x-rays of the cervical spine are indicated when atlanto-axial subluxation is suspected if the patient complains of severe pain and painful movements of the neck, occipital pain or electric shock-like sensations when bending. A space of 4 mm or more between the dens axis and atlas in flexion is pathological and an indication for specialist consultation.
- If the patient has symptoms in the fingers, wrists or MTP joints, x-rays of the hands and feet should be taken at 2–3 year intervals in order to detect erosions.
- A symptomatic hip joint should be followed up with x-rays, because eventual arthroplasty should be performed before the roof of the acetabulum is broken.

Need for rehabilitation, orthoses and patient education

- The most common orthoses include
  - wrist splints B [1]
  - neck splint for car travel if the patient has neck symptoms from the cervical spine
  - appropriate footwear  [1]

- A physiotherapist or an occupational therapist should visit the patient at home and assess the need for help and orthoses. This visit should be offered to a patient whose activities are limited by the disease.
- Daily exercises should be discussed with the patient and repeatedly instructed.
- Patient education in groups C [2 3 4] may be beneficial, but the efficacy in general is not proven for pain or disability C [5 6].
- Multi-disciplinary team care programmes are effective in the short term, but proof of long-term efficacy is scanty B [7 8].
- Re-education and financial help in the occupational career can be discussed with the local authorities.

Specialist consultations

- Most working-age patients visit hospital outpatient clinics.
- The primary care physician can be responsible for a planned follow-up of the patient.
- Specialist consultation is always recommended if the disease is continuously active, a change to more efficient medication is needed, or if complications develop.
  - Active synovitis implies the risk of permanent damage to the joints and should be treated with effective disease-modifying and anti-inflammatory therapies.
  - If disease activity does not decrease within 4–6 months of a change of drugs, a further change should be considered.
  - Remember the indications for rheumatoid arthritis surgery (21.22).

References

1. Egan M, Brosseau L, Farmer M, Ouimet MA, Rees S, Wells G, Tugwell P. Splints and Orthosis for treating rheumatoid arthritis. Cochrane Database Syst Rev. 2004;(2):CD004018.
2. Riemsma RP, Kirwan JR, Taal E, Rasker JJ. Patient education for adults with rheumatoid arthritis. Cochrane Database Syst Rev. 2004;(2):CD003688.
3. Taal E, Rasker JJ, Wiegman O. Group education for rheumatoid arthritis patients. Semin Arthr Rheum 1997;26:805–16.
4. The Database of Abstracts of Reviews of Effectiveness (University of York), Database no: DARE-970867. In: The Cochrane Library, Issue 4, 1999. Oxford: Update Software.
5. Superio-Cabuslay E, Ward MMM, Lorig KR. Patient education interventions in osteoarthritis and rheumatoid arthritis: a meta-analytic comparison with nonsteroidal anti-inflammatory drug treatment. Arthritis Care & Research 1996;9:292–301.
6. The Database of Abstracts of Reviews of Effectiveness (University of York), Database no.: DARE-965403. In: The Cochrane Library, Issue 4, 1999. Oxford: Update Software.
7. Vliet Vlieland TP, Hazes JM. Effect of multidisciplinary team care programs (MTCP) in rheumatoid arthritis. Seminars in Arthritis and Rheumatism 1997;27:110–122.
8. The Database of Abstracts of Reviews of Effectiveness (University of York), Database no.: DARE-985127. In: The Cochrane Library, Issue 1, 2000. Oxford: Update Software.

21.22 Rheumatic surgery

Editors

Basic rule

- Rehabilitation with the help of a physiotherapist significantly contributes to the benefit gained from an operation.

Acute or urgent surgery

- Nerve compression caused by synovitis or tenosynovitis (the median nerve in the carpal tunnel, the ulnar nerve in the elbow region).
- Incipient or apparent tendon rupture.
- Atlantoaxial subluxation accompanied by neurological symptoms.
- A deformity severe enough to interfere with the patient's daily life (e.g. washing).
- Severe ankylosis or dislocation of the jaw.
- Bursitis that interferes with the patient's functional ability, and rheumatic nodules, which show a tendency to ulcerate.

Relative indications for surgery

- Therapy-resistant synovitis, tenosynovitis or bursitis. (For example, a trigger-finger not responding to corticosteroid injections or a significant limitation of movement due to tenosynovitis of the flexor tendons)
- Severe and protracted pain or ache
- Severe limitation of joint movement
- Severe deformity

Synovectomy

- The number of surgical synovectomies of the large joints has decreased considerably.
- Most synovectomies are performed by arthroscopy.
- After synovectomy, active and effective physiotherapy is of crucial importance for regaining joint function.

The most important sites and indications for synovectomy

- The metacarpophalangeal and proximal interphalangeal joints of the hands
- Flexor tenosynovitis of the fingers
- Tenosynovitis of the palmar or dorsal side of the wrist
- The tendons of the ankle region
- The metatarsophalangeal joints
- Knee and elbow joints

Reconstructive rheumatic surgery

Prosthetic surgery

- Increasingly used for all limb joints

Arthrodeses

- The ankle
- The first metatarsophalangeal joint
- The finger joints
- The wrist

Indications for, and results of, surgery

Atlantoaxial subluxation

- Neurological deficiency symptoms are decisive when surgery is considered.
- A basilar impression, i.e. protrusion of the dens into the foramen magnum may be life threatening.
- An anterior luxation of more than 9 mm and severe cervical and occipital pain may necessitate surgery.

The shoulder joint

- Improved diagnostic methods (ultrasound examination, magnetic resonance imaging) have offered better opportunities for early (soft tissue) surgery.
- Prosthetic surgery (according to Neer, for example) relieves pain effectively, but functional outcome depends on the integrity of the rotator cuff and is not always satisfactory.

The elbow joint

- Synovectomy relieves pain at least partially.
- Removal of the radial head
- Liberation of the ulnar nerve
- The results of prosthetic surgery have improved.

The wrist

- Carpal tunnel syndrome should be identified and treated. (It may be overlooked in a rheumatoid arthritis patient because of other forms of pain.)
- Dorsal tenosynovectomies prevent tendon ruptures.
- Arthrodesis can be a good alternative if the wrist is used in heavy work and if there is severe wrist instability caused by refractory rheumatoid arthritis.
- Partial arthrodesis improves stability and spares the range of motion partially.

The hand

- Tenosynovitis of the flexor tendons is primarily treated by corticosteroid injections, the efficacy of which always has to be evaluated. Tenosynovectomy should be performed before a nodular tendon-damaging synovitis develops.
- Synovectomies of the metacarpophalangeal and proximal interphalangeal joints are still performed commonly.
- Early boutonnière or swan-neck deformities are always treated with a dynamic splint.

The hip joint

- In rheumatoid arthritis, protrusion of the femoral head into the acetabulum commonly occurs (in about 15 percent of all patients). Because the condition may progress within a few months, surgery of the hip joint is more urgent in RA than in osteoarthritis.

The knee joint

- Arthroscopic synovectomies are becoming more common but long-term results are still unavailable.
- The results for prosthetic surgery on the knee are even better than those for the hip joint.

The ankle joint

- The subtalar joints are more often damaged than the talocrural joint. A so-called triple arthrodesis is a helpful procedure.
- Ankle joint prosthesis has been improved in the recent years and seems to yield better results in RA than in arthrosis.

The foot

- For inflammation in the metatarsophalangeal joints, early synovectomy can be recommended rather than late-phase metatarsal bone resections.
- Resection gives effective pain relief, but with regard to function the result is poor.

21.30 Psoriatic arthropathy

Editors

Basic rule

- Chronic arthritis in a psoriatic patient should be considered psoriatic arthropathy if the clinical features do not clearly suggest another disease.

Epidemiology

- 5–7% of psoriatic patients also have arthritis. In severe psoriasis as many as 40% of the patients have arthritis.

- Susceptibility to the disease is determined by genetic factors. HLA-B27-positive patients have often sacroilitis or spondylitis. Psoriatic arthropathy as such is not associated with HLA-B27.

Diagnosis

- The arthritis may commence before the psoriatic rash. In such cases family history and nail affection may give a clue of the diagnosis.
- The characteristics of psoriatic arthropathy include
  - psoriatic nails
  - negative rheumatoid factor
  - involvement of DIP joints (often DIP + PIP)
  - dactylitis (sausage finger or toe)
  - insertitis or enthesopathy (inflammation of tendon insertions)
  - sacroilitis or spondylitis
  - erosions in limb joints without concomitant osteoporosis
  - asymmetric oligoarthritis.

Treatment

- The same drugs and same doses apply as in the treatment of rheumatoid arthritis:
  - NSAIDs
  - Methotrexate and sulphasalazine are the most effective drugs (B) [1]. Methotrexate is also effective in the treatment of the psoriatic rash.
  - Systemic steroids and antimalarials may worsen the rash.
  - Parenteral gold is more effective than peroral gold.
  - Also azathioprine alleviates psoriatic arthropathy.
  - Cyclosporin is effective against skin symptoms and also controls arthritis.
  - Intra-articular steroids are effective.
- The prognosis is often better than in rheumatoid arthritis, but severe forms of the disease exist.

Reference

1. Jones G, Crotty M, Brooks P. Interventions for treating psoriatic arthritis. Cochrane Database Syst Rev. 2004;(2):CD000212.

21.31 Reactive arthritis and rheumatic fever

Editors

Aims

- Reactive arthritis should be considered in all patients under 60 years of age who fall ill with acute arthritis. For the timing of diagnostic procedures, see 21.1.
- All patients in whom the causative agent has been found in bacterial cultures are treated with antimicrobial drugs. There is no need to start antimicrobial therapy if the cultures are negative. A chlamydia infection is treated even if the diagnosis is based merely on serological grounds.
- Single inflamed joints are treated with local corticosteroid injections (21.10).
- The patient should avoid new infections that may precipitate reactive arthritis (appropriate dietary habits while travelling) (2.3).
- Diagnose carditis in a patient with fever and migrating polyarthritis (auscultation of the heart, ECG, chest x-ray, eventually echocardiography).
- Do not determine streptococcal serology if the clinical presentation of the patient does not suggest rheumatic fever (avoid false positive results).

Epidemiology

- The annual incidence is about 3/10 000 in the adult population.
- The average age of the patients is 20–30 years.
- There is no sex predilection but symptoms tend to be more severe in males.
- Established causative agents are the bacteria Yersinia (half of the cases of enteroarthritides), Salmonella, Shigella and Campylobacter. Uroarthritis is precipitated by chlamydia and the gonococcus. There is no difference between the occurrence of entero- and uroarthritis.
- 80% of patients with enteroarthritis and 60% of those with uroarthritis are HLA-B27 positive.

The clinical picture

- The onset is usually acute. A fulminant disease is accompanied by fever and a marked elevation of the ESR and the serum CRP concentration. Involvement of many joints helps to differentiate reactive arthritis from bacterial arthritis.
- In most patients with enteroarthritis, but not in all, the precipitating infection is obvious (diarrhoea, abdominal pain). In males, an infection in the urogenital tract usually causes symptoms (urethritis), but in females it may pass with no or only mild symptoms. A gonococcal infection may often cause inflammatory joint symptoms, but so-called postgonococcal arthritis is probably most often precipitated by a concurrent chlamydia infection.
- The joints of the lower limbs are almost always involved.
- Arthritis in the upper limbs is seen in about one half of all cases.
- Extra-articular manifestations are frequent:
  - Enthesopathy, peritendinitis in 30–50% of patients
  - Clinically evident sacroiliitis in 20–30% of all patients
  - Balanitis in 10–25% of all patients. (Balanitis circinata is characterized by ring formed lesions of the glans.)
  - Conjunctivitis in 20–35% of all patients
  - Uveitis in 2–4% of all patients

- Abnormal ECG in 5–15% of all patients
- Erythema nodosum

Diagnostic procedures

- Faecal cultures, isolation of chlamydia (PCR), ESR, CRP and ECG at the first visit always when there is a suspicion of reactive arthritis.
- Gonococcal culture at the first visit when there are urogenital symptoms and arthritis.
- At the first visit or after 1–3 weeks if the clinical picture is compatible with reactive arthritis
  - Anti-Yersinia antibodies
  - Anti-Salmonella antibodies
  - Anti-Campylobacter antibodies
  - Anti-Chlamydia PCR (better than antibodies)
  - Anti-streptolysin if there is suspicion of rheumatic fever
  - Anti-Borrelia antibodies (1.29)
- Investigations may be carried out stepwise so that anti-Yersinia antibodies are tested first (best diagnostic yield) and other antibodies tested as a second step.
- Bearing the possibility of sarcoidosis in mind, chest radiographs should be taken. X-rays of the joints are normal in the early phase of the disease.
- ECG, because the patient may suffer from (usually symptom-free) carditis.
- Testing for HLA-B27 has no place in the primary diagnostic work-up.

Treatment

- See 8.44.
- Antimicrobial drugs against the causative agent should always be given when bacterial cultures are positive. Treatment of a chlamydia infection requires only serological or PCR confirmation. The duration of treatment is 10 days (except in chlamydia infection; see below).
  - Yersinia, Salmonella, Shigella: ciprofloxacin 500 mg twice daily
  - Campylobacter: erythromycin 500 mg twice daily
  - Chlamydiae: doxycycline 150 mg once daily. For the primary infection, antimicrobial drugs should be given for 14 days. If arthritis persists, therapy is continued (up to 3 months, if needed).
- Treatment of the acute phase of arthritis
  - Non-steroidal anti-inflammatory drugs (NSAIDs)
  - Peroral prednisolone if symptoms are severe
  - Corticosteroid injections are recommended for local treatment of single inflamed joints.
  - Rest, physical therapy to preserve muscle strength and joint mobility
  - In prolonged symptoms sulphasalazine, or some other antirheumatic drug

Prognosis

- Usually reactive arthritis subsides within 3 to 5 months

Table 21.31 Diagnostic criteria of rheumatic fever (the Jones criteria)

Major criteria	Minor criteria
♦ Migrating polyarthritis	♦ Fever
♦ Carditis	♦ Joint pain
♦ Erythema marginatum	♦ History of rheumatic fever
♦ Chorea	♦ Prolonged P–R interval in the ECG
♦ Subcutaneous nodules	♦ Elevated ESR, increased serum CRP or leucocytosis

- About 15% of the patients will develop a chronic arthritis, chronicity is more often seen in uroarthritis than in enteroarthritis.

Prevention

- A patient who has had a reactive arthritis or has a positive family history for HLA-B27-associated arthropathies should avoid enterobacterial or chlamydial infections.
  - While travelling, the use of antimicrobial drugs to prevent gastrointestinal infections is recommended (2.3).

RHE

Rheumatic fever

- A disease triggered by pharyngeal beta-haemolytic group A streptococcus with features of reactive arthritis
- Not associated with HLA-B27

The clinical picture

- The most common manifestation is arthritis, which is usually migratory.
- Carditis (pancarditis) may be expressed as valvulitis or pericarditis or as heart failure after myocarditis.
- The other major diagnostic symptoms (see Table 21.31) are very rare.

Diagnosis

- Two major criteria or one major and two minor criteria are needed for a definite diagnosis (see Table 21.31). In addition, **evidence of a prior streptococcal infection is a prerequisite for the diagnosis** (increased AST titre, positive throat streptococcal culture, recent scarlatina).

Antibiotic prophylaxis

- Indicated if the patient has had carditis
- Give long-acting penicillin C [1] for five years. A cephalosporin is suitable for patients allergic to penicillin.

Reference

1. Manyemba J, Mayosi BM. Penicillin for secondary prevention of rheumatic fever. The Cochrane Database of Systematic

Reviews, Cochrane Library number: CD002227. In: The Cochrane Library, Issue 3, 2002. Oxford: Update Software.

21.32 Ankylosing spondylitis

Editors

General considerations

- Inflammation of the insertions of the ligaments of the spine, the facet joints and the sacroiliac joints is an integral feature of the disease.
- The condition affects almost exclusively HLA-B27 positive individuals and belongs to the group of seronegative spondylarthropathies together with
  - reactive entero- and uroarthritides and Reiter's syndrome (21.31)
  - type 2 (late onset) juvenile oligoarthritis (32.56)
  - psoriatic spondylitis (21.30)
  - arthropathy associated with chronic inflammatory bowel disease.
- In the same family, several of the above mentioned diseases may be seen and all of them may lead to ankylosing spondylitis.
- The disease is classified as ankylosing spondylitis when it has become chronic and no causative agent has been detected.

Epidemiology

- Ankylosing spondylitis is nearly as common as rheumatoid arthritis. There is no sex predilection, but most patients with severe ankylosing spondylitis are males.
- The incidence peaks at 20 years of age but the diagnosis is often delayed.

The clinical picture

- Sacroiliitis: Lumbosacral and gluteal pain, which awakens the patient in the morning
- Stiffness after rest and sitting
- Peripheral arthritis mainly of the large joints of the lower limbs
- Enthesopathies are common in the lower limbs (heel pain)
- Dactylitis ("sausage" finger or toe)
- Attacks of acute uveitis in 20 percent of cases (may be the first manifestation of the disease)
- Occasionally aortitis and conduction disturbances of the heart (auscultation, electrocardiography)
- Ankylosing spondylitis needs to be remembered as a diagnostic possibility when the patient presents with protracted pain in the lumbosacral region and buttocks: morning stiffness and an increased ESR are helpful diagnostic hints.

Diagnosis

- The history (as above)
- Clinical findings
  - Tenderness on pressing, palpating and testing the movements of the sacroiliac joints
  - Fingertip–floor distance while bending forwards
  - Schober distance (normal more than 5 cm)
  - Lateral flexion of the lumbar spine C [1 2]
  - Occiput–wall distance (normal 0)
  - Chest movements during respiration (normal increase in maximal inspiration compared to maximal expiration more than 5 cm at the level of the mamillae).
- In most patients, ESR and serum CRP concentration are elevated.
- X-rays are taken of the lumbar spine, the lowest thoracic vertebra and the sacroiliac joints. It takes 2–8 years for radiological signs of sacroiliitis to develop.
- Prior to the radiological abnormalities, an increased joint uptake may be detectable on scintigraphy, but there are many potential causes for false positive findings.

Differential diagnosis

- Osteitis condensans ilii on x-rays
- Degenerative diseases of the spine
- Diffuse idiopathic skeletal hyperostosis (DISH) on x-rays
- Other forms of spondylarthropathy
  - Reiter's disease
  - Psoriatic arthropathy
  - The arthropathy associated with chronic inflammatory bowel disease
- Sciatica

Treatment

- Physiotherapy C [3] is crucial (particularly during inflammatory phases and immediately after them) in order to prevent a stiff back. Active exercises are an integral part of the physiotherapy!
- Non-steroidal anti-inflammatory drugs
- Sulphasalazine induces a response in about half of the patients. In severe cases cytotoxic drugs or combinations of drugs have been tried.
- Peripheral arthritides and enthesopathies are treated with local corticosteroid injections.

References

1. On the accuracy of history, physical examination, and erythrocyte sedimentation rate in diagnosing low back pain in general practice. Spine 1995;20:318–327.

2. The Database of Abstracts of Reviews of Effectiveness (University of York), Database no.: DARE-978022. In: The Cochrane Library, Issue 4, 1999. Oxford: Update Software.
3. Dagfinrud H, Hagen K. Physiotherapy interventions for Ankylosing Spondylitis. Cochrane Database Syst Rev. 2004;(2): CD002822.

21.40 Scleroderma

Tom Pettersson

Basic rules

- Scleroderma is characterized by small vessel injuries, immunological abnormalities, and thickening and scarring of the connective tissue.
- The disease is classified into a systemic and a local form.

Epidemiology

- The prevalence of scleroderma is 100–200 cases per one million people.
- The incidence is highest in women aged 30–50 years.

The clinical picture

- Raynaud's phenomenon (see 21.4) can be observed in almost every patient. The condition may lead to ulcerations and scars on the fingertips.
- Skin changes occur, especially in the face, hands and feet. First there is swelling of the skin, then thickening and finally atrophy (Figures 21.40.1, 21.40.2 and 21.40.3).
- Telangiectasies may be seen.
- 20–30% of all patients have arthralgia and myalgia.
- There may be gastrointestinal symptoms, particularly dysphagia and reflux oesophagitis.
- Lung fibrosis, pulmonary hypertension
- Heart failure, arrhythmias
- Renal symptoms: proteinuria, renal failure, hypertension, scleroderma renal crisis

Laboratory findings

- The ESR is usually moderately increased. The serum CRP level is normal or mildly increased.
- The blood count is usually normal.
- In the systemic form of the disease, anti-nuclear antibodies can be detected in 90% of patients, rheumatoid factor in 30% and anti-Scl-70 antibodies in 30% B [1 2].

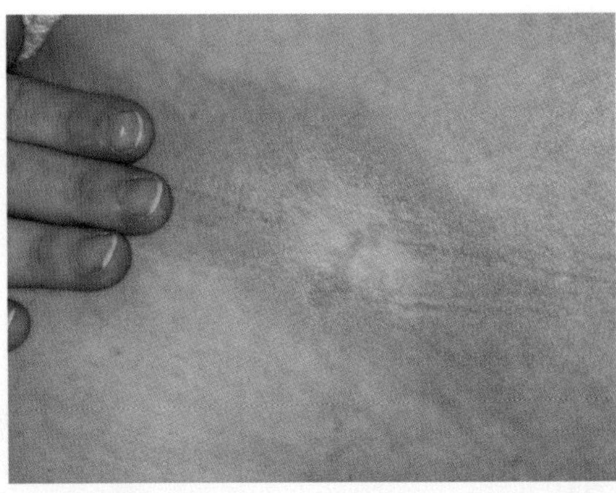

Figure 21.40.1 Scleroderma circumscripta or morphea is an autoimmune disease, limited to the skin. A pale, whitish, often glistening, inelastic and hardened central area is surrounded by a reddish-lilac diffuse ring. The lesions may be multiple. The diagnosis can be confirmed by biopsy. Photo © R. Suhonen.

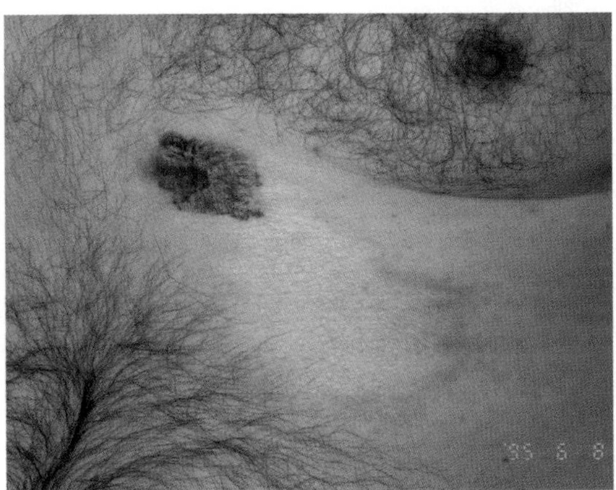

Figure 21.40.2 Scleroderma circumscripta or morphea is a patchy skin-hardening disease. A markedly pale, whitish, inelastic, hardened central area is typically surrounded by a reddish-lilac diffuse ring. The red spot in the uppermedial region is an ecchymosis. There is no specific cure, but penicillin (orally, for one month) combined with topical calci(po)triol for a few months may be tried. Photo © R. Suhonen.

- Anti-centromere antibodies occur in the CREST syndrome (calcinosis, Raynaud's phenomenon, oesophageal hypomotility, sclerodactyly, teleangiectasies) B [1 2].

Diagnosis

- The clinical picture (skin changes, Raynaud's phenomenon)
- Involvement of the inner organs
- Serological findings B [1 2]
- Skin biopsy as required

Treatment

- The patient should try to protect her skin, avoid cold and stop smoking.

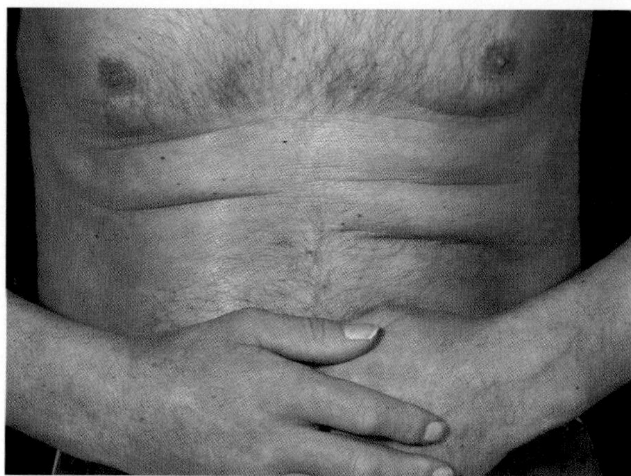

Figure 21.40.3 Diffuse scleroderma (progressive systemic sclerosis, PSS) is an autoimmune disorder affecting the whole skin/body. The skin is thickened and inelastic, the fingers swell ("sausage-deformity"), leading to difficulty in the use of the hand. Raynaud's phenomenon and involvement of the inner organs are common findings. Photo © R. Suhonen.

- Non-steroidal anti-inflammatory drugs for arthralgia and myalgia.
- Corticosteroids in the inflammatory phase of the disease.
- Calcium inhibitors and nitroglycerin ointment for peripheral circulatory disturbances.
- Angiotensin converting-enzyme inhibitors are preferred as antihypertensive medication.
- I.v. iloprost is effective **B** [3] and prazosin is moderately effective **C** [4] for Raynaud's phenomenon in progressive systemic sclerosis.

Prognosis

- Favourable when the disease is confined to the skin.
- Respiratory or renal failure signifies a poor prognosis.

References

1. Spencer-Green G, Alter D, Welch HG. Test performance in systemic sclerosis: Anti-centromere and Anti-Scl-70 antibodies (review). Am J Med 1997;103:242–248.
2. The Database of Abstracts of Reviews of Effectiveness (University of York), Database no.: DARE-971190. In: The Cochrane Library, Issue 4, 1999. Oxford: Update Software.
3. Pope J, Fenlon D, Thompson A, Shea B, Furst D, Wells G, Silman A. Iloprost and cisaprost for Raynaud's phenomenon in progressive systemic sclerosis. Cochrane Database Syst Rev. 2004;(2):CD000953.
4. Pope J, Fenlon D, Thompson A, Shea B, Furst D, Wells G, Silman A. Prazosin for Raynaud's phenomenon in progressive systemic sclerosis. Cochrane Database Syst Rev. 2004;(2):CD000956.

21.41 Systemic lupus erythematosus (SLE)

Marianne Gripenberg-Gahmberg

Definition

- SLE is a syndrome characterized by clinical diversity, changes in the disease activity over time and by aberrant immunological findings.

Epidemiology

- The prevalence of SLE worldwide is 4–250 per 100 000. The incidence is most frequent in women aged 15–25 years.

Clinical presentation

- The clinical presentation varies between different patients, and in a single patient the disease activity varies over time.
- General symptoms such as fatigue and fever are common.
- A vast majority of the patients have arthralgia, mostly of the hands.
- About one-half of the patients have cutaneous features, such as butterfly rash and discoid lupus (Figures 21.41.1 and 21.41.2) as well as photosensitivity.
- About one-third of the patients have oral ulcerations.
- About 50% of the patients have nephropathy, which varies from mild proteinuria and microscopical haematuria to end-stage renal failure.
- About 20–40% of the patients have pleurisy. Acute pneumonitis and chronic fibrotising alveolitis are relatively rare.
- Pericarditis is somewhat less common than pleuritis. T-wave changes in the ECG are usual.
- Depression and headache are the most common neuropsychiatric symptoms. Grand-mal seizures and organic psychoses are rare. Peripheral neuropathy is observed in about 10% of the patients and as many patients get a thromboembolic or haemorrhagic complication of the brain.
- The lymph nodes may enlarge especially when the disease is active.
- There is a risk of first and second trimester foetal losses and of premature birth.

Laboratory findings

- Laboratory findings are diverse.
- ESR is usually elevated, the CRP value is often normal.
- Mild or moderate anaemia is common. A clear-cut haemolytic anaemia is seen in less than 10% of the patients.

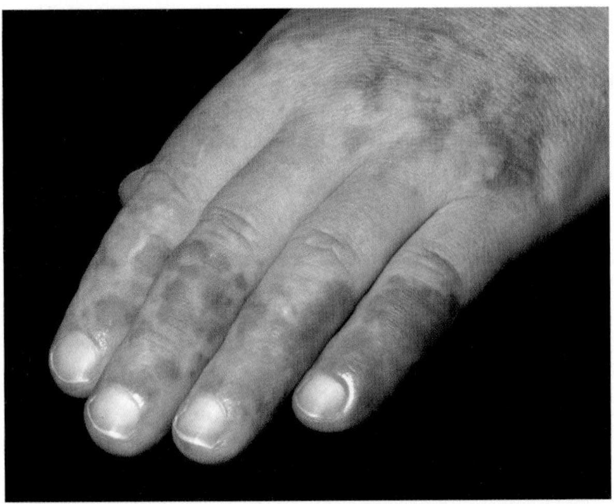

Figure 21.41.1 The skin symptoms in systemic lupus erythematosus (SLE) are variable. The skin in distal fingers, especially in nail folds, shows telangiectasias. Purpuric vasculitis lesions are not uncommon. Photo © R. Suhonen.

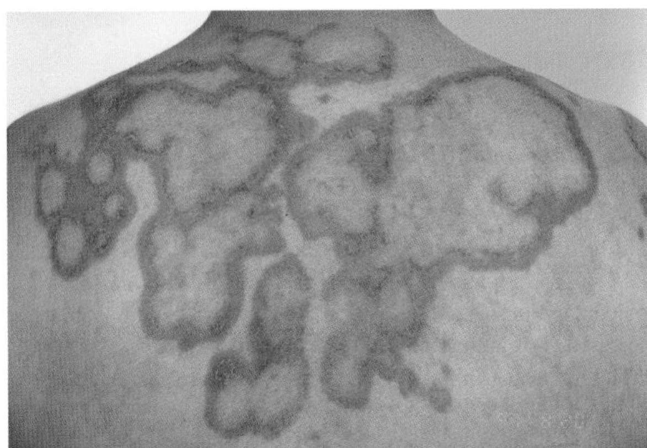

Figure 21.41.2 Very typical picture of subacute cutaneous lupus erythematosus (SCLE). Anti-Ro (SS-A) antibodies are positive in this disease in 9 out of 10 patients. In this female patient antimalarials were ineffective, but the symptoms healed completely in a few weeks by oral acitretin. Photo © R. Suhonen.

- Leucocytopenia (lymphocytopenia)
- Mild thrombocytopenia
- Antinuclear antibodies are found in over 90% of the patients.
- Anti-DNA antibodies (in 50–90% of the patients)
- Polyclonal hypergammablobulinaemia
- Decreased complement values (C3 and C4)
- Antiphospholipid antibodies
- Proteinuria, microscopic haematuria, decreased creatinine clearance

Diagnosis

- There is no single symptom or finding that is sufficient in itself for making the diagnosis.
- When SLE is suspected the basic laboratory investigations are:
  - blood count
  - platelets
  - ESR
  - anti-nuclear antibodies
  - dipstick test of the urine and urinanalysis.
- The diagnosis is based on the clinical symptoms and the laboratory findings and on the ARA classification criteria (1982).
- The patient should be referred to a specialist for confirmation of the diagnosis.

Treatment

- The treatment is always individual and depends on the manifestations and activity of the disease. There is no need for treatment solely on the basis of the immunological findings.
- The patients should be encouraged to restrain from sunbathing and to use sunscreens.
- The most important drugs are:
  - non-steroidal anti-inflammatory drugs
  - hydroxychloroquine C [1 2]
  - corticosteroids
  - immunosuppressive drugs (e.g. azathioprine, cyclophosphamide).
- Hydroxychloroquine and non-steroidal anti-inflammatory drugs are used in the treatment of mild symptoms such as cutaneous manifestations and arthralgia. When the response is insufficient or when the patient has fatigue or fever a low dose of corticosteroids (prednisolone 5–7.5 mg/day) can be added.
- In the treatment of pleuritis or pericarditis larger amounts of corticosteroids (about 30 mg prednisolone per day) are used.
- In the treatment of severe CNS symptoms and of severe glomerulonephritis, thrombocytopenia and haemolytic anaemia large corticosteroid doses and other immunosuppressive drugs are used A [3 4 5].
- The differential diagnosis between an infection and a flare of the SLE is of utmost importance.
- Other drugs that the patient might need, such as antihypertensive treatment, should be remembered.
- If there are signs of renal manifestations the patient should be referred to a nephrologist for a renal biopsy.
- The patients are often allergic to a variety of antibiotics, especially sulfonamides.

Primary antiphospholipid syndrome

- A syndrome manifesting as recurrent venous or arterial thrombotic events, recurrent miscarriages, thrombocytopenia and antiphospholipid antibodies, but without other features of SLE.

References

1. The Canadian Hydroxychloroquine Study Group: A randomized study of the effect of withdrawing hydroxychloroquine in systemic lupus erythematosus. N Engl J Med 1991;324:150–154.
2. Wallace DJ. Antilamarial agents and lupus. Rheum Dis Clin North Am 1994;20:243–263.
3. Bansal VK, Beto JA. Treatment of lupus nephritis: a meta-analysis of clinical trials. Am J Kidney Dis 1997;29:193–199.
4. The Database of Abstracts of Reviews of Effectiveness (University of York), Database no.: DARE-970317. In: The Cochrane Library, Issue 4, 1999. Oxford: Update Software.
5. Flanc RS, Roberts MA, Strippoli GFM, Chadban SJ, Kerr PG, Atkins RC. Treatment for lupus nephritis. The Cochrane Database of Systematic Reviews, Cochrane Library Number: CD002922. In: Cochrane Library, Issue 1, 2004. Chichester, UK: John Wiley & Sons, Ltd.

21.42 Mixed connective tissue disease (MCTD)

Tom Pettersson

Definition and epidemiology

- Mixed connective tissue disease (MCTD) is a rare disorder, that shows features of rheumatoid arthritis, SLE, polymyositis and scleroderma and that is characterized by anti-ribonucleoprotein antibodies in high titre.
- The clinical picture is variable. Over several years the disease tends to resemble scleroderma more and more.
- Most patients are women aged 30–40 years.

The clinical picture

- Almost all patients have arthritis or arthralgia
- Swelling of the fingers and Raynaud's phenomenon
- Skin changes resembling those seen in SLE
- Muscle symptoms, which resemble those seen in polymyositis
- Pleuritis, carditis and nephritis occur but are more common in SLE

Laboratory findings

- Elevated ESR
- Anaemia, leucopenia
- Speckled pattern of anti-nuclear antibodies, high titre
- Rheumatoid factor positive in 50% of the patients
- Antibodies against extractable nuclear antigens reacting with nuclear ribonucleoprotein

Treatment

- Non-steroidal anti-inflammatory drugs for arthritis
- Small-dose corticosteroids for general symptoms
- Large-dose corticosteroids for severe organ manifestations
- As in SLE, treatment should be adjusted according to the clinical picture

21.43 Sjögren's syndrome

Editors

Aim

- To identify patients with Sjögren's syndrome among all people suffering from dry eyes and dry mouth.

Basic rules

- Reduced function of exocrine glands is manifested as dryness of the eyes (keratoconjunctivitis sicca) and mouth (xerostomia).
- May occur as a primary disease or secondary to rheumatoid arthritis, or rarely to SLE or scleroderma.
- 10–15% of patients with rheumatoid arthritis suffer from sicca symptoms.
- Presence of autoantibodies is typical in Sjögren's syndrome. Their absence in patients suffering from dryness of the eyes and mouth speaks against the diagnosis.

The clinical picture

- A gritty sensation in the eye, sensitivity to light and eye fatigue.
- Dryness of the mucosa of the oral cavity causing dysphagia.
- Decreased gustatory and olfactory sensation.
- Fissures in the tongue and lips.
- Recurrent swelling of the parotid glands may occur.
- Crustae on the nasal mucosa, dry cough, recurrent respiratory tract infections.
- Dry skin
- Dysphagia, atrophic gastritis may occur.
- Other autoimmune phenomena such as thyroiditis, pernicious anaemia, coeliac disease.
- Dryness of the vulva and vagina, dyspareunia.
- Fatigue, joint pain and Raynaud's phenomenon are common manifestations.
- Rarely acute pancreatitis, hepatomegaly.
- Concurrent primary biliary cirrhosis may occur but is rare (9.23).
- Elevated erythrocyte sedimentation rate
- Increased risk of lymphomas

Diagnostic criteria

- To establish the diagnosis of Sjögren's syndrome, four of the following criteria should be fulfilled. Exclusion criteria include lymphoma, HIV infection, sarcoidosis and graft-versus-host disease.
  - Eye symptoms: dry eyes for more than 3 months or a sensation of a foreign body in the eye.
  - Oral symptoms: dry mouth for more than 3 months or permanently swollen parotid glands.
  - Eye findings: in Schirmer's test a paper slip is moistened less than 5 mm in 5 minutes.
  - Salivary gland biopsy of the lower lip: focal sialoadenitis.
  - Changes in the salivary glands: diminished saliva secretion or changes visible on sialography or scintigraphy.
  - Autoantibodies: Anti-SSA or Anti-SSB antibodies, anti-nuclear antibodies or rheumatoid factor.

Therapy

- Artificial tears
- Treatment of dry mouth, see 7.10.

21.44 The vasculitides

Tom Pettersson, Markku Ellonen

Aim

- Vasculitis has to be taken into account when the patient presents with systemic symptoms

Basic rules

- The vasculitides are a rare and heterogeneous group of clinical syndromes characterized by inflammation and injury of blood vessels.
- They are often serious but still treatable disorders.
- Because of a variable clinical picture the diagnosis may be delayed.
- The size and the localization of the affected blood vessel determine the clinical picture.

Symptoms and signs of vasculitis

- Fever and weight loss
- Palpable purpura, livedo reticularis
- Myalgia, myositis, arthralgia, arthritis
- Mononeuritis multiplex, stroke
- Epistaxis, sinusitis, haemoptysis, pneumonitis, asthma
- Myocardial infarction, hypertension, intermittent claudication, weak peripheral pulses
- Abdominal pain, melena
- Glomerulonephritis
- Elevated ESR, high serum CRP value, anaemia, leucocytosis, thrombocytosis, proteinuria, haematuria, anti-nuclear cytoplasmic antibodies (ANCAs)

Classification of the vasculitides

Large vessel vasculitis

- Temporal arteritis (21.46)
- Takayasu's arteritis

Small and medium-sized vessel vasculitis

- Polyarteritis nodosa
- Microscopic polyangiitis
- Wegener's granulomatosis
- Churg-Strauss syndrome
- Kawasaki disease (32.57)

Small vessel vasculitis

- Henoch-Schönlein purpura (32.53)
- Associated with connective tissue diseases
- Mixed cryoglobulinaemia
- Associated with infections
- Associated with drug allergy
- Associated with malignant tumours

Temporal arteritis

- See 21.46.

Takayasu's arteritis

- Most common in young women of Asian descent. Damages the aorta and its main branches.
- In the early phases, nonspecific symptoms such as malaise, arthralgias and myalgias are frequent. Increased ESR and serum CRP concentration.
- Signs of narrowing of the arteries develop gradually.
- Weakened pulses in the upper extremities and difficulty measuring the blood pressure.
- Central nervous system manifestations
- The diagnosis is confirmed by arteriography.

Polyarteritis nodosa

- A serious disease that most frequently affects middle-aged males.

- General symptoms: fever, weight loss, malaise
- Arthralgia and myalgia occur frequently.
- Gastrointestinal symptoms, such as vomiting, diarrhoea and abdominal pain are seen in about half of the patients. Haematemesis, melena and intestinal perforation may occur.
- Coronary arteritis occurs in more than 70% of the patients.
- Renal disease, most often renal arteritis, which manifests as haematuria, proteinuria, renal insufficiency and hypertension
- Mononeuritis multiplex is the most typical neurological manifestation and occurs in one-half or more of all cases.
- Cerebral haemorrhage occurs in 10% of patients.
- Occasionally eye manifestations, such as episcleritis, uveitis and retinal haemorrhages are present.
- Cutaneous manifestations, such as exanthema and purpura are seen in 30% of all cases.
- The ESR and serum CRP level are elevated. Anaemia, neutrophilic leucocytosis, thrombocytosis, proteinuria, haematuria and a raised serum creatinine concentration are frequent findings.
- In the classic form of the disease anti-nuclear cytoplasmic antibodies are rarely seen.
- Hepatitis B surface antigen and antibody have been found in more than 15% of patients.
- The diagnosis is based on the clinical picture and on evidence of vasculitis obtained at biopsy or arteriography.

Microscopic polyangiitis

- A vasculitis that preferentially affects small arteries and arterioles.
- In more than 90% of the cases there is a focal segmental necrotizing glomerulonephritis, which may be the only manifestation of the disease.
- Other manifestations include lung infiltrates, haemoptysis, arthralgia, myalgia, purpura and fever.
- ANC-antibodies (most commonly p-ANC/MPO-antibodies) are found in most patients.
- The diagnosis is based on the clinical picture, biopsy findings and a positive ANCA test.

Wegener's granulomatosis

- Patients typically present with fever, weight loss and upper respiratory tract symptoms such as sinusitis and bloody nasal discharge.
- There may be episcleritis, conjunctivitis and arthritis or arthralgia.
- During the course of the disease, a cough with purulent or bloody sputum develops. Chest x-rays show single or multiple nodular infiltrates.
- Renal involvement is common and varies from mild focal segmental glomerulonephritis to rapidly progressive crescentic glomerulonephritis.
- There may be cutaneous and peripheral nervous system manifestations.
- The ESR and serum CRP concentration are elevated.
- Anaemia, neutrophilic leucocytosis and thrombocytosis are frequent findings.
- Patients with renal involvement have proteinuria and urinary red cells and red cell casts.
- c-ANC/PR3-antibodies are remarkably specific for Wegener's granulomatosis C [1 2] and the titre has been used as a marker of disease activity.
- The diagnosis is based on the clinical picture, the ANCA test and biopsy findings.
  - Biopsy of the nasal mucosa or of the lung may show a granulomatous inflammation.
  - Histological examination of a kidney biopsy typically shows a necrotising focal or diffuse crescentic glomerulonephritis.
- The ANCA test should not be used as a screening test in cases where the probability of Wegener's granulomatosis is low.

Churg-Strauss syndrome (allergic granulomatosis and angiitis)

- A rare disease, which occurs in patients with asthma or a history of allergy.
- General symptoms: fever and weight loss
- Glomerulonephritis and joint symptoms tend to be less severe than in polyarteritis nodosa.
- Mono- and polyneuropathies. Cardiac involvement.
- Marked blood eosinophilia and an elevated serum CRP concentration and ESR. ANC-antibodies of the p-ANC/MPO type.
- Lung infiltrates on chest x-ray
- The diagnosis is based on the clinical picture, a history of asthma or allergy, blood eosinophilia, lung infiltrates and typical biopsy findings.

Henoch-Schönlein purpura

- See 32.53.
- Henoch-Schönlein purpura or anaphylactoid purpura is most commonly seen in children, but may also occur in adults.
- In 90% of all patients an upper respiratory tract infection has preceded the vasculitic symptoms by 1–3 weeks.
- Articular, intestinal and renal symptoms may occur.
- There is usually a spontaneous remission within a week but relapses may occur.
- A chronic glomerulonephritis occurs rarely.
- The diagnosis is based on the clinical picture. Skin biopsy shows a leucocytoclastic vasculitis with IgA and C3 precipitated in the vessel walls. The serum IgA concentration tends to be high.

Mixed cryoglobulinaemia

- There may be an underlying infection, connective tissue disease, lymphoproliferative disease or liver disease.
- Essential forms occur, the great majority of which are probably caused by hepatitis C virus. Hepatitis B virus may be the causative agent in a minority of cases.

- Mixed cryoglobulins have the properties of an immune complex vasculitis.
- General symptoms: fatigue, weakness
- Cutaneous manifestations in almost all patients: purpura, Raynaud's phenomenon, skin necrosis, leg ulcers
- Other manifestations include arthralgias, proteinuria, haematuria, renal failure, hypertension, hepatomegaly, mono- or polyneuropathy and abdominal pain.
- Elevated ESR, high titre of rheumatoid factor and low concentration of complement (particularly C4).

Differential diagnosis of vasculitides

- Infections such as septicaemia and endocarditis
- Malignant tumours
- Embolizations, such as atheromatous cholesterol embolization, mycotic aneurysms, atrial myxoma
- Thrombotic conditions such as DIC, TTP and the antiphospholipid syndrome

Principles of treatment of vasculitides

- The management of patients with vasculitis is best performed in specialized hospitals.
- Corticosteroids and cytotoxic drugs constitute the basis of the therapy.

References

1. Rao J, Weinberger M, Oddone E, Allen N, Landman P, Feussner JR. The role of antineutrophil cytoplasmic antibody (c-ANCA) testing in the diagnosis of Wegener granulomatosis: a literature review and meta-analysis. Ann Intern Med 1995;123:925–932.
2. The Database of Abstracts of Reviews of Effectiveness (University of York), Database no.: DARE-968019. In: The Cochrane Library, Issue 4, 1999. Oxford: Update Software.

21.45 Polymyalgia rheumatica

Editors

Aims

- To identify those patients with musculoskeletal pain who can be offered a successful treatment.
- To prevent loss of vision when temporal arteritis is associated.

Aetiology

- Unknown

Epidemiology

- The annual incidence among people over 50 years of age is about 50/100 000.
- The incidence peaks at 70 years of age.
- 70% of all patients are women.

Symptoms

- Pain and stiffness in the neck, shoulder and lumbar regions. Symptoms are exacerbated by exercise. No tenderness on palpation as in fibromyalgia and myositis.
- The onset is usually acute: the patient is able to tell the exact day when the symptoms started.
- In more severe forms of the disease, general symptoms include fever, weight loss, fatigue, depression and anorexia.
- Concurrently with polymyalgia rheumatica the patient may have temporal arteritis (giant cell arteritis) (21.46), which may cause severe headache.

RHE

Findings

- Tenderness (although not always) of the superficial temporal artery in the case of arteritis. Loss of vision may be the first symptom in these patients.
- There may be an arthritis resembling rheumatoid arthritis. In elderly people, rheumatoid arthritis may have a polymyalgic onset.
- In addition to temporal arteritis, there may be an arteritis of extracranial vessels causing other ischaemic organ symptoms.

Laboratory investigations

- The ESR is markedly elevated: usually exceeds 40 mm/h, but may be more than 100 mm/h (unlike in fibromyalgia). Serum CRP concentration is also markedly increased and liver specific serum alkaline phosphatase concentration is mildly raised in 30% of all patients. In very few patients (1–2%) ESR is not elevated. The ESR is a good screening test when polymyalgia rheumatica is suspected to be the cause of musculoskeletal pain and temporal arteritis the cause of headache.
- Rheumatoid factor is not detectable. Serum creatine kinase concentration is normal (unlike in polymyositis).

Diagnosis

- Can usually be based on clinical findings: a typical clinical picture, elevated ESR and rapid response to corticosteroids.
- Biopsy of the superficial temporal artery may confirm the diagnosis of temporal arteritis. There may be arteritic

changes even if there is no headache or tenderness of the artery. The arteritis may also be focal, which is why absence of inflammatory findings in the biopsy sample does not exclude temporal arteritis. Biopsy is recommended if temporal arteritis can be suspected on clinical grounds. Typical changes may still be visible several days after institution of corticosteroid therapy.

Differential diagnosis

- Fibromyalgia, viral myalgia, rheumatoid arthritis, polymyositis, osteoarthritis, multiple myeloma, depression, hypothyroidism, infectious diseases and malignant tumours.

Treatment and prognosis

- In principle the disease is self-limiting, wherefore several mild cases probably pass undiagnosed.
- The symptoms are relieved by corticosteroids within a few days.
  - It is essential to give corticosteroids to those patients who have an arteritis and impending severe complications (loss of vision etc.).
  - Prednisolone is given in a dose of 10–20 mg daily depending on the severity of the disease. Symptoms should disappear within 3–5 days. The diagnosis has to be re-evaluated if the symptoms persist.
  - The prednisone dose may be tapered gradually after 2–3 weeks, depending on the symptoms and the ESR.
  - Treatment is usually given for (6)–12–24 months. Some patients require corticosteroid therapy for several years. Corticosteroids abolish the symptoms quickly but the duration of the disease is not reduced.
  - The prednisone dose is tapered by 2.5 mg monthly. The maintenance dose ranges from 5 to 7.5 mg daily. In temporal arteritis much higher corticosteroid doses are used and treatment is continued for a longer period of time.
  - Cytostatics (methotrexate, azathioprine) are sometimes needed in addition to corticosteroids
- If treatment is stopped too early and there is an activation of the disease, reinstitution of corticosteroids will have favourable effect.
- There is a tendency to relapse. The patient is usually able to identify the symptoms and seek medical advice.

21.46 Temporal arteritis

Tom Pettersson

- Polymyalgia rheumatica, see 21.45.

Objectives

- To remember the possibility of temporal arteritis as a cause of headache, visual disturbances and disturbances in brain circulation.
- To prevent serious complications, such as loss of vision.

Basic rules

- Giant cell arteritis is called temporal arteritis or cranial arteritis when it manifests in the arteries of the head, and polymyalgia rheumatica, when muscular pain and stiffness characterize the clinical picture.
- The disease must be diagnosed and treated rapidly because of visual disturbances. Most visual disturbances are caused by infection and consequent ischaemia in arteria ophthalmica and its branches. Also the aorta and the big vessels emerging from the aorta may become affected. Neurological deficiency symptoms caused by brain infarction may develop.
- The aetiology is unknown.

Epidemiology

- Temporal arteritis has been considered a rare disease but the prevalence seems to be increasing (or it is diagnosed better than earlier).
- In a Finnish study, on the basis of biopsies, positive findings were seen in about 12/100 000/year in patients aged 50 years or more.
- There is a female preponderance, and the patients are elderly (most of them 60 to 70 years old).

Symptoms

- General
  - Fatigue
  - Weight loss, loss of appetite
  - Fever
  - Depression
- Symptoms of temporal arteritis
  - Severe headache, localized in one or both temples, stabbing or sometimes throbbing, temporal tenderness of the scalp.
  - Masseter claudication (pain in the jaw provocated by chewing, stiffness of the masseter muscles), pain in the muscles of the tongue and the pharynx.
  - Visual disturbances: partial or total, temporary or permanent, loss of vision in one or both eyes, double vision, scintillating cloud, scotomata, cortical blindness (temporary visual disturbances resemble amaurosis fugax and migraine).
  - Sometimes there are other symptoms from cranial nerves, such as vertigo and tinnitus.
- Other symptoms resembling TIA or stroke, confusion

- Symptoms from the systemic circulation are rare: disturbances in the circulation of the heart, extremities, lungs and spinal cord.
- Symptoms of polymyalgia rheumatica
  - Ache, stiffness and pain of the neck, pectoral and pelvic girdles.

Clinical signs

- Swelling, tenderness, nodularity, weak or absent pulse over the temporal artery or other superficial artery of the head (facial or occipital artery)
- Visual signs
  - Blurred vision, scotomata
  - Ocular paresis, internuclear ophthalmoplegy
  - At ophthalmoscopy, swelling and paleness of the optic nerve may be observed, if the lesion is in the anterior part of the nerve.
  - Bleeding or paleness of the retina in case of occlusion.

Laboratory findings

- ESR is usually elevated, at least 50 mm/h, often >100 mm/h (normal in 1–2% of patients)
- Serum CRP is elevated
- Leucocytosis
- Normochromic normocytic anaemia
- Alkaline phosphatase may be elevated.

Confirming the diagnosis with biopsy

- Biopsy is an outpatient procedure but requires prior training. The biopsy should be taken from the part of the artery with most pathological changes. Arteritis is segmental and it is possible that there are no changes in the artery where the biopsy is taken. If the clinical signs strongly suggest the diagnosis, biopsy from the other side should be considered if the finding is negative.
- After confirmation of the diagnosis, the disease rapidly responds to corticosteroid treatment. In case of severe symptoms, corticosteroid treatment may be indicated even before the biopsy, which preferably should be taken within a few days.

Treatment

- Corticosteroids, usually prednisone. Initial dose is 40–80 mg/day; high doses e.g. methylprednisolone 1 g i.v. on 3 consecutive days are given especially if the patient has had visual disturbances.
- If the disease has caused loss of vision, the patient should lie in bed with feet slightly elevated to assure the best possible circulation in the eye.
- Symptoms alleviate and laboratory findings are normalized within a few weeks and the dose of prednisone is tapered gradually. Headache is relieved within days. Temporary and partial visual disturbances often disappear, total loss of vision is irreversible.
- The dose of prednisolone is based on the clinical response and laboratory findings. Usually it is 7.5–10 mg/day.
- Especially in older patients, a prolonged corticosteroid treatment causes adverse effects. A careful diagnosis, verified with a biopsy is therefore necessary.
- If the response to prednisone is poor, methotrexate can be added to it. In one study, combination therapy was found to reduce the number of disease recurrences and decrease the need for prednisone **C** [1].

Prognosis

- The inflammatory process of arteritis often subsides within months or years, but relapses occur even after many years. Treatments are long, 1 to 2 years.
- Symptoms may flare when corticosteroid use is tapered or stopped.
- It is important that the physician treating the patient is aware of the disease, otherwise the symptoms can be assigned to arteriosclerosis.

RHE

Reference

1. Jover JA, Hernandez-Garcia C, Morado IC, Vargas E, Banares A, Fernandez-Gutierrez B.Combined treatment of giant-cell arteritis with methotrexate and prednisone. a randomized, double-blind, placebo-controlled trial. Ann Intern Med 2001 Jan 16;134(2):106–14.

21.50 Gout

Editors

Basic rules

- Gout is an important cause of joint inflammation, for which a specific treatment is available: tests for gout should always be included in the work-up for (mono)arthritis in the adult.
- If gout is suspected and synovial fluid can be aspirated, the fluid should always be examined for the presence of crystals.
- The serum urate concentration should be measured but a diagnosis of gout should not be made (or excluded) on the basis of the result.
- When gout occurs in a patient on diuretic drugs, withdrawal of the diuretic should be considered as the first step.
- Dietary instructions should be given to all patients suffering from gout.
- The aims of therapy are to relief symptoms and to lower the serum urate concentration to the reference range (below 400 μmol/l).

Causes and epidemiology

- In the elderly and in women, diuretic therapy is the most common cause of gout.
- In persons using alcohol, several mechanisms account for a rise in serum urate concentration.
- In young women and in children, gout is extremely rare.
- The symptoms start in middle age.
- Causes of secondary gout include dehydration, renal failure, myeloproliferative diseases.

Symptoms and signs

- The most characteristic symptom is inflammation with pain and redness of the first metatarsophalangeal joint. Symptoms may be exacerbated by exposure to cold and are often worse during the night.
- The large joints of the lower or upper limbs are more infrequently involved.
- During the acute attack the patient may be mildly febrile.
- There is often fluid in the joint but on palpation the synovium does not appear thickened.
- During an attack of gout, there may be a marked elevation of ESR and serum CRP.
- The number of cells in synovial fluid is usually greatly increased (up to 30,000/mm^3) with a predominance of granulocytes.
- Using a microscope with a polarisation filter, anisotropic urate crystals can be seen. Evidence of phagocytosis of crystals by leucocytes confirms the diagnosis. For handling of synovial fluid samples and further analyses, see 21.11.
- The serum urate concentration is usually above 300 μmol/l. (The theoretical solubility limit of urate is 450 μmol/l.)
- Radiographic findings are usually normal when the first symptoms occur (compare with chondrocalcinosis (21.52), where intra-articular calcifications are seen). In advanced gout, erosions and shadows representing accumulations of urate (tophi) are seen close to the joint.

Investigations

- Serum urate
  - Seldom normal during an acute attack of gout
- Serum creatinine (renal failure may be a cause of gout and it influences the choice of therapy)
- Haemoglobin, leucocytes, platelets, ESR (haematological malignancies may be a cause of gout)

Treatment

An acute attack

- The joint is aspirated and methylprednisolone is injected locally (21.10), for example 0.2 ml in the first metatarsophalangeal joint.
  - If the possibility of an infection seems remote, installation of the corticosteroid may be injected with the same needle used to take the diagnostic sample.
- Rest, ice packages
- Pain is relieved effectively with non-steroidal anti-inflammatory drugs. Indomethacin and diflunisal increase the excretion of urate and may therefore be more recommendable than acetylsalicylic acid, piroxicam and tenoxicam. The dose of indomethacin may be raised to 150 mg per day, when necessary.

Reduction of the concentration of uric acid in serum

- Withdrawal of diuretic therapy should be considered.
- Dietary restrictions to prevent gout (not needed if withdrawal of diuretics is sufficient)
- If the serum urate concentration remains above 420 μmol/l and the patient accepts a continuous medication, allopurinol is initiated after the third attack of arthritis.
  - According to some authors, to avoid exacerbation of symptoms, allopurinol should not be started until the attack has subsided. The initial dose is small (100–150 mg per day) and the dose should be increased to the therapeutic level (300 mg per day) within two weeks. Later on, if the effect persists, the dose may be halved.
  - If the serum urate concentration has not been reduced within two weeks, the dose may be increased to 600 mg per day.
  - In renal failure (serum creatinine 160–560 μmol/l) the dose is halved. In severe renal failure the maximal dose is 50–100 mg per day.
  - The most common side effects are rash and liver dysfunction. Bone marrow suppression is rarely seen. Allopurinol should not be used in combination with azathioprine.
- Attacks of gout may still occur 2–3 months after initiation of allopurinol.
- If the patient has renal stones, raised serum creatinine or polyarticular gout, allopurinol should be started immediately. Allopurinol inhibits the formation of renal stones (both urate and oxalate stones).
- If the patient does not tolerate allopurinol, an alternative is probenecid 500 mg twice daily (initial dose 250 mg twice daily). Probenecid predisposes for renal stone formation. A prerequisite for probenecid therapy is normal renal function. When probenecid is started, sodium bicarbonate 3 g daily for at least one month is required to prevent renal stones.
- Non-steroidal anti-inflammatory drugs may also be of prophylactic value.
- Provided serum urate is within normal limits, withdrawal of allopurinol may be attempted after one year. If serum urate increases again to the level where symptoms occurred, allopurinol medication should be resumed.
- Allopurinol has not been proved to be effective for symptom-free hyperuricaemia. Here, dietary therapy is the primary form of treatment.

21.51 Dietary treatment of gout

Editors

- The aim is to avoid foods that contain large amounts of purines. Purines are metabolized to uric acid, which may be injurious to health.

Foods to be avoided

- All alcoholic beverages, particularly beer
- Internal organs, such as liver, kidney, thymus

Foods to be eaten in restricted amounts

- Fish (roe, baltic herring, sardines, etc. larger fish may be eaten)
- Crustaceans
- Meat (beef, pork, poultry, beef stock, etc.)
- Some vegetables (peas, beans, asparagus, mushrooms)

Freely consumable foods

- Cereals (bread, porridge, bran, etc.)
- Dairy products (milk, sour milk, cheese)
- All fruits and fruit juices
- Eggs
- Fat (cooking oil, margarine, butter, etc.)
- Coffee, tea, chocolate
- Most vegetables (potatoes, salad, cabbage, tomato, cucumber, pumpkin, onion, carrot, beetroot, radish, celery)
- Sugar (causes an increase in weight!)
- Spices

Other recommendations

- The metabolic disturbances are aggravated by obesity. Thus, maintaining a normal body weight is important. Overzealous fasting may, however, lead to accumulation of urate in the blood and precipitate an attack of gout.
- The intake of fluid should be adequate.

21.52 Chondrocalcinosis (pseudogout)

Editors

Basic rules

- Differentiate the disease from gout and other arthritides on the basis of the analysis of synovial fluid cells and radiological findings.

Causes and epidemiology

- Pyrophosphate crystals accumulate in the joint as a result of local metabolic disturbance.
- Often a complication of osteoarthritis.
- Occurs most often in the elderly.
- Some forms of the disease are hereditary.

Symptoms

- Pain, swelling and effusion of the knee, or rarely of the ankle.
- The symptoms are paroxysmal.

Diagnosis

- The clinical picture
- Calcified cartilage is seen on x-rays.
- Arthrosis at the "wrong" location may be pyrophosphate arthropathy.
- Pyrophosphate crystals can be identified in the synovial fluid (They are more difficult to recognize than urate crystals).
- Conditions predisposing to pyrophosphate arthropathy are ruled out (hyperparathyroidism 24.21, haemochromatosis 24.65).

Treatment

- Rest
- Conservative treatment of osteoarthritis
- Local steroid injection in a joint with effusion (21.10)
- NSAIDs.

21.70 Complex regional pain syndrome (Reflex sympathetic dystrophy)

Martina Bachmann, Pertti Pere

Aim

- To prevent complex regional pain syndrome (CRPS) by adequate mobilization of all limb injuries, such as radial fracture (18.25).

RHE

Pathophysiology

- The pathophysiology is not well understood. The central nervous system, peripheral nervous system, sympathetic nervous system and local muscle tissue are all involved in the development of the pain syndrome.

Definition and diagnosis

- All four criteria must be fulfilled.
  - A precipitating injury or disease, which has led to the immobilization of an extremity.
  - Constant pain and disproportionately severe pain on slight stimuli (touch etc.). Pain is aggravated by stress, changes in temperature and movement of the affected limb.
  - Swelling of the painful area, a change in the peripheral circulation (a change in the temperature and colour of the skin), sudomotor changes or abnormal motor functions.
  - The severity of the symptoms and dysfunction cannot be explained by any other cause.
- The aetiology of the syndrome is unknown. At least in some cases the provocative event is a reaction precipitated by sympathetic nervous system activity (see section Pathophysiology).
- The pain usually starts several weeks after the injury. The pain is constant and burning in character. The extremity will initially swell, become red and show increased sweating (1–3 months). Later on the skin will atrophy, become cool to the touch and cyanotic. Deeper tissues and muscles will also atrophy (3–6 months). Without treatment the condition may become chronic and the symptoms may spread to the opposite limb.
- Radiographically detectable osteoporosis is a characteristic finding in advanced cases. In these cases the condition may be irreversible.

Prevention and treatment

Prevention

- After an injury the limb should be elevated in order to avoid swelling.
- Adequate exercise therapy should be applied to any free joints in upper limb fractures in a plaster cast:
  - If a patient with a fracture of the radius complains of hand pain and swollen fingers, treatment should consist of repeated extension and flexion exercises of the fingers with the limb elevated, not of prolonged immobilization.
  - As soon as the immobilization ends, the immobilized area must be mobilized with professional input (physiotherapy).
  - Adequate pain relief

Treatment

- Often requires cooperation between a physician, psychologist and physiotherapist.
- Intensified exercise therapy and analgesia should be introduced as soon as symptoms appear. Analgesia should be similar to the one indicated for neuropathic pain.
- Other treatment modalities, such as medium-dose, short-term steroids or regional sympathetic blockade, have been tried for severe symptoms.
- Calcitonin may be beneficial.

Geriatrics

Evidence Based Medicine Guidelines. Edited by the Duodecim Editorial Team
 ISBN: 0-470-01184-X

22.1 Falls of the elderly

Editors

Aims

- The cause of the fall has to be identified and eliminated.
- The risks and dangers of falls must be evaluated and minimized.

Risk factors for falls

Internal

- Medications, alcohol
  - Hypnotics and sedatives C [1 2 3 4]
  - Neuroleptics C [1 2 3 4]
  - Tricyclic antidepressants C [1 2 3 4]
  - Pharmaceuticals lowering blood pressure and nitroglycerine, digoxin, type IA anti-arrhythmics, and diuretics C [5 6]
  - Antiparkinson and antiepileptic medicines
  - Alcoholism
- Acute disorders
  - Infections
  - Disorders of water and sodium balance (diuretics)
  - Heart failure
  - Arrhythmia
  - Transient ischaemic attack and other cerebrovascular diseases
- Chronic diseases
  - Epilepsy
  - Vascular dementia, sequelae of stroke
  - Orthostatic hypotension
  - Parkinsonism
  - Diabetes
  - Anaemia, insidious gastrointestinal bleeding
- Disabilities
  - Poor vision
  - Osteoarthritis of the lower extremities, muscular weakness and clumsiness
  - Peripheral neuropathy
  - Deformities of the feet
- Forgetting regular medication or incorrect dosage

External

- Slippery surface, poor lighting, rough surface, obstacles, need to reaching for objects
- Poor shoes, unsuitable assistive devices
- History indicates the cause of the fall. The patient, caregivers, eye witnesses should be interviewed.
  - In what situation did the patient fall?
    - Getting out of bed, while walking, in the toilet, reaching out, at rest or during exertion?
  - What other symptoms were associated with the fall?
    - Dizziness, loss of bladder control, chest pain (hypotensive collapse caused by nitroglycerin), arrhythmia, unconsciousness before or after the fall?
    - Convulsions?
  - Did the patient get up without help, how soon, and what was the state of consciousness?
  - Have there been changes in the state of health lately?
  - Does the aged person use medicines?
  - How much does the aged person eat and drink?

Physical examination

- Blood pressure in supine and standing position
- Heart sounds, ECG and Holter monitoring
- Auscultation of carotid bruits
- Vision
- Orientating neurological status (gait; weakness or numbness of limbs, trunk or face; Romberg test)
- Digital rectal examination, blood haemoglobin

Management

- Check the medications, including over the counter drugs. Remove the unnecessary ones A [7].
- Consult the ophthalmologist when needed.
- Treat acute illnesses.
- Promote physical exercise B [8 9] (muscle strengthening and balance training A [7])
- Check how chronic diseases are managed.
- Medicines for dizziness are useless for falls.
- If you cannot find the cause of the fall and eliminate it, identify, evaluate and minimize the risk factors A [7].

Reducing the risk factors

- Table 22.1.

Improving the home safety

- A home visit is often needed: the patient and the caregiver should check with a doctor, physiotherapist or home nurse what arrangements are needed at home.
  - Lighting: adequate general lighting, a light in the staircase and a night light in the bedroom and the toilet.
  - Clear access: in the apartment, in the staircase, in the yard, removal of snow and ice in the wintertime
  - Low-edged carpets, anti-sliding friction material underneath, removal of doorsteps and carpets when needed
  - Toilet and bathroom: handles, non-slip floor and bathtub bottom and a raised toilet seat. A lock on the door of the toilet should also open from the outside.
  - Steady and high enough chairs and bed.
  - Kitchen: Items should be accessible without having to reach.
  - Appropriate shoes (low, non-slip heal)

Table 22.1 Falls of the elderly-reducing the risk factors

Risk factor	Intervention
Impaired vision	Correcting the refractive error, management of cataracts, improving lighting
Impaired sense of balance	Removing medicines affecting balance
Dementia	Removing unnecessary medicines, optimal treatment of chronic diseases, improving home safety, walking exercises
Foot problems	Management of callus and hallux valgus, appropriate shoes
Orthostatic hypotension	♦ Checking medicines, sufficient intake of fluids, rest after dining, raising the head end of the bed, slow rising to upright position ♦ Possible medicines (dihydroergotamine, etilefrine hydrochloride, fludrocortisone)
Degeneration of the cervical spine	Personal belongings at an easy reach
Musculoskeletal disorders	Walking aids, non-slip spikes on soles and on the cane, improved home safety

- If the safety of the patient (and the caregiver) seems to be insufficient, consider arranging for a home nurse or home aid to follow up the patient and obtaining a safety telephone in case of further falls.
- Multifactorial programmes for screening the elderly at risk and the removal of both internal and external risk factors are effective in the prevention of falls (A) [7]. External hip protectors (B) [10] [11] can prevent 60% of hip fractures in high-risk persons.
- High-dose vitamin D combined with calcium intake (B) [12] [13] [14] [15] [16] may reduce the incidence of fractures.

References

1. Leipzig RM, Cumming RG, Tinetti ME. Drugs and falls in older people: a systematic review and meta-analysis: I. Psychotropic drugs. J Am Ger Soc 1999;47:30–39.
2. The Database of Abstracts of Reviews of Effectiveness (University of York), Database no.: DARE-990250. In: The Cochrane Library, Issue 2, 2000. Oxford: Update Software.
3. Hanlon JT, Cutson T, Ruby CM. Drug-related falls in the older adult. Topics Geriatr Rehabilitation 1996;11:38–54.
4. The Database of Abstracts of Reviews of Effectiveness (University of York), Database no.: DARE-965365. In: The Cochrane Library, Issue 4, 1999. Oxford: Update Software.
5. Leipzig RM, Cumming RG, Tinetti ME. Drugs and falls in older people: a systematic review and meta-analysis: II. Cardiac and analgesic drugs. J Am Ger Soc 1999;47:40–50.
6. The Database of Abstracts of Reviews of Effectiveness (University of York), Database no.: DARE-990251. In: The Cochrane Library, Issue 2, 2000. Oxford: Update Software.
7. Gillespie LD, Gillespie WJ, Robertson MC, Lamb SE, Cumming RG, Rowe BH. Interventions for preventing falls in elderly people. Cochrane Database Syst Rev. 2004;(2): CD000340.
8. Province MA, Hadley EC, Hornbrook MC, Lipsitz LA, Miller JP. Mulrow CD. The effects of exercise on falls in the elderly: a preplanned meta-analysis of the FICSIT trials. JAMA 1995;273:1341–7.
9. The Database of Abstracts of Reviews of Effectiveness (University of York), Database no.: DARE-954030. In: The Cochrane Library, Issue 4, 1999. Oxford: Update Software.
10. Kannus P, Parkkari J, Niemi S, Pasanen M, Palvanen M, Järvinen M, Vuori I. Prevention of hip fractures in elderly people with use of a hip protector. N Engl J Med 2000;343:1506–1513.
11. Lauritzen JB, Petersen MM, Lund B. Effect of external hip protectors on hip fractures. Lancet 1993;341:11–13.
12. Gillespie WJ, Avenell A, Henry DA, O'Connell DL, Robertson J. Vitamin D and vitamin D analogues for preventing fractures associated with involutional and post-menopausal osteoporosis. Cochrane Database Syst Rev. 2004;(2):CD000227.
13. Lips P, 2002fsmans WC, Ooms ME et al. Vitamin D supplementation and fracture incidence in elderly persons. A randomised, placebo-controlled trial. Ann Intern Med 1996;124:400–6. Comment in ACP Journal Club 1996;July/August:16.
14. Chapuy MC et al. Effect of calcium and cholecalciferol treatment for three years on hipfractures in elderly women. BMJ 1994;308:1081–2.
15. Dawson-Hughes B et al. Rates of bone loss in postmenopausal women randomly assigned to one of two dosages of vitamin D. Am J Clin Nutr 1995;61:1140–5.
16. Trivedi DP, Doll R, Khaw KT. Effect of four monthly oral vitamin D3 (cholecalciferol) supplementation on fractures and mortality in men and women living in the community: randomised double blind controlled trial. BMJ 2003; 326(7387):469.

22.2 Delirium in the elderly

Kaisu Pitkälä

Objectives

- To recognize delirium in the elderly on medical wards, for example by carefully reading reports written by nurses. According to studies only about half of delirious patients are noticed, diagnosed and adequately managed. The prognosis of delirium is poor.
- To detect and manage the underlying illness causing delirium.
- To manage anxiety and restlessness symptomatically.

Definition and symptoms

- Delirium is a global disturbance of the brain which has an underlying organic aetiology. Symptoms start abruptly and resolve in the course of time.
- It is a disorder of attention: patients are less aware of their surroundings and have difficulties in concentrating. A common feature is disorganized thinking.
- Often the consciousness is disturbed, and cognitive functions are abruptly impaired.
- There may be perceptual disturbances: misinterpretations and hallucinations (less than 50% of patients), disturbance of sleep-wake cycle, or increased or decreased psychomotor activity.
- Clinical features develop over a short period of time and tend to fluctuate over the course of the day.

Predisposing factors

- Advanced age, impaired function
- Dementia, cancer, severe illnesses
- Impairment of vision and hearing
- Sleeplessness, unfamiliar environment, darkness, physical restraints
- Surgery

Causes

- A variety of underlying conditions can cause delirium C [1 3 4 5].
- Infections
  - Urinary infection, pneumonia (often without fever in the elderly), septicaemia, meningitis, encephalitis, HIV
- Cerebrovascular diseases
  - Cerebral infarction, TIA; haemorrhage, subarachnoid haemorrhage
- Vascular diseases
  - Heart failure, myocardial infarction, arrhythmias, pulmonary embolism, hypotension, etc.
- Metabolic disorders
  - Disorders in acid-base balance; disorders in fluid and electrolyte balance; hypoalbuminaemia; hypophosphataemia; insufficiency of the liver, kidneys or lungs; hypo- or hyperglycaemia; hypo- or hyperthyroidism; disorders of calcium balance; deficiencies of different B-vitamins; anaemia; other endocrinological disorders.
- Others
  - Traumas (head injury, subdural haematoma, burns, hip fracture, etc.)
  - Epilepsy, postictal state
  - Tumours (intracerebral, pulmonary), myeloma
  - Poisoning
  - Extensive life stress (especially with dementia patients)
- Medications
  - Drugs with anticholinergic properties, levodopa, antihistamines, digitalis, diuretics, neuroleptics, tricyclic antidepressants, sedatives, lithium, NSAIDs, oral hypoglycaemics, histamine-2 receptor blockers, hypertensives, antiepileptic drugs, steroids, narcotics, many antibiotics
  - Abrupt discontinuation of regularly used medication (e.g. sedative-hypnotics, antidepressants, steroids) or discontinuation of alcohol usage.

Investigations

- History: When was the patient last well? Course of symptoms? Cognition before the illness? Usage of medications? Usage of alcohol?
  - Careful physical examination
- CRP, (ESR), blood count, sodium, potassium, creatinine, blood glucose, urine sample, ECG
- Glytamyltransferase, alkaline phosphatase, TSH, free T_4, vitamin B_{12}, erythrocyte folate and arterial blood gas analysis when needed
- Chest x-ray
- Analysis of cerebrospinal fluid, CT scan of brain, EEG when needed
- Further tests when needed. An underlying causal factor is found in 80–90% of cases when investigated carefully.

Differential diagnosis

- Dementia
  - Insidious onset and slow course of symptoms
  - Level of consciousness is normal, and attention intact until late stages
- Psychotic disorders
  - Level of consciousness is normal, cognitive functions are not globally disturbed. Speech is not totally disorganized.
  - Auditory hallucinations are common in psychosis, whereas visual hallucinations are more common in delirium.
- Dementia and delirium are often seen in same patient.

Prevalence and prognosis

- The prevalence and incidence of delirium in hospitalized elderly are together about 25–40%. Physicians recognize only 30–50% of them.
- The patient may recover from delirium that has endured several weeks.
- Mortality is 25–40% on average; about 40% are institutionalized within 1 year.
- Patients should not be institutionalised before the cause of delirium is diagnozed and managed and the patient's condition is stabilized.

Management

- Management of the underlying causal factor.
- Management of the general condition: fluid and oxygen balance, prevention of urinary obstruction, management of bowel movements, discontinuation of unnecessary

medication, prevention of bedsores, rehabilitation, adequate lighting, familiar objects C [47] [48] [49]

- Control of restlessness
  - Haloperidol in severe agitation 2.5–5 mg i.m. or 0.5–2 mg orally. This may be repeated every 30 minutes until sedation is sufficient. In mild cases 0.5–5 mg × 1–2 for seven days orally may be sufficient.
  - Haloperidol should be given to dementia patients with caution, as it often provokes extra-pyramidal side effects.
  - As alternatives, risperidone 0.25–0.5 mg × 1–2 or olanzapine 2.5–5 mg × 1 may be used. In addition, diazepam 2.5–5 mg intravenously or lorazepam 0.5–1 mg intramuscularly may be used for sedation, repeated if needed.
  - Often sleeping pills are needed to normalize diurnal rhythm: short or medium half-life benzodiazepine (e.g. temazepam 10–20 mg).
  - A peaceful, well-lit room; the patient should be approached unhurriedly and conversation should be informative.

References

1. Britton A, Russell R. Multidisciplinary team interventions for delirium in patients with chronic cognitive impairment. Cochrane Database Syst Rev. 2004;(2):CD000395.
2. Inouye SK, Charpentier PA. Precipitating factors for delirium in hospitalized elderly persons. Predictive model and interrelationship with baseline vulnerability. JAMA 1996;275:852–7.
3. O'Keeffe ST, Lavan JN. Predicting delirium in elderly patients: Development and validation of a risk-stratification model. Age and Ageing 1996;25:317–21.
4. Inouye SK. The dilemma of delirium: Clinical and research controversies regarding diagnosis and evaluation of delirium in hospitalized elderly medical patients. Am J Med 1994;97:278–287.
5. Cameron DJ et al. Delirium: A test of the diagnostic and statistical manual III criteria on medical patients. J Am Geriatr Soc 1987;35:1007–10.
6. Johnson JC et al. Using DSM-III criteria to diagnose delirium in elderly general medical patients. J Gerontology 1990;45:M113–9.
7. Schor JD et al. Risk factors for delirium in hospitalized elderly. JAMA 1992;267:827–31.
8. Pompei P et al. Delirium in hospitalized older persons: Outcomes and predictors. J Am Geriatr Soc 1994;42:809–15.
9. Erkinjuntti T et al. Dementia among medical patients. Evaluation of consecutive 2000 admissions. Arch Intern Med 1986;146:1923–6.
10. Cole MG et al. Systematic intervention for elderly inpatients with delirium: a randomized trial. Can Med Assoc J 1994;151:965–70.
11. O'Keeffe S, Lavan J, The Prognostic significance of delirium in Older hospitalized patients. J Am Geriatr Soc 1997; 45:174–8.
12. Williams MA et al. Predictors of acute confusional states in hospitalized elderly. Res Nurs Health 1985;8:31–40.
13. Gustafsson Y et al. Acute confusional states in elderly patients treated for femoral neck fracture. J Am Geriatr Soc 1988;36:525–30.
14. Rogers MP et al. Delirium after elective orthopedic surgery: Risk factors and natural history. Int J Psychiatr Med 1989; 19:109–21.
15. Williams-Russo P et al. Post-operative delirium: predictors and prognosis in elderly orthopedic patients. J Am Geriatr Soc 1992:40:759–67.
16. Marcantonio ER et al. A clinical prediction rule for delirium after elective noncardiac surgery. JAMA 1994;271: 134–9.
17. Inoye SK et al. A predictive model for delirium in hospitalized elderly medical patients based on admission characteristics. Ann Intern Med 1993;119:474–81.
18. Williams-Russo et al. Cognitive effects after epidural vs. general anesthesia in older adults. A randomized trial. JAMA 1995;274:44–50.
19. Francis J. Delirium in older patients. J Am Geriatr Soc 1992;40:829–39.
20. Perez EL, Siverman M. Delirium: The often overlooked diagnosis. Int J Psychiatr Med 1984;14:181–8.
21. Inouye SK et al. Clarifying confusion: The confusion assessment method, a new method for detection of delirium. Ann Intern Med 1990;113:941–8.
22. Gustafsson Y et al. Underdiagnosis and poor documentation of acute confusional states in elderly hip fracture patients. J Am Geriatr Soc 1991;39:760–5.
23. Thomas RI et al. A prospective study of delirium and prolonged hospital stay. Arch Gen Psychiatr 1988;45:937–40.
24. Rockwood K. Acute confusion in elderly medical patients. J Am Geriatr Soc 1989;37:150–4.
25. Francis J et al. A prospective study of delirium in hospitalized elderly. JAMA 1990;263:1097–101.
26. Levkoff SE et al. Delirium. The occurrence and persistence of symptoms among elderly hospitalized patients. Arch Intern Med 1992;152:334–40.
27. Jitapunkl S et al. Delirium in newly admitted elderly patients. A prospective study. Q J Med, New Ser 1992;83: 307–14.
28. Koponen H et al. A prospective study of delirium patients admitted to a psychiatric hospital. Psychol Med 1993;23:103–9.
29. Breibart W et al. A double-blind trial of haloperidol, chlorpromazine, and lorazepam in the treatment of delirium in hospitalized AIDS patients. Am J Psychiatr 1996;153:231–7.
30. Owens JF, Hutelmyer CM. The effect of postoperative intervention on delirium in cardiac surgical patients. Nurs Res 1982;31:60–2.
31. Schindler et al. Beneficial effects of psychiatric intervention on recovery after coronary artery bypass graft surgery. Gen Hosp Psychiatr 1989;11:358–64.
32. Cole MG et al. Systematic intervention for elderly inpatients with delirium: a randomized trial. Can Med Assoc J 1994;151:965–70.
33. Williams-Russo MA et al. Reducing acute confusional states in elderly patients with hip fractures. Res Nurs Health 1985;8:329–37.
34. Gustafsson Y et al. A geriatric-anesthesiologic program to reduce acute confusional states in elderly patients treated for femoral neck fractures. J Am Geriatr Soc 1991;39: 655–62.
35. Wanich CK et al. Functional status outcomes of a nursing intervention in hospitalized elderly. Image 1992;24:201–7.

GER

36. Marcantonio ER, Flacker JM, Wright RJ, Resnick NM. Reducing delirium after hip fracture: a randomized trial. J Am Geriatr Soc 2001;49:678–9.
37. Inoye SK, Bogardus ST, Charpentier PA et al. Multicomponent intervention to prevent delirium in hospitalized older patients. N Engl J Med 1999;340:669–76.
38. Cole MG, Primeau FJ, Elie LM. Delirium: prevention, treatment and outcome studies. Journal of Geriatric Psychiatry and Neurology 1998;11:126–137.
39. Cole MG. McCusker J. Bellavance F. Primeau FJ. Bailey RF. Bonnycastle MJ. Laplante J. Systematic detection and multidisciplinary care of delirium in older medical inpatients: a randomized trial. CMAJ 2002;167(7):753–9.

22.3 Delusional symptoms in the elderly

Pirkko Hiltunen, Tuula Saarela

Definition

- Delusional disorder often manifests as exaggerated and comprehensive mistrust and suspicion of the motives of other people, with increased alertness and observation.
- Suspicion can be limited or comprehensive.
- Thoughts are distorted: the person is convinced of the correctness of his/her beliefs.
- Delusions can also direct the course of action.

Prevalence

- Delusions can be found in 2–4% of the elderly in the community.
- It is more common in women than in men.
- It is more common in patients with cognitive dysfunction than in others.
- Deficiency of senses predispose to delusional problems.
- Elderly people with paranoid symptoms are more socially isolated than other elderly in the community.

Symptom features

- Unwarranted mistrust of others and increased sensitivity leads to misinterpretation of environmental stimuli.
- Delusions are often persecutory in nature and may influence the patient's behaviour.
- Partition delusions are common. They are beliefs that people, material, radiation etc. can pass through a structure, such as the door, ceiling or the walls, that normally constitutes a barrier to such passage.
- Agitation or anger may be present.
- In dementia the simple delusions of theft and suspicion are common, however, jealousy delusions may also occur.

Clinical assessment

History

- How long has the problem been present and how did it develop?
- The patient's account of her or his experience may be unreliable or difficult to understand. It is often worthwhile to find out the opinions of family members and neighbours.
- Make sure you have an objective assessment of the situation: could the patient really be the victim of malevolence?
- Why is an assessment necessary now? How has the situation changed?

Psychiatric examination

- Communication and co-operation. Can the patient discuss the situation?
- Cognitive functions: memory, observation?
- Thought: content of thought, conclusions, ability to question his/her own account of events?
- Affect: depression, anxiety, elation, agitation, defensive, aggressive?
- Functional capacity?

Physical assessment

- Could delusions be associated with a somatic illness?
- Does the patient have acute somatic illnesses?

Social and environmental assessment

- Is the patient unattended, dirty, hungry?
- Is the accommodation adequate?
- Is there a need for home care? Are the caretakers exhausted?
- Is the patient willing to receive help (home nursing)?

Assessment of urgency of care

- Is the patient anxious, fearful, depressed or agitate?
- Is the patient able to take care of him/herself?
- Is the patient able to cooperate?
- Does the patient have acute somatic illnesses?
- Does the patient pose such a risk to him/herself or to others that admission to hospital is warranted? The patient may be dangerous if he/she feels threatened. A person with good memory and strong suspicions or jealousy who possesses weapons is potentially dangerous.

Delusional disorder and diagnostic alternatives

- Sudden onset of symptoms with disorientation and fragmented delusions: delirium. Cause?
- Transient delusional symptoms, memory impairment, global impairment in functioning: dementia
- Long history of mental illness, organized persecutory delusions, hallucinations, odd behaviour, drug-side effects: schizophrenia

- Depressive mood:hopelessness, submission, often somatic delusions: depression
- Long-term predisposition to distrustfulness: paranoidic personality disorder
- Bizarre delusions, somatic symptoms resembling delusions, no significant dementia: late-onset schizophrenic psychosis.
- Lack of social contacts, no noteworthy problems with personal care or environment, no schizophrenia, no dementia, no depression, a recluse style of life: no psychiatric diagnosis

Management

Immediate aims of management

- Optimizing the physical condition
- Relieving anxiety and fear
- Is there a need for compulsory assessment and treatment in the interests of the patient's health and safety or for the protection of others?

Long-term aims of management

- Try to establish and maintain treatment compliance.
- Reduce mental suffering.
- Moderate tolerance of symptoms.
- Combat isolation, offer support by the social service.
- Support the family and inform persons in contact with the patient.
- A paranoid elderly rarely has insight into his delusions, which often just disappear spontaneously or the patient becomes accustomed to them.

Antipsychotic medication

- There are no rapid solutions. Start with the lowest possible dose in order to avoid side effects. Elderly with late-onset paranoid psychosis do not seem to tolerate as high doses of neuroleptics as elderly with early-onset schizophrenia.
- There is no real evidence that any particular drug is more effective than another in this group of patients. The choice of drug for each individual patient should thus be based on considerations of concomitant physical illness and other treatments received.
- Other medications and acute somatic problems are assessed. Does the patient have hypotension or tendency for extrapyramidal symptoms?
- Recommendations for neuroleptics
  - Haloperidol 0.5–2–4 mg/d
  - Perphenazine 2–4(–8) mg/d
  - Risperidone 0.25–1–2 mg/d
  - Olanzapine (2.5)–5–(10) mg/d
  - Quetiapine 12.5–25 mg × 1–2/d with dose increments to up to 75 mg × 2/d.
- New generation atypical neuroleptics cause fewer side effects and should be preferred when long-term medication is necessary.
- Pay attention to side effects in patients with memory impairment. Neuroleptics are used for psychotic symptoms with individual dosing and follow-up of the response.
- Injections are used if the patient behaves violently:
  - Haloperidol 2.5–5 mg × 2–3/day i.m.
  - Haloperidol decanoate 25(–50) mg i.m.; the effect lasts 4 weeks
  - Zuclopenthixol acetate 25(–50) mg i.m. has an effect lasting several days
  - Zuclopenthixol decanoate 100(–200) mg i.m. every 3 to 4 weeks
- Treatment with long-acting (depot) preparations is started with the lowest dose of the oral preparation.
- Long-acting neuroleptics should not be started for psychosis before the suitability of the drug has been verified by using the short-acting form of the preparation first. A review of side-effects should be carried out after every injection.
- The physician in charge for care should assess the patient at 3-month intervals at the most.
- If delusions are caused by psychotic depression, the patient is treated with antidepressives combined with a neuroleptic or electroconvulsive therapy (ECT).

Management and follow-up

- Local health care centre or ward.
- Home care: home nursing services (doctor, nurse, home help), psychiatric outpatient service.
- Day hospital.
- Psychiatric hospital: inpatient if acute severe psychosis.
- Psychogeriatric nursing home or ward.

When should the general practitioner refer to the psychiatrist?

- The diagnosis is not clear.
- Compulsory admission to psychiatric care is considered.
- Finding the correct medication is problematic.

22.4 Depression in old age

Tuula Saarela

Objectives

- To recognize depression in an elderly person. It is often an underdiagnosed and undermanaged illness.
- To manage acute depression with the aim to alleviate all symptoms.
- To improve the patient's quality of life by offering support and providing medications in such a way that the adverse effects are minimized.

GER

Background and epidemiology

- The incidence of serious depression declines with age. The prevalence of serious depression is 2–3% in men and 3–5% in women over 64 years of age.
- The incidence of mild depression increases with age: the prevalence is about 15–22% in men and 19–30% in women over 64 years of age.
- Ageing is associated with reduced opportunities, losses and frailty. Difficulties in adjusting to these changes predisposes a person to depression. Acute life events such as bereavement (loss of a spouse or another family member) are also common precipitating factors.
- A previous history of a depressive disorder and a physical illness are significant predisposing factors.

Symptoms

- The symptoms are diverse, partly overlapping with the signs and symptoms of physical illnesses and often difficult to recognize as depression.
- Major symptoms suggestive of depression include low spirits of at least two weeks' duration, loss of interest or pleasure in normal daily activities, tiredness and decreased energy levels.
- Symptoms such as apathy and poor motivation may resemble dementia.
- Patients often have difficulties in managing daily activities and feel unmotivated particularly in the mornings.
- Other symptoms include: irritability, tearfulness, anxiety, pessimism, feeling of worthlessness, self-accusations, suicidal thoughts, loneliness, fearfulness and dependence on other people.
- Physical symptoms often mask depression: diverse aches and pains, hypochondria, disturbed sleep, lack of appetite, weight loss and weariness.

Differential diagnosis

- Grief as a normal reaction to bereavement.
- Dementia (testing see 22.21, or trial with antidepressant medication). Note, however, that dementia patients may also have depression.
- Chronic pain
- Hypothyroidism, hyperparathyroidism
- Parkinson's disease
- Deficiency of vitamin B_{12}
- Adverse effects of drugs (methyldopa, beta-blockers, diuretics, L-dopa, indomethacin, digoxin, steroids, neuroleptics, medicines causing hypoglycaemia)
- Alcoholism

Diagnosis

- Discuss the symptoms and current life situation with the patient. If available, someone close to the patient may contribute valuable information.
- History: previous psychiatric history, current medication
- Physical and mental examination
- Screening test for depression (22.21)
- Dementia test
- Laboratory tests (for exclusion): TSH, free thyroxine, blood count, differential count, vitamin B12, calcium, liver enzymes, electrolytes and creatinine
- ECG

Management

- Provide education about depression for the patient and his/her family and carers, i.e. depression can be treated.
- Treat comorbid somatic illnesses and try to reduce or compensate the effects of disability; good management of physical illnesses serves to treat depression at the same time.
- Map the patient's psychosocial status and the support network.
- With an elderly depressed person the doctor-patient relationship should be active, encouraging and supportive.
- There is good evidence on the effectiveness of psychological interventions (cognitive psychotherapy, interpersonal therapy, brief psychodynamic therapy) with motivated elderly depressed patients.
- Allow the patient to mourn normally after a bereavement but be aware of the possibility of depression when symptoms persist or become intense.
- The patient may find physiotherapy both supportive and a positive intervention.
- Medication:
  - When selecting an antidepressant, assess the symptomatology (apathetic–excited) and ensure that the drug is suitable for the patient's comorbidities and other drug therapies.
  - There are no differences in the effectiveness between the various drugs **A** [1 2 3 4 5 6 7 8].
  - Selective serotonin re-uptake inhibitors activate the patient. They include citalopram, sertraline, paroxetine and fluvoxamine. The MAO-A-inhibitor moclobemide is also often used for depression in the elderly.
  - Tricyclic antidepressants are contraindicated if the patient has cardiac conduction defects, glaucoma, orthostatic hypotension, a predisposition to urine retention or a tendency to fall. In these cases mianserin may be useful (risk of neutropenia, frequent blood counts are warranted).
  - Mirtazapine, with a starting dose 15–30 mg/day, is a good option in depression combined with anxiety or sleep disturbance.
  - Tricyclic antidepressants, amitriptyline or doxepine are not recommended for the elderly because of their anticholinergic adverse effects. Nortriptyline may be a good option in apathetic depression. Tricyclic antidepressants are usually not recommended for patients over 75 years of age, but they may be considered for patients treated in psychiatric units.
  - Venlaflaxine (37.5–150 mg/day) may be effective in depression resistant to other drugs.
  - If depression is associated with paranoid/psychotic features, try an antipsychotic agent (primarily atypical

anti-psychotics such as risperidone or quetiapine). Consider consulting a psychiatrist.
  - An effect of medication usually becomes apparent within 4–8 weeks. If there is no effect, or the effect is only slight, increase the dose or, if dosage is optimal, try another medicine from another group of antidepressants.
  - Continue medication for 1/2–2 years after patient has recovered. If depression recurs, the elderly person should be managed with medication for several years.
- Suicidal tendencies in an elderly patient are an indication for in-patient care.

Summary

- Caring for an elderly depressed person may be difficult and challenging both for nursing staff and carers. The patient may have given up hope, be bitter, blaming, dependent and emotionally labile.
- Staff support groups and family counselling for carers and close family members may be helpful.
- Consult a psychiatrist with diagnostic problems or when a patient continues to be depressed despite treatment. Several antidepressants may be combined in severe cases. ECT (electro convulsive therapy) is safe and effective in severe cases.
- Severely depressed and suicidal patients should be treated in a psychiatric hospital.

References

1. Selective serotonin reuptake inhibitors (SSRIs) in the treatment of elderly depressed patients: a qualitative analysis of the literature on their efficacy and side-effects. International Clinical Psychopharmacology 1996;11:165–175.
2. The Database of Abstracts of Reviews of Effectiveness (University of York), Database no.: DARE-973205. In: The Cochrane Library, Issue 1, 2000. Oxford: Update Software.
3. Mittman N, Herrmann N, Einarson TR et al. The efficacy, safety and tolerability of antidepressants in late life depression: a meta-analysis. J Affect Disorders 1997;46(3):191–217.
4. Song F, Freemantle N, Sheldon TA et al. Selective serotonin reuptake inhibitor: meta-analysis of efficacy and acceptability. BMJ 1993;306:683-7. Comment in ACP Journal Club 1993; 119:45.
5. Wilson K, Mottram P, Sivanranthan A, Nightingale A. Antidepressants versus placebo for the depressed elderly. Cochrane Database Syst Rev. 2004;(2):CD000561.
6. Banerjee S, Shamash K, Macdonald AJ, Mann AH. Randomized controlled trial of effect of intervention by psychogeriatric team on depression in frail elderly people at home. BMJ 1996;313:1058–61.
7. Gerson S, Belin TR, Kaufman A, Mintz J, Jarvik L. Pharmacological and psychological treatments for depressed older patients: a meta-analysis and overview of recent findings. Harvard Review of Psychiatry 1999:7;1–28.
8. The Database of Abstracts of Reviews of Effectiveness (University of York), Database no.: DARE-994490. In: The Cochrane Library, Issue 1, 2002. Oxford: Update Software.

22.5 Nutritional disorders in the elderly

Kaisu Pitkälä

Basic rules

- Chronic diseases are the most common causes of malnutrition. Malnutrition should be treated more actively than what is often the practice.
- Moderate weight loss by increasing physical activity is important in the treatment of diabetes, heart failure, high blood pressure and osteoarthritis. Otherwise, moderate overweight is rarely an indication for a slimming diet in the aged.
- To prevent osteoporosis ensure that the patient gets enough calcium (1.5 g/day). Institutionalised elderly people often suffer from vitamin D deficiency B [1 2 3 4 5]. Vitamin D supplementation is recommended for all persons over 70 years of age to prevent osteoporosis.
- If an elderly person has vitamin B_{12} or iron deficiency, suspect a gastrointestinal disorder.
- Routine use of vitamins or other trace elements has not been proven effective D [6 7 8 9 10 11 12].

Prevalence of malnutrition

- In the aged population the prevalence is 5–10%
- In over 80-year-olds it is 10–20%
- In hospitalized elderly malnutrition occurs in 27–65%
- Among permanently institutionalized elderly 30–80% suffer from malnutrition

Predisposing factors

- Problems in obtaining food
  - Economic (low pension income, stinginess)
  - Problems with mobility
  - Fixed habits, alcoholism
- Difficulty with chewing and swallowing
  - Stroke, parkinsonism, missing teeth
- Increased need for nourishment
  - Infections
  - Trauma, surgery, particularly hip fracture patients
- Disorders causing cachexia
  - Cancer, chronic infections (e.g. tuberculosis)
  - Alzheimer's disease
- Impaired utilization of nutrients
  - Malabsorption (intestinal disorders)

GER

- Other causes
  - Psychological causes (depression, paranoia)
  - Medications
  - Decreased taste or smell
  - Decreased sense of thirst
- Immobility
- Physiological changes related to ageing
  - Slowing of basal metabolism and reduction in physical activity lowers the need for calorie intake; in elderly women calorie intake is often below 1500 kcal. This is considered the risk level for insufficient intake of several trace elements.
  - With ageing, muscle tissue diminishes and the proportion of adipose tissue increases.
  - Decreasing glucose tolerance
  - Susceptibility to disorders of fluid balance

Consequences of malnutrition

- Increased morbidity and mortality are associated with malnutrition.
- Prolonged hospitalization
- Impaired immune function, slower wound healing, increased risk of infections
- Muscle function and strength diminishes, risk for falls and fractures increases

Diagnosis of malnutrition

- Clinical findings are not sensitive indicators of malnutrition.
- The most commonly used indicators are low body weight or BMI, thickness of the triceps and upper arm, serum albumin, haemoglobin and lymphocytes, interview on the contents of the diet, intake of vitamins, clinical examination, weight loss.
- The so-called Mini Nutritional Assessment (MNA) is currently considered the most reliable measure of malnutrition. It has been validated in several countries.

Treatment of malnutrition

- Protein malnutrition, in particular, is a problem affecting the elderly with a disease and it should be addressed more actively than what is now the practice.
- Protein supplements have been found to shorten hospital stays and to reduce complications A [13].
- An elderly person should receive 1–1.2 g of protein per kg of body weight daily; a sick person needs even more.
- With age the proportion of protein in the diet should increase.

Other common nutritional disturbances

- Deficiencies of particular nutrients
- Anaemias (iron, vitamin B12); look for an underlying gastrointestinal disease
- Osteoporosis and osteomalacia. Vitamin D deficiency is a common condition in institutionalized elderly and those who stay mainly indoors. Routine vitamin D supplementation is well justified. At the dose 800 IU daily, vitamin D has been shown effective in the prevention of fractures B [1 2 3 4 5] The recommended dose 800 IU daily for all elderly.
- Night-blindness
- Neuropathies (B vitamins)
- Obesity
  - Metabolic disorders (diabetes)
  - Physical limitations in mobility
  - Skin infections (intertrigo)
  - Cardiovascular diseases
- Attempts to lose weight should be cautious. Weight loss easily leads to loss of muscle tissue and increase of the relative share of fat tissue.

References

1. Gillespie WJ, Avenell A, Henry DA, O'Connell DL, Robertson J. Vitamin D and vitamin D analogues for preventing fractures associated with involutional and post-menopausal osteoporosis. Cochrane Database Syst Rev. 2004;(2):CD000227.
2. Lips P, 2002fsmans WC, Ooms ME et al. Vitamin D supplementation and fracture incidence in elderly persons. A randomised, placebo-controlled trial. Ann Intern Med 1996;124:400-6. Comment in ACP Journal Club 1996;July/August:16.
3. Chapuy MC et al. Effect of calcium and cholecalciferol treatment for three years on hipfractures in elderly women. BMJ 1994;308:1081–2.
4. Dawson-Hughes B et al. Rates of bone loss in postmenopausal women randomly assigned to one of two dosages of vitamin D. Am J Clin Nutr 1995;61:1140–5.
5. Trivedi DP, Doll R, Khaw KT. Effect of four monthly oral vitamin D3 (cholecalciferol) supplementation on fractures and mortality in men and women living in the community: randomised double blind controlled trial. BMJ 2003; 326(7387):469.
6. Jha P, Flather M, Lonn E, Farkouh M, Yusuf S. The antioxidant vitamins and cardiovascular disease: a critical review of epidemiologic and clinical trial data. Annals of Internal Medicine 1995;123(11):860–72.
7. Pahor M, Applegate WB. Recent advances in geriatric medicine. BMJ 1997;315:1071–4.
8. Sano M et al. A controlled trial of selegiline, alfa-tocopherol, or both as treatment for Alzheimer's disease. The Alzheimer's disease cooperative study. N Engl J Med 1997;336:1216–22.
9. Clark LC et al. Effects of selenium supplementation for cancer prevention in patients with carcinoma of the skin. A randomised controlled trial. Nutritional Prevention of Cancer Study Group. JAMA 1996;276:1957–63.
10. Helzlsouer KJ et al. Prospective study of serum micronutrients and ovarian cancer. J Natl Cancer Inst 1996;88:32–7.
11. Hennekens CH et al. Lack of effect of long-term supplementation with beta-carotene on the incidence of malignant neoplasm and cardiovascular disease. N Engl J Med 1996;334:1145–9.
12. Omenn GS et al. Effects of a combination of betacarotene and vitamin A on lung cancer and cardiovascular disease. N Engl J Med 1996;334:1150–5.

13. Milne AC, Potter J, Avenell A. Protein and energy supplementation in elderly people at risk from malnutrition. Cochrane Database Syst Rev. 2004;(2):CD003288.
14. Guigoz Y, Vellas B, Garry PJ. Assessing the nutritional status of the elderly: the Mini Nutritional Assessment as part of the geriatric evaluation. Nutrition Rev 1996;54:(11)559–565.

22.6 Urinary incontinence in the elderly

Reijo Tilvis

Principles

- The prevalence of urinary incontinence rises rapidly with age. It is most prevalent in institutionalised, frail elderly women and in elderly with dementia.
- In primary care incontinence is often a hidden symptom. Polite questions are needed for eliciting the symptom and making the diagnosis.
- In identifying the causes of incontinence the patient's cognitive functions should be examined. It is important to exclude iatrogenic causes, e.g. medication.
- Management is often successful. In order to succeed, several different medications may need to be tried.

Causes explaining the prevalence of urinary disturbances in the elderly

- Changes connected with ageing
  - Decreased kidney concentrating ability
  - Diminished capacity of the urinary bladder
  - Deteriorating function of the detrusor muscle (amount of residual urine increases)
  - Anatomic changes in the pelvic region (atrophy, enlargement of prostate hyperplasia)
- Diseases causing incontinence
  - Diseases of the central nervous system, e.g. delirium, dementia, stroke, etc.
  - Infections
  - Constipation
- Iatrogenic causes
  - Medications (e.g. loop-diuretics taken in the evening)
  - Invasive procedures and operations
  - Barriers to normal urination in institutional care (e.g. immobilization etc.)

Examining the urinary incontinence of the aged

- Temporary or continuous?
  - The DIAPPERS rule of incidental incontinence:
    - D = delirium
    - I = infection
    - A = atrophy
    - P = pharmaceutical, medications
    - P = psychological causes
    - E = endocrinological causes of polyuria
    - R = restricted mobility (normal micturition prevented?)
    - S = stool impaction (severe constipation)
- Is incontinence caused by a central nervous system?
  - The cause of deteriorating incontinence in 60–80% of cases.
- Could the symptoms be due to retention?

Classification of urinary incontinence in the aged

- Stress incontinence
  - Atrophy
- Urge incontinence
  - Motor (common in the aged)
  - Sensory
- Reflex incontinence
- Overflow incontinence

Management of incontinence

Objective: causal management

- The muscles of the pelvic region should be strengthened by a following special exercise programme. In elderly women atrophy should be managed by oestrogens.
- Manage the causes of retention.
  - Enlarged prostate
- Manage the causes of temporary incontinence.
  - Treat urinary tract infection (but do not treat symptomless bacteriuria).
  - Check medications (diuretics, alfa-adrenolytics).

Experimental medications, if the causes are not manageable

- Control the detrusor muscle
  - Anticholinergic (A) [1] and other drugs that restrict contractions of the bladder
    - tolterodine
    - oxybutynin
    - emeprone
    - propantheline
    - imipramine
    - doxepine
    - flavoxate
    - nifedipine
    - inhibitors of prostaglandin synthesis
  - Anticholinergic medications may worsen memory problems and decrease the threshold for delirium.

- Try medications that improve the closing mechanism of the urinary tube
  - Alfa-adrenergic medications B [2]
  - Drugs that stimulate the sphincter
    - phenylpropanolamine
    - ephedrine
    - imipramine
    - baclofen
- Try antidepressants that have both anticholinergic and alfa-adrenergic effects
  - Imipramine
  - Secondary depression may be alleviated at the same time.
- Sometimes prostaglandin inhibitors may help.
  - Remember the risk of gastrointestinal side effects.
- Combine different medications, if possible.

Overflow incontinence

- Find the cause of the obstruction.
- Stimulating the atonic bladder is possible with cholinergic agents.
  - Drugs that improve bladder contractions.
    - carbachol
    - bethanechol
    - distigmine
    - neostigmine
    - prostaglandin E2
  - Remember contraindications!
- Consultation with the urologist is often indicated.
- Clean intermittent catheterization is also possible with the aged.
- An indwelling urethral catheter is not justified in the management of incontinence.
- Consider specialist investigation if (URINE-rule):
  - U = unsuccessful. Management is not successful.
  - R = Recurrent complications.
  - I = Incontinence does not improve after prostate surgery.
  - N = Non-response. None of the medications help.
  - E = Excessive residual.
- Ensure that the patient has the necessary help and devices.
  - Nappies
  - Collecting containers and urinals
  - Toilet renovation
  - Others

References

1. Hay-Smith J, Herbison P, Ellis G, Moore K. Anticholinergic drugs versus placebo for overactive bladder syndrome in adults. Cochrane Database Syst Rev. 2004;(2):CD003781.
2. Alhasso A, Glazener CMA, Pickard R, N'Dow J. Adrenergic drugs for urinary incontinence in adults. Cochrane Database Syst Rev. 2004;(2):CD001842.

22.7 Infections in old age

Editors

Basic rules

- Cell-mediated immunity and part by also humoral immunity diminish in old age.
- Age-related diseases and associated conditions as well as immunosuppressive medications all affect defence mechanisms.
- Symptoms of infections are often atypical. Even mild infections may cause decompensation of different organs.
- Fever is often absent. CRP is a useful marker of infection.

Pneumonia

- Predisposing factors for pneumonia in old age B [1] are:
  - impaired cough reflex
  - possible neurological diseases causing impaired functioning of the pharynx and susceptibility to aspiration
  - obstructive pulmonary diseases
  - immobilization
  - heart failure.
- The temperature of a pneumonic patient may be normal. Pneumonia may manifest as symptoms of impaired general condition and functioning, confusion, or even chest pain caused either by irritation of the lungs or by aggravation of coronary heart disease.
- The most common agent causing pneumonia in non-institutional care is Streptococcus pneumoniae (pneumococci), and the first-line antibiotic for this is G penicillin.
- During an influenza epidemic there are often secondary bacterial pneumonias, which are usually caused by Staphylococcus aureus. In this case cefuroxime is a justifiable choice for antibiotic.
- The length of treatment for pneumonia is 10 days.
- Preventing pneumonia by pneumococcal vaccination B [2] or influenza vaccination is worthwhile. Amantadine may be used as protective medication for influenza in patients who have not been vaccinated, but one must bear in mind the side effects (1.40).
- In prolonged lung infection the probability of tuberculosis is higher (skin test, sputum cultures).

Urinary tract infections and pyelonephritis

- Women are predisposed to urinary tract infections because of age-related atrophy of the vaginal mucosa or prolapses of the vagina or uterus. Men are predisposed because of prostate hyperplasia. The most important external factor predisposing for urinary tract infection is catheterization.

- The cause of recurrent infections should be defined and treated. If the cause is not found, periodic prophylactic treatment with nitrofurantoin or trimethoprim may be used as one dose at night.
- Symptomless bacteriuria of the elderly should not be managed with antibiotics unless some specific (dysuria, incontinence) or non-specific (confusion, falls) symptoms of infection appear.
- In institutional care management is sometimes given for the smell related to infections. This practice is not recommended. The treatment does not reduce bed wetting. In this case the treatment should be short lasting, and the drug should be mild (e.g. single-dose nitrofurantoin at night).
- Cefuroxime intravenously is the first-line management of pyelonephritis. When the general condition improves or when the temperature normalizes, oral medication may be substituted for the i.v. drug. The length of treatment is 2 weeks.
- Patients with indwelling catheter should not be given prophylactic medication. Taking samples from the catheter for follow-up is not worthwhile.

Gastrointestinal and intra-abdominal infections

- Because the sense of visceral pain is decreased with ageing, acute appendicitis and biliary tract infections may be difficult to diagnose. They may silently lead to perforation or acute abdominal catastrophe.
- Diverticulosis and diverticulitis are age-related diseases.
- Serum CRP and blood leukocytes, repeated clinical examination and exclusion infections affecting other organs help to reach the correct diagnosis.

References

1. Riquelme-R et al. Community-acquired pneumonia in the elderly: A multivariate analysis of risk and prognostic factors. Am J Respir Crit Care Med 1996;154:1450–5.
2. Örtqvist Å et al. Randomized trial of 23-valent pneumococcal capsular polysaccharide vaccine in prevention of pneumonia in middle-aged and elderly people. Lancet 1998;351:399–403.

22.8 Reviewing an elderly patient's medications

Kaisu Pitkälä

Basic rules

- Nearly all medicines may cause side effects in elderly patients, and certain medications frequently cause adverse effects (long half-life benzodiazepines, oral hypoglycaemics, medications with anticholinergic properties, anti-inflammatory analgesics, etc.).
- In addition to underlying illness, medicines must be considered as a cause of disorders C [1].
- As much as elderly patients tend to over-use medication, they are prone to under-use potentially beneficial therapy (e.g. thrombolytic treatment in acute myocardial infarction, preventive medications, and management of pain).
- Reduction of medication should be carried out tactfully and in good understanding between the doctor and patient.

Assessment of medication

Compliance

- Find out when and why the medicines have been prescribed and how the patient uses them. Is there over- or underuse of prescribed medicines? Is the patient taking medicines prescribed by other physicians? Is the patient taking over-the-counter drugs (including dermatological products, vitamins and eyedrops)?
- Make use of the patient's history, information from relatives, home nurses or carers.
- A visit to the patient and assessment of medication found in his/her home gives a more accurate picture of the use of drugs.

GER

Selecting the right medication

- Clarify what needs to be treated. The various symptoms of the elderly patient must be assessed carefully. All the symptoms cannot be cured. However, all the symptoms in elderly patients are not due to ageing alone.
- Assess the inconvenience the symptoms cause to the patient. Would a possible medication and its adverse effects create more problems than what the symptoms are causing?
- Assess the whole "metabolism" of medication: memory, compliance, dependence on medicines, diet, fluid intake, malabsorption, liver and kidney function.
- For elderly persons the dose is usually half of that for a middle-aged person. This is particularly relevant in psychiatric pharmacotherapy.
- Always start a drug at the lowest possible dose, monitor the effects and side effects carefully (view any new symptoms and signs as possible drug side effects). Raise the dose very slowly.
- Manage the patient's medication as a whole; take into account the interactions of different medicines.

How to reduce medication

- Reports from trials are inconsistent.
- Explain to the patient that the symptoms may be side effects caused by used drugs.
- Find out how dependent (physically or psychologically) the patient is on his/her medicines.

- Propose a trial period during which the patient stops taking a medicine, observes his/her condition and reports it to the doctor.
- It may be necessary to check all the medicines found at the patient's home and dispose of non-essential drugs. The home nurse could do this, respecting the opinions of the aged patient.
- If the symptoms are serious, refer the elderly person to a hospital, withdraw all suspected medicines, and then start only the necessary medication with careful follow-up.

Increasing the safety of medication

- Organize a regular medication round in the nursing home and on the ward. In particular, antipsychotics, analgesics and sleeping pills tend to remain on the patient's chart long after the condition has resolved.
- The medications should be given as infrequently as possible, even if effectiveness must be compromised.
- Arrange for the medication to be the same every day.
- Give clear, written instructions always when there are more than two drugs at the time.
- Ensure that the written instructions for medication are available to all people taking care of the elderly person.
- Drug dispensing boxes should be for administering the daily medication.
- Ask home nurses and caregivers to report on the real use of medicines.
- In the most extreme cases medicines may be stored at the home nurse's office. However, do not infringe the patient's right to self-determination

Drugs that are inappropriate or ineffective for the elderly

- In 1997[24] and 2003[25], a US expert panel developed a list of drugs that are potentially inappropriate for the elderly.
  - Amitriptyline and doxepine are highly anticholinergic drugs that may cause confusion, memory impairment, urinary retention, constipation and aggravations of glaucoma.
  - Long-acting benzodiazepines (diazepam, nitrazepam) accumulate in the adipose tissue and may cause sedation and fallings.
  - The dose of short acting benzodiazepines is less than half of the normal dose.
  - Dextropropoxyphene has a narrow therapeutic range.
  - The risk of CNS and GI side effects are higher with indomethasine than with other NSAID drugs.
  - Meprobamate and barbiturates cause sedation and involve the risk of developing drug dependency.
  - Disopyridamide is strongly anticholinergic.
  - For the elderly the dose of digoxin should not exceed 0.125 mg.
  - Old sedative antihistamines, and GI tract antispasmodics are strongly anticholinergic and often quite sedative.
  - The efficacy of dihydroergotamine has not been shown.
  - A necessary drug may sometimes be replaced by another drug with fewer side effects, for example
    - long-acting benzodiazepine by short-acting one
    - NSAID by paracetamol or a COX2 inhibitor
    - anticholinergic trisyclic antidepressant by other antidepressant
    - rigidity-causing low-dose neuroleptic by riseperidone or olazepine
- Do not use symptomatic medications for dizziness in the elderly.

Under-use of potentially beneficial therapy

- Old age alone should never be a contraindication for potentially beneficial therapy.
- Typical examples of underused therapy:
  - Thrombolysis in acute myocardial infarction is often avoided in the elderly, the major concern being the risk of haemorrhage. The absolute risk of death from myocardial infarction increases sharply with advancing age as does the risk of haemorrhage. However, the absolute number of deaths prevented by thrombolysis also increases even more, making therapy worthwhile.
  - Analgesic therapy is underused: chronic pain, the management of cancer pain and the pain experienced by patients in long-term care settings are underestimated **B** [13 14 15 16 17 18 19 20 21 22 23].

References

1. Mannesse CK, Derkx FHM, de Ridder MAJ et al. Adverse drug reactions in elderly patients as contributing factor for hospital admission: cross sectional study. BMJ 1997;315: 1057–8.
2. Kroenke K, Pinholt EM. Reducing polypharmacy in the elderly: a controlled trial of physician feedback. J Am Geriat Soc 1990;38:31–6.
3. Meyer TJ, Van Kooten D, Marsh S, et al. Reduction of polypharmacy by feedback to clinicians. J Gen Intern Med 1991;6:133.6.
4. Lipton HL, Bero LA, Bird JA, et al. The impact of clinical pharmacists´ consultations on physicians´ geriatric drug prescribing: a randomized, controlled trial. Med Care 1992;30:646–58.
5. Hanlon JT, Weinberg M, Samsa GP, et al. A randomized controlled trial of a clinical pharmacist intervention to improve inappropriate prescribing in elderly outpatients with polypharmacy. Am J Med 1996;100:428–37.
6. Smith DH, Christiansen DB, Stergachis A, et al. A randomized controlled trial of a drug use review intervention for sedative hypnotic medications. Med Care 1998;36:1013–21.
7. Fillit HM, Futterman R, Orland BI, et al. Polypharmacy management in Medicare managed care: changes in prescribing by primary care physicians resulting from a program promoting medication reviews. Am J Manag Care 1999;5:587–94.

8. Soumerai SB, Avorn J. predictors of physician prescribing change in an educational experiment to improve medication use. Med Care 1987;25:210–21.
9. Avorn J, Soumerai SB. Improving drug-therapy decisions through educational outreach: a randomized controlled trial of academically based "detailing". N Engl J Med 1983;308: 1457–63.
10. Steele MA, Bess DT, Franse VL, et al. Cost effectiveness of two interventions for reducing outpatient prescribing costs. DICP 1989;23:497–500.
11. Pitkälä KH, Strandberg TE, Tilvis RS. Is it possible to reduce polypharmacy in the elderly? Drugs Aging 2001;18: 143–9.
12. Gilchrist WJ. Lee YC, Tam HC, et al. Prospective study of drug reporting by general practitioners for an elderly population referred to geriatric service. BMJ 1987;294:289–90.
13. Cleeland CS, Gonin R, Hatfield AK, et al. Pain and its treatment in outpatients with metastatic cancer. N Engl J Med 1994;330:592–6.
14. Zenz M, Willweber-Strumpf A. Opiophobia and cancer pain in Europe. Lancet 1993;341:1075–6.
15. Larue R, Colleau SM, Brasseur L, et al. Multicentre study of cancer pain and its treatment in France. Br Med J 1995;310:1034–7.
16. Bernabei R, Gambassi G, Lapane K, et al. Management of pain in elderly patients with cancer. SAGE study group. Systematic assessment of geriatric drug use via epidemiology. JAMA 1998;279:1877–82.
17. Cleeland CS, Gonin R, Baez L, Loehrer KJ. Pain and treatment of pain in minority patients with cancer. The eastern cooperative oncology group monirity outpatient pain study. Ann Intern Med 1997;127:813–6.
18. Cleeland CS. Undertreatment of cancer pain in elderly patients. JAMA 1998;279:1914–5.
19. Feldt KS, Ryden MB, Miles S. Treatment of pain in cognitively impaired compared with cognitively intact older patients with hip fracture. J Am Geriatr Soc 1998;46:1079–85.
20. Ferrell BA, Ferrell BR, Osterweil D. Pain in the nursing home. J Am Geriatr Soc 1990;38:409–14.
21. Won A, Lapane K, Gambassi G, et al. Correlates and management of non-malignant pain in the nursing home. SAGE study group. Systematic assessment of geriatric drug use via epidemiology. J Am Geriatr Soc 1999;47: 936–42.
22. Fox PL, Raina P, Jadad AR. Prevalence and treatment of pain in older adults in nursing homes and other long-term care institutions: a systematic review. CMAJ 1999;160: 329–33.
23. Pitkälä KH, Strandberg TE, Tilvis RS. Management at nonmalignant pain in the home-dwelling elderly: a population-based survey. J Am Geriatr Soc 2002;50:1861–1865.
24. Beers HH. Explicit criteria for determining potentially inappropriate medication use by the elderly. An update. Arch Intern Med 1997;57:1531–6.
25. Fick DM, Cooper JW, Wade WE, Waller JL, Maclean JR, Beers MH. Updating the Beers criteria for potentially inappropriate medication use in older adults: results of a US consensus panel of experts, Arch Intern Med 2003;163: 2716–24.

22.10 Hypertension in elderly patients

Timo Strandberg

Introduction

- The treatment of hypertension in an elderly patient is beneficial regardless of the medication used.
- The treatment should be introduced cautiously to avoid the risk of disturbances in cerebral circulation and subsequent falls.
- The target of the treatment should be normotension (less than 140/90), unless prevented by orthostatic problems or impairment of renal function.

An elderly person and blood pressure

- Systolic blood pressure increases with age whereas diastolic blood pressure starts to decrease after the age of 60 years.
- Isolated systolic hypertension (ISH) is often seen in the elderly population. Associated diseases not only make treatment more difficult but also hamper the comparison of relevant hypertension treatment studies.
- Treatment reduces, in particular, the incidence of stroke and heart failure. The effect on coronary heart disease is small. Treatment initiated before the onset of old age may prevent the incidence of Alzheimer's disease. This benefit might be dependent upon the drug choice.
- The following factors should be taken into account in the treatment of hypertension:
  - non-steroidal anti-inflammatory drugs reduce the efficacy of ACE inhibitors and may further damage the kidneys in renal disease
  - renovascular hypertension is difficult to normalize without compromising renal function.
- A very wide pulse pressure may indicate aortic regurgitation. The target should be to normalize both the systolic and diastolic pressure.
- There is no definite evidence of the overall benefit of initiating drug treatment in patients aged 80–85: the incidence of strokes will decrease but mortality remains unchanged. The decision on whether to start treatment or not, and which drug to use, should be made in relation to any co-existing illnesses and the general health of the patient.

Diagnosis

- Almost 20% of the elderly have pseudohypertension where atherosclerotic arteries do not compress under the cuff, resulting in falsely high readings.
- "White coat" hypertension is also common in the elderly. Home measurements are warranted.

- In order to diagnose orthostatic hypotension, blood pressure must also always be measured with the patient standing up; an asymptomatic drop of systolic pressure by 20 mmHg is common and acceptable.
- Co-existing illnesses and medication that may reduce blood pressure include:
  - parkinsonism and its medication
  - psychiatric medication, particularly antipsychotics
  - diabetic neuropathy
  - nitrates.

Treatment

- Life style modifications are usually not effective when treating hypertension in an elderly patient; the illnesses of this age group are usually no longer related to lifestyle.
- The treatment should be initiated cautiously with a small dose which is increased gradually. The target is not always achieved but even a small reduction in blood pressure is beneficial.
- The patient should be advised to get out of bed slowly, and the symptoms of presyncope should be explained.
- The drug choice should be made taking any co-existing illnesses into consideration.
- A diuretic is often the first line drug, unless an associated disease requires the use of an ACE inhibitor or an angiotensin-II receptor antagonist (particularly if the patient suffers from a cough as an adverse effect to an ACE inhibitor).
- A small dose of a thiazide is sufficient for blood pressure reduction.
  - An excessive dose of a diuretic may easily cause orthostatic hypotension in a small-sized elderly person.
- If the elderly patient also has diabetes, coronary heart disease or heart failure, a diuretic alone will not be sufficient.
  - A combination of an ACE inhibitor or an angiotensin-II receptor antagonist with a diuretic is effective in blood pressure reduction, but may cause orthostatic problems and increased serum creatinine concentrations.
  - An ACE inhibitor or an angiotensin-II receptor antagonist should not be combined with a potassium-sparing diuretic (risk of hyperkalaemia). A combination product should be prescribed instead. A possible exception is the combination of an ACE inhibitor and spironolactone in the treatment of heart failure.
- Beta-blockers are of no particular benefit.
  - Their efficacy may be improved with the addition of a vasodilating calcium-channel blocker; however, this combination may lead to orthostatic problems as the beta-blocker prevents the required increase in heart rate.
  - A beta-blocker is indicated in coronary heart disease and chronic heart failure.
- Calcium-channel blockers may be used. Concomitant use with a diuretic is not usually recommended due to the possibility of hypovolaemia.
- An ACE inhibitor or an angiotensin-II receptor antagonist is usually indicated if the patient has co-existing chronic heart failure, history of myocardial infarction or type 2 diabetes.
  - The monitoring of renal function is important (creatinine, K, Na), particularly if the patient uses concomitant non-steroidal anti-inflammatory drugs.
  - A slight increase in the concentration of serum creatinine does not usually prevent the use of an ACE inhibitor or angiotensin II receptor antagonist (unless serum creatinine concentration rises above 30% over baseline during the first 2 months or hyperkalaemia develops).

22.20 Health checks for the elderly

Jaakko Valvanne

Aims

- Functional ability and health are maintained for as long as possible.
- Quality of life is insured and safety is increased.
- Social ties are strengthened.
- The elderly are provided information about health services and normal ageing.
- Mortality is reduced.

Basic rules

- The most convincing proof of the efficacy of preventive measures in the elderly has been obtained for the following interventions: breast cancer screening, smoking cessation, treatment of hypertension, increasing the amount of exercise, vaccinations and preventing falls.
- Results on the efficacy of non-targeted screening are contradictory, despite the fact that various undiagnosed diseases may be found.
- Screening performed by health care providers (community nurse, personal physician) during the patient's visits to the health centre might be more beneficial. It is well suited for population-based primary care. Screening can be performed by any health care professional, with a more thorough health check performed by a physician when necessary.
- Only those diseases or disabilities for which an effective treatment exists and which could be considered for the elderly should be sought for.

Screening of own patients

- Individuals who require a more detailed assessment should be identified.
- The main emphasis should be on functional ability (ability to move, cognitive function, managing daily activities), not only on disease.

♦ Incipient functional disability is an indication for detailed assessment as it is often a sign of somatic disease.

Content of screening in primary care

♦ No consensus exists on the content of a feasible screening programme.
♦ Scientific proof of the efficacy of the following screening measures is available:
  • Measuring blood pressure
  • Mammography
  • Touch by rectum, faecal blood and sigmoidoscopy (for detecting colon cancer)
♦ The following measures have also been suggested
  • Managing daily activities; ADL (Activities of Daily Living) (22.21) and IADL (Instrumental Activities of Daily Living; shopping, finance, preparing food, using the telephone)
  • Hearing: history or whispering 20 cm from the ear
  • Mood (examined e.g. with a depression test: Zung, GDS, DEPS)
  • Test for dementia –only if memory disturbances occur
  • Visual acuity, intraocular pressure
  • Blood glucose, cholesterol, thyroid function
  • ECG
  • Nutritional state examined with a MNA questionnaire (Mini Nutritional Assessment)
  • Bone density measured with densitometry
  • Ability of getting into and out of a chair and ability of walking (patients at increased risk of falling or with a history of previous falls)
♦ However, it has been found that
  • screening the visual acuity of asymptomatic elderly persons does not improve vision C [1]
  • health survey including medical examination seldom leads to detection of new important findings in general elderly population
  • routine use of questionnaires for detecting psychiatric disorders (depression, anxiety) does not increase the detection rate or improve the prognosis of emotional disturbances
  • interventions aimed at reducing the risk of falling should be targeted at patients most likely to benefit from them.
♦ There is no settled view on the significance of prostate palpation and/or PSA in the screening of prostate cancer.

Whom to screen and how often?

♦ The above-listed screening measures or some of them can be recommended to be carried out at 1 to 5 year intervals if the test results influence the actions taken by the physician.
♦ Setting an upper age limit to screening is difficult; however, the meaningfulness of screening asymptomatic over 85-year-old persons for diseases has been questioned.
♦ In institutionalized elderly, focus should be on preventing pressure sores, urinary incontinence and falls and in maintaining the ability to move. Yearly laboratory investigations are not considered justified in these patients.
♦ Evaluating the potential benefits is particularly problematic when
  • there is no cure for the disease
  • earlier examinations have been negative
  • the person in question has a severely limited functional ability or is demented
  • the expected quality or duration of life is limited because of some other cause.
♦ Although the age of 85 years is considered the upper limit of screening, the individual differences in personality and need for care must be taken into account.

Reference

1. Smeeth L, Iliffe S. Community screening for visual impairment in the elderly. Cochrane Database Syst Rev. 2004;(2):CD001054.

22.21 Assessment of physical and mental functioning

Kaisu Pitkälä

GER

Functional ability

♦ Many different tests and methods are used in the assessment of physical and cognitive functioning of the elderly. There is no international consensus of which tests are most suitable for assessment of the elderly.
♦ Scales may be used for
  • assessment of need for institutional care
  • screening of functional disability and diseases
  • setting objectives for rehabilitation and management and following up their effects
  • longitudinal follow up of physical functioning of the elderly in long-term care settings and comparison of different care places
  • epidemiological research.
♦ Different scales suit these different functions.
♦ Below, four scales are introduced. The first is the Barthel index (Table 22.21.1), which is widely used on home-dwelling elderly.
♦ This scale is easy and rapid to use, and it is well validated. It is reliable and quite sensitive to changes in physical functioning.
♦ It may be used on the elderly in home care whose need for institutional care needs to be assessed as well as on elderly patients undergoing rehabilitation. This scale has been recommended by Scandinavian professors of geriatrics.

Table 22.21.1 The Barthel Index–a scale for measuring physical functioning

1. Feeding	Unable to eat independently	0
	Needs help cutting, spreading butter etc. or requires modified diet	5
	Independent	10
2. Transfers (from bed to chair and back)	Unable, no sitting balance	0
	Major help (one or two people, physical), can sit	5
	Minor help (verbal or physical)	10
	Independent	15
3. Grooming	Needs help with personal care	0
	Independent face/hair/teeth/shaving (implements provided)	5
4. Toilet use	Dependent	0
	Needs some help, but can do something alone	5
	Independent (on and off toilet seat, dressing, wiping)	10
5. Bathing	Dependent	0
	Independent (or in shower)	5
6. Mobility on level surfaces	Immobile or <50 m	0
	Wheelchair independent, including corners, >50 m	5
	Walks with help of one person (verbal or physical) >50 m	10
	Walks independently 50 m, may use any aid, for example a stick)	15
7. Ascending or descending stairs	Unable to walk up/down stairs	0
	Needs help (verbal, physical or carrying aid)	5
	Independent	10
8. Dressing and undressing	Dependent	0
	Needs help but can do about half unaided	5
	Independent (including buttons, zips, laces, etc.)	10
9. Bowels	Incontinent (or needs to be given enemas)	0
	Occasional accident	5
	Continent	10
10.Bladder	Incontinent, or catheterised and unable to manage alone	0
	Occasional accident	5
	Continent	10
max 100 points		

Table 22.21.2 Katz's ADL index for assessment of activities of daily living

Bathing	Receives no assistance (gets in and out of tub on own if tub is the usual means of bathing)	Receives assistance in bathing only one part of the body (such as back or leg)	*Receives assistance in bathing more than one part of the body (or not bathed)*
Dressing	Gets clothes and gets completely dressed without assistance	Gets clothes and gets dressed without assistance except for assistance in tying shoelaces	*Receives assistance in getting clothes or in getting dressed, or stays partly or completely undressed*
Toileting	Goes to lavatory, cleans self, and arranges clothes without assistance (may use object for support such as cane, walker, or wheelchair and may manage night bedpan or commode, emptying same in morning)	*Receives assistance in going to lavatory or in cleaning self or arranging clothes after elimination or in use of night bedpan or commode*	*Does not go to the lavatory for the elimination process*
Transfer	Moves in and out of chair as well as in and out of bed without assistance (may be using object for support such as cane or walker)	*Moves in and out of bed or chair with assistance*	*Does not get out of bed*
Continence	Controls urination and bowel movement completely by self	*Has occasional "accidents"*	*Supervision helps keep urine or bowel control; catheter is used or is incontinent*
Feeding	Feeds self without assistance	Feeds self except for getting assistance in cutting meat or buttering bread	*Receives assistance in feeding or is fed partly or completely by using tubes or intravenous fluids*

The patients are divided according to their functional ability to independent (on the left side) and dependent ones (on the right side, marked with italics typeset), which is used to classify the patients into different Katz classes.

Classification of patients into different classes of dependence according to their functional ability:

A–Independent in all six functions.

B–Independent in all but one of these functions.

C–Independent in all but bathing and one additional function.

D–Independent in all but bathing, dressing and one additional function.

E–Independent in all but bathing, dressing, toileting and one additional function.

F–Independent in all but bathing, dressing, toileting, transferring and one additional function.

G–Dependent in all six functions.

Other–if patient cannot be classified using the classes above.

Table 22.21.3 IADL scale (Instrumental activities of daily living), Lawton

1. Ability to use telephone	1	Operates telephone on own initiative; looks up and dials numbers etc.
	1	Dials a few well-known numbers
	1	Answers telephone but does not use it to make calls
	0	Does not use telephone at all
2. Shopping	1	Takes care of all shopping needs independently
	0	Shops independently for small purchases only
	0	Needs to be accompanied on any shopping trips
	0	Completely unable to shop
3. Food preparation	1	Plans, prepares and serves adequate meals independently
	0	Prepares adequate meals if supplied with ingredients
	0	Heats and serves prepared meals, or prepares meals but does not maintain adequate diet
	0	Needs to have meals prepared and served
4. Housekeeping	1	Maintains house alone or with occasional assistance (e.g. "heavy work"–domestic help)
	1	Performs light daily tasks such as dishwashing and bedmaking
	1	Performs daily tasks but cannot maintain acceptable level of cleanliness
	1	Needs help with home maintenance tasks
	0	Does not participate in any housekeeping tasks
5. Laundry	1	Does personal laundry completely
	1	Launders small items–rinses socks, stockings, etc.
	0	All laundry must be done by others
6. Mode of transport	1	Travels independently on public transport or drives own car
	1	Arranges own travel via taxi, but does not otherwise use public transport
	1	Travels on public transportation when assisted or accompanied by others
	0	Travel limited to taxi or car with assistance of another person
	0	Does not travel at all
7. Responsibility for own medications	1	Is responsible for taking medications in correct dosages at correct time
	0	Takes responsibility if medication is prepared in advance in separate dosages
	0	Is not capable of dispensing own medications

(*continued overleaf*)

Table 22.21.3 (*continued*)

8. Ability to handle finances	1	Manages financial matters independently (budgets, writes cheques, pays rent and bills, goes to bank), collects and keeps track of income
	1	Manages day-to-day purchases, but needs help with banking, major purchases, etc.
	0	Incapable if handling money

Table 22.21.4 Geriatric depression screening scale, GDS

Directions to Patient: There questions concern everyday mood, attitudes and feelings. Please choose the best answer for how you have felt over the past week. I shall read the questions and would like you to answer "yes" or "no".

	Yes	No
1. Are you basically satisfied with your life?	0	1
2. Have you dropped many of your activities and interests?	1	0
3. Do you feel that you life is empty?	1	0
4. Do you often get bored?	1	0
5. Are you hopeful about the future?	0	1
6. Are you bothered by thoughts that you cannot get out of your head?	1	0
7. Are you in good spirits most of the time?	0	1
8. Are you afraid that something bad is going to happen to you?	1	0
9. Do you feel happy most of the time?	0	1
10. Do you often feel helpless?	1	0
11. Do you often feel restless and fidgety?	1	0
12. Do you prefer to stay at home rather than going out and doing things?	1	0
13. Do you frequently worry about the future?	1	0
14. Do you feel you have more problems with memory than most?	1	0
15. Do you think it is wonderful to be alive now?	0	1
16. Do you often feel downhearted and blue?	1	0
17. Do you feel pretty worthless the way you are now?	1	0
18. Do you worry a lot about the past?	1	0
19. Do you find life very exciting?	0	1
20. Is it hard for you to get started on new projects?	1	0
21. Do you feel full of energy?	0	1
22. Do you feel that your situation is hopeless?	1	0
23. Do you think that most people are better off than you are?	1	0
24. Do you frequently get upset over little things?	1	0

(*continued overleaf*)

Table 22.21.4 (*continued*)

25. Do you frequently feel like crying?	1	0
26. Do you have trouble concentrating?	1	0
27. Do you enjoy getting up in the morning?	0	1
28. Do you prefer to avoid social occasions?	1	0
29. Is it easy for you to make decisions?	0	1
30. Is your mind as clear as it used to be?	0	1
Total score	0–10	Normal
	11–20	Mild depression
	21–30	Severe depression

- ♦ The Katz ADL index (Table 22.21.2) is widely used in institutional settings and it is not very sensitive in assessing the functional impairment of elderly patients living at home. However, it is widely used in the assessment of elderly home care patients.
- ♦ Tests measuring IADL functioning (instrumental activities of daily living) add to the picture of functional impairment of aged persons living at home. In following the Lawton and Brody IADL test is also introduced (Table 22.21.3).

Dementia test

- ♦ Cognitive functioning may be assessed by e.g. MMSE (Mini-Mental State Examination) B [1]. The test is not specific for dementia: for example, acute delirium may affect the score. The test is not suitable for patients with dysphasia.

Screening for depression

- ♦ Many tests are used to screen for depression. One of the most commonly used is the Geriatric Depression Screening Scale (GDS), see Table 22.21.4.

References

1. Mulligan R, Mackinnon A, Jorm AF et al. A comparison of alternative methods of screening for dementia in clinical setting. Arch Neurol 1996;53:532–6.
2. Mahoney FL, Barthel DW. Functional evaluation: The Barthel Index. Maryland State Med Y 1965;(Felor):61–5.
3. Lawton MP, Brody EM. Assessment of older people: self-maintaining and instrumental activities of daily living. Gerontologist 1969;9:179–86.
4. Yesavage JA, Brink TL. Development and validation of a geriatric depression screening scale: a preliminary report. J Psychiatr Res 1983;17:37–49.
5. Katz S, Downs TD, Cash HR, Grotz RC. Progress in development of the Index of ADL. Gerontologist 1970;10:20–9.

22.30 Organisation of elder care–Intermediate services

Editors

General

- ♦ Intermediate services in elder care form a heterogeneous group of activities in the border and between outpatient care and institutional care. In the Table 22.30 describing the present organization of elder care these activities are marked with an asterisk (*).
- ♦ Other intermediate services might include
  - a shared care cooperation between home services, home health services, and hospital services, resembling a hospital at home–"hospital-based home care".

Table 22.30 Organization of the services for the elderly

Social services	Health services
Individual social work ♦ guidance, counselling ♦ welfare payments	Health centre care ♦ health counselling ♦ general practise consultations ♦ dental care ♦ rehabilitation ♦ home health services (*)
Home services ♦ home help ♦ transportation services ♦ financial support for caregivers ♦ day centre activities (*) ♦ day care (*)	
Supported living ♦ service apartments (*) ♦ small renovations	Mental care services
Assisted living ♦ group homes (*)	
Nursing home care ♦ day care (*) ♦ short term care (*) ♦ periodic care (*) ♦ special units for dementia care (*) ♦ regular long-term care	Community hospital ♦ day hospital (*) ♦ night care (*) ♦ week hospital (*) ♦ periodic care (*) ♦ terminal (hospice) care ♦ acute care ♦ geriatric assessment ♦ rehabilitation ♦ long-term care Specialist hospital ♦ acute care ♦ diagnostic evaluations ♦ rehabilitation ♦ psychiatric care ♦ psychogeriatric care ♦ (long-term care)

- psychogeriatric day activities
- day care activities for special groups (e.g. demented patients).

♦ The development of intermediate services is encouraged by several social trends:
  - An increasing proportion of the population needing institutional care
  - High costs of institutional care, and economic difficulties experienced by health care providers
  - The elders' increasing demand for good services.

Service apartments

♦ Enable independent living even for disabled persons
♦ Provide security for the elderly living alone, as round-the-clock help is available.
♦ Equipment standards
  - The size of a service flat for a single person should be about 42–45 m^2.
  - It should be possible to get in, and move about in, the apartment with mobility aids, e.g. a wheelchair.
  - Round-the-clock availability of assistance can be enabled by alarm systems.
  - Shared facilities are needed for the use of the inhabitants and for the personnel (either the house's own or for community home care services).

Group homes

♦ A form of assisted living based on maximizing living autonomy for the elderly in need of round-the-clock supervision and assistance
♦ Bedrooms (or suites) situated close to shared facilities (which include work and social space for the personnel)
♦ In home-like environment with a small group of people living together a cognitively impaired person manages better than in most larger institutions.
♦ A demented person needs continuous supervision and a safe environment, where doors can be locked.
♦ Group homes have benefited demented persons in particular, and also those elderly who previously needed psychiatric inpatient care.
♦ Especially a unit designed for dementia care should be small (8–10 patients), and it should be prepared to care for 1 or 2 patients with challenging behavioural problems.

Week hospital

♦ A hospital ward providing care during weekdays is suitable for rehabilitation and geriatric assessment services. The patients must be able to cope at home over the weekends.
♦ Sharing the care between the home and hospital improves the patients' motivation for rehabilitation.

Hospital-at-home

♦ Hospital-at-home means medical care given by health care professionals at the home of the patient that would otherwise require care on a hospital department.
♦ Evidence on the effectiveness of hospital-at-home care is scarce Ⓐ [1].

Short-term care and periodic care in nursing homes

♦ The goal is to
  - maintain the ability of the elderly to live at home by providing access to periodic care and evaluation.
  - postpone and prevent institutionalization by relieving the burden of the caregivers (respite care) Ⓓ [2,3].

♦ The care should be included in a service and care plan made well in advance.

Night care

♦ Night care may benefit a small group of patients or their caregivers, such as those needing frequent lifting.

GER

Designs for the future

♦ Institutional care must be seen as a support service for home care.
♦ Resources should be allocated to enhance the autonomy and coping of individuals and communities.
♦ The organizations of health and social services need to be coordinated to facilitate the development of intermediate services.
♦ The quality of care given in institutions should be improved.
♦ Services for demented persons are still a major challenge for the care of the elderly.
♦ Expertise of dedicated general practitioners, geriatricians and old age psychiatrists is required at crucial points in the life of a disabled elderly person, especially when permanent institutional living is considered.
♦ The target is that 90% of those aged 80 or more could live at home with the help of various services.

References

1. Shepperd S, Iliffe S. Hospital at home versus in-patient hospital care. Cochrane Database Syst Rev. 2004;(2):CD000356.
2. Flint AJ. Effects of respite care on patients with dementia and their caregivers. Int Psychogeriatrics 1997;7:505–517.
3. The Database of Abstracts of Reviews of Effectiveness (University of York), Database no.: DARE-973434. In: The Cochrane Library, Issue 4, 1999. Oxford: Update Software.

22.31 Assessment of the need for institutionalization

Annamaija Sutela

Basic rules

- An aged person should not be taken into institutional care without a careful medical and psychosocial assessment and consideration of the possible effects of rehabilitation and care. The possibility of returning back to outpatient care should be evaluated even after admission to institutional care.
- Determination of psychological and functional abilities using set tools systematically is always a part of the assessment. The patient's state of health and living conditions are also important factors. The possibilities offered by primary care should be considered and the opinions of the patient and the caregivers should be taken into account.
- Cooperation of different working groups in social care and health care is required in the assessment.

Assessment group

- Assessment of need for institutional care in the community should be carried out by a centralized group (in a large community, several groups), that specializes in this activity Ⓐ [1]. The composition of the group may vary. The following health care professionals might belong to the group:
    - geriatrician or physician responsible for long-term care
    - home nurse or nurse familiar with the patient
    - social worker
    - psychologist
    - physiotherapist
    - occupational therapist.
- Often different specialist consultations are needed, for example neurologist, orthopaedic, psychiatrist, physiatrist, ophthalmologist or ENT specialist.

Assessment of the patient

- The psychological and functional abilities must be defined in order to find the right level of care. The state of health and living conditions are also important factors.

Functional assessment

- Different scales and indicators can be used when defining the functional disability of an aged person. Katz's ADL index is widely used. It is quite insensitive for estimating the functional disabilities of patients in non-institutional care (22.21). One should add the IADL (Instrumental Activities of Daily Living) assessment to it. This assesses how the aged person manages with shopping, cooking, using the telephone, cleaning the house, finances and taking care of medications (22.21).

Cognitive impairment and psychiatric symptoms

- Cognitive function
    - Cognitive function can be assessed, for example with the Folstein's Mini-Mental Status examination. An American test developed by CERAD for assessing memory impairment and early dementia contains more tasks and is recommended by some experts. Before assigning an elderly person to institutional care, dementia should be diagnosed correctly and possible therapy for dementia should be tested and found appropriate (36.22).
- Depression
    - In addition to the clinical picture, the DSM-III criteria are suitable for diagnosing depression. GDS (geriatric depression scale) is widely used for screening for depression (22.21)
    - Many other scales are also suitable for assessing functional or psychological disabilities in an elderly person, but one must be thoroughly acquainted with the chosen scale.

State of health

- The effects of diseases on the functional ability of the aged person and the subsequent need for care should be assessed when the state of health of an elderly person is examined. When choosing the place of care one should consider following question:
    - Stability of the condition
        - Behavioural disturbances in a demented person, poor treatment balance in diabetes, severe heart failure or COPD are examples of conditions involving instability.
    - Long-term prognosis of the disease
        - When arranging long-term care in an institution, the effect of the disease on functional capacity must be taken into account in advance. Aggravation of dementia or Parkinson's disease and progression of cancer are examples of conditions that require planning in advance.
        - The prognosis should influence the choice of the place of care.
    - Need for treatment
        - The need for special treatment procedures should be taken into account, such as multiple-injection insulin therapy, stoma, bed or leg sores, need for suction, management of pain, terminal care.
        - The need for aids, such as oxygen concentrator, wheelchair or mechanical lifter, should be considered.

- Safety risks
  - Does the aged person escape from the ward, use alcohol or drugs, smoke?

Social situation

- ♦ Many social factors determine the urgency of finding a care place.
  - The patient's living conditions are significant. An apartment with convenient facilities and an elevator permits living at home longer than a property with no running water or central heating.
  - Financial matters should not be the only cause preventing living at home.
  - The social network of the elderly has a significant role when living at home is supported. Living alone without close relatives or friends may cause the person to move to institutional care earlier. On the other hand, trouble in relationships (e.g. an aggressive, heavy-drinking next of kin) may lead to a need for institutional care.
  - It is important to listen to the opinions of the patient and the caregiver and to assess their ability to cope with the situation. The various possibilities for placement naturally have an influence on selection of the care place.

Prolonging home-based care

- ♦ In all phases of assessment the possibility of continuing home-based care should be evaluated. A home visit by a physician may give the best picture of the conditions in which the elderly person is living.
  - Could home appliances or renovation of the dwelling help the elderly person to manage longer at home?
  - Has respite care sufficiently relieved the caregivers' stress?
  - Could the elderly person manage better at home if home care and home aid were intensified? Individually tailored home care may prolong living at home.

Purpose-built apartments for elderly people

- ♦ Living in this type of accommodation is similar to living at home, with basic services nearby. In some apartment buildings 24-hour help is available.

Residential care

- ♦ In some residential care certain services are included, and in others residents buy services.

Nursing homes

- ♦ Along with board and lodging personnel help with activities of daily living and with medicines. Some nursing homes may have separate units for the demented.

Hospitals and hospital-based long-term care

- ♦ For the somatically ill and of the severely demented. Possibilities for rehabilitation are often better than in the above-mentioned institutions.

Hospital-at-home

- ♦ Is defined as a service that provides effective care given by health-care professionals in the patient's home in situations when in-patient hospitalization would be otherwise necessary. Such treatment is always meant to continue for only a limited period.
- ♦ There is no evidence supporting the development of hospital at home services as a cheaper alternative to in-patient care. Early discharge schemes for patients recovering from elective surgery and elderly patients with a medical condition may have a place in reducing the pressure on acute hospital beds, providing the views of the carers are taken into account (A) [2].

Choosing the place of care

- ♦ When physical functioning, grade of dementia, state of health, social situation and resources are known, the choice is made between institutional care and home-based care. Persons knowledgeable in geriatrics and gerontology should make the decision.
- ♦ The persons making the decision should be well acquainted with the quality of the care services for the elderly and should have a system for evaluating these services.
- ♦ The aim is to make individually tailored decisions with the right timing. Cooperation with the patient and the next-of-kin is important.
- ♦ In most cases dementia eventually leads to institutional care. However, care at home can often be extended with the help of supportive actions and by foreseeing the development of the condition. Institutional care too early is harmful for the elderly person.
  - Incipient dementia may require minor support for the family. Giving family members information about the condition is important.
  - In moderately severe dementia, the patient often manages at home, sometimes even if he/she lives alone. Regular daily rhythm is important and it can be supported by day hospital or day care activities.
  - A severely demented elderly needs a place in institutional care. Home care is sometimes successful with the help of the family. In such cases the family members must be given sufficient support.

GER

References

1. Stuck A E, Siu A L, Wieland G D, Adams J, Rubenstein L Z. Comprehensive geriatric assessment: a meta-analysis of controlled trials. Lancet 1993;342:1032–6.
2. Shepperd S, Iliffe S. Hospital at home versus in-patient hospital care. Cochrane Database Syst Rev. 2004;(2):CD000356.

22.32 Day hospital care of the elderly

Kaisu Pitkälä

Purpose of care

- To rehabilitate and maintain functioning
- To diagnose and manage diseases
- To decrease the caregiver's burden
- To carry out different procedures, to start administration of a new medicine, to educate patients
- To manage patients socially and psychologically. To provide recreational activities and other management if the community does not have a day centre.
- The aims of the management of each patient as well as the length of the management period should be decided upon in advance. The effects of management should be evaluated afterwards. Day hospital care is as costly as inpatient hospital care.

Arrangements

- The elderly person is transported to the day hospital 1–5 times a week. The length of the management period is agreed upon at the beginning.
- Services may include:
  - transportation
  - meals
  - opportunity to rest
  - medical examination, laboratory tests and radiography, procedures and therapies
  - nursing
  - physiotherapy, occupational therapy, speech therapy
  - health education
  - recreational therapy, group activities
  - bathing and laundry services
  - chiropody, hairdressing
  - assessment of efficacy and tolerability of medications, starting a new medication
  - assessment of need for institutional care.

Different types of day hospitals

- Day hospitals are often part of a larger geriatric unit or the department of medicine in an inpatient hospital. They are intense assessment and rehabilitation units with good staff resources (especially physiotherapy and occupational therapy) and good opportunities for specialist consultation.
- Dementia day care centres give caregivers an opportunity to rest.
- Day centres usually do not have medical staff. Day centres are intended to provide lonely, depressive elderly people with recreation. They also provide continuous care for day hospital patients, and day care for elderly patients whose caregivers need rest.

Effectiveness of care

- Studies concerning cost-effectiveness show that the most efficient units are either those with good resources (A) [1] and geriatric expertise or day care units for dementia patients. Geriatric assessment units have been shown to be effective, and in dementia day care costs are so low that even a small reduction in other hospital care results in savings.
- Day hospital care is well liked by many patients, and it improves the quality of life (A) [1]. However, it does not suit all patients because of the transportation involved.

References

1. Foster A, Young J, Langhorne P for the Day Hospital Group. Medical day hospital care for the elderly versus alternative forms of care (Cochrane Review). Cochrane Database Syst Rev. 2004;(2):CD001730.
2. Engedal K. Day care for demented patients in general nursing homes effects on admissions to institutions and mental capacity. Scan J Prim Health Care 1989;7:161–166.
3. Stuck AE, Siu AL, Wieland 6D et al. Comprehensive geriatric assessment: a meta-analysis of controlled trials. Lancet 1993;342:1032–1036.

Diabetes

Evidence Based Medicine Guidelines. Edited by the Duodecim Editorial Team
 ISBN: 0-470-01184-X

23.1 Diabetes: definition, differential diagnosis and classification

Hannele Yki-Järvinen, Tiinamaija Tuomi

Definitions

- The diagnosis of diabetes is based on elevated fasting glucose level (plasma glucose ≥ 7.0 mmol/l) or on a glucose level measured two hours after glucose tolerance test (plasma glucose ≥ 11.0 mmol/l) (Table 23.1). Whole blood glucose + approximately 1 mmol/l = plasma or serum glucose. Patients with slightly elevated fasting glucose levels are now considered a separate risk group.
- Impaired glucose tolerance (IGT) refers to normal fasting values with an elevated 2-hour value (plasma glucose ≥ 7.8–11.0 mmol/l).
- Glycosylated haemoglobin, HbA_{1c} is well suited for monitoring long term glucose control in diabetic patients; however, with the current methods the test is not sensitive enough for diagnostic purposes.
- Unless the patient shows signs of **type 1 diabetes** (insulin-dependent diabetes mellitus, i.e. IDDM) (polydipsia, polyuria, weight loss, markedly elevated blood glucose values and ketones in both blood and urine) the patient is most likely to have type 2 diabetes.
- The term **type 2 diabetes** (non-insulin-dependent diabetes mellitus, i.e. NIDDM) usually refers to diabetes diagnosed after the age of 35 years. Even though these patients can survive without insulin it is often prescribed in order to prevent organ damage caused by hyperglycaemia.
- The age of onset is not always indicative of the type of diabetes. At diagnosis, 10–15% of type 1 diabetic patients are over the age of 30 years. The so-called MODY (Maturity Onset Diabetes of Youth) type of diabetes often begins before the age of 30 years, as occasionally does type 2 diabetes.
- Some patients (approximately 10%) appear to have type 2 diabetes, but develop a significant insulin deficiency within a few years. GAD antibodies are usually detected in these patients. These patients are classified as having type 1 diabetes according to the latest WHO classification. This condition is also referred to with the following non-established terms: LADA "Latent Autoimmune Diabetes in Adults" and "type $1\frac{1}{2}$ diabetes".

Table 23.1 Diagnostic threshold values of glucose concentration (mmol/l) during fasting and 2 hours after glucose tolerance test with 75 g of glucose (WHO 1999)

Result	Fasting/ 2-hours	Plasma, venous	Whole blood, venous
Development Programme for the Prevention and Care of Diabetes in Finland 2000–2010			
Normal	Fasting value	≤6.0	≤5.5
	2-hour value	≤7.7	≤6.6
Impaired fasting glucose (IFG)	Fasting value	6.1–6.9	5.6–6.0
	2-hour value	<7.8	<6.7
Impaired glucose tolerance	Fasting value	<7.0	<6.1
	2-hour value	7.8–11.0	6.7–9.9
Diabetes mellitus	Fasting value	≤7.0	≤6.1
	2-hour value	≤11.1	≤10.0

Signs and symptoms suggestive of type 1 diabetes (ICD-10: E10)

- The patient is usually thin or of normal weight.
- Unintentional weight loss
  - Significant unintentional weight loss during the few weeks preceding the diagnosis usually suggests insulin-dependent diabetes.
- Ketoacidosis at the time of diagnosis
  - Ketones clearly present in the urine and/or serum
  - Metabolic acidosis
- Low C-peptide concentration (=i.e. endogenous insulin production impaired)
  - **Serum C-peptide** low at the time of diagnosis (<0.2–0.3 nmol/l), later undetectable (usually <0.1 nmol/l). Note! The C-peptide level is dependent on the blood glucose level (increased with high glucose levels and decreased with low glucose levels).
- Islet cell or glutamate decarboxylase (GAD) antibodies (positive in 70–80% of the patients at the time of diagnosis, determination is usually not necessary in patients under 20-years of age).
- Onset usually under the age of 30 years; however, in some patients (10–15%) the illness appears at a later stage.

Signs and symptoms suggestive of type 2 diabetes (ICD-10: E11)

- The most common type of diabetes (70–80% of all diabetic patients).
- 80% of the patients are overweight.
- **Insulin resistance syndrome (metabolic syndrome)** often precedes the illness: obesity, elevated blood pressure, abnormal lipid levels (high triglycerides (2–3 mmol/l, rarely >5 mmol/l) and low HDL cholesterol) and often elevated serum urate concentration.
- Usually diagnosed in adulthood (after 35 years of age).
- Atherosclerosis is the most significant complication of the illness, i.e. coronary heart disease, arteriopathies of the lower limbs and brain and other macrovascular diseases (stroke).
- The patients have a considerable family history of diabetes, hypertension and coronary heart disease.

Other types of diabetes

- **MODY** (Maturity Onset Diabetes of Youth) (ICD-10: E14.9)
  - Can be confused with both type 1 and type 2 diabetes.
  - Includes several subtypes caused by mutations in genes which regulate insulin secretion.
  - Typical features of MODY diabetes include
    - early onset (often <25 years of age, large variation!)
    - dominant inheritance pattern (diabetes present in several generations– important to investigate other members of the family)
    - insulin deficiency of varying degree
    - insulin sensitivity, i.e. an increased risk of hypoglycaemia
  - Some patients manage with a diet or oral medication while others may require multiple-injection regimes if insulin.
  - If MODY is suspected, the patient should be referred to a diabetic clinic (genetic counselling, for example, may be indicated).
- **Mitochondrial diabetes** is a **rare genetic defect**, which is passed from the mother to the next generation (both males and females). Comorbidities include other organ changes, such as hearing defects. The severity of insulin deficiency varies.
- **Secondary diabetes (E13)**
  - May develop after pancreatitis (9.32). May also be associated with hypercorticoidism (cortisone medication or Cushing's syndrome) or with over-excretion of the growth hormone (acromegaly). The patients often have a positive family history of type 2 diabetes.
- **Diabetes following pancreatectomy (E89.1)**
  - Develops after complete pancreatectomy and is associated with an increased proneness to hypoglycaemia.

Gestational diabetes

- Diabetes during pregnancy (see 26.1)
- 20–40% of patients will later develop type 2 diabetes, a small proportion will develop type 1 diabetes.

Oral glucose tolerance test

- Necessary for detecting impaired glucose tolerance.
- Diabetes can also be detected from a fasting blood sample.
- The patient is given 75 g of glucose in a 10% or 20% solution after an overnight fast.
- The blood glucose level is determined immediately before and 2 hours after ingesting the solution.
- The patient must eat normal amounts of carbohydrates for the three days preceding the test except during the night before the test.
- For interpretation of the values, see 23.1.

23.10 Hypoglycaemia in a diabetic patient

Liisa Hiltunen, Minna Koivikko

Goals

- The possibility of hypoglycaemia should be considered with every unconscious diabetic patient, especially with type I diabetics.
- To avoid hypoglycaemic attacks the insulin dosing should be checked every time the patient has
  - symptoms of hypoglycaemia
  - low plasma blood sugar levels (<3.3 mmol/l) in home tests.
- Low values at night (plasma glucose < 3.3 mmol/l) are particularly dangerous.
- Treatment of the elderly patients with sulphonylureas should be undertaken with great care.

Criteria for hypoglycaemia

- Low levels of blood or plasma glucose (<3.0 mmol/l or 3.3 mmol/l, respectively, in severe hypoglycaemia <2.5 mmol/l or 2.8 mmol/l).
- Symptoms indicating hypoglycaemia (can be absent, see below).
- The symptoms disappear after giving glucose

END

The symptoms of sudden adrenergic hypoglycaemia

- Symptoms
  - Heart palpitation
  - Sweating
  - Hunger
  - Tremor of hands
  - Restlessness
- Note that these symptoms may disappear with the duration of diabetes or if glucose balance has been tight and the patient has had repeated hypoglycaemic attacks. In the latter case, increasing blood glucose levels may for some weeks or months restore the warning symptoms.
- If the blood glucose level has been high for a long period, some patients may develop symptoms of hypoglycaemia even when the blood glucose level is normal. This may be partly due to physiological adaptation, which is correctable by improving the glucose balance. Often the reason is the patient's fear of hypoglycaemias due to earlier experiences. Discussion of the problem with the patient is recommended.

Neuroglucopenic symptoms

- Signs of severe hypoglycaemia
  - Headache
  - Confusion
  - Visual disturbances, especially double vision
  - Behavioural and personality disturbances
  - Unconsciousness and convulsions

Patients at risk

- The risk of hypoglycaemia is greatest in diabetic patients who
  - have tight glucose balance and who lack symptoms of hypoglycaemia
  - have very low nocturnal blood sugar levels (the morning fasting level can even be high)
  - exercise actively and irregularly
  - neglect their treatment, in particular because of alcohol misuse
  - have previously had serious hypoglycaemias
  - have other medications that can possibly mask the symptoms of hypoglycaemia
- Remember treatment of the elderly with sulphonylureas and insulin as a risk factor.

Treatment

- Mild symptoms suggesting hypoglycaemia should be treated with snacks containing 10g of rapidly absorbed glucose-containing ingredients. If the symptoms have not disappeared after 10 minutes another snack should be taken.
- Recommended snacks include
  - syrup or strong sugar solution (10 lumps of sugar in warm water) given with a spoon
  - 1 dl (half a glass) of fruit juice
  - 2 dl (a glass) of milk or curdled milk
  - 1 piece of fruit
  - 1 dl of lemonade with sugar
  - 1 dl of ice cream
  - 3–5 pieces of sugar
  - 1 tablet of fructose (10g)
  - 1 tablespoon of honey
  - 20 g of chocolate
- In obvious hypoglycaemia give one ampoule of glucagon (1 mg). The dose is the same for adults and children. The content of the ampoule is dissolved in the solvent in the package and injected subcutaneously or intramuscularly.
- For unconscious patients a 10% glucose solution is rapidly infused until the patient reaches consciousness. A glucagon injection can be given as first aid. An unconscious patient must not be forced to drink, however, strong sugar solution can be offered by spoon if there is no other treatment available.

Further treatment

- The medication of the diabetic patient must be checked and the reason for hypoglycaemia investigated.
  - If the patient is confused, intoxicated or in bad condition, he should be put under hospital observation to avoid recurrence of hypoglycaemia.
  - After follow-up the patient can be discharged if his condition has improved and his ability to recognize and treat hypoglycaemia is considered sufficient. The insulin dose should be reduced. An additional appointment with the doctor or nurse should be arranged so that the reasons for hypoglycaemia can be found and the treatment controlled. The patient needs clear instructions.
  - The patient should carry a bar of chocolate at all times. An ampoule of glucagon should be kept nearby in case of need.
  - The effect of sulphonylureas is long lasting. The hypoglycaemias caused by sulphonylureas should be observed for at least 24 hours.
  - A small child should be put under hospital observation and the avoidance of further fits discussed with the parents.
- If the patient does not regain consciousness despite normalization of blood glucose a referral to hospital must be made. This could be a case in
  - Brain damage due to hypoglycaemia or
  - Another aetiological explanation for unconsciousness.

23.11 Diabetic ketoacidosis

Liisa Hiltunen, Minna Koivikko

Goals

- Always remember to measure plasma/blood glucose in insulin-treated diabetic patients showing symptoms of any kind.
- Check for an acute disease needing treatment (infection) as the reason for plasma glucose increase.
- Ketoacidosis must always be treated in hospital. If the hyperglycaemic, non-ketotic patient is not admitted to hospital for observation, make sure that
  - the patient is given insulin and the plasma glucose begins to decrease.
  - the patient is able to take care of himself and gets immediate help if he feels any worse.

The most common reasons for ketoacidosis

- The cause of diabetic ketoacidosis is a lack of insulin which can be due to
  - recent onset of diabetes
  - interruption of insulin treatment for any reason
  - acute infection
  - sudden (acute) severe illness such as myocardial infarction
  - insulin pump therapy. If the pump is malfunctioning and alternative methods are not immediately used, the patient may become ketotic because insulin is not stored under the skin.

Symptoms and findings

- Reduced consciousness
- Thirst
- Diuresis
- Nausea
- Stomach and chest pains
- Tachycardia
- Weight loss
- Fever (infection)
- Deep hyperventilation (Kussmaul's respiration)
- Smell of acetone in breath

Laboratory findings

- Plasma glucose usually >15 mmol/l
- The urine dipstick test for ketones is positive
- Increased ketones
- Metabolic acidosis

Differential diagnosis

- Hypoglycaemia
- Hyperosmolaric coma
- Lactic acidosis
- Diabetic uraemic coma
- Intoxication, injury, cerebral circulation disorders, cardiac causes
- Ketoacidosis in alcoholics without hyperglycaemia

Tests and treatment

Clinical examinations to find infection sites

- Auscultation of lungs
- Skin, especially between the toes and on the legs (erysipelas)

Laboratory tests

- Plasma glucose
- Serum sodium and potassium
- Urine strip tests and culture
- CRP and blood leukocytes
- Acid–base balance, if available
- Serum creatinine
- ECG
- Chest x-ray

Treatment with fluids

- Give isotonic salt solution. If the patient has hypernatraemia (serum sodium > 155 mmol/l), a 0.45% NaCl solution should be given.
- For the elderly and patients with heart failure the dosing should be more cautious, adjusted to the patient's condition and response being approx. 50% of the following doses:
  - 1000 ml of 0.9% NaCl during the first 30 mins
  - 500 ml of 0.9% NaCl during the following 30 mins
  - 500 ml of 0.9% NaCl/hour, until blood glucose is approx. 12 mmol/l
  - 500 ml of 5% glucose/hour, until dehydration has been corrected.

Treatment with insulin

- Short-acting insulin is given intramuscularly once an hour (the effectiveness of subcutaneous absorption is unknown)
- With severely dehydrated patients a continuous intravenous infusion is used (no boluses because of the short half-life of insulin)
- Intramuscular dosing
  - Starting dose 10–20 units
  - Continuing with 6–8 units every hour
  - When plasma glucose is approx. 12 mmol/l and the dehydration has been treated, the patient can be managed with subcutaneous dosing giving 10–15 units of short-acting insulin (long-acting insulin can also be started at this stage).
  - If the plasma glucose level has not decreased within 2 hours of starting fluid and insulin treatment the patient should be moved to i.v. insulin treatment with 12 units/h.
- Intravenous dosing
  - Starting dose 8–10 units as a bolus
  - Over the first hour 6–12 units (in the beginning some of the insulin is absorbed into the walls of the infusion tubes)
  - Continuing with 4–6 units/h
  - Insulin can be given with a regulator, see table 23.11. The solution is 1000 ml of 0.9% NaCl + 5 ml (200 units) of rapid-acting insulin = 0.2 units/ml (20 gtt).
  - If the blood glucose level does not decrease within 2 hours of the start of treatment, increase the dose to up to 16 units/hour i.v.

Treating acidosis

- Acidosis is normally corrected by giving insulin. The treatment of severe acidosis with bicarbonate requires checking the dosing and by observing the response by following the acid–base balance (Astrup).

Table 23.11 Intravenous administration of insulin in diabetic ketoacidosis.

Insulin units/hour	Infusion ml/hour	Infusion gtt/minute
2	10	3
4	20	7
6	30	10
8	40	13
10	50	17
12	60	20
14	70	23
16	80	27

The prevention and treatment of potassium depletion

- Potassium substitution is started if there are no signs of hyperkalaemia (high positive T waves on ECG, a shortened QT interval, widening of QRS complex, patient oligouric or in shock.)
  - During the first hour 20 mmol KCl added to the salt solution
  - if after this serum potassium is
    - <3 mmol/l, increase KCl to 35 mmol/h
    - <4 mmol/l, increase KCl to 25 mmol/h
    - <5 mmol/l, diminish KCl to 15 mmol/h
    - >5 mmol/l, do not give potassium.
- Important: Because of the risk of arrhythmia potassium cannot be infused rapidly as a pure concentration.
- Potassium substitution should be continued for a week after stopping infusion.
- The reason for ketoacidosis should always be investigated and the patient's awareness of, and ability to manage, his/her diabetes should be checked.

23.12 Non-ketotic, hyperglycaemic, hyperosmolaric coma

Liisa Hiltunen, Minna Koivikko

Aims

- Manage a febrile patient with hyperglycaemia before he/she enters coma
- Do not confuse this condition with ketoacidosis.

Symptoms and findings

- The patient usually has type 2 diabetes. Hyperosmolaric coma may sometimes be the first manifestation of diabetes.
- Plasma/blood glucose usually >25 mmol/l
- Either no ketosis or a mild ketosuria
- Fever is a common finding
- Signs of dehydration
- Thirst, polyuria, fatigue, decreased level of consciousness.

Predisposing factors

- Hyperglycaemia-inducing medication (diuretics, corticosteroids)
- Operations and comparable stress-creating situations
- Acute severe infections
  - Pneumonia
  - Diabetic gangrene
  - Pyelonephritis
  - Sepsis
  - Gastroenteritis leading to dehydration
- Chronic diseases and excessive diuretics
  - Renal failure
  - Heart failure
- Low fluid intake and dehydration because of various underlying causes
- Neglecting the treatment of diabetes.

Treatment

- Febrile hyperglycaemia can be treated in primary care while coma requires hospitalization.
- Principles of therapy
  - Recognize the condition immediately (coma involves an approx. 50% mortality).
  - Provide sufficient (re)hydration with 0.45% NaCl solution.
  - Manage the electrolyte imbalance (usually hypernatraemia).
  - Correct hyperglycaemia with short-acting insulin.
  - Treat infection effectively after samples have been obtained (urine and blood cultures, etc).
  - Prophylactic therapy for thrombosis with low-molecular-weight heparin is often indicated.

Implementing fluid and insulin therapy

- Water deficiency (6–10 l) should be corrected with hypotonic salt solution (=0.45% NaCl)
  - 2 litres within the first 2 hours
  - Thereafter 500 ml/hour until plasma glucose < 15 mmol/l
  - 3.5% glucose solution until dehydration has resolved
- Insulin
  - Starting dose 20 units i.v. or 20–25 units i.m.
  - 5–7 units i.v. or 6–8 units i.m. at 1-hour intervals
  - When plasma glucose reaches 12–15 mmol/l add long-acting insulin
  - After acute phase treatment and stabilization the patient can be managed by oral medication or even with a controlled diet

- Potassium
  - When diuresis starts, 20–25 mmol of potassium is given over one hour.

23.20 Primary and follow-up examinations in diabetes

Liisa Hiltunen, Minna Koivikko

When diabetes is first diagnosed

- Clinical examination
  - Weight, body mass index
  - Blood pressure
  - Heart and large arteries
  - Peripheral nerves
    - Ankle tendon reflexes
    - Sense of vibration
  - Feet
  - Visual acuity
  - Ophthalmoscopy
- Laboratory examinations
  - Fasting plasma blood glucose
  - HbA_{1c}
  - Overnight urine albumin excretion (CU-alb-MI or U-albumin/creatinine)
  - Serum creatinine
  - Serum cholesterol, HDL cholesterol, LDL-cholesterol, triglycerides

Clinical examinations on visits to physician

- Enquire about the patient's well-being
- Weight
- Results of home monitoring
- Insulin doses used
- Hypoglycaemias and hypoglycemia unawareness
- Blood pressure measurement on every visit, if the patient or a close relative has hypertension or the patient has been diagnosed as having albuminuria
- Foot examination, if the patient has symptoms or previous problems with feet

Other examinations to be performed once a year

- Ophthalmoscopy (through dilated pupils) and or fundus photography and visual acuity (23.40)
- Blood pressure is measured in a lying position and after standing for 2–3 minutes.
- Feet and sense of vibration
- Knee and ankle tendon reflexes
- Injection sites

Laboratory measurements

On every examination (at 3–6 month intervals)

- $GHbA_{1c}$
- Review the results of self-monitoring of plasma glucose (SMPG).

Measurements to be performed once a year or when needed

- Serum cholesterol, HDL cholesterol, LDL-cholesterol, triglycerides, creatinine, overnight urine albumin excretion (CU-alb-MI) or U-albumin/creatinine
- To check the accuracy of the patient's glucose meter plasma glucose measurement simultaneously from a sample obtained by the patient's own glucose meter and from a sample drawn in the laboratory.

Home monitoring

- Weight
- Plasma glucose (SMPG) (monitored regularly, see below)
- Follow-up notebook is used to educate and advise the patient.

Blood glucose measurements

- Sufficient information on the 24-hour glucose profile can usually be obtained from four samples:
  - Fasting plasma glucose value to determine whether the dose of the long-acting evening insulin is sufficient. A high fasting value suggests an insufficient dose and a low value suggests a too high a dose. Fasting hyperglycaemia, see also 23.21.
  - The adequacy of the dose of rapid acting insulin is evaluated from the plasma glucose levels measured 1.5–2 hours after a meal.
  - Samples before lunch, dinner and bedtime to determine whether the dose of short-acting insulin (if used) or the morning long-acting insulin is sufficient. High values usually suggest the need to increase the dose of short-acting insulin before meals or the long-acting morning insulin.
- In a stable phase of the disease two measurements a day at 2–3 day intervals may be sufficient.

Blood pressure

- Blood pressure should remain below 140/90 mmHg or at the same (lower) level it was before hypertension required medication.

- Therapy is necessary if
  - systolic blood pressure is at least 140 mmHg and diastolic is at least 90 mmHg
  - blood pressure rises permanently above a level measured earlier or if microalbuminuria is detected, even if the pressures do not exceed the above given threshold values
  - a patient with microalbuminuria has a family history of hypertension (therapy should be started early)
- Non-pharmacological therapy is the primary option
  - salt intake is restricted to less than 6 g daily
  - alcohol intake is restricted
  - regular exercising is started
  - smoking is stopped.

Pharmacotherapy for hypertension

- ACE inhibitors or ATR inhibitors are the drugs of choice if the diabetic patient has nephropathy or microalbuminuria
- Selective beta-blockers
- Small dose thiazide diuretic
- Calcium antagonists in pharmacotherapy of hypertension, see 4.25
- Individual tailoring of pharmacotherapy, see 4.26
- Diabetic nephropathy, see 23.41

23.21 Insulin treatment of type 1 diabetes

Tero Kangas, Liisa Hiltunen

Basic rules

- The target range for HbA_{1c} is 7.0–7.5% (reference range 4.0–6.0%). In order to avoid diabetic complications, HbA_{1c} should be as near to normal as possible A [1 2]. This is not always feasible in practice, and a value below 8% can be considered good. However, if the value of HbA_{1c} is below 7%, the risk of hypoglycaemia increases A [3 4].
- The target range for plasma/blood glucose in home measurements is 4.4–6.7 mmol/l after fasting and before meals, and 6.1–8 mmol/l 90–120 minutes after a meal. Plasma glucose must never fall below 4.0 (3.0) mmol/l (23.32).
- Hypoglycaemia should be avoided.
- The target level should always be chosen individually.

Cornerstones of insulin therapy

- Understanding and mimicking the physiology of insulin excretion.
- Uninterrupted insulin effect = life-maintaining replacement therapy in type 1 diabetes.
- Insulin therapy is planned around the patient's daily rhythm.
- Carbohydrate intake is counted.
- Insulin sensitivity is tested.
- Self-monitoring of plasma glucose (SMPG) is the key to understand the principles of therapy and to succeed in treatment.
- Innovative approach to the planning of insulin therapy.

Principles of insulin therapy

- A sufficient dose of basal insulin must be ensured for 24 hours a day.
- To obtain (near-normal) normal blood glucose level in the morning after an overnight fast.
- A sufficient amount of insulin must be ensured for basic metabolism.
- The treatment must cover hyperglycaemia caused by meals, and restore a (near) normal blood glucose level before the following injection.
- Insulin therapy must not cause severe hypoglycaemia.
- The patient should change his insulin dosage according to SMPG. The dose ranges for mealtime and bedtime insulin should be determined together with the patient.
- Insulin administration should be adjusted to the life rhythm.
- The mealtime insulin and carbohydrate intake must match.
- The patient should be instructed to estimate carbohydrate intake.
- Independent and flexible adjusting of the mealtime insulin requires carbohydrate counting and SMPG.

Assessing the need for insulin

- The daily dose of insulin determines the $GHbA_{1c}$ level.
- The premeal plasma blood glucose values depend on the correctness of the basal insulin dose if the mealtime insulin doses match carbohydrate intake. When assessing the premeal blood glucose levels, the different duration of action of short- and long-acting insulin must be taken into account (short-acting insulin also contributes to the effect of basal insulin).

Principles of insulin administration

- The dose of basal insulin should cover 50–60% of the daily dose; over 70% is too much.
- Insulin glargine is usually given in one daily dose and NPH basal insulin should be given in at least two, preferably three, or up to four doses to obtain the best and most even action possible.
- Mealtime insulin doses should be adjusted according to the intake of carbohydrates.
- Do not change the insulin treatment regimen if it works!
- If $GHbA_{1c}$ is high and all plasma glucose levels are high, increase the daily dose (particularly basal insulin doses if they are too low).
- Then correct the overnight fasting glucose levels to meet the target by adjusting the timing and rhythm of dosing long-acting insulin.

- Next, correct the premeal blood glucose levels to target levels starting with lunchtime.
- If $GHbA_{1c}$ still continues to be too high, following matters should be checked
  - Reliability of blood glucose monitoring technique and measurements
  - Injection technique and sites (lipohypertrophy)
  - Glucose levels after meals and around midnight
  - Mealtime insulin and carbohydrate intake
  - The proportion of basal insulin of the daily dose
  - The adequacy of the total daily dose
- The lowest dose that works is the correct daily dose.
- When SMPG repeatedly shows target glucose levels, the used daily dose is (usually) sufficient and the timing of the administration needs to be corrected.
- When SMPG shows hypoglycaemic values, the daily dose (usually) needs to be decreased.

Injection techniques

- Raise a skin fold to ensure subcutaneous (and NOT intramuscular) injection.
- Avoid hardened areas on the skin.
- Do not change the injection site irregularly, but follow a set plan.
- Do not inject in the arm.
- Inject rapid-acting insulin analogue under abdominal skin just before the meal or immediately after it. In children, after-meal injection is a good option, as the real amount of food consumed is then known. Inject short-acting insulin 20–30 minutes before the meal, Long-acting insulin should be injected in the thigh or buttocks.
- The accelerating effect of exercise and heat on the absorption of insulin and the slowing effect of cold should be explained to the patient.
- The same syringe and needle can be used 4–6 times or for 2–3 days. If rapid- or short- and long-acting insulin are injected separately, different needles should be used (not the same needle alternatively for either rapid- or short- or long-acting insulin).
- Needle-free injectors are not recommended, as the absorption of insulin varies too much.

Methods of insulin administration

Principles

- Multiple injections are the therapy of choice.
- Two or three injections can be used if the patient does not want multiple injections and an acceptable plasma blood glucose level is achieved.
- Tight plasma blood glucose control increases the risk of hypoglycaemia (A) [3 4]. Weight gain is common with excessive insulin dosage.

Twice or thrice daily therapy?

- **Three times daily injection** therapy should be substituted for the twice daily regime if morning blood glucose levels are high or postprandial hyperglycaemia occurs. Only short-acting insulin is injected before the main meal, and long-acting (an if necessary also short-acting) insulin is injected in the morning and before bedtime. Three times daily injection therapy allows free timing of the day meal.

Multiple injection therapy

- Multiple injection therapy is the best method of insulin administration. Rapid-acting or short-acting insulin is injected 3–4 times before meals, and long-acting NPH or determin insulin is taken in two doses before bedtime and in the morning (2/3 of the dose in the morning).
- Insulin glargine is usually injected once daily.

Insulin analogues

- Starting with or changing short-acting insulin into an insulin analogue (e.g. lispro insulin) offers flexibility to patients who must change their timing of meals because of work.
- The effect of lispro and aspart insulin starts almost immediately after the injection. The injection should be taken just before meal.
- Optimal dosing of basal insulin is particularly important.

Short-acting insulin

- Short-acting insulin is injected 3–4 times before meals, and long-acting insulin is taken in two doses before bedtime and in the morning (2/3 of the dose in the morning).
- A small amount of short-acting insulin is often added into the morning and night dose of long-acting insulin. If an evening meal is the habit, the blood glucose is often high during the first half of the night. At first, a mixture of two insulins can be used, later a ready-made mixture is often more convenient.
- The interval between injections of short-acting insulin should not exceed 5–6 hours. Even if a meal is neglected, a small amount of insulin is still indicated.

Insulin pump

- Continuous subcutaneous infusion of insulin with portable pump is effective in achieving good outcomes in type 1 diabetic patients but the effect is comparable to intensive schedules with multiple injections (B) [5 6].
- The risk of ketoacidosis is moderately increased in insulin pump therapy; plasma blood glucose monitoring during hyperglycaemia and infections is important and particularly when the pump fails to function normally.

Glargine insulin

- The long-acting human analogue insulin glargine is usually injected once daily and it offers a steadier insulin delivery with less hypoglycaemias than NPH insulin.
- When changing from NPH to insulin glargine the dosing of rapid-acting mealtime insulin should be checked.

ENL

- The role of the new long-acting insulin analogue insulin detemir will be clarified in the near future.

The effect of hypoglycaemia

- Symptoms occur generally at plasma blood glucose values below 33 mmol/l. Adrenergic warning symptoms may be absent if the disease has lasted for a long time, blood glucose control has been poor for long or the control is extremely tight.
- Hypoglycaemia may decrease insulin sensitivity for as long as 12 hours after the hypoglycaemic episode.

Causes for hypoglycaemia

- Excessive or ill-timed insulin dose
- Occasional dosing error
- Diet "error": delay of a meal, insufficient amount of carbohydrates, or a missed meal
- Physical exercise without reducing insulin dose or increasing calorie intake
- Changing injection techniques or site
- Accidental intramuscular or intravenous injection
- Excessive consumption of alcohol or withdrawal symptoms (hangover).
- Decreased need of insulin during a remission period, because of weight loss, renal insufficiency or endocrine disorders such as hypothyroidism or adrenal insufficiency.

Prevention and treatment of hypoglycaemia

- Adequate patient counselling is essential in the prevention of hypoglycaemia.
- Physical exercise during the day is an indication for reducing the basic evening insulin dose with 2–4 units according to the patient's insulin sensitivity and experience.
- Treatment of hypoglycaemia, see 23.32.

Causes for increased insulin requirement

- Weight gain. If weight gain is caused by excessive insulin dose both the dose and the amount of calories should be reduced.
- Acute infections may significantly increase the requirement of insulin
  - If plasma glucose concentration is repeatedly above 13 mmol/l and the patient has ketonuria, the dose of rapid or short-acting insulin is increased by 1 unit for each mmol of plasma glucose value in excess of 13 mmol/l. Plasma glucose concentration should be monitored at 1-hour intervals.
  - Nausea and vomiting are not indications for reducing the insulin dose. "A gastroenteritis" may be a symptom of ketoacidosis: always check plasma glucose and urine ketones in a diabetic patient with abdominal pain. Ensure intake of insulin, carbohydrates and fluid.
- Medicines: corticosteroids, sympathomimetics
- Hyperthyroidism
- Other acute systemic diseases

Morning hyperglycaemia

- Insulin deficiency causing morning hyperglycaemia can result from the following causes:
  - Insufficient effect of insulin due to early morning decrease of insulin sensitivity
  - The effect of afternoon or evening insulin dose does not last to the next morning
  - High plasma glucose concentration before sleep
  - Having a meal just before going to bed without injecting insulin
  - A too high a dose of evening insulin
  - Reactive hyperglycaemia following nightly hypoglycaemia
- Determining the cause of morning hyperglycaemia
  - Measure plasma glucose in the evening, in the morning, and once at night 4 hours before waking up.
  - It is important to find out whether the plasma glucose is high or low in the early morning (at 2–4 o'clock), and whether it is high already at midnight.

Causes for brittle diabetes

- Poor control of treatment, lack of knowledge and skill
- Inappropriate adjustment of meals, exercise and insulin dosage
- Changing the treatment continuously
- Psychological factors: lack of motivation, conflicts, rarely manipulation of insulin dose
- Irregular, heavy exercise
- Inappropriate dosing, e.g. excessive doses (over-treatment of hyperglycaemia) and reactive hypoglycaemia
- The need for insulin often increases, but in some patients decreases before menstruation.
- Severe comorbidities (renal failure, GI tract dysfunction)
- Endocrine disorders: hypo- or hyperthyroidism, Addison's disease.
- Anorexia or bulimia
- Insulin antibodies may cause unexpected hypoglycaemias. Insulin antibodies should be determined if no other cause for hypoglycaemia is evident.
- Systemic diseases
- Idiopathic lability. The typical patient is a young, obese woman.

Investigations for brittle diabetes

- Take a thorough history of living habits (exercise, meals) and insulin dosage
- Consider family background and social situation.
- Ask the patient's opinion.

- Analyse carefully the patient's home monitoring diary.
- Look for signs of an endocrine disorder (determine serum TSH, potassium, sodium, cortisol)
- Monitor plasma glucose systematically over a long period of time. Living habits and treatment should be held constant during monitoring.
- Consider referral to an internal medicine specialist if the reason for lability is not resolved (observation in hospital?).
- For plasma glucose determinations at home, see 23.20.

Insulin dosage when travelling across time zones

Travelling west

- Before the flight the normal injection schedule is followed (the morning and lunch injections at the time of the country of departure), the lunchtime dose is changed if necessary.
- During the flight rapid or short-acting insulin is injected at a rate of 2–4% of the total daytime insulin dose for each hour of time difference.
- After arrival the normal injection schedule is followed (supper and night injections) at the time of the destination country; the doses are changed according to plasma blood glucose determinations.

Travelling east

- Before departure the normal injection schedule is followed (morning, lunch and supper injections), and the normal evening dose of long-acting insulin is taken during the flight; as a meal (supper) is served at the beginning of the flight, extra 2–6 units of rapid or short-acting insulin are often required.
- Before landing a meal (breakfast) is served. The normal morning dose of rapid or short-acting insulin is injected, but the dose of morning long-acting insulin is reduced 3–5% for each hour of time difference.
- After landing the normal schedule is followed (supper and evening injections), the doses are changed according to blood glucose determinations; the lunchtime injection is not needed.

References

1. Lawson ML, Gerstein HC, Tsui E, Zinman B. Effect of intensive insulin therapy on early macrovascular disease in young individuals with type 1 diabetes: a systematic review and meta-analysis. Diabetes Care 1999;22(Suppl 2):B35–B39.
2. The Database of Abstracts of Reviews of Effectiveness (University of York), Database no.: DARE-990495. In: The Cochrane Library, Issue 3, 2000. Oxford: Update Software.
3. Egger M, Smith GD, Stettler C, Diem P. Risk of adverse effects of intensified treatment of insulin-dependent diabetes mellitus: a meta-analysis. Diabetic Medicine 1997;14:919–928.
4. The Database of Abstracts of Reviews of Effectiveness (University of York), Database no.: DARE-971430. In: The Cochrane Library, Issue 1, 2000. Oxford: Update Software.
5. Pons JMV. Continuous subcutaneous infusion of insulin with portable pump in diabetes type 1 patients. Barcelona: Catalan Agency for Health Technology Assessment (CAHTA). CAHTA. IN01/2000. 2000. 53.
6. The Health Technology Assessment Database, Database no.: HTA-20000896. In: The Cochrane Library, Issue 1, 2001. Oxford: Update Software.

23.22 Type 1 diabetes: dietary treatment and exercise

Editors

- Type 2 diabetes, see 23.33

Principles of dietary treatment

- The number of calories should be adjusted to the patient's needs and meals should be scheduled according to the needs of the day.
- The amount of fat should not exceed 30% of the total energy supply. The amount of the amount of saturated fat should not exceed 10% and polyunsaturated fat should be at least 10% of the total energy supply, and other lipids should be mono-unsaturated (for example, rapeseed or olive oil).
  - In practice, the use of milk fat, hard plant fats and meat products rich in fat should be restricted and the intake of unsaturated fat and fish should be increased.
- Protein should provide approximately 15% of the total energy supply.
- Due to the restriction of fat and protein, carbohydrates should provide approximately 55% of the total energy supply.
  - The use of carbohydrates rich in fibre is recommended.
  - The most suitable carbohydrates are those that release sugar slowly: roots, potatoes and rice. Bread should contain wholemeal flour, preferably wholegrain.
  - Carbohydrates rich in fibre should be preferred (wholegrain bread, vegetables, pea plants, fruits).
  - The use of sucrose should be avoided. Small amounts (approximately 10 g) are allowed, if they can be included in the total energy amount. Fruit and berries may be used in moderate amounts.
- Food should be low in salt.
- Alcohol should be used in moderation. Sweet drinks should be avoided.

Exercise

- Exercise improves physical fitness and mood and has a positive effect on blood lipids, obesity and insulin sensitivity.
- During intensive exercise the insulin dose should be lowered or the number of calories ingested increased.

- The dosage of insulin and carbohydrates should be adjusted using plasma blood glucose measurements.
- If exercise is scheduled in the evening, the insulin dose may need to be reduced, because the plasma blood glucose lowering effect of exercise may last for 12 hours.
- Plasma blood glucose falls
  - if there is no lack of insulin during exercise
  - if the exercise is prolonged (30–60 minutes) or intensive
  - if the interval between the preceding meal and exercise is long (over 3 hours)
  - if no extra snack is eaten before or during exercise.
- The blood glucose will remain unchanged if
  - the exercise is brief
  - a sufficient amount of food has been eaten before or during exercise.
- The blood glucose value rises if
  - insulin deficiency occurs during the exercise
  - muscle work is intensive
  - too big a snack has been eaten before exercise.

23.31 Newly diagnosed type 2 diabetes

Hannele Yki-Järvinen

Aims

- Explain the permanent nature and severity of the illness to the patient– the condition is more an arterial illness than an illness of the glucose metabolism.
- Explain the importance of self-care. Emphasize the importance of weight reduction to overweight patients. However, other lifestyle modifications will also form a part of the treatment, even when they do not lead to weight reduction (exercise, smoking cessation, avoidance of dietary fat).
- In addition to hyperglycaemia, identify and treat effectively other risk factors of atherosclerosis (smoking, hypertension, dyslipidaemia).

Investigations at diagnosis

- History, note especially:
  - Lifestyle (amount of physical exercise, consumption of alcohol, fat and salt as well as smoking, see 23.33).
  - Symptoms of coronary heart disease are often already present at the time of diagnosis.
  - Family history (type 1 or 2 diabetes, CHD, hypertension?). Siblings have a 40% risk of developing type 2 diabetes– investigation of family members is recommended.
- Clinical examination
  - Weight, height, body mass index (weight/height^2)
  - Blood pressure (target level 130/85 mmHg)
  - Heart and large arteries: auscultation
  - Peripheral arteries: palpation
  - Feet (sense of vibration, sense of touch, suitable footwear, calluses, see 23.44)
  - Visual acuity
  - Ophthalmoscopy
- Laboratory investigations
  - Fasting blood glucose
  - HbA_{1C}
  - Urine ketones (usually negative in type 2 diabetes)
  - Serum cholesterol, HDL cholesterol, triglycerides, LDL cholesterol
  - ECG
  - Serum creatinine
  - Overnight urine for albumin excretion (<20 µg/min normal, 20–200 µg/min microalbuminuria, >200 µg/min macroalbuminuria)
  - Determine serum fasting C-peptide level if there is uncertainty about the type of diabetes. A very low level (below 0.2–0.3 nmol/l) strongly suggests insulin deficiency and the possibility of a rapidly developing need for insulin therapy. The patient may not have typical type 2 diabetes (see 23.1). On the other hand, severe hyperglycaemia (>15 mmol/l) at the onset may reduce the excretion of insulin temporarily, i.e. even a low C-peptide level may normalize when hyperglycaemia is treated. Determining the level again may be indicated to assess the further need of insulin therapy. A high C-peptide level is difficult to interpret. It often suggests insulin resistance. Glucagon tolerance test is not necessary.
  - GAD antibodies if the patient's age is less than 40 years, if the C-peptide level is below 0.2–0.3 nmol/l or the patient has atypical type 2 diabetes (symptoms of autoimmunity, the patient is particularly slim, the symptoms have developed rapidly).

Principles of patient education

- See Lifestyle education in type 2 diabetes 23.33

23.32 Treatment and follow-up in type 2 diabetes

Hannele Yki-Järvinen

Objectives

- The main objective of the treatment is to prevent the development or worsening of vascular complications. The treatment strategy should be targeted at correcting hyperglycaemia, hypertension, dyslipidaemia and increased coagulability.

- The fasting blood glucose target should be below 6.7 mmol/l (4–6 mmol/l with regimens using bedtime NPH (isophane) insulin, and 4–5 mmol/l with regimens using insulin glargine).
- HbA_{1C} target is <7.0%, with insulin therapy <7.5% (NPH insulin), <7% (insulin glargine)
- Treat hypertension aggressively B [1] (target level 130/85).
- The target levels for lipids are defined roughly by the 123 rule, i.e. HDL cholesterol > 1, triglycerides < 2, LDL cholesterol < 3 mmol/l. In 50–70% of the patients drug therapy for hyperlipidaemia is necessary to achieve target levels.
- Prescribe aspirin (100 mg) for all patients with type 2 diabetes, unless it is contraindicated.
- Encourage smokers to stop smoking.
- The target for BMI is below 25 kg/m^2, but 25–27 kg/m^2 is acceptable.

I Treatment of hyperglycaemia

- Treatment of hyperglycaemia reduces the incidence of microvascular complications and symptoms. In type 2 diabetes the symptoms of hyperglycaemia usually develop slowly, and the patient may be unaware of them (tiredness, need to take naps, depression, weakness). These symptoms may co-exist with the classical symptoms (unintentional weight loss, increased urinary frequency, thirst). The diagnosis of type 2 diabetes is often delayed because of the scarcity of symptoms. Weight loss, tiredness and depression lower the patient's motivation and ability to receive lifestyle education, and drug therapy should therefore always be prescribed in severe hyperglycaemia. Drug therapy must not replace lifestyle education and it may be withdrawn if education proves to be successful.

Principles of treating hyperglycaemia

- HbA_{1c} 6–8% at the time of diagnosis
    - Lifestyle education (23.33) for 6 months, if this is unsuccessful, prescribe one oral antidiabetic drug (metformin or sulphonylurea or glitazone or glinide).
- HbA_{1c} 8–10% at the time of diagnosis
    - Lifestyle education and one oral antidiabetic drug (metformin or sulphonylurea or glitazone or glinide) (23.33)
    - If the target level of 6–8% is not achieved within 6 months (i.e. fasting blood glucose < 6.7 mmol/l) prescribe another oral antidiabetic drug (23.34)
- HbA_{1c} 10–12% at the time of diagnosis
    - Lifestyle education and two oral antidiabetic drugs (e.g. metformin and sulphonylurea)
- HbA_{1c} > 12% at the time of diagnosis
    - Lifestyle education and two antidiabetic oral drugs (e.g. metformin and sulphonylurea) and once-daily (bedtime) insulin (23.35).
- Note that insulin treatment once prescribed is not necessarily permanent. It can be withdrawn, as can oral medications, if lifestyle education proves successful.

II Treatment of hypertension

- 40–60% of patients with type 2 diabetes are already hypertensive at the time of diagnosis.
- The UKPD study showed that effective treatment of hypertension significantly reduces both macrovascular and microvascular complications associated with diabetes (also the progression of diabetic retinopathy).
- Target blood pressure is 130/85 mmHg.
- All diabetic patients should be educated about the principles of non-pharmacological treatment (weight loss, reduction of salt intake, physical exercise).
- Vascular events have been shown to be prevented with:
    - a low-dose diuretic (12.5–25 mg hydrochlorothiazide)
    - a selective beta-blocker
    - an ACE inhibitor (or angiotensin II inhibitor if ACE inhibitor is not suitable)
    - a calcium channel blocker
- Effective treatment of hypertension often requires the use of more than one drug.
- The patient's comorbidities affect the choice of hypertensive medication.
    - Coronary heart disease
        - selective beta-blocker
    - Intermittent claudication, chronic bronchitis or asthma:
        - diuretic
        - ACE inhibitor (or angiotensin-II receptor antagonist)
    - Impotence:
        - ACE inhibitor (or angiotensin-II receptor antagonist)
    - Metabolic syndrome and marked dyslipidaemia:
        - ACE inhibitor (or angiotensin-II receptor antagonist)
    - Diabetic nephropathy:
        - ACE inhibitor (or angiotensin-II receptor antagonist)

Treatment of hypertension in a patient without nephropathy

1. Lifestyle modification:
    - reduction of salt intake and excessive consumption of alcohol, regular exercise, weight reduction in overweight patients as well as smoking cessation
2. Start with a small dose of a thiazide diuretic, an ACE inhibitor or selective beta-blocker. Take into consideration other diseases and adverse effects when choosing the drug.
3. If necessary, add another drug. Effective combinations are e.g. a diuretic and an ACE inhibitor as well as a diuretic with a selective beta-blocker.

4. If necessary, add a calcium-channel blocker as the third drug, for example, a diuretic + ACE inhibitor + long-acting dihydropyridine group calcium-channel blocker or a diuretic + selective beta-blocker + calcium-channel blocker.
5. If no response is achieved with a particular drug, it should be stopped and another drug prescribed from a different drug group.
6. Before prescribing a new drug, check patient compliance and the dose that he/she has been taking.
7. Following parameters should be monitored after starting medication (see also 4.25):
   - Thiazides: potassium, urate, glucose, and lipids
   - Beta-blockers: glucose and lipids (e.g. 3 months from starting)
   - ACE inhibitors: creatinine and potassium during the first weeks of treatment. Avoidance of salt increases the effect.

Treatment of hypertension in a patient with nephropathy

- The target is 130/85 mmHg (125/75 mmHg, when protein excretion into urine exceeds 1 g/24 h).
- ACE inhibitor (reduce the dose if creatinine is increased) or angiotensin-II receptor antagonist.
- If necessary, add a small dose of a thiazide diuretic. If serum creatinine concentration is >200 µmol/l replace the thiazide diuretic with a loop diuretic.
- If necessary, add a selective beta-blocker.
- If necessary, add an antihypertensive drug belonging to another drug group.

III Treatment of dyslipidaemias

Target level

- Patients with type 2 diabetes have such a high risk of vascular complications that drug therapy for hyperlipidaemia is necessary in order to achieve target levels (the 123 rule) even if the patient does not have clinical signs of vascular complications. Precise target levels for lipids are shown in Table 23.32.1.

Treatment strategy

1. Lifestyle modifications are sufficient if they reduce the concentration of LDL cholesterol to below 3 mmol/l.
   - Weight reduction, diet (low-fat diet in particular), increased physical exercise and cessation of smoking
2. Improving diabetic control
   - Correction of hyperglycaemia reduces the triglyceride concentration; however, the concentration of LDL cholesterol is usually not affected.
3. Drug therapy
   - Should be started if other forms of treatment do not lower the LDL cholesterol to below 3 mmol/l.
   - If LDL cholesterol is over 4 mmol/l and the patient belongs to a high-risk group, drug therapy should be started simultaneously with diet therapy.
   - A triglyceride level >10 mmol/l is an indication for immediate (fibrate) medication due to the risk of pancreatitis.
   - Note that markedly elevated triglyceride concentration (>5 mmol/l) is usually not caused by diabetes alone.

Table 23.32.1 Precise target levels for lipid concentrations in diabetic patients (the 123 rule)

Lipid	Target level
HDL cholesterol	>1.1mmol/l
Serum triglycerides	<1.7 mmol/l
LDL cholesterol	<2.6 mmol/l

Choosing drug therapy

- The principles of choosing drug therapy are shown in Table 23.32.2.
- Comparison of the efficacy of different statins: simvastatin 10 mg = lovastatin 20 mg = pravastatin 20 mg = fluvastatin 40–60 mg. Atorvastatin 10 mg = simvastatin 20 mg.
- For dosage, see 24.56

IV Aspirin

- Aspirin at 100 mg/day is beneficial for all patients with type 2 diabetes, also for those who have no clinical signs of macrovascular disease.
- Aspirin is contraindicated in patients with haemophilia, active bleeding of the gastrointestinal tract or the urinary tract, or retinopathy with associated bleeding.

Interpretation and treatment of microalbuminuria

- Definition: overnight albumin excretion 20–200 µg/min.
- Microalbuminuria with concurrent retinopathy can be a sign of incipient nephropathy.
- If the patient does not have retinopathy, microalbuminuria is likely to reflect a high risk of cardiovascular disease. A patient with microalbuminuria can have either normal or elevated blood pressure.

Table 23.32.2 Choosing a drug for the treatment of dyslipidaemia in type 2 diabetes

Lipid disorder	Drug of choice
LDL cholesterol > 3 mmol/l and triglycerides < 2 mmol/l	1. Statin
LDL cholesterol > 3 mmol/l and triglycerides 2–4.4 mmol/l	1. Statin 2. Fibrate or statin + fibrate
Triglycerides ≥ 4.5 mmol/l	1. Fibrate 2. Fibrate + statin

In combination treatment the doses of the drugs should be reduced and the possibility of myocyte damage should be kept in mind.

- Microalbuminuria may result from causes other than diabetic nephropathy.
- Treatment consists of 1) tight blood pressure control, i.e. reduced salt intake and use of antihypertensive drugs, 2) cessation of smoking, 3) tight glucose control, 4) treatment of dyslipidaemia.
- Elevated serum creatinine/nephrosis
  - If serum creatinine > 150 µmol/l, 50% of renal function is lost, in an elderly patient even more. The patient should be referred to a nephrologist.
  - The patient should also be referred if proteinuria exceeds 3.5 g/day (threshold of nephrosis).

Treatment of coronary heart disease

Diagnosis

- The routine follow-up of patients with type 2 diabetes includes an ECG at 1-year intervals.
- Clinical exercise testing should be considered if the patient has
  - symptoms (typical or atypical clinical picture)
  - abnormal resting ECG
  - other arterial disease
  - several risk factors.
- Indications for coronary artery angiography (4.64).

Treatment of myocardial infarction

- The benefits of thrombolytic therapy in diabetic patients are at least as good as in non-diabetic patients.
  - Diabetic retinopathy is not a contraindication to thrombolytic therapy.
- The benefits of beta-blockers in diabetics who have had a myocardial infarction (MI) are even greater than in non-diabetic patients with an MI.
  - $Beta_1$-selective blockers do not mask the symptoms of hypoglycaemia and have less metabolic adverse effects than nonselective beta-blockers.
- In the acute phase of an MI, ACE inhibitors are particularly beneficial for diabetic patients.
- Secondary prevention should be intensive. Statins should be started immediately when LDL cholesterol exceeds 4 mmol/l.

Examinations during routine visits

At every visit

- Symptoms
  - Physical performance: coronary heart disease/intermittent claudication?
  - Fatigue and poor treatment compliance may also result from poor glucose control.
  - Episodes of hypoglycaemia (rare in overweight patients)
- Examinations
  - Weight
  - Blood pressure (target 130/85 mmHg)
  - Examine the feet especially carefully if the patient has any of the following:
    - Earlier lesion or amputation
    - Neuropathy (deficient sense of monofilament touch, sense of vibration or Achilles tendon reflex)
    - Arteriosclerosis of the lower limbs (claudication, absent pulses, skin lesions)
    - Malpositions and calluses
  - HbA_{1c} (in tablet and diet treatment the target is <7.0%, if above 8.0% -> glucose control is poor and insulin treatment should be considered).
  - Fasting blood glucose (in tablet and diet treatment the target is <6.7 mmol/l, with bedtime insulin treatment the target is 4–5 mmol/l. If fasting glucose concentrations are approximately 6 mmol/l, the HbA_{1c} level will be around 7.5%).
- Encourage the patient to adopt and maintain a healthy lifestyle.
- Medication
  - Dose of drugs (blood pressure/glucose/lipids)
  - Does the patient take aspirin (100 mg)?

Annual examinations

- ECG
- Photograph of the fundus of the eye (dilate pupils) at 1–3-year intervals, alternatively ophthalmoscopy. The photograph can be taken every 3 years, if glucose control is good (HbA_{1c} < 7.5%) and the funduscopic findings are normal.
- Blood pressure (target 130/85 mmHg)
- Examination of the feet
- Examination of injection sites
- LDL cholesterol, HDL cholesterol and triglycerides
- Clean-voided urine, serum creatinine
- Urine albumin excretion. Strip test is sufficient; if the result is abnormal, measure overnight urine albumine excretion.

Home monitoring

- Weight
- Blood pressure (it is recommended that the patient has his own device)
- Self-monitoring of blood glucose. Explain the purpose of monitoring as it varies depending on the type of treatment:
  - Patients on diet treatment learn to identify the factors which regulate the blood glucose level in everyday life.
  - In patients on tablet treatment, there is the additional purpose of documenting the occurrence of hypoglycaemia.
  - Patients on insulin treatment are the most important group to be taught self-monitoring with the aim of learning self-adjustment of the insulin dose (see 23.35). When bedtime insulin is started, fasting glucose levels should be monitored daily. When the target has been achieved, a few times a week is sufficient.

Reference

1. Adler AI, Stratton IM, Neil HAW, Yudkin JS, Matthews DR, Cull CA, Wright AD, Turner RC, Holman RR on behalf of the UK Prospective Diabetes Study Group. Association of systolic blood pressure with macrovascular and microvascular complications of type 2 diabetes (UKDPS 36): prospective observational study. BMJ 2000;321:412–419.

23.33 Lifestyle education in type 2 diabetes

Hannele Yki-Järvinen

Principles

- Every primary care unit should be prepared to provide lifestyle education for patients with type 2 diabetes (either as a group or individual basis).
- Successful lifestyle education has a beneficial effect on all metabolic abnormalities in type 2 diabetes **A** [1 2].
- The primary aim is to introduce permanent lifestyle changes.
- Weight reduction is not the only goal; increasing the amount of physical exercise without a weight change is also beneficial as are changes in the content of the diet even if weight reduction is unsuccessful **C** [3 4]
- A very low energy diet (VLED) is no better than other methods. Prevention of relapses after dieting is essential. Medication (orlistat) may be beneficial.

The progress of lifestyle education

1. Assess the present situation

- Requires a personal visit by the patient to the nurse, doctor or a group meeting.
- Clinical examination and laboratory investigations to determine:
  - what is the primary problem, i.e. hypertension/hyperglycaemia/dyslipidaemia/obesity.
  - the patient's motivation and functional capacity
  - the possibility of gestational diabetes
- Lifestyle assessment
  - Eating habits (ask the patient what he/she eats and drinks at each meal, does he/she snack between meals or eat whilst preparing meals?)
  - Salt intake (does the patient add salt at the table, consume foods high in salt–crisps, sausages, pickles; use of salt in cooking?)
  - Smoking
  - Physical exercise, how strenuous is the exercise (how many times a week does the patient become short of breath and sweat, for how long at a time, physical exercise at work, exercise during free-time?)
  - Alcohol consumption (estimate the number of units per week, see Table 23.33). Alcohol is high in calories; 1 gram of alcohol provides 7 kcal. A typical value is 75 kcal for a glass of wine.

Table 23.33 As a general guideline the following drinks contain one unit of alcohol (a unit is equivalent to 8 gm or 10 ml (1cl) of pure alcohol).

- $\frac{1}{2}$ pint (284 ml) of ordinary strength beer, lager or cider
- 1 glass (125 ml) of wine (9% AbV)
- 1 pub measure (25 ml) of spirits
- 1 small glass (50 ml) of any fortified wine (e.g. sherry, martini or port)

Note

- A 125 ml glass of wine at 11-12% AbV contains approximately 1.5 units
- A 330 ml bottle of strong beer/lager/cider contains about 1.5 units
- A 330 ml bottle of an alco pop at 4 or 6% AbV contains 1.3 or 2 units respectively

The recommended maximum amount of alcohol for men is up to 21 units per week (three units per day) and for women up to 14 units per week (two units per day)

2. Discuss the aims

- Weight reduction is usually a desired aim (see 24.2).
- Any targets should be set by the patient him/herself and should be something he/she perceives as important. The targets should be small rather than large, they should be attainable and easily measurable, and associated with behavioural modifications **C** [5 6].
  - For example, changing to skimmed milk, halving the amount of cheese and fatty snacks and becoming familiar with low-fat products, experimenting with oil in cooking or prolonging the evening walk by 10 minutes. Write down any agreed targets.
- If weight reduction is desired consider the following:
  - Reduction of fat intake (see 24.55)
  - Reduction of total food intake
  - For most patients reduction in the intake of fat and fat-containing foods and changing to low-fat products is sufficient.
  - Regular physical exercise predicts good long-term results, whereas rapid weight loss at the beginning does not.
  - Orlistat (24.2) combined with a low-calorie, low-fat diet enhances weight loss. After successful initial weight reduction the drug can also be used to prevent relapses.
  - Morbidly obese patients (BMI > 40) can be offered the possibility of laparoscopic gastric banding. After the operation the size of a meal will be reduced down to about 250 ml. Referral to surgery does not guarantee that

it can be performed. Contraindications include bulimia and alcohol abuse.

- VLCD (very low calorie diet) and lifestyle modifications C [5 6]
  - A VLCD does not reduce the need for lifestyle education but rather increases its need as a VLCD alone will only produce temporary weight loss.
  - Transition to a normal diet is carried out gradually.
  - Diet education is needed particularly at the time when the patient stops eating formulas and moves on to regular food as the patient has to learn new eating habits; resumption of old eating habits will lead to weight gain.
  - In addition to a weight-reducing diet, orlistat can be used to control calorie intake.
- Stopping smoking
  - Always important
  - See advice for smoking cessation 40.20
- **The aim is to improve the quality of the diet and/or increase physical activity, and to attain normal weight**
  - Essential modifications:
    - Increasing physical activity
    - Improving the quality of dietary fat, see 24.55
    - Reducing the intake of fat (more carbohydrates instead)
    - Minimizing the use of alcohol, see 40.3
    - Reducing salt intake
    - Increasing the intake of fruit and vegetables
    - Maintaining or increasing the intake of whole grain products
    - Reducing the intake of food as diabetic control improves
    - Stopping smoking, see 40.20

3. Offer guidance to achieve personal targets

- **Recommended diet**
  - Energy intake according to target weight.
  - Not more than 10% of energy intake from hard (saturated) fats.
  - Less than 25–35% of energy from fat. If the amount of fat is greater, the proportion of monounsaturated fatty acids can be increased whilst carbohydrate intake is decreased.
  - 5–10% of energy from polyunsaturated fatty acids
  - 1% of energy intake from n-3 fatty acids
  - 50–60% of energy intake from carbohydrates
  - 15% of energy intake from protein
  - Less than 5 g/day of salt
  - At least 25 g of fibre daily
  - Minimize alcohol intake
- **How to keep to the recommended diet**
  - Advice the patient to choose varying and colourful food
    - Plenty of grain products, especially whole grain
    - Moderate amounts of low-fat or fat-free dairy products (approx. 500 ml/day)
    - Potatoes in varying forms without added fat
    - Plenty of vegetables, berries and fruit every day
    - Fish to be used frequently (a couple of times a week); lean meat
    - Fat to be used sparingly: vegetable margarine or fat mixture on bread, oil for cooking and oil-based dressings for salads
    - Sugar in moderation
  - Meal size in proportion to weight
    - Weight changes indicate whether meal sizes are correct.
    - Estimate the energy need.
    - Provide a sample meal or a picture of a recommended meal.
  - Meals are to be enjoyed without hurrying.
  - Fixed meal times in order to support weight control
    - Hunger will easily lead to extra snacks or to a larger meal than had been planned, or to uncontrolled eating, during the next meal.
    - Most patients are comfortable eating a light breakfast, lunch and evening meal as well as a small evening snack. A piece of fruit in the afternoon may help to control hunger.
- **Increasing physical activity**
  - Consider how the patient's activity level can be increased during normal daily activities. This will increase energy consumption and facilitates weight reduction as much as planned exercise. Suitable forms of exercise include brisk walking, jogging, cycling, cross-country skiing, rowing, swimming, aerobics-type exercise and some ball games.
  - The recommended amount of exercise is at least three times a week for 30 minutes at a time. Several shorter periods of exercise give almost the same benefit as one longer period. The patient may be motivated to keep on exercising regularly, for example by keeping an exercise diary.
  - Discuss the various ways to increase the patient's exercise level when discussing the aims of the treatment, and set targets with the patient.

4. Follow-up

- Follow-up visits are necessary, as prescribing a weight-reducing diet alone will not lead to permanent results.
- Orlistat (24.2) may help to prevent relapses after successful weight loss.
- See 24.2, 24.55, 4.24 for basic principles of follow-up.

References

1. Brown SA. Studies of educational interventions and outcomes in diabetic adults: a meta-analysis revisited. Patient Educ Counsel 1990;16:189–215.
2. The Database of Abstracts of Reviews of Effectiveness (University of York), Database no.: DARE-952486. In: The Cochrane Library, Issue 4, 1999. Oxford: Update Software.

3. Brown SA, Winter M, Upchurch S, Ramirez G, Anding R. Promoting weight loss in type II diabetes. Diabetes Care 1996;19:613–624.
4. The Database of Abstracts of Reviews of Effectiveness (University of York), Database no.: DARE-961033. In: The Cochrane Library, Issue 4, 1999. Oxford: Update Software.
5. Ciliska D, Kelly C, Petrov N, Chalmers J. A review of the weight loss interventions for obese people with non-insulin-dependent diabetes mellitus. Can J Diab Care 1995;19:10–15.
6. The Database of Abstracts of Reviews of Effectiveness (University of York), Database no.: DARE-975275. In: The Cochrane Library, Issue 2, 2000. Oxford: Update Software.

23.34 Oral antidiabetic drugs in the treatment of type 2 diabetes

Hannele Yki-Järvinen

- Note that oral antidiabetic drugs are only one aspect of the treatment strategy in type 2 diabetes (glucose control, lipids, hypertension, coagulation) (23.32).

Objectives

- Oral medication should be introduced at an early stage, when drug therapy is still effective. In the absence of contraindications, medication should be considered when the HbA_{1c} value exceeds 7.0% despite non-pharmacological intervention. If one antidiabetic drug does not lower the HbA_{1c} value to below 7.0%, add another antidiabetic drug unless there are contraindications.
- Insulin therapy must be initiated at the latest when HbA_{1c} remains over 7.5% (reference range 4.0–6.0%) despite oral medication.

Summary of oral antidiabetic drugs

- See Table 23.34

Metformin

- Metformin is the drug of first choice for overweight patients Ⓐ [1 2 3 4 5 6 7 8]. It can be combined with sulphonylureas and a single injection of insulin at bedtime. It is also suitable for patients of normal weight. In long-term use, metformin decreases cardiovascular disease.
- Metformin does not stimulate insulin excretion, but reduces blood glucose levels by inhibition of hepatic glucose production. Metformin does not induce hypoglycaemia, and it has a more beneficial effect on weight than other antidiabetic drugs Ⓐ [1 2 3 4 5 6 7 8] (as monotherapy it produces a weight loss of a few kg; combined with sulphonylureas and a single injection of insulin at bedtime it also counteracts weight gain).
- To produce an effect the dose must be adequately high (2–2.5 g/day). The treatment is begun with, for example, 500 mg/day followed by increases of 500 mg/week to up to the maximum dose of 2–2.5 g/day.
- Abdominal pain is the most disturbing adverse effect of metformin, leading to discontinuation of the treatment in approximately 10% of the patients. In order to eliminate the risk of lactic acidosis metformin must not be given to patients with
  - hepatic impairment

Table 23.34 Oral antidiabetic drugs

Product	Dose (minimum-maximum)	Number of doses per day	Reduction in HbA_{1c}	Weight gain	Risk of hypoglycaemias	Binding to proteins	Active metabolites (liver)
Inhibitors of hepatic glucose production							
Metformin	500–2000 mg	2	1.5–2.0%	No	No	No	No
Enhancers of insulin excretion							
Sulphonylureas							
Glimepiride	1–6 mg	1		++	++	>98%	Yes
Glibenclamide	1.75–14 mg	2	1.5–2.0%	++	++	>98%	Yes
Glipizide	2.5–15 mg	2	1.5–2.0%	++	++	>98%	Yes
Phenylalanine derivatives							
Nateglinide	60–360 mg	3	1.5–2.0%		++	>98%	Yes
Repaglinide	0.5–12 mg	3	1.5–2.0%	++	++	>98%	Yes
Glitazones							
Rosiglitazone	4–8 mg	1	1.5–2.0%	++	++	>98%	Unknown
Pioglitazone	15–45 mg	1	1.5–2.0%	++	++	>98%	Unknown
Drugs affecting carbohydrate absorption							
Guar gum	5–15 g	3	0.5%	No	No	No	No

- creatinine concentration above 150 μmol/l
- proteinuria above 0.5 g/day
- alcohol abuse
- obvious cardiac insufficiency or other conditions leading to hypoxia

- Advanced age does not prevent the use of the drug; however, creatinine concentration should be normal before and during the therapy in the elderly
- Metformin treatment must be interrupted during severe infections, elective surgery and trauma. If the patient is to undergo a procedure involving the administration of intravenous contrast medium, ensure that renal function is normal prior to the procedure.

Sulphonylureas

- Sulphonylureas reduce blood glucose levels by enhancing insulin excretion, and decrease microvascular, and possibly also macrovascular, changes in long-term use.
- The starting dose may be small, but the dose should be increased rapidly up to the maximum doses (daily dose of glimepiride 6 mg, glibenclamide 10–14 mg, glipizide 15 mg, gliclazide 320 mg). With these doses HbA_{1c} can be expected to decrease by 1.5–2.0%. If the HbA_{1c} value is above 10%, diabetic control will not be achieved by prescribing only one oral antidiabetic drug (A) [9 10].
- Adverse effects are quite rare. Prolonged hypoglycaemia, however, is seen particularly in the elderly. Glimepiride is administered once daily, glibenclamide twice daily and glipizide three times daily. Glipizide is shorter acting than glibenclamide.
- Severe renal insufficiency is a contraindication to sulphonylurea therapy.
- There are many drug interactions.

Nateglinide and repaglinide

- Nateglinide and repaglinide are short-acting phenylalanine derivatives that increase insulin secretion and should be taken before meals. The effects on diabetic vascular changes have not been studied.
- Convincing evidence of benefits (fewer episodes of hypoglycaemia?) as compared with older sulphonylureas is lacking.
- An effect comparable to that of glibenclamide (10 mg) is obtained with nateglinide 120 mg three times daily or with repaglinide 4 mg three times daily.
- Particularly suitable for patients with high postprandial blood glucose values but only slightly elevated fasting blood glucose.
- Repaglinide is excreted mainly in bile, which means it can be used in patients with moderate renal insufficiency.

Glitazones

- Glitazones are insulin sensitizers i.e. they improve insulin sensitivity especially in the liver. The effects on diabetic vascular changes have not been studied.
- Indicated for the treatment of hyperglycaemia as monotherapy or in combination with metformin or sulphonylurea.
- When starting the treatment, the patient must not have signs or symptoms of cardiac failure.
- Fluid retention (oedema) occurs in ~5% of patients. Clinically insignificant decrease in hemoglobin (5–10 g/l) occurs in most patients.

References

1. Johansen K. Efficacy of metformin in the treatment of NIDDM: meta-analysis. Diabetes Care 1999;22:33–37.
2. The Database of Abstracts of Reviews of Effectiveness (University of York), Database no.: DARE-990116. In: The Cochrane Library, Issue 1, 2002. Oxford: Update Software.
3. Campbell IW, Howlett HCS. Worldwide experience of metformin as an effective glucose-lowering agent: a meta-analysis. Diabetes-Metabolism Reviews 1995;11(suppl 1): 57–62.
4. The Database of Abstracts of Reviews of Effectiveness (University of York), Database no.: DARE-952803. In: The Cochrane Library, Issue 4, 1999. Oxford: Update Software.
5. Campbell IW, Howlett HCS. Worldwide experience of metformin as an effective glucose-lowering agent: a meta-analysis. Diabetes-Metabolism Reviews 1995;11(suppl 1):57–62.
6. The Database of Abstracts of Reviews of Effectiveness (University of York), Database no.: DARE-952803. In: The Cochrane Library, Issue 4, 1999. Oxford: Update Software.
7. Melchior WR, Jaber LA. Metformin: an antihyperglycemic agent for treatment of type II diabetes. Ann Pharmacother 1996;30:158–164.
8. The Database of Abstracts of Reviews of Effectiveness (University of York), Database no.: DARE-960475. In: The Cochrane Library, Issue 4, 1999. Oxford: Update Software.
9. Campbell RK. Glimepiride: role of a new sulfonylurea in the treatment of type 2 diabetes mellitus. Annals of Pharmacotherapy 1998;32:1044–1052.
10. The Database of Abstracts of Reviews of Effectiveness (University of York), Database no.: DARE-981850. In: The Cochrane Library, Issue 3, 2000. Oxford: Update Software.

23.35 Insulin therapy in type 2 diabetes

Hannele Yki-Järvinen

Objectives

- Glucose control in type 2 diabetes is improved with additional insulin, self-monitoring of blood glucose and self-adjusting of the insulin dose.

- Insulin therapy can be safely started in primary care.
- A combination of evening insulin and is the therapy of choice in most patients.
- A realistic target in type 2 diabetics is to reduce the HbA_{1c} level to 7.5% or below.

Indications for insulin treatment

- Insulin treatment should be started when other methods to treat hyperglycaemia have not been successful $HbA_{1c} >$ 7.5%.
- Temporarily increased need for insulin
  - Transient, serious diseases (e.g. infections, myocardial infarction, aggravation of asthma, etc.) and surgical procedures may worsen insulin resistance and increase blood glucose levels so much that temporary insulin treatment is necessary for correcting the imbalance.
  - Insulin treatment should be started if blood glucose level before meals is repeatedly over 10 mmol/l in the above-mentioned conditions.

Practical algorithm to start insulin therapy

Principles

- Comparative studies and meta-analyses support combination therapy with oral agents and evening insulin as the insulin treatment regimen of choice in type 2 diabetes.

Evening insulin treatment

- Can be carried out by taking basal insulin in the evening between 9 and 11 p.m. The dose may vary greatly between patients (8–170 IU, mean doses: 70 kg 14 IU, 80 kg 24 IU, 90 kg 36 IU, 100 kg 50 IU). The patient should learn to adjust the insulin dose. See follow-up in insulin treatment (below).
- Compared with the combination of sulphonylurea and evening insulin or 2-injection insulin alone, the combination of metformin and evening insulin is better in preventing weight gain and reducing the incidence of hypoglycaemias. Weight gain during insulin treatment is mainly caused by the correction of hyperglycaemia ("calories lost in urine are now retained in the body") and the higher the blood glucose level before the start of insulin treatment, the greater the gain.
- For diabetic patients who do not tolerated metformin, evening insulin combined with sulphonylurea is an option.
- 10 IU in the evening is a safe starting dose for all patients. See Table 23.35. Insulin glargine may be injected in the morning, before dinner or in the evening. Self-adjustment of the dose is still based on the fasting blood glucose level.
- Give written instructions on how to adjust the dose on the basis of fasting blood glucose measurements carried out at home (see follow-up of evening insulin therapy).

Table 23.35 Starting dose for evening insulin

Fasting blood glucose	Starting dose
8–20 mmol/l	8–20 units
>20 mmol/l	20 units

- In evening insulin combination treatment a fasting blood glucose level of 6 mmol/l corresponds to a HbA_{1c} value of 7.5%. This is why fasting blood glucose must be below 6 mmol/l, if the target value of $HbA_{1c} < 7.5\%$ is to be reached. According to present knowledge, the recommended evening insulin is the medium long-acting NPH insulin. Maximum effect on blood glucose is seen 4–6 hours from the injection, and the total duration of effect is approx. 15 hours. Insulin glargine is a long-acting insulin analogue that has no peak in action profile with an effect lasting for 24 hours. Insulin glargine causes 50% less night-time hypoglycaemias compared with NPH insulin and lowers daytime blood glucose levels more than NPH insulin. This is why the fasting blood glucose target can be set at 4–5 mmol/l and HbA_{1c} at <7% with insulin glargine without fear of hypoglycaemias.
- In lifestyle education, emphasis should be on learning self-adjustment and on motivation.
- Snacks are not a part of insulin therapy in type 2 diabetes. The diet does not need to be changed when evening insulin therapy is started if the patient already follows a healthy diet (see 23.33).

Two-injection treatment

- If the patient has renal insufficiency or some other contraindication to oral diabetes drugs, 2-injection treatment with, e.g., premixed insulin (30% of short-acting or rapid-acting and 70% of long-acting) is an option.
- Two-injection treatment with premixed insulin is also an alternative for patients who do not tolerate oral medications.
- When the twice-daily regimen with premixed insulin is used, the morning injection is taken before breakfast and the second before dinner. Starting dose: morning injection and dinnertime injection = fasting blood glucose mmol/l (see Table 23.35). On average the dose is the same in the morning and evening (see above). The dose is determined on the basis of the fasting blood glucose level (dose of the injection before dinner) and the blood glucose level measured before dinner (dose of the morning injection).

Follow-up of insulin treatment

- Successful and safe insulin treatment in type 2 diabetes requires self-monitoring of blood glucose.
- During combination therapy with evening insulin treatment and oral agents a fasting blood glucose measurement in the morning and when hypoglycaemia symptoms appear is sufficient.

- Because the need for insulin varies in type 2 diabetes, **the patient must be instructed to adjust the dose of evening insulin her/himself**.
  - **If the fasting glucose level exceeds 10 mmol/l on three consecutive measurements, the dose is increased by 4 units and if it exceeds 6 mmol/l the dose is increased by 2 units.**
  - If the physician alone adjusts the dose, good glycemic control is not achieved and both the patient and the doctor may become frustrated. Good glycaemic control is not achieved overnight – it usually takes 6 to 12 months or more before glycaemic targets are reached.
- In evening insulin combination treatment the target of HbA_{1c} is below 7.5% with NPH insulin (fasting blood glucose 5–6 mmol/l) and below 7.0% with insulin glargine (fasting blood glucose 4–5 mmol/l).
- In the beginning of treatment it is important to give the patient the possibility of contacting the nurse or the doctor by phone or otherwise.

23.36 Metabolic syndrome (MBS)

Mauno Vanhala

The aim

- Primary and secondary prevention of type 2 diabetes (B) [1 2], cardiovascular disease (hypertension, CHD, stroke, claudication), and Alzheimer's disease.

Definition and signs of MBS

- MBS is a clustering of many insulin resistance-associated cardiovascular risk factors such as obesity, central adiposity, increased sympathetic activity, hypertension, hypertriglyceridaemia, low high density lipoprotein (HDL) cholesterol, abnormal glucose metabolism, hyperinsulinaemia, and microalbuminuria.
- The clustering of risk factors results in a higher risk of diabetes and cardiovascular disease than what would be estimated on the basis of the solitary risk factors.
- In insulin resistance the biological response of adipose and muscle tissues and the liver to insulin is lowered, resulting in the appearance of the risk factors and their clustering simultaneously in one individual. Clustering of insulin resistance, compensatory hyperinsulinaemia and dyslipidamiea is the metabolic core of the syndrome.

The signs of MBS

1. Familial component, at least one first-degree relative with type 2 diabetes.
2. Obesity: body-mass-index (BMI) $\geq$30 kg/m^2.
3. Central adiposity: waist-to-hip ratio (WHR) $\geq$1.00 in men, and $\geq$0.88 in women
4. Hypertension: a systolic blood pressure of 140 mmHg or more, and/or a diastolic blood pressure of 90 mmHg or more, or antihypertensive drug treatment
5. Hypertriglyceridaemia: fasting serum triglycerides $\geq$1.70 mmol/l
6. Low HDL-cholesterol: <1.00 mmol/l in men, <1.20 mmol/l in women
7. Abnormal glucose metabolism (impaired glucose tolerance or type 2 diabetes according to WHO criteria)
8. Hyperuricaemia: fasting serum urate $\geq$450 μmol/l in men, $\geq$340 μmmol/l in women
9. Hyperinsulinaemia: $\geq$78 pmol/l ($\geq$13.0 mU/l)
10. Microalbuminuria: $\geq$20 mg/24 hours
11. Sleep apnoea, depression, and Alzheimer's disease may also be associated with MBS.

National Cholesterol Education Program Adult Treatment Panel III criteria

- A diagnosis of metabolic syndrome is made when 3 or more of the risk determinants are present:
  - Fasting blood glucose $\geq$6.1mmol/l
  - Blood pressure $\geq$130/85 mmHg
  - Serum triglycerides $\geq$1.7 mmol/l
  - Serum HDL-cholesterol <1.0 mmol/l (men); <1.3 mmol/l (women)
  - Abdominal obesity (waist circumference >102 cm in men; >88 cm in women)

Diagnosis

- Central obesity (obesity associated with central adiposity) is the most characteristic sign of MBS (which is seen extremely rarely in lean persons).
- MBS can be identified by anamnesis, anthropomethric measurements, blood pressure measurements and by examination of
  - serum lipids
  - blood or plasma glucose (2-hour glucose tolerance test (or plasma (blood) glucose after a meal if fasting glucose level is normal).
  - Serum urate should be investigated in patients with high blood pressure, obesity, or obvious central adiposity.
- **Probable metabolic syndrome**; the subject has at least three (any three) of the above-listed ten abnormalities
- **Obvious metabolic syndrome**: the subject has dyslipidaemia (hypertriglyceridaemia and/or low HDL cholesterol) and at the same time at least one of the abnormalities 7–10.
- Measurements of the fasting plasma insulin level and microalbuminuria are necessary only if this knowledge affects the choice of drug treatment (antihypertensive etc.).
- C-peptide level reflects the insulin secretion capacity of pancreas and is often increased in chronic hyperinsulinaemia. It is, however, not as good as fasting plasma insulin in revealing insulin resistance.

Prevalence

- In a Finnish population study of subjects aged 40–55 years, the prevalence of MBS was 17% (95% CI 13%–20%) in men and 7% (95% CI 6%–11%) in women. The prevalence of MBS was statistically significantly ($p < 0.01$) higher in men compared with women.
- About one half of hypertensive patients are hyperinsulinaemic and have insulin resistance. In a Finnish middle-aged hypertensive population, the prevalence of MBS was 35% in men and 25% in women, the prevalence in men being statistically significantly ($p < 0.01$) higher than in women.
- Among subjects with central obesity (the subjects having simultaneously BMI ≥30 kg/m_2 and WHR >1.00 in men and >0.88 in women), the prevalence of MBS was 55% in men and 40% in women. In the non-obese subjects without central adiposity the prevalence of MBS was 2–4%.

Treatment

- The basic treatment is always non-pharmacological (23.33).

Non-pharmacological treatment

- Increasing physical activity
- Weight reduction
- Change of eating habits, increasing the intake of fibre and decreasing that of fat (particularly saturated fat) and rapidly metabolized carbohydrates (highly refined).
- Quit smoking
- Avoid drinking of alcohol more than two drinks per day

Drug treatment

- MBS should be taken into account in the prevention and treatment of hypertension, type 2 diabetes and coronary heart disease.
- If a hypertensive has MBS, it is important to avoid non-selective beta-blockers and high-dose diuretics, as these drugs may worsen insulin resistance. However, if a patient has coronary heart disease or he/she has suffered from myocardial infarction, the use of beta-blockers may be necessary. The following drugs can be used for hypertension
  - Superselective beta-blockers that apparently do not affect insulin sensitivity
  - ACE inhibitors
  - Alpha1 receptor blockers
  - Calcium channel blockers
  - Angiotensin II receptor antagonists (losartan, valsartan, eprosartan, candesartan).
- If hypertriglyceridaemia is repeatedly >5.0 mmol/l in spite of non-pharmacological treatment, dyslipidaemia should be treated with fibrates. If a patient has coronary heart disease, the pharmacological treatment should be started if the level of triglycerides exceeds 2.3 mmol/l and total-cholesterol/HDL-cholesterol ratio is higher than 5, or HDL-cholesterol is lower than 0.9 mmol/l.
- Biguanides, acarbose and guar gum may correct insulin resistance and thus are feasible as a first hand drug for an obese type 2 diabetic patient.
- Orlistat or sibutramine may be indicated if the BMI is >30 kg/m^2. These drugs lower weight and reduce adipose fat in particular.
- Thiazolidinediones (rosiglitazone, pioglitazone, and related drugs) are insulin sensitizers that may appear to have a role in the treatment of diabetes associated with MBS.

Follow-up

- It is important to motivate the patient and to follow up possible changes in lifestyle.
- A physician should follow up patients who are on drug therapy (antihypertensives, antilipaemic drug etc.). Regular visits to the doctor are often important for motivation.
- Patients without drug treatment should be followed up by a public health nurse for motivation of lifestyle changes, measurements of BMI, WHR, blood pressure and control of lipids and fasting glucose when needed. If the lipids are abnormal, the 2-hour glucose tolerance test should be performed. A doctor should be consulted if
  - blood pressure is repeatedly >160/95 mmHg
  - total cholesterol:HDL cholesterol ratio is >5
  - fasting serum triglyceride level is repeatedly is ≥2.30 mmol/l
  - fasting plasma glucose is ≥7.8 mmol/l and
  - the patient gets symptoms of some other disease (gout, etc.).

References

1. Tuomilehto J, Lindström J, Eriksson JG, Valle TT, Hämäläinen H, Ilanne-Parikka P, ym. Prevention of type 2 diabetes mellitus by changes in lifestyle among subjects with impaired glucose tolerance. N Engl J Med 2001;344:1343–50.
2. Knowler WC, Barrett-Connor E, Fowler SE, Hamman RF, Lachin JM, Walker EA, Nathan DM; Diabetes Prevention Program Research Group. Reduction in the incidence of type 2 diabetes with lifestyle intervention or metformin. N Engl J Med 2002;346:393–403.

23.40 Diabetic eye disease, with special reference to diabetic retinopathy

Leila Laatikainen, Paula Summanen

Aims

- To understand the importance of regular fundus examination in diabetics B [1 2 3 4], to be able to assess the fundus changes with an ophthalmoscope or preferentially from fundus photographs, to refer the patients to ophthalmologist in time; and to motivate the patient to maintain good glycaemic control for the sake of eye health.

Epidemiology

- The most common systemic disease affecting the eye, mainly the retina and primarily its smallest vessels, the capillaries (microangiopathy).
- Affects other parts of the eye as well (see cataract 37.33; and may cause recurrent corneal erosions).
- The estimated frequency of diabetes is up to 3% in Western populations.
- Diabetic retinopathy is the leading cause of acquired blindness in people of working age in all industrialized countries and the third most common cause of impaired vision in patients aged 65 and over (after age-related macular degeneration and glaucoma).
- The prevalence and severity of diabetic retinopathy depends on the type of the disease (type I or II), its duration, and the level of glycaemic control. Other risk factors are systemic and diastolic hypertension, dyslipidaemias, nephropathy, and infections. Puberty, pregnancy and socioeconomic factors also have an influence.
- Some retinopathy occurs in almost all (80–95%) patients with type I diabetes after 15 to 20 years of diabetes and about half of them have proliferative retinopathy. Some changes occur in almost 70–80% of patients with type II diabetes after 15 years, and about 20% already have some changes at the time of diagnosis of diabetes mellitus.
- About 20% of those on insulin therapy and less than 10% of those on diet or peroral medication develop proliferative retinopathy in type II diabetes.
- Clinically significant macular oedema (see below) occurs in between 10% and 25% of diabetics after 20 years duration of diabetes.

Pathogenesis

- Retinal vascular changes are caused by hyperglycaemia and influenced by high blood pressure and dyslipidaemia, which alter blood components, the endothelial cells of the capillary wall (active hormonal tissue, responsible for the blood-retinal barrier), pericytes (contractile tissue) and the basal membrane (skeleton). Vessel walls become weak and leaky and allow plasma and whole blood to escape into the retina causing oedema, lipid exudation and haemorrhages. Weakness and death of pericytes allow outward bulging of capillaries, leading to microaneurysms. Closure of capillaries may be caused by erythrocytes (increased rigidity), thrombocytes and leucocytes (increased adherence). Since the fibrinolytic system is impaired in diabetes, capillaries remain occluded leading to a locally visible irregular capillary bed, intraretinal microvascular abnormalities (IRMA), venous beading and microinfarcts ("cotton wool spots"), and eventually to angiogenesis and new vessels growing on the optic nerve head or on the retina towards the occluded areas suffering from hypoxia. The new vessels leak and cause the collapse of the vitreous humour which then detaches from the retina. This causes traction on the new vessels growing on the posterior surface of the vitreous humour and some vessels may break and bleed. This also causes traction on the retina, especially if these fibrovascular proliferations are extensive. They may cause traction retinal detachment. A detached retina and large areas of capillary closure also cause angiogenesis and new vessel formation in the anterior chamber angle and lead to neovascular glaucoma.

Clinical picture

- None of the changes (microaneurysms, haemorrhages, oedema, lipid exudates, IRMA, retinal microinfarcts, venous beading, new vessels on the optic nerve head or on the retina, vitreous haemorrhage, fibrovascular proliferation) are pathognomonic of diabetic retinopathy but do create typical clinical pictures of diabetic retinopathy which can be divided into two main groups: background retinopathy (or nowadays nonproliferative retinopathy) characterized by all other changes in varying combinations except the appearance of new vessels and their sequelae); and proliferative retinopathy (with new vessels and the corresponding sequelae).
- Can be observed through a well dilated pupil with an ophthalmoscope or assessed from fundus photographs.

Classification of retinopathy

1. No diabetic retinopathy (no changes attributable to diabetes)
2. Mild nonproliferative diabetic retinopathy (microaneurysms only- and/or small haermorrhages indistinguishable from microaneurysm (modification))
3. Moderate nonproliferative diabetic retinopathy (more than just microaneurysms but less than severe nonproliferative diabetic retinopathy)
4. Severe nonproliferative diabetic retinopathy (previously called preproliferative retinopathy; any of the following lesions present consistent with the 4-2-1 rule: more than 20 intraretinal haemorrhages in each of 4 quadrants; definite venous beading in 2+ quadrants; prominent intraretinal microvascular abnormalities in 1+ quadrant; and no signs of proliferative retinopathy)
5. Proliferative retinopathy (mild, moderate, or severe with high-risk characteristics (HRC) for visual loss)
6. Advanced diabetic eye disease (vitreous haemorrhage, traction retinal detachment, neovascular glaucoma)

Classification of macular oedema

1. Macular oedema apparently absent
2. Macular oedema apparently present
    - Mild diabetic macular oedema (some macular thickening or hard exudates in posterior pole but distant from the centre of the macula)
    - Moderate diabetic macular oedema (retinal thickening or hard exudates approaching the centre of the macula but not involving the centre)

- Severe diabetic macular oedema (retinal thickening or hard exudates involving the centre of the macula)

Treatment

I Glycaemic control

- Good glycaemic control in patients with both type I and II diabetes decreases the incidence and progression of diabetic retinopathy. This has been well shown in both primary and secondary prevention groups.

II Other medical therapies

- There is some evidence that ACE-inhibitors have benefial effect on retinal vessels, endothelial cells, and do slow the progression of diabetic retinopathy. This effect is independent of the blood pressure lowering effect. However, this is not yet an indication per se to start ACE-inhibitor medication.
- Blood pressure should be lowered by medication if the pressure is repeatedly 135/85 mmHg or higher.
- Acetosalicylic acid (ASA) did not have any clear effect on the progression of diabetic retinopathy either alone or with dipyridamole. The same is true with ticlopidine even if the occurrence of microaneurysms was slightly decreased in the treatment group. It is, however, important to note that there are no contraindications for ASA in patients with diabetic retinopathy when it is required for cardiovascular disease.
- New peroral drugs affecting vasoendothelial growth factor, VEGF, which is associated with both increased permeability of the vessels and angiogenesis in diabetic retinopathy, staurosporin and LY 333531 are undergoing clinical trial. They are selective inhibitors of protein kinase C beta through which VEGF functions. Preliminary results have been promising.

III Laser treatment

- Regular eye examinations necessary to identify patients in need of laser treatment **B** [1 2 3 4].
- Timely laser treatment for proliferative retinopathy prevents visual impairment and blindness in 95% of patients with HRC for visual loss **B** [1 2 3 4].
- Indications for laser treatment
  - Clinically significant macular oedema (CSME) (See below.)
  - Proliferative retinopathy: urgently when risk factors for severe visual loss are present
  - Consider also in severe nonproliferative retinopathy, in patients with type I diabetes and with type 2 diabetes, if regular check-ups are not possible.
- Definition of clinically significant macular oedema
  - Thickening of the retina (oedema) with or without lipid exudates at least within 500 μm from the centre of the fovea (about: 1/3 disc diameter).
  - Thickening of the retina, at least one disc diameter in size and involving the region within one disc diameter from the centre of the fovea.
- Definition of high risk characteristics for visual loss
  - New vessels on the optic disc or within one disc diameter of it, covering at least one third of the disc area.
  - New vessels on the disc smaller than above, or elsewhere in the retina when at least one half of the disc area in size, with preretinal or vitreous haemorrhage.
  - Preretinal or vitreous haemorrhage, at least one disc diameter in size.
- In diabetic maculopathy tens to hundreds laserspots are given, in proliferative retinopathy 1000 or even several thousand spots are needed. In patients with high-risk characteristics for visual loss full panretinal photocoagulation is carried out, and in others with mild to moderate proliferative retinopathy, under and around sectoral or modified panphotocoagulation.
- The effect of laser treatment has been shown in several prospective, randomized, multicentre studies.
- In diabetic maculopathy the results are not always as marked as in proliferative retinopathy, but laser treatment succeeds in stopping the visual impairment in about 60% of patients, vision improves in about 20% and deteriorates in spite of therapy in 20%.
- It is estimated that about ten million diabetics have retained their eyesight due to laser treatment. This effect can at present not be achieved by any other means.
- With vitrectomy it is possible to restore vision in most patients with persistent vitreous haemorrhage or those with traction retinal detachment threatening the macula. If the macula has been detached for a long period of time or the fundus and/or the optic nerve is atrophic, or the macula is damaged with extensive capillary and arteriolar closure, the outcome may be poor even if the optic media remains clear.

IV Indications for vitreoretinal surgery

- Unresorbable vitreous haemorrhage
- Traction retinal detachment threatening the macula
- A combination of the above two indications
- Inability to complete laser treatment
- Aggressive proliferative retinopathy inspite of panretinal photocoagulation.

Screening

- Diabetic retinopathy fulfils all the criteria for a disease to be effectively screened: a defined population, a well known clinical course, and availability of effective treatment **B** [1 2 3 4].
- The fundi of all diabetics must be examined regularly, preferably with photography (ophthalmoscopy is insensitive, especially when done by nonophthalmologists).

Frequency of examination

- Rule of thumb: at diagnosis of diabetes and annually thereafter.
- With some important specifications:
  - In children, retinopathy is uncommon before puberty. Annual examinations are started when the first signs of

puberty are seen as a practical rule from the age of 10 years onwards. Picture without any retinopathy are a positive message to the young patient.
  - In adult type I diabetics and type II diabetics on insulin therapy, regular examinations every year or every second year until the first changes are detected, then annually, or more often if risk factors are present (poor glycaemic control, nephropathy, dyslipidaemias). During pregnancy, once in every trimester.
  - In type II diabetics on peroral medication with no fundus changes (confirmed by high quality photographs): at two year intervals.
  - In those with dietary therapy and no changes (confirmed by high quality photography): at three year intervals.
  - In those with some changes: annually or more often if severe nonproliferative retinopathy or risk factors are present.
- Do not wait for visual impairment to occur before referring the patient to ophthalmologist for check-up or treatment.
- The regular fundus examination may be carried out by the diabetologist until more than mild nonproliferative retinopathy has been detected. Then refer the patient to an ophthalmologist.
- In photographic screening, there must be consultation between the diabetologists, general practitioners and an ophthalmologist.

References

1. Bachmann MO, Nelson SJ. Impact of diabetic retinopathy screening on a British district population: case detection and blindness prevention in an evidence-based model.
2. The Database of Abstracts of Reviews of Effectiveness (University of York), Database no.: DARE-988259. In: The Cochrane Library, Issue 4, 1999. Oxford: Update Software.
3. Bachmann M, Nelson S. Screening for diabetic retinopathy: a quantitative overview of evidence, applied to the populations of health authorities and boards. Health Care Evaluation Unit 1996;1–46.
4. The Database of Abstracts of Reviews of Effectiveness (University of York), Database no.: DARE-978032. In: The Cochrane Library, Issue 4, 1999. Oxford: Update Software.

23.41 The diagnosis and treatment of diabetic nephropathy

Leo Niskanen

Basic rule

- Control microalbuminuria and blood pressure yearly and treat them effectively.

General principles

- Nephropathy is a common and severe complication of diabetes. About every third patient with type 1 diabetes is affected after diabetes has lasted for 15–20 years. Of type 2 diabetics about 20% have microalbuminuria and 3% have macroalbuminuria at the time of diagnosis.
- Nephropathy signifies poor prognosis and decreased life span. The negative effect on prognosis is mainly associated with a markedly increased risk for cardiovascular complications.
- The number of new dialysis treatments for type 2 diabetes patients is rising and has exceeded the number of treatments for type 1 patients
- The earliest sign of nephropathy is microalbuminuria.
- The progression of nephropathy can be slowed by treatment.
- In type 2 diabetes microalbuminuria may be a sign of vascular damage and a part of metabolic syndrome.

Prevention

- The progression of microalbuminuria can be delayed by
  - good control of diabetes
  - effective treatment of hypertension
  - reducing the amount of protein in the diet 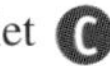 [1]
  - stopping smoking
  - treatment of dyslipidaemia.
- These measures may be of importance when the aim is to prevent the development and progression of renal failure.

Screening for diabetic nephropathy

- Microalbuminuria is the earliest sign of nephropathy.
- In type 1 diabetes the development of nephropathy is very uncommon during the first 5 years of the disease.
- In children nephropathy is hardly ever diagnosed before puberty.
- Some type 2 diabetics have microalbuminuria already at the time of diagnosis.
- Screening of microalbuminuria is recommended yearly for all patients with type 1 diabetes after the diabetes has lasted for 5 years, and for patients with type 2 diabetes from the time of diagnosis.

Microalbuminuria and diabetic nephropathy

- **Microalbuminuria** is defined as the secretion of albumin between 20 and 200 μg/min (nocturnal urine) or between 30 and 300 mg daily (24-h urine collection). As occasional albuminuria may have several causes, a positive result must be controlled twice at 6–12 week intervals. The diagnosis of microalbuminuria is made if 2 out of 3 samples are positive.
- In children the threshold level for diagnosing early nephropathy is set at the secretion of 12 $\mu g/min/m^2$ of albumin or 20 $\mu g/min/1.73\ m^2$.

- Nephropathy is defined as an overnight albumin secretion of above 200 µg/min.
- Nephropathy is nearly always associated with diabetic retinopathy especially in type 1 patients. If the patient has no retinopathy, it is possible that the proteinuria is not caused by diabetes.

Determination of microalbuminuria

Collection of night urine

- Measuring albumin secretion during night rest
  - The patient empties his/her bladder in the evening and records the time with the precision of one minute.
  - In the morning the patient voids into a collection container and records the time. The minimum duration of urine collection is 6 hours.
  - The laboratory must be informed of the height and weight of a child because albumin secretion is adjusted to body surface.
- The specimen is collected in a clean container and stored in a cool place; albumin remains intact for 2 weeks in a refrigerator. Freezing is not recommended because part of the albumin may be degraded.

Single urine sample

- Urine collection can be substituted by the determination of albumin:creatinine ratio from the first voiding in the morning or other single urine sample. However, overnight urine albumin collection is preferred.
  - In microalbuminuria the ratio is 3.4–34 mg/ml (30–300 mg/g).
  - A positive result must be verified by determining albumin secretion rate from urine collected overnight.

Test method

- Dipstick tests for microalbuminuria can be used for screening from a single urine sample with some precautions, but they are not suitable for the quantification of microalbuminuria.
- Note that Albustix® is positive only at concentrations of 300 mg/l and above. The test is not suitable for sensitive screening; positive results are naturally significant.
- Cystatine C in serum is a new and promising marker in early diagnosis of diabetic nephropathy. Its use has not been established.

Treatment of hyperglycaemia

- The target value of HbA_{1c} is 7.0–7.5%.

Treatment of hypertension

- The treatment of hypertension in a diabetic patient should be started if the diastolic pressure is repeatedly 90 mmHg or higher. If the patient has diabetic retinopathy, drug treatment should be started at diastolic pressure of 85 mmHg. The target blood pressure is below 130/80–85 mmHg.
- If microalbuminuria is detected in a normotensive patient, starting an ACE inhibitor should be considered, at least if the diastolic pressure is between 85 and 90 mmHg. ACE inhibitors decrease microalbuminuria independently of the blood pressure level (A) [2].
- An ACE inhibitor is always the drug of choice for type 1 patients. Angiotensin-II type 1 receptor blockers (ARB) are good options when ACE inhibitors are not suitable and are primary for type 2 patients. Also thiazide diuretics (12.5–25 mg of hydrochlorothiazide), calcium antagonists and selective beta-blockers can be used. A combination of these is often needed.
- Remember that renal artery stenosis is common in diabetic patients, and measure serum creatinine to detect eventual rapid increase in serum creatinine concentration after starting an ACE inhibitor.
- If the patient has oedema due to high proteinuria, start a loop diuretic (furosemide). Small doses of thiazide diuretics can be used for type 1 diabetic patients with normal renal function in combination with other groups of antihypertensive drugs.
- In the majority of patients with type 2 diabetes elevation of blood pressure is associated with obesity, and non-pharmacological therapy should always be preferred. The treatment includes weight reduction, reducing salt intake (5–6 g daily), reducing the consumption of alcohol and increasing exercise.
- Autonomic neuropathy is common in patients with diabetic nephropathy. Orthostatic hypotension should be prevented.

Diet

- The diet has an influence on the following factors that are of importance in diabetic nephropathy:
  - Diabetes control
  - Blood pressure
  - Serum lipids
  - Obesity
  - Renal function and amount of proteinuria

Targets

- The proportion of fat in the total energy intake should not exceed 30 energy per cent (E%), and the proportion of saturated fat should not exceed 10 E%. Monoenic and polyunsaturated fatty acids should constitute about 20 E%.
- Carbohydrates are the most important source of energy (50–55%).
- The proportion of protein in the total energy intake should be 10–20 E%. A sufficient amount of protein for an adult with normal body weight is 0.8 g/kg body weight daily.

Protein restriction

- The restrictions adjusted to body weight refer to normal body weight.

- Good patient compliance is a prerequisite for the application of protein restriction and poor application predisposes the patient to malnutrition.
- Protein restriction is not necessary for elderly patients with type 2 diabetes.
- Protein restriction always includes a phosphate restriction of 0.8–1 g/day.
- There is some evidence of short-term effectiveness of protein restriction on renal function in patients with microalbuminuria **C** [1].

Protein restriction in different stages of nephropathy

1. Microalbuminuria (night urinary albumine secretion 20–200 μmol/l)
   - Protein intake less than 1 g/kg daily in adults
2. Clinically evident diabetic nephropathy (proteinuria > 0.5 g daily or creatinine in serum > 200 μmol/l)
   - Recommended daily intake of protein is 0.6–0.8 g/kg
3. Serum creatinine > 400 μmol/l
   - Other treatments for uraemia determine the diet.
   - Individualized protein restriction (<0.6 g/kg daily) is indicated in conservative therapy.

Diet therapy in practice

- Instead of protein and animal fat, low-protein starch, sucrose, small amounts of fructose, and unsaturated vegetable fat are consumed as sources of energy. Carbohydrates rich in fibre are recommended.
- Consultation by a dietitian is recommended.

Indications for consultation of a nephrologist

- Serum creatinine concentration increases rapidly.
- Serum creatinine is at or above 200 μmol/l.
- Nephrotic syndrome (proteinuria 3 g daily or more)
- Active treatment of uraemia should be started early in patients with diabetic nephropathy.
- Renal transplantation is usually the treatment of choice for patients under 45 years of age. If coronary artery bypass surgery or angioplasty is needed, it should be performed before the transplantation.
- Continuous ambulatory peritoneal dialysis (CAPD) is a suitable treatment for many patients. Insulin is administered in the dialysis solution.

Drug therapy in diabetic nephropathy

- Particularly the use of glibenclamide in the elderly (serum creatinine > 160 μmol/l) may cause prolonged and severe hypoglycaemia. In renal insufficiency insulin treatment is recommended but glimepiride and glipizide can also be used.
- Metformin should be avoided if serum creatinine is above 150 μmol/l because of the risk of lactic acidosis.
- Of the statins, fluvastatine and pravastatine are to recommended in patients with renal failure.
- The dose of gemfibrozil and fenofibrate should be reduced to 50% in moderate renal insufficiency and to 25% in severe insufficiency. Bezafibrate should not be used even in moderate renal insufficiency. In general the use of fibrates in patients with renal insufficiency should be carefully considered.
- NSAIDs may affect glomerular filtration.

Other renal and urinary tract problems in patients with diabetes

- The benefits of antimicrobial treatment of asymptomatic bacteriuria are disputable **B** [3].
- The incidence of pyelonephritis is increased in diabetic patients. They should be treated well.
- Neurogenic bladder and increased residual urine predispose to urinary tract infections and may cause incontinence.
- Diabetic patients have an increased risk of acute renal failure associated with surgery, trauma or systemic infections.
- Contrast media may cause acute renal failure. If a contrast medium investigation must be performed, the dose should be as small as possible, and adequate hydration must be ensured.

END

References

1. Waugh NR, Robertson AM. Protein restriction for diabetic renal disease. Cochrane Database Syst Rev. 2004;(2):CD002181.
2. Lovell HG. Angiotensin converting enzyme inhibitors in normotensive diabetic patients with microalbuminuria. Cochrane Database Syst Rev. 2004;(2):CD002183.
3. Harding GKM, Zhanel GG, Nicolle LE, Cheang M, for the Manitoba Diabetes Urinary Tract Infection Study Group. N Engl J Med 2002;347:1576–1583.

23.42 Diabetic neuropathy

Esa Mervaala

- Polyneuropathies, see 36.90

General

- Occurrence of some form of neuropathy among all diabetics
  - Approximately 25% have symptoms.
  - 75–80% have subclinical neuropathy (diagnosed in clinical examinations or as abnormalities in ENMG).

- The diagnosis of diabetic neuropathy is based on the diagnosis of diabetes, typical symptoms and clinical findings, as well as exclusion of other causes leading to neuropathy. Neuropathy can be verified objectively by ENMG.
- Neuropathy may be the first sign of type 2 diabetes.

Symmetric and asymmetric polyneuropathy

- Pains beginning predominantly distally, paraesthesias and dysaesthesias
- Muscle cramps
- Tendon reflexes are weak or absent
  - The Achilles tendon reflex is the first to be affected.
- Sensory disturbances
  - Vibration and position sense in lower limbs are affected at first, other sensory modalities later on. Sense of touch is investigated with monofilament examination.
- Muscle weakness when the disease progresses
- Restless legs

Diabetic amyotrophy (= proximal neuropathy)

- There is usually asymmetric weakness and muscle atrophy in the hip and the femoral region accompanied by dorsal and femoral pains.
- The patient is typically a middle-aged or an older man, whose diabetes is in poor control. The condition is relieved remarkably within 6–18 months by regaining good treatment balance.

Diabetic thoracal radiculopathy

- The condition has been poorly recognized, but it is not uncommon.
- Begins at the age of 50–70 years in type 2 diabetes.
- Symptoms
  - The leading symptom is a severe unilateral pain in the thoracic region, which reaches maximal intensity within a few days.
  - There may be a sensory defect in the affected region, and sometimes a regional weakness in the thoracic or abdominal muscles.
  - No motor symptoms or findings in the extremities.
  - The patient often loses weight.
- Cardiac and abdominal diseases must be taken into account in the differential diagnosis.
- The disease often resolves spontaneously.

Mononeuropathy and multiple mononeuropathy

- The most typical mononeuropathies caused by diabetes are:
  - painful neuropathy of the femoral nerve, causing weakness of the quadriceps muscle, which resolves spontaneously.
  - neuropathy of the oculomotor nerve without pupillomotor defect.
- Disturbances may also occur in other peripheral nerves as single or multiple mononeuropathies. These are usually resolved within weeks or months.

Diabetic ophthalmoplegia

- A disturbance in the ocular movements caused by diabetic neuropathy. See 36.7, 36.8.
- The nerve most often affected is the oculomotor nerve, more rarely the abducent nerve or trochlear nerve.
- Often heals spontaneously.

Autonomic neuropathy

Symptoms and findings

- Diminished or abolished pulse rate variability
- Postural hypotension
- Disturbances in intestinal function, diarrhoea, constipation
- Disturbances in gastric motility, gastroparesis, nausea after meals
- Urinary disturbances
- Impotence
- Sweating disturbances, changes in the skin
- Weakening or disappearance of hypoglycaemic symptoms
- Altered renal sodium handling, diabetic oedema, arrhythmias

Diagnosis

- History (symptoms, control of diabetes, alcohol)
- Clinical examination
  - Muscle atrophies
  - In the orthostatic test a rise in pulse rate is absent or systolic blood pressure decreases more than 20 mmHg.
  - A resting pulse rate above 90/min may indicate autonomic neuropathy.
- Several diagnostic tests are used, the most useful being decrease of pulse rate variability during forced inhalation and exhalation and the orthostatic test.

Treatment of diabetic neuropathy

- Optimal control of diabetes is the basis of the prevention and treatment of diabetic neuropathy.
- Mononeuropathy and radiculopathy usually resolve spontaneously.
- Tricyclic antidepressants (and analgesics) are used in the treatment of neuropathic pain **A** [1 2 3 4]. Carbamazepine and gabapentine may be useful **B** [5]. Levomepromazine may be a good choice in the evening in small doses

(5–25 mg) because of its sedative effect. The efficacy of physical treatments has not been verified. See also 17.40.

- Topical capsaicin may be effective **B** [6,7].
- The treatment of autonomic neuropathy is usually symptomatic.
  - Sufficient fluid volume should be assured in orthostatic hypotension by a mineralocorticoid.
  - Gastroparesis is relieved by metoclopramide or cisapride (only to be started by a specialist as this drug causes marked prolongation of the QT time and consequent risk of arrhythmias), or if these cause diarrhoea, by erythromycin in small doses.
  - For treatment of impotence, see 11.40.
- Smoking aggravates neuropathy.

References

1. Kingery WS. A critical review of controlled clinical trials for peripheral neuropathic pain and complex regional pain syndromes. Pain 1997;73:123–139.
2. The Database of Abstracts of Reviews of Effectiveness (University of York), Database no.: DARE-980065. In: The Cochrane Library, Issue 4, 1999. Oxford: Update Software.
3. McQuay JH, Tramer M, Nye BA, Carroll D, Wiffen PJ, Moore RA. A systematic review of antidepressants in neuropathic pain. Pain 1996;68:217–227.
4. The Database of Abstracts of Reviews of Effectiveness (University of York), Database no.: DARE-978044. In: The Cochrane Library, Issue 4, 1999. Oxford: Update Software.
5. Wiffen P, McQuay H, Carroll D, Jadad A, Moore A. Anticonvulsant drugs for acute and chronic pain. The Cochrane Database of Systematic Reviews, Cochrane Library number: CD001133. In: The Cochrane Library, Issue 2, 2002. Oxford: Update Software. Updated frequently.
6. Zhang WY, Li Wan Po A. The effectiveness of topically applied capsaicin: a meta-analysis. Eur J Clin Pharmacol 1994;46:517–522.
7. The Database of Abstracts of Reviews of Effectiveness (University of York), Database no.: DARE-968401. In: The Cochrane Library, Issue 4, 1999. Oxford: Update Software.

23.43 Diabetic macroangiopathy

Editors

General

- The primary aim of treatment for type 2 diabetes is to prevent the development of atherosclerotic vascular disease **B** [1] by managing hyperglycaemia, hypertension, hyperlipidaemia and coagulation disorders (23.32).

Manifestations

- Coronary heart disease is an early complication of type 2 diabetes. Newly diagnosed diabetic patients already have 2–3 times more often coronary heart disease compared with age-matched non-diabetic persons. Even impaired glucose tolerance increases the risk of coronary heart disease.
- The occurrence of cerebrovascular disease and especially that of peripheral arterial disease depends on the duration of the diabetes.
- High blood pressure, increased serum insulin level during fasting, insulin resistance, high serum triglyceride level, and low HDL-cholesterol concentration are known risk factors for atherosclerosis among type 2 diabetic patients. Together with central obesity they are the features of metabolic syndrome (23.36).
- Asymptomatic myocardial infarctions are more common among diabetic patients than among their non-diabetic counterparts. This is due to diabetic autonomic neuropathy.
- Heart failure is 2–5 times more common among diabetic patients compared with the general population. This cannot be explained solely by the occurrence of coronary heart disease or hypertension. One explanation may be diabetic heart disease due to a metabolic disturbance in the cardiac muscle, arteriolar changes, cardiac fibrosis and autonomic neuropathy.

Treatment

- See article 23.32.

Reference

1. Gaede P, Vedel P, Larsen N, Jensen GVH, Parving HH, Pedersen O. Multifactorial intervention and cardiovascular disease in patients with type 2 diabetes. N Engl J Med 2003;348:383–393.

23.44 Treatment of the diabetic foot

Editors

Goals

- The diabetic patient's feet should be examined regularly. In particular, patients at risk should be followed up.
- A podiatrist takes part in the treatment of the diabetic patient's feet and patient education **C** [1].
- Skin infections should be treated early and effectively.

- Walking cast or some other relief of weight-bearing helps in chronic wounds (B) [2].
- Critical ischaemia should be recognized and treated with vascular surgery.
- Charcot's neuroarthropathy should be recognized and treated quickly.

Screening for foot problems and recognition of patients at risk

- The feet of all diabetic patients should be examined once a year.
  - It is particularly important to examine the feet of type 2 diabetic patients and those of type 1 diabetic patients aged 30 years or over, whose disease has lasted for more than 15 years.
  - A podiatrist or a diabetes nurse specialist should perform the screening examination and educate the patient (C) [1].
- Patients at risk should be recognized on the basis of the findings and they should be followed up frequently (also by a physician, not by nursing staff only).
  - Previous ulcers and infections
  - Callus (the risk of an ulcer is increased of there are dark haemorrhage in the callus)
  - Macerations and bullae of the skin
  - Deformities of the feet and toes.
    - Pes transversoplanus predisposes to a callus or ulcer in the middle of the ball of the foot
    - Hammer toes
    - Hallux valgus
    - Prominent metatarsal bones in the base of the foot
  - Decreased sense of touch (neuropathy)
  - Decreased circulation in the feet, previous vascular surgery
  - The risk of a foot lesion is also increased by:
    - poor glucose control
    - retinopathy which threatens eyesight
    - nephropathy
    - smoking
    - poor foot hygiene.
  - The heels of a bedridden diabetic patient should be prevented from developing pressure ulcers by paddings and position treatment. The skin should be checked daily.

Examination of a diabetic patient's feet

1. Search for signs of neuropathy (B) [3] [4]
   - Tingling, paraesthesias, cramps, restlessness, lack of sensation, pain, and hyperaesthesia are the signs of sensory neuropathy.
   - Disappearance of the sense of vibration, absence of the Achilles tendon reflexes and weakened sense of touch are the most easily recognized signs of neuropathy (23.42).
2. The examination of the shoes and their suitability.
   - Are the shoes worn those used on weekdays or shoes that are used only occasionally?
   - Is the shoe big enough (= the length of the foot + 1–1.5 cm)? Are there distensions around the first and second toes? Where is the lining worn?
   - Are the socks of a suitable size and made of soft cotton?
3. Examine the circulation
   - Are there symptoms of claudication?
   - Cold feet and a thin, gleaming and reddish skin suggest poor arterial blood flow.
   - The femoral arteries should be auscultated and the peripheral arteries should be palpated. Marked macroangiopathy can be excluded only if peripheral pulses are clearly palpable.
   - Autonomic neuropathy increases the arteriovenous shunting, which makes the foot feel warm to the hand and the veins full. In spite of a seemingly good blood flow the oxygen supply of the tissues is decreased.
   - A Doppler stethoscope can be used in the evaluation of peripheral blood flow (5.20) Decreased ankle pressure is always a notable finding. Erroneously high ankle pressure can be measured when media sclerosis is present, but a slow (low frequency) and one phase pulse sound indicates poor blood flow. The ischaemia is critical if the ankle pressure is below 60 mmHg or the ankle–arm pressure ratio is below 0.50 and the patient has pain or an ulcer. For lower limb ischaemia, see (5.60).
4. Look for signs of tarsal deformities, changes in the skin, changes in the nails, ulcers and lacerations (also between the toes), and infections.
   - A fungal culture should be taken if Candida is suspected.
   - Thickening of the skin in the pressure areas.
   - The podiatrist's mirror or a pedography will help in recognizing pressure sites.

The treatment of position deformities

- Suitable shoes, special factory-made or tailor-made when needed
- Skin hygiene and regular moisturizing.
- Foot exercises and walking
- Insoles giving relief of weight bearing or designed to stimulate the foot biomechanically
- Orthoses, toe splints, paddings
- Regular removal of callosities
- Surgical treatment: correction of hammer toe, removal of hallux valgus, metatarsal resections.

Superficial fungal and bacterial infections

- The diagnosis of fungal infection (13.50) should be based on fungal culture, which is performed after the healing of any bacterial infection.

- Topical treatment is applied to the spaces between the toes (imidazole or terbinafine).

- Onychomycosis and the so-called moccasin foot (tinea pedis) require oral medication (terbinafine or itraconazole) (13.50). Onychomycosis that is limited to the tip of the nail (outer one third) can be managed with amorolfine nail varnish.
- Infections eczema is often preceded by a fungal infection.
  - A pustular eczema between the toes and on the metatarsus with a sudden onset
  - Antibiotics targeted at staphylococci are started as early as possible (e.g. cephalexin 500 mg × 3).
  - Potassium permanganate baths (1:10 000) and, in the pustular phase, a cream containing corticosteroid and an antibacterial agent with a moist compress of physiological saline on top. The compress is changed or moistened every 4–6 hours.
- Paronychia (with ingrowing toenail) in a diabetic patient requires serious attention. Wrongly cut nails or tight shoes are usually the cause.
  - Antibiotics (e.g. cephalexin 500 mg × 3) are indicated in the early phase.
  - Potassium permanganate baths. Neomycin and bacitracin should be avoided because of the risk of allergy.
  - If paronychia becomes chronic, the edge of the nail should be cut and the nail root should be phenolized (13.80). Possible granulation in excavated. The procedure cannot be performed under local anaesthesia if the circulation in the foot is clearly impaired.
  - The patient is instructed to cut his nails in another way. A podiatrist can correct the growth of the nail with a spring or some other device.

Indications for hospital treatment of a foot ulcer

- A deep ulcer, which possibly extends to the bone or the joint
- Fever or poor general condition
- Cellulitis more than 2 cm diameter around an infected ulcer
- Difficult (critical) ischaemia
- The patient is unable to follow the advice for treatment of the wound
- Poor conditions for the treatment (hygiene, family situation)
- The indications for a specialist consultation are as follows:
  - The ulcer does not show signs of healing within two weeks.
  - The pulses are not palpable in the foot with the ulcer.

Treatment of a foot ulcer

- Even small injuries should be treated and followed up.
- The blood glucose level is kept as normal as possible.
- A neuropathic ulcer often arises at the site of a callus or clavus and is surrounded by hyperkeratotic skin.
  - Alleviation of the pressure load is the most important treatment.
  - The ulcer will heal in approximately 1–1.5 months with a walking cast. The treatment is carried out in a unit with experience of the condition. A deep infection requiring drainage, difficult ischaemia, broken skin on the foot or leg, severe oedema of the foot, often accompanied by poor cooperation, poor vision, problems with balance and obesity are contraindications for cast treatment.
  - An insole giving relief of weight bearing is an alternative, and can be prepared by a podiatrist or and orthopaedic technician.
- An ischaemic ulcer is situated in the tip of the toes, between the toes, at the lateral edge of the foot or on the heel. The surrounding skin is thin.
  - The possibility of vascular surgical treatment must be assessed immediately in critical ischaemia.
  - An insole giving relief of weight bearing or special shoe may be needed.
  - A walking cast treatment can also be used for an ulcer on the edge or tip of the foot.
  - The recognition of osteitis in deep ulcers is important (see later).

Topical treatment

- A hyperkeratosis around a neuropathic ulcer must be removed as often as once weekly.
- The black base of the ulcer, the necrotic tissue, is removed with pinchers and a knife or scissors. If necessary, topical anaesthetic is used.
- Healing of a purulent deep ulcer is accelerated with enzyme preparations (Varidase® or Iruxol®). These are administered in a compress of physiological saline that is changed or moistened at 8(–12)-hour intervals.
- Potassium permanganate bathing (1:10 000) is a good topical antimicrobial therapy.
- Deep wounds can be drained with dextranomer paste (e.g. Debrisan®) B [5] or with gauze (e.g. Sorbact®). After the ulcer is dry, cadexomer iodine (e.g. Iodosorb®) can be used for further treatment.

Antibiotic treatment

- Indicated at least in all ulcers reaching the muscle layer and in ulcers surrounded by infection of the soft tissue (clear redness of the skin).
- Perform the bacterial culture on the fluid excreted from tissue at the base of deep ulcers after the necrotic tissue and pus have been removed.
- The antibiotic must be effective against staphylococcus and streptococcus.
  - Cephalexin or cefadroxil 500 mg × 3 or
  - Clindamycin 150 mg × 3 or
  - Cloxacillin 500 mg × 4.

Deep infections (osteitis and cellulitis)

Osteitis

- The depth of the ulcer (the bone can be detected by a sound at the bottom of the ulcer), fistula passage and copious secretion indicate osteitis.
- The changes of osteitis become visible on the radiograph only after 2–6 weeks, sometimes even later.
- Sonding and x-ray are often adequate as primary examinations.
  - If the sound hits the bone, treat the ulcer as if it were osteitis.
  - If the bone cannot be reached by the sonde, an antibiotic is given, as in soft tissue infections. Repeat x-ray and evaluate the treatment after two weeks. If osteitis is seen on the x-ray or the ulcer is still secreting, the ulcer should be treated as osteitis.
- CRP will increase in an acute infection. In chronic osteitis, CRP is often normal and the erythrocyte sedimentation rate slightly increased.
- A specialist should be consulted regarding the treatment of osteitis.
  - In acute phase, the treatment is, for example, clindamycin 450 mg × 4 i.v. + ciprofloxacin 500 mg × 2 orally.
  - The treatment can be continued with clindamycin 150 mg × 4 orally.
  - The antibiotic treatment should be continued after clinical healing and closure of the ulcer for 1–2 months, sometimes even for years.

Cellulitis

- Cellulitis with high fever, resembling erysipelas, should always be treated in hospital with i.v. antibiotics.
  - In difficult cases the treatment is imipenem or a third generation cephalosporin + clindamycin in a central hospital.
  - In milder cases the treatment is cefuroxime 1.5 × 3 i.v. + clindamycin 150–300 mg × 4 orally in the health centre patient ward. The treatment can be continued orally (clindamycin) after the fever has decreased and the infection has subsided (CRP is useful). The total duration of the antibiotic treatment is 2–4 weeks.
  - Penicillin G (13.20) can be used in the treatment of mild erysipelas, if no diabetic neuro- or macroangiopathy is present in the patient's feet.

Charcot's neuroarthropathy

- This condition often involves rapidly progressing fragmentation of the bones, injury of the joints, a predisposition to subluxation and luxation, and can appear in a non-ischaemic foot of a patient with long-standing diabetes.
  - The first symptoms are oedema, mild pain, raised temperature and sometimes redness of the foot. Radiographic changes are visible in the late stage of the disease. A collapsed arch due to destruction of the TMT joint is typical.
- CRP and erythrocyte sedimentation rate are normal; serum alkaline phosphatase may be increased.
- The diagnosis can be verified by a bone scan, where an abundant uptake can be seen, resembling a snowball.
- The treatment is 6–9 months' immobilization with a cast and crutches.
- For treatment after amputation, see 20.94.

Treatment advice for the diabetic patient

- The shoes must be suitable.
- Minor injuries should be avoided.
- Walking bare foot outside should be avoided.
- The feet should be kept clean.
- Artificial warming is harmful.
- The nails should be treated carefully.
- Fungal infections should be prevented effectively.
- The formation of callus should be prevented.
- Regular moisturizing is important.

Quality criteria

- The completion of foot examination of the diabetic patients
- The availability of podiatric services
- The availability of specialist care
- The hospital treatment days of serious foot infections
- The number of cases requiring amputation.

References

1. Valk GD, Kriegsman DMW, Assendelft WJJ. Patient education for preventing diabetic foot ulceration. Cochrane Database Syst Rev. 2004;(2):CD001488.
2. Spencer S. Pressure relieving interventions for preventing and treating diabetic foot ulcers. Cochrane Database Syst Rev. 2004;(2):CD002302.
3. Mason J, O'Keeffe C, McIntosh A, Hutchinson A, Booth A, Young RJ. A systematic review of foot ulcer in patients with type 2 diabetes mellitus I: prevention. Diabetic Medicine 1999;16:801–812.
4. The Database of Abstracts of Reviews of Effectiveness (University of York), Database no.: DARE-992284. In: The Cochrane Library, Issue 3, 2001. Oxford: Update Software.
5. Smith J. Debridement of diabetic foot ulcers. Cochrane Database Syst Rev. 2004;(2):CD003556.

Endocrinology

Evidence Based Medicine Guidelines. Edited by the Duodecim Editorial Team
 ISBN: 0-470-01184-X

24.1 Assessment of an obese patient

Pertti Mustajoki

Basic rules

- Determine the degree of obesity
  - In adults the body mass index (BMI) is a suitable measure.
  - In children the relative weight adjusted to height given in the growth chart or age-adjusted BMI-curves are suitable measures.
  - Mild obesity does not usually necessitate treatment. Treatment is usually indicated if the BMI exceeds 30 kg/m^2. The more overweight the person is, the more active measures are necessary.
- Identify central obesity
  - The diagnosis is based on mere inspection or on measuring waist circumference or waist/hip ratio.
  - Weight reduction should be considered even in mild obesity ("overweight", BMI 25–30) if the waist circumference exceeds 102 cm in men or 88 cm in women, or if the waist/hip ratio exceeds 1.0 in men or 0.90 in women.
- Assess disorders associated with obesity.
  - Treat the patient actively if he or she has a disease that is related to obesity and that can be alleviated by weight reduction.
- Consider the patient's age when planning the treatment
  - The younger the patient the more active the treatment should be.
  - Patients above the age of 65 should be treated only if there are compelling indications.

Body mass index and waist circumference

- Weight (kg) divided by square of height (m)
  - For example, 78 kg/(1.70 m × 1.70 m) = 27.0 kg/m^2
- See Table 24.1.
- Waist circumference is measured with the patient standing. The correct place of measurement is the area between the iliac crest and the lowest rib, which is easily identified also in fairly obese patients. The measurement becomes more accurate if the right level is marked on both sides by a pen and the measure passes over these marks. In women waist circumference > 88 cm and in men > 102 cm increases considerably the risk of cardiovascular disease.

Investigating an obese patient

- Aetiology
  - The most common cause is excessive energy intake in relation to consumption.

Table 24.1 According to the WHO classification BMI 25-29.9 is "overweight" and BMI 30 or more is "obesity". In some classifications BMI 40 or more is named "morbid obesity". From clinical point of view this may be too rough, for which reason here the obesity classes are defined for every 5 BMI-units.

Index	Class	160 cm	170 cm	180 cm
<18.5	underweight	<52	<58	<65 kg
18.5–25	normal range	52–64	58–72	65–81 kg
25–30	mild obesity, "overweight"	64–77	72–87	81–97 kg
30–35	moderate obesity	77–90	87–101	97–113 kg
35–40	severe obesity	90–102	101–116	113–130 kg
>40	morbid obesity	>102	>116	>130 kg

  - Metabolic diseases are rare
    - Hypothyroidism (24.34), Cushing's syndrome (24.40), hypothalamic disorders
    - If there are no clinical signs suggesting these diseases the hormone assays need not be performed.
    - Many psychiatric drugs increase body weight.
- Associated diseases
  - Must be identified because they influence the treatment approach.
  - The most important associated diseases include
    - Diabetes
    - Hypertension
    - Sleep apnoea (loud intermittent snoring, day-time fatigue) (6.71)
    - Hyperlipidaemias
    - Menstruation disorders and/or infertility.
- Others
  - Osteoarthrosis
  - Heart failure
- Psychosocial factors
  - Binge eating is common in obese persons (uncontrolled episodes of binge eating weekly). Severe eating disorder should be treated before weight reduction is attempted.
  - Many psychosocial problems in obese persons are caused by obesity and not vice versa.
  - In a stressful life situation (economical problems, divorce etc.) weight reduction should be postponed.
  - Motivation: Is the patient ready to make personal commitment to reduce weight and willing to do permanent life style changes for maintenance.
- Habits of life
  - Interview by nurse
    - Amount and type of food, meal times, snacks, use of alcohol
    - Eating behaviour: evening and night meals, eating for sorrow, binge eating
    - Type and amount of exercise.
- Laboratory investigations

- Blood pressure, fasting blood glucose, serum cholesterol, HDL cholesterol, and triglycerides are determined to screen for associated diseases.

24.2 Treatment of obesity

Pertti Mustajoki

Assessment of the need of treatment

- Overweight (mild obesity): body mass index (BMI) 25–30 kg/m^2
  - Usually no treatment is indicated.
  - Treatment (A) [1,2] is indicated in central obesity, metabolic syndrome (23.36), or non-insulin-dependent diabetes.
  - In children even mild obesity should be treated.
- Moderate obesity: BMI 30–35 kg/m^2
  - Treatment (A) [1,2] is always indicated if the patient has diabetes, hypertension, hyperlipidaemia, or other associated disease (B) [3,4].
  - A young obese person with good health should be treated. The treatment of middle-aged persons is decided individually according to the available resources.
- Severe obesity: BMI > 35 kg/m^2
  - Must always be treated.

Selecting the method of treatment

1. Basic treatment consisting of a gradual and permanent change in living habits by counselling and guidance.
   - Well suited for patients with mild and moderate obesity, and for the majority of patients with severe obesity; **should always be included in other forms of conservative treatment.**
2. Basic treatment and a very low calorie diet
   - Well suited for morbid and severe obesity.
   - A choice in moderate obesity if the basic treatment has been unsuccessful and there is a strong indication for reducing weight (associated diseases).
3. Drugs (orlistat or sibutramine)
   - Do not automatically help all patients.
   - An alternative especially if other approaches have been failed.
   - Life-style counselling must also be included.
4. Surgical treatment
   - Suitable only for selected patients with morbid obesity (see criteria below).

Basic treatment

Organisation

- **Group treatment** is less costly and as effective as individualised treatment
  - At least 10 meetings are arranged with about one-week intervals.
  - The group leader is a nurse or a dietician with special training in the treatment of obesity.

Goals that can be measured

- **The optimal rate of weight reduction is 0.5 kg/week.** As the adipose tissue contains about 30 MJ (7000 kcal)/kg a daily reduction of 2100 kJ (500 kcal) in the energy intake will result in this rate of weight reduction.
- The goal is to reduce weight by 5–10%, which already results in significant benefit in the treatment of diseases associated with obesity.
- A permanent result is always aimed at. This means that the changes in living habits must be permanent.
- In growing children weight should be kept constant so that the growth of height corrects the relative weight.
- There are many treatments with no proven efficacy. Appetite-suppressant drugs may result in a moderate weight reduction but the effect is transient.

Aims and contents of counselling

- Changes in knowledge and attitudes
  - Human energy consumption is reduced if the body weight is reduced. In order to sustain the weight that has been achieved **the changes in living habits must be permanent.**
- Changes in meals (A) [5,6]
  - Find out the present contents of meals.
  - Reduce intake by about 2000 kJ (500 kcal) daily.
  - The main emphasis is on the reduction of fat intake (B) [7].
  - Remember alcohol as a cause of obesity.
  - Small daily changes are effective in the long run.
  - Keep three daily meals.
- Changes in physical exercise (A) [5,6]
  - The advice depends on the degree of obesity.
  - Exercise during daily activities should be encouraged (climbing up stairs, walking or cycling to work.)
- Changes in eating behaviour
  - The most common goal is to change behaviour, not to "hunt kilograms".
  - Identify the circumstances that trigger eating.
  - Reduce temptations (no food in sight!).
  - Do nothing else when eating (such as watch TV, read magazines.)
  - Eat slowly.

Very low calorie diet (VLCD)

- Constituents

- 1700–2100 kJ (400–500 kcal) of energy, a maximum of 3300 kJ (800 kcal) daily
- Protein as needed (at least 50 g daily)
- Essential fatty acids, trace elements and vitamins as needed

♦ Schedule

- Ready-made commercial formulas should be used as the only food continuously for 8–10 weeks in severe obesity, and for a shorter period in milder obesity, but usually for a minimum of 6 weeks.
- The patient is followed up at 1–2 week intervals.
- Suitable for patients with non-insulin-dependent (type 2) diabetes and hypertension. Insulin treatment is stopped or the dose is reduced considerably, and the dose of sulphonylureas is halved (risk of hypoglycaemia!) before starting VLCD. The doses of other drugs need not be reduced.
- The rate of weight reduction is about 1.5–2 kg/week, and the short-term weight reduction is 2–2.5 times that on basic treatment.
- A VLCD alone does not yield permanent results. Basic treatment for permanent life-style changes is applied in the normal fashion.

Weight-reducing drugs

- ♦ Orlistat **B** [8, 9] is a lipase inhibitor. The most common side effects are bloating and diarrhoea after fatty meals.
- ♦ Sibutramine **A** [10, 11] is a centrally acting appetite suppressant. Side effects are slight increase of blood pressure and pulse rate, dry mouth and constipation.
- ♦ With both drugs mean weight reduction is 4–5 kg better than with placebo.
- ♦ Stopping of a drug leads to relapse, i.e. permanent result needs continuous use.
- ♦ Do not use alone. Life-style counselling is always needed, and with orlistat reduction of food fat content is mandatory.
- ♦ Drugs are not a firsthand treatment of obesity. They can be used if other approaches have failed.
- ♦ If no significant weight reduction can be seen over 2–3 months, stop the drug.

Surgical treatment

Criteria

- ♦ Age below 60 years.
- ♦ BMI at least 35–40 kg/m^2.
- ♦ An efficient conservative treatment strategy has been tried.
- ♦ The patient is cooperative.
- ♦ There is no abuse of alcohol or drugs.

Method

- ♦ Gastroplasty, gastric banding **B** [12, 13, 14, 15, 16, 17] or gastric bypass so that the patient can eat only slowly and small amounts at a time. There are several surgical techniques, including laparoscopic procedures.
- ♦ The operation is not sufficient alone. Adequate preoperative investigations, patient counselling, and organized follow-up are mandatory.
- ♦ The outcome of successful surgical treatment is much better than that of conservative treatment **A** [18, 19, 20, 21, 22, 23, 24, 25, 26, 27, 28]: the patients reduce 30–40 kg of their weight, and the result is long lasting **A** [1, 2].
- ♦ Some patients experience complications after surgery.

References

1. Glenny A, O´Meara S. Systematic review of interventions in the treatment and prevention of obesity. CRD Report 1997;10:1–149.
2. The Database of Abstracts of Reviews of Effectiveness (University of York), Database no.: DARE-971098. In: The Cochrane Library, Issue 4, 1999. Oxford: Update Software.
3. Douketis JD, Feightner JW, Attia J, Feldman WF. Periodic health examination, 1999 update: 1. detection, prevention and treatment of obesity. Canadian Medical Association Journal 1999;160:513–525.
4. The Database of Abstracts of Reviews of Effectiveness (University of York), Database no.: DARE-998429. In: The Cochrane Library, Issue 3, 2000. Oxford: Update Software.
5. Miller W, Koceja DM, Hamilton EJ. A meta-analysis of the past 25 years of weight loss research using diet, exercise or diet plus exercise intervention. Int J Obesity 1997;21: 941–947.
6. The Database of Abstracts of Reviews of Effectiveness (University of York), Database no.: DARE-971214. In: The Cochrane Library, Issue 4, 1999. Oxford: Update Software.
7. Pirozzo S, Summerbell C, Cameron C, Glasziou P. Advice on low-fat diets for obesity. Cochrane Database Syst Rev. 2004;(2):CD003640.
8. Development and Evaluation Committee. Orlistat for the treatment of obesity. Southampton: Wessex Institute for Health Research and Development. Wessex Institute for Health Research and Development. DEC Report No. 101. 1999.
9. The Health Technology Assessment Database, Database no.: HTA-20008151. In: The Cochrane Library, Issue 1, 2001. Oxford: Update Software.
10. McNeely W, Goa KL. Sibutramine: a review of its contribution to the management of obesity. Drugs 1998;56:1093–1124.
11. The Database of Abstracts of Reviews of Effectiveness (University of York), Database no.: DARE-990113. In: The Cochrane Library, Issue 3, 2001. Oxford: Update Software.
12. Schneider WL. Laparoscopic adjustable gastric banding for clinically severe (morbid) obesity. Edmonton, AB, Canada: Alberta Heritage Foundation for Medical Research. Health Technology As. 2000.33.
13. The Database of Abstracts of Reviews of Effectiveness (University of York), Database no.: DARE-20018109. In: The Cochrane Library, Issue 3, 2002. Oxford: Update Software.

14. Chapman A, Game P, O'Brien P, Maddern G, Kiroff G, Foster B, Ham J. A systematic review of laparoscopic adjustable gastric banding for the treatment of obesity (update and re-appraisal). Australian Safety and Efficacy Register of New Interventional Procedures - Surgical (ASERNIP-S). 2002. 149. Australian Safety and Efficacy Register of New Interventional Procedures - Surgical (ASERNIP-S). www.surgeons.org/asernip-s/.
15. Health Technology Assessment Database: HTA-20030005. The Cochrane Library, Issue 1, 2004. Chichester, UK: John Wiley & Sons, Ltd.
16. Newer techniques in bariatric surgery for morbid obesity. Chicago IL: Blue Cross Blue Shield Association Assessment Program, Vol. 18, No. 10, September 2003. Blue Cross Blue Shield Association (BCBS). www.bcbs.com.
17. Health Technology Assessment Database: HTA-20031130. The Cochrane Library, Issue 1, 2004. Chichester, UK: John Wiley & Sons, Ltd.
18. Colquitt J, Clegg A, Sidhu M, Royle P. Surgery for morbid obesity. Cochrane Database Syst Rev. 2004;(2):CD003641.
19. Clegg A J, Colquitt J, Sidhu M K, Royle P, Loveman E, Walker A. The clinical effectiveness and cost-effectiveness of surgery for people with morbid obesity: a systematic review and economic evaluation. Health Technology Assessment Vol.6: No.12. 2002. 153. The National Coordinating Centre for Health Technology Assessment (NCCHTA) on behalf of Southampton Health Technology Assessments Centre(SHTAC), Southampton. www.ncchta.org.
20. Health Technology Assessment Database: HTA-20020727. The Cochrane Library, Issue 1, 2004. Chichester, UK: John Wiley & Sons, Ltd.
21. Special report: the relationship between weight loss and changes in morbidity following bariatric surgery for morbid obesity. Chicago IL: Blue Cross Blue Shield Association. 2003. 25. Blue Cross Blue Shield Association (BCBS). www.bcbs.com.
22. Health Technology Assessment Database: HTA-20031129. The Cochrane Library, Issue 1, 2004. Chichester, UK: John Wiley & Sons, Ltd.
23. Gastric restrictive surgery for morbid obesity. Bloomington, MN: Institute for Clinical Systems Improvement (ICSI). 2000. Institute for Clinical Systems Improvement (ICSI). www.icsi.org.
24. Health Technology Assessment Database: HTA-20030550. The Cochrane Library, Issue 1, 2004. Chichester, UK: John Wiley & Sons, Ltd.
25. Newer techniques in bariatric surgery for morbid obesity. Chicago IL: Blue Cross Blue Shield Association Assessment Program, Vol. 18, No. 10, September 2003. Blue Cross Blue Shield Association (BCBS). www.bcbs.com.
26. Health Technology Assessment Database: HTA-20031130. The Cochrane Library, Issue 1, 2004. Chichester, UK: John Wiley & Sons, Ltd.
27. Nilsen E M. Surgery for morbid obesity. Oslo: The Norwegian Centre for Health Technology Assessment (SMM). 2003. The Norwegian Centre for Health Technology Assessment (SMM).
28. Health Technology Assessment Database: HTA-20030502. The Cochrane Library, Issue 1, 2004. Chichester, UK: John Wiley & Sons, Ltd.

24.10 Hypokalaemia

Editors

Basic rules

- The potassium level of patients using diuretics, particularly the elderly, should be monitored yearly (to detect either hypo- or hyperkalaemia).
- Identify and correct hypokalaemia in patients with diarrhoea and vomiting.
- If the patient has unexplained hypokalaemia remember renal diseases, subtle vomiting and bulimia as well as primary aldosteronism, i.e. Conn's syndrome.
- Consider magnesium deficiency as a cause of therapy-resistant hypokalaemia.

Reference values

- Serum potassium 3.5–5.1 mmol/l
- 24-hour urine potassium 60–90 mmol/l
- Note the reference value of the particular laboratory you are using (there is a difference between plasma and serum reference values).

END

Aetiology

- Diuretics
  - The most common cause of hypokalaemia: often mild in patients treated in primary care.
  - To prevent hypokalaemia associated with diuretic therapy: if the patient has serum potassium < 3.7 mmol/l, cardiac disease or uses digoxin, combine a potassium chloride or potassium-sparing diuretic (usually amiloride, triamterene, spironolactone). After starting diuretics determine serum potassium after 1–3 months, and thereafter annually.
  - Concurrent use of ACE inhibitors prevents hypokalaemia.
- Eating disorders
  - If a young, healthy woman has normal blood pressure and unexplained hypokalaemia, the most probable diagnosis is vomiting associated with bulimia (34.10) or anorexia nervosa (34.10), possibly also the use of laxatives (hypokalaemic, hypochloraemic alkalosis, 24-hour urine chloride is low).
  - Alcoholism and/or malnourishment.
  - Licorice syndrome: the patient is often a young woman presenting with high blood pressure and low serum potassium and plasma renin and aldosterone.
- Gastroenteritis

- Because patients with vomiting and diarrhoea may lose considerable amounts of potassium, monitor serum potassium and sodium in such patients.

♦ Renal diseases

- In particular, tubular disorders are associated with hypokalaemia; usually renal failure leads to hyperkalaemia.

♦ Rare diseases, often with hypertension, that usually require specialist consultation for diagnosis and treatment.

- **Primary aldosteronism** (24.41) caused by an aldosterone-producing adrenocortical adenoma or (rarely) carcinoma. A clue to the diagnosis is a combination of hypertension and hyperkalaemia (without diuretic treatment) or marked tendency to hypokalaemia in patients on diuretics.
- **Secondary hyperaldosteronism** is associated with heart failure, cirrhosis of the liver and renovascular hypertension and relevant medication.
- **Cushing's syndrome** (24.40)

Symptoms of hypokalaemia

♦ In patients with mild hypokalaemia (serum potassium > 3 mmol/l) symptoms are usually associated with the underlying disease.

♦ Fatigue and muscular weakness occur in more severe hypokalaemia.

♦ ECG abnormalities occur at serum potassium levels below 3 mmol/l: Flattening or inversion of the T wave, emergence of a prominent U wave, which may resemble the T wave (and give the impression of a prolonged QT interval). The condition may result in severe ventricular arrhythmias particularly in patients using digoxin and in those with severe cardiac disease.

Further investigations

♦ Further investigations are indicated if the cause of hypokalaemia is not evident on the basis of the underlying disease and medication.

♦ Initial investigations include serum sodium and creatinine, ECG and blood pressure.

♦ 24-hour urine potassium, sodium and chloride

- Normal or increased potassium excretion (24-h urine potassium > 30 mmol) despite a low serum potassium concentration with a diet rich in sodium (a sodium excretion of 200 mmol/24 h) suggests hyperaldosteronism or renal hyperkalaemia.
- If 24-hour urine potassium excretion is low, potassium loss occurs via another route (the gastrointestinal tract).

♦ Hypertension associated with hypokalaemia suggests hyperaldosteronism, hypercortisolism, renal hypertension or licorice syndrome.

♦ A low 24-hour chloride excretion suggests vomiting.

Treatment

♦ The intensity of treatment depends on whether the hypokalaemia is acute or chronic.

♦ Serum potassium > 3 mmol/l

- Oral substitution is usually sufficient.
- The dose is 2–4 g/day unless the patient is losing a lot of potassium continuously.
- Potassium tablets may cause gastric irritation. In such cases a liquid form should be tried.

♦ Serum potassium < 3 mmol/l irrespective of aetiology

- Serum potassium below 2.5 mmol/l corresponds to a deficiency of 200–400 mmol in the body.
- For substitution infuse 40–80 mmol/day in 5% glucose or (0.45%) saline. Because of the risk or arrhythmias, a higher dose may be necessary.
  - 40–60 mmol of potassium chloride can be added to one litre of infusion fluid when infusing via a peripheral vein. The maximum infusion rate is 20 mmol/h. If necessary, a central venous catheter can be applied.
- Adjust the dosage according to serum potassium levels.

♦ Diarrhoea and vomiting in a child

- See article 32.23.

♦ A patient on diuretics whose serum potassium is not sufficiently corrected by adequate substitution

- Consider adding magnesium (24.14) (a combination of potassium chloride–magnesium hydroxide is available).
- Serum magnesium can be determined but the result does not reliably mirror body magnesium balance, as most magnesium, like potassium, is in the intracellular space.
- Remember to rule out hyperaldosteronism.

24.11 Hyperkalaemia

Editors

Basic rules

♦ Monitor serum potassium in patients using potassium preparations, potassium-sparing diuretics, ACE inhibitors or angiotensin II receptor blockers (ARB).

♦ Hyperkalaemia is often present in renal failure.

♦ Avoid false diagnosis of hyperkalaemia associated with haemolysis, thrombocytosis, leucocytosis, or prolonged stasis during blood sampling, which lowers the sample pH.

Reference values

- Serum potassium 3.5–5.1 mmol/l
- 24-hour urine potassium 60–90 mmol

Aetiology of hyperkalaemia

- Renal failure
  - Hyperkalaemia is nearly always present in acute renal failure.
  - In chronic renal failure serum potassium remains within the reference limits for a long time because of compensatory mechanisms.
  - Remember obstructive uropathy as a cause for hyperkalaemia.
- Diuretics
  - Spironolactone may cause severe hyperkalaemia, particularly if the patient is taking ACE inhibitors or potassium.
  - Other potassium-sparing diuretics (amiloride, triamterene) are always combined with a thiazide or furosemide. Even these preparations may cause hyperkalaemia if the patient has renal failure.
- ACE inhibitors and ARB
  - Serum potassium increases slightly. In the elderly the increase may be significant if the patient has renal disease. Diabetics may also be susceptible.
- NSAIDs in renal disease
- Severe systemic diseases resulting in acidosis
  - Acute circulatory failure
  - Tissue hypoxia
  - Extensive trauma
  - Rhabdomyolysis
- Addison's disease
  - Hyperkalaemia is often associated with dark skin pigmentation, low blood pressure and many systemic symptoms (24.42).

Symptoms of hyperkalaemia

- ECG
  - High T waves with serum potassium values in the range 5.5–6 mmol/l
  - Widened QRS complex and disappearance of P waves in severe hyperkalaemia (up to 7–8 mmol/l).
  - The risk of ventricular fibrillation and asystole is increased in severe hyperkalaemia.
- Muscle weakness
  - Similar to hypokalaemia

Treatment of hyperkalaemia

- Serum potassium < 6 mmol/l, no ECG changes
  - Discontinue potassium preparations and drugs causing hyperkalaemia.
  - Rehydrate, if necessary.
- Serum potassium 6–7.5 mmol/l, high T wave in ECG
  - Treat the underlying cause.
  - 20–50 g of a cationic exchange resin mixed with drinks is administered 3–4 times a day.
  - If urgent treatment is indicated, dissolve 50 g of the resin in water and administer as an enema. Leave the resin in the rectum for 30 minutes.
- Serum potassium > 7.5 mmol/l or widened QRS complex, atrioventricular block, or ventricular arrhythmias
  - Infuse 50–100 ml of 7.5% sodium bicarbonate intravenously over 5 minutes. Repeat after 10–15 minutes if necessary.
  - Infuse glucose with insulin: 200–500 ml of 10% glucose with 5 units/100 ml of rapid-acting insulin is infused over 30–60 min. 5% glucose should be infused next in order to prevent hypoglycaemia.
  - 10% calcium gluconate antagonizes the cardiac effects of potassium (10–30 ml slowly i.v.). Digitalized patients are treated with extreme caution. Note! The drug must be administered via another route than $NaHCO_3$ (calcium carbonate will precipitate).
  - Hyponatraemic or hypovolaemic patients can be given 2.5% NaCl solution at the rate of 200–400 ml/30 min to prevent cardiotoxic effects of potassium (contraindicated in oliguria, heart failure and severe hypertension).
  - Cationic exchange resin in given as instructed above.
  - NaCl fluid therapy and furosemide (20–40 mg i.v.)
  - If necessary, haemo- or peritoneal dialysis, especially if the patient has renal failure or rhabdomyolysis.
  - Serum potassium should be monitored after treatment, at the latest on the next day.
- Chronic hyperkalaemia
  - Furosemide is the treatment of choice if hyperkalaemia is caused by renal failure.
  - ACE inhibitors and spironolactone are avoided.

END

24.12 Hyponatraemia

Markku Ellonen

Goals

- Consider hyponatraemia as a cause of obscure fatigue, convulsions, confusion or even unconsciousness. Both hyponatraemia and mismanagement of the condition may be dangerous to the patient.
- Avoid iatrogenic hyponatraemia: hypotonic hydration of a seriously ill patient may lead to severe hyponatraemia.
- Avoid too rapid correction of hyponatraemia (risk of central pontine demyelinization).

- Thiazide diuretics are the most common cause of the syndrome of inappropriate antidiuretic hormone (SIADH). The risk patient is an elderly small woman using thiazide; giving water to drink or infusing hyponatraemic solutions may cause severe hyponatraemia.

General

- Hyponatraemia is seldom caused by sodium deficiency. Most often the cause is excess water.
- Mild hyponatraemia (serum sodium approximately 125–135 mmol/l) is a fairly common accidental finding in patients with severe heart disease. The prevalence increases with age and the number of diseases and is suggestive of poor prognosis. Adding salt to food is of no benefit.
- The patient is considered to have hyponatraemia when sodium is below 125 mmol/l. The condition is considered severe when sodium is below 115 mEq/l.
- There are several obscure and complicated mechanisms to hyponatraemia. Some are idiopathic.
- Iatrogenic hyponatraemia is caused by hypotonic hydration of a patient p.o. or i.v. with diminished water diuresis capacity.
- Hyponatraemia may follow from excessive drinking combined with desmopressin therapy (nocturia in children and the elderly).
- Excessive drinking of fluids by athletes during prolonged exercise.
- Mild hyponatraemia is usually corrected by treating the primary cause, if the condition is treatable.

Normal values

- Serum sodium 135–145 mEq/l
- Serum osmolality 285–300 mOsm/kg H_2O

Causes

- The aetiology is most often evident immediately. In some cases finding out the underlying cause can be a difficult clinical problem and some even remain idiopathic.
- The most common mechanism of hyponatraemia is the retention of fluid in the body, when the patient is normo- to hypervolaemic. Loss of salts is a rarer cause. In these cases the patient is hypovolaemic and hypotonic (urine sodium < 20 mmol/l, physiological saline corrects hyponatraemia).
- Heavy drinking of alcohol often leads to symptomatic hyponatrenia and hypokalaemia.

Retention of water (hyper- or normovolaemic patient)

- The syndrome of inappropriate antidiuretic hormone secretion (SIADH) is mainly caused by a thiazide-amiloridine diuretic with simultaneous polydipsia. The patient at risk is an elderly slender woman. Carbamazepin is the second most common cause of SIADH. More rare causes of SIADH include chemotherapeutic agents, neuroleptics and antidepressants, also SSRI.
- The most common diseases causing SIADH are pneumonia and lung cancer. Rarer diseases include other malignancies, CNS disorders. Postoperative state and anaesthesia are very common causes of mild hyponatraemia.
- SIADH often remains idiopathic.
- The most common serious diseases causing hyponatraemia by retention of water and salt are congestive heart failure, cirrhosis and nephrotic syndrome. Tendency for retention of water and sodium is associated with these conditions, suggesting poor prognosis. Accompanying hyponatraemia is usually asymptomatic and not severe. Large doses of furosemide are often used to treat these conditions; however, it is not considered the cause of hyponatraemia. Activated renin-angiotensin-aldosterone system increases the secretion of anti-diuretic hormone (ADH).
- Water intoxication (acute polydipsia) is usually psychogenic. Low urine osmolality (<150 mOsm/kg) and polyuria suggest polydipsia.

Sodium depletion (hypovolaemic patient)

- Renal loss of sodium: diuretics, glucocorticoid deficiency (Addison's disease), osmotic diuresis of severe hyperglycaemia; urine sodium > 20 mmol/l.
- Extrarenal causes: diarrhoea, vomiting, burns.

Symptoms

- Neurological symptoms usually appear when serum sodium falls below 115 mEq/l. The severity of symptoms depends on how rapidly the condition develops.
- If the change in sodium concentration is rapid, symptoms may occur already at Na values of 125 mEq/l.
  - Symptoms of elevated intracranial pressure: confusion, headache, nausea, vomiting, and lethargy progressing to unconsciousness and convulsions.
- The symptoms of slowly developed or chronic hyponatraemia are vague and mild. The patient may be only fatigued and confused.

Diagnosis

- History: drugs, vomiting, diarrhoea, thirst, water drinking, urine volume and mental health (polydipsia).
- Clinical evaluation: hyper-, normo- or hypovolaemia.
- Initial laboratory tests: Serum sodium, potassium, creatinine and blood glucose. Later tests: Serum and urine osmolality, urine sodium. Clearly elevated triglyceride or paraproteinaemia causes pseudohyponatraemia where serum osmolality is normal.
  - Elevated serum potassium is a sign of glucocorticoid deficiency.
  - Elevated serum creatinine is a sign of renal disease or hypovolaemia.

Table 24.12 Differential diagnosis of hyponatraemia

Urine sodium secretion	Hypovolaemia	Normo- or hypervolaemia
	Lack of salt	Decreased effective plasma volume
<20 mmol/l	♦ vomiting ♦ diarrhoea	♦ cirrhosis of the liver ♦ nephrotic syndrome ♦ heart failure
	Renal salt loss	
>20 mmol/l	♦ diuretics ♦ mineralocorticoid deficiency ♦ renal disease ♦ osmotic diuresis	♦ over-excretion of ADH ♦ glucocorticoid deficiency ♦ hypothyroidism ♦ thiazides

- Very high blood glucose decreases serum sodium: a 5 mmol/l elevation in glucose lowers sodium by 2 mmol/l.
- Urine sodium is important in diagnosing the aetiology of hyponatraemia (urine sodium < 20 mmol/l suggests hypovolaemia).
- Serum osmolality is lowered in true hyponatraemia. It can be calculated as follows: S-osmol = 2 × serum Na + blood glucose. A value below 275 mOsm/l is of clinical importance.
- Urine osmolality < 150 mOsm/kg in hyponatraemia suggests polydipsia.
- Diagnosis of hyponatraemia, see Table 24.12

Principles of therapy

Hyponatraemia with neurological symptoms (water intoxication)

- Infusing hypertonic NaCl solution (3% = 513 mmol/l) at the rate of 0.05 ml/kg/min (150 ml/h/50 kg) corrects serum Na by 1–2 mEq/h. The correction may be carried out with half the rate if water intoxication has developed slowly. Serum sodium may not rise by more than 24 mmol in two days.
- Combine furosemide (40–80 mg i.v.) to infusion for rapid diuresis.
- Serum Na is raised only to the level 120–125 mmol/l. Thereafter treatment of the basic cause usually normalizes hyponatraemia.
- Rapid correction is stopped when neurological symptoms alleviate.
- Do not correct a slowly developed hyponatraemia too rapidly as this will aggravate neurological symptoms.

Accidentally detected hyponatraemia with mild symptoms

- The condition has usually developed slowly.
- Sodium is usually over 120 mmol/l. The condition does not require active management, but rather diagnostic work-up.
- A patient with SIADH is often hypervolaemic. Manage by treating the underlying cause, by stopping medication (thiazide!) and by restricting water intake to 500–700 ml/day.
- Heart failure combined with high doses of diuretics causes mild-scale hyponatraemia with serum sodium at the level 125–130 mmol/l. The condition may be corrected by adding an ACE inhibitor to drug therapy.
- In addition to oedema, mild hyponatraemia (130 mmol/l), which is considered a sign of poor prognosis, is often associated with severe heart failure, cirrhosis and nephrotic syndrome. (It needs no treatment.) The condition is reversed by treating the underlying cause, if possible.
- In Addison's disease and other corticoid deficiencies the patient is hypovolaemic and hypotonic (rarely has neurological symptoms). The condition is treated with physiological NaCl solution and corticoids.
- In central hypocortisolism, hyponatraemia results from disturbance in water excretion and is corrected with corticosteroids.
- Salt loss (diarrhoea, vomiting) is substituted for with 0.9% sodium chloride often with additional potassium.

Follow-up and prophylaxis

- Monitor symptoms, fluid balance, serum potassium and sodium.
- Acute cases require management in hospital and frequent follow-up.
- Thiazide-induced hyponatraemia has a high probability of recurrence, because the drug causes a sense of thirst is these patients with consequent polydipsia. Thiazide should not be started again in these patients.
- Patients at risk for thiazide-induced SIADH are often slender elderly women. Mild and almost symptomless SIADH is common in the elderly. The condition becomes symptomatic if hypotonic fluids are administered in large amounts.
- Drinking ample amounts of water may be dangerous for risk patients (elderly patients on thiazide, carbamazepine or desmopressin).
- Iatrogenic hyponatraemia
  - Desmopressin used for nocturia in children and the elderly may lead to water intoxication if the patient drinks much.
  - Routine infusion of hypotonic fluids after surgery is dangerous: because of SIADH, the patient is unable to excrete the water excess.
  - May lead to severe brain damage. The risk of hyponatraemia is avoided:
    - by identifying risk patients (slender elderly patients, those on thiazide, carbamazepine or desmopressin)
    - by avoiding routine use of hypotonic fluids without serum sodium determination
    - by considering hyponatraemia as a possible aetiology in confusion and other cerebral symptoms.

24.13 Hypernatraemia

Editors

Basic rule

- Prevent hypernatraemia by adequate fluid therapy in patients with fluid loss.
- Ensure that fluid intake (1.5–2 l/day) is monitored in elderly patients with inadequate thirst control.

Reference values

- Serum sodium 136–146 mmol/l
- 24-hour urine sodium excretion 150–220 mmol

Symptoms of hypernatraemia

- Thirst, dehydration, hypotension
- From the central nervous system: confusion, somnolence, loss of consciousness, convulsions.

Causes of hypernatraemia

- Insufficient fluid intake (the elderly and demented patients)
- Fluid loss through the skin
  - Perspiration, fever, burns
- Fluid loss through the gastrointestinal tract
  - Vomiting, diarrhoea (salt loss is often associated)
- Fluid loss by the kidneys
  - Diabetes insipidus, rarely hypernatraemia if the patient is allowed to drink water
  - Disturbances of thirst control (dementia).
  - Low urine osmolality (<300) in a hypernatraemic patient suggests diabetes insipidus.

Treatment

- Water deficiency can be calculated quantitatively from the equation $0.6 \times$ weight (kg) $\times 1 - (140/\text{S-Na})$.
- 5% glucose or hypotonic (0.45%) fluid is administered perorally or intravenously, for example 200 ml/h. If blood pressure is low, start with 0.9% saline. The ideal correction rate is 1 mmol/h and 10 mmol over the first 24 hours.
- **Excessively rapid fluid administration may worsen the central nervous system injury caused by hypernatraemia.**

24.14 Magnesium deficiency

Markku Ellonen

Essential

- The significance of magnesium deficiency and its therapy is a debated issue. The significance of magnesium is obscured by its complicated relationship with other electrolytes (K, Na, Ca) and the acid-base balance.
- Only 2% of total body magnesium is in the serum, which makes it difficult to use serum magnesium as a measure of magnesium deficiency. Low serum magnesium usually signifies deficiency of total body magnesium. Normal serum magnesium does not rule out deficiency. The reference value of serum magnesium is 0.7–1.1 mmol/l.
- The most important physiological significance of magnesium is its calcium antagonist action in nerve tissue.

Causes of magnesium deficiency

- Use of large doses of diuretics; amiloride, triamteren and spironolactone spare magnesium.
- Diarrhoea, malabsorption, nasogastric suction
- Prolonged fluid therapy and parenteral nutrition
- Alcoholism
- Poorly controlled diabetes with excessive diuresis.

Conditions probably associated with magnesium deficiency

- Therapy-resistant arrhythmias (including atrial fibrillation)
- Hypokalaemia, hyponatraemia, hypocalcaemia
- Muscle weakness, leg cramps, tetany, tremor, accelerated reflexes.

Treatment

- Indications for treatment have not been established. Magnesium deficiency is considered an under-diagnosed condition.
- Treat the underlying cause.
- The peroral or parenteral dose is 10–50 mmol/day.
- Patients on parenteral nutrition need substitution with 4–8 mmol/day.
- Hypokalaemia caused by diuretics can sometimes be corrected only by adding magnesium.
- Magnesium is used in the following conditions without confirmed magnesium deficiency: eclampsia (the effectiveness is proven), arrhythmias, leg cramps. Magnesium is no longer used in the acute phase of myocardial infarction.

Reference values

- Serum magnesium 0.7–1.0 mmol/l

24.20 Hypocalcaemia, hypoparathyroidism and vitamin D deficiency

Editors

Basic rules

- Make sure that the patient does not have pseudohypocalcaemia caused by hypoalbuminaemia (when serum albumin is reduced by 10 g/l, serum calcium in reduced by 0.2 mmol/l. This explains why mild asymptomatic hypocalcaemia is associated with severe diseases and malnutrition; in these cases the level of serum ionized calcium is normal).
- Start a slow infusion of intravenous calcium in patients with evident symptoms of acute hypocalcaemia (tetany, long QT interval on the ECG) without waiting for laboratory results.
- Determine and treat the cause of hypocalcaemia.

Aetiology of hypocalcaemia

Hypoparathyroidism

- Parathormone deficiency
  - Usually postoperative after thyroid or parathyroid surgery.
  - Rarely a familial disease as a component of the APECED (autoimmune polyendocrinopathy-candidiasis-ectodermal dystrophy) syndrome (24.63)

Deficiency of vitamin D

- Leads to secondary hyperparathyroidism and osteomalacia. Mild deficiency (25-(OH)-D-vit < 37 nmol/l) increases the risk of osteoporosis (reference values are 25–125 nmol/l; concentration varies greatly with the time of year).
- Causes in adults
  - Lack of sunlight and poor diet (in institutionalized elderly people)
  - Coeliac disease, malnutrition
- Phenytoin and carbamazepine used in the treatment of epilepsy may cause or worsen vitamin D deficiency by inducing its metabolism.
- Abnormal metabolism of vitamin D (hepatic disease, renal insufficiency)
- Symptoms include bone pain, muscular weakness, fractures, deformities.
- Prophylaxis: 600–800 IU/day of vitamin D to institutionalized elderly.

Renal insufficiency

- Active production of vitamin D (1,25OH)2-D-vitamin, calcitriol) decreases. This results in hypocalcaemia and secondary hyperparathyroidism, which is treated with calcium carbonate and alphacalcidol (10.21).

Other rare causes

- Magnesium deficiency
- Convalescent phase of a metabolic bone disease (great need for calcium after an operation of the thyroid gland)
- Septicaemia, shock, pancreatitis and other severe diseases requiring intensive care.

Symptoms for hypocalcaemia

- Usually symptomless when serum calcium ion > 0.8 mmol/l.
- Tetany, muscle cramps (finger paresthesia, cramps in the hands, face and larynx)
- Paraesthesias
- Brisk tendon reflexes
- The Chvostek sign: Buccal muscle spasm can be elicited by snapping the cheek lightly with a reflex hammer.
- The Trousseau sign: The pressure in a blood pressure cuff is raised slightly above systolic blood pressure while the patient hyperventilates. A tetanic spasm can be observed in the hand after 2–3 minutes.
- Encephalopathy, psychiatric symptoms, papilloedema are possible symptoms of severe disease
- Changes on the ECG: prolonged QT interval; arrhythmias; QT interval measurement can be helpful in diagnostics!

Differential diagnosis of hypocalcaemia

- See Table 24.20.

Treatment

Patients with acute symptoms (often following thyroid gland operation)

- The symptoms depend on the rapidity of development of the condition (after thyroid or parathyroid surgery, in association with pancreatitis).
- 10 ml of 10% calcium gluconate should be infused intravenously over at least 10 minutes.

Table 24.20 Differential diagnosis of hypercalcaemia

	Serum phosphate	Serum alkaline phosphatase	Serum parathormone (PTH)	24-hour urine calcium
Hypoparathyroidism	Increased	Normal	Decreased	Normal/decr.
Osteomalacia	Decreased	Increased	Increased	Decreased
Renal insufficiency	Normal/ increased	Normal/ increased	Increased	Decreased

- If necessary, give a continuous infusion (100 ml 10% calcium gluconate in 1 l 5% glucose at a rate of 10–15 drops/min).
- A calcium infusion can be started without waiting for laboratory results in a patient with clinically suspected hypocalcaemia (tetany).

Chronic hypocalcaemia in hypoparathyroidism

- If serum calcium is above 1.8 mmol, prescribe calcium salts at a dose of 1–3 g of calcium/day.
- Severe hypocalcaemia should be treated with derivatives of vitamin D in addition to calcium salts.
  - The initial dose of dihydrotachysterol is 1–2 mg/day, and the maintenance dose is 0.2–0.6 mg/day. A specialist should start treatment for severe hypoparathyroidism.
- The target level of serum calcium is 2.00–2.25 mmol/l; higher levels are associated with the risk of hypercalciuria.
- Avoid rapid changes in treatment. Take care not to induce hypercalcaemia (which can be triggered by adding dihydrotachysterol in the medication).
- Avoid hypercalciuria (renal calculi, nephrocalcinosis).
- A stable diet (milk products).
- Regular laboratory tests should be performed monthly at first, then at 2–3 month intervals, and later at 6-month intervals.
  - Serum calcium, 24-hour urine calcium excretion (for the assessment of risk of nephrocalcinosis) and serum magnesium should be determined.
- Inform the patient about the symptoms of hypercalcaemia (nausea, obstipation, abdominal pain, fatigue, headache, thirst, increased urine output).
- For the treatment of renal failure, see article 10.21.

Deficiency of vitamin D

- Vitamin D should be prescribed. Prophylaxis 400–800 IU/day, in the winter more, laboratory controls not necessary.
- Simultaneous correction of calcium and phosphate deficiencies.

24.21 Hypercalcaemia and hyperparathyroidism

Ritva Kauppinen-Mäkelin

Basic rules

- Identify hypercalcaemia as the cause of the patient's symptoms
- Assay serum intact PTH (parathyroid-dependent or parathyroid-independent?)
- How urgent is the need for the treatment of hypercalcaemia?
- Determine the cause of hypercalcaemia
- Treat the cause of hypercalcaemia

Definition and prevalence of hypercalcaemia

- Serum calcium concentration exceeds 2.65 mmol/l (serum ionized calcium > 1.3 mmol/l repeatedly). Reference ranges vary in various central hospitals. Do not confuse these with the decision-making threshold.
- The prevalence of primary hyperparathyroidism in postmenopausal women is > 1%. See below the prevalence of hypercalcaemia in cancer patients. Otherwise hypercalcaemia is quite rare.

Common causes of hypercalcaemia (most common causes in bold type)

Parathyroid-dependent hypercalcaemia

- **Primary hyperparathyroidism**
- Tertiary hyperparathyroidism
- Familial hypocalciuric hypercalcaemia

Parathyroid-independent hypercalcaemia

- **Tumours**
  - In cancer, serum calcium concentration increases because of either lytic bone metastases or hormone-like transmitters

secreted by the cancer. Hypercalcaemia is detected in about 20% of patients with breast cancer, about 10–15% of patients with lung or renal cancer, 10–30% of patients with multiple myeloma, and 10% of patients with leukaemia or lymphoma.

- **Sarcoidosis**, other granulomatous diseases, certain types of lymphoma
- Hyperthyroidism, Addison's disease (mild hypercalcaemia)
- Acute renal failure, recovery phase
- Rhabdomyolysis, recovery phase
- Pharmaceuticals
  - Vitamin D overdose
  - Thiazide diuretics (promote the expression of mild hyperparathyroidism)
- Immobilization

Symptoms of hypercalcaemia

- The severity of the symptoms varies from asymptomatic to severe systemic symptoms. Usually asymptomatic when serum calcium concentration is <2.8 mmol/l. Today primary hyperparathyroidism is often detected incidentally. It may also be found in patients with chronic aches, constipation or depressive symptoms, or when looking for the cause of urinary calculi or osteoporosis. Rapidly progressing symptoms and poor general condition indicate a malignant tumour.
- Systemic symptoms
  - Fatigue, loss of appetite
- Gastrointestinal symptoms
  - Nausea, constipation, abdominal pain, peptic ulcer, pancreatitis
- Kidneys and fluid balance
  - Urinary and kidney calculi
  - Polyuria, polydipsia, dehydration
  - Renal insufficiency
- Bones and joints
  - Arthralgia, bone aches, pain, fractures
  - Radiological changes (in hyperparathyroidism, malignancies)
- Neuropsychiatric symptoms
  - Inability to concentrate, depression, dementia
  - Confusion, psychosis
- Cardiovascular symptoms
  - Short QT interval and arrhythmias
  - Hypertension

Laboratory investigations

- Serum calcium and albumin, or serum ionized calcium. A 10 g/l change in serum albumin causes a 0.2 mmol/l change in the same direction in serum calcium. Ionized calcium is more useful than calcium if there are serum protein disturbances.
- Serum intact PTH levels can be used for differential diagnosis between parathyroid-dependent and parathyroid-independent hypercalcaemia.
  - In parathyroid-dependent hypercalcaemia, PTH concentration is increased or near the upper limit of the normal range.
  - In parathyroid-independent hypercalcaemia, PTH concentration is decreased or too low to measure.
  - Please note: Secondary hyperparathyroidism caused by insufficient intake or malabsorption of dietary calcium and/or vitamin D is a common cause for elevated PTH levels. In this case serum calcium levels are either normal or low.
- Specific tests to discover the cause of hypercalcaemia are selected according to the suspected aetiology. Primary hyperparathyroidism can be diagnosed if serum calcium or ionized calcium levels are increased and serum intact PTH concentration is increased or close to the upper limit of the normal range, and 24-h urinary calcium level is normal or increased (consult specialized health care). In parathyroid-independent hypercalcaemia we usually look for a malignant tumour with bone metastases or sarcoidosis (investigations in specialised health care).

Treatment

Urgency

- If serum calcium (ionized calcium) is
  - <3.25 mmol/l (<1.6 mmol/l), immediate treatment is rarely indicated
  - >3.5 mmol/l (1.75 mmol/l) treatment of hypercalcaemic crisis is usually indicated

Treatment of hypercalcaemic crisis

- Correct dehydration (starting with 0.9% sodium chloride solution) and ensure diuresis (furosemide will increase urinary calcium excretion). Give potassium and magnesium supplements as needed.
- Lower serum calcium concentrations by giving a single intravenous dose of bisphosphonate (4 mg zolendronate in 50 ml 0.9% sodium chloride solution over 15 min or 60–90 mg pamidronate in 250–500 ml of 0.9% sodium chloride solution at a rate not exceeding 30 mg/2 h) or calcitonin (5–10 IU/kg/day in 500 ml 0.9% sodium chloride solution / 6 h). Repeat the calcitonin dose on the following 2–3 days, if necessary. Bisphosphonates reduce calcium concentrations more efficiently than calcitonin. Calcitonin takes effect slightly sooner, but the effect is weaker and short-lived. Calcitonin is safer than bisphosphonates in patients with kidney failure but bisphosphonates are not contraindicated in moderate kidney failure. Kidney failure is most often corrected by fluid therapy and as serum calcium levels decrease. Corticosteroids are useful in myeloma, sarcoidosis, vitamin D overdose and hypercalcaemia related to lymphomas.

Primary hyperparathyroidism

- The only curative treatment is surgery. Indications of surgical treatment:
  - Serum calcium > 2.85 mmol/l or serum ionized calcium > 1.5 mmol/l
  - Increased serum creatinine
  - Kidney or urinary calculi
  - Osteoporosis detected by bone densitometry
  - Age <50 years
  - Impaired cognitive functions
- If surgical treatment is not indicated in primary hyperparathyroidism or surgery is not performed for some other reason, serum calcium (ionized calcium) levels should be monitored twice annually. If serum calcium levels increase the need for surgery should be re-assessed. Serum calcium levels often remain unchanged year after year–particularly in elderly women. There is no need to restrict dietary calcium intake, however, calcium supplements are not recommended. Intake of vitamin D tends to aggravate hypercalcaemia. Prevention of osteoporosis should be considered.

Other causes

- The basic cause of hypercalcaemia should be treated appropriately.

24.24 Osteoporosis: diagnostics and pharmacotherapy

Editors

Basic rules

- The aim of prevention is to reduce the occurrence of upper femur, vertebral and wrist fractures.
- Prevention is primarily targeted at patients who already have had an osteoporotic fracture, as an earlier fracture predicts new fractures.
  - A radial fracture should always be suspected to be osteoporotic, and the patient should be referred for evaluation of possible osteoporosis. The responsibility for referral lies on the physician treating the fracture(s) and on primary health care. The evaluation can be performed in primary health care.
  - Secondary prevention yields the best benefit, which is why these patients should be identified and treated (National Institutes of Health Consensus Development Panel, 2001).

Table 24.24.1 Conditions warranting bone density measurement

	Condition
1.	History discloses a low-energy fracture with suspected osteoporotic aetiology. This patient group has a particularly high risk of a new fracture, which can often be prevented by pharmacotherapy for osteoporosis.
2.	The patient is a woman aged over 65 years who does not use oestrogen therapy and who has other risk factors • Hip fracture in previous generation (mother) • Sedentary lifestyle, prolonged immobilization • Heavy smoking • Low calcium intake • Slender physique.
3.	The patient has other diseases and factors that increase the risk of osteoporosis, such as • Menopause before the age of 45 years and no oestrogen therapy • Prolonged amenorrhoea • Long-term (>6 months) glucocorticoid therapy • Primary hyperparathyroidism • Vitamin D deficiency • Organ transplantation • Chronic renal failure • Cushing's syndrome • GI disease: coeliac disease, ulcerative colitis, Crohn's disease, post-gastrectomy state, and severe lactose intolerance unless the patient uses calcium supplementation • Chronic liver disease • Rheumatoid arthritis and related diseases • Medications: phenytoin, carbamazepine, thyroxin in large doses as used for cancer of the thyroid gland, long-term heparin therapy.
4.	Suspicion of osteoporosis on the basis of radiography (change in vertebra or impression of lowered calcium concentration). In patients with fracture of the vertebra, bone density measurement is not always necessary for initiation of therapy. Excluding secondary osteoporosis may be more important.
5.	Loss of stature (over 4–5 cm), thoracic kyphosis

- Early diagnosis of osteoporosis is the responsibility of primary care. Bone density measurements targeted at risk groups should be available for diagnosis, see Table 24.24.1.
  - General, non-targeted screening is not indicated **B** [1 2 3 4].
  - Bone density measurements are usually not needed in women on postmenopausal hormone replacement therapy for postmenopausal symptoms and in those who do not have any risk factors.
- Causes of secondary osteoporosis should be identified and treated accordingly (hyperparathyroidism, hyperthyroidism, Cushing's syndrome, hypogonadism, uraemia, coeliac disease, glucocorticoid therapy, smoking, rheumatoid arthritis).
- Elderly patients (>80 years) with a hip fracture who are in poor physical condition usually do not benefit from examinations for osteoporosis. They should be treated with calcium + vitamin D. Safety of the living environment

should be ensured and the patient should wear hip protectors (22.1).

Definitions

- **Osteoporosis** is defined as a condition where bone density is decreased (amount of bone tissue/volume unit). Bone strength is thus compromised and susceptible to osteoporotic fractures. Most common fracture sites include upper femur (femoral neck and trochanters), wrist and thoracic vertebrae.
- **Osteomalacia** is a disturbance of mineralization of the bone matrix. Occasionally, osteomalacia and osteoporosis are simultaneously present.

Prevention

- **Calcium** should be available in the diet in sufficient quantities (see Table 24.24.2), in the risk groups as much as 1–1.5 g/day (A) [5 6 7 8 9 10].
  - Four glasses of fat free milk or buttermilk contain one gram of calcium; the same amount is obtained from 100 g of cheese.
  - Sufficient calcium intake should be assured in children and adolescents.
  - The available amount of calcium in calcium preparations varies; larger doses than are recommended are not beneficial in either prevention or treatment.
  - There is not enough information available on the effect of calcium on the bones of men.
- The recommendation for the daily intake of vitamin D in Northern and temperate climate is presented in Table 24.24.2.
  - The most important source of vitamin D is fish.
  - Over 70-year-olds are a risk group for inadequate vitamin D intake.
  - Vitamin D substitution (400 IU daily) may be indicated during the winter season as prevention of fractures in both men and women (B) [11 12 13 14 15].
  - Institutionalized elderly can be given vitamin D (600–800 IU/day) and calcium supplementation throughout the year.
  - Substitution of vitamin D and calcium is also recommended for patients on long-term corticosteroid therapy. (B) [16 17 18]

Table 24.24.2 Recommended calcium and vitamin D intake

Age or life circumstances	Calcium, mg	Vitamin D, IU[1)]
Growth	900	200
21–60 years	800	200
>60 years	800[2)]	400
Pregnancy and breast-feeding	900	400

1. 40 IU = 1μg
2. Increasing the intake of calcium in the diet to 500–1000 mg of calcium daily may have some effect in preventing osteoporosis in women.

- **Physical exercise** is preventive for osteoporosis (A) [19 20 21 22 23 24 25 26] and for hip fractures (C) [27 28]. Exercise is necessary in childhood and adolescence; however, exercise can still increase bone density at the age of 40 years.
- **Postmenopausal hormone substitution** used for treatment of postmenopausal symptoms is beneficial in the prevention of osteoporosis, especially during the first 10 years.
  - Even after that period hormone replacement therapy has beneficial effects and is known to decrease the risk for vertebral fractures.
  - In patients younger than 75–80 years a reduction in the occurrence of upper femoral fractures is also probable.
  - However, because of the risk of breast cancer and thromboembolism, HRT is not indicated for the prevention or treatment of osteoporosis in women who do not need HRT for postmenopausal symptoms.
- **Bisphosphonates** (A) [29] should be considered for patients on long-term corticosteroid therapy in addition to the basic therapy (calcium and vitamin D) (B) [16 17 18].

Bone density measurements

- Comparison groups (B) [1 2 3 4]
- Early diagnosis of osteoporosis is possible only by **measurement of bone density**. The recommended methods are based on low energy x-ray radiation (Dual Energy X-Ray Absorptiometry, DEXA). These can be used to measure bone density in vertebral bodies and the femoral neck.
  - The results are compared with bone density values from healthy 20–40-year-old persons (maximum value, T-score). When decisions on treatment are made, the patient's bone density is compared with age-based reference values (Z-score).
  - The findings are considered significant for osteoporosis if the bone density is less than 2.5 SD (ca. 25%) below the maximum value. Decreased bone density is an independent **risk factor for fractures**. A decrease of 1 SD (osteopenia) measured at the femoral neck more than doubles the risk of fractures (B) [30 31 32 33]. See Table 24.24.3.
  - Osteoporosis is considered severe if bone density is more than 2.5 SD below the maximum value and the patient already has a complication of osteoporosis.
  - Evaluation of results is difficult and requires experience. In the elderly, osteoarthritic changes of the spine complicate the evaluation of osteoporosis. Plain x-rays are necessary for evaluation. In patients with spondylarthrosis, bone density should be measured at the upper end of the femur.
  - At present, the availability of bone density measurement is limited in many countries.
- **Ultrasound measurement** (C) [34 35] of the calcaneus is a new, rapid and non-radiating screening method.
  - It is not a density measurement and does not replace DEXA.
  - Correlation with bone density is only moderate and is better in older women.

END

Table 24.24.3 Diagnostic criteria of osteoporosis by the WHO working group. The absolute threshold values are based on large patient material collected by device manufacturers and consisting of Caucasian women.

Classification	Criteria
Normal	Bone mass/mineral density (BMD) in the range corresponding to the average bone density of healthy 20–40-year-olds (peak bone density) ±1 SD
Low done density, i.e. osteopenia	BMD is 1–2.5 SD lower than peak bone density ($-2.5 <$ T-score ≤ -1) ♦ Lumbar spine: Lunar < 1.08 g/cm^2, Hologic < 0.94 g/cm^2 (L1–L4) ♦ Femoral neck: Lunar < 0.86 g/cm^2, Hologic < 0.74 g/cm^2
Osteoporosis	BMD is 2.5 SD or more lower than peak bone density (T-score ≤ -2.5) ♦ Lumbar spine: Lunar < 0.90 g/cm^2, Hologic < 0.77 g/cm^2 (L2–L4) ♦ Femoral neck: Lunar < 0.68 g/cm^2, Hologic < 0.57 g/cm^2
Severe osteoporosis	In addition to the criteria of osteoporosis, the patient has one or more osteoporotic fracture(s).

- Ultrasound measures also other factors and it may have implications in evaluating fracture risk.

Indications for bone density measurements

- See Table 24.24.1.
- **Bone density measurements should not be used**
  - When oestrogen therapy is started for reasons other than osteoporosis prevention if the patient has no risk factors (25.51).
  - As a primary investigative method in the evaluation of pain patients.
  - In diagnostics when sufficient evidence of osteoporosis, such as osteoporotic fractures of the vertebrae, already exists.
  - In persons older than 80 years even with fractures, therapeutic options are limited and measurement in the degenerated spine is ambiguous. Basic care consists of calcium and vitamin D.

Screening of bone density

- Unselected bone density screening has not been found to be scientifically justifiable (SBU-report 1995).
- Bone density measurements are increasingly performed for the purpose of evaluating the individual risk of fractures in patients with one or several risk factor(s) when prolonged treatment is considered. The same device that is used for diagnosis should also be used for follow-up. Additional justification has been found in favourable results of reversing osteoporotic changes with new drugs and in the reduction of the risk for fractures.

Laboratory testing in suspected osteoporosis

- At present, no laboratory tests are available for diagnosing primary osteoporosis. The tests aim at revealing secondary osteoporosis, osteomalacia and at ruling out other causes of bone pain. In men and premenopausal women osteoporosis is in most cases secondary and warrants specialist consultation.
- Primary laboratory investigations
  - ESR, blood count, serum calcium, urine 24-hour calcium, serum alkaline phosphatase, serum creatinine, in men serum testosterone. Antibody determinations to detect coeliac disease (transglutaminase and endomysium antibodies) should be performed readily.
  - Urine 24-hour calcium measures malabsorption and often also vitamin D deficiency. Low serum calcium is often associated with low serum albumin in a sick elderly person.
- Low or normal levels of serum calcium in combination with low levels of serum phosphate points to malabsorption and osteomalacia. The bone-related serum alkaline phosphatase level is elevated under these circumstances, and the serum parathyroid hormone level is secondarily increased. The total level of serum alkaline phosphatase is not useful in the diagnostics of primary osteoporosis.
- Laboratory tests for detecting secondary osteoporosis are chosen on the basis of history and clinical findings (hyperthyroidism, hyperparathyroidism, vitamin D deficiency, Cushing's syndrome, uraemia, coeliac disease, lactose intolerance, myeloma, rheumatoid arthritis, possibly castration for prostate cancer).
- When primary hyperparathyroidism is suspected
  - The serum parathyroid hormone and serum calcium levels are elevated; serum creatinine and albumin levels are normal. N.B. A secondary rise in serum parathyroid hormone is common in coeliac disease and in calcium and vitamin D deficiencies.
- When serum vitamin D deficiency is suspected
  - Serum 25-OH vitamin D is low. Serum alkaline phosphatase levels are increased or near normal, serum calcium level is decreased or normal urine 24-hour calcium level is normal or decreased, the serum parathyroid hormone level may be secondarily increased.
  - Vitamin D deficiency is common in the elderly during the dark season and is often the cause for a slight elevation in serum alkaline phosphatase.
  - Serum vitamin D concentration depends heavily on season and the amount of sunlight, complicating the interpretation of results, as the reference range is wide.
  - In children vitamin D deficiency causes rickets, in adults osteomalacia.

- Radiography
  - Interpretation of mild osteoporosis is difficult and only the probability of the condition can be evaluated.

Pharmacotherapy of osteoporosis

- See Table 24.24.4.
- Calcium and vitamin D constitute basic therapy in all cases. For the elderly this therapy is often sufficient and also indicated B [11 12 13 14 15].
- Indications for other than basic therapy include osteoporotic fractures or decrease of bone mineral density despite basic anti-osteoporotic treatment: T-score $\leq$ 2.5 SD or Z-score $\leq$ 1 SD.
- Nowadays, three groups of medication are available: bisphosphonates, calcitonin A [36 37], and oestrogen-receptor modulators and oestrogens B [38 39 40]. They act as inhibitors of osteoclastic activity. Bone build-up is promoted by testosterone and androgens, which are well suited for clinical use.
- Bisphosphonates are the drugs of choice for patients who do not need oestrogens for postmenopausal symptoms
  - Alendronate, etidronate A [41] or risedronate A [42].
- In patients with menopausal symptoms, oestrogens are recommended (25.51).
  - For a small group of women oestrogen is not sufficient for therapy. Bisphosphonates enhance the effect of oestrogen.
- Other options include
  - raloxifene (selective oestrogen receptor modulator)
  - calcitonin A [36 37]
  - testosterone (male hypogonadism).

Vitamin D + calcium

- A combination of calcium and vitamin D is recommended as the basic therapy for corticosteroid-treated patients B [16 17 18]. Patients belonging to risk groups should also take bisphosphonates.
- In young patients vitamin D therapy is indicated if laboratory tests reveal evidence of vitamin D deficiency, such as low levels (in the lower range of reference values or lower) of serum calcium and phosphate, decreased calcium urinary excretion, and increased levels of bone-related serum alkaline phosphatase. Vitamin D deficiency can be confirmed by determining the level of serum 25-OH vitamin D level (depends on the amount of sunlight and is often difficult to interpret). Persons eating only vegetarian food are a risk group.
- The effectiveness of vitamin D alone in the prevention of osteoporosis-associated fractures in postmenopausal women is unclear D [43].

Calcitonin

- Painful osteoporotic fractures are a special indication for calcitonin.

Table 24.24.4 Prevention and treatment of osteoporosis

Intervention	Implementation
Prevention and basic therapy	♦ Sufficient intake of calcium and vitamin D ♦ Regular physical activity ♦ Avoidance of smoking
Pharmacotherapy	
Oestrogens	♦ Oral oestradiol or topical oestradiol valerate 1–2 mg transdermally, a transdermal patch releasing 25–50 μg of oestradiol/day or 0.5–1.5 mg of oestradiol gel twice weekly on the skin depending on the product. ♦ Progestin for 12–14 days once every 1–3 months is combined with oestradiol (not if the patient has undergone hysterectomy) ♦ Combination therapy that does not cause continuous bleeding: oestrogen as instructed above + a low dose of progestin continuously (norethisterone acetate 1 mg or medroxyprogesterone acetate 2.5–5 mg/day)
Raloxifene	♦ 60 mg orally once daily
Bisphosphonates	♦ Alendronate 10 mg in the morning half an hour before breakfast with ample water; the patient must remain upright for the half hour before breakfast; or 70 mg once a week. ♦ Etidronate 400 mg/day for 14 days every three months initially 2 hours after a meal and 2 hours before the next meal. ♦ Risedronate 5 mg/day taken as alendronate or 2 hours after a meal and 2 hours before the next meal; or 35 mg once a week.
Calcitonin	♦ 200 IU daily intranasally: a lower dose is sufficient for pain relief
Testosterone (only for men)	♦ 250 mg testosterone esters every 2–3 weeks intramuscularly ♦ A patch releasing 2.5–5 mg of testosterone/day on the skin once daily

  - The duration of the treatment is usually one to two months.
  - Calcitonin usually improves cancellous bone density in the spine. An intranasal dosage of 200 IU is used. There is some evidence that long-term medication may prevent fractures C [44 45].
- Bisphosphonate and oestrogen can be combined with calcitonin.

END

Bisphosphonates

- Of the bisphosphonates, alendronate (10 mg/day) and risedronate (5 mg/day) **A** [42] have been shown to improve osteoporosis and to prevent occurrence of osteoporotic fractures in the wrist, upper femur and spine **C** [46 47]. Intermittent use of etidronate **A** [41] (400 mg × 1 for two weeks at a time every three months) has been shown to prevent osteoporotic fractures of the spine.
- Oesophagitis is a potential side effect of alendronate; thus the drug should be taken in an upright position with a sufficient amount of water. Alendronate is available as a 70 mg tablet that is taken once a week.

Long-term use of bisphosphonates and calcitonin

- Long-term use of these drugs is expensive; thus the diagnosis of osteoporosis must be confirmed and the therapeutic effect must be evaluated.
- The above drugs are indicated in women who do not wish to take oestrogens for postmenopausal symptoms or in whom oestrogens are contraindicated. In addition, patients on long-term corticosteroid treatment may benefit from bisphosphonates **A** [29] and possibly from calcitonin **B** [48]. Calcitonin and bisphosphonates may also be administered to patients in whom bone loss is not caused by oestrogen or androgen deficiency.

Raloxifene

- Raloxifene has an oestrogen-like effect on bone and cholesterol metabolism, but no effect on hypothalamus, uterus or breast.
- The recommended dose is 60 mg × 1.
- Raloxifene is indicated for the prevention of vertebral fractures in postmenopausal women with increased risk of osteoporosis. There is no evidence of the prevention of other than vertebral fractures. Raloxifene has no effect on menopausal symptoms.
- Based on a rather short-term follow-up, raloxifene does not increase the risk of uterine cancer and may reduce the risk of breast cancer.
- Contraindications include thromboembolic diseases and hepatic insufficiency, uterine bleeding of unknown origin and, for the time being, cancer of the body of the uterus and breast cancer.
- The most common adverse effects include vasodilatation (hot flushes), leg cramps and peripheral oedema. The risk of thromboembolism is probably similar to that of hormone replacement therapy.

Other medications

- **Anabolic steroids** (testosterone 250 mg i.m. every third week) are indicated in male hypogonadism. They have been administered in special cases to men undergoing cortisone therapy. They are not recommended for use in females, not even in low doses.
- **Fluorides** are currently not recommended for treatment of osteoporosis. Fluoride supplementation may even increase non-vertebral fractures **B** [49].
- **Calcitriol** is an active vitamin D, used in patients with renal disorders. It is under investigation for use in the treatment and prevention of osteoporosis in the elderly. Problem areas include the need for exact dosage and adverse consequences of overdosage.
- **Thiazides** decrease urinary excretion of calcium and protect against osteoporosis **C** [50 51], which has to be taken into account when choosing a medication for hypertension or cardiac insufficiency.

Effects of drugs in reducing risk of fractures

- The first osteoporotic fracture strongly predicts new fractures. This is why secondary prevention is more effective than primary prevention and why the target group for treatment are those who have already had one fracture.
- The effects of oestrogen in the prevention of vertebral and hip fractures have been shown in primary and secondary prevention **B** [38 39 40].
- Alendronate, risedronate and ethidronate have been shown to be effective in secondary prevention in patients with manifest osteoporosis or related complications, reducing the risk of fractures. Calcitonin has also been shown effective in secondary prevention at the dose 200 IU/day.
- Prevention of a new fracture with bisphosphonates (secondary prevention) is effective, and the NNT numbers are much lower than in primary prevention.
- The fracture risk reduction has been more difficult to confirm than the effect of on bone density. However, reduced bone mineral density is a risk factor for fractures and thus a therapeutic indication. The essential problem in primary prevention is to identify patients needing bone density measurement and treatment.
- Oestrogens have been shown to still have beneficial effects in 75-year-old women and bisphosphonates in 65-year-olds. In principle, the treatments of osteoporosis are intended to be used for long periods if risk factors cannot be eliminated.
- In over 80-year-olds osteoporosis is no longer a main risk factor for fractures. At that age neurological and cardiological diseases that cause falls constitute the main risk. Falls should be prevented and at the same time the patient should be protected from fractures by wearing hip protectors, as primary prevention of falls (22.1) is often difficult.

Combination medication and duration of therapy

- If basic therapy for primary osteoporosis has been started and oestrogen is used, adding other drugs to the regimen does not usually provide additional benefits. In 20% of women oestrogen alone is, however, not sufficient, and these patients need also bisphosphonate. An exception to this rule is a painful vertebral fracture where calcitonin is indicated at least for a limited period of time.

Follow-up

- The therapeutic effects are evaluated on the basis of bone density measurements. The patient is examined with the same DEXA device two years after the initial investigation; even with the same device a 2–3% precision error is common.
- NTx allows the evaluation of the effect already after 1–3 months.
- If osteopenia is initially left untreated, the situation should be reassessed after 2 years.
- At the population level, a decrease in the incidence of complications should be monitored.

References

1. University of York. NHS Centre for Reviews and Dissemination. Screening for osteoporosis to prevent fractures. Effective Health Care 1992;1:12.
2. The Database of Abstracts of Reviews of Effectiveness (University of York), Database no.: DARE-950029. In: The Cochrane Library, Issue 4, 1999. Oxford: Update Software.
3. Hailey D, Sampietro-Colom L, Marshall D, Rico R, Granados A, Asua J. The effectiveness of bone density measurements and associated treatments for prevention of fractures: an international collaborative review. Int Technol Assess Health Care 1998;14:237–254.
4. The Database of Abstracts of Reviews of Effectiveness (University of York), Database no.: DARE-988678. In: The Cochrane Library, Issue 4, 1999. Oxford: Update Software.
5. Welten DC, Kemper HC, Post GB, van Staveren WA. A meta-analysis of the effect of calcium intake on bone mass in young and middle aged females and males. J Nutrition 1995;125:2802–2813.
6. The Database of Abstracts of Reviews of Effectiveness (University of York), Database no.: DARE-963246. In: The Cochrane Library, Issue 4, 1999. Oxford: Update Software.
7. Mackerras D, Lumley T. First- and second year effects of calcium supplementation on loss of bone density in postmenopausal women. Bone 1997;21:527–533.
8. The Database of Abstracts of Reviews of Effectiveness (University of York), Database no.: DARE-980076. In: The Cochrane Library, Issue 4, 1999. Oxford: Update Software.
9. Cumming RG, Nevitt MC. Calcium for prevention of osteoporotic fractures in postmenopausal women. Journal of Bone and Mineral Research 1997;12:1321–1329.
10. The Database of Abstracts of Reviews of Effectiveness (University of York), Database no.: DARE-983068. In: The Cochrane Library, Issue 3, 2000. Oxford: Update Software.
11. Gillespie WJ, Avenell A, Henry DA, O'Connell DL, Robertson J. Vitamin D and vitamin D analogues for preventing fractures associated with involutional and post-menopausal osteoporosis. Cochrane Database Syst Rev. 2004;(2):CD000227.
12. Lips P, 2002fsmans WC, Ooms ME et al. Vitamin D supplementation and fracture incidence in elderly persons. A randomised, placebo-controlled trial. Ann Intern Med 1996;124:400-6. Comment in ACP Journal Club 1996;July/August:16.
13. Chapuy MC et al. Effect of calcium and cholecalciferol treatment for three years on hipfractures in elderly women. BMJ 1994;308:1081–2.
14. Dawson-Hughes B et al. Rates of bone loss in postmenopausal women randomly assigned to one of two dosages of vitamin D. Am J Clin Nutr 1995;61:1140–5.
15. Trivedi DP, Doll R, Khaw KT. Effect of four monthly oral vitamin D3 (cholecalciferol) supplementation on fractures and mortality in men and women living in the community: randomised double blind controlled trial. BMJ 2003; 326(7387):469.
16. Homik J, Suarez-Almazor ME, Shea B, Cranney A, Wells G, Tugwell P. Calcium and vitamin D for corticosteroid-induced osteoporosis. Cochrane Database Syst Rev. 2004;(2): CD000952.
17. Amin S, LaValley MP, Simms RW, Felson DT. The role of Vitamin D in corticosteroid-induced osteoporosis: a meta-analytic approach. Arthritis and Rheumatism 1999;42: 1740–1751.
18. The Database of Abstracts of Reviews of Effectiveness (University of York), Database no.: DARE-991644. In: The Cochrane Library, Issue 1, 2001. Oxford: Update Software.
19. Kelley G. Aerobic exercise and lumbar spine bone mineral density in postmenopausal women: a meta-analysis. J Am Ger Soc 1998;46:143–152.
20. The Database of Abstracts of Reviews of Effectiveness (University of York), Database no.: DARE-980339. In: The Cochrane Library, Issue 2, 2000. Oxford: Update Software.
21. Kelley GA. Exercise and regional bone mineral density in postmenopausal women: a meta-analytic review of randomized trials. Am J Phys Med Rehab 1998;77:76–87.
22. The Database of Abstracts of Reviews of Effectiveness (University of York), Database no.: DARE-980338. In: The Cochrane Library, Issue 2, 2000. Oxford: Update Software.
23. Ernst E. Exercise for female osteoporosis: a systematic review of randomised clinical trials. Sports Medicine 1998;25: 359–368.
24. The Database of Abstracts of Reviews of Effectiveness (University of York), Database no.: DARE-981288. In: The Cochrane Library, Issue 2, 2000. Oxford: Update Software.
25. Kelley GA. Aerobic exercise and bone density at the hip in postmenopausal women: a meta-analysis. Preventive Medicine 1998;27:798–807.
26. The Database of Abstracts of Reviews of Effectiveness (University of York), Database no.: DARE-998371. In: The Cochrane Library, Issue 3, 2001. Oxford: Update Software.
27. Joakimsen RM, Magnus JH, Fonnebo V. Physical activity and predisposition to hip fractures: a review. Osteop Int 1997;7:503–513.
28. The Database of Abstracts of Reviews of Effectiveness (University of York), Database no.: DARE-980126. In: The Cochrane Library, Issue 4, 1999. Oxford: Update Software.
29. Homik J, Cranney A, Shea B, Tugwell P, Wells G, Adachi R, Suarez-Almazor M. Bisphosphonates for steroid induced osteoporosis. Cochrane Database Syst Rev. 2004;(2): CD001347.
30. Marshall D, Johnell O, Wedel H. Meta-analysis of how well measures of bone mineral density predict occurrence of osteoporotic fractures. BMJ 1996;312:1254–1259.

31. The Database of Abstracts of Reviews of Effectiveness (University of York), Database no.: DARE-968218. In: The Cochrane Library, Issue 4, 1999. Oxford: Update Software.
32. Ringertz H, Marshall D, Johansson C, Johnell O, Kullenberg RJ, Ljunhall S, Saaf M, Wedel H, Hallerby N, Jonsson E, Marke LA, Werko L. Bone density measurement: a systematic review. J Int Med 1997;241(suppl 739):1–60.
33. The Database of Abstracts of Reviews of Effectiveness (University of York), Database no.: DARE-970472. In: The Cochrane Library, Issue 4, 1999. Oxford: Update Software.
34. Homik J, Hailey D. Quantitative ultrasound for bone density measurement. Health Technology Assessment Report. HTA 11. 1998. 1–41.
35. The Database of Abstracts of Reviews of Effectiveness (University of York), Database no.: DARE-998389. In: The Cochrane Library, Issue 1, 2001. Oxford: Update Software.
36. Cardona JM, Pastor E. Calcitonin versus etidronate for the treatment of postmenopausal osteoporosis: a meta-analysis of published clinical trials. Osteoporosis Int 1997;7: 165–174.
37. The Database of Abstracts of Reviews of Effectiveness (University of York), Database no.: DARE-970814. In: The Cochrane Library, Issue 4, 1999. Oxford: Update Software.
38. Torgerson DJ, Bell-Syer SE. Hormone replacement therapy and prevention of nonvertebral fractures. A meta-analysis of randomized trials. JAMA 2001;285:2891–2897.
39. Nelson H D. Hormone replacement therapy and osteoporosis. Rockville, MD: Agency for Healthcare Research and Quality (AHRQ). 2002. 47. Agency for Healthcare Research and Quality (AHRQ). www.ahrq.gov.
40. Health Technology Assessment Database: HTA-20031089. The Cochrane Library, Issue 1, 2004. Chichester, UK: John Wiley & Sons, Ltd.
41. Cranney A, Welch V, Adachi JD, Guyatt G, Krolicki N, Griffith L, Shea B, Tugwell P, Wells G. Etidronate for treating and preventing postmenopausal osteoporosis. Cochrane Database Syst Rev. 2004;(2):CD003376.
42. Cranney A, Waldegger L, Zytaruk N, Shea B, Weaver B, Papaioannou A, Robinson V, Wells G, Tugwell P, Adachi JD, Guyatt G. Risedronate for the prevention and treatment of postmenopausal osteoporosi.s Cochrane Database Syst Rev 2003(4):CD004523.
43. Gillespie WJ, Henry DA, O´Connell DL, Robertson J. Vitamin D and vitamin D analogues for preventing fractures associated with involutional and post-menopausal osteoporosis. The Cochrane Database of Systematic Reviews, Cochrane Library number: CD000227. In: The Cochrane Library, Issue 2, 2002. Oxford: Update Software. Updated frequently.
44. Kanis JA, McCloskey EV. Effect of calcitonin on vertebral and other fractures. QMJ-Monthly Journal of the Association of Physicians 1999;92:143–149.
45. The Database of Abstracts of Reviews of Effectiveness (University of York), Database no.: DARE-990697. In: The Cochrane Library, Issue 2, 2001. Oxford: Update Software.
46. Karpf DB, Shapiro DR, Seeman E, Ensrud KE, Johnston CC, Adami S, Harris ST, Santora II AC, Hirsch LJ, Oppenheimer L, Thompson D. Prevention on nonvertebral fractures by alendronate: a meta-analysis. JAMA 1997;277:1159–1164.
47. The Database of Abstracts of Reviews of Effectiveness (University of York), Database no.: DARE-978299. In: The Cochrane Library, Issue 4, 1999. Oxford: Update Software.
48. Cranney A, Welch V, Adachi JD, Homik J, Shea B, Suarez-Almazor ME, Tugwell P, Wells G. Calcitonin for preventing and treating corticosteroid-induced osteoporosis. Cochrane Database Syst Rev. 2004;(2):CD001983.
49. Haguenauer D, Welch B, Shea B, Tugwell P, Wells G. Fluoride for treating postmenopausal osteoporosis. Cochrane Database Syst Rev. 2004;(2):CD002825.
50. Jones G, Nguyen T, Sambrook PN, Eisman JA. Thiazide diuretics and fractures: can meta-analysis help?. J Bone Mineral Res 1995;10:106–111.
51. The Database of Abstracts of Reviews of Effectiveness (University of York), Database no.: DARE-988096. In: The Cochrane Library, Issue 4, 1999. Oxford: Update Software.

24.30 Laboratory testing of thyroid function

Editors

Basic rules

- Clinical examination should be the first step in the evaluation of thyroid function (with thyroid stimulating hormone, TSH).
- The following strategy of laboratory diagnostics should be followed:
  - TSH is the first-line test of thyroid function
  - further tests are performed if
    - confounding factors exist
    - controversial results are obtained
    - a thyroid disease is confirmed (an abnormal TSH).

Thyroid function tests

TSH assay as the first-line test

- The screening for both hypo- and hyperthyroidism can be carried out by the primary care physician.
- The measurement allows the detection of subclinical primary hypothyroidism (TSH is increased, free T4 is still normal).
  - If TSH concentration is above 10 mU/l treatment is almost always indicated C [1] [2]. (Individual consideration must be given to patients with COPD or angina pectoris.)
  - If TSH concentration is repeatedly slightly increased (5–10 mU/l) in a patient with symptoms suggestive of hypothyroidism a trial treatment with thyroxine (50–100 μg/day) should be scheduled for 6 months. See article 24.34.

- Very low TSH concentrations do not always indicate hyperthyroidism in the following conditions:
  - Treated Graves' (Basedow's) disease
  - Euthyroid nodular goitre and some autonomous adenoma
  - Some systemic diseases
  - Certain drugs, e.g. high-dose corticosteroids
- In hyperthyroidism, TSH may remain within the reference range in the presence of heterophilic antibodies.
- Disadvantages
  - The measurement of TSH alone will not detect rare forms of hypothyroidism caused by pituitary dysfunction. The signs and symptoms of hypothyroidism are often minor in these cases; usually the first sign is gonadotrophin deficiency.
  - No information is obtained as regards the active hormone (T4 or T3).
  - In hospitalised patients with severe systemic illnesses TSH concentration may temporarily be abnormal (either decreased or increased) without co-existing thyroid disease. In these cases, the concentration of free T4 will often be close to the lower limit of the reference range.
  - TSH measurements change slowly (4–6 weeks). If any changes are evident, free T4 should also be measured.

Other thyroid tests

- If TSH concentration is abnormal, free T4 should be measured (the laboratory should perform the assay automatically).
  - Unlike total T4, the concentration of free T4 is not significantly influenced by changes in the concentration of the binding proteins, by pregnancy (during the last quarter of pregnancy the concentration may decrease slightly), or by the use of oestrogen or other drugs, with the exception of carbamazepine and phenytoin (which may decrease free T4 and free T3 concentrations).
  - Even if free T4 is within the reference range in subclinical hypothyroidism, treatment with thyroxine may still be warranted (24.34).
- If hyperthyroidism is suspected on the basis of symptoms and a low TSH concentration, but free T4 is normal, free T3 should be measured in order to detect T3-hyperthyroidism.
- The presence of thyroid peroxidase antibodies or microsomal antibodies should be tested if hypothyroidism (chronic thyroiditis), goitre or a solitary nodule is diagnosed.

Monitoring replacement therapy

- TSH is the most important test to be used. It is acceptable to have TSH concentration close to the lower limit of the reference range, if free T4 is within the reference range and the patient has no symptoms of hyperthyroidism.
- When the treatment for hypothyroidism has been established, measurements every few years will suffice. The increased risk of autoimmune diseases must be borne in mind.
- Thyroxine medication must not be taken in the morning of the day when free T4 and TSH are to be measured.

References

1. Helfand M, Redfern CC. Clinical guideline, part 2: screening for thyroid disease: an update. Annals of Internal Medicine 1998;129:144–158.
2. The Database of Abstracts of Reviews of Effectiveness (University of York), Database no.: DARE-988963. In: The Cochrane Library, Issue 3, 2000. Oxford: Update Software.

24.31 Enlarged or nodular thyroid gland

Editors

Basic rules

- Goitre in a euthyroid patient needs no treatment if it does not cause cosmetic problems or compression symptoms or show signs of growth.
- Consider the possibility of carcinoma in patients with a solitary nodule detected clinically or ultrasonographically. A multinodular goitre may contain a carcinoma.
- Risk factors for malignancy include
  - Male gender
  - Age below 20 or over 70 years
  - Solidity of the nodule
  - Growth of the nodule
  - Irradiation to the neck.
- Thyroid nodules and cysts are common incidental findings in ultrasonographic examinations.

Diagnostic and treatment strategy

- Investigate ESR, serum free thyroxine, and TSH in all patients with one or more thyroid nodules. Possible functional disturbance is corrected.
- After correction of functional disturbance, all patients should be examined by ultrasound of the neck and fine-needle biopsy.
  - If several nodules are detected in ultrasound, fine-needle biopsy is taken from the largest nodule and from any suspect nodules.
- A cyst with a diameter less than 4 cm should be aspirated during ultrasound examination and the contents should be examined cytologically.
- A cyst with a diameter over 4 cm should be removed surgically.
- Follow-up examination is always indicated after detection of a thyroid gland nodule or cyst.

- If growth of the nodule is suspected, repeating ultrasound and fine-needle biopsy in 3–6 month's time is indicated.
- If the patient has multinodular goitre or cyst that appears benign and does not grow, the situation can be followed up after one year. If the finding is normal, further follow-up is not necessary.

Investigations

Ultrasound

- The primary investigation. The examination is most useful in cases where a solitary nodule turns out to be multinodular goitre, which is usually a benign condition. However, fine-needle biopsy is indicated.
- A fine-needle biopsy can be taken during ultrasound investigation.
- Benign and malignant changes cannot be reliably differentiated. Malignancies are found most often in hypoechogenic nodules. A cystic nodule may, however, be malignant.

Needle biopsy

- An accurate examination in experienced hands. False negative or non-diagnostic results are often a problem.
- Fluid obtained from a cyst in fine-needle biopsy does not confirm the benign nature of the cyst; a carcinoma may grow on the cyst wall. The number of cells aspirated from a cyst is often small and the finding is not diagnostic.
- Needle size: 25 G.

Indications for surgical treatment

- A history of neck irradiation (predisposes to malignancy).
- The nodule is large (over 4 cm) or it causes compression symptoms.
- The nodule grows continuously or recurs after repeated aspiration.
- The nodule is hard in consistency.
- The patient is young.
- The patient is worried.
- Cytological finding is class III.

Treatment of diffuse goitre

- Exclude thyroiditis (24.33) and functional disturbances (24.30).
- Find out possible goitre-producing substances (iodine, amiodarone, lithium, carbamazepine, phenytoin).
- Thyroxine can also be tried. It reduces the size of the goitre in chronic thyroiditis, but rarely in cases with other aetiology.
- Surgery is indicated if the goitre causes tracheal compression or cosmetic harm or grows.

24.32 Subacute thyroiditis

Editors

Basic rule

- Identify subacute thyroiditis as a cause of neck pain and high ESR that can be easily treated with corticosteroids.

Symptoms

- A systemic disease with neck pain and an enlarged thyroid gland or part of it (histologically, giant cell thyroiditis).
- Sometimes neck pain is minimal ("silent thyroiditis"), and the diagnosis can only be suspected afterwards.

Laboratory findings

- The ESR is always elevated, as is CRP.
- Initial hyperthyroidism is followed in 20% of cases by hypothyroidism 1–2 months after treatment. Permanent hypothyroidism develops in 2–3% of the patients.
- Anti-thyroid antibodies may be detected transiently. The determination of antibodies is not necessary.
- Scintican, isotope uptake scintigraphy and ultrasonography are not necessary.
- The diagnosis of giant cell thyroiditis can be confirmed by fine-needle biopsy.
- Diagnosis: tender thyroid gland, clinical picture of hyperthyroidism, elevated ESR and CRP, rapid response to corticosteroid therapy.

Course of the disease

- Thyroiditis can be managed in primary care.
- If left untreated the disease usually lasts for 3–4 months, rarely more than one year.
- The disease responds to corticosteroid treatment within days (the fever comes down, thyroid pain lessens). If there is no response consider alternative diagnoses: lymphadenitis with fever, acute bacterial thyroiditis (a rarity).
- The symptoms tend to recur if corticosteroids are reduced too early.

Treatment and follow-up

- Administer a glucocorticoid, e.g. prednisolone at 40 mg for 3 days, 30 mg for 3 days, 20 mg for one week, 15 mg for one week, 10 mg for 2 weeks, 5 mg for 2 weeks, and 5 mg every second morning for 2 weeks.
- NSAIDs at normal doses may be sufficient in mild cases.

- Hyperthyroidism is treated with beta-blockers.
- TSH and free T4 levels should be monitored; e.g. 3, 6 and 12 months after treatment. Transient hypothyroidism at the beginning rarely needs treatment, but if it persists for 4–6 months it is probably permanent, and thyroxine substitution is indicated. Substitution is not necessarily life long.

24.33 Chronic autoimmune thyroiditis

Editors

Forms of clinical presentation

- Hypothyroidism (subclinical and clinical)
- Goitre (Hashimoto's disease)
- Solitary thyroid nodule (rare)
- Rarely neck pain (in contrast to subacute thyroiditis)

Diagnosis

- The consistency of the thyroid gland is solid on palpation.
- The ESR may be slightly elevated (in contrast to subacute thyroiditis where ESR is markedly elevated).
- Anti-thyroid antibodies are often present in high titres.
- Fine-needle biopsy may be necessary if the presenting problem is enlargement of the thyroid. It is always indicated in the case of a solitary nodule unless the patient is referred for surgery immediately.
- Classification on the basis of fine-needle biopsy finding
  - Hashimoto (most common)
  - Primary hypothyroidism, i.e. chronic atrophic thyroiditis
  - Juvenile thyroiditis
  - Asymptomatic autoimmune thyroiditis
- The patient is frequently euthyroid. Both hypo- and hyperthyroidism are possible. Sometimes the patient has eye symptoms resembling Basedow's disease.

Treatment

- The treatment for chronic thyroiditis is thyroxine. The initial dose is 50 μg/day for 1–2 weeks, and 100–150 μg/day thereafter
  - for the treatment of hypothyroidism
  - to decrease the size of goitre, serum TSH should be decreased to the lowest reference value
  - not for the treatment of elevated antibody titres alone (found in 10–15% of the general population).
- If the goitre or nodule does not decrease in size during treatment, question the diagnosis. Ultrasound and fine-needle biopsy are necessary to confirm the diagnosis and the rule out neoplasm.
- The patients have a higher than normal incidence of autoimmune diseases. Careful annual follow-up is necessary in the beginning. Transient hyperthyroidism that requires treatment often occurs after childbirth.

24.34 Hypothyroidism

Editors

Basic rules

- Identify hypothyroidism as the cause of the patient's symptoms: the symptoms are often mild but obvious if the diagnosis comes into mind. Remember the specific symptoms.
- Remember that hypothyroidism can be the cause of high cholesterol levels.

Causes of hypothyroidism

Permanent hypothyroidism

- Autoimmune thyroiditis (atrophy or goitre)
- Rarely irradiation of the neck, developmental anomalies of the thyroid gland, hypopituitarism

Transient hypothyroidism

- Subacute thyroiditis
- Postpartal hypothyroidism 1–3 months after delivery
- Lithium, amiodarone, iodine

Transient or permanent

- Thyroid surgery
- Radio-iodine therapy
- Basedow's disease
- Thyrostatic medication

Symptoms and diagnosis of hypothyroidism

- The symptoms and their severity vary in different individuals.
- In advanced hypothyroidism the systemic symptoms include lack of initiative, fatigue and somnolence, memory problems, slow motor functions and speech, coarse voice,

feeling cold, decreased perspiration, constipation, weight gain, and generalized oedema. The skin symptoms include a dry, rough, cold or pale skin. Periorbital oedema may occur. Hair may become rough, and there is hair loss. Pulse rate becomes slower. In severe hypothyroidism the weakening of the achilles reflex and movements is a valuable specific finding.

- Mild hypothyroidism is often associated with symptoms of the nervous system such as tremor and irritability that may rise suspicion of hyperthyroidism.
- In subclinical hypothyroidism the patient feels normal but serum TSH is increased. However, the patient may have subtle symptoms such as decreased tolerance to cold weather and depression that respond to treatment with thyroxine.
- In the elderly the clinical picture is often atypical with slowing and depression that may simulate dementia or it may manifest only as atrial fibrillation.
- In young women the first symptom may be amenorrhoea or infertility.
- Central hypothyroidism (with a low TSH concentration) is often mild and the deficiencies of other hormones affect the patient more than deficiency of thyroxine.

Thyroxine treatment

- Make sure that the TSH concentration is increased before commencing substitution. If TSH concentration is low or in the reference range in a patient with hypothyroidism, pituitary disease is probable and investigations by a specialist is necessary. (Such patients often have deficiencies of other hormones, too.)
- Thyroxine substitution is always indicated if the TSH concentration is increased and the patient has symptoms. In asymptomatic patients treatment is indicated if serum TSH is above 10 mU/ml and the patient has anti-thyroid antibodies.
- Many patients have a slightly increased serum TSH concentration (5–10 mU/l) and a serum free thyroxine concentration at the lower limit of the reference range (subclinical hypothyroidism). At the lower limit of the reference range the result is distorted by the determination methods, leading to higher values. Thyroxine substitution can be tried.
  - In these patients a therapeutic trial of 50–100 μg thyroxine once daily can be performed without any harm. Antibody positivity speaks if favour of a treatment trial. If the treatment does not improve the patient's condition it can be discontinued. After discontinuation, transient symptoms of hypothyroidism may occur for up to one month while the thyroid gland gradually restarts functioning.
  - A treatment trial for subclinical hypothyroidism is a debated issue and often ends disappointingly: In many cases cholesterol levels and unspecific symptoms are corrected or alleviated only a little B [1].
- In young patients the initial dose is 50–100 μg/day. TSH is assessed 6–8 weeks from the initiation of therapy.
- In the elderly and in patients with ischaemic heart disease the initial dose is 12.5–25 μg/day, and the dose should be increased slowly and carefully monitoring heart rate. If necessary, beta-blockers should be used. Cardiac patients may not be given too high doses of thyroxine.
- The response to treatment is evaluated on the basis of clinical symptoms, serum TSH and free T4. TSH is the most important examination. The patient should not take thyroxine in the morning of the day when free T4 is measured. In long-term follow-up it is, however, justified to occasionally examine both TSH and free T4. TSH may be below the reference range, which is acceptable if free T4 is within the normal range and the patient is well. In some cases, the subjective condition of the patient is a more important guideline for dosing than laboratory tests.
- After a change in the dose of thyroxine serum free T4 and TSH are determined after 8 weeks at the earliest because the concentration of TSH changes slowly. When the dose has been established, TSH is determined at a few years' interval.
- In controversial cases (e.g. in possibly transient hypothyroidism) serum TSH should be determined 6 weeks after discontinuation of treatment. If serum TSH rises above the reference range permanent thyroxine substitution is indicated.
- Remember the possibility of concurrent Addison's disease if the patient does not improve or has low blood pressure, high potassium, low sodium, tendency for low blood glucose or pigmentation. In Addison's disease, 25% have concurrent hypothyroidism (Do not confuse with panhypopituitarism).

Treatment during pregnancy

- Thyroxine requirement is increased by 25–50 ug.
- Euthyroidism is important to the well-being of the mother and thus also for the foetus, particularly in early pregnancy.
- Certain drugs, particularly iron supplementation, disturb the absorption of thyroxine; the drugs must be taken at different times.

Thyroxine in the long-term treatment of thyroid carcinoma

- Usually the thyroid gland has been operated and treated with radio-iodine.
- Serum TSH should be kept undetectably low (TSH is believed to stimulate the growth of papillary and follicular carcinomas). The required dose is usually 150–250 μg of thyroxine.
- Serum free T3 should be monitored and kept in the normal range (free T3 correlates better with the symptoms of thyrotoxicosis).
- Thyroglobulin is the best marker for papillary and follicular thyroid cancer. Its concentration should be undetectable. Consult a specialist if thyroglobulin is detected in the serum.
- The dose of thyroxine can be reduced after 10 years.

Reference

1. Chu JW, Crapo LM. The treatment of subclinical hypothyroidism is seldom necessary. J Clin Endocrinol Metab 2001;86:4591–9.

24.35 Hyperthyroidism

Editors

Basic rules

- The final treatment plan is generally outlined by a specialist in internal medicine.
- Start beta-blockers and consider thyrostatic medication as you refer the patient to a specialist.
- In cases of Basedow's disease and pregnancy-induced hyperthyroidism, refer promptly to a specialist.
- Hyperthyroidism should not be treated unless the patient clearly shows clinical symptoms, the serum level of free thyroxine (FT4 or FT3) is considerably raised, and the serum level of TSH low. In uncertain cases, begin only with a beta-blocker.
- Remember that after radioiodine or surgical treatment the patient must be followed up throughout his life for hypothyroidism.

Causes of hyperthyroidism

- Basedow's disease (Grave's disease)
  - The most common cause
  - Age at onset 30–40 years
  - The majority of patients is women
- Toxic nodular goitre or adenoma
- Subacute thyroiditis (especially "silent thyroiditis")
- Subacute autoimmune thyroiditis (often following pregnancy, "painless thyroiditis")
- Other causes
  - Overdosage of thyroxine
  - Excessive consumption of iodine (seaweed)
  - Use of amiodarone; hypothyroidism is also possible
  - Radiation thyroiditis as a result of radioiodine treatment; treat with corticosteroids

Symptoms of hyperthyroidism

- General symptoms
  - Hypersensitivity to heat and sweating
  - Fatigue, muscular weakness, deterioration of general condition
  - Increased appetite, weight loss
  - Thirst, polyuria
- Thyroid gland is often enlarged
- Skin symptoms
  - Warm and moist skin
- Psychological symptoms
  - Lability, nervousness, irritability
- Cardiac symptoms
  - Tachycardia and arrhythmias, particularly atrial fibrillation, systolic hypertension
- GIT symptoms
  - diarrhoea and abdominal discomfort
- Optical symptoms
  - Only in Basedow's disease
- Symptoms vary between patients. The elderly are often monosymptomatic (e.g. atrial fibrillation, diarrhoea or fatigue alone) or their symptoms are masked (those already on beta-blocker treatment).
- The probability of hyperthyroidism is lower if the patient has cool hands, enjoys warmth, gains weight and has a normal thyroid gland.

Diagnostics

- TSH below and free T4 above the normal range.
- If TSH is below the normal range and the level of free T4 is normal, test free T3 for hyperthyroidism.
- If TSH is normal but FT4 and FT3 are above the reference range, the patient may have heterophilic antibodies to TSH and hyperthyroidism.
- If TSH is below the normal range but both free T4 and T3 are normal and the patient has symptoms, consider treatment. An asymptomatic patient is tested again after 6 months.
- If the patient has a nodus on palpation, consider scintiscan for the diagnosis of toxic adenoma.

Basic rules for treating hyperthyroidism

- Radioiodine is the primary treatment. Patients with mild hyperthyroidism and good general condition may be started immediately on radioiodine with beta-blocker cover alone; other patients should first be made euthyroid with a short course of thyrostatic medication. The dose of radioiodine determines the final treatment result. The aim can be set at uncomplicated hypothyroidism.
- Prolonged thyrostatic treatment (12–18 months) is given to the pregnant and to children if the thyroid gland is small or if the patient has eye symptoms.
- Surgery if the thyroid is large (A) [1 2] or carcinoma is suspected.
- A patient with eye symptoms is always treated at a specialist unit: TSH is lowered, surgery after recurrence.

- Thyrostat treatment can be continued for years if the patient does not wish other forms of treatment.
  - Basedow's disease is self-limiting.
  - In toxic nodular goitre permanent treatment results cannot be expected.

Implementing pharmacotherapy for hyperthyroidism

Symptomatic treatment

- Beta-blockers B [3]
  - Propranolol, 40 mg × 3
  - Metoprolol, 50 mg × 2

Starting preventive treatment

- A thyrostat (generally carbimazole 15–40 (–60 mg)) should be given alone or preferably combined with a beta-blocker.
- The leucocyte count should be controlled one week after the beginning of treatment and thereafter at one-month intervals. Give directions in case agranulocytosis occurs (instruct the patient to seek medical advice if there is fever or a sore throat).

Long-term preventive treatment

- Initiated if the patient has a small thyroid gland or eye symptoms. The duration is 18 months B [4].
- After euthyroidism has been achieved, use a combination of the thyrostat carbimazole (20 mg/24 h) and thyroxine (50–100 μg/24 h). The aim is to lower TSH and prolong the interval of control visits without causing fear of hypothyroidism. Combination therapy 'as the only right' treatment has been criticized
- In euthyroidism monitor TSH, free T4 and leucocytes at 2–3-month intervals. In euthyroidism, free T4 is within the normal range and TSH is either within or below the normal range.
- When the treatment is stopped, a recurrence is seen in half of the patients with Basedow's disease and in all patients with toxic nodular goitre.

Problems associated with treatment

Side effects of thyrostat

- Agranulocytosis (induced by all thyrostats)
  - Fever and sore throat are the first signs
  - Develops in 0.5% of patients.
  - Treat by stopping the pharmacotherapy immediately, see 15.5.
- Complete remission is rarely achieved in multinodular goitre.

Disadvantages of radioiodine treatment

- The risk of thyroid cancer or leukaemia is not increased.
- Permanent hypothyroidism develops in 60–70% of the patients; demands life-long surveillance. Hypothyroidism is sometimes a desired 'disturbance' that is easy to treat.
- Transient radiation thyroiditis.
- Eye symptoms may worsen; operation is the primary treatment option after a recurrence if eye symptoms are severe.

Disadvantages of surgery

- Requires an 8–10 week initial treatment with a tyrostat (TSH must be low).
- Permanent hypothyroidism; requires life-long surveillance.
- Recurrent nerve paresis and hypoparathyroidism develop in 2–4% of operated patients.

References

1. Palit TK, Miller CC, Miltenburg DM. The efficacy of thyroidectomy for Graves' disease: a meta-analysis. Journal of Surgical Research 2000, 90(2), 161–165.
2. The Database of Abstracts of Reviews of Effectiveness (University of York), Database no.: DARE-20001132. In: The Cochrane Library, Issue 2, 2002. Oxford: Update Software.
3. Henderson JM, Portmann L, Van-Melle G, Haller E, Ghika JA. Propranolol as an adjunct therapy for hyperthyroid tremor. European Neurology 1997;37:182–185.
4. Abraham P, Avenell A, Watson WA, Park CM, Bevan JS. Antithyroid drug regimen for treating Graves' hyperthyroidism. Cochrane Database Syst Rev 2003(4):CD003420.

24.40 Cushing's syndrome

Editors

Basic rules

- Recognize Cushing habitus in a hypertensive patient.
- Diagnose or rule out Cushing's syndrome in primary care with the 1–1.5-mg dexamethasone test.
- Monitor the development of Cushing symptoms in patients receiving peroral corticosteroids.

Causes of hypercortisolism

- Pituitary (most common) or adrenocortical tumour
- Primary nodular adrenocortical hypertrophy (very rare)
- Ectopic ACTH produced by an extra-pituitary tumour
- Use of corticosteroids or ACTH. See article on pharmacological glucocorticoid treatment 24.43.

Symptoms (% of the patients)

- Typical appearance: moon face, bull neck in almost 100%
- Weight gain in 90%
- Muscular weakness (proximal myopathy) in 90–95%
- Hypertension in 80%
- Hirsutism in 80%
- Striae in 70%
- Altered personality in 70%

Laboratory diagnosis

- Short 1.0–1.5 mg dexamethasone test
  - Suitable as primary investigation in primary care
  - The baseline sample for assay of serum cortisol is taken at 8 a.m. At 11 p.m. the patient takes 1–1.5 mg of dexamethasone. In children the dose is 1 mg/1.72 m^2. The second serum sample for cortisol assay is taken at 8 a.m. the next day.
  - Reference values
    - In a healthy person, S-cortisol decreases below 100 nmol/l after the administration of dexamethasone
  - False positive findings can be seen during drug therapy (phenytoin, carbamazepine, barbiturates, contraceptive pills and other oestrogens), and sometimes in acutely or chronically ill patients, and in obese or depressive patients.
- Further investigations are performed in an endocrinology unit. 24-hour urine cortisol is usually determined first. It is useful both as a diagnostic test and as a follow-up examination.

Treatment

- The treatment is surgical with the exception of iatrogenic hypercortisolism.
- Eventual postoperative hypocortisolism is treated by substitution, and followed up as in Addison's disease (24.42).

24.41 Primary aldosteronism (Conn's syndrome)

Editors

Basic rules

- Assay serum potassium as an initial examination in patients with hypertension.
- Suspect Conn's syndrome in a patient with hypertension and
  - serum potassium < 3.5 mmol/l **or**
  - clear tendency towards hypokalaemia (<3.0 mmol/l) during low-dose diuretic treatment
  - poor response to antihypertensive medication or good response to spironolactone.

Aetiology

- The cause of primary aldosteronism is usually adrenocortical adenoma (rarely carcinoma) or idiopathic hyperplasia.

Symptoms

- Hypertension in association with hypokalaemia; hypokalaemia may sometimes be mild or even within the normal range (3.5–4.0 mmol/l).
- Excessive (>30 mmol/day) secretion of potassium in the urine in relation to low serum potassium concentration while on a diet rich in sodium (24-hour urine sodium > 200 mmol)

Differential diagnosis

- Other causes of the syndrome of hypokalaemia and hypertension
  - Diuretic treatment of hypertension (high serum renin)
  - Renal hypertension (high serum renin)
  - Cushing's syndrome (normal serum renin)
  - Over-consumption of liquorice (low serum aldosterone and renin)

Initial investigations in primary care

- Serum sodium, potassium, acid-base balance (if available)
- Urine 24-h potassium and sodium

Further investigations

- Plasma aldosterone and renin are assayed at a specialized unit. Spironolactone should be discontinued for 4–6 weeks, and ACE inhibitor for 2 weeks before the determination of renin concentration (ACE inhibitor reduces sensitivity). Intake of salt should be sufficient.
  - Primary aldosteronism is probable if the basic aldosterone/renin ratio is > 800 and concurrent plasma aldosterone is > 400.

Strategy for investigation and treatment (hypertensive hypokalaemic patient)

- Serum potassium is 3.5–3.6 mmol/l and the patient has mild hypertension
  - There is no need for further investigation if the serum potassium concentration becomes normal during follow-up.

- If the serum potassium concentration does not return to normal, and particularly if the patient is old, diagnosing aldosteronism is not essential. Spironolactone (25–50 mg × 3/day) can be tried. If the serum potassium concentration becomes normal and blood pressure remains under control with this treatment further investigations are not necessarily needed. Serum potassium should be monitored monthly at first, but in a stable situation it is sufficient to determine serum potassium yearly at control visits for hypertension.

- Serum potassium is 3.0–3.4 mmol/l
  - Primary investigations are performed in primary care. An ophthalmologist should be consulted if the findings suggest aldosteronism.
  - The cause of hypokalaemia must always be identified (24.10).
- Serum potassium < 3.0 mmol/l (severe hypokalaemia).
  - Further investigations are indicated. Standard determination of plasma renin and aldosterone determinations are the main investigations.
  - In a later phase CT is indicated if laboratory tests suggest Conn's syndrome.

24.42 Hypocortisolism

Editors

Basic rules

- Suspect hypocortisolism in a patient with weight loss, fatigue, skin pigmentation, and hypotension. The disease may also present with an acute Addison's crisis.
- Advise patients on substitution to increase the dose of hydrocortisone prophylactically in stressful conditions.

Aetiology

- Adrenocortical disease (Addison's disease)
  - Caused by autoimmune adrenalitis, tuberculosis, haemorrhage, or metastases or appearing as a manifestation of APECED syndrome (24.63)
- Pituitary or hypothalamic disease
  - Tumour, trauma, infection, or circulatory disorder (in the elderly)
  - No skin pigmentation or hyperkalaemia because there is no mineralocorticoid deficiency.
- Long-term steroid treatment causes glucocorticoid depression (24.43)

Symptoms

Slowly developing symptoms (percentage of patients with Addison's disease)

- Fatigue almost 100%
- Loss of appetite, nausea 90%, weight loss 80%
- Hypotension (<110/70 mmHg) 90%, initially only postural
- Skin or mucosal pigmentation 80%
  - Note that the skin is pale in hypocortisolism caused by hypopituitarism.
- More rarely
  - Abdominal pain, diarrhoea, constipation
  - Salt hunger, collapsing tendency, vitiligo

Laboratory findings

- Electrolyte disturbances
  - Hyponatraemia is the first electrolyte disturbance in Addison's disease.
  - In secondary hypocortisolism (ACTH deficiency) the electrolyte levels are often normal but hyponatraemia may occur.
  - In advanced Addison's disease the findings also include hyperkalaemia and hypercalcaemia.
- Hypoglycaemia, even neuroglycopenia
- Normocytic anaemia and eosinophilia

Diagnostic laboratory examinations

- Serum cortisol
  - Cortisol deficiency is probable if morning serum cortisol is under 180 nmol/l or under 500 nmol/l in a patient with severe disease during stress.
- If the diagnosis is not certain a short ACTH test should be performed.
- If the results of these tests suggest Addison's disease refer the patient to a specialist for further investigation and planning of treatment.
- Glucocorticoid depression can be evaluated towards the end of the tapering period of cortisol therapy from a sample taken on a day off the medication. The level should be > 200 nmol/l.

Addison's crisis

- An acute situation with severe symptoms of hypocortisolism. Consider the possibility of Addison's crisis if the patient has severe fatigue and asthenia, low blood pressure, nausea and vomiting, and an impaired level of consciousness. Addison's crisis may affect a patient with hypocortisolism during an infection or severe stress.

Treatment

- Substitution
  - Examine haematocrit, serum potassium, serum sodium, blood glucose, serum creatinine, plasma cortisol (save a

sample for later determination), and ECG immediately the diagnosis is suspected. Tests of infection and a chest x-ray are also often indicated. Start hydrocortisone substitution (100–200 mg i.v. without waiting for test results).
- Further treatment **on the first day** consists of an infusion of 100 mg hydrocortisone over 6 hours, and thereafter 50–100 mg every 6 hours. The total dose is 400 mg.
- **On the second day** give 200 mg hydrocortisone i.m. or i.v., divided into 4 doses.
- **On the third day** give hydrocortisone at 25 mg × 3 per os or 50 mg × 3 i.m. or i.v.
- Thereafter the dose is 30 mg/day (20 + 10 mg).

♦ Fluid therapy
  - Aim at correcting hypovolaemia and dehydration, and eventual hyponatraemia and hypoglycaemia.
  - 1000 ml of glucose-saline is infused over 2 hours. The total amount of fluid **should not exceed 3000 ml** on the first day.

♦ Antibiotics should be started if there are signs of a bacterial infection.

♦ During the acute phase, haematocrit, serum potassium and blood glucose should be monitored.

Substitution treatment

♦ Hydrocortisone at 25–30 mg/day divided into 2 or 3 doses (8 a.m.–6 p.m.), or prednisone at 5–7.5 mg at bedtime, and (if necessary) hydrocortisone at 5–10 mg in the afternoon. The smallest adequate doses should be used. Laboratory follow-up is not necessary.

♦ A mineralocorticoid (Florinef®) at 0.05–0.2 mg/day is administered in one dose. Follow up potassium, sodium, blood pressure and oedemas.

Treatment in special circumstances

♦ Give the patient written advice. The patient should carry a medical alert card (necklace, wristband) noting his condition.

♦ Double the dose of hydrocortisone during an infection with fever.

♦ Advise the patient to increase the mineralocorticoid dose and salt intake if rapid sodium loss (perspiration, diarrhoea) is expected.

Substitution during surgery

♦ Small elective procedures
  - 100 mg hydrocortisone before the operation
  - 20 mg hydrocortisone after the operation per os

♦ Minor operations
  - 100 mg hydrocortisone every 8 hours on the day of operation

♦ Major operations or severe stress (e.g. myocardial infarction)
  - Hydrocortisone at 100 mg every 8 hours for 3 days

Follow-up

♦ Yearly examination
  - Clinical examination
  - Weight
  - Blood pressure
  - Serum sodium and potassium
  - Ask about salt hunger (implies need for mineralocorticoids), and determine serum ACTH and renin, if necessary.

♦ The probability of other autoimmune diseases (type 1 diabetes, hypothyroidism, pernicious anaemia, hypogonadism) is increased in patients with autoimmune adrenalitis.

24.43 Pharmacological glucocorticoid treatment

Ritva Kauppinen-Mäkelin

Aims

♦ Utilize the effect of glucocorticoids to suppress inflammation and immune response.

♦ Minimize adverse effects (correct administration and dosage).

♦ Consider for which disease or symptoms the glucocorticoid is intended and how the activity of the disease or the efficacy of the treatment will be monitored.

♦ Remember that the ability to withstand stress may be decreased for several months after the cessation of long-term glucocorticoid treatment.

Indications

♦ Polymyalgia rheumatica and temporal arteritis

♦ Severe rheumatoid arthritis and other collagen diseases, certain immunological liver diseases

♦ Severe asthma, where the symptoms are not controlled by inhaled corticosteroids or other asthma medication

♦ Subacute thyroiditis

♦ Facial nerve paresis, acute optic neuritis

♦ Basedow's eye disease

♦ Severe dermatological diseases, such as pemphigus and pemphigoid

♦ Adjuvant therapy in certain haematological diseases and cancers

♦ Immunosuppression after organ transplantation

♦ Increased intracranial pressure (usually symptomatic treatment of a malignant disease, which means that the long-term adverse effects of glucocorticoids are less important)

Choice of drug

- Intermediate acting prednisone, prednisolone and methylprednisolone are the best choices for long-term treatment because of their negligible mineralocorticoid action.
- In patients with liver disease prednisolone is preferred, as prednisone requires conversion in the liver to the biologically active prednisolone.
- Dexamethasone is suitable if the activity of the pituitary is to be slowed down. Dexamethasone is the first-line corticoid in the treatment of increased intracranial pressure.
- Hydrocortisone is used for physiological replacement therapy only.

Implementation of drug therapy

- Start the treatment with the correct dose (high doses, if necessary).
- Use the lowest possible dose for maintenance therapy.
- Consider the possibility of topical treatment.
- Give detailed instructions to the patient.

Timing of administration

- Usually the steroid is given as a single dose in the morning. The daily dose is divided into two doses if ACTH suppression is desired (e.g. in rare congenital adrenal hyperplasia) and often in diabetic patients, because only by dividing the daily dose can a constant level of blood glucose be achieved.

Equivalent doses

- 5 mg prednisone – 4 mg methylprednisolone – 0.75 mg dexamethasone – 20 mg hydrocortisone

Adverse effects of glucocorticoid treatment

- Acute
  - Mental disturbances, hyperglycaemia, fluid retention
- Chronic
  - Glucocorticoid suppression, osteoporosis, hypertension, gastrointestinal ulceration, cataract and glaucoma, infections, iatrogenic Cushing's syndrome (24.40), myopathy, atherosclerosis, acne

Glucocorticoid suppression

- Is due to the inhibition of ACTH secretion
- Becomes significant if treatment is stopped abruptly or if the patient is subjected to severe stress while on low or moderate maintenance doses (withdrawal syndrome such as Addison's crisis (24.42))
- Clinically significant risk is
  - unlikely if the steroid treatment has been of a short duration (<10 days)
  - possible if doses of 10–20 mg/day have been given for several weeks
  - probable if doses of >20 mg have been given for a long time.
- Inhaled steroids may cause glucocorticoid suppression at daily doses of >1500 µg in adults or >400 µg in children **A** [1].
- Because of the risk of glucocorticoid suppression long-term steroid treatment should be tapered off gradually. At 5 mg daily doses of prednisone the dosage can be reduced further to 5 mg every other day until the patient copes without steroid substitution.

Estimation of stress tolerance

- The degree of glucocorticoid suppression can be evaluated by measuring morning concentrations of serum cortisol. If the serum cortisol level in the morning (8 a.m.) is
  - >500 nmol/l, the hypothalamic-pituitary-adrenal axis functions normally and no substitution is needed even in severe stress
  - 200–500 nmol/l, the patient's own cortisol production is good and steroid substitution can safely be withdrawn but adequate cortisol production cannot be guaranteed in severe stress (a short ACTH test should be conducted as necessary)
  - 100–200 nmol/l, stopping of the steroid treatment is probably not possible yet, and glucocorticoid substitution will be needed at least in stress
  - <100 nmol/l, the patient suffers from glucocorticoid suppression and substitution is needed.
- As prednisone, prednisolone and methylprednisolone affect serum cortisol assay, the patient should not take these during the 47 hours before serum cortisol assay. If needed, substitute short-acting hydrocortisone for prednisone, prednisolone or methylprednisolone, and leave the afternoon/evening dose of hydrocortisone off before measuring serum cortisol concentration next morning. Oestrogen replacement will also affect serum cortisol assay.
- Indications for ACTH test
  - The patient is about to stop steroid treatment and you wish to know whether he or she will need substitution therapy in a stress situation.
  - Steroid treatment has been stopped, the patient is going to have an operation, and it is important to know whether he or she will need substitution therapy during the operation.

Substitution therapy during stress

- Substitution therapy during stress is needed if the patient is on steroid therapy and suppression is evident or probable.
- If the patient is on continuous high-dose steroid therapy, no additional treatment is needed.

Table 24.43 Recommended glucocorticoid dosage in a stressful situation in patients with adrenal insufficiency

Procedure or clinical state	Glucocorticoid dosage
Minor procedure or illness ♦ Repair of inguinal hernia ♦ Colonoscopy ♦ Mild febrile illness ♦ Mild gastroenteritis	♦ Usual replacement dose + 25 mg hydrocortisone or 5 mg prednisolone on the day of the procedure/illness ♦ Return to usual replacement dose within 1–2 days
Moderate procedure or illness ♦ Cholecystectomy ♦ Hemicolectomy ♦ Pneumonia ♦ Severe gastroenteritis	♦ Usual replacement dose or an equivalent dose of hydrocortisone or methylprednisolone + ♦ 50–75 mg hydrocortisone or 10–15 mg methylprednisolone i.v. on the day of the procedure/illness ♦ Return to usual replacement dose within 1–2 days
Major procedure or illness ♦ Bypass surgery ♦ Hepatic resection ♦ Pancreatectomy ♦ Pancreatitis	♦ Usual replacement dose or an equivalent dose of hydrocortisone or methylprednisolone + ♦ 100–150 mg hydrocortisone or 20–30 mg methylprednisolone i.v. on the day of the procedure/illness ♦ Return to usual replacement dose within 1–2 days
Critically ill ♦ Sepsis ♦ Shock	♦ 100 mg hydrocortisone i.v., to be followed by 50–100 mg i.v. every 6–8 hours ♦ Dose gradually decreased ♦ In shock, also fludrocortisone 50 µg/day, until condition improves

♦ Recommendations for substitution therapy are presented in Table 24.43.

Prevention of osteoporosis

♦ The prevalence of osteoporosis during long-term glucocorticoid treatment (fractures in 2–45%, decreased bone density in 70%) depends on the underlying disease, duration of treatment and common risk factors. Glucocorticoids affect basically all regulatory factors in the bone and calcium metabolism.
♦ Prevention
- Additional calcium (total dose 10 µg = 1500 mg/day)
- Additional vitamin D (400 IU/day)
- Substitution if there is a deficiency of any of the following: vitamin D, oestrogens, testosterone
- Bisphosphonates (alendronate, risedronate), as necessary

♦ Treatment
- Bisphosphonates (alendronate 70 mg once a week or risedronate 35 mg once a week)
- Calcitonin 100 U/day as a nasal spray if the patient is in pain or cannot tolerate bisphosphonates. The drug is expensive and its efficacy is not as well documented as that of bisphosphonates but it has the benefit of an analgesic effect. If calcitonin is used for pain, treatment should be continued until pain subsides, and calcitonin should then be replaced by a bisphosphonate.
- Thiazides if the patient has definite hypercalciuria. This treatment is still experimental.

Reference

1. Sharek PJ, Bergman DA, Ducharme F. Beclomethasone for asthma in children: effects on linear growth. Cochrane Database Syst Rev. 2004;(2):CD001282.

24.50 Classification of hyperlipidaemias

Timo Strandberg, Hannu Vanhanen

END

Ordinary hypercholesterolaemia

♦ Develops as a result of the combined effect of diet, excessive energy intake (obesity), and hereditary susceptibility (often apoprotein E4 phenotype).

Familial hypercholesterolaemia

♦ Inherited autosomal dominantly
- Prevalence in heterozygotes 1:500
- Prevalence in homozygotes 1:1 000 000

♦ The most typical clinical manifestations are tendon xanthomas in the Achilles tendon (detected most easily by ultrasonography), knees, and extensor tendons of the fingers.
♦ Arcus lipoides and xanthelasmas (Figure 24.50.1) are relatively common.
♦ A greatly increased serum cholesterol concentration (usually > 8 mmol/l) is the most important lipid abnormality.
♦ Some patients have a slightly decreased serum HDL cholesterol concentration.
♦ Early-onset ischaemic heart disease (IHD) is nearly always present in the family.

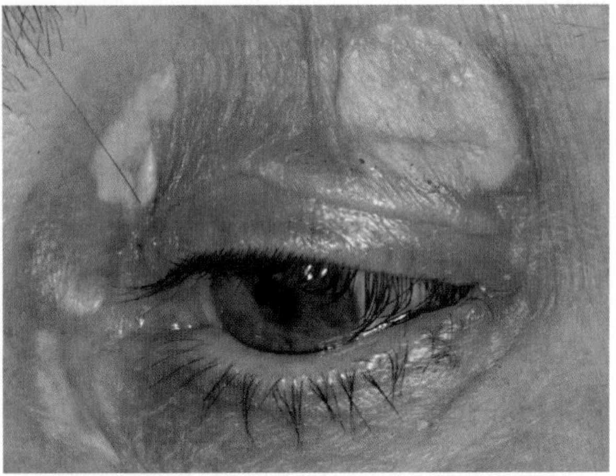

Figure 24.50.1 In xanthelasma, a disturbance in the lipid metabolism is found in 50% of patients. There are several therapeutic alternatives, including surgery and cryotherapy with liquid nitrogen spray. Photo © R. Suhonen.

Familial combined hypercholesterolaemia

- Often manifests in adult age.
- The most important lipid abnormality is excessive production of apoprotein B (the major binding protein for cholesterol and triglycerides)
- Early development of arterial disease may be the only clinical manifestation. Early-onset IHD is present in the family. The lipid abnormalities are variable and may vary in members of the same family.
- Arcus lipoides and xanthelasmas are sometimes observed.
- The diagnosis is based on the familial occurrence of IHD.

Type III hyperlipoproteinaemia (dysbetalipoproteinaemia)

- A rare abnormality
- Serum cholesterol and triglycerides are moderately or markedly increased (both at 7–10 mmol/l).
- The catabolic products of VLDL accumulate.

Hypertriglyceridaemia

- Mild hypertriglyceridaemia (2.0–5.0 mmol/l) is usually associated with living habits alone (obesity, alcohol consumption) and results from the combined effect of several genes and the environment.
- About 1% of the population have primary (autosomal dominantly) inherited primary hypertriglyceridaemia.
- A patient with mild hypertriglyceridaemia has no symptoms.
- A markedly increased serum triglyceride concentration is associated with risk of acute pancreatitis and eruptive xanthomatosis. Articular symptoms caused by gout may sometimes occur.

Table 24.50 Secondary hyperlipidaemias

Hypercholesterolaemia	Hypertriglyceridaemia	Hypercholesterolaemia + hypertriglyceridaemia
Hypothyroidism Nephrotic syndrome	Alcohol Obesity	Hypothyroidism Nephrotic syndrome
Cholestasis Anorexia Acute intermittent porphyria Hypopituitarism	Insulin resistance Diabetic ketosis Type 2 diabetes Uraemia Cushing's syndrome Paraproteinaemias	Hepatic diseases (Type 2 diabetes)

Metabolic syndrome

- Metabolic syndrome (23.36) is often, but not always, associated with hypertriglyceridaemia. Special attention should be paid to this cluster of risk factors, which is probably a hereditary metabolic disorder. The manifestations of metabolic syndrome include
  - central obesity
  - insulin resistance that can be detected years before the development of non-insulin-dependent diabetes mellitus
  - tendency for hypertension
  - low serum HDL cholesterol
  - increased serum triglyceride concentration.

Secondary hyperlipidaemias

- See Table 24.50.
- The most important disease to identify is hypothyroidism.

24.51 Investigations in patients with hyperlipidaemia

Hannu Vanhanen, Timo Strandberg

Basic rules

- Identify patients with familial hypercholesterolaemia and their relatives.
- Identify secondary hyperlipidaemia (most commonly caused by hypothyroidism, either overt or subclinical).
- Identify hyperlipidaemia associated with other risk factors (with special emphasis on persons with ischaemic heart

disease or other arterial diseases, familial history of cardiovascular diseases, high blood pressure, diabetes, metabolic syndrome (23.36), and smokers).

Investigations in patients with lipid concentrations indicating treatment

History

- Atherosclerotic diseases and cholesterol values in the family
- Symptoms of arterial disease
- Dietary habits

Clinical examination

- Blood pressure
- Auscultation of the heart and the large arteries
- Doppler stethoscope examination of the lower extremities if peripheral ischaemia is suspected
- Examination of the skin in order to detect xanthelasmas (around the eyes) and tendon xanthomas (in the Achilles tendons)
  - In a patient with suspected familial hyperlipidaemia, ultrasonographic examination may reveal xanthomas in the Achilles tendon.

Laboratory examinations

- Serum cholesterol, HDL cholesterol, triglycerides; and serum LDL cholesterol that can be calculated from the former: LDL = total cholesterol−HDL−0.45 × serum triglycerides.
- Serum TSH at least in all cases where pharmacological medical treatment is planned
- Blood glucose
- Urine test (proteinuria?)

24.52 Strategies and priorities in screening for hyperlipidaemia

Timo Strandberg, Hannu Vanhanen

Basic rules

- Secondary prevention should be carried out by effectively treating hyperlipidaemia in all patients with ischaemic heart disease or other atherosclerotic disease (cerebral or peripheral arterial disease) Ⓐ [1 2] as well as in diabetics.
- Identify patients with familial hypercholesterolaemia.
- Primary prevention should be directed at people at greatest risk (among working-aged adults with several risk factors such as high blood pressure, smoking, or metabolic syndrome, and diabetics).

Phase I: people with markedly increased risk

1. The benefit of treatment for hyperlipidaemia in patients with ischaemic heart disease, other arterial disease or diabetes has been clearly proven in several long-term trials, especially with statins Ⓐ [3]. A marked decrease in mortality and in the complications of ischaemic heart disease was observed in studies in the statin groups. Also strokes were decreased Ⓐ [4 5 6 7].
2. Identify individuals with familial hypercholesterolaemia.
   - People with an atherosclerotic disease (ischaemic heart disease, cerebrovascular disease, or lower extremity ischaemia at a young age (men below 55 years, women below 65 years).
   - Close relatives of individuals with ischaemic heart disease at young age (children, brothers and sisters).
   - People with earlier high concentrations of serum cholesterol (at least 8 mmol/l)
   - Close relatives of individuals with a markedly increased serum cholesterol.

Carrying out the screening

- Also women and elderly are screened, especially patients with markedly increased risk.
- Propose the checking of all lipid values (serum cholesterol, HDL cholesterol, LDL cholesterol and triglycerides) when the patient visits the doctor's surgery for any reason.
- Check the latest lipid levels from computerized patient registers and patient files. Add a reminder to determine lipid concentrations at the next visit.
- Relatives and family members can usually be contacted by the index patient.

Phase II: People with other risk factors

- Screening for lipid levels in the whole population is not the primary goal in the prevention of atherosclerotic disease. The main emphasis on the population level should be on the promotion of healthy diet and living habits, complemented by action in the community (e.g. in public restaurants).
- If screening is planned it should be directed at working-aged people with other risk factors.
  - Overweight (body mass index >25 kg/m^2). In particular, patients with metabolic syndrome (24.50) associated with central obesity should be identified.
  - Smokers
  - People with hypertension
  - Early-onset coronary heart disease in the family.
- The screening of lipid levels is indicated in all working-age men.

END

Carrying out the screening

- Propose the checking of all lipid values (serum cholesterol, HDL cholesterol, LDL cholesterol and triglycerides) when the patient visits the surgery.
- Occupational health care and normal health checks can be used to contact people in this group.
- The screening should include the assessment of other risk factors (hypertension, smoking, obesity).
- Screening is not recommended for symptomless elderly or for children. For hypercholesterolaemia in children see article 32.83.

References

1. Gould AL, Roussouw JE, Santanello NC, Heyse JF, Furberg CD. Impact of cholesterol reduction on total mortality. Circulation 1995;91:2274–2282.
2. The Database of Abstracts of Reviews of Effectiveness (University of York), Database no.: DARE-950830. In: The Cochrane Library, Issue 4, 1999. Oxford: Update Software.
3. Scandinavian Simvastatin Survival Study Group. Randomized trial of cholesterol lowering in 4 444 patients with coronary heart disease: The Scandinavian Simvastatin Survival Study (4S). Lancet 1994;344:1383–9.
4. Hebert PR, Gaziano JM, Chan KS, Hennekens CH. Cholesterol lowering with statins and risk of stroke. JAMA 1997;278:313–321.
5. The Database of Abstracts of Reviews of Effectiveness (University of York), Database no.: DARE-978231. In: The Cochrane Library, Issue 4, 1999. Oxford: Update Software.
6. Bucher HC, Griffith LE, Guyatt GH. Effect of HMGcoA reductase inhibitors on stroke. Ann Intern Med 1998;128: 89–95.
7. The Database of Abstracts of Reviews of Effectiveness (University of York), Database no.: DARE-988130. In: The Cochrane Library, Issue 4, 1999. Oxford: Update Software.

24.53 Lipid measurements and their sources of error: LDL cholesterol

Hannu Vanhanen, Timo Strandberg

Number and timing of measurements

- One lipid assay is not sufficiently reliable. Before starting treatment of hyperlipidaemia the lipid concentrations must be determined at least 2 or 3 times.
- Blood sampling should be performed after 12 hours of fasting. A meal has a negligible effect on serum total cholesterol but a considerable effect on serum triglyceride concentration.

Diseases reducing serum cholesterol and HDL cholesterol

- Acute myocardial infarction
- Trauma
- Surgery
- Acute infections

Secondary hyperlipidaemia

- If a high serum cholesterol concentration is detected remember the causes of secondary hyperlipidaemia (24.50).
  - Hypothyroidism (even subclinical); the most important cause of secondary hyperlipidaemia.
  - Non-insulin-dependent diabetes mellitus
  - Renal disease
  - Liver disease
  - Alcoholism
  - Antihypertensive drugs

Calculating serum LDL concentration (Friedewald's equation)

- Serum LDL cholesterol is best determined by calculating it according to the Friedewald's equation. Direct assays are not well standardised or are laborious.
- A precondition for the use of the equation is a serum triglyceride concentration under 4 mmol/l. The lipid concentrations should be determined after 12 hours of fasting.
- **Serum LDL cholesterol = serum cholesterol −serum HDL cholesterol −0.45 × serum triglycerides**
- Example:
  - Serum cholesterol = 7.0 mmol/l
  - Serum HDL cholesterol = 1.0 mmol/l
  - Serum triglyceride = 3.1 mmol/l
  - Serum LDL cholesterol = 7.0 −1.0 −0.45 × 3.1 = 4.6
- The target serum LDL concentration is below 3.0 mmol/l (in high risk individuals below 2.5 mmol/l)

24.54 Treatment of hyperlipidaemia: aims and selection

Timo Strandberg, Hannu Vanhanen

Basic rules

- The goals are:
  - Secondary prevention of arterial disease. (The most important patient group to be treated are patients with diagnosed arterial disease.)

- Decreasing the risk of atherosclerotic arterial disease guided by the total risk (combined effect of risk factors). The assessment of the risk for arterial disease may be facilitated by the use of different risk calculators.

- Changing living habits is the primary target in all patients.
- Rule out secondary hypercholesterolaemia before starting drug treatment (serum TSH, fasting blood glucose, urine test).
- The aim of treatment is to maintain
  - serum cholesterol under 5.0 mmol/l (under 4.5 mmol/l in high-risk individuals)
  - serum LDL cholesterol under 3.0 mmol/l (in high-risk individuals under 2.5 mmol/l).
  - serum HDL cholesterol over 1.0 mmol/l
  - serum triglyceride under 2.0 mmol/l
  - serum cholesterol: serum HDL cholesterol ratio under 4.0
- The treatment of a low HDL cholesterol concentration and a high serum triglyceride concentration is probably beneficial at least in patients with non-insulin-dependent diabetes mellitus.
- The serum triglyceride concentration should be under 10 mmol/l, to minimize the risk of pancreatitis.

Patients with ischaemic heart disease

- The risk of myocardial infarction or cardiac death increases sharply with rising serum cholesterol concentrations in patients with IHD.
- The effectiveness of drug treatment has been clearly shown in controlled studies (A) [1]. The target serum cholesterol concentration is under 4.5 mmol/l (LDL cholesterol under 2.5 mmol/l).
- See Table 24.54.1.

Patients with other atherosclerotic diseases (cerebrovascular disease, peripheral arterial disease)

- See above.

Table 24.54.1 Hypercholesterolaemia in patients with ischaemic heart disease

Serum cholesterol (mmol/l)	LDL cholesterol (mmol/l)	Risk of disease progression	Action
♦ 5.0 or higher	3.0 or higher	Greatly increased	Improve diet, change living habits, control cholesterol levels in 2 months. Reduce risk by modifying other risk factors. Drug therapy is always indicated if target levels are not reached.

Symptomless individuals

- The target serum cholesterol level is under 5.0 mmol/l (LDL cholesterol under 3.0 mmol/l). When considering indications for intervention the age and sex and total risk of the patient should be taken into account. (Those of working age are the most important group.) See Table 24.54.2.

Elderly patients (>80 years)

- There are no randomized prognostic studies in this age group.

Table 24.54.2 Hypercholesterolaemia in asymptomatic individuals

Serum cholesterol (mmol/l)	LDL cholesterol (mmol/l)	Risk of disease progression	Action
8.0 or higher	6.5 or higher	Greatly increased	Assess risk factors. Improve diet and change living habits. Control cholesterol levels in 2–3 months. Drug therapy is indicated if values near the target levels are not reached. The probability of an inherited disorder is high. Relatives should be investigated.
6.5–7.9	5.0–6.4	Moderately increased	Assess risk factors and start dietary therapy. Control cholesterol levels in 6 months. Further measures (drug treatment) according to outcome of dietary therapy and other risk factors. Hereditary disorders of lipid metabolism are possible (and should be treated in the same way as patients with serum cholesterol above 8 mmol/l).
5–6.4	3.0–4.9	Slightly increased	Counselling on healthy diet and assessment of risk factors. Further measures according to other risk factors. Control of serum cholesterol after about 5 years.

END

- The biological age and the general prognosis should be taken into account when deciding on treatment.
- The principles of treatment are the same as in younger patients.

Reference

1. Scandinavian Simvastatin Survival Study Group. Randomized trial of cholesterol lowering in 4 444 patients with coronary heart disease: The Scandinavian Simvastatin Survival Study (4S). Lancet 1994;344:1383–9.

24.55 Diet therapy for high serum cholesterol levels

Hannu Vanhanen, Timo Strandberg

Basic rules

- Advise the patient to:
  - reduce the intake of saturated fat
  - increase the intake of polyunsaturated fat and monoenes (vegetable fat) instead of saturated fat (A) [1 2 3 4]. Rape seed oil is the best choice.
  - reduce the intake of cholesterol
  - reduce weight
  - increase the intake of dietary fibre (A) [5 6 7 8] (gel-forming fibre can be added if indicated (24.56)).
- Stanol/sterol margarine can be used (overweight individuals should use diet margarine (40% fat) or nothing).
- If target serum lipid values are not reached with diet therapy start drug treatment (instead of just ordering further control measurements).

Recommendations

- Fat < 30 E% of total energy
  - Saturated < 10 E%
  - Monoenes and polyunsaturated 20 E%
- Diet cholesterol
  - 250–300 mg/day
- Plenty of soluble fibre (A) [5 6 7 8]
  - >20 g / 1000 kcal
- Weight reduction in obese persons
- Avoidance of boiled coffee
- Reduction of alcohol consumption if the patient has
  - overweight
  - high blood pressure
  - hypertriglyceridaemia.
- Reduction of salt intake if the patient has high blood pressure.

Expected effectiveness of diet therapy

- Fasting serum cholesterol may decrease by 15% in some patients, but on the average the effect is only 3–6% (A) [9 10].
- In some individuals the decrease in cholesterol level may exceed 30%.

Diet therapy in practice

- A thorough diet history, preferably by diary, is the basis of diet counselling.
- Reduce animal and milk fat. Advise the patient to:
  - use fat-free milk or sour milk
  - prefer other low fat milk products
  - use vegetable margarine, diet margarine, or plant stanol/sterol margarine
  - prefer low fat meat products, fish, skinless poultry, and sausages low in fat.
- Avoid foods rich in cholesterol.
  - Meat products rich in fat and milk fat
  - Internal organs
  - Egg yolk
- Reduce overweight by hypocaloric diet (or very-low-calorie diet, if necessary) and exercise.
- Increase the intake of vegetable fibre (A) [5 6 7 8]. Prefer
  - vegetables, roots, leguminous plants
  - berries and fruit
  - whole-grain cereals.
- Prepare food without adding fat or by using vegetable oils or vegetable margarines. Suitable oils include canola (most favourable content of fatty acids), olive, sunflower, soy, and maize oil.
- Use filtered coffee instead of boiled.
- As the proportion of fat as energy source is reduced it is substituted by carbohydrates: potatoes, cereals, rice, pasta, fruit, berries, vegetables, and roots.

Plant stanol/sterol margarine as treatment for hypercholesterolaemia

- A daily 25 g dose of sitostanol margarine (2 g of sterol) decreases serum cholesterol by 10% and LDL cholesterol by 15% more than ordinary margarine. The concentrations of HDL cholesterol and triglycerides remain unchanged.
- Sitostanol margarine may be suitable as the only treatment for mild hypercholesterolaemia in addition to other diet therapy. Patients that remain hypercholesterolaemic can be treated with a combination of sitostanol and statins.
- Some patients with familial and other hypercholesterolaemia may be able to avoid hypocholesterolaemic drugs or reduce their doses by using sitostanol margarin.

- Remember the high energy content of vegetable stanols/sterols (overweight persons should use low fat modifications where plant stanols/sterols are added).
- Monitor the outcome and weight of the patient.

References

1. Clarke R, Frost C, Collins R, Appleby P, Peto R. Dietary lipids and blood cholesterol: quantitative meta-analysis of metabolic ward studies. BMJ 1997;314:112–117.
2. The Database of Abstracts of Reviews of Effectiveness (University of York), Database no.: DARE-978007. In: The Cochrane Library, Issue 4, 1999. Oxford: Update Software.
3. Gardner CD, Kraemer HC. Monounsaturated versus polyunsaturated dietary fats and serum lipids. Arteriosc Thrombosis Vasc Biology 1995;15:1917–1927.
4. The Database of Abstracts of Reviews of Effectiveness (University of York), Database no.: DARE-963287. In: The Cochrane Library, Issue 4, 1999. Oxford: Update Software.
5. Brown L, Rosner B, Willett WW, Sacks FM. Cholesterol-lowering effect of dietary fiber: a meta-analysis. Am J Clin Nutr 1999;69:30–42.
6. The Database of Abstracts of Reviews of Effectiveness (University of York), Database no.: DARE-990275. In: The Cochrane Library, Issue 2, 2000. Oxford: Update Software.
7. Olson BH, Anderson SM, Becker MP, Anderson JW, Hunninghake DB, Jenkins DJ, LaRosa JC, Rippe JM, Roberts DC, Stoy DB, Summerbell CD, Truswell CD, Wolever TM, Morris DH, Fulgoni VL III. Psyllium-enriched cereals lower blood total cholesterol and LDL cholesterol, but not HDL cholesterol, in hypercholesterolemic adults: results of a meta-analysis. Journal of Nutrition 1997;127:1973–1980.
8. The Database of Abstracts of Reviews of Effectiveness (University of York), Database no.: DARE-983021. In: The Cochrane Library, Issue 1, 2000. Oxford: Update Software.
9. Tang JL, Armitage JM, Lancaster T, Silagy CA, Fowler GH, Neil HA. Systematic review of dietary interventions to lower blood total cholesterol in free-living subjects. BMJ 1998;316:1213–1220.
10. The Database of Abstracts of Reviews of Effectiveness (University of York), Database no.: DARE-988475. In: The Cochrane Library, Issue 4, 1999. Oxford: Update Software.

24.56 Drug treatment for hyperlipidaemias

Timo Strandberg, Hannu Vanhanen

Basic rules

- Make sure that an effective diet has been implemented, and start drug therapy without delay if clearly indicated.
- People with atherosclerotic disease or diabetes are the most important target groups.
- Determine serum cholesterol, triglycerides, and HDL cholesterol, and calculate serum LDL cholesterol according to the Friedewald equation before commencing drug treatment.
- Rule out secondary hypercholesterolaemia. If the cause of secondary hypercholesterolaemia cannot be managed treat the patient as if he had primary hypercholesterolaemia.
- Identify patients with familial hypercholesterolaemia (serum cholesterol usually above 8 mmol/l, xanthomas, family history) in order to screen family members.
- If an increased serum LDL cholesterol concentration is the most important lipid abnormality a statin is the drug of choice **A** [1 2 3 4].
- If an increased triglyceride concentration (>4.5 mmol/l) and a low HDL cholesterol concentration are the most important abnormalities a fibrate may be the drug of choice.

General principles on the choice of drug

- Of the drugs in common use pravastatin, simvastatin, lovastatin, cholestyramine and gemfibrozil have been tested in randomized double-blind trials lasting at least 5 years **A** [5]. There are long lasting trials on atorvastatin and fluvastatin, as well.
- A statin is the drug of choice **A** [1 2 3 4] unless the main abnormality is hypertriglyceridaemia in combination with a low HDL cholesterol concentration.
- Resins and guar gum are safe during pregnancy and in children because they are not absorbed from the intestine. Their adverse effects may cause problems.

END

Choice of drug according to the type of hyperlipidaemia

- See Table 24.56.

Statins

- The most important group of antihyperlipidaemic agents.

Mechanism of action

- Based on the inhibition of HMG-CoA reductase resulting in the inhibition of cholesterol synthesis in hepatocytes. The number of LDL receptors on hepatocytes is increased, and the elimination of LDL from the blood is enhanced. Part of the action may be through VLDL or even other mechanisms.

Effectiveness

- LDL is decreased by 30–40%.
- HDL is increased by 5–15%.
- Triglycerides are decreased by 10–30%.
- Combining statins with resins results in additive effects **C** [6 7].

Table 24.56 Selection of lipid lowering drug according to the type of hyperlipidaemia

Dyslipidaemic (pheno)type	Drug of choice
Hypercholesterolaemia alone (familial hypercholesterolaemia)	Statin or a combination of statin and ezetimibe or a combination of a statin and a resin (the dose of resin < 20 g to avoid adverse effects).
Both cholesterol and triglycerides increased	♦ Statin if serum triglycerides < 4.5 mmol/l. ♦ Fibrate + statin if increasing the dose of statin is not sufficient (the need for combination treatment should be evaluated by a specialist).
Pure hypertriglyceridaemia	♦ Reducing weight and limiting alcohol consumption is essential before drug treatment is considered. Control of diabetes should be improved. ♦ Fibrate.
Hypothyroidism	Thyroxine substitution normalizes the lipid abnormality if it is caused by hypothyroidism.

Adverse effects

- Statins are usually well tolerated, even by elderly patients.
- Serum aminotransferase concentrations rise in about 2% of the patients.
- Serum creatine kinase need not be determined routinely. The test is indicated if the patient has unexplained myalgias or muscular symptoms. Concentrations 10 times above the upper limit of the reference value are significant. The incidence of myopathy is about 0.5%.
- The incidence of notable muscular side effects is <0.1%
- The risk of myopathy is increased by
  - simultaneous cyclosporine, fibrate, macrolide or conazole medication
  - very high age
  - multiple diseases
  - operations
  - hypothyroidism.
- Individual cases of polyneuropathy have been described in connection with statin treatment.

Dosage

- Adjust the dose (A) [8 9 10 11] according to response. Doubling the dose provides a further decrease of serum cholesterol by 7%.
- Lovastatin: 20–80 mg
- Pravastatin: 20–40 mg/day
- Simvastatin:10–80 mg
- Fluvastatin: (20)–40–80 mg/day
- Atorvastatin:10–80 mg/day
- Rosuvastatin: 10-40 mg/day

Resins (cholestyramin, cholestipol)

Mechanism of action

- The resins adsorb bile acids in the intestine, prevent their reabsorption, and increase their excretion in the faeces.
- They do not increase the excretion of neutral steroids or cause fat malabsorption.
- The enhanced excretion of bile acids results in increased metabolism of cholesterol into bile acids and further in an increase in the number of LDL receptors and intake of cholesterol into hepatocytes.

Effectiveness

- Serum total and LDL cholesterol concentration decrease by 15–30%.
- Serum triglyceride concentration may increase slightly.

Dosage

- Cholestyramin 16–32 g/day
- Cholestipol 20–40 g/day

Adverse effects

- Bowel symptoms: constipation, flatulence, nausea, epigastric pain
- Deficiency of fat-soluble vitamins and folic acid

Interactions

- The absorption of the following drugs may be affected. These drugs should be taken at least 1 hour before or 4 hours after the resin.
  - Digoxin
  - Thyroxine
  - Warfarin
  - Thiazide diuretics

Guar gum

Mechanism of action

- Guar gum is an unabsorbable dietary fibre, galactomannan. The mechanism of action is similar to that of resins. Guar gum also increases the excretion of neutral steroids in the faeces.

Effectiveness

- Serum total cholesterol and LDL cholesterol are decreased by 10–15%. HDL and triglyceride concentration remain unchanged.
- Guar gum is a suitable alternative in hypercholesterolaemia associated with diabetes as a supplement to diet or in severe hypercholesterolaemia in combination with statins or fibrates.

Dosage

- 5 g 2–5 times a day

Adverse effects

- About 30% of the patients have adverse effects
- Abdominal distention, flatulence, diarrhoea

Fibrates (gemfibrozil, bezafibrate and fenofibrate)

Mechanism of action

- Fibrates act through the nuclear PPAR (peroxisome proliferator activated receptor) system that regulates lipid metabolism.

Effectiveness

- Triglyceride concentration is decreased by 20–70%.
- HDL cholesterol is increased by 10–25%.
- LDL cholesterol is decreased if the initial concentration is high.

Adverse effects

- Mild abdominal and bowel irritation
- Myalgia and an increase in serum creatine kinase concentration
- Possible formation of gallstones
- Increase in serum transaminase levels
- Retention of water, growth of mammary tissue and impotence are rare.

Interactions

- Protein-bound drugs are released and their concentrations are increased (warfarin, sulphonylureas)

Contraindications

- Severe renal or hepatic dysfunction, diseases of the gallbladder.

Dosage

- Gemfibrozil: 600–1200 mg/day divided into 2–3 doses
- Bezafibrate: 400 mg × 1 at lunch
- Fenofibrate: 200 mg × 1 with meal

Ezetimibe

- For patients whose hypercholesterolaemia cannot be treated with statin or when the effect is insufficient, ezetimibe is a good choice.

Mechanism of action

- Prevents cholesterol from being absorbed in the small intestine.
- Effect is additive to statins which prevent cholesterol synthesis.

Effectiveness

- Alone diminishes the concentration of LDL cholesterol 18–19%, triglycerides 4–11% and increases the concentration of HDL cholesterol 2–3%
- Combining etzetimibe with statin is additive and equals a large dose of statin in reducing cholesterol level.

Dosage

- 10 mg/day

Side effects

- The studies conducted so far show little side effects.

Follow-up of a patient on cholesterol-lowering drugs

- Lipid concentrations should be controlled after 1–2 months, then after 3–6 months and thereafter annually, if necessary.
- Before changing the drug wait for the effect for 3–6 months.
- Make sure that the target lipid levels (24.54) are achieved.

END

Laboratory tests

- Statins: serum ALT should be determined after 1–2 months. A slight increase (ad 2 x) in serum ALT concentration is an indication for follow-up, not necessarily for discontinuation of the drug. If unexplained myalgia occurs determine serum creatine kinase.
- Fibrates: ALT or AST and alkaline phosphatase are determined after 1–2 months, and thereafter at 6–12-month intervals. If used in combination with statins, ALT should be determined at 3–4 month intervals. If myalgia occurs serum creatine kinase should always be examined.

Indications for specialist consultation

- Need for a drug combination
- A lipid disorder associated with another complicated disease
- Serum triglyceride concentration is primarily above 10 mmol/l or remains above 5 mmol/l despite treatments.
- Very high serum cholesterol concentration (above 15 mmol/l).
- Ischaemic heart disease or xanthomas occur in childhood or in adolescents or young adults.

References

1. Bucher HC, Griffith LE, Guyatt GH. Systematic review on the risk and benefit of different cholesterol-lowering

interventions. Arteriosclerosis, Thrombosis and Vascular Biology 1999;19:187–195.
2. The Database of Abstracts of Reviews of Effectiveness (University of York), Database no.: DARE-993524. In: The Cochrane Library, Issue 4, 2000. Oxford: Update Software.
3. Ross S D, Allen I E, Connelly J E, Korenblat B M, Smith M E, Bishop D, Luo D. Clinical outcomes in statin treatment trials. Archives of Internal Medicine 1999;159:1793–1802.
4. The Database of Abstracts of Reviews of Effectiveness (University of York), Database no.: DARE-999402. In: The Cochrane Library, Issue 1, 2002. Oxford: Update Software.
5. Scandinavian Simvastatin Survival Study Group. Randomized trial of cholesterol lowering in 4 444 patients with coronary heart disease: The Scandinavian Simvastatin Survival Study (4S). Lancet 1994;344:1383–9.
6. Schectman G, Hiatt J. Dose-response characteristics of cholesterol-lowering drug therapies. Ann Intern Med 1996: 125:990–1000.
7. The Database of Abstracts of Reviews of Effectiveness (University of York), Database no.: DARE-978010. In: The Cochrane Library, Issue 4, 1999. Oxford: Update Software.
8. Illingworth DR, Tobert JA. A review of clinical trials comparing HMG-CoA reductase inhibitors. Clin Ther 1994;16:366–384.
9. The Database of Abstracts of Reviews of Effectiveness (University of York), Database no.: DARE-940339. In: The Cochrane Library, Issue 4, 1999. Oxford: Update Software.
10. Hsu I, Spinler SA, Johnson NE. Comparative evaluation of the safety and efficacy of HMG-CoA reductase inhibitor monotherapy in the treatment of primary hypercholesterolemia. Ann Pharcother 1995;29:743–759.
11. The Database of Abstracts of Reviews of Effectiveness (University of York), Database no.: DARE-952141. In: The Cochrane Library, Issue 4, 1999. Oxford: Update Software.

24.60 Excessive hair growth (hirsutism)

Editors

Basic rules

- Polycystic ovary syndrome (PCO) (25.15) is the most common cause of excessive androgen production.
- Other androgen-producing tumours are rare.
- Adrenocortical enzyme deficiencies are also rare.
- Cushing's syndrome is associated with both hypertrichosis of hair and hirsutism.

Investigations

- History of the development of hirsutism: age, weight gain, discontinuation of oral contraceptives
- Localisation of hirsutism and differentiation from hypertrichosis
- Signs of virilism
- Menstrual cycle and fertility

Androgen-mediated hair growth

- Female hyperandrogenism is suggested by hair growth in the following areas:
  - Face: moustache, beard, cheeks
  - Chest: midline between breasts and scapulae
  - Abdomen: midline above the navel
  - Pubic area
  - Extremities: hair growth on the internal aspects of the thighs is abnormal.

Pathogenesis

Hyperandrogenism

- Increased androgen production by the ovaries or adrenal cortex or both
- Use of androgenic and anabolic steroids

Peripheral hirsutism (hypertrichosis)

- Genetic and ethnic factors
- Begins after puberty
- Exacerbates with weight gain and after discontinuing oral contraceptives

Clinical signs suggesting virilism

- Menstrual disorders; the diagnosis of PCO is based on ultrasonography.
- Lowering of the pitch of the voice
- Hypertrophy of the clitoris
- Male-type hair growth, temporal baldness

Investigation and treatment strategy

- Examine whether the location of the hair suggests androgen-mediated hirsutism.
  - If the hair is located on the legs and arms (non-androgen-dependent hirsutism), the menstrual cycle is normal, and there are no signs of virilism, no further investigations are needed. Treatment options: no treatment, local treatment, or oestrogen + antiandrogen.
  - If the hirsutism is androgen-mediated, determine serum testosterone. If the menstrual cycle is irregular, determine also serum prolactin. Rule out Cushing's syndrome.
  - In practice, serum testosterone < 6 nmol/l and DHEAS < 20 μmol/l rule out an androgen-producing tumour.
- Perform further investigations in case of
  - progression of hair growth
  - signs of virilism

- menstrual cycle irregularities
- infertility
- markedly abnormal laboratory results
- clinical suspicion of Cushing's disease (a dexamethasone test is indicated).

♦ Suspicion of Cushing's syndrome or a rare tumour
- Refer to an endocrinologist.

♦ Increased serum testosterone, menstrual cycle abnormalities, infertility
- Refer to a gynaecologist.

Treatment options

♦ Often limited
♦ Local treatment (shaving hair does not accelerate its growth)
♦ Weight reduction; reduces risk factors
♦ Drug treatment is often unsatisfactory.
♦ Surgery

Drug therapy

♦ Oestrogen + antiandrogen (cyproterone acetate) C [1]. If the patient has an irregular menstrual cycle she may also have infertility problems. In such cases a specialist consultation is indicated.
♦ Treatments by a specialist
- Dexamethasone (congenital adrenocortical hyperplasia)
- Spironolactone D [2]
- Ketoconazole

References

1. Van der Spuy ZM, le Roux PA. Cyproterone acetate for hirsutism. Cochrane Database Syst Rev 2003(4):CD001125.
2. Farquhar C, Lee O, Toomath R, Jepson R. Spironolactone versus placebo or in combination with steroids for hirsutism and/or acne. Cochrane Database Syst Rev. 2004;(2):CD000194.

24.61 Male hypogonadism and hormone replacement

Ritva Kauppinen-Mäkelin

Aims

♦ Differentiate between primary and secondary hypogonadism. In secondary hypogonadism, also treat the underlying cause.
♦ Prescribe testosterone as hormone replacement therapy, unless it is contraindicated.

Regulation of male sex hormone levels

♦ Luteinising hormone (LH) stimulates testosterone secretion in Leydig cells.
♦ Follicle-stimulating hormone (FSH) stimulates the function of testicular Sertoli cells, which have an important role in the production of spermatozoa.

Symptoms of hypogonadism (testosterone deficiency)

♦ The onset of hypogonadism before puberty results in eunuchoidism, i.e. long extremities, high-pitched voice, asthenic muscles, infantile genitals.
♦ Adult-onset hypogonadism results in decreased libido, impotence and weakening of secondary sex characteristics.

Main causes of hypogonadism

♦ Primary (testicular, hypergonadotropic) hypogonadism
- Klinefelter's syndrome
- Cryptorchidism
- Orchitis
- Irradiation, toxic substances, pharmaceuticals
- Certain systemic diseases (liver cirrhosis, uraemia)

♦ Secondary (central, hypogonadotrophic) hypogonadism
- Congenital causes
- Acquired: trauma to the pituitary gland or hypothalamus, tumours, infiltrating disease, pituitary apoplexy, sequelae of pituitary surgery or radiotherapy, pharmaceuticals (oestrogens in the treatment of prostate cancer), hyperprolactinaemia, undernourishment, anorexia nervosa

♦ Subclinical hypogonadism
- The number of Leydig cells decreases with age.

Klinefelter's syndrome (47,XXY)

♦ Incidence approx. 1:500
♦ Small, firm testes
♦ Long extremities
♦ Puberty delayed to a varying degree
♦ In some boys testosterone production is relatively good during puberty. Later on, serum testosterone levels decrease and LH levels increase (FSH levels are also increased), resulting in decreased libido, impotence, gynaecomastia, weakening of secondary sex characteristics, and infertility. The patient may seek treatment for any of these symptoms.
♦ Some patients suffer from slightly subnormal intelligence, diabetes or pulmonary disease.

END

Investigations

- Serum testosterone and SHBG (sex hormone binding globulin) (or free testosterone), LH and prolactin.
  - Normally only 2% of testosterone is free, i.e. in a biologically active form, the rest is bound to SHBG.
- If serum testosterone is at the lower end of the reference range and
  - SHBG is low, free testosterone is normal
  - SHBG is high, free testosterone is low.
- SHBG concentration will increase with advanced age, in hyperthyroidism and by the influence of oestrogens; androgens will decrease SHBG concentration.
- In case of hypergonadotrophic hypogonadism, cytogenetic analysis (in specialist health care) is indicated if Klinefelter's syndrome is suspected.
- In case of hypogonadotrophic hypogonadism magnetic resonance imaging of the sella region is indicated (in specialist health care).

Treatment

- Testosterone replacement therapy for both primary and secondary hypogonadism
- In patients with secondary hypogonadism, gonadotropin treatment may restore sperm production.
- In secondary hypogonadism, the cause of hypogonadism must also be treated (for example by surgical treatment of a pituitary tumour).

Testosterone replacement therapy

- Intramuscular testosterone esters (e.g. Sustanon® 250 mg) every 2–4 weeks
  - The patient's subjective feeling of well-being is the best indicator of suitable dosing interval.
- Testosterone patches, 2.5–5 mg/day
  - The usual dosage is one 5 mg patch every night on the skin (not on the scrotum). Dosage is appropriate if morning testosterone concentrations fall well within the reference range. Testosterone concentrations can be measured 3 days after the beginning of treatment with the patches.
  - Treatment with the patches is considerably more expensive than intramuscular injections.
- Testosterone gels (e.g. Testogel® 50 mg/dose) once daily.
- During testosterone treatment, the size of the prostate, PSA concentrations, serum lipid levels and the blood count should be monitored.

Contraindications to testosterone treatment

- Prostate cancer
- Untreated prostatic hyperplasia causing bladder outlet obstruction
- High hematocrite (>52%)

When should testosterone be prescribed?

- Replacement therapy is indicated if serum testosterone concentration is below 10 nmol/l and the patient has signs and symptoms of hypogonadism.
- Replacement therapy may also be of benefit in subclinical hypogonadism (serum testosterone >10 nmol/l and LH >6 U/l). An experimental course of testosterone can be prescribed if the patient is symptomatic and there are no contraindications for the treatment.

24.62 Gynaecomastia

Editors

Basic rules

- Differentiate physiological breast enlargement and "normal variant" from pathological conditions in order to avoid unnecessary investigations.
- Refer patients with quickly developing or symptomatic gynaecomastia for further investigations or perform at least the initial investigations.

Physiological breast enlargement

- In the neonate maternal and placental oestrogens regulate the growth of the breasts. The phenomenon disappears during the first weeks of life but may sometimes last longer.
- At puberty many boys have breast growth that is often asymmetric. The growth starts on average at the age of 14 and ceases by the age of 20. The condition is probably associated with variation of androgen and oestrogen levels during puberty.
- As many as 40% of elderly men have gynaecomastia, caused by androgens metabolised into oestrogens in peripheral tissues.

Pathological breast enlargement

- For gynaecomastia of puberty, see article 28.42.
- **Hormonal** breast growth is caused by oestrogen-androgen disequilibrium in men.

- **Testosterone deficiency** is caused by congenital or acquired hypogonadism (24.61). The causes for hypogonadism include
  - gonadotrophin deficiency
  - hyperprolactinaemia
  - testicular disease
  - hypersecretion of oestrogen.
- **Increased oestrogen production** is caused by
  - adrenocortical, testicular and other tumours producing oestrogens and human chorionic gonadotrophin (hCG)
  - cirrhosis of the liver
  - hyperthyroidism
  - many drugs: spironolactone, oestrogens, androgens, digoxin, isoniazid, phenothiazines, amphetamine, marijuana, tricyclic antidepressants, diazepam, ketoconazole, penicillamine, cytotoxic drugs, and herbal drugs.
- **Local nonendocrine gynaecomastia** may be caused by a primary tumour or a metastasis.

Diagnostic assessment

- Observe the following signs and history
  - Sexual function (impotence, decreased libido)
  - Size of the testes (small testes indicate hypogonadism, asymmetry suggests a tumour)
  - Hair growth (masculine or feminine?)
  - Milk or other discharge when squeezing the breasts
  - Signs of liver disease
  - Drug history

Further investigations

- For gynaecomastia of puberty, see article 28.42.
- Because gynaecomastia is often transient and the aetiology can be determined in only about half of all cases, not all patients need hormone assays. Investigations are indicated if the drugs used by the patient do not explain the gynaecomastia, and
  - the breast is tender (a sign of rapid growth) or
  - the diameter of the breast tissue is >4 cm.
- In other cases the need for investigations is decided individually. For example, gynaecomastia associated with signs of androgen deficiency should always be investigated.

Laboratory investigations

- The following tests are always indicated
  - Serum testosterone and sex-hormone binding globulin (SHBG) (or serum free testosterone)
  - Serum luteinizing hormone (LH)
  - Serum TSH

Interpretation of the laboratory results

- If serum LH concentration is increased and serum testosterone concentration decreased the patient probably has testosterone deficiency caused by testicular dysfunction.
- If both tests are normal the patient probably has hypogonadotrophic hypogonadism or increased oestrogen production.
- If both serum LH and free testosterone concentrations are increased the patient has androgen resistance or a rare gonadotrophin-secreting tumour of the pituitary gland.
- Serum beta-hCG concentration is increased in testicular trophoblast tumours.
- In problematic cases the following tests can be performed according to specialist advice:
  - Serum SHBG
  - Serum oestrone
  - Serum estradiol
  - Serum prolactin
  - Serum beta-hCG
  - Liver function tests
  - Karyotype
  - Mammography or breast ultrasonography in order to determine breast structure or detect eventual tumours.

Treatment

- In transient gynaecomastia the breast usually decreases in size spontaneously after the underlying cause has been corrected.
- Tamoxifen is the drug of choice.
- Cosmetic harm and malignant tumours are indications for surgery.

END

24.63 APECED (autoimmune polyendocrinopathy -candidiasis -ectodermal dystrophy)

Jaakko Perheentupa

- Synonyme: Autoimmune Polyendocrine Syndrome/Disease type 1

Basic rule

- Suspect the disease in all children and young adults with otherwise unexplained
  - persistent or recurrent oral candidiasis (in mild cases rhagades of the corners of mouth)
  - hypoparathyroidism or Addison's disease
  - alopecia
  - chronic keratoconjunctivitis
  - autoimmune hepatitis of a child
  - flashing erythema with fever of a child
  - chronic diarrhoea or severe obstipation

- The suspicion is strengthened by presence of
  - enamel hypoplasia of permanent teeth
  - pitted nail dystrophy

Epidemiology

- Autosomal recessive inheritance: mutations of both AIRE genes (chromosome 21q22.3)
- Occurs in all populations; so far most frequently recognized in people of Finnish, Sardinian and Iranian Jewish origin
- The clinical picture and course are highly variable.

Symptoms

- The symptoms are highly variable, depending on the disease components present. Most frequently the first symptoms are sore mouth corners, symptoms of hypocalcaemia (clumsiness, vague tetany, convulsions, often in connection to febrile infection), or weakness, fatigue and weight loss. However, none of these is constant. The first components usually appear before the age of 15 years, but sometimes only in adulthood. New components may develop throughout life.
- See Table 24.63.

Treatment and follow-up

- An endocrinologist should be consulted in suspected cases, and must supervise the management of the patients
- The development of endocrinopathies should be monitored by means of appropriate laboratory tests.
- The treatment of each component disease is similar to the therapy of that disease when occurring alone. However, the endocrine components may affect each other.

Table 24.63 Prevalence (%) of disease components of APECED at ages 10 and 40 years in Finnish series of 89 patients

Component	at 10 years	at 40 years
At least one endocrinopathy	74	100
Hypoparathyroidism	64	86
Addison's disease	39	79
Diabetes mellitus	3	23
Hypothyroidism	1	18
Ovarian atrophy		72
Male hypogonadism		26
Pernicious anaemia	2	31
Hepatitis	11	17
Chronic diarrhoea	11	18
Severe obstipation	6	21
History of flashing erythema with fever	9	11
Mucocutaneous candidiasis	79	100
Keratoconjunctivitis	16	22
Alopecia	15	40
Vitiligo	8	26

- Oral candidiasis must be effectively controlled, because it is carcinogenic. Follow-up by a specialist of oral medicine is recommended.

24.64 Clinical use of vitamins

Editors

Basic rules

- The vitamin requirement of the human body is usually met by adequate nutrition. Vitamin supplementation is of no proven efficacy in the prevention of diseases.
- Risk groups for vitamin deficiencies include small children, the elderly with inadequate food intake, alcoholics, and patients suffering from severe systemic diseases. In these groups the prophylactic use of vitamins may be beneficial, and diagnosed vitamin deficiencies should be actively treated.
- Consider vitamin deficiency as a possible cause of vague or non-specific symptoms (such as aches, loss of strength, rashes) in the risk groups.

Prophylactic vitamin D for children

- The preparations should contain vitamin D only. The need for vitamin A is always met by the normal diet.
- Vitamin D preparations are not indicated after the age of 2 years.
- For dosage see Table 24.64

The most important indications for vitamin substitutions

- Vitamin B_1 should be given to alcoholics in the treatment and prevention of Wernicke's encephalopathy (36.73).

Table 24.64 Dosage of vitamin D in children in Northern climate

Group	Dosage
Age 2 weeks–1 year	
♦ Solely on breast milk or breast milk substitutes only occasionally (maximum 1–2 dL daily)	10 μg (400 IU)/day
♦ Breast milk substitutes as the main or sole food	6 μg (240 IU)/day
♦ Breast milk substitutes continuously and in large amounts (more than 10 dL daily)	None
Age 1–2 years	10 μg (400 IU)/day
Dark-skinned immigrants up to the age of 4–5 years	10 μg (400 IU)/day

- Vitamin B_{12} should be given in established deficiency. The risk groups include patients with atrophic gastritis or post-gastrectomy state.
- Vitamin D should be given to elderly institutionalised patients for the prevention of osteoporosis especially in the winter, to patients with malabsorption, to those adhering to a vegan diet, to patients on anti-epileptic drugs, to patients with renal insufficiency and osteomalacia if vitamin D deficiency has been diagnosed, and as deemed necessary to patients with osteoporosis in combination with calcium. Vitamin D is also safe for premenopausal women for building up bone mass (deficiency need not be proven or followed up).
- Vitamin K should be given prophylactically to the newborn to prevent intracerebral haemorrhage.
- Folic acid prophylaxis in early pregnancy is indicated in special cases (26.1).
- Vitamin C deficiency has been found in elderly persons who live at home and have an unbalanced diet. Recommendations for daily need are not uniform.

The most important therapeutic uses of vitamins

- Treatment of vitamin deficiencies (e.g. vitamin B_{12}, folate)
- Vitamin K for warfarin overdose (15.31)

Preventing excessive intake of vitamin A

- During pregnancy and while trying to become pregnant do not eat liver products.

24.65 Haemochromatosis

Matti Vuoristo

Introduction

- Haemochromatosis refers to an excessive and harmful accumulation of iron in the body.
- The most common manifestation is primary or hereditary haemochromatosis which is a relatively common and probably underdiagnosed disease.
- Early diagnosis is important in order to prevent serious late complications from developing.
- Primary haemochromatosis should be considered particularly in middle-aged men with intense fatigue, lowered libido, loss of body hair, diabetes, hepatomegaly, joint symptoms, excessive skin pigmentation or an unexplained rise in serum aminotransferase.
- Secondary haemochromatosis is usually seen in chronic anaemias which are associated with reduced erythropoiesis and repeated red cell transfusions.

Definitions

- Primary haemochromatosis is a hereditary iron storage disorder in which iron absorption is increased in relation to the total body iron content. Large amounts of iron accumulate in tissues causing fibrotic changes predominantly affecting the liver, pancreas and heart.
- Secondary or acquired haemochromatosis is usually seen in patients with chronic anaemia (e.g. sideroblastic anaemia or beta-thalassaemia) and in patients who have received repeated blood transfusions for reasons other than iron deficiency anaemia.

Genetics of haemochromatosis

- Most cases of haemochromatosis are due to two mutations (C282Y and H63D) of the HFE gene.
- HFE is a cell membrane protein which is associated with the regulation of iron absorption. In Europe most cases of haemochromatosis are due to two point mutations of the HFE gene, i.e. C282Y and H63D. These mutations have particularly high prevalence in Northern Europe, and approximately five in a thousand Europeans are estimated to be homozygous for the C282Y mutation. However, not all cases of mutation lead to haemochromatosis. The HFE gene is located at the short arm of chromosome 6.
- In men, the disease usually develops after the age of 20 and, in women, after the age of 40. However, an earlier manifestation is also possible.
- Haemochromatosis is approximately 5 times more common in men than in women.

Symptoms and clinical findings

- Hepatomegaly. Signs of chronic liver disease such as jaundice, ascites and portal hypertension are infrequent.
- Two-thirds of the patients develop diabetes, which may lead to retino-, nephro- or neuropathy.
- Pigmentation of the skin. Skin may appear metallic gray ("bronze diabetes").
- Lowered libido, testicular atrophy. Insufficiency of the pituitary, the thyroid or the parathyroid gland and Addison's disease are rare.
- Fatigue
- Cardiac involvement, right heart failure, arrhythmias.
- Arthralgia
- As many as one-third of patients with cirrhosis develop hepatoma

Diagnosis

- A serum iron concentration exceeding 27 µmol/l and transferrin iron saturation exceeding 60% in men, and 50% in women, strongly suggest haemochromatosis.

- Increased serum ferritin concentration (350–500 μg/l). Because ferritin is an acute phase protein its concentration is also elevated in many other diseases, particularly inflammatory and hepatic diseases.
- Liver function tests are seldom useful in diagnosis, unless the disease has progressed to cirrhosis. Serum aminotransferases usually rise only a little (<100 U/l; ALT > AST).
- Liver biopsy with iron staining is a diagnostic test. Liver iron content is usually over 150 μmol/g of dry weight (normal reference range 5–40 μmol/g). The iron content can also be estimated by computed tomography or magnetic resonance imaging.
- A definite diagnosis can be obtained by testing the patient for HFE gene mutation.
- First-degree relatives of patients who are homozygous for C282Y or combined C282Y/H63D heterozygotes should be screened with the HFE mutation test.
- Screening of the general population with DNA testing is not recommended at present.

Treatment

- The treatment aims at removing excessive iron. The amount of iron overload varies between 10 and 45 g.
- Venesection is the most effective and safest form of treatment. Aim at removing 500 ml of blood by venesection once or twice weekly. Monitor blood count values (haemoglobin and haematocrit once a week) and iron content (serum iron, transferrin and ferritin every 3 months).
- Because 500 ml of blood contains 250 mg of iron, removing excess iron by weekly venesections will take 2–3 years before the blood iron concentration and haemoglobin are reduced. Ferritin should be kept at around 25–50 μg/l. If necessary, complete depletion of iron can be verified by liver biopsy.
- Venesection once every 3 months is usually sufficient for maintenance.
- Reducing the iron stores of patients with anaemia, hypoproteinaemia or cardiac disease poses a problem. In these cases, the use of iron chelating desferrioxamine may be helpful, but the daily removal of iron is only 10–20 mg.
- The use of excessive amounts of vitamin C and alcohol should be avoided.

Prognosis

- The most severe complications are insulin-dependent diabetes, heart disease, cirrhosis and hepatoma.
- Prognosis is poor for untreated patients, but improves significantly with treatment. Five-year survival is 70–90%.
- Removing iron does not reduce the risk of hepatoma in patients with haemochromatosis and cirrhosis.

24.66 Acute porphyria

Pertti Mustajoki

Prevalence and aetiology

- Acute intermittent porphyria, porphyria variegata, and to a lesser degree hereditary coproporphyria can all cause acute symptoms.
- The symptoms begin after puberty, most often between the ages of 20 and 40 years.
- Symptoms may be triggered by drugs, alcohol, menstruation, infection, or fasting. All precipitating factors should be eliminated during acute symptoms.
- Porphyrias are inherited dominantly and autosomally. Family members should be interviewed for cases of the disease.

Symptoms and diagnosis

- Nearly all patients have abdominal pain. The abdomen may be tender to palpation, but there is no defence.
- Vomiting and obstipation are common.
- Other symptoms include red colour of urine, limb pain, psychiatric symptoms, tachycardia, hypertension, and hyponatraemia.
- Peripheral neuropathy (muscle weakness, paresis) in advanced cases.
- When porphyria is suspected, urine porphobilinogen should be determined. A quick test is available, but the diagnosis should always be confirmed by a quantitative method.
    - A markedly increased excretion of porphobilinogen is diagnostic of acute porphyria.
    - In a symptomatic patient the excretion rate is more than 10–30 times the reference value.

Specific treatment

- Triggering factors should be eliminated.
- Treatment consists of heme arginate 3 mg/kg for 4 days C [1], and plenty of carbohydrates (glucose intravenously 400 g daily or a carbohydrate-rich diet).

Other treatments

- Opiates for severe pain
- Beta-blockers for hypertension
- A neuroleptic (e.g. chlorpromazine) for psychotic symptoms
- Vigorous physiotherapy for pareses.

Reference

1. Herrick AL, McColl KE, Moore MR, Cook A, Goldberg A. Controlled trial of haem arginate in acute hepatic porphyria. Lancet 1989: 1295–7.

24.67 Pituitary tumours

Ritva Kauppinen-Mäkelin

Epidemiology

- Relatively common; found in about 10–20% of autopsies. Clinically insignificant areas of decreased or increased density in the pituitary gland, possibly representing small microadenomas, are seen as incidental findings in cranial imaging in about 5–10% of patients.

Symptoms indicating pituitary tumour

- Symptoms of hormone deficiency
  - In men, loss of libido and impotence, for example; in women secondary amenorrhea (gonadotropin deficiency); abnormal fatigue with hyponatraemia and/or normochromic anaemia (hypocortisolism)
- Symptoms of excessive hormone secretion
  - Symptoms of hyperprolactinaemia such as galactorrhea and amenorrhea, acromegalic habitus, features of Cushing's syndrome
- Compression symptoms in surrounding tissues
  - Most commonly visual symptoms (visual field defect, impaired vision, paresis of muscles moving the eyeball)
  - Headache
- Nasal CSF leakage
- Enlarged sella as an incidental radiological finding
- Pituitary apoplexy

Remember the possibility of pituitary tumour

- As a cause of hypothyroidism (disproportionately low TSH level)
- As a cause of hyponatraemia (hypocortisolism)
- As a cause of normochromic anaemia

Hypopituitarism

- Hormone deficiencies usually develop in the following order:
  - Growth hormone
  - Gonadotropins, resulting in hypogonadism
    - In women menstrual disturbances, amenorrhea
    - In men decreased libido, impotence, decreased beard growth, muscle weakness, decreased energy, decreased haemoglobin concentrations
  - TSH, resulting in mild hypothyroidism
    - TSH level disproportionately low for hypothyroidism. In patients with hypothyroidism even TSH levels that fall within the reference range are disproportionately low, suggesting a central defect.
  - ACTH, resulting in hypocortisolism
    - Symptoms milder than in Addison's disease
    - Often hyponatraemia

Findings indicating hypothalamic disorder

- ADH deficiency, resulting in diabetes insipidus
- Hyperprolactinaemia resulting from damage to the pituitary stalk (hyperprolactinaemia often relatively mild, >600 mU/l; prolactinoma is a more common reason for hyperprolactinaemia, leading to more clearly elevated prolactin levels).

Symptoms of excessive hormone secretion

- Prolactinoma is the most common pituitary tumour
  - In microadenoma serum prolactin levels are usually 1000–4000 mU/l, in macroadenoma clearly elevated (>5000 mU/l)
  - In women galactorrhea and hypogonadotropic hypogonadism resulting in menstrual disturbances, amenorrhea and infertility
  - In men loss of libido, impotence and infertility
  - Hypothyroidism and use of drugs causing hyperprolactinaemia (nearly all psychotropic drugs, metoclopramide, but not benzodiazepines) must be excluded.
  - Hyperprolactinaemia caused by psychotropic drugs is often mild (serum prolactin level at 1000–2000) and insignificant if there are no symptoms.
  - Symptomless hyperprolactinaemia may be caused by macroprolactinaemia (prolactin as an inactive polymer, can be determined).
- Acromegaly
  - Enlargement of distal parts of the body (chin, hands, feet)
  - Hypertension
  - Sweating and fatigue, snoring, arthralgia, headache
- Cushing's disease
  - Typical habitus (central obesity, proximal muscle atrophy, thin skin, bruising tendency)
  - Hypertension, diabetes based on insulin resistance
  - Osteoporosis
  - Menstrual disturbances
  - Mental sensitivity

Diagnostics

- In case of suspected hypopituitarism assay the concentrations of appropriate peripheral hormones and regulating

pituitary hormones (for example free T4 and TSH; morning serum cortisol, plasma ACTH, serum testosterone and serum LH)
- In case of suspected excessive hormone production
  - Prolactinoma: serum prolactin
  - Acromegaly: serum GH, serum IGF-1; 2-hour glucose challenge test, if necessary, with blood glucose and serum GH. (Because evaluation of the results requires specialization, the patient should normally be referred to specialized care.)
  - Cushing's disease: as screening tests 1-mg dexamethasone test and/or 24-h urinary free cortisol (in patients taking oestrogen 24-h urinary free cortisol, as oestrogen will interfere with serum cortisol assay), confirmation by further tests in specialized health care
- Imaging
  - MRI of the sellar region (in specialized care)

Treatment

- Surgical resection of the tumour
- Pharmacological treatment
  - Cabergoline, bromocriptine, quinagolide for prolactinoma
  - Octreotide, lanreotide, cabergoline, bromocriptine for acromegaly
- Radiotherapy in selected cases

24.68 Rare endocrine tumours (pheochromocytoma and insulinoma)

Editors

Pheochromocytoma

- Pheochromocytoma is a rare tumour excreting catecholamines (the yearly incidence is 1:400 000). High blood pressure is caused by pheochromocytoma in about 0.1% of patients with hypertension.
- Some cases are associated with endocrinological syndromes (MEN2a, MEN2b).

Symptoms

- High blood pressure, often with atypical features
  - Very high blood pressure readings at times
  - Poor response to treatment and worsening of the condition during beta-blocker treatment
- During paroxysmal elevations of the BP the patient often has general symptoms: perspiration, palpitations, chest or abdominal pain, nausea, pallor or flushing.

Diagnosis

- Metanephrine and normetanephrine in 24 h urine. Collection should be started during a symptomatic attack or just afterwards (give a sampling container to the patient; urine collection should be started immediately at the onset of symptoms).
- If the results are normal, investigation should be continued only if the clinical suspicion is strong. Further investigations are performed at an endocrinological unit.

Treatment

- The tumour is located by CT scan of the adrenal gland or by octreotide scanning.
- Surgical removal of the tumour.

Follow-up

- Blood pressure is followed up annually in patients who have undergone surgery.

Insulinoma

- Rare pancreas tumour that secretes insulin. Incidence 1–2 /million/year.
- Symptoms of hypoglycaemia (blood glucose $<$ 2.5 mmol/l): disturbances of consciousness, visual disturbances, lack of concentration, convulsions, feeling of hunger, sweating.
- Symptoms occur in the morning, during long breaks between meals and in physical strain.
- The diagnosis is made on basis of a serum insulin sample (or C-peptide sample) taken during hypoglycaemia: the result is disproportionately high.
- Often the patient must be referred on clinical grounds without prove of high insulin/glucose ratio. In such cases a long fasting test is needed in specialized care.
- Acute hypoglycaemias are managed as in diabetics. When the patient recovers, a thorough history of medications must be elicited (sulphonylureas, insulin).
- Differential diagnostic alternatives: prolonged hunger, use of alcohol, suicide attempt using diabetes medication, endocrine diseases (hypocortisolism, hypopituitarism, hypothyroidism), rare functional disturbances of the liver or kidneys.
- Insulinoma is localized by CT or MRI.
- Surgical treatment.

Other tumours

- Gastrinoma
  - Rare tumour of the pancreas or upper gastrointestinal tract that causes multiple ulcers in the duodenum (Zollinger-Ellison syndrome).
- Diagnosed by secretin stimulation test
- Vipoma, glucagonoma

Gynaecology

Evidence Based Medicine Guidelines. Edited by the Duodecim Editorial Team
© 2005 John Wiley & Sons, Ltd ISBN: 0-470-01184-X

25.1 Pap (cervical) smear and endometrial biopsy

Pekka Nieminen

Pap smear

Indications

- Diagnosis of cervical cancer and precancerous lesions
- In addition, clinically valuable information is obtained about
  - gynaecological infections and reactive conditions
  - the hormonal stage at the time of sampling (however, hormone assays are more accurate in the diagnosis of hormonal dysfunction)
  - the efficacy of treatment.
- Routine screening with cervical smears should be carried out at 5 year intervals. Samples should be taken more often (at least annually or in specific cases even more frequently) from symptomatic women and from those in high risk groups, e.g. with a history of human papillomavirus (HPV) infection.

Sampling

- Provide a sufficient amount of clinical details with the request form (at least the date of the last menstrual period and the duration of the cycle, history of abnormal smear results and any subsequent treatment).
- Collect three samples on the same slide
  - Vaginal sample with the rounded end of the spatula
  - External cervix sample with the convex end of the spatula
  - Internal cervix (endocervix) sample with a cytobrush A [1].
- Spread the material collected over the slide with a single smooth stroke motion (not with to and fro movements) to avoid damaging the cells. It is important to rotate the brush on the slide.

Fixation

- Fix the sample as soon as possible.
- Use an appropriate fixation spray, and keep a sufficient distance when spraying to avoid damage to the sample.
- Immersing the slide in 85–90% ethanol for 10 minutes results in even better fixation.

Sensitivity of the Pap smear

- Squamous cell carcinoma of the uterine cervix 85–95% A [2 3]
- Cancer of the body of the uterus (corpus uteri) only 50–60%
- The Pap smear is not useful in the diagnosis of cancer of the ovary.

Reporting of Pap smears

The Bethesda system

- The Bethesda system is an internationally accepted reporting system, and its latest version was updated in 2001.
- The 2001 Bethesda System (TBS) (see Table 25.1.1) is the recommended reporting system; however, some laboratories still use the old Papanicolaou classification system or other descriptive versions of reporting.

Papanicolaou classification

- Class I
  - Normal
- Class II
  - Benign cell atypia usually caused by inflammation, viral infection, regeneration or metaplastic process. Mild HPV infections and mildly atypical glandular cells.
- Class III
  - A borderline finding, slight suspicion of malignancy. Early premalignant epithelial atypias (mild and moderate dysplasia) are usually reported as class III.
- Class IV
  - The sample contains cells with a high suspicion of malignancy, severe dysplasia or carcinoma in situ.
- Class V
  - A high probability of cancer.

Interpreting the results

- Measures and follow-up (see Table 25.1.2)

Infection

- **Clue cells** are typical of **bacterial vaginosis (BV)**. Symptomatic patients should be treated. Asymptomatic patients should be treated particularly during pregnancy.
- **Mixed flora** is reported in about 10% of the samples. Mixed flora needs no treatment unless it is associated with inflammatory cell changes.
- The diagnosis of **trichomonas** is reliable. Trichomonas must be treated.
- The diagnosis of **fungal organisms** is less accurate. However, the presence of fungal hyphae (approx. 4% of samples) is suggestive of Candida. Usually only symptomatic patients need treatment.
- **Actinomyces** is usually only seen in conjunction with an IUD. The treatment consists of the removal of the IUD. If needed, a new IUD may be inserted after a few months. Actinomyces requires treatment. If there are signs of infection, order a course of penicillin and metronidazole, in addition to removal of the IUD.
- **Herpes** may be detected by a Pap smear, which is specific but not very sensitive.

Table 25.1.1 The 2001 Bethesda system

Classification	Result
Sample type	Conventional smear, Liquid-based smear
Adequacy of the specimen	Satisfactory for evaluation Satisfactory for evaluation, no glandular cells Satisfactory, but limited by... (specify reason) Unsatisfactory for evaluation... (specify reason)
General categorisation	Negative for intraepithelial lesion or malignancy Epithelial cell abnormality Other, see report
Abnormal microbes	BV, clue cells Mixed flora Fungal organisms Actinomyces Trichomonas vaginalis Herpes
Reactive changes	Inflammation Regeneration Radiation Change caused by intrauterine contraceptive device (IUD)
Other non-neoplastic changes	Endometrial cells in a woman > 50 years of age Glandular cells after hysterectomy Atrophy Cytolysis
Squamous cell abnormalities	ASC-US - atypical squamous cells of undetermined significance (formerly ASCUS) ASC-H – atypical squamous cells, cannot exclude high-grade squamous intraepithelial lesion (HSIL) LSIL – low-grade squamous intraepithelial lesion HSIL – high-grade squamous intraepithelial lesion Squamous cell carcinoma
Glandular cell abnormalities	Of endocervical origin, of undetermined significance Of endocervical origin, favour neoplastic Of endometrial origin, of undetermined significance Of endometrial origin, favour neoplastic Of undetermined origin, of undetermined significance Of undetermined origin, favour neoplastic Adenocarcinoma in situ Adenocarcinoma
Hormonal evaluation	Maturation index....../....../ Compatible with age and history Incompatible with age and history (specify) Hormonal evaluation is not possible due to...
Report	

- **HPV infection** and associated cellular changes are reported as atypical epithelial cells according to their severity; HPV is a significant factor in the development of atypical changes.
- For the treatment of vaginitis, see 25.30.

Hormonal evaluation

- Evaluation is only suggestive. The use of hormonal preparations has an influence on the results.
- The maturation index is used for reporting the percentage of parabasal cells/intermediate cells/superficial cells.
  - The higher the **oestrogen** concentration, the higher the number of superficial cells (e.g. near ovulation 0/30/70, in an amenorrhoeic hypo-oestrogenaemic patient 80/20/0).
  - After ovulation the intermediate cells become more abundant (e.g. 0/80/20).
  - In postmenopausal women the parabasal cells prevail (typical postmenopausal atrophy: 100/0/0).
  - **The progesterone or luteal phase** is visible in the Pap smear 3–4 days after ovulation on the days 19–24 of the menstrual cycle.
- The hormonal evaluation, particularly that of the luteal phase, is more accurate if two samples are taken, one in mid-cycle and the other at the end of the cycle.
  - If a postmenopausal woman without hormonal replacement therapy appears to have a markedly high oestrogen concentration the possibility of a hormonally active ovarian neoplasm should be considered.

Sources of error

- One of the most common problems is the inadequacy of clinical details provided.
- Insufficient number of cells: if a cervical sample contains endocervical cells it is likely that the sample collection has been correct.
- Incorrect sampling, particularly slide material too thick or insufficient, is the largest error source.
- Infection, blood and cytolysis may disturb the hormonal evaluation, and so does recent topical treatment.
- Lubricants may also affect the interpretation, and only normal saline should be used for lubrication.

Endometrial biopsy

- The condition of the endometrium can be assessed with the use of an endometrial biopsy, for example in bleeding disorders.
- The collection of the biopsy is relatively easy, and may be carried out at a primary care facility. The diagnostic yield of the examination may be improved with a concurrent intravaginal ultrasound examination.

Indications

- Postmenopausal bleeding in a patient with an unclear history ("slightly brown discharge", "a bit of spotting") and also if the patient gives a definite history of a bleed.

Table 25.1.2 Measures and follow-up in various Pap smear findings.

Finding	Measures	Follow-up
Satisfactory for evaluation, no glandular cells	Consider taking a new sample	
Evaluation unreliable	Consider taking a new sample	
Unsatisfactory for evaluation	Take a new sample	
Negative for intraepithelial lesion or malignancy		
Infection	If necessary, microbe-specific therapy and repeat sample after 1-6 months	
Regeneration	A repeat sample after 1–3 months; colposcopy if strong evidence of regeneration persists	
Atrophic vaginitis	Local oestrogen therapy and repeat sample during therapy. Further treatment according to findings.	
Change caused by radiation	Repeat sample after 4–12 months; colposcopy if the change is significant.	Annual smear test
Epithelial cell abnormality		
ASC-US (atypical squamous cells of undetermined significance, former ASCUS)	Repeat sample after 6-12 months, colposcopy if the change recurs three times during 24 months. Further treatment according to findings.	Annual smear test
ASC-H (as above but cannot exclude high-grade squamous intraepithelial lesion)	Colposcopy within 6 months. Treatment is warranted if dysplasia is detected, in other cases repeat samples at 6 month intervals until the finding is normal.	Annual smear test
LSIL (low-grade squamous intraepithelial lesion)	Colposcopy within 6 months. Treatment is warranted if dysplasia is detected, in other cases repeat samples at 6 month intervals until the finding is normal.	Annual smear test
HSIL (high-grade squamous intraepithelial lesion)	Colposcopy within 1 month. Treatment is warranted if dysplasia is detected, in other cases repeat colposcopy after 6 months and take repeat samples at 6 month intervals until the finding is normal.	Annual smear test
Squamous cell carcinoma	Colposcopy, loop excision and treatment of the carcinoma according to the degree of invasion.	Follow-up at an oncology clinic
Atypical glandular cells of endocervical origin	Suspected neoplasm– colposcopy within 1 month. Undetermined significance– repeat smear within 6 months.	Annual smear test
Atypical glandular cells of endometrial origin	Vaginal ultrasound and endometrial biopsy	Postmenopausal endometrial follow-up
Adenocarcinoma	Colposcopy, treatment of the carcinoma	Follow-up at an oncology clinic
Other malignancy	Colposcopy and histological samples	Follow-up at an oncology clinic
Hormonal state inconsistent with age and history	Depending on the case (N.B. oestrogen-secreting tumours after menopause)	

- Slight but recurring bleeding disorder in a woman below 40 years of age.
- Recurring bleeding disorder in a woman using progestogen-only or combined contraceptives.
- The determination of endometrial response during long-term hormone replacement therapy.

Techniques

- Both disposable and multiple use catheters are available. No local anaesthesia is necessary.

1. Perform pelvic examination to determine the position of the uterus.
2. Clean the cervix with saline solution.
3. Grasp the cervix with a tenaculum and gently pull outwards in order to straighten the uterocervical angle, thus facilitating the insertion of the uterine sound.
4. The distance from the fundus to the external cervical os can be measured if necessary.
5. Insert the biopsy catheter into the uterine cavity. Aspirate whilst twisting the catheter 360 degrees against the uterine walls.
6. Once the tissue sample is collected the sample is placed in a container with buffered formalin solution for a histological examination.
   - If the sample is scant or if the pathologist so wishes the sample could be placed into a container with ethanol for cytological examination.

References

1. Martin-Hirsch P, Jarvis G, Kitchener H, Lilford R. Collection devices for obtaining cervical cytology samples. Cochrane Database Syst Rev. 2004;(2):CD001036.

2. Fahey MT, Irwig L, Macaskill P. Meta-analysis of Pap test accuracy. Am J Epidemiol 1995;141:680–689.
3. The Database of Abstracts of Reviews of Effectiveness (University of York), Database no.: DARE-950964. In: The Cochrane Library, Issue 4, 1999. Oxford: Update Software.

25.2 Gynaecological ultrasound examination

Pertti Palo

Introduction

- To perform gynaecological ultrasound (US) examinations a general practitioner must receive training under specialist guidance, acquire sufficient experience and have proper equipment at his/her disposal.

Equipment

- The improved resolution of ultrasound equipment brought about by improvements in transducer technology and computer capacity for image processing, combined with concurrent reductions in the cost of equipment, has made US a routine gynaecological examination. In skilled hands it yields important information.
- Gynaecological ultrasound investigation consists of **both a transvaginal sonography (TVS) and a transabdominal sonography (TAS)** Ⓐ [1 2]. A gynaecological US examination is not recommended if a transvaginal probe is not available. On the other hand, large pelvic tumours may be missed if only TVS is carried out, since the resolution of high-frequency vaginal probes remains good only up to the depth of 60–80 mm.
- The patient's bladder should usually be empty as this allows easy transvaginal examination of the ovaries and the uterus (large tumours can be seen with an abdominal probe even if the patient has an empty bladder). A full bladder is used as an "acoustic window" when examining children, young women with an intact hymen or very old patients. Rectal ultrasound examination may also be carried out if the transvaginal approach is not possible.

Menstrual cycle and infertility

Endometrial development

- The cyclic changes of the endometrium during the menstrual cycle can be imaged with US. If the uterus is stretched, the imaging of the endometrium is not always successful.
- The thickness of the endometrium usually is expressed as the double wall thickness including both the anterior and posterior endometrial walls.
- Immediately after menstruation the endometrium is homogenous, 1–4 mm thick. As the oestrogen concentration rises the proliferative endometrium changes into a triple-layer structure and its thickness increases to 7–10 mm. After ovulation, the echogenicity of the endometrium begins to increase starting from the basal area, and in the luteal phase it has become hyperechogenic throughout with a thickness of 8–16 mm.

Follicle and corpus luteum

- Several 2–5 mm follicles may be seen in the ovaries with TVS. One or more of the follicles will grow during the early cycle.
- Around cycle days 9–10 the leading follicle can be identified; it has a diameter of about 10 mm. Thereafter it grows rapidly, and by ovulation it is 20–24 mm in diameter.
- After ovulation the follicle collapses and as the corpus luteum develops, the content of the cyst may have a slightly heterogeneous consistency. The wall is sometimes seen as a rather thick formation with low-level echoes. Occasionally, corpus luteum forms a homogeneous hypoechogenic thin-walled structure. The diameter of a normal follicle or corpus luteum does not usually exceed 30 mm.

Monitoring of infertility treatment

- In infertility treatment the growth of the follicle and the development of the endometrium can be monitored during hormone stimulation. With US the developing follicles can be counted, the dosage of hormone treatment adjusted and the timing of interventions, such as insemination during ovulation, determined.
- US can be used to recognise ovarian hyperstimulation syndrome, which is a rare but serious complication of gonadotrophin stimulation used for infertility treatment. After stimulation and follicle puncture the ovaries can be 60–70 mm in diameter and multicystic. In hyperstimulation syndrome the ovaries are often over 80 mm in diameter, and in severe cases there is fluid in the peritoneal cavity.

Localisation of an IUD

- US can be used to verify the presence and proper intrauterine localisation of an IUD.
- A copper IUD gives a strong echo and is easy to detect.
- The presence of a hormone-releasing IUD might be more difficult to verify. Only the ends of the plastic arm of the device are detectable with US. Moreover, being a foreign body it produces dark extrauterine shadows which differ according to projections used.
- If an IUD is positioned correctly, i.e. high enough in the uterus, the difference between the upper portion of the IUD and the outer edge of the fundus should not exceed 20 mm in a normally sized uterus.

- It is usually impossible to detect an IUD that is located outside the uterus with an US.

Bleeding disorders

Fertile age

- The most common causes
  - Functional bleeding disorder of hormonal origin.
    - Deviation from the normal structure of the endometrium in the different phases of the menstrual cycle described above is not sufficient for making a diagnosis.
    - Endometrial thickness of more than 18 mm suggests endometrial disease.
  - Endometrial polyp.
    - An echodense, well-defined, round mass in the uterine cavity, which is best visualised during the proliferative phase. It may have a cystic structure.
    - The polyp can be imaged even better should any liquid be present in the uterine cavity, or if fluid is introduced with an insemination catheter. The blood vessel supplying the polyp may be visualised with colour Doppler.
  - Submucotic myoma
    - A submucotic myoma gives a low echo as compared with a polyp. It is usually possible to differentiate a submucotic myoma from a polyp.

Postmenopausal bleeding disorders

- Bleeding or bloody discharge in a postmenopausal woman should be considered as a sign of endometrial cancer until otherwise proven.
- An endometrium more than 10 mm in thickness in a postmenopausal patient strongly suggests endometrial cancer.
- Endometrial cancer is seen extremely rarely when the endometrium is less than 5 mm thick.
- US alone is not sufficient for making a diagnosis. A histological sample of the endometrium is always needed.

Sonohysterography

- In sonohysterography 5–15 ml of saline solution is injected into the uterine cavity with, for example, an insemination catheter. The saline solution gives a contrast in the uterine cavity which allows the best visualisation of any polyps in the uterine corpus and submucotic myomas protruding into the cavity. A histological sample should be taken before performing sonohysterography.

Salpingosonography

- Salpingosonography may be used as a primary investigation for infertility instead of laparoscopic chromopertubation. Agitated saline is injected into the uterine cavity with an insemination catheter. The air bubbles in the saline act as a contrast, and the fallopian tubes can be visualised. The procedure is markedly reliable compared with chromopertubation. The flow through the tubes can be confirmed as well as tubular patency.

Gynaecological tumours

- Bimanual palpation is the basic examination, which sometimes reveals a tumour of the pelvic region. It may also be sufficient for differential diagnosis of uterine myomas. Palpation may, however, be greatly hindered by the patient's obesity.
- US examination is indicated to verify diagnosis when
  - diagnosing a pelvic mass is otherwise difficult
  - an adnexal tumour is detected
  - the findings on examination are not clear and the patient has symptoms in the pelvic region and lower abdomen (swelling, pain, bleeding, bladder symptoms)
  - the patient has a family history of ovarian cancer.

Myoma and adenomyosis

- A myoma is often seen as a more hypoechogenic mass when compared with the normal myometrium. It has well defined margins and a thin wall may be visible. Cyst formation can often be seen in rapidly growing or degenerating myomas.
- A pedunculated myoma or a multimyotic massively enlarged uterus may be difficult to differentiate from ovarian cancer even with US.
- The ring like vascularisation on the outer border of a myoma may be visualised with colour Doppler. Vascularisation of the inner structures is scant. Profuse vascularisation may be suggestive of a malignant myoma, i.e. sarcoma.
- Adenomyosis, in which the benign cystic structures of the endometrium grow diffusely into the uterine wall, may be seen as focuses that resemble myoma, but are not clearly discernible from the muscular layer of the uterus.

Endometrial cancer

- Cancer of the uterine corpus is always diagnosed from a histological sample.
- Endometrial cancer is often seen as non-homogenous thickening of the endometrium (14–15 mm).
- The depth of invasion can often be determined rather precisely with US.
- In most cases, cervical cancer cannot be diagnosed by US.

Ovarian cysts

- Functional cysts are mostly detected as incidental findings in US, sometimes also when US is performed because of diffuse pelvic pains or suspicious findings on bimanual examination.
- Functional cysts have typically thin and smooth walls without internal echoes.
- A haemorrhagic cyst or a corpus luteum cyst may have variable internal structures, which disappear during follow-up.

- Functional cysts are usually less than 60 mm in diameter.
- Even postmenopausal women may have benign ovarian cysts, which are less than 50 mm in diameter and may disappear during follow-up.
- Verifying the disappearance of a functional cyst by a follow-up examination after 3–4 months is indicated. If the cyst grows, its removal is indicated (see ovarian tumours 25.44).
- Patients with a hormone releasing IUD may have a higher than normal incidence of ovarian cysts which usually disappear without surgical intervention.

US diagnosis of ovarian tumours

- It is not always possible to differentiate between a benign and a malignant ovarian tumour by US.
- An ovarian cyst less than 60 mm in diameter, with no internal echoes and a smooth internal surface is extremely seldom malignant.
- A malignant tumour may
  - have a tumour wall of over 3 mm in thickness or tumour septa
  - have papillary growth inside the inner walls
  - be multilocular
  - have a complex structure of solid and cystic components (the probability of cancer is then over 60%)
  - have poorly organised and profuse vasculature
  - be accompanied with ascites.
- Particular types of an ovarian tumour include
  - mucinous tumours with a "snowstorm" echo pattern
  - endometriomas which are thin-walled cysts with homogenous granular inner material, but their presentation may also be atypical.
  - dermoid tumours often contain fine granular sebaceous material, which may consist of the more solid bone or cartilage components, which can cause acoustic shadowing. Hypoechogenic cysts may also occur.

Pelvic infection

- An acute pelvic inflammatory disease may cause a tubo-ovarian abscess. This is seen in US examination as a multilocular, thick-walled mass that contains echo-dense fluid collections. This type of mass is usually void of vasculature.
- When the infection subsides, the infectious complex may disappear or it may turn into a sactosalpinx, which is an elongated multilocular mass causing a torsion of the fallopian tube. The torsion is easily identifiable from different projections, and the ovary will be seen as a separate structure.
- Actinomyces may cause inflammatory foci that resemble a tumour.
- Periappendicular abscess may sometimes be mistaken for a tumour around the right ovary.

Differential diagnosis

- Dilated bowel loops may sometimes simulate a cystic adnexal mass in a patient with abdominal pains that are connected to a bowel motility disturbance. However, the movement of the bowel contents and peristalsis will confirm the nature of the finding.
- Venous plexuses near the uterus, associated with pelvic vein varices, may sometimes be very large and resemble a cystic ovarian tumour. If differential diagnosis is difficult, a colour Doppler investigation will yield a typical image of venous circulation.
- Sometimes multiple nabothian cysts in the uterine cervix may be mistaken as a cystic ovarian tumour.

Gynaecological ultrasound examination in the diagnosis of acute abdomen

- The most common gynaecological reasons for acute abdomen include:
  - Rupture of an ovarian cyst
    - The cyst may appear irregular and free fluid may be detected in the peritoneal cavity.
  - Ovarian hyperstimulation syndrome
    - See above.
  - Torsion of an ovarian cyst/tumour
    - The onset of lower abdominal pain is acute, the ovary may appear oedematous with fluid cavities of various sizes. In multiple torsion, colour Doppler usually fails to detect vascularity in the ovarian tissue.
  - Ectopic pregnancy
    - If the serum human chorionic gonadotrophin concentration is $\geqslant$1000 units/l, the pregnancy should be detectable in the uterus. If the uterine cavity is empty, or only contains a small fluid cavity (pseudogestational sac), an ectopic pregnancy should be suspected. The most common manifestations are tubal or ovarian pregnancy. A typical view resembles that of a millstone; the homogenous placental tissue forms a thick ring around an anechoic central cavity. A minute foetus or pulsating heart may sometimes be detected within the central cavity.
    - The detection of an abdominal pregnancy with ultrasound examination may be very difficult, or impossible, in early pregnancy.
    - An ectopic pregnancy may also be located in the cervical canal or uterine cornua.
  - Infection. See above.
  - Pain caused by ovarian tumour
    - As an ovarian tumour grows it may bleed either inside the tumour itself or to the surrounding tissues. The tumour may become twisted. Malignant tumours are often associated with ascites which may cause sudden and significant swelling of the abdomen.
  - Pain caused by uterine tumour
    - A necrosed myoma may cause severe pain, for example during pregnancy. Its shape and structure may change and it may shrink.

References

1. Smith-Bindman R, Kerlikowske K, Feldstein VA, Subak L, Scheidler J, Segal M, Brand R, Grady D. Endovaginal ultrasound to exclude endometrial cancer and other endometrial abnormalities. JAMA 1998;280:1510–1517.
2. The Database of Abstracts of Reviews of Effectiveness (University of York), Database no.: DARE-989095. In: The Cochrane Library, Issue 3, 2000. Oxford: Update Software.

25.10 Dysmenorrhoea

Päivi Härkki

Epidemiology

- All women complain of occasional dysmenorrhoea of some degree.
- 10–40% complain of severe dysmenorrhoea.

Symptoms

- Lower abdominal pain 100%
- Nausea, vomiting 90%
- Tiredness 80%
- Lower back pain 60%
- Dizziness 60%
- Diarrhoea 60%
- Headache 40%

Primary dysmenorrhoea

Symptoms

- Cramping lower abdominal pains emerge with the onset of menstrual bleeding and radiate to the back and thighs.
- Pain lasts for about 24 hours.
- Pain is associated with the ovulatory cycle.
- The problem first emerges 6–12 months after menarche.

Aetiology

- Pain is caused by prostaglandins.
- The production of prostaglandins increases after ovulation.
- Prostaglandins cause uterine cramps and decreased blood flow leading to ischaemic uterine pain.
- Prostaglandins released into the circulation cause the systemic symptoms.

Diagnosis

- Usually obvious on the basis of history.
- No abnormalities found during a gynaecological examination.
- No need for laboratory investigations.

Treatment

- In mild cases, an explanation of the reasons behind the symptoms is sufficient.
- Drugs that inhibit prostaglandin synthesis are effective:
  - they inhibit the action of the cyclo-oxygenase enzyme thus blocking prostaglandin synthesis
  - medication must be taken immediately at symptom onset
  - the duration of medication is 24–48 hours
  - provide pain relief in 80–90% of cases
  - reduce the contractility of the uterus
  - reduce the amount of blood loss by 20–30% if taken throughout the menstrual period.
- Combined oral contraceptives:
  - prevent ovulation and associated pain
  - thin the endometrium and reduce the production of prostaglandins
  - reduce menstrual bleeding
  - may be prescribed even if contraception is not needed
  - remember contraindications
  - may be combined with analgesics
- Hormone-releasing intra-uterine devices:
  - thin the endometrium and reduce the production of prostaglandins
  - reduce menstrual bleeding
  - provide pain relief
  - not suitable for very young patients
  - an ordinary intra-uterine device will worsen dysmenorrhoea

Secondary dysmenorrhoea

Symptoms

- Previously painless menstruation becomes painful
- Pain emerges before menstruation commences
- Pain lasts for the entire duration of menstrual bleeding
- Condition attributable to a gynaecological condition
- Pain also partially attributable to prostaglandins

Aetiology

- Adenomyosis (25.42), causes pain in 70–100% of cases
- Endometriosis (25.42), causes pain in 50–90% of cases
- Myoma (25.44), causes pain in 20–80% of cases
- Sequela of an infection, causes pain in 10–50% of cases
- Menorrhagia (25.13) causes pain in 20–30% of cases
- Intra-uterine device (27.4), causes pain in 0–20% of cases

Diagnosis

- Gynaecological examination, blood tests and swabs to diagnose possible infection (25.41) and cervical smear (25.1).
- Transvaginal ultrasonography (25.2) if a gynaecological illness is suspected.
- Laparoscopy in severe pain.

Treatment

- Symptomatic treatment
- If an intra-uterine device is causing dysmenorrhoea it should be removed.
- Prostaglandin synthesis inhibitors might be of benefit.

25.11 Premenstrual syndrome (PMS)

Päivi Härkki

Definition

- Premenstrual syndrome (PMS) denotes repeatedly occurring physical and emotional symptoms at the latter part of the menstrual cycle in women of reproductive age.

Incidence

- Almost all women suffer from premenstrual symptoms at some point in their lives.
- The incidence of severe PMS is less than 10%.
- Symptoms are worst in women aged 30–40 years, but they may occur before the age of 20. Symptoms usually lessen after the age of 45.

Aetiology

- The aetiology remains unknown.
- Ovarian functioning is a prerequisite for PMS.
- Central nervous system neurotransmitters are thought to play a role in the development of the syndrome, and altered serotonergic transmission is currently considered to be a significant factor behind PMS.

Symptoms

- Emotional: depression, irritability, mood changes, outbursts of anger, confusion, concentration difficulties, tiredness, insomnia, changes in appetite, social withdrawal.
- Physical: breast tenderness, bloating, headache, swelling and pain of the hands and feet.

Diagnosis

- At least one emotional and one physical symptom for five days before menstruation.
- Symptoms disappear within three to four days after the start of menstruation and return no earlier than on day 12 of the menstrual cycle.
- Symptoms recur during two consecutive cycles; an isolated cycle may be symptom free.
- Symptoms interfere considerably with everyday life.
- Laboratory tests are of no benefit.
- Gynaecological examination is normal.
- The breasts are normal on palpation.

Differential diagnosis

- Depression
- Personality disorder
- Eating disorder
- Mastopathy and other causes of breast pain (25.20)
- Systemic illnesses causing oedema
- Hypothyroidism (24.34)
- Perimenopause (25.50)

Treatment

- Often an explanation of the syndrome, and its relation to normal hormonal functioning, is sufficient.
- Avoidance of coffee and alcohol, and increasing the amount of exercise, may lessen the symptoms.
- Selective serotonin re-uptake inhibitors have proved to be effective in the treatment of PMS, either administered continuously or cyclically, starting midway through the cycle until the start of menstruation. The dose is smaller than that used in the treatment of depression.
- An occasional patient may gain benefit from cyclic progestogens on days 15–24 of the cycle. There is no evidence of the benefit.
- Some patients gain benefit from a levonorgestrel-releasing intra-uterine device.
- Combined oral contraceptives prevent ovulation and may lessen the symptoms in some patients.
- Pyridoxine (vitamin B_6) has been tried (up to 100 mg/day) but there is only little evidence available on the benefit.
- Bromocriptine (2.5 mg/day) from mid-cycle until the start of menstruation may lessen breast tenderness.
- Spironolactone (25–100 mg/day) can be prescribed for severe oedema.
- Gonadotrophin-releasing hormone agonists (GnRH-A) will depress ovarian functioning and result in a postmenopausal hormonal state. This in turn will reduce PMS symptoms. Any subsequent menopausal symptoms can be lessened by adding oestrogen/progestogen to the treatment regime.

25.12 Altering the time of menstruation

Anneli Kivijärvi

Introduction

- It is possible to postpone menstruation by using a progestogen with a good anti-oestrogenic effect.

- It is preferable to alter the time of menstruation before a journey or other event and not during it (avoids the need to take medication during a journey).

Women not using oral contraceptives

- The safety of progestogen during early pregnancy is not known. Pregnancy is therefore a contra-indication. Contraception (IUD, condom, abstinence) must be used during the treatment.

Products

- Norethisterone
  - 5 mg twice daily (three times daily if spotting occurs) for a maximum of 14 days. Treatment is started at least three days before anticipated onset of menstruation. Bleeding starts 2–3 days after cessation of treatment.
- Lynestrenol
  - 10 mg daily (usually a sufficient dose)
  - When longer period of amenorrhoea (over 14 days) is required.
  - Two tablets in the evening. Treatment is started 4–5 days before anticipated onset of menstruation. Treatment is continued as long as amenorrhoea is required. If breakthrough bleeding occurs, the dose can be increased to 15 mg per day for 3–5 days.

Women using oral contraceptives

- **Users of monophasic combined oral contraceptives** can continue taking the tablets from the next strip, omitting the usual tablet-free period.
  - It is possible to continue taking the tablets without a break for as long as amenorrhoea is required, for example two entire strips could be taken one after the other followed by a 7-day tablet-free period.
  - Bleeding starts 2–4 days after the last tablet. After a 7-day break the product can be used as usual.
- **Users of sequential, biphasic or triphasic combined oral contraceptives** can continue to take the tablets as described above but when a new strip is started the tablets from towards the end of the strip should be used as they contain more progestogen. This will prevent the onset of menstruation.
- The amount of progestogen in the **oral progestogen-only contraceptives** ("minipill") is too small to be relied on to postpone menstruation, and users should take norethisterone as described above. However, they should also continue to take their daily progestogen as usual.
  - Users of oral progestogen-only contraceptives may also change to a combined oral contraceptive for the duration of the journey, provided that there are no contraindications to oestrogen.
- **Users of other hormonal contraception.**
  - Hormone-releasind IUD: a combined oral contraceptive containing ethinylestradiol with levonorgestrel should be added for the required time, provided that there are no contraindications to oestrogen. Lynestrenol may also be used in the same way as in women not using oral contraceptives.
  - Implants: If the patient has an etonogestrel implant, menstruation may be postponed by using a combined oral contraceptive containing either ethinylestradiol with norethisterone or ethinylestradiol with desogestrel. If the patient has a levonorgestrel implant, menstruation may be postponed with a combined oral contraceptive containing ethinylestradiol with levonorgestrel, provided that there are no contraindications to oestrogen. Lynestrenol may also be used.

25.13 Abnormal menstrual bleeding

Ritva Hurskainen

Introduction

- A detailed history of menstrual bleeding is often more important than the pelvic examination.
- Differentiate between organic and hormonal causes.
- Differentiate between anovulatory and ovulatory bleeding.

Normal menstrual cycle

- The average age of menarche (the first menstrual period) is 12.5 years.
- The menstrual cycle varies from 23 to 36 days, usually from 26 to 30 days.
- Uterine bleeding usually lasts 2–7 days, and the normal blood loss during one cycle is 25–40 ml with the upper limit of normal being 80 ml.

Associated terminology

- Amenorrhoea
  - Absence of menstrual bleeding
    - Primary– no menstrual bleeding ever
    - Secondary– no menstrual bleeding for at least 6 months
- Oligomenorrhoea
  - Menstrual cycle more than 36 days
- Polymenorrhoea
  - Menstrual cycle less than 23 days

- Menorrhagia
  - Regular bleeding, but more profuse than normally
- Metrorrhagia
  - Irregular bleeding with varying length and amount
- Dysfunctional bleeding
  - Abnormal uterine bleeding without any organic pathology, pregnancy or general bleeding disorder

Menorrhagia or hypermenorrhoea

- Excessive bleeding (>80 ml) that occurs at regular menstrual intervals.
- According to blood volume measurements, the prevalence among women of reproductive age is 9–14%. However, approximately one in three women suffer from excessive bleeding at some stage of their lives.

The most common causes

- Systemic causes (5–15%)
  - von Willebrand's disease
  - impaired thyroid function, uncontrolled diabetes
  - anticoagulation therapy, not properly carried out
- Uterine causes (40–50%)
  - Polyps of the uterine cavity and submucous myomas (25.44)
  - Adenomyosis (invasion of myometrium by endometrial tissue)
  - Standard intrauterine device (IUD)
  - Infection (25.41)
  - Endometrial carcinoma (the cause of menorrhagia only in 0.08% of cases) (25.44).
- Essential menorrhagia (approximately 50%)
  - No cause can be identified with current diagnostic methods. Caused by a multitude of mechanisms.

History

- It is difficult, but important, to estimate the amount of blood loss. Objectively, only about half of those complaining of heavy bleeding lose more than 80 ml. Pictoral blood assessment chart (PBAC) can be used to estimate the blood loss. The patient gives herself points by comparing her own sanitary towels/tampons and blood loss/clots to pictures.
- The patient can also be asked whether the bleeding interferes with her work and leisure time activities, does she need to use more protection now than before, does she need to change protection overnight, are there any clots, and does she feel tired or dizzy during her periods (the estimation will remain fairly rough).
- A recent onset of symptoms may be suggestive of a uterine cause, whereas symptoms of long duration are more suggestive of a systemic cause or essential origin.
- Menorrhagic bleeding is regular, and usually of normal duration. Anovulatory bleeding is irregular with long cycles and long duration.

Investigations

- Pelvic examination
  - Size of the uterus, tenderness, myomas
- Ultrasound examination (25.2) will reveal polyps and submucous myomas in 50–90% of cases.
  - Sonohysterography (25.2) will give more accurate information (comparable to hysteroscopy).
- Hysteroscopy, if clear diagnosis not achieved with ultrasound examination.
- Serum ferritin, full blood count
  - Haemoglobin correlates fairly poorly with the amount of blood loss.
- If necessary (only if supported by other findings)
  - Infection parameters
  - Clotting studies (von Willebrand factor activity, Ristocetin cofactor activity (vWF:Rco), clotting factor VIII)
  - TSH and free T4
- Endometrial curettage seldom gives more information
- Endometrial biopsy (25.1) should be considered to exclude malignancy if the patient has mid-cycle bleeding or other risk factors (age > 45 years, obesity > 90 kg, diabetes).

Treatment

- Systemic causes
  - von Willebrand's disease
    - Oral contraceptives, desmopressin, hormone-releasing IUD, thermal balloon endometrial ablation
- Uterine causes
  - Polyps and submucous fibroids
    - Polypectomy and resection of submucous myomas hysteroscopically
  - Adenomyosis
    - Drug therapy (see below under treatment of essential menorrhagia)
    - Hormone-releasing IUS
    - Endometrial ablation
    - Hysterectomy
  - Removal of the IUD
  - Tranexamic acid or a non-steroidal anti-inflammatory drug if the patient wants to keep the IUD
- Essential menorrhagia
  - Tranexamic acid 2–3 tablets (1–1.5 g) 3 times daily for 2–3 days, administered when (A) [1] bleeding is most heavy, will reduce bleeding by about 50%.
  - Non-steroidal anti-inflammatory drugs (not aspirin), such as mefenamic acid 500 mg 3 times daily, naproxen 500 mg twice daily, diclofenac 50 mg 3 times daily or ibuprofen 400 mg 4 times daily, taken when bleeding is most heavy, will reduce bleeding by about 30% (A) [2] and alleviate menstrual pain.
  - Combined oral contraceptives reduce bleeding by 40–50% (D) [3]. Alleviates also menstrual pain and guarantees good contraception. Remember smoking and obesity.

GYN

- A hormone-releasing IUS will reduce bleeding by more than 90%. It also alleviates menstrual pain, pre-menstrual symptoms and guarantees contraception to the level of sterilization **B** [4].
- Endometrium can be resected or destroyed by thermal ablation. The success rate is 70–97%. During a four year follow-up the need for further treatment is 38%.
- Hysterectomy may be carried out transvaginally, laparoscopically or by open surgery **A** [5 6]. The patient should be informed of the need for surgery and given time for consideration.

Metrorrhagia

- Irregular uterine bleeding with varying length and amount. Metrorrhagia is usually functional in a younger woman, unless she has an infection or pregnancy-related problems. The possibility of an organic cause increases with age.

Causes

- Functional causes
  - Disturbance in the hormonal regulation of the hypothalamus, pituitary gland and ovaries
  - Luteal hormone insufficiency
  - Ovulation bleeding
- Uterine causes
  - Problems associated with pregnancy, see 26.10, 26.11
  - Infection, such as endometritis or salpingo-oophoritis (25.41)
  - Submucous myomas (25.44)
  - Adenomyosis, endometriosis (25.42)
  - Cervical and endometrial polyps (25.44)
  - Cervical and uterine cancers (25.44)
- Other causes
  - An IUD
  - Dysfunction of the thyroid gland, hyperprolactinaemia, diabetes or obesity
  - Hepatic cirrhosis
  - Cardiovascular diseases that cause heart failure or venous stasis
  - Dysfunction of clotting factors or anticoagulant treatment
  - Certain drugs, such as doxycycline, metoclopramide

About functional causes

- Ovulatory bleeding disorders
  - Young, slightly overweight girls may have frequent (<22 days) but regular bleeding. There seems to be no hormonal disturbance and no treatment is needed.
  - Premenstrual spotting may occur due to a functional disturbance of the corpus luteum. The histological finding from an endometrial biopsy will show "irregular shedding" and "irregular ripening".
  - Some women have regular bleeding associated with ovulation. The bleeding lasts from a few hours to 1–2 days, and requires no treatment. The cause of the bleeding is the rapid decrease in the oestrogen levels after ovulation.
- Anovulatory bleeding disorders
  - Usually in young girls (so-called metropathia juvenilis) or in premenopausal women (hyperplasia cystica glandularis).
  - Hypothalamic disturbance is usually the causative factor of temporary anovulation in young women (e.g. excessive stress, strenuous exercise, slimming, systemic illnesses or polycystic ovaries (25.15)). Dysfunction of the ovaries is the usual cause after the reproductive age. If the condition is prolonged it may lead to endometrial hyperplasia.

Diagnosis and examination

- Careful history and physical examination are most important.
- The choice of diagnostic methods is dependent on the patient's age and history.
  - Exclude pregnancy and infection. Cervical smear from everyone.
    - Pregnancy test either from the urine or blood.
    - Swabs for bacterial culture or PCR (Chlamydia, gonorrhoea if necessary), CRP and blood counts.
  - Vaginal ultrasound (25.2) should be carried out on all patients if feasible. Very accurate in the diagnosis of submucous myomas, endometrial polyps and endometrial hyperplasia but does not substitute an endometrial biopsy (25.1).
  - Endometrial biopsy should be obtained from older women (>45 years) (25.1) particularly if there are risk factors for uterine cancer (25.44) (age, obesity, diabetes).
  - Hysteroscopy if diagnosis remains unclear after the ultrasound examination or if an endometrial biopsy is required of a particular area.
  - Laboratory tests as required: TSH, prolactin, clotting factor studies

Stopping dysfunctional bleeding

- If no organic cause has been found to explain the abnormal bleeding and the symptoms are transient, no treatment is needed.
- The IUD may be removed (remember contraception) or if the patient so wishes a watchful wait may be instigated, provided that no organic cause has been identified.
- Tranexamic acid may be useful in reducing the amount of blood loss (dose 1–1.5 g three times daily).
- Bleeding can usually be stopped with progestogens, the most suitable ones being norethisterone (5 mg three times daily), norethisterone acetate (10 mg twice daily) and lynesterol (10 mg twice daily). They should be administered for 10 days. After stopping the medication the patient will have withdrawal bleeding (inform the patient).
- Oestrogen and progestogen given together for 7–14 days is the most effective way to stop hormonal bleeding at the extreme ends of reproductive age. Oral contraceptives

(monophasic) three tablets per day for one week should be prescribed for young women. If the patient feels unwell the dose should be reduced. Ethinylestradiol 2 mg daily, combined with a progestogen, should be prescribed for older women and for those who have contraindications for synthetic oestrogen. A withdrawal bleeding will follow after the medication is stopped. If the withdrawal bleeding is profuse it can be treated with a prostaglandin inhibitor or tranexamic acid.
- The daily administration of oral contraceptives is introduced according to the packet instructions. Otherwise, the treatment of functional bleeding is continued with cyclical progestogen on days 15–24 of the cycle for 3–6 months. Weaker progestogens and lower doses can be used.
- Endometrial curettage is not usually needed. Endometrial hyperplasia as a result of anovulatory states requires curettage. Polyps and submucous fibroids should be removed hysteroscopically. In some cases curettage is diagnostically important, but in most cases it can be replaced by an endometrial biopsy, which has high accuracy.

References

1. Lethaby A, Farguhar C, Cooke J. Antifibrinolytics for heavy menstrual bleeding (Cochrane review) In: The Cochrane Library Issued 2003, Oxford: Update Software.
2. Lethaby A, Augood C, Duckitt K. Nonsteroidal anti-inflammatory drugs for heavy menstrual bleeding. Cochrane Database Syst Rev. 2004;(2):CD000400.
3. Iyer V, Farquhar C, Jepson R. Oral contraceptive pills for heavy menstrual bleeding. Cochrane Database Syst Rev. 2004;(2):CD000154.
4. Lethaby AE, Cooke I, Rees M. Progesterone/progestogen releasing intrauterine systems for heavy menstrual bleeding. Cochrane Database Syst Rev. 2004;(2):CD002126.
5. University of Leeds, Nuffield Institute for Health, University of York, NHS Centre for Reviews and Dissemination. The management of menorrhagia: what are the effective ways of treating excessive regular menstrual blood loss in primary and secondary care. Effective Health Care 1995;9:1–14.
6. The Database of Abstracts of Reviews of Effectiveness (University of York), Database no.: DARE-952731. In: The Cochrane Library, Issue 4, 1999. Oxford: Update Software.

25.14 Amenorrhoea and oligomenorrhoea

Helena Tinkanen

Basic rules

- **Amenorrhoea** is defined as the absence of menstruation.
- **Primary amenorrhoea** is the failure to establish menstruation.
- **Secondary amenorrhoea** is the absence of menstruation for six consecutive months or, if the menstrual cycle is clearly longer than normal, the absence of three consecutive menstrual periods.
- In **oligomenorrhoea** the menstrual cycle is longer than 36 days.

Aims

- The aetiology of amenorrhoea must be established.
- Treat the cause.
- The treatment will have repercussions on the woman's health throughout the rest of her life.

Primary amenorrhoea

- Investigate further if
  - no signs of puberty have emerged by the age of 13–14 or
  - menstruation has not started by the age of 16, even though puberty has otherwise progressed normally.

Causes

- The cause in 45% of cases is irreversible ovarian failure; often no onset of puberty.
  - Usually associated with chromosomal abnormalities, e.g. Turner's syndrome
  - Other ovarian defect (dysgenesis).
- The cause in 15% of cases originates from the central nervous system; often no onset of puberty.
  - Pituitary tumour (often prolactinoma), other brain tumour, pituitary insufficiency, Kallman's syndrome
- In 13% of cases the cause is physiological; pubertal changes often lacking.
  - Constitutional delay
  - Anorexia
  - Excessive physical exercise
- In 17% of cases the cause is structural; development of puberty otherwise normal
  - Rare: transverse vaginal septum, absent cervix or agenesis of the uterus.
  - Rare: androgen insensitivity syndrome, i.e. an XY female, female external genitalia and body habitus, short vagina, absent internal genitalia.
- In 10% of cases primary amenorrhoea is caused by a systemic illness.
  - Hypothyroidism, untreated coeliac disease, Cushing's syndrome, adrenal hyperandrogenism etc.
  - Obesity.

Diagnosis and treatment

- Specialist referral (a referral both to a paediatrician and gynaecologist)

- The referral should include the patient's growth charts, past medical history and the history of the parents' puberty.

Secondary amenorrhoea

- A normal functioning of both the hypothalamus-pituitary-ovary axis and endometrium are prerequisites for a regular menstrual cycle.

History

- Previous menstrual history, contraception
- Pregnancies, deliveries and associated procedures
- Weight loss or weight gain (assess the significance of the weight change in relation to baseline weight, i.e. if BMI is 18, a weight loss of a few kg may cause amenorrhoea)
- History of increased physical exercise, recent stress, medication (25.21)
- Any other symptoms associated with amenorrhoea (sudden sweating, vaginal dryness etc.)

Status

- Height, weight, blood pressure
- Fat distribution (truncal obesity)
- Striae, abnormal pigmentation of external genitalia and armpits
- Hirsutism, greasy skin, acne
- Thyroid gland
- Breasts, possible galactorrhoea
- Gynaecological examination: state of the vaginal epithelium, size of the uterus and ovaries.

Diagnosis and treatment

- Exclude **pregnancy**
- **Serum prolactin**
  - Galactorrhoea? (25.21). If yes, examine visual fields.
  - If increased prolactin and amenorrhoea, ask about antipsychotic medication (25.21)
  - Pituitary and hypothalamic tumours are possible (24.67).
  - **Hyperprolactinaemia** without a clear cause (lactation, antipsychotic medication) warrants a referral for further investigation.
- **Serum TSH**
  - Hypothyroidism (24.34) is a more common cause of abnormal menstrual bleeding than hyperthyroidism (24.35).
- **Progestogen challenge test** for 7–10 days (e.g. dydrogesterone 10–20 mg/day or medroxyprogesterone 10 mg/day)
  - If withdrawal bleeding occurs within two weeks of the last tablet, the level of oestrogen is sufficient to proliferate the endometrium. If no bleeding occurs, the level of oestrogen is low or the endometrium is nonresponsive.
- **If no withdrawal bleeding occurs**, measure **estradiol, FSH and LH.**
  1. **Low estradiol with low FSH and LH**
     - Hypothalamic/pituitary aetiology
     - Anorexia, refer to a psychiatric team
     - Excessive exercise, inform the patient about the risk of osteoporosis and consider oral contraceptives or hormone replacement therapy.
     - If the amount of exercise and low body weight offer no explanation for the finding, refer the patient for further investigation, since the possibility of hypothalamic or pituitary tumour must be excluded.
  2. **Low estradiol with high FSH and LH**
     - Ovarian insufficiency
     - The aetiology and treatment (e.g. risk of osteoporosis) in a woman less than 40 years of age should be evaluated at an appropriate hospital.
     - Early menopause (familial tendency in 30–50% of cases) (25.50), (25.51)
     - Polyendocrinopathy
     - Iatrogenic aetiology (surgery, chemotherapy)
  3. **Normal estradiol with normal FSH and LH**
     - The aetiology is related to endometrial response
     - Presence of intrauterine adhesions, e.g. after curettage, (Asherman's syndrome)
     - Referral to a specialist
  4. **Systemic illness may cause amenorrhoea**
     - Hyperthyroidism, hypothyroidism, renal or hepatic insufficiency, severe untreated coeliac disease (8.84) etc. Usually no withdrawal bleeding after progestogen challenge test.
- **If withdrawal bleeding occurs** the patient is normoestrogenic and anovulatory.
  1. **Ask about possible stress factors** (problems with personal relationships, recent changes in employment status, death of a close family member etc.). The condition is transient.
     - Treat with cyclical progestogen (dydrogesterone 10 mg on days 15–24 of the cycle) for three months.
     - If normal menstrual cycle is not achieved without medication, refer the patient to a gynaecologist.
  2. **Measure serum testosterone**, if the patient gives a history of weight gain, truncal obesity, acne, hirsutism.
     - **Polycystic ovarian syndrome**, see 25.15.
     - Ovulation disturbed by **obesity** alone, treated with cyclical progestogen until weight normalizes to avoid the risk of endometrial hyperplasia (25.44), (25.13)
     - Rare: Cushing's syndrome (24.40).
     - If there are clear signs of **virilism** (alopecia, marked hirsutism, enlargement of the clitoris, deepening of the voice) and serum testosterone level is increased, the patient must be referred to a gynaecologist. The patient may have an androgen-producing adrenal or ovarian tumor.
     - Note! If the testosterone level is very high, no withdrawal bleeding will occur after the progestogen challenge test.

25.15 Polycystic ovary syndrome (PCOS)

Laure Morin-Papunen

Basic rules

- Polycystic ovary syndrome is not purely a gynaecological problem.
- Diagnosis can be made if the patient has two of the following: menstrual disorder, hyperandrogenism, polycystic ovaries.
- Polycystic ovary syndrome is associated with reduced insulin sensitivity which may lead to increased health risks.

Prevalence and consequences

- The prevalence of PCOS is estimated to be 5–10% in women of reproductive age.
- PCOS will mean increased morbidity at various stages throughout the woman's life.

Gynaecological problems

- Patients usually present with menstrual irregularities, hirsutism and infertility problems.
- Pregnancies appear to be associated with a higher risk of miscarriage, hypertension and diabetes. The increased risk is, however, likely to be associated with obesity rather than with PCOS as such.
- Long-term lack of luteal hormone activity are known to predispose the endometrium to hyperplasia and thus increase the risk of uterine cancer. It has been reported that the risk of uterine cancer is increased five-fold in women with PCOS as compared with the general population. However, it is difficult to distinguish between the increased risk caused by obesity and that by PCOS, and large-scale epidemiological studies are needed.
- There is no evidence of a link with breast cancer.

Metabolic disturbances

- Women with PCOS often have reduced insulin sensitivity which is associated with truncal obesity and disturbances in lipid metabolism.
- Half of the women with PCOS are overweight.
- Insulin resistance and the resulting compensatory increased concentration of insulin are more marked in overweight patients with PCOS than in otherwise overweight controls.
- Typical findings include low serum HDL-cholesterol concentration and hypertriglyceridaemia.
- PCOS appears to increase the risk of developing type 2 diabetes at a considerably early age (the risk is 2–5-fold) and, at a later age, hypertension (the risk is 2–3-fold).
- Even though it has been suggested that women with PCOS have a manyfold risk of developing ischaemic heart disease, no definite evidence exists to support the claim.
- The risk of complications associated with cerebrovascular disease and diabetes is increased.

Diagnosis

- Diagnosis is based on the history, clinical findings (menstrual irregularities, male pattern of hair distribution, acne) and, if necessary, on hormone studies.
- A gynaecological ultrasound examination is used to verify the diagnosis; polycystic morphology of the ovaries is evident.
- Two of the following criteria must be present for PCOS diagnosis:
  - anovulation characterized by menstrual irregularities
  - clinical (male pattern of hair distribution or acne) or biochemical (serum testosterone > 2.7 nmol/l) signs of hyperandrogenism
  - polycystic morphology of the ovaries, verified by ultrasound examination (presence of 12 or more follicles in each ovary measuring 2–9 mm in diameter, and/or increased ovarian volume > 10 ml).
- Exclude thyroid disease, hyperprolactinaemia, androgen-secreting tumours and disturbances in adrenal function.
  - If the patient presents with menstrual irregularities, measure serum TSH and prolactin to exclude other causes.
  - If the patient presents with hirsutism and/or acne, measure serum testosterone.
  - Serum FSH, LH and estradiol are not usually of diagnostic benefit.
- Due to the risk of metabolic disturbances the following screening is indicated, particularly in overweight patients:
  - blood glucose, lipids and blood pressure at regular intervals (for example every two years)
  - glucose tolerance testing in conjunction with the first visit followed by regular testing (for example every two years).

Treatment

- The most important treatment form is weight reduction down to the patient's normal weight. Weight reduction may
  - regularize the menstrual cycle through restoring ovulation
  - significantly reduce the risk of miscarriage during early pregnancy as well as other pregnancy-associated risks
  - enhance the safety and efficacy of ovulation induction treatments and reduce the risk of late complications associated with PCOS, such as type 2 diabetes and coronary heart disease.
- Exercise reduces insulin resistance.
- Smoking cessation is important due to the increased risk of vascular diseases.

Hormone treatment

- Oral contraceptives restore the normal menstrual cycle. In order to improve hirsutism and to minimize the harmful effects on lipids, contraceptive agents containing progestogens which are as little androgenic as possible should be chosen. Choose, for example, drospirenone, cyproterone or desogestrel containing product. However, so far, no studies comparing the metabolic and antiandrogenic effects of oral contraceptives in PCOS patients are available.
- To prevent endometrial hyperplasia cyclic progestogen has to be prescribed (for example, for 10 days on days 15–24 of the cycle or for 14 days every 2 or 3 months).
- If hirsutism is unacceptable despite oral contraceptives an antiandrogen may be added (50 mg of cyproterone on the first 10 days of the cycle).

Spironolactone

- If oral contraceptives are contraindicated, hair growth may be suppressed by using spironolactone (100–200 mg/day). Monitor serum electrolytes (Na and K) at regular intervals, for example after the first 3 months after instigating treatment and annually thereafter.

Metformin

- Metformin is effective for inducing ovulation in PCOS (A) [1], and there is some evidence of its beneficial effects on metabolic risk factors.
- Consider metformin if the patient wishes to conceive. Refer a patient with PCOS to a gynaecologist with infertility expertise at an earlier stage than normal.
- Consult a gynaecologist before prescribing metformin.
  - Even though it is considered that metformin may reduce the risk of gestational complications, such as miscarriage in early pregnancy, pre-eclampsia and gestational diabetes, no adequately large placebo-controlled studies exist so far. Metformin should not be administered routinely to all women with PCOS who have problems conceiving. There is not enough evidence on the benefits of metformin in PCOS women with normal weight.

Treatment of anovulation

- All other ovulation induction treatment is carried out by a gynaecologist who has expertise in fertility treatment.
- Clomifene citrate is the drug of choice (A) [2 3]. It is an oral anti-oestrogen, which increases the gonadotrophin release from the pituitary gland which, in turn, will initiate the development of an ovarian follicle in the ovary and induce ovulation. The effect of treatment should be monitored either with an ultrasound on days 11–13 of the cycle or by measuring the progesterone concentration midway through the luteal phase.
- The dose may be increased up to 100 mg/day (maximum dose is 150 mg/day). Ovulation occurs in approximately 80% of patients and the rate of conception is approximately 25–50%, depending on the patient group. Treatment may be continued for the duration of up to six ovulatory cycles.
- If clomifene treatment is unsuccessful the patient will be given gonadotrophins. Gonadotrophin treatment is expensive and more problematic than clomifene treatment. Gonadotrophins are injected daily, and ovulation induction may take a long time. The treatment requires repeated ultrasound examinations, but the risk of multiple pregnancy or hyperstimulation cannot be totally excluded.
- Ovarian cauterisation (drilling), which is carried out laparoscopically, has recently regained popularity along with the newer techniques. Treatment costs are considerably lower than those of gonadotrophin treatment, and the method has been found to be equally effective. It also reduces the risk of multiple pregnancy.
- If conception does not occur with ovulation induction, in vitro fertilization is considered.

References

1. Lord JM, Flight IHK, Norman RJ. Insulin-sensitising drugs (metformin, troglitazone, rosiglitazone, pioglitazone, D-chiro-inositol) for polycystic ovary syndrome. Cochrane Database Syst Rev. 2004;(2):CD003053.
2. Hughes E, Collins J, Vandekerckhove P. Clomiphene citrate for ovulation induction in women with oligo-amenorrhoea. The Cochrane Database of Systematic Reviews, Cochrane Library number: CD000056. In: The Cochrane Library, Issue 2, 2002. Oxford: Update Software. Updated frequently.
3. Hughes E, Collins J, Vandekerckhove P. Clomiphene citrate for unexplained subfertility in women. Cochrane Database Syst Rev. 2004;(2):CD000057.

25.20 Physical examination of the breasts: diagnosing a lump and pain in the breasts

Editors

Inspection

- The sitting patient holds the arms first at the sides and then over the head.
  - The breasts must move symmetrically and their contour must be regular when the arms are moving.
- Observe
  - abnormal variation in breast size
  - retractions of the skin (Starting from rest, the patient contracts the pectoralis muscles. A tumour fixed to the fascia causes slight retraction of the skin.)
  - lumps
  - "the orange peel sign"
  - ulcerations

- eczema of the nipple
- nipple retraction
- discharge from the nipple

Palpation

- Palpation is performed with the patient supine and arms both abducted and at the sides.
- The breasts are palpated all over one quarter at a time or by moving the hand in circles over the breast.
- Palpation only with the fingertips is unreliable. The breast must be palpated with the whole length of 2–5 fingers and the palm. A rotary or swinging movement of the hand gives better contact.
- The retraction of the skin can often be demonstrated by lifting the suspected skin area between the fingers.
- The axillary region is palpated while holding the patient's upper arm tightly so that the muscles relax and it is easy to move the arm. The axillary region must also be palpated against the chest wall, to get an impression of the lymph nodes that are situated high up in the axilla.
- In premenstrum the breasts can be tense or tender and the examination is therefore unreliable. In these cases re-examine the patient after menstruation.
- Palpation of large breasts in unreliable.

Further examination

- Every lump found by palpation or a suspected change noticed during inspection (retraction, change of the skin) must be diagnosed by mammography and/or by ultrasonography and, if necessary, by fine-needle or core needle biopsy, and in unclear cases eventually by lumpectomy.
  - If there is tenderness and diffuse nodularity in the breasts before menstruation, wait and palpate the breasts again after menstruation. If the finding is still abnormal, refer the patient for further examination.
- Discharge from the nipple, see 25.21.
- Screening by mammography, see 16.20.

Mastalgia (mastodynia, painful breast)

- Mastalgia can be on uni- or bilateral, cyclic (about 70%) or constant (about 25%). In about 5% of cases mastalgia turns out to be costochondral pain in the region of the mammae.
- Mastalgia in breast cancer is unilateral and constant.
- Pain is the primary symptom of cancer in up to 10–15% of the cases.

Examination

- A good history
- Clinical examination of the breasts
- Mammography and ultrasonography when necessary.

Treatment

- If no cancer is found, most of the patients are happy when they hear that the condition is benign.
- After consultation with a specialist, you can in rare cases try danazol 200–400 mg daily or if that does not help, bromocriptine 2.5 mg daily beginning on the 14th day of the cycle.

25.21 Galactorrhoea and other discharge from the nipple

Editors

Basic rules

- Rule out a local tumour by sufficient investigations in all cases with serous or bloody unilateral discharge. Milky discharge or discharge from more than one mammary duct does not suggest breast cancer.
- Prolactin and TSH assays are indicated in galactorrhoea in adult women. Children and men must be investigated further and more thoroughly.

GYN

Aetiology

- **Unilateral serous or bloody discharge** is caused by mammary duct ectasias, cystic mastopathy, intraductal papilloma, or carcinoma. Cancer is found in about 1% of the patients.
- **Several drugs** may cause **galactorrhoea**
  - Phenothiazines and other neuroleptic agents such as sulpiride.
  - Tricyclic antidepressants
  - Tamoxifen
  - Oral contraceptives
  - Medroxyprogesterone
  - Metoclopramide
  - Verapamil
  - Isoniazid
  - Antihistamines
- There are several **endocrinological** causes of galactorrhoea.
  - Prolactin-secreting adenoma (the most common cause)
  - Other tumours of the pituitary gland and its vicinity
  - Thyroid disorders (particularly hypothyroidism)
  - Hormone-secreting tumours in other parts of the body (very rare)
- **Mechanical or other prolonged irritation** of the breast may cause galactorrhoea (touching, massage, shingles).

History

- Unilateral or bilateral discharge?
- Local pain or tenderness in the breast (recent or past)
- Pregnancy and lactation (has lactation persisted after the baby was weaned?)
- Menstrual cycle (amenorrhoea?)
- Headache
- Visual disturbances (diplopia, difficulties in dim light)
- Disturbances of the sense of smell
- Disorders of general condition, appetite, body weight, heat tolerance, and sexual function
- Medication
- Recurrent irritation of the skin on the breasts

Clinical examination

- Palpation and squeezing to find out whether the discharge is unilateral or bilateral. This is particularly important if the patient reports that the discharge is unilateral.
- The investigations for unilateral or bloody discharge include:
  - Palpation of the breasts (looking for nodules and the orifice of the duct where the discharge comes from; discharge originating from one single duct suggests papilloma).
  - Mammography, echography and ductography
- The investigations for bilateral milky discharge include:
  - Palpation of the breasts
  - A targeted neurological examination, particularly the visual fields, ocular fundi, and cranial nerves
  - Serum prolactin (Do not rely on one determination because intercourse, squeezing the breasts, and stress may temporarily increase the prolactin levels.)
  - Serum TSH.

Indications for further investigations

- In the newborn a milky discharge up to the age of a few weeks is a normal phenomenon that does not require investigations.
- Milky discharge in men, children, or adolescents is always an indication for specialist consultation.
- Bilateral galactorrhoea in an adult woman with normal laboratory results, normal menstrual cycle, and no abnormal clinical signs can be followed up for one year in primary care. If the discharge continues, the patient should be referred to a specialist for further pituitary function tests. For the investigations of amenorrhoea see 25.14.

Treatment

- Lactation after delivery can be stopped with a single 1-mg dose of cabergoline. The drug may lower the blood pressure for 3–4 days. Cabergoline has fewer side effects than bromocriptine.
- Milk secretion other than that following delivery should not be treated before specialist investigations.
- If hyperprolactinaemia is associated with the use of neuroleptics, a change of the preparation can be tried. Medication to suppress galactorrhoea is not indicated.

25.22 Mastitis

Editors

Basic rules

- Antibiotic treatment of a nursing mother must begin as soon as possible in order to prevent complications.
- Mastitis of a non-lactating woman needs always further examination.

Aetiology

- Mastitis is usually a staphylococcal infection. However, not all mastitis is bacterial.
- Nipple erosion and a poorly emptying breast predispose to inflammation.

Symptoms

- High fever, often up to 40°C
- Redness and tenderness of the breast

Treatment

- Laboratory tests are usually not necessary for making the decision on treatment; the clinical picture is sufficient.
- Treatment with antibiotics must begin at once if the patient has fever.
- Follow-up and emptying of the breast are sufficient if the patient does not have fever and there is no evident breast abscess. The cause is probably milk that has accumulated in the glands. Warming of the breast (e.g. with a hair dryer) is a good treatment. The mother is asked to contact the clinic immediately if she gets fever.
  - Treatment by emptying: The baby should always be fed from the affected breast first. The breast can be emptied with a mechanical suction device and then the baby can suck the remaining milk. If possible, the mother should keep the infected part of the breast higher than the nipple while nursing (so that the infected fluid can drain).

Antibiotic therapy

- Choose an antibiotic effective against staphylococci. The treatment should last (7–)10 days.

- A first generation cephalosporin
  - Cloxacillin or dicloxacillin 500 mg × 4
  - Cephalexin or cefadroxil 500 mg × 3
- A macrolide
  - Erythromycin 400–500 mg × 4
  - Roxithromycin 150 mg × 2

Other treatment

- Encourage the mother to nurse normally from the infected breast or to empty the breast regularly with a suction device. This reduces the pain in the breast, improves drainage of the pus and prevents abscess formation.
- If an abscess develops (10%), proper incision often requires general anaesthesia and placement of a rubber slip to drain the abscess.

Follow-up

- If the nursing mother becomes asymptomatic, she does not need follow-up.
- Mastitis in a non-lactating woman is treated in the same way as for a lactating woman, but **mammography must always be scheduled after treatment in order to find a possible carcinoma.**
- Remember the possibility of carcinoma also in nursing mothers, particularly in recurrent cases or if a lump remains in the breast after inflammation.

25.23 Breast cancer

Kaija Holli

Epidemiology

- Breast cancer is the most common type of cancer in women (one woman in ten is affected).
- The disease becomes more prevalent after 45 years of age. It is rare in women under 30 years of age (0.3% of all).
- Men can also have breast cancer (0.1% of all cancers in men).

Aetiology

- The aetiology is not known in detail, but hormonal imbalance is somehow involved.
- An inherited gene defect ($BRCA_1$, $BRCA_2$) predisposes to breast cancer. Genetic breast cancers account for 5–10% of all cases.

Risk factors

- Nulliparity
- Early menarche
- Late menopause
- Long-term (>5 years) use of oestrogens or oestrogen-progestin combinations
- Proliferative mastopathy
- Atypical lobular hyperplasia
- Breast cancer in the family
- Postmenopausal obesity
- The effect of oral contraceptives is controversial 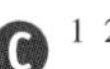 [1 2].

Factors lowering the risk of breast cancer

- Stopping ovarian hormone production premenopausally (ovariectomy, pharmacotherapy)
- Multiparity
- First delivery at a young age
- Bilateral (prophylactic) mastectomy
- Antioestrogen
- Physical activity 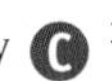 [3]

Symptoms

- A painless lump in the breast (in about 80% of the patients); sometimes the lump is tender.
- Retraction of the skin or nipple
- Eczematous skin changes near the nipple (Paget's disease)
- Discharge from the nipple
- Vague pain, pricking, or heaviness may also be initial symptoms.
- Lump in the armpit
- Symptoms caused by metastases

Diagnosis

- History, family, nature and duration of symptoms, and the patient's own observations.
- Clinical examination B [4 5], including inspection and palpation (25.20).
- Mammography and eventual supplementary imaging such as ultrasound, magnification imaging, galactography, and MRI
- The sensitivity of mammography is better in older age groups compared with the younger ones
- Ultrasonography is used as an initial investigation supplementing mammography, mainly for differentiating cysts from solid tumours.
- Fine-needle or large-core needle biopsy can be performed during mammography or ultrasonography or afterwards. Uncertain diagnoses must be confirmed, and negative cytology is not reliable if the results of other investigations are suggestive.
- Benign lesions such as mastopathy and fibroadenoma should be considered in the differential diagnosis.
- Laboratory investigations are of no use in the initial stage unless advanced disease is suspected.

GYN

Histology

- The main types of breast cancer are ductal and lobular carcinomas. About 75–80% of invasive breast cancers are of the ductal type, and 15–15% are of the lobular type. Inflammatory carcinoma is a clinical diagnosis, not a separate histological type. In situ forms of both types occur. The ductal in situ carcinoma is a precancerous lesion, whereas the lobular in situ lesion is merely a risk factor for carcinoma.
- In addition to the above-mentioned types there are a number of other histological types such as tubular, papillare, medullar, and mucinous carcinoma. Paget's disease of the nipple is also classified separately.

Initial treatment

1. Surgical removal of the tumour (mastectomy or lumpectomy). A sparing operation can be performed if the diameter of the tumour is <2 cm (in a large breast even a tumour 4 cm in diameter can be removed by a lumpectomy) A [6 7]. In other cases a modified radical mastectomy and axillary clearance is performed. In some cases, however, biopsy of the sentinel node is sufficient for excluding spread to the axillary nodes. Breast reconstruction can be performed in the same operation or later. Immediate TRAM (transverse abdominal muscle flap) is becoming increasingly common but requires a plastic surgeon.
2. Chemotherapy C [8 9] and/or irradiation A [10] are nowadays given before surgery (neoadjuvant therapy) with the aim of diminishing tumour size which would allow using a sparing technique also in larger tumours.

Postoperative problems

- A seroma (fluid collection) in the operated area can be emptied in primary care by puncture with a sterile needle.
- Leakage of lymph in the axilla causes swelling, pain, heaviness, erythema, induration and locally elevated skin temperature, all of which are symptoms suggesting an infection. A puncture may be required to confirm that the fluid does not contain pus. No antibiotics are indicated.
- A haematoma must be punctured and drained.
- Phlebitis in the superficial veins of the axillar region cause tension under the skin during elevation of the arm and are visible as linear bulging of the skin. The condition is self-limiting.
- Pain, tingling, and paraesthesia of the shoulder and axillar region is caused by transsection (permanent) or stretching (transient) of intercostal nerves during the operation.

Postoperative treatment

1. Radiotherapy (5–6 weeks) is always indicated after lumpectomy A [11 12]. In other cases the size, TNM stage and other characteristics of the tumour determine the need for radiotherapy.
2. Adjuvant chemotherapy is given in certain situations after the operation. Either cytostatics or hormones can be used as adjuvant treatment. The selection of the adjuvant treatment is based on the evaluated risk of recurrence (>10%), age and hormonal state of the patient and the hormone receptor status of the tumour.
   - Chemotherapy is the primary therapy in premenopausal patients A [13 14]. The duration of treatment is usually 4–6 months. Hormone receptor-positive patients are also treated with tamoxifen for 5 years. A [15 16 17 18 19].
   - Postmenopausal patients can also be treated with chemotherapy (4–6 months), and patients with hormone receptor-positive tumours can also be treated with anti-oestrogens (tamoxifen or toremifen). Hormone receptor-positive patients can also be treated with anti-oestrogens alone for 5 years.
   - Aromatase inhibitor can be used in adjuvant setting instead of anti-oestrogens especially if there is some contraindication for anti-oestrogen.

Treatment of recurrent or advanced breast cancer

- About 70% of recurrences and metastases are detected within three years of the operation. Recurrence may, however, occur very late, even after 20 asymptomatic years. Some tumours are very aggressive and spread rapidly whereas others grow very slowly.
- About one third of first recurrences occur in the operated area, in the skin or subcutaneous tissue of the chest and local lymph nodes. Distant metastases occur in the skeleton, lungs, pleura, abdominal cavity, liver, and the brain.
- Radiotherapy can be used in bone and brain metastases of solitary and local recurrent tumours. Radiotherapy is effective against painful skeletal metastases.
- Single or combined chemotherapy is used in the treatment of advanced disease B [20 21]. The treatments are repeated at predetermined intervals. The medications are usually administered intravenously, but peroral chemotherapy can also be used. The medicine can also be injected locally, for example in the pleural space.
- Hormonal treatment is used in receptor-positive advanced breast cancer B [20 21]. Hormonal treatments are often administered perorally, but subcutaneous or intramuscular preparations also exist. Extinction of ovarian activity (either by surgeon, irradiation or chemicals) can also be used as hormonal treatment in premenopausal women B [22 23].
- Bisphosphonates reduce the risk of skeletal events in women with advanced breast cancer and clinically evident bone metastases and prevent hypercalcaemia A [24].
- Aromatase inhibitors (anastrozole, letrozole, exemestane) are more efficient and less harmful than progestines. They are also efficient in patients who no longer respond to anti-oestrogens. B [25]

Rehabilitation

- Physiotherapy of the upper arm and shoulder joint must be started as soon as possible after the operation, and the patient must continue with the exercises for the rest of her life. Swelling and scar formation are thus prevented after removal of axillary nodes.

- Mobilizing exercises
- Intermittent pressure treatment (can be carried out in primary care)
- Lymphatic massage is an alternative to intermittent pressure treatment.

- Breast prosthesis should be used at home after ablation to ensure symmetrical weight-bearing on the shoulders.
- Breast reconstruction can be performed one year after the primary operation. After total radiotherapy the reconstruction should be postponed by two years.

Follow-up

- The aim of the follow-up is to identify and treat adverse effects of the primary treatment, detect recurrences or contralateral breast cancer, and support the patient's ability to cope by organizing rehabilitation and psychosocial support.
- Giving adjuvant therapy also to patients with a low risk of recurrence and the use of new medications warrant more attention to the long-term adverse effects of the therapies. These include cardiac adverse effects and second cancers.
- The follow-up of a breast cancer patient can be carried out in primary health care; however, the specialist unit in charge of the treatment must give individually tailored instructions on the content of follow-up. Because breast cancer is such a heterogeneous disease, similar follow-up protocol for all patients is not justified B [26].
  - Paying attention to the patient's symptoms and clinical examination of the affected site is most important.
  - Mammography is indicated at two-year intervals, complemented regularly with ultrasound when necessary. In patients below 50 years of age the recommended interval is 1–1.5 years.
  - Other diagnostic investigations are performed as deemed necessary.
  - In patients with ductal carcinoma in situ follow-up of the breasts and close areas is sufficient. In lobular invasive cancer the sites of recurrences are often very different from those seen in ductal cancer (contralateral breast, retroperitoneum, etc.) and attention should be paid to these sites.

Pregnancy

- Radiotherapy is contraindicated throughout pregnancy. Chemotherapy is not recommended during the first two trimesters of pregnancy.
- Pregnancy should be postponed for two years after the treatment of breast cancer because the risk for recurrence is highest in this period. Pregnancy after treatment is not a risk factor of recurrence. Chemotherapy or radiotherapy for breast cancer has not been observed to increase the risk of malformations if the pregnancy starts after the treatment has been discontinued.
- After lumpectomy lactation is usually not possible from the operated breast. The treatment does not affect lactation of the contralatcral breast.

Postmenopausal oestrogen treatment

- Caution should be exercised when initiating hormone replacement therapy in women who have survived breast cancer. The results of a recent randomized study (HABITS) show that oestrogen treatment of two years duration significantly increased the risk of recurrence of breast cancer B [27].
  - Should uncomfortable symptoms warrant the introduction of hormone replacement therapy the patient must be thoroughly informed of the benefits and risks.
  - In breast cancer patients, the fist-line treatment should consist of non-hormonal alternatives.
- Tibolone has not been found to affect the mammary gland in animal studies, and density is not seen on mammography in the breasts of a woman using tibolone.

References

1. Collaborative Group on Hormonal Factors in Breast Cancer. Breast cancer and hormonal contraceptives: collaborative reanalysis of individual data on 53,297 women with breast cancer and 100,239 women without breast cancer from 54 epidemiological studies. Lancet 1996;347:1713–1727.
2. The Database of Abstracts of Reviews of Effectiveness (University of York), Database no.: DARE-968506. In: The Cochrane Library, Issue 4, 1999. Oxford: Update Software.
3. McTiernan A, Koopenberg C, White E et al. Recreational physical activity and the risk of breast cancer in postmenopausal women. The Women's Health Initiative Cohort Study. JAMA 2003;290:1331–1336.
4. Barton MB, Harris R, Fletcher SW. Does this patient have breast cancer: the screening clinical breast examination: should it be done: how. JAMA 1999;282:1270–1280.
5. The Database of Abstracts of Reviews of Effectiveness (University of York), Database no.: DARE-999724. In: The Cochrane Library, Issue 3, 2001. Oxford: Update Software.
6. Morris AD, Morris RD, Wilson JF et al. Breast-conserving therapy vs mastectomy in early-stage breast cancer: a meta-analysis of 10-year survival. Cancer Journal from Scientific American 1997;3:6–12.
7. The Database of Abstracts of Reviews of Effectiveness (University of York), Database no.: DARE-970773. In: The Cochrane Library, Issue 4, 1999. Oxford: Update Software.
8. Colleoni M, Coates A, Pagani O, Goldhirsch A. Combined chemo-endocrine adjuvant therapy for patients with operable breast cancer: still a question? Cancer Treatment Reviews 1998;24:15–26.
9. The Database of Abstracts of Reviews of Effectiveness (University of York), Database no.: DARE-980868. In: The Cochrane Library, Issue 2, 2000. Oxford: Update Software.

10. Early Breast Cancer Trialists' Collaborative Group. Radiotherapy for early breast cancer. Cochrane Database Syst Rev. 2004;(2):CD003647.
11. Early Breast Cancer Trialists' Collaborative Group. Effects of radiotherapy and surgery in early breast cancer: an overview of the randomized trials. N Engl J Med 1995;333:1444–1455.
12. The Database of Abstracts of Reviews of Effectiveness (University of York), Database no.: DARE-953281. In: The Cochrane Library, Issue 4, 1999. Oxford: Update Software.
13. Hall PD, Lesher BA, Hall RK. Adjuvant therapy of node-negative breast cancer. Ann Pharmacotherapy 1995;29: 289–298.
14. The Database of Abstracts of Reviews of Effectiveness (University of York), Database no.: DARE-952083. In: The Cochrane Library, Issue 4, 1999. Oxford: Update Software.
15. Early Breast Cancer Trialists' Collaborative Group. Tamoxifen for early breast cancer. Cochrane Database Syst Rev. 2004;(2):CD000486.
16. Early Breast Cancer Trialists' Collaborative Group. Tamoxifen for early breast cancer: an overview of the randomised trials. Lancet 1998;351:1451–1467.
17. The Database of Abstracts of Reviews of Effectiveness (University of York), Database no.: DARE-988598. In: The Cochrane Library, Issue 2, 2000. Oxford: Update Software.
18. Crump M, Sawka CA, DeBoer G, Buchanan RB, Ingle JN, Forbes J, Meakin JW, Shelley W, Pritchard KI. An individual-based meta-analysis of tamoxifen versus ovarian ablation as first line endocrine therapy for premenopausal women with metastatic breast cancer. Breast Cancer Research and Treatment 1997;44:201–210.
19. The Database of Abstracts of Reviews of Effectiveness (University of York), Database no.: DARE-970997. In: The Cochrane Library, Issue 4, 1999. Oxford: Update Software.
20. Fossati R, Confalonieri C, Torri CV, Ghislandi R, Penna A, Pistotti V, Tinazzi A, Liberati A. Cytotoxic and hormonal treatment (CHT) for metastatic breast cancer. J Clin Oncol 1998;16:3439–3460.
21. The Database of Abstracts of Reviews of Effectiveness (University of York), Database no.: DARE-981765. In: The Cochrane Library, Issue 2, 2000. Oxford: Update Software.
22. Early Breast Cancer Trialists' Collaborative Group. Ovarian ablation in early breast cancer: overview of the randomised trials. Lancet 1996;348:1189–1196.
23. The Database of Abstracts of Reviews of Effectiveness (University of York), Database no.: DARE-978204. In: The Cochrane Library, Issue 4, 1999. Oxford: Update Software.
24. Pavlakis N, Stockler M. Bisphosphonates for breast cancer. Cochrane Database Syst Rev. 2004;(2):CD003474.
25. Johnston S, Stebbing J. Selective aromatase inhibitors for breast cancer in postmenopausal women. Clinical Evidence 2000;4:1005–1006.
26. Rojas MP, Telaro E, Russo A, Fossati R, Palli D, Rosselli Del Turco M,Confalonieri C, Liberati A. Follow-up strategies for women treated for early breast cancer. Cochrane Database Syst Rev. 2004;(2):CD001768.
27. Holmberg L, Anderson H, for the HABITS steering and data monitoring committees. HABITS (hormonal replacement therapy after breast cancer– is it safe?), a randomised comparison: trial stopped. Lancet 2004;363:453–455.

25.30 Vaginitis

Editors

Introduction

- Treatment should be directed at the most likely cause of the infection.
- It is usually possible to obtain a diagnosis of sufficient accuracy by gynaecological examination and basic laboratory tests.

Symptoms

- Increased vaginal discharge without pelvic pain or systemic symptoms.
- Itching and a burning sensation, usually in the external genital organs.
- Characteristic "fishy" smell.
- Dysuria; experienced at the urethral orifice.

Aetiology

- Candida species (Candida albicans, C. glabrata)
- Anaerobic bacteria (Gardnerella vaginalis, Bacteroides species etc.)
- Trichomonas vaginalis
- Aerobic bacteria (for example, group G beta-haemolytic streptococcus, E.coli)
- Actinomyces (ALO, actinomyces-like organisms) are sometimes isolated from patients with an intra-uterine device (IUD) (>3 years).

Diagnostics

Clinical examination

- Itching and a burning sensation usually indicate vaginal mycosis (candidiasis). The discharge is lumpy, whitish and sticks to the vaginal wall.
- A malodorous, homogeneous, greyish discharge sticking to the vaginal wall is typical of bacterial vaginosis.
- A frothy, greenish discharge indicates trichomoniasis. It is quite rare nowadays.
- A copious, yellowish, odourless discharge is suggestive of vaginitis caused by aerobic bacteria.
- The vaginal mucous membranes of postmenopausal women become thinner, and they bleed and become irritated easily due to the lack of oestrogen (atrophic vaginitis). Remember that slightly brownish discharge can be the first symptom of uterine cancer (take an endometrial biopsy).
- The uterus and adnexa are not tender in vaginitis. Purulent discharge from the cervix should be examined for gonococci and chlamydia (see pelvic inflammatory disease 25.41).

Strategies for investigation

- Symptoms and clinical picture are usually sufficient to diagnose vaginal mycosis.
- If the clinical picture does not match mycosis, perform a potassium hydroxide test: a couple of drops of potassium hydroxide are placed onto the used speculum; a strong odour of fish indicates bacterial vaginosis.
- It is also possible to take a bacterial culture to identify mycosis or trichomoniasis, as well as clue cells. The culture results should be available on the following day.
- If a microscope is available:
  - put one drop of discharge on a glass slide, add one drop of saline and examine with 400-fold magnification.
- See Table 25.30.1.
- In typical bacterial vaginosis there are clue cells, but only a few leucocytes. If a large number of leucocytes are seen together with clue cells, suspect concurrent cervicitis (remember chlamydia!).
- Fungi can be identified as threads, spores (budding, small, clear and homogeneous cells) or both. There may be a large number of polymorphonuclear leucocytes.

Treatment

Vaginal mycosis

- Treat according to clinical manifestation.
- Possible balanitis of the partner must also be treated (e.g. with a cream).
- Treat with pessaries for 1–3 days or with an oral antimycotic as a single close A [1 2 3].
- Vaginal mycosis during pregnancy is treated topically A [4].
- If the patient has a history of vaginal mycosis and typical symptoms recur, for example during antibiotic treatment, a prescription can be given for "a reserve" or over the telephone to the pharmacy.

Table 25.30.1 Microscopic investigation of vaginal discharge

Infection	Physiological discharge
A large number of leucocytes (the majority of cells, grouped together, minimum 10/visual field)	A few leucocytes/visual field
A large number of small round bacteria	Rod-like bacilli, some of which are very long (rods of Döderlein) Epithelial cells
Bacterial vaginosis epithelial cells containing and surrounded by bacteria (clue cells) **Mycosis** budding, small, clear and homogeneous cells **Trichomoniasis** actively mobile protozoa	

- Recurrent mycosis can result from antibiotics, the contraceptive pill or increased blood glucose.
- Recurrent mycosis may require prophylactic treatment (a single dose of an antimycotic once a week), for example for 2–3 weeks. Remember dietary advice (sugar, chocolate!).

Bacterial vaginosis

- Common with IUD use.
- Treat with metronidazole 400 mg two or three times daily for 5–7 days C [5 6].
- Topical treatments available include metronidazole pessaries or 2% clindamycin cream; these are also suitable during pregnancy A [7 8]. Oral metronidazole is also safe A [9] during pregnancy.

Atrophic vaginitis

- Treat with topical oestrogen (nightly for a week and thereafter twice a week).

Vaginitis caused by aerobic bacteria

- Known also as desquamative inflammatory vaginitis (DIV).
- Symptoms include treatment resistant, yellowish, odourless vaginal discharge that smears underwear.
- The vaginal mucosa may be ulcerous, irritated and inflamed. It may even be sore to touch and show erythematous lesions.
- A cervical smear often shows mild atypia and severe inflammatory reaction.
- A microscopic examination of the discharge is characteristic: marked leucocytosis and parabasal cells. No specific diagnostic test exists.
- In differential diagnosis, erosive lichen planus should be taken into consideration.
- If in doubt take a sample for bacterial culture and treat according to the results.
- Metronidazole is not effective; clindamycin cream (for 7 days) may be beneficial in some cases.

Trichomoniasis

- Treat with a single dose of metronidazole 2 g, or 400–500 mg twice or three times daily for 5–7 days A [10].
- The partner must always be treated A [10].
- Exclude other sexually transmitted diseases.

Actinomyces

- Sometimes isolated in the cervical smear of patients with an IUD in situ (>3 years)
- May predispose the patient to pelvic inflammatory disease.
- The best treatment form is the removal of the IUD, a new one can be inserted after a few months.
- If the patient shows signs of infection, a course of penicillin and metronidazole should be prescribed.

Differential diagnostics of vaginitis

- See Table 25.30.2.

Table 25.30.2

Clinical parameter	Normal	Mycosis	Trichomoniasis	Bacterial vaginosis
Discharge	Unhomogeneous, white	Lumpy, white	Purulent, frothy	Homogeneous, pasty, malodorous
pH	⩽4.5	⩽4.5	>4.5	>4.5
KOH test	–	–	+	++
Plain microscopy	Epithelial cells, rods	Fungal threads	Mobile trichomonads	Clue cells

References

1. Watson MC, Grimshaw JM, Bond CM, Mollison J, Ludbrook A. Oral versus intra-vaginal imidazole and triazole anti-fungal treatment of uncomplicated vulvovaginal candidiasis (thrush). Cochrane Database Syst Rev. 2004;(2):CD002845.
2. Reef SE, Levine WC, McNeil MM, Fisher-Hoc S, Holmberg SD, Duerr A, Smith D, Sobel JD. Treatments for vulvovaginal candidiasis: 1993. Clin Infect Dis 1995;20(suppl 1):pp. 80–90.
3. The Database of Abstracts of Reviews of Effectiveness (University of York), Database no.: DARE-950851. In: The Cochrane Library, Issue 4, 1999. Oxford: Update Software.
4. Young GL, Jewell D. Topical treatment for vaginal candidiasis (thrush) in pregnancy. Cochrane Database Syst Rev. 2004;(2):CD000225.
5. Joesoef MR, Schmid GP. Bacterial vaginosis: review of treatment options and potential clinical indications for therapy. Clin Infect Dis 1995;20(suppl 1);S72–S79.
6. The Database of Abstracts of Reviews of Effectiveness (University of York), Database no.: DARE-950850. In: The Cochrane Library, Issue 4, 1999. Oxford: Update Software.
7. McDonald H, Brocklehurst P, Parsons J, Vigneswaran R. Antibiotics for treating bacterial vaginosis in pregnancy. Cochrane Database Syst Rev. 2004;(2):CD000262.
8. Ugwumadu, A, Manyonda I, Reid F, Hay P. Effect of early oral clindamycin on late miscarriage and preterm delivery in asymptomatic women with abnormali vaginal flora and bacterial vaginosis: a randomized controlled trial. Lancet 2003;361:983–988.
9. Forna F, Gülmezoglu AM. Interventions for treating trichomoniasis in women. Cochrane Database Syst Rev. 2004;(2): CD000218.
10. Gülmezoglu AM. Interventions for trichomoniasis in pregnancy. Cochrane Database Syst Rev. 2004;(2):CD000220.

25.31 Bartholinitis: Bartholin's duct abscess and cyst

Pentti K. Heinonen

Principles

- An acute abscess is incised as an on-call procedure (do not treat with antibiotics or refer for a procedure later on).
- Refer to a gynaecologist a patient with symptomatic cysts.

Anatomy

- Bartholin's glands are located posterolaterally to the vaginal orifice, embedded in the posterior part of the vestibular bulb. There are two glands that are about 1 cm in size. The duct from the glands is 2 cm in length and runs downward and inward opening at the introitus below the hymen but above the attachment of the posterior end of the labium minus. The gland is not normally felt on palpation but the orifice of the duct is often visible.

Abscess

- In a mild infection, pus excreted from the duct is the only symptom.
- In a more severe infection the duct is blocked and an abscess is formed in the gland. The abscess is painful and prevents the patient from sitting and walking. The patient may have fever as a general symptom.

Cyst

- A Bartholin's duct cyst usually develops as a sequela of an infection.
- It may also result from trauma or from damage to the duct in episiotomy.
- A Bartholin's cyst is often an accidental finding.
- If the cyst grows large it may cause swelling and dyspareunia. The cyst may also become infected and form a secondary abscess.

Differential diagnosis

- Infectious haematoma in the vulva.
- Infection of paraurethral (Skene's) glands, which are located anteriorly in the distal urethra.

Aetiology

- Mostly a mixed infection cause by both aerobic and anaerobic bacteria. E. coli is the most frequent facultative aerobic microbe causing bartholinitis and Bacteroides and Prevotella species are the most common anaerobic bacteria isolated from abscesses.

- Neisseria gonorrhoeae and Chlamydia trachomatis rarely cause bartholinitis.

Sampling

- The sample for microbial cultures can be taken from the contents of the Bartholin's abscess or from discharge from the infected cyst.
- If venereal disease is suspected, specimens of N. gonorrhoeae and C. trachomatis should also be obtained.

Treatment

Abscess

- A mature, fluctuating abscess is incised and drained through the mucosa after applying a local anaesthetic. Abscesses are often lobulized and all the lobules have to be drained. A rubber slip can be placed in the abscess, but it often fails to stay in place.
- Antimicrobial treatment is recommended if
  - the abscess is large
  - it has extended outside the gland or
  - the patient has fever.
- Recommended antimicrobial regimen
  - Orally cephalosporin (e.g. cephalexin or cephadroxil) 500 mg × 3
  - **and** metronidazole 400 mg × 3 for 10 days.
  - For chlamydia, doxycycline 100 mg × 2 or erythromycin 500 mg × 3 for 7–10 days.
- If an abscess is not yet fluctuating an antimicrobial drug can be administered without attempting drainage. The patient should, however, be told that the development of an abscess is likely and that eventually the abscess may have to be incised.

Cyst

- The cyst is actually a distension of the duct and does not involve the gland. Therapy is directed towards resumption of gland function. This is accomplished by cyst excision or marsupialization, which provides the duct with a new opening (the edges of the cyst lining are everted and sutured to the surrounding skin and mucous membrane) .
- During pregnancy an abscess is treated normally. During pregnancy procedures are complicated by the increased blood flow in the outer genitals and a cyst can be aspirated by a needle. Cyst excision should be scheduled after delivery.

Follow-up

- The patient returns for follow-up 1 month after incision. Perform gynaecological examination and palpation and enquire about symptoms. Refer patients with a symptomatic cyst to a gynaecologist.
- Remember the possibility of a malignant neoplasm of Bartholin's gland in a postmenopausal woman with recurrences.

25.32 Vulvodynia

Jorma Paavonen

Basic rules

- An underdiagnosed syndrome with pain and burning of the female external genital organs. In general gynaecological practice, up to 15% of women admit having experienced vulvar pain at some stage of their lives.
- A complicated clinical problem which may cause significant physical incapacity and psychological distress as well as sexual and marital problems.
- Acknowledgement of the multi-dimensional character of the condition and an empathetic approach are the cornerstones of successful management.
- There is very little evidence-based research data on the condition.

Symptoms and diagnosis

- General points
  - A patient with vulvodynia will find a gynaecological examination painful. A speculum examination, cervical smear or bimanual palpation are not necessary for the diagnosis, and are often difficult to perform.
  - Vulvodynia is often associated with vaginismus which relates to involuntary muscle spasms or tension of the pelvic floor muscles.
  - Ask the patient whether she has any symptomless days. Does the pain vary according to her menstrual cycle? Is the pain associated with intercourse?
  - Exclude the possibility of underlying premalignant and malignant conditions. Consider taking a biopsy of any vulvar lesions, under local anaesthesia, and consult a dermatologist if necessary.
- Vulvar vestibulitis syndrome:
  - The most common subtype of vulvodynia.
  - The vestibule is painful to touch (e.g. during intercourse).
  - Sensitivity to pain may also be distributed more diffusely around the vulvar area.
  - The pain is easy to localize, for example with the aid of a cotton-tipped swab. Test the vestibular point tenderness with the tip of a moistened swab.
  - Sharp pain is usually experienced at the 5 and 7 o'clock positions in the posterior vestibule or in the paraurethral area at the anterior vestibule, or both.

- The sites of point tenderness in the posterior vestibule may coincide with erythema which correspond to the position of vestibular glands.
- The aetiology of vulvar vestibulitis syndrome is unknown. Some cases seem to be provoked by recurrent fungal or bacterial infections, use of oral contraceptives, laser treatment or cryotherapy.

♦ Cyclic vulvovaginitis

- Pain as above but it is cyclical and worses just before menstrual bleeding.
- Pain typically becomes exacerbated after intercourse, and is worst on the following day.
- Cyclic vulvovaginitis is suspected to be a hypersensitivity reaction to a Candida antigen.

♦ Dysaesthetic vulvodynia (essential vulvodynia)

- Differs from the above conditions in that the patients are usually older (typically over 40 years of age), the pain is continuous and diffuse around the entire vulvar region, and the pain may radiate to the anal area, lower back and thighs. The condition is usually not associated with dyspareunia.
- Also known as pudendal neuralgia.
- Palpating with a cotton-tipped swab will not elicit pain in the vestibule only, but sharp pain may be felt throughout the vulvar region and even in areas outside the vulvar region.
- Hyperaesthesia is believed to result from altered innervation of the skin and mucous membranes. The pain is neuropathic in origin (similar to pain in postherpetic neuralgia).

Differential diagnosis

♦ Genital herpes, other ulcerative vulvar conditions
♦ Vulvovaginitis (e.g. Candida)
♦ Desquamative inflammatory vaginitis (rare, purulent vaginitis caused by aerobic bacteria)
♦ Vulvar dermatoses (e.g. lichen planus or lichen sclerosis; referral to a dermatologist).

Treatment

♦ Empathy and support.

- Talk about possible dyspareunia. Has the condition affected sexual relations or the patient's mood?
- Help the patient to understand the condition and the variable nature of the symptoms.
- Explain the relevant anatomy, with the aid of a mirror and drawing if possible.

♦ Treatment to be carried out at home:

- Skin oil (from a pharmacy) to be applied to the painful areas at bedtime, with the aid of a mirror at the beginning.
- Pelvic floor exercises. It is important that the patient learns to identify the pelvic floor muscles and how to relax them. A physiotherapist with expertise in the pelvic floor rehabilitation is able to advise and offer guidance; biofeedback training will improve results.
- It is often advisable to involve the partner in discussions.
- At a later stage lubricants or anaesthetic gels may ease coitus.
- Basic care: wash the genital area only once a day using water alone, loose clothing, no underwear at night.

♦ Set simple and realistic goals. Improvement will take a long time, emphasize the importance of following instructions. Avoid "doctor shopping" if possible.

♦ Make a follow-up appointment; every 1–2 months until the condition has improved.

♦ Vulvar vestibulitis syndrome:

- The condition may remain unchanged for years, but the severity of the symptoms will vary. Spontaneous remission is possible.
- Few effective treatment choices are available. Good information is an integral part of the treatment and will help the patient to cope with her condition.
- Suggest temporary withdrawal of oral contraceptives (e.g. for 6 months).
- If pelvic floor vaginismus is present refer the patient to a physiotherapist.
- If there is no response to the above treatment, refer the patient to a specialist for vestibulectomy.

♦ Cyclic vulvovaginitis

- Topical or oral antifungal drugs (consider prophylaxis, e.g. fluconazole 150 mg once weekly for up to 6 months).

♦ Dysaesthetic vulvodynia

- Treatment consists of tricyclic antidepressants, usually amitriptyline, with a low dose initially (e.g. 10 mg at bedtime) followed by dose increases every few weeks until the pain disappears.
- Amitriptyline 20–40 mg at bedtime is usually a sufficient maintenance dose.
- Since response is slow to develop treatment should be continued for several months after which dose reduction could be attempted.
- If the patient does not tolerate amitriptyline (or other tricyclic antidepressants), consider gabapentin 300 mg TID, gradually increasing the dose.
- Surgical treatment (vestibulectomy) is contraindicated since the pain is neuropathic in origin.

25.40 Lower abdominal pain of gynaecological origin

Editors

Basic rule

♦ The cause of lower abdominal pain is more often intestinal (8.9) than gynaecological.

- Cyclic pain, bleeding disorders or a foul-smelling vaginal discharge suggests a gynaecological cause.

Status

- Remember abdominal palpation (consider appendicitis in differential diagnosis).
- When assessing the gynaecological status observe for the following
  - purulent cervical discharge
  - does moving the cervix produce pain
  - resistance next to the uterus.

Laboratory tests

- Pregnancy test, urine test, C-reactive protein, blood count, chlamydia and gonorrhoea (first-void urine sample).

Other investigations

- Ultrasound (26.3) (25.2)

Patients of fertile age

Infection

- Pelvic inflammatory disease (25.41)
- Acute endometritis
  - Infection after recent childbirth, spontaneous or induced abortion or the insertion of an IUD or other instrumentation.
  - Aetiological organisms are most commonly those of normal vaginal flora, aerobic or anaerobic cocci.
  - A foul-smelling discharge is an indicator of an anaerobic infection.
  - Symptoms
    - Acute illness a few days after insertion of the device or childbirth
    - Cold shivers
    - Lower abdominal pain
    - Tiredness
    - Fever, 39–40°C
    - Sometimes malaise
    - Sometimes headache or aching of the muscles
  - Signs
    - Pain on palpation in the lower abdomen around the uterus and the adnexa of the uterus. The upper abdomen is soft and painless.
    - In the pelvic examination the uterus is tender, firm and moveable.
    - Adnexa are of normal size.
  - Diagnosis
    - History of a procedure on the internal genitalia, and a typical clinical picture.
  - Treatment
    - Antibiotics (cephalosporin and quite often also metronidazole), often in hospital (25.41)
- Chlamydial infection often causes only few symptoms.

Extrauterine pregnancy

- See 26.10.
- The severity of pain and bleeding varies.
- The previous cycle may have been irregular, or there may have been extra bleeding. Amenorrhoea does not always occur.
- Should always be considered when the pregnancy test is positive but there is no ultrasonographic evidence of pregnancy inside the uterus.

Ovulation

- An acute, often unilateral pain in the middle of the cycle that usually subsides in 24 hours.

Torsion or rupture of an ovary or an ovarian cyst

- See article 25.44.
- The history may include twisting of the body, eg. bowling, belly dancing or washing the floor on the knees.
- Rupture of the corpus luteum
  - The symptoms are similar to extrauterine pregnancy yet the pregnancy test is negative.
  - There is blood in the peritoneal cavity.
  - Treatment is operative if the pain is severe.
- Rupture of an endometriosis cyst
  - The symptom is an acute and very severe irritation of the peritoneum.
  - Treatment is usually an acute operation.
- Rupture of a dermoid cyst
  - Rare
  - Very painful because the sebum causes strong irritation in the peritoneal cavity.
- Torsion of the ovary or the tube
  - The cause is usually a cyst.
  - Gynaecological investigation reveals a tender, possibly moveable mass.

Ovarian hyperstimulation syndrome (OHS)

- An excessive reaction of the ovaries to the hormones used in the treatment of infertility.
- All medicines used for the induction of ovulation, such as clomiphene, gonadotrophins, GnRH and its analogues, may cause OHS.
- The syndrome typically begins 3–10 days after the induction.
- The symptoms are abdominal pain, oedema and nausea.
- The risk is increased in women aged below 35, with low body weight and use of a GnRH analogue.

- When OHS is suspected, ultrasound (25.2) and blood count are the basic tests, and C-reactive protein is used for differential diagnosis.
- **In strong suspicion of OHS, gynaecological investigation is contraindicated** (pressing may damage the brittle ovaries).
- Refer readily to hospital or to the doctor in charge of the fertility treatment.
- OHS is severe if the patient has
  - severe nausea, diarrhoea or weight gain
  - even a mild dyspnoea
  - leucocytes over 10×10^9/l or haematocrit over 0.45
  - the size of the ovaries is over 10 cm by ultrasound.

Rupture and necrosis of a pedunculated uterine myoma

- The symptom is cyclic pain resembling childbirth.
- The myoma may grow into the vagina through the cervix.
- CRP is usually elevated.

Malignant neoplasms

- See 25.44.
- May cause acute pelvic pain when they rupture or bleed, although this is rare.
- The patient has a tender mass in the lower abdomen and often ascites.

Labour

- Sudden severe acute pelvic pain may originate from a labour without the pregnant woman or her parents knowing of the pregnancy. Sometimes the pregnant female (usually a schoolgirl) knows but her mother does not.

Perforation of the vagina

- The most common aetiologies are intercourse (the patient is often drunk) or trauma caused by a foreign body.

Young patient without menses

- See 25.14.

Structural anomalies

- The normal route for bleeding is blocked.
- Symptoms
  - The pain is preceded by milder cyclic lower abdominal pain, and sometimes cyclic retention of urine.
  - Sudden severe pelvic pain, strong peritoneal irritation
- Cause
  - The most common is an unperforated hymen.
  - Various anomalies of the uterus (e.g. a bifurcated uterus, one of part emptying into the vagina while blood collects in the other.)
- The treatment is operative.

Torsion or rupture of an ovarian cyst

- Sudden pain
- The treatment is operative

Postmenopausal women

- See 25.44.

Purulent endometritis (pyometra)

- The cause is tightness of the cervix that is often due to treatment of the cancer of the cervix (e.g. loop electrosurgical, cryo- or laser-conization).
- Symptoms
  - Begins gradually.
  - The condition becomes acute when a bloody and purulent discharge appears, and pain and fever begins.
- Treatment
  - Depends on a specialist consultation.

Malignant neoplasm of the uterus

- See 25.44.
- The symptoms are bleeding and pain.

Ovarian neoplasm

- See 25.44.
- The symptoms are abdominal pain, bleeding disorders, internal haemorrhage and urine disorders.

Chronic lower abdominal pain

Endometriosis

- See 25.42.
- Symptoms
  - Gradually worsening pains are usually felt in the premenstrual phase when cycling, sitting in the car, exacerbated by jolts.
  - Defecation and intercourse may be painful.
  - If endometriosis has grown to the surface of the bladder or bowel, symptoms occur around these areas.

Neoplasms

- See 25.44.

Chronic cervicitis

- Gives rise to indefinite pains and a whitish discharge.
- Examine for infection and venereal diseases.

Varicose veins of adnexes

- Cause indefinite pains, which get worse during the day, especially while standing.

Premenstrual tension

- See 25.11.
- Premenstrual symptoms are irritation, nausea, and aching and swelling of the abdomen.

25.41 Diagnosis and treatment of acute pelvic inflammatory disease (PID)

Klaus Teisala

Aims

- Early diagnosis and treatment reduce the late sequelae of PID:
  - Infertility
  - Ectopic pregnancy
  - Chronic abdominal pain

Epidemiology

- PID generally occurs only during the reproductive years, and its annual incidence is about 1% in fertile women.

Pathophysiology and clinical manifestations of acute PID

- PID typically begins after menstruation.
- PID is usually an ascending infection from cervicovaginal flora via the mucosal surface to the uterus, fallopian tubes and into the peritoneal cavity, causing endometritis and salpingitis.
- Perihepatitis and periappendicitis may also occur. A tubo-ovarian abscess and pelvioperitonitis are serious sequelae of acute PID.

Aetiology of acute PID

- The nature of acute PID is usually polymicrobial. The sexually transmitted microbes Chlamydia trachomatis and/or Neisseria gonorrhoeae are isolated in many cases of acute PID.
- Many other facultative and anaerobic bacteria (non-haemolytic streptococci, Escherichia coli, Haemophilus influenzae, peptococci, peptostreptococci and Bacteroides species) often occurring in normal cervicovaginal flora are found in acute PID. Mycoplasmas and possibly viruses are also associated with acute PID.
- PID is usually caused by several microbes at the same time.

Symptoms of acute PID

- Bilateral abdominal pain worsened by vibration
- Abnormal discharge
- Possibly bleeding disturbances
- Fever
- The severity of symptoms appears to vary between patients and the disease can even be asymptomatic (particularly chlamydia).

Clinical findings

- Cervical and uterine tenderness
- Adnexal swelling or mass and tenderness
- The right upper abdomen is tender in cases of perihepatitis
- Mucopurulent discharge

Laboratory investigations

- CRP (elevated)
- Urine analysis (important for differential diagnosis)
- HCG (differential diagnosis)
- Chlamydia trachomatis and Neisseria gonorrhoeae (first-void urine sample)
- Possibly also PAP smear for detecting abnormal cytology

Special investigations in hospital

- Laparoscopy
- Endometrial biopsy
- Transvaginal ultrasound

Differential diagnosis

- Appendicitis
- Ectopic pregnancy
- Ovarian cyst
- Endometriosis
- Urinary tract infection

Treatment

- IUD is removed

Antimicrobial treatment

- Inpatient treatment is started intravenously in hospital, particularly for the young and nullipara.
- Outpatient treatment is targeted primarily against chlamydia: oral doxycycline 150 mg once daily or 100 mg twice daily for at least 10 days (12.1).
- If gonorrhoea is suspected (obvious purulent discharge from the cervix), start the treatment with a single oral dose of norfloxacin 800 mg or ciprofloxacin 500 mg and continue with doxycycline (12.2).

- If the patient has bacterial vaginosis or an intrauterine device (IUD), metronidazole is combined the treatment. Metronidazole should not be used routinely in the treatment of mild PID.
- If chlamydial and gonococcal infections are excluded and the infection recurs, for example, after insertion of an IUD, start treatment with a combination of cephalexin 500 mg and metronidazole 400 mg three times daily.
- All male sexual partners should be examined and samples for chlamydia and gonorrhoea should be taken.

Treatment results

- Patients normally recover fairly quickly from the acute phase of PID. Aspiration of a possible abscess speeds recovery.
- Most problems are caused by the long-term sequelae of acute PID: lower abdomen pain, recurrences of the infection, infertility, and ectopic pregnancy.

25.42 Endometriosis

Päivi Härkki

Definition

- The presence of tissue resembling endometrium at sites outside the uterine cavity, for example on:
  - the peritoneal surfaces
  - the ovaries
  - the area between the vagina and the rectum (rectovaginal endometriosis).
- Pathogenesis remains unclear; the peritoneal tissue transforms to resemble endometrial tissue.
- The natural defence mechanisms of affected individuals are weakened making it possible for endometriosis to develop.
- Adenomyosis (which is not discussed in this article) is defined as an ectopic occurrence of endometrial tissue in the muscle layer of the uterus (myometrium).

Epidemiology

- Since endometriosis is an oestrogen-dependent condition it only affects women in their reproductive years; symptoms are rarely seen after menopause.
- Affects about 10% of women of reproductive age,
- 5% of women who have been sterilized and
- 25% of patients with fertility problems.
- Almost 50% of patients with endometriosis suffer from infertility.

Signs and symptoms

- The most common symptom is dysmenorrhoea that starts several days before the onset of menstrual bleeding.
- Dyspareunia and pain induced by shaking or vibration.
- Abnormal vaginal bleeding.
- Dysuria, pain on defecation, blood in stools.
- Infertility.
- Lower abdominal mass.
- Symptoms are usually cyclical.

Diagnosis

- Typical gynaecological findings include pain in the posterior uterine ligaments, a tender uterus during examination and in some cases, the presence of bluish endometriosis in the vagina.
- An ultrasound examination will only reveal major changes, such as ovarian endometrial cysts, i.e. endometriomas.
- Diagnosis can be verified by laparoscopy.
- If the patient has pain on urination or defecation, cystoscopy and colonoscopy are warranted.
- Pelvic MRI scan should be reserved for special cases.

Treatment

- In endometriosis, either the pain or infertility is treated; it is not possible to treat both simultaneously.
- No curative treatment exists.
- Pharmacotherapy aims to prevent the action of oestrogen on the endometrial tissue. Symptoms will return when treatment is withdrawn.
- Surgical treatment aims to remove any ectopic endometrium and to restore normal anatomy.

Treatment of pain

- Non-steroidal anti-inflammatory drugs are the first choice medication in mild cases.
- Combined oral contraceptives (3–6 packs can be used consecutively without a break, resulting in only 2–4 menstrual bleeds per year).
- A continuous administration of luteal hormones for several months will induce therapeutic amenorrhoea and provide pain relief (medroxyprogesterone acetate 10–50 mg/day or lynestrenol 5–15 mg/day).
- The popularity of synthetic steroids (danazol) has reduced, due to their androgenic adverse effects.
- A levonorgestrel-releasing uterine device or a continuous administration of progestins for several months (if the treatment is continued for longer, hormone replacement therapy with oestrogen and progestogens should be added).
- Surgical treatment aims to remove endometriosis tissue, thus leading to pain relief. Aggressive surgery may be considered in advanced disease, i.e. hysterectomy and bilateral salpingo-oophorectomy and, if necessary, bowel resection and excision of the urinary bladder.

- In some cases aromatase inhibitors, which inhibit peripheral oestrogen synthesis, may be tried after radical surgery or menopause.

Treatment of infertility

- Hormonal medication used to manage pain will prevent a woman from conceiving.
- Laparoscopy is indicated if endometriosis is suspected in a patient with fertility problems.
- Surgical resection in minimal or mild endometriosis appears to enhance fecundity.
- If infertility is prolonged, or the disease is advanced, in vitro fertilization should be considered.
- Pregnancy will lessen symptoms and, in some cases, mild symptoms may even disappear altogether.

25.43 Gynaecological hernias

Juha Mäkinen

- Urinary incontinence, see 11.4.

Basic rules

- As long as the patient is operable, protruding changes causing symptoms are to be corrected surgically.
- Permanent changes after pregnancy and childbirth can be prevented by intensive training of the muscles of the pelvic floor (especially during the postpartal recovery time, i.e. 6 months).

Definition

- Protruding changes that distend into the parturition canal and out of it; they can be called gynaecological hernias. The bottom of the abdominal cavity gives way through the pelvic floor (parturition canal or vagina) and urogenital organs are pushed out of place, even out of the parturition canal. These changes may occur as (respective organ)
    - uterine descensus (uterus)
    - cystocele (urinary bladder)
    - urethrocele (urethra)
    - rectocele (rectum)
    - enterocele (small intestine) and
    - eversion/prolapse of the vagina after a hysterectomy.
- Descent of the uterus out of the vaginal introitus is called a prolapse. Note! A prolapse of the rectum or the urethra is not pushed out of the parturition canal and thus are not gynaecological "hernias".

Grades of severity

- Gradus I: The organ slides to the outer third of the vagina at the furthest.
- Gradus II: The organ comes into sight in the external female genitalia, i.e. at the introitus level.
- Gradus III: The organ pushes clearly out of the vaginal introitus.
- Gradus IV: The organ, the uterus in particular, has completely slidden out of the vagina (total prolapse of the uterus).

Frequency

- It is estimated that every fifth gynaecological operation involves some kind of repair of gynaecological protrusions through the pelvic floor.

Aetiology

- Descensus and prolapses are associated with ageing. Most problems occur in postmenopausal women.
- The decrease in oestrogen secretion in the menopause makes the connective tissue, the mucosa, and the muscles of the pelvis weaker, and their ability to support the genital organs decreases.
- The connective tissue can be permanently damaged in a difficult childbirth (forceps, vacuum, or a very fast delivery).
- Also multiparity may overdistend the pelvic floor, as well as heavy work, chronic cough, constipation, ascites and large tumours in the pelvis.
- About 5% of prolapses are caused by congenital weakness of the connective tissue, which sometimes causes a uterus prolapse, even in quite young women who have not given birth.

Symptoms

- In the early stage
    - A feeling of a burden in the lower part of the abdomen, which grows worse towards the evening and disappears when the patient lies down.
    - The patient has low back pain and she feels a downward tension.
- If the patient often seeks for treatment when a clear distension is felt or can be noticed protruding out of the vagina. At this stage the patient usually also has other symptoms of this disorder:
    - Difficulties in sexual intercourse
    - Problems with the urinary bladder
        - increased frequency (pollakisuria and nocturia)
        - urgency
        - stress incontinence
        - a feeling of residual urine
        - a weak or prolonged urinary jet

  - difficulty in beginning and/or ending micturition
  - the patient facilitates emptying of the bladder either by hand or by changing position
  - urinary retention
- Problems with the rectum
  - compulsion in defaecation
  - pain in defaecation
  - difficulty in defaecation
  - a feeling of incomplete emptying of the rectum
  - the patient facilitates the emptying with the finger
  - soiling with faeces
  - flatus incontinence
  - incontinence of loose faeces
  - incontinence of solid faeces

Examination

- Evaluate the type and severity of the change. The urinary bladder and the rectum should be empty. The provocation (e.g. Valsalva) is performed with the patient lying down or half sitting (so that the state from which the patient suffers when she is standing up is reproduced as much as possible).
- On inspection the low perineum and a clear protrusion coming out of the introitus can be seen.
- During the examination with speculum the disappearance of the anterior fornix can be noticed as the first sign indicating a defect/weakness in the anterior wall.
- After removal of the speculum the anterior wall is supported with an elevator and the disappearance of the posterior fornix can be seen, which indicates an incipient enterocele or a distending rectocele lower down.
- The poor status of the muscles in the pelvic floor, which in general is associated with a prolapse, is tested rectovaginally when the patient contracts the muscles in question. The weak contracticity of the sphincter of the anus is also examined.
- The severity of prolapse of the uterus in particular can be confirmed when the patient strains or by pulling the cervix further down with an instrument.
- The differential diagnosis excludes prolapse-like distensions such as divertuculum of the urethra, congenital cysts of the Gartner's duct, metastases of malignant tumours or a rare intestinal hernia pushing into the area.

Treatment

Conservative treatment

- Strengthening the muscles of the pelvic floor (written instructions), assisted by the guidance of a physiotherapist, and if necessary electrostimulation of the muscles.
- An aid or instrument of suitable size and shape (ball, tube, cone) placed in the vagina can gradually increase the muscle power of the pelvic floor (the patient feels the resistance when contracting the muscles).
- In slight changes the above-mentioned treatment reduces the symptoms and the patient may even avoid operative treatment.
- The check-up after childbirth should include instruction about muscle training.
- For postmenopausal females muscle training should be initiated, as should local oestrogen treatment, continued permanently to thicken the mucosa strengthen the muscles and fascias and increase the blood flow in the urogenital area.

Surgical treatment

- Implemented if
  - the change is severe (grade III–IV)
  - the symptoms are difficult
    - pain
    - protrusion in the introitus
    - micturition disorders
    - functional disorders of the intestine/rectum
    - problems with sexual intercourse
  - there are other problems associated with the prolapse
    - ulceration of the vagina or cervix
    - repeated urinary tract infection
    - urinary retention
- The operation is traditionally performed via the vagina, but nowadays also a laparoscopic operation is possible. Promising results have been achieved, for example in laparoscopic treatment of uterus prolapse with artificial supportive material(s) or mesh(es) when uterine removal should be avoided.
- In connection with the repair of a prolapse, especially, in postmenopausal females, a vaginal hysterectomy is always recommended. If a young patient wishes to become pregnant, a so-called Manchester operation is available.
- For recurrent plastic repair of the vaginal area a mesh application is currently available.

Contraindications for surgical treatment

- The patient refuses an operation
- Pregnancy and puerperium (6 months)
- A young patient (especially radical or ablative surgery)
- Absolute contraindications for an operation (partial closure of the external female genitalia can nevertheless be performed under local anaesthesia).

First aid

- The prolapse is repositioned in order to prevent complications (e.g. urinary retention) and is kept inside vagina (with a ring or tampon) above the level of the introitus.
- If the patient uses a prolapse ring (made of vulcanized rubber), she must also use some vaginal creme containing antiseptic agent and oestrogen.
- The above-mentioned aids are used only until the operation. They are used as the actual treatment only in exceptional cases (for patients in very poor condition).

25.44 Gynaecological tumours

Pentti K. Heinonen

Principles

- Diagnose tumours of the genital organs.
- Early diagnosis and treatment of the cancer improves the prognosis of, for example, ovarian cancer significantly.
- Most benign and all malignant tumours and their precancerous forms need the attention of a specialist.
- Do not treat the patient's symptoms. Always perform a pelvic examination on all patients including elderly women (or refer the patient to a centre where a pelvic examination can be done).

Tumours of the uterine cervix

Symptoms and diagnosis

- The symptoms are increasing vaginal or bloody discharge, and postcoital spotting. Specific symptoms cannot always be found, but changes will be seen by routine examination.
- Vaginal cytology (Pap smear) (25.1) is the most important examination.
- Further examinations are colposcopy and biopsies and/or endocervical curettage.

Benign changes of the uterine cervix

- A **Nabothian cyst** is caused by occlusion of the lumina of glands in the mucosa of the uterine cervix. A large cyst can be opened with, for example, the top of a ball forceps.
- The symptom of a **cervical polyp** is bloody discharge, often postcoital. The size of polyps varies from a few millimeters to 2 cm. Stalked polyps originate in the endocervix. A polyp can be removed by avulsion with uterine packing forceps. Cervical polyps are mainly benign, but it is wise to submit the removed tissue for microscopic examination. Polyps often recur. In cases of recurrence endocervical curettage can be useful.
- **Condyloma** associated with the human papillomavirus (HPV) infection of the uterine cervix can be either an outward growing tumour or a so-called flat condyloma, found in cytological smear of the cervix (12.4).
  - If cytological smear suggests condyloma a follow-up can be scheduled e.g. at 6 months.
  - Exophytically growing condylomas can be operated on.
  - About half are cured spontaneously within 6 months.
  - The diagnosis of cell changes that need colposcopy is based on the histological finding: the premalignant stages are classed as mild dysplasia (CIN I) (CIN = cervical intra-epithelial neoplasia), moderate dysplasia (CIN II) and severe dysplasia and carcinoma in situ (CIN III) (25.1).
  - If there are dysplastic changes in the uterine cervix, the treatment is vaporization with a laser or conization of the cervix by laser or electrical loop. Follow-up usually takes place in the gynaecology outpatient clinic every 6 months for 1–2 years after which the Pap smears can be taken once a year in primary health care.

Carcinoma of the uterine cervix

- Mass screening (Pap test) and effective treatment of precancerous states have lowered the incidence. Cervical cancer is common in many developing countries and causes mortality.
- Remember that cervical carcinoma also affects young women (30–35 years).

Symptoms and diagnosis

- Bloody or malodorous vaginal discharge or postcoital spotting. Most patients have no symptoms.
- Detected mainly by a Pap test. The extent and depth of invasion are determined by biopsy, conization, curettage and radiological, MRI and ultrasound examinations.
- Most cases are squamous cell carcinomas, but about 20–25% are adenocarcinomas that are not detected by a Pap test as well as the squamous cell carcinomas.
- If there is discrepancy between the clinical status and the Pap test a biopsy must be taken.

Treatment

- Depends on the extent and depth of invasion, as determined by radiological, MRI and ultrasound examinations.
- In cases of microinvasive carcinoma, hysterectomy is often sufficient.
- Invasive carcinomas and tumours limited to the uterus are treated by preoperative intra-uterine radiation therapy, radical hysterectomy, Wertheim's operation and, if necessary, by postoperative external radiation therapy to the pelvis minor and sometimes also to the para-aortic region **B** [1 2] or by combination radiation therapy.
- More severe cases are treated only by radiotherapy **A** [3 4], sometimes together with cytotoxic medication **A** [5]. In some cases, a simple hysterectomy may be performed after radiotherapy.

Follow-up

- Mainly in the gynaecology outpatient clinic for 3–5 years, after that once a year in primary health care.
- Pap test, colposcopy, and, when necessary, blood tests and radiological examinations (chest radiograph every 1 or 2 years)

Prognosis

- The 5-year survival rate for patients with cancer limited to the uterus (Stage I) is 90%, 65% for those with Stage II and 35% for those with Stage III.

Tumours of the uterine corpus

Symptoms

- Abnormal bleeding is the most common symptom. In 10–15% of patients the cause of postmenopausal bleeding is carcinoma of the endometrium.

Diagnosis

- Endometrial biopsy or a cytological test (25.1) are taken before the treatment. Vaginal ultrasonography is useful: the thickness of the endometrium can be determined and possible polyps and myomas found (25.2). After menopause, an endometrium thickness of under 5 mm is rarely malignant, but over 10 mm is abnormal and calls for a biopsy. In malignancies, ultrasound findings show an uneven endometrium with an average thickness of 15 mm. In women of reproductive age an endometrium thickness of over 18 mm is abnormal and calls for further investigations (biopsy/curettage).
- The cause of postmenopausal bleeding must always be established before treatment. In this case a normal Pap test result does not exclude carcinoma of the endometrium.

Clinical status

- An enlarged tumourous uterus usually suggests myomas.

Benign tumours

- An endometrial polyp can cause prolonged, heavy menstrual bleeding or spotting. Polyps can be seen by ultrasound or found by biopsy of the endometrium. They are treated in hysteroscopy by extraction or curettage. Polyps are rarely malignant (1%), but concomitant endometrial hyperplasia is more common (10%).

Endometrial hyperplasia

- The cause is an excessive effect of oestrogen or deficient or short-lived action of progesterone. It usually occurs in premenopause, when there is an increase in the number of anovulatory cycles.
- The diagnosis is made by endometrial biopsy or curettage:
  - Cystic hyperplasia of the endometrium (hyperplasia simplex) is the most common (risk of cancer is 2–3%).
  - In the premenopause, the treatment consists of cyclic progestin (e.g. medroxyprogesterone acetate 10 mg on the days 14–25 day of the cycle), as long as the patient has bleedings. If the bleeding is profuse and difficult, hysterectomy is considered.
- Adenomatous hyperplasia (hyperplasia complex) is a more severe condition. 20–30% of untreated patients develop cancer. The treatment is hysterectomy in peri- and postmenopausal women, and continuous high-dose progestational therapy (e.g. MPA 100 mg/day) and control endometrial biopsy in fertile-aged women.
- Atypical hyperplasia is even a more severe condition. Without treatment 50% will develop carcinoma of the endometrium within 5 years. The treatment is hysterectomy in most cases.

Myoma of the uterus

- Every third woman in fertile age has a myoma.
- Most are benign; about 0.1% are leiomyosarcomas.
- Myoma is the most common indication for hysterectomy.
- The size of myomas varies greatly.
- Submucous myomas, which are under the mucous membrane of the uterus, cause heavy bleeding followed by anaemia.
- Detected by pelvic examination and verified by ultrasound.
- Note: It can be difficult to differentiate between a myoma and an ovarian tumour.
- Treatment
  - Hysterectomy when there are many myomas in the uterus and the patient is not planning a pregnancy.
  - Enucleation of the myomas if the uterus is spared.
  - Submucous myomas can be removed in hysteroscopy.

Carcinoma of the endometrium

- Most often an adenocarcinoma of the endometrium.
- The usual symptom is irregular bleeding.
- The risk increases with obesity, diabetes, high blood pressure, anovulatory cycles, late menopause, nulliparity and family history.
- The median age at diagnosis is 65 years.

Diagnosis

- Diagnosis as in tumours of the fundus uteri
- Regular endometrial biopsy enables early detection.
- The extent of the disease is preoperatively determined by curettage, hysteroscopy, and ultrasound and MRI examinations.
- Staging according a surgical-pathological staging system (FIGO)

Treatment

- The most usual treatment is total hysterectomy and bilateral salpingo-oophorectomy (the disease is most often restricted to the uterus). The pelvic and sometimes also the para-aortic lymph nodes are removed as well.
- If the cancer is superficial and well differentiated, the patient may be given postoperative vaginal radiotherapy (A) [6 7].
- If the cancer is more extensive and/or poorly differentiated, the patient is given external radiotherapy to the pelvis minor, and in selected cases medication (cytotoxic or hormonal).

Follow-up

- Follow-up at the gynaecology outpatient clinic for 3–5 years and thereafter yearly in primary health care.

- Clinical examination, Pap test, chest x-ray and ultrasound.
- Usually recidivation is found in the vagina.

Prognosis

- Two-thirds of the patients have grade I cancer, for which the 5-year survival rate is over 80%.

Tumours of the ovary

- Ovarian tumours are common in all age groups. 85% are benign.
- Most of the malignant tumours occur in postmenopausal women.
- At childbearing age functional ovarian tumours are common, but in women over 50 years old almost half are malignant.

Symptoms

- Most ovarian tumours cause no symptoms and are discovered during clinical examination.
- Hormonally active tumours can cause menstrual disturbances.
- Large tumours can cause pressure, abdominal swelling and increased urinary frequency.

Diagnosis

- Pelvic examination is important. Use ultrasound if possible.
- All ovarian tumours must be removed, because cancer can be determined only by histological examination of the removed tumour.
- As a complementary investigation a tumour marker, e.g. CA 125, can be used, although it is not specific because, for example, both endometriosis and infections raise the value.
- Early diagnosis of ovarian cancer is especially important and improves the prognosis. Three out of four ovarian cancers are first discovered when the cancer has spread into the abdominal cavity.
- An ovarian tumour in a postmenopausal woman is most likely a cancer.

Pathology

- The origin and the structure of ovarian tumours vary, but most are epithelial. Tumours can be benign, malignant or so-called borderline tumours.
- Some are hormonally active.

Benign ovarian tumours

- Epithelial tumours (serous, mucinous) are the most common (80%).
- During the menstrual years functional ovarian cysts are very common: follicle cysts and corpus luteum cysts. (If unilocular and smaller than 5 cm, they will disappear spontaneously.)
- Some cysts (e.g. corpus luteum cysts) rupture, cause heavy bleeding, and require immediate surgery (25.40).
- Torsion-causing tissue ischaemia can occur, and also requires an operation.
- Other cysts are parovarian cysts and dermoid cysts, which are treated surgically, mostly by laparoscopy.
- If a round cyst, smaller than 5 cm in diameter, is found in a premenopausal woman by ultrasound, and there is no papillar structure or septum, follow up after 2–4 months that the cyst has disappeared. All other cysts require specialist attention.

Ovarian cancer

- The peak incidence is at the age of 65 years.

Symptoms

- In most cases there are no symptoms and the disease is first diagnosed when it has spread into the abdominal cavity.
- About half of the patients have abdominal swelling and sense of pressure. Ascites develops readily.

Diagnosis

- See ovarian tumours above. Investigate by ultrasound: if the tumour is multilocular and/or partly solid, and/or there are papillar structures, promptly refer the patient for further investigations.
- Remember that malignant ovarian tumour is more common in a postmenopausal woman.

Treatment

- Generally surgical **B** [8 9]. The aim is to remove, as far as possible, the cancer tissue from the abdominal cavity. Hysterectomy, resection of the omentum and removal of all visible lymph nodes, possibly also the para-aortic lymph nodes.
- Further treatment consists of chemotherapy and in a minority of cases, radiotherapy **B** [8 9]. Paclitaxel/carboplatin regimen has become the standard postoperative treatment for patients with advanced ovarian cancer. Platinum-based chemotherapy is probably more effective than non-platinum therapy **B** [10]. Further cytoreductive surgery may be necessary **C** [11 12] as well as neoadjuvant chemotherapy.

Follow-up

- In the gynaecology outpatient clinic for 3 years after completing the treatment, then in primary health care: clinical status, an irrigation specimen from the abdominal cavity, ultrasound and radiological examinations, and tumour markers.

Prognosis

- It is important to remember that 80% of patients whose cancer is limited to the ovaries survive. However, most cases are found in the extended stage, with a 5-year survival rate of 30% and for stage IV disease under 10%.

GYN

Tumours of the vulva and the vagina

- Benign tumours are the most common.
- Condyloma is common in young women.
- Carcinoma of the vulva is a disease of the elderly.

Symptoms

- Some patients do not have any specific symptoms.
- Some have vulvar irritation, or pruritus in the genitals.

Diagnosis

- Pap test and, when necessary, biopsy.

Benign tumours

- **Condyloma** is the most common tumour of the external female genitalia and vagina (12.4). Some of the condylomas are exophytic, but a flat condyloma is most often invisible to the naked eye.
- Single condylomas are treated with podophyllotoxin or imiquimode cream. The use of this treatment is restricted to condylomas on external genitalia. It is not to be used during pregnancy.
- Single condylomas can be removed with scissors or by freezing.
- Recurrent tumours and large lesions require specialist treatment (CO_2 laser or freezing).
- If there are **precancerous changes** in lesions of the external genitals (vulvar intraepithelial neoplasia, VIN), the patient must be referred to a specialist.
- Further investigations are usually colposcopy and biopsy.
- Epithelial changes in the skin include **haemangiomas**, **naevi** and **cysts**.
- A cystic swelling of the vaginal wall is **Gardner's cyst**, which can be punctured or opened with a knife.
- A cyst can develop into the duct of the Bartholin's gland (25.31).
- Sometimes **endometriosis** can be seen in the vagina.
- **Lichen sclerosus** is associated with the thinning of the skin and easily causes pruritus and irritation.
  - There are light areas on the external genitals, often with small wounds. The diagnosis is made by biopsy.
  - The condition is not curable. Treatment possibilities include cortisone ointments, vitamin A and an operation.
  - Some lesions can become malignant.

Cancer of the vagina

- Extremely rare (adenocarcinoma or melanoma).

Cancer of the vulva

- Rare
- More than 80% of cases are found in women over 65 years of age (the peak incidence is at 75 years).

Symptoms

- Irritation and pruritus of the external genitals, sometimes a bloody discharge.
- Note that carcinoma of the vulva develops more frequently in women who have had lichen sclerosus in their external genitalia.
- Important: Never treat irritation and pruritus of the external genitals in an elderly person without first examining the patient.

Diagnosis

- Verified by biopsy.

Treatment

- Radical surgery C [13]. Further treatment can consist of radiotherapy or chemotherapy.

Follow-up

- In the gynaecology outpatient clinic for 3–5 years, after that in primary health care.

Prognosis

- The 5-year survival rate is 50%, or 70% if the cancer was localized.

Carcinoma of the fallopian tube

- Gives no specific symptoms and is usually first found by laparotomy.
- Treatment as in ovarian cancer.

Gestational trophoblastic diseases

- In a hydatidiform mole the villi of the placenta transform into moles and the entire placenta consists of tissue comprised of liquid-filled moles. Usually there is no embryo.
- The aetiology is unknown.

Classification

- Complete and partial hydatidiform mole (molar pregnancy)
- Invasive mole
- Choriocarcinoma (carcinoma of the placenta)

Frequency

- The incidence of molar pregnancy is 1/1000 pregnancies.
- It is preceded by a molar pregnancy, abortion or extrauterine pregnancy, but it can also occur after normal delivery.

Symptoms

- Uterine bleeding early in the pregnancy
- Excessive nausea and vomiting

Diagnosis

- The uterus is larger than expected in a normal pregnancy of the same duration and softer than usual.
- By ultrasound the inside of the uterus resembles snowfall and there is no foetus.
- The serum hCG value is very high.

Treatment and follow-up

- Molar pregnancy: empty the uterus effectively. Weekly follow-up of the serum hCG value until it is no longer detectable (usually two months). If the hCG value rises again, further investigations are needed (relapse or invasive mole).
- Pregnancy should be avoided for a year. Prescribe an oral contraceptive (combination pills) for birth control.
- An earlier molar pregnancy increases the risk of a new molar pregnancy by 20-fold. Ultrasound to confirm a normal pregnancy.
- Invasive mole and choriocarcinoma are treated with chemotherapy.
- Metastases can develop in the vagina, lungs, liver and brain.

Prognosis

- The 5-year survival rate is 80–100%.
- Liver and brain metastases worsen the prognosis.

References

1. The Swedish Council on Technology Assessment in Health Care. Cervical cancer (cervix uteri). Acta Oncologica 1996;2 (suppl 7):57–80.
2. The Database of Abstracts of Reviews of Effectiveness (University of York), Database no.: DARE-978129. In: The Cochrane Library, Issue 4, 1999. Oxford: Update Software.
3. Shueng PW, Hsu WL, Jen YM, Wu CJ, Liu HS. Neoadjuvant chemotherapy followed by radiotherapy should not be a standard approach for locally advanced cervical cancer. International Journal of Radiation Oncology, Biology, Physics 1998;40:889–896.
4. The Database of Abstracts of Reviews of Effectiveness (University of York), Database no.: DARE-980606. In: The Cochrane Library, Issue 1, 2000. Oxford: Update Software.
5. Green J, Kirwan J, Tierney J, Symonds P, Fresco L, Williams C, Collingwood M. Concomitant chemotherapy and radiation therapy for cancer of the uterine cervix. Cochrane Database Syst Rev. 2004;(2):CD002225.
6. The Swedish Council on Technology Assessment in Health Care. Uterine cancer (corpus uteri). Acta Oncologica 1996; 2(suppl 7):pp. 81–85.
7. The Database of Abstracts of Reviews of Effectiveness (University of York), Database no.: DARE-978130. In: The Cochrane Library, Issue 4, 1999. Oxford: Update Software.
8. The Swedish Council on Technology Assessment in Health Cae. Ovarian cancer. Acta Oncologica 1996;2(suppl 7): 86–92.
9. The Database of Abstracts of Reviews of Effectiveness (University of York), Database no.: DARE-978131. In: The Cochrane Library, Issue 4, 1999. Oxford: Update Software.
10. Advanced Ovarian Cancer Trialists Group. Chemotherapy for advanced ovarian cancer. Cochrane Database Syst Rev. 2004;(2):CD001418.
11. Bristow RE, Lagasse LD, Karlan BY. Secondary surgical cytoreduction for advanced epithelial ovarian cancer: patient selection and review of the literature. Cancer 1996;78:2049–2062.
12. The Database of Abstracts of Reviews of Effectiveness (University of York), Database no.: DARE-961861. In: The Cochrane Library, Issue 4, 1999. Oxford: Update Software.
13. Ansink A, van der Velden J, Collingwood M. Surgical interventions for early squamous cell carcinoma of the vulva. Cochrane Database Syst Rev. 2004;(2):CD002036.

25.50 Menopausal complaints

Aila Tiitinen

Definitions

- **Climacterium** is the entire period during which the function of the ovaries diminishes (ovulation and oestrogen production) and finally ceases totally.
- Menopause means cessation of menstrual bleedings in the menopause age.
- Perimenopause covers the time preceding menopause and one year after it.
- **Menopause** appears on average at the age of 51 years (range 45–55 years).
- The criterion for menopause is amenorrhoea lasting more than one year.
- About 75% of menopausal women suffer from symptoms affecting the autonomous nervous system, such as hot flushes and nocturnal sweating, but not all women seek help from a doctor.

Aetiology

- With the decrease in the number of ovarian follicles the production of oestrogen ceases almost totally in menopause. At the same time the secretion of luteinizing hormone (LH) and follicle stimulating hormone (FSH) increases.
- Low levels of oestrogens and the activation of the hypothalamus may cause climacteric symptoms in premenopause years before cessation of menstrual bleedings.

Physiological changes

- The vaginal epithelium becomes atrophic, i.e. thin and dry. Vaginal pH rises and Pap smear shows parabasal cells and lymphocytes.
- The changes in the urethral mucosa cause dysuria and pollacisuria.
- Some women may experience urge incontinence due to atrophy of the epithelium of the trigonum.
- The skin loses its elasticity; wrinkling of the skin occurs due to reduction of collagen content.
- The size of the breasts diminishes and their shape alters.
- With the decline in oestrogen, age-related osteoporosis progresses more rapidly. The prevalence of ischaemic cardiovascular diseases also increases after the menopause and in fertile-aged women who have undergone ovarectomy.

Symptoms

- As a rule the symptoms affecting the autonomous nervous system persist for 2 to 5 years, in some patients up to 10–20 years.
- Hot flushes and night sweats
  - The most common climacteric complaints. Palpitation is sometimes associated with these symptoms.
  - Experience of climacteric complaints varies between women. Women whose oestrogen secretion ceases abruptly, as after ovariectomy, have the most severe symptoms.
  - Hot flushes occurring by day are experienced as socially unpleasant. However, night sweats may affect the quality of life even more by causing frequent interruptions of sleep.
- Sleep disorders
  - Insomnia is associated with night sweats. However, the quality of sleep can deteriorate also without this symptom.
- Psychological symptoms
  - Tiredness, irritability, changes in mood, depression, lack of initiative and self-esteem are common features associated with climacterium. It is important to distinguish depression from climacteric melancholy.
  - The correlation of the symptoms with oestrogen deficiency is not established.
- Sexual changes
  - Loss of sexual interest may occur.
  - Pain on intercourse may occur as the result of thinning of vaginal mucosa.
- Gynaecological symptoms
  - In premenopause, bleedings may be profuse or scanty and irregular.
  - In postmenopause, the symptoms are mainly related to the thinning of vaginal mucosa and weakening of pelvic floor tissues.
- Urogenital symptoms
  - Urethral syndrome includes pollakiuria and dysuria without infection.
  - Recurrence of urinary tract infections may occur.
  - Trigonitis can cause urge incontinence.
- Skeletal symptoms
  - Joint pains and tenderness, and muscle aches
  - Remember rheumatoid arthritis in the differential diagnosis.

Treatment

- See postmenopausal hormone replacement therapy 25.51.

25.51 Postmenopausal hormone replacement therapy

Aila Tiitinen

Principles

- Tell the patient the basic facts, the advantages and disadvantages of the treatment as well as the health benefits and risks of long-term use. The final decision about starting the treatment should be left to the patient.
- The younger the patient is at the onset of menopause, the more readily the treatment should be started.
- Add progestogen to the oestrogen therapy for women with an intact uterus.
- The only indication for postmenopausal hormone replacement therapy (HRT) is the treatment of menopausal symptoms – not disease prevention.

Indications of HRT

- Menopausal symptoms (hot flushes, urogenital disorders)
- Osteoporosis prophylaxis only in patients who have concomitant menopausal symptoms requiring treatment. In other patients bisphosphonates may be a better option.

Initiation of treatment

- Oestrogen therapy should not be introduced too early, preferably not until the menstrual cycles are infrequent, or have ceased, and the patient has clear menopausal symptoms.
- In unclear cases a progestogen challenge test (e.g. medroxyprogesterone acetate MPA, 10 mg daily for ten days) should be carried out. If the patient has withdrawal bleeding (which normally occurs within a week after discontinuing therapy)

cyclical progestogen treatment should be continued between days 15 and 25 of the cycle as long as regular uterine bleedings continue.

- In women without a uterus the serum level of follicle-stimulating hormone (FSH) can be measured. Values above 30 IU/l signify oestrogen deficiency.
- Absence of bleeding or very scant bleedings mean deprivation of endogenous oestrogen production and oestrogen can be added to the treatment.
- In amenorrhoeic women below the age of 45 other causes of amenorrhoea than the menopause should be considered. Following tests are useful in differential diagnosis: serum prolactin, TSH, FSH, and progestogen challenge test. Determination of serum oestradiol level alone is not valuable.

Clinical investigations

- Before starting treatment
  - A gynaecological and breast examination
  - Pap smear (25.1) and mammography (previous results from the last two years are acceptable)
  - blood pressure and weight
  - assessment of possible contraindications (remember family history).

Contraindications for HRT

- Breast cancer. Caution should be exercised when initiating hormone replacement therapy in women who have survived breast cancer. The results of a recent randomised study (HABITS) show that oestrogen treatment of two years duration significantly increased the risk of recurrence of breast cancer **B** [1].
- Endometrial carcinoma (not absolute, evaluation by a gynaecologist is needed)
- Difficulty to manage heart disease
- Severe liver disease
- History of deep vein thrombosis, pulmonary embolism **C** [2 3 4 5 6 7] or known coagulation disturbance (not absolute).
- Treatment-resistant hypertension (antihypertensive medication as such is not a contraindication).
- Systemic lupus erythematosus (SLE) when blood antiphospholipid antibodies are present (risk of thrombosis). However, SLE patients need osteoporosis prophylaxis because of corticosteroid treatment (specialist consultation).
- Undiagnosed vaginal bleeding

Principles of treatment

- Treatment is started with a cyclical combined oestrogen/progestogen preparation **A** [8 9] or with oestrogen, which is given continuously and progestogen is added for the first 12–14 days of each calendar month.
- If the woman wants to avoid uterine bleeding, continuous combined regimens may be used where both oestrogen and progestogen are given daily. However, it is recommended that this treatment form is not prescribed until 12 months after the menopause, when cyclic therapy has reduced uterine bleeding. It may also be prescribed for osteoporosis prophylaxis at a later age.
  - The therapy is started with a low dose of oestrogen, e.g. estradiol 1 mg, or a 25 μg patch, combined with a low oral dose of progestogen or a progestogen-releasing intrauterine device. The doses can be tailored at a later stage according to response or adverse effects.
- Tibolone may be used as a bleeding-free treatment form (not within 12 months of last menstrual period).
- In hysterectomized women oestrogen only is used.

The choice of treatment regimen and mode of administration

Oestrogens

- Estradiol is the most commonly used oestrogen, and is administered orally or via a patch or gel. Mode of administration should be decided according to the convenience of use.
- Tablet form may be preferred for a patient with unfavourable lipid profile, whereas for patients with a family history of coagulation disorders administration via a patch or gel may be more suitable. The latter modes of administration are also suitable for patients with migraine and those taking antiepileptic agents.
- The lowest effective dose to treat menopausal symptoms should be prescribed. Follow-up according to clinical response; oestrogen measurements are usually of no benefit.
- If treating urogenital symptoms alone, topical treatment with oestrogen creams or pessaries is the best choice **A** [10 11 12]. For elderly patients who are unable to administer topical treatment themselves an oestrogen-releasing vaginal ring can be inserted. Topical estriol treatment does not need to be combined with cyclical progestogen. The cause of any uterine bleeding must be identified.

GYN

Progestogens

- The modes of administration of progestogens are oral, transdermal (combined with oestrogen) and topical hormone-releasing IUD).
- The subjective adverse effects of different progestogens may vary.
- The 19-norprogestogens have a stronger antiproliferative effect on the endometrium than the natural progesterone or dydrogesterone and 17-alpha-hydroxyprogesterone derivatives. They are therefore effective in bleeding disorders (menorrhagia) but should be used in higher daily doses (5–10 mg of norethisterone daily for 12 days per cycle).

Adverse effects of HRT

- During the first few months of HRT, adverse effects, such as bloating and breast tenderness, are common.

- Progestogenic adverse effects include headache and psychogenic symptoms. There is no evidence that HRT causes weight gain A [13].
- If adverse effects are severe or persist for more than 3 months the dose should be reduced.
- The ways to reduce progestogenic adverse effects include the use of the lowest effective dose and the change of the mode of administration to a transdermal patch or intrauterine system.

Uterine bleeding

- The aim is for the bleeding to occur during the treatment-free week, or after the end of the progestogen phase in cyclical treatment. The amount and duration of bleeding should be normal. During treatment of several years duration, the amount of bleeding will diminish in many women, or cease altogether.
- With bleeding-free regimens the bleeding should cease totally within 4–6 months from the start of the therapy.
- The cause of irregular bleeding always has to be investigated (Pap smear, ultrasonography (25.1), endometrial biopsy (25.2)).
- Transvaginal ultrasonography is very sensitive in detecting endometrial hyperplasia, submucous myomas and polyps.
- Endometrial biopsy is easy to obtain during a general appointment, curettings are rarely needed.

Follow-up of the treatment

- A follow-up visit is recommended within 12 months of starting HRT.
- During the first year attention should be paid to the disappearance or persistence of the symptoms, occurrence of any adverse effects and to the patient's satisfaction with the treatment.
- During annual follow-up visit blood pressure should be recorded and a gynaecological and breast examination carried out.
- Mammography and a Pap smear are recommended at 2-year intervals (remember the timing of screening programmes).

Advantages and disadvantages of HRT

- The benefits of HRT in the treatment of menopausal symptoms are well established.
- HRT clearly reduces the atrophy and inflammation of the urogenital region.
- Oestrogen treatment prevents the development of menopause-related osteoporosis and osteoporotic fractures.
- Oestrogens have both direct and indirect (lipids) effects on the vascular system. Epidemiological studies have suggested a decreased risk of myocardial infarction during the use of HRT. However, during a controlled study (the HERS study), in which the combination of oestrogen and progestogen was used for secondary prevention of CHD, the number of cardiovascular events in the treatment group increased during the first twelve months, but decreased towards the end of the follow-up period B [14]. The results of another randomized controlled study showed that HRT does not reduce the recurrence of stroke in women who have suffered a previous stroke or transient ischaemic attack.
- During the WHI study, combination HRT started on average at the age of 63 years increased the risk of coronary heart disease, stroke, pulmonary embolism, and breast cancer, but reduced the incidence of osteoporosis A [15].
- HRT may be beneficial for the treatment of menopausal depressed mood C [16 17], but it does not improve cognitive function in asymptomatic women C [18 19 20].
- Both oestrogen and oestrogen/progestogen therapies are associated with an increased risk of venous thromboembolism C [2 3 4 5 6 7]. The extra risk is calculated to be 1 per 10 000 oestrogen users and the risk of death from pulmonary emboli is calculated to be 1 per 100 000. The risk of thromboemboli appears to be greatest at the start of treatment. Family history and previous thromboembolic episodes, severe obesity and immobilization should be taken into consideration when planning the introduction of HRT. The absolute risk (attributable risk) is, however, small (3.2×10^{-4} women years).
- The disadvantages of HRT are the occurrence of hormonal adverse effects and bleeding, and the mildly increased risk of breast cancer.
    - According to meta-analyses, the relative risk of breast cancer is 1.35 in women who have used HRT for at least 5 years D [21 22 23 24]. Between 50 and 65 years of age the cumulative incidence of breast cancer is 45 per 1000 women who have never used HRT. Use of HRT for ten years causes an excess risk (attributable risk) of six cases per 1000 women (confidence interval, 3–9). According to the WHI study, the risk of breast cancer may not be increased in hysterectomized patients using oestrogen alone B [25].
- According to epidemiological studies, prolonged use (>10 years) of oestrogen therapy may be associated with an increased risk of developing ovarian cancer C [26 27 28 29]. The risk has not been noted to be elevated when progestogen has been added to the treatment.
- The risk of endometrial cancer is not increased if adequate progestogen is added to the treatment C [30 31 32 33].
- The combination of oestrogen and progestogen reduces the risk of colon cancer A [15], but the cancers of HRT users may be more advanced which offsets the benefit.
- Postmenopausal HRT is associated with a 1.8-fold increase in the risk of cholecystitis.

References

1. Holmberg L, Anderson H, for the HABITS steering and data monitoring committees. HABITS (hormonal replacement therapy after breast cancer – is it safe?), a randomised comparison: trial stopped. Lancet 2004;363:453–455.

2. Douketis JD, Ginsberg JS, Holbrook A, Crowther M, Duku EK, Burrows RF. A reevaluation of the risk for venous thromboembolism with the use of oral contraceptives and hormone replacement therapy. Arch Intern Med 1997;157:1522–1530.
3. The Database of Abstracts of Reviews of Effectiveness (University of York), Database no.: DARE-978272. In: The Cochrane Library, Issue 4, 1999. Oxford: Update Software.
4. Oger E, Scarabin PY. Assessment of the risk for venous thromboembolism among users of hormone replacement therapy. Drugs and Aging 1999;14:55–61.
5. The Database of Abstracts of Reviews of Effectiveness (University of York), Database no.: DARE-990307. In: The Cochrane Library, Issue 1, 2001. Oxford: Update Software.
6. Miller J, Chan BKS, Nelson H. Hormone replacement therapy and risk of venous thromboembolism. Rockville, MD: Agency for Healthcare Research and Quality (AHRQ). 2002. 54. Agency for Healthcare Research and Quality (AHRQ). www.ahrq.gov.
7. Health Technology Assessment Database: HTA-20031088. The Cochrane Library, Issue 1, 2004. Chichester, UK: John Wiley & Sons, Ltd.
8. Udoff L, Langenberg P, Adashi EY. Combined continuous hormone replacement therapy. Obst Gynecol 1995;86:306–316.
9. The Database of Abstracts of Reviews of Effectiveness (University of York), Database no.: DARE-952043. In: The Cochrane Library, Issue 4, 1999. Oxford: Update Software.
10. Cardozo L, Bachmann G, McClish D, Fonda D. Meta-analysis of estrogen therapy in the management of urogenital atrophy in postmenopausal women: second report of the hormones and urogenital therapy committee. Obstetrics and Gynecology 1998;92:722–727.
11. The Database of Abstracts of Reviews of Effectiveness (University of York), Database no.: DARE-981730. In: The Cochrane Library, Issue 3, 2000. Oxford: Update Software.
12. Suckling J, Lethaby A, Kennedy R. Local oestrogen for vaginal atrophy in postmenopausal women. Cochrane Database Syst Rev 2003(4):CD001500.
13. Norman RJ, Flight IHK, Rees MCP. Oestrogen and progestogen hormone replacement therapy for peri-menopausal and post-menopausal women: weight and body fat distribution. Cochrane Database Syst Rev. 2004;(2):CD001018.
14. Hulley S, Grady D, Bush T, Furberg C, Herrington D, Riggs B, Vittinghoff E. Randomized trial of estrogen plus progestin for secondary prevention of coronary disease in postmenopausal women. Heart and Estrogen/progestin Replacement Study (HERS) Research Group. JAMA 1998;280:605–613.
15. Writing Group for the Women's Health Initiative Investigators. Risks and benefits of estrogen plus progestin in healthy postmenopausal women. Principal results from the Women's Health Initiative Randomized controlled trial. JAMA 2002;288:321–333.
16. Zweifel JE, O'Brien WH. The effect of hormone replacement therapy upon depressed mood. Psychoendocrinology 1997;22:189–212.
17. The Database of Abstracts of Reviews of Effectiveness (University of York), Database no.: DARE-973496. In: The Cochrane Library, Issue 1, 2000. Oxford: Update Software.
18. Hogervorst E, Yaffe K, Richards M, Huppert F. Hormone replacement therapy for cognitive function in postmenopausal women. Cochrane Database Syst Rev. 2004;(2):CD003122.
19. Leblanc E, Chan B, Nelson H D. Hormone replacement therapy and cognition. Rockville, MD: Agency for Healthcare Research and Quality (AHRQ). 2002. 49. Agency for Healthcare Research and Quality (AHRQ). www.ahrq.gov.
20. Health Technology Assessment Database: HTA-20031090. The Cochrane Library, Issue 1, 2004. Chichester, UK: John Wiley & Sons, Ltd.
21. Haskell SG, Richardson ED, Horwitz RI. The effect of estrogen replacement therapy on cognitive function in women: a critical review of the literature. J Clin Epidemiol 1997;50: 1249–1264.
22. The Database of Abstracts of Reviews of Effectiveness (University of York), Database no.: DARE-971511. In: The Cochrane Library, Issue 4, 1999. Oxford: Update Software.
23. Yaffe K, Sawaya G, Lieberburg I, Grady D. Estrogen therapy in postmenopausal women: effects on cognitive function and dementia. JAMA 1998;279:688–695.
24. The Database of Abstracts of Reviews of Effectiveness (University of York), Database no.: DARE-988294. In: The Cochrane Library, Issue 2, 2000. Oxford: Update Software.
25. Anderson GL, Limacher M, Assaf AR, Bassford T, Beresford SA, Black H, Bonds D, Brunner R, Brzyski R, Caan B, Chlebowski R, Curb D, Gass M, Hays J, Heiss G, Hendrix S, Howard BV, Hsia J, Hubbell A, Jackson R, Johnson KC, Judd H, Kotchen JM, Kuller L, LaCroix AZ, Lane D, Langer RD, Lasser N, Lewis CE, Manson J, Margolis K, Ockene J, O'Sullivan MJ, Phillips L, Prentice RL, Ritenbaugh C, Robbins J, Rossouw JE, Sarto G, Stefanick ML, Van Horn L, Wactawski-Wende J, Wallace R, Wassertheil-Smoller S,. Effects of conjugated equine estrogen in postmenopausal women with hysterectomy: the Women's Health Initiative randomized controlled trial. JAMA 2004;291(14):1701–12.
26. Garg PP, Kerlikowske K, Subak L, Grady D. Hormone replacement therapy and the risk of epithelial ovarian carcinoma: a meta-analysis. Obstetrics and Gynecology 1998;92:472–479.
27. The Database of Abstracts of Reviews of Effectiveness (University of York), Database no.: DARE-981528. In: The Cochrane Library, Issue 1, 2001. Oxford: Update Software.
28. Lacey JV, Mink PJ, Lubin JH, Sherman ME, Troisi R, Hartge P, Schatzkin A, Schairer C. Menopausal hormone replacement therapy and risk of ovarian cancer. JAMA 2002;288: 334–341.
29. Anderson GI, Judd HI, Kaunitz AM, Barad DH, Beresford SAA, Pettinger M, Liu J, McNeeley SG, Lopez AM. Effect of estrogen plus progestin on gynecologic cancers and associated diagnostic procedures. JAMA 2003;290:1739–1748.
30. Grady D, Gebretsadik T, Kerlikowske K, Ernster V, Petitti D. Hormone replacement therapy and endometrial cancer risk: a meta-analysis. Obst Gynecol 1995;85:304–313.
31. The Database of Abstracts of Reviews of Effectiveness (University of York), Database no.: DARE-950328. In: The Cochrane Library, Issue 4, 1999. Oxford: Update Software.
32. Pickar JH, Thorneycroft I, Ehitehead M. Effects of hormone replacement therapy on the endometrium and lipid parameters: a review of randomized clinical trials, 1985 to 1995. Am J Obst Gyn 1998;178:1087–1099.
33. The Database of Abstracts of Reviews of Effectiveness (University of York), Database no.: DARE-980991. In: The Cochrane Library, Issue 2, 2000. Oxford: Update Software.

25.60 Care of a rape victim

Editors

Basic rules

- Collect forensic specimens.
- Offer postcoital contraception.
- Prevent infections.
- Provide counselling.

Investigations

- The doctor should preferably have a nurse assisting in the examination of the patient.
- The patient may have someone with her for mental support.
- Document the history precisely. However, an excessively detailed history may result in discrepancies with the police report and can cause problems in criminal proceedings.
  - Time of assault
  - Number and identity of the assailants
  - Type of force and use of weapons
  - Attempts of vaginal, rectal or oral penetration
  - Digital penetration or penetration with objects
  - Did the victim observe an ejaculation?
  - Did the victim do something that may have destroyed or altered the evidence after the assault: bathing, douching, wiping, use of tampons, dental hygiene, defecation, changing clothes?
- Document the presence of any injuries, including those of the genitalia and oral cavity.

Contraception

- Postcoital contraception when necessary (27.6).

Prevention, treatment and follow-up of infections

- Always take specimens for chlamydia and gonococci.
- HIV serology and HbsAg. Hepatite B vaccination should be offered to victims who wish to have it if they are HbsAg negative.
- HIV prophylaxis if the assailant is know to be HIV positive.
- A tetanus booster is indicated if the patient has wounds (do not forget vaginal and rectal wounds!).
- The victim is instructed to use a condom until all venereal diseases have been excluded.
- The doctor should see the victim after 3–4 weeks.
  - Chlamydia and gonococci specimens
  - HbsAg and HB-IgM
  - Syphilis serology 4–8 weeks after the rape
  - An asymptomatic rape victim can be given a single dose medication against chlamydia and gonorrhoea (12.1) (12.2).
- HIV serology (3–) 6 months after the rape

Emotional support and follow-up

- If possible the patient should have an escort when she is discharged.
- The victim should have an opportunity to express her thoughts and worries soon after the incident, and she should know how to contact a professional if needed (give written instructions on whom to contact).
- A psychological assessment (by a doctor or a psychologist) is indicated after 1–2 weeks. It is very important that the victim is allowed to express her feelings of anger openly. Expression of anger is an important step in regaining self-esteem and self-reliance.
- If the victim is under age, a consultation by a child psychiatrist is always indicated.
- The patient should preferably be assessed three months after the psychological trauma. A psychiatrist should write a statement on the assessment.

Obstetrics

Evidence Based Medicine Guidelines. Edited by the Duodecim Editorial Team
© 2005 John Wiley & Sons, Ltd ISBN: 0-470-01184-X

26.1 Antenatal clinics and specialist care: consultations, referrals, treatment guidelines

Jukka Uotila

In general

- Familiarize yourself with the referral criteria submitted by your local maternity hospital.
- In unclear cases, consult an appropriate specialist either by telephone or in writing.
- If possible avoid an emergency referral, and make an appointment for the patient. This will ensure that adequate hospital staff and equipment will be available, and the hospital staff will have time to consult the appropriate literature should it be necessary.
- Send the patient as an emergency if the state of the mother or foetus requires immediate assessment or treatment. The problems of an emergency referral are many: waiting times at the hospital might be long, investigations and treatment may be carried out in haste, the referral may cause unnecessary worry for the patient and the credibility of the antenatal clinic might even be questioned.
- See also 26.2.

Referral at the pregnancy pre-planning stage

- Pre-planning the pregnancy together with specialist teams might be necessary if the patient has
  - a chronic illness which is classified as serious or the prognosis of which is unclear
  - a history of a serious complication during a previous pregnancy the character of which was inadequately evaluated during postnatal examination
  - a family history of a hereditary illness and she is not aware of the incidence rate or the availability of screening.
- If required, the patient will be invited to attend an obstetrics clinic, a genetics clinic or another specialist clinic. Treatment guidelines will be drawn up by the primary care team and the hospital together.

Diabetes mellitus

- It is important that diabetes is well controlled at conception as well as during early pregnancy in order to reduce the risk of malformations.
- The mother should discuss pregnancy plans with her own doctor. Insulin should be introduced in tablet controlled diabetes, and insulin therapy should be intensified in type 1 diabetes.
- If the patient's diabetes is already complicated (nephropathy, renal impairment, severe retinopathy, coronary disease) the additional risks of pregnancy should be considered and specialist consultation sought when required.

Other chronic illnesses

- Illnesses warranting pregnancy risk assessment and pre-planning of pregnancy include significant heart disease, severe hypertension or renal disease, thromboembolic illness or severe autoimmune illness.
- Investigations at the pre-planning stage might also be warranted for some very rare illnesses.

Hereditary illnesses

- A referral to genetic counselling (or obstetrician) should be considered if the patient is not fully aware of the character of the hereditary illness or if carrier status studies of the genetic defect have not been performed.

Referral during early pregnancy–based on medical history

Mother's chronic illness

- See also 26.15.
- The timing of the referral depends on the severity of the illness and on the extent to which relevant treatment guidelines and the effect of the pregnancy are known.
- Insulin or tablet controlled diabetes
  - Refer immediately after the pregnancy has been confirmed.
  - The aim is to maintain good control before conception as well as during early pregnancy.
- Thromboembolic predisposition or a history of venous thrombosis
  - The timing and method of thrombosis prophylaxis depends on the following factors: in what situation and location was the previous venous thrombosis and how severe is the thrombotic predisposition, whether congenital or acquired, according to laboratory findings.
  - Even if the thrombosis prophylaxis is not commenced until late pregnancy the patient should be referred for an obstetric consultation during her early pregnancy for additional investigations and information.
- Congenital or acquired cardiac disease
  - Illnesses which are poorly tolerated during pregnancy are cardiac defects with NYHA class III–IV symptoms, Marfan's syndrome with dilatation at the aortic root, Eisenmenger's syndrome and other pulmonary hypertension.
  - During the pregnancy the cardiological status should be monitored as well as the mother's functional capacity. A

birth plan is drawn up and prophylactic medication should be decided upon, e.g. anticoagulation, antiarrhythmic agents and cover against endocarditis.
- The treating obstetrician should be made aware of the pregnancy, and an appropriate referral should be made in early or mid pregnancy.

♦ Autoimmune illness
- The course of the illness or its treatment (medication) might alter during pregnancy.
- The illness may affect the pregnancy, particularly in the presence of phospholipid or ENA antibodies.
- The mother should usually be referred to the care of an obstetric team in early pregnancy unless the illness is particularly mild, well investigated and problem free.

♦ Chronic hypertension (26.14)
- If hypertension is severe and complicated consideration should be given to referring the patient in early pregnancy.
- If hypertension is not complicated and requires no medication, three routine antenatal appointments should suffice: early/mid pregnancy, weeks 28–32 and late pregnancy.
- The patient should, however, be referred to an obstetrician if her blood pressure shows significant increase or other complications arise.

♦ Chronic renal disease
- A well controlled renal disease does not require more than regular check-ups at early, mid and late pregnancy. The potential risks involved include the development of associated pre-eclampsia, worsening of the renal disease and disturbances in the foetal growth.

♦ Bleeding disorder
- The most common bleeding disorder is von Willebrand's disease. Specialist consultation is required to ascertain the severity of the condition and to obtain information regarding the birth.

♦ Epilepsy or other neurological disease
- Referral to an obstetrician and a neurologist should be done in early pregnancy. Due to the increased risk of malformations, an accurate anomaly screening should be carried out, and medication and treatment plans should be drawn up for the pregnancy and delivery. Folic acid supplementation (A) [1], see 26.2.

♦ Chronic intestinal illness
- The patient should first be referred to the treating physician. If the illness is severe, symptomatic or newly diagnosed the patient should also be referred to an obstetrician. Long-term medication may need to be instigated during pregnancy. An active intestinal illness increases the risk of preterm birth.

♦ Lung disease, e.g. brittle asthma
- The patient should first be referred to the treating physician. During pregnancy, medication should be adequate to maintain optimal lung function.
- Asthma medication has not been shown to be harmful during pregnancy.

♦ Treated malignant tumour
- A structural ultrasound examination should be carried out by the specialist team, particularly if the principles regarding the monitoring of the pregnancy and the tumour remain unclear.

♦ Thyroid dysfunction
- Mild hypothyroidism in early pregnancy may be harmful to foetal development, and hypothyroidism in early pregnancy should therefore be corrected.
- Untreated hyperthyroidism may be dangerous both to the mother and the foetus. The medication for chronic hypothyroidism often needs adjustment during pregnancy.

♦ Psychiatric illness
- If the pregnant mother has a significant psychiatric illness, a multidisciplinary approach must be adopted, including a psychiatrist, the treating physician and an obstetrician.
- These patients often need a great deal of input during their pregnancy and appointments with an obstetrician might be beneficial even when the pregnancy progresses without actual problems.

♦ Chronic infections, see "Infections" in this chapter.

Genital malformation and uterine myomas

♦ Potential risks include increased likelihood of miscarriage, slowed foetal growth, preterm birth, obstruction to delivery or prolonged parturition.

Previous pregnancies with complications

GYN

♦ The patient should be referred to an obstetrician during early pregnancy if she has a history of
- three or more consecutive miscarriages
- very preterm births
- foetal death or severe foetal developmental problems
- early and severe pre-eclampsia

♦ The patient should be referred at a later stage, as considered necessary, if she has a history of
- abnormal delivery with problematic labour, e.g. emergency caesarean section, difficult vacuum extraction, heavy blood loss, inadequate pain relief or problems with the newborn.
- other problems of late pregnancy.

Increased risk of foetal malformation or hereditary illness

♦ If the results of screening or other investigations suggest that the risk of foetal abnormality is increased the mother should be referred for a specialist consultation should she so wish.

Substance abuse

♦ See 26.18.

- If it is noted or suspected during antenatal appointments and guidance that the mother suffers from substance addiction (alcohol, illegal drugs or use of medicinal products for a non-therapeutic effect) she should be referred to the care of a specialist team because
  - the treatment of the addiction and the mother's motivation is likely to be enhanced by the referral
  - substance abuse is associated with multidisciplinary problems
  - the hospital team will prepare themselves for problems associated with the delivery and puerperium, both for the mother and newborn.
- Definitions
  - Experimentation; if tried drugs at some stage of life
  - Drug addiction; if used drugs more than 10 times
  - Current substance addiction; if less than 12 months from stopping regular use or continues to use on an irregular basis
  - Excessive alcohol consumption; the consumption of more than 10 units of alcohol per week or binge drinking of more than 5 units at a time (criteria for pregnancy).

Consultation in case of disorder or abnormality

A. Maternal reasons for referral

Hyperemesis gravidarum (intractable vomiting)

- It is sometimes difficult to tell the difference between mild and severe vomiting during pregnancy. The mother should be sent to hospital if ketosis, weight loss (5%, >2 kg/week) or dehydration is present. The mother should also be sent to hospital if the condition becomes prolonged or is intolerable for her. In the hospital, intravenous fluids are usually administered to restore normal fluid balance.
- Treatment of nausea at the antenatal clinic, see 26.2.

Maternal blood loss

- Bleeding will usually originate from the uterine cavity, but may also be caused by inflammation, ulceration or tumour of the vagina or cervix.
- Maternal blood loss in early pregnancy (before week 22) (26.11) signifies impending miscarriage. No effective treatment is available. Rest can be considered. If emergency curettage is not feasible due to the extent of blood loss or pain, an ultrasound examination (26.3) should be carried out on the following working day to determine the character of the pregnancy.
- Maternal blood loss can originate from
  - a normal intrauterine pregnancy
  - intrauterine pregnancy where the embryo or foetus has died (missed abortion)
  - intrauterine pregnancy where the embryo fails to develop (blighted ovum, "anembryonic pregnancy")
  - inevitable miscarriage where the cervix opens and the uterine contents are expelled. It is likely that at the time of the examination only fragments of the pregnancy tissue remain in the uterus.
  - extrauterine pregnancy
- Maternal blood loss in late pregnancy (after week 22) might originate from
  - the uterine mucous membranes as the cervix ripens, the uterus contracts or labour begins
  - placenta praevia or placental abruption.
- The blood is usually maternal but could also partly be foetal.
- Because blood loss may be indicative of a serious danger to the foetus, and rapid measures might be needed to save the foetus, the mother must be sent to a maternity hospital urgently.

Increased blood pressure or pre-eclampsia

- See also 26.14 and 26.15.
- Blood pressure at rest is considered to be abnormally high if repeated measurements show
  - systolic pressure over 140 mmHg
  - diastolic pressure over 90 mmHg
  - systolic pressure increased more than 30 mmHg from baseline
  - diastolic pressure increased more than 15 mmHg from baseline
- Proteinuria is considered significant if the concentration is over 0.3 g/l in a 24-hour urine sample (strip test + or ++).
- Other symptoms associated with pre-eclampsia include: oedema, upper abdominal pain, nausea, headache, visual disturbances and other neurological symptoms.
- A non-urgent referral for an obstetric consultation should be made for an asymptomatic patient with elevated blood pressure or with significant proteinuria. The patient should receive an appointment within a week of the referral.
- A symptomatic patient or a patient who presents with proteinuria and acutely increased blood pressure might warrant an urgent referral to a maternity hospital.
- Acute upper abdominal pain associated with a rise in blood pressure, however small, and/or the presence of proteinuria may be indicative of the HELLP syndrome. In this case the mother must be sent to hospital urgently.

Abnormal glucose tolerance (gestational diabetes)

- Screening at the antenatal clinic is based on risk factors and a glucose tolerance test (GTT).
- A GTT should be carried out between weeks 26 and 28 if the mother
  - has glucose in morning urine (one positive result is enough)
  - is overweight (BMI > 25 kg/m^2)
  - has previously given birth to a child with a birthweight of over 4.5 kg
  - is over 40 years of age
  - has a macrosomic foetus.

Table 26.1 GTT upper limits for normal glucose values (mmol/l)

Sample	0 hr	1 hr	2 hrs
capillary whole blood or venous plasma	4.8	10.0	8.7
capillary plasma	5.3	10.9	9.5

- The mother has gestational diabetes if one or more of the results of an oral 75 g glucose challenge (2 hours) is abnormal, see Table 26.1.
- GTT should be carried out earlier if the mother presents with repeated glycosuria or if she has a history of gestational diabetes. Even if the earlier test is normal it should nevertheless be repeated between weeks 26 and 28.
- If the GTT is abnormal (approximately 5% of all pregnant women) the mother should be referred for specialist care in order to assess the need for further investigations and follow-up.
- Some hospital districts will refer only those mothers who either have at least two abnormal blood results in the GTT, an abnormal fasting value or who have other risk factors.
- Foetal macrosomia must, however, be always detected early enough and appropriate delivery plans put into action.

Cholestasis of pregnancy (hepatosis)

- If the mother complains of pruritus, blood is taken for ALT and bile acids. If one of these values is elevated the mother is referred to an obstetrician.
- If the pruritus is severe and intolerable the patient must be sent to hospital urgently, without waiting for the laboratory results. Likewise, if a patient with hepatosis complains of an acutely worsening pruritus she must be sent to hospital urgently.

Anaemia

- See also 15.22.
- The mother will need specialist consultation if
  - her Hb is <10.0 g/dl despite iron substitution of three weeks
  - her Hb is <9.0 g/dl.

Premature contractions or impending preterm birth

- See also 26.13.
- Premature contractions are very common. The majority of women who suffer from premature contractions will go on to deliver full term.
- The cervix is assessed either manually or measured with an ultrasound to assess the risk of preterm birth.
- Send the mother to hospital urgently if
  - the contractions are painful and regular (lasting for more than 2 hours and occurring <10 minutes)
  - contractions are accompanied by bloody, mucous or watery discharge
  - contractions are associated with significant pain or feeling of pressure
  - frequent contractions occur together with a significantly ripe cervix, considering the weeks of gestation.
- A non-urgent referral may be considered if the risk of preterm delivery is not imminent but specialist consultation is required to clarify treatment guidelines; for example, the mother's need for tocolytic medication, corticosteroids for foetal lung development or the mother's need for hospitalisation.
- After the mother completes 34 full weeks of pregnancy no other active measures except rest are offered; the benefit of such measures has not been established. The closer the mother is to completing the full 34 weeks the less urgency there is to send her for a specialist consultation.
- A non-urgent referral should be considered if
  - contractions remain frequent despite primary care interventions (sickness leave, rest, treating of infections)
  - considering the weeks of gestation, the cervix appears markedly ripe.

Rupture of the membranes

- Suspected or confirmed rupture of the membranes requires an urgent referral to hospital.
- Rupture of the membranes often leads to the onset of labour. It might also signify an existing infection or lead to an infection.
- As the membranes rupture the placental circulation usually alters and the umbilical cord may become compressed.
- If the mother describes a very small and uncertain loss of fluid and if, based on speculum examination and the history, rupture of the membranes does not appear likely it is safe to wait and observe.

Formation of antibodies

- In many countries the blood of the mother is tested for antibodies against the foetal red cells at a national transfusion laboratory. The laboratory will advise the antenatal clinic staff regarding the necessity for repeat samples.
- The presence of antibodies is reported both to the antenatal clinic and to the appropriate maternity hospital. The hospital will arrange any necessary follow-up studies and instigate appropriate treatment guidelines.
  - The maternity hospital staff must prepare themselves for the correct monitoring of the newborn and the possibility of blood transfusions.
  - Some of the more severe antibody formations against red cells or thrombocytes might require specialist procedures which need to be carried out during the pregnancy.
- The majority of the antibody formations, however, are mild and require no intervention during the pregnancy.

Abnormal uterine growth or abnormal amount of amniotic fluid

- Uterine growth is measured using the symphysis–fundal height (SFH).
- Usually the growth of the uterus coincides with a given reference curve. The growth of the uterus of a particularly

small- or large-sized woman might obviously deviate from the reference curve.

- An ultrasound examination (26.3) is warranted if
  - the SFH deviates over 2 cm from the reference curve
  - the SFH deviates over 2 cm from the patient's own curve.
- A referral for an obstetrician should be considered if
  - the amount of amniotic fluid is particularly large (single deepest amniotic fluid pocket measurement over 8 cm)
  - the amount of amniotic fluid is particularly low (largest amniotic fluid pocket measurement less than 3 cm)
  - the foetus is exceptionally small or large (see later "Foetal reasons for referral").

Method of delivery

- If the method of delivery has not been decided upon, this should be done during the last pregnancy month by the treating obstetric team. By this time realistic assessments can be made regarding the predicted size of the foetus, its presentation, the ripening of the cervix and other relevant factors.
- If the patient is highly anxious or very worried about the birth, an earlier consultation could be considered, see below.
- A referral in order to draw up a birth plan should be considered if
  - the patient has a history of a complicated delivery
  - the uterus has been operated on
  - a narrow pelvis is suspected
  - a disproportionately large foetus is suspected.

Post-term pregnancy

- The first assessment appointment is usually made with the maternity hospital 10–12 days after the expected date of delivery has passed, unless there are other indications to refer the mother earlier.
- The mother should be informed that the appointment is merely for the assessment of the maternal and foetal condition and not necessarily for the purposes of inducing labour.
- The term "overdue" should not be used until week 42 has been completed.

Fear of childbirth

- The antenatal staff should discuss the most common reasons behind any fears. It is important for the success of the future delivery that all fears are recognised and addressed. Special questionnaires may be used to recognise any fears.
- A mother who is particularly afraid of the birth should be referred to the care of the maternity hospital by week 30, at the latest, so that any relevant issues can be discussed.

B. Foetal reasons for referral

Multiple pregnancy

- There is regional variability regarding the referral system and the workload division between primary care and the maternity hospital.
  - As soon as a triplet pregnancy is diagnosed the mother should be referred to the care of an obstetric team.
  - After a twin pregnancy is diagnosed the possibility of a monoamniotic or monochorionic pregnancy should also be assessed during the early pregnancy (the presence and thickness of inter-twin membrane, lambda sign).
  - As soon as a monoamniotic or monochorionic twin pregnancy is diagnosed the mother should be referred to the care of an obstetric team.
  - In a monochorionic twin pregnancy the uterine growth might be fast during the second trimester, causing stretching of the uterus. Should the mother present with such symptoms an urgent referral should be made in order to diagnose and treat a possible twin-to-twin transfusion syndrome.
  - In all twin pregnancies, the state of the cervix and the growth of the foetuses should be monitored at regular intervals. Preterm birth and developmental problems of one or both foetuses are common in twin pregnancies. The monitoring of twin pregnancies is usually carried out by an obstetrician.

Abnormally large foetus

- The assessment of the size of the foetus should always take the size of the mother into account.
- If the foetus is assessed to be large (26.3) (weight assessment or abdominal circumference > 75–90 percentile) and there is a suspicion of foeto-pelvic disproportion, the mother should be referred early enough, preferable by weeks 37–38, for the drawing up of a birth plan.
- Glucose metabolism investigation should be considered if the foetus is not symmetrically macrosomic, particularly if the body is prominent.
- An asymmetrically macrosomic foetus is more likely to require obstetric intervention than a symmetrically macrosomic foetus.

Delayed foetal growth

- A low SFH measurement, or a measurement which falls below its own curve, may be indicative of delayed foetal growth. Likewise, an ultrasound examination carried out in primary care (26.3) might reveal a small-for-gestational-age foetus.
- An abnormal growth of the foetus may be indicative of structural or functional abnormality. A foetus whose development is delayed is also more prone to either acute or chronic asphyxia.
- Delayed foetal growth (weight assessment or abdominal circumference < 10–25 percentile) is an indication for further investigations (the possibility of infectious aetiology, chromosome and structural abnormalities or an insufficiency of the placenta) and monitoring by an obstetrician.

Abnormal presentation

- External cephalic version for breech or transverse presentation and the mode of delivery are usually considered around week 36 (B) [2].

Suspected or confirmed foetal structural abnormality

- The mother should be referred for confirmation and further management of the situation.
- The mother should be given an appointment as soon as possible when the necessary expertise and relevant diagnostic investigations are available at the hospital.

Abnormal foetal heart rate

- Persistent bradycardia (heart rate < 100–120/min) or tachycardia (heart rate > 160–180/min) might be indicative of foetal arrhythmias or other complications of the pregnancy.
- A persistent abnormal rhythm might have haemodynamically serious consequences and such patients should be sent to hospital urgently, even if the possibility to carry out further investigations were not immediately available.
- A short-term (lasting for a few minutes) bradycardia or tachycardia might indicate a predisposition to arrhythmias. Usually, however, an arrhythmia of this type is merely a healthy indication of foetal activity or mother's supine position. If necessary, an appointment could be considered for further investigations of the structure and functioning of the foetal heart.
- Occasional foetal ectopic beats are normal, and occur in all foetuses. Should ectopic beats occur frequently a non-urgent referral should be considered in order to have the structure and functioning of the foetal heart further investigated.
- If an abnormal foetal heart beat is associated with other problems, e.g. abnormally few foetal movements, delayed foetal growth or a known maternal risk, contact the on-call obstetric team.

Slowing down of foetal movements

- If the mother counts less than 10 foetal movements for one hour, including the particularly active times of the day, foetal distress should be considered.
- Foetal movements should be recounted and if there is no change the mother should be sent urgently to the maternity hospital for the evaluation of the state of the foetus.

Foetal death

- A suspected or confirmed foetal death must be referred to the maternity hospital urgently.

C. Maternal infectious diseases

Herpes simplex

- See 12.5.
- The incidence of neonatal herpes simplex is approximately 2 per 10000 births. Maternal primary infection during pregnancy is more than one hundred times as likely to infect the foetus than a recurrent infection. Antibodies of a recurring herpes infection offer protection to the foetus.
- Herpesvirus nucleic acid testing is used to diagnose primary herpes infection.
- Aciclovir (200 mg five times daily for five days) can be used particularly in primary infection, but also in recurrent infection, to alleviate the mother's symptoms and to provide the foetus with potential protection. Prophylactic treatment, or the introduction of aciclovir on symptom onset, should be considered in late pregnancy. The aim is to reduce the activity of genital herpes during labour.
- When the mother is admitted for her delivery she should inform the hospital staff of the occurrence of genital herpes during pregnancy.
- If primary herpes is suspected, or recurrent infection is particularly problematic, a referral is made for an obstetric consultation.

Chickenpox

- See 31.50.
- The risk of varicella embryopathy between the pregnancy weeks 12 and 24 is 2–3%, and very small at the other stages of pregnancy.
- In practice there is no risk if the mother herself has had chickenpox, antibodies are demonstrable or the illness is herpes zoster (shingles).
- If a seronegative mother comes into contact with chickenpox aciclovir medication (800 mg, five times daily for 7 days) should be considered 7–9 days post contact.
- If the mother is diagnosed with chickenpox before week 24, a foetal anomaly investigation may be considered after the illness, and, in some cases, foetal infection can be determined with nucleic acid testing of amniotic fluid.
- Chickenpox can be a serious illness for a pregnant woman. If hospitalisation is required the mother should be treated on a medical ward.

Parvovirus infection

- See 31.53.
- Should the foetus become infected, hepatitis and myelosuppression are possible which, in turn, may be fatal for the foetus.
- Antibody assays are used to diagnose a parvovirus infection.
- If the antibody assay is positive a referral should be made for a specialist team who will organise appropriate monitoring to determine foetal infection status or detect signs of anaemia.

Toxoplasmosis

- An acute toxoplasma infection is diagnosed with antibody assays, see 1.62.
- If the antibody assay is positive a referral should be made for a specialist team who will organise further investigations to determine foetal infection status and organise treatment for mother and foetus.

Hepatitis and HIV

- See 9.20 and 1.45.
- Newly diagnosed hepatitis or HIV require a referral for specialist care.
- Drug treatment in HIV is particularly important to prevent mother-to-child transmission.
- The maternity hospital must be made aware of a mother's chronic hepatitis.

Listeriosis suspicion

- See 1.23.
- A possible exposure to Listeria monocytogenes does not warrant a referral for specialist care.
- A clinically significant listeriosis in a pregnant woman manifests itself as a septic febrile disease or severe enteritis.
- Listeriosis, and its consequences, is the most serious septic illness for a pregnant woman, but other bacteria are also capable of infecting the foetus and foetal membranes, leading to an early induction of labour.
- If the mother's pyrexia is of unknown origin the mother should be sent urgently to hospital for a specialist consultation regarding the diagnosis, treatment and the foetal status.

Indications for emergency referral

- Suspicion of deteriorating foetal status
  - Decreased foetal movements (less than 10 movements per hour whilst the foetus is at its most active)
  - Persistent bradycardia or tachycardia
  - Suspected or confirmed foetal death
- Impending (preterm) birth
  - Maternal blood loss after week 22
  - Suspected rupture of the membranes
  - Regular contractions
  - Severe abdominal pain
- Blood pressure complications
  - Increased blood pressure together with abnormal headache, visual disturbances, dyspnoea, upper abdominal pain
  - Increased blood pressure together with decreased or weak foetal movements
  - Acutely high blood pressure (>160/105 mmHg)
  - Increased blood pressure together with marked proteinuria
  - Suspected HELLP syndrome: upper abdominal pain and malaise with an increase in blood pressure, however small
- Severe, intensive pruritus
- Severe nausea
- Suspected venous thrombosis or pulmonary embolus
- High-grade pyrexia
- Any other condition where emergency measures are considered appropriate.

References

1. Lumley J, Watson L, Watson M, Bower C. Periconceptional supplementation with folate and/or multivitamins for preventing neural tube defects. Cochrane Database Syst Rev. 2004;(2):CD001056.
2. Hofmeyr GJ, Kulier R. External cephalic version for breech presentation at term. Cochrane Database Syst Rev. 2004;(2): CD000083.

26.2 Antenatal clinics: care and examinations

Jukka Uotila

- The tasks of antenatal clinics
  - Provide the expectant mother with information and guidance regarding the pregnancy, childbirth and care of the newborn.
  - Offer a wide range of psychosocial support and identify the need of such support.
  - Identify any health risks to the foetus or mother so that any problems can be duly attended to, either at the antenatal clinic or by specialist intervention.
  - Provide routine care of various illnesses and complaints. Identify situations which require specialist health care.
  - See also 26.1.
- Co-operation between the physician and midwife, and a mutually agreed workload division, is important in the provision of antenatal care. When appropriate, the following tasks associated with medical examinations can be carried out by the midwife.

First medical examination during weeks 10–15

- Assessment of gestational age
  - Date and character of last menstrual period?
  - Was the menstrual cycle regular or irregular?
  - Had the patient used oral contraceptives (up to conception)?
  - Date of positive pregnancy test?
- Gestational age is marked in the patient's records using the number of full weeks + additional days.
- If the assessment of the gestational age is not straightforward, an ultrasound scan should be carried out (26.3) to support the assessment **B** [1 2]. A scan should also be considered in cases where problems with post-term pregnancy or low birthweight are anticipated (complications with a previous pregnancy, hypertension, smoking).
- The accuracy of an ultrasound scan in early and mid-pregnancy is +/− 7 days. If the discrepancy between the ultrasound estimate and last menstrual period is more than 7 days the ultrasound dating is to be used to determine the gestational age.

- How has the early pregnancy progressed (mood, general health)?
- Are there any chronic illnesses (26.15) (referral criteria for specialist consultation, see 26.1)?
- Any other problems (for example obesity, frequent urinary tract infections, uterine anomalies)?
- The course of previous pregnancies and the health of the newborn children?
- Any hereditary illnesses?
- Any medication use during early pregnancy?
- Smoking (40.20)?
- Alcohol consumption or substance abuse (26.18)?
- Any allergies?
- Character of employment; does the work pose possible risks to the foetus (if problems are anticipated, specialists in occupational health should be consulted)?
- Any psychosocial problems?
- See criteria for screening tests. Screening for foetal, chromosomal abnormalities varies widely, check your practice in your area.

Investigations

- A pelvic examination is usually carried out at the first appointment. The main objective is to identify possible infections.
  - At the beginning of pregnancy the vaginal membranes swell, and it might be more difficult than usual to see the external uterine orifice. The amount of physiological vaginal discharge is increased throughout pregnancy.
  - The vagina and the cervix are examined for signs of infection (25.30). Findings suggestive of infection include erosions and offensive or otherwise abnormal discharge. In addition to the clinical picture, a sample of vaginal discharge may be tested for the release of fishy odour on adding alkali. The sample may also be tested for yeasts, Trichomonas or clue cells, either microscopically or by culture. If there is discharge from the cervical canal or the patient's history so indicates, samples should be taken for chlamydial infection (12.1) and gonorrhoea (12.2).
  - A pelvic examination is used to determine whether the size of the uterus corresponds with the period of amenorrhoea (see Table 26.2). Should any discrepancy exist, the patient should be referred for an ultrasound scan.
  - Should a suspicion of uterine or ovarian tumour arise during the pelvic examination, the patient must be referred for an ultrasound scan or for a specialist consultation.
  - It is also possible to conduct a pelvic examination during late pregnancy if it is carried out carefully and without irritating the cervix. An examination is necessary particularly if the patient complains of contractions or feeling of pressure, which may both be indicative of impending preterm labour. Possible dilatation of the cervix and membrane bulging can also be detected during speculum examination.
- Blood pressure should be measured at each appointment. Urinary protein and glucose as well as haemoglobin/haematocrit are also easy to check during most appointments.

Table 26.2 Size of the uterus during pregnancy

Weeks of gestation	Size of the uterus
6	No noticeable growth
8	9 cm
12	12 cm
16	Halfway between symphysis and umbilicus
20	Up to umbilicus

- Screening tests during the first trimester
  - Blood group and blood group antibodies
  - VDRL test
  - Hepatitis B surface antigen
  - HIV antibodies

Second medical examination in week 28 (±2 weeks)

- The objectives of this appointment include the identification of the risk of preterm birth, disturbances in the uterine growth, gestational diabetes and early pre-eclampsia. The forthcoming childbirth is approaching and the patient may wish to obtain information regarding the rest of the pregnancy and the delivery. Issues relating to the possible fear of childbirth should be addressed at this stage at the latest.
- Ask how the mother is coping at work. Sick notes should be issued whenever necessary, even for short time periods.
- Status
  - The size of the uterus (a deviation of over 2 cm from the reference curve or from patient's own curve)
  - Cervix: the presenting part deep within the pelvis and the softening, shortening and opening of the cervix as well as the alignment of the cervix in relation to the vagina are signs of impending delivery.
  - The size of the foetus is estimated either by weight or by the following criteria: s = small for gestational age, n = normal for gestational age, l = large for gestational age.
  - The amount of amniotic fluid is estimated, i.e. normal, excessive or small amount.
  - Abnormal weight gain (does the patient have pre-eclampsia, abnormal foetal growth, excessive amniotic fluid, gestational diabetes?).

Third medical examination in week 36 (±1 week)

- The objectives of this appointment include the detection of abnormal presentation, verification of foetal growth, assessment of issues relating to delivery, detection of genital herpes and the identification of expectant mothers whose delivery needs specialist pre-planning.
- Ask the mother about
  - foetal movements
  - possible contractions, feeling of pressure
  - oedema

GYN

- pruritus – if hepatic cholestasis of pregnancy is suspected, blood is taken for ALT and fasting bile acids.
- ♦ Status
  - Size of the uterus and foetus
  - Foetal presentation
  - Status of the cervix
  - External genital organs (herpes suspicion, see later in this chapter)

Postnatal examination 5–12 weeks after delivery

- ♦ How is the mother managing with breast feeding and caring for the infant?
- ♦ How does she feel about her pregnancy and delivery?
- ♦ How is her mood? How is she coping? Note any signs of depression. Should the mother have negative feelings about her delivery or if some relevant issues are not clear to her a referral could be written for the relevant obstetric team.
- ♦ Gynaecological status
  - Mucous membranes are often thin and erythematous before the return of hormonal activity and the menstrual cycle. The situation will correct itself, but, should the patient complain of discomfort, topical oestrogen may be prescribed in the form of pessaries or creams. The episiotomy wound may be tight and tender, but this complaint will also heal itself with time.
  - Cervical ectopy is common and does not need treatment at the postnatal appointment. Cervical smear is taken when the menstrual cycle returns (25.1). If the ectopy is later associated with excessive mucous discharge, which the patient finds uncomfortable, the area can be treated with electrocoagulation.
  - Any infections are to be diagnosed and treated. Fever, abnormal discharge and a tender uterus are suggestive of endometritis (25.41) which is treated with a course of antibiotics (e.g. cephalosporin for 7 days + metronidazole for 5 days). If offensive discharge is the only symptom anaerobic bacteria are likely to be the causative agent, and metronidazole alone will suffice for the treatment.
  - Postnatal discharge (lochia) will usually persist for 4–6 weeks after the delivery. If the discharge remains heavy the possibility of retained placental fragments, poor contractility of the uterus and infection should be borne in mind.
  - A good time for cervical smear is during the postnatal period after the return of the normal menstrual cycle.
- ♦ Important points
  - The need and method of contraception (27.2). An intrauterine device can be inserted when the uterus has returned to its normal size, but usually not until menstruation has commenced (27.4). The "minipill" can be taken during lactation. Combined oral contraceptives or a vaginal ring can be introduced towards the end of lactation when breast milk no longer forms the baby's main source of nutrition (27.3). Sterilization is an option for women aged over 30 years who already have many children and who are eligible for sterilization according to legislation.
  - If blood pressure was elevated, has it now normalised itself and has proteinuria disappeared? If risk factors relevant to the patient's future health (high blood pressure, obesity, gestational diabetes) were noted during the pregnancy, possible life style changes and other measures to prevent morbidity in later life are discussed. Follow-up appointments in primary care are agreed on.
  - Is there urinary or faecal incontinence? Involuntary escape of flatus? Pelvic floor exercises are encouraged should the patient suffer from urinary incontinence (11.4). Consideration should be given for follow-up appointments or specialist intervention.
  - Any signs of postnatal depression (35.13)?

Antenatal screening programmes

Blood group antibodies

- ♦ Each mother's blood is grouped during the first trimester, and tested for blood group antibodies, at a national transfusion laboratory. If antibodies are present the concentrations are measured every 4 weeks.
- ♦ Even if Rh-negative mothers have no antibodies during the first trimester their blood is tested again during each trimester for the presence of antibodies.
- ♦ The presence of antibodies is reported both to the antenatal clinic and to the appropriate maternity hospital. If the presence of antibodies is significant the hospital will invite the patient for follow-up studies and plan the delivery accordingly (26.1).

Screening for syphilis, HIV and hepatitis B

- ♦ A non-specific VDRL-test is used to test for syphilis. Positive results are confirmed with a TPHA assay (12.3) and the patient is referred for specialist care.
- ♦ Drug treatment of a confirmed HIV infection (1.45) considerably reduces the risk of the foetus or newborn contracting the virus.
- ♦ If the expectant mother is HBsAg-positive, the newborn is to be offered protection immediately after birth with hepatitis B immunoglobulin and by vaccination.
- ♦ The incidence of hepatitis C has increased lately, particularly among drug abusers. The mother-to-child transmission of hepatitis C cannot be prevented by medical measures. The medical staff should be alert for blood born contamination (9.20) when caring for patients with hepatitis B and C and HIV. Patients with a history of drug abuse should have their blood tested for hepatitis C.

Blood pressure monitoring

- ♦ See also 26.14 and 26.15.

- Sitting blood pressure is checked at each antenatal appointment, after making sure the mother has rested for at least 15 minutes, by using a cuff of sufficient length and width.
- The presence of protein in the urine is also checked.
- Other non-specific signs of pre-eclampsia include oedema (oedema without an increase in blood pressure is not, however, indicative of pre-eclampsia), headache, upper abdominal pain, visual disturbances and slowed uterine growth.
- If the diastolic blood pressure is repeatedly more than 90 mmHg or blood pressure has increased from the early pregnancy readings by more than 30/15 the patient is to be referred to an obstetrician. The degree of proteinuria, the severity of the patient's symptoms or a suspicion of problems with the foetal health will determine the urgency of the referral.

Screening for diabetes mellitus

- Gestational diabetes mellitus is diagnosed by a 75 grams glucose tolerance test (GTT) (see 26.1).
- The GTT is carried out between weeks 26 and 28 if the patient presents with the following risk factors:
  - glucose in morning urine sample
  - previous child with a birthweight of over 4.5 kg
  - age over 40 years
  - foetal macrosomia.
- The GTT should be carried out in early pregnancy if the patient has
  - a history of gestational diabetes
  - recurring glucosuria.
- If the GTT is normal during the early pregnancy, it must nevertheless be repeated between weeks 26 and 28.
- If gestational diabetes is confirmed with the GTT (one or more blood glucose values above the upper limit) the patient is to be given dietary advice at the antenatal clinic.
- Whether or not the patient is referred to a specialist team varies between hospital districts –some districts will refer all patients, some only those who either had at least two abnormal blood results in the GTT, an abnormal fasting value or who have other risk factors.
- Foetal macrosomia must be detected early enough and appropriate delivery plans put into action.
- The dietary treatment of gestational diabetes aims to reduce big fluctuations in blood glucose levels. Therefore, regular, small and fairly frequent meals are recommended and the consumption of quickly absorbed carbohydrates is to be avoided.

Screening and treatment of anaemia

- See also 15.22.
- Maternal anaemia does not in general cause problems to the foetus.
- Anaemia during pregnancy is usually caused by iron deficiency since the body's iron stores are being utilised during pregnancy. A small size of red cells and low serum ferritin are indicative of iron deficiency.
- If the Hb remains below 10.0 g/dl despite iron supplementation, consideration should be given to a referral for further investigations to rule out rarer complications and to instigate any specialist procedures.
- Iron supplementation is recommended if the Hb is below 12.0 g/dl, particularly if the patient complains of tiredness, lack of energy or other symptoms suggestive of anaemia. A dose of 50 mg of Fe++ is usually sufficient.
- Should the patient's diet not be sufficiently balanced, folic acid supplementation can also be considered. See section "Nutrition".

Growth of the uterus

- A normal growth of the uterus mirrors a normal size of the foetus and a normal amount of amniotic fluid.
- The measurement of symphysis–fundal height (SFH) is carried out with the patient in a gynaecological position. The urinary bladder must be empty.
- A deviation of over 2 cm from the reference curve, or from the patient's own sequential SFH measurements, warrants further investigations but only after technical errors have been excluded.
- Foetal size and the amount of amniotic fluid should also be assessed by abdominal palpation. The results must be adjusted for maternal height and weight.

Monitoring of foetal movements

- Whilst resting, the mother counts the number of foetal movements in one hour. The counting should be carried out whilst the foetus is particularly active.
- If the number of movements is less than 10, counting is continued for a further hour.
- If the mother's recognition of foetal movements remains less than 10 it is recommended that, during the following 24 hours, she visits an obstetric outpatients' clinic for further investigations.

Foetal heart auscultation ("listening for the heartbeat")

- Hearing the foetal heartbeat confirms that the foetus is alive. Auscultation of foetal heartbeat during a routine antenatal visit will not yield much information regarding possible foetal distress, but foetal arrhythmias can be detected.
- Isolated ectopic beats are common and harmless.
- Should ectopic beats occur frequently and be regular (every third beat or more) a non-urgent referral should be considered for further investigations of the foetal heart and its functioning.
- Persistent tachycardia (over 180/min) and bradycardia (less than 100/min) are rare. These situations may be indicative of obstetric complications requiring immediate intervention and an urgent referral for a specialist team might be warranted.

Infections during pregnancy

Infections of vagina and cervix

- See also 25.30.
- Yeasts are the most common causative agents of vaginitis. Vaginal thrush has not been shown to be harmful to the foetus. Symptomatic thrush is treated with topical medication.
- Signs and symptoms of bacterial vaginosis (BV) are greyish, malodorous discharge and the release of fishy odour on adding alkali, or clue cells on direct microscopy.
- BV is associated with preterm birth. However, due to modest treatment outcomes routine screening for BV is not recommended.
- According to the Cochrane review, treating BV, as compared with placebo or not treating it, significantly reduced symptoms and lowered the rate and tendency of preterm birth within the entire group. A mother attending an antenatal clinic should therefore be asked about the presence of offensive discharge, and during a speculum investigation attention should be paid to signs of BV.
- If signs suggestive of BV are present the infection should be treated, for example with topical metronidazole. No follow-up is necessary after the treatment. However, the treatment may be repeated should the symptoms recur.
- Cervicitis caused by gonorrhoea or chlamydial infection, or an asymptomatic carrier status, increase the risk of preterm birth, premature rupture of the membranes and infections of the newborn. Should the signs, symptoms or the patient's history suggest the presence of these infections, they should be diagnosed or excluded, for example with a urine test (12.1 and 12.2). A diagnosed infection must be treated.
- Recurrent, symptomatic genital herpes (12.5) should be treated with oral aciclovir (200 mg, five times daily for five days).
- If the episodes of herpes are frequent, prophylactic medication with aciclovir should be considered, 400 mg b.d., towards the end of the pregnancy, or the patient should at least be recommended to start medication immediately on the occurrence of symptoms.
- In cases of primary gestational genital herpes the diagnosis must be confirmed and medication with aciclovir commenced. Specialist consultation should also be considered.

Urinary tract infections

- See also 10.10.
- Asymptomatic bacteriuria during pregnancy leads to pyelonephritis in 30% of the cases and is a risk factor for preterm birth.
- Treatment of asymptomatic bacteriuria reduces the risk of pyelonephritis and preterm birth.
- Urine is tested with a strip test during antenatal appointments. Urine is sent for bacterial culture if infection is suspected.
- If the patient complains of premature contractions, the possibility of urinary tract and vaginal infections should be borne in mind.
- The treatment of asymptomatic bacteriuria is the same as that for symptomatic urinary tract infection, i.e. antibiotics for 5–7 days.
- Follow-up after treatment
- Should the patient suffer from two infections during the pregnancy, prophylactic treatment should be considered for the rest of the pregnancy, usually with nitrofurantoin.

Listeria

- See also 1.23.
- Listeria may cause a serious uterine and foetal infection, which is strongly associated with a risk of losing the foetus (miscarriage, death of the foetus or newborn).
- Even though Listeria is a common bacteria of the soil, epidemics caused by contaminated foodstuffs comprise the most significant health threat.
- Listeriosis, which poses a hazard to the foetus, is very unlikely without a maternal, symptomatic infection. In practice, listeriosis should be considered in patients with pyrexia of unknown origin or in febrile patients with intestinal or uterine complaints. These febrile patients must be sent urgently to a hospital for further investigations and treatment.
- There is no need to carry out antibody assays at the antenatal clinic.

Group B Streptococcus, Streptococcus agalactiae

- Group B Streptococcus (GBS) can be isolated from the normal flora of the vagina and rectum in some women.
- Some countries have introduced a wide range of screening programmes to reduce the risk of early-onset GBS sepsis in the newborn.
- Maternity hospitals carry out bacterial cultures in cases of early rupture of the membranes or impending preterm birth.
- The "treatment" of GBS colonisation during pregnancy does not reduce the incidence of perinatal exposure or improve the outcome of the pregnancy.
- There is no evidence to suggest that individual patients should be screened for GBS at antenatal clinics or that bacterial culture should be repeated after a course of antibiotics.

Other infections

- A systemic infection of the mother increases the risk of preterm birth, even when the infection does not originate from the genital area.
- Moreover, septic infections can be transferred to the foetus via the placenta.
- Only a few microbes are known to possess teratogenic potential. These include all herpes viruses, rubella virus (31.52), Toxoplasma (1.62) and parvovirus (31.53).
- When a pregnant mother presents with pyrexia of unknown origin the possibility of pregnancy complications must be

borne in mind, i.e. are there any signs of sepsis or an infection of the uterus, or is there anything to suggest preterm labour?

- Consider consulting a specialist in case of an infection. It is also noteworthy that a generalised infection during pregnancy, e.g. chickenpox (31.50), might be of a particular severity and require hospitalisation on an infectious diseases ward.

Treatment guidelines for common ailments of pregnancy

Nausea

- Almost every pregnant mother complains of nausea. It usually starts in weeks 5–7 and is at its worst during weeks 9–11. Cessation of symptoms is usually reported by week 14.
- Nausea might be alleviated by certain medication (vitamin B6 10–25 mg t.d.s., antihistamines, prochlorperazine, metoclopramide), but no strong evidence exists of their efficacy **B** [3]. In primary care, non-pharmacological interventions should be sought and offered whenever possible.
- Such measures include adequate rest, avoidance of irritant smells, tastes and situations, regular small snacks and psychiatric support.
- Hospitalisation is required in severe cases of hyperemesis gravidarum.

Heartburn

- Heartburn is common towards the end of the pregnancy as the growing uterus exerts mechanical pressure on the stomach and the gastroesophageal sphincter relaxes.
- Often all that is needed is an intake of non-irritant foods during small but frequent meals.
- In severe cases antacids, sucralfate or H2-receptor antagonists can be prescribed for a short time.

Constipation

- Pregnancy causes a relaxation of the smooth muscles, and may thus increase the tendency towards constipation.
- An adequate amount of exercise and a fibre rich diet are recommended.
- Bulk-forming laxatives and, if necessary, osmotic laxatives such as lactulose and milk of magnesia may also be used.

Cramps

- There is very little good study data, but many patients have reported an improvement with the use of calcium (500–100 mg/day) or magnesium (250–500 mg/day).

Headache and migraine

- As is the case with most ailments in pregnancy, the first-line recommendation should be a non-pharmacological intervention: rest, healthy life style, avoidance of irritants, neck and shoulder massage and other measures offered by physiotherapy.
- In severe cases, medication should be considered. Paracetamol, either alone or combined with codeine, is the first-line analgesic. Ibuprofen and ketoprofen can also be used temporarily. However, large doses should be avoided in late pregnancy.
- Ergotamine products are contraindicated, and there is insufficient experience in the use of triptans to warrant their recommendation.
- Drugs used for the treatment of nausea, such as metoclopramide and vitamin B6, may also alleviate migraine. The use of metoprolol, nifedipine or magnesium can be considered for migraine prophylaxis.

Depression

- During the development of a normal pregnancy the mother often also experiences fear, worry and low spirits. However, pathological anxiety, panic disorders or depression during pregnancy must be identified, and appropriate therapy offered.
- The warning signs include sleep disturbances with early waking up, consistent lack of appetite and nausea, excessive pessimism and feelings of guilt as well as an inappropriately nonchalant attitude or impaired orientation.
- If medication is needed to treat depression, citalopram is the most used medication during pregnancy.

Allergic rhinitis

- Topical preparations which are applied to eyes or nostrils can be used during pregnancy.
- Of the conventional antihistamines, hydroxyzine has been used widely without any reported serious adverse events. It does, however, cause tiredness.
- There is little experience of the use of the new antihistamines, and their use cannot therefore be recommended. However, the use of cetirizine could be considered, since it is a metabolite of hydroxyzine.

Backache

- Physiotherapy and ergonomic counselling is beneficial for the treatment and prevention of backache.
- Women with lower back pain have sometimes been treated successfully with stability enhancing support belts.
- If the pain is worse at night, a wedged pillow, which gives support to the abdomen, could be tried.

Nutrition, lifestyle, smoking and substance abuse

Nutrition

- Energy requirements are usually met by eating a normal balanced diet. Attention should be paid to the nutritional

value of the diet to ensure an adequate intake of trace elements.
- Special attention and dietary advice should be given to women whose diet is restricted or who are undernourished, who follow a special diet or are overweight.
- The mother should not put herself on an antigen avoidance diet in an attempt to prevent an allergy from occurring in her child.
- Conflicting opinions prevail regarding prophylactic iron supplementation. Routinely administered iron supplementation during pregnancy reduces the incidence of low Hb perinatally and 6 weeks postnatally, but there is no data regarding the well being of the mother and child.
- Iron stores of approximately one third of pregnant women are significantly low, and iron supplementation should be considered at least for this patient group (15.22).
- Folic acid intake is usually adequate if the diet consumed is balanced and sufficient (A) [4].
- Folate supplementation is required for the prevention of neural tube defects in the following cases:
  - Daily folic acid supplementation of 0.4 mg (tablets)
    - Folic acid deficiency can be caused by certain antiepileptics, such as phenytoin and barbiturate derivates, long-term use of sulphonamides, disturbances of intestinal absorption (e.g. coeliac disease), excessive alcohol consumption or an unbalanced diet.
    - Folic acid supplementation can also be considered for women with Type 1 diabetes and in association with clomifene, valproate and carbamazepine treatment. It can also be considered if there is a past family history of neural tube defects.
  - Daily folic acid supplementation of 4 mg (tablets)
    - If the risk of having a child with neural tube defects is higher than average.
    - If there is a close family history (an affected child of the parents or an affected child of one of the parents with another partner or the mother or father affected themselves) of neural tube defects.
  - High risk families should be referred to genetic counselling as soon as a pregnancy is planned.
- Supplementation must occur under medical supervision. The patient must be checked for vitamin B12 deficiency before and, as necessary, during the supplementation.
- The dose of the prescribed supplementation must be clearly marked on the prescription sheet since the tablet sizes available vary greatly.
- Folic acid supplementation is commenced during the menstrual cycle after which conception is planned, and is continued until the end of week 12 of gestation.
- In international studies folic acid reduced the incidence of neural tube defects whereas the consumption of multivitamin products had no effect (A) [5].
- Vitamin D supplementation, 10 μg/day, is recommended for all pregnant mothers during the winter months, particularly in sunless climates.

Exercise

- Exercise during pregnancy should be a pleasant activity with the aim to maintain the mother's fitness level.
- The mother should be advised to "listen to her body". Activities to be avoided, particularly during late pregnancy, include high risk sports and exercise forms which may compress the uterus or expose it to bouncing movements.
- Should the mother suffer from complications, the amount of exercise might have to be restricted.

Sex life

- Sexual intercourse is not hazardous during normal pregnancy.
- Intercourse is not recommended if the mother suffers from vaginal bleeding or her medical history suggests a risk of preterm birth.

Smoking

- Nicotine crosses the placenta readily, and the foetus is exposed to the same concentration as the mother.
- The neonates of smoking mothers are often fretful and tend to cry a lot.
- In boys, foetal exposure to nicotine has been shown to reduce future sperm production which in turn may lead to later problems in conception.
- Cigarettes impair the placental functioning and increase the risk of placental abruption. Smoking cessation is of particular importance in situations where disturbances in placental functioning and a low weight of the foetus are noted.
- Nicotine replacement therapy can be used during pregnancy. Short acting preparations are recommended (40.20).

Alcohol

- See also 26.18.
- One standard drink at the most once a week has not been shown to be harmful during pregnancy.
- Alcohol crosses the placenta readily and the foetal concentrations may rise even higher than those of the mother.
- Heavy alcohol consumption and especially drunkenness during early pregnancy may lead to cardiac and limb malformations.
- Continuation of heavy alcohol consumption after discovery of pregnancy (after first trimester) may lead to foetal alcohol syndrome (FAS) which is characterised by growth deficiencies, microcephaly, various neurological symptoms, developmental disabilities and abnormal facial features.
- Specialist consultation should always be borne in mind.

Other substance abuse

- See also 26.18.

- Substance dependence (alcohol, illegal drugs and use of medicinal products for a non-therapeutic effect) is a significant psychosocial problem and should be addressed, particularly during pregnancy.
- Substance abuse is often associated with psychiatric problems and problems with personal relationships. At a later stage, issues relating to child protection should also be addressed.
- The mother should be referred to the care of an obstetrician.
- Hashish and marijuana
  - The active ingredient is tetrahydrocannabinol, which crosses the placenta readily.
  - The risk of malformations or miscarriage has not been shown to increase.
  - Placental circulation, and therefore foetal nutrition, will be reduced leading to increased risk of a low birthweight infant.
- Amphetamines
  - May cause cardiac problems, developmental abnormality of the head and brains as well as cleft palate.
  - A risk of undernourishment and unbalanced diet.
  - Placental circulation will be impaired leading to retarded foetal growth.
  - An increased risk of elevated blood pressure, premature membrane rupture, preterm birth and infection.
- Cocaine
  - May cause an atrophy of the optic nerve and other developmental abnormalities of the eyes.
  - Placental circulation will be impaired leading to retarded foetal growth.
  - An increased risk of preterm birth and placental abruption.
- Opioids
  - The child will have an increased risk of physical and mental disability.
  - An increased risk of maternal blood loss and placental abruption.
  - The foetus will be at an increased risk of oxygen starvation.
  - An increased risk of early membrane rupture, preterm birth and infections.
  - The newborn might suffer from severe withdrawal symptoms.

References

1. Aymerich M, Almazan C, Jovell AJ. Assessment of obstetric ultrasonography for the control of normal pregnancies in primary care. Barcelona: Catalan Agency for Health Technology Assessment. Catalan Agency for Health Technology Assessment (CAHTA). IN97007. 1997. 44.
2. The Health Technology Assessment Database, Database no.: HTA-988952. In: The Cochrane Library, Issue 1, 2001. Oxford: Update Software.
3. Jewell D, Young G. Interventions for nausea and vomiting in early pregnancy. Cochrane Database Syst Rev. 2004;(2):CD000145.
4. Mahomed K. Folate supplementation in pregnancy. Cochrane Database Syst Rev. 2004;(2):CD000183.
5. Lumley J, Watson L, Watson M, Bower C. Periconceptional supplementation with folate and/or multivitamins for preventing neural tube defects. Cochrane Database Syst Rev. 2004;(2):CD001056.

26.3 Ultrasound scanning during pregnancy

Ari Ylä-Outinen

Basic rules

- Training under a specialist is essential (exceptions: foetal pulse on weeks 7–9 of pregnancy and presentation in late pregnancy).
- Do not hesitate to consult a specialist.

Aims

- Expected date of confinement, EDC (the most important and easiest to carry out)
- Number of foetuses
- Position of the placenta
- Foetal structures, morphology
- Presentation, when needed (easy to carry out)
- Growth if deviation is suspected
- The time of the first routine scan is agreed upon locally and depends on the mode of trisomy screening.

GYN

Recognizing pregnancy

Amniotic sac

- An intrauterine amniotic sac can be identified as early as on the 5th week of pregnancy (WOP) with a transvaginal scan (TVS). The sac is visualized as a round clear area in the uterine cavity.
- With a transabdominal scan (TAS) the amniotic sac can be seen much later, usually between the 7th and 9th WOP depending on the thickness of mother's abdominal wall and the position of the uterus.
- In practice, visualization of an intrauterine amniotic sac rules out the possibility of an extrauterine pregnancy.

The embryo

- First seen as a small dense echo within the amniotic sac.

- The foetal heart beat can be detected as a barely visible flutter already when the foetus in only a few mm long.
- The yolk sac is seen as a separate ring-like structure in the amniotic sac.

Multifoetal pregnancies

- A twin pregnancy can be determined in early pregnancy. One embryo can, however, be aborted, which manifests as bleeding in early pregnancy.
- It is possible to predict the chorionicity of a twin pregnancy in several ways: the placental tissue penetrating between the layers of the placental insertion of the separating membrane ("twin peak" or lambda sign) indicates dichorionicity. If the thickness of the separating membrane is less than 2 mm, monochorionicity is likely. It may sometimes be possible to count the number of layers of the separating membrane (two in mono- and four in dichorionitic twins).

Corpus luteum cyst

- On WOP 7–11 a separate unilocular clear, thin, walled cyst measuring 2–4 cm is often seen beside the uterus. This vanishes later on and needs no intervention.

Estimation of gestational age

- Ultrasound scan before 20 WOP is the most reliable method for determining EDC.
- Accuracy is best on 10–12 WOP ±3–4 days, at other times ±7 days. If the time determined by ultrasound differs from that determined from menstruation by more than one week, EDC should be corrected.
- The crown-rump-length (CRL) is used to estimate gestational age before 13 WOP .
- After 11 WOP biparietal diameter (BPD) or the length of the diaphysis of the femur (femur length) or both are used.
- The gestational age corresponding to the obtained measures is given in tables that are programmed in to many ultrasound devices. Such devices give both the gestational age and EDC automatically.

Foetal structures (morphology)

- The most appropriate time for routine scanning of foetal structures is 16–20 WOP.
- The structures are examined systematically.

1. The head and spinal canal

- In the transverse plane the foetal skull is seen as an ellipsoid structure with a symmetric mid-echo. BPD is measured in this plane. If a good BPD cannot be achieved, anencephaly should be suspected.
- Normally, symmetrical dense echoes, choroid plexuses, are seen on both sides of the mid-echo. If the echoes are asymmetrical or non-homogeneous and the duration of gestation counted from menstruation and femur length differs clearly from that estimated from BPD, further investigations are warranted.
- In the sagittal plane the profile of the foetal face, skull and nuchal area can be seen and encephalocoele can be ruled out.
- The spinal canal forms a zip-like structure and should be inspected for possible meningocoele. Additionally, a lemon-shaped skull indicates a neural tube defect.
- The neck region is examined for possible cysts and nuchal oedema. Every fourth foetus with abnormal nuchal translucency seen (on weeks 11–13) in subcutaneous tissue has a chromosomal deviation (most commonly trisomy, with 21 trisomy causing Down's syndrome being the most frequent finding). Nuchal translucency screening allows to detect up to 60–80% of foetuses with Down's syndrome (29.20).
- The scan is most reliable, when the fetal crown-rump length (CRL) is between 45 and 85 mm (gestational age 11–13 weeks). An analogue 95th percentile scale is used for an abnormal nuchal translucency (NT): the cut-off point for a 45 mm CRL fetus being 2.0 mm, for a 60 mm CRL fetus 2.5 mm and for a 85 mm CRL fetus 3.0 mm. A single cut-off point 2.5 mm is also widely used. The higher the NT, the greater is the risk for an abnormal karyotype.
- NT is measured from the inner edge of the skin to the outer edge of the underlying tissue, i.e. the shortest distance as possible. The best possible side profile and image magnification should be used.
- Strongly deflected fetal head can give a false positive finding. A loose amniotic membrane at the dorsal side of the fetus can also be a source for misinterpretation.
- Fetal nasal bone is possible to see during the same scan. If this can be seen, the risk for a trisomy 21 is very low.

2. The outline of the foetal body

- Any abnormality on the dorsal side is usually seen upon inspection of the spinal canal.
- In the ventral outline, attention should be paid to the insertion of the umbilical cord for possible omphalocele or gastrochisis in the abdominal wall.
- A greater magnification is used to look for sacral teratoma.
- Foetal body movement should be noted.

3. The thorax and heart

- In the transverse plane of the thorax the normal heart gives a four chambered view. The synchronized function of the atria, ventricles and valves should be noted. The heart is located near the midline and takes up about one third of the total area of the thoracic cavity.
- Small echo-dense spots (golf balls) in the area of the papillary muscles suggest a slightly increased risk of trisomy.
- The pulmonary tissue is homogenous in echodensity.
- The points of departure of the great vessels are difficult to distinguish before 20th WOP.

4. The abdominal cavity

- The ventricle forms an echo-free, bean-shaped structure beneath the diaphragm and this finding also indicates a patent oesophagus.
- Liver and kidneys are not easy to identify before 20 WOP. A fluid-filled bladder at the caudal end of the cavity indicates normal function of at least one kidney and ureter. If the bladder cannot be visualized but the amount of amniotic fluid is normal, control the finding.
- Fluid accumulation in the abdomen, other than the ventricle and bladder, indicate further investigation.
- Echo-dense intestines and/or mild pyelectasia suggest increased risk of trisomy.

5. The extremities

- In addition to biparietal length, the length of the femur is an important measure when determining gestational age on weeks 15–19 of pregnancy. A considerable discrepancy between these measures warrants further investigations.
- The outline of the limbs, hands and feet, the position of the wrists and ankles should be noted.
- Foetal body movement should be noted.

6. The placenta, umbilical cord and amniotic fluid

- A low-lying placenta is a common finding in early and mid-pregnancy. The position of the placenta needs to be determined on weeks 25–27. However, as the isthmic portion of the uterus usually grows more than the other parts, the placenta seems to "migrate" upwards.
- The identification of the lower end of the placenta is easier with full maternal bladder.
- A back-wall placenta is seen better with transvaginal ultrasound.
- In early pregnancy the amniotic fluid is formed by the amniotic membranes and the foetus can move freely in ample fluid.
- In mid- and late pregnancy the fluid results from foetal metabolism, predominantly urine. Severe oligohydramnios in mid-pregnancy, irrespective of the aetiology, is associated with poor prognosis due to the fact that a sufficient amount of amniotic fluid is essential for foetal pulmonary maturation.
- The amount of amniotic fluid is considered to be normal when the diameter of the deepest pocket measures 3–8 cm. Amniotic fluid index (AFI) is considered a more extensive measure of the amount of amniotic fluid. In this investigation the gestational sac is divided into four equal-sized blocks and the deepest pocket in each block is measured. AFI is the sum of these measures. On the second and third trimesters, AFI between 8 and 24 is regarded normal.
- An abnormal amount of amniotic fluid is an indication for further investigations.
- In a cross-section of a normal umbilical cord, three vessels can be seen. A single umbilical artery can be associated with other vascular (or urinary) anomalies and warrants careful examination of foetal structures.

7. The cervix

- In early and midpregnancy, the cervix is quite easy to see if the maternal bladder is full. If the length of the cervical canal is less than 30 mm, or the proximal part is dilated, cervical incompetence should be suspected.

8. Gender

- There are very few clinical indications for identifying foetal sex.
- Labia suggest a female foetus and echo-dense testes that have descended to the scrotum and penis suggest a male. Umbilical cord between the legs easily causes false interpretations of gender.

Ultrasound markers for trisomy in mid-pregnancy

- As single findings, the following markers increase the risk for trisomy only slightly. However, if two or more markers are present in one foetus, foetal karyotyping should be considered.
  - Plexus choroideus cysts
  - Flat profile
  - Echo-dense dots in the papillary muscles of the foetal heart ("golf balls")
  - Echo-dense intestine
  - Mild hydronephrosis
  - Growth retardation
  - Short femur
  - Umbilical cord cysts.

GYN

Foetal growth

- On the latter half of pregnancy the growth and development are followed up in addition to foetal structures.
- Routine ultrasound screening in late pregnancy is not necessary in low-risk pregnancies or without a clear target B [1].
- Rapidly growing BPD may suggest hydrocephalus and slowly growing microcephaly or some other CNS disease.
- Retarded growth of the foetal abdominal circumference with normally growing BPD is often a sign of impaired function of the placenta. Excessive growth of the body may suggest foetal hydrops.
- Retarded growth of the limbs warrants further investigations.

Estimation of weight

- Measurement of abdominal circumference is the most important parameter for weight estimation. This should be measured as symmetrically as possible from the plane of the foetal liver, sinum umbilicalis and ventricle. Several measurements should be made and the average should be used in the final estimation.
- Many programs give an estimate automatically on the basis of abdominal circumference and BPD.

- In the beginning of the third trimester, BPD correlates well with foetal weight, however, towards the end and, especially if foetal gigantism is suspected, femur length is a more accurate measure.
- In a large-sized foetus, small BPD and great abdominal circumference indicate an increased risk of getting stuck at the shoulders at birth.
- Before week 30, a weight estimate has little significance.

Presentation

- After the 35th WOP anything other than a cephalic presentation is an indication for an obstetric consultation.

Post-term pregnancy

- Decreasing amniotic fluid volume is considered to correlate better with deteriorating placental function than structural changes (calcification and lobularity) in the placenta.

Doppler ultrasound of the umbilical artery

- There is some evidence that doppler ultrasound of the umbilical artery may reduce perinatal deaths in risk pregnancies (B) [2 3].

References

1. Bricker L, Neilson JP. Routine ultrasound in late pregnancy (after 24 weeks gestation). Cochrane Database Syst Rev. 2004;(2):CD001451.
2. Goffinet F, Paris J, Nisand I, Breart G. Utilite clinique du doppler ombilical: resultats des essais controles en population a haut risque et a bas risque. Journal de Gynecologie, Obstetrique et Biologie de la Reproduction 1997;26:16–26.
3. The Database of Abstracts of Reviews of Effectiveness (University of York), Database no.: DARE-973300. In: The Cochrane Library, Issue 1, 2000. Oxford: Update Software.

26.5 Counselling and problems of breastfeeding

Editors

Principles

- Frequent breastfeeding on demand during the very first days is essential to successful breastfeeding: frequent breastfeeding promotes lactation.
- Some mothers are worried about the baby's intake of nutrition during the first days. Healthy babies are born with a "fluid load" and initial weight loss is natural. The neonate needs only very small portions: just what is obtained from the mother.
- Bottle-feeding during the first days will fill the baby's stomach too easily, which may reduce the eagerness to suckle, thus resulting reduction in lactation.
- Poor lactation can also be corrected later on by increasing the frequency of breastfeeding.

Breastfeeding counselling

- Breastfeeding support should be a part of routine health care provision (A) [1].

Good breastfeeding position

- There are many good positions for breastfeeding. The mother needs to be in a relaxed and comfortable position and the baby needs to get a good hold of the breast. Breastfeeding both sitting up and lying down should be practised from the start in order for the breasts to be emptied evenly.
- For the baby to get a good hold of the breast, he or she needs to be held closely (with the infant's belly against the mother's body).

Good sucking hold

- The baby has a firm hold of the breast and the areola is almost completely in the baby's mouth.
- Swallowing is both visible and audible.
- If the infant seems to want to feed almost continuously, the sucking hold should be checked. An ineffective hold will not stimulate the breast and the amounts of milk obtained remain small.

Dummy and feeding bottle

- It is advisable to avoid using dummies and feeding bottles, in particular during the first two weeks.
  - The child may begin to prefer the bottle, which yields milk more easily than the breast.
  - The manner of sucking may change and the skill of sucking the breast may become rusty.
  - Mothers with low and inverted nipples in particular should avoid using these "competitors".
- Once the infant masters sucking the breast and the amount of milk has been stabilized, a dummy may be given if the parents find it necessary.

Problems related to breastfeeding

Low nipples

- Showing the correct sucking hold and position is important. Various breastfeeding positions are worth trying; sometimes "under-the-arm-feeding" may help.

- The nipple may be stimulated either by twisting with the fingers or by means of a manual breast pump. Breast shields are useful to some mothers.
- Some milk may be pumped into the baby's mouth, so that the baby will not be so easily frustrated. Holding the baby against the chest skin to skin will help the baby to become acquainted with the breast and encourage him or her to try and grip the breast.

Abrasion of nipples

- The areolas may be abraded in particular at the beginning, making breastfeeding painful. The nipples may be treated with oily basic ointment after breastfeeding.
- The reason for this may be too long breastfeeding sessions. Some babies like to continue sucking for pleasure, and this should be discouraged if the breasts do not tolerate it. Breastfeeding sessions of 15 to 20 minutes are enough to provide sufficient nutrition, and breastfeeding may be stopped by inserting the little finger between the breast and the baby's upper gingiva.

Engorgement of the breast and duct blockades

- The breasts may become engorged within 1 to 3 days of delivery due to milk production.
  - Frequent breastfeeding started during the infant's first 24 hours and a correct breastfeeding position prevent breast engorgement due to swelling.
  - The treatment includes emptying of the breast, either by breastfeeding or by pumping as often as possible. Pumping just 5 to 10 ml relieves tightness of the breast and the infant can get a better hold of the breast.
  - A damp, cool gauze cloth may alleviate tightness.
  - The breasts are pumped by hand.
- Later on, engorgement may be related to the baby's ineffective sucking, infrequent breastfeeding sessions, stress, tight clothing or abundant lactation.
  - A warm shower or a warm bandage will help to induce the oxytocin reflex. Mild massage of the breast will do the same.
  - Breastfeeding as often as the infant will suckle.
  - If the baby is unable to suck, the breast should be emptied manually or by means of a breast pump. Even pumping small amounts may help the situation so that the infant is able to get hold of the breast and suck.

Mastitis

- See 25.22.

Neonatal breast milk jaundice

- In some breastfed babies, breast milk jaundice may occur even after the neonatal period.
- These infants are in a good condition and alert.
- Jaundice is due to competition of breast milk with the excretion of bilirubin.
- This breast milk jaundice is not harmful and, therefore, breastfeeding should not be discontinued.
- Infections and other general illnesses of the infant should, however, be excluded (at least midstream-urine, CRP).

Breast rejection (sucking strike)

- Reasons for rejection of the breast and treatment suggestions:
  - The baby is ill. If the baby is unable to suck, the mother should resort to pumping.
  - Nasal congestion → Instil drops of physiological saline in the nostrils.
  - Mouth tenderness → Check the mouth and treat any candidiasis. Teething may cause tenderness; in this case, administration of pumped milk can be tried.

Difficulties in sucking technique may be due to various reasons

- Use of dummy and feeding bottle.
- The baby is not allowed to suck freely, for example the mother interferes by guiding from the back of the head, the sucking hold is not correct or the breastfeeding time is limited → counselling of the mother.
- Scanty lactation → Frequent breastfeeding sessions.
  - How is the mother? → Ask about her rest, eating, drinking.
- Too abundant lactation
  - The baby sucks frequently but ineffectively, resulting in increased amount of milk → Empty the breast a little by pumping before breastfeeding and teach a correct sucking hold.
  - Suggest that the mother start to donate breast milk. The location of the closest breast milk centre is given.
  - Lactation is tapered: only one breast is given to the baby and about 20 ml less than on the previous day's sessions is pumped from the other breast.

GYN

Reference

1. Sikorski J, Renfrew M J, Pindoria S, Wade A. Support for breastfeeding mothers. Cochrane Database Syst Rev. 2004;(2):CD001141.

26.10 Ectopic pregnancy

Juha Mäkinen

Basic rule

- Always suspect an ectopic pregnancy in a woman of fertile age with pains in the lower part of the abdomen and/or abnormal bleeding, if a pregnancy is possible at all (regardless of the method of contraception).

Epidemiology

- The highest incidence is in women aged 25–34 years.
- In the 1980s a large increase in incidence was reported in Western countries, associated with pelvic inflammatory disease (PID) and subsequent infertility, the large post-World War II birth cohorts, increased use of intrauterine devices, improved diagnosis, and increased use of infertility treatment.
- By the 1990s the incidence had fallen.
- In 1994 the incidence was 155/100 000 women between the ages of 15 and 44 (or 2.8/100 deliveries, 2.0/100 pregnancies), and in 2000 only 84/100 000 women, in Finland.

Location

- Most (98%) occur in the uterine tube. Abdominal, ovarian and cervical pregnancies are very rare.

Risk factors

- Previous PID
- Previous operation on the uterine tube
- Previous ectopic pregnancy
- Use of copper intrauterine device (IUD) (not hormonal IUD) C [1 2]
- A history of infertility and treatment of infertility (e.g. IVF)
- (Endometriosis)
- (Anomalies)

Complications

- An actively growing pregnancy mass may rupture (by week 10 of the pregnancy at the latest) causing a life-threatening haemorrhage into the abdominal cavity.
- A so-called persistent ectopic pregnancy begins to grow after management.

Symptoms

- Abnormal bleeding (the amount varies) and/or pains in the lower part of the abdomen. The patient does not necessarily have a clear amenorrhoea (e.g. IUD patients).
- Nowadays most patients have only slight symptoms (no acute risk of shock), because the patients present early for examination and treatment.
- If the pregnancy focus bursts and causes bleeding in the abdominal cavity, the patient often faints at home or work.
- Shoulder pain in severe cases.

Diagnosis

- In cases of bleeding and pains, first check whether the patient is pregnant.
    - It is recommended that serum is used for the pregnancy test.
    - The most sensitive tests (hCG 10–20 IU/ml) are positive as early as one week before menstruation stops.
    - A urine pregnancy test is less sensitive: a positive result is significant, but a negative one does not eliminate an ectopic pregnancy with certainty.
    - On clinical examination
        - See Figure 26.10.1
        - Vaginal discharge does not contain remnants of tissue, the external os of the uterus is closed, and usually the uterus is not enlarged (as in spontaneous abortion).
        - Pain on palpation and muscle guarding suggest a serious condition
        - (Elevated pulse and/or low blood pressure suggest also a serious condition).
- When the pregnancy test is positive the location of the pregnancy is confirmed by ultrasound:
    - Examination with a vaginal probe at around 41 days after the last menstruation (the menstruation being about 2 weeks late) confirms an intrauterine pregnancy (the heart beat can be seen intrauterinally) with almost 100% certainty.
- Together, the quantitative level of hCG and an ultrasounds scan help in the differential diagnosis:
    - When the hCG level in the serum rises above 1 000 IU/ml and no intrauterine pregnancy can be detected by ultrasound an ectopic pregnancy is approximately 95% certain.
- With a good ultrasound device an experienced gynaecologist may detect an ectopic pregnancy in up to 90% of the cases. If the ultrasound does not verify the diagnosis, the location, size and nature of the ectopic pregnancy are in general confirmed by laparoscopy (risk of rupture).

Treatment

- Patients in poor condition (at risk of shock) are immediately put on an i.v. drip. When the haemodynamics allow, they are quickly operated on. Nowadays only 5% need a laparotomy because of severe haemoperitoneum.
- The patient's own decision, as well as the size and the nature of the pregnancy, affect the choice between surgical treatment and other treatment. The final decision is most often made in laparoscopy.
    - **Radical treatment** (extirpation of the uterine tube) is advisable if the uterine tube is badly ruptured, the extrauterine pregnancy has recurred in the same place, the patient is not planning further pregnancies (it is possible to carry out sterilization at the same time), the pregnancy has started after sterilization, or IVF treatment is currently used or planned.
    - **Conservative surgical treatments** can be performed laparoscopically if the patient wants to become pregnant in the future and a sparing operation is technically possible C [3 4]. The most common of these is tubal section (salpingostomy).

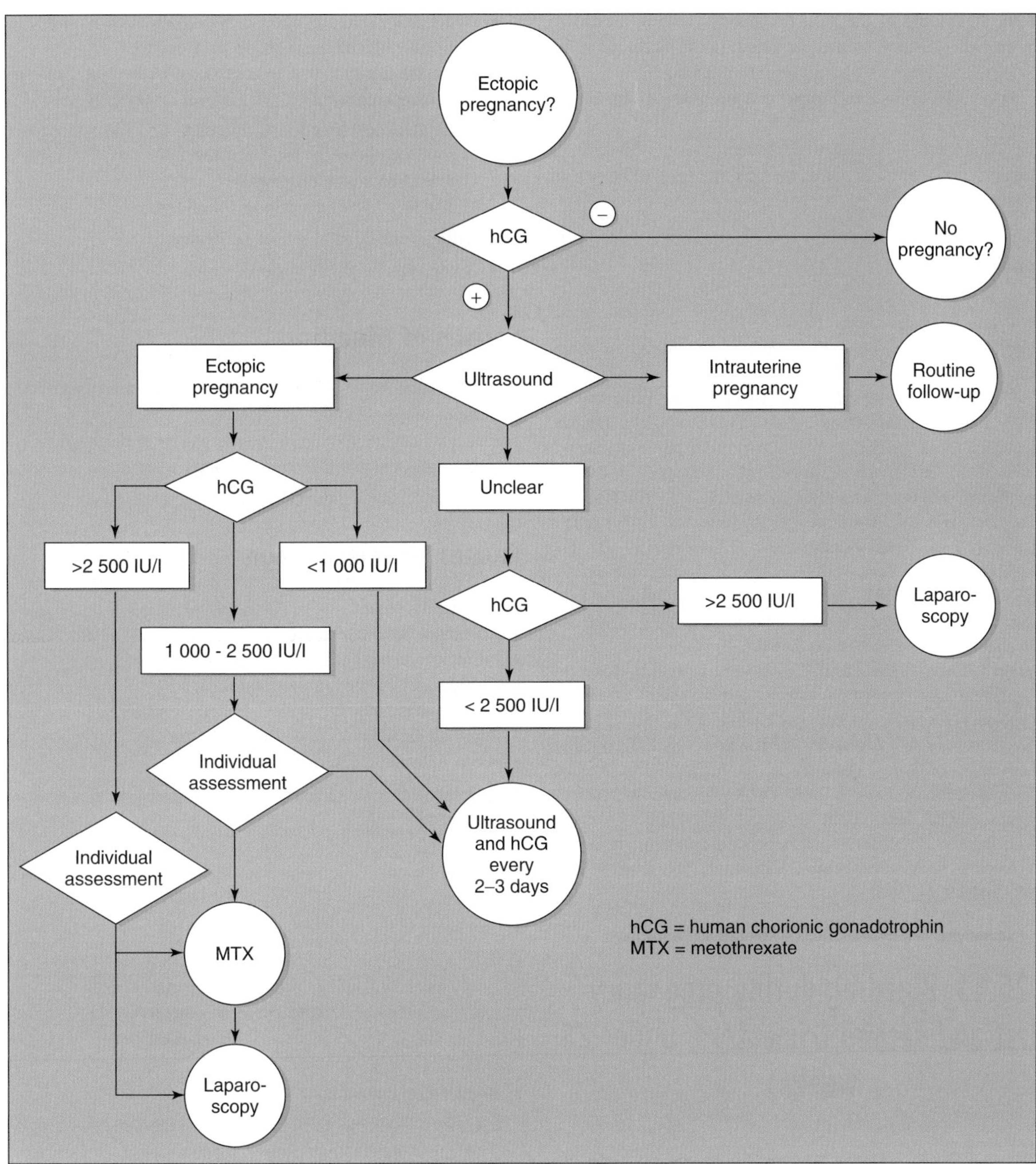

Figure 26.10.1

- **Medicines** can induce resorption of the pregnancy tissue. The best results (>90%) have been achieved with methotrexate injected laparoscopically into the pregnancy sac. Methotrexate can also be given systematically intramuscularly C [5] [6] [7] together with folic acid as a treatment in series or as one single treatment. 70–90% of ectopic pregnancies have been managed successfully with a single i.m. injection of methotrexate. The outcome is better if the serum hCG level is low C [8].
- In some cases (18–33%) mere **follow-up** is sufficient (low level of hCG, small pregnancy focus). Then the decrease in hCG level must be confirmed by repeated measurements, and the patient must be followed up by a doctor.

Further treatment and prognosis

- The final effect of conservative treatments is confirmed by follow-up of hCG (ad < 10 IU/l).
- If hCG falls slowly or there is a suspicion that the primary treatment has failed, methotrexate can be given i.m. as a booster.

- At the beginning of the next pregnancy there is a need to confirm the location of the pregnancy at an early stage by hCG measurement and transvaginal ultrasound.
- A copper IUD is not recommended because of the risk of recurrence.
- The prognosis for further pregnancies is good with a conservative operation and/or medical treatment; the risk of recurrence is 5–15%.

References

1. Mol BW, Ankum WM, Bossuyt PM, van der Veen F. Contraception and the risk of ectopic pregnancy: a meta-analysis. Contraception 1995;52:337–341.
2. The Database of Abstracts of Reviews of Effectiveness (University of York), Database no.: DARE-960198. In: The Cochrane Library, Issue 4, 1999. Oxford: Update Software.
3. Clausen I. Conservative versus radical surgery for tubal pregnancy: a review. Acta Obst Gynecol Scand 1996;75:8–12.
4. The Database of Abstracts of Reviews of Effectiveness (University of York), Database no.: DARE-960339. In: The Cochrane Library, Issue 4, 1999. Oxford: Update Software.
5. Hajenius PJ, Mol BWJ, Bossuyt PMM, Ankum WM, Van der Veen F. Interventions for tubal ectopic pregnancy. Cochrane Database Syst Rev. 2004;(2):CD000324.
6. Parker J, Bisits A, Proietto AM. A systematic review of single-dose intramuscular methotrexate for the treatment of ectopic pregnancy. Aust N Z J Obst Gyn 1998;38:145–150.
7. The Database of Abstracts of Reviews of Effectiveness (University of York), Database no.: DARE-981085. In: The Cochrane Library, Issue 2, 2000. Oxford: Update Software.
8. Lipscomb GH, McCord ML, Stovall TG, Huff G, Portera SG, Ling FW. Predictors of success of methotrexate treatment in women with tubal ectopic pregnancy. N Engl J Med 1999;341:1974–1978.

26.11 Bleeding during pregnancy (first and second trimesters, under 28 weeks)

Mika Nuutila

Basic rules

- The borderline between when to refer patients to a gynaecology outpatient clinic and when to refer them to an obstetric outpatient clinic is agreed locally.
- Bleeding before 22nd week of pregnancy
  - Consider rest, if bleeding is minimal and contractions are few. The usefulness of rest is not proven. Ultrasound is performed, if possible (a living foetus is a good prognostic sign).
  - Acute referral to a gynaecology outpatient clinic is needed if profuse bleeding or severe pain occurs.
  - Refer the patient to a gynaecology outpatient clinic the next working day if
    - spontaneous abortion is complete and the patient is in good condition and has not fever
    - a dead foetus is observed
    - bleeding increases during follow-up.
- Bleeding after 22nd week of pregnancy
  - Acute referral to an obstetric clinic.

Causes of bleeding

- Miscarriage
- Ectopic pregnancy (26.13)
- Placental causes (placenta previa, placental detachment)
- Vaginal or cervical infections, polyps or damage
- Trophoblastic disease (hydatid mole)

Causes of miscarriage

- Foetal abnormalities
- Chromosomal abnormalities
- Immunological rejection
- Uterine and cervical abnormalities
- Endocrinological imbalance, diabetes and hyperthyroidism, impaired function of the corpus luteum
- Viral infections, listeriosis, toxoplasmosis
- An intrauterine pregnancy sac but no foetus (blighted ovum, or ovum abortivum)

Status

- General condition
  - If you suspect a feverish infection or the patient has bled profusely, immediately refer the patient to a gynaecological department as an emergency. If necessary, measure body temperature, blood pressure, pulse (blood picture and C-reactive protein).
- Gynaecological status
  - Uterus: Does the size correlate with the number of weeks of pregnancy? Tenderness? Contractions? Is the length of the cervix decreased or is the cervix dilated? Is there bleeding, and is it profuse?
  - Foetus: Can you see the foetus or is it already expelled? If the cervix is not dilated, can you hear heart sounds (after the 12th week of pregnancy) or can you observe the heart function with ultrasound or palpate movements (after weeks 16–18 of pregnancy)?

Threat of miscarriage (abortus imminens)

- Minimal vaginal bleeding and pains. Good general condition. The size of the uterus is increased and the cervix is

not dilated. Heart function can be observed by doppler or ultrasound.
- Repeat ultrasound after 1–2 weeks.
- Investigate for chlamydia or gonorrhoea if necessary (part of the examination routine in many maternal care centres).
- Rest may be indicated, and physical exertion should be avoided. Sick leave may be necessary.
- Advise the patient to avoid sexual intercourse (could act as a local stimulus).
- As the efficacy of drug treatment is poorly verified, do not prescribe betasympathomimetics routinely.

Missed abortion (abortus inhibitus)

- The foetus is dead and begins to be resorbed but the uterus remains closed with the foetus inside. The patient feels a weight in the pelvic region. The size of the uterus is not increased. Blood is present as a brownish and watery discharge. Missed abortion can usually be diagnosed by ultrasound early in the pregnancy (usually <12th week).
- Referral to hospital the next working day for vacuum evacuation B [1] and abrasion.

Miscarriage (abortus incipiens: incompletus, completus)

- Miscarriage is inevitable (incipiens), and the cervix is open. Bleeding is often profuse, and there are cramps in the lower abdomen while the uterus contracts. Blood clots may come out.
- Loss of the foetus is observed by ultrasound.
- If bleeding is profuse, insert an intravenous drip and arrange patient transportation to a hospital.
- Treatment consists of vacuum evacuation and abrasion of the uterus. Expectant management is a good option B [2 3 4].
- Miscarriage is complete (completus), when the uterus is totally empty. In this case curettage is seldom needed. The practice is agreed locally.
- Miscarriage is incomplete (incompletus) when not all pregnancy tissue has been expelled from the uterine cavity. In case of slight bleeding the patient may be referred to hospital on the following day for curettage.

Septic miscarriage

- Caused by microbes passing from the vagina to the uterus. Usually the result of incompletely induced abortion in unsterile conditions. Profuse bleeding and pain often occur, possibly with symptoms of toxic shock. The most common causative organisms are E. coli and Streptococcus faecalis.
- Acute referral to hospital. May need treatment for sepsis.

Recurrent miscarriage (abortus habitualis)

- Three or more spontaneous miscarriages. Women wishing to conceive can be referred for further investigations at an earlier stage (26.12).

Risk of preterm delivery (>22nd gestational week)

- In cases of mild contractions, follow-up, rest and leave from work when needed (at least from physical work) are usually sufficient.
- Acute referral to a prenatal clinic (26.13) is needed if
  - regular or painful contractions occur
  - the cervix is dilated or shortened
  - the presenting part is low in the delivery channel
  - the membranes bulge out
  - blood and mucus are present.

References

1. Forna F, Gülmezoglu AM. Surgical procedures to evacuate incomplete abortion. Cochrane Database Syst Rev. 2004;(2):CD001993.
2. Geyman JP, Oliver LM, Sullivan SD. Expectant, medical, or surgical treatment of spontaneous abortion in first trimester of pregnancy: a pooled quantitative literature evaluation. Journal of the American Board of Family Practice 1999;12:55–64.
3. The Database of Abstracts of Reviews of Effectiveness (University of York), Database no.: DARE-993574. In: The Cochrane Library, Issue 1, 2002. Oxford: Update Software.
4. Luise C, Jermy K, May C, Costello G, Collins WP, Bourne TH. Outcome of expectant management of spontaneous first trimester miscarriage: observational study. BMJ 2002;324:873–5.

GYN

26.12 Recurrent miscarriage

Eero Varila

Basic rules

- At least three miscarriages in succession is defined as recurrent miscarriage. This is the latest time to start investigations to find the cause.
- Investigate even earlier in cases where there is a high risk of recurrence or if the pregnancy started after assisted fertilization.

Epidemiology

- A casual abortion occurs in 15–20% of pregnancies.
- Recurrent miscarriage is experienced by 0.4–1% of fertile-aged women.
- The risk of recurrence is not increased after one miscarriage. After two miscarriages the risk is 17–35% and after three it is 25–49%.
- 75% of miscarriages occur before the 13th gestational week.
- 77% of miscarriages are ovum abortivum pregnancies.

Causes of recurrent abortion

- Unknown (37–79%)
- Genetic error (6–60%)
- Endocrinological disturbance (impaired function of the corpus luteum, diabetes, impaired thyroid function) (8–35%)
- Immunological cause (1–40%)
- Anatomical abnormality (uterine anomaly, myoma, polyp, syndrome of Asherman) (2–15%)

Investigations

- Recurrent miscarriages are stressful both physically and mentally. The aim is to clarify the causes and possible treatments and estimate the chance of succeeding with the next pregnancy. Otherwise the couple might not dare to try again.
- There is no evidence-based knowledge about effect of investigations and treatments. The following strategy is the author's own:
  - Investigation or careful follow-up is always needed when there is a clinical impression of a surprising miscarriage (e.g. if a living, healthy-looking foetus was observed by ultrasound).
  - After two miscarriages the next pregnancy should be followed early and carefully, preferably from the 6th gestational week. This is the only way to observe the development of the amniotic sac, embryo, etc.
  - At the latest after a third miscarriage the appropriate investigations should be performed.
- **History**
  - Diseases, especially endocrinological and autoimmune
  - On what week did the miscarriage occur? Early abortion suggests a genetic problem, which is difficult to treat; a later miscarriage may be easier to manage.
  - Was it an ovum abortivum pregnancy or was the foetus observed? If a living foetus was observed, it might be useful to perform the investigations that are possible in the primary health care centre, already after one miscarriage.
  - Have there been miscarriages or developmental abnormalities in the family?
- **Clinical examination**
  - Physical examination to identify underlying diseases, particularly endocrinological and autoimmune diseases.
  - Gynaecological examination: palpation, infections; at a specialist clinic ultrasound and hysteroscopy
- **Laboratory tests**
  - Thyroid function at the primary health care centre
  - In secondary care, chromosome analyses from the blood (both parents), phospholipid antibodies in the serum and a test for factor V mutation.

Treatment

- Usually there is no treatment. The prognosis is good: the probability of delivering a healthy child is over 50% even without treatment.
- There is no treatment for genetic disorders and chromosomal abnormalities. In vitro fertilization makes it possible to choose the embryos that are transferred into the uterus. With the development of preimplantation diagnostics it is possible to investigate the chromosomes of the embryo in this phase and to transfer into the uterus an embryo that has normal chromosomes.
- Organic abnormalities in the uterus such as polyps or partition are treated by hysteroscopy. Laparotomy is rarely needed.
- There are no good randomized controlled trials for treatment of impaired function of the corpus luteum. Natural progestogen has been used at 300–600 mg per day for 10 days after ovulation or sometimes even up to the 10th gestational week. Placental gonadothropin (hCG) is also used.
- In cases of autoimmune disease (especially with phospholipid antibodies) prednisone (30–60 mg/day), acetylsalicylic acid (75–225 mg/day) and heparin (5 000 IU twice a day) has been given from the detection of pregnancy until delivery. Intravenous immunoglobulin has also been used. Randomized controlled trials on these therapies are needed.

26.13 Threatening premature labour

Editors

Imminent premature labour

- The likelihood of premature labour becomes greater when several of the following signs can be identified. (Signs 1–3 are the easiest to identify and, when seen together, often indicate the start of actual premature labour.):
  - Regular uterine contractions less than 10 minutes apart.
  - The contractions are painful.
  - The cervix is ripe and at least 1–2 cm dilated.

- The cervix is shortened or effaced.
- The presenting part of the foetus has descended to the spinous stage or even lower.
- Bulging of foetal membranes is diagnosed.
- Light bleeding takes place.

- Irregular and weak uterine contractions are common during normal pregnancy.
- Inhibition of premature labour is usually not needed if the duration of pregnancy is at least 35 weeks (limit of full-term pregnancy is 37 weeks).

Inhibition of premature labour

- Bed rest
- Pharmaceutical treatment
  - Atosiban is an oxytocin receptor antagonist that competes with oxytocin for the receptors in the myometrium.
  - A single bolus injection of 6.75 mg over 1 min is sufficient for transferring the woman to a maternity hospital.
  - Betasympathomimetics, e.g. 10 mg of ritodrine hydrochoride intramuscularly have been used, but it has not been shown to improve perinatal outcome C [1 2].
  - Alternatives to betamimetics are prostaglandin synthase inhibitors such as sulindac, 200 mg tablets given twice in 24 hours. PG-inhibitors are only recommended before 32 weeks of pregnancy and the duration of treatment should not exceed 48–72 hours. PG-inhibitors may induce contraction and closure of the foetal ductus arteriosus.

Treatment of immature foetal lungs with corticosteroids

- Corticosteroids should be used to increase the synthesis of surfactant in foetal lungs on weeks 24–34 of pregnancy A [3]. If considered necessary the treatment can be started already on week 22.
  - 12 mg betamethasone is given intramuscularly and the dose is repeated after 24 hours. This treatment has no risks, even if the pregnancy continues uneventfully. An obstetrician may be consulted regarding this treatment. Other corticosteroids can also be used.

Transport to hospital

- The mother is transported to hospital in a lateral lying position, especially if the foetal membranes are ruptured and there is a risk of protrusion of the umbilical cord.

References

1. Gyetvai K, Hannah ME, Hodnett ED, Ohlssson A. Tocolytics for preterm labour: a systematic review. Obstetrics and Gynecology 1999;94:869–877.
2. The Database of Abstracts of Reviews of Effectiveness (University of York), Database no.: DARE-992142. In: The Cochrane Library, Issue 1, 2001. Oxford: Update Software.
3. Crowley P. Prophylactic corticosteroids for preterm birth. Cochrane Database Syst Rev. 2004;(2):CD000065.

26.14 Pregnancy and blood pressure

Anneli Kivijärvi

Aims

- Detect pre-eclampsia as early as possible.
- Follow up pregnancy-induced hypertension carefully.
- Follow up a pregnant woman with pre-existing hypertension with care.

Definitions

- High blood pressure during pregnancy is defined as pressure > 140/90 or an increase in systolic pressure > 30 mmHg or an increase in diastolic pressure > 15 mmHg.
- Hypertension is chronic when the pressure is increased before pregnancy or before the 20th gestational week.
- Gestational hypertension occurs after the 20th gestational week.
- The definition of pre-eclampsia includes both increased blood pressure and proteinuria simultaneously after the 20th gestational week.
- Proteinuria (0.3 g/day) may occur in normal pregnancy; however, for the diagnosis of pre-eclampsia proteinuria must be 0.5 g/day.
- At the onset of pre-eclampsia there may be a phase when the kidneys are not yet damaged and the blood pressure is increased without proteinuria.
- Associated pre-eclampsia occurs when chronic hypertension is accompanied by proteinuria after the 20th gestational week.

General points

- Detection of pre-eclampsia as early as possible is the most important aim of prenatal care.
- Hypertension in pregnancy is a major cause of maternal morbidity and perinatal morbidity and mortality.
- The risk of perinatal death is clearly higher in second or further pregnancies of mothers with pre-existing hypertension who develop attached pre-eclampsia than primigravidas who develop pre-eclampsia without earlier hypertension.

GYN

Blood pressure during pregnancy

- In normal pregnancy systolic blood pressure remains slightly below the level before pregnancy most of the time.
- Diastolic blood pressure remains below the level before pregnancy until the last trimester when it reaches the prepregnancy level.
- Blood pressure decreases moderately in the second trimester in almost half of all gravidas.
- This physiological change is not easily detected in prenatal care, and in most cases blood pressure seems to rise mildly and evenly throughout pregnancy.

Follow up of blood pressure in prenatal care

- It is important to monitor the level initially and the direction of changes during pregnancy.
- Blood pressure must be measured at every visit; it can rise very quickly in a short time.
- It should be measured from a bare right upper arm after a rest of at least 15 minutes; for obese patients a mantle long and wide enough should be chosen.
- For tense mothers, recommend using a meter at home: it helps if more intensive follow up is needed when the blood pressure is over 140/90 mmHg or the mother is at risk.
- In the second trimester diastolic pressure > 85 mmHg is a risk factor.
- Raised blood pressure at night suggests increased risk.
- Estimate the risk of high blood pressure and pre-eclampsia at the beginning of pregnancy.
- In cases of increased risk, follow-up must be intensified after the 20th gestational week (a 4-week interval is too long!).

Risk factors for pre-eclampsia

- First pregnancy
- Multiple foetuses
- Pre-eclampsia in the family
- Age < 20 years or >40 years
- Obesity
- Chronic hypertension
- Diabetes
- Chronic nephropathy

Follow up of proteinuria

- The urine is tested for albumin at every visit.
- Teach patients with elevated blood pressure how to test their urine at home with dipsticks after the 24th gestational week (1–3 times per week depending on the situation).

Other laboratory tests (at prenatal outpatient clinics)

- Haematocrit
- Haemoglobin
- Serum ALT
- Platelets
- Blood urea nitrogen
- The haematocrit might rise due to haemoconcentration associated with pre-eclampsia.
- An increase in transaminases, a decrease in platelets and a rise in blood urea nitrogen suggest an abnormal condition.

Treatment of blood pressure during pregnancy

- Salt restriction and rest
- Antihypertensives are prescribed when the diastolic pressure is 100 mmHg or more (A) [1].
- In cases of diabetes or disease of the kidneys medication is often prescribed at lower blood pressures.
- Treatment is prescribed after specialist consultation.
- None of the treatments used increase foetal blood circulation. A large decrease in blood pressure might impair uterine circulation (B) [2 3]. The chosen drug must be safe for the foetus.
- Labetalol (an alpha-beta-blocker) (C) [4] is commonly used in doses of 100–400 mg three times a day.
- ISA-blockers (B) [5 6 7], nifedipine (C) [4], clonidine, verapamil or prazosine can be used.
- Avoid ACE-blockers, diuretics, reserpine and diazoxide (C) [4].
- Calcium supplementation is beneficial for women at high risk of gestational hypertension (A) [8].

Prophylaxis of pre-eclampsia

- Mini-ASA (50–75 mg/day) starting at the end of the first trimester for a gravida in the risk group might improve the prognosis of the foetus (A) [9].

Referral to prenatal outpatient clinics

- Refer for pregnancy planning those who suffer from chronic renal disease, severe hypertension or hypertension of nephrological origin.
- Refer those with pre-existing hypertension preferably in early pregnancy for estimation of need for medication.
- Refer those whose blood pressure is raised before the 24th gestational week for differential diagnosis between essential and secondary hypertension as early as possible.
- Refer as acute cases patients with hypertension and pre-eclampsia when symptoms ares seen (26.1).

References

1. Abalos E, Duley L, Steyn DW, Henderson-Smart DJ. Antihypertensive drug therapy for mild to moderate hypertension during pregnancy. Cochrane Database Syst Rev. 2004;(2):CD002252.

2. von Dadelszen P, Ornstein MP, Bull SB, Logan AG, Koren G, Magee LA. Fall in mean arterial pressure and fetal growth restriction in pregnancy hypertension: a meta-analysis. Lancet 2000, 355, 87–92.
3. The Database of Abstracts of Reviews of Effectiveness (University of York), Database no.: DARE-20008014. In: The Cochrane Library, Issue 2, 2002. Oxford: Update Software.
4. Duley L, Henderson-Smart DJ. Drugs for treatment of very high blood pressure during pregnancy. Cochrane Database Syst Rev. 2004;(2):CD001449.
5. Magee LA, Duley L. Oral beta-blockers for mild to moderate hypertension during pregnancy. Cochrane Database Syst Rev. 2004;(2):CD002863.
6. Magee LA, Elran E, Bull SB, Logan A, Koren B. Risks and benefits of beta-receptor blockers for pregnancy hypertension: overview of the randomized trials. European Journal of Obstetrics, Gynecology, and Reproductive Biology 2000:88;15–26.
7. The Database of Abstracts of Reviews of Effectiveness (University of York), Database no.: DARE-2000. In: The Cochrane Library, Issue 1, 2002. Oxford: Update Software.
8. Atallah AN, Hofmeyr GJ, Duley L. Calcium supplementation during pregnancy for preventing hypertensive disorders and related problems. Cochrane Database Syst Rev. 2004;(2):CD001059.
9. Duley L, Henderson-Smart DJ, Knight M, King JF. Antiplatelet agents for preventing pre-eclampsia and its complications (Cochrane Review). In: The Cochrane Library, Issue 1, 2004. The Cochrane Database of Systematic Reviews: CD004659. Chichester, UK: John Wiley & Sons, Ltd.

26.15 Systemic diseases in pregnancy

Seppo Saarikoski

General

- Poorly treated or untreated systemic disease impairs fertility; adequate management effectively restores fertility.
- Preconception examination and counselling by both the specialist treating the systemic disease and an obstetrician is essential for assessing individual risks of pregnancy and delivery.
- Systemic disease must be monitored closely throughout gestation in a high-risk pregnancy. Good collaboration between the prenatal clinic and maternity hospital is essential.

Heart and vascular diseases

- Cardiac output begins to rise during the first trimester of pregnancy and increases by 30–50%. This means an increased circulatory burden for the heart. Both heart rate and stroke volume increase, and peripheral vascular resistance falls.
- The ability of the cardiovascular system to react to physical strain is limited, especially during the third trimester.
- The axis of the heart shifts horizontally and slightly to the left because of the rise of the diaphragm, increasing the tendency of ectopic beats.
- During pregnancy the uterus causes obstruction of the vena cava in the supine position. This diminishes venous return. Therefore, a pregnant woman must be placed in a left lateral recumbent position for every examination or treatment that lasts for long.

Hypertension

- See 26.14 and 26.1.
- Arterial blood pressure does normally not exceed 140/90 mmHg in pregnancy.
- Hypertension during pregnancy is associated with pre-eclampsia in 70% of patients, and chronic hypertension in 30% of patients.
- The incidence of chronic hypertension in Northern Europe is about 2–4%. The risk of hypertension increases after the age of 30 years.
- Foetal risks are connected with chronic placental insufficiency, e.g. small-for-gestational-age newborn and foetal hypoxia. The maternal risks in very severe hypertension are circulatory brain disturbances, heart failure and complications resulting from superimposed pre-eclampsia.
- A slight or moderate rise of arterial blood pressure without albuminuria is not an indication of high risk. Close monitoring of the pregnancy in the outpatient clinic of the maternity hospital is important. If albuminuria occurs, the expectant mother must be admitted to the hospital.
- Most antihypertensive drugs are also useful during pregnancy. Of all the adrenergic beta-receptor blocking agents, labetolol is the most used and is the drug of choice. Atenolol can cause foetal growth retardation. Nifedipine is useful.
- ACE-blocking agents are forbidden during pregnancy. They can increase the risk of foetal malformations. They also inhibit normal gestational development of the vascular system. Diuretic drugs are also not recommended because decreased plasma volume is associated with chronic hypertension and especially with pre-eclampsia.

Heart diseases

- The increased load of pregnancy is most serious in connection with a pressure load, for example in mitral stenosis, but also in congenital heart diseases with hypoxia. Mothers with mitral stenosis have an increased risk for atrial flimmer and acute failure in the form of pulmonary oedema.
- Maternal mortality risk in cases of Marfan's syndrome as well as in Eisenmenger's syndrome and in cardiomyopathy is about 50%.
- Obstetric patients with heart disease are not at risk if the functional capacity of the heart is classified into NYHA Classes I or II (4.72).
- Maternal mortality in cases of NYHA Class III–IV heart disease is about 10%, especially if a full assessment of

cardiac status and medical management was not performed prior to the pregnancy. The risk level is the same in pregnancy after myocardial infarction.

- Medical treatment is chosen according to the cardiac disease and the condition of the patient.

Thrombotic complications

- The risk of recurrence of deep vein thrombosis or pulmonary embolism increases greatly during pregnancy.
- As basic laboratory tests, AT_{III}, protein-C and protein-S, as well as APTT, are needed to detect lupus anticoagulant syndrome.
- When earlier deep vein thrombosis or pulmonary embolism was associated with a lack of AT_{III}, protein-C or protein-S, thrombosis prophylaxis has to be started on gestational week 6, and continued throughout pregnancy until 3 months since delivery. AT_{III} concentrate is also useful during labour.
- If an earlier thrombosis has occurred without a lack of AT_{III}, protein-C or protein-S, the prophylactic treatment is started on gestational weeks 20–24 and ended 6–12 weeks after delivery.
- The drug of choice is low molecular weight heparin administered once daily C [1 2]. Monitoring of the treatment is not needed. After the 24th week of gestation a double dose is needed as also when the mother weighs more than 75 kg.
- Subcutaneous heparin as a dose of 75 000–125 000 IU can also be used, its use has declined. This treatment needs normal monitoring. Both low molecular weight heparin and subcutaneous heparin treatment have to be stopped for the time of labour, 12 hours before induction of labour.
- Warfarin is known as a teratogenic agent. Therefore, it is not useful in thrombosis prophylaxis during pregnancy except in patients with a cardiac prosthetic valve.

Metabolic disorders

Diabetes

- The number of mothers with impaired glucose tolerance is about 10-fold higher than that of women with type 1 diabetes.
- Pregnancy complicated by insulin-dependent diabetes is one of the most important risk groups in obstetrics today. Due to the low number of cases, diabetic control should be concentrated at university and central hospitals.
- Diabetes involves an increased risk of malformation but this may be reduced by good periconceptional glucose balance. Cooperation between obstetricians and internists throughout pregnancy is important.
- Careful monitoring at the prenatal clinic continues from the first trimester of pregnancy at 1–2 week intervals and a short stay in the antenatal ward of the obstetric department according to an individual plan is indicated for every patient.
- The maternal risks later in pregnancy are renal failure, disturbances in glucose balance, aggravation of diabetic retinopathy, increased risk of pre-eclampsia and polyhydramnios. The foetal risks are malformations, spontaneous abortion and premature labour, intrauterine death, macrosomia with shoulder dystocia and Erb's paresis. Neonatal adaptation problems are increased, including hypoglycaemia, hypocalcaemia, hyperbilirubinaemia and respiratory distress syndrome.
- Insulin therapy is given as a multi-injection treatment. Peroral treatment with an antidiabetic drugs is not possible because of foetal malformation risk.
- Very tight diabetic control may lead to maternal hypoglycaemia and is no more effective than tight control of diabetes during pregnancy C [3].
- Vaginal delivery is planned near to term if obstetrically possible. Indications for Caesarean section are obstetric, such as pelvic disproportion, foetal distress in the first stage of labour, worsening pre-eclampsia, and abnormal foetal presentation. Maternal proliferative retinopathy and renal failure are also indications for Caesarean section.

Hypothyroidism

- Untreated hypothyroidism causes reduced fertility and increases risk of miscarriage.
- Thyroxine is needed throughout pregnancy, usually in a higher dosage than before pregnancy. Biochemical monitoring is essential: TSH, free thyroxine, T_4, and T_3.
- Therapeutic balance is estimated before conception, during the first prenatal visit and possibly also in gestational weeks 16–20 and 28–32. Slight hyperthyroidism is not dangerous for the foetus or the mother. After an operation for thyroid gland cancer, TSH concentrations must remain undetectable.
- After delivery, thyroid substitution therapy can be reduced into the pregestational level.

Hyperthyroidism

- Undiagnosed and untreated hyperthyroidism may cause a spontaneous abortion or premature labour.
- Hyperthyroidism is difficult to identify in pregnancy because many of the symptoms and signs are similar to the changes in normal pregnancy (tachycardia, anxiety, peripheral vasodilatation, goitre, slight exophthalmus).
- Biochemical monitoring as in hypothyroidism, plus the level of serum thyroid-stimulating antibodies. Those antibodies can cross the placenta, and increase the risk of hypothyroidism of the newborn.
- A thyrostatic drug (carbimazole) is the most important treatment. Biochemical monitoring is essential to keep the serum free thyroxine level at a level slightly higher than normal. The risk of foetal goitre is only 1% in such cases.
- Partial thyroidectomy is sometimes needed. Treatment with radioiodide is not possible.

Obesity

- A maternal pregestational body weight of more than 90 kg is associated with a 4-fold risk of gestational hypertension and a 1.5-fold risk of gestational diabetes compared with normal-weight women.

- Obesity also increases the risk of thromboembolic complications, especially if bed rest during pregnancy or puerperium is needed.
- Foetal risk for macrosomia increases, which in turn is associated with prolonged labour, increased need for Caesarean section, and shoulder dystocia.
- The acceptable weight gain for obese expectant mothers is not more than 4–9 kg. Heavy slimming during pregnancy is not recommended.

Neurological diseases

Epilepsy

- Good preconceptional control of the antiepileptic medication is important.
- The general principle in antiepileptic medication is monotherapy, if possible. Drugs used before conception are usually continued during pregnancy.
- Children of epileptic mothers run a 1.5–2 times higher risk of major malformations than controls. Some teratogenity is associated with antiepileptic drugs. For example, valproate is a cause of spina bifida in 1% of infants. Because of hypoxia an epileptic grand mal seizure is always more dangerous for the foetus than drug treatment.
- Serum concentrations of folic acid and antiepileptic drugs must be measured monthly throughout pregnancy. Drug levels are often below the usual ranges because of increased plasma volume. Risk of convulsive seizure increases only slightly because the decrease in concentration of freely circulating drug is small. The dosage of antiepileptic drug should be increased near term due to increased risk of seizure during labour.
- Daily administration of folic acid is especially important during the first trimester.
- Vaginal delivery is possible. The indications for Caesarean section are obstetric, but the incidence of operative delivery is about twice that of controls. Vitamin K injection is essential for the offspring.
- Breastfeeding is usually possible. Large doses of phenemal and diazepam may cause somnolence in the newborn because of a high drug concentration in the breast milk.

Migraine

- Tension headache is more common than migraine during pregnancy.
- The incidence of migraine seizure is highest during the first and third trimester, seldom during the second trimester.
- Close to the delivery pre-eclampsia-like symptoms (vision disturbances, high blood pressure, headache and subdiaphragmatic pain) cause differential diagnostic problems.
- Prostaglandin synthesis inhibitors and acetylsalicylic acid can be used during the first trimester of pregnancy, as well as prochlorperazine. Ergotamine derivatives are prohibited.
- Prostaglandin synthesis inhibitors are not used after week 32 of gestation because the foetal ductus arteriosus may close intrauterinally.
- $5HT_1$ antagonists (triptans) are not used during pregnancy and lactation because of insufficient experience of their use.
- Adrenergic beta-receptor blocking agents, such as propranolol, may be suitable for prophylaxis in severe cases.

Disturbances of cerebral circulation

- Risk of thrombotic stroke is increased about tenfold during pregnancy. The number of spontaneous subarachnoid haemorrhages is also increased during gestation, as is the rupture of cerebral angiomas and aneurysms.
- Treatment of cerebral vascular disorders does not differ during pregnancy compared with non-pregnant patients. When the aneurysm is operated on, a subsequent pregnancy does not increase the risk of a cerebral attack. In non-operated patients pregnancy and delivery are relative contraindications because of increased risks. The indications for Caesarean section are obstetric. The delivery should be managed so that the mother has no need to strain or push.

Renal diseases

- Renal blood flow and glomerular filtration increase by 30–50% during gestation. Renal tubular function also changes. Uric acid and creatinine clearance increase and the concentration of serum creatinine decreases. The normal level of serum creatinine is <80 μmol/l. A degree of hydronephrosis and hydroureter also occurs, especially on the right side.
- When chronic renal failure with an increased level of serum creatinine, high blood pressure and proteinuria develops, the pregnancy is complicated. Pregnancy is not recommended when the non-pregnant diastolic blood pressure exceeds 90 mmHg and the concentration of serum creatinine is 120–175 μmol/l.
- In all cases, renal function, as well as the obstetric antenatal situation, must be observed closely in collaboration with a physician specializing in renal diseases.
- Hypertension and albuminuria occur in over 50% of even less severe cases of renal insufficiency, followed by poor placental function, growth retardation of the foetus and premature labour.
- The prognosis of the pregnancy is greatly affected by lupus nephropathy, membranous glomerulonephritis and scleroderma, even if the renal function tests are near normal. In such cases pregnancy is relatively contraindicated.
- Untreated asymptomatic bacteriuria is a cause of pyelonephritis in about 40% of cases. Therefore, antibiotic treatment with nitrofurantoin, cephalosporins or mecillinam should be given during the first trimester of pregnancy.
- A patient with feverish pyelonephritis is best cared for in an obstetric antenatal ward. The antibiotic therapy is started parenterally, for example with cephalosporins, until

the sensitivity of urinary bacteria to antibiotics has been determined. Peroral antibiotic therapy is continued for 3 weeks. The risk of recurrence is quite high during pregnancy and in puerperium. Therefore, in these cases long-term maintenance therapy for the remainder of the pregnancy and puerperium is needed: nitrofurantoin 50 mg, cephalexin 250 mg or mecillanam 200 mg in the evening.

- Pregnancy is not recommended earlier than 1–2 years after renal transplantation, if there are no problems with renal function or immunosuppressive therapy. Very close follow-up is needed, starting before conception.

Rheumatic disorders

- The most problematic rheumatic disorders during pregnancy are rheumatoid arthritis and systemic lupus erythematosus, SLE.
- Pregnancy suppresses rheumatoid arthritis. 75% of women with rheumatoid arthritis have less pain and other symptoms already at the end of the first trimester in comparison with non-pregnant patients. Following delivery, the symptoms recur in 90% of cases and are usually more serious.
- Acetylsalicylic acid, prostaglandin inhibitors, sulphasalazine and glucocorticoids are useful treatments. Gold, hydroxychloroquine, D-penicillamine, azathioprine and cyclophosphamide are not recommended.
- SLE is always an extremely serious threat to pregnancy. The probability of an exacerbation is more than 30%; no improvement of the disease is seen during pregnancy. The prognosis of the mother and the foetus is especially poor in cases with circulatory antibodies to phospholipids (e.g. cardiolipin or lupus anticoagulant antibodies) because of increased risk of thrombotic disorders (arterial thrombosis, fibrotic placenta, placental infarction, spontaneous abortion, foetal growth retardation and intrauterine foetal death).
- When SLE is in an active phase, any treatment has only a minimal influence on the prognosis. There is no preferred management approach. Prednisone 20–40 mg daily is given orally throughout pregnancy as well as miniaspirin at a dose of 50 (–100) mg daily or miniheparin treatment. SLE is so rare that no good controlled studies are available on the comparison between different treatment schedules.

Psychiatric problems

- Some psychiatric drugs, e.g. phenothiazines, may reduce the likelihood of conception by increasing prolactin production. Sexual problems associated with emotional disorders may also be a reason for delayed conception.
- Pregnancy, delivery and the postpartum period are always times of psychological stress for women. Earlier severe psychiatric disorders before pregnancy or during an earlier pregnancy, delivery or puerperium present a major risk in subsequent gestation and puerperium. The risk is also increased when the husband has a history of psychopathology.
- The need for drug treatment should be reconsidered in pregnant women with the well-being of the mother and child taken into account. Drugs should not be interrupted suddenly! Lithium may increase the risk of congenital heart malformations. Phenothiazines and thioxanthines are considered safe. There is some doubt concerning the use of tricyclic antidepressants, butyrophenones and benzodiazepines in the first trimester of gestation.
- There is a suspected link between congenital cleft lip and palate and administration of benzodiazepine derivatives during the first 40–60 days of gestation. The risks are not obvious later in gestation.
- Tranquillizers taken close to the birth depress the newborn and cause somnolence and muscular atony.

Bronchial asthma

- The prevalence of asthma in pregnancy is reported to be about 1%. The condition is worsened in every third woman during pregnancy, but improves in the same proportion of cases. Bronchial asthma is a minor problem in the normal course of gestation.
- The use of inhaled beta$_2$-agonists, theophylline, inhaled glucocorticoids, as well as cromolyn and some antihistamines is not known to be associated with congenital malformation. Oral corticosteroids are sometimes also needed for short periods.
- Status asthmaticus during labour is a problem, as poor maternal oxygenation can result in foetal hypoxia. The treatment is similar to that in non-pregnant patients. The risk of Caesarean section is increased because of hypoxia.

Cancer in pregnancy

- The prevalence of carcinoma during pregnancy is about 1:1000–2000 deliveries, i.e. similar or lower than in non-pregnant women of comparable age.
- The most common type of cancer during pregnancy is breast cancer, followed by leukaemias, and uterine cervical, ovarian and intestinal cancer.
- Transplacental transmission of carcinoma cells is possible only in malignant melanoma.
- All procedures (surgery, radiotherapy and administration of cytotoxic drugs) are dangerous for the foetus during the first trimester. Cytotoxic drugs are especially teratogenic during organogenesis of the foetus, as is radiotherapy treatment if given below the diaphragm. Risk of spontaneous abortion is also increased during that time.
- It is important to treat every case individually, in collaboration with the patient.
- The outcome is mainly seen in 2 years: if the prognosis is good no signs of recurrence of the cancer are seen; if it is poor, symptoms and signs of cancer recur.
- After surgery for breast cancer, pregnancy should be avoided for 2 years. (Previous recommendation: 5 years.) There

is no evidence that pregnancy itself affects the prognosis; however, examination of the breasts is more difficult in pregnant than in non-pregnant women.

References

1. Ensom MH, Stephenson MD. Low-molecular weight heparins in pregnancy. Pharmacotherapy 1999;19:1013–1025.
2. The Database of Abstracts of Reviews of Effectiveness (University of York), Database no.: DARE-991717. In: The Cochrane Library, Issue 4, 2000. Oxford: Update Software.
3. Walkinshaw SA. Very tight versus tight control for diabetes in pregnancy. Cochrane Database Syst Rev. 2004;(2):CD000226.

26.16 Bleeding in late pregnancy

Mika Nuutila

Introduction

- Do not carry out pelvic examination on a pregnant woman who is bleeding.
- Always send a pregnant woman with vaginal bleeding immediately to a maternity hospital.

Most common reasons for bleeding

- Bleeding associated with onset of labour, contractions and opening of the cervix.
- Bleeding caused by recent pelvic examination
- Post-coital bleeding
- Bleeding caused by a cervical polyp
- Bleeding caused by trauma (see Premature detachment of the placenta)
- Bleeding mucous membranes caused by vaginitis
- Placenta praevia
- Premature detachment of the placenta.

Investigations

- A careful history is important. Avoid bimanual examination, only carry out a speculum examination if necessary.
- Check the state of the foetus: verify the presence of heart sounds either with a Doppler or an ultrasound.
- If the bleeding is heavy, insert an intravenous cannula and promptly send the patient by ambulance, accompanied by an escort, to a hospital.

Placenta praevia

- Predisposing factors include previous uterine procedures, e.g. curettage and caesarean section.
- Placenta praevia may be either
  - complete (obstructs the internal os completely),
  - partial (obstructs the internal os only partially) or
  - marginal (placenta encroaches on the internal os).
- Bleeding usually starts without a clear provoking cause.
- The bleeding is bright red and the mother is usually pain free.
- At the maternity hospital the diagnosis is confirmed with an ultrasound examination and treatment decisions are based on the maternal and foetal state, the amount of blood loss and the number of gestational weeks.
- If the bleeding is not particularly heavy, and the mother and foetus are both well, and, in particular, if the pregnancy is not near term a decision is often taken only to observe the situation.
- If the bleeding is heavy and uncontrolled, a caesarean section will be indicated (partial or complete placenta praevia).

Premature detachment of the placenta (abruptio placentae)

- Predisposing factors include:
  - trauma to the abdominal area
  - a sudden reduction in the uterine volume (for example, in association with a rupture of the foetal membranes)
  - maternal pre-eclampsia or diabetes.
- The risk is also increased in alcohol and drug abuse as well as in patients with a previous history of placenta praevia or premature detachment of the placenta.
- Symptoms vary according to the extent and severity of the detachment.
- The most common signs and symptoms include pain and a taut and tender uterus.
- Even when the mother presents with symptoms of shock vaginal bleeding may remain fairly slight (extensive retroplacental bleeding).
- Foetal ECG will show signs of hypoxia.
- Clinical diagnosis is most important, and ultrasound examination is usually not needed.
- At the maternity hospital the treatment usually consists of a caesarean section, either urgently or as an emergency, as well as the treatment of the haemorrhagic shock of the mother.

26.18 Substance abuse in pregnancy

Erja Halmesmäki

Basic rules

- People tend to understate the amount of alcohol and drugs they use, and the maternal health service is no exception to

this rule. Pose direct questions about the use of intoxicating substances and aim at an open and confidential discussion.
- The pregnancies of women who abuse alcohol or drugs are risk pregnancies, and these women should be referred as early on as possible to a maternal outpatient clinic for management and follow-up.

Limits of moderate use of alcohol

- One to two standard drinks per week are considered moderate use during pregnancy.
- With less than two standard drinks a week, adverse effects on the course of the pregnancy and on the health of the mother or the foetus have not been observed.
- Ten drinks a week is considered the limit of excessive alcohol use during pregnancy.

Identifying alcohol abuse in maternal health service

- Spontaneous discussion about alcohol is the best way to find out how much alcohol a pregnant women drinks.
- The use of alcohol is culture-dependent. In many countries drinking alcohol is considered a normal part of life and in these cultures the doctor should not take a strong stand against the use of alcohol in general. A neutral discussion about the risks of alcohol use during pregnancy is favoured.
- The following questions can be used for assessing the amount of alcohol consumed by a pregnant woman:
  - How many glasses of wine or bottles of beer do you usually drink in a week?
  - What is your favorite drink?
  - Do you drink alcohol at home with your husband or friends or when you go out?
  - Do you ever get a hangover and have you needed a drink to make you feel better the next day?
- A pregnant mother often says that she drinks a little alcohol or none at all. It is useful to ask her to be precise about the meaning of "a little", i.e. how many portions or alcohol per week counted as bottles of beer or glasses of wine.
- Sometimes a structured questionnaire may help to discuss the use of alcohol (e.g. Alcohol Use Disorders Identification Test, AUDIT).

The risks of alcohol during pregnancy

- Excessive use of alcohol causes
  - the risk of miscarriage
  - the risk of infection of the uterus and foetal membranes
  - foetal growth retardation
  - risk of malformation
  - underdevelopment of the brain
  - oxygen insufficiency and resulting possible brain damage and foetal death.
- Foetal alcohol syndrome and foetal alcohol effects (partial FAS) (29.15)

Referral

- Every woman attending a maternal health check should be interviewed thoroughly.
- If a pregnant woman discloses that she uses alcohol regularly a few times a week or every weekend, she should be referred to a maternal outpatient clinic.
- At the clinic the woman is encouraged to participate in the follow-up programme regularly by explaining her the consequences of intoxicant use and lifestyle on the course of the pregnancy and the well being of the child.
- Frequency of follow-up should be tailored individually and depend on the woman's condition.

Identifying the use of drugs in maternity care

- The use of drugs is always a risk during pregnancy.
- The majority of drug users do not tell voluntarily about their addiction to the maternal health service staff.
- Questions concerning drug use must be posed directly. Asking about possible experimenting with drugs is easiest when done immediately after asking about smoking.
- If a pregnant woman has never tried even hashish, it may, nevertheless, be useful to ask about the use of other drugs or medicines.
- If the woman tells that she has experimented, ask when was the last time and whether she has used amphetamine and in what form.
- A targeted interview may reveal small matters that may in turn help to determine how experienced a drug user the patient possibly is.

Cannabis drugs: hashish and marijuana

- The active agent is tetrahydrocannabinol (THC) that passes through the placenta easily.
- THC has not been shown to cause malformations in the foetus or to increase the risk of miscarriage; however, it does increase the incidence of low weight-for-age in newborns.

Amphetamine

- Foetal exposure to amphetamine may cause heart defects, microcephalia and mental retardation.
- A mother using amphetamine gains little or no weight at all, which easily leads to the undernourishment of both the mother and the newborn.
- Withdrawal symptoms are common in newborns: elevated blood pressure, abnormal crying voice, difficulty with suckling, and vomiting.

Opioids: heroin and buprenorphin

- An opioid-dependent drug addict acts fairly normally after receiving a drug dose.

- The use of opioids has been associated with occasional anomalies of the urinary tract, brain and heart.

Referral

- If a pregnant woman discloses that she has experimented with drugs, consider seriously referring her to a maternal outpatient clinic.
- The role of the maternal outpatient clinic is to give the patient detailed information on the effects of drugs on the pregnancy and on the foetus as well as to follow-up the growth, development and well being of the foetus.
- The pregnant woman should be motivated to participate in a withdrawal programme either as an outpatient or in a withdrawal unit.
- In some countries the legislation may include a paragraph on involuntary treatment when voluntary measures cannot be applied or have proven inadequate and the health or the life of the patient is at risk.
- Short-term involuntary treatment may sometimes be indicated as the mother often understands the consequences of the abuse better after she has been forced to sober up and may then be better motivated to try withdrawal.

26.20 Causes of infertility

Outi Hovatta

General

- About 15% of couples suffer from infertility at some point in their lives.
- The cause of infertility can be found in the female alone in (approximately) 30% of cases, in the male in 30%, and in both partners in a further 30% of cases. In 10% it remains unexplained.

Causes of female infertility

- Ovulatory disturbances, about 30% of all cases
  - Polycystic ovaries (PCOS, probably genetic)
  - Weight-related anovulation (over- and underweight, eating disorders)
  - Hypogonadotrophic hypogonadism
    - Kallmann's syndrome
    - Idiopathic
    - Weight-related
  - Hyperprolactinaemia
    - Prolactinoma
    - Pharmaceutical (psychopharmaca)
  - Hypothyroidism
  - Premature ovarian failure
    - Turner's syndrome
    - FSH receptor failure
    - APECED
    - Other genetic
    - Autoimmune
    - Galactosaemia
    - Chemotherapy or radiotherapy
    - Sequelae of surgery (tumours, severe endometriosis)
- Endometriosis, in about 20% of cases
- Tubal dysfunction, in about 15% of cases
  - Salpingitis
  - Salpingitis isthmica nodosa
  - Sequela of ectopic pregnancy
  - Sequela of appendicitis or other abdominal infections C [1 2]
  - Adhesions in the abdominal cavity
  - Tubal sterilization
- Uterine causes
  - Congenital anomalies
  - Myomas (especially submucous) and adenomyosis
  - Endometrial polyps
  - Intrauterine adhesions (Asherman's syndrome)
  - Sequela of malignant tumours (hysterectomy and radiotherapy)
  - Sequela of severe infection (tuberculosis)
- Sexual problems
  - Vaginism
  - Intercourse more seldom than once a week

GYN

Causes of male infertility

- Undescended testes (if treated after 4 years of age)
- Orchitis (parotitis)
- Varicocoele
- Hypogonadotrophic hypogonadism
  - Kallmann's syndrome
  - Tumour
  - Vascular, traumatic
  - Idiopathic
  - Other causes
- Hyperprolactinaemia
- Klinefelter's syndrome
- 47,XYY males, 46,XX males
- Deletions on the Y chromosome
- Autosomal rearrangements
- Gonadal dysgenesis of various causes
- FSH receptor mutations
- LH receptor mutations
- Androgen insensitivity (receptor mutations, enzyme defects)
- Sertoli-cell-only syndrome
- Spermatogenic arrest

- APECED
- Cystic fibrosis (31.23)
- Leydig cell hypoplasia or aplasia
- Chemotherapy or radiotherapy
- Testicular cancer
- Pesticides (DBCP), heavy metals, solvents
- Alcohol abuse
- Pharmaceuticals (sulfasalazine, calcium antagonists, antiandrogens such as ketoconazole, anabolic steroids)
- Antisperm antibodies
- Structural abnormalities in spermatozoa (immotile cilia syndrome, i.e. Kartagener syndrome, globozoospermia, fibrous sheath abnormalities)
- Systemic diseases
- Blockage of epididymis and vas deferens (infection, congenital anomalies, hernia operations, vasectomy, cystic fibrosis)
- Anejaculation or retrograde ejaculation (spinal cord injury, pelvic operations and traumas, pelvic lymphadenectomy, diabetic neuropathy, other neurological causes, unknown aetiology)
- Erectile impotence
- Poor sperm quality of unknown cause.

References

1. Mob BWJ, Dijkman B. Wertheim P, Lijmer J, Vanderveen F, Bossuyt PMM. The accuracy of serum chlamydial antibodies in the diagnosis of tubal pathology: a meta-analysis. Fertil Steril 1997;67:1031–1037.
2. The Database of Abstracts of Reviews of Effectiveness (University of York), Database no.: DARE-970778. In: The Cochrane Library, Issue 4, 1999. Oxford: Update Software.

26.21 How to investigate and treat infertility

Outi Hovatta

Principles

- Investigate the causes of infertility if the couple has had unprotected intercourse for a year, and pregnancy has not occurred.
- If one of the partners has a history of a disorder that is known to cause infertility, such as clearly irregular periods, salpingitis or endometriosis, or in the male partner, undescended testes or orchitis, the investigations should be carried out without the 1-year delay. The age of the female partner should be noted. It does not usually take a whole year for a 40-year-old woman to become pregnant; however, the time to pregnancy increases with age.

History of infertility

- Both partners should visit the clinic together.
  - History and clinical examination of both partners.
  - Factors regarding the relationship.

History of the female partner

- Menstrual periods
- Earlier pregnancies
- Earlier contraception
- Infections
- Pelvic pain (endometriosis)
- Gynaecological and other operations
- Sexual history

History of the male partner

- Descent of the testes
- Pubertal development
- Operations (herniae, varicocoele, hydrocoele, etc.)
- Parotitis
- Other infections (sexually transmitted diseases, epididymitis, prostatitis)
- Traumatic injuries to the genital area
- Possible exposure to pesticides, other chemicals, heavy metals and irradiation
- Use of drugs and alcohol
- Erection, ejaculation

Issues relevant to both partners

- Feelings, expectations and frustrations connected with infertility
- Effects on sex life
- Possible problems in the relationship

Investigations

- Systematic investigation, bearing in mind that one cause does not exclude another.
- A general practitioner can take the history and carry out the primary investigations, and then decide where to refer the couple for treatment.
- The GP will remain an important support for the couple and a member of the specialist team during the subsequent treatment.
- The treatments are given in specialized units that can also offer assisted reproduction.

The female partner

Primary investigations

- Gynaecological examination
- Pelvic ultrasound scan

- Serum concentration of progesterone on the 21st day of the menstrual cycle
- Serum concentrations of prolactin and thyroid stimulating hormone (TSH)
- Sonosalpingography or hysterosalpingography 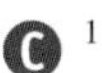 [1 2]

Further investigations (special clinic)

- Hormone measurements (gonadotrophins, oestradiol, progesterone, androgens, thyroid hormones)
- Follow-up of follicle development
- Structure of the uterus using an ultrasound scan
- Hysteroscopy
- Laparoscopy if necessary
- Endometrial and ovarian biopsies if necessary
- Chromosomes if necessary
- Genetic tests if necessary

The male partner

Primary investigations

- Andrological examination
  - Hair growth (beard, pubes, axillary hair)
  - Possible gynaecomastia (suggests Klinefelter's syndrome, hyperprolactinaemia or testicular tumours)
  - Scrotum, possible varicocoele
  - Testes (size, consistence, possible tumours); small testes indicate severe disturbances in sperm production
  - Epididymides, vasa deferentia (agenesis refers to cystic fibrosis)
  - Prostate
- Semen analysis (including antisperm antibodies) 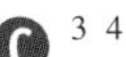 [3 4]

Further investigations (specialist clinic)

- Semen analysis combined with sperm preparation C [3 4]
- Hormone measurements (gonadotrophins, testosterone, sex hormone binding globulin, prolactin, TSH, thyroid hormones)
- Ultrasound scan of the testes (and prostate if necessary)
- Chromosome analysis, measurement of Y-chromosomal deletions
- Other gene tests
- Testicular biopsy (needle biopsy)

Treatment of infertility

- There are no age limits for infertility treatment with the exception of normal menopause (at about 50 years).
- The general practitioner remains a member of the specialist team and helps in treating the infertility crisis.
- Infertility treatments are given in specialized units.

Female infertility

- Ovulation induction A [5 6 7 8]
  - Clomiphene citrate [9]
  - Gonadotrophins (FSH rather than hMG [10 11])
  - GnRH agonists B [12 13] and antagonists
- Optimization of weight in over- and underweight women
- Treatment of other endocrine abnormalities
- Laparoscopical treatment of endometriosis C [14], sometimes laparotomy in severe endometriosis. Danazol is not recommended D [15].
- Laparoscopic adhesiolysis and reversal of sterilization
- Assisted reproduction
  - Intrauterine insemination A [16 17], often combined with ovulation induction A [5 6 7 8]
  - In vitro fertilization (IVF) C [18 19 20]
    - Use of donated eggs is possible
    - Gestational surrogacy in cases of a non-functional uterus

Male infertility

- Treatment of endocrine disorders
  - Hypogonadotrophic hypogonadism
  - Prolactinomas
  - Disorders in thyroid function
- Percutaneous embolization of obvious varicocoeles. The benefit of treating subclinical varicocoeles is controversial D [21 22].
- Microsurgical vasectomy reversal, possibly vasoepididymostomy
- Insemination
  - Often combined with ovulation induction
  - Prepared sperm (density gradient, swim-up) for intrauterine insemination, IUI
  - Spouse's sperm if there are more than 1 million motile spermatozoa in the sperm preparation
  - Donor sperm if no sperm are found (in semen or testicular biopsy)
- In vitro fertilization, if four attempts at IUI have failed to induce pregnancy
- Intracytoplasmic sperm injection, ICSI
  - Fewer than 1 million prepared spermatozoa
  - Low motility
  - High percentage of spermatozoa with abnormal forms
  - Failed fertilization in previous IVF
  - Spermatozoa obtained by aspiration from the epididymis, or from testicular biopsy
  - Electroejaculated sperm in cases of anejaculation

References

1. Swart P, Mol BW, Vanderveen F, Vanbeurden M, Redekop WK, Bossuyt PMM. The accuracy of hysterosalpingography in the diagnosis of tubal pathology: a meta-analysis. Fertil Steril 1995;64:486–491.
2. The Database of Abstracts of Reviews of Effectiveness (University of York), Database no.: DARE-952533. In: The Cochrane Library, Issue 4, 1999. Oxford: Update Software.

3. Coetzee K, Kruge TF, Lombard CJ. Predictive value of normal sperm morphology: a structured literature review. Hum Reproduction Update 1998;4:73–82.
4. The Database of Abstracts of Reviews of Effectiveness (University of York), Database no.: DARE-980952. In: The Cochrane Library, Issue 2, 2000. Oxford: Update Software.
5. Hughes EG. The effectiveness of ovulation induction and intrauterine insemination in the treatment of persistent infertility: a meta-analysis. Human Reprod 1997;12:1865–1872.
6. The Database of Abstracts of Reviews of Effectiveness (University of York), Database no.: DARE-971299. In: The Cochrane Library, Issue 4, 1999. Oxford: Update Software.
7. Citrate de clomifene ou hMG: quelle stimulation ovarienne choisir avant inseminations intra-uterines? Les apports d'une meta-analyse. Contraception Fertilite Sexualite 1995;23: 115–121.
8. The Database of Abstracts of Reviews of Effectiveness (University of York), Database no.: DARE-950677. In: The Cochrane Library, Issue 1, 2000. Oxford: Update Software.
9. Hughes E, Collins J, Vandekerckhove P. Clomiphene citrate for unexplained subfertility in women. Cochrane Database Syst Rev. 2004;(2):CD000057.
10. Daya S, Gunby J, Hughes EG, Collins JA, Sagle MA. Follicle-stimulating hormone versus human menopausal gonadotropin for in vitro fertilization cycles: a meta-analysis. Fertil Steril 1995;64:347–354.
11. The Database of Abstracts of Reviews of Effectiveness (University of York), Database no.: DARE-951968. In: The Cochrane Library, Issue 4, 1999. Oxford: Update Software.
12. Soliman S, Daya S, Collins J, Hughes EG. The role of luteal phase support in infertility treatment: a meta-analysis of randomized trials. Fertil Steril 1994;61:1068–1076.
13. The Database of Abstracts of Reviews of Effectiveness (University of York), Database no.: DARE-941139. In: The Cochrane Library, Issue 4, 1999. Oxford: Update Software.
14. Jacobson TZ, Barlow DH, Koninckx PR, Olive D, Farquhar C. Laparoscopic surgery for subfertility associated with endometriosis. Cochrane Database Syst Rev. 2004;(2): CD001398.
15. Hughes E, Tiffin G, Vandekerckhove P. Danazol for unexplained infertility. Cochrane Database Syst Rev. 2004;(2): CD000069.
16. Goldberg JM, Mascha E, Falcone T, Attaran M. Comparison of intrauterine and intracervical insemination with frozen donor sperm: a meta-analysis. Fertility and Sterility 1999;72:792–795.
17. The Database of Abstracts of Reviews of Effectiveness (University of York), Database no.: DARE-992209. In: The Cochrane Library, Issue 2, 2001. Oxford: Update Software.
18. Pandian Z, Bhattacharya S, Nikolaou D, Vale L, Templeton A. In vitro fertilisation for unexplained subfertility. Cochrane Database Syst Rev. 2004;(2):CD003357.
19. Corabian P, Hailey D. The efficacy and adverse effects of in vitro fertilization and embryo transfer. Journal of Technology Assessment in Health Care 1999;15:66–85.
20. The Database of Abstracts of Reviews of Effectiveness (University of York), Database no.: DARE-999294. In: The Cochrane Library, Issue 2, 2001. Oxford: Update Software.
21. Marsman JWP, Schats R. The subclinical varicocele debate. Human Reproduction 1994;9:1–8.
22. The Database of Abstracts of Reviews of Effectiveness (University of York), Database no.: DARE-940036. In: The Cochrane Library, Issue 4, 1999. Oxford: Update Software.

26.22 Infertility crisis

Outi Hovatta

Basic rules

- Infertility causes a psychological crisis for those involved. The severity depends on many personal factors, but no one can completely escape it. Parenthood is part of the identity of every adult. Giving up the natural, probably largely biological, desire to have children leads to sorrow, which has to be dealt with. This sorrow has been described as due to the loss of unborn children who have lived in the minds of the persons involved.

Crisis stages

- The first stage is usually denial of infertility. Better treatment options and clinics are usually sought at this stage.
- In the reactive phase of the crisis, feelings of unexplained guilt and shame are common. Spouses tend to blame themselves, each other or the treatment unit for the problems. Depression and anxiety are common. Meeting friends and relatives who have children may be difficult, and leads to isolation. Sexual difficulties may occur. At this stage it is important that these feelings can be discussed with the personnel responsible for infertility treatment. It may be reassuring to hear that the feelings are a natural aspect of infertility, and resolve little by little.
- At the resolution phase, the couples accept that a full life is possible without biological children. Alternatives, such as adoption, can be considered. Successful resolution of the infertility crisis often improves the relationship, and explains why children born to such couples have fewer problems than children born to parents without a period of infertility.

26.30 Management of delivery (outside hospital)

Editors

- When a baby is born unexpectedly outside hospital the delivery is usually uncomplicated. The baby is delivered spontaneously without any special assistance needed.

Table 26.30 The Apgar scoring system

Features evaluated	0 Points	1 Point	2 Points
Heart rate	0	<100	>100
Respiration effort	Apnoea	Irregular, shallow, or gasping respiration	Vigorous and crying
Colour	Pale, blue	Pale or blue extremities	Pink
Muscle tone	Absent	Weak, passive tone	Active move-ment
Reflex irritability	Absent	Grimace	Active avoidance

Is the child in good condition?

- Limbs in good flexion, good muscle tone
- Reacts immediately to stimulation.
- Begins to breathe spontaneously or cries within 1 minute of birth.
- The heart beats more than 100 times per minute.
- The skin colour is reddish or only slightly bluish.

The Apgar score

- See Table 26.30.
- The scores are usually assessed at the age of 1 and 5 minutes.

Suction and clearance of the airways

- If the amniotic fluid is clear and there is no mucus in the airways, suction is not needed.
- If the amniotic fluid is green in colour and contains meconium or blood, immediate suction of the airways is obligatory to avoid aspiration of meconium or blood by the child.
- If the amniotic fluid is thick with meconium-like porridge, suction of the ventricle is also obligatory.

Cutting the umbilical cord

- The umbilical cord is clamped with two sterile Kocher instruments and cut using sterile scissors.
- The stump is swabbed with antiseptic solution (e.g. chlorhexidine containing alcohol) and closed with rubber or plastic clamps in hospital. Outside hospital clean string or thread can be used.
- Try to take a sample of umbilical blood with a syringe from the placental side of the umbilical vein for analysis of thyrotropin (thyroxin stimulating hormone, TSH).

Is resuscitation needed?

- If the child does not begin to breathe, is pale and limp, and if the pulse rate is less than 100 per minute on auscultation, resuscitation is needed.
  - In the majority of cases ventilation with a mask is sufficient.
  - Heart massage is given by pressing the breastbone to a depth of approximately 1 cm about 120 times per minute (ventilation/heart massage 1:3).

Keep the child warm

- Wipe the child with a soft towel as quickly as possible.
- The baby can be put on the mothers bare belly.
- Cover the baby with a blanket to keep it warm. Do not forget to observe the colour, breathing (normally 40–70 times per minute) and heart rate (normally 120–160 times per minute).

Contraction of the uterus and delivery of the placenta

- After delivery of the baby the mother is given 5 IU of oxytocin intravenously in order to stimulate uterine contraction and avoid excessive bleeding.
- If the mother does not bleed there is no urgency to deliver the placenta, it can be delivered later by a midwife in hospital.
- If the placenta has been delivered and the mother is bleeding, she is given 0.2 mg of methylergometrine intramuscularly to further stimulate uterine contractions and prevent bleeding. Methylergometrine is not recommended before delivery of the placenta because it also contracts the lower parts of the uterus and may thus complicate placental removal.

Birth Control

Evidence Based Medicine Guidelines. Edited by the Duodecim Editorial Team
© 2005 John Wiley & Sons, Ltd ISBN: 0-470-01184-X

27.1 Contraception: first examination and follow-up

Anneli Kivijärvi

- The choice of method and follow-up are both equally important for the success of contraception.
- Prior to starting contraception, pay attention to
  - possible diseases
  - current medication
  - familial risk factors (e.g. venous thromboses, high blood pressure, cardiovascular diseases)
    - If a close family member has had venous thrombosis, exclusion of resistance to activated protein C by a blood test is indicated.
  - smoking
  - gynaecological history (regularity of menses and amount of bleeding, pains)
  - obstetrical history (toxaemia, ectopic pregnancies, hepatic cholestatis of pregnancy, caesarean sections).
- At every follow-up visit, examine the following regardless of the method used
  - weight
  - blood pressure
  - gynaecological examination (abnormal anatomy, infections)
  - palpation of the breasts
- Take a Pap smear from everyone prior to starting contraception (from young women one year after intercourses have started) and every two or three years (as other women of the same age). It is better to screen for infection (chlamydia, gonococci) too often than too seldom.
- Monitor the haemoglobin level for one year after the insertion of an IUD.

27.2 Choice of contraception method

Anneli Kivijärvi

Matters to be taken into account

- Age
- Common state of health (chronic diseases, overweight)
- Smoking
- Parity–nulliparity
- Duration and amount of menstrual bleeding, pains during menses
- Required duration of contraception, plans for future pregnancies
- Required effectiveness of contraception
- Lactation (see Table 27.2), time since last delivery
  - Lactation itself gives about a 98% protection from pregnancy if the time since delivery is less than 6 months, menses have not begun and the child is breast-fed only B [1].
- The relationship of the couple (frequency of intercourse, varying partners or a stable relationship?)
- The woman's motivation and her own preferences concerning the contraception method

The suitability of the contraceptive methods for different situations

- Check the contraindications and more precise details from articles describing the methods.
- The advantages of the **combined pills** (27.3) make them the primary and superior method of contraception for women,
  - who are young (no limit for teenagers) and nulliparous
  - whose menses are either irregular, of long duration, profuse or painful
  - who have problems associated with the menstrual cycle
  - who suffer from acne, greasy hair or skin, or hirsutism
  - who are inclined to develop ovarian cysts.
- Consider contraception with **minipills** (27.3) when combination pills are contraindicated:
  - high blood pressure or blood pressure that increases during use of combination pills
  - smoking and the age above 35 years (a combination containing natural oestrogen is an alternative)
  - lactating women
- **Contraceptive implants** (27.3) are suitable for women of any age,
  - who need contraception for a long period
  - who do not have contraindications for progestogens
  - who have contraindications for other contraceptive methods and do not want sterilization.
- **Injectable medroxyprogesterone acetate**
  - Injected deep into muscle every 3 months
  - An alternative to a progestogen-only contraception method for women in whom oestrogen is contraindicated or causes side effects.
  - Injection is a hindrance but can be an advantage for women who easily forget to take the pills.
- A **hormone-releasing intrauterine device** (27.4) is a good alternative for a parous woman who
  - wants an IUD, but
  - has profuse menstrual bleeding, or
  - bleeding that increases with a copper IUD.
- A **copper IUD** (27.4) is a safe and effective method for a parous woman with a stable relationship.

Table 27.2 Contraception for a breast-feeding woman

Method	Start after childbirth	Noteworthy
Lactation	Immediately	♦ First six months, if ♦ breast milk is the only nutrition for the baby, and ♦ menstruation has not begun
Barrier methods	Immediately	Reliability? (During lactation-induced amenorrhoea, condom is a secure method)
IUD	8 weeks	
Hormone-releasing IUD	8 weeks	
Contraceptive implants	Follow-up examination, 6 weeks	
Minipills (progestin only)	1 week	
Progestin injection	Follow-up examination	Seldom used postpartum
Sterilization	1–3 days	Irreversible
Postcoital contraception		♦ Necessary only if menstruation has started ♦ Levonorgestrel-only regimen might be safer (oestrogen may reduce milk secretion) ♦ To minimize the hormonal effect on the baby, skip one lactation after taking the pills
Not recommended		
Combination oral contraceptive pills	First menstruation or 6 months	♦ Choose the pills with the lowest hormone content ♦ May reduce milk secretion ♦ Long-term effects on the baby?
Hormone-releasing vaginal rings and skin patches	First menstruation or 6 months	♦ Might be a better option than combination pills (steady hormone release) ♦ May reduce milk secretion ♦ Long-term effects on the baby?

- The **condom** (27.5) is the only method that completely prevents infection. It should therefore always be used in new and casual relationships, even if another contraception method is used simultaneously.

Reference

1. Van der Wijden C, Kleijnen J, Van den Berk T. Lactational amenorrhea for family planning. Cochrane Database Syst Rev 2003(4):CD001329.

27.3 Hormonal contraception (combined oral contraceptives, progestogen-only pills, skin patch and vaginal ring, hormone-releasing intrauterine device)

Anneli Kivijärvi

Combined oral contraceptives

- There are usually two types of combined oral contraceptives (COCs) on the market:
  - **Monophasic pills**, in which every pill contains the same amount of oestrogen and progestogen.
  - **Bi- or triphasic pills**, in which every pill contains both oestrogen and progestogen but the amounts vary in different phases of the menstrual cycle. There is no significant difference in efficacy or adverse effects between monophasic and biphasic pills (C) [1].
- Start with low dose products independent of the age of woman unless there is some contraindication. (The amount of ethinyloestradiol is 20–30 μg; the so-called ultra-light combination pill contains 20 μg of ethinyloestradiol.)
- For a woman with acne or hirsutism select a product with desogestrel or cyproterone acetate as the progestogen.
- For a woman over 40 years old start with a biphasic product in which the progestogen part is cyproterone acetate and the oestrogen part is so-called natural oestrogen (oestradiol valerate). A 40–50 year old healthy non-smoking woman of normal weight can also use any other low dose combination pill.

Absolute contraindications COCs

- Any past proven arterial or venous thrombosis (C) [2 3]
- Focal and crescendo migraine (the classical type)
- Age above 35 years and smoking
- Hypertension
- Serious liver diseases
- History of cholestatic hepatitis of pregnancy
- Systemic lupus erythematosus

- Undiagnosed genital tract bleeding
- Carcinoma of the ovary or breast
- Suspicion of pregnancy
- Lactation
- Absolute contraindications to COCs are based on the risks, which are known to correlate with the use. The risk of myocardial infarction, a thromboembolic process **C** [4 5 6 7 8 9] or stroke **B** [10 11] is increased with the use of currently available products. The risk of combined pills probably correlates with both the oestrogen and progestogen part of the pill. There is evidence that smaller amounts of hormones produce smaller risks.
- New trials prove that the progestogen (desogestrel, gestodene, norgestimate) of third generation drugs may increase the risk of venous thromboembolism approximately twofold compared with first or second-generation products **B** [12 13 14 15] (tables 27.3.1, 27.3.2).
    - Desogestrel and gestodene are contraindicated if the woman is obese (BMI > 30), immobilized or has varicose veins or if there has been a thromboembolisms in the family.
- The increased risk of myocardial infarction with oral contraceptives was earlier associated with the oestrogen but recent reports also implicate progestogens.
- As risk factors, the use of oral contraceptives, smoking and age are synergistic; smoking increases the risk of myocardial infarction more than the use of pills. The risk of myocardial infarction in a woman on oral contraceptives is approximately 350–800-fold higher for a smoker aged 41–45 than for a non-smoker aged 27–37 years.

Benefits of combined pills

- High effectiveness
- Reduction in

Table 27.3.1 Odds ratios for venous thromboembolism

	Odds ratio (95% confidence interval)
All OCs v. no current use	4.0 (3.1–5.3)
First generation drugs v. no current use	5.7 (3.4–9.4)
Second generation drugs v. no current use	3.2 (2.3–4.3)
Third generation drugs v. no current use	4.8 (3.4–6.7)
Products containing levonorgestrel v. no current use	3.0 (2.0–3.9)
Third generation products v. second generation products	1.5 (1.1–2.1)
Products containing gestodene v. second generation products	1.5 (1.0–2.2)
Products containing desogestrel v. second generation products	1.5 (1.1–2.2)

Table 27.3.2 Odds ratios for venous thromboembolism in Europe and in developing countries

Progestogen generation (low oestrogen)	Europe OR (95% CI)	Developing countries (OR (95% CI)
First	3.37 (1.44–7.93)	0.00
Second	3.61 (2.55–6.13)	2.79 (2.08–3.75)
Third	7.36 (4.20–12.90)	12.93 (4.76–31.43)

    - ectopic pregnancies
    - functional ovarian cysts
    - dysfunctional bleeding
    - dysmenorrhoea **D** [16]
    - symptoms of premenstrual tension
    - pelvic inflammatory disease
    - cancer of the ovaries
    - cancer of the endometrium
    - myomas
    - mastopathy
- Reduced androgen production
- Regular bleeding
- Less heavy bleeding
- Timing can be controlled
- For special indications for combination pills see 27.2.

Contraception with progestogen

- Hormonal contraception is possible with minipills (contain only progestrogen) and hormone-releasing products such as subcutaneous implants, progestogen injections and hormone-releasing intrauterine devices.
- Contraception with progestogen-only avoids the disadvantages of oestrogen. Use of the progestogen-only pill is associated with less severe side effects but the relation between the benefits and risks is not as well documented as for combination pills.

Contraindications to contraception with progestogen

- Suspicion of pregnancy
- Severe active hepatic diseases
- Breast cancer
- Cholestatic hepatosis of pregnancy
- Earlier ectopic pregnancy
- Undiagnosed genital tract bleeding

Progestogen-only pills

- For special indications for contraception with progestogen-only pills (POP) see 27.2.

- During the use of POP
  - bleeding disorders are quite common
  - risk of ectopic pregnancy is increased.

Contraceptive implants

- Two different products are available
  - A product with two implants releasing levonorgestrel effective for 5 years (4 years in women weighing more than 60 kg).
  - A product with one implant releasing etonogestrel effective for 3 years
- Implants are an effective method of contraception, although the effect might be decreased in women weighing more than 75 kg. Women of every age who need long-term contraception and who do not have contraindications to progestogens can use implants. In practice implants are an alternative for women who cannot use other methods and do not want sterilization.
- It is important to insert the implants subcutaneously and not into the fat tissue where absorption is lower and from where they are difficult to remove. Removal is more difficult than insertion but is made easier by injecting the local anaesthetic cautiously under the ends of the implants so that the implants are raised and can be easily seen.
- The most common side effects include bleeding disorders (amenorrhoea, spotting, which most often resolve during the first year of use). Pregnancy is rare. If a pregnancy does occur, it can be continued but the implants must be removed.

Injectables

- An injection (1 ml) containing 150 mg medroxyprogesterone acetate is given intramuscularly at 12-week intervals, with the first injection given during the first 15 days of the menstrual cycle.
- It is possible to give the injection during the first five days after labour if the woman is not going to lactate. Otherwise it is given six weeks post-partum.
- Can be used at any age when progestogen contraception is desired.
- Lactation is not a contraindication.
- The most common side effects include bleeding disorders, nausea, headache and weight gain.
- Some women consider the regular injections a disadvantage but others appreciate not having to remember to take oral contraceptives every day.

Skin patch

- Low dose combined contraceptive that releases ethinyloestradiol 20 μg/day and norelgestromin 150 μg/day.
- Dosage form is a thin, skin coloured patch (size 45 mm × 45 mm).
- Has similar effects to contaceptive pills, also similar indications and contraindications, advantages and disadvantages A [17].
- Simple and easy to use: when started for the first time, the patch is administered on the first day of the menstrual cycle. Patch regimens include 21 dosing days (3 consecutive 7-day patches) followed by 1 dose-free week when the bleeding appears.
- Skin patch is an alternative to contraceptive pills and suitable for those who wish to avoid daily pills.

Vaginal ring

- A combined hormone contaceptive that contains 2.7 mg ethinyloestradiol and 11.7 mg etonogestrel.
- Flexible and translucent vaginal ring the diameter of which is 54 mm and cross diameter is 4 mm.
- The effects of the ring are the same as those of combined pills, contraindications are the same, and the advantages and disadvantages are the same.
- Vaginal ring releases 15 μg ethinyloestradiol daily and 120 μg etonogestrel daily for 3 weeks, which makes it a low dose combined contraceptive.
- The ring is inserted into the vagina for three weeks. This is followed by a week without the ring then a new ring is inserted etc. Bleeding appears during the week without the ring.
- Vaginal ring is an alternative to combined pill. It suits especially those who do not or do not want to remember daily contraception.

GYN

Hormone releasing IUD

- The effect of a levonorgestrel-releasing IUD lasts five years.
- It is a good alternative A [18] for a parous woman who wants an IUD, but has heavy bleeding or bleeding increases with a copper IUD. A hormone-releasing IUD decreases the menstrual bleeding, sometimes to amenorrhoea A [18].
- An effective method of contraception.

Follow-up of hormonal contraception

- The first check-up should take place 3–6 months after the start of contraception and thereafter annually. Follow up young women (<18 years) more often. Regarding laboratory tests, only a Pap smear is needed, as for other women of the same age. Test for chlamydia routinely in young women who have just started on contraception at the first follow-up visit.

Side effects of hormonal contraception

- Bleeding disorders
    - If spotting continues after the initial phase, switch to a triphasic pill or to one with more progestogen. The next step is a pill also containing more oestrogen.
    - Check for chlamydia as it is often the cause of bleeding.
- Headache
    - Switch to a pill with a different progestogen. If this does not help, choose a pill with less oestrogen. If the headache appears only during the one-week pill-free interval advise the woman to use two (monophasic regimen) rounds after each other and then have break for one week. The last alternative is a POP.
- Nausea
- Lost libido
    - Change the progestogen.
- Irritation
- Depression
- Numbness of extremities
- Tenseness of the breast tissue
- Changes in weight
- Swelling of the lower abdomen
- Pains in the lower back or abdomen
- Difficulties in using contact lenses
- Increase in blood pressure
- Acne
- Objectively observable side effects are: change in weight, increase in blood pressure and sometimes acne. Ask the woman about other side effects.
- If problems occur, change the product. If this does not help, some of the side effects can be treated.
    - Depression and irritation can sometimes be helped by regularly used pyridoxine (vitamin B_6).
    - For mild migraine prescribe prostaglandin inhibitors.
- **If blood pressure rises above 140/90** change the regimen or switch from combined pills to, for example, progestogen-only pills.
- **If weight gain exceeds 5 kg and dieting is not effective**, consider another method.
- Regarding combined pills and risk of venous thromboembolism see 5.41.
- When continuous contraception is needed hormonal contraception can be used for years.

References

1. Van Vliet HAAM, Grimes DA, Helmerhorst FM, Schulz KF. Biphasic versus monophasic oral contraceptives for contraception. Cochrane Database Syst Rev. 2004;(2):CD002032.
2. Koster T, Small RA, Rosendaal FR, Helmerhorst FM. Oral contraceptives and venous thromboembolism: a quantitative discussion of the uncertainties. J Intern Med 1995;238:31–37.
3. The Database of Abstracts of Reviews of Effectiveness (University of York), Database no.: DARE-951917. In: The Cochrane Library, Issue 4, 1999. Oxford: Update Software.
4. Douketis JD, Ginsberg JS, Holbrook A, Crowther M, Duku EK, Burrows RF. A reevaluation of the risk for venous thromboembolism with the use of oral contraceptives and hormone replacement therapy. Arch Intern Med 1997;157:1522–1530.
5. The Database of Abstracts of Reviews of Effectiveness (University of York), Database no.: DARE-978272. In: The Cochrane Library, Issue 4, 1999. Oxford: Update Software.
6. Oger E, Scarabin PY. Assessment of the risk for venous thromboembolism among users of hormone replacement therapy. Drugs and Aging 1999;14:55–61.
7. The Database of Abstracts of Reviews of Effectiveness (University of York), Database no.: DARE-990307. In: The Cochrane Library, Issue 1, 2001. Oxford: Update Software.
8. Miller J, Chan B K S, Nelson H. Hormone replacement therapy and risk of venous thromboembolism. Rockville, MD: Agency for Healthcare Research and Quality (AHRQ). 2002. 54. Agency for Healthcare Research and Quality (AHRQ). www.ahrq.gov.
9. Health Technology Assessment Database: HTA-20031088. The Cochrane Library, Issue 1, 2004. Chichester, UK: John Wiley & Sons, Ltd.
10. Gillum LA, Mamidipudi SK, Claiborne Johnston S. Ischemic stroke risk with oral contraceptives: a meta-analysis. JAMA 2000;284:72–78.
11. The Database of Abstracts of Reviews of Effectiveness (University of York), Database no.: DARE-20008335. In: The Cochrane Library, Issue 3, 2001. Oxford: Update Software.
12. Spitzer WO, Lewis LA, Heinemann LAJ, Thorogood M, Macrae KD. Third generation oral contraceptives and risk of venous thromboembolic disorders: an international case-control study. BMJ 1996;312:83–8.
13. World Health Organization Collaborative Study of Cardiovascular Disease and Steroid Hormone Contraception. Venous thromboembolic disease and combined oral contraceptives: results of international multicentre case-control study. Lancet 1995;346:1572–82.
14. World Health Organization Collaborative Study of Cardiovascular Disease and Steroid Hormone Contraception. Effect of different progestogens in low oestrogen oral contraceptives on venous thromboembolic disease. Lancet 1995;346:1582–8.
15. Jick H, Jick SS, Gurewich V, Myers MW, Vasilakis C. Risk of idiopathic cardiovascular death and nonfatal venous thromboembolism in women using oral contraceptives with differing progestagen components. Lancet 1995;346: 1589–93.
16. Proctor ML, Roberts H, Farquhar CM. Combined oral contraceptive pill (OCP) as treatment for primary dysmenorrhoea. Cochrane Database Syst Rev. 2004;(2):CD002120.
17. Gallo MF, Grimes DA, Schulz KF. Skin patch and vaginal ring versus combined oral contraceptives for contraception. Cochrane Database Syst Rev. 2004;(2):CD003552.
18. French R, Cowan F, Mansour D, Morris S, Hughes D, Robinson A, Proctor T, Summerbell C, Logan S, Guillebaud J. Hormonally impregnated intrauterine systems (IUSs) versus other forms of reversible contraceptives as effective methods of preventing pregnancy. Cochrane Database Syst Rev. 2004;(2):CD001776.

27.4 Intrauterine device

Anneli Kivijärvi

- A copper-releasing IUD is a safe and effective method of contraception for a parous woman living in a faithful, stable relationship.
- There is little difference in effectiveness or safety of various IUDs.

Advantages of an IUD

- Continuous and successful use of the method is independent of the motivation of the woman.
- Older women who are smokers can use an IUD.
- An IUD can be used during lactation and it does not affect milk production.
- An IUD can also be used for postcoital contraception. In this case it must be inserted within 6 days of unprotected intercourse.

Contraindications of copper IUD use

Absolute

- Pregnancy (or suspicion of it)
- Current or very recent active pelvic inflammatory disease
- Undiagnosed genital tract bleeding
- Suspected or observed malignancy of the cervix or endometrium
- Disorders of blood coagulation
- Wilson's disease or known true allergy to copper
- Abnormal anatomy of the vagina, cervix or corpus of uterus, which prevents successful insertion and use of an IUD (e.g. fibroids, intrauterine septum)

Relative

- Previous ectopic pregnancy, if a later pregnancy is desired
- Anaemia
- Profuse bleeding or very painful menstruation
- Less than two months from childbirth
- High risk of sexually transmitted infections
- A nulliparous woman under the age of 25

Insertion of an IUD

- The Pap smear (at the most one year old) should be class I; possible infections are treated; the haemoglobin level is measured if needed.
- Insert the IUD preferably after the menstrual flow (within 10 days after the beginning of bleeding). An IUD can be inserted immediately after abortion **B** [1].
- Follow the insertion instructions of the manufacturer and use aseptic technique.
- After insertion, cut the threads to the standard length (2.5–3 cm).
- There is no need for antibiotics **B** [2] or abstinence from intercourse after insertion.
- There is no use in advising the woman to check for the presence of the threads herself.

Disadvantages of an IUD and follow-up

- The problems associated with an IUD are increased bleeding and duration of menses, pain and expulsions. Change the IUD if side effects appear (an uncorrectly positioned IUD in the uterine cavity may cause problems).
- Treat heavy bleeding and pain caused by the IUD with prostaglandin inhibitors.
- A hormone-releasing IUD decreases menstrual bleeding, see 27.03.
- Monitor haemoglobin during the first year to detect possible iron deficiency anaemia.
- Although all IUDs tend to descend, total expulsion is rare. It is acceptable for an IUD to descend 2 cm from the fundal position, but an IUD positioned partly or totally in the cervix must be changed. Threads always cut to the same length help to reveal any change in position.
- Sometimes the threads disappear. With ultrasound (25.2) it is possible to check whether the IUD lies in the uterine cavity. IUD hook and curved uterine forceps are good instruments for removing the IUD with lost threads. If removal is difficult, refer the patient to a hospital outpatient clinic.
- Bacterial vaginosis (a foul-smelling vaginal discharge caused by anaerobic bacteria and Gardnerella vaginalis) occurs four times more often in IUD users than in others. Treat with metronidazole, tetracyclines or locally applied clindamycin cream for a week. In frequently recurrent infections remove the IUD, and after a couple of months insert a new one.
- If pregnancy occurs with an IUD, remove the IUD.
- If the IUD has to be removed because of side effects, remember the possibility of pregnancy if there has been intercourse during the previous week without some other protection. If for some reason the IUD has to be removed acutely, give the patient postcoital hormonal contraception.
- Routine follow-up 3 and 12 months after insertion, and thereafter once a year. Advise the patient to contact the doctor if problems occur.

References

1. Grimes D, Schulz K, Stanwood N. Immediate postabortal insertion of intrauterine devices. Cochrane Database Syst Rev. 2004;(2):CD001777.
2. Grimes DA, Schulz FK. Antibiotic prophylaxis for intrauterine contraceptive device insertion. Cochrane Database Syst Rev. 2004;(2):CD001327.

27.5 Barrier methods for contraception

Anneli Kivijärvi

- The barrier methods are the condom (for men) and for women the sponge, diaphragm, different contraceptive vagitories and jellies.
- All barrier methods are quite efficient (85–98%) when used correctly. They are suitable for those who need contraception infrequently or casually. Most women use them after childbirth during lactation.
- The condom is the only method of contraception that offers total protection from infection. That is why it should always be used in casual and new relationships, even if another method of contraception is used. The need and usefulness of condom cannot be overemphasized.
- Some oil-based lubricants and vaginal medications may rapidly damage the condom. The use of baby oils, vaseline and topical clindamycin, miconazole or oestrogen reduce the safety of a condom.
- Persons using barrier methods should be advised about the possibility of postcoital contraception.

27.6 Postcoital contraception

Anneli Kivijärvi

Hormonal postcoital contraception

Levonorgestrel alone

- The regimen of choice for postcoital contraception
- Drug
  - Levonorgestrel 750 µg
- Dosage
  - 2 tablets (2 × 0.75 mg) is taken as soon as possible, preferably within 12 hours and at the latest 72 hours after intercourse. B [1]
- Pregnancy starts in 1.1%
- Contraindications
  - No other contraindications than pregnancy
- Adverse effects
  - Mild nausea

Levonorgestrel + ethinyloestradiol (Yuzpe regimen)

- Drug
  - Levonorgestrel 0.25 mg + ethinyloestradiol 50 µg No. IV
- Dose
  - Two pills immediately or at the latest 72 hours after intercourse C [2] [3], and the next two pills 12 hours later
- Pregnancy begins in 3.2% B [1]
- Contraindications
  - Pregnancy
  - Ongoing focal migraine attack
  - Active porphyria
  - Sickle cell crisis
  - Earlier serious thrombosis
- Adverse effects
  - Nausea and vomiting
- Bleeding
  - Occurs within three weeks

Postcoital contraception during breastfeeding

- Lactation is not a contraindication; however, the infant should be protected from the exogenous steroids by discontinuing breastfeeding for 24 hours after starting the medication.

An intrauterine device as postcoital contraception

- A copper IUD (not a hormone-releasing IUD) can be inserted up to six days after unprotected intercourse and be left in place and used for continuous contraception when needed.

References

1. Task Force on Postovulatory Methods of Fertility Regulation. Randomised controlled trial of levonorgestrel versus the Yuzpe regimen of combined oral contraceptives for emergency contraception. Lancet 1998;352:428–33.
2. Trussell J, Ellertson C, Rodriquez G. The Yuzpe regimen of emergency contraception: how long after the morning after? Obst Gynecol 1996;88:150–154.
3. The Database of Abstracts of Reviews of Effectiveness (University of York), Database no.: DARE-961127. In: The Cochrane Library, Issue 4, 1999. Oxford: Update Software.

27.8 Contraception in patients with systemic diseases

Seppo Saarikoski

Cardiovascular diseases

Vascular diseases (including mitral valve prolapse)

- Subcutaneous progestogen implants and progestogen pills are options, as well as a progestin and copper IUD (in a stable sexual partnership).

- Combined oral contraceptives (COCs) are not recommended because of the increased risks of thromboembolism.

Chronic hypertension

- Copper or progestogen IUDs, or progestogen-only as pills, implants or injections are the alternatives.
- COCs are contraindicated.

Thromboembolic diseases

- COCs are contraindicated.
- Laboratory tests of haemostasis are indicated in cases with a family history of thromboembolism, even without earlier thromboembolic complication in the patient.

Metabolic diseases

Diabetes

- COCs may impair the response to insulin. Therefore, it is important to control glucose balance soon after beginning to take a COC.
- Low-dose COCs are safe in young, nulliparous women.
- A copper and hormone-releasing IUD or sterilization are alternatives for parous and older women.

Dyslipidaemia

- A desogestrel- or gestoden-containing COC as well as a hormone-releasing IUD or copper IUD and progestogen-containing subcutaneous implant are suitable.

Polycystic ovarian syndrome (PCOS)

- COCs with desogestrel, gestodene or cyproterone acetate as the progestogen derivative are suitable. See 25.15.

Serious liver diseases

- Copper IUD and barrier methods

Thyroid disorders

- All contraceptive methods are possible.

Neurological diseases

Migraine

- COCs worsen the symptoms of migraine in every third patient. An IUD is the best choice in such cases.
- COCs are not recommended for patients with focal symptoms associated with migraine attacks.

Epilepsy

- A copper IUD is the best choice.
- Phenobarbital, phenytoin, carbamazepine and paramethadione induce steroid-metabolizing enzymes. This increases the risk of pregnancy because of too low steroid concentrations. Therefore, high-dose COC tablets are indicated or the daily dose of COC must be doubled.
- Patients taking benzodiazepines or valproate can safely take a COC.

Psychosis, drug addiction

- Copper and hormone-releasing IUDs are preferred because of their reliability and easiness of use.
- COCs may increase the tendency to depression in some patients. However, they are not contraindicated.

Other diseases

Rheumatic diseases

- COCs may relieve symptoms in rheumatoid arthritis as pregnancy does.
- COCs can worsen symptoms in SLE. Therefore, an IUD is the best choice in SLE. Progestin-only methods are also possible.

Cancer

- COCs might increase the risk of recurrence of hormone-dependent breast cancer or promote the spread of the disease.
- A COC is not contraindicated in patients with cervical carcinoma.

Renal diseases

- Hypertension associated with renal disease may affect the choice of contraceptive method.

Asthma

- All contraceptive methods can be used.

Child and School Health Services

Evidence Based Medicine Guidelines. Edited by the Duodecim Editorial Team
 ISBN: 0-470-01184-X

28.1 Medical examinations at Child Health Clinics

Ilkka Kunnamo, Elina Hermanson

In general

- In Finland, all the children are routinely examined by a paediatrician before being discharged from the maternity hospital. At a Child Health Clinic a doctor re-examines all children at 6–8 weeks, 8 months, 18 months and 5 years, and whenever possible at 4 months and 3 years. These examinations are described in this article.
- The aims of scheduled examinations at a Child Health Clinic should include not only the screening for diseases and abnormalities but also the health promotion of the entire family. Although this article will concentrate mainly on the physical signs and symptoms, attention should also be paid to the child's mental status, his/her social environment (family) and risk factors; any concerns should be addressed.
- A health visitor should be available at each visit. If the policy of the clinic is such that a doctor will only examine children at 4 months and 3 years when referred by a health visitor, enough time must be allocated for these examinations. A doctor running a Child Health Clinic is expected to be able to identify deviations from normal. He must therefore be well versed in the normal development of children of all ages, even if he does not routinely examine children of a particular age group.
- According to Finnish guidelines, a health visitor sees the child and his/her family more often than the physician: at least monthly, until the child is six months old, and thereafter annually. Frequent visits are necessary, for example to monitor the child's growth and to deal with issues relating to health promotion (dietary advice, counselling regarding upbringing, vaccinations). These issues are not covered in this article.
- The task allocation between the doctor and health visitor during a scheduled visit should be decided on carefully, taking into account the experience and expertise of both professionals. The main task of the doctor is to draw up a conclusion of any suspected abnormalities, risk factors, resources and the child's overall situation. He should then explain his findings to the child and the family and work together with the family to plan any necessary further measures.
- Before a clinic the doctor and health visitor should together familiarize themselves with the case notes of the families attending the clinic.

6–8 weeks

Goals

- Diagnosis of developmental dysplasia of the hip by this age at the latest
- Detection of congenital cataract
- Detection of congenital hearing impairment
- Detection of severe cerebral palsy and severe visual impairment
- Any problems in the interaction between the child and parent should be noted, as should possible depression in the mother

Medical examination

- Read any notes entered by the health visitor (family situation, general observations) as well as the obstetrician's notes from the maternity hospital. Note the duration of the pregnancy, any observed abnormalities and risk factors.
- Talk to the parent. Postnatal depression is common and intervention is warranted, for the benefit of the mother and the infant since interaction problems may have far reaching implications. Make a new appointment if necessary (35.13).
- If the examination suggests an abnormality in the child's development the examination should be repeated after a short time interval (two weeks).
- Before examining the child check the progression of the child's length, weight and head circumference from the measurements obtained by the health visitor.
- The child should lie supine on the examination table
  - General impression, muscle tone, alertness. A referral for further investigation is warranted if the child's general health shows abnormal features (urgent referral) or weight gain is poor. Signs suggestive of cardiac problems in an infant include exhaustion whilst feeding, atypical pallor and sweating as well as increased respiratory rate (over 40 bpm).
  - Interaction and contact with the parent. The child should look comfortable on the lap and respond to a smile. The parent's responses to the infant should be empathetic and warm.
  - Observe and ask about oral motor functions and note any vocalising: the child should be able to suck without problems and make short vowel sounds.
  - Observe fixation of the eyes towards light. The child should be able to make brief eye contact and follow with his/her eyes for at least 90 degrees from one side to another and across the midline. Absent fixation or nystagmus may indicate visual impairment.
  - Check pupil size and reaction to light and confirm the presence of red reflex with an ophthalmoscope (28.5).
  - Auscultate the heart and palpate the femoral pulses. Absence of the femoral pulses is an indication for blood pressure measurement in the lower limbs (28.3), (28.4).
  - Palpate the head and cranial sutures, as well as abdomen: liver, spleen, possible masses. Inspect the skin.
  - Palpate the testes or inspect the vulval region. If the testes are undescended, inform the parents and examine the testes again at the next checkup (28.14).
  - Observe the posture of the child (remember that asymmetric tonic neck reflex is a normal phenomenon) and spontaneous movements. Examine the muscle tone by flexing the body, and the tone of the limbs by flexing the joints. Make sure that the ankles can be flexed with

gentle pressure with the hips and knees extended, and that the hips can be passively fully flexed. Inspect the feet for possible structural anomalies (28.13).

- Holding the child under the arms, check the support and stepping reflexes. Ability to support the whole body weight is not necessarily a sign of hypertonia.
- Check head control: a healthy and alert child will be able to hold his/her head up when the body is supported at 45 degrees from the horizontal. The child should also be able to hold his head momentarily when supported in a sitting up position. Failure to hold the head to any extent needs further investigation by a child neurologist.
- Observe whether the child is able to lift head from prone position so as to free his/her nose.
- Observe and ask about opening the hand from a fist. This should occur from time to time.
- Carry out the Ortolani test (28.5) and a provocation test for dislocation of the hip. Observe leg length discrepancy and asymmetry of skin folds. If either one is suspected but the Ortolani test is negative, perform the heel-buttock test. Even the slightest suspicion of congenital dislocation of the hip is an indication for specialist consultation (28.10).
- Check whether the child responds to noise (small bell etc.) with a startle, blinking his/her eyes or stopping to listen. If no reaction is evident ask about reactions to noise at home (during light sleep). If any suspicion arises or if the parents suspect hearing impairment re-examine the child in 1–2 weeks and refer for further investigations to an ENT specialist if necessary.

Four months

Goals

- ♦ Detection of hypertonia, abnormal body posture or movements, or asymmetry in order to commence physiotherapy.
- ♦ Identify any jerky movements which occur immediately upon awakening suggesting infantile spasms. If such are suspected, refer the child for further investigation.
- ♦ Identify the family's possible need for extra support and organize help as necessary.
- ♦ It is possible for a health visitor to manage all the above problems. Local arrangements may therefore be agreed on whereby, for example, the doctor reads the case notes of all the children coming up to their four month's check and will then only examine those he considers necessary. The doctor should discuss the children and their families with the health visitor and give the health visitor support to ensure that any problems and risk factors are addressed as early as possible.

Medical examination

- ♦ Talk to the parent first about the situation at home and ask whether the parents have any particular concerns.
- ♦ Check the progression of the child's length, weight and head circumference and read any notes entered by the health visitor (vaccinations, general observations).
- ♦ If the examination suggests an abnormality in the child's development the examination should be repeated after a short time interval (four weeks).
  - General impression and alertness.
  - Interaction and contact with the parent. The child should smile in response to a smile or a voice. He/she should be able to babble, squeal and laugh out loud as well as make various sounds in response to talk.
  - The child should lie supine and undressed. Check the child's ability to fixate his/her eyes by moving a red object or your own face across his/her visual field. If the child fails to follow with his/her eyes ask the mother about her observations regarding eye contact. The child's inability to follow an object during the examination, or according to parenteral observation, is an indication of an abnormality warranting further investigation (28.5).
  - Check the light reflex (Hirschberg test) and the red reflex. Strabismus and absence of red reflex warrant specialist intervention.
  - Check hearing (stops to listen to a small bell etc.). Pay special attention to hearing if the child vocalizes little, the parents suspect a hearing impairment or the family or pregnancy history (prematurity, asphyxia, infections) suggest the risk of a hearing defect.
  - Auscultate the heart and palpate the femoral pulses (28.3), (28.4).
  - Observe and ask about the use of the upper extremities: hands not in fist when resting, hands together when supine, puts hands into mouth, reaches for an object and tries to grasp objects with a half open hand.
  - Check head control by pulling the child up to about 45 degrees from the horizontal. The head should follow the body or lag behind no more than 10–15 degrees. The child should be able to hold his/her head and upper body steady when fully supported in a sitting position. If the head control is poor the examination should be repeated soon, and if no improvement is observed the child should be referred.
  - Observe the posture of the child and check for neonatal reflexes (the Moro reflex, grasp reflex, asymmetric tonic neck reflex and the stepping reflex). If these reflexes can be clearly elicited, further investigations are indicated. Test the muscular tone of the limbs and make sure that the ankles can be flexed with gentle pressure with the hips and knees extended (29.6). Any suggestion of mild hypertonia, hypotonia or asymmetry warrants a medical examination at 5 months.
  - Inspect the skin. Food allergy (milk) must be excluded as the causative agent of any persistent, extensive or worsening atopic eczema. As far as other skin and intestinal complaints are concerned, evaluate first whether the symptom is abnormal and requires further investigation or whether it is a manifestation of normal infancy.
  - Palpate the abdomen: liver, spleen, and possible masses. Examine the vulval region or testes. If one testicle remains undescended, observe. If both are undescended, refer the child to the care of a paediatric surgeon.
  - Place the child in the prone position and observe how he supports his/her upper body. Normally the child can

PAE

support himself so that the elbows are positioned in a vertical line with the shoulder joints or in front of them. Flexion of the elbows and upper extremities under the abdomen is an indication for referral.
- Check the abduction of the hips and carry out the Ortolani test (28.10). If stiffness is noted in the hips (the knees cannot be abducted towards the examination table) or the abduction is clearly asymmetric, leg length discrepancy is apparent or a "click" is heard on the Ortolani test, the child should be referred to a paediatric surgeon.

Eight months

Goals

- ♦ Detection of undescended testes by this age at the latest.
- ♦ Detection of motor abnormalities in order to introduce (sufficiently early) physiotherapy. Asymmetry should have already been diagnosed!
- ♦ Detection of strabismus
- ♦ Detection of impaired vision or hearing (health visitor test).
- ♦ Detection of preverbal problems. The child should be able to eat food that is of fairly coarse consistency, imitate sounds and vocalize in a polysyllabic fashion. If necessary may be referred to a speech therapist, provided that the child's hearing is normal.
- ♦ Detection of severe interaction disorders. Note whether the child avoids contact with the parent (whilst being held, eye contact); possible indication of abnormal parent–child interaction or psychosocial deprivation.
- ♦ Identify the family's possible need for extra support and organize help as necessary.

Medical examination

- ♦ Talk to the parent first about the situation at home and ask whether the parents have any particular concerns .
- ♦ Check the progression of the child's length, weight and head circumference and read any notes entered by the health visitor (vaccinations, general observations).
- ♦ If the examination suggests an abnormality in the child's development, appropriate professionals should be consulted (e.g. a physiotherapist). They are often able to give the parents advice regarding the child's development. The examination should be repeated after a short time interval (four weeks). An isolated finding is rarely of great significance.
  - General impression and alertness.
  - Observe the child's ability to interact: desire to be held, eye contact, responsive vocalisation, differentiation between familiar and unfamiliar people.
  - Observe and ask about oral motor functions and note any vocalising: the child should be able to eat from a spoon, chew and swallow. Responsive polysyllabic vocalisation (28.6).
  - Hirschberg's test and cover test to detect strabismus. If strabismus is detected or suspected, refer the child to an ophthalmologist (28.5). Check the ability to follow with eyes by moving an object up, down and to the sides.
  - Observe and ask about firmly grasping objects with both hands. Ability to transfer objects from hand to hand. Putting things in the mouth. Asymmetry in use of hands is so rare at this age that, if observed, the child should be referred for further investigations.
  - Auscultation of the heart (28.3, 28.4).
  - Inspect the skin and palpate the abdomen, testes. If a high scrotal testis or cryptorchidism is detected the examination should be repeated at the age of ten months. Alternatively the child can be referred immediately (28.14).
  - Observe whether the ankles are symmetrically dorsiflexed spontaneously while the hips and knees are extended (often only passive dorsiflexion is elicited during the examination while spontaneous dorsiflexion must be asked about). Absent or asymmetric dorsiflexion is an indication for referral (29.6).
  - Observe whether the child can support the upper body with straightened upper extremities when lying prone, and whether he can move the weight onto one hand when reaching for an object with the other (able to grasp the toy without losing balance). If this is unsuccessful, further investigations are indicated.
  - Examine the protective reflexes of the head forwards and to the sides. If the protective reflexes are totally absent the test should be repeated after one month, and if they are still absent the child should be referred for further investigations. If the child sits solidly on the floor unsupported with straight back and head up, this is sufficient and no further investigations are needed.
  - Weight bearing on straight legs. Observe for symmetry and whether the child supports his/her body weight on the soles of the feet or just on the toes and whether the legs cross each other. Standing on the toes occurs in about 10% of normal children at this age, but crossing of the legs and adduction spasm are always abnormal. If the child does not support his/her weight normally the examination should be repeated, and if there is no improvement a referral is warranted.
  - Test hearing by observing whether the child turns his/her head towards a noise coming obliquely from behind. If the child does not respond to the sound of a miniature audiometer, test hearing using a small bell. If the child has difficulties localizing the source of sound the test should be repeated after 1–2 weeks. Inspect the tympanic membranes. If the problem persists, and no fluid is seen behind the tympanic membranes, the child should be referred to an ear specialist.
  - Vision: the child should follow an object falling from the table, reach for a toy, and focus on an 8 mm ball at a distance of 30 cm (28.5).

18 months

Goals

- ♦ Detection of strabismus.

- Detection of major abnormalities in mental development.
- Detection of delayed speech with early intervention.
- Re-evaluation of any food restrictions imposed on a child with allergies. Many restrictions may be lifted from this age onwards.
- Identify the family's possible need for extra support and organize help as necessary.

Medical examination

- Talk to the parent first about the situation at home and ask whether the parents have any particular concerns.
- Check the progression of the child's height, weight and head circumference and read any notes entered by the health visitor (vaccinations, general observations).
  - General impression and alertness.
  - Observe the child's ability to interact: desire to be held, eye contact. The child shows distress with strangers at this age at the latest.
  - Speech: the child should have a few appropriately used words (28.6).
  - Uses a spoon to eat and chews without problems (parenteral observation).
  - Pincer grasp.
  - Builds a tower with two bricks (any problems may be associated with muscle tone, impaired hand-eye coordination or inability to imitate).
  - Appropriate handling of objects.
  - Interest in a new toy (nonspecific sign of visual observation and processing ability).
  - Ability to interact (a ball game, or "give and take" game).
  - Check the ability to follow with eyes and strabismus: move an object up, down and to the sides.
  - Hirschberg's test (28.5).
  - Sound localisation response. The child should turn his/her head towards the person who whispers his/her name.
  - Ability to walk without support.
  - Ability to stand up without support, e.g. when picking up a ball from the floor.
  - Spontaneous movements, sitting posture, muscle tone: pay particular attention to asymmetry and torticollis due to visual problems.
  - Skin, state of upper front teeth, heart sounds (28.3), abdomen, femoral pulses, testes.

Three years

Goals

- Detection of strabismus at the latest
- Detection of minor abnormalities of mental development
- Detection of linguistic problems
- Detection of chronic diseases affecting growth. Identify the family's possible need for extra support and organize help as necessary.
- It is possible for a health visitor to manage all the above problems. Local arrangements may therefore be agreed on whereby, for example, the doctor reads the case notes of all the children coming up to their 3 year's check and will then discuss the children and their families with the health visitor. The aim should be for the doctor to give the health visitor support who would otherwise have the whole responsibility of monitoring the child's development, and addressing any risk factors, between the ages of 18 months and 5 years. A medical examination should be carried out in all unclear cases.
- If a physician participates in the examination, it is wise to carefully decide on the task allocation between the doctor and health visitor. The health visitor will examine sight and hearing, measure height and weight and often also carry out the various tests involving drawing, building with bricks and understanding speech. The doctor's main tasks should involve the assessment of the tests carried out by the health visitor and the overall evaluation. The doctor will also assess gross motor skills, the child's ability to communicate and physical status. He should then draw an appropriate conclusion.

Medical examination

- Talk to the parent first about the situation at home and ask whether the parents have any particular concerns.
- Check the progression of the child's height, weight and head circumference and read any notes entered by the health visitor (vaccinations, general observations, notes regarding the child's skills). Any notes received from the child's day carers should also be taken into account.
- If the child does not pass a particular screening test it might be due to temper, tiredness or another transient factor. The test should therefore be repeated at a later stage. If the child attends a day care facility, the staff may need to be contacted.
  - General impression, abnormal movements.
  - Psychosocial development: the child should be able to wait for a short time and tolerate a short absence of the parent. He/she should be able to talk about incidents relating to himself/herself (narrative self; me, myself, I), show interest in other children, tell the difference between reality and fiction and be able to use the words "he" and "she" correctly.
  - Gross motor skills: gait, walking on toes, standing on one leg, jumping and throwing a ball. Walking should be directional, rhythmical, bouncy and relaxed. The child should be able to keep the direction even when looking around. If an abnormality is detected in at least three subtasks, when testing gross motor skills, the child should be referred to a physiotherapist or paediatric neurologist for further assessment. If the child fails two subtasks the examination should be repeated after a short time interval. An assessment can also be made in other sub-areas by using the same approach.
  - Speech comprehension: obeys simple commands, able to point to limbs and parts of the face (28.6).
  - Speech production: uses short sentences with correct basic grammar (28.6).

- Speech comprehension and perception: able to tell the difference between big and small in a picture, able to place different coloured bricks in their allocated place. (The test may be carried out by the health visitor).
- Hearing comprehension: understands the meaning of similar words that mean different things. (The test may be carried out by the health visitor).
- Hand-eye coordination: able to stack seven bricks, copy a circle and a horizontal and vertical line, able to unscrew a lid. (The test may be carried out by the health visitor).
- Vision: check near and distance vision with an appropriate vision chart (e.g. LH or LEA chart). (The test may be carried out by the health visitor. If the child is not co-operative, the test may be carried out at the next visit). Check for strabismus both visually and by cover test and Hirschberg's test (28.5).
- If the child exhibits problems in comprehending or producing speech, check hearing with a miniature audiometer or by whispering the child's name from a distance of approximately 2 m, from both sides of the child. Refer the child to a speech therapist if his/her speech is unclear or scant, if he/she has problems understanding short commands, changes the subject instead of replying to questions or is unable to concentrate on listening.
- Skin, state of upper front teeth, facial symmetry, heart auscultation (28.3), abdomen, femoral pulses, testes (28.14).

Five years

Goals

- ♦ This a good age to treat minor physical abnormalities surgically. The child is now mentally mature enough, for example, to tolerate a short separation from his/her parents.
- ♦ Assessment of the child's maturity to cope with school and identification of special needs. Many neurological problems which could lead to learning difficulties at school are evident at this age and appropriate support should be commenced.
- ♦ Detect and start the treatment of nocturnal enuresis.
- ♦ Identify the family's possible need for extra support and organize help as necessary.

Examination

- ♦ A questionnaire for the parents should be included in the procedure. Parents should complete the questionnaire before the examination; ideally it should have been posted to the home. In addition to questions, the form should have a description of the behaviour of a normal five-year-old child.
- ♦ If the child attends a day care facility, the staff may be included in discussions regarding the child's status, skills and possible problems.
- ♦ A health visitor will conduct most of the examination. The doctor will carry out the physical examination and assess the gross neurological status. However, the main task of the doctor is to draw up a conclusion of any suspected abnormalities, risk factors, resources and the child's overall situation. The doctor should then explain his/her findings to the child and the family and work together with the family to plan any necessary further measures.

Examination by a health visitor

1. General impression; height, weight and head circumference.
2. Gross motor skills: walking on heels and toes, walking on toes along a straight line for 5 m, standing on one leg (at least 10 seconds without marked swaying) and skipping on one leg (should be able to do at least 10 times rhythmically). Should be able to throw and catch a beanbag from the distance of 2 m with arms clearly off the body.
3. Interaction, attention and motivation: should be able to concentrate continuously on the tasks of the examination (approx. 25–30 minutes). Speech should be adequate, taking both parties into consideration. Inability to move on from task to task may also be indicative of an attention deficit.
4. Speech and language skills are preferably tested with an appropriate, standardized test. Assess descriptive speech, speech comprehension (sentence structure, tense) speech motor control, serial auditory memory, sentence memory and word images, naming objects and articulation as well as the understanding of basic concepts and various instructions. Speech impediment involving one or two sounds is not a cause for concern if the speech is otherwise fluent and language skills are appropriate for age.
5. Visual perception: the child should be able to rebuild a six brick structure.
6. Hand-eye coordination: able to copy patterns (a triangle and a combination of a triangle and a square), able to cut out a circle with scissors, able to thread 5–6 beads (1 cm) onto a plastic thread in a minute.
7. Vision: check near and distance vision with an appropriate chart (e.g. LH or LEA chart, see 28.5). Check visually for strabismus. Normal visual acuity is above 0.7 (monocular and binocular testing) and the test result should not differ more than one line between the two eyes.
8. Check hearing with an audiometer. Normal hearing is 20 dB at 0.25–4 kHz.
9. Blood pressure.

Examination by a doctor

- ♦ Familiarize yourself with medical notes and test results, interview the parents and examine the child. Some of the above tests might be included in the medical examination, particularly if the health visitor has been unsure of the outcome of a particular test.
- ♦ If the child has an ongoing problem (e.g. enuresis) it should naturally be addressed during this visit. Address the reasons for, as well as the necessity of, possible avoidance diets.
  - General impression; the progression of height, weight and head circumference.
  - Diadochokinesia (able to repeat five times with the same tempo without moving the upper arm).
  - Finger-to-nose test (should be able to perform without tremor or compulsive movements).

- Vision: check results from visual acuity testing, cover test, Hirschberg's test (28.5), convergence.
- Skin, state of upper front teeth, facial symmetry, heart auscultation (28.3), abdomen, femoral pulses, testes (28.14).
- Chat to the child: how does he/she perceive his health, who are his/her friends, what are his/her favourite games. It is important to listen to the child's opinions and to evaluate his/her ability to interact and concentrate. The child should be able to follow simple rules, concentrate on one game at a time for 10–15 minutes and enjoy role playing.
- Draw a conclusion regarding any suspected abnormalities, risk factors, resources and the child's overall situation. Plan any necessary further measures together with the family.

Equipment

Necessary

- Stethoscope
- Spatula
- Spot light (an otoscope without an earpiece)
- Ophthalmoscope
- Headlamp
- Pneumatic otoscope + a series of earpieces
- Instruments for cleaning wax from the ears
- Reflex hammer
- Sphygmomanometer (5 cm and 7.5 cm cuffs)
- Chart for visual examination (e.g. with LEA symbols)
- Equipment for hearing examination: small bell, miniature audiometer
- Equipment for neurological examination (e.g. books, pictures, red ball of wool, bell, rattle, bricks, ball, beanbag, pencil, scissors, raisins)

Recommended

- Doppler stethoscope
- Tympanometer or acoustic reflectometer

28.3 Heart auscultation and blood pressure recording in children

Ilkka Kunnamo

Heart auscultation

- The heart should be auscultated both precordially and between the scapulae at every child health surveillance visit.
- Pay attention to the following:
  - Loudness of the possible murmur
  - Punctum maximum (PM) where the murmur is best heard
  - Timing of the murmur (systolic or diastolic?)
  - Nature of the murmur (crescendo or decrescendo)
  - Tone (vibratory, coarse, softly hissing)
- The second heart sound (S2) should be auscultated at the pulmonary area. Observe accentuation and splitting and whether splitting is constant (pathological) or present only during inspiration (normal).
- If a clear murmur can be heard at the back further investigations should always be performed to rule out coarctation of the aorta (a murmur on the left side of the spine), patent ductus arteriosus, or pulmonary stenosis (a murmur on both sides).
- For murmurs see 28.4.

Recording the blood pressure

Equipment

- Blood pressure is recorded with a normal stethoscope. A Doppler stethoscope (5.20) or an oscillometric manometer (e.g. Dinamap®) can also be used.

When to record blood pressure in children

- Blood pressure should be recorded
  - in all children at the age of 5–6 years and always regardless of age in children with
    - 2nd degree murmur
    - even a weak murmur at the back, or
    - a weak or unpalpable femoral pulse.

Recording and interpretation of the result

- Children below 6 months of age are examined in a supine position. Older children should sit on the lap of a parent, because the child should be calm during the recording (crying raises blood pressure).
- Place the cuff around the upper arm when recording blood pressure from the upper extremity.
  - Auscultate with stethoscope at the cubital area. If a doppler stethoscope is used, auscultate the radial pulse.
- When recording lower extremity pressure place the cuff around the thigh when the pressure is measured by auscultating the popliteal artery with an ordinary stethoscope. If a Doppler stethoscope or oscillometer is used place the cuff around the leg proximal to the malleoli. Auscultate the pulse from the tibialis posterior or dorsalis pedis arteries.
  - Normally the blood pressure measured in the lower extremity is at least as high as that measured in the upper arm (even in a supine position). When the measurements are compared, remember that the first value is higher than subsequent values because of the child's possible anxiety.

- If there is no difference in the blood pressures the recording should be repeated later.
- If the pressure measured by the ankle is even slightly lower than the upper arm pressure record the pressures from all four limbs.
- If the average blood pressure measured at the lower limb is more than 5 mmHg lower than the higher of the values obtained from the upper arms, refer the child to a paediatrician C [1].

Reference

1. Rahiala E, Tikanoja T. Suspicion of aortic coarctation in an outpatient clinic: how should blood pressure measurements be performed? Clin Physiol 2001;21:100–104.

28.4 Cardiac murmur in a child

Eero Jokinen

General principles

- Murmurs suggestive of organic disease should be identified; 1% of children have a congenital heart defect.
- A vibratory sound is heard in at least every fifth child, and occasionally in more than half of the children (for example during fever).
- Blood pressures from the right arm and the leg should be measured in each child with a systolic murmur to rule out aortic coarctation.

Signs of congenital heart disease

- Poor sucking, paleness, easy sweating and rapid breathing (>40/min) may be signs of cardiac failure in an infant.
- Often the clinical condition of the child is quite normal in spite of a congenital heart malformation that requires surgery.
- Cyanosis only around the mouth is usually an innocent finding caused by abundant venous vascularity in that area and slow peripheral circulation.
- Cyanosis associated with congenital heart disease is always seen also in the trunk, face and tongue if the child is not anaemic.

Systolic murmurs

- The tone of an **innocent murmur** is mostly vibratory and of the ejection type (crescendo–diminuendo pattern). It is usually heard best in the third intercostal space on the left side of the sternum. The murmur is clearly less audible in the standing position.
- In **ventricular septal defect** (VSD), the murmur begins with the first heart sound and is often pansystolic but may end in midsystole when the defect is small. The sound is often whistling. The punctum maximum of the murmur is usually located in the 3rd–4th intercostal space.
- In **atrial septal defect** (ASD), the punctum maximum is usually in the second to third i.c. space on the left side. The second heart sound is permanently split, also during expiration. ECG shows partial right bundle branch block.
- A cardiac murmur high on the right side of the sternum is suggestive of a **bicuspid aortic valve** or **aortic stenosis**. Echocardiography is indicated.
- The tone of a murmur caused by **pulmonary stenosis** is harsher than that associated with an ASD or that of a physiological ejection sound. The closure of the pulmonary valve is delayed leading to constant but mobile splitting of the second heart sound. The murmur is easily audible on both left and right sides in the back.
- No systolic murmur should be regarded as physiological before the possibility of **aortic coarctation** is ruled out. In addition to palpation of femoral pulses blood pressures must be measured in right arm and in thigh (with sphygmomanometer) or leg (oscillometric device). Normally the systolic BP is at least as high in the leg as in the arm. A murmur caused by aortic coarctation is usually easily heard left of the spine on the back. In an infant with heart failure and low cardiac output there may be hardly any murmur audible.
- A physiological ejection murmur is a diagnosis of outruling.

Murmurs heard both in systole and diastole

- A diastolic murmur is rarely innocent. Venous hum is the only benign diastolic murmur. This soft murmur is heard both in systole and diastole under the clavicles, usually better on the right side. The murmur disappears when the jugular veins are compressed, the head is turned or when the child lies down.
- Patent ductus arteriosus causes a murmur that is heard in systole and also continues to be heard after the second heart sound (continuous murmur). The punctum maximum is under the left clavicle. The murmur is often heard also in the back.

What to do when a murmur is heard for the first time

- All cardiac murmurs heard, perhaps excluding very soft murmurs of I/VI grade, should be reported to the parents. A murmur heard during fever is usually a physiological ejection murmur, which may not be audible in other circumstances. This is why a murmur heard during infection is not something to be alarmed about; it is enough to agree with the parents over when and where the child's heart will be auscultated next time.
- When you give information about the murmur, it is best to mention that innocent murmurs are very common and that

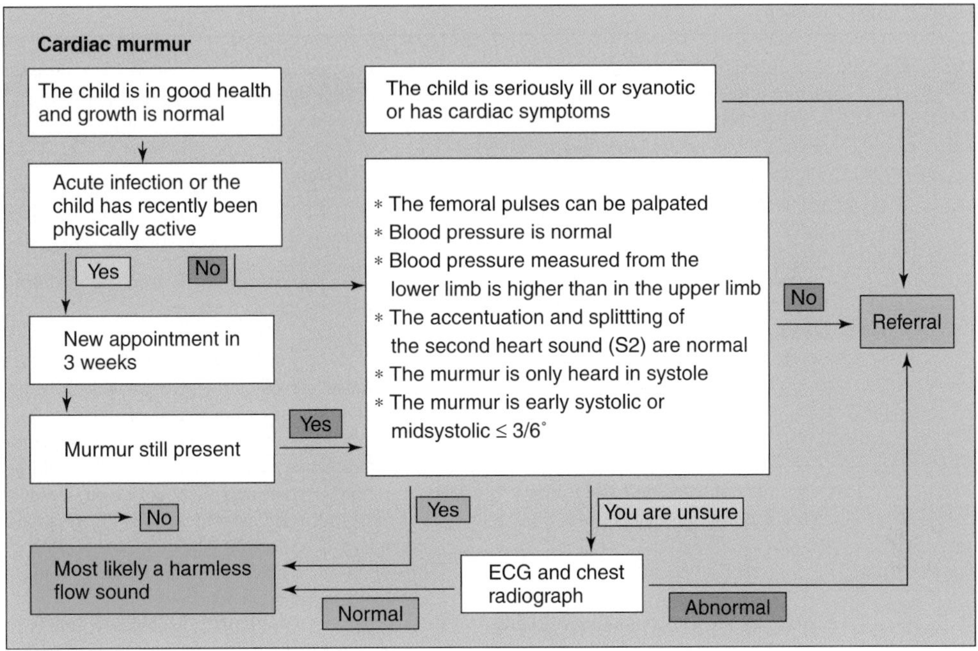

Figure 28.4.1

aortic coarctation has been ruled out in a child with normal blood pressures.

- If a heart defect is suspected the child should be referred for further studies.
  - Terms like 'a hole in the heart' should not be used. Neither should comments about cardiac surgery be made.
  - No restrictions for physical activities are given unless it is necessary for quite obvious reasons.
- If the child is in good health and heart defect has been ruled out, referral for further studies is not necessary. These children can be followed up on normal child health clinic visits. However, majority of significant structural heart defects is found during the first months of life, so murmurs heard in infancy should be well investigated.

Prophylaxis for endocarditis

- See also recommendations on endocarditis prophylaxis 4.81.
- To prevent endocarditis a single dose of antibiotics is given in conjunction with a procedure that causes laceration of the mucous membranes resulting in iatrogenic temporary bacteraemia. In persons with congenital heart disease the basic guidelines of antibiotic therapy are otherwise the same as in all other persons.
- The need for endocarditis prophylaxis is always decided by a specialist. Prophylaxis is usually given to patients with any congenital heart disease, ASD being an exception to the general rule. Usually the prophylaxis is given also after surgical treatment of the defect (excluding the closure of patent ductus arteriosus).

28.5 Examination of the eyes and vision as a part of paediatric health care

Lea Hyvärinen

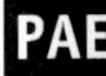

Examination scheme

- See Table 28.5.

Investigations

Red reflex

- Should be examined before the 6th week of life.
- Congenital cataract, structural abnormalities of the eyes, and abnormal pupillary reaction to light are indications for further investigation.

Hirschberg's test

- Perform the test at each visit from the age of 3–4 months.
- Keep a penlight in front of your eyes at a distance of about 50 cm from the child's face.
- If the child has no strabismus, the light is reflected from the centre or slightly off-centre of the pupil, symmetrically in

Table 28.5 Paediatric vision screening

Age	Observations	Indications for referral
Newborn	Structure of the eyes; size and light reaction of the pupils at penlight examination, red reflex with an ophthalmoscope	Structural abnormalities of the eyes, strabismus
6–8 weeks	Eye contact, symmetry of eye movements. Record eye and vision problems in the family (amblyopia, refractive errors, strabismus, tumours).	Roving nystagmus, strabismus
3 months	Social smile. The child fixates on the small fixation target picture, smooth tracking, convergence, Hirschberg's test.	Irregular tracking, constant or intermittent strabismus or problems with early interaction
6 months	As at the age of 3 months + cover test	As at the age of 3 months, constant or intermittent strabismus (may not be present during the examination!); refer constant strabismus without delay if the eyes have previously been aligned (retinoblastoma!). Children at risk (= with a family history of amblyopia) should be referred.
9–12 months	As above at 6 months (test one eye at a time); test also pincher grasp!	As at 6 months strabismus (may not be present during the examination); refer without delay if the eyes have previously been straight. Children at risk (with a family history of amblyopia) should be referred to an ophthalmologist if not referred earlier.
3–4 years	Visual acuity binocularly and monocularly with LEA symbol charts (10-row chart[1]). Eye movements, cover test and stereotest (TNO).	♦ Less than 0.5 (20/40, 6/12) binocularly, unless near visual acuity is 0.5 or better (= myopia), or a difference of more than one line between the eyes. ♦ Latent squint, manifest strabismus, abnormal head posture.
5–6 years	Visual acuity and stereovision as in children at the age of 3–4 years; (LEA symbol chart, 15-row chart or a translucent chart) cover tests	Less than 0.8 binocularly (unless near visual acuity is 0.8) or a difference of more than one line in both distant and near vision tests; visual perception problems in neurological screening tests

both eyes. Asymmetry of reflexes suggests strabismus that can be further assessed with the cover test.

Cover test

- If the visual acuity of the child is asymmetrically impaired (amblyopia, lazy eye) the cover test is abnormal even if the Hirschberg's test was normal.
- The child looks at a fixation target (a picture or a small toy) at a distance of 30 cm from the eyes.
- If the child reacts asymmetrically to the covering of each eye in turn, further investigation is indicated even if no strabismus is detected.
- If movement of an eye is observed when the examiner's hand covers the other eye, the child has strabismus. (The eye with strabismus does not fixate on an object when both eyes are used. When the dominant eye is covered, the deviating eye fixates on the object, and thus moves away from the deviated position.)
- Stereovision tests are useful for the detection of deficient stereoscopic vision in children aged 3–6 years.

Actions to be taken

- Strabismus is always an indication for referral to an ophthalmologist. Particularly strabismus manifesting between the ages of 6 months and 3 years may result in permanently impaired vision in the squinting eye if left untreated.
- A family history of all abnormalities in the development of senses (amblyopia, strabismus, hearing impairment) and hereditable diseases should be recorded in the health record during the first visit. Children at risk should be referred to an ophthalmologist at latest at the age of 7–9 months.
- The eyes of children at risk should be examined and possible refractive errors diagnosed during early development. In particular, esotropia should be diagnosed before it has become permanent in order to ensure the development of binocular vision.
- The eyes and vision of preterm infants, as well as those of children with developmental delay, hearing impairment or multiple abnormalities, should be carefully examined at the time of the primary diagnosis because these children often have asymptomatic eye problems requiring treatment.

Reference

1. http://www.lea-test.fi.

28.6 Speech and language development

Ritva Kalenius

Introduction

- Children deviating from the age-related development path should be referred to a speech therapist for assessment **B** [1 2].
- Observation of early interaction is important: how does the adult make contact with the child; what is the developmental stage of the child's emotional life; what is the psychosocial situation?
- Delayed speech and language may be the first signs of a particular verbal problem (dysphasia), dyslexia, impaired hearing, mental retardation, autism or other conditions associated with contact problems, motor disorder (dyspraxia), deprivation, interaction problems within the family or complicated psychosocial problems encountered in children from a multicultural background.
- Family history of language or attention difficulties warrant a closer than normal monitoring of the development of the child's language skills and communication.

Referral to a speech therapist at different ages

- First year of life
  - Little vocalizing and babbling
  - Poor contact with adults
  - Suspicion of impaired hearing
  - Orientation, sucking, and swallowing reflexes are poorly developed; difficulties in eating
  - Short frenulum of the tongue (28.13)
- Children aged 1–2 years
  - No words or attempted words or other attempts at expressing oneself (gestures)
  - Suspicion of poor speech comprehension or does not obey commands (remember recurrent otitis media as a cause of impaired hearing)
  - Poor alertness
  - Difficult to make contact with the child
  - Speech is scant or not clear after the second birthday.
- Children aged 3–4 years
  - Speech is defective or not clear (phonemes or syllables change place, long words are shortened)
  - Major grammatical errors
  - Poor vocabulary, difficulty in finding words
  - Little speech, no or only a few sentences
  - Inadequate answers, "own language"
  - Stammering continues or starts after the physiological stammering age (at about 3 years)
  - Poor contact, the child does not stop to listen
  - Difficulties in following short instructions.
- Children aged 5–6 years
  - Pronunciation errors (r, s, l, k etc.) should be corrected before school age **B** [3]
  - Non-fluent speech (stammering, slurred speech) **B** [3]
  - Language or speech is scant or poorly developed in relation to age
  - The overall speech is not clear, which may be due to problems with motor and/or phonological fluency or difficulties in the ability to comprehend spoken language.
- Children aged 7–15 years
  - All the above mentioned problems if they have not been investigated before.

References

1. Law J, Boyle J, Harris F, Harkness A, Nye C. Screening for speech and language delay: a systematic review of the literature. Health Technology Assessment 1998;2:1–184.
2. The Database of Abstracts of Reviews of Effectiveness (University of York), Database no.: DARE-989012. In: The Cochrane Library, Issue 2, 2000. Oxford: Update Software.
3. Law J, Garrett Z, Nye C. Speech and language therapy interventions for children with primary speech and language delay or disorder. Cochrane Database Syst Rev. 2004;(2):CD004110.

28.10 Congenital dislocation of the hip

Ilkka Kunnamo

PAE

Aim

- To identify congenital dislocation of the hip in a neonate by examining the hips carefully both at the maternity hospital and at the first child health clinic check-ups in order to start abduction splinting as early as possible.

Epidemiology

- Congenital dislocation of the hip is present in about 0.7% of newborns.
- Familial occurrence is common.

Examination of the hips

- The hips must be examined carefully at the first scheduled child health clinic (well-baby clinic) examinations after birth and examination is recommended also on further visits until the child has learned to bear weight.

- In the **Ortolani's test** the lower extremities are abducted while the child is lying on the back. If the hip is dislocated it returns to its normal position with an audible snap.
- **Provocation test** is performed by attempting to dislocate the femoral head first by applying pressure on the medial aspects of the thighs. Perform the Ortolani's test after the provocation test.
- If the Ortolani's test is positive either without or with provocation, refer the child to a specialist. At the age of 4 months the Ortolani's test is no longer always positive even if the hip is dislocated. Instead there is abduction rigidity, which is also an indication for referral.
- **Length discrepancy** of the lower extremities may indicate dislocation. The discrepancy is best observed when both the hips and the knees are flexed 90°. Asymmetric inguinal skin folds may suggest dislocation; however, they are 10 times more common than actual dislocation.
- The heel–buttock test is often abnormal in dislocation: Flex the knees and extend the hips with the child lying prone so that the heels touch the buttocks. The heel on a dislocated side crosses the midline and touches the opposite buttock.
- Congenital dislocation may be bilateral. In such cases tests for asymmetry do not disclose the dislocation. The Ortolani's test and the provocation test are also positive in bilateral cases.

28.11 Screening for secretory otitis media at the child health clinic

Ilkka Kunnamo

- Ear examination need not be carried out in asymptomatic children C [1 2 3].
- The appearance and mobility of the tympanic membranes should be examined if the child has
  - prolonged symptoms of respiratory tract infection
  - wheezing or cough
  - frequent crying at nights
  - recurrent episodes of acute otitis media
  - observed or suspected impairment of hearing
  - difficulties in speech perception or no spoken words at the age of 18 months.
- If the tympanic membrane looks inflamed and the child has symptoms of otitis media, prescribe antibiotics and re-examine the ears after 3–4 weeks (31.42).
- Asymptomatic serous or secretory otitis media can be followed up for at least three months before the child is referred to an ENT specialist. For nasal insufflation therapy see 31.44.

References

1. New Zealand Health Technology Assessment. Screening for the detection of otitis media with effusion and conductive hearing loss in pre-school and new entrant school children: a critical appraisal of the literature. NZHTA. Report 3. 1998. pp. 1–161.
2. The Database of Abstracts of Reviews of Effectiveness (University of York), Database no.: DARE-989040. In: The Cochrane Library, Issue 2, 2000. Oxford: Update Software.
3. Butler CC, van der Linden MK, MacMillan H, van der Wouden JC. Screening children in the first four years of life to undergo early treatment for otitis media with effusion. Cochrane Database Syst Rev. 2004;(2):CD004163.

28.12 Lacrimal duct stenosis in an infant

Ilkka Kunnamo

Basic rule

- Wait for spontaneous recovery for at least 6 months.

Symptoms

- About 2–5% of newborns have symptoms of lacrimal duct stenosis.
- The stenosis makes the eye wet from the age of two weeks.
- The stenosis predisposes the infant to conjunctivitis (37.22).

Treatment

- 80% of stenoses are canalized spontaneously before the age of 8 months.
- The treatment of an eye with conjunctival discharge is as follows:
  - Press the medial corner of the eye with a cotton-tipped swab or the little finger (with the nail cut short) 4–5 times a day, wipe off the discharge that eventually emerges from the lacrimal canal, and apply a drop of topical antibiotic to the conjunctival sac. Pressing the lacrimal sac often succeeds best if the child is approached from above while he/she is sleeping or drinking from the bottle. Show the correct location of the lacrimal sac to the parents, who often tend to press the wrong site. The lacrimal sac is under a ligament inserted in the medial corner of the eye, and the pressure applied must be sufficiently great.
- The treatment is repeated every time the eye produces purulent discharge. Topical antibiotics should be applied only if there is marked discharge, and redness or swelling of the conjunctiva.

- Referral to a specialist is indicated only if symptomatic stenosis is present after the age of 6–8 months.

28.13 Structural anomalies in children (extremities, trunk, genitals, frenulum of the tongue)

Ilkka Kunnamo

Basic rule

- None of the abnormalities listed below requires systematic screening in primary care or at the child health clinic (with the exception of foot disorders). However, a GP should be familiar with the approach to these conditions in case he/she or the parents or a nurse detects such a condition.

Structural anomalies of the extremities

- **Club foot (talipes equinovarus)** can always be diagnosed immediately after birth.
- **Talipes calcaneovalgus congenitus,** with the foot of the newborn inverted to a valgus position and dorsiflexion, seldom needs treatment other than mobilization performed by the parents.
- **Talipes metatarsus adductus** is characterized by internal rotation of the forefoot visible as an inverted curvature of the medial side of the forefoot. A cast, plaster, or surgery may sometimes be needed.
- **Flat foot** is an innocent finding if the forefoot can be freely mobilized into inversion and eversion, and the valgus angle disappears when the child stands up on the toes.
- **Walking with the feet rotated externally or internally** is a normal condition that does not need treatment.
- **Genu varum (bandy-leg)** is an indication for specialist consultation if it is unilateral or becomes worse after the second year of life.
- **Genu valgum (knock-knee)** is an indication for specialist consultation if it is unilateral (Blount's disease) or if the distance between the malleoli continues to be at least 10 cm at school start. Bilateral genu valgum is a normal condition and is usually most evident around the age of 3 years.
- Toes lying on each other seldom need surgical treatment.
- **Syndactylia** of the hands should be evaluated by a paediatric surgeon soon after birth if the first and second finger are involved. In other cases surgical correction should take place at the age of 4–5 years. All cases of syndactylia need evaluation by a pediatric surgeon. **Syndactylia of the foot** usually needs no treatment.

Anomalies of the trunk

- A **phimosis** is an indication for circumcision if the child has recurrent balanitis or even one urinary tract infection, if there are scars in a tight foreskin, or if the child has episodes of paraphimosis (the foreskin is trapped behind the glans). Bulging of the preputium during urination is not alone an indication to surgery.
- An **umbilical hernia** should probably be treated surgically if a finger can be passed through the hernia canal after the age of one year (i.e. the canal is at least 1.5 cm in diameter). All children with an umbilical hernia remaining at the age of 5 years should be referred to a paediatric surgeon.
- An **inguinal hernia** is always an indication for referral. The parents are told that a bulging hernia itself is not dangerous, they are instructed how to reduce the hernia, and are advised to consult a doctor if the hernia cannot be reduced and the child cries continuously.
- A **hydrocele** need not be operated on before the age of three years. In younger children it can be followed up in primary care (11.23).
- Occasional **pigmented spots** are usually harmless (Figure 28.13.1).
- A **haemangioma** may grow during the first year of life. The parents should be told this, and assured about its tendency to regress spontaneously (Figure 28.13.2).
- A "pseudotumour" of the sternocleidomastoid muscle (torticollis of an infant) can be treated by changing the lying position and by physical therapy. If the muscle remains contracted, surgery may be indicated at the age of 10–12 years.
- **Pectus carinatum** is not an indication for surgery. **An exceptionally severe pectus excavatum** may require surgery.

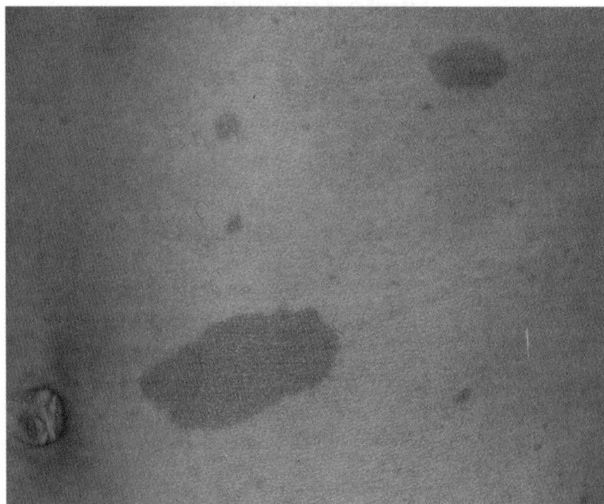

Figure 28.13.1 Occasional, small, evenly coloured brown patches-cafe au lait spots - have no clinical significance. If more numerous and larger - as shown here - the possibility of neurofibromatosis should be considered. Photo © R. Suhonen.

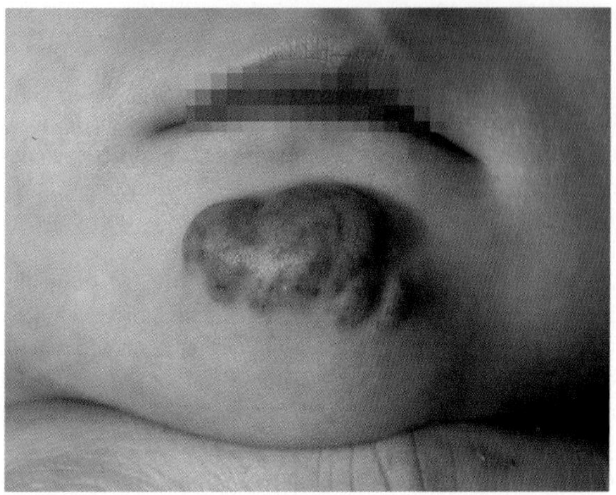

Figure 28.13.2 In medical literature this type of tumour may be called a capillary or cavernous haemangioma. The prominent vascular tumour may be present at birth or develop during the first weeks to months. It may ulcerate. Most commonly no therapy is needed, but the haemangioma retracts spontaneously during childhood, leaving a pale scar. Photo © R. Suhonen.

Frenulum of the tongue

- A **frenulum of the tongue** does not require an operation unless it prevents the tip of the tongue from touching the upper teeth, hampers eating or is associated with speech problems in children aged above 4 years.
- An ENT specialist performs the operation.

28.14 Undescended testicle

Seppo Taskinen

Principles

- If left untreated, the amount of germ cells in an undescended testis decreases with time. Even when treated, the undescended testes are usually smaller at adult age than testes that have descended normally.
- Approximately one half of undescended testes observed at birth descend spontaneously during the first year of life.
- In pre-school age, a movable testis (testis saltans) is very common. The underlying cremaster reflex usually subsides by school age, but in some cases the testis may retract again.
- Examine the testes at every health check in pre-school and school age.
- Refer to a paediatrician children with
  - undescended testis or testes at the age of one year
  - earlier if absence of both testes is suspected (particularly if there is any abnormality in the external genitalia)
  - also later if the testis is constantly out of the scrotum.

Table 28.14 Dosage of human chorionic gonadotrophin

Age	Single dose
1–3 years	1 500 IU
3–6 years	3 000 IU
>6 years	5 000 IU

Examination of the testicles

- Inspect the testes calmly with the child standing or sitting on a parent's lap in the taylor's position with the legs crossed. (The testis often bounces up when the examining hand approaches).
- The testes are palpated either in the taylor's position or in supine position. The testis is 'milked' down from the inguinal fold with one hand and taken hold of with the other hand.
- Note whether the testis can be pulled to the bottom of the scrotum and whether it remains there.

Treatment

- The aim is to treat an undescended testis during the second year of life to minimize permanent damage.
- Uncertain cases may require follow up before a decision on treatment can be made.
- The treatment of a true undescenced testis is surgical.
- Hormone treatment can be considered in mild cases if the testis can be pulled to the scrotum with difficulty and does not remain there. The safety of hormone treatment especially in children below 2 years of age as regards to the development of the testes has been questioned.
  - The drug used for hormone treatment is human chorionic gonadotrophin (HCG) Ⓐ [1,2] given in three injections at one-week intervals, see Table 28.14.

References

1. Pyörälä S, Huttunen NP, Uhari M. A review and meta-analysis of hormonal treatment of cryptorchidism. J Clin Endocr Metab 1995;80:2795–2799.
2. The Database of Abstracts of Reviews of Effectiveness (University of York), Database no.: DARE-952666. In: The Cochrane Library, Issue 4, 1999. Oxford: Update Software.

28.15 Enuresis in a child

Ilkka Kunnamo

Basic rules

- Examine a urine specimen in all children with daytime enuresis and refer them to a paediatrician.

- Treat nocturnal enuresis in primary care (with an alarm device and temporarily with desmopressin) from the age of 5 years.

Epidemiology

- 15–20% of children aged 5 years have enuresis, and two thirds of these children have only nocturnal enuresis.

Aetiology

- The development of bladder control is a complex skill that usually develops before the age of 4 years.
- Delays and disturbances in bladder control are common. At the age of 7 years about 10% of children have enuresis at least occasionally.
- Enuresis as such does not indicate a psychological disturbance, but as bladder control is vulnerable to external disturbances, exciting events and life changes may cause enuresis in a child who has already achieved bladder control. Enuresis should not be called a disease but an annoyance.

Timing of treatment

- Nocturnal enuresis need not be treated in children below 5 years of age nor in children who have enuresis no more than once a week.
- The child's own desire to become dry is a prerequisite for successful treatment.

Selecting the method of treatment

- An **enuresis alarm device** is the recommended method (A) [1 2 3]. Its use requires that both the child and the parents are sufficiently motivated.
- **Desmopressin** nasal spray can be used as a temporary treatment (A) [4]; during travelling for example. In long-term treatment desmopressin is an alternative to an alarm device if this is not effective or if the child does not wake up when the device sounds.
- After desmopressin spray or tablets have been taken the child should not drink because of the risk of water intoxication.
- Tricyclic antidepressants are effective but their use is limited by side effects (A) [5].

Principle of operation and use of an alarm device

- The sensor of the alarm device placed in the bed or in the clothing triggers a loud alarm when it becomes wet.
- Every alarm is a "teaching opportunity": the child learns to become aroused and stop voiding when spontaneous voiding begins.
- After the alarm wet clothing and bedclothes should be changed but the child need not go to the lavatory if he or she does not want. For learning it is useful to have another alarm during the same night. Because the results are based on learning there will be no dry nights at the beginning but only after a couple of weeks or more.
- It is important to teach the child and the parents how the device functions and what its effects are based on. It is preferable that the child takes part in the preparations (making the bed and setting the alarm). The alarm blanket should be placed in the middle of the bed, and if possible, the child should sleep without clothing on the lower part of the body to allow the alarm blanket to become wet as early as possible. A trouser-like alarm device (Rapidosec®) is also on the market.
- The parents should keep a diary (did the bed get wet, was the alarm triggered?) and they should be able to contact a nurse by telephone. The alarm device should be returned after 3 months at the latest. On return, the diary is examined and the response to treatment is assessed.
- If enuresis recurs later the alarm device can be taken into use again.

Investigating and treating daytime enuresis

- A urine specimen (dipstick test and bacterial culture) should be examined in all children with daytime enuresis.
- Daytime enuresis is an indication for specialist consultation. Renal ultrasonography should always be performed, complemented by mictiocystography (isotope method or radiographs) if vesicoureteral reflux is suspected.
- Daytime enuresis can often be treated by bladder schooling and oxybutynin medication according to the results of cystometry.
- For a child psychiatrist's approach to enuresis see 33.9.

References

1. Glazener CMA, Evans JHC, Peto RE. Alarm interventions for nocturnal enuresis in children. Cochrane Database Syst Rev. 2004;(2):CD002911.
2. NHS Centre for Reviews and Dissemination. A systematic review of the effectiveness of interventions for managing childhood nocturnal enuresis. York: NHS Centre for Reviews and Dissemination (NHSCRD). 1900640104. CRD Report 11. 1997. 173.
3. The Health Technology Assessment Database, Database no.: HTA-998340.In: The Cochrane Library, Issue 1, 2001. Oxford: Update Software.
4. Glazener CMA, Evans JHC. Desmopressin for nocturnal enuresis in children. Cochrane Database Syst Rev. 2004;(2): CD002112.
5. Glazener CMA, Evans JHC, Peto RE. Tricyclic and related drugs for nocturnal enuresis in children. Cochrane Database Syst Rev. 2004;(2):CD002117.

28.16 Recurrent infections and immunodeficiencies

Ilkka Kunnamo

Reasons for recurrent infections

Related to the child

- An overwhelming majority of children suffering from recurrent infections have a normal immune system, and there is no need for special investigations or treatments. The following features suggest normal immune system:
  - Only respiratory infections
  - The infections are caused by viruses
  - Recovery from individual infections is normal
  - Normal growth and development
  - Normal physical status and chest x-ray
  - No family history of increased sensitivity to infections
- Some children have dysfunctional problems of the middle ear, the Eustachian tube or on the adenoids. Children with gastro-oesophageal reflux tend to have frequent lower respiratory infections.
- Atopy as such does not predispose to infections, and there are no indications for prescribing antibiotics to atopic children with less strict criteria than to other children. Children with respiratory wheezing, "asthma-like symptoms" or airway hyper-reactivity will easily become misclassified as children with recurrent infections because they often have prolonged cough and rhonchi.
- True immunodeficiencies (see below) are very rare.

Environmental factors

- Frequent contact with infections
  - Small children in public day care have 1.5–3-fold more infections compared with those cared for at home.
- Passive smoking
  - Exposure to environmental tobacco smoke may increase the number of infections by twofold.

Primary investigations

- History
  - The number and duration of infections (5–10 infections a year may be considered normal in children younger than 3 years of age)
  - Form of day care
  - Exposure to environmental tobacco smoke
- Ears should be examined with a pneumatic otoscope or a tympanometer (glue ear).
- The size of the adenoid may be deduced from mouth breathing and snoring. A x-ray is not indicated.
- Children over 4 years of age will need a sinus x-ray or ultrasound.
- Chest x-ray, if indicated.

Treatment

- Continuing doctor–patient relationship
- Advice to parents
- Consider changing form of day care
- Chewing xylitol-containing chewing gum between meals decreases middle ear infections in 4–5-year-olds.
- Adenoidectomy and tympanostomy
- Antibiotics my be beneficial in prolonged rhinosinusitis B [1].

Adenoidectomy and tympanostomy

- Indications for consulting a specialist
  - Continuous rhinitis or cough
  - Recurrent middle ear infection and sinusitis
  - Glue ear and obstruction of the Eustachian tube
  - Mouth breathing, snoring and disturbed sleep
  - Dental malocclusion and delayed growth of the maxilla
- The adenoid of a child may grow larger as a result of respiratory infections, but rarely obstructs the nasopharynx totally. The bacteria colonizing the adenoid act as a reservoir during viral infections, increasing the risk of complications.
- Measuring the size of the adenoid before the procedure with x-ray is only rarely indicated.
- Adenoidectomy should be considered when there is no other obvious cause for the above symptoms (remember asthma in the coughing child); however, there is scant evidence on the benefits of adenoidectomy in preventing recurrent infections or in treating glue ear.
- Insertion of tympanostomy tubes is often performed on children with glue ear that has not healed within 3 months. Operative treatment should be considered also after 3 (–5) documented acute middle ear infections.
- Usually the lower age limit is set at 9–12 months, and the lower weight limit at 8 kg.
- In an adult nasopharynx, any adenoid tissue should be considered tumorous, until its benign nature has been documented.

Indications for special investigations

- Characteristics suggesting immunodeficiency:
  - Recurrent purulent or invasive bacterial infections (skin infections, pneumonias etc.). Immunodeficiency should be suspected in a child with at least 10 suppurative middle ear infections that continue even after insertion of tympanostomy tubes.
  - The child has infections caused by unusual organisms (fungi, Pneumocystis carinii).
  - The child fails to thrive, and has prolonged diarrhoea or dermatitis.
  - There is a family history of problematic infections.

Immunodeficiencies

- IgA deficiency does not always increase proneness to infections.
- IgG subclass deficiency, where total IgG may be normal, increases the risk of infections caused by encapsulated bacteria.
- Severe humoral or cell-mediated immunodeficiencies are very rare.

Other biochemical deviations related to infection proneness

- Cystic fibrosis (31.23)
- Alfa-1-antitrypsine deficiency
  - Proneness to chronic lung disease, pulmonary infections and liver cirrhosis usually becomes manifest first in adulthood.

Investigations

- If immunodeficiency is suspected on the basis of symptoms listed above, the child should be referred to a paediatric unit.
- Specialist investigations include
  - sweat test
  - serum IgG, IgM, IgA
  - serum alfa-1-antitrypsine
  - serum electrophoresis
  - estimating the size of the thymus on chest x-ray.
- Further investigations may include IgG subclass determination, and other immunological measures, and diagnostic workup on gastro-oesophageal reflux.

Reference

1. Morris P, Leach A. Antibiotics for persistent nasal discharge (rhinosinusitis) in children. Cochrane Database Syst Rev. 2004;(2):CD001094.

28.17 Allergic diseases in the child health clinic

Ilkka Kunnamo

Indications for further examinations and specialist consultation

Dermatitis

- The child has a widespread dermatitis that does not respond to topical treatment.
- Sensitization to main foodstuffs is suspected (cow's milk, common cereals).

Respiratory and rhinitis symptoms

- Allergic rhinitis that does not respond to a mild medication
- Allergic rhinitis for which hyposensitization is considered (NB local treatment guidelines for hyposensitization: age at least 5 years, IgE-mediated allergy)
- Suspicion of asthma:
  - Recurring obstructive bronchitis (more than 2–3 episodes)
  - First case of obstructive bronchitis if a first-degree family member has asthma or if the child has been shown to have an IgE-mediated food allergy or atopic dermatitis
  - Prolonged cough in addition to allergic rhinitis during pollen season
  - Prolonged cough (lasting more than 6–8 weeks), particularly if the family history is positive
  - Prolonged night-time coughing every night.
  - The child is unusually tired and out-of-breath when playing, particularly if wheezing is heard on breathing.
  - Chest pain when physically active

28.40 The premature infant

Anna-Liisa Järvenpää

Definitions

- **Prematurity** denotes preterm delivery before the 37th week of pregnancy. Most premature infants weigh less than 2500 g, which has also been considered a criterion for prematurity. Premature infants may be small (small for gestational age (SGA), small for date), normal (appropriate for gestational age (AGA)) or large (large for date), as all other neonates.
- A **very low birthweight infant** denotes an infant weighing less than 1500 g. Most problems occur in infants weighing less than 1000 g ("extremely low birthweight infants").
- The **corrected age** is calculated from the estimated date of gestation determined according to the ultrasonography in early pregnancy or according to the last menstruation. The corrected age corresponds to the biological age better than the calendar age. The development of the premature infant should be assessed according to the corrected age as long as the difference is important in practice. If the child was born before the 28th week of pregnancy the correction is necessary at the age of one year, and possibly at the age of two years, but not any more at the age of three.

Growth

- The growth of premature infants is assessed according to the corrected age.

- Growth charts starting two months before the estimated time of birth are available. The charts also allow the monitoring of weight without relating it to unreliable (at this age) height.
- Monitoring of still earlier growth is based on intrauterine growth charts.
- Infants weighing more than 1500 g at birth grow evenly after they have attained birth weight (in 10–14 days).
- The growth is almost invariably retarded in very premature infants because of suboptimal conditions after birth. As soon as nutrition is adequate a catch-up growth starts both in these infants and in infants with intrauterine growth disturbance (small for date). Absence of the catch-up growth indicates continued problems with nutrition or body functions, or some underlying disease.

Nutrition

Energy, proteins, minerals

- The growth rate of premature infants is faster than that of full-term infants, resembling foetal growth. Thus the weight-adjusted need for nutrients and energy is higher in premature infants during the first weeks and months of life compared with full-term infants. Catch-up growth also increases the need for nutrients and energy. On the other hand, the stores obtained from the mother are small. Because of respiratory problems the amount of fluids may have to be restricted even to less than half of the normal weight-adjusted amount.
- Infants weighing more than 1800 g at birth grow well on a diet similar to that of full-term infants.
- Special arrangements are necessary for very low birthweight infants: in the hospital or after discharge until the child has either become "full-term" or has attained the weight of 3000–3500 g, breast milk needs to be fortified with proteins and minerals, or special preterm formulas that contain more energy, protein and trace elements than regular formulas are used. These formulas can also be used to supplement breast milk. Instructions concerning the use of these nutrients are given by the hospital.

Iron

- Premature infants need more iron than in children born at term because their blood volume and iron stores are small and their relative growth is rapid. Most of iron is transferred from the mother to the foetus during the last few weeks of pregnancy. The total iron intake in premature infants can be determined by birth weight:
  - birth weight < 1000 g: 4 mg/kg/day
  - birth weight 1000–1500 g: 3 mg/kg/day
  - birth weight 1500–2500 g: 2 mg/kg/day
  - or supplementary iron 2mg/kg/day and maximally 15 mg/kg/day.
- Additional iron is recommended up to the age of 12–15 months. Written instructions are provided for the parents. When iron solutions are used for children who have teeth, special attention should be paid on dental hygiene.

Vitamins

- The vitamin stores of premature infants are small, and a surplus of vitamins is required during the first weeks because of rapid growth. The need for vitamin D is, however, normal. i.e. 400 IU/day. Additional vitamin D should be administered up to the age of three years to prevent rickets. Infants with a very dark skin need supplementation up to the age of 5 years in Finland.
- Special vitamin preparations containing vitamins A, B_{12}, E, and folic acid are available for premature infants.
- The need for vitamins depends on the type of milk or milk formula.
  - Infants on breast milk
    - A special vitamin preparation for premature infants.
    - Vitamin D up to the age of three years even in summer.
  - Infants on special formulas for premature children
    - A special vitamin preparation for premature infants is not needed
    - Vitamin D is given if the amount of vitamin D-containing formula is <400 ml/day
    - Hospital staff advises on the use of other vitamin supplements.

Additional foods

- The child begins to receive other foodstuffs at the age of 4 months like full-term children. However, to ensure adequate nutrition, very premature children, particularly those weighing less than 1000 g at birth may require additional food earlier than this, already at 3–3.5 months.

Vaccinations

- The BCG vaccination is usually given after the weight of 2.5 kg has been reached.
- The rest of the immunization schedule can be carried out according to the chronological age (and not according to the corrected age).

Diseases

- During the first year of life, premature infants need more medical services than full-term infants. The smaller the child the more care is needed. The most common causes are respiratory infections, inguinal hernias and need for rehabilitation

Bronchopulmonal dysplasia (BPD)

- BPD is defined as a chronic pulmonary disorder caused by oxygen and ventilator therapy in very premature infants. BPD usually manifests before the age of four weeks or 36th gestational weeks.

- The clinical symptoms include rales, dyspnoea, and obstructive wheezing, and often, prolonged need of oxygen. In addition to the clinical symptoms the diagnosis is based on typical abnormalities on a chest x-ray and a typical history.
- The treatment of the most severely affected infants consists of inhaled corticosteroids, and bronchodilators during infections. If diuretics have been used, the medications are aimed to be stopped before the infant is discharged home as well as the fluid restriction is cancelled. Ensuring sufficient nutrition is important. The follow up of BPD infants is organised by the hospital.

Sensory defects

- Premature infants are subject to therapies that involve the risk of a hearing defect. The hearing of these children should be monitored carefully during childhood as some of the defects appear only later. New methods, such as otoacoustic emission and brainstem evoked potentials, help to identify infants who need special follow up and to detect hearing impairment early.
- Retinopathy affects nowadays the very smallest premature infants with the risk being highest in those born before gestational week 27. In addition to prematurity itself, oxygen therapy predisposes to retinopathy. The eyes of all infants born before week 32 are examined for retinopathy. The most severe cases are treated with laser or cryotherapy. Mild retinopathy can later result in myopia. Strabismus is more common in premature children compared with full-term children.

Psychomotor development

- The neurological development is monitored according to the same principles as in children born at term. During the first 18 months the corrected age is used for assessment of the developmental stage; in children born before week 30 it can be used up to the age of 18–24 months. In children born later using the correction can be discontinued earlier. Obvious developmental abnormalities require special investigations and assessment by a specialist.
- A typical problem of very premature children is cerebral palsy, particularly diplegia. In children with a birth weight over 1 500 g or born after week 30 the prevalence of neurological problems is clearly lower. However, most cases of cerebral palsy are not associated with prematurity.
- Problems with concentrating and cognitive skills are also more common among premature children compared with full-term children. Approximately one third of children with birth weight below 1 000 g need special support at school.
- However, the majority of infants weighing less than 1 500 g at birth develop normally although the risk of defects is increased.

28.41 Growth disturbances in children

Elina Hermanson

Basic rules

- Analysing the growth curves of children is essential for diagnosis of growth disturbance.
- Diagnose or rule out treatable conditions (thyroid disorders, coeliac disease, growth hormone deficiency, hypercortisolism).
- Anticipate the psychosocial consequences of growth disturbance and be prepared to hasten growth even in cases where there is no treatable cause.
- Consult a specialist early in all disturbances of height increase requiring assessment and treatment.

Anthropometric indexes

- The growth charts and classification systems vary from country to another. Remember to check that the reference population is applicable to your patient. In Finland, the anthropometric indexes used are length/height-for-age (L/A), head circumference-for-age (HC/A), weight-for-age (W/A), and weight-for-length/height (W/L or W/H). L/A, HC/A and W/A are expressed in standard deviation (SD) units (= z-scores) and W/L in percent-of-median.
- The use of L/A abolishes age and sex differences in the assessment of height. The use of W/L helps to identify situations where increases in weight are disproportional to increases in height.
- The expected L/A can be calculated from the equation
  - (average of parents' heights in cm)–171)/10
  - e.g. if the father is 185 cm and the mother is 165 cm the expected L/A of the child is ((185 + 165/2)–171)/10 = 4/10 = 0.4 SD units (z-score).
  - 171 is the average height of men and women in the finnish population and can be replaced by another figure if that is known to be more appropriate.
- Alternatively, some growth surveillance data sheets have nomograms to assess the expected L/A.
- Expected L/A should only be used for evaluation of growth and not for prediction of final height, for which it is an inaccurate estimate. If expected L/A greatly deviates from the average, similar deviations in the observed L/A should be accepted.

Growth between birth and adolescence

- Growth proceeds to its "channel" usually during the first year of life. Thereafter, L/A should remain fairly stable.

PAE

- After the first year the growth velocity decreases steadily until the spurt at adolescence. In some children there is a slight increase in growth velocity between the ages of 6 and 8 years.
- For growth in adolescence see 28.42.

Screening rules

Screening rule for height

- The limits of allowed relative height L/A
  - Deviation from expected L/A ± 2.3 SD
  - If the expected L/A is not known ± 2.7 SD
- See Tables 28.41.1 and 28.41.2

Screening rule for weight

- See Tables 28.41.3 28.41.4 28.41.5 28.41.6.

Table 28.41.1 Accepted variation in relative height (SD) in L/A (SD) in children below 2 years of age.

Age, years	During the preceding 0.25 years	During the preceding 0.5 years	During the preceding 1.0 years
0.25	1.7		
0.5	1.1	2.1	
0.75	0.9	1.6	
1.0	0.9	1.5	2.3
1.25	0.8	1.4	1.9
1.5	0.7	1.3	1.7
1.75	0.6	1.2	1.6
2.0	0.6	1.0	1.5

The values of acceptable change in L/A (decrease and increase) are given for the period preceding the ages when height is measured. The headings indicate the length of time between controls.

Table 28.41.2 Accepted variation in L/A (SD) in children aged 2–12 years.

Age, years	During the preceding 1 year	During the preceding 3 years	During the preceding 5 years
2	1.5		
3	1.4		
4	1.2	1.8	
5	0.9	1.5	
6	0.9	1.2	1.9
7	0.9	1.1	1.7
8	0.7	0.9	1.4
9	0.6	0.9	1.3
10	0.6	0.9	1.3
11	0.7	1.0	1.3
12	0.7	1.1	1.3

The values of acceptable change in L/A (decrease and increase) are given for the period preceding the ages when height is measured. The headings indicate the length of time between controls.

Table 28.41.3 Accepted W/L (% of median) in children, height 50–100 cm

Height, cm	50	60	70	80	90	100
–	15	15	15	15	15	15
+	20	20	20	20	20	20

Table 28.41.4 Accepted W/L (% of median) in children, height 80–170 cm

Height, cm	80	90	100	110	120	130	140	150	160	170
–	15	15	15	15	15	20	20	20	25	25
+	20	20	20	20	20	25	25	25	30	30

Table 28.41.5 Accepted variation in W/L (% of median) in children, height 55–100 cm

Height, cm	During the preceding growth of 5 cm	During the preceding growth of 5 cm	During the preceding growth of 20 cm	During the preceding growth of 20 cm
55	−16	+18		
60	−14	+16		
65	−12	+14		
70	−12	+14	−26	+28
75	−12	+14	−26	+28
80	−10	+12	−26	+26
90	−10	+12	−22	+22
100	−10	+12	−18	+20

The columns with a minus sign denote the limits for decrease and the columns with a plus sign the limits for increase during the growth period (5 or 20 cm) preceding the height stated in the column.

Table 28.41.6 Accepted variation in W/H (% of median) in children, height 80–150 cm

Height, cm	During the preceding growth of 5 cm	During the preceding growth of 5 cm	During the preceding growth of 20 cm	During the preceding growth of 20 cm
80	−10	+12	−26	+26
90	−10	+12	−22	+22
100	−10	+12	−18	+20
110	−10	+12	−16	+18
120	−12	+14	−16	+18
130	−14	+16	−18	+20
140	−14	+16	−20	+22
150	−14	+16	−20	+22

The columns with a minus sign denote the limits for decrease and the columns with a plus sign the limits for increase during the growth period (5 or 20 cm) preceding the height stated in the column.

Causes of short stature

Congenital growth disturbances

- Small growth reserve (inherited short adult height) and a slow pace of growth (growth is distributed over a period longer than usual) are mutually independent, hereditary factors resulting in short stature in childhood. The largest group of children with growth problems have both these factors (they are "double-minus" variants).

- A small growth reserve is characterized by growth that has a consistent L/A score. The skeletal age is normal. In differential diagnosis remember osteochondrodysplasias (sitting height greated than normal), chromosomal abnormalities, prenatal disturbances, and short stature syndromes (Russel–Silver and Noonan syndromes).
- A slow pace of growth is associated with a decrease in L/A during the first years of life. The growth pattern resembles that in chronic diseases, which have to be ruled out before a diagnosis of slow pace of growth can be made.

- Cystic fibrosis is associated with respiratory problems and steatorrhoea that can lead to severe growth delay during the first year of life (see 31.23).
- With growth disturbances in children under one year, consider metabolic and neurodegenerative diseases, especially if there are associated developmental delays.
- There are tens of skeletal diseases (dysplasias), mostly hereditary. They all decrease adult height by 40–50 cm. The most common osteochondrodysplasia is achondroplasia (autosomal dominant).
- The most common chromosomal abnormalities in phenotypic females include Turner's syndrome (45,X and its karyotype variants such as 45,X/46,XY).
- Prenatal growth disturbances may be caused by infections, placental dysfunction or maternal abuse of alcohol, narcotics, or other drugs.

Acquired growth disturbances

- In hypothyroidism the L/A shifts downwards, and the relative weight W/L shifts simultaneously upwards. Skeletal age is delayed even in relation to the child's height.
- Hyperglucocorticoidism (often an adverse effect of drug therapy) is also associated with an increase of the W/L and a decrease of the L/A. The retardation in L/A is not as marked as in hypothyroidism.
- A psychosocial growth disturbance (emotional deprivation) may result in marked growth retardation, probably because the secretion of growth hormone decreases.
- Rickets is associated with a growth disturbance resulting in short limbs.
- The diagnoses of cystic fibrosis and growth hormone deficiency should be made by appropriate specialist paediatricians.
  - The degree of growth hormone deficiency varies from mild to total.
  - The prevalence of growth hormone deficiency is about 1:4000 in school-aged children.
  - Most cases are idiopathic, or the deficiency may be related to pre- or perinatal injury. Other causes include radiotherapy of the hypothalamic area, a craniopharyngeoma, or other tumour.
  - The birth length is usually normal, even if the growth hormone deficiency is congenital. Later, L/A shows a progressive decrease.
  - Under the age of 2 years about one in four patients have symptoms of hypoglycaemia. In older children such symptoms are rare.
  - Typical features are a large head, thick subcutaneous fat, particularly in the abdomen, and a relative body weight greater than normal.

Investigations of short stature

- Analyse the growth curve carefully (check the original reading dates of measurements). It is essential to determine whether the growth disturbance is congenital (growth follows the curve) or acquired (growth shifts downwards on the curve). In clinical examination, pay attention to heart and circulation, lungs, skin, body proportions and any abnormal lineaments.
- Declining L/A
  - An increase of the W/L associated with decreased growth suggests hypothalamic injury (growth hormone deficiency), hypothyroidism, or hyperglucocorticoidism. A decrease of the W/L suggests malnutrition (cystic fibrosis, coeliac disease) or other systemic disease.
  - Hypothyroidism and coeliac disease should be ruled out by laboratory tests (TSH, serum free thyroxin, anti-gliadin, -reticulin, and/or -endomysial antibodies).
  - Determine blood count, ESR, sodium, potassium, calcium, phosphorus, creatinine, and blood pH to rule out systemic diseases.
  - Cystic fibrosis, see 31.23.
  - Growth hormone deficiency should be considered only after hypothyroidism, coeliac disease, and growth disturbance resulting from psychosocial causes (which can cause secondary growth hormone deficiency) have been ruled out.
- Growth follows the curve
  - Investigate the growth of parents and close relatives (if a similar growth pattern is found in the family the child is probably a normal variant).
  - Measure sitting height (particularly among short members of the family).
  - Look for a developmental disorder and abnormal appearance.
  - Determine the karyotype in girls (Turner's syndrome and its variants).

Treatment of short stature

- The psychosocial consequences of short stature may be serious.
- People tend to evaluate a child according to his/her height rather than his/her age.
- The aim of treatment is to influence the attitudes of other people and to promote the child's self-esteem and enhance growth.

- Synthetic growth hormone (A) [1] is available. The decision as whom to treat should be made by a paediatric endocrinologist. The indications for treatment are not clear-cut. The treatment is very expensive and long-standing.

Causes and treatment of tall stature

Growth follows the normal chart

- The most common abnormality is a hereditary normal variant.
  - Knowledge of the heights and growth patterns of family members is essential for diagnosis.
  - Normal body proportions and normal skeletal age differentiate the condition from pathological conditions.
- Excessive growth of the limbs (reduced relative sitting height) is typical of Marfan's syndrome and homocystinuria. In suspected Marfan's syndrome, dislocation of the lens and mitral prolapse should be sought.
- Klinefelter's syndrome and its variants result in slightly excessive growth, particularly in the limbs of affected males. The karyotype is diagnostic.
- Anomalies and atypical features may suggest Sotos' or Beckwith-Wiedeman syndrome.

Growth deviated upwards from the normal chart

- Obesity is usually associated with slight acceleration of growth and skeletal maturation. Obesity associated with a decrease in L/A is a worrying sign (see above).
- Precocious puberty (28.42) is associated with accelerated growth and even more accelerated skeletal maturation, followed by the appearance of secondary sexual characteristics.
- Androgen excess is the cause of accelerated growth in congenital adrenal hyperplasia. The signs of sexual maturation do not follow the normal pattern in either boys or girls.
- In hypothyroidism accelerated growth and skeletal maturation may precede the diagnosis by years. A concomitant decrease in W/H is pathognomonic.

Prevention of excessive height

- Tall stature may cause serious harm to the mental health of girls.
- Adult growth should be predicted.
- Accelerating female puberty by oestrogen treatment given by a paediatric endocrinologist reduces adult height as much as 10 cm if the treatment is started at a skeletal age of 10 years. Remaining growth potential can be reduced by about one third. In Finland, a predicted height exceeding 185 cm has been considered an indication for treatment in girls.

Obesity

- About 6% of teenage children are obese (W/H exceeding 20% of the median).
- A 10%-of-median units increase of W/H in a year or a 5%-of-median units increase in a shorter period calls for attention.
- Risk factors of childhood obesity include
  - obesity in parents
  - life crisis
  - mental retardation.
- In less than 10%, an underlying disease is found to be the cause of obesity.
- Obesity in infancy increases the risk of obesity at school age by a factor of 2.5. However, 80% of obese infants have normal body weight by the time they reach school age.
- Both increased appetite and the consumption of sweets, sweet drinks, and snacks are associated with obesity.
- Obese girls have an early start of puberty, whereas puberty is often delayed in obese boys.

Treatment

- Prevention (C) [2] of an increase in body weight is most practical when marked obesity has not yet developed.
- It is sufficient to keep the body weight stable while the increase in height corrects obesity.
- Food items rich in fat should be replaced by other items, and sedentary behaviour should be discouraged (B) [3].
- The whole family must take part in the treatment. Counselling of the parents should be carried out first (C) [4, 5].
- Increasing exercise is a primary goal when reducing body weight is desired in adolescents (C) [6, 7].

Endocrine obesity

- Acquired endocrine obesity (hypothyroidism, growth hormone deficiency, hypercortisolism) is nearly always associated with short stature or a reduction in L/A. Analysis of the growth chart is essential in diagnosis.

Hypothalamic obesity

- Associated with two congenital syndromes
  - Prader-Willi syndrome (deletion of chromosome 15) is associated with hypotonia in the neonate (learning to walk at an average age of 2–2.5 years), mental retardation, typical facial appearance (narrow forehead, antimongoloid eyes, epicanthus, small chin, abnormal ear lobes), small hands, clino- and syndactyly. Boys usually have undescended testes. Obesity starts at the age of 2 years and becomes marked.
  - Laurence–Moon–Biedl syndrome is an inherited autosomal recessive syndrome. Obesity developing by the 4th year of life, short stature, mental retardation, and poly- and syndactyly, pigmented retinopathy, and genital hypoplasia are typical features of the syndrome.

Determination of skeletal age

X-rays

- See Table 28.41.7.

Table 28.41.7 X-rays necessary for the determination of skeletal age

Expected skeletal age (y) Boys	Girls	X-rays
0–0.2	0–0.2	Both knees and ankles (lateral projection)
0.2–2.0	0.2–1.0	Left shoulder, elbow, hand, hip, knee and foot (anteroposterior), ankle (lateral)
2.0–5.0	1.0–3.0	Left hand (anteroposterior)
5.0–8.5	3.0–7.0	Left hand and elbow (anteroposterior)
8.5–	7.0–	Left hand (anteroposterior), elbow (anteroposterior and lateral)

Interpretation

- Before the appearance of epiphyseal nuclei in the hands the skeletal age is determined according to Elgenmark, and thereafter according to Creulich and Pyle.
- Rules of interpretation see Table 28.41.8.

Normal percentages of sitting height (95% confidence interval)

- See Table 28.41.9.

Table 28.41.8 Some hints for determination of skeletal age from x-rays

Parameter	Skeletal age Boys	Girls
Appearance of medial epicondyle of the humerus	6.25	3.4
Appearance of head of radius	5.2	3.9
Appearance of elbow	9.7	8.0
Appearance of lateral epicondyle of the humerus	11.2	9.2
Incipient fusion of the elbow in lateral view	13.5	11.5
Completed fusion of the elbow in lateral view	14.5	12.5

Table 28.41.9 Normal percentages of sitting height (95% confidence interval) vs. total height

Age (y)	Boys and girls	Age (y)	Boys	Girls
0.25	60.0–72.5	9.0	50.5–55.5	50.7–55.8
0.50	60.7–71.4	10.0	49.9–54.9	50.2–55.5
1.0	60.3–68.2	11.0	49.5–54.6	50.0–55.3
1.5	59.3–66.1	12.0	49.1–54.1	49.9–55.1
2.0	58.3–64.2	13.0	48.8–53.8	50.1–55.0
2.5	57.2–62.5	14.0	48.8–53.7	50.5–55.0
3.0	56.1–61.3	15.0	48.9–53.7	51.1–55.1
4.0	54.5–59.5	Adult	51.1–55.9	51.6–56.4
5.0	53.4–58.3			
6.0	52.5–57.3			
7.0	51.8–56.6			
8.0	51.2–56.1			

References

1. Bryant J, Cave C, Milne R. Recombinant growth hormone for idiopathic short stature in children and adolescents. Cochrane Database Syst Rev 2003(4):CD004440.
2. Campbell K, Waters E, O'Meara S, Kelly S, Summerbell C. Interventions for preventing obesity in children. Cochrane Database Syst Rev. 2004;(2):CD001871.
3. Summerbell CD, Ashton V, Campbell KJ, Edmunds L, Kelly S, Waters E. Interventions for treating obesity in children. Cochrane Database Syst Rev. 2004;(2):CD001872.
4. Jelalian E, Saelens BE. Empirically supported treatments in pediatric psychology: pediatric obesity. Journal of Pediatric Psychology 1999;24:223–248.
5. The Database of Abstracts of Reviews of Effectiveness (University of York), Database no.: DARE-993984. In: The Cochrane Library, Issue 2, 2001. Oxford: Update Software.
6. Friedenreich CM, Courneya KS. Exercise in treating obesity in children and adolescents. Clin J Sports Medicine 1996;6: 237–244.
7. The Database of Abstracts of Reviews of Effectiveness (University of York), Database no.: DARE-964209. In: The Cochrane Library, Issue 4, 1999. Oxford: Update Software.

28.42 Pubertal development and disturbances

Editors

Aim

- To identify abnormal pubertal development.

Stages of pubertal development (according to Tanner)

Breasts

- M1
  - As in a child: only the nipple is elevated.
- M2
  - Budding stage: The breast and the nipple are slightly elevated, and some glandular tissue is felt on palpation. The areola is enlarged.
- M3
  - The breast and the areola are further enlarged, and their contour forms an even arch when inspected from the side.
- M4
  - The areola is elevated from the surroundings.

PAE

- M5
  - A mature breast: Only the nipple is elevated, and the areola aligns the contour of the breast.

Pubic hair

- P1
  - As in a child: The pubic hair does not differ from the hair of the abdomen.
- P2
  - Some long, slightly pigmented, sometimes slightly curved hair in the labia major or at the base of the penis.
- P3
  - Darker, stronger, and more curved hair spreading slightly on the pubic arch.
- P4
  - Adult-type hair but on a clearly smaller area. Does not spread on the inner aspect of the thighs.
- P5
  - The hair spreads also towards the navel.

Male genitals

- G1
  - The testes (<20 mm by length), the scrotum, and the penis are as in early childhood.
- G2
  - The scrotum and the testes are enlarged (>20 mm), the skin over the scrotum is slightly erythematous and thinner, but the penis is not yet enlarged.
- G3
  - The penis has grown longer, and the scrotum and the testes are further enlarged.
- G4
  - The penis has grown also in diameter. The glans has developed, and the testes and the scrotum are further enlarged. The colour of the scrotal skin is dark.
- G5
  - The genitals are the same size and shape as in adults.

Screening rules for pubertal development

- See Table 28.42.
- A parental deviation of at least 1.0 year from the average development schedule (menarche in the mother at the age of 13.0 years, fastest growth in the father at the age of 14.0 years) allows a further deviation of 1.0 year in the development of the child. It is important to inform the adolescent about the situation.

Table 28.42 Screening rules for pubertal growth

	Not before	At the latest
Girls		
M2	8.0 yrs	13.0 y, 1.25 yrs after P2
P2	9.0 yrs	13.5 yrs
Growth spurt	9.0 yrs	13.5 yrs
Menarche	10.5 yrs	15.5 yrs, 4.5 yrs from M2
Boys		
G2	9.5 yrs	13.5 yrs
P2	10.0 yrs	14.0 yrs
Growth spurt	10.5 yrs	15.5 yrs

Normal growth at puberty

- Pubertal growth has three stages.
  - Slow growth in early puberty
  - A growth spurt lasting about two years
  - Final slowing and cessation of growth
- The fastest spurt occurs in girls at the average age of 12 years, and in boys at the average age of 14 years.
- The fastest growth in girls usually occurs at stage M3. In about a quarter of girls the growth spurt begins before the pubic hair develops, but always before menarche. After menarche the height increases by 3–11 cm, on average 7 cm.
- In boys the spurt occurs only after the boy has pubic hair. In three quarters of the boys the spurt occurs at stage G4. If the penis had not yet grown thicker and the glans has not developed, a growth of 12–30 cm is still to be expected.

Precocious puberty

- The assessment should be performed at a specialized unit. The history should be taken and a clinical examination performed in primary care to determine whether the condition is abnormal and whether indications for referral exist. The investigations should be started without delay.
- Determine the maturation schedule of close family.
- Use of sex hormones, cranial trauma, symptoms of increased intracranial pressure, vaginal bleeding
- Analysis of growth: normal, constantly increasing growth velocity (suggesting a congenital abnormality) or a change in growth velocity.
- Thorough examination of pubertal status
- X-rays to determine skeletal age (28.41)
- Special examinations: hormone assays, neurological examination, visual fields, ultrasonography of the ovaries and uterus, etc.

Classification and investigations according to the findings

- Pure growth of the breasts (telarche) in girls (without hair growth and accelerated skeletal maturation): Inform the child and the parents and follow up.

- Pure effects of androgens (pubic and armpit hair, sebaceous transformation of the skin, acne, and/or acceleration of growth velocity and skeletal maturation without development of the breasts or testes): The cause should be determined with hormone assays. Usually the child has benign hypersecretion of adrenal steroids (isolated adrenarche), but an androgen-secreting tumour and a late manifestation of an enzyme defect must be ruled out.
- Pure vaginal bleeding: Colposcopy should be performed to rule out a foreign or body botryoid sarcoma.
- True precocious puberty: The cause is classified as central or peripheral according to the results of the hormone assays (GnRH stimulation test). Imaging studies are performed thereafter (hypothalamus, abdomen).
- No aetiological factor is detected even during extended follow-up in 8/10 girls and in 1/3 boys with true precocious puberty.

Gynaecomasty of puberty in boys

- Gynaecomasty is associated with normal puberty and it is usually a transient phenomenon of unknown aetiology. It usually occurs at the stage of fastest growth and genital development.
- The breasts are often tender on palpation, which even disturbs sport activities.
- The areola is not pigmented, and the glandular tissue is only detected on palpation (diameter < 3 cm).
- The glandular tissue often disappears in a few months. The larger the glandular tissue is originally the slower the rate of regression.

Delayed puberty

- Although most cases fall within the limits of normal variance (2.5% of adolescents develop two years later than average) counselling and support for the adolescent are always indicated to prevent harm to the developing personality.
- Acceleration of development with hormonal treatment is often indicated.
- Hypogonadic adolescents should be identified early and the substitution treatment should be started before they differ too much from their companions.

Primary investigations

- Can be performed in primary care but a specialist should always be consulted.
- The growth and maturation schedule of close family members (there is often a hereditary component in slow maturation)
- Signs of chronic disease (e.g. coeliac disease, Crohn's disease)
- Hypogonadism or impaired sense of smell in the relatives
- Orchitis, testis surgery, cerebral trauma, chronic disease
- Long-term corticosteroid treatment, irradiation, or treatment with cytotoxic drugs
- Analysis of growth, skeletal age, body proportions (sitting height)
- Pubertal status, size of the testes, gynaecomasty
- Investigation of the sense of smell and colour vision
- Neurological examination, including fundoscopy and visual fields

Further investigations

- Always indicated if the history or primary investigations suggest a cause other than normal delayed maturation.
- Hormone assays, karyotype, imaging
- The most common cause of primary hypogonadism in boys is Klinefelter's syndrome (prevalence 1:400). The syndrome is suggested by increased height (particularly of the limbs) before puberty (a decreased proportion of sitting height). The testes initially enlarge (as large as 30 mm) but then regress over a few years.
- In girls the most common cause of hypogonadism is Turner's syndrome, which should be identified on the basis of abnormal, slowing growth in childhood.

28.52 Doctor's check-ups in school health care

Juhani Laakso

PAE

Objectives

- Health check-ups provide school health care personnel with information about the general health status both of individual pupils and of the entire age class.
- Effort is made to determine each pupil's health and well-being holistically, taking the physical, mental and social state into account.
- The purpose of check-ups is to support pupils' healthy growth and development, to reveal health risks and deviations, and to refer pupils for any necessary additional examinations and treatment.

Timing of doctor's check-ups

- The recommendation is to perform at least one doctor's check-up for each level of comprehensive school.
- At the lower level of comprehensive school, in addition to the check-up done when pupils first come to school, pupils have a doctor's check-up
  - in the 5th class (at the age of 11 years)
  - at the upper level of comprehensive school, in the 8th class

- in the 1st or 2nd class of senior secondary school
- in the 1st class of a vocational education institute.

♦ In addition to these check-ups, an extra doctor's check-up is done in the following cases:

- the pupil has been absent from school for a long time, or is frequently absent from school
- the pupil is newly moved from another locality
- an additional check-up if necessary for choosing an occupation
- a pupil with a chronic illness, a disability or health risks needs special monitoring
- before transferring the pupil to a special school.

Content of check-ups

♦ At least 30 minutes should be reserved for the check-up, and the presence of parents is desirable in the more extensive check-up of lower level comprehensive school pupils.

♦ Each doctor's check-up takes the following considerations into account:

- The pupil's previous data are important.
- Special attention is paid to the transfer of data from one level of the school system to another.
- Aside from data provided by the pupil, preliminary data are acquired from the nurse, teachers, parents and, possibly, from friends.
- In addition to the preliminary data forms, the pupil should always be interviewed.
- The child should always have a careful general check-up where particular attention is paid to the problems typical of the age group in question.
- The growth charts drawn by the nurse are shown to the pupil, too; visual acuity, hearing acuity and blood pressure are checked. The results of other possible screening tests are also shown to the pupil.
- The doctor, the pupil and his/her parents discuss the pupil's prior illnesses, health-related habits, family structure, difficulties at home and with friends, hobbies and school achievement.
- The doctor also gives health guidance. Anti-intoxicant education is topical at all levels of the school system.

♦ At the end of each doctor's check-up, the pupil's current situation is summarised and a plan for any additional examinations and treatment is made.

♦ If the check-up uncovers nothing out of the ordinary, the pupil should be told this, too!

For particular attention at the lower level of comprehensive school

♦ The most important objective of the **doctor's check-up when the pupil first comes to school** is to ensure the pupil's adjustment to school work.

- Learning difficulties, which in comprehensive school occur among some 10–15% of pupils, often surface during the early phase of going to school or can be predicted already on the basis of the check-ups done at child-care clinics.
- The somatic check-up follows the guidelines for check-ups administered to the age group of 5–6 year-olds at child-care clinics (28.1).

♦ **The doctor's check-up done near the end of the lower level of comprehensive school (usually around 11 years)** is marked by puberty, which is then approaching or has begun.

- During the somatic check-up, attention is paid to the stage of puberty.
- Look for signs of atopic diseases on the skin or in the respiratory organs.
- Unclear heart murmurs are grounds for ultrasonography.
- Of the musculoskeletal diseases, e.g. Osgood–Schlatter disease (32.63), Sever's disease, osteochondrosis dissecans (20.47), chondromalacia patellae (20.40), Perthes disease (32.62) and epiphysiolysis of the hip (32.61) (32.54) begin to surface at this age.
- If a boy has a very tight, scarred phimosis, surgery is considered. Other phimoses can be treated during the upper level of comprehensive school if they aren't corrected spontaneously.
- Already at the lower level of comprehensive school, the cause of growth disturbance may be post-thyroiditic hypothyroidism, coeliac disease, Crohn's disease and Turner syndrome or a general disease, such as diabetes, rheumatic disease, asthma and kidney ailment (28.41).
- Attention is paid to the pupil's ability to make contact and to the pupil's speech and general outward manner.
- With regard to mental, intellectual and social development, it is important to form an opinion as to whether the pupil is able to make the transition to the regular upper level of comprehensive school, whether the pupil should be placed in a special class, or whether the pupil needs other support measures.

For particular attention at the upper level of comprehensive school

♦ Puberty is associated with a dramatic change in physical, mental and social state

- A central consideration is the adolescent's uncertainty about his/her own identity.
- From the perspective of health, many show risk behaviour.
- Increasing numbers of adolescents come from a broken home or have experienced the recent death of a close relative.
- Some are dating for the first time.
- Use of intoxicants, lifestyle, depression, and anxiety should be noted.
- Inquire about leisure time activities and the circle of friends.

♦ During the somatic check-up, scoliosis and kyphosis (e.g. Scheuermann's disease), in particular, as well as spondylolisthesis, should be kept in mind.

- Now, at the latest, phimoses are treated. Any varicocele should be noted and treated if testicular growth begins to slow down.
- Of the dermatological ailments, acne and atopic eczema are common.
- Anorexia, bulimia and obesity are becoming more widespread.
- School performance, learning difficulties and plans for the future are recorded.
- Health restrictions affecting the occupational selection should be noted, e.g. poor colour vision and atopy.
- An adolescents' health certificate is filled in (either for everyone or for those who need a certificate).
- Important aspects of health education include the prevention of substance abuse and, in some pupils, contraception and protection from STD.

For particular attention in senior secondary school and vocational school

- Studying is more goal-oriented and more independent than before.
- The personality is more mature and more independent of friends than that of a pupil in the upper level of comprehensive school.
- Some pupils live away from home to go to school.
- Central issues are attitudes pertaining to one's own body, sexuality, the future and becoming an adult.
- The importance of one's own health increases; health guidance gains in emphasis.
- During the check-up, special attention is paid to the progression of puberty. Signs of puberty should be determined among all. If menstruation has not begun, effort must be made to determine the reason.
- Many adolescents experience repeated headache, neck and shoulder pain, general fatigue and tension symptoms.
- Eating disorders become more common and mental health problems increase. Particular attention should be paid to early signs of isolation. Effort should be made to recognise depression and, in extreme cases, a tendency towards self-destruction.
- The priorities of health guidance are favourable nutritional and physical exercise habits, preventing the use of intoxicants C [1], protection against sexually-transmitted diseases C [2] [3] and birth control.
- The adolescents' health certificate is checked and updated.
- At vocational education institutes, the initial check-up is important.
  - Any health-related obstacles to the line of work in question are determined (usually at the nurse's check-up)
  - A doctor's check-up in the beginning and at fixed intervals for those exposed to work involving a particular risk of illness.
  - Activities are guided by the legislation on occupational safety and occupational diseases.
  - If a student at a vocational education institute has to interrupt studies for health reasons, the possibility of occupational disease should be investigated; occupational guidance and retraining should be provided, with appropriate benefits.

References

1. Sowden A, Arblaster L. Community interventions for preventing smoking in young people. The Cochrane Database of Systematic Reviews, Cochrane Library number: CD001291. In: The Cochrane Library, Issue 2, 2002. Oxford: Update Software. Updated frequently.
2. Kirby D, Short L, Collins J, Rugg D, Kolbe L, Howard M, Miller B, Sonenstein F, Zabin LS. School-based programmes to reduce sexual risk behaviours: a review of effectiveness. Public Health Reports 1994;109:339–360.
3. The Database of Abstracts of Reviews of Effectiveness (University of York), Database no.: DARE-940275. In: The Cochrane Library, Issue 4, 1999. Oxford: Update Software.

28.54 Occupational guidance in school health care

Eija-Liisa Ala-Laurila

Objectives

- Health factors limiting the choice of occupation are determined and information about them is provided.
- Support is given for the pupil's realistic career plan, in co-operation with the pupil, the school guidance counselling, parents and, if necessary, with other bodies.

PAE

Pupil-specific examinations at set times in the upper level of comprehensive school

- Through a questionnaire form completed in advance and discussion, the examination occurring in the 8th class determines
  - the pupil's chronic diseases and symptoms
  - hopes and plans for further education.
- The following are checked
  - visual acuity and colour vision (the nurse's check-up around 13–14 years)
  - hearing acuity (the nurse's check-up at the age of 14)
  - the clinical examination of the doctor's check-up (14 years)
- A stand on health limitations is taken
  - As necessary, follow-up of a symptom or illness and a re-examination at the age of 15

- Additional examinations as necessary (e.g. more precise examination of colour vision, allergy tests)
- Information provided to the pupil, the parents, the study counsellor, specialised health care.

Health factors limiting the choice of occupation

Allergies

- The limitations should be considered on an individual basis (type of symptoms, severity, the pupil's known sensitisations, need for medication and other treatment).
- All pupils with symptoms are given information about work involving risk.
- A mere atopic tendency without symptoms is not cause for limitations.
- A pupil with asthma or allergic rhinitis should avoid work involving exposure to flour dust, cattle and animal tending, textile work, carpentry and barbering-hair dressing.
- Owing to the risk of allergic respiratory ailments, a pupil with atopic eczema should avoid work involving exposure to flour dust as well as cattle and animal tending.
- A pupil who has, or has had, eczema on the hands should take the following limitations into account:
- Line of work–Suitability of the work
  - Hair-dressing–not suitable
  - Care-giving, nursing–not suitable (with reservations)
  - Foods industry–not suitable
  - Animal tending–with reservations
  - Cleaning–not suitable/with reservations
  - Exposure to chemicals–with reservations
- Contact allergy is a limitation for tasks that involve dealing with contact allergens causing symptoms (rubber, nickel, fruits, vegetables and spices cross-reacting with leaf-tree allergy).
- Hairdressing and the cleaning sector are also risk-prone lines of work, owing to the intense exposure to chemicals.

Vision defects

- Defective vision correctable with eyeglasses in general is not a limitation. Some jobs have detailed visual requirements: e.g.
  - deck staff of ships
  - railway engine drivers
  - professional pilots
  - police and certain duties in the defence forces.
- Defective colour vision: The screening test done in the scope of school health care determines whether colour vision is normal or defective.
- Completely normal colour vision is required for the following lines of work:
  - deck staff of ships
  - railway engine drivers
  - professional pilots.
- Colour vision is of importance
  - in electrical, telecommunications, electronic and instrument fitting
  - in producing illustrations in the graphic industry
  - in the work of painters, laboratory assistants, cosmetologists, hair-dressers and fashion designers.
- If the screening test indicates defective colour vision and the pupil aspires to one of these sectors, an ophthalmologist's determination of the degree of the defect in colour vision is needed, and a stand on the choice of occupation is taken on the basis of it.

Hearing defects

- Weakened hearing is a limitation if coping on the job or general safety require a certain level of hearing or if the work, owing to the level of noise, poses a risk of weakened hearing among individuals with a hearing defect of inner-ear origin.
- Good hearing determined in detail is a prerequisite in certain transport tasks in navigation and air traffic, on the railway and in professional traffic.
- If the pupil has a hearing defect of inner-ear origin and is considering a line of work involving exposure to noise (e.g. the automobile body, wood, metal or process industry, building construction), the opinion of an otologist is recommended.

Epilepsy

- A clear limitation: not suited to be a professional driver in land, water or air traffic nor to be a driver of heavy vehicles on land.
- Other restrictions are relative, specific to the individual and specific to the work.
- Epileptic attacks: not suited for work involving accident risk (falling, hazardous machinery, danger of electrical accident or fire)

Other limiting factors and diseases

- Diabetes, rheumatic disease, heart defects, neurological handicaps, rare diseases require individual solutions and often call for co-operation with the body responsible for treatment.
- In cases of mental disease or learning difficulties, the load involved in the course of study and in the future work should also be considered.

Co-operation in occupational guidance

- Together in discussions with the school guidance counselling (the pupil's counsellor, the nurse, the doctor as needed)
  - The pupil's specific problems are determined.
  - Agreement is reached on further measures, e.g.
    - the employment office's occupational guidance
    - consultation with vocational education institutes.

- Co-operation with the employment office's occupational guidance is called for particularly in the case of pupils with a chronic disease or handicap.
  - As needed, the pupil is referred to the occupational guidance psychologist for
    - guidance discussion
    - aptitude tests
    - work and educational trials.
- It is important to agree on the division of tasks with specialised health care personnel, and to provide information about observations made in school health care.

Doctor's statements

- A written account to the pupil, stating the health limitations affecting the choice of occupation.
  - The account can be a free-form statement or an adolescent's health certificate.
  - Diseases and handicaps noteworthy with respect to the choice of occupation, their treatment, the job types in which they hinder working, and the types of work that can make them worse are pointed out.
  - If necessary, a statement is compiled for the employment office's occupational guidance.

PAE

Paediatric Neurology

Evidence Based Medicine Guidelines. Edited by the Duodecim Editorial Team
 ISBN: 0-470-01184-X

29.1 Headache in children

Helena Pihko

Basic rules

- A thorough history, clinical examination, selection of suitable medication, and sufficient follow-up are the cornerstones of treatment.
- Neuroradiological examinations should be considered in small children, in children with a short history of headaches, and in children with vomiting or abnormal clinical findings.

Primary investigations

- Thorough history
  - School and friends. The occurrence of headache increases at school start (C) [1].
  - Hobbies
  - Eating and sleeping habits
  - The child's usual reactions to stressful situations
  - Family history of headache
  - Other diseases and their medications
- Careful somatic and neurological examination
  - Blood pressure determination
  - Examination of vision and fundoscopy
  - Assessment of growth using the growth chart
  - Growth chart of the head circumference in small children
- Examination of the maxillary sinuses (ultrasonography or radiographs) particularly if the child has allergic symptoms affecting the airways or a tendency for recurrent infections.
- Serum CRP (and ESR) in children with symptoms of an infection.

Further investigations

- The majority of children with headache can be managed in primary care if sufficient attention is paid on their condition.
- If the history of headaches is short the patient should be followed up for a few months to make sure that the symptom is not progressive.
- Indications for computed tomography or magnetic resonance imaging include:
  - a headache during the night and in the morning associated with vomiting, which can occur also without the headache
  - impaired consciousness associated with the headache
  - progressive headache (over a few weeks or months)
  - alteration of the behaviour or the mood of the child
  - retardation of normal development or growth
  - abnormal clinical findings (strabismus, impaired visual acuity, visual field defect, diplopia, blurred optic disks, difficulties in swallowing, equilibrium or coordination, or clonic tendon reflexes)
- Imaging should also be considered in the following cases:
  - The age of the child is below 5 years.
  - Physical exercise or coughing worsens the headache.
- Consultation of an ophthalmologist
  - may be indicated to search for concealed strabismus and refractory errors.
- Examination by a dentist
  - Infections of the teeth or jaw, correcting devices for dental alignment
- EEG
  - Indicated if epilepsy is suspected.

Migraine

- The time of onset often coincides with starting preschool or school (C) [1]. At school age the prevalence of migraine and headache increase steadily until early puberty.
- There is a strong hereditary disposition.
- During typical attacks the child is definitely ill, he/she prefers to stay in a dark, quiet room, and does not want to play. After the attack has subsided the child is quite normal.
- Visual disturbances, difficulties in speech, paraesthesias, or paralyses may also be associated with migraine in children. If an aura or abnormal neurological signs are associated with an attack they precede the attack and disappear after the headache has started. In epilepsy and cerebral tumours the neurological symptoms occur simultaneously with the headache.
- The attacks may also occur at night. In such cases imaging is usually indicated to exclude increased intracranial pressure.
- The highest frequency of the attacks is usually about twice a week. Daily attacks are not typical of migraine.
- The diagnosis is made by exclusion and sufficient follow-up.

Tension headache

- Tension headache is caused by continuous contraction of the muscles of the neck and is usually associated with psychological or physical stress. The onset of headache is often insidious, and it occurs in the afternoon or evening after school. Rest alleviates tension headache.
- Tension headache can also occur in children who have typical attacks of migraine. A clear distinction between migraine and tension headache cannot always be made.
- The attacks occur rarely during weekends or holidays.
- Rest and relaxation usually help better than medicine.

Other types of headaches

Psychogenic headache

- Continues from day to day, is described more vaguely, and does not affect normal activities as much as migraine or tension headache.

- Severe psychological problems such as school phobias, depression, and sleeplessness are often associated with the headache.
- Long-term professional help is often needed.

Headaches of ocular or dental origin

- Concealed strabismus and refractive errors may cause a headache in the forehead and temporal region that disappears after the child is given spectacles.
- Devices for dental alignment may cause daily headaches that disappear as soon as the device is removed.
- Patients with bruxism or dental malocclusion who have even mild daily or frequent headaches should be referred to a dentist.

Sinusitis

- The headache is often located on the forehead and cheeks but may also be generalized.
- Other signs of infection may be scant.

Cerebral tumours and blockage of cerebrospinal fluid circulation

- A headache associated with malignant intracranial tumours usually progresses rapidly and does not cause differential diagnostic problems.
- Benign intracranial tumours (often in the posterior fossa or in the midline) may cause symptoms from increased intracranial pressure for 1–2 years before the diagnosis is made.
- A slowly developing hydrocephalus caused by obstruction of the aqueduct may cause headache after the second or third year of life.
- The symptoms of increased intracranial pressure include:
    - headache occurring in the morning or before noon, vomiting in the morning
    - strabismus, disturbance of balance.
- A tumour in the sellar region may cause growth retardation.

Sleep apnoea

- See 29.5.
- Continuous snoring is a sign of obstruction in the pharynx and in the respiratory passages.
- Night-time hypoxaemia may cause headache in the daytime, tiredness in the morning, and difficulties with concentration.
- Adenoidectomy, and possibly also tonsillectomy, is indicated.

Idiopathic intracranial hypertension (pseudotumor cerebri)

- The intracranial pressure is elevated without disturbance of c.s.f. circulation or a space-occupying process.
- The ventricles are normal-sized and upon lumbar puncture the c.s.f. pressure is elevated.
- Papiloedema
- Known causative factors are obesity, tetracycline and various hormonal changes. Often the cause is unknown.
- If the causative factor is known, it is corrected first. Pharmacological treatments; acetazolamide, glycerol and furosemide.

Non-pharmacological treatment

- Informing the child and the parents that there is no serious illness may bring the necessary relief.
- Stress, fasting, fatigue, irritation by light or noise, and head traumas for example in ball games may trigger attacks of migraine.
- The parents should keep a diary of the headaches and think of possible causes for the headache.
- Regular exercise may be of benefit.
- The personal standards of performance set by the child or the parents may be too high and the ability to tolerate disappointment may be low. In such cases counselling may be necessary to help the family adopt a more realistic expectations regarding school and hobbies.
- Sufficient sleep, regular meals and avoiding unnecessary hurry are important aspects of therapy.

Pharmacological treatment

- If the symptoms continuously affect everyday life, pharmacological treatment is indicated.
- The most common problems with the treatment are a delay in the administration of the drug and insufficient doses.

Treatment of a migraine attack

- Administer a sufficient dose of the drug, and repeat the dose after 1 hour if necessary.
- Dissolved tablets and mixtures are absorbed more rapidly than ordinary tablets.
- Suppositories are an option if there is vomiting.
- Drugs against nausea and vomiting may promote the absorption of analgesics. Their infrequent adverse effects include extrapyramidal and dystonic reactions that disappear after the drug has been discontinued.
- See Table 29.1.
- Specific migraine drugs are not yet used for children.

Prophylactic treatment for migraine

- Indicated if the attacks are severe or they recur several times a month.
- Propranolol is used in doses of 2–4 mg/kg/day **B** [2 3 4], and carbamazepine or valproate in doses used for epilepsy.
- The maximum duration of the prophylactic treatment should be 6 months at a time.

PAE

Table 29.1 Treatment of migraine attacks in children

Drug	Single dose mg/kg/day	Highest allowed dose mg/kg/day	Mode of administration
Analgesics			
Paracetamol	10–15	60	Mixture, dissolving tablet, tablet, suppository
Ibuprofen	10–20	40	Mixture, dissolving tablet, tablet, suppository
Ketoprofen	2.5	5	Tablet/capsule, suppository
Naproxen	5–7	10–15	Grains for mixture, mixture, tablet, suppository
Drugs against nausea and vomiting			
Metoclopramide	0.15–0.30	0.5–1.0	Mixture, tablet, suppository
Prochlorperazine	0.10–0.30	0.4–0.5	Tablet, suppository

References

1. Anttila P, Metsahonkala L, Sillanpaa M. School start and occurrence of headache. Pediatrics 1999;103:e80.
2. Hermann C, Kim M, Blanchard EB. Behavioural and prophylactic pharmacological intervention studies of pediatric migraine: an exploratory meta-analysis. Pain 1995;60:239–56.
3. Hermann C, Kim M, Blanchard EB. Behavioural and prophylactic pharmacological intervention studies of pediatric migraine: an exploratory meta-analysis. Pain 1995;60:239–256.
4. The Database of Abstracts of Reviews of Effectiveness (University of York), Database no.: DARE-950740. In: The Cochrane Library, Issue 4, 1999. Oxford: Update Software.

29.2 Treatment of acute seizures and status epilepticus in children

Eija Gaily

Basic rules

- First secure vital functions and then proceed to medication immediately.
- All first seizures in a child necessitate further investigations. The only exception is a short symmetric febrile seizure (fever over 38.5°C) in a child aged 6 months to 4 years with a family history of febrile seizures. Recurrence of febrile seizures usually warrants further investigation.
- Before discharging a child after a seizure, the possibility of a serious acute disease, such as bacterial meningitis, must be excluded.

First aid

- Secure vital functions.
  - Remove any airway obstruction if present (use suction when needed). Position the patient on her/his side and supply extra oxygen.
  - Measure blood pressure and pulse.
- Lower body temperature.
  - Undress the child and cool physically, e.g. with a wet towel to the skin.
  - Give antipyretic drugs (29.3) only after anticonvulsive medication (see below) has been administered.
- Start an intravenous line.
  - Start an intravenous line when beginning treatment only if it can be done quickly. It is usually advisable to give the first medication rectally.
  - Use any physiological salt solution without glucose (unless the child is hypoglycaemic).
  - Avoid excess fluids.

Medication

Benzodiazepines

- Start medication with rectal **diazepam**, which is available as a ready-made commercial preparation and thus the quickest drug to administer. Give as a single dose of diazepam 0.5 mg/kg (up to 20 kg body weight). A therapeutic serum concentration is achieved within about 5 minutes after administration. Suppositories are absorbed poorly–do not use them! B [1].
- Diazepam may also be given intravenously.
  - The single i.v. dose is 0.2–0.3 mg/kg (infants 1–2 mg, preschool-age 3–5 mg, school age 6–10 mg). The maximum cumulative dose (p.r. plus i.v.) is 1 mg/kg up to 20 mg.
- If the seizure does not stop within 5–10 minutes after the first diazepam dose, the treatment is continued with **lorazepam** B [2] or **clonazepam** D [3], if available (in other cases, repeat the diazepam treatment). The advantage of clonazepam and lorazepam compared with diazepam is the longer duration of action B [2].
  - The single dose of lorazepam i.v. or p.r. is 0.05–0.1 mg/kg with a maximum of 2 mg/single dose.
  - The single dose of clonazepam i.v. or p.r. is 0.05–0.1 mg/kg ad 2 mg, e.g. 0.25–0.5 mg to an infant, 0.5–1 mg to a preschool-age child and 1–2 mg to a school-aged child.
  - The maximum cumulative dose of both drugs is 1 mg in infancy, 2 mg at preschool age and 4 mg at school age.
  - Both drugs may be given rectally; use the i.v. solution as such, dilute it with physiological saline or mix it with paraffin 1:1–2.

- Keep in mind that all benzodiazepines may cause respiratory depression especially when administered quickly p.r. or i.v. These drugs should always be given slowly within 2–3 minutes. Pay attention to the patient's breathing and be prepared to assist ventilation, if necessary. The risk of respiratory arrest is highest in infants with an acute serious illness.

Laboratory tests and other procedures needed immediately

- Determination and correction of blood glucose
  - If the child has hypoglycaemia (blood glucose below 4 mmol/l), infuse 10% glucose solution i.v. 2 ml/kg within 3–4 minutes. Avoid hyperglycaemia.
- Lower body temperature
  - If fever exceeds 38°C, cool physically and administer paracetamol (10–) 15 mg/kg rectally (suppository).
- Laboratory tests
  - Serum CRP, sodium, potassium, blood haemoglobin, leukocytes, serum calcium, blood gases (Astrup)
  - Do not wait for test results before transporting the patient to a hospital!
  - In short febrile seizures, determining serum CRP may be sufficient.
- Hypocalcaemia
  - If there is a strong suspicion of hypocalcaemia, 10% calcium gluconate may be given i.v. (dose 0.5 ml/kg infused over 5 minutes) after the blood sample for determining serum calcium has been taken. Always monitor ECG during calcium infusion.

Treatment of prolonged seizures

- If the seizure continues despite maximum benzodiazepine dose, lowering of temperature and treatment of hypoglycaemia and hypocalcaemia (if present), continue with the following medication:
  - **Fosphenytoin** (prodrug of phenytoin, Pro-Epanutin®, a solution containing 75 mg/ml of fosphenytoin, which is equivalent to 50 mg/ml of phenytoin). The loading dose is 22.5–30 mg/kg of fosphenytoin (15–20 mg/kg in FE or phenytoin equivalents) i.v., with an infusion rate of 3–4.5 mg/kg/min of fosphenytoin (= 2–3 mg/kg/min FE) to a maximum of 225 mg/min of fosphenytoin (= 150 mg/min FE). The advantage of fosphenytoin compared with i.v. phenytoin is less tissue irritation and better compatibility with intravenous fluids D [4]. ECG monitoring is necessary during i.v. infusion. Fosphenytoin may also be given i.m. at the same dose, a maximum of 10 ml to one injection site. With this mode of administration the maximum therapeutic concentration is achieved about 30 min from dosing. This is suitable for children of all ages, even new-borns.
  - Intravenous **phenobarbitone** is an alternative when fosphenytoin is contraindicated. The loading dose is 15–20 mg/kg, half of which is given slowly i.v. and half i.m. (maximum speed 100 mg/min). The maximum single dose is 500 mg.
  - If the seizure lasts longer than 20 minutes, start prevention of cerebral oedema:
    - mild restriction of fluids (75% of the basic requirement),
    - do not give hypotonic solutions
    - give furosemide 1 mg/kg i.v.
    - raise the patient to a slightly elevated position (30 degrees).
- Start arranging for transport to intensive care in a hospital simultaneously with the procedures described above. As a seizure lasting longer than 1–2 hours may cause permanent brain damage C [5], there is an urgent need for more effective treatment (usually thiopental infusion).

Transport to hospital

- Further care and investigations at a hospital are almost always necessary even after brief seizures if the patient has not had seizures before. After a prolonged seizure or if the seizure is not stopped by the means described above, immediate transport to a hospital is always necessary.
- Especially after prolonged seizures, the patient should be accompanied during transportation by a person who is competent in treating seizures (preferably a physician).
- The patient should be positioned on his/her side during the transport to minimize the risk of aspiration. Vital functions should be monitored.
- The means for suctioning airways, cardiopulmonary resuscitation, supplying extra oxygen and administering additional drugs should be provided for the transport.

PAE

Further investigations

- After the first seizure, a paediatric neurologist or a paediatrician should always examine the child to establish aetiology and plan the prevention of further seizures. The only exception from this rule is a short typical febrile seizure (age 6 months to 4 years and fever over 38.5°C required for diagnosis) in a child with a family history for febrile seizures (29.3). Instructions concerning first aid and a prescription for rectal diazepam solution may be sufficient in that situation. Recurrence of febrile seizures usually warrants further investigation.
- If the child is known to have epilepsy, he/she may be discharged home after a short seizure that was typical to the child, provided that he/she has fully recovered from the seizure. Otherwise it is advisable to refer the patient to hospital for further care.
- If the child is discharged home after a seizure, it is important to exclude any serious illness such as meningitis, encephalitis or a systemic disease. The child should always be given a careful physical examination and kept under observation until he/she has fully recovered from the seizure. Laboratory tests such as serum CRP and examination

of cerebrospinal fluid should be carried out whenever necessary.

References

1. Knudsen FU. Plasma-diazepam in infants after rectal administration in solution and by suppository. Acta Paediatr Scand 1977;66:563–7.
2. Appleton R, Sweeney A, Choonara I, Robson J, Molyneux E. Lorazepam versus diazepam in the acute treatment of epileptic seizures and status epilepticus. Dev Med Child Neurol 1995;37:682–8.
3. Congdon PJ, Forsythe WJ. Intravenous clonazepam in the treatment of status epilepticus in children. Epilepsia 1980;21:97–102.
4. Morton LD. Clinical experience with fosphenytoin in children. J Child Neurol 1998;13(Suppl 1):S19–22.
5. Eriksson KJ, Koivikko MJ. Status epilepticus in children: aetiology, treatment, and outcome. Dev Med Child Neurol 1997;39:652–8.

29.3 Febrile convulsions

Editors

Basic rules

- ♦ Give effective first aid for an acute attack (29.2).
- ♦ Advise the parents about first aid for a new attack and provide them with rectal diazepam.
- ♦ Refer children with atypical convulsions (see criteria below) or recurrent convulsions.

Causes for convulsions associated with fever

- ♦ Benign febrile convulsions
- ♦ Epileptic seizure triggered by fever
- ♦ Central nervous system infection (meningitis, encephalitis)
- ♦ A metabolic disorder triggered by an infection (hypoglycaemia, hyponatraemia)
- ♦ Benign febrile convulsions are by far the most common.

Criteria for "typical" febrile convulsions

1. The age of the child is between 6 months and 4 years.
2. The child has a fever above 38.5°C. Often the fever is not detected before the convulsion.
3. The convulsions are grand-mal type, with symmetric twisting and stiffening of the upper or lower limbs or both.
4. The convulsions last no longer than 10 minutes.
5. The patient is awake after the convulsions, and there are no local signs such as pareses.
6. Members of the extended family have a history of febrile convulsions.
   - Epileptic seizures triggered by fever occur in children of all ages. The convulsions are often prolonged, lasting for more than 30 minutes. Convulsions can recur as short repetitive convulsions. They are often asymmetric and have a focal beginning. In many cases there is epilepsy in the family.
   - Any infection may trigger febrile convulsions. A rapid rise in the body temperature and a high temperature increase the risk of convulsions. The risk is highest at the beginning of the fever.
   - Febrile convulsions occur in 2–3% of all children. About two thirds are short, typical febrile convulsions.

Indications for referral and special examinations

- ♦ EEG 1–2 weeks after the convulsions is indicated if
  - the child had a prolonged or atypical seizures, or
  - the child has had 2 or 3 typical febrile convulsions (EEG is not indicated after 1 or 2 typical convulsions).
- ♦ If the parents phone the doctor about febrile convulsions that have already ceased, it is essential to make sure that the convulsions were short and symmetric and that the child can be contacted fully after the seizure. Convulsions may be a symptom of bacterial meningitis of encephalitis; therefore the child should be examined if there is a slightest doubt.
- ♦ If the child has had an ordinary febrile seizure and is well after the attack referral is not necessary.

Preventing febrile convulsions

- ♦ A febrile seizure recurs in 20–30% of the children in association with new episodes of febrile infection. The parents should be advised to lower high fever as in any child using physical methods and antipyretics (paracetamol (10 -) 15 mg/kg body weight four times a day C [1] or naproxen 5 mg/kg twice a day). Rectal diazepam should be available at home, and the parents should be instructed how to use it.
- ♦ Prophylactic diazepam (0.3–0.4 mg/kg every 8 hours) or clobazam (0.5 mg/kg daily divided into 1–2 doses) can be given during the first two febrile days for children who have had febrile convulsions, but its efficacy is uncertain. Suppositories are poorly absorbed and they are not recommended.

Reference

1. Meremikwu M, Oyo-Ita A. Paracetamol for treating fever in children. Cochrane Database Syst Rev. 2004;(2):CD003676.

29.4 Epilepsy in children

Editors

Basic rules

- Children with prolonged (>15 min) or frequently recurring seizures are examined and treated in hospital as emergencies.
- Identify patients with suspected infantile spasms and refer them immediately to hospital.
- "Atypical" seizure symptoms are identified as possible epilepsy, and the child is referred to a paediatric neurologist for further examinations.
- A blood sample for determining drug concentrations should be taken immediately after prolonged seizures or if the seizures worsen.

Partial (locally initiated or partial) seizures

Uniform seizures

- The patient is conscious.
- The patient has motor (tonic, clonic, or tonic-clonic), sensory, autonomous, or psychological symptoms and sensations.

Polymorphic (psychomotor)

- Consciousness is impaired already at the beginning or during the course of the seizure (which may sometimes be difficult to recognize).
- Often compulsive, inadequate actions: fiddling with things, making smacking noises, swallowing, taking one's clothes off and putting them on, laughing, crying, restless movements, visual and auditory sensations, sensations and symptoms in internal organs, etc.
- The seizure usually lasts for more than 30 secs.
- The patient is usually tired after the seizure.

Medication

- Oxcarbazepine 20–40 mg/kg/day in 2–3 doses, or carbamazepine 15–20 mg/kg/day in 2–3 doses.
- Alternative drugs are sodium valproate 20–40 mg/kg/day in 2–3 doses, new antiepileptic drugs, or in difficult cases phenytoin.

Generalized seizures

- The initial symptoms always originate from both cerebral hemispheres. The motor symptoms are bilateral from the start. Unconsciousness is usually the first symptom.

Absence seizures

- Duration <30 s, typically 10–15 s.
- Dozens of seizures often occur in one day.
- A staring gaze, blinking of the eyes or deviation of the eyes upwards, or both.
- Automatisms may occur in longer attacks.
- No tiredness after the attack.
- Preceding activities continue after the attack, and the patient usually maintains balance.

Medication

- Ethosuximide 20–40 mg/kg/day (250–1000 mg/day) in two doses.
- Sodium valproate 20–40 mg/kg/day in 2–3 doses.

Motor seizures

- Clonic
- Tonic
- Tonic-clonic
- Myoclonic
- Atonic

Medication

- The drug of choice is usually sodium valproate 20–40 mg/kg/day. In tonic, clonic and tonic-clonic seizures alternative drugs are oxcarbazepine 20–40 mg/kg/day or carbamazepine 15–20 mg/kg/day.
- Benzodiazepines should only be used temporarily.

Epilepsy syndromes in childhood

Rolandic epilepsy

- The seizures typically start at the age of 5–10 years.
- The most common type of epilepsy starting at this age.
- The seizures usually start at night. They are localized in the oral region, but may sometimes become generalized.
- The prognosis is good.
- Susceptibility to the disease is inherited dominantly.

Infantile spasms

- Flexion and extension attacks of the extremities and body occur in series after waking up or when the child is tired.
- The development is often halted or retarded when the seizures start.
- Cessation of normal development may be the first symptom of the disease.
- The seizures start at the age of 1–11 months (usually at the age of 4–7 months).
- Hypsarrhythmia is a typical finding on the EEG. The absence of hypsarrhythmia does not rule out infantile spasms.
- If infantile spasms are suspected the child should be investigated and treated in a paediatric neurological unit within days (make a phone call!).
- Immediate treatment (vigabatrin C [1] [2], ACTH) improves the prognosis.

PAE

Lennox syndrome

- Many types of seizures: drop attacks, absences, convulsions, myoclonia, partial seizures.
- Usually starts before school age.
- The prognosis is varying. The disease often results in cognitive retardation.

Prognosis

- If there are no neurological signs, development is consistent with the patient's age, and the results of the investigations (magnetic resonance imaging, metabolic screening) are normal, the seizures will be cured in 80% of patients.
- Of retarded or neurologically abnormal children about 40% will be cured.
- Symptoms starting before the age of one year have a worse prognosis.

Indications and urgency for specialist referral

Refer immediately

- First seizure (to rule out an acute disease of the brain)
- Prolonged seizure (>15 min)
- Frequently recurring short seizures
- Suspicion of infantile spasms
- Retardation of development without evident cause in infants (may be the first sign of infantile spasms)

Urgent referral (investigations within 2–4 days)

- Symptoms arousing suspicion of epilepsy (that have lasted for weeks). Immediate referral is indicated if abnormal signs or general symptoms are detected.

Referral not always necessary

- A single, short febrile convulsion. (For indications for referral in febrile convulsions, see 29.3.)

Seizures during antiepileptic medication

- Prolonged seizures should be treated like status epilepticus (29.2).
- In prolonged seizures and if the seizures become more frequent or severe it is important to take a blood sample for the determination of drug concentrations immediately (the blood should be centrifuged and the serum separated).
- Other questions
    - Does the child take his/her medication?
    - The type of seizure (a thorough history)
    - Triggering factors (fever? staying awake late?)
    - Psychological well being of the family

References

1. Hancock E, Osborne JP. Vigabatrin in the treatment of infantile spasms in tuberous sclerosis: a literature review. Journal of Child Neurology 1999;14:71–74.
2. The Database of Abstracts of Reviews of Effectiveness (University of York), Database no.: DARE-990436. In: The Cochrane Library, Issue 4, 2000. Oxford: Update Software.

29.5 Sleep disorders in children

Pertti Rintahaka

Aims

- Parents are given information on normal sleep and sleep behaviour in children and told that parasomnias are usually harmless.
- Disorders of sleep rhythm in infants are identified early at the child health clinic and parents are instructed how to correct abnormal sleep behaviour **C** [1].
- The use of a sleep diary should be promoted in investigating sleep disorders.
- Serious sleep disorders (for example apnoea and narcolepsy) and seizures during sleep require hospital investigations.

Normal sleep in children

- The need for sleep in children ranges widely and decreases with advancing age from 20 hours sleep in an infant aged less than six months to an average of nine hours in a teenager.
- Daytime naps are a fundamental part of daily total sleep in infancy. The naps gradually become shorter. At the age of a few months, infants usually nap two or three times per day. Naps are taken until the age of four or five years.
- The longest uninterrupted period of sleep is usually two to four hours during the first weeks of life. At its shortest it can even be half of this. From the age of six weeks, the continuous uninterrupted period of sleep increases to six hours and mostly occurs during night-time.
- Sleeping through the night has been defined as sleep from midnight to 5 a.m. for at least four weeks. Sleep periods of the newborn are distributed evenly throughout the day and night. From the age of three months, children normally sleep most of their 14–15-hour sleep at night.

Disorders of sleep rhythm

- The most common sleep disorders in infants and toddlers are
    - difficulty in falling asleep

- interrupted sleep
- waking up too early

♦ Waking up two to four times per night over a one-week period is considered to be a sleep problem.

Parasomnias

♦ Parasomnias are disturbances of arousal, partial arousal or transitions between sleep stages.

♦ **Body rocking and head banging** start from the age of six months. No treatment is needed if the infant is developing normally. These children do not usually have any neurological or psychological problems. Repeated jerks or twitches, especially if they occur in series, may be signs of infantile spasms. Children with suspected infantile spasms should urgently be referred to a paediatric neurology department.

♦ **Tooth grinding** means noisy biting or rubbing of the teeth against each other. If the child repeatedly bites his/her tongue at night, epileptic seizures should be suspected.

♦ **Pavor nocturnus**, like other parasomnias, usually starts one to two hours after falling asleep. The child sits up in bed with an appearance of fear and may vocalize or scream. The pulse is quick. The duration of the attack ranges from a few to 20 minutes. No treatment is needed. There is no reason to wake the child up. Sudden waking in the early morning may sometimes be caused by epileptic seizures.

♦ **Sleepwalking** lasts from few minutes to half an hour. The sleepwalker should be taken back to his/her bed. The surroundings of a sleepwalker should be safe, to minimize the risk of an accident.

♦ **Sleep talking** is seen during various stages of sleep. The symptom does not need to be treated. Sleep talking should be differentiated from nocturnal epileptic seizures, which are usually associated with other kinds of vocalization.

♦ **Snoring** is also classified as a parasomnia. In most instances, snoring is benign. If snoring is associated with excessive daytime tiredness, behavioural or learning disorders, it necessitates further investigations.

♦ **Nightmares** are associated with dreaming. The child seems to be fearful, as in pavor nocturnus. Yet in most cases, the child remembers nightmares. It is advisable to wake the child up. Parental reassurance is important. A calm evening routine helps to prevent nightmares.

Apnoeas

♦ Respiratory pauses during sleep (apnoeas) are significant sleep disorders in children.

♦ **Obstructive sleep apnoea** (OSAS) is the most common. In most cases, airway obstruction is caused by enlargement of the adenoids or the tonsils. Physical obstruction combined with decreased muscle tone prevents free airflow.
  - Symptoms include excessive daytime tiredness, sleeplessness, morning headaches, hyperactivity and learning difficulties.
  - Removal of the adenoid tissue usually may relieve the symptoms, although there is no evidence from randomized trials of its efficacy (D) [2]. The size of the adenoid tissue does not always correlate with the severity of apnoea.
  - If apnoea still persists, tonsillectomy is performed.
  - In doubtful cases, the diagnosis of apnoea and the outcome of operation should be documented by a whole-night polysomnography.

♦ **Brief central apnoeas** are normal in small infants. Both central and obstructive apnoeas lasting more than 15 seconds require detailed investigations because they can precede sudden infant death syndrome.

Excessive daytime tiredness

♦ Infants usually sleep enough. Excessive daytime tiredness is rare, because an infant falls asleep when he/she is tired. The infant should be alert when awake.

♦ Of the causes of excessive daytime tiredness, obstructive sleep apnoea is the most important. Narcolepsy is rare and may be manifested at school age as restlessness and hyperactivity. Later symptoms include involuntary falling asleep and cataplexy. Narcolepsy (36.9) usually starts at the age of 15–20 years. The diagnosis is often delayed by many years.

Examination of the child

♦ In the beginning, it is important to know what parents mean by a sleep disorder.

♦ Detailed history of sleep.

♦ In interrupted sleep of recent onset, remember to check the eardrums.

♦ As routine laboratory tests, a blood cell count and urinary tests are performed to exclude anaemia and infection.

♦ Use of a sleep log.

Using a sleep log

♦ If the cause of the sleep problem is not obvious, the parents fill in a sleep log for two to three weeks. In the sleep log, time to bed, observed or assumed time of falling asleep, nightly awakening and duration of wakefulness, night feeding or eating at night, naps and eating times during the day are marked as accurately as possible with symbols.

♦ With the history and sleep log it is possible to clarify whether the child has dysfunctional sleep habits, faulty sleep associations or a serious disorder requiring hospital investigations, or whether the parents have unrealistic expectations about sleep quality. Falling asleep too early or too late and waking up too late or too early are revealed by the sleep log, as are regular but inappropriate, and completely irregular sleep habits.

Treatment of sleep disorders

♦ The sleep routines and associations of infants should be modified. If the child is used to company or other entertainment immediately after waking, a sleep problem may arise in the family.

- The best way to prevent sleep disorders in children is to follow as regular living habits and sleep routines as possible C [1].
- Sleeping in the same bed as the parents makes it more difficult for the child to transfer to his/her own bed. A child should not be taught to fall asleep in a brightly lit room, or when held, rocked or fed, or to feed the child immediately after waking.
- The sleep surroundings should be quiet. Soft sleep toys are recommended from infancy onwards.
- The best and most gentle method to treat disturbances of the sleep-wake rhythm is a gradual change of sleep rhythm, although the quickest results have been reached by letting the child cry himself or herself asleep.

Scaling of treatment and indications for consultation

- Most sleep disorders are investigated and treated by general practitioners.
- If epilepsy is suspected, examination by a paediatric neurologist and an EEG are necessary.
- Obstructive sleep apnoea is treated by an ENT specialist.
- If central apnoeas or narcolepsy are suspected, the child should be referred for university hospital investigations.
- Because of parents' exhaustion it is sometimes necessary to refer the child to a hospital to change the sleep-wake rhythm.
- For bed-wetting see 28.15.

References

1. Renfrew MJ, Lang S. Interventions for influencing sleep patterns in exclusively breastfed infants. The Cochrane Database of Systematic Reviews, Cochrane Library number: CD000113. In: The Cochrane Library, Issue 2, 2002. Oxford: Update Software. Updated frequently.
2. Lim J, McKean M. Adenotonsillectomy for obstructive sleep apnoea in children. Cochrane Database Syst Rev 2003(1): CD003136.

29.6 Detection of neurological disorders in children

Editors

Aims

- Refer all children with developmental stagnation for further investigations without delay.
- Treatment of cerebral palsy should be started as soon as abnormal movement patterns are detected C [1,2]. The aetiology should be determined if possible.
- Refer for further investigation all children
    - with hypotonia, however mild, if the tendon reflexes are absent, in order to exclude myopathies
    - with marked hypotonia and developmental delay even if tendon reflexes are normal (suspicion of a developmental disability)
    - with symptoms suggestive of infantile spasms or other types of seizures.

Basic rules

- An accurate diagnosis is not needed before the parents can be given instructions on how to care for their child or before physiotherapy is started. A deviation in motor function in infancy should not be labelled cerebral palsy (CP) before adequate investigations and follow-up.
- Consider referring all children with any abnormality, detected by the doctor or suspected by the parents.

Clinical examination

- **Gross motor** development gives an idea of the child's general stage of development. Any delays or mild abnormalities may be due to psychosocial factors, but in some cases they may be suggestive of hereditary illnesses, developmental disability, delayed development due to other reasons or, at a later age, learning difficulties.
- An evaluation of **fine motor** functions may assist in the detection of the following conditions, illnesses or problems:
    - General developmental delay/mental retardation (prevalence 10/1000)
    - Some cases of cerebral palsy (prevalence of cerebral palsy 2.5/1000)
    - Regression in the child's development
    - Cerebral fine motor disorders with associated motor coordination problems (prevalence of fine motor disorders, including Attention Deficit Hyperactivity Disorder (ADHD), 70/1000 children aged 5–10 years).
    - Some cases of learning difficulties (10–15% of school-aged children suffer from learning difficulties).
- An evaluation of **perception** abilities may assist in the detection of the following conditions, illnesses or problems:
    - General developmental delay/mental retardation
    - Regression in the child's development
    - Cerebral fine motor disorders with associated perception problems (approximately 5% of children aged 5–10 years)
    - Narrow, specific perception problems (2–3% of school aged children)
    - Some cases of learning difficulties
- In **mental retardation** the child will show delayed development of fine motor functions and language as

well as problems with perceptual and observational skills.

- An assessment for **cerebral palsy** involves an evaluation of fine motor skills together with an evaluation of gross motor skills and a basic neurological examination (muscle tone, tendon reflexes, range of movement).
- In **diseases leading to developmental regression** (for example aspartylglycosaminuria and other lysosomal storage diseases) the first symptoms include loss of hand skills and observational powers (a child's decreased interest in the surroundings).
- For detailed information about the clinical examinations, see 28.1.
- For development of the speech, see 28.6.
- Does the developmental stage correspond with the age of the child (motor functions, grasping, contact, vocalizing, following with eyes etc.)?
- The muscle tone and activity of an infant are usually symmetrical. Persistent asymmetry is usually abnormal. Does the developmental stage correspond with the age of the child (motor functions, grasping, contact, vocalizing, following with eyes etc.)?

Motor function abnormalities requiring physiotherapy

- A definite tendency for extension that increases towards the age of 4 months (between the ages of 3–6 months preterm infants in particular may have a transient tendency for extension).
- Hypertonicity or alternating muscle tone (dystonia) in an infant.
- Asymmetry of muscle tone or activity in the extremities.
- Hypotonia associated with delayed or dissociated development (delayed gross motor function but normal fine motor function).

Conditions requiring further investigation

Suspicion of infantile spasm or other forms of epilepsy

- The parents of children aged 3–7 months should be asked whether the child has jerky movements.
- Infantile spasms should be suspected and further investigations carried out if the child has rapid jerky movements when awake, particularly upon awakening, characterized by forward-bending of the neck and abduction of the upper limbs or flexion of the elbows, and throwing the legs upwards when lying supine.
- Early onset of treatment is likely to improve the prognosis of infantile spasms.
- All seizures (also those other than infantile spasms) require investigation and treatment without delay.
- The Moro reflex (up to the age of 3 (–4) months) and sleep jerks during REM sleep are normal phenomena.

Muscular hypotonia

- Mild hypotonia is usually benign, and often familial.
- Examine the tendon reflexes in children with muscular hypotonia. Absence of the reflexes may be a sign of a muscular disease and an indication for further investigation. A high serum creatine kinase concentration suggests myopathy.
- Remember that many developmental disabilities are associated with muscular hypotonia. If developmental disability of any type is suspected the diagnosis and the aetiology should be verified as soon as possible in order to start genetic counselling etc.

Muscular hypertonicity

- See above.

Asymmetric muscle tone or activity of the limbs

- Always an indication for referral

Stagnation or retardation of development

- Infantile spasms
- Metabolic disorders
- Developmental disability
- Neuromuscular diseases
- Diseases affecting general health

References

1. Darrah J, Fan JS, Chen LC, Nunweiler J, Watkins B. Review of the effects of progressive resisted muscle strengthening in children with cerebral palsy: a clinical consensus exercise. Pediatr Phys Ther 1997;9:12–17.
2. The Database of Abstracts of Reviews of Effectiveness (University of York), Database no.: DARE-975092. In: The Cochrane Library, Issue 4, 1999. Oxford: Update Software.

PAE

29.7 Hydrocephalus and complications of cranial shunts

Editors

Basic rules

- Recognize abnormal head growth at the child health clinic.
- Recognize shunt complications at an early stage.

Epidemiology

- Hydrocephalus associated with meningomyelocoele: 1:4000
- Other causes: 1:2000

Screening during child health surveillance

- The diagnosis of hydrocephalus is based on the monitoring of head growth.
- If the head circumference grows by one standard deviation more than what is the normal growth curve in 1–2 months time refer the child for further investigations immediately.
- Refer all children whose head circumference is above + 2 SD.
- If the head circumference has grown one standard deviation more than the normal growth curve over a period of 6 months or longer, follow-up can be performed in primary care provided that the accelerated growth gradually subsides and the development of the child is otherwise normal.

Symptoms

- Enhancement of extracranial veins, increased tonus of the fontanelle
- Opening of the cranial sutures
- Sunset gaze (a gaze directed downwards) is rare.
- Irritability
- Failure to thrive and eat
- Vomiting
- Psychomotor retardation (Poor support of the head may be the initial symptom.)
- Symptoms of high intracranial pressure in children above 2 years of age: headache (particularly in the morning), vomiting, and convulsions.

Indications for head imaging

- Ultrasonography is always indicated in small children when the head circumference increases abnormally.
- Computed tomography or magnetic resonance imaging should be performed in older children who have symptoms or signs of high intracranial pressure or whose head circumference growth is accelerated or exceeds + 2 SD.

Symptoms and signs suggesting a shunt complication and indicating immediate referral

- Oedema around the shunt, erythema or skin infection
- Vomiting, headache, or irritability
- Abdominal pain
- Neck stiffness, opisthotonus
- Painful head or eye movements
- Abnormal eye movements on examination
- Strabismus with sudden onset
- Recurring convulsions
- Headache/nausea in the afternoon
- Impaired consciousness (Puncture the shunt before referral as the condition may deteriorate very rapidly during transportation.)
- Unexplained fever
- **Immediate sterile shunt puncture with removal of 20–30 ml of cerebrospinal fluid is indicated in the following situations:**
    - Impaired consciousness without an obvious cause other than increased intracranial pressure
    - Extensor rigidity
    - Large or non-responding pupils
    - Respiratory arrest
- Consult the specialist clinic by telephone about shunt puncture.
- Lumbar puncture is dangerous and contraindicated. The absence of papillar stasis on fundoscopic examination does not rule out high intracranial pressure.

29.8 ADHD and MBD syndromes

Hannu Westerinen

Definitions

- A cluster on problems that includes attention deficit, hyperactivity and lack of impulse control is nowadays called attention deficit/hyperactivity disorder (ADHD) in international literature.
- The term minimal brain dysfunction (MBD) is no longer included in ICD-10, and all special problems should be referred to with the proper terms.
- The term MBD has largely been replaced by DAMP (Deficits in Attention, Motor Coordination and Perception).
- Particularly in the USA the term used is ADHD, which is included in the psychiatric disease classification system DSM-IV. A set of questions has been defined for diagnostic purposes and these questions can be used to determine whether the child has only attention deficit disorder or hyperactivity/impulse control problem or a combination of these.
- CNS symptoms, such as learning difficulties and motor clumsiness, are often associated with ADHD, in which case ADHD and MBD are identical concepts.
- The term MBD is used when problems in other areas are associated with the attention deficit disorder:
    - Motor coordination: hyperactivity, slowness of movement, fine and gross motor clumsiness.
    - Perception: difficulties are observed mainly in vision, hearing, feeling and perceiving space and body positions.
    - Language: different problems that manifest in various ways.
    - Learning: in addition to the above-mentioned difficulties problems may be caused by difficulty in concentrating, short attention span or memory dysfunction.
    - Behaviour: behavioural disorders and emotional problems are either directly caused by MBD or are a secondary consequence of malfunctioning social interaction.

- The concept of MBD and other diagnostic definitions underline the weaknesses of a child. According to several studies it is rather a question of balance between weaknesses or risk factors and counteracting protective factors. The amount of psychosocial support that the child receives correlates strongly with the degree of difficulties at school, even more strongly than biological risk factors.

Epidemiology and prognosis

- At least 5% of children have an attention deficit/hyperactivity disorder, problems of motor coordination and perception difficulties at school start: every class has at least one hyperactive child.
- Problems are more common in boys than in girls; however, in girls less apparent problems may remain undiagnosed.
- One third of these children have such considerable difficulties that treatment and rehabilitation are necessary already in pre-school age, while the rest need supportive measures at school age.
- At school age motor problems often alleviate, yet about one third still suffer from clumsiness in adulthood.
- Problems with attention deficit may continue to adulthood and require care.

Examinations and procedures

- Early detection is important for targeting rehabilitation correctly.
- Diagnosis is set after special examinations (paediatric neurologist and if necessary psychiatrist, occupational therapist, speech therapist, psychologist, etc) and rehabilitative measures are determined by the diagnosis.
- Rather than delay school start, the child should go to school for longer if necessary. These children commonly need special educational programmes or extra tuition in some subjects. Adjusted curriculum may be the best option.
- Factors that stress children in general, such as marital problems, neglect in divorce, violence in the family, etc. are also found in the lives of children with MBD. Their harmful effects are more marked in these children with special difficulties and the health care staff should seek to identify these factors actively in a way that promotes cooperation with all parties.
- Families benefit from adjustment programmes, holidays for parents or for the family, social support, good written information, peer group activities of parental groups, and sometimes from family psychotherapy.
- Expertise is needed also in career choice guidande and planning of studies. The important transition from childhood to adulthood requires special attention.

Medication

- The best-documented short-term effect for symptoms of hyperactivity is obtained with psychostimulants (methylphenidate B [1] [2] [3] [4], dextroamphetamine and magnesium pemoline).
- Psychostimulant therapy may be most beneficial for children who suffer from severe hyperactivity, whose attentiveness is abnormal in relation to their intelligence and who don't have simultaneous emotional disturbances.
- The clinical response to drug therapy is hard to predict and treatment is always started as a trial.

References

1. Shukla VK, Otten N. Assessment of attention-deficit/hyperactivity disorder therapy: a Canadian perspective. Ottawa: Canadian Coordinating Office for Health Technology Assessment/ Office Canadien de Coordination de l'Evaluation des Technologies de la Santé. Alberta Heritage Foundation for Medical Research (AHFMR). 12039012. Technology Overview.
1999. 11.
2. The Health Technology Assessment Database, Database no.: HTA-998360. In: The Cochrane Library, Issue 1, 2001. Oxford: Update Software.
3. Jadad AR, Boyle M, Cunningham C, Kim M, Schachar R. Treatment of attention-deficit/hyperactivity disorder. Rockville, MD, USA: Agency for Healthcare Research and Quality. Evidence Report/Tech. 1999. 1–341.
4. The Database of Abstracts of Reviews of Effectiveness (University of York), Database no.: DARE-20008341. In: The Cochrane Library, Issue 1, 2002. Oxford: Update Software.

29.12 Encountering the family of a child with a neurological disability

Matti Sillanpää

Basic rules

- Place yourself in the position of a parent in family with a disabled child and treat the family accordingly.
- Be understanding and helpful yet at the same time realistic. Act according to your conviction as a doctor and do not allow anything else but the facts to guide your actions.

General rules

- The hopes and dreams set on a child are devastating when a developmental defect or a long-term illness exists.
- The blow experienced by the parents is often very hard and may affect their attitude towards the child for the rest of the child's life.

- Information given to the parents and the rest of the family should be honest, discreet, and consistent. The standpoint of the family should guide the approach, and the ability of the family to receive information should be taken into account.
- Handling a crisis is not just giving information, but rather facing and going through the crisis together with the family.

Behaviour of the family members

- In difficult situations all families apparently go through the various stages of a crisis in the order outlined by the crisis theory.
- The stages through which families progress in their own pace include denial of the problem, depression or resorting to aggression, acknowledging the problem and hoping for any kind of help and finally stabilization and fact-like and calm acceptance of the situation with arrangements for the treatment and habilitation of the child so that they become a part of the daily life.
- The duration and difficulty of the process depend on the ability of both the treating doctor and the family members to encounter a crisis. Guilty feelings of the parents should be addressed seriously. In most cases they are totally unfounded, and even if the parents had contributed to the situation, nothing can be gained by blaming them.
- Feelings of guilt can only add to the already threatening danger of overprotection for the child. To avoid overprotection the parents must be told from the beginning that they should expect the child to manage all age-related daily activities that he/she is known to manage, although extra time may be needed, for example, for dressing or undressing.
- Feelings of success give the disabled child self-esteem, which is often fragile and easily damaged. The doctor's caring and empathetic, yet strongly factual attitude and behaviour give family members a sense of security.
- The parents are often very worried about the child's future. The doctor should not raise or support totally unfounded hopes, however, the biological variation and inter-individual differences in seemingly very similar situations should also be kept in mind.

Nature of the disability

- It makes a difference whether the child's disability is visible or not. A visible disability, e.g. a motor one, is not questioned and thus need not be explained.
- It has been found that the people around the child have a more positive attitude towards a disability that is visible than towards, for example, a disorder of language development, as a visible disability is easier to understand.

Doctor's attitude

- The doctor should be able to relate to the parents' emotional states and their fluctuations. What is yet more important is that the doctor continues to maintain a kind and warm but strictly professional role towards the family.
- The professional should be able to tolerate the aggressive feelings of the family even when those are directed towards the doctor himself.
- The behaviour of the parents is often led by a feeling of guilt.
- Subconsciously, the parents may test whether the doctor can put up with their anxiety. They need that information to be able to trust the doctor.
- Educational background of the parents has no effect on their behaviour. Yet, it is important for the doctor to be aware of the background of the family in order to know what kind of expressions and terminology can be used in discussions.

When and how to tell the suspicions to the parents

- When the family doctor first begins to suspect a developmental defect or chronic disease, he/she first notices isolated symptoms suggesting the condition. These symptoms can be discussed with the parents, assessing the need and possibilities of treatment.
- In most cases the family only needs to be instructed to carry on taking care of the child as usual and to follow up the development both at home and on visits to the doctor.
- If the child's muscle tone is found to be abnormal, he/she can be referred to a physiotherapist's consultation and, if necessary, habilitation.
- A diary for following up the child's development is often very helpful. If suspicions of a defect grows, follow-up visits are scheduled more frequently and the child is referred to investigations in a hospital and for multi-professional assessment.
- Discussing the child's symptoms with the parents should be left to the treating doctor. If too many persons are involved in talking to the parents about the diagnosis, the risk of contradictory information and misunderstandings increases. If this happens, or if the child responds slowly to habilitation, the parents may, as the last resort, seek for a second opinion from various professionals.
- The doctor should not discourage this; nevertheless, he/she should be frank about the realistic possibilities that may exist and about the costs that may incur to the parents.

Diagnosis

- The diagnosis should not be set before the disability has been ascertained. Discussing the matter carelessly, "this could be cerebral palsy" is detrimental to the doctor–patient relationship and should be avoided.
- However, the diagnosis should be told as soon as it is certain, and the doctor must offer all the support to the family when he/she gives this information.
- The doctor who is in charge of the treatment of the child is responsible for the diagnosis and for making sure that it

is correct. He/she is thus also the right person for telling the diagnosis to the family. This must be done so that the family understands the diagnosis and what it signifies.

- The information is necessary for all those involved in the treatment and habilitation of the child both in primary and specialist care and naturally also for the family.
- Many questions arise later at home. Therefore, it is important that the parents know whom they can contact. The family may also acquire more information of the disorder from the patient organization, parent groups, the Internet and other sources.
- It is important to be able to tell about the child's problems to neighbours, family, and friends. These people also need to understand the nature and the causes of the disability to accept the child's behaviour.
- All bad behaviour is not just the result of a failed upbringing.

Treatment

- The treatment of the child and the family starts already when the first isolated symptoms are discussed. When the diagnosis has been clarified the causes underlying the problem can be discussed.
- When the family has accepted the inevitable, the family members need to be able to do something for the child's habilitation on a daily basis to feel that they are trying to do their best.
- The instructions on habilitation given by therapists often need to be rather detailed. All information on the particular disability is important. Skills needed in daily life, such as how to handle the child when changing the nappy, dressing, feeding, holding in different positions are important acts of habilitation.
- However, it is also important to emphasize the right of the parents to parenthood without taking the role of a habilitation therapist. The child is to be taken to routine well-baby check-ups, given the normal vaccinations and other services provided by the well-baby centre or clinic, like any other child.

Prognosis

- The family ought to be told at the very beginning of the treatment that, despite treatment and management, the child's development will be slower than normal but he/she will make progress anyway. The actual defect cannot be treated, but the functional and social limitations can be reduced significantly.
- Care should be taken when explaining the prognosis, as biological variation is considerable. Certain hopefulness should be encouraged, as a positive attitude towards the child and his/her disability has a dramatic effect on the results of rehabilitation.
- Encouraging reports of real-life cases give the family strength to believe that their child may also make it through the life.

29.15 Foetal alcohol syndrome (FAS)

Erja Halmesmäki

Aims

- To make an early diagnosis of FAS or the milder form of the syndrome FAE (foetal alcohol effects).
- To ensure that a child with FAS/FAE receives individualized treatment and rehabilitation as well as the necessary support from the various health and welfare services.

Diagnostic criteria

- FAS = symptoms from all three groups
- FAE = symptoms from two groups and a history of exposure to alcohol.
  - **Pre- and postnatal growth retardation**
    - Birth weight, height and head circumference below the 10th normal percentile curve value.
  - **Central nervous system dysfunction**
    - Neurological symptoms
    - Delay in development
    - Mental retardation
  - **Typical facial features**, at least two of the following:
    - Microcephalia
    - Microphthalmia and/or narrow palpebral fissures
    - Poorly developed philtrum, narrow upper lip and/or low maxilla
    - Broad dorsum of the nose, pointed tip of the nose.

Prevalence

- As little as 8–10 standard doses of alcohol per week slows foetal development

Growth retardation

- Of children born to alcoholics, approximately 80% are small for gestational age at birth.
- Catching-up growth after birth does not occur.
- The suck reflex of the newborn is poorly developed or absent.
- Microcephalia is the most severe concrete finding in a newborn and it is not corrected with age, instead the growth of the head circumference follows the −2–−3 SD or even the −4 SD curve.

Neurological and other symptoms

- The degree of alcohol exposure affects the severity of the symptoms (26.18).
- The children are often impatient, easily irritated and restless.

- Motor functions develop slower than normal and speech development is also delayed.
- Hearing impairment is possible, which is why the hearing of all FAS-FAE children should be examined thoroughly at an early stage.
- At preschool age and school age the children suffer from attention deficit disorders that do not resolve with age. Only one out of five children with FAS-FAE manages in a normal school class without supportive measures or without being transferred to a special education class.
- In mild cases the child has learning difficulties and perception disorders.
- The average I.Q. of children with FAS is 60–70, however, the range is rather large.
- Children most severely affected by FAS are seriously mentally retarded with hearing and visual impairment and are usually placed in an institution.

Rehabilitation and prognosis of a child with FAS

- The environment of a child with FAS-FAE greatly affects the prognosis.
- In severe cases placement in a foster home before the age of 6 months clearly improves prognosis.
- The rehabilitation and treatment of the child are organized individually.
- Small children with FAS usually need both physiotherapy and speech therapy.
- The child should be placed in a school class that corresponds to his/her skills, and, if necessary, school start should be postponed.
- Sometimes it is in the child's interest that special education is given from the beginning or the child is placed in a special class, as changing from a normal class to a special education class at a later point would further affect the child's self-esteem, which is poor in many cases.
- The prevention and treatment of psychological and behavioural disorders should be arranged early on, although this may be difficult if the child lives in an alcoholic family.

29.20 Down's syndrome

Hannu Westerinen, Maija Wilska

Aims

- Patients with Down's syndrome (DS) should be treated in the normal health care system for the usual diseases of childhood and later age.
- However, they should be directed to seek help from special services for problems that are typical to DS.
- These typical disorders, such as congenital heart diseases, eye, ear and thyroid problems, should be diagnosed early to diminish their impact on the patient's developmental progress.

Epidemiology

- The incidence of Down's syndrome in the Western world is 1/600–1/900; at maternal age of 40, about 1/100.
- The most common cause is 21-trisomy, occasionally mosaicism, and in 1–2% the underlying cause is translocation of parental origin.

Diagnosis and primary prevention

- The definitive prenatal diagnosis is made by amniocentesis or placental biopsy. In cases of parental translocation or one previous child with DS, prenatal diagnosis is available in most countries. However, there is great variation between communities in policies concerning screening methods and prenatal chromosomal studies associated with maternal age.
- The clinician has to be able to give to the family unbiased, thorough information about DS and services available to these children.
  - Various health problems are frequently present.
  - Most people with DS have moderate intellectual disability, however, their intellectual level may vary from profoundly to mildly impaired. With assistance some may even keep up with the normal elementary school curriculum, at least for a few years.
  - Most people with DS live a happy life, particularly if they are trained and supported to live as competently as possible. Thus, the "prevention" of DS is only seldom targeted against the suffering of the affected individual, as is the case in, for example, severe progressive metabolic diseases. It is rather a question of how the parents and other people concerned react, and involves also economic aspects of care and rehabilitation.
- The decision on continuation or termination of pregnancy must be left entirely to the family. They may wish to prepare for the birth of a handicapped child or to terminate the pregnancy if they feel that for social or financial reasons they could not care for a child with DS.

Early rehabilitation

- Breastfeeding an infant with DS is important, not only for the intimacy of the early contact between the mother and the child, but also for developing the oral musculature and motor function and for providing protective antibodies through mother's milk. If the baby has problems with sucking, specialized personnel at child health clinics or speech therapists can give helpful instructions.
- Early intervention may be very helpful in supporting and optimizing the child's development. Such a programme is ideally followed by home visits by professionals trained in the developmental problems of handicapped young children. They also provide the necessary training for the family,

who can then actively participate in the programme. Early intervention often follows the framework of a special method, such as Portage. Day care should also be involved in carrying out the programme. Physiotherapy is sometimes indicated.

- Early provision of communication therapy is important. Non-verbal communication, such as sign language has been proven beneficial to language development. Contrary to a frequent misconception, the latter does not delay acquisition of speech and may in fact aid it.

Typical health problems associated with Down's syndrome

Growth

- Persons with trisomy 21 are shorter and have a smaller head circumference compared with general population. Modified growth charts for children with DS are available from doctors specialised in managing intellectually disabled children.
- Individuals with DS have tendency to be overweight. The main reason is low metabolic rate, but dietary habits, inactivity and hypothyroidism may contribute to it. The target weight is given in weight curves for healthy children of equal height.

Sensory systems

- Ophthalmological problems are common, including:
  - Accommodation problems, myopia, hyperopia and amblyopia
  - Alternating esotropia occurs frequently.
  - Congenital cataracts are occasionally seen and with increasing age, cataracts become rather common, and may require surgery.
  - About 5% develop keratoconus later in life, which may also require surgery.
  - Nystagmus is occasionally seen as a maturation problem.
  - An ophthalmologist should evaluate the vision of children with DS before the age of 1 year because of the high incidence of disturbances.
- Problems with ears
  - The outer auditory canal is narrow, especially in children, and is often obstructed by wax. Regular cleaning with wax-dissolving preparations is recommended.
  - Secretory otitis media, accompanied by a conductive hearing disorder is observed in 60–70% of children with DS. Therefore regular follow-up by an ENT specialist is often necessary, particularly because the narrowness of the outer auditory canal may lead to incorrect diagnoses and treatments if special instruments are not used during the examination.

Central nervous system

- Alzheimer-type changes in the brain are seen microscopically by the age of 40 years, although clinical dementia is rarely manifested at that age. Generally, the symptoms are milder if the individual is provided with appropriate stimulation and the activity level is kept up.
- In differential diagnostics the possibility of pseudodementia associated with hypothyroidism should be kept in mind.
- Infantile spasms are seen in 1% of the children; however, the prognosis is better than in other children. The incidence of epilepsy increases with the aging of the brain.

Psychiatry

- Autistic features are found in up to 10% of persons with Down's syndrome.
- Depression is 2–3 times more common than in other developmentally disabled persons. Serotonergic drugs are the primary therapy.

Endocrine disorders

- Hypothyroidism is common.
  - The clinical picture cannot be relied upon in follow-up, making regular monitoring of laboratory values necessary. High prevalence of subclinical hypothyroidism is a special feature of Down's syndrome (TSH is elevated, but free T4 is normal in as many as 30%). In one third, subclinical hypothyroidism resolves spontaneously. Follow-up regimen:
    - TSH determination from umbilical cord blood
    - TSH at the age of one year. If the result is normal, follow-up every 2 years throughout life.
  - If TSH is elevated, free T4 must be added to the regimen.
    - Low free T4 → start thyroxine substitution
    - Normal free T4 and TSH 6–10: TSH, free T4 and TPOAb annually
    - Normal free T4 and TSH > 10: TSH, free T4 and TPOAb every 6 months.
- The risk of diabetes is increased.

Gastrointestinal disorders

- Congenital anomalies, especially atresias are common, requiring early surgery.
- Constipation is very common and is managed with diet and medications. It may result in anal fissures that may cause discomfort and pain leading to behavioural problems and worsening of the symptoms.
- Hirschprung's disease must be kept in mind as a possible cause of constipation.
- The risk of coeliac disease is 6–7% in screened persons, however only 0.8–3% of persons with Down's syndrome suffer from the symptoms at some point in life. Screening is indicated at any age in the presence of even slight symptoms. The same methods that are generally used to screen for coeliac disease are applied. Determining the HLA-antigens limits the need for further tests to 30%.

Urinary tracts

- Congenital anomalies may be underlying causes of urinary tract infections.

Genitalia

- Cryptorchidism is common, and its surgical correction before school age is recommended (otherwise the risk of testicular cancer is increased).
- Reproductive capability of men with DS is weak.
- Many women with DS are fertile, and the need for contraception should be kept in mind.

Musculoskeletal and connective tissues

- Joints are abnormally mobile and muscles hypotonic.
  - Early weight bearing in the standing position should be avoided.
  - A sturdy shoe with laces is recommended. If flat feet cause pain, arch supports are necessary. If the foot, knee and/or hip become painful inspite supports, it is necessary to consult a specialist.
  - Atlantoaxial instability is rather common and should be kept in mind before anaesthesia and contact sports are considered (risk of spinal cord compression!).
  - Patellar and pelvic luxations do not usually cause disability.
  - Dislocation of the hip may occur also after the age of 7–8 years and requires consultation with an orthopaedist.

Cardiovascular system

- Congenital heart anomalies are observed in 40–50% of children with DS. Every child with DS has to undergo ultrasound examination during the first 1–3 months of life because the common occurring atrioventricular canal requires surgery at 3–6 months of age. Indications for surgical correction are the same as for other children. Remember prophylactic antibiotics prior to dental procedures such as removal of dental calculus.
- Peripheral circulation may be poor in older individuals with DS in whom it may result in bluish feet.

Immune and haematological disorders

- The risk of leukaemia is increased, particularly in those children who had a transient leukemoid reaction (leucocytosis, myeloblasts and hepatosplenomegaly) as neonates/infants. Its treatment and prognosis are the same as in other children.
- Susceptibility to infections is increased, and may be due to a cellular immune deficiency. Mucous discharge, congestion and wheezing may result from the narrow airways with thick productive mucous membranes rather than from infection.
- Leucocyte function abnormality is associated with a strong tendency for gingivitis.

Skin disorders

- Dry skin is common, especially on the cheeks. Heel sores necessitating the use of ointments may develop.
- Seborrhoeic eczema is common.
- Tinea may occasionally be aggressive.

The significance of antioxidant therapy

- The benefits of antioxidant therapy (selenium, zinc, vitamins E and B6) are controversial.
- In theory, these substances slow down premature degeneration of the tissues caused by free radicals.
- However, their effectiveness has not been demonstrated as yet in practice or in controlled studies. Appropriate dietary supplementation should be given in obvious cases of deficiency.
- Using large doses of vitamins does not bring any benefits.
- Enthusiastically offering antioxidant therapy, which fails to meet the expectations, can only reinforce denial of the child's condition.
- For more information contact your local authorities on the care and support of the handicapped.

29.22 Treating psychological problems of the intellectually disabled in primary health care

Hannu Westerinen

Aims

- To recognize conditions requiring a more specific assessment of a possible mental disease or psychiatric disorder.
- To identify possible somatic causes and treat them.
- To provide psychiatric first aid care when necessary.
- To ensure further evaluation and treatment of the patient in an appropriate unit.

Psychological problems

- Intellectual disability (ID) is defined as subaverage intellect. Common comorbidities (epilepsy, physical handicap, sensory defects) cause additional problems.
- The prevalence of mental diseases and psychological disorders in the intellectually disabled is as high as in the normal population. However, because of the different appearance and behaviour of the ID people it is sometimes difficult to detect these diseases.

Mood disorders

- The patient may not necessarily be able to tell of his/her moods, experience of self-esteem or hopes. Variation in mental alertness observed by others may give clues to changes in mood.
- Periodical variation manifesting as lack of energy and restlessness may suggest bipolar mood disorder.

- Sometimes an intellectually disabled person may speak openly of suicidal ideation.
- Depression continues to be underdiagnosed in the ID population.

Mannerism, stereotypy

- Autistic conditions, in particular, may include various kinds of "strange" behaviour and mannerism without any underlying mental disease.
- For example a blind person may use the sense of smell to orientate to the environment or a person with poor eyesight may look at a bright light and wave fingers in front of his eyes.

Nocturnal enuresis

- Treatment consists of an enuresis alarm, imipramine, desmopressin nasal spray (Minirin) (note contraindications).

Physical and psychological violence, sexual abuse

- Discrimination/abuse is not rare; verifying the events is often difficult.

Rumination

- The symptom may be associated with reflux oesophagitis requiring treatment.

Restlessness, behaviour disorders, aggression

- May be associated with somatic diseases, mental disorders or problems of social interaction; these will be discussed later.

Self-injurious behaviour

- Underlying cause may be somatic. Extensive examination is necessary, particularly if the behaviour has not occurred earlier. Banging the head and tearing off nails were initially almost the only symptoms of a 17-year-old autistic girl after the perforation of the gall bladder.
- The situation is often improved by an extensive rehabilitation programme.
- If necessary, a behaviour therapeutic teaching programme should be planned (C) [1 2].

Disturbing sexuality

- Masturbation in the presence of other people can often be eradicated by teaching proper intimacy and by setting clear borders/limits.
- Arranging creative activities, work and hobbies is usually very beneficial.

Other problems

- Some special conditions (fragile X syndrome, Prader–Willi syndrome) are associated with particular psychological problems.

Special challenges in the psychological development of an intellectually disabled person

- A possible brain damage affects learning skills, comprehension and personality.
- Aetiological assessment, additional handicap, physical handicap, sensory handicap, difficulties in communication, epilepsy and other diseases make the person the target of constant observation and physical contact in different ages.
- Because of treatment in hospital the patient is repeatedly separated from his/her parents.
- Identity is based on the diagnosis, which may be difficult to comprehend.
- The early life of an ID child is shadowed by disappointed and depressed parents–the ability of a family to recover from the shock varies.
- The fact that the child needs help daily affects the way the concept of independence is perceived.
- Affective bonds are sometimes distorted and may involve pity, admiration of the performance of the child in spite of the handicap, experiences of rejection or feelings of shame of the parents, hiding the child from others and direct violence. In opposite cases the child is given the role of a pet or a mascot.
- Sexual relationships are complicated, and finding a suitable partner may be difficult. Other people may not accept dating and sexuality. Having children is usually out of the question, even if the person considers him/herself suitable for parenthood and is fond of children.

Assessing somatic causes

- Restlessness in an ID person may result from somatic pain (remember the following causes: hip (sub)luxation, fractures, gastro-oesophageal reflux or peptic ulcer, disorders of the dentition or sinuses).
- Aggression occurring in attacks or other behavioural disorders may be associated with epilepsy: the disease may only have started or may have been diagnosed earlier but presents with new symptoms ⇒ the patient is referred to a neurologist.
- Sometimes epilepsy medication can cause psychological symptoms. Carbamazepine and clonazepine may cause symptoms of toxicity even at therapeutic doses. Antiepileptics have several interactions. Erythromycin increases the concentration of carbamazepine and tetracyclines increase that of phenytoin to toxic levels.
- Dysfunction of the thyroid gland is often associated with Down's syndrome; malfunction causes depression, whereas overproduction easily leads to agitation–follow up the clinical picture, not just the TSH levels!
- Even if the cause of intellectual disability has been determined, symptoms can result from a new intracranial process.

PAE

- Evaluate medication carefully: polypharmacy can cause psychological side effects, e.g. anticolinergic side effects may accumulate (imipramine + neuroleptic + parkinsonism medication).

Is everything well? Even minor help can improve the quality of life

- The life of an ID person often differs from the normal in many ways and may be disturbingly different in the eyes of a healthy person. The ID person, however, may be grateful for even minor help and does not compare his/her situation with the ideals set by other people. When planning an extensive rehabilitation programme, look for areas where help can be arranged.
- Problem-solving approaches, behaviour therapeutical methods, psychodynamic individual and group therapies and various forms of creative activity have been used successfully in treating mental disturbances and other problems.

The symptoms of an ID person are a part of the community

- Often the ID person has a carefully protected place or position in a social group; unsettling this position may lead to symptoms.
- The group creates a set of rules with power struggles; identifying and discussing power struggles may set free from wrong bonds.
- Unclear expectations and limits or inconsistent policy (one member of the personnel may be strict while another gives in) may need unifying.

Learning is associated with symptoms

- Restlessness or other symptoms may be a way to get around real learning difficulties.
- Symptoms may be the best way of achieving a pleasant goal or just to get attention.

Life crises

- The effects of a crisis may extend over a long period of time, the person cannot understand the events, symptoms may occur long after
    - a period of active rehabilitation when the person begins a more independent life.
    - changes in the family, a baby, sickness or death.
    - leaving home, moving to new housing facilities, supported housing, etc.
    - a crisis has made the person more aware of his/her handicap and of being different.

How are others coping?

- For those around, intellectual disability is often both physically and mentally hard in everyday life. Burn-out of parents, family members or immediate care givers may first manifest as symptoms of the ID person. Sense of duty may prevent others of talking/admitting their tiredness. Sometimes many of the family members make enormous sacrifices because of the ID family member.
    - Show concern for the family, care givers and ask how they are coping.
    - Is someone depressed?
    - How does the family live, do they have other people to visit them, do they see others as they used to, how much time and in what way do the family members spend with the ID person?
    - Does everyone have the desired amount of time for own recreation?
- Special health care services and organizations for the ID offer services and adaptation training courses, short-term care, camps, supportive personnel and group activities. These may help the family to cope.

Principles of rational medication

- Define the target symptom clearly so that the change can be evaluated (e.g. "morning toilet takes 2 hours", "30-min fits of rage three times daily").
- The main rule is to prescribe only one psychopharmaceutical drug at a time. If polypharmacy is justified, try only one new drug at a time in order to be able to evaluate the effect. Follow up long enough (weeks, months).
- Do not prescribe two neuroleptics at the same time (particularly similar ones).
- Treat obvious mental diseases and severe mental disorders with drugs according to the principles used for treating people with normal intelligence.
- Do not prescribe a strong, long-term psychopharmaceutical for restlessness before trying other methods used in the care of the ID.
- Restlessness, aggression and behaviour disorders can be treated e.g. with the following preparations:
    - Carbamazepine (slow, gradual changes in dosage, use the same serum concentrations as in epilepsy)
    - Neuroleptics (use drugs that you are familiar with)
    - Propanolol (slow, gradual changes in dosage, follow-up of pulse and blood pressure)
    - Lithium (as in mania)
    - Antidepressives
- When evaluating the effects and side effects of treatment consider the opinion of preferably three persons: the patient him/herself, family member or staff and representative of the school or work place.
- Remember to follow-up pharmaceutical treatment –ensure that the goals are achieved, adjust dosage and stop inefficient treatments.

References

1. Didden R, Duker PC, Korzilius H. Meta-analytic study on treatment effectiveness for problem behaviours with individuals who have mental retardation. Am J Ment Retard 1997;101: 387–399.
2. The Database of Abstracts of Reviews of Effectiveness (University of York), Database no.: DARE-973364. In: The Cochrane Library, Issue 4, 1999. Oxford: Update Software.

PAE

Paediatric Infectious Diseases

Evidence Based Medicine Guidelines. Edited by the Duodecim Editorial Team
© 2005 John Wiley & Sons, Ltd ISBN: 0-470-01184-X

31.1 Child with fever but no localizing symptoms

Editors

Principles

- Identify diseases requiring immediate treatment (septicaemia, meningitis (31.70)) and diseases requiring urgent treatment in less than 1 day (urinary tract infection, pneumonia). If the general condition is affected, or the child is irritable on touching, a referral to a hospital is indicated.
- Children below the age of 3 months should be referred to a paediatrician.
- Use serum CRP determination to rule out bacterial infection in children who could be discharged home on the basis of their good general condition. However, CRP may be increased also in viral diseases.
- Careful follow-up, e.g. by frequent telephone contacts with the same doctor is necessary if the symptoms continue.
- Exanthema subitum is the most common innocent cause of fever and urinary tract infection is the most common disease requiring specific treatment.

Assessing the general condition

- Signs of a serious bacterial infection include
  - impaired general condition
  - unwillingness to drink
  - irritability on touching (even a gentle touch makes the child cry)
  - lethargy
  - continuous complaining
  - impaired consciousness
  - petecchiae on the skin (red or brown spots that do not disappear under pressure).

Investigations

- When assessing the general status pay particular attention to the general condition, the skin (31.3), the respiratory tract and the lymph nodes.
- Examine the ears with pneumatic otoscope or tympanometer testing to detect acute otitis media.
- A urine sample (clean bag urine or middle stream sample) should be taken from all children with a high fever but no clear focus of infection.
- Determine serum CRP, urine test and blood count if there is the slightest suspicion of a serious disease. If the general condition is good, urine test is sufficient as the first examination. CRP and blood count are determined if the fever continues. However, CRP will not yet be elevated even in bacterial infections, if the child is brought to investigations only hours after the onset of fever.
- Examine the maxillary sinuses by ultrasonography (38.30) or x-ray in children above 6 years of age.
- A chest x-ray in necessary in children whose respiratory rate is more than 40/min, whose general condition is impaired, or who have respiratory difficulty other than expiratory stridor alone. See 31.22 for the indications of a chest x-ray.

31.2 Treatment of fever in children

Sirkka Keinänen-Kiukaanniemi

Aims

- To identify serious cases that require urgent treatment or investigation.
- To diagnose the primary disease causing the fever.
- To evaluate the need and possibilities of treating the underlying cause.
- To evaluate the need for and implementation of the treatment of symptomatic fever.

Causes of fever

- Infectious disease is the most common cause of fever for children in outpatient care.
- Other possible causes of fever are inflammatory intestinal, joint and connective tissue diseases, allergic reactions, malignant tumours and haematological diseases.

Objectives in the symptomatic treatment of fever

- When reducing body temperature, normothermia need not be the quantitative objective; the aim can be so-called optimal antipyresis.
  - The increased body temperature is reduced to the extent that subjective symptoms alleviate but the beneficial effects remain.
  - In practice this usually means that the body temperature decreases by 1–1.5°C 1–2 hours after drug administration.

Indications for symptomatic treatment of fever

- Fever is associated with other symptoms that cause considerable discomfort, such as muscle pains, headache, nausea, aches, a feeling of nausea and noticeable tiredness.

- The fever is markedly high (over 39–39.5°C measured from the rectal site A [1 2]).
- The child has a tendency for febrile convulsions. (The rise of fever is prevented by giving antipyretic drugs in time. In recurrent febrile convulsions diazepam medication has also been used; however, the benefits of prophylactic therapy have been questioned (29.3)).
- The child has a serious primary disease, for example severe heart, lung or kidney disease. In these cases fever may be harmful.

Treatment of fever

General treatment

- Sufficient fluid intake, see Table 31.2.
- Light, tasty food
- Avoidance of physical strain. Absolute bed rest is not needed.
- Reducing the room temperature artificially or removing clothing to the point of discomfort is unnecessary and even harmful.

Medical treatment

- The antipyretic should be taken only when necessary. Regular use of fever medication should be avoided in all other children except those prone to febrile convulsions.
- Paracetamol is the primary medicine.
  - The single dose is (10–) 15 mg/kg, which brings a decrease in temperature of about 1.5°C within 1–2 hours of ingestion.
- The maximum daily dose is 60 mg/kg/24h (e.g. 10 mg/kg × 6 or 15 mg/kg × 4).
- Other suitable antipyretics for children in special circumstances include ibuprofen and naproxen. Their antipyretic effect is at least as good as that of paracetamol and they are the effect lasts longer.
  - The dose for ibuprofen is 6–10 mg/kg, with maximum daily dose 40 mg/kg.
  - The dose for naproxen is usually 5 mg/kg, the maximum daily dose is 15 mg/kg.

Table 31.2 Need of fluid intake in a febrile child.

Child's weight (kg)	Amount of fluid (ml/24h)[1)]
5	500
10	1000
15	1250
20	1500
30	1700
40	1900
Add 12%/°C	
39 °C	+12%
40 °C	+24%

1. Cool drinks (juice, milk). Sugar containing drinks if eating is poor. Vomiting and diarrhoea increase the need for fluids.

- Using ibuprofen and naproxen instead of paracetamol should be considered only when fever is caused by
  - disease that clearly has an inflammatory component
  - the child has pains associated with infectious disease, in which the effect of paracetamol is weak.
- Aspirin should not be used as the primary antipyretic drug for children because it has more side effects than paracetamol. The side effects include gastric irritation and pain, nausea, bleeding tendency, and occasionally allergic reactions. It has also been reported that use of Aspirin in connection with fever diseases can cause so-called Reye's syndrome, a rare but serious side-effect.
- Advantages of paracetamol compared with other antipyretic drugs:
  - It is well tolerated.
  - It causes few or no serious side effects when taken in the recommended doses.
  - It does not affect bleeding or coagulation factors.
  - Allergies are rare.
  - The fever-reducing effect has been proven and is well documented.

Situations requiring special attention

- Fever without any clear focal symptoms or focal findings
  - Keep in mind the possibility of septicaemia of pneumococcal or other aetiology.
- Fever in a child below 3–6 months of age
  - Remember the possibility of serious fulminant disease.
  - Observe the child's general condition, neurological symptoms, and alertness. Hospital level investigations are usually necessary. If the patient is cared for in primary care, arrange follow-up and ensure that the parents can contact a doctor easily.
- Fever and rash (31.3)
  - Meningococcal septicaemia, Kawasaki disease
- Fever, stomach pain and vomiting
  - Keep in mind appendicitis, and urinary tract infection.
- Fever and neck pain
  - Remember the possibility of a CNS infection.
- Fever and joint pain
  - Consider purulent joint infection.
- Prolonged fever
  - Arrange for further investigations.

PAE

References

1. Duce JS. A systematic review of the literature to determine optimal methods of temperature measurement in neonates, infants and children. 1996, 124 pages (source not stated in more detail).

2. The Database of Abstracts of Reviews of Effectiveness (University of York), Database no.: DARE-978207. In: The Cochrane Library, Issue 4, 1999. Oxford: Update Software.

31.3 Fever and rash in a child

Editors

Basic rules

- Differentiate petechiae from other spots (meningococcal sepsis!)
- Identify septic bacterial infections, Kawasaki disease, and leukaemia, that require immediate hospitalization.
- In addition to the former refer to hospital patients with idiopathic thrombocytopenic purpura (ITP), Henoch–Schönlein purpura with clear symptoms, Stevens–Johnson syndrome, and systemic juvenile rheumatoid arthritis (Still's disease).
- Identify allergic reactions (itching or urticarial rash and serum sickness) to avoid future (drug) exposure. Unnecessary diagnoses of drug allergy should not be made!

Aetiology, clinical picture, and typical symptoms

- See Table 31.3.
- **Serum CRP should always be assayed when the aetiology is not evident on the basis of the clinical picture** and if the child is not referred immediately on the basis of poor general condition. If the symptoms have lasted for less than 12 hours a low CRP concentration does not exclude septic infection.

31.10 Tonsillitis and pharyngitis in children

Marjukka Mäkelä

Basic rules

- Antibiotics are indicated in infections caused by group A streptococci diagnosed by culture or rapid antigen test. Symptomatic treatment is indicated in other cases.
- Identify mononucleosis.
- Identify and treat a streptococcal epidemic.

Aetiology

- Adenoviruses are the most common aetiological agents.
- Streptococcal pharyngitis is rare in children below 3 years of age.

Symptoms and signs

- Clinical diagnosis is unreliable.
  - Adenoviruses and other viruses can cause exudative tonsillitis.
  - In two thirds of school-aged children with streptococcal tonsillitis there is no exudate.
- Sore throat with rash is often caused by adenoviruses or other viruses.
- Ear pain may radiate to the tonsillar region (and vice versa).
- Streptococcal pharyngitis may cause abdominal pain.

Diagnostics

- Diagnosis should be based on the detection of streptococci in pharyngeal secretions by culture or rapid antigen test. Bacteria other than streptococci need not be sought.
- A rapid culture method (Streptocult®) will give a result the next morning (38.21). If a rapid antigen test is used a negative result should be verified by culture. (In children below 3 years of age streptococcal tonsillitis is so rare that a negative antigen test need not be controlled by culture.)

Treatment

- Fever and pain are best treated with paracetamol. Naproxen and ibuprofen are alternatives. Infections caused by group A streptococci should be treated with penicillin V, 70 mg/kg/day (100 000 units/kg/day), or (in patients with penicillin allergy) cephalexin, 50 mg/kg/day, in two doses for 10 days (A) [1 2]. Because of infectiousness the child should be isolated from day care or school for one day after the onset of antibiotic treatment. The length of absence from day care or school is determined by the general condition and not by the aetiological agent.

References

1. Deeter RG, Kalman D, Rogan M, Chow SC. Therapy for pharyngitis and tonsillitis by group A beta-hemolytic streptococci: a meta-analysis comparing the efficacy and safety of cephadroxil monohydrate versus oral penicillin V. Clin Therap 1992;14:740–754.
2. The Database of Abstracts of Reviews of Effectiveness (University of York), Database no.: DARE-953519. In: The Cochrane Library, Issue 4, 1999. Oxford: Update Software.

Table 31.3 Fever and rash in a child–diagnostic clues

Dominant symptom, diseases	Typical features	Laboratory findings
Petechiae (small, non-blanching red spots)		
Meningococcal sepsis	Irritability, hypotonia, poor general condition	CRP concentration high
Henoch–Schönlein purpura (32.53)*	Petechiae on the buttocks and lower extremities, joint and abdominal pain	CRP low, normal platelet count
ITP (32.2)	Good general condition, usually no fever	Low platelet count
Leukaemia	Often fatigued and pale, occasionally bone pain	Low platelet count, abnormal leukocyte count, low haemoglobin concentration
Enlarged lymph nodes, conjunctival erythema, oral or pharyngeal symptoms		
Kawasaki disease (32.57)	Irritability, other criteria of the disease	High CRP concentration, leukocytosis
Scarlet fever*	Tonsillitis	Streptococcal culture positive
Mononucleosis*	Often tonsillitis sometimes hepatosplenomegaly. Rash may follow a course of amoxycillin.	Often lymphocytosis; mononucleosis rapid test positive in children above 4 years of age
Rash with fine spots (<3 mm)		
Exanthema subitum (31.54)*	Fever precedes the rash by 2–4 days	Low CRP concentration
Other firal exanthema*		Low CRP concentration
Drug reaction*	Preceding medication (may have been stopped a few days earlier)	
Kawasaki disease (see above)		
Red maculae on the cheeks		
Erythema infectiosum* (31.53)	Mild fever, pharyngitis, headache, good general condition	Low CRP concentration
Vesicles on the skin or mucosa		
Chickenpox*	Usually a recent infectious contact can be recalled	
Hand, food and mouth disease	Vesicles on the hands, feet and often on the oral mucosa	
Stevens–Johnson syndrome	Mucosal symptoms, erythema multiforme	
Primary herpes infection*	If the patient has stomatitis both the oral mucosa and the skin on the lips are affected	
Cough and rhinitis		
Adenovirus	2–8% of the patients have a rash	
Urticaria		
Viral infection*	Other local symptoms of infection	Low CRP concentration
Type I drug reaction*	Preceding medication	Low CRP concentration
Urticaria with arthritis* (serum sickness) (32.52)	Joint swelling and erythema, preceding antibiotic treatment (often cefaclor or penicillin)	Low CRP concentration
Oscillating fever, macular rash during fever		
Kawasaki disease		
Systemic juvenile rheumatoid arthritis (Still's disease)	The rash often appears on the upper part of the body	High CRP concentration and ESR, leukocytosis

♦ Italics: immediate hospitalization, *: can usually be treated in primary care.

31.11 Sinusitis in children

Anne Pitkäranta, Jouko Suonpää

Basic rules

- Suspect sinusitis if a child has prolonged rhinitis, headache and a cough after a (viral) respiratory infection.
- X-rays and ultrasound examinations of the paranasal sinuses are not reliable until the child is 7–8 years old.
- Sinusitis leads to complications more often in children than in adults. Swelling of the eyelids or cheek (orbit) is a warning sign.

Development of the maxillary sinuses

- The maxillary sinuses are bean-sized at birth, and their lower edge parallels the attachment point of the inferior concha.

PAE

During the first three years of life the sinuses grow laterally and posteriorly. After the permanent teeth have developed the growth increases in the direction of the palate, and by the age of 10–12 years the lower edge of the maxillary sinus parallels the lower edge of the nasal meatus. The maxillary sinuses reach their final size at the age of 15–18 years.

Sinusitis

- In children, acute sinusitis denotes an infection of the mucosa, and it is very common. In infants whose sinuses are widely open to the nasal cavity the prognosis is good, and the infection usually resolves spontaneously as rhinitis subsides and the ciliary function is restored.
- As the child grows, the ostium of the maxillary sinus becomes narrower in relation to the size of the sinus. At the same time the importance of sinusitis increases.

Aetiology

- Although an infection of paranasal mucosa is nearly always of viral origin, sinusitis itself is usually a bacterial infection.
- Streptococcus pneumoniae, Haemophilus influenzae, and Moraxella catarrhalis are the most common causative agents in children.
- If the ciliary activity of the sinus is sufficient to remove bacterial debris and other secretions, the infection will heal spontaneously. If this is not the case the proteases liberated by bacteria may damage the deeper layers of the mucosa and prevent normal ciliary activity. Prolonged retention of secretions may cause a chronic infection and tissue damage to the sinus mucosa.
- Cystic fibrosis, see 31.23.

Symptoms and diagnosis

- Because the illness usually occurs in association with other upper respiratory tract infections, the symptoms often originate outside the sinuses. In small children persistent rhinitis and a wheezing cough are the most common symptoms. In older children persistent rhinitis, a feeling of pressure over the cheeks and the temporal region, headache and nausea are common. Sometimes symptoms are totally absent.
- If sinusitis is suspected, the nasal cavity and the pharynx should always be carefully inspected. A purulent discharge may be visible in the nasal cavity, and sometimes a trickle of purulent exudate from under the middle concha is evident. In a small child, a diagnosis of sinusitis is based on clinical findings, i.e. symptoms (nasal discharge, cough, fever) have persisted and worsened over the period of more than (10)–14 days. Nasal polyps in children warrant a referral to an ENT specialist to exclude cystic fibrosis, choanal polyp and meningocoele.

X-ray and ultrasonography

- Imaging of paranasal sinuses in children requires a conservative approach.
- Sinus x-rays are difficult to interpret in small children, and the findings must be related to the whole clinical presentation. Mucosal oedema of variable degree is common even in healthy children. In an older child, a fluid level is a certain sign of an inflammation. Furthermore, a totally opacified sinus requires treatment or further assessment. Unerupted teeth may cause diagnostic problems.
- In older children, ultrasonography is particularly beneficial in the follow-up of fluid retention and in recurrent sinusitis. A simple A-image yields little information on the type and course of mucosal oedema. The findings must always be related to the symptoms, which ultimately determine the need for treatment.
- Clinical presentation (temperature and general status) is decisive.

Treatment

- If the sinuses have become inflamed during an acute respiratory infection they usually recover when rhinitis subsides and the ciliary function is resumed. No special treatment is necessary. Prolongation of the symptoms, persistent cough, rhinitis and headache are an indication for an examination of the sinuses.
- Antibiotics (B) [1] (usually amoxicillin 40 mg/kg/day in two divided doses) and nasal decongestants are the preferred treatment forms. If the patient has true penicillin allergy a broad-spectrum macrolide, such as clarithromycin or azithromycin, is recommended.
- A bacterial culture taken from under the middle concha may help in the selection of antibiotic. If the response to the first antibiotic is insufficient, amoxicillin+clavulanic acid may be prescribed. If the patient has true penicillin allergy, a combination of sulphonamides and trimethoprim may be prescribed.

Recurrent and persistent sinusitis

- The treatment of recurrent and persistent sinusitis should be carried out by an ENT specialist or a physician specialized in paediatric infectious diseases. The underlying factors should be identified and treated. The lymphatic tissue in the pharynx of a child reacts strongly to inflammatory irritants. In addition to the enlarged adenoids and tonsils, the lymphatic tissue in the posterior wall of the pharynx will enlarge. Enlarged adenoids on their own may cause breathing difficulties and obstruct the passage of mucus. A vicious circle develops easily, and it can only be broken by adenoidectomy.
- Allergies should be identified and any allergens eliminated if possible. In addition to allergies, all factors irritating the nasal mucosa such as dust, pollutants, recurrent infectious contacts etc. may contribute to the development of sinusitis. The prognosis of sinusitis is good if the underlying factors

can be eliminated. A CT scan can be used to evaluate the structural anatomy (abnormality) of the paranasal sinuses.

- FES (functional endoscopic sinus surgery) is effective in cases resistant to pharmacotherapy, and the complication rate is low C [2 3].

Complications of sinusitis

- Pyogenic material in a closed space tends to spread into the surroundings. Cellulitis of the cheek or eyelids may be the first symptoms of complicated maxillary or ethmoid sinusitis. During the first years of life the site of infection is unusually the ethmoid sinuses, sometimes resulting in periorbital oedema. Eyelid oedema associated with rhinitis should be considered a complicated sinusitis and the child should be referred to hospital.

References

1. Morris P, Leach A. Antibiotics for persistent nasal discharge (rhinosinusitis) in children. Cochrane Database Syst Rev. 2004;(2):CD001094.
2. Hebert RL. Bent JP. Meta-analysis of outcomes of pediatric functional endoscopic sinus surgery. Laryngoscope 1998;108: 796–799.
3. The Database of Abstracts of Reviews of Effectiveness (University of York), Database no.: DARE-981077. In: The Cochrane Library, Issue 4, 2000. Oxford: Update Software.

31.12 Wheezing in children

Editors

Aims

- Identify the following conditions requiring **immediate treatment**:
  - Foreign body in the respiratory tract
  - Epiglottitis
- Differentiate between laryngitis and obstructive bronchitis or asthma.
- Treat acute obstructive bronchitis with inhaled salbutamol administered by nebulizer (Figure 31.12.1).
- Refer the child to hospital if breathing difficulties continue after initial treatment.

Clues for differential diagnosis

- If a previously well child develops difficulty in breathing during an infection, the cause may be a foreign body in the respiratory tract or an obstructive respiratory tract infection.
- The aspiration of a foreign body causes a sudden burst of cough with varying degrees of difficulty in breathing. Most often, but not always, the parents suspect a foreign body. A suspicion of foreign body aspiration is an indication for urgent brochoscopy.
- There are two types of obstructive respiratory tract infections.
  - Difficulty in inspiration
    - Epiglottitis
    - Laryngitis
    - Laryngotracheitis
    - Bacterial tracheitis
  - Difficulty in expiration
    - Obstructive bronchitis
    - Bronchiolitis

Epiglottitis

- See article 31.16.
- The typical patient is a preschool-aged child presenting with a few hours of high fever, hoarseness, difficulty in breathing and salivation.
- Salivation, anxiety and the absence of cough differentiate the condition best from laryngitis.
- Hib vaccination reduces the incidence of epiglottitis in children efficiently.

Laryngitis

- See 31.15.
- Inflammation in the larynx and upper part of the trachea may cause the well-known triad:
  - Hoarseness
  - Barking cough
  - Inspiratory stridor
- Patients can be divided into two subgroups according to the clinical presentation: laryngotracheitis and spasmodic croup (Laryngitis simplex)
  - **Laryngotracheitis** usually begins insidiously and is associated with rhinitis, cough and fever for 1–3 days before the onset of dyspnoea.
  - **A spasmodic croup** is characterized by a rapid onset of the symptoms–often in the middle of the night–without prior signs of infection. Most patients (80%) are boys, and the disease often recurs.

Obstructive bronchitis

- See 31.13
- The diagnosis is often easy: a coughing child with rapid and noisy breathing.
- The expirium is prolonged and wheezing can be heard on auscultation.
- In moderate obstruction, mostly expiratory rales are often heard rather than wheezing.

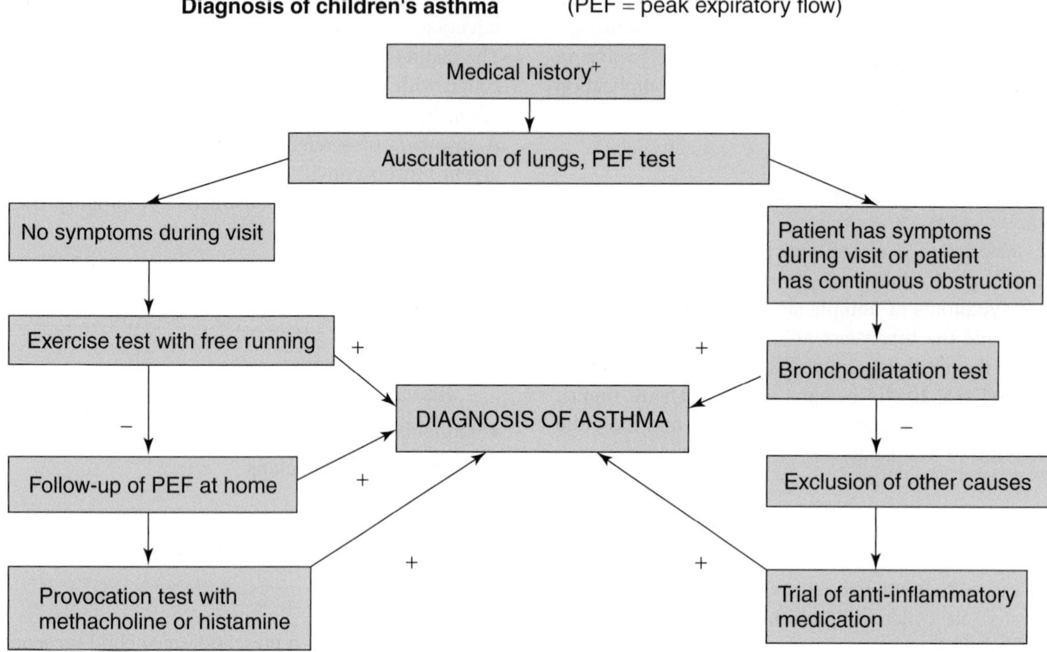

Figure 31.12.1 Diagnosis of asthma in children

- In severe obstruction the auscultation findings may be betrayingly normal because of shallow breathing. It is essential to assess respiratory function comprehensively by inspection and auscultation.
- Mild obstruction does not cause visible dyspnoea but only rales or wheezing detectable by auscultation.
  - The situation may be interpreted as "incipient bronchitis", and the child may receive a course of antibiotics, when he needs brochodilators.
  - It is important to identify those children with obstruction who have repeated rales and secretion of mucus from the respiratory tract, and treat them with inhaled steroids **A** [1] [2] under the supervision of a paediatrician. The most common mistake is to treat these children with repeated courses of antibiotics.

The diagnosis of asthma in children

- See article 31.14
- If the child has asthmatic symptoms during the consultation, a clinical diagnosis can be made immediately. The symptoms and expiratory rales disappear, and the peak expiratory flow (PEF) increases after inhalation of a sympathomimetic.
- If the obstruction is not relieved by inhaled sympatomimetics during consultation, a running test and home PEF monitoring are used to reach the diagnosis. In uncertain cases methacholine or histamine inhalation provocation test or a therapeutic trial with glucocorticoids can be performed.

Criteria for asthma in children

- See 31.14
- See algorithm on the diagnosis of asthma in children (Figure 31.12.1).

References

1. Calpin C, Macarthur C, Stephens D, Feldman W, Parkin PC. Effectiveness of prophylactic inhaled steroids in childhood asthma: a systematic review of the literature. J All Clin Immunol 1997;100:452–457.
2. The Database of Abstracts of Reviews of Effectiveness (University of York), Database no.: DARE-971295. In: The Cochrane Library, Issue 4, 1999. Oxford: Update Software.

31.13 Treatment of obstructive bronchitis and acute asthma in children

Minna Kaila

Aims

- To treat acute symptoms so that hospitalization can be avoided.
- To recognize early symptoms of asthma so that regular drug therapy can be started in time.

General treatment

- Good general treatment, with rest according to the condition of the child, antipyretics, if necessary, and appropriate fluid intake.

Symptoms and examinations

- Expiratory dyspnoea and wheezing.
- Symptoms frequently begin over a period of several days and their severity is underestimated B [1].
- Inspection, auscultation, PEF, infection focuses, skin.
- Staging of the asthma attack, see Table 31.13.1.

Medication

- Bronchodilatating medication
  - Mild obstruction
    - Salbutamol inhalation is the first line drug treatment B [2].
    - From the age 2 years on, inhalation aerosol and spacer are as effective as a nebulizer A [3 4]. Dosing: 200 µg two to several puffs. When using nebulizer, solution 0.15 mg/kg (max 5 mg), see Table 31.13.2.
    - The dose can be repeated after 20–30 min (in case of side effects (hand tremor, tachycardia, considerable anxiety): reduce the dose by half).
  - If the child has an asthma diagnosis and regular medication: ensure correct inhalation technique and patient compliance, add an inhaled corticosteroid or boost the dose of inhaled corticosteroid (basic principle: double the daily dose for 1–2 weeks).
  - A child with asthma must have written instructions! D [5]
- Obvious obstruction
  - Repeated salbutamol inhalations with a spacer (or a nebulizer)
  - If the child lives near a hospital, consider treatment at outpatient clinic: repeated inhalations at 2–4-hour intervals for a few times.
  - A child with asthma is given prednisolone p.o. (2 mg/kg initially, thereafter 2 mg/kg divided into two daily doses as a course of 3–5 days) A [6 7].
  - If the child already has an asthma diagnosis and medication, remember boosting of the dose.
- Recurring or prolonged obstruction
  - Repeated salbutamol inhalations
  - For infants and when arranging instructions on how to take/administer the inhaled medication is not feasible, consider salbutamol p.o. in solution or tablet form 0.2–0.3 mg/kg daily divided into three doses. Rule of thumb: the daily dose (ml) must be less (50–75%) than the patient's weight in kilograms when the concentration of the solution is 0.4 mg/ml.
  - In addition, prednisolone p.o. (2 mg/kg starting dose, thereafter 2 mg/kg divided into two doses for 3–5 days)
  - If repeated courses of corticosteroid are needed, a doctor's appointment should be made for careful evaluation of the child's condition, e.g. by the GP or the paediatrician treating the child.
  - If the child already has an asthma diagnosis and medication, remember boosting.
  - Arrange for a control visit at the GP or pediatrician treating the child.
- Severe obstruction
  - Salbutamol inhalation in oxygen C [8] with a tight-fitting mask.
  - Prednisolone p.o. or i.v. 2 mg/kg
  - Adrenaline (concentration **NOTE!** 1:1 000) 0.01 ml/kg or 0.1 ml/10 kg s.c. or i.m (max 0.3 ml)
  - The dose can be repeated after 20–30 min (thereafter repeat the dose at the same 20–30 min intervals, but reduce the dose by half).

Table 31.13.1 Staging the asthma attack of a child

Symptom	Mild	Moderate	Severe
General status	Normal	Normal	Normal / reduced
Skin colour	Normal	Pale	Pale / cyanotic
Ability to speak	Unhindered	Partial sentences	1–2 words
Respiratory frequency/min	Normal	Normal / <50	>50
Respiratory distress	No/mild	Moderate	Severe
Intercostal/ jugulum retraction	Not usually	Moderate	Severe
Tightness of the sternocleido (mastoid) muscle	Not usually	Moderate	Severe
Auscultation	Wheezing at the end of expiration	Wheezing on inspiration + expiration	Quiet respiratory sounds
PEF (% of normal/earlier best result)	70–90	50–70	<50

Table 31.13.2 Dosing of salbutamol with a nebulizer (concentration 5 mg/ml); the dose given below is diluted to 2 ml with 0.9% NaCl

Weight (kg)	Salbutamol (ml)
<10	<0.3
11–15	0.3–0.4
16–20	0.5–0.6
21–25	0.7–0.8
26–30	0.8–0.9
31–35	0.9–1.0
36–40	1.0
41–	1.0

PAE

- Intravenous theophylline should not be used routinely, but it may be of some benefit in severe asthma B [9 10].
- Referral to the hospital

Indications for hospitalization and specialist consultation

- First-line treatment of acute obstruction and complicated asthma in primary health care.

Emergency referral

- Severe obstruction
- Obstruction does not respond to bronchodilators even at repeated dosage.
- Obstruction continues for a long time (temporal relief), and the child starts to become exhausted.
- The smaller the child, the lower the threshold for hospitalization.
- Parents are worried about the child.

Normal referral

- After the second or third clear episode of obstruction.
- Should be considered already after the first episode if it has been preceded by mild symptoms (mucus discharge, cough for more than 6 weeks, milder wheezing, symptoms provoked by physical exertion or cold weather).
- Consider already after the first episode if the child has risk factors: strong tendency for atopy, asthma in a first-degree relative, smoking at the home of the child.
- Written treatment instructions reduce the risk of hospitalization of a child with asthma C [11].

References

1. Kolbe J, Ferguson W, Garrett J. Rapid onset asthma: a severe but uncommon manifestation. Thorax 1998:53;241–7.
2. Chavasse R, Seddon P, Bara A, McKean M. Short acting beta agonists for recurrent wheeze in children under two years of age. Cochrane Database Syst Rev. 2004;(2):CD002873.
3. Cates CJ, Rowe BH. Holding chambers versus nebulizers for beta-agonist treatment of acute asthma. Cochrane database of systematic reviewa, Issue 1, 2000.
4. Amirav I, Newhouse MT. Metered-dose inhaler accessory devices in acute asthma: efficacy and comparison with nebulizers: a literature review. Arch Pediatr Adolesc 1997:151;876–82.
5. Toelle BG, Ram FSF. Written individualised management plans for asthma in children and adults. Cochrane Database Syst Rev. 2004;(2):CD002171.
6. Rowe BH, Keller JL, Oxman AD. Effectiveness of steroid therapy in acute exacerbations of asthma: a meta-analysis. Am J Emerg Med 1992:10;301–10.
7. Rowe BH, Spooner CH, Ducharme FM et al. Corticosteroids for preventing relapse following acute exacerbations of asthma. Cochrane Library, Issue 4, 1999. Oxford: Update Software.
8. Keeley D. Asthma in children. Clinical Evidence 2002;7: 244–261.
9. Mitra A, Bassler D, Ducharme FM. Intravenous aminophylline for acute severe asthma in children over 2 years using inhaled bronchodilators. Cochrane Database Syst Rev. 2004;(2):CD001276.
10. Goodman DC, Littenberg B, O'Connor GT, et al. Theophylline in acute childhood asthma: a meta-analysis of its efficacy (see comments). Pediatr Pulmonol 1996:21;211–8.
11. Lieu T, Quesenberry CP, Capra AM, et al. Outpatient management practices associated with reduced risk of pediatric asthma hospitalization and emergency department visits. Pediatrics 1997:100;334–41.

31.14 Diagnosis and treatment of childhood asthma

Minna Kaila

- For treatment of acute asthma see 31.13.

Aims

- Early detection and accurate diagnosis of asthma
- Good therapeutic control of asthma, allowing the child to lead a normal life
- An arrangement whereby one physician is responsible for the care of the child's asthma
- Periodic review of therapy for ensuring that unnecessary treatment is withdrawn

Epidemiology

- Asthma is the most common chronic illness in children.
- According to recent population surveys, 4 to 7% of children have medically treated asthma and a similar proportion have asthma-like symptoms.
- Prognostic factors for the development of asthma and for the chronicity of symptoms include asthma in parents (especially the mother), atopic dermatitis in the child, and recurrent airway obstruction especially in the absence of respiratory infection.
- Cystic fibrosis, see 31.23.

Symptoms

- Recurrent expiratory difficulty and wheezing
- Reduced exercise tolerance, conscious avoidance of physical exertion (cough, dyspnoea)
- Patient woken up at night by cough and/or dyspnoea

- Continuous excessive production of mucus, rales
- In addition: history of atopy (food allergy, atopic dermatitis, allergic rhinoconjunctivitis)
- Prolonged coughing (over 6 weeks) associated with dyspnoea

Diagnosis

- History:
  - From patient, family and health/medical records
  - Current symptoms: onset, frequency, recurrence, severity, aggravating and alleviating factors, especially seasonal variations and symptoms related to certain locations.
- Family history
- Environmental factors: smoking, exposure to animals, other exposures
- Number of antibiotic treatments (including those for bronchitis contrary to recommendations)
- Physical examination (emphasis on the most relevant findings – starting with careful inspection)
  - Record growth development in growth curve
  - Posture, chest
  - Appearance of breathing
  - Auscultation, also during forced expiration
  - Measurement of peak expiratory flow (PEF) (mastery of expiration technique is important; measurement may be attempted from four to five years of age)
  - Mouth, throat, nose, ears
  - Skin (presence of rash compatible with atopic dermatitis)
- Examinations
  - Symptom diary
  - Bronchodilation test (e.g. salbutamol 200 μg, two puffs): PEF measurement before and after bronchodilator administration (for calculations see 6.7)
  - Therapeutic trial with a bronchodilator (teach correct inhalation technique)
  - Running-exercise test
    - Preferably outdoors, six minutes of hard running is sufficient (heart rate monitoring)
    - Auscultation of breath sounds, measurement of forced expiratory volume in 1 second (FEV_1) and/or PEF from the age of five: before running, immediately after running and 10 (15 and 20) minutes after running
    - Exercise-induced asthmatic symptoms typically emerge 5–10 minutes after the end of exercise, and they subside without medication in about one hour.
    - Be prepared to administer a bronchodilator as required.
    - The test is diagnostic if the symptoms are compatible with asthma or the expiration volumes are reduced by 15% and then restored with bronchodilatory medication.
    - Reductions of 10 to 15% are suggestive of asthma.
  - PEF monitoring at home
    - Teach correct technique.
    - Three measurements in the morning, three measurements in the evening, all values recorded
    - The best result of the three measurements is marked on a PEF chart.
    - During the first week, PEF is measured without medication. During the second week, PEF is measured before and 15 min after bronchodilator administration.
    - PEF should also be measured when there are symptoms and whenever a bronchodilator is used.
    - Repeated 20% fluctuations within 24 hours or 15% improvements with a bronchodilator are diagnostic of asthma. (Note: Fluctuations may also be caused by a faulty expiration technique.). For calculations see 6.7.
  - Spirometry
    - Use if available, in school-age children.
    - The results of metacholine or histamine provocation tests should be interpreted according to the clinical situation.
  - Allergy tests
    - History
    - Skin prick tests for relevant airborn allergens (if the necessary skill exists in the primary health care unit).
- See Figure 31.12.1

Diagnostic criteria for childhood asthma

1. Symptoms or signs compatible with asthma:
   - Recurrent (at least three times) expiratory difficulty
   - Expiratory wheezing or
   - Prolonged (>6 weeks) or recurrent cough. Cough without dyspnea should be carefully assessed to avoid over diagnosis.
2. At least one of the following:
   - Significant (at least 20%) diurnal fluctuation in PEF values
   - An increase (of at least 15%) in PEF values during therapeutic trial
   - Significant improvement in FEV_1 or PEF (or mid-expiratory flow at 50% of forced vital capacity, MEF_{50}) in a bronchodilation test
   - Significant reduction in FEV_1 or PEF (or MEF_{50}) in an exercise test
   - Demonstration of bronchial hyperresponsiveness in histamine or metacholine provocation tests
   - Or, in a small child, expiratory wheezing during airway inflammation, allergen exposure or exercise test
3. Absence of other reasons (such as sinusitis, bronchitis, bronchiolitis, pertussis, laryngeal, tracheal or bronchial constriction or malacia, oesophageal reflux, foreign body, bronchiectasis, cystic fibrosis, psychogenic aetiology) for a child's cough or respiratory problems

- If the above criteria (1 and 2 and 3) are met, a diagnosis of asthma can be made.

Criteria for initiating regular daily drug therapy

- Regular drug therapy should be considered if the child has symptoms weekly.

PAE

- The more symptoms the child has, and the lighter the symptom-provoking exercise is, and the more severely atopic the child is, and the more suggestive for asthma the family history is, the stronger is the indication for starting medication with inhaled corticosteroids.
- A school-age child can be started on regular drug therapy within primary health care, provided that the physician knows what he/she is doing.

Drugs

- Symptomatic bronchodilatory medication as needed
  - Salbutamol
  - Terbutaline
- Anti-inflammatory medication–as periodic courses or as regular long-term therapy
  - Inhaled corticosteroid (A) [1, 2]
    - Beclomethasone
    - Budesonide
    - Fluticasone
  - Cromones have good safety profile, but evidence of effectiveness is lacking (B) [3].
- Only as complementary drugs in children at the discretion of a specialised physician
  - Long-acting bronchodilator
    - Formoterol
    - Salmeterol (C) [4]
  - Leukotriene antagonist (C) [5]
- Adequate treatment of allergies is started at a young age, for instance by medication during the pollen season.
  - Eye symptoms (eyedrops)
    - Cromoglycate
    - Nedocromil
    - Antihistamine eyedrops
  - Nasal symptoms (nasal spray)
    - Cromoglycate
    - Nedocromil
    - Antihistamine
    - Corticosteroid
  - In small children, oral antihistamine can be used during the pollen season.

Basic principles of drug therapy

- The goal is the minimal dosage needed to control symptoms. Make sure that the child is not avoiding physical exertion to avoid symptoms.
- Symptoms rare and mild: symptomatic bronchodilatory medication as needed
- Symptoms weekly: low dose of inhaled corticosteroid (200 to 400 µg/day or less, fluticasone 100 to 200 µg/day or less)
- Symptoms frequent and severe: inhaled corticosteroid
- Compliance and sufficient guidance at the start of therapy!
- Written instructions on drugs, doses and the procedures to be followed when symptoms worsen
- Diagnosed irritants (e.g. animals) should be avoided individually.
- Parents who smoke should be motivated to stop smoking.
- Patient education (A) [6]
  - Basics of diagnosis
  - Nature of asthma (= an inflammatory disease)
  - Basic principles of drug therapy, especially the purposes and differences of maintenance treatment and bronchodilator treatment
  - Technique of drug administration
  - Monitoring (symptoms, PEF)
  - Primary site of care, physician responsible for the care, specialised care
  - Information on patient organisations
  - Avoidance of triggering factors: smoking in all patients, allergens on an individual basis
- Drug therapy should be withdrawn when the child has been without symptoms for a long period of time (e.g. symptom-free over a whole season, which has previously been difficult).

Referral to specialised medical care for diagnosis

- A physician who is not familiar with the diagnosis and management of paediatric asthma should refer all paediatric patients with asthmatic symptoms.
- Patients who are below school age
- Patients whose symptoms are not brought under control by drug therapy
- Patients in whom low-dose corticosteroid treatment is insufficient or whose growth is retarded (B) [7, 8, 9]
- Patients in whom the actual daily dose of inhaled corticosteroid starts to exceed 800 µg budesonide or 800 µg beclomethasone or 400 µg fluticasone
- According to local agreements

Follow-up and shared care

- Children below school age and on regular medication always followed up by a paediatrician
- Referral to a paediatrician for consultation on additional drug requirement
- Spirometry once a year is recommended, but not as often if the result has initially been normal (school-aged children).
- Patients followed up within primary health care:
  - Older children using normal doses of corticosteroids
  - All patients whose symptoms are limited to the pollen season
- It is important to withdraw unnecessary maintenance therapy (trial after an asymptomatic period of about six months; not at the start of the pollen season in patients with pollen allergy).

Task list for follow-up visits

- Interview on the patient's condition: detailed account of exercise tolerance, nocturnal symptoms, need for bronchodilator
- Review of symptom diary or PEF monitoring at home
- Respiratory infections (awareness of the possibility to step up asthma medication)
- Medication: name of drug, dosage, actual use (compliance)
- Growth curve (physician's responsibility)
- Any food allergies or special diets
- Physical examination: skin, general status, posture, chest, examination of ears, nose and throat, PEF, auscultation
- Future medication (written instructions = medication card): Is the drug still needed?
- Further follow-up: where and when?
- Need for spirometric tests
- Always review drug administration technique; need for other guidance
- Bringing certificates etc. up to date
- Transfer of information to other health care professionals treating the child.

References

1. Calpin C, Macarthur C, Stephens D, Feldman W, Parkin PC. Effectiveness of prophylactic inhaled steroids in childhood asthma: a systematic review of the literature. J All Clin Immunol 1997;100:452–457.
2. The Database of Abstracts of Reviews of Effectiveness (University of York), Database no.: DARE-971295. In: The Cochrane Library, Issue 4, 1999. Oxford: Update Software.
3. van der Wouden JC, Tasche MJA, Bernsen RMD, Uijen JHJM, de Jongste JC, Ducharme FM. Inhaled sodium cromoglycate for asthma in children. Cochrane Database Syst Rev. 2004;(2):CD002173.
4. Keeley D. Asthma in children. Clinical Evidence 2002;7: 244–261.
5. =Keeley D. Asthma in children. Clinical Evidence 2002;7: 244–261.
6. Wolf FM, Guevara JP, Grum CM, Clark NM, Cates CJ. Educational interventions for asthma in children. Cochrane Database Syst Rev. 2004;(2):CD000326.
7. Sharek PJ, Bergman DA. Beclomethasone for asthma in children: effects on linear growth. The Cochrane Database of Systematic Reviews, Cochrane Library number: CD001282. In: The Cochrane Library, Issue 2, 2002. Oxford: Update Software. Updated frequently.
8. Allen ADB, Mullen M, Mullen B. A meta-analysis of the effect of oral and inhaled corticosteroids on growth. J Allergy Clin Immunol 1994;93:967–976.
9. The Database of Abstracts of Reviews of Effectiveness (University of York), Database no.: DARE-953418. In: The Cochrane Library, Issue 4, 1999. Oxford: Update Software.

31.15 Laryngitis in children

Editors

Basic rules

- Patients with mild symptoms are treated at home.
- More severe cases of spasmodic croup are treated with glucocorticoid, and when necessary, racemic adrenalin may be also be given as first aid.
- Refer to hospital patients with
  - retraction on inspiration, severe inspiratory stridor
  - suspected bacterial tracheitis or pneumonia complicating laryngitis.

History and clinical findings

- The symptoms of laryngitis include sudden-onset hoarseness, dull cough, and inspiratory stridor.
- Try to observe the degree of breathing difficulty and chest wall motions when the child is not scared and crying. The best moment is in the beginning of the consultation before the child starts to "cry because of the doctor".
- The patient's history is helpful. A slowly developing laryngotracheitis is also alleviated more slowly than laryngitis that starts rapidly.
- In patients with recurring laryngitis, the severity of earlier episodes predicts the severity of the present episode.
- Suspect pneumonia (or bacterial tracheitis) if a child with laryngitis has persistent fever and does not respond to treatment; serum CRP is often increased in such cases.

PAE

Treatment

- Laryngitis is caused by viruses and there is no specific treatment. Parainfluenza virus is the cause in 70% of the cases.
- Cool, moist air is beneficial: weather permitting, the child should be taken outdoors.
- The traditional symptomatic treatment consists of vapour breathing given with a vaporizer at the doctor's office or emergency department. At home the bathroom should be filled with moist vapour by showering on the floor and walls with warm water. The parent should stay in the bathroom with the child for about 15 min at a time. Generation of vapour from a coffee pan or kettle is not recommended because of the risk of burns.
- Although vapour breathing is an established mode of therapy, there is no scientific evidence on its effect in resolving dyspnoea C [1 2]. It is recommended only if it can be performed without scaring the child and without force.

Table 31.15 Dosage of racemic adrenaline

Weight of child	Dose
<10 kg	4.5 mg
10–20 kg	6.8 mg
>20 kg	9.0 mg

- **Dexamethason** is effective in spastic croup at a dose of 0.6 mg/kg p.o or i.m. (max 10 mg) **A** [3 4 5 6 7 8]. The dose can later be repeated 1–2 times. The effect starts slowly. Inhaled steroid (e.g budesonide 1 mg) or oral methylprednisolone 2 mg/kg are alternatives.
- In severe stridor **racemic adrenalin** 0.5–1.0 mg/kg during 5–10 min, see Table 31.15) can be given with a nebulizer **B** [8 9]. Because the stridor often recurs after 1–2 hours, these children should be referred to hospital after first aid or at least they should be followed up at the office for that time.

Indications for referral to hospital

- The severity of the breathing difficulty determines where the child is managed.
- Hoarseness and laryngeal cough can be treated at home.
- Children with inspiratory stridor but no retraction recover quickly. The disease worsens markedly in only 1% of these patients.
- About 50% of children with marked retraction of the intercostal spaces and use of auxiliary respiratory muscles get worse, and a small proportion may need intensive care. These children should be referred.
- A feverish child with treatment-resistant "laryngitis" should be referred as a suspected case of bacterial tracheitis.

References

1. Bourchier D, Dawson KP, Fergusson DM. Humidification in viral croup: a controlled trial. Aust Paediatr J 1984;20:289–91.
2. Henry R. Moist air in the treatment of laryngotracheitis. Arch Dis Child 1983;58:577.
3. Russell K, Wiebe N, Saenz A, Ausejo Segura M, Johnson D, Hartling L, Klassen TP. Glucocorticoids for croup. Cochrane Database Syst Rev. 2004;(2):CD001955.
4. Ausejo M, Saenz A, Pham B, Kellner JD, Johnson DW, Moher D, Klassen TP. The effectiveness of glucocorticoids in treating croup: meta-analysis. BMJ 1999;319:595–600.
5. The Database of Abstracts of Reviews of Effectiveness (University of York), Database no.: DARE-999674. In: The Cochrane Library, Issue 4, 2000. Oxford: Update Software.
6. Cruz MN, Stewart G, Rosenberg N. Use of dexamethasone in the outpatient management of acute laryngotracheitis. Pediatrics 1995;96:220–3.
7. Super DM, Cartelli NA, Brooks LJ, Lembo RM, Kumar ML. A prospective randomized double-blind study to evaluate the effect of dexamethasone in acute laryngotracheitis. Journal Of Pediatrics 1989;115:323–9.
8. Kuusela AL, Vesikari T. A randomized double-blind, placebo-controlled trial of dexamethasone and racaemic epinephrine in the treatment of croup. Acta-Paediatr-Scand 1988;77:99–104.
9. Westley CR, Cotton EK, Brooks JG. Nebulized racemic epinephrine by IPPB for the treatment of croup: a double-blind study. Am J Dis Child 1978;132:484–7.

31.16 Epiglottitis in children and adults

Editors

Basic rules

- If there is strong suspicion of epiglottitis do not try to open the mouth and examine the pharynx but calmly escort the (child) patient to hospital (carried by a parent).
- If epiglottitis is unlikely but possible on the basis of the symptoms, inspect the pharynx and epiglottis before discharging the patient for treatment at home.
- If there is imminent airway obstruction, mask ventilation should be tried first.
- If mask ventilation is not successful the doctor should try either intubation or tracheal puncture with a thick infusion needle (6.60).
  - A thick infusion needle and a ventilation bag that can be attached to it should be easily available as a single package at all first aid units.

Symptoms

- A preschool-aged child has a high fever for a few hours, hoarseness, dyspnoea and salivation.
- Cough is usually not present in epiglottitis, but salivation and restlessness are present more often than in laryngitis.
- Swallowing pain is a typical symptom of adult epiglottitis.
- Perform indirect laryngoscopy and examine the epiglottis in adults complaining of severe pain on swallowing, particularly if the clinical findings on inspection of the pharynx are minimal.

Aetiology and epidemiology

- As the result of Hib vaccinations epiglottitis has become rare in children.
- The proportion of cases in older age groups is increasing.

First aid and emergency care

- Avoid all procedures causing oral or pharyngeal irritation or scaring the child.
- Escort the patient (carried by a parent) to a hospital with facilities for intubation and intensive care. Administer oxygen with a mask held near the mouth if this can be accomplished without scaring the child. An adult patient is transported in a sitting or half-sitting position.
- In imminent airway obstruction:
  - Try ventilation with a mask and pharyngeal tube. Often increasing air pressure in the upper respiratory tract is sufficient for opening the airway.
  - If mask ventilation is not successful try intubation with a small tube (never thicker than the patient's little finger). If intubation is not successful in 10–20 seconds, or if the doctor has little experience in intubation, the trachea should be punctured between the thyroid and cricoid cartilages by inserting a thick (e.g. Viggo®) infusion needle perpendicularly into the trachea. Attach a 2 ml syringe to the needle and the connector of the ventilation bag to the syringe. Ventilate the patient with 100% oxygen through the catheter.

Antibiotic treatment

- Cefuroxime i.v. is effective against Haemophilus and betahaemolytic streptococci, which are the most common aetiological agents in adults.

31.17 Prolonged cough in children

Editors

Basic rule

- A child with continuous cough without an obvious cause should be referred to a paediatrician, so that investigations for allergy, pulmonary function tests, and possibly also investigations for gastro-oesophageal reflux, bronchoscopy and histological examination of airway mucosa can be performed.

Causes of prolonged cough

Recurrent infections

- The cough is not caused by a single episode of disease as the parents may remember, but rather by frequently occurring new infections associated, e.g. with the beginning of day care.
- A careful history of the symptoms and the conditions in the family and in day care is often helpful.

An infectious focus

- Cough may be the only significant symptom of silent otitis media with effusion in small children or subacute sinusitis in older children.
- In sinusitis cough is often present during the night or in the morning. It is not merely the result of mucus 'running down' to the throat, but both the middle ear and the sinuses have cough receptors that cause the cough. Ultrasonography of the maxillary sinuses is a safe method also for repeated examinations of maxillary sinus fluid retention.
- The tympanic membranes should be examined with a pneumatic otoscope or by acoustic impedance testing. Mere visual inspection is not sufficient.
- Indications for chest x-ray are considered carefully; repeated radiographic examinations during the same cough episode are usually unnecessary.

Whooping cough, mycoplasma, chlamydia

- See the article about whooping cough for the clinical manifestations 31.19.
- Cough associated with pulmonary mycoplasma and chlamydia infections may be prolonged and continue for weeks, in the manner of whooping cough.

Hyper-reactivity after an infection

- Bronchial hyper-reactivity lasting for weeks is common after viral or mycoplasma infections. The most important symptom are bouts of cough during exercise and in cold weather.

Asthma

- Asthma manifests most often as difficulty in breathing arising from mucosal oedema and brochospasm. The diagnosis is easy in such cases.
- Cough is another manifestation of bronchial hyper-reactivity in asthma.
- The patients typically have cough during the night, during exercise and in cold weather.
- It is important to evaluate the child's condition clinically on several occasions: What are the child's symptoms, how does expiration appear and sound (if the child is old enough, always auscultate forced expiration).
- All symptoms or their absence are recorded.
- In children above 5 years of age, a 1–2-week follow-up of PEF values with a simple instrument at home is a useful examination (31.14).
- A bronchodilatation test or a free exercise test can also be performed (31.12).
- Asthma should be suspected if
  - Wheezing is heard repeatedly on auscultation of expiration
  - PEF values are lower than gender- and height-adjusted reference values.
  - PEF values are paroxysmally reduced by 20%.

- PEF values decrease by 15% under exertion and increase by at least 15% after the inhalation of a sympathomimetic drug.

- The frequency of symptoms and the circumstances in which they appear as well as the efficacy of a possible trial medication can be follow up by using a symptom diary.
- In small children a trial medication with inhaled corticosteroids is often the only possibility. Education for the proper administration of the inhaled medicine must be arranged.

A foreign body in the respiratory tract

- The patient may have had symptoms for weeks or months, without a foreign body being suspected.
- When taking the history of a coughing patient it is always worthwhile to ask specifically for the possibility of a foreign body.
- If the foreign body is radio-opaque (which is rare) the diagnosis can be made by chest radiography. In other cases a bronchoscopy is indicated.

Other causes of cough

- Children subjected to cigarette smoke at home may suffer from continuous cough.
- Gastro-oesophageal reflux may associate with prolonged cough. The history may reveal a considerable tendency for rumination in infancy. The child should be examined in specialist care by using pH registration and, in necessary, endoscopy.
- Typical manifestations of psychogenic cough include hawking, speaking with a loud voice and coughing in specific situations. In 10% of children with prolonged cough the condition is psychogenic.

31.19 Whooping cough

Matti Uhari, Jussi Mertsola

Objectives

- To identify whooping cough as a cause of persistent cough in school children and spells of cough and whooping in infants.
- To treat the patient with macrolide antibiotics and to administer medication prophylactically to the entire family if there is another child in the family aged below 6 months **C** [1 2].

Causative agent

- Bordetella pertussis
- Similar picture can also be caused by B. parapertussis, possibly also by Chlamydia and adenovirus.
- B. pertussis is extremely contagious.

Prevalence

- Prevalence varies and depends on how well the population is protected by immunization.
- Infants: Maternal vaccination in childhood is not sufficient to protect the neonate.
- School children: Immunity conferred by vaccination lasts only 3–6 years.

Clinical picture

- Incubation period 1–2 weeks.
- Clinical diagnosis based on history.
- In unvaccinated infants during the **catarrhal phase** (1–2 weeks) there is slight cough, red eyes and rhinitis, sometimes also mild fever.
- During the **coughing phase** there are spells of coughing. In infants these may be associated with inspiratory stridor or whooping. The spells of coughing occur at night in particular, and often conclude with vomiting of mucus. The spells continue at regular intervals for 1–4 weeks and then become less frequent. They may recur during a new respiratory infection.
- During the coughing phase the patient is afebrile. CRP and ESR are usually normal. Fever or elevated CRP and ESR suggest some other infection or a secondary bacterial infection.
- A school child with whooping cough is usually brought for consultation because of cough that has lasted for weeks or months. The cough is usually described as being exceptionally severe, and almost always occurring in spells. When enquiry is made as to whether the child has ever had this kind of cough and the answer is no, a diagnosis can often be reached. Whooping is not always present in school children.
- Stress, cigarette smoke and changes of temperature (eating ice cream, for example) can trigger a spell of coughing. Such hyper-reactivity of the airways can last for 3–6 months, and asthma may be suspected.
- Whooping cough also occurs in adults.
- Whooping cough may in unvaccinated infants cause leucocytosis, in particular lymphocytosis to develop.

Diagnostic strategy

- Epidemics are usually only detected after the patients have been coughing for weeks or months. In such patients, diagnosis is usually made on the basis of one serum sample, as IgM and IgA antibodies increase to diagnostic levels 3–4 weeks after symptoms commence. A further sample may be taken if necessary after 4 weeks.

- Negative serological findings do not exclude whooping cough, because the sensitivity of the test is only 50–60%.
- Fresh cases (duration of symptoms less than 4 weeks) in the area can be sampled for PCR and cultures can be undertaken. For cultures, samples should be taken via the nostrils from the posterior larynx, using a metal-shafted calcium alginate pin. Samples should be cultured immediately on fresh media (carbon cephalexin dish). For PCR, a Dacron pin is more appropriate (can be used for cultures as well). Culture dishes and sample pins can be ordered from microbiological laboratories.
- After diagnosis has been confirmed on the basis of results of tests relating to one patient or several patients, treatment decisions relating to contacts can be made on the basis of their clinical symptoms.

Treatment

- Infants and unvaccinated children should be referred readily to hospital for treatment.
- For infants the recommended drug is erythromycin 50 mg/kg/day for 2 weeks. For vaccinated and older children other macrolides can be used at normal doses C [1 2]. Prophylactic medication is always recommendable if there is a child under 6 months of age in the same family as a whooping cough sufferer. The entire family should always be treated simultaneously.
- Alternative medications are roxitromycin, claritromycin, azithromycin and sulpha-trimethoprim.
- The primary aim of treatment is to reduce infectivity and spread. For treatment to affect symptoms it should be started 1–2 weeks after symptoms commence. In practice, treatment should be started immediately after a sample is taken for culture, or a clinical diagnosis is reached on the basis of symptoms and the epidemiological situation suggesting whooping cough. If the patient has exhibited symptoms for over one month, treatment is not usually worthwhile. Repeated courses of antibiotics are of no benefit.
- The period of isolation should be 5 days from the start of antibiotic treatment. If symptoms have lasted for more than 3 weeks, isolation is unnecessary.
- Contacts below 7 years of age should also undergo PDT vaccination if seroprotection has remained insufficient.

References

1. Dodhia H, Miller R. Review of evidence for the use of erythromycin in the management of persons exposed to pertussis. Epidemiology and Infection 1998;120:143–149.
2. The Database of Abstracts of Reviews of Effectiveness (University of York), Database no.: DARE-983483. In: The Cochrane Library, Issue 2, 2000. Oxford: Update Software.

31.20 When should a child with a cough be treated with antibiotics?

Editors

The aetiology of bronchitis and rationale for antibiotic treatment

- Coughing is one of the most common causes for unnecessary antibiotic treatment. Antibiotics should not be prescribed for bronchitis in children. A typical candidate for a course of antibiotics is a child aged 1–5 years with fever, cough and rhinorrhoea for 3–6 days, and bronchial rales on auscultation.
- Pathogenic bacteria (Pneumococci, Haemophilus or Moraxella) can often be isolated from the bronchial secretions of children with a cough. However, tracheobronchitis is nearly always a viral disease, not a primary or secondary bacterial disease. Only mycoplasmae, Bordetella pertussis, and chlamydiae are considered significant pathogens in the aetiology of bronchitis in children. The probability of a secondary bacterial infection is small.
- In the majority the diagnosis "acute bacterial bronchitis" is an unnecessary precaution. However, it is important to identify children with bronchial hyper-reactivity who have recurrent wheezing or rales. In such children treatments for asthma should be considered after consultation with a paediatrician. It is a mistake to treat these children with recurrent courses of antibiotics.

PAE

Antibiotics are not indicated

- for a cough associated with and following a common cold and lasting for 1–2 weeks.
- for a child with fever, rhinitis and a cough that has lasted at least 4 days. (The child probably has a prolonged viral infection.)
- for a child who is recovering from symptoms of an infection but who has bouts of coughing, especially in cold weather or after exercise. (The child probably has hyper-reactivity of the airways during convalescence.)
- for a child with bronchial rales on auscultation and a history of frequent antibiotic courses for incipient bronchitis. (The child probably has obstructive bronchitis with mild symptoms.)
    - Sometimes a look at the face confirms the diagnosis: the child has dry skin and signs of atopic dermatitis on the cheeks and under the eyes.

Antibiotics are indicated

- if the findings on auscultation or on a chest x-ray are typical of pneumonia.

- if the child has sinusitis (verified by ultrasonography or radiography in children aged 4 years or above, or suspected on the basis of a prolonged (>10 days) wet cough at nights and in the morning).
- if the child has otitis media.
- if several members of the family are affected and there is an epidemic of mycoplasma infections.
- Bacterial bronchitis and bacterial tracheitis may exist but they are rare and do not indicate routine antibiotic treatment for a child with fever and cough.

31.21 Treatment of pneumonia in children

Editors

Basic rule

- Treat with antibiotics all children with pneumonia diagnosed on the basis of auscultation or chest radiography.

Diagnosis by auscultation

- It is not always easy to differentiate obstructive rales from pneumonic rales. The latter are dry and fine.
- Unilaterally diminished breathing sounds are a significant finding.
- Antibiotic treatment can be started on the basis of auscultation if the general condition of the child is good. For indications for chest radiography, see 31.22.

Choice and dosage of antibiotic

- If the general condition of the child is good there is no need for hospitalization.
- The drug of choice for children **below school age** is amoxicillin, 40 mg/kg/day, in three doses for 7 days.
  - Amoxicillin is effective against the most probable bacterial pathogens, pneumococci and Haemophilus influenzae.
  - Erythromycin can be used as an alternative, particularly if mycoplasma pneumonia is suspected.
- At **school age** the drug of choice is erythromycin, 40 mg/kg/day, in three doses for 10 days, or other macrolides. Macrolides are effective against the most probable pathogens, pneumococci and mycoplasma.

Follow-up of treatment

- If pneumonia is treated in primary care it is essential to follow-up the response to treatment, e.g. by asking the parents to telephone on the next day. If the patient is definitely ill and does not show signs of improvement in 2–4 days the doctor should reassess the situation and consider referral to a hospital.
- Follow-up chest x-ray should be carried out if there has been lobar infiltration or atelectasis, or if recovery is slow.
- Remember that the radiographic picture normalizes slowly. If the general condition of the child is good, control x-ray should not be carried out before 4–6 weeks have elapsed.
- At one month about 20% of the patients continue to have abnormalities on the x-ray that gradually disappear.

Indications for hospitalization

- The child should be referred to hospital if he or she has
  - impaired general condition
  - dyspnoea
  - widespread pneumonic infiltration
  - pleuropneumonia (pleural effusion).
- Children below the age of 6 months should always be hospitalized.

31.22 Indications for and interpretation of chest x-ray in a child with symptoms of an infection

Editors

Indications for chest x-ray

- An ill-looking child with unilaterally diminished breathing sounds.
- An ill-looking child who has lower respiratory tract symptoms (e.g. tachypnoea) whether or not auscultation suggests pneumonia.
- There are signs of bacterial infection (fever and a markedly increased serum CRP concentration) but the focus of infection is unknown.
- Foreign body aspiration is suspected. (Many foreign bodies are not seen in x-ray but they may result in atelectasis, signs of infection, or hyperinflation.)

Interpretation of a chest x-ray

- If a chest x-ray is taken from a child with fever and a cough the findings are abnormal in up to 70% of the cases. The most common findings are peribronchial enhancement, hyperinflation of the lungs, atelectasis, and hilar lymphadenopathy.

- Children with bronchial discharge very often have **peribronchial enhancement** that can be interpreted as central pneumonia by an inexperienced observer. The definition of pneumonia is often obscure.
- Another pitfall is **atelectasis**. Mucus easily obstructs small airways, which results in linear or even larger opacities. The differentiation from pneumonic consolidation is not easy, and atelectasis and pneumonia often coexist.
  - A decrease in lobar volume and wedge-like narrowing of opacity towards the periphery is typical of pure atelectasis.
- The interpretation of **hyperinflation of the lungs** is often subjective. A flat diaphragm and "funnel" appearance in lateral view suggest hyperinflation, but the phase of respiration also influences the interpretation. However, hyperinflation is an important finding because it suggests lower respiratory tract infection and obstruction, e.g. in bronchiolitis the picture is diagnostic.
- In a child with obstruction and secretions, both hyperinflated and atelectatic areas can be seen simultaneously.
- **The aetiology of pneumonia cannot be identified according to the radiological appearance**: both viral and bacterial pneumonias may result in lobar density, although this finding is more common in bacterial pneumonia.

31.23 Cystic fibrosis

Erkki Savilahti

Essentials

- In the UK, cyctic fibrosis (CF) is the most common cause of severe chronic lung disease in childhood and accounts for most cases of exocrine pancreatic insufficiency.
- Sweat test is of vital importance in the diagnosis, but it should be performed by specifically trained technicians in controlled hospital settings.

Epidemiology

- CF is the most common hereditary, metabolic disease among most Caucasian populations; among them its incidence varies from 1 in 2000 newborn infants (Great Britain) to 1 in 20,000 (Finland).
- The disease is autosomal and recessive. The affected genes codes for a molecule that facilitates the transport of chloride ions across apical cell membranes. Mutations in the gene lead to variable alterations in the concentration of electrolytes and the water content of fluids on cell surfaces. More than 1000 mutations have been described.
- Respiratory disease is caused by failure of local innate defence system and exaggerated inflammatory response.
- Exocrine secretory system of pancreas is destroyed in 85% of patients before or shortly after birth by own proteolytic enzymes activated in the duct system.
- Excretory defects cause liver disease in 70% (fatty infiltration) and aspermia in 98% of men. In females, the reproductive capacity is impaired due to dehydrated cervical mucus.

Clinical picture

- CF has a wide spectrum of manifestations which may relate to the mutant genotype.
- Meconium ileus causes intestinal obstruction in up to 15% of newborn children with CF.
- Clinically obvious pancreatic insufficiency occurs in up to 85% of cases during infancy.
- Failure to thrive is common. Chronic diarrhoea (steatorrhea) with malabsorption due to pancreatic failure leads to severe growth retardation. It sometimes appears only after reduction of breastfeeding, because milk contains lipase.
- Recurrent rectal prolapse may be the sole presenting feature.
- Salt deficiency with metabolic alkalosis is common at diagnosis and may occur at times of copious sweating.
- In neonates and infants, other symptoms include hepatitis, oedema (due to protein deficiency), disorders due to deficiency of fat soluble vitamins (A-, E-, K-).
- After infancy, the most prominent symptoms are respiratory. A chronic or recurrent cough is usually the first symptom. Acute pneumonias due to Staphlococcus aureus, Haemophilus influenzae and Pseudomonas aeruginosa are common.
- Pneumonia is often followed by chronic colonization by these microbes and gradual destruction of the lung tissue.
- Sinusitis is common, and 10–30% of the patients develop nasal polyps.
- Destruction of pancreatic islets may lead to diabetes.
- Males have drastically reduced fertility, but some may be able to father children.

Diagnosis

- The quantitative measurement of sweat electrolytes (chloride) following stimulation by pilocarpine iontophoresis is vital in the diagnosis.
- The sweat test can be performed 2 weeks after birth in infants greater than 3 kg who are normally hydrated and without significant systemic illness.
- A sweat chloride of less than 40 mmol/l is normal; a result above 60 mmol/l supports the diagnosis. The analysis should always be repeated.

- Gene mutation analysis is useful particularly in patients with mild or atypical phenotype where sweat chloride concentration may be intermediate (test locally prevalent mutations).
- Pancreatic function defect: Decreased amount of elastase or chymotrypsin in feaces (finding present in ca. 90%).

Treatment and prognosis

- CF patients should be treated in dedicated CF clinics.
- The treatment of pancreatic disease includes adequate replacement therapy with pancreatic enzymes and nutritional therapy with extra doses of fat soluble vitamins C [1].
- Intensive antibiotic treatment is needed when infection or colonization with S. aureus, H. influenzae or P. aeruginosa is diagnosed.
- The patients may also need anti-inflammatory treatment (e.g. inhaled steroids), mucolytic treatments (e.g. inhalation of saline, DNAse C [2]) and mechanical removal of mucus (physical treatment of lungs, increased physical activity).
- Lung transplantation is an option to some patients.
- Median age of death in 2000 in US was 32 years. Considerably longer lifetimes may be expected for infants born today.

References

1. Beckles Willson N, Elliott TM, Everard ML. Omega-3 fatty acids (from fish oils) for cystic fibrosis. Cochrane Database Syst Rev. 2004;(2):CD002201.
2. Jones AP, Wallis CE, Kearney CE. Recombinant human deoxyribonuclease for cystic fibrosis. Cochrane Database Syst Rev. 2004;(2):CD001127.

31.30 Oral candidiasis in children

Editors

Self-care by parents

- If there are no ulcers in the mouth the parents can apply for example lemon juice.

Drug treatment

- Mild oral candidiasis requires no drug treatment.
- Antimycotics (miconazole, nystatin, or natamycin drops) after each meal are the primary therapy.

31.31 Stomatitis in children

Editors

Aetiology and clinical presentation

Gingivostomatitis

- See 7.21.
- Herpes simplex virus is the causative agent.
- The general symptoms of a primary infection include fever, malaise, and headache.
- Herpetiform vesicles can be detected on the buccal mucosa, lips, and tongue; the vesicles often break and result in a small erosion.
- The gingivae are red, swollen, and often bleeding. The mouth is extremely sore, and the child does not want to eat.
- The patient recovers spontaneously: the fever disappears after the fourth day, and the vesicles resolve a couple of days later.

Herpangina

- See 7.21
- The causative agent is a coxsackievirus.
- Vesicles can be detected in the posterior part of the mouth, on the palate, tonsils, and posterior pharynx.
- The vesicles burst more easily than in herpes infection. The general symptoms include fever, mouth pain, and unwillingness to eat.

Hand, foot, and mouth disease

- See 7.21.
- The disease is caused by a coxsackievirus. Vesicles can be found in the mouth, and on the hands and feet.
- Diagnostic difficulties are caused by the fact that the mouth and skin lesions do not always occur simultaneously.
- Other enteroviruses may also result in vesicles in the mouth and on the skin.
- Unlike herpesviruses, the enteroviruses rarely cause gingivitis (and gingival bleeding).
- The disease is most prevalent in late summer.

Aphthous stomatitis

- The condition is characterized by recurring painful ulcers in the mouth.
- The aetiology is unknown. L-forms of Streptococcus sanguis have been isolated from the lesions, but their role as causative agents is not clear. An autoimmune aetiology has also been suggested.
- Usually there are 1–5 very painful ulcers in the mouth.
- Unlike herpes infection, there are no blisters at the onset or general symptoms (e.g. fever).

Treatment

- Occasionally viral stomatitis becomes prolonged, resulting in a disturbance of fluid and electrolyte balance so that hospitalization is necessary.
- Gargling the mouth with lidocaine solution before eating often allows the child to take enough fluids and energy. A single dose of 5–15 ml is safe even if the child swallows the solution.
- There is some evidence that acyclovir (and valacyclovir) may shorten the duration of symptoms in stomatitis caused by herpes. It can be used on patients with severe symptoms within three days after onset of symptoms. When using a 40 mg/ml solution orally the dose is 5 ml × 5 for over 2-year olds and 2.5 ml × 5 for children between 3 months and 2 years of age.
- Aphthous stomatitis is also treated with a local anaesthetic ointment or solution.

31.39 Prevention of otitis media in children

Terho Heikkinen

Essential

- As otitis media in children is almost invariably a complication of a viral upper respiratory infection, all measures to reduce viral infections would probably also reduce the incidence of otitis.

Influencing risk factors

- Day care outside the child's home is the most important environmental risk factor for otitis. Moving a child suffering from recurring episodes of otitis from a day-care centre to care at home or in another family would be a logical solution.
- However, the efficacy of such an intervention in preventing otitis has not been proven by research.
- Avoidance of exposure to tobacco smoke is also justified, but here also evidence on the effect of avoidance is lacking.
- Limiting the use of a dummy (pacifier) has some effect in reducing the incidence of otitis.
- Breastfeeding continued for longer than 3 months may have some protective effect; however, this effect is probably very small.

Antimicrobial medications

- Long-term antibiotic prophylaxis that is continued for months probably prevents the incidence of otitis somewhat. The clinical significance of long-term prophylaxis is, however, questionable, as it has been estimated that to prevent one episode of otitis a child would need a 9-month course of antibiotics. Because of increasing bacterial resistance to antibiotics, initiation of long-term prophylaxis requires critical consideration.
- Starting a course of antibiotics as soon as symptoms of a common cold have appeared does not prevent the development of otitis media effectively.
- Almost half of all episodes of otitis associated with influenza virus infection can be prevented with oseltamivir if the medication is started within 48 hours of the appearance of symptoms.

Other medications

- Nasal decongestants or combinations of an antihistamine and decongestant have not been shown effective in the prevention of otitis media.

Xylitol

- Xylitol chewing gum administered five times daily has been shown to reduce the incidence of acute otitis media by about one third during a 3-month follow-up. There are no data on the efficacy of xylitol with less frequent dosing or longer use. Xylitol taken only during a respiratory tract infection does not prevent the development of otitis.

Surgery

- Adenoidectomy is often performed to prevent otitis media. However, there is no evidence on the effect of this intervention in preventing otitis media in young children. The evidence currently available rather suggests that adenoidectomy has no significant role in the prevention of otitis.
- Tympanostomy tubes have been shown to have some effect in preventing otitis, although the main indication for the tubes is chronic OME ("glue ear").

Vaccinations

- Vaccination against influenza has succeeded in preventing the majority of otitis episodes associated with influenza and at the same time about one third of all episodes of otitis during an influenza epidemic.
- The vaccination can be given from the age of 6 months onward, and it can be justifiably recommended to children suffering from recurring episodes of otitis.
- A new protein-conjugated pneumococcal vaccine has reduced the incidence of AOM caused by serotypes included in the vaccine by half; however, because of the wide spectrum of causative agents, the efficacy of the vaccine in the prevention of all episodes of otitis is only approximately 6%.

Passive immunization

- Various immunoglobulin products have not been shown to have significant efficacy in the prevention of acute otitis media in children.

31.40 Otitis media in children: definition, epidemiology and diagnosis

Terho Heikkinen

Aims

- The diagnosis of acute otitis media (AOM) is based on findings on inspection of the tympanic membrane.
- Over-diagnosing AOM must be avoided; using diagnostic devices is helpful (31.43).

Definition

- **Acute otitis media (AOM)**
  - Effusion in the middle ear
  - Tympanic membrane does not appear normal, see Table 31.40.
  - The child has symptoms of acute infection.
- **Otitis media with effusion (OME)**
  - There is effusion in the middle ear, but the child lacks symptoms of acute infection.
- In **myringitis** the child has symptoms and the tympanic membrane is hemorrhagic or bullous but its mobility is normal.

Epidemiology

- AOM is the most common bacterial infection in children and the reason for most courses of antimicrobial drugs.
- The incidence is highest between the ages of 6 months and 2 years Ⓐ [1 2 3 4 5].
- By the age of one year 40%, and by the age of two years 70% of children have had at least one episode of AOM Ⓐ [6 7 8].
  - Every fifth child has at least three episodes of AOM.
- The incidence is highest in the winter, lowest in the summer.

Risk factors

- AOM is generally preceded by viral upper respiratory tract infection which can be considered the main risk factor for AOM Ⓐ [9 10 11].
  - The peak of occurrence is on the third or fourth day from the appearance of symptoms of infection.
- Other known risk factors include
  - Young age
  - Day care outside the home Ⓐ [12 13 14]
  - Occurrence of otitis in other family members Ⓐ [12 13 14]
  - Having at least one sibling Ⓐ [12 13 14]
  - Exposure to cigarette smoke Ⓑ [15 16 17 18 19 20 21 22 23 24]
  - Using a dummy (pacifier).
- Breast-feeding for a short period or not at all may have some effect in increasing the occurrence of AOM Ⓑ [25 26 27 28 29 30 31 32 33 34 35 36 37 38 39]
- Evidence on the role of allergy as a risk factor for AOM is very contradictory.

Table 31.40 Tympanic membrane findings in a healthy child and in acute otitis media

Characteristics of the tympanic membrane	Normal finding	Finding suggesting otitis media
Colour	Pearly grey	Red, yellowish or white
Transparency	Transparent	Cloudy
Shape	Concave	Flat or bulging
Light reflex	Narrow, clear boundaries	Widened or absent
Mobility	Normal	Decreased or absent

Examination of the ears

- When the ear is examined, an adult holds the child firmly on his/her lap and supports the child's head towards his/her own chest.
- Both ears are examined even if the child complains only one ear. Begin by examining the healthy ear.
- Earwax in the outer auditory canal should be removed to allow an unhindered view of the tympanic membrane.

Removing earwax

- Removing earwax is often the most difficult phase in the examination of a young child's ears.
- The wax should be removed as gently as possible without hurrying as the skin of the outer auditory canal is very thin and sensitive.
- Holding the child's head steadily towards the chest of the accompanying adult is the prerequisite of successful removal of wax.
- Soft wax clots lining the auditory canal can usually be removed easily with a cotton stick, which is inserted behind the wax clot and then pulled back pressing it gently towards the ear canal.
- Running wax can often be removed easily by suction.

- Dry wax clots or wax that blocks the ear canal entirely are best removed with a small curet or probe.
- To remove a tightly fastened wax clot that blocks the entire canal, softening eardrops can be inserted into the ear canal about 30 minutes before the procedure.

Symptoms

- The unspecific symptoms commonly associated with AOM are much the same as those of a normal respiratory tract infection without otitis; therefore, the diagnosis of otitis cannot be made reliably on the basis of symptoms B [40 41 42].
- Earache is a quite specific symptom suggesting AOM, however, it is present in only more than half of children with otitis A [43 44 45 46].
- Sudden loss of hearing during a respiratory tract infection suggests otitis D [47], but this is often difficult to notice in young children who cannot yet express themselves clearly.
- Nocturnal restlessness occurs in AOM slightly more often than in respiratory infections without AOM, but its predictive value in the clinical setting is not sufficient B [48 49].
- Ear pulling is common in young children, and does not suggest AOM if respiratory infection is not present.

Findings on the tympanic membrane

- Both ears are examined with a pneumatic otoscope.
- A pneumatic otoscope and a head mirror or an otomicroscope are good instruments for the examination of the ear, but their use requires training.
- The mobility of the tympanic membrane cannot be evaluated reliably unless the otoscope fits the ear canal completely airproofly.
- The diagnosis of otitis media is based on tympanic membrane findings (see Table 31.40) A [50 51]
  - There may be one or more findings suggesting otitis
  - Differences between the tympanic membranes support the diagnosis of otitis D [52 53].
- Mild redness of the tympanic membrane is usual in a crying or feverish child and is not as such a sufficient sign for making the diagnosis of otitis.
- If the child has tympanostomy tubes, the diagnosis of AOM is based on observation of secretion flowing through the tube to the ear canal.

Diagnostic devices

- Tympanometer (31.43) is an easy-to-use and quick device for estimating the mobility of the tympanic membrane B [54 55 56].
- Tympanogram can be abnormal also in the absence of AOM; however, if the result is normal, AOM is highly unlikely.
- The results of a tympanometry performed on an infant younger than 6 months or on a crying child are often unreliable. Perform tympanometry before removing ear wax or using the pneumatic otoscope, i.e. before the child begins to cry.
- Acoustic reflectometer is a new and even easier device for examining the ear (31.43)
  - Does not require airproof closing of the ear canal like the tympanometer
  - Accuracy is more or less the same as that of tympanometer.

References

1. Pukander J, Karma P, Sipilä M. Occurrence and recurrence of acute otitis media among children. Acta Otolaryngol 1982;94:479–86.
2. Lundgren K, Ingvarsson L. Epidemiology of acute otitis media in children. Scand J Infect Dis 1983; Suppl 39:19–25.
3. Sipilä M, Pukander J, Karma P. Incidence of acute otitis media up to the age of 1≪ years in urban infants. Acta Otolaryngol (Stockh) 1987;104:138–45.
4. Alho O-P, Koivu M, Sorri M, Rantakallio P. The occurrence of acute otitis media in infants: a life-table analysis. Int J Pediatr Otorhinolaryngol 1991;21:7–14.
5. Teele DW, Klein JO, Rosner B. Epidemiology of otitis media during the first seven years of life in children in Greater Boston: a prospective, cohort study. J Infect Dis 1989;160:83–94.
6. Sipilä M, Pukander J, Karma P. Incidence of acute otitis media up to the age of 1≪ years in urban infants. Acta Otolaryngol (Stockh) 1987;104:138–45.
7. Alho O-P, Koivu M, Sorri M, Rantakallio P. The occurrence of acute otitis media in infants: a life-table analysis. Int J Pediatr Otorhinolaryngol 1991;21:7–14.
8. Teele DW, Klein JO, Rosner B. Epidemiology of otitis media during the first seven years of life in children in Greater Boston: a prospective, cohort study. J Infect Dis 1989;160:83–94.
9. Henderson FW, Collier AM, Sanyal MA, ym. A longitudinal study of respiratory viruses and bacteria in the etiology of acute otitis media with effusion. N Engl J Med 1982;306:1377–83.
10. Ruuskanen O, Arola M, Putto-Laurila A, ym. Acute otitis media and respiratory virus infections. Pediatr Infect Dis J 1989;8:94–9.
11. Arola M, Ruuskanen O, Ziegler T, ym. Clinical role of respiratory virus infection in acute otitis media. Pediatrics 1990;86:848–55.
12. Uhari M, Mäntysaari K, Niemelä M. A meta-analytic review of the risk factors for acute otitis media. Clin Infect Dis 1996;22:1079–83.
13. Sipilä M, Karma P, Pukander J, Timonen M, Kataja M. The Bayesian approach to the evaluation of risk factors in acute and recurrent acute otitis media. Acta Otolaryngol (Stockh) 1988;106:94–101.
14. Alho O-P, Koivu M, Sorri M, Rantakallio P. Risk factors for recurrent acute otitis media and respiratory infection in infancy. Int J Pediatr Otorhinolaryngol 1990;19: 151–61.
15. Ståhlberg M-R, Ruuskanen O, Virolainen E. Risk factors for recurrent otitis media. Pediatr Infect Dis 1986;5: 30–2.

16. Pukander J, Luotonen J, Timonen M, Karma P. Risk factors affecting the occurrence of acute otitis media among 2–3-year-old urban children. Acta Otolaryngol (Stockh) 1985;100:260–5.
17. Owen MJ, Baldwin CD, Swank PR, Pannu AK, Johnson DL, Howie VM. Relation of infant feeding practices, cigarette smoke exposure, and group child care to the onset and duration of otitis media with effusion in the first two years of life. J Pediatr 1993;123:702–11.
18. Stenstrom R, Bernard PAM, Ben-Simhon H. Exposure to environmental tobacco smoke as a risk factor for recurrent acute otitis media in children under the age of five years. Int J Pediatr Otorhinolaryngol 1993;27:127–36.
19. Teele DW, Klein JO, Rosner B. Epidemiology of otitis media during the first seven years of life in children in Greater Boston: a prospective, cohort study. J Infect Dis 1989;160:83–94.
20. Sipilä M, Karma P, Pukander J, Timonen M, Kataja M. The Bayesian approach to the evaluation of risk factors in acute and recurrent acute otitis media. Acta Otolaryngol (Stockh) 1988;106:94–101.
21. Alho O-P, Koivu M, Sorri M, Rantakallio P. Risk factors for recurrent acute otitis media and respiratory infection in infancy. Int J Pediatr Otorhinolaryngol 1990;19: 151–61.
22. Kero P, Piekkala P. Factors affecting the occurrence of acute otitis media during the first year of life. Acta Paediatr Scand 1987;76:618–23.
23. Uhari M, Mäntysaari K, Niemelä M. A meta-analytic review of the risk factors for acute otitis media. Clin Infect Dis 1996;22:1079–83.
24. Etzel RA, Pattishall EN, Haley NJ, Fletcher RH, Henderson FW. Passive smoking and middle ear effusion among children in day care. Pediatrics 1992;90:228–32.
25. Teele DW, Klein JO, Rosner B. Epidemiology of otitis media during the first seven years of life in children in Greater Boston: a prospective, cohort study. J Infect Dis 1989;160:83–94.
26. Alho O-P, Koivu M, Sorri M, Rantakallio P. Risk factors for recurrent acute otitis media and respiratory infection in infancy. Int J Pediatr Otorhinolaryngol 1990;19: 151–61.
27. Pukander J, Luotonen J, Timonen M, Karma P. Risk factors affecting the occurrence of acute otitis media among 2–3-year-old urban children. Acta Otolaryngol (Stockh) 1985;100:260–5.
28. Owen MJ, Baldwin CD, Swank PR, Pannu AK, Johnson DL, Howie VM. Relation of infant feeding practices, cigarette smoke exposure, and group child care to the onset and duration of otitis media with effusion in the first two years of life. J Pediatr 1993;123:702–11.
29. Kero P, Piekkala P. Factors affecting the occurrence of acute otitis media during the first year of life. Acta Paediatr Scand 1987;76:618–23.
30. Chandra RK. Prospective studies of the effect of breast feeding on incidence of infection and allergy. Acta Paediatr Scand 1979;68:691–4.
31. Saarinen UM. Prolonged breast feeding as prophylaxis for recurrent otitis media. Acta Paediatr Scand 1982;71:567–71.
32. Fleming DW, Cochi SL, Hightower AW, Broome CV. Childhood upper respiratory tract infections: to what degree is incidence affected by day-care attendance? Pediatrics 1987;79:55–60.
33. Tainio V-M, Savilahti E, Salmenperä L, Arjomaa P, Siimes MA, Perheentupa J. Risk factors for infantile recurrent otitis media: atopy but not type of feeding. Pediatr Res 1988;23:509–12.
34. Rubin DH, Leventhal JM, Krasilnikoff PA, ym. Relationship between infant feeding and infectious illness: a prospective study of infants during the first year of life. Pediatrics 1990;85:464–71.
35. Uhari M, Mäntysaari K, Niemelä M. A meta-analytic review of the risk factors for acute otitis media. Clin Infect Dis 1996;22:1079–83.
36. Paradise JL, Elster BA, Tan L. Evidence in infants with cleft palate that breast milk protects against otitis media. Pediatrics 1994;94:853–60.
37. Bauchner H, Leventhal JM, Shapiro ED. Studies of breast-feeding and infections: how good is the evidence? JAMA 1986;256:887–92.
38. Duncan B, Ey J, Holberg CJ, Wright AL, Martinez FD, Taussig LM. Exclusive breast-feeding for at least 4 months protects against otitis media. Pediatrics 1993;91:867–72.
39. Aniansson G, Alm B, Andersson B, ym. A prospective cohort study on breast-feeding and otitis media in Swedish infants. Pediatr Infect Dis J 1994;13:183–8.
40. Niemelä M, Uhari M, Jounio-Ervasti K, Luotonen J, Alho O-P, Vierimaa E. Lack of specific symptomatology in children with acute otitis media. Pediatr Infect Dis J 1994;13:765–8.
41. Heikkinen T, Ruuskanen O. Signs and symptoms predicting acute otitis media. Arch Pediatr Adolesc Med 1995;149:26–9.
42. Kontiokari T, Koivunen P, Niemelä M, Pokka T, Uhari M. Symptoms of acute otitis media. Pediatr Infect Dis J 1998;17:676–9.
43. Niemelä M, Uhari M, Jounio-Ervasti K, Luotonen J, Alho O-P, Vierimaa E. Lack of specific symptomatology in children with acute otitis media. Pediatr Infect Dis J 1994;13:765–8.
44. Heikkinen T, Ruuskanen O. Signs and symptoms predicting acute otitis media. Arch Pediatr Adolesc Med 1995;149:26–9.
45. Uhari M, Niemelä M, Hietala J. Prediction of acute otitis media with symptoms and signs. Acta Paediatr 1995;84: 90–2.
46. Kontiokari T, Koivunen P, Niemelä M, Pokka T, Uhari M. Symptoms of acute otitis media. Pediatr Infect Dis J 1998;17:676–9.
47. Niemelä M, Uhari M, Jounio-Ervasti K, Luotonen J, Alho O-P, Vierimaa E. Lack of specific symptomatology in children with acute otitis media. Pediatr Infect Dis J 1994;13: 765–8.
48. Heikkinen T, Ruuskanen O. Signs and symptoms predicting acute otitis media. Arch Pediatr Adolesc Med 1995;149: 26–9.
49. Kontiokari T, Koivunen P, Niemelä M, Pokka T, Uhari M. Symptoms of acute otitis media. Pediatr Infect Dis J 1998;17:676–9.
50. Karma PH, Penttilä MA, Sipilä MM, Kataja MJ. Otoscopic diagnosis of middle ear effusion in acute and non-acute otitis media. I. The value of different otoscopic findings. Int J Pediatr Otorhinolaryngol 1989;17:37–49.
51. Arola M, Ruuskanen O, Ziegler T, ym. Clinical role of respiratory virus infection in acute otitis media. Pediatrics 1990;86:848–55.

52. Arola M, Ruuskanen O, Ziegler T, ym. Clinical role of respiratory virus infection in acute otitis media. Pediatrics 1990;86:848–55.
53. Jero J, Virolainen A, Virtanen M, Eskola J, Karma P. Prognosis of acute otitis media: factors associated with poor outcome. Acta Otolaryngol (Stockh) 1997;117:278–83.
54. Puhakka H. Pieni tympanometri parantaa lasten välikorvantulehdusten diagnostiikkaa avohoidossa, Suom Lääkäril 1991; 46:2708–11.
55. van Balen FAM, de Melker RA. Validation of a portable tympanometer for use in primary care. Int J Pediatr Otorhinolaryngol 1994;29:219–25.
56. Koivunen P, Alho O-P, Uhari M, Niemelä M, Luotonen J. Minitympanometry in detecting middle ear fluid. J Pediatr 1997;131:419–22.

31.42 Treatment and follow-up of acute otitis media in children

Terho Heikkinen

Aims

- Pain in the acute phase is treated efficiently.
- Symptoms and middle ear effusion disappear in a reasonable time.
- Prolonged middle ear effusion (chronic otitis media with effusion) is detected.
- Normal hearing is resumed.

Starting therapy

- In the initial management of painful otitis media, adequate pain relief is essential C [1 2].
  - Paracetamol (acetaminophen) 15–20 mg/kg × 4
  - Ibuprofen 10 mg/kg × 3
  - Naproxen 5 mg/kg × 2
  - Anaesthesizing eardrops C [3]
- There is no hurry to start treatment with antibiotics and the child need not to be brought in at night-time to see a doctor for the initiation of antibiotic therapy.
- The pain usually alleviates within a few hours by itself. The disappearance of pain does not rule out the possibility of otitis, which is why examining the ears on the next day is warranted in any event.

Treatment with antibiotics

- In a substantial proportion of children, otitis media resolves within a few weeks without any treatment; however, some children clearly benefit from antibiotic therapy A [4 5 6 7 8 9] (disappearance of effusion B [10 11 12], alleviation of symptoms B [13 14 15 16 17 18 19]).
- As individual factors that would predict the need for antibiotic therapy are presently not known, the recommendation is to treat otitis media primarily with antibiotics D [20].
- The optimal duration of antibiotic therapy is 5–7 days.
  - In practice, 5-day courses have yielded the same results as courses lasting more than one week B [21 22 23].

Selecting the antimicrobial agent

- The recommended drug of choice is amoxicillin at 40 mg/kg daily or penicillin V 100 000 IU/kg daily, both divided into two doses.
- If the clinical response is poor or if the bacterial culture of the middle ear effusion reveals a beta-lactamase-producing bacterium, amoxicillin-clavulanic acid may be the most recommendable choice as the second-line antibiotic.
- In penicillin allergy, trimethoprim-sulphonamide, azithromycin or clarithromycin can be used. In other patients, second-line drugs include e.g. cefaclor and cefuroxime axetil.
- Intramuscularly administered single dose of ceftriaxone is an option, particularly when, for example, vomiting disturbs oral administration.

Other medications

- Antihistamines, decongestants or NSAIDs are not beneficial in otitis A [24].
- Decongestants can be used for a few days as they may make the nasal breathing of a child with rhinitis easier and thus improve sleep.

Tympanocentesis

- Tympanocentesis does not speed recovery in the primary treatment of acute otitis media (AOM) and has therefore no role in the routine treatment of uncomplicated otitis B [25 26 27].
- Tympanocentesis may sometimes be indicated as first aid of severe earache or to clarify the aetiology of otitis in special circumstances:
  - generalized disease (e.g. mastoiditis or meningitis)
  - immunodeficiency
  - hospitalisation for severely impaired general condition.

Local anaesthesia for the tympanic membrane before tympanocentesis

- A lidocaine-prilocaine ointment (Emla®) is the drug of choice.

PAE

- A piece of cotton wool is soaked with the anaesthetic.
- If an alligator forceps is available, the piece of cotton wool can be placed directly on the tympanic membrane. If only an ordinary forceps is available, a tail in the piece of cotton wool should be left so that the piece can be removed easily.
- The tympanic membrane is anaesthesized in 30–60 min.

Supportive care

- Keeping the head end of the bed elevated may help the breathing of a child with nasal congestion.

Follow-up

- If the symptoms do not alleviate within a few days from the onset of antibiotic therapy, the ears should be re-examined already during the treatment.
  - If the tympanic membrane does not show signs of healing, changing to another antibiotic is often justified.
- The primary aim of follow-up is to identify children in whom the effusion and consequent hearing impairment continue for more than 3 months.
- A suitable time for a follow-up examination is about one month from the start of antibiotic therapy.
- Tympanometry (31.43) is a highly recommendable method for follow-up.
- In AOM, middle ear fluid normally remains for an average of 3–4 weeks (B) [28] [29] (Figure 31.42.1).
  - The range is from a few days to several months.
  - Approximately 10% of children still have fluid after 3–4 months.

No fluid in the middle ear

- If the tympanic membrane is normal, the child is asymptomatic and hears normally, there is no need for further follow up.

Fluid in the middle ear

1. If the child is asymptomatic, do not start a new course of antibiotics, but arrange for a new follow-up appointment 4 weeks later. If fluid persists and the child continues to be asymptomatic, reschedule a third follow-up visit one month from the second one. If the fluid has not disappeared in three months, refer the child to an ENT specialist for further treatment.
2. If the child has symptoms suggesting otitis (other that impaired hearing), start a new course of antibiotics with a second-line drug. Follow-up at one month, and, if necessary, as instructed in point 1.

Indications for specialist consultation

- Suspicion of a complication of otitis media (e.g. mastoiditis or facial paralysis).
- Discharge (31.45) from the middle ear that has continued for longer than 7 days (either through a tympanostomy tube or perforation) despite appropriate antibiotic therapy.
- Bacterial culture grows pseudomonas.
- Symptomatic otitis continues after a second-line antibiotic.
- The fluid has persisted for more than three months.
- Repeated AOMs (more than three within the last 6 months or more than four within the last year).
- The child had a hearing impairment already before the infection.

Chronic otitis media with effusion (OME)

- According to the commonly used definition, chronic OME is a condition in which there is effusion in the middle ear continuously for at least 2–3 months (Figure 31.42.1) without the symptoms or findings of acute infection.
- Up to several per cent of school-aged children have been found to have chronic OME.
- In the majority of the cases the condition develops as a consequence of AOM. In these cases, the effusion does not disappear from the middle ear in the course of a few weeks as usual. With prolonged secretion, the number of mucus-secreting cells on the epithelium of the middle ear increases, resulting in viscous, glue-like secretion.
- In some children, OME develops without an obvious preceding AOM.
- In about one-third of cases, bacteria can be cultured from the effusion.
- Diagnosing OME by otoscopy is often difficult, as the tympanic membrane may look misleadingly normal.
- The mobility of the tympanic membrane is, however, reduced or absent, and often also the transparency is diminished and the light reflex widened. Occasionally, air bubbles are detected behind the tympanic membrane.
- Tympanometer is a highly recommended device for diagnosing OME.
- As in the case of AOM, spontaneous cure is common also in OME.

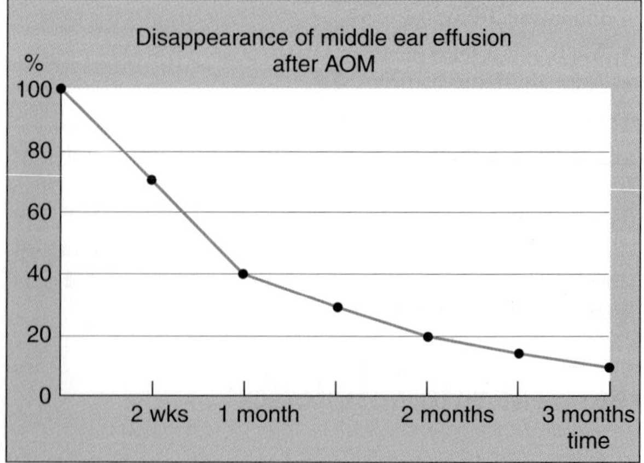

Figure 31.42.1 Disappearance of middle ear effusion after AOM

- If the child is found to have effusion in the middle ear without any symptoms and the tympanic membrane appears normal, antibiotics are not needed even if the child has other symptoms of acute respiratory infection.
- If the effusion persists in the middle ear for more than 3 months, the child should be referred to an ENT specialist for insertion of tympanostomy tubes **A** [30 31].
- In older children nasal balloon therapy may be tried (31.44)
- Antihistamines, decongestants or mucolytic agents have no effect in the treatment of OME.

References

1. Bertin L, Pons G, d'Athis P, ym. A randomized, double-blind, multicentre controlled trial of ibuprofen versus acetaminophen and placebo for symptoms of acute otitis media in children. Fundam Clin Pharmacol 1996;10:387–92.
2. Varsano IB, Volovitz BM, Grossman JE. Effect of naproxen, a prostaglandin inhibitor, on acute otitis media and persistence of middle ear effusion in children. Ann Otol Rhinol Laryngol 1989;98:389–92.
3. Hoberman A, Paradise JL, Reynolds EA, Urkin J. Efficacy of Auralgan for treating ear pain in children with acute otitis media. Arch Pediatr Adolesc Med 1997;151:675–8.
4. Glasziou PP, Del Mar CB, Sanders SL, Hayem M. Antibiotics for acute otitis media in children. Cochrane Database Syst Rev. 2004;(2):CD000219.
5. Rosenfeld RM, Vertrees JR, Carr J, Cipolle RJ, Giebink GS, Canafax DM. Efficacy of antimicrobial drugs for acute otitis media. J Pediatr 1994;124:355–367.
6. The Database of Abstracts of Reviews of Effectiveness (University of York), Database no.: DARE-940081. In: The Cochrane Library, Issue 4, 1999. Oxford: Update Software.
7. Damoiseaux RA, van Balen FA, Hoes AW, Melker RA. Antibiotic treatment of acute otitis media in children under two years of age: evidence-based?. British Journal of General Practice 1998;48:1861–1864.
8. The Database of Abstracts of Reviews of Effectiveness (University of York), Database no.: DARE-989715. In: The Cochrane Library, Issue 3, 2000. Oxford: Update Software.
9. Damoiseaux RAMJ, van Balen FAM, Hoes AW, Verheij TJM, de Melker RA. Primary care based randomised, double blind trial of amoxicillin versus placebo for acute otitis media in children aged under 2 years. BMJ 2000;320:350–354.
10. Damoiseaux RA, van Balen FA, Hoes AW, Melker RA. Antibiotic treatment of acute otitis media in children under two years of age: evidence-based?. British Journal of General Practice 1998;48:1861–1864.
11. Kaleida PH, Casselbrant ML, Rockette HE, ym. Amoxicillin or myringotomy or both for acute otitis media: results of a randomized clinical trial. Pediatrics 1991;87:466–74.
12. Burke P, Bain J, Robinson D, Dunleavey J. Acute red ear in children: controlled trial of non-antibiotic treatment in general practice. BMJ 1991;303:558–62.
13. Halsted C, Lepow ML, Balassanian N, Emmerich J, Wolinsky E. Otitis media: clinical observations, microbiology, and evaluation of therapy. Am J Dis Child 1968;115:542–51.
14. Laxdal OE, Merida J, Jones RH. Treatment of acute otitis media: a controlled study of 142 children. Can Med Assoc J 1970;102:263–8.
15. Del Mar C, Glasziou P, Hayem M. Are antibiotics indicated as initial treatment for children with acute otitis media? A meta-analysis. BMJ 1997;314:1526–9.
16. Mygind N, Meistrup-Larsen KI, Thomsen J, Thomsen VF, Josefsson K, Sörensen H. Penicillin in acute otitis media: a double-blind placebo-controlled trial. Clin Otolaryngol 1981;6:5–13.
17. van Buchem FL, Dunk JHM, van't Hof MA. Therapy of acute otitis media: myringotomy, antibiotics, or neither? A double-blind study in children. Lancet 1981;ii:883–7.
18. Kaleida PH, Casselbrant ML, Rockette HE, ym. Amoxicillin or myringotomy or both for acute otitis media: results of a randomized clinical trial. Pediatrics 1991;87:466–74.
19. Burke P, Bain J, Robinson D, Dunleavey J. Acute red ear in children: controlled trial of non-antibiotic treatment in general practice. BMJ 1991;303:558–62.
20. Jero J, Virolainen A, Virtanen M, Eskola J, Karma P. Prognosis of acute otitis media: factors associated with poor outcome. Acta Otolaryngol (Stockh) 1997;117:278–83.
21. Kozyrskyj AL, Hildes-Ripstein GE, Longstaffe SEA, Wincott JL, Sitar DS, Klassen TP, Moffatt MEK. Short course antibiotics for acute otitis media. Cochrane Database Syst Rev. 2004;(2):CD001095.
22. Kozyrskyj AL, Hildes-Ripstein GE, Longstaffe SE, Wincott JL, Sitar DS, Klassen TP, Moffatt ME. Treatment of acute otitis media with a shortened course of antibiotics: a meta-analysis. JAMA 1998;279:1736–1742.
23. The Database of Abstracts of Reviews of Effectiveness (University of York), Database no.: DARE-988673. In: The Cochrane Library, Issue 3, 2000. Oxford: Update Software.
24. Flynn CA, Griffin G, Tudiver F. Decongestants and antihistamines for acute otitis media in children. Cochrane Database Syst Rev. 2004;(2):CD001727.
25. van Buchem FL, Dunk JHM, van't Hof MA. Therapy of acute otitis media: myringotomy, antibiotics, or neither? A double-blind study in children. Lancet 1981;ii:883–7.
26. Engelhard D, Cohen D, Strauss N, Sacks TG, Jorczak-Sarni L, Shap M. Randomised study of myringotomy, amoxycllin/clavulanate, or both for acute otitis media in children. Lancet 1989;2(8655):141–143.
27. Kaleida PH, Casselbrant ML, Rockette HE, ym. Amoxicillin or myringotomy or both for acute otitis media: results of a randomized clinical trial. Pediatrics 1991;87:466–74.
28. Teele DW, Klein JO, Rosner BA. Epidemiology of otitis media in children. Ann Otol Rhinol Laryngol 1980;89:5–6.
29. Marchant CD, Shurin PA, Turczyk VA, Wasikowski DE, Tutihasi MA, Kinney SE. Course and outcome of otitis media in early infancy: a prospective study. J Pediatr 1984;104:826–31.
30. University of York. Centre for Reviews and Dissemination. The treatment of persistent glue ear in children. Effective Health Care 1992;1:pp. 12.
31. The Database of Abstracts of Reviews of Effectiveness (University of York), Database no.: DARE-950032. In: The Cochrane Library, Issue 4, 1999. Oxford: Update Software.

PAE

31.43 Acoustic impedance testing

Ilkka Kunnamo

Tympanometry

Indications

- Confirming the diagnosis of otitis media (B) [1, 2].
- Initial screening of children with upper respiratory tract symptoms
- Diagnostics of secretory otitis media
- Diagnostics of myringitis (a red tympanic membrane with a normal tympanogram)
- Follow-up of otitis media
- Verifying the patency of ventilatory tubes

Principles of operation

- The ear canal is sealed with the instrument, and the pressure in the ear canal is first elevated then lowered. The compliance of the tympanic membrane (the reciprocal figure of acoustic impedance) is recorded using a tone generator (normally 226 Hz) and a microphone.
- The horizontal position of the peak of the resulting graph indicates the pressure in the middle ear (the compliance is highest at this pressure). The height of the peak indicates the mobility of the tympanic membrane. If the middle ear is filled with fluid and the tympanic membrane is immobile, the resulting graph is a straight line.
- The instrument also measures the volume of the ear canal.

Recording technique

- An earpiece of appropriate size is inserted gently but tightly into the orifice of the ear canal and is held in place for the duration of the recording (usually 1–3 seconds). A drop of ultrasonic jelly on the outer edge of the earpiece allows to achieve ear-tightness with less insertion pressure.

Interpretation

- A straight line (B curve) is probably due to fluid in the middle ear (sensitivity 65–85%, specificity 95%).
- A markedly negative pressure peak (< −200 dPa) indicates subatmospheric pressure in the middle ear and dysfunction of the eustachian tube.
- An extreme negative pressure peak (<−300 dPa) is an indication for a follow-up examination within 2–4 weeks.
- In the initial phase of acute otitis media, a positive pressure peak (>+ 30 dPa) is occasionally seen.
- If the ventilatory tubes are patent, the instrument either indicates that ear tightness is not achieved or prints a B graph with a high ear canal volume (usually above 2 ml).
    - A peaked graph indicates that the tube is not patent, but the middle ear is normally ventilated through the eustachian tube.
    - A flat graph with a small volume (below 1-0–1.5 ml) indicates that the tube is not patent and there is fluid in the middle ear.

Sources of error

- If the child struggles or cries during the recording, an artefact graph of irregular shape is obtained. It is less likely that the child will cry if tympanometry is performed as the first step before otoscopic examination.
- Identical graphs in repeated measurements suggest that the result is reliable.
- The examination is usually not possible if the earpiece is pressed against the ear canal or an earwax clot, although a B-curve is sometimes obtained.
- A thickened tympanic membrane in healing otitis media may yield a flat graph, although some mobility of the tympanic membrane can be detected by pneumatic otoscopy.
- A small amount of fluid does not yield a B-curve; however, the peak is often wide.
- Compliance (the peak height) changes with age: in infancy the lower threshold is 0.1 cm^3, in pre-school age 0.2 cm^3 and in adolescence and adulthood 0.3 cm^3.

Choosing the examiner

- Nursing personnel can learn to perform tympanometry as an initial examination of children with symptoms of upper respiratory tract infection. A normal graph indicates a normal middle ear, and pneumatic otoscopy is not always necessary. In the case of a flat graph, a physician should examine the ear.

Acoustic otoscope (reflectometry)

- The instrument is cheaper and easier to transport than a tympanometer.

Uses

- See tympanometry above.

Principles of operation

- A tone is directed into the ear canal, and the reflection of the tone is investigated. The result is the amount of reflected sound (reflectivity reading) and in newer models a spectrum of the reflected sound with the peak angle defined.
- A mobile tympanic membrane reflects a small amount of sound energy, and low (normal) reflectivity is recorded. If the tympanic membrane is immobile, a lot of sound is reflected, and high (abnormal) reflectivity is recorded.

- In contrast to tympanometry, the crying of the child does not interfere with the recording (the instrument only records during pauses in crying).

Recording technique

- The ear canal is straightened by gently pulling the ear lobe upwards and backwards.
- The earpiece is held rather tightly to the orifice of the ear canal, and the axis of the tone emitter is rotated in different directions (a straight "listening view" of the ear drum is sought for) while the tone trigger knob is pressed continuously. The (repeatedly) highest reflectivity reading is recorded.
- After the examination the ear canal must be inspected to exclude total obstruction by cerumen (a wax prop obstructing up to three quarters of the ear canal does not yet prevent recording).

Interpretation

- Reflectivity 7–9: fluid in the middle ear is probable.
- Reflectivity 5 (6): borderline case; pneumatic otoscopy is necessary.
- Reflectivity 1–4: normal mobility of the tympanic membrane.
- In the ear with a ventilatory tube a reflectivity of 1–4 indicates patency of the tube or a normal middle ear with expulsion of the tube.

Sources of error

- If the earpiece is too far from the orifice of the ear canal, a falsely low reflectivity is recorded.
- If the ear canal is not straightened, reflectivity may be falsely low.
- Eardrops in the ear canal can result in falsely low reflectivity.

Choosing the examiner

- Nursing personnel can learn to perform acoustic reflectometry as an initial examination of children with symptoms of upper respiratory tract infection. The use of the instrument requires more experience than the tympanometer, as false negative results can be obtained with inappropriate recording techniques.

References

1. van Balen FAM, de Melker RA. Validation of a portable tympanometer for use in primary care. Int J Pediatr Otorhinolaryngol 1994;29:219–25.
2. Koivunen P, Alho O-P, Uhari M, Niemelä M, Luotonen J. Minitympanometry in detecting middle ear fluid. J Pediatr 1997;131:419–22.

31.44 Treating low middle ear pressure with nasal insufflation

Jouko Suonpää

Low middle ear pressure

- Low middle ear pressure observed after acute otitis media or at a routine health check is caused by impaired function of the Eustachian tube. If the condition persists the risk of serous or secretory otitis media increases (31.40). The peak at tympanometric recording is observed between −200 and −400 dPa.
- The most important measures to manage the condition are prevention and adequate treatment of respiratory tract infections and the removal of fluid from the middle ear.
- If the symptoms of acute otitis media are absent a follow-up of a few months is indicated. During the follow-up period, opening of the Eustachian tube can be promoted by repeated Valsalva manoeuvres or by using a nasal insufflation balloon.
- Children above 3 years of age can learn to perform insufflation with a nasal balloon. The treatment normalizes the pressure in the middle ear and promotes the healing of secretory otitis media (C) [1].

Techniques

- After inspiration one nostril is closed and the balloon is insufflated to a diameter of 15–20 cm with the nose piece placed in the other nostril. Another person can also fill the balloon.
- Next the balloon is allowed to deflate into the nose, and the child attempts to swallow several times.
- The procedure is repeated three times a day, and the ear is re-examined after 3 weeks. The method can be used on any occasion when the child feels that the ear is obstructed.
- Insufflation should not be carried out during an attack of acute otitis media.
- The low pressure tends to recur after common colds, and long-term follow-up of the middle ear is indicated. (The mobility of the tympanic membrane is examined with a pneumatic otoscope or tympanometer.)
- If no response is observed after 2–3 months the child should be referred to an otorhinolaryngology specialist.
- Nasal balloon insufflation can also be used in adults with recurrent Eustachian tube obstruction or barotitis (38.41).

Reference

1. Reidpath DD, Glasziou PP, Del Mar C. Systematic review of autoinflation for treatment of glue ear in children. BMJ 1999;318:1177–1178.

PAE

31.45 Otorrhoea in children with tympanostomy tubes

Terho Heikkinen

Aim

- To stop otorrhoea effectively and ensure the patency of the tube.

General

- Insertion of tympanostomy tubes is the most frequent ENT operation on children.
  - The primary indication is chronic OME ("glue ear").
  - Tympanostomy tubes also have some effect in preventing recurring episodes of otitis.
  - The tubes facilitate the diagnosis of otitis and enable bacteriological sampling without tympanocentesis.
- The tubes usually remain patent for 8–12 months.
- 20–50% of children with tympanostomy tubes have at least one episode of otorrhoea.
- The diagnosis is based on the detection of otorrhoea through the tube, other findings related to the tympanic membrane are not diagnostically significant in this context.
- If the ear with a tube is painful without discharge, blocking or loss of the tube should be suspected primarily.

Otorrhoea immediately after insertion of the tubes

- Otorrhoea on the days following insertion of the tubes is quite common.
- The discharge usually stops spontaneously without any treatment.
- If pathogenic bacteria are cultured from the secretion, the child can be treated with an antibiotic selected according to the sensitivity tests.

Acute otorrhoea

- Acute otitis media that develops in connection with an upper respiratory tract infection is the main cause of otorrhoea through tympanostomy tube.
- In such case, the causative bacteria are usually the same as in any episodes of AOM, and oral antibiotics can be selected according to the same principles as in normal AOM (31.42).
- A sample for bacterial culture should always be taken from the secretion before starting antibiotics.
  - The culture results are needed if the otorrhoea does not stop in a few days as was expected.
  - Bacterial culture is particularly important when concomitant symptoms of viral respiratory infection are lacking.
  - The cause of prolonged otorrhoea can be for example Pseudomonas aeruginosa or Staphylococcus aureus.
  - Coagulase-negative staphylococci, which are occasionally found in culture, belong to the normal bacterial flora of the ear canal and are most probably innocent contaminants.
- The significance of eardrops in the management of acute tube otorrhoea is rather small.
  - Their effective use would require daily cleaning of the ear canal at a doctor's surgery.
  - The use of ototoxic eardrops should be restricted to the most difficult situations.
- Otorrhoea usually stops with oral antibiotics within 3 days.
- A short course of steroid as an adjunctive to antibiotics (e.g. prednisolone 2 mg/kg/daily for a maximum of 3 days) clearly shortens the duration of otorrhoea; however, steroids must not be given to children during the incubation period of chickenpox.
- Soon after the otorrhoea has discontinued, the ear should be examined to ensure that it is cured and that a blockage of the tube did not bring about the end of discharge.
- The patency of the tube can be examined with tympanometry (31.43).

Prolonged otorrhoea

- If otorrhoea persists for more than one week despite antibiotics selected according to the bacterial sensitivity tests, or if pseudomonas grows on culture, the child should be referred to an ENT specialist.
- In addition to bacterial infection, other causes can prolong otorrhoea (for example granulation tissue, polyps).
- In prolonged otorrhoea the bacterial spectrum can vary greatly from that in acute otorrhoea, often changing as the condition persists.

31.50 Chickenpox

Editors

Basic rules

- Prevent chickenpox in immunocompromized patients with Zoster hyperimmunoglobulin and treat symptomatic disease with antiviral drugs.
- Give antiviral medication to chronically ill or severely atopic persons as well as to persons on peroral corticosteroids.

Clinical picture

- There are no prodromal symptoms.
- A maculopapular rash starts suddenly and quickly develops into vesicles.
- Body temperature is slightly elevated.
- Pneumonia (cough, opacity in chest x-ray) is rare in children but occurs in 15–30% of adults. The risk is increased during pregnancy and in smokers.
- Streptococci and staphylococci can cause secondary bacterial infections.
- Meningoencephalitis is rare (1:3000–10 000).
- 10% of all cases of Reye's syndrome are associated with chickenpox. Aspirin and possibly also other NSAIDs should be avoided in patients with chickenpox.
- Post-infectious transient thrombocytopenia may be associated with chickenpox, sometimes with haemorrhagia.
- Post-infectious cerebellitis presents as cerebellar symptoms (ataxia, disturbance of balance) after chickenpox infection.

Contagiousness

- Chickenpox is easily spread by droplets already one day before the emergence of the rash, and for one week thereafter (until the vesicles have dried).
- The incubation period is 12–16 (10–20) days.

Chickenbox in pregnant women and at the time of delivery

- **If a woman gets chickenpox 0–5 days before delivery or during the first two days after delivery** there is a high risk of infection of the foetus or neonate. About 17% of such neonates are clinically infected, with a mortality as high as 31%. Therefore **all exposed neonates should be treated with Zoster hyperimmunoglobulin (ZIG)**.
- If one of the neonate's sisters or brothers gets chickenpox the neonate need not be treated with ZIG.
- Chickenpox may be dangerous for a pregnant woman. Chickenpox in a pregnant woman or chickenpox exposure in a pregnant woman who has not had the disease is an indication for immediate consultation with a gynaecologist or specialist in internal medicine. Decisions on treatment are made in the hospital individually.

Vaccine

- A vaccine containing live attenuated virus is available. Its efficacy is best in healthy children. About 5% of them have a mild exanthema after the vaccination. In children with cancer the vaccine fails more often. The vaccine does not afford full protection.
- In most countries the vaccine is not yet included in vaccination programmes, but combining it with the MMR (measles-mumps-rubella) vaccination is investigated. See separate article on vaccinations 3.1. The vaccine can be prescribed for children aged 12 months or above whose parents ask for it.

Treatment

- ZIG should be given to a patient exposed to chickenpox who has **leukaemia, lymphoma, or congenital or acquired immunodeficiency, and who has not had chickenpox before or the history is unclear.** Exposure is defined as a case of chickenpox or herpes zoster in the family, or chickenpox in a companion (with whom the patient has been in the same room for at least one hour). In a hospital, exposure is defined as a case in the same room. ZIG should be given within 72 hours of exposure. However, there is no absolute limit in this regard.
- **If an immunocompromised child gets chickenpox he/she should receive acyclovir in a hospital**. Varicella virus is less susceptible to acyclovir than herpes simplex virus. Hence acyclovir should be administered intravenously (45 mg/kg/day). In mild cases, oral valacyclovir therapy is sufficient.
- There are no established recommendations on the treatment of healthy children with acyclovir B [1]. Treatment is clearly indicated if the child has a chronic disease or severe atopy or if he/she is on peroral corticosteroids. The dose is 20 mg/kg × 4 × 5 perorally in mixture form. The treatment should be started within 24 hours of onset of the rash.
- Itch can be treated with hydroxyzine. Secondary bacterial infections of the skin (erythema of the skin around crusts, impetigo) can be treated, for example, with cephalexin (50 mg/kg/day perorally).

PAE

Reference

1. Klassen TP, Belseck EM, Wiebe N, Hartling L. Acyclovir for treating varicella in otherwise healthy children and adolescents. Cochrane Database Syst Rev. 2004;(2):CD002980.

31.52 Rubella

Editors

Infectivity

- The incubation period is 14–21 days.
- Infectiousness starts about 2 days before the onset of symptoms and lasts for one week.
- Rubella is nowadays extremely rare in countries in which it is included in the vaccination programme.

Symptoms

- Mild catarrhal symptoms
- Fever (may be absent)
- Enlarged lymph nodes in the neck and jaw angles already before the rash
- A macular rash spreads from the face onto the trunk and extremities, and disappears in 2–3 days.

Diagnosis

- The clinical picture is not sufficient for diagnosis.
- The diagnosis should be verified by paired serum samples, which should always be taken for epidemiological reasons (monitoring of epidemics and the effectiveness of rubella vaccinations).

Complications

- Risk of foetal injury. Termination of pregnancy is indicated if a woman has rubella during the first 16 weeks of pregnancy.
- Symptoms in the joints are common in adolescents and adults.
- Thrombocytopenic purpura (rarely).
- Encephalitis (rarely).
- The administration of gammaglobulin does not help to prevent the disease after exposure.

Vaccination

- Rubella vaccination (3.1) prevents the disease effectively.
- If a pregnant woman has no rubella antibodies she should be vaccinated after delivery.

31.53 Erythema infectiosum

Editors

Definition

- Erythema infectiosum (fifth disease) is an exanthematous disease caused by parvovirus. It affects most often children aged 5–15 years and occurs as epidemics in the spring.

Symptoms

- The most typical symptom is a macular or slightly elevated rash starting from the face ("slapped cheek") (Figure 31.53.1). The cheek lesions are flushing red but they are not tender.

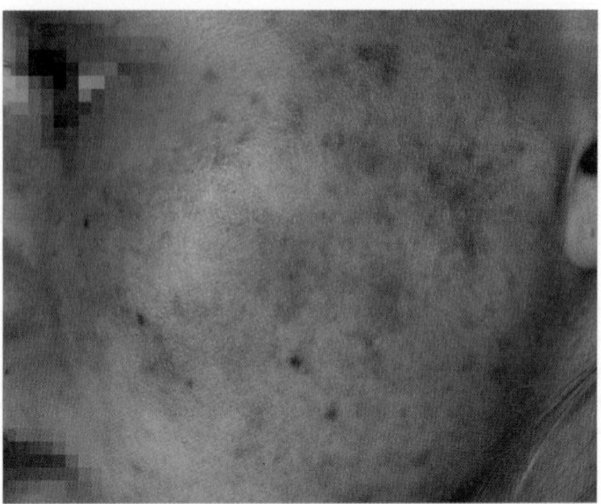

Figure 31.53.1 In parvovirus infection ("5th disease") the skin on the cheeks is unevenly red, like "slapped"; similar erythema is often visible on the lateral aspects of the upper arms and on the trunk. Parvovirus B19-3 is considered to be the causative agent. The disease is cured spontaneously. Photo © R. Suhonen.

- Lack of tenderness, symmetry, and good general condition differentiate the disease from bacterial cellulitis.
- A maculopapular rash follows the cheek lesions within 1–4 days. The rash starts from the extensor surfaces of the upper limbs and spreads in a reticular pattern predominantly on the limbs.
- The rash lasts typically 3–7 days, but it can disappear and reappear over several weeks.
- A part of the patients have fever, headache, pharyngitis and myalgia before the rash appears.
- During the rash, 15–30% have fever. Arthralgia and arthritis are rare in children, but more common in adults.
- Incubation time is 6–16 days. School-aged children are mostly affected, and several members of the same family may fall ill. In the rash-phase infectivity is low, and children can attend day care of school
- The infection is asymptomatic in many patients.

Diagnosis and treatment

- The diagnosis is based on the clinical picture.
- Serological diagnosis (IgM) is available, but not necessary in practice.
- The treatment is symptomatic.

Complications

- Parvovirus infection during pregnancy often causes an infection in the foetus. The virus has not been found to cause malformations.
  - Infection of the foetus may cause hepatitis and bone marrow depression, which can lead to abortion (in about 10%).
  - The parvovirus infection is diagnosed serologically. After serological confirmation, the patient is referred to a

prenatal clinic. The clinic then organises fetal monitoring in order to detect infection of the foetus and possible signs of anaemia.

- The virus may cause aplastic crisis in a patient with malignant haematological disease.

31.54 Exanthema subitum

Editors

Basic rule

- More serious diseases should be ruled out as the cause of fever.

Aetiology

- Human herpesviruses (HHV) 6 and 7

Clinical picture

- Children aged 6 months –2 years are affected. The infection probably spreads when the baby is held in arms.
- The disease starts with fever that lasts for 3–5 days, after which a rash appears. In a small proportion of the children the rash starts during the fever, and in an equal proportion there is an interval of one day between the fever and the rash. The rash lasts from a few hours to a couple of days.
- Separate, small, red macules or maculopapular lesions start around the ears and spread on the face, neck and trunk.
- Additional findings include conjunctivitis, eyelid oedema, small spotlike papules in the uvula and palate, lymphadenopathy in the neck and occipital area and bulging fontanelle.
- Only a minority of children with HHV infection develop the typical exanthema subitum. In most cases the infection manifests a high fever without obvious localizing symptoms.
- Febrile convulsions, which occur in 10–15% of infants with the infection, are the most important complication.

Differential diagnosis

- See the article about child with fever without localizing symptoms 31.1.
- A urine sample is necessary to rule out pyelonephritis.
- A low CRP concentration helps to rule out bacterial infection if the disease has lasted for more than 12 hours.
- In exanthema subitum CRP hardly rises at all, whereas in a septic infection it is clearly elevated.
- CRP determination at the first encounter is not necessary if
  - the general condition is good
  - the child drinks well
  - the child is not tender to touch.

31.60 Urinary tract infection in a child

Matti Uhari

Basic rules

- The diagnosis of urinary tract infection (UTI) in children must always be based on bacterial culture from one sample that has been taken by direct puncture of the bladder or from two samples of cleanly voided urine.
- The treatment of urinary tract infections is aimed at preventing sepsis and permanent kidney damage.
- Investigating children after their first urinary tract infection results in the detection of treatable structural anomalies at an early stage.

Epidemiology

- The incidence is 7/1000 in infants below 1 year of age. Boys and girls are equally affected at this age.
- At a later age mainly girls are affected.

Aetiology

- Escherichia coli is by far the most common aetiological agent.
- Klebsiella, enterococci, and Pseudomonas are infrequent. The less frequent bacteria are usually isolated in patients with structural abnormalities, or prolonged or recurrent UTI.
- The same E. coli strain can nearly always be isolated from both the urine and the faeces. The bacterial counts that are mentioned later are applicable to E. coli; however, even smaller counts of other bacteria may sometimes imply an infection.

Symptoms and signs

- Fever without respiratory symptoms in infants, particularly if the child is irritable and the general condition is affected. See 31.61.
- Poor weight gain, vomiting, frequent crying, or poor appetite in an infant.
- In older children the symptoms include frequent voiding, newly started enuresis, dysuria, and abdominal pain after voiding.
- The parents' observation that the smell of the urine has become foul.

Diagnosis

- The diagnosis of a child's first UTI should be reliable because a false positive diagnosis leads to unnecessary further investigations and follow-up.
- The diagnosis must always be based on bacterial culture.
- The bladder should always be punctured (31.61) if a UTI is suspected and a cleanly voided urine specimen cannot be obtained, or if the treatment must be started before the result of the bacterial culture is available. Puncture is relatively easy to perform, and complications are very rare. If ultrasonography is available, confirming that the bladder is full before puncture is attempted is easy.
- If a bacterial count of 10^5/ml or more is detected in a cleanly voided or bag urine specimen a UTI is probable. A count around 10^3/ml does not rule out infection if the urine has not been in the bladder for a minimum of 4 hours.
- For the decision on the necessity the treatment, the probability of a UTI must be estimated on the basis of a dipstick test or microscopy.
  - A dipstick test positive for nitrites is a reliable indicator of a UTI, but the usefulness of the test is limited by the fact that enterococci, Staphylococcus saprophyticus, and some Acinetobacter species do not produce nitrites. In infants the urine does not always stay in the bladder for long enough.
  - The sensitivity of the dipstick test for leucocytes is high, and a positive result for leucocytes must be confirmed by microscopy (5 or more leucocytes/high-power field in the sediment is significant, corresponding to 25 leucocytes or more per mm^3 of fresh uncentrifuged urine in a counting chamber).
  - If several uniform bacteria per high-power field are seen at microscopy of a fresh uncentrifuged urine specimen a UTI is probable.
- Start the treatment of a symptomatic child after the samples for confirming the diagnosis have been obtained (either one sample from bladder puncture, or two cleanly voided urine samples). If the suspicion of a UTI turns out to be false the treatment is stopped and the parents are informed that the child did not have a UTI. Further investigations are not performed.
- The most important source of error is the technique of sampling. Voided urine is always contaminated by perineal bacteria, and the sample is never sterile. The method of sampling should be taken into account when the reference value for bacterial growth is determined. A cleanly voided urine specimen is the best non-invasive form of urine sampling. The sample can be obtained from children using a chamber pot by placing the sampling vessel in the front part of the pot so that a sample of mid-stream urine hits the vessel.

Determining the level of infection

- The child has pyelonephritis if the serum CRP concentration is above 40 mg/l or the child has fever of at least 38.5°C.
- All infants below 3 months of age should be considered to have pyelonephritis irrespective of the above-mentioned criteria.

Principles of treatment

- Place of treatment
  - Children below 2 years of age who have fever should be initially treated in a hospital.
  - Children above 2 years of age should be referred to a hospital if they have serious general symptoms. In most cases ambulatory care is appropriate for children below school age with a UTI, and for children above school age who also have fever.
- Before culture results are available, the treatment should be directed against E. coli because it is the most common aetiological agent.
- An infant with high fever, a high serum CRP concentration, and irritability, should be treated parenterally in a hospital, and parenteral treatment should be continued as long as the child has fever or the CRP concentration remains high. Further peroral treatment is often indicated thereafter.

Antibiotic treatment

Perorally

- Even a renal infection in children below and at school age can be treated perorally with trimethoprim-sulfamethoxazole or 2nd or 3rd generation cephalosporins.
- Cystitis can also be treated with trimethoprim-sulfamethoxazole. Other suitable drugs include pivmecillinam, cephalosporins, and trimethoprim alone.
- Amoxicillin and nitrofurantoin are effective against enterococci.

Parenteral treatment in a hospital

- Cephalosporins are effective against gram-negative rods. Cefuroxime (100 mg/kg/24 h), cefotaxime (100 mg/kg/24 h), ceftriaxone (80 mg/kg/24 h), and ceftazidime (100 mg/kg/24 h) are good choices for parenteral treatment. The price is the only practical difference between the drugs in addition to the fact that ceftriaxone can be administered only once daily.
- Aminoglycosides are effective against E. coli and they are excreted in the urine in high concentrations. There are no significant differences in the toxicity of different aminoglycosides, and it is obvious that they are safe in the treatment of UTI in children.
- If enterococci are isolated from the urine, amoxycillin should be given.

Duration of treatment

- The duration of treatment varies according to the severity of the infection, the age of the child, and the causative agent.

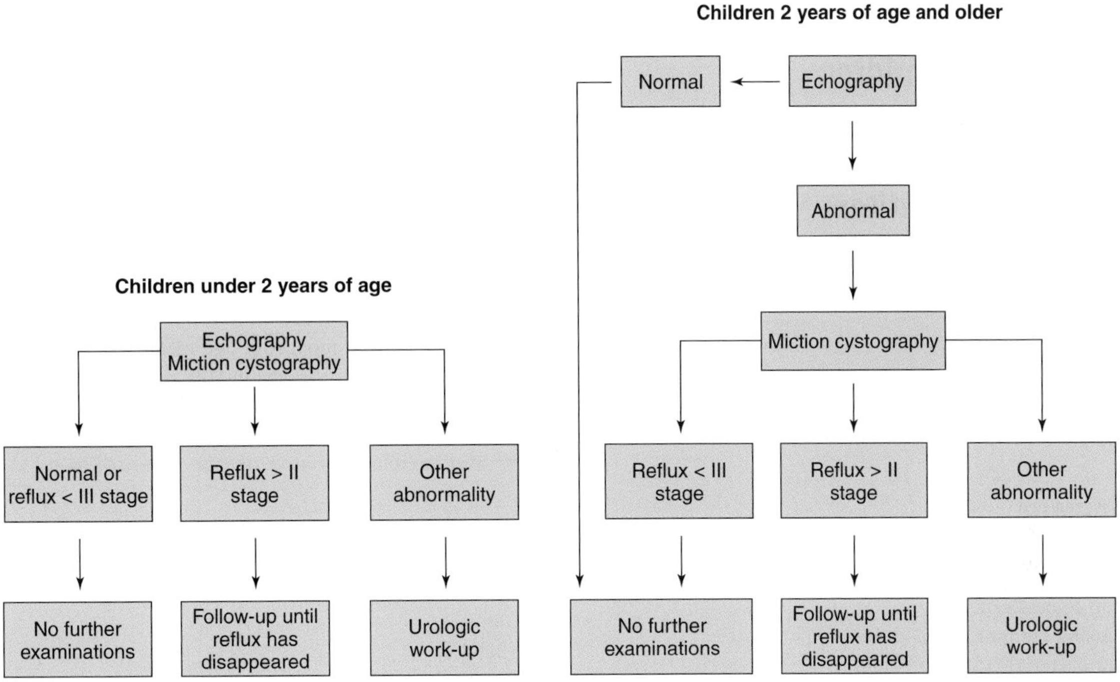

Figure 31.60.1 Further investigations in children with urinary tract infection

- Infants should be treated for 10 days.
- Infections in older children should be treated for at least 5 days to prevent early recurrence.

Treatment of constipation

- Severe constipation may increase the risk of UTI. Constipation should always be diagnosed and treated in a child who has had a UTI.

Further investigations

- See Figure 31.60.1
- As the value of Tc^{99}DMSA scintigraphy is not yet known it is not recommended for routine use.
- Vesicoureteral reflux is the most important underlying condition.
- Other structural anomalies include
  - hydronephrosis
  - ureterocele
  - urethral valve in boys.
- A structural anomaly requiring surgical treatment or follow-up is detected in nearly 25% of the patients.
- Recurrence of a UTI is most common in children with cystitis without structural anomalies.

Follow-up

- A monthly urine specimen should be taken for 6 months after the infection from all children with vesicoureteral reflux who have had a UTI. Bag urine samples are adequate in infants, and cleanly voided urine samples in older children. If the test suggests a UTI, the diagnosis should be confirmed with a new sample, or if necessary, with bladder puncture.
- If a UTI has not recurred within 6 months and the child does not have a vesicoureteral reflux (>grade II) dilating the renal pelvis, the follow-up can be discontinued.

PAE

Prophylactic medication

- If the child has a vesicoureteral reflux of grade III–V, prophylactic medication is indicated after the first UTI C [1]. The medication should be continued until the reflux has disappeared or improved so that there is no dilatation of the renal pelvis during miction.
- Nitrofurantoin (1–2 mg/kg/day) is the drug of choice B [2].
- During prophylactic medication a urine test should be performed four times a year, and always if the child has symptoms suggesting a UTI.

References

1. Smellie JM, Barratt TM, Chantler C, Gordon I, Prescod NP, Ransley PH, Woolf AS. Medical versus surgical treatment in children with severe bilateral vesicoureteral reflux and bilateral nephropathy: a randomised trial. Lancet 2001;357:1329–1333.
2. Williams GJ, Lee A, Craig JC. Long-term antibiotics for preventing recurrent urinary tract infection in children. Cochrane Database Syst Rev. 2004;(2):CD001534.

31.61 Urine aspiration sampling in children

Editors

Indication

- Verifying urinary tract infection

Equipment

- 20 ml syringe
- A thin injection needle
- Cleansing equipment, bandages
- Urine bacterial culture medium
- Blood bacterial culture bottle

Performing the aspiration

1. Lidocaine–prilocaine gel anaesthesia is recommended (the skin is anaesthesized in 30–45 minutes). Infiltration anesthesy is not indicated.
2. The bladder should be as full as possible. In an acute situation, a one-hour wait after urination is often enough. The child should drink during the wait.
3. The child lies supine with the legs straight, held by a safe and calm adult.
4. Disinfect the skin over the bladder with an antiseptic (e.g. 0.01% chlorhexidine solution). If an ultrasonography device is available the doctor should check the filling and position of the bladder before the procedure. **At this point a sterile container should be kept available for a "flying sample" in case the child begins to urinate.**
5. Take some 3 ml of air in the syringe before the puncture to make it easier to observe the urine flow into the syringe. Insert the needle perpendicularly to the skin through the transverse skin fold above the symphyse (or where ultrasonography indicates that the bladder is closest to the skin) and aspirate a sample (10–15 ml). If no urine is obtained after inserting the needle rather deep, retract the needle slowly and aspirate gently. Sometimes a specimen is obtained at this stage.
6. Remove the needle and cover the puncture site with a small dressing. If no sample was obtained try again after 30 min.
7. Take both an ordinary urine culture sample, and inject urine into a blood bacterial culture bottle.

31.70 Meningitis in children

Heikki Peltola

Aetiology

- In children above 3 months of age meningococci and pneumococci are causative agents in 90% of cases. Haemophilus has almost disappeared because of vaccinations.
- In the newborn, group B streptocci, E. coli and Listeria are the most common causative agents.

Symptoms suggesting meningitis in the newborn

- Irritability
- Disturbances of consciousness
- Difficulty in breathing
- Hypotonicity
- Crying
- Jaundice
- Poor eating
- Diarrhoea and vomiting
- Neck stiffness is by far less common in children below 6 months than in older children. Irritability, or its opposite, lethargy, are prominent symptoms; the child is awake but does not react when approached, and no normal contact can be made with him.

Symptoms of meningitis in the older child

- Fever and headache ("has never before had such headache")
- Vomiting
- Neck stiffness
- Disturbances of consciousness
- Petecchiae and purpura

Councelling by telephone

- Find out the following three things:
  - Can you get contact with an infant normally?
  - Does an older child have neck stiffness (which can be tested by asking him to touch his knees with his nose)?
  - Does the child have red spots (petecchiae)?
- If the answers are negative, and the child eats and drinks normally, and particularly if the child has respiratory symptoms, observation at home is safe.

First aid for a child with suspected meningitis

- If the patient is in shock, immediately infuse sterile **Ringer solution** or **4% albumin** 20 ml/kg for 15 minutes and monitor the response (pulse, blood pressure, peripheral temperature). If there is no response to the infusion, repeat with the same volume.
- If the patient is not clearly in shock, infuse sterile Ringer solution 10 ml/kg for 15–30 minutes, continue according to response.
- Maintenance fluid therapy consists of **5% glucose** with 0–20 mmol/l of sodium chloride, and 20–50 mmol/l of potassium chloride according to the duration of the condition.
    - Do not give pure glucose solution, because it may cause hyponatraemia and increase cerebral oedema; avoid volume overload.
- Convulsions should be treated with diazepam (0.5 mg/kg ad 10 mg) either as a rectal solution or an intravenous injection (29.2).
- Impaired consciousness and convulsions are signs of increased intracranial pressure, which can be treated with efficient mask ventilation during transportation to the hospital.

Timing of antibiotics

- Antibiotics are usually started in the hospital. The first doses may liberate bacterial toxins that worsen the patient's condition.
- If there is a strong suspicion on meningitis (an infant with poor general condition and bulging fontanelle, or an older child with neck stiffness, impaired consciousness or petecchiae) and the journey to the hospital takes at least 1 (-2) hours, start intravenous fluids, give dexamethasone 0.15 mg/kg intravenously (A) [1 2 3 4 5 6], and start a slow infusion of penicillin G (0.5–1 million units per hour). There is a good theoretical basis for this practice, but little clinical documentation.
- Before antibiotics are started, a blood bacterial culture should be obtained, and preferably also a lumbar puncture should be performed. However, it must not delay the fastest available transportation to a specialized care unit.

References

1. Prasad K, Haines T. Dexamethasone treatment for acute bacterial meningitis: how strong is the evidence for routine use. J Neurol Neurosurg Psych 1995;59:31–37.
2. The Database of Abstracts of Reviews of Effectiveness (University of York), Database no.: DARE-951931. In: The Cochrane Library, Issue 4, 1999. Oxford: Update Software.
3. McIntyre PB, Berkey CS, King SM, Schaad UB, Kilpi T, Kanra GY, Perez CM. Dexamethasone as adjunctive therapy in bacterial meningitis: a meta-analysis of randomized clinical trials since 1988. JAMA 1997;278:925–931.
4. The Database of Abstracts of Reviews of Effectiveness (University of York), Database no.: DARE-978360. In: The Cochrane Library, Issue 2, 2000. Oxford: Update Software.
5. de Gans J, van de Beek D; European Dexamethasone in Adulthood Bacterial Meningitis Study Investigators. Dexamethasone in adults with bacterial meningitis. N Engl J Med 2002 Nov 14;347:1549–56.
6. van de Beek D, de Gans J, McIntyre P, Prasad K. Corticosteroids in acute bacterial meningitis. Cochrane Database Syst Rev 2003(3):CD004305.

31.71 Encephalitis in children

Editors

Basic rules

- Suspect encephalitis on the basis of clinical symptoms and refer the child to a hospital for diagnostic assessment.
- All children with suspected herpes encephalitis should be treated with acyclovir in hospital.

Symptoms

- Acute or subacute neurological symptoms suggesting brain parenchymal affection (coma, convulsions, focal symptoms or altered mental state) are typical of encephalitis.
- Symptoms suggesting encephalitis include
    - headache
    - nausea and vomiting
    - fever
    - impaired consciousness
    - ataxia
    - altered mental state
    - convulsions
    - positive Babinski's reflex
    - muscular hypotonia
    - meningism
    - altered tendon reflexes
- The symptoms of encephalitis are not always dramatic. The essential clues for diagnosis are obtained from the history as related by the parents and by adequate neurological examination.
- Varicella encephalitis usually manifests about two weeks after the initial illness with ataxia and disturbance of balance (caused by cerebellitis).

Causes of encephalitis

- Since universal vaccination has almost eradicated measles and mumps, the most important aetiological agents are
    - varicella

PAE

- enteroviruses
- adenoviruses.

- Herpes simplex causes only about 6% of all cases of encephalitis.
- Arboviruses cause encephalitis in several areas, e.g. tick-borne encephalitis in the Baltic region and in Central Europe, and Japanese encephalitis (2.32) (spread by mosquitoes) in Eastern and South-Eastern Asia.

Treatment

- Treatment that covers herpes virus, bacteria causing meningitis and borrelias (intravenous acyclovir + ceftriaxone) is immediately started for all patients with a suspicion of encephalitis (symptoms from central nervous system associated with an infection and without other cause, or EEG findings suggesting encephalitis).

Prognosis

- The prognosis is good with the exception of herpes encephalitis and Japanese encephalitis. About 70% of patients with herpes encephalitis recover fully, about 20% remain permanently affected and about 10% die. The prognosis is worst in children below one year of age and in those who present in an unconscious state.

31.81 Infections in immunocompromized children

Jukka Rajantie

Aims

- Early recognition of
  - septicaemia or risk of it
  - severe viral illnesses
  - Pneumocystis carinii pneumonitis.

Centralization of treatment

- Cytostatic treatment for children is provided by hospitals with paediatric haemato-oncologists or oncologically trained paediatricians. Therefore, families have been advised to contact directly the hospital responsible for the treatment of their child.

Signs of septicaemia

- Fever during neutropenia due to bone marrow suppression: contact immediately the nearest paediatric hospital. In cases with a blood neutrophil count $< 0.5 \times 10^9$/l, blood culture is taken and broadspectrum antibiotics started i.v.
- Abdominal pain and diarrhoea can be the first signs of septicaemia.
- Focal infections without fever (otitis, sinusitis) can be treated normally if the general condition of the patient is good.

Viral infections

- Children undergoing chemotherapy for malignancy (especially leukaemias and lymphomas) need to have a zoster hyperimmunoglobulin injection (2 ml i.m. if the child weighs less than 20 kg and 4 ml i.m. if the weight is more) within 72 hours of contact with a person with varicella or varicella zoster if the patient's varicella disease history is negative. If a patient, however, already has symptoms he/she should be treated with i.v. acyclovir at hospital.
- Consult the specialist unit if a child undergoing chemotherapy becomes sick with measles. Usually chemotherapy needs to be discontinued for the duration of the disease. The child does not always need hospitalization.

Pneumocystis carinii

- Most children with cancer chemotherapy have trimethoprim-sulphamethoxazole prophylaxis to prevent P. carinii pneumonia. If, however, such a patient is suffering from a low-grade fever and frequent and superficial breathing they should be admitted to a paediatric hospital for chest x-ray and arterial blood oxygen measurement. The diagnosis is confirmed by a lung biopsy.

Splenectomized children

- Such children are usually vaccinated against Streptococcus pneumoniae, Neisseria meningitidis and Haemophilus influenzae at least one month before the operation. In cases of high fever, however, blood culture should be taken and the patient hospitalized for appropriate antibiotic therapy i.v.

31.83 Mumps

Editors

Contagiousness

- The incubation period is 14–21 days.
- The contagious period begins as a highly infective droplet infection 1–2 days before and ends about 7 days after the onset of clinical symptoms.
- The disease is nowadays extremely rare in countries in which it is included in the vaccination programme.

Symptoms

- Fever
- Unilateral or bilateral swelling of the parotid salivary glands spreading above the jaw angle and in front of the ear which differentiates the disease from lymphadenopathy
- Pain on swallowing
- Meningoencephalitis begins within a few days from the onset of other symptoms with headache, nausea, and vomiting.
- Encephalitis is far less frequent, and usually develops more than one week after the onset of other symptoms.
- 30–40% of men who get mumps after puberty are affected by orchitis
  - Swelling, increased temperature, and tenderness of the testis
  - Both testes are affected in 20% of the patients.
  - 2% of men who had bilateral orchitis become infertile.
- Pancreatitis, thyroiditis, salpingitis, mastitis, and hearing impairment are rare manifestations.

Diagnosis

- The clinical picture with fever and bilateral parotid swelling is characteristic in unvaccinated patients. Other causes of parotid swelling must be considered if the patient has been vaccinated against mumps.
- Paired serum samples at 2 week intervals are recommended in suspected mumps patients for seroepidemiological reasons in areas where vaccination is universal.

Treatment

- Bed rest reduces headache during the fever.
- Analgesics.

Vaccination

- See 3.1.

31.84 Discharging BCG scars in infants

Eeva Salo

Normal vaccination reaction

- The BCG vaccination contains live bacteria. An induration that develops at the vaccination site 2–6 weeks after the vaccination and that may burst and discharge for a few weeks is a normal and desired reaction to the vaccine.
- The discharging vaccination site should be covered with clean dressings. Slight swelling of the local lymph nodes is often associated with the reaction.

Atypical reactions to the vaccine

- Fluctuating abscess and large lymph node in the groin are indications for referral to a specialist. Antimicrobial medication and/or incision may be necessary.
- A discharging ulcer remaining for several months after the vaccination may be caused by secondary bacterial infection. Take bacterial culture and treat with first-generation cephalosporin. A deep, crater-like ulcer is an indication for referral.

Paediatrics

Evidence Based Medicine Guidelines. Edited by the Duodecim Editorial Team
 ISBN: 0-470-01184-X

32.1 Anaemia in children

Jukka Rajantie

Aims

- Distinguish leukaemias and acute haemolytic anaemias as these conditions require immediate referral to a paediatric hospital with haematological experience.
- Reveal the underlying cause of iron deficiency.
- Ensure an adequate response to iron medication.

Examinations in primary health care

- Note the age-dependent variation of blood haemoglobin concentration
  - at birth > 150 g/l
  - 1–4 months > 100 g/l
  - 5 months–5 years > 105 g/l
  - 6–15 years > 115 g/l
- Register the general condition, colour of the eyes (conjunctivae), jaundice, signs of infection, pains, lymph nodes, size of liver, spleen and testes, cardiovascular functions, signs of bleeding, oedema.
- Laboratory tests in mild anaemia: haemoglobin (Hb), mean corpuscular volume (MCV), white blood cell count (WBC), platelets (reticulocytes, if possible).
- If haemoglobin < 100 g/l: also test leucocyte differentials, blood cell morphology, sedimentation rate (and red (blood) cell size distribution width (RDW), if technically possible). The appearance of small erythrocytes in the peripheral blood is the first sign of iron deficiency. Their appearance during early disease and disappearance in response to therapy can be seen only on histogram or by microscopy. The MCV can be normal.
- If the MCV is not small (normocytic or macrocytic anaemia), consult a paediatric haematologist or paediatrician (usually a direct Coombs test, liver and kidney function tests, folate and vitamin B12, and faecal and urinary blood search are recommended).
- If a child has a pure anaemia with normal other blood cells, the direct Coombs test is negative and he/she is not bleeding, prompt action is unnecessary.
- If other cell lines are also deviant, suspect leukaemia and refer the child immediately to a hospital with preparedness for bone marrow examination and treatment of leukaemia.

Treatment of iron deficiency anaemia

- If the haemoglobin and MCV values are low, but in line with each other, the child usually has iron deficiency anaemia. Start oral ferrous sulphate (Fe++) at a dose of 4 mg/kg/day in 1–3 doses, preferably taken into an empty stomach with orange juice.
- Follow up haemoglobin after two weeks, and if possible, reticulocyte count (plus histogram or red blood cell morphology by microscopy). The diagnosis was correct if a treatment response is observed. Reticulocytosis is a clearly more rapid measure of successful iron therapy than the raised haemoglobin value.
- **Continue iron medication for at least three months after haemoglobin has normalized.**
- When the diet has provided too little iron, correcting the child's nutrition is an important part of therapy. Consumption of milk should be limited to a maximum of 500 ml per day.

Clarify the cause of iron deficiency

- Iron deficiency is merely a symptom, not a disease. Find its cause. In cases of poor response to iron medication, think again! Look for dietary causes for insufficient intake of iron (especially in small children), for malabsorption and for blood loss due to bleeding (in older children in particular).
  - Diet history (too much milk?) and, if necessary, a diary of one week's meals
  - Colour of stools (black?)
  - Growth curves; relevant antibodies in the serum for the detection of coeliac disease, if indicated.
  - Tests for blood in urine and stool (blood is examined from three stool samples)
  - Refer to a paediatric hospital if blood is detected in the stools (sedimentation rate, endoscopies, Meckel scan). Possible diagnoses include Meckel's diverticulum or terminal colitis, in older children ulcerative colitis or Crohn's disease.
  - Sometimes anaemia of a pre-school-aged child results from occult gastrointestinal bleeding associated with excessive intake of cow's milk. The child may also have hypoproteinaemia that responds to iron medication. Usually the child drinks large amounts of milk, and reduction of milk consumption can be recommended on the basis of history alone. Total abstinence is not necessary.

Investigations and treatment of anaemia at the hospital

- If a direct Coombs test is positive: the child has autoimmune haemolytic anaemia (AIHA). Start prednisolone immediately with 2–4 mg/kg/day in three doses. RBC transfusion is given only in emergency.
- If the child has Coombs-negative haemolytic anaemia, and spherocytes are seen on a blood film during the neonatal period, the newborn's and mother's blood groups (ABO; Rh) should be examined. From older children take family history and RBC osmotic fragility test (also after a 24-hour incubation time) or AGLT (acidified glycerol lysis test). Patients with congenital spherocytosis (CS) may need RBC transfusions if the haemoglobin concentration falls clearly below 80 g/l. Serum bilirubin and haptoglobin might give additional information on the degree of haemolysis. High plasma haemoglobin level, disappearance of

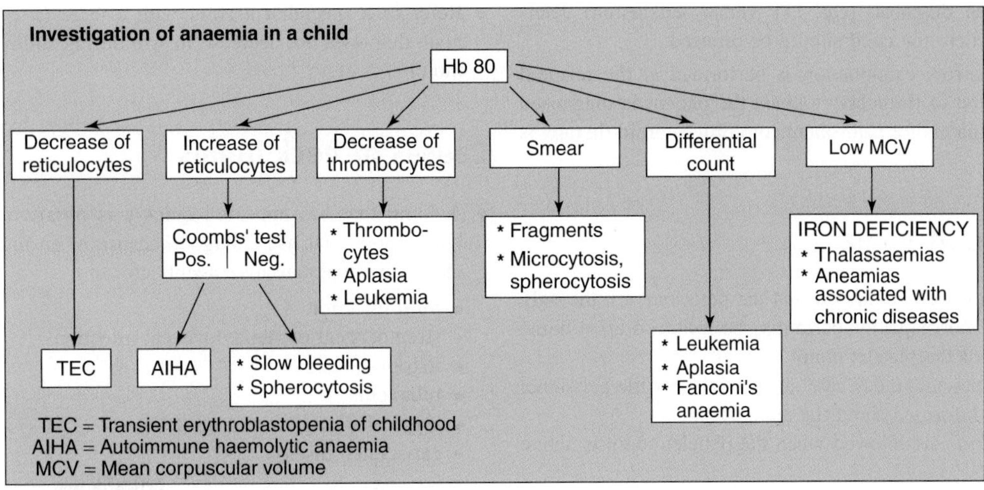

Figure 32.1.1

haptoglobin binding capacity, and the presence of RBC fragments in the blood smear indicate intravascular haemolysis.

- If there is also thrombocytopaenia, ask about intestinal symptoms and check the urine and serum creatinine for possible haemolytic uraemic syndrome.
- If the reticulocyte count is low despite anaemia and the MCV normal or enlarged, these may be due to bone marrow hypoplasia. Check for other blood cell lines and ensure that the child does not have congenital spherocytosis (aplastic crisis usually after erythema infectiosum). Transient erythroblastopenia of childhood (TEC) is the most probable aetiology. Keep also in mind rare inborn syndromes: Diamond-Blackfan anaemia (infants) and Fanconi's anaemia (older children). Bone marrow examination is usually indicated. If leukaemia is suspected (abnormalities in other blood cell lines) refer the patient to a paediatric hospital the same day for bone marrow examination.
- Thalassaemia minor and haemoglobinopathies (Hb S, C, E) are examples of microcytic anaemias that do not respond to iron medication. Take family history, verify ethnic background, examine parents' haemoglobin and MCV, and consider haemoglobinelectrophoresis and haemoglobin isoelectric focusing of the child's erythrocytes.

32.2 Bruises and purpura in children: ITP and its differential diagnosis

Jukka Rajantie

Clinical characteristics

- Idiopathic thrombocytopenic purpura (ITP) in children is an acute autoimmune disorder, with normal or increased platelet production in the bone marrow but shortened platelet survival in the peripheral blood.
- ITP typically appears in early childhood with bruises, petechiae and isolated thrombocytopenia. Half of the patients have had an acute (usually viral) infection or have been vaccinated (MMR) 2–3 weeks earlier.
- If a patient has high fever and the general condition is poor, suspect another disease (meningococcal septicaemia, leukaemias); see 31.3. See also Henoch–Schönlein purpura 32.53.

History

- Any medicines (e.g. valproate, acetylsalicylic acid)
- Signs or symptoms of infections in the patient or people in physical contact with the patient
- Vaccinations
- Urine or stool blood
- Headache
- Abdominal complaints (Henoch–Schönlein syndrome)
- Joint symptoms (Henoch–Schönlein syndrome)
- Family history (autoimmune diseases?)

Investigations

- Signs of infections or bleeding
- Liver and spleen size
- Tumours
- Giant haemangiomas (may use up thrombocytes, Kasabach–Merritt syndrome)
- Auscultation of the head, neck and abdominal area (AV malformations, etc.)
- Haemoglobin, RBC indices and morphology, white blood cell count (WBC) and differentials, platelets and CRP can be investigated in primary care (on call) mainly in cases when
  - the child has few bruises and petechiae and the diagnosis is uncertain (normal values may make referral unnecessary).

- the initial diagnosis (e.g. ITP versus leukaemia) determines where the child should be referred.
- A bone marrow examination is performed at the hospital if in addition to thrombocytopenia the patient is diagnosed with anaemia and/or neutropenia or corticosteroid therapy is initiated.

Follow-up at home

- When it has been confirmed that the petechiae are the only sign of haemorrhage, the child may be followed up at home regardless of the platelet count.
- The child can attend day care and school after the personnel have been informed about the condition.
- Contact sports are allowed when the platelet count is above 50×10^9/l.
- Aspirin is absolutely contraindicated. Other NSAIDs and fish oil can also prevent agglutination of thrombocytes.
- Haemoglobin, thrombocyte count, urine erythrocytes and stool blood (if considered necessary) should be checked at 1–4-week intervals. The interval is prolonged when the platelet count begins to rise. Follow-up is stopped when the count has been twice above 150×10^9/l.
- In most children, thrombocytopenia will resolve by itself within few months, but in a minority of patients (15 to 20%) it becomes chronic and will last over 6 months. In such cases, consult a paediatric haematologist.

32.3 Enlarged lymph nodes and other neck lumps in children

Editors

Basic rules

- Bilateral lymph node enlargement on the neck that begins to diminish during a few weeks' follow-up: calm the parents and do the follow-up without laboratory investigations.
- A unilateral lymphadenitis of the neck is an indication for pharyngeal group A streptococcal culture.
- The following laboratory investigations can be performed on a child with fever: haemoglobin, leucocytes, differential white cell count, platelets, CRP, ESR and mononucleosis test.
- A unilateral, tender, or erythematous lymph node or an infected salivary gland: treat as a bacterial infection.
- Refer the child to a hospital if the general condition is impaired, there is respiratory distress, or the lymph node is fluctuating or it is large and situated in an unusual place (e.g. the subclavicular fossa) or the blood picture is abnormal.
- Refer to a specialist a child with a large (>2 cm) lymph node that does not decrease in size during follow-up of one month.

Causes of neck lumps

- A lump that has appeared quickly is almost invariably a lymph node that has enlarged because of an infection. The most important causative agents are
  - viral infection
  - streptococcal or staphylococcal infection
  - toxoplasmosis
  - tularaemia
  - atypical mycobacterial infection
  - cat-scratch disease
- During the first few weeks of life a haematoma of the sternocleidomastoideus muscle is a common cause of neck lump.
- Dermoid cyst
- Bacterial infection of a salivary gland (situated on the jaw margin)
- Dental abscess
- Kawasaki disease (fever, rash, conjunctivitis) (32.57)
- Tumours originating from the thyroid gland, parotid glands, or neuronal tissues
- Lymphoma or leukaemia

A neck lump that has appeared acutely

- In the majority of the cases an acute bilateral lymph node enlargement is lymphadenitis associated with a viral infection (particularly adenovirus, Ebstein-Barr virus and cytomegalovirus). Less frequently the cause is streptococcal tonsillitis, which typically results in enlargement of the lymph nodes in the jaw angles.
- An acute unilateral neck lump is a bacterial lymphadenitis caused by Staphylococcus aureus or group A betahaemolytic streptococci in 40–80% of the cases; rarely an anaerobic or mixed infection. The lymph node is 2.5–6 cm in diameter, tender, warm, and red. Fever and other systemic symptoms are often absent. A solitary enlarged lymph node is a typical finding in Kawasaki disease and in the rare cat-scratch disease.

A neck lump that has been there for a long time

- Long-lasting lumps in the jaw angles and beside the sternocleidomastoideus muscle are almost invariably innocent. More than a half of school-aged, asymptomatic children have at least one lymph node exceeding 1 cm in diameter.
- It is important to observe the size of the lymph node and its enlargement during 2–4-week follow-up. Most lymph nodes detected by parents are "residuals" of an infection and they become smaller during follow-up.

- Be much more careful with lymph nodes that are situated in places other than near the jaw angle (particularly the subclavicular fossa). If a suspicion of malignancy arises refer the child to a paediatric unit immediately.
- The most common infectious causes of chronic lymphadenitis of the neck are toxoplasmosis, atypical mycobacteria, and cat-scratch disease.
- In toxoplasmosis (1.62) a single enlarged, non-tender, and fluctuating lymph node is situated in the posterior part of the neck. Most patients are otherwise asymptomatic. A serum IgG avidity test is the most important diagnostic investigation (the more recent the infection, the weaker the avidity).
- Atypical mycobacteria often cause unilateral lymphadenitis. Lymph node enlargement is at first rapid, but it ceases within 2–3 weeks. The skin over the enlarged lymph node may be erythematous, and as the infection continues the skin may adhere to the gland.
- Cat-scratch disease is most commonly caused by the bacterium Bartonella henselae. In about 50% of the cases a cat bite or scratch precedes the onset, which is characterized by erythema and induration at the site of the wound within 7–14 days, and the lymphadenitis that follows. Diagnosis can be made from a histological specimen.

Treatment

- Bilateral acute lymphadenitis needs no treatment, with the exception of lymphadenitis associated with group A streptococcal infection.
- Treatment of a unilateral acute neck lump is directed against the most common causative agents, staphylococci and streptococci. The recommended drugs include cephalexin, erythromycin (40 mg/kg/day in 3 doses), cloxacillin, and clindamycin. Because most staphylococci produce beta-lactamase, penicillin V is not recommended. A clinical response can be observed within 36–48 hours if the treatment is successful.

32.10 Interpretation of ECG in children

Eero Jokinen

General principles

- ECG must always be interpreted in respect to the age of the child.
- Modern recorders of twelve lead ECG often give a summary of the findings. The reliability of the interpretation varies markedly depending on the reference values used. The interpretation may be misleading, especially when the rhythm is evaluated. The summary often includes a comment like "possible hypertrophy". This may be due to high voltage measured in the recording of a single lead. Thus, the physician must always evaluate the ECG as an entity.
- Because of large individual variation and changes occurring with age the reference intervals are rather wide. ECG in children is not a very sensitive and accurate method for evaluating, for example, ventricular hypertrophy (B) [1].

Heart rate

- Table 32.10.1

Conduction intervals and QRS axis

- The ECG of a newborn and of an infant always shows right ventricular dominance and the electrical axis of the heart is to the right. The electrical axis will shift to the left as the child grows. In 8 to 12 year olds, the ECG may show rather strong left ventricular dominance and the QRS-axis may be more to the left than in adults. Not until teenage will the ECG resemble that of an adult.
- Table 32.10.2

QT interval

- Corresponds to the systole of the heart. The duration of this interval depends on heart rate.
- Table 32.10.3

ST segment and T wave

- ST segment may normally be elevated or depressed by one mm from the baseline in limb leads and slightly more in precordial leads.

Table 32.10.1 Heart rate

Age	Reference limits, beats per min (mean)
1–11 mo	105–185 (130)
1–2 yrs	90–150 (120)
3–7 yrs	65–140 (105)
8–15 yrs	60–130 (90)

Table 32.10.2 Conduction intervals (s) and QRS axis in different age groups

	Neonate	0.5–3 yrs	3–15 yrs
P wave (sec)	<0.09	<0.09	<0.10
PR interval (sec)	<0.14	<0.16	<0.18
QRS duration (sec)	<0.07	<0.08	<0.11
QRS axis (degrees)	+60 – +165 (+130)	+5 – +110 (+60)	0 – +110 (+60)

PAE

Table 32.10.3 The longest normal QT interval at various heart rates (sec)

Heart rate (/min)	Longest normal QT interval (sec)
50	0.49
60	0.44
70	0.42
80	0.39
100	0.35
120	0.32
150	0.28
170	0.27

Table 32.10.4 Physiological T inversions in precordial leads in children

Lead	Age
V1	ad 16 yrs
V2	ad 12 yrs
V3	ad 10 yrs
V4	ad 5 yrs
V5	ad 15 h
V6	ad 8 h

- T wave is normally always positive in leads I and II. It may be positive or negative in lead III and it is normally negative in lead aVR.
- T wave is negative in right-sided precordial leads throughout childhood until ca. 16 years of age (Table 32.10.4). In infants and in children of preschool age, a positive T wave in lead V1 suggests right ventricular hypertrophy.

Estimation of ventricular hypertrophy

- It is easiest to evaluate the degree of ventricular hypertrophy in precordial leads. However, deviation of the electrical axis to the right is suggestive of right ventricular hypertrophy and deviation to the left is suggestive of left ventricular hypertrophy.
- However, when assessing ventricular hypertrophy, it must be kept in mind that in 8 to 12 year olds both the R and S waves are 0.5 to 1 mV (5 to 10 mm when the amplification is 10 mm/mV) higher than in adults. Thus, in children of this age, the ventricular hypertrophy cannot be reliably measured from the sum of Q, R and S waves alone.
- When assessing ventricular hypertrophy, check the amplification used in the ECG recording: 5 mm/mV or 10 mm/mV?

Electrical axis

- Count the sum of R and S peaks in two limb leads (for example, lead I = horizontal axis and aVF = vertical axis; R = positive value, S = negative value). Draw a vector (the length of which is equivalent to the RS sum measured) on each of the two respective axis. Draw lines that are in 90° angles in respect to the tips of these vectors. Then draw a line that connects the starting point of the vectors and the crossing point of these lines. The sum vector drawn in this manner shows the electrical axis.

Right ventricular hypertrophy

- RV1 is higher than normally by age
- SV6 is deeper than normally by age
- Positive T wave in lead V1 during childhood after the first week of life
- QR complex in V1
- QRS complex with RSR' morphology in V1; an R' greater than 1 mV (10 mm) is suggestive of either right ventricular hypertrophy or right bundle branch block or both.
- Reference values for different age groups 32.10.5.

Left ventricular hypertrophy

- RV6 is higher than normally by age
- SV1 is deeper than normally by age
- Negative T wave in leads V5–V6 after the first day of life
- Deep Q in left sided precordial leads (in infants younger than 1 year, a Q wave deeper than 3 mm, in 1 to 5 year olds, a Q wave deeper than 3, 5 mm).
- Reference values for different age groups 32.10.5.

Biventricular hypertrophy

- The criteria for both right and left ventricular hypertrophy are fulfilled separately.
- Tall QRS complexes (R + S > 50 mm) in leads V3–V4

Right atrial hypertrophy

- High (>2.5 mm) and sharp P waves in leads II, III, aVF and V1

Left atrial hypertrophy

- Broad-P waves in leads I and II (P mitrale) and broad biphasic P wave that has a negative terminal portion in V1

Congenital heart malformations that may cause findings suggestive of right ventricular hypertrophy in ECG

- Pulmonary stenosis
- Various defects with left to right shunts and with increased pulmonary vascular pressure
- Coarctation in a neonate (usually)

Table 32.10.5 Upper limits for QRS voltages in children (mm)

Interpretation	Lead	Age < 1 mo	Age 1–12 mos	Age 1–15 yrs
Right ventricular hypertrophy	R V1	27	20	18
Left ventricular hypertrophy	S V6	10	7	6
	S V1	23	18	25
Right and left ventricular hypertrophy	R V6	16	23	27
	R+S V4	53	62	54

- Partial right bundle branch block, almost invariable in connection with atrial septal defect.

Congenital heart malformations that may cause findings suggestive of left ventricular hypertrophy in ECG

- Aortic stenosis
- Aortic coarctation in an older child (usually the ECG finding is minor)
- Patent ductus arteriosus (usually the ECG finding is minor).

Congenital heart malformations that may cause findings suggestive of biventricular hypertrophy in ECG

- Ventricular septal defects (either of the ventricles may dominate depending on pressure and flow circumstances)

Arrhythmias

Breathing variation

- In many children, phases of inspiration and expiration cause marked variance in beat intervals. If the P wave precedes the QRS-complex with a normal conduction interval, this irregularity in pulse rate is totally normal phenomenon.

Tachycardias

- Approximately one child in five hundred is congenitally predisposed to supraventricular tachyarrhythmias. The pulse rate is usually "uncountable" during the attack, with ECG showing mostly a pulse rate exceeding 200/min.
- If the tachycardia first appears already during infancy, the child almost certainly has a re-entry tachycardia even if no delta-waves are found in ECG.
- In Wolff-Parkinson-White syndrome, the anomalous pathway is able to conduct the impulse from the atria to the ventricles, and a delta wave is often visible during sinus rhythm.
- In such cases, an atrial arrhythmia may cause a dangerously rapid ventricular response, and a paediatric cardiologist should assess the patient for treatment. In tachycardias caused by either an extra pathway or by a so called duplicated AV node, eventual catheter ablation is preferably postponed until school age, if possible.

Long QT syndrome

- ECG must be registered in every child presenting with an attack of unconsciousness or an epileptiformic attack to exclude prolonged QT interval.
- Long QT-syndrome is a hereditary repolarisation disorder that predisposes to ventricular tachycardia. The disorder usually becomes symptomatic at school age or during young adulthood, presenting as a sensation of tachycardia or as a sudden syncope associated with physical exercise, excitement or startle. If a child with sudden unconsciousness or suspected epileptic seizure has a QT-interval longer than appropriate for pulse rate (Table 32.10.3; best assessed in leads V4–5 and II), further examinations are absolutely necessary.

Reference

1. Davignon A, Rautaharju P, Boisselle E, Soumis F, Megelas M, Choquette A. Normal ECG standards for infants and children. Pediatr Cardiol 1979;1:123–31.

32.11 Hypertension in children

Eero Jokinen

- Essential hypertension is rare in childhood or adolescence. A secondary cause behind the raised blood pressure should therefore be searched, e.g. renal disease, aortic coarctation, endocrine causes, raised intracranial pressure etc. Blood pressure medication should not be commenced before aetiological examinations have been conducted in specialist care.
- Further examinations conducted by a specialist are needed if the blood pressure values measured in a child exceed the 95th percentile values repeatedly (Table 32.11).

Clinical examination

- The diagnosis of systemic hypertension should be based on repeated blood pressure measurements within a few days. BPs from the right arm should be measured at least three times. The cuff bladder should cover 75% of the circumference of the arm. Using too narrow cuffs leads to incorrectly high BP recordings. Diastolic BP is defined as the disappearance of Korotkoff sounds (K5). If the sounds do not disappear, the point where they soften (K4) is recorded.
- Oscillometric devices for BP measurements may yield BP values slightly differing from those obtained with a sphygmomanometer (which is the standard method). Therefore, at least in borderline cases, sphygmomanometers should be used.

Table 32.11 95th percentiles for systolic and diastolic blood pressure

Age (yrs)	95th percentile (mmHg)
<1	110/60
1–5	115/75
6–10	125/85
11–18	140/90

PAE

- Crying elevates BP. Sometimes it is necessary to make arrangements that allow measurements of the BP when the child is asleep (28.3).
- If a child has high BP and a systolic murmure it is always essential to measure BP also from the thigh (sphygmomanometer) or leg to rule out or to confirm aortic coarctation. When an oscillometric device is used, lower limb BP is measured from the leg above the malleolar level. Normally the systolic pressure measured from the leg is at least as high as the systolic pressure measured from the upper arm C [1].
- Auscultation of the heart
- Palpation of the abdomen (renal cysts, tumours)
- Check for signs of endocrinological diseases (habitus typical of Cushing's syndrome, pigmentation) and signs of Turner's syndrome (short stature).

Aetiology and differential diagnosis

Neonates and infants

- Aortic coarctation
- Congenital malformations of the kidneys
- Renal artery stenosis (or thrombosis)

1–10-year-olds

- Renal parenchymal disease
- Aortic coarctation
- Renal artery stenosis

11–18-year-olds

- Renal parenchymal disease
- Aortic coarctation
- Essential hypertension (rare; secondary hypertension must always be excluded!)
- See also articles 4.22, 28.3.

Reference

1. Rahiala E, Tikanoja T. Suspicion of aortic coarctation in an outpatient clinic: how should blood pressure measurements be performed? Clin Physiol 2001;21:100–104.

32.20 Investigating a child with abdominal symptoms

Ilkka Kunnamo

Aims

- Diseases requiring surgical treatment are identified immediately.

Diseases

- Unnecessary laboratory investigations should be avoided: history and clinical examination are usually sufficient for preliminary diagnosis.

Acute appendicitis

- By far the most common cause of abdominal pain requiring urgent treatment.
- The diagnosis is based on local tenderness, provocation tests (jumping, coughing, rebound tenderness) and, in unclear cases blood tests B [1] [2]. Often follow-up in a hospital is needed to confirm the diagnosis.

Pyloric stenosis

- Suspect this condition if a child below 2 months of age vomits violently.

Intussusception of the small bowel

- Suspect this condition if a child below 2 years of age has cramping pain and poor general condition.

Non-surgical diseases

- Of non-surgical diseases urgent treatment is indicated in **severe bacterial infections** (pyelonephritis, meningitis) that should be remembered as potential causes of fever and vomiting.
- Most abdominal symptoms in children can be treated by the general practitioner. The most common one is 'dolores abdominis NUD' that has no known aetiology but apparently is a disease in its own.

History

- Age
- How acutely did the symptoms begin and how long have they lasted?
- Type of pain (continuous or paroxysmal?)
- Associated symptoms

Physical examination

Palpation of the abdomen

- If the child is frightened the examination is best performed with the child lying in the parent's arms on his back with his knees flexed.
- Testing for local tenderness should be started as far as possible from the expected site of pain.
- Defence of the abdominal wall is a sign of tenderness. The sign should be elicited several times to confirm its presence and location.

Digital rectal examination

- May be a frightening and painful experience for the child. Hence the examination should not be performed without an indication.

- If the suspicion of appendicitis is so strong that the child is referred to a hospital in any case, there is no need for digital rectal examination by the referring physician.
- Tenderness on the right side suggests appendicitis.
- Digital rectal examination is useful for assessing the quality of the faeces if invagination (children < 2 years of age) or severe constipation (usually in older children) is suspected.

General physical examination

- Ears and respiratory tract (infections)
- Genitals (testes), inguinal region (hernias)
- Skin (Henoch–Schönlein purpura)
- Weight loss should always be estimated in a child who is vomiting or has diarrhoea. In addition to the physical examination, measurements performed at the child health clinic should be used for reference (by extrapolating from the growth sheet, if necessary).

Laboratory investigations

Urine test

- A few per cent of children presenting with abdominal pain have a urinary tract infection.
- A dipstick test for the presence of leucocytes and nitrites is sufficient as a screening examination.
- Microscopy and bacterial cultures are performed if necessary. The diagnosis of a urinary tract infection must always be based on bacterial culture, preferably from two different samples (31.60).
- Some patients with appendicitis have pyuria but the presence of nitrites always suggests urinary tract infection.

Blood leucocytes and serum CRP

- Important examinations in cases where the symptoms have started rather acutely if they are mild but appendicitis is not ruled out.
- The clinical picture and its development in follow-up are the most important grounds for referral or treatment decisions, and a child with severe symptoms should never be discharged home even if the results of the laboratory tests are normal.
- If both serum CRP and blood leukocytes (B) [1 2] are normal, the pain has lasted for at least 12 hours, and is not severe, acute appendicitis is unlikely, and the child can be followed up at home.
- If one or both test results are abnormal the child should be referred to a hospital.
- If the pain has only lasted for a short time even normal laboratory results do not rule out appendicitis. On the other hand, advanced disease is improbable, and a few hours of follow-up is usually safe.
- Comparing axillar and rectal temperatures is of no use in the diagnosis of appendicitis.
- In painful constipation the blood leucocyte count may be high but serum CRP is normal.

ESR, haemoglobin, faecal blood, and serum endomysium or transglutaminase antibodies

- Indicated if a child with recurrent abdominal pain has
  - fever
  - diarrhoea
  - abnormal growth.

Lactose provocation test

- Should only be performed with strict indications in children below seven years of age (32.22).

Ultrasonography

- For indications see article 32.22.

References

1. Hallan S, Asberg A. The accuracy of C-reactive protein in diagnosing acute appendicitis. Scand J Clin Lab Invest 1997;57:373–380.
2. The Database of Abstracts of Reviews of Effectiveness (University of York), Database no.: DARE-971078. In: The Cochrane Library, Issue 4, 1999. Oxford: Update Software.

32.21 Acute abdominal symptoms in children

Ilkka Kunnamo

PAE

Diagnostic clues

- The most important specific causes and diagnostic clues for abdominal pain in different age groups are presented in the Table 32.21. Diseases requiring surgical treatment are indicated in bold type.

Pyloric stenosis

- Develops gradually from the second week of life and causes jet-like vomiting.
- The child should be referred to hospital at the latest when weightgain stops.

Invagination

- Typical symptoms include severe, paroxysmal cramping attacks between which the child can be almost asymptomatic.
- The general condition deteriorates rapidly.
- Watery, blood-stained stools ("meat water") is a typical finding.

Table 32.21 The most important specific causes of abdominal pain, and diagnostic clues in different age groups

Age group	Cause of pain	Diagnostic clues
0–2 y	**Pyloric stenosis**	Jet-like vomiting; age 2–8 weeks
	Invagination	Paroxysmal pain, some diarrhoea, "meat water" at DRC
	Hernia	Reposition is neither easy nor successful
	Testis torsion	Visible swelling (but intra-abdominal torsion is possible in retention)
	Gastroenteritis	Diarrhoea or vomiting are the first and dominant symptoms
	Otitis media	Ear status
	Urinary tract infection or other serious infection	Fever and vomiting without evident diarrhoea; urine test
3–11 y	**Appendicitis**	Transfer of pain, pin-point tenderness, jumping test
	Dolores abdominis NUD	The most common entity; important to differentiate from appendicitis
	Mesenterial lymphadenitis	Clues do not differ from those of appendicitis
	Gastroenteritis	Diarrhoea at onset, non-existent or slight tenderness on palpation
	Constipation	History, hard stools; pain is often severe
	Pneumonia	Cough, findings on auscultation, chest radiograph
	Sinusitis	Local symptoms, ultrasonography, sinus radiograph
	Tonsillitis	Inspection of the pharynx
	Urinary tract infection	Urine test
	Henoch–Schönlein purpura	Petechial rash
>11 y	**Appendicitis**	See above
	Gastroenteritis	See above
	Salpingitis	Only in the sexually active
	Ovarian cyst	May burst at exertion
	Urinary tract infection	Urine test

Diseases needing surgical treatment are indicated in bold type.

- A sausage-like abdominal mass is often felt on palpation (right and upper mid-abdomen).
- On digital rectal examination the rectal ampoule is empty or there may be a small amount of watery and bloody stools.
- Repositioning of the bowel in a radiological procedure with air or contrast media is usually successful.

Incarcerated hernia

- Typically seen in children below 1 year or age, rarely in older children.
- The main symptom is pain, and in prolonged condition vomiting and symptoms of occlusion.
- The most important finding is a tender, hard, reddish mass in the area of the inguinal canal above the inguinal ligament.
- Scrotal hydrocoele may be associated with incarcerated hernia.
- Reposition of an incarcerated hernia
    - Press the hernia from its peak with three fingers towards the inguinal canal. The pressure can be considerable, as the risk of rupturing the incarcerated intestine is minimal. Continue to press for several minutes until the hernia retracts.
    - Refer the patient to hospital for surgical correction that should take place within a few days. The child should be transferred to a paediatric surgery unit immediately if the hernia is not repositioned.
- Differential diagnosis of incarcerated hernia
    - Tight or acute hydrocoele or funicocoele
    - Inguinal lymphadenitis
    - Testicular torsion

Acute testis

- Differential diagnoses
    - Testicular torsion
    - Acute hydrocoele
    - Torsion of appendix testis
    - Epididymitis/epididymo-orchitis
- The peaks of incidence are in the neonates and prepubertal boys.
- Torsion of the epididymis and epididymitis are more common than testicular torsion.
- Frequently the initial symptom is abdominal pain.
- In all above-listed conditions inspection and palpation of the testes reveals swelling and tenderness. In testicular torsion the testis is usually retracted to the upper part of the scrotum or the opening of the inguinal canal.
- Acute scrotum requires urgent surgery unless torsion is excluded with certainty.

Gastroenteritis

- A common cause of abdominal pain in children.
- Gastroenteritis is the most probable diagnosis if diarrhoea and vomiting are the main symptoms, and (mild) oscillating abdominal pain presents simultaneously.
- There is usually no tenderness on palpation.

Respiratory infections

- Pneumonia, sinusitis, otitis media, and sometimes also tonsillitis may cause abdominal pain.

- Upper respiratory tract and ear status and readily also chest and sinus x-rays or sinus ultrasonography are indicated if findings suggesting appendicitis are not quite clear.

♦ In particular, pneumonia of the right lower lobe may cause referred pain at McBurney's point.

Urinary tract infection and other serious bacterial infections

♦ Infections often present with fever and vomiting.
♦ Do not make a diagnosis of gastroenteritis if the child does not have obvious diarrhoea.

Acute appendicitis

♦ The initial symptom is nearly always pain in the umbilical region.
♦ Location of the pain in the right lower quadrant suggests a more advanced disease causing peritoneal irritation.
♦ If there is palpable tenderness at McBurney's point in a very small area (pin-point tenderness), appendicitis should be highly suspected.
♦ Pain elicited by movements and vibration is typical of appendicitis.
♦ Jumping is a good provocation test: ask the child to jump on both heels, or down from a small chair. If this does not cause any pain appendicitis is improbable.
♦ Vomiting is a typical symptom in appendicitis. Unlike gastroenteritis it usually begins only after the pain has lasted for a relatively long time.
♦ Diarrhoea is less frequent than vomiting, and it is never profuse.

Constipation

♦ Strong pains are most often associated with acute constipation; in chronic constipation they are rare.
♦ The pain is fluctuating and is felt in mid-abdomen.
♦ In acute constipation a palpable mass of retained faeces is usually not felt. On digital rectal examination the rectal ampoule is however filled with hard faeces.
♦ The initial treatment of painful coprostasis is one enema (bisacodyl mini-enema or a 120 ml enema). Large-volume water enemas should be avoided. In addition to dietary advise, other therapy is usually not needed.

Anal fissure

♦ The main symptom is pain on defecation and bright blood on the faeces or on the toilet paper.
♦ The fissure is visualized by inspection of the borderline of skin and mucosa; digital rectal examination is painful and is not necessary for diagnosis. Contrary to adults, in children an anal fissure can be located anywhere on the anal circumference.
♦ Painful defecation makes the child afraid of defecating, which results in constipation and delays the healing of the fissure as large hard faeces tear the fissure open repeatedly.
♦ Anal fissure is quite often the cause of constipation also in infants.
♦ Almost all fissures are cured with conservative therapy that consists of bulk laxatives (e.g. lactulose) and ointments to protect the anus (e.g. white vaseline). Haemorrhoid and fissure ointments intended for adults should not be used for children.
♦ Very rarely (<5%) does a fissure become chronic in a child necessitating surgical treatment. Dilatation of the anus alone is not sufficient for a chronic fissure.

Henoch–Schönlein purpura

♦ The initial symptom is paroxysmal abdominal pain.
♦ A papular, and later petechial rash on the buttocks and lower extremities is a clue to the diagnosis.
♦ Invagination is a rare complication of the disease.

Other causes

♦ A teenaged, sexually active girl may pose a diagnostic problem. Potential causes of abdominal pain include
  - appendicitis
  - causes of genital origin
  - rupture of a cyst in the ovary (causes sudden abdominal pain, sometimes associated with physical exertion. The pain subsides during follow-up and laboratory test results are normal.)
  - extrauterine pregnancy.

PAE

32.22 Recurrent abdominal pain in children

Ilkka Kunnamo

Definition

♦ Abdominal pain is defined recurrent when it lasts for at least 3 months and interferes with the child's normal activity.

Symptoms and aetiology

♦ Most common at the age of 6 to 12 years.
♦ Nausea or even vomiting, loose stools, heartburn, and, in older children, headache, may be associated.
♦ Although in the majority of cases recurrent abdominal pain in children is functional, the cause is quite often organic (e.g. gastritis, oesophagitis).

- Lactose intolerance rarely develops before the age of 3–4 years. The symptoms resemble those of adults: abdominal swelling, flatulence, and diarrhea. The symptoms are maximal about 2 hours after a meal containing milk products.
- Constipation may cause abdominal pain.
- At least one child in three has psychosocial problems (33.2). The assessment of these problems may require consultations with the whole family and specialized services.
- Most children with recurrent abdominal pain come from quite normal families, and comparative studies have not found any psychogenic aetiology.
- Rare causes of recurrent abdominal pain include
  - food intolerance
  - coeliac disease
  - gastro-oesophageal reflux
  - inflammatory bowel disease
  - hypothyroidism
  - disorders of the urinary tract (hydronefrosis is detected in 1% of children with recurrent abdominal pain).

Examinations

- Palpation of the abdomen and digital rectal examination
- Blood count, ESR, lactose provocation test, and endomysium or transglutaminase antibodies.
  - Lactose provocation test is indicated in children below school age if the history clearly suggests that the symptoms are associated with milk ingestion, and particularly if family members have lactose intolerance. Interprete the test positive only if the child gets symptoms during the test, and the rise in blood glucose is pathologically small.
  - The serological tests for coeliac disease are sensitive. The diagnosis must be verified by small bowel biopsy.
- Consult a specialist if the pain is exceptionally annoying or often recurring.
- Abdominal ultrasonography is useful in the diagnosis of (obstructive) urinary tract problems. It should be performed if the pain is colicky, severe, and disturbs the child.
- The determination of helicobacter antibodies or a helicobacter breath test may be indicated if there is a patient with peptic ulcer in the family.

32.23 Diarrhoea and vomiting in children

Per Ashorn, Ilkka Kunnamo

Aims and basic rules

1. Make a diagnosis
   - Usually a viral gastroenteritis
   - Exclude all other causes (e.g. intussusception, serious bacterial infections, etc.)
   - History and clinical examination are usually sufficient, laboratory tests are seldom needed.
2. Assess the degree of dehydration in per cent and grams
   - Mild 4%, moderate 8%, severe 12%
   - In a child below 1 year 5–10–15%, in an adult 3–6–9%, respectively
   - Dry mucous membranes, decrease in tears and oliguria suggest mild dehydration
   - Above-listed signs combined with cool periphery, loss of skin elasticity and prolonged (> 2 seconds) capillary refill time on the palmar surface of the distal fingertip suggest moderate dehydration (B) [1]. The loss of skin elasticity is shown in the "tent" phenomenon: when a fold of abdominal skin is pinched and raised, it remains raised like a tent and does not immediately retract back like it normally would.
   - Above-listed signs and deep, gasping breathing, ice-cold periphery and poor general condition suggest severe dehydration.
   - Observed or estimated weight loss should also be used to estimate dehydration in grams (in acute disease dehydrations almost equals weight loss).
3. Choose the place of care
   - Usually the child's home; see indications for referral to hospital below.
4. Plan and instruct how to give treatment (see next section)
5. Plan and instruct how to implement follow-up
   - Improvement in general condition
   - Sufficient urine excretion
   - Weight gain
6. Give a prognosis
   - Viral gastroenteritis usually continues for 4–7 days, rotavirus disease sometimes even longer.

Treatment

1. Rehydrate the child with oral rehydration solution (ORS) (A) [2 3]. Give 4/3 of the amount of fluid deficit over a period of 6–10 hours.
   - The fluid can be given from a bottle, drinking glass, by spoon or syringe.
   - Most children prefer to take the fluid cold
2. After the rehydration phase a normal diet is resumed.
3. If diarrhoea or vomiting continues, advise the parents to make sure the child has adequate fluid and salt intake. This can be achieved through normal feeding, but if the child is suffering from anorexia, additional fluid intake should be encouraged. Fluids with very low (e.g. water) or very high (e.g. soft drinks) osmolarity should be avoided as the only diet during viral gastroenteritis, since their excessive use may lead to disturbances in salt balance or aggravation of diarrhoea in the patient.

- The adequacy of fluid intake can be judged from a number of easily observable clinical signs. A child, whose tongue looks damp, who passes a reasonable amount of urine and who sheds tears when crying is normally adequately hydrated.

Indications for referral to hospital

- The child is referred if even one of the following criteria is met:
  - Age below 6 months
  - Profuse diarrhoea or vomiting, poor general condition
  - Dehydration of 8% or more (at least moderately severe dehydration)
  - Diarrhoea lasting for more than 5 days (the general condition and loss of weight are decisive factors)
  - Colicky abdominal pain (and sudden ceasing of the diarrhoea)–intussusception?
  - Bloody diarrhoea
  - Suspicion of hypo- or hyperosmolalic dehydration based on the clinical picture or foregoing treatment
  - Inability to treat the child at home
- If the child is in shock when referred, infuse Ringer solution 20 ml/kg in 15 minutes.

References

1. Steiner MJ, DeWalt DA, Byerley JS. Is this child dehydrated. JAMA 2004;291:2746–2754.
2. Gavin N, Merrick N, Davidson B. Efficacy of glucose-based oral rehydration therapy. Pediatrics 1996;98:45–51.
3. The Database of Abstracts of Reviews of Effectiveness (University of York), Database no.: DARE-961213. In: The Cochrane Library, Issue 4, 1999. Oxford: Update Software.

32.25 Foreign body in the gastrointestinal tract of a child

Risto Rintala

- The type, consistency, and form of a swallowed foreign body determine the intensity of attempts to locate and remove it. The guidelines are based on the following principles:
  - A mercury battery may perforate the bowel or cause serious mercury poisoning.
  - A foreign body stuck in the oesophagus may cause severe symptoms.
  - A foreign body that has passed through the oesophagus into the stomach usually exits spontaneously without causing symptoms.

Guidelines

1. If the swallowed object is known to be a mercury battery the child should immediately be referred to a hospital where the battery can be removed endoscopically. In unclear cases a neck, chest and abdominal plain x-ray can be taken in the referring unit to confirm the presence of a foreign body.
2. Round mini-sized alkali batteries, especially if they are still highly charged, can adhere to the gastric mucosa and cause a deep chemical burn. If an alkali battery does not exit the stomach in 24 hours, it should be removed endoscopically.
3. Symptomatic (gagging etc.) patients should be referred immediately without imaging in the referring unit.
4. If the swallowed object is known to be non-radio-opaque and the patient is asymptomatic the child should be reviewed again at a control visit and referred to a hospital if symptoms develop.
5. Neck and chest and abdominal plain x-ray should be taken of all patients who have swallowed a radio-opaque or unidentified foreign body.
6. If the foreign body is visible in the upper part of the oesophagus the patient should be referred immediately for endoscopic removal.
7. If the foreign body is visible below the oesophagogastric junction or it is not visible at all, it is most probably harmless. Asymptomatic children do not need follow-up if the foreign body is small. Large objects and coins sometimes remain in the stomach where they can become attached on the mucosa. These children should be followed up by radiography (within 1–2 weeks) and the foreign body removed endoscopically, if necessary.

32.30 Ingestion of a caustic substance in a child

Matti Nuutinen

PAE

Basic rules

- Caustic substances include acids (60–80% vinegar, acid detergents, battery acid, fiberglass hardener) and alkali with a pH $\geqslant$ 12 (lye, dishwasher detergent, ammonia, sodium hydroxide).
- Washing the mouth and drinking fluid is an adequate first aid.
- In general children without symptoms can be followed up at home, but those with symptoms should be referred to a hospital (B) [1 2 3 4].

First aid at home

- Wash the mouth and pharynx with water as soon as possible.
- Give fluid (water, milk) to dilute the corrosive substance.

- Do not induce vomiting.

First aid in primary care

- **Asymptomatic children** can be sent home for follow-up. The parents are advised to contact the doctor if symptoms develop (see below).
- **Dysphagia** (the child does not want to drink or eat), drooling, vomiting, or respiratory distress are indications for immediate referral to a hospital B [1 2 3 4].
- Also refer to hospital children who have ingested **lye** or an **unknown** corrosive substance.
- Laboratory tests, radiographic examinations, corticosteroids B [5] or antibiotics are not indicated.

Treatment in the hospital

- If the child has dysphagia, drooling, vomiting, or respiratory distress, follow-up in a hospital or, if necessary, on an intensive care unit is indicated.
- The child can take fluid and food freely if there is no vomiting or dysphagia preventing drinking and eating (in the latter case intravenous fluids should be administered).
- No routine diagnostic investigations such as oesophagoscopy, laboratory tests or radiographs are indicated. Oesophagoscopy is performed no earlier than after 24–36 hours on children who have had salivation and pain on swallowing for 12–24 hours B [1 2 3 4].
- Endotracheal intubation may be indicated because of respiratory distress.

References

1. Wason S. The emergency management of caustic ingestions. J Emerg Med 1985;2:175–82.
2. Howell JM. Alkaline ingestions. Ann Emerg Med 1986;15:820–5.
3. Nuutinen M, Uhari M, Karvali T, Kouvalainen K. Consequences of caustic ingestion in children. Acta Paediatr 1994;83:1200–5.
4. Christesen HB. Prediction of complications following unintentional caustic ingestion in children. Is endoscopy always necessary? Acta Paediatr 1995;84:1177–82.
5. Anderson KD, Rouse TM, Randolph JG. A controlled trial of corticosteroids in children with corrosive injury of the esophagus. N Engl J Med 1990;323:637–40.

32.31 Adder (Vipera berus) bite

Arno Vuori

Basic rules

- An adder bite may be dangerous to a child. If a bite is suspected refer the child to a hospital.
- The symptoms are variable. Severe symptoms occur in about 15% of viper bites. Anaphylactic reactions also occur.
- The bite wound may be typical or atypical.
- The venom is "injected" deep in the tissues. It is no use trying to remove the venom.

Venom

- The venom is pharmacologically complex, and its composition varies:
  - several enzymes (causing tissue destruction, fibrinogen degradation, etc.)
  - other proteins and peptides
  - free amino acids.
- The most important effects are on the circulatory system and blood coagulation.
- The body's reactions may further complicate the situation.
  - The liberation of bradykinin, histamine, etc. causes vasodilatation and collapse.
- The venom is slowly mobilized in the tissues.

Effects of the venom

- Rapid increase in capillary permeability lasting 2–3 days
  - Local swelling and pain
  - Skin discolouration (skin turns dark and purple), petechiae
  - Fluid extravasation leading to shock
  - Platelet extravasation
- Cell destruction
  - Liberation of histamine and other vasoactive substances leading to vasodilatation and shock
- Central nervous system symptoms are common
  - Impaired consciousness, convulsions, headache
- Gastointestinal symptoms are common
  - Vomiting, diarrhoea, abdominal pain
- Kidneys
  - Oliguria or anuria which can often be avoided with sufficient fluid therapy
- Lungs
  - ARDS
  - Often preventable if shock has been avoided
- Blood
  - Haemolysis leading to free haemoglobin in the plasma
  - Platelet destruction and extravasation
  - Degradation of some clotting factors
  - Disseminated intravascular coagulation
- Heart
  - Sometimes bradycardia or negative T waves.

Other symptoms

- Sweating
- Allergic symptoms

- Exanthema, urticaria, angioneurotic oedema, bronchospasm, anaphylaxis, etc.

♦ Delayed symptoms
- Toxic neuropathy of the extremities (sensory disturbance lasting for months)
- Secondary infections
- Large bullae, necroses
- Skin discolouration may last for 1–2 months.

Treatment

At the site of the bite accident

♦ Self-help package (containing e.g. 150 mg of hydrocortisone)
- In theory, stabilizes cell membranes and decreases the liberation of vasoactive substances.
- The efficacy has not been proven.
- Incisions and sucking of blood from the wound are ineffective.

♦ Tourniquet
- May be beneficial if transportation takes a long time D [1].
- Must be opened for five minutes every hour.

♦ Immobilization
- Important! D [1]
- Immobilize with a splint and carry the patient from the site of the accident, when possible.

First aid

♦ I.v. infusion (physiological saline) as soon as possible

♦ Methylprednisolone 2–3 mg/kg i.v.
- The efficacy has not been proven.

♦ Treatment of anaphylaxis if necessary (14.1)

♦ Transportation to a hospital, preferably with an escort.

Treatment in the hospital

♦ Follow-up
- Adults should be followed up for hours, children for 1–2 days. The follow-up should be intensive for small children.

♦ If systemic symptoms develop the patient should be transferred to an intensive care unit.

♦ Fluid therapy in the beginning (during the first 2–4 days) is important.
- Ringer's lactate (large amounts if necessary)
- The infusion rate is determined by the clinical response (peripheral circulation, diuresis, haematocrit, heart rate, acid-base balance).

♦ Methylprednisolone i.v. in doses of 2 mg/kg once or several times.
- The efficacy has not been proven.

♦ Treatment of the kidneys
- Fluid therapy and diuretics if necessary.

♦ Evaluate the need for antibiotic prophylaxis
- E.g. Penicillin i.v. 250 000 units/kg/day.

♦ Tetanus immunization

♦ Pain relief: paracetamol 20 mg/kg every 6 hours. Starting dose for children rectally up to 40 mg/kg, maximum daily dose for adults 6 g, for children 100 mg/kg. Anti-inflammatory drugs should be avoided because of possible kidney damage.

♦ Snake antiserum C [2 3]
- The indications for snake antiserum include
  - rapidly progressing or disseminated oedema
  - recurrent or therapy-resistant cardiovascular symptoms
  - prolonged or recurrent intensive abdominal pain and vomiting
  - angioneurotic oedema and risk of obstruction of the respiratory passages.
- In controversial cases the decision to start antiserum therapy is supported by the following laboratory findings: early leucocytosis ($>15-20 \times 10^9$/l) C [4], metabolic acidosis, haemolysis, ECG abnormalities, disturbances of blood coagulation.
- Administer the antiserum with corticosteroids to avoid allergic reactions.
- The antiserum should be given as soon as possible after indications have been established.
- Viperatab® is a new, fragmented antiserum, which should be preferred.
- Zagreb and Pasteur Ipser Europe are horse antisera.
- The dose is per bite, not per kilogram.

♦ The vital functions should be monitored and supported by means of intensive care.

♦ Blood component therapy as necessary: red cells, coagulation factors, platelets, etc.

♦ The site of the bite should be kept dry. Do not break any vesicles.

♦ Symptomatic treatment for pain, excitation, oedema, convulsions.

PAE

Follow-up

♦ Always
- Body weight, limb circumference, heart rate, blood pressure, diuresis

♦ In mild systemic symptoms
- As above + blood count, blood group, urine protein, urine red cells and haemoglobin

♦ In moderate systemic symptoms
- As above + acid-base balance, serum sodium and potassium, cross test, chest radiograph, ECG

♦ In severe systemic symptoms
- As above + serum urea, creatinine, bleeding time, APTT, thromboplastin time (INR), serum calcium, osmolality, protein, creatine kinase, reservation of transfusable blood, urine sodium and potassium, urine osmolality

References

1. Howarth DM. Lymphatic flow rates and first-aid in simulated peripheral snake or spider envenomation. Med J Aust 1994;161:695–700.
2. Karlson-Stiber C, Persson H. Antivenom treatment in Vipera berus envenoming– report of 30 cases. J Int Med 1994;235: 57–61.
3. Smith D, Reddi KR, Laing G et al. An affinity purified ovine antivenom for the treatment of Vipera berus envenoming. Toxicon 1992;30:865–71.
4. Grönlund J, Vuori A, Nieminen S: Adder bites. A report of 68 cases. Scand J Surg 2003;92(2):171–174.

32.40 Nappy rash

Editors

Epidemiology

- Occurs most commonly between the ages of 9 to 12 months. The condition has become rare in Western countries.
- More common in children on cow's milk than on breast milk.
- More common in children with reusable rather than disposable nappies.

Clinical picture

- The rash is erythematous, irritated, often moist, and does not affect skin folds.
- In therapy-resistant cases consider the following diseases in differential diagnosis:
  - atopic dermatitis complicated by candida or bacterial infection
  - histiocytosis (which also occurs at the bottom of skin folds)

Treatment

- Use disposable nappies with good absorbing capacity.
- Minimize the time of contact between moisture, urine, faeces, and the skin.
- Change the nappy at least 8 times a day.
- Protect the skin with a barrier cream.
- Zinc paste or zinc dioxide cream is often more effective than a barrier cream or a corticosteroid cream.
- Hydrocortisone-chlorhexidine cream should be tried if the aforementioned treatments fail.

32.41 Itch in a child

Editors

Clinical picture and differential diagnosis

- **Scabies** lesions (see also 13.40) are papular or papulovesicular. Furrows are often found if they are sought in the palms and soles of the feet. The lesions break easily resulting in crusts. Large bullous lesions suggest a secondary bacterial infection.
- **Atopic dermatitis** presents with dry, scaling skin. The response to local hydrocortisone and barrier creams is usually favourable.
- **Chickenpox** is characterized by vesicles, fever, and a rapid course.
- **Urticaria**, particularly dermographism, starts abruptly. In dermographism hives are not visible but they can be triggered by scratching the skin bluntly.
- In children, infections easily trigger urticaria, which should be differentiated from pox diseases.
- **Hypersensitivity** may present only with itch. Known causes include citrus fruit, fresh strawberries, and cocoa.
- In the summer an itch may be a symptom of hypersensitivity to light.
- **Mastocytosis** (urticaria pigmentosa) is a rare cause of an itch.

Treatment of scabies

- See 13.40.

Treatment of atopic dermatitis

- See 32.43.

32.42 Atopic dermatitis in children: clinical picture and diagnosis

Sakari Reitamo

- Treatment of atopic dermatitis in children (32.43).

Clinical picture

Infants (below 1 year of age)

- Atopic dermatitis = infantile eczema

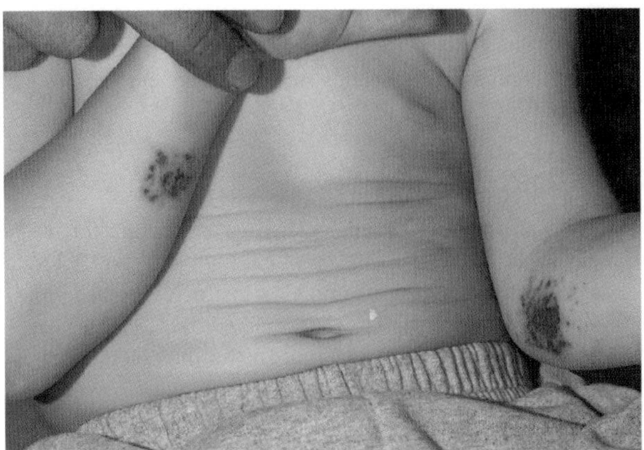

Figure 32.42.1 Nummular dermatitis may also affect children, where it is a feature of atopic dermatitis. The weeping, crusted, itchy nummular dermatitis is often rather resistant to therapy. Photo © R. Suhonen.

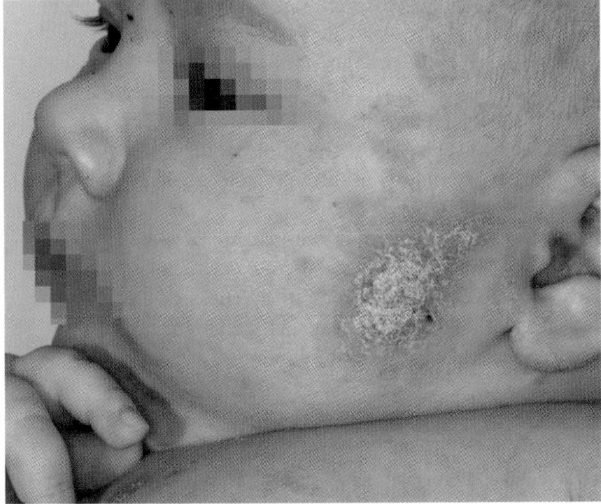

Figure 32.42.2 The exudative and crusted facial atopic dermatitis (crusta lactea) in a small child is commonly misdiagnosed as bacterial infection. In most cases of atopic dermatitis, Staph. aureus is in fact found in bacterial culture. Low potency topical corticoid creams with moist dressings relieve the symptoms effectively. Photo © R. Suhonen.

- **Seborrhoeic type infantile eczema** appears as scaling of the scalp already during the first few weeks of life. It also appears as dermatitis in the skin folds, and may develop into erythroderma.
- **Nummular type infantile eczema** (Figures 32.42.1 and 32.42.2) begins as patchy, often crusty dermatitis on the cheeks, buttocks and/or extremities usually at the age of 2–6 months. This type of dermatitis can also develop into erythroderma.

Preschool-aged children

- Infantile eczema disappears in about 50% of the children before two years of age. In the other half, dermatitis continues but tends to move to the skin folds.

School-aged children

- At school age, dermatitis is predominantly found in the skin folds. Special forms of dermatitis affect volar sides of the hands and plantar surfaces of the feet (juvenile palmar and plantar dermatoses). Hand and feet symptoms are at their worst in wet and cold weather, and they may even disappear during a sunny summer.
- When diagnosing foot dermatoses, remember that dermatophytosis is very rare in children. Avoid misdiagnosis and unnecessary treatment.
- Atopic dermatitis in the buttocks and the inner sides of the thighs usually begins 1–2 years before school age and usually ends in adolescence.

Clinical examination

- Clinical picture is usually sufficient for diagnosis.
- Skin prick testing is indicated if
  - an infant has moderate or severe dermatitis.
  - there is widespread dermatitis at any age (erythrodermic or pre-erythrodermic).
  - there are acute episodes of dermatitis.
  - dermatitis is located in the eyelids, lips and perioral area.
  - in addition to dermatitis, the patient also has respiratory or gastrointestinal symptoms.
  - the patient is allergic to pollens.
- Skin prick tests include both food and respiratory allergens. The tests are performed by a specialist.
- RAST is an alternative method for detecting respiratory allergies but in many cases of food allergy skin prick tests give more reliable result.
- The results of skin tests and RASTs are more reliable the younger the child is.
- Patch testing for foods are also performed. Opinion of the reliability of these tests is not uniform.
- Elimination diet and peroral food challenges are usually needed to confirm the diagnosis of food allergy particularly to cereals and milk.
- Remember that breast milk may also be allergenic.

32.43 Treatment of atopic dermatitis in children

Sakari Reitamo

- Atopic dermatitis in children: clinical picture and diagnosis (32.42).

Diet

- The following foods evoke symptoms in 80% of all atopic children and should therefore be avoided by all children with atopic dermatitis:

- citrus fruits, either fresh or as juice
- chocolate and cocoa
- fresh strawberries.

♦ Other diets should be based on allergy testing (14.8). It is worth remembering that food allergies in children usually disappear with age. No child should be placed on a lifelong avoidance diet.

Reduction of trigger factors

♦ Measures to reduce house dust are necessary only if the child also has respiratory symptoms or if allergy to house dust mite has been verified by RAST, skin prick or patch tests. Dust-proof bedding may be of benefit.

♦ Animal dander (dandruff) can aggravate atopic dermatitis. In such cases the allergy is apparent in RAST and skin prick tests. The family should not give up pets "just in case", as this may cause other problems.

Topical treatment

♦ Corticosteroid creams and ointments comprise the primary therapy.

♦ Emollients should be changed when the preparation starts to irritate the skin. Emollients do not alleviate the inflammation of atopic dermatitis, but they do reduce the evaporation of moisture from the skin.

♦ A moderate amount of washing, i.e. showering the skin quickly with lukewarm water 2–7 times a week, does not cause any harm. Soaps and wash liquids are indicated in the treatment of dermatitis with secondary infection and crusts.

♦ Sweating may aggravate itching.

Children below 2 years

♦ 1% hydrocortisone cream for 1–3 weeks at a time.

♦ Emollients for at least 10 days between the hydrocortisone courses.

♦ Showering or bathing daily.

Children 2–6 years

♦ Mild corticosteroid cream for 1–3 weeks at a time or

♦ Moderately potent corticosteroid cream for 1–2 weeks at a time.

♦ Emollients for at least 10 days between the corticosteroid courses.

♦ If no response is achieved with the corticosteroid creams, pimecrolimus (Elidel®) or tacrolimus (Protopic® 0.03%) creams may be used as alternatives. Both can be used as continuous treatment with intermittent administration.

♦ Pimecrolimus is licensed for the treatment of moderate, and tacrolimus for moderate to severe, atopic dermatitis.
  - The cream is applied initially twice a day for two weeks, then reduced to once daily until symptoms resolve.
  - During treatment, exposure to sunlight should be minimized by avoiding excessive time spent in the sun, using sun creams and by wearing protective clothing.
  - Treatment should by initiated by a dermatologist or a physician with extensive experience in the use of immunomodulating agents in the treatment of atopic dermatitis.

School-aged children

♦ Mild to moderately potent corticosteroid cream for 1–3 weeks at a time.

♦ Potent corticosteroid cream only as instructed by a dermatologist.

♦ The scalp tolerates topical steroids better than other sites of the skin.

♦ If no response is achieved with conventional treatment, pimecrolimus (Elidel®) or tacrolimus (Protopic® 0.03%) may be used, administered intermittently until symptoms resolve.

Other treatments

♦ Phototherapies are used in patients with widespread dermatitis and poor response to conventional topical corticosteroid therapy. Even infants can be treated. Selective ultraviolet phototherapy (SUP) can be used for children of any age. UVA solariums benefit some children. UVB phototherapy is usually given to adolescents or older patients.

♦ There is no evidence that antihistamines alleviate pruritus other than through their sedative effect.

♦ There is no evidence of the effectiveness of gammalinoleic acid, vitamins or trace elements, and these should not be prescribed as "treatment" to children.

32.50 Clinical examination of a child with arthritic symptoms

Ilkka Kunnamo

Principles

♦ The diagnosis of arthritis is made on clinical grounds: swelling or limitation of motion with
  - warmth
  - tenderness, or
  - pain in motion.

♦ Morning stiffness is typical of arthritis whereas pain after exercise is more common in non-inflammatory joint affection.

♦ If the history suggests arthritis but there are no clinical findings the child should be re-examined when the symptoms recur.

Examination of the joints

- The following joint examination can be performed in less than 10 minutes:
- Observe the **gait when the child walks and runs**. A limp in a small child is an important clue as regards pain or stiffness. The parents' observations about a limp are usually correct, even if the child has no limp during examination.
- Inspect the joints for **swelling**.
- Try the temperature of the skin over the knees and ankles with the dorsal side of your fingers and **observe temperature differences**. Asymmetric arthritis in these joints almost always causes a temperature difference.
- Test the **mobility of joints.** Observe pain (muscle guarding, resistance) at the ultimate range of motion in cases where the range of motion is normal.
  - Move the ankles in different directions and observe asymmetry.
  - Flex the knees
    - Normally the heels touch the buttocks without difficulty.
  - Extend the knees maximally with the child supine
    - Observe asymmetry.
  - Test the internal rotation of the hip joints. The child should be lying supine, with the hips and knees flexed 90 degrees. While keeping the knees together, move the legs outwards.
    - Almost all diseases of the hip first affect internal rotation.
  - Flex and extend both elbows and observe asymmetry.
  - Test maximal extension of the wrists
    - The ranges should be symmetrical and at least 80 degrees.
  - Flex every finger separately at the PIP and DIP joints so that the MCP joint is kept straight. You can also ask the child to flex four fingers maximally, first touching the distal palmar fold with the fingertips, then touching the palm as proximally as possible (in the former position the MCP joints are straight, in the latter they are flexed). The former test is usually sufficient.
    - Normally the fingers can easily touch the palm.
    - Marked restriction of flexion is usually easily detected even in cases where there is no visible swelling.
- Detect **knee hydrops**. Dislocate the fluid from the suprapatellar recessus with a flat hand and observe the bulging on both sides of the patella using your index finger and thumb.
- **Provoke pain** at the sacroiliac joint by pressing the pelvic girdle firmly from both sides. Pain originating from the sacroiliac joints radiates to the buttocks.
- **Pain at the MTP and MCP joints** can be provoked by pressing the hand or foot from the sides.
- Examine **rotation of the cervical spine** (normally 90 degrees) and backwards extension. Observe pain, limitation of motion and asymmetry.

32.51 Diagnosis and epidemiology of arthritis in children

Ilkka Kunnamo

- Arthritis can usually be differentiated from other conditions on the basis of the clinical examination (32.50). This article deals with the diagnostic approach to a condition that has been diagnosed as arthritis on clinical grounds.

Urgency of the diagnosis

1. Immediate
   - Septic infection
2. 1–7 days
   - Malignancy (leukaemia)
   - Fracture
   - Slipped epiphysis of the hip
3. 2–4 weeks
   - Juvenile rheumatoid arthritis (iridocyclitis!)
   - Perthes disease

Primary diagnosis

- The following guidelines for primary diagnosis are based on the urgency of diagnosis and easily available diagnostic methods.
  - Identify **septic infections and malignancies** immediately (perform phase I diagnostic tests). Severe pain on motion, fever above 38.5°C, or a serum CRP concentration above 20 mg/l in monoarthritis suggests a bacterial infection. Severe pain at rest and abnormal blood count suggest leukaemia. If these diseases are suspected refer the patient immediately to a hospital.
  - Identify the following conditions on the basis of the clinical picture:
    - Transient synovitis of the hip (32.54). (The diagnosis should be confirmed by ultrasonography if available.)
    - Henoch-Schönlein purpura (32.53)
    - Urticaria with arthritis (serum sickness) (32.52)
  - Suspect the following diseases on the basis of the clinical picture:
    - Juvenile rheumatoid arthritis (32.56)
    - Enteroarthritis (32.55)
  - and after two weeks from the onset of symptoms (or immediately in selected cases) determine serology for
    - Yersinia, Salmonella (and Campylobacter)
    - Antinuclear antibodies
    - Borrelia
- A delay of two weeks is a good "diagnostic test" because two thirds of all cases of arthritis are cured during that time and no further investigations are needed.

PAE

- The interpretation of Borrelia serology and decisions on treatment, as well as further investigations in suspected juvenile rheumatoid arthritis, should always be performed by a specialist.

Investigations in the differential diagnosis of arthritis in children

- See Table 32.51.1.

Differential diagnosis

- The sensitivity of the combination of fever of at least 38.5° and serum CRP concentration above 20 mg/l for septic arthritis is almost 100%. A high sensitivity is necessary because septic arthritis must always be treated. Arthrocentesis is not usually indicated if neither of the above-mentioned conditions are present.
- A normal blood leucocyte count does not rule out a septic infection but an increased count supports the diagnosis. The ESR rises more slowly than CRP but is better than CRP in the differentiation of any inflammatory condition from non-inflammatory (orthopaedic) causes of joint symptoms.
- Because leukaemia may initially manifest as joint symptoms (usually severe pain at night) the differential leucocyte count should be included in the initial investigations of arthritis.
- Beta-haemolytic group A streptococci may be detected in a throat smear in Henoch-Schönlein purpura (32.53) and some other forms of acute arthritis. It should always be eradicated with antibiotics. The possibility of rheumatic fever should be considered on the basis of the clinical presentation (fever and migratory polyarthritis) if group A streptococci are detected.

Table 32.51.1 Investigations in the differential diagnosis of arthritis in children

Patient group	Test
All children with joint symptoms (Phase I)	• **CRP** • **ESR** • **Leucocyte count**, differential count, haemoglobin, platelet count. Streptococcal throat smear. Urine test.
• Arthritis lasting for more than two weeks or suspicion of enteroarthritis (Phase II)	• (Antinuclear antibodies) • **Yersinia** and Salmonella serology (>5 yrs) • Faecal bacterial culture (>5 yrs) • Borrelia serology
Investigations by a specialist	• Antinuclear antibodies • Rheumatoid factor • Antistreptolysin • Chlamydial serology • Viral antibodies

- The investigations in bold type must always be performed.

Table 32.51.2 Epidemiology of arthritis in children

Aetiology	Percentage of all arthritides
Septic arthritis	6%
Acute transient arthritis	72%
- **Transient synovitis of the hip** (32.54)	48%
- **Urticaria arthritis (serum sickness)** (32.52)	5%
- **Henoch–Schönlein purpura** (32.53)	14%
- **Others**	14%
Prolonged arthritis	22%
- Juvenile rheumatoid arthritis (32.56)	17%
- Enteroarthritis (32.55)	5%
Others	<1%
- Malignancy (e.g. leukaemia)	
- Rheumatic fever	

- Diseases in bold type can be treated by a general practitioner.

- The urine test may be abnormal in Henoch-Schönlein purpura, systemic lupus erythematosus (haematuria), and enteroarthritis (pyuria).
- The causative agents for enteroarthritis (32.55) should be searched for in all patients aged five years or over with the clinical presentation suggesting enteroarthritis or with arthritis lasting for more than two weeks.
  - Stool bacterial culture should be taken from such patients at an early phase.
- Antinuclear antibodies and borrelia antibodies should be determined in all cases of arthritis lasting for more than two weeks.
- Rheumatoid factor is rarely present in juvenile rheumatoid arthritis (32.56). It should not be included in the initial examinations of arthritis in children but rather postponed until further assessment and classification of prolonged arthritis is performed.
- The antistreptolysin test is useless as an initial examination because "false positive" results are common and rheumatic fever is rare.

Epidemiology

- The incidence of arthritis in children is about 1/1000/year. A practical classification divides arthritis into four groups (Table 32.51.2).

32.52 Urticaria and arthritis (serum sickness)

Ilkka Kunnamo

Basic rule

- Identify a drug reaction as the cause of the condition and avoid unnecessary examinations.

Symptoms and diagnosis

- Urticaria and arthritis is a serum sickness-like disease usually caused by drugs. The presenting symptoms include
  - urticarial (or sometimes maculopapular) rash and
  - polyarticular erythema, swelling and pain on motion. Typical sites are the dorsum of the foot and the MTP joints.
- The patient may have mild fever and a slightly elevated ESR, and rarely also a slightly elevated serum CRP concentration.
- The symptoms commence suddenly after a course of antibiotics (usually cefaclor or penicillin) and disappear in a week.

Treatment

- Stop the medication (and avoid it in the future), and relieve the itch with antihistamines, e.g. hydroxyzine 1–2 mg/kg/day. Rest is recommended for joint pain.

32.53 Henoch-Schönlein purpura

Ilkka Kunnamo

Basic rule

- Rule out severe infections and haematological disease before setting the diagnosis of Henoch-Schönlein purpura.

Symptoms and signs

- The disease most commonly affects children aged 2–10 years.
- Papules that develop into petecchias appear on the lower extremities and buttocks (Figure 32.53.1).
- Periarticular swelling and tenderness is observed in the ankles, knees, and sometimes also wrists and elbows.
- Abdominal pain is common.
- Microscopic haematuria is a common finding at the early stage of the disease and often confirms the diagnosis together with a normal platelet count.
- Overt nephritis is rare, and occurs at a later stage of the disease.

Differential diagnosis

- Consider another disease if
  - the patient has a fever exceeding 38.5 °C
  - the serum CRP concentration exceeds 20 mg/l or the ESR is above 35 mm/h

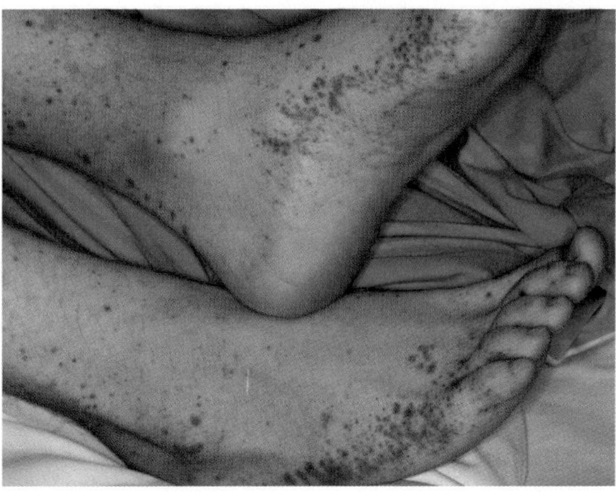

Figure 32.53.1 Young (teenage) boys are the most common targets for Henoch-Schönlein's purpura, also called allergic purpura. There is no thrombocytopenia. Usually no specific causative agent is found, although infections and drugs may be suspected. The main risk is renal involvement. Rest is needed, and the opinions of the benefit of oral corticoid therapy are not unanimous. Photo © R. Suhonen.

  - the platelet count is decreased or anaemia or leukopenia is detected.
- Remember that meningococcal sepsis causes petecchias and sometimes also joint symptoms. If the platelet count is low (<100) the patient may have ITP or a haematological malignancy.

Complications

- The acute complications of the disease include intestinal intussusception, melena, and rarely bleeding in other parts of the body.

PAE

Treatment and follow-up

- Patients without intestinal symptoms can be treated at home, but those with abdominal pain or melena should be referred to a hospital.
- If microscopic haematuria continues after the acute stage of the disease several urine samples should be taken over 6 months. Consult a specialist if proteinuria or symptoms of nephritis are observed during this period.
- If there is renal involvement initially, and particularly if the renal symptoms are severe and last for more than one month, the patient's renal function must be followed up throughout life, as the risk of renal failure is significant. All women who had even mild renal symptoms at onset of Henoch-Schönlein purpura should be carefully observed during and after pregnancy.

32.54 Transient synovitis of the hip

Ilkka Kunnamo, Pentti Kallio

Basic rule

- Diagnose transient synovitis of the hip on the basis of typical symptoms and by exclusion of leukaemia, septic arthritis and Perthes' disease. Avoid unnecessary examinations.

Symptoms and signs

- The disease is the most common cause of acute limp in a child aged below 10 years
- The child limps or refuses to walk and complains of pain in the hip or knee, and keeps the hip in position of flexion and external rotation.
- Painful and limited internal rotation of the hip is a typical clinical finding.
- The ESR may be slightly elevated.
- An effusion of the hip joint is easily detected by ultrasonography.
- The patient probably has another disease (and should be referred to hospital) if
  - the symptoms have lasted for more than 2 weeks
  - the patient is younger than 2 or older than 10 years of age
  - the patient has fever
  - the serum CRP concentration exceeds 20 mg/l or the ESR exceeds 35 mm/h.

Differential diagnosis

- Perthes' disease (32.62) and epiphysiolysis (32.61), septic arthritis, osteomyelitis, juvenile rheumatoid arthritis, osteoid osteoma, and malignant diseases should be considered in differential diagnosis.
- The disease may occasionally be bilateral. If joints other than the hip are affected the patient has another disease.
- A plain x-ray of the hips should be taken if the symptoms persist or the clinical picture is atypical. **In children above 10 years of age x-ray should not be delayed**, in order to detect epiphysiolysis.

Treatment

- Keep the child at rest with the hip flexed.
- Joint aspiration in a hospital is necessary only if septic arthritis is suspected or the pain is severe.
- The prognosis is good.

32.55 Enteroarthritis, borrelia and other acute forms of arthritis in children

Ilkka Kunnamo

Enteroarthritis

- An enterobacterial infection (yersiniosis, salmonellosis, campylobacter infection) is occasionally followed by severe arthritis that may be difficult to differentiate from septic arthritis. About 10% of children have joint symptoms after a salmonella infection.
- Typical clinical features of enteroarthritis include the following:
  - The disease is polyarticular (which is rare in septic arthritis).
  - Children below school age are very rarely affected.
  - The large joints of the lower extremities (knees, ankles) are most commonly affected, but small joints of the toes and hands may also be affected.
  - The patient often has fever.
  - ESR, and serum CRP concentrations may be considerably increased (even up to 100).
  - Preceding diarrhoea or abdominal pain is recalled by only about half of the patients.
- Enteroarthritis may also present as a more insidiously developing monoarthritis.

Borrelia arthritis

- A tick-bite is recalled by a minority of the patients.
- Borrelia serology should be determined in all cases of prolonged arthritis (>2 weeks) in children.
- The interpretation of Borrelia serology and the treatment of Borrelia infection should be reserved for a specialist.

Other acute forms of arthritis

- Many cases of acute arthritis that do not have a diagnostic clinical presentation (32.52), (32.53), (32.54) and that cannot be included in the aforementioned categories will be left without more specific diagnosis.
- Arthritis may be associated with viral infections (rubella, chickenpox, parvovirus, adenovirus).
- The determination of viral antibodies is seldom indicated because quick spontaneous recovery is the rule.
- Chlamydial serology should be determined in prolonged arthritis of unknown aetiology. Always consult a specialist.

32.56 Juvenile rheumatoid arthritis

Ilkka Kunnamo

Aims

- Examine the joints systematically (32.50) in all children with suspected arthritis.
- Diagnose juvenile rheumatoid arthritis (JRA) at an early stage with minimal symptoms in order to detect asymptomatic iridocyclitis.
- The diagnosis of JRA should be confirmed and decisions on treatment made at a specialized unit. A general practitioner should follow up the child's pharmacotherapy in cooperation with the specialist unit.
- Adequate physiotherapy should be arranged near the patient's home.

Definition

- Arthritis lasting for more than 3 months is considered JRA if other causes of arthritis have been ruled out with sufficient certainty.

Symptoms and signs

- Morning stiffness and a limp are the most common initial symptoms.
- Prolonged neck pain and torticollis may be an early symptom of JRA.
- Often clinical signs can be elicited only by systematic joint examination (32.50).
- In systemic JRA (Still's disease) oscillating fever and erythematous macular rash on the upper trunk during fever may be the only symptoms for a long time (31.3).

Sub-types of JRA

- Five sub-types have been defined. 20% of patients with oligoarticular onset develop polyarthritis during follow-up. In 2% of all cases the symptoms start before the first birthday.
- Early onset oligoarthritis (about 50% of all cases)
  - Occurs in children aged 1–5 years.
  - 85% of the patients are girls.
  - In most cases the knee and the ankle are initially affected.
  - Antinuclear antibodies (ANAs) are detected in 80%.
  - Almost 50% of the patients have chronic, usually asymptomatic iridocyclitis that may result in loss of vision if left untreated.
  - The prognosis is good.
- Late onset oligoarthritis (10–15% of all cases)
  - Large joints of the lower limbs, including the hips, are affected.
  - Occurs in children aged 8–15 years.
  - 90% of the patients are boys.
  - HLA-B27 is present in 75%.
  - Insertitis (enthesitis) is a common clinical feature.
- Seronegative polyarthritis (about 30% of all cases)
  - Occurs in children aged 1–15 years.
  - In addition to large joints, small joints, the temporomandibular joints and the cervical spine are affected.
  - 90% of the patients are girls.
  - Antinuclear antibodies are detected in 25%.
- Seropositive polyarthritis (<10% of all patients)
  - Occurs in children aged 8–15 years.
  - Is the same disease as seropositive rheumatoid arthritis in adults.
  - 80% of the patients are girls.
  - The rheumatoid factor is positive.
  - The prognosis is often poor.
- Systemic JRA (<10% of all cases)
  - Fever and rash are the initial symptoms. Joint symptoms develop later, and are sometimes totally absent.
  - Leucocytosis, high ESR and CRP are nearly always detected.
  - Tests for ANAs and rheumatoid factor are negative.
  - About 50% of the patients develop severe polyarthritis.

Principles of treatment

- Non-steroidal anti-inflammatory drugs should be taken regularly (naproxen, 10–15 mg/kg/day; diclofenac, 1–3 mg/kg/day; ibuprofen, 20–40 mg/kg/day).
- Local steroids should be injected in joints with hydrops or moderate or severe symptoms. (The doctor in charge of the treatment usually gives the injections.)
- Hydroxychloroquine is often used in early onset oligoarthritis.
- Methotrexate (B) [1] administered weekly in small doses has become the drug of choice in the treatment of children with significant symptoms.
- Alternatives to methotrexate include sulphasalazine and parenteral gold (i.m). (nowadays extremely rare).
- In severe cases that do not respond to methotrexate a combination of several long-acting drugs or tumour-necrosis factor antagonists can be tried.
- Laboratory tests for monitoring drug safety (21.60) are performed in ambulatory care.
- Physiotherapy should be regular (1–3 times a week).
- Vaccinations should be given during remission: no live viral vaccinations for patients on large-dose glucocorticoid and/or cytotoxic therapy.
- Coping with the disease at school requires cooperation with teachers and parents. Career choice counselling is important in adolescence if the child continues to have symptoms.

PAE

Reference

1. Takken T, Van der Net J, Helders, PJM. Methotrexate for treating juvenile idiopathic arthritis. Cochrane Database Syst Rev. 2004;(2):CD003129.

32.57 Kawasaki disease

Eeva Salo

Pathology

- Kawasaki disease is an acute febrile vasculitis affecting infants and young children with coronary artery dilatation as a possible complication.
- The aetiology is unknown, but it is possibly triggered by an infectious agent.

Aims

- Early diagnosis and intravenous immunoglobulin treatment lessen the risk of coronary aneurysms (A) [1].
- Kawasaki disease should be suspected and the child referred to hospital if four of the six criteria listed below are fulfilled, irrespective of how long the symptoms have lasted. See also Child with fever and rash 31.3 and Febrile child without local symptoms 31.1.
- The disease should also be kept in mind when a small child has a febrile disease that does not respond to antibiotic treatment and fulfils three of the six criteria listed below.

Diagnosis

- Diagnosis is based on the clinical picture. The diagnosis can be made if five of the following six criteria are fulfilled:
  1. Fever over 38°C for 5 days or more
  2. Conjunctival injection; no discharge or exudate
  3. Changes in the mouth (at least one of the following): strawberry tongue, erythema of the pharynx and oral mucosa, and red and cracked lips.
  4. Changes in the peripheral extremities (at least one of the following): swelling of the hands and feet, erythema of the palms and soles, peeling of the skin of the hands and feet about two weeks after the onset of the disease.
  5. Rash, which can be very diverse, most commonly erythematous or urticarial.
  6. Enlargement of a cervical lymph node over 1.5 cm.
- Children below 6 months of age may lack some of the symptoms. Kawasaki disease should be suspected in an infant with unexplained febrile illness.
- All symptoms are not always present at the same time; take a good history from the parents.
- About half of the patients have additional symptoms, such as otitis media, diarrhoea or abdominal pain. Twenty-five per cent have aseptic meningitis, joint pain or arthritis.
- Other illnesses causing similar symptoms should be ruled out (for example measles).
- Children with Kawasaki disease are usually clearly ill. Infants are especially irritable, difficult to console and they show tenderness on touching.

Laboratory findings

- Fit any bacterial illness
  - CRP and sedimentation rate clearly elevated
  - Leucocytosis and left shift in differential white cell count
  - Often sterile pyuria

Complications

- In about 20% of untreated patients coronary artery enlargement or aneurysms develop. These may be thrombosed and lead to myocardial infarction and sudden death. Some of the aneurysms regress spontaneously; others leave stenoses, obstructions or tortuosity.
- Coronary aneurysms can be detected in cardiac ultrasonography. It should be carried out at once when Kawasaki disease is suspected, and repeated at least once to detect possible changes about a month after the onset of the disease.

Treatment

- High-dose intravenous immunoglobulin in one dose (A) [1]. The treatment efficiently prevents coronary enlargement and brings prompt alleviation of symptoms.
- Treatment should be started as soon as possible when Kawasaki disease is suspected, preferably within a week of disease onset. Hence it is important to suspect the disease and send the children to hospital in time for early treatment.

Reference

1. Oates-Whitehead RM, Baumer JH, Haines L, Love S, Maconochie IK, Gupta A, Roman K, Dua JS, Flynn I. Intravenous immunoglobulin for the treatment of Kawasaki disease in children. The Cochrane Database of Systematic Reviews, Cochrane Library Number: CD004000. In: Cochrane Library, Issue 1, 2004. Chichester, UK: John Wiley & Sons, Ltd.

32.60 A child with a limp or refusing to walk

Editors

Aims

- Diagnose bacterial infections of bones and joints immediately.
- Diagnose aseptic synovitis of the hip without unnecessary investigations.
- Diagnose epiphysiolysis within one week and Perthes disease within one month.

- A limp or refusal to walk for one week is an indication for specialist consultation.

History

- Type of onset (sudden, associated with a trauma, subtle) and course (continuous, recurrent). If the symptom was associated with a trauma, was there an asymptomatic period?
  - Late onset juvenile rheumatoid arthritis may manifest with pain at tendon insertions (enthesitis) (32.56).
- General symptoms. (A fever may suggest bacterial infection, and a respiratory infection may precede aseptic synovitis of the hip.)
- Pain at rest (often a symptom of a bone infection or tumour)
- Morning stiffness (a symptom of arthritis, particularly juvenile rheumatoid arthritis)

Clinical examination

- Proceed slowly so that the child's fear and crying do not hinder the assessment of tenderness. Small children should sit in their parent's arms.
- If the child has a limp the first thing to find out is which leg is affected: the child avoids bearing weight on the affected extremity and climbs the stairs with the healthy leg first. Observe the side to which the pelvis tilts during walking. The Trendelenburg sign is elicited by letting the child stand on each leg alternately. (When standing on the healthy leg the opposite side of the pelvis is raised, and when standing on the affected leg the opposite side of the pelvis is lowered.)
- Start the examination of the extremity by inspection (swelling of the knee or ankle, signs of trauma) and by assessing the temperature difference of the knees and ankles (32.50). Do not forget to inspect the soles (foreign body, wart).
- Because the most common cause for a limp in a child aged 2–10 years is aseptic synovitis of the hip (32.54), the examination should be started with rotation of the hips (32.50): asymmetry in the range of internal rotation and tenderness suggest hip disease.
- Tenderness in joints and ligaments can be elicited by flexing the joints passively. Tenderness in bones and joints can also be observed by compressing the long bones or the whole extremity in a longitudinal direction and avoiding bending. Find out whether there is a swelling or a hydrops in the (hip or ankle) joint.

Examination strategy

- A rule of thumb: the cause of the limp is in the hip until confirmed otherwise.
- If the tenderness or limitation of motion has been located in a joint, perform a systematic joint examination (32.50) to assess whether the child has arthritis, and treat or refer according to the urgency of the condition (32.51).
- X-rays are indicated if
  - a fracture is suspected
  - the symptoms in the hip last for more than a week or
  - recur more than one week after the first occurrence of the symptom.
  - Boys aged over 10 years with hip symptoms should be investigated by radiography within 2 days. Ask for a consultation by a radiologist as Perthes disease or epiphysiolysis at an early stage may be difficult to diagnose from the x-ray.
- Ultrasonography is useful in the diagnosis of hip synovitis. The examination can even be performed in primary care.
- A specialist consultation is indicated if
  - the clinical presentation or laboratory findings suggest a septic infection or malignancy (immediate referral)
  - epiphysiolysis (32.61) or Perthes disease (32.62) is suspected
  - a limp or refusal to walk of unknown aetiology lasts for more than a week
  - a neurological disease is suspected.

32.61 Epiphysiolysis of the femoral head

Pentti Kallio

PAE

Basic rule

- Early diagnosis and surgical treatment should be pursued. If left untreated the medial and posterior shift of the femoral head increases and the function of the hip becomes impaired. In moderate and severe cases there is an increased risk of early secondary osteoarthritis.

Definition

- The epiphysis of the femoral head slides aside in relation to the femoral neck.
- The condition is defined as stable if the epiphysis is fixed in a new position. The patient is able to walk. Instability means that the epiphysis is not fixed and the hip is very painful.

Epidemiology and symptoms

- Occurs at the age of 10–16 years (somewhat earlier in girls), often in association with obesity. The male/female ratio is 2.5.
- Both hips are affected in 20–30% of patients.

- Limping and pain on weight-bearing in the knee, thigh, and inguinal area. The patient typically holds the lower extremity in slight external rotation.

Diagnosis

- X-rays show a posterior shift of the epiphysis. If the disease is suspected (hip symptoms at a typical age) both anterioposterior and Lauenstein projections of both hips should be assessed.
- The indentation caused by a recent dislocation can be seen well by ultrasonography. If effusion is detected in ultrasonography the epiphysiolysis is unstable.

Treatment

- The treatment is always surgical. The epiphysis is usually stabilized with a single screw. The smaller the dislocation the better the outcome.
- Prophylactic fixation of the contralateral asyptomatic hip should be considered if the patient is very young or has an endocrinological or metabolic underlying disease (in 7% of the cases).

32.62 Perthes' disease (Legg–Calvé–Perthes disease, pseudocoxalgia)

Pentti Kallio

Basic rules

- Make the diagnosis in an early phase and treat the tendency for subluxation.
- The prognosis is good if sphericity of the femoral head can be maintained.

Definition

- Aseptic necrosis of the femoral head resulting in a symptomatic subchondral stress fracture within 4–8 months. The fracture and delay in the ossification of the femoral head cartilage result in softening of the epiphysis. If left untreated the femoral head may become flattened.

Epidemiology and symptoms

- Occurs mostly in boys aged 2–12 years. The male–female ratio is 5:1.
- The condition is bilateral in 10% of the cases, but both femoral heads are usually not affected simultaneously.
- A limp is the main symptom. The disease resembles transient synovitis of the hip (32.54) but starts more insidiously and becomes prolonged or recurs.
- The pain is located at the region between the inguinal fold and the knee.
- ESR, serum CRP, and blood leucocyte count are normal.
- The skeletal age (28.41) is usually delayed by about 2 years.

Diagnosis

- The diagnosis is based on x-rays: the first sign is subchondral irregularity of the bony structure, followed by cysts and epiphyseal flattening.

Treatment

- The prognosis is good in young children (below 6 years of age).
- If no clear indication for treatment exists initially, follow-up and control x-rays are indicated.
- Abduction mobility of the hip should be more than 30 degrees on clinical examination during follow-up.
- An observed tendency towards subluxation on x-rays or limitation of hip motion are indications for treatment. The cause of limited mobility can be determined in arthrography performed under anaesthesia.
- Measures to improve the geometry of the hip joint, such as abduction splints or operation (femoral or pelvic osteotomy or both), are needed in about 20% of the cases.

32.63 Osgood–Schlatter disease

Editors

Basic rule

- Spontaneous healing is promoted by avoiding excessive strain.

Definition

- Repetitive strain injury in the apophysis of the tibial tuberosity. The onset of symptoms coincides with prepubertal growth spurt.

Symptoms

- Pain is experienced in the upper part of the lower leg or in the knee when running or jumping. When the child runs the pain is more intense at the moment of heel touch than at take-off (physiology of the extensor apparatus of the knee!).

Signs

- The tibial tuberosity is prominent and sensitive on palpation.
- X-ray shows a fragmented tuberosity. In a typical case a x-ray is not necessary.

Treatment

- Explain the condition to the patient and the parents.
- The patient should avoid painful exertion (avoid school gymnastics involving running or jumping, for 3 months).
- Consult an orthopaedic specialist if the symptoms are severe (treatment options include cast immobilization for 4–6 weeks and excision of a very prominent tibial tuberosity after growth has ceased.)

32.64 Back problems in children and adolescents

Editors

Basic rules

- Diagnose spondylolisthesis in symptomatic patients and monitor its progress.
- Prevent the development of excessive kyphosis by extension exercises in patients with Scheuermann's disease; a supportive corset should be used if the kyphosis angle exceeds 40 degrees **B** [1 2].
- Identify and treat scoliosis before a permanent deformity develops.

Spondylolisthesis

- The most common cause for prolonged or recurrent back pain in adolescents.
- Low back pain triggered by exercise and often radiating in the thighs may be a symptom of spondylolisthesis. The clinical signs include
  - exaggerated lumbar lordosis
  - palpable "threshold"
  - elevated spinous process.
- The diagnosis is based on the detection of vertebral shift in a lateral x-ray (an anterio-posterior x-ray need not be taken)
- The progress of spondylolisthesis in monitored by x-rays 2–3 times a year (and consultation by a paediatric surgeon) in children who have symptoms.
- Maximal strain (weight-lifting, gymnastics) should be avoided.
- Bone-fusion surgery is indicated if
  - the patient has recurrent symptoms
  - the olisthesis increases
  - the olisthesis exceeds 1/3 of the sagittal diameter of the vertebra.

Scheuermann's disease

- Scheuermann's disease is an osteochondritis affecting the anterior part of the vertebral cartilage occurring in late puberty (at the age of 13–15 years in girls, 15–17 years in boys). The disease is four times more common in girls than in boys.
- Pain in the thoracic spine, stiffness of the back and tightness of the hamstring muscles are the most common symptoms.
- The diagnosis is based on x-rays showing
  - wedge-shaped vertebrae that are flattened anteriorly
  - deformed end plates of the vertebrae; Schmorl's prolapses (indentations towards the vertebral body) develop in a later phase.
- Differential diagnosis: tuberculosis, fractures
- The treatment consists of avoiding excessive flexion strain (e.g. weight-lifting), and corset treatment in severe cases (with a thoracic kyphosis exceeding 45°).

Scoliosis

- Scoliosis is idiopathic and progressive in 85% of cases, and functional in 15%.
- Scoliosis is a disease, not a bad posture. Gymnastics does not help.
- The disease develops at the phase of rapid growth (at the age of 10–12 years in girls, a couple of years later in boys).
- Screening is based on inspection of the spine from behind as the child bows down with the knees extended. Scoliosis is present if one scapula rises higher than the other.
- Mild or controversial cases should be followed up at 6-month intervals.
- The severity of scoliosis is assessed from x-rays by determining the maximum scoliosis angle. An x-ray is indicated if a clinically evident scoliosis is detected.
- Treatment
  - Under 20°: follow-up
  - 20–40°: corset treatment **B** [1 2]
  - Over 40°: surgery

Calvé's disease (vertebra plana)

- A rare disease of children aged 2–10 years with total collapse of a vertebra.
- The clinical features include local tenderness, increased ESR, sometimes leucocytosis. Tuberculosis should be considered in the differential diagnosis. Refer patients with

suspected Calvé's disease to hospital for further investigations.

Discitis

- Usually aseptic but may also be caused by bacteria.
- Difficulty in walking and sitting is a typical clinical presentation for a child below school age.
- The diagnosis is based on local tenderness and painful movements of the spine. The diagnosis can be confirmed by a technetium bone scan.
- The child should be hospitalized for further investigations.
- In most cases the condition is benign and heals spontaneously.

References

1. Rowe DE, Bernstein SM, Riddick MF, Adler F, Emans JB, Gardner-Bonneau D. A meta-analysis of the efficacy of non-operative treatments for idiopathic scoliosis. J Bone Joint Surg 1997;79A:664–674.
2. The Database of Abstracts of Reviews of Effectiveness (University of York), Database no.: DARE-970689. In: The Cochrane Library, Issue 4, 1999. Oxford: Update Software.

32.65 Innocent leg aches in children

Editors

Basic rules

- Diagnose innocent leg aches ("growing pains") on the basis of the clinical presentation and rule out arthritis. Suspect other causes of pain if the child is below 4 years of age.
- The psychosocial situation should be assessed particularly if there are other symptoms (headache, abdominal pain).

Epidemiology

- Recurrent pain with no organic cause in the limbs of growing children
- One child in two suffers from leg aches at some point in childhood.
- The aches usually start around the age of 4 years. The peak incidence is at the ages of 6 to 11 years.
- Familial occurrence is common.

Clinical presentation

- The knee, leg, and thigh are the most common sites of the pain. Upper limbs are rarely affected.
- The pain is usually felt symmetrically in both lower limbs or it shifts from one limb to the other.
- The pain is usually present in the evening, during bedtime, or during the night, but not in the morning (in contrast to arthritis causing morning stiffness).
- The pain is felt during rest, but not during exercise.
- The pain lasts 0.5–5 hours.
- The child may also have a tendency for headaches or abdominal pain.
- Another cause for the pain should be considered if the child has
    - continuous unilateral pain
    - associated symptoms (e.g. a limp or the general condition is affected)
    - symptoms in the morning or during the day.

Investigations

- If the presentation is not typical, blood count and erythrocyte sedimentation rate should at least be determined.

Treatment

- Self-care by massage, warm bath, etc. is commonly used; only a minority of the parents consult a doctor.
- Clinical examination (32.50) to rule out other diseases and explaining the nature of the symptoms to the parents is often all that is required.
- Paracetamol can be used temporarily.

32.70 Injuries in children: lacerations and incisions

Editors

Basic rule

- Prefer tissue glue to sutures (most wounds in children are recent and yet nonbleeding, and thus suitable for closing without sutures) Ⓐ [1].
- Conservative treatment is as effective as suturation in hand lacerations less than 2 cm in length Ⓑ [2]

Epidemiology

- Superficial lacerations of the skin are the most common wounds.
- Lacerations are usually located on the head, and excoriations on the extremities.
- A child with a wound appears at the first aid clinic more quickly after injury than a child with an excoriation.

Lacerations

- Lacerations normally cease bleeding before arrival at the first aid clinic. Usually the laceration is along the cleavage lines of the skin and only transsects the corium, saving deeper structures. Therefore most lacerations in children can be closed without sutures.
- There is no need for surgical revision of a fresh wound. Wound infection is rare. No antibiotic prophylaxis is indicated in fresh wounds A [3 4].
- Wound care starts with cleansing. Tap water is suitable, but physiological saline may be less irritating. Antiseptics should be water-based: chlorhexidine and povidone-iodide can be used as dilute solutions.
- After drying the wound with gentle pressure, the margins are pressed together and the wound is closed with tissue glue (Histoacryl®).
  - Contraindications for its use include exceptionally lacerated wound margins, tissue defects, continuous bleeding, and visible contamination.
  - After closing with tape or tissue glue, or both, the wound should be kept dry for one week. The blue colour of the glue disappears in three weeks.
  - The method saves the patient from pain. Unnecessary use of materials and a follow-up visit are avoided as well.
  - Unsuccessful results are caused by incorrect techniques: the glue is inserted into the wound before the margins are pressed together, the glue bottle tip is held in the wound, or the glue is not dropped onto the wound.
- Oral lacerations usually need no treatment. A patient with a deep laceration of the tongue should be referred, as general anaesthesia may be required to allow treatment (ligation of the lingual artery). Consult a dentist on dental injuries (7.33).

Lacerations of the fingertips

- The potential for healing is good.
- A fingertip that has been detached from the rest of the finger at a cleavage near the base of the nail should be apposed with a piece of tape (e.g. Steri-Strip®) placed over the fingertip from the volar to dorsal aspect of the finger, or with a couple of lateral sutures. The wound is wrapped with a grease mesh and the finger is placed in an aluminium cast with the neighbouring finger.
- The fingertip may become black or blue but the sense of touch may remain.
- With time (after several weeks) the superficial tissues are detached as a crust, and the remaining minifinger is more functional than an amputated stump.

Incisions

- Incisions are uncommon.
- If the incision was caused by glass, make sure that there are no nerve injuries. Nerve injuries should be treated with primary suturation performed by a specialist. Even interdigital nerves can be sutured.
- Even long incisions are well suited for treatment with tissue glue and tape. If a foreign body of glass is suspected to remain in the wound, ultrasonography may help in diagnosis.

References

1. Farion K, Osmond MH, Hartling L, Russell K, Klassen T, Crumley E, Wiebe N. Tissue adhesives for traumatic lacerations in children and adults. Cochrane Database Syst Rev. 2004;(2):CD003326.
2. Quinn J, Cummings S, Callaham M, Sellers K. Suturing versus conservative management of lacerations of the hand: randomised controlled trial BMJ 2002; 325: 299–231.
3. Cummings P, Del Beccaro MA. Antibiotics to prevent infection in simple wounds: a meta-analysis of randomized studies. Am J Emerg Med 1995;13:396–400.
4. The Database of Abstracts of Reviews of Effectiveness (University of York), Database no.: DARE-952075. In: The Cochrane Library, Issue 4, 1999. Oxford: Update Software.

32.71 Excoriations and bite injuries in children

Editors

Cleansing the wound

- Wash an excoriation with water D [1], isotonic saline, and disinfectant. Only definitely necrotic tissue should be excised.
- Soil and dirt should be removed meticulously–using local anaesthesia and brushing if necessary, as tattooing caused by dirt is much more difficult to treat.

Applying a bandage

- An excoriation should be covered with a greasy bandage held in place by a piece of gauze dressing fixed at its corners. Avoid use of sticking plasters. No antibiotics are indicated.

Further treatment

- The parents should observe for eventual signs of infection–pain, exudate, and elevated temperature. If no exudate is visible the dressing should be left in place.
- An infection should be treated by rinsing repeatedly with warm water. Oral penicillin can be used if necessary.

PAE

Complications

- A joint effusion resulting from an excoriation should be considered as arthritis unless it is reliably excluded. Bacterial arthritis must be treated in a hospital.
- In excoriations of the vulva make sure that the patient is able to void. A small-energy injury such as falling off a bicycle hardly ever causes significant injuries in the urogenital area.

Animal bites

- An animal bite should be considered heavily contaminated and left open after cleansing.
- Cover the wound with a saline compress, administer intravenous cefuroxime as prophylaxis against infection, and re-examine and eventually suture the wound within 24 hours.
- Antibiotic prophylaxis has been used traditionally, but there is little evidence of its efficacy. Prophylaxis can be recommended in human bites. Amoxicillin-clavulanic acid is a good alternative to penicillin.
- Check tetanus immunization status and give a booster if indicated.
- If any bite injury in the face is larger than minimal refer the patient to a specialist (plastic surgeon) without delay.

Viper's bite

- See article 32.31.

Reference

1. Fernandez R, Griffiths R, Ussia C. Water for wound cleansing. Cochrane Database Syst Rev. 2004;(2):CD003861.

32.73 Fractures in children

Editors

Principles

- The general practitioner can treat most fractures in children.
- Difficult diagnosis, rapid healing, and spontaneous correction of malpositions are typical of fractures in children. Conservative treatment is almost always sufficient. Surgery is indicated in about 2% of cases.
- Treatment of pain is the main purpose of immobilization; the fracture itself would heal spontaneously.

Diagnosis

- Diagnosis is based on history, clinical examination, and x-rays.
- The x-ray should be examined for
  - periosteal wrinkles
  - irregularities of trabecular bone
  - fissures.
- If interpretation of the x-ray is difficult it should be compared with a x-ray of the contralateral side.
- Certain fractures may even be treated without a x-ray (see below).

Treatment

- The fractured extremity is immobilized to alleviate the pain.
- Most fractures in children would heal even without immobilization and without resulting in malposition or growth disturbance.

Fractures that can be treated in primary care

- Fracture of the clavicle
  - Clinical diagnosis is sufficient; children hardly ever have complicated fractures.
  - Treatment involves use of a sling.
- Fracture of a toe
  - Clinical diagnosis is sufficient.
  - Treatment involves use of a hard-soled shoe.
- Fracture of the wrist without dislocation
  - An x-ray is necessary.
  - Treatment involves use of a dorsal cast.
- In angulated fractures of the arm the dorsal periosteum should be broken to prevent reangulation that often develops during healing. The procedure can be performed under local anaesthesia in a calmed child. Treatment involves use of an angular cast of the upper and lower arm combined with a volar cast of the arm. A control x-ray is indicated after one week. If the angulation has returned the child should be referred to a specialist.
- Fracture of a finger without dislocation or joint subluxation
  - An x-ray is necessary.
  - The treatment involves use of a finger cast.
- Fracture of the proximal humerus without dislocation
  - The treatment involves use of a sling.
- Fissure of the tibia without dislocation can even be treated without immobilization, especially if the fracture is already several days old at the first consultation.

Indications for referral to a specialist

- Elbow fractures with clear dislocation, and injuries of the elbow region with diagnostic difficulties.
  - An undislocated supracondylar fracture can be treated with an angular cast for 3 weeks.
  - Condylar fracture of the humerus may become dislocated.

- Fractures of the long bones of the lower extremity with clear dislocation.
- Fractures traversing the joint surface
- Impression fractures of the skull.

Immobilization

- The immobilization times for fractures in children are shorter than those in adults.
- In the most common fractures (clavicula, wrist, proximal humerus), immobilization for 2–3 weeks results in a good outcome.
- Malpositions of joints (equinus position of the ankle, extension of the MCP joints) need not be avoided as carefully as in adults.
- Joint mobility is quickly resumed. Systematic follow-up of recovery of mobility, or physical therapy is seldom required.

32.74 Joint and ligament injuries in children

Editors

Subluxation of the head of the radius

- A typical injury in the age group 1 to 5 years.
- Pulling or suspending the child by one hand causes the injury.
- A fresh injury can easily be repositioned by first rotating the arm into supination, and then pushing the head of the radius through the annular ligament "like a screw into the wall". A snap can be heard, and the symptoms alleviate in a moment.
- Reposition is often unsuccessful in older injuries. In such cases the treatment consists of a few days in a supporting mitella bandage. The symptoms disappear spontaneously.

Sprained ankle

- Rupture of the anterior fibulotalar ligament is the most common tendon injury. The draw test is positive if pulling forward brings about a sensation of the foot separating from the leg. Instability is an indication for immobilization with a cast (5 weeks) or, very rarely, for surgical repair.

Luxation of the patella

- The most common luxation in teenagers is luxation of the patella.
- A laterally shifted patella should be repositioned as soon as possible. For further treatment see 18.32.

32.75 Central nervous system injuries in children

Editors

Principles

- Central nervous system injuries are common. Usually they are low-energy injuries caused, for example, by falling or by colliding with another child, and can be classified as concussions.
- Follow-up of symptoms and level of consciousness is essential.
- Bed rest is not necessary after concussion.

Investigations

- History and clinical examination concentrating on
  - assessing the level of consciousness
  - spontaneous activity
  - pupillary size and reaction to light.
- A skull x-ray is of little benefit. It may show an impression fracture that can usually be suspected on clinical grounds, or a fissure suggesting a hard blow on the skull that may require follow-up in a hospital.

Follow-up

- A doctor should follow up a child recovering from a head injury for at least a couple of hours. The clinical examination should be repeated and the findings recorded before discharge.
- The aim of the follow-up is to make sure that eventual symptoms (short period of unconsciousness, somnolence, paleness, amnesia) are not caused by intracranial haemorrhage.
- Intracranial bleeding in children is usually extradural, and soon results in deterioration of consciousness or lateralizing symptoms, 6–12 hours after the injury at the latest.
- The child can be discharged when he or she is red-cheeked, tired of waiting, playing, or reading. In infants a retracted fontanelle pulsating in time with respiration indicates normal intracranial pressure.
- A person who knows the child well should continue with follow-up at home.
- Advise the parents to give only liquids (to avoid risk of aspiration of solid food), and to wake the child up during the night for assessing his or her general condition.

- Later symptoms are not common in children. Bed rest is of no benefit.

Severe brain contusion

- Brain contusion is more common than intracranial haematoma. It is the most common single cause of death after the age of 4 years.
- Impaired consciousness and neurological symptoms are usually present from the time of injury.
- The child should be transported to a facility where CT, intensive care, and neurosurgery are available. During transportation adequate ventilation must be ensured to prevent and treat brain oedema.

32.76 Intra-abdominal injuries and bleeding in children

Editors

Principles

- A child with suspected visceral trauma (symptomatic contusion injury of the trunk) should always be referred to a hospital. Thus a vomiting child without preceding concussion should always be followed up in hospital.
- Bleeding from visceral organs is not uncommon in children. Sometimes bleeding results from a relatively minor trauma such as falling off a bicycle. If an ultrasonograph is available, the (general) practitioner on duty can look for fluid in the abdominal cavity of a child who will not be referred to a hospital immediately on the basis of symptoms or type of accident.

Symptoms

- Signs of bleeding in children may differ from those of adults.
- Low blood pressure or rapid pulse as signs of arterial insufficiency are not always evident in children with hypovolaemia, but significant blood loss is always associated with decreased peripheral circulation. Therefore, in the assessment of an injured child note the temperature of the extremities, paleness of the skin, and mood.
- Cold hands and legs, greenish-grey paleness, and excited mood indicate adrenal hyperactivity that may correct blood pressure and mask hypovolaemia.
- The diagnosis of internal bleeding is made on the basis of clinical examination. Haematocrit can be used to follow up bleeding. A single haematocrit determination is often not helpful in the diagnosis of bleeding. The white cell count correlates with the severity of bleeding.

Treatment

- Rapid transport to a unit with facilities for surgery is essential in internal bleedings ("load and go") (17.3).
- First aid consists of physiological saline infusion if the infusion route can be established without delay. Intraosseal infusion is an alternative in emergencies: insert a thick needle in the marrow cavity of the proximal tibia.
- A symptomatic child has lost about one quarter of his or her blood volume (20 ml/kg of body weight). At least this amount of saline can be infused rapidly without substituting totally for the loss in circulating volume.
- The adequacy of volume correction can be assessed by observing skin temperature and urine volume: urine output of 1 ml/h per kg of bodyweight is the target. The fluid infusion is too rapid if the respiratory rate increases. Systolic blood pressure need not be raised to the normal level.

32.77 Suturing a wound

Editors

Basic rules

- Small wounds in children should be treated conservatively with tissue glue (A) [1].
- Conservative treatment is as effective as suturation in hand lacerations less than 2 cm in length (B) [2]

Selection of thread and suturing techniques

- Use 5-0 or 4-0 monofilament thread (nylon or polypropylene) attached to a skin needle (3/8 bending, triangular cross-sectional shape).
- Avoid all tension when apposing the margins of the wounds by sutures. Tension is painful and results in a scar. A clean, fresh (facial) laceration can also be sutured with intradermal continuous suture by a doctor experienced in the technique.
- Interrupted sutures should be removed from the face after 4–5 days and replaced by tape if necessary.

Bleeding wounds

- Compress the wound to control the bleeding. Compression should be effective and last long enough. The best motivated person to perform compressing is the adult accompanying the patient.
- If the bleeding continues after compression, the wound must be sutured. Place the sutures near each other to stop the bleeding. A loose X-suture circumferencing the bleeding site from both sides is even more effective in stopping the bleeding.

- Locating and ligating a bleeding vessel is very seldom necessary (and usually unsuccessful if performed by an inexperienced physician).

Contaminated wounds

- If the wound is contaminated, prescribe penicillin V, 100 000 IU/kg/day for 3–4 days.

References

1. Farion K, Osmond MH, Hartling L, Russell K, Klassen T, Crumley E, Wiebe N. Tissue adhesives for traumatic lacerations in children and adults. Cochrane Database Syst Rev. 2004;(2):CD003326.
2. Quinn J, Cummings S, Callaham M, Sellers K. Suturing versus conservative management of lacerations of the hand: randomised controlled trial BMJ 2002; 325: 299–231.

32.80 Incidental glucosuria in children

Jukka Rajantie

Aims

- Detect possible insulin-dependent diabetes mellitus as the cause of incidental glucosuria and arrange for care immediately.
- Investigate whether glucosuria results from a prediabetic state and arrange follow-up.

Causes

- Blood glucose is elevated because of diabetes or some other cause
  - About 6% of children with asymptomatic glucosuria later develop type 1 diabetes.
- Stress factors
  - Infections
  - Traumas
  - Burn injuries
  - Hypoxia
  - Hypothermia
  - Surgery
- Low renal threshold
- Hyponatraemic dehydration caused by diarrhoea
- Certain medications can cause glucosuria in high doses
  - Cephalosporins
  - Penicillin G
  - Nalidixic acid
  - Nitrofurantoin
  - Anti-inflammatory agents
  - Ascorbic acid

Investigation strategy in cases of symptomless glucosuria

1. Determine blood glucose concentration immediately
   - If the fasting level is examined and the plasma level exceeds 7.0 mmol/l or postprandial level exceeds 11.1 mmol/l (in venous blood 6.7 or 10 mmol/l respectively) diabetes is probable and the child should be referred urgently to further investigations (oral glucose tolerance) and treatment.
   - If only postprandial glucose levels can be examined and the result is below 11.1 mmol/l, the fasting value should be examined on the next morning. If the level is above 7.0 mmol/l, action is taken as instructed above.
2. If blood glucose level is <6.7 mmol/l, further investigations can be performed in primary care.
   - A control urine sample on the next morning or at the latest when a known stress factor, for example, infection has disappeared.
   - Glycosylated haemoglobin determination
   - Diabetes type I associated autoantibodies
3. If the results of these investigations are normal and there are no type 1 diabetics in the family, further investigations are not necessary and follow-up is not needed.
4. Further investigations are indicated
   - **immediately** if
     - glucosuria is detected repeatedly
     - HbA_{1c} exceeds reference values
   - within 2–3 weeks if
     - autoantibodies are detected
     - a family member has type 1 diabetes
5. Further investigations should be performed in a paediatric specialist unit
   - The parents follow-up the child's morning urine glucose levels and contact the paediatric unit if need arises.

32.82 Rickets

Editors

Aetiology

- Insufficient intake of vitamin D (failure to give a vitamin preparation to the child)
  - More than 90% of all cases

PAE

- Families with a negative attitude to vitamins (and often also vaccinations), and children of immigrants with pigmented skin (whose requirement of vitamin D is particularly high) living in Northern countries carry the greatest risk.
- For dosing of vitamin D, see 24.64.

♦ Associated with malabsorption (e.g. untreated coeliac disease)

♦ Resistance to vitamin D

♦ Deficiency of phosphate (X-linked hypophosphataemic rickets, paraneoplastic rickets and osteomalacia, Fanconi's syndrome, renal acidosis)

Clinical course of rickets due to deficiency of vitamin D

1. A hypocalcaemic phase usually lasts for a few days, but it can become prolonged at the age of 2–9 months and result in tetany and convulsions.
2. A phase of hyperparathyroidism, normocalcaemia, and hypophosphataemia
3. A phase of hypocalcaemia and severe bone disease, with associated predisposition to infections and muscular weakness.

Diagnosis

Diagnosis of rickets

♦ Clinical presentation
- Symptoms associated with hypocalcaemia (tetany)
- Bone abnormalities and growth disturbance (rachitic rosary of the costochondral junctions, growth disturbance of distal epiphyses, decelerating increase in height, retarded psychomotor development, muscular hypotonia)

♦ Radiology
- The distal ends of the diaphyses of the radius and ulna lose their clear outline, are cup-shaped, and show spotty or fringed rarefaction.

♦ Laboratory findings
- Increased serum alkaline phosphatase, decreased 25-OH-D_3, and in tetany decreased serum calcium and silicon.

Discovering the aetiology

♦ History of vitamin D intake, signs of malabsorption

♦ A specialist should always be consulted.

♦ Rickets is managed with vitamin D. Further investigations to detect rarer forms of rickets are necessary only if vitamin D does not bring cure.

Treatment

Treatment of hypocalcaemia

♦ Generalized convulsions
- Calcium gluconate (10%) intravenously
  - Loading dose 0.2 ml/kg slowly
  - Continuous infusion 4–6 ml/kg/24 h

♦ Prolonged hypocalcaemia
- Alphacalcidol 0.06–0.1 μg/kg/day perorally or intravenously for a few days in hospital if necessary

♦ Peroral calcium
- Calcium lactate 50 mg Ca^{2+}/kg/day divided in 4–6 doses for 2 weeks.

Vitamin D treatment

♦ Vitamin D (drops, 80 units/drop)

♦ 2000 units/day perorally for one month simultaneously with the recommended normal daily intake of vitamin D (which must be ensured continuously)

32.83 Diagnosis and treatment of childhood hypercholesterolaemia

Matti Salo

Aim

♦ To identify children with hypercholesterolaemia on the basis of a family history (parents) of coronary heart disease and high blood lipid levels. Screening the entire child population is not recommended.

Directing screening at risk families

♦ Hypercholesterolaemia should be searched for in families with precocious coronary heart disease.
- Father or grandfather at age < 55 years, or mother or grandmother at age < 65 years, or
- hyperlipidaemia
  - serum cholesterol ⩾ 8.0 mmol/l or
  - serum LDL cholesterol ⩾ 6.0 mmol/l or
  - serum triglycerides ⩾ 5.0 mmol/l or
  - milder hyperlipidaemia with low (<0.9 mmol/l) serum HDL cholesterol.

♦ At screening every family member older than 2 years of age should have their fasting serum cholesterol, HDL cholesterol and triglycerides measured after a 12-hour fast, and LDL cholesterol calculated with Friedewald's formula (24.53).

♦ Increased values measured at screening should be double-checked.

♦ Secondary hyperlipidaemias should be excluded by measuring serum free T_4, serum TSH, serum ALT and urine albumin before commencing therapy.

Table 32.83 Classification of hypercholesterolaemias in childhood)

	Serum cholesterol (mmol/l)	Serum LDL cholesterol (mmol/l)
Not increased	<5.5	<4.0
Increased	5.5–6.9	4.0–5.4
Significantly increased	⩾ 7.0	⩾ 5.5

- Young patients with coronary heart disease and hyperlipidaemias should be informed of the importance of having their children and grandchildren examined. A general practitioner or an internist may initiate directed screening. Departments of internal medicine and paediatrics should agree on examination of the children and coordinate assessment of results.
- If the family history indicates frequent coronary heart disease, the finding of hyperlipidaemia may be a cause of anxiety for the nearest relatives. As accurate evaluation of the family history often requires informing and assessing persons living in various parts of the country, a consultation at a genetic unit can be considered.

Classification of hypercholesterolaemia

- See Table 32.83

Therapy: indications and practice

- Serum cholesterol of less than 5.5 mmol/l (LDL < 4.0), does not require further action.
- With an increased serum cholesterol, it usually suffices to commence a diet and follow up the child at 3, 6 ja 12 months. If a diet maintained for 6–12 months does not decrease serum cholesterol to below 5.5 mmol/l or LDL cholesterol below 4.0 mmol/l, the child should be remitted to a paediatric clinic for assessment by a paediatric endocrinologist or a paediatrician familiar with therapy of hyperlipidaemias. If necessary, a dietician should be used for dietary instructions.
- A child with significantly increased serum cholesterol should be remitted directly to a paediatric clinic.
- The need for drug therapy is decided mainly on family history of coronary heart disease. Drug therapy (a resine is the first-line drug B [1 2 3]; a statin may be used as an alternative) is initiated by an experienced paediatrician.
- Drug therapy is rarely needed before puberty, and very rarely before school age.

Diet

- Diet is the single most important treatment for hyperlipidaemia, and it may be sufficient even for familial hypercholesterolaemia in childhood. The diet should be followed from the age of two years. It is most important to decrease the amount of saturated fat.
  - Reduction in the use of dairy fat.
    - Skim milk or 1% fat milk
    - No- or low-fat dairy products and cheeses
  - Sitostanol- and sitosterol containing margarine or vegetable oil-based margarine on bread.
  - Reduction in the use of fatty veal or pork.
  - Use of fibre-rich and full corn products, oatmeal and fish is encouraged.
  - To maintain adequate calcium intake total abstention from dairy products is not recommended.

References

1. Kwiterovich PO Jr. Identification and treatment of heterozygous familiar hypercholesterolemia in children and adolescents. Am J Cardiol 1993 Sep 30;72(10):30D–37D.
2. Ballantyre CM. Familiar hypercholesterolaemia: Optimum treatment strategies. Int J Clin Pract Suppl. 2002 Jul;(130):22–26.
3. Wiegman A, Hutten BA, de broot E et al. Efficacy and safety of statin therapy in children with familiar hypercholesterolaemia: a randomized controlled trial. JAMA 2004;21:377–378.

32.91 Guidelines regarding sudden unexpected death in infancy

Pertti Rintahaka

PAE

Aims

- To prevent sudden infant death syndrome (SIDS) by instructing parents not to let the infant sleep in the prone position and not to clothe the infant too warmly.
- To perform necessary studies to find out the most common causes of sudden death in infancy.
- To support the family.
- To give the first information on SIDS.

Definition

- The definition of SIDS includes every sudden unexpected infant death that remains unexplained after post-mortem examinations.

Diagnosis

- It is necessary to start looking for the causes leading to the need of resuscitation already during the procedure.
- Attention is paid to the following:
  - State of health of the infant
  - Events before death
  - Possible illnesses and symptoms

- Time, when the infant was last seen alive
- The place where the infant was found lifeless
- Possible vomit in bed or on clothes.

♦ In addition to detailed background information and physical examination, the following laboratory tests are performed:
- Complete blood cell count
- Blood glucose
- Blood sodium, potassium and calcium
- Urea nitrogen
- Blood and urinary culture
- Viral antibodies
- Urinary glucose, cells and bacteria
- Bacterial and viral isolation from the upper respiratory tract and stool.

♦ If trauma or battering is suspected (bruises, abrasions, possible old or recent fractures etc.) whole body x-ray is performed.

♦ With these examinations it is possible to
- recognise or to raise suspicion of several diseases (for example sepsis, hypoglycaemia, electrolyte disturbances) which may cause sudden death.
- explain factors contributing to death or triggering factors (for example mild respiratory tract infection or mild diarrhoea) and their severity.

♦ Microbial specimens taken at autopsy are almost always contaminated. For this reason, samples taken immediately after death are more reliable. This also applies to blood glucose and electrolyte levels, where post-mortem changes make interpretation even more difficult.

♦ The physician in charge informs the police immediately about a sudden death. The police decides whether a forensic autopsy is necessary and asks for a referral if needed.

♦ If SIDS is suspected, it is necessary to give or arrange immediate support to the family as described below. Part of this information may also be applied in cases of sudden death due to various known causes.

Immediate support of the family

♦ Although the infant's life cannot be saved, the family needs support in this dramatic situation and support should start immediately. Drugs do not substitute for information.

♦ The parents should be offered the possibility to stay with the dead infant as long as they want. This helps them to accept the reality of death and shortens the mourning process and associated reactions.

♦ In the shock stage of the mourning process, the mere presence of the physician in charge makes the situation easier for the parents.

♦ A discussion including both parents and preferably also all siblings is important. The first information should be simple and focused on basic things, because the parents' ability to understand is limited in the shock stage. Some information should also be given on the mourning process.

♦ It is necessary to make it clear to the parents that the examination of a sudden death also includes a police investigations and this does not mean that the parents are suspected. According to the law, all sudden deaths require detailed investigations and autopsy. Investigations also serve as legal protection for the parents. Absolute refusal of autopsy usually means that the parents have not yet accepted the death.

♦ If the sudden infant death syndrome is suspected, especially the following should be made clear for the parents:
- SIDS is the most common single type of death after the neonatal period.
- The cause(s) of SIDS is (are) unknown.
- SIDS is not predictable.
- SIDS occurs during sleep. It is painless and silent.
- Suffocation on bed clothing or vomit is usually not the cause of death although stomach contents may be seen around the infant.
- Mild illness, for instance rhinitis, may preceed death, it is not a cause of death, however.
- SIDS is not contagious, and it is rare after the age of six months. It does not threaten the other children in the family.
- Recurrence in the family is rare.
- The death was nobody's fault and was not due to neglect.

♦ Check the patient information resources available in your country/district and have handouts ready for this emergency.

Continuation of the family's treatment

♦ The family is seen again on the following day after death. This meeting should also include sisters and brothers of the dead infant.

♦ The next meeting with the family takes place latest after the forensic pathology results are available.

♦ Sometimes the parents are worried because there has been talk of SIDS, although the death certificate gives another diagnosis, such as suffocation, aspiration of stomach contents, mild pneumonia etc. In these situations, a consultation with the forensic pathologist may be necessary.

♦ The recommended frequency of seeing the family is two weeks, one month, three and six months and one year after death. In this way it is possible to start treatment in time if the family has difficulties in the mourning process.

♦ It is preferable that whenever possible the physician in charge of the acute situation continues to see the family. If this is not possible, another person (a social worker, family physician or a health care nurse) should take the responsibility of follow-up visits with the family. If needed, a physician should explain once more the autopsy results.

♦ During follow-up visits, the parents often again ask questions discussed earlier. This does not necessarily mean that the information has been unclear or inadequate, but it reflects the limited ability to understand in the shock stage of mourning.

♦ In the normal mourning process, the parents start to use the past tense when they talk about the infant and to remember also happy events. The most difficult times are for example the birth day and the death date of the infant. The mourning process is usually completed in a year from the death.

- Alarming signs indicating that the mourning process is not successful are repeated denial of death, failure to come to the funeral or to visit the grave, strong feelings of guilt, or blaming the husband/wife, caretaker or even sisters or brothers, other family problems, inability to work, problems reflected by sisters and brothers etc.
- Do not recommend a new pregnancy to the parents. The couple should make this decision by themselves.
- Production of breast milk may be stopped by cabergoline if necessary.

Treatment of the sisters and brothers

- SIDS has an inevitable effect on the dead infant's sisters and brothers. The recently adopted role of big brother or sister ends abruptly, and the child is unable to understand the cause(s) or meaning of the event. The child can deny the death, stay apparently unconcerned or develop various behavioural disturbances or psychosomatic symptoms, if he/she does not get adequate support or information.
- The ability of children to understand death varies with age; children less than five years see death as reversible. Not until the age ten years do children recognize death as an irreversible event. Children aged 5 to 10 years often think that somebody is responsible for the death. Not until puberty do children have a mourning process similar to adults.
- It is important to explain to the sisters and brothers that SIDS occurs only in infancy. SIDS is not caused by anybody and the good health of sisters and brothers is emphasized. The siblings should be told about the death of infant and the powerful emotions caused by sorrow should not be hidden. There is no reason to be angry with children for apparent lack of mourning, because this only shows that they do not understand the finality of death. Sisters and brothers should also be taken to the funeral.
- Failure of the mourning process of the family can be expressed as various symptoms in the other children. More detailed examination is indicated if the parents are overprotective towards their other children. If there are any obvious problems, a child psychiatrist should be consulted.

Paediatric Psychiatry

Evidence Based Medicine Guidelines. Edited by the Duodecim Editorial Team
 ISBN: 0-470-01184-X

33.1 Babies with a tendency to cry – from the point of view of a child psychiatrist

Leena Launis

General principles

- Objective
  - To break the negative cycle that is often connected to a baby's crying with a sufficiently accurate estimate and treatment. Prerequisites for the creation of safe attachment, which is the basic foundation for the child's entire development, are thus strengthened.
- Differential diagnosis is essential.
  - It is always essential to rule out or treat somatic illnesses. Often, when a baby's tendency to cry is strong, the problem is neither somatic nor psychological. Somatic symptoms always include psychological ones and psychological problems are often manifested as somatic symptoms. In practice it is often useless to contemplate what constitutes the cause and what is a consequence. Often many different approaches are necessary. All means of healing should be eagerly used to put an end to the vicious cycle.
- Especially in the case of babies it is often impossible to distinguish between somatic and psychological problems - this developmental stage constitutes the very source of psychosomatics. Babies sense holistically with their entire being both positive and negative feelings, and they express themselves primarily through physical means.
- If a child is clearly ill or injured, it is easy to explain crying as a reaction. It is essential, however, to keep in mind that somatic and mental factors are interrelated. Caring for a sick child is always more demanding than caring for a healthy one. It is often more difficult and less rewarding. Parents must be more persistent, and it is often more difficult to detect coherence in the child's reactions. Sometimes there may be little hope for the future. It is also possible that the child's traumatic experiences, such as painful manoeuvres or separation during hospital care, are reflected, for example, in the care of the child as panic, difficulty to calm down and an increased tendency to cry.
- All of the aforementioned is linked to the interaction between the mother and baby and the development of attachment. Problems related to early interaction are a common cause of a baby's tendency to cry. The problems with interaction can be more a result of either the mother's or the child's actions, but both are always part of the dilemma. The father also has an important role in the child's life from the very beginning, even though it is partly indirect in his support of the mother; the baby does, however, start to create a relationship with the father at the very beginning.

Reasons for a baby crying

- Babies never cry out of maliciousness or to tease or manipulate their parents, even though it may feel like it to the parents. Babies do not want to be in charge; they need determined parents that take responsibility for what happens. Nor do babies accuse their parents or think they are useless or hate them, as parents often assume; rather babies simply do not feel good for some reason: they feel unsatisfied or uncomfortable or are in pain. Babies may also feel bad because they do not feel they are mentally supported in an insecure, controversial and unpredictable or indifferent relationship. When babies do not experience life as safe in the hands of adults, they are forced to support themselves. This effort often manifests itself as physical tension or the rejection of physical contact, the turning away from a parent, refusal to eat, or the like. Often the symptoms include sleeping disorders, hyperactivity, a low threshold for stimuli, difficulty in expecting satisfaction and relief in accordance to their age and a low ability to endure frustration.
- Crying is a natural way for babies to express themselves, and it is their essential means of communication. The quantity and intensity of crying are relative matters; the parents' views can differ considerably and also deviate from norms. In some families babies are not allowed to cry at all. It is also a cause of concern if babies do not cry at all (babies who have given up or are depressed).
- A strong tendency for a baby to cry is always a problem for the entire family. A crying baby may, for example, be made a scapegoat when the relationship of the parents escalates into a crisis. Older siblings may also suffer unreasonably because of a screaming younger brother or sister. Sometimes a child may be labelled as difficult and demanding for the rest of his or her life if the situation is not dealt with in due time by analysing the different beliefs and projections that parents generally have concerning their difficult baby.
- A tendency of a baby to cry may also originate from the mother's mental problems. A mother may have a background of depression or psychosis, but a clear mental disturbance is not always the cause. Many different kinds of problems may lie behind the crying of a baby, for example, early trauma experienced by the mother, difficulties that the mother has had in her relationship with her own mother or problems with the present or earlier pregnancies, childbirths or the perinatal stage of the child. A primigravida may sometimes be extremely insecure as a mother, but with adequate support at the beginning and with experience she may quickly become more sure of herself. When the crying of a baby alarms an anxious mother, it is impossible for her to calm her baby, who feels insecure. A baby is extremely sensitive to the mother's state of emotion, and also reacts accordingly.

Evaluation of problems with interaction

- Evaluation requires the opportunity to observe the child and mother together. Even a considerably short time can give an

adequate impression, although a reliable estimate calls for lengthier and repeated observation. The physician should trust his or her impressions and have the courage to initiate discussions about the possible causes of concern.
- Somatic problems
- Psychiatric problems of the mother (33.15)

Evaluation of the child's role

- Is the psychophysical development of the child within normal variation or are there signs of deviation, defective motor skills or the lack of ability to make contact, cessation or abuse? Is breastfeeding normal? Has a baby over 4 months of age developed a regular rhythm and schedule?
- Does the child appear calm, willing to make contact (eye contact, reciprocal smile and voices), interested in the surroundings, comfortable in the mother's arms, and reactive and communicative towards the mother? OR Is the child restless, motorically uneasy, gesticulating and tense in motion and presence, over-sensitive to stimuli, easily excitable into fierce crying, difficult to calm, uncomfortable in the mother's arms, aversive to the mother's attempts at contact (turns head away, shuts eyes, falls asleep), concerned and fatigued in facial expressions?
- What does the character of the crying and facial expressions reveal (hunger, pain, fatigue, desolation, powerlessness)?

Evaluation of the mother's role

- Is the mother interested in her baby; does she attempt to make contact with the baby? Does she talk to the child? How does she speak and what does she say? Is the mother capable of empathising with the baby's situation? Is the mother capable of distinguishing between the nuances and meanings of different kinds of cries? How successful in general is the mother in caring for the baby and carrying out everyday routines? Are the mother's actions adequate with respect to the situation? Are her speech, voice and grip harmonious, or does she express great insecurity or aggression, for example, in handling the baby? Does the mother give up easily? Is she disappointed, if the baby does not immediately react positively towards her initiatives? Is she offended by the baby? Does the mother also express compassion towards her baby regardless of her own fatigue or is she openly hostile? What impression does the mother give of her child? Is it mainly positive or negative? It is not unusual that mothers sometimes have very negative impressions of their children, for example, as a teaser or a user.
- Remember to evaluate the personal state of the mother as well. Does the mother appear to be exhausted, serious, disoriented or does she cry easily? Does she complain of physical feelings of illness? Does she appear to be over-concerned or indifferent? Is she afraid that the baby may be seriously ill or constantly hungry or in serious pain? Is she afraid of what other people might say or that something awful may happen? Whatever the mother conveys about caring for her baby or being a mother, it is essential that her experiences be taken seriously and without belittlement. Mere encouragement does not suffice!

Evaluation of parenting skills

- Some questions that the mother or parents can be asked:
  - How would they describe their child; what kind of baby is John/Jill?
  - Has parenthood been what they expected, or has something in particular surprised them?
  - What has been most difficult in parenthood? What has been best in parenthood?
  - Has the mother/father had prior experiences with babies?
  - Do the parents have a similar concept of the baby's crying?
  - Are the parents able to deal with their possible disagreements?
  - Do they have a good relationship? Has the birth of the baby made them closer, or has it made them grow apart?
  - What kind of a supportive network does the family have? Can they ask grandparents, relatives or friends to help, and do they have the courage to do so?
  - Does the mother have contact with the outside world or has she cocooned herself in the home?
  - Does the mother have contacts with other women? What is the mother's relationship with her own mother like (indicates the way the mother is able to become attached to her own child)?
  - What, in the mother's opinion, would best help her cope in the exhausting situation? Determine the need for home aid and the willingness of the mother to receive outside help. Investigate the need for support from child welfare services.
  - What is the parents' worst scenario about what might happen if the baby continues to cry as constantly as in the current situation? (Risk of abuse?)
  - In the end, parents tend always to have some idea of why their baby cries, even if it may sound inconceivable. It is always useful to ask.
  - Whatever problems may surface during the discussion, ask the mother if she has had an opportunity to discuss the situation with someone also from the point of view of her own ability to cope.

Actions and treatment

- Encourage the mother to speak about negative and even conflicting feelings and let her know that other mothers feel the same way. Tell her that it is also possible to get expert help with these problems from psychologists or child psychiatrics at the child health clinic.
- Sometimes the mother is in need of intense guidance that would support her strengths rather than in need of detailed instructions on child care. Such guidance can free the mother to see her child more realistically and open up to the baby's messages.
- Sometimes the mother-baby twosome is in need of help from an expert therapist or what can be called "child care through the parent".
- Mother-child discussion groups have proved helpful. They offer mothers an opportunity to share their feelings with

women in the same situation, explore different solutions, get a more realistic idea of child care and make use of the group process under the guidance of therapists. There may be groups, organised by different societies in your area that may benefit the mother and child. Even if a municipality cannot offer any forms of special support, the child health clinics can bring parents and babies with similar problems together and possibly provide facilities, for example, for groups that are arranged by the parents themselves.

- It is important to support the relations of the mother to the outside world in general, for example, by encouraging her to participate in mother-baby groups at playgrounds or in local church congregations, mother-baby gymnastics, musical playschools for babies, and the like when she is in danger of becoming secluded at home.
- Sometimes the mother is in need of a separate evaluation by a psychiatrist and possible individual therapy and or medication. In the case of clear postnatal depression or psychosis, the examination and treatment coincides with normal treatment policies for depression and psychosis, with the addition that special effort must be made to preserve the connection between the baby and mother and it must be ensured that the adult who takes care of the baby is safe and able to make contact.
- Some parents need therapeutic support to cope in their relationship (e.g., family clinics, family counselling centres and the like).
- When there is great concern about the baby's health, a simple thorough examination by a paediatrician can ease the situation considerably.
- An overactive crying baby may often respond to physical relaxation, for example, baby massage, which, at the same time, is combined with interaction with the mother. Child health centres can often provide written instructions and even counselling on the subject. A tight, secure grip on the child is important and gives the baby a safe feeling of "holding together". Often a mother must be encouraged to speak and sing to her child. A "silent" mother is often a depressed mother. The mother may also have to be helped to realise that the child actually reacts to her voice. The importance of eye contact should be emphasised.
- Carrying the baby in a babysling even at home promotes a feeling of closeness and contact with the mother, and it can also relax the baby. The baby can also be carried upright, which often eases stomach pains.
- Home visits are often welcomed and useful for families with babies, and the visits can facilitate a more vivid idea of the family's situation and everyday life.
- Trust your impressions and do not hesitate to ask questions, as long as you are discrete.
- Do not jump to conclusions. Reserve enough time for the meeting when you know that you will be examining a baby with a tendency to cry.
- Do not seek to solve the situation in one meeting. Make an appointment for another meeting even if all efforts to ease the crying of the baby seem to have been exhausted.

33.2 Recurring psychogenic stomach-aches and headaches among children

Irma Moilanen

Basic rules

- Most problems can be treated in primary health care.
- A somatic examination is important to rule out organic causes. At the same time it is possible to chart the psychological state of the child and family.

Background

- Recurring stomach-ache is a child's way of responding to emotional stress at home and in school.
- Children who suffer from psychogenic stomach-aches are typically shy, conscientious and sensitive. They set high standards for themselves, and they may have difficulties in expressing their feelings.
- Recurring stomach-aches and headaches are often typical also for the family members of these children.
- Psychogenic stomach-aches and headaches appear in the same children and adolescents.

Treatment

- A somatic examination is always important, and many are relieved by having a somatic cause for the problem ruled out.
- The child and family may be encouraged to express their feelings verbally, and they may be subtly guided to see the possible connection of symptoms with moods and atmospheres.
- If common methods do not help, psychologist or a child psychiatrist should be consulted.

33.3 Childhood depression

Kaija Puura

Objective

- To identify depression in a child, with symptoms that are complex and often irritant.

What is depression like in a child?

- Depression in a child is a state of melancholy that enervates experiences.
- The ability to be interested and to feel joy and satisfaction disappears.
- Depressive children feel rejected. They think that nobody cares for them. It is also hard for them to accept offers of help.
- A depressive child often appears unhappy and miserable.

Prevalence of depression in children

- The prevalence of severe depression is 0.1–2% in school-age children and 2.5–6% in adolescents.
- Milder, clinically important depression occurs in about 4% of children, and about 10–40% of children have depressive experiences.

Diagnostics; symptoms at different ages

- Depression in the infant
  - There are no official criteria for depression in the infant. Studies have shown that infants develop symptoms in response to unsatisfactory interaction.
  - Depression in the infant is usually due to interaction with a depressive parent.
    - A depressive parent does not seek eye contact with the infant or talk to the infant (no baby talk).
    - Handling of the baby is rare, often mechanical, or the baby is held at a distance.
    - The parent is exhausted, and baby care seems laborious and difficult.
    - The parent is often worried and anxious about his/her ability to care for the baby.
    - In the worst case, the parent may have ideations relating to suicide or killing the baby.
  - A depressive infant avoids eye contact.
  - The infant's ability to be interested in the environment and other people is impaired.
  - The infant is passive.
  - The infant's cry is muted, querulous.
  - Sleeping and eating disorders often occur in depressive infants.
  - Both cognitive and motor development are retarded and may even regress.
  - In the extreme case, the infant may lose his/her lust for life.
- Depression in toddlers
  - Depression is often manifested by irritability, dissatisfaction and boredom.
  - The child has lost his/her joy of life, and the child does not like to play.
  - Lack of concentration may manifest as restlessness
  - The child can be tired.
  - The child can have difficulty in falling asleep or may wake up in the middle of the night.
  - In some cases, depression can manifest itself as violent temper tantrums or as inability to play with others.
  - Self-destructive tendencies (33.14) associated with depression may manifest as attempts to run away from home and as proneness to accidents.
  - Psychosomatic symptoms such as encopresis, headache, and abdominal pain can be signs of depression.
  - Changes in appetite can be signs of depression.
- Depression in school-age children
  - Depression often manifests as irritability and boredom.
  - Decreased interest in the environment and lesser enjoyment of life lead to fewer leisure time activities or to withdrawal from such activities.
  - Concentration problems manifest as restlessness.
  - The child may be tired and sleep much or wake up early in the early hours of morning.
  - School performance is impaired.
  - The child thinks that he or she is worthless, a failure, and has feelings of guilt.
  - Feelings of worthlessness can be hidden by taking the role of a clown: The child masks his or her hopelessness by making others laugh.
  - Prolonged depression can lead to social withdrawal and isolation, and the child is susceptible to bullying at school both as a bully and as a bullying target.
  - A child's depression can even lead to thoughts of self-destruction and, in the extreme case, acts of self-destruction.
  - Children's suicides are violent and often mistakenly interpreted as accidents.

Differential diagnosis

- Depression in children may coincide with anxiety disorder, school phobia and disturbances of conduct.
- In children and adolescents, depression is often associated with various somatic disorders. On the other hand, sick children may also appear quiescent and depressed.
- Normal children can also be sad, tired and exhausted, and a short-lived depressive reaction may be a developmental phenomenon, possibly associated with an experienced loss or change.
- If depression unfavourably affects the child's psychosocial coping, e.g. when with friends or at school, or mental development, it has to be treated appropriately.

Evaluation of a depressive child

- The diagnostics or treatment of depression usually requires child-psychiatric evaluation or consultation.
- When the depressive child seen by a doctor, at a guidance centre or by a school nurse is evaluated, not only the child should be interviewed but also the parent(s) and possibly other important adults, such as the child's teacher(s).

- When the child is interviewed, it is useful to ask about symptoms of depression (Do you sleep well?) and use words that are familiar to the child.
- If suicidal tendencies are suspected, direct questions should be asked (Have you felt so bad lately that you have thought of hurting yourself or killing yourself?).
- If the child answers affirmatively, the parents should be asked if they know how bad the child is feeling and that there is a risk of suicide.
- In addition to the interview, attention should be paid to the child's appearance and any interaction between the child and the parent(s), especially when evaluating infants or toddlers.
- When a child's depression is evaluated and treated, the family's entire life situation should be mapped, because depression may be associated with certain events in the family, and parents always have an important role in the treatment of the child.
- Questionnaires (such as Children's Depression Inventory (CDI)) can be used to map depression in school-age children and adolescents.

Treatment of depression

General principles

- A depressive child needs support from an adult who is able to cope with the child's feelings of desolation, helplessness, anger and bitterness safely and without anxiety, and who can also show interest in and take care of the child and his or her needs.
- Parents or childminders must always participate in the treatment, because the child is an inseparable part of the family.
- The severity of the depression, the family situation and the treatment facilities made available by the system determine the treatment chosen.

Depression in infants and toddlers

- It is extremely important that the child has sufficient satisfactory interaction with an adult. This can be made possible by treating the parent's depression and supporting parents in interaction, or, if this is not possible, by providing a childminder for the infant or toddler. In severe cases, interaction therapy may be indicated.
- University hospitals are equipped to provide psychiatric treatments for infants and toddlers.

Depression in school-aged children

- Short-term depressions as responses to a change
  - can be treated at a guidance centre or the school health care unit in cooperation with the family.
  - require adequate follow-up to determine if the depression has receded or if prolonged depression requires continued treatment at a specialist level.
- Indications for medical specialist care or other specialist care (child psychiatric clinic or family guidance centre)
  - Prolonged depression (duration more than 2 months), even with mild symptoms
  - Severe depression affecting the functional capacity of the child.
  - Depression associated with multiple or severe disturbances of conduct.

Choosing treatment

- Family therapy is indicated especially for younger children when the parents or one of the parents is depressive, or the child has evidently been neglected.
- Individual therapy is especially suitable for adolescents, but in some cases also for younger children (B) [1 2].
- Children at suicidal risk should immediately be referred to a special hospital treatment. The primary aim of treatment is to ensure physical safety, which can be done on an outpatient basis or in a hospital ward.
- Inpatient treatment is also indicated in children whose depression considerably affects their school performance and other psychosocial coping.
- Selective serotonin reuptake inhibitors (SSRIs) can be used as medical treatment (33.20) for severe or prolonged depression in children. In the latest studies their efficacy has been weaker than what was reported earlier and suicidal thoughts have been connected to SSRIs in some studies.
- The use of medical treatment should always be carefully considered by a child psychiatrist and the treatment should be monitored with frequent follow-ups.
- Tricyclic antidepressants are not beneficial (B) [3] in primary-school pupils.

Prognosis of depression in a child

- The probability of recovery from the first episode of depression is almost 100%.
- Severe depression in a child is often prolonged, and relapses are common.
- Childhood depression increases the risk for depression and suicide in adolescence and adulthood.

References

1. Harrington R, Whittaker J, Shoebridge P. Psychological treatment of depression in children and adolescents: a review of treatment research. Br J Psychiatr 1998;173:291–298.
2. The Database of Abstracts of Reviews of Effectiveness (University of York), Database no.: DARE-981790. In: The Cochrane Library, Issue 2, 2000. Oxford: Update Software.
3. Hazell P, O'Connell D, Heathcote D, Henry D. Tricyclic drugs for depression in children and adolescents. Cochrane Database Syst Rev. 2004;(2):CD002317.

33.4 Adjustment disorders in childhood

Kirsti Kumpulainen

General information

- In adjustment disorders the patient has difficulties in adapting to a certain identified psychosocial stress factor and, as a result, he/she begins to experience psychological symptoms. In other words it is a reactive disorder associated with the patient's life situation.
- Anxiety caused by an emotional disturbance and a normal state alternate.
- The individual predisposition and vulnerability of the child plays an important role in the aetiology of the disorder.
- Changes in life circumstances, losses, separation from family, bullying at school or illness can lead to an adjustment disorder.

Epidemiology

- The prevalence of adjustment disorders is not clear but according to some studies it is about 4%.
- Substantial number of adolescents (about 40%) referred to emergency units for psychiatric evaluation suffer from adjustment disorders.

Symptoms and clinical picture

- Symptoms appear within 1–3 months after the stressful situation or traumatic event.
- If the symptoms are present longer than 6 months after the stress factor has disappeared, it is likely that there is some other psychiatric disturbance in question.
- Symptoms are similar to many other mental disorders. Clinical picture is strongly dependent on the child's age and development.
- The reactions of parents and other individuals close to the child as well as their abilities and possibilities to support the child probably play a role in the occurrence of the disorder.
- When making the diagnosis other mental disorders must be excluded.

Characterization of adjustment disorders

- Brief depressive reaction
- Prolonged depressive reaction
- Mixed anxiety and depressive reaction
- With predominant disturbance of other emotions (for instance, regressive behaviour)
- With predominant disturbance of conduct
- With mixed disturbance of emotions and conduct

Treatment

- Little scientific information is available.
- Changing the child's environment and giving support and guidance to both the child and the family is helpful. Mild adjustment disorders can be treated in primary health care using the principles mentioned.
- Cognitive therapies have been reported to be effective in the treatment of more severe forms of adjustment disorders.
- According to the current knowledge, children recover from the adjustment disorder well. Early diagnosis and treatment are considered to be important in respect of the recovery.
- Especially, if the traumatic event is also experienced to be difficult to handle by the parents of the child and taxes their emotionals resources as guardians, the need for individual psychological support and treatment has to be assessed carefully.
- Children can also have acute reactions to stress and post-traumatic stress disorders (PTSD) (adults', see 35.36). These disorders must be treated because children do not forget the traumas they experience. Instead they often need help in handling them. The debriefing technique has been applied also to children, but it is often not enough, especially for children under school age.

33.5 Childhood panic disorder

Saija Roine

Basic rules

- If a child has inexplicable somatic symptoms that fit those of panic disorder, consultation with a child psychiatrist is imperative.
- An early as possible diagnosis is essential to prevent the child from adopting a role of illness within the family or larger social network.

Epidemiology

- Over 10% of children have some sort of anxiety symptoms that coincide with the criteria for anxiety disorders or subclinical phobias.
- According to several studies 1.7–7.6% of school-aged children suffer from school phobias.

General information

- It is thought that panic disorder is inherited through an autosomal dominant gene.
- The triggering of a panic disorder is often preceded by the death of someone close, illness, or a break up with a girl or boy friend in adolescence.

- As a result of an undiagnosed and untreated panic disorder, a child can develop disabling forms of avoidance behaviour, of which dropping out of school is the most common.

Symptoms

- Usual age of onset between 5 and 10 years.
- Pounding heart rate
- Weakness
- Shaking
- Feelings of dying and becoming mad
- Shortness of breath
- Dizziness
- Tightness and pain in the chest
- Prickling of fingers and face
- Feeling of suffocation
- Sweating
- Hot and cold flushes
- Blurriness of sight
- Somatic examinations often sought first.

Differential diagnosis

- Asthma
- Hyperthyroidism
- Neurological disorder
- Heart disease
- Side effect of medication (salbutamol)
- Effect of caffeine

Treatment

- A diagnosis of panic disorder requires examinations by specialists, and, even more importantly, the medication should be initiated in the care of specialized personnel.
- Both biological and psychological treatments are used.
- Good results have been attained with both clomipramine and imipramine. Currently the safer serotonin-specific reuptake inhibitors, fluoxetine and citalopram are used for treatment.
- Behavioral therapy is recommended for treating the secondary symptoms of panic disorder. Especially information given to parents and people who care for the child has proved to be important to the success of treatment.

33.6 Obsessive-compulsive disorder in children

Kirsti Kumpulainen

General information

- Ritualistic behavior without any further remarkable problems is often normal during childhood before puberty.

Epidemiology

- Obsessive compulsive disorders (OCD) are fairly rare.
- The prevalence among children and adolescents has been found to be between 0.3%–3% depending on the sample and age group studied.
- About 30–50% of adult OCD cases have already begun in childhood.
- The obsessive-compulsive disorder has a tendency to become chronic.
- The delay in seeking psychiatric evaluation and care has been estimated to be long which might impact the prognosis. Early intervening is recommended.
- Early onset is currently considered to be associated with increased genetic loading in etiology.
- Studies have shown that close relatives of the affected child display elevated rates of OCD and tic disorders when compared to the general population.

Etiology

- Etiology and pathogenesis of OCD still unknown but considered to be multifactorial including both biological and psychological factors. Currently, neurobiological models are more preferred.
- According to genetic studies predisposition to OCD is genetic. The disorder is often associated with tic disorders and both of these disorders are more common in members of the immediate family than in the population in general.
- Fronto-temporal dysfunction as well as dysfunction of the basal ganglia is suggested to play a part in etiology.
- Neurotransmitter dysregulation (e.g. serotonin, dopamine and glutamate) has been associated to the pathogenesis of OCD.
- According to the psychological theories OCD is associated with depression and the superego of individuals with OCD is considered to be unreasonably severe and restrictive.
- OCD affects and is affected by family functioning. Traits of perfectionism are common in the families of affected individuals.

Symptoms

- The disorder manifests as recurrent
  - compulsive thoughts and obsessions
  - compulsions
- Typical compulsive thoughts include various recurrent thoughts, incitements and fantasies that are compulsively in mind. Typical compulsive behavior includes e.g. continuous washing of the hands, repeated ensuring and checking that various tasks are completed, e.g. that the electric equipment has been turned off or the door is closed. Compulsive ritualistic behavior associated with going to bed, rising up, dressing and going to school are common in children.
- Symptoms are significantly time-consuming, cause marked distress, or result in significant impairment in daily routines like social, academic, or occupational functioning.

- The individual at some point recognizes the obsessions and compulsions displayed as unreasonable. However, young children might not have this kind of insight due to their immature cognitive development.
- Studies have identified impairments in executive, memory and visuospatial functioning in affected individuals.
- Childhood onset OCD is very often associated with other psychiatric disorders, such as tics, and Tourette's syndrome, severe depression, anxiety disorder and behaviour disorder.
- A beta-haemolytic streptococcal infection may cause symptoms of obsession in some children, and therefore it is worthwhile to obtain a history of infections and take a throat culture.
- Early diagnosis and onset of therapy is suggested to be essential in respect of good prognosis.

Treatment

- Various methods of psychotherapy as well as pharmacotherapy have been used in the treatment.
- Cognitive behavioral therapy (CBT) is currently considered to be the most effective psychotherapy approach.
- Medication with serotonergic activity is demonstrated to be effective. However, it is important to be born in mind that these drugs have no official approval for paediatric use.
  - Earlier clomipramine was commonly used but due to the side-effect profile it is not currently recommended to be used as a first line pharmacological agent.
  - The selective serotonin reuptake inhibitors (SSRIs) which have fewer side-effects than clomipramine have also been proven to be effective. Clinical response and relief of OCD symptoms might be ascertained only after 6-10 weeks, and higher dosages than in other disorders medicated with SSRIs are commonly needed.
  - Some patients need medication for longer periods of time.
- Combination of CBT and pharmacotherapy is currently recommended. It is also hypothesized that this combination of treatment modalities leads to greater improvement as well as to lower relapse rates.
- Children and adolescents with OCD easily involve the family in their symptoms, which is why working with the family is also essential.
- The course of the disorder is variable. Relapses of symptoms are common.

33.7 Learning disorders

Heikki Lyytinen

Objective

- Learning disorders must be treated with expertise and as early as possible.

Readiness for school

- The cognitive and motor skills of a school beginner can vary considerably. A small number of children are permitted to start school a year early, or a year late. This decision is made in a consultation between the child's parents and specialists who assess readiness for school.
- It may be difficult to decide to delay school attendance because school may well prove to promote the child's development by offering stimuli and experiences that cannot be attained at home.
- A kindergarten-like environment is often beneficial for a child whose school attendance has been delayed. Almost one fourth of children are in need of special individual attention during kindergarten age and early school years due to developmental delays in cognitive or motor domain.
- A learning disorder in family members is a risk to the child which can, however, be reduced by early preventive measures.

Disturbances in reading and writing

- Difficulties in reading (dyslexia), spelling and writing (dysgraphia) often co-occur.
- These disturbances are not equivalent to retardation.
- Over 10% of children have difficulties learning basic scholastic skills and the most common challenge is reading acquisition.
- Almost 6% of adults have dyslexia and/or dysgraphia.
- Dyslexia can often be explained genetically. Over 60% of individuals with dyslexia have a close relative who also has problems with reading and spelling.

Special disturbances in arithmetic skills

- About 10–15% of schoolchildren have problems learning mathematics, and about 3% of these children have severe developmental dyscalculias.
- Dyscalculia is a developmental failure to understand basic numerical concepts, expressed, e.g., as difficulty to make numerical comparisons, to remember arithmetic facts and to learn and process numerical symbols.

Special disturbances in speech and language

- In dysphasia, the learning of speech and language is abnormal already in the early stages of development.
- If a child does not use single word expressions by the age of 24 months or sentences by the age of 32 months, dysphasia should be suspected.
- From the point of view of differential diagnostics, it is essential to differentiate between a developmental language disorder and a hearing disorder.
- Language impairment can continue into adulthood as difficulties to use or understand language.

- Approximately 3% of the population suffers from dysphasia.
- The risk of language impairment is highest in a child with a delay in language development at the age of 2–5 years and a family history of language impairment, e.g. dyslexia.
  - Interventions to support language development should be started as early as possible.

Developmental disturbances in motor functions

- About 2–5% of children suffer from developmental coordination disorders, dyspraxia.
- Developmental coordination disorder manifests itself as unusual motor clumsiness that is not related to intellectual retardation or general medical conditions.
- Motor clumsiness is often a part of a larger developmental problem, such as the MBD syndrome (nowadays often titled ADHD, attention deficit hyperactivity disorder).

Diagnosis and treatment

- Diagnosis requires examination both by a psychologist, preferably a neuropsychologist, and a special education teacher.
- Learning disorders can be treated with special teaching. Computer supported drilling of skills in need of intensive training may be very helpful if it has been made enjoyable enough for keeping the child interested until the learning goals have been achieved.
- Untreated special learning disorders will affect the child's future harmfully.
- If the child does not receive the necessary encouragement to motivate him or her to make a special effort, learning disorders can lead to other, more extensive difficulties and, at worst, to early dropping out of school.
- Early support for learning difficulties has been found to prevent the generation of secondary problems effectively.

33.8 Conduct disorders of children and adolescents

Irma Moilanen

Basic rules

- Recurring antisocial or aggressive behaviour, such as stealing, temper tantrums, violence, destroying property or bullying others is typical of conduct disorders.
- Conduct disorders are often associated with other psychological disorders, of which the most common are attention deficit hyperactivity disorder (ADHD), learning disorders and depression.

Types of problems

Conduct disorders confined to the family context

- The prognosis is more positive than for other types of disturbances.

Socialized conduct disorder

- The child also has good relationships with his/her companions and an ability to feel empathy towards them. His/her superego may deviate from the norms of the society but meet those of a gang.

Unsocialized conduct disorder

- The child has no positive relationships or ability to feel empathy.

Oppositional defiant disorder

- Usually found only in children below the age of 10 years.
- The child's conduct is typically disobedient without being seriously aggressive.

Diagnosis

- An established model of conduct is required for diagnosis. Single asocial or criminal acts do not justify a diagnosis.

Differential diagnosis

- Attention deficit hyperactivity disorder
- Motor clumsiness, difficulties in drawing and speech disorders may indicate a generalized developmental disorder.

Risk factors in the family exposing a child or adolescent to conduct disorders

- Lack of rules, agreements and regularity. Children do not know what they are allowed to do or what they are expected to do.
- Parents do not monitor what their children are doing or feeling.
- Consequences – appraisals and punishments – are inconsistent.
- Ability to negotiate and solve problems is poor.
- Parents' relationship is unstable.
- The border between generations is missing or weak.

Treatment

- When needed, a general practitioner can, in cooperation with other health care personnel, help the parents to develop their skills in parenting and help them learn to express their feelings verbally **B** [1].
- Problem solving therapies are often successful.
- If the problem is not solved by these methods, the GP should consult either a family guidance centre or a psychiatric clinic for children.
- Children with the most difficult conduct disorders should be directly referred to a psychiatric clinic for children.
- Some children who are over 12 years of age are referred to special foster homes or reform schools that cooperate with psychiatric clinics for children or adolescents.

Reference

1. Woolfenden SR, Williams K, Peat J. Family and parenting interventions in children and adolescents with conduct disorder and delinquency aged 10–17. Cochrane Database Syst Rev. 2004;(2):CD003015.

33.9 A child psychiatrist's view of enuresis

Irma Moilanen

Basic rules

- Psychological factors need to be considered when the type and timing of treatment are chosen for enuresis; these factors influence the prognosis of wetting.

Enuresis caused by psychological factors

- Psychological factors promote the recurrence of enuresis in a child that was already toilet-trained, as well as the delay of learning for many children whose genetic maturing would already imply tidiness.
- Enuresis can affect the well-being of the child.
- Parents depict the characteristics of night wetters with words that fit mental immaturity: sloppy, impatient, easily angry.
- Inner factors that expose the child to enuresis include a fear of being abandoned, or difficulty of growing. Enuresis manifests a regression in the child's development that can be seen as an appeal for a better environment for mental growth.
- According to parents, children who wet themselves during day have the lowest self-esteem and the most fears and feelings of inferiority. These characteristics can also be secondary and actually be caused by teasing by peers, for example.

Treatment of enuresis

- Careful attention to the child's and his or her family's problem during the examination has been experienced therapeutic. A good relation with a family physician promotes learning to be dry.
- A diary kept by the child increases his or her own responsibility and therefore promotes dryness.

Enuresis alarms

- A behavioral therapeutic system used also in the family physician and family guidance system **A** [1 2 3].
- The enuresis alarm system (28.15) seems to be most successful in cases in which the child is independent, has many hobbies, has good relationships at home, and in cases in which the treatment has succeeded earlier (in recurring cases). If the child is emotionally immature, huddling under the mother's wing, this method does not seem to help.

Desmopressin

- Taken in the evening, the medicine "matures" the child's antidiuresis, even in the case of a night wetter, so that the effect is the strongest at night, during which the amount of urine secreted decreases **A** [4].
- Desmopressin is recommended especially in situations in which the child feels ashamed for wetting, for example, during camps and trips. The drug is effective, but its effect lasts only for the night it is taken. Some studies report positive long-term effects in helping a child to become dry; this may also refer to a normal maturing process and a good doctor-patient relationship and the responsibility created by the child's own diary keeping. Combining alarm and drug therapy was found to be superior to alarm treatment alone.

Tricyclic antidepressants

- Has a three-sided effect: it is anticholinergic and antidepressive and it also lightens sleep. Because of side-effects, tricyclic antidepressants are currently used only in special cases for depressive night wetters and together with psychotherapy. The contraindications include a tendency to have convulsions, an obstruction of the urinary tract and refluxing **A** [5].

Psychotherapy

- Is recommended when the child has psychological problems, such as sleeplessness, tension, or anxiety. This type of treatment can also be useful when a stress factor (such as a family crisis) causing the secondary enuresis is still ongoing.

- The psychotherapy of a wetting child can involve two different strategies: When enuresis is caused by an unconscious fear of being abandoned, the problem should be brought to the awareness of the child, and it should also be discussed with the parents. In this way the child could be realistically strengthened. On the other hand, independence, self-action, and the development of the child's own responsibilities is emphasized in the treatment of enuresis.
- A child psychiatrist or a psychologist who has worked with children should determine the form and length of the psychotherapy usually at a family counselling clinic, in the private sector or at a psychiatric clinic for children.
- Enuresis, see 28.15.

References

1. Glazener CMA, Evans JHC, Peto RE. Alarm interventions for nocturnal enuresis in children. Cochrane Database Syst Rev. 2004;(2):CD002911.
2. NHS Centre for Reviews and Dissemination. A systematic review of the effectiveness of interventions for managing childhood nocturnal enuresis. York: NHS Centre for Reviews and Dissemination. NHS Centre for Reviews and Dissemination (NHSCRD). 1900640104. CRD Report 11. 1997. 173.
3. The Health Technology Assessment Database, Database no.: HTA-998340.In: The Cochrane Library, Issue 1, 2001. Oxford: Update Software.
4. Glazener CMA, Evans JHC. Desmopressin for nocturnal enuresis in children. Cochrane Database Syst Rev. 2004;(2):CD002112.
5. Glazener CMA, Evans JHC, Peto RE. Tricyclic and related drugs for nocturnal enuresis in children. Cochrane Database Syst Rev. 2004;(2):CD002117.

33.10 Encopresis

Irma Moilanen

General information

- Toilet training requires both neurological maturity and psychological development.
- More than half of all children are toilet-trained by the age of 18–24 months, and almost all children learn the skill before they are 2.5 years of age.
- Four years of age is a limit after which soiling one's clothes or bed is considered abnormal and is called encopresis.

Epidemiology

- Encopresis is more common among boys than among girls. According to the parents of 8–9-year-old boys, 0.6% soil their clothes or bed weekly, and 4.3% do it more seldom. The respective figures for girls are 0.1% and 2.1%.

Symptoms

- In many ways, encopresis is different from wetting oneself. Encopresis happens generally during the day, wetting happens during the night.

Classification according to symptom

- Control of the movement of the bowels is incomplete.
  - The child is not always aware of the soiling.
  - The problem may be connected with a delay in intellectual development, neurological disorders, or social aggression.
  - The failure to be toilet-trained may be caused by incorrect or insufficient teaching or psychological stress during the period when control of the movement of the bowels should be learned.
- The child is able to control the physiological process of defecation, but he/she defecates in improper places.
  - The symptom may be regressive and entreating in nature. The child may lose his/her control of the movements of the bowels when psychological stress occurs. Learning not to soil may return after the stress has ceased if the matter is understood and handled properly.
  - On the other hand, a child may irritate the family by soiling and manifest aggression by doing so.
- Soiling may be caused by constipation, the gathering of faecal masses in the bowels and the running of soft faeces around the masses because of the block.
  - The cause may be an ongoing fight between parent and child concerning toilet training or painfulness of defecation, for example, because of an anal fissure.
- From the psychological point of view encopresis can be seen as a regressive or aggressive symptom. Some children may manifest depression by soiling; they are indifferent of cleanliness or their own general development. Sometimes encopresis may be an expression of fear of or even horror towards the toilet seat.

Differential diagnosis

- Aganglionic megacolon
- Spina bifida
- Anal fissure
- Diarrhoea

Examinations

- Anamnesis examines the possible organic factors, the developmental history of the child and family, the toilet-training and the child's toilet behaviour.
- In the determination of somatic status the level of neurophysiological maturity and possible signs of ADHD are investigated, the abdominal wall is palpated (megacolon), the area of the anus is examined, and the anus is given a digital rectal examination (length of the anal canal)

- The feet should be examined: pes cavus muscular hypotonia and sensory or reflex deficits may suggest a spinal disorder. Skin abnormalities or pits in the lumbar midline are an indication for spinal imaging.
- In addition, the ordinary psychiatric status is examined.

Treatment

- Components of the treatment that are emphasized according to the situation are
  - searching for possible constipation and its treatment
  - a behavioral therapeutic programme to regularize defecation **C** [1]
  - treatment of parents
  - hospital care to initiate effective treatment
  - regular, sufficiently long lasting treatment, because the tendency to recur is great.
- If the problem is a failure in toilet training, which is typical for small children, a learning programme, including follow-up scale and small prizes is necessary. If this does not give results in a few months under the guidance of primary heath care personnel, the child is best referred to the care of special personnel. If the relationship between the parent and child is tense because of the symptom, a short period of hospital care is in order, especially in cases in which the treatment of constipation requires enemas.

Reference

1. Brazzelli M, Griffiths P. Behavioural and cognitive interventions with or without other treatments for defaecation disorders in children. Cochrane Database Syst Rev. 2004;(2):CD002240.

33.11 Tic disorders in childhood

Editors

Basic rules

- Prolonged (over 2 months) tics require consultation with a child psychiatrist.

Definition

- Tic disorder means sudden, repeated and unintentional convulsion-like twitches or vocal symptoms of the same muscle or muscle group. It is important that the movements and sounds are discharging, repetitive and arrhythmic, and that the symptoms are unintentional.

Classification

- Tics are divided into transient tics, chronic tics and the Tourette's syndrome.
- Chronic tics and the Tourette's syndrome are thought to have a similar background, the only difference being the level of severity of the disease. The diagnostic criteria of both diseases are that the symptoms have begun before the patient has reached the age of 21.
- Opinions of the causes of transient tics vary.

Epidemiology

- The prevalence of chronic tics is over 4%.
- The incidence of the Tourette's syndrome is less than 1% of the entire population.
- The average age for the beginning of chronic motor tics is about 7 years, and, for the Tourette's syndrome the same or slightly older. Usually the symptoms begin at the age of 4–15 years, but the Tourette's syndrome has even occurred in children below the age of 1 year.

Clinical picture

- Tics may occur all over the body, usually in the area of the head, especially in the muscles of the face and upper body.
- The most usual types of motor tics are shaking the head, grimacing, raising the eyebrows, winking the eye, wrinkling the nose, twitching the mouth, raising the shoulders, and flexing the limbs.
- Vocal tic symptoms include sighing, yawning, coughing, sniffling, grunting, snorting and barking.
- More complex symptoms of vocal tics include sudden bursts of obscene words and phrases (coprolalia), from which 30% of the Tourette's syndrome patients suffer.
- Tics are generally connected with a large number of other behavioural disorders, such as disturbances in attention, learning disorders, stuttering and other speech disorders, conduct disorders, obsessive-compulsive symptoms, panic attacks, phobias, etc.

Differential diagnostics

- Extreme motor activity or restlessness of small children
- Hyperkinesia
- Chorea and athetosis in their mild forms
- Compulsive movements that are connected to CP symptoms (36.6)

Background of tics

- Attempts have been made to explain the background of tics with factors of individual psychology, family psychology, and also with biological factors.
- Tourette's syndrome is thought to be inherited single-gene disorder. It is estimated that 1.2% of the population would have this gene and that about one-half of these individuals would manifest some form of symptoms.

- In addition to having tics, people who have the Tourette's syndrome have attention disorders 10 times, conduct disorders 17 times, panic attacks 13 times, and depression 11 times more often than healthy individuals.
- In addition to heritability, other factors are thought to promote the symptoms. Especially situations that cause anxiety, as well as emotional stress, increase symptoms in vulnerable persons.

Treatment

- The course of tics and the Tourette's syndrome can vary greatly. Spontaneous remissions occur, and the symptom can easily be followed up for a couple of months. Supportive and informing discussions with the child and family are clearly useful. If the symptom continues for a long time, special examinations and treatment are necessary.
- Difficult cases are treated with psychotherapy and medication. Before the treatment is initiated, the diagnosis is confirmed by a thorough child psychiatric and psychosocial investigation that is complemented by neurological examinations.
- Of the actual psychotherapies, behavioral therapies have provided the best results. In addition to therapy, related information, advice and guidance are essential.
- Haloperidol and pimozide are used as medication. Also clonidine has been used to treat tics, but it is not thought to be as effective as the aforementioned drugs.
- Before medication is initiated, a child who suffers from tics must be referred to examinations conducted by a specialist in child psychiatry, and the medication must be implemented under the guidance of a child psychiatrist.

33.12 Selective mutism

Kirsti Kumpulainen

General information

- Selective mutism is a form of abnormal behaviour in which the child refuses to speak in a certain or several social situations after having learned to speak properly.
- Temperamental factors and anxiety components have a substantial role in selective mutism.
- Relatives of selectively mute children more commonly have anxiety disorders than individuals in the general population.

Epidemiology

- The prevalence of selective mutism has been estimated to be at 0.2–0.8%; the disorder is most common among 5–7-year-olds when they start day care or school.
- Selective mutism is considered to be resistant to change, particularly in cases of long duration and therefore early intervening is important.

Symptoms

- Emotional factors are important in the aetiology.
- The child refuses to speak in certain social situations (in which the individual is expected to speak, such as at school) although the child is capable of speaking in other situations so has no organic inability to understand the language or lack of knowledge of the spoken language. The disturbance commonly begins gradually.
- The child may speak at home, but refuse to do so elsewhere. Reverse situations are rare.
- Approximately 70% of mute children also have other psychological problems, such as anxiety, encopresis, enuresis, hyperactivity or tics.

Treatment

- Children with selective mutism need psychiatric assessment.
- The treatment is based on the comprehensive assessment that addresses both primary and comorbid problems.
- Various approaches in the treatment of selective mutism like for example family therapy, play therapy, behavioral therapy, speech therapy and group therapy have been adopted.
- Currently behavior modification and other cognitive methods, together with co-operation with the family and the school or day care personnel, are recommended.
- Selective serotonin reuptake inhibitors, especially fluoxetine, have recently been reported to be helpful when treating selectively mute children. At the moment, pharmacotherapy cannot be recommended as the treatment of first choice but if other methods of treatment are not effective, medication can be included in the treatment scheme. These drugs, however, do not have an official approval for pediatric use.
- The child will probably continue to be shy and be apt to suffer from symptoms of anxiety in certain situations even after successful treatment.

33.13 Autism

Sirkka-Liisa Linna

Objective

- An autistic child should be referred to rehabilitation as early as possible to ensure optimal results.

General information

- Autistic disorders include a group of children's mental disorders in which the child's social ability to function, and his or her language and play are disproportional to the child's general development and are thus highly abnormal.

Epidemiology

- Begins at an early age, generally before the age of 3 years.
- Is four times more common among boys than among girls.
- The prevalence of autism is estimated to be 2–20 cases per 10 000 children. Some autistic characteristics are said to have a 7 times greater prevalence.

Background

- Autism is biological in origin. There is no known specific causal factor.
- Heredity probably plays an important role in the appearance of autism.
- In a small group of children, autism is known to be caused by a dysfunction of the brain as a result of, for example, measles during pregnancy, neonatal herpes encephalitis, chromosomal abnormalities, fragile-X syndrome, or a metabolic disease. MMR vaccination is not associated with autism.

Symptoms

- Symptoms of autism differ, and the condition prevails throughout life, even if its forms change with age.
- Underdevelopment in social interaction.
  - Remains to him- or herself in the company of others.
  - Lacks the skill to imitate.
- Underdevelopment in communication and speech.
  - No babbling, focusing of vision, facial expressions, or spoken language
  - Very abnormal nonverbal communication, no desire to be held, no smiling
- Very limited ability to function and few objects of interest.
  - Repeated body movements such as swaying or banging of the head
  - Persistent attachment to parts of objects
  - Notable anxiety due to small changes in the environment
- Other abnormal symptoms.
  - Fears, sleeping and eating disorders
  - Fits of rage, aggression or self-destructiveness
- Three out of four autistic children are intellectually retarded.

Diagnosis

- Based on typical abnormalities in behaviour and a careful clinical examination.

Differential diagnosis

- Asperger's syndrome
  - Asperger's syndrome and autism differ in that the patients with Asperger's syndrome are not intellectually retarded nor do they have a language disability; their other symptoms resemble those of autism, however.
- Rett's syndrome
  - A neurogenerative disease that is assumed to be inherited in the X chromosome and is found in girls.
  - Begins with autistic symptoms, but advances to include the musculoskeletal system and leads to total disability.
- Disintegrative disorders (Heller's disease)
  - An extensive developmental disorder in which a child whose earlier development has been normal changes rapidly and starts to have neurological symptoms and also symptoms that resemble autism.

Treatment and rehabilitation

- Purposeful and effective rehabilitation can reduce autistic symptoms.
- The aim of rehabilitation is to help the child to manage everyday activities.
- Every autistic child needs an individual rehabilitation programme; such programmes are the most successful if the families, day-care personnel and therapists collaborate.
- Autistic children need a personal assistant during day care and at school to help them carry out an individualized learning programme, to support their play and to assist them in personal and group activities.
- Holding therapy has proved to be effective in some autistic children. In the treatment the child is taught to look into the eyes of the holder and discover eye contact with another person, usually the mother.
- The treatment can include communication therapy, learning therapy, music therapy, or riding therapy.

PAE

The family and the autistic child

- Having an autistic child as a family member is heavy burden for a family.
- The autistic child ties the entire family to the home because the child cannot be left alone.
- Parents usually feel they get the most help and support from people they are in contact with daily, such as instructors, speech therapists, and occupational therapists.
- Temporary care and a personal assistant are important forms of support for the family.
- Parent training may provide benefits to both children and parents in the treatment of autism spectrum disorders C [1].

Reference

1. Diggle T, McConachie H R, Randle V R L. Parent-mediated early intervention for young children with autism spectrum disorder. Cochrane Database Syst Rev. 2004;(2):CD003496.

33.14 Suicidal behaviour in childhood and adolescence

Kirsti Kumpulainen

General information

- Children plan and might carry out suicidal acts in many ways, such as by jumping or charging into the middle of traffic, but also by hanging or shooting themselves, or by consuming poisonous substances, including medicines and alcohol.
- Because of the methods used by children and adolescents, their suicides are probably often classified as accidents or other mishaps.
- Suicides committed by youngsters are not recommended to be reported in newspapers and lectures concerning suicidal behaviour should not be addressed to minors.

Epidemiology

- Suicidal thoughts are common in children and adolescents and by no means always associated with other symptoms of psychopathology.
- Suicidal ideation and suicidal behaviour of children have increased during the last few decades. Suicides before puberty are rare but thereafter they become increasingly frequent through adolescence.
- Boys commit suicides more commonly than girls.
- Children referred to the emergency unit for psychiatric consultation commonly display suicidal behaviour.
- The risk of suicidal acts to be repeated later in life is in general high, but the risk of an individual child or adolescent is difficult to assess.

Background

- Suicidal children are generally depressed and often come from chaotic families.
- Difficult experiences and a stressful life situation in general like parental divorce, loss of a loved one, ending of a romantic relationship, various problems at school as well as with parents predispose the youngster to act in suicidal ways.
- Further risk factors are the use of alcohol and drugs, earlier suicidal acts, minority sexual orientation as well as having experienced physical or sexual abuse.

Symptoms

- Suicidal behaviour includes thoughts and expressed wishes to die as well as suicidal attempts and completed suicides.
- Children and adolescents in general overestimate the lethality of different suicidal methods, so the youngster with a significant degree of suicidal intent may fail to carry out a lethal act.
- Suicidal ideation and behaviour expressed by children and adolescents should always be taken seriously. Manipulative threats of suicidal acts are not always easy to separate from serious suicidal ideation.
- In young children suicidal attitude can manifest as running away or accident proneness.
- Disruptive disorders, asocial behaviour, substance abuse as well as separation anxiety and mood disorders are associated with children's and, especially, adolescents' suicidal ideation (34.12).
- Children who threaten with suicide want their environment to realise how desperate they are, and, if their situation is not noted, they may carry out their plans.

Treatment

- Includes both the acute assessment and intervention as well as the psychiatric treatment of associated mental disorders carried out later. A suicidal youngster should always be referred for a psychiatric consultation.
- Always pay attention to the possibility of depression or other psychiatric symptoms and disorders as well as to the use of alcohol and drugs.
- The seriousness of the suicidal behaviour has to be assessed using the following information:
    - Does the youngster understand what suicide means?
    - What are the symptoms of suicidality and in which situations are they displayed by the youngster?
        - Has the child or adolescent planned the suicidal act in detail?
    - Does the youngster display anxiety or is he/she agitated?
    - Is the family capable of protecting the youngster from suicidal impulses at all times?
    - Evaluation of risk factors known to be associated with suicidal ideation and attempts.

- **Emergency admission** to the hospital is needed if
  - Suicidal ideation or behaviour are displayed constantly during consultation
  - The psychological state of the youngster concerned is deviant and his/her unstable condition makes behaviour unpredictable
  - Parents cannot guarantee a safe environment and constant supervision until the consultation in the mental health services takes place
  - Parents are not able to support the youngster because of their own psychological reactions.
- If emergency admission is not needed
  - Refer the youngster for psychiatric consultation as soon as possible. Verify by phone that the consultation will take place without delay.
  - Discuss about the safe environment with the parents and verify that no guns, alcohol, drugs or other harmful materials are available at home.
  - Advise the parents to contact the emergency unit if needed.
  - Have contact with the family for example by phone until the consultation in the mental health services takes place. It is important to support the family in carrying out the planned actions because the tendency to deny the suicidal ideation of the youngster is high if the suicidal symptoms to some extent alleviate.
- The treatment is individually planned and generally initiated as crisis therapy, in outpatient or inpatient hospital care, and it is continued as individual or family therapy.

33.15 Psychiatric illness of a parent with respect to the child

Anne-Maria Vartiovaara

General information

- The psychiatric illness of a parent is a significant risk factor with respect to a child's mental health because of hereditary factors, direct and indirect effects of the illness and other ramifications of the illness. The risk to the child's mental health increases as problems accumulate.
- The situation of children and the help they may need must be taken into account in the psychiatric care of a parent.
- In a severe psychiatric crisis of a parent, children should be offered crisis therapy.
- In addition to a psychiatric illness, the parent may have an alcohol or drug problem, or be suicidal or violent, the other parent may also have mental problems, the parents may have problems in their relationship, or the family may face economic difficulties.
- As the result of a parent's psychiatric illness, the quality of parenting suffers, and, at times, the conditions are not conducive for sufficient parenthood. On the other hand, children who live with schizophrenic mothers do not suffer from mental illness more often than those who have been separated from their schizophrenic mothers and families.
- The evaluation of a child's mental wellbeing requires the co-operation of a network of professionals who also take into consideration the viewpoints of day care and school personnel.

Psychiatric illness of a mother with respect to her baby

- The biological development of the brain continues after birth and is dependent on the quality of early interaction.
- In their interaction with their babies psychotic mothers have been found to be more nervous and less attentive than mentally healthy mothers. They also smile and make eye contact and other contact less while playing with their babies and are less sensitive to their babies' needs.
- In their interaction with their mothers, the babies have been found to smile and make sounds less often and to make less social or eye contact with them.
- The absence of shyness in a baby may relate to the mother's nervousness or insecurity or unpleasant feeding situations and the crying of the baby.
- Disturbed attachment of a one-year-old baby to the parent may be related to the negative and divergent nature of his or her early interaction.
- Serious and recurrent depression of the mother and her significantly diminished functional capacity and ability to avail herself are great risks for the child, especially during the child's early years.
- Mothers who bring their children to be examined for depression are often depressed themselves or have other, often unattended, mental problems (C) [1].
- Mothers who suffer from an eating disorder feed their babies differently from healthy mothers, and it is suspected that these abnormal eating habits expose the children, especially daughters, to eating disorders (C) [2].

Treatment

- The quality of interaction between a psychotic mother and her baby should always be assessed and help, mother-child

PAE

psychotherapy, psychoeducative counselling, and possibly an immediate caretaker should be offered. The situation should be followed up closely.

- The mother and child can be admitted to a mother-baby bed on a psychiatric ward, or they can be met in a working group for treating psychiatric infant outpatients. If necessary, the baby can be placed on the infant ward of a children's home and the mother can be involved in intensive daily interaction therapy.
- The other parent must be supported in taking the responsibility of childcare, and the mother must have a contact person whom she can contact whenever needed.
- An expert must evaluate the sufficiency of the parenting to ensure the mental health of the child.

Immediate intervention is necessary when

- the baby is withdrawn, uninterested in communication, does not make contact.
- the baby is depressed, apathetic, very tearful, unattended.
- the physical health and development of the baby is at risk.
- the functional level of the mother's parenting is not sufficient.
- the attitude of the mother is hostile and the relationship "abusive".

The child's risk is increased due to the psychiatric illness of a parent

- the mother's interactive and empathetic skills and her ability to recognise her child's needs are inadequate.
- the mother is recurrently admitted to hospital during the child's early years.
- the child is placed in an institution rather than in a foster family during the mother's hospital care.
- the mentally ill mother has no supportive network.
- the symptoms of the illness directly affect the child.
- the relationship to the sick parent is entangled or too intense and the child is the object of symptoms (e.g., hostility).
- the parent's have problems with their relationship or with other matters.
- the basic resources of the child are diminished.
- the child lacks the presence of a close adult or a sufficient supportive network.
- the child takes on too much responsibility in the family and is left internally alone.

The child's need for therapy must be assessed when

- the child displays significant mental symptoms (micropsychotic states of mind, delusions, shares the world of the psychotic adult, is depressed, talks of suicide).
- the parent has attempted or committed suicide.
- the parent's illness is severe and chronic.
- the problems or symptoms of the parent's illness are directed towards the child,
- there is violence, substance abuse or sexual abuse of the child within the family.
- the child has become parentified beyond his or her resources.

Treatment

- The family of a psychiatric patient should undergo a child-oriented family examination, in which the situation of the child, the parental resources and the child's need for help are evaluated. The family can be directed into family therapy in the family ward, and the child can attend child psychiatric consultation if needed. Traumatic events may have also taken place within the family.
- If the child shares the delusionary world of the parent, it is recommended that the child and parent be separated. Some children become parentified and carry the burden of responsibility within the family.
- The child can be informed about the parent's illness, the guilt of family members can be diminished, the parentification of the child can be lessened and the supportive network can be activated to support the child.

Supportive actions of social welfare services

- Depending on the services available, the family can receive domestic help and acquire a family social worker to support the child, permanent day care can be arranged as a supportive action, a supportive family or a support person for an older child can be arranged through social services. The child can also receive support in his or her hobbies.

References

1. Ferro T, Verdeli H, Pierre F, Weissman MM. Screening for depression in mothers bringing their offspring for evaluation or treatment of depression. Am J Psychiatry 2000;157:375–9.
2. Agras S, Hammer L, McNicholas F. A prospective study of the influence of eating-disordered mothers on their children. Inj J Eat Disorder 1999;25:253–62.

33.20 Psychopharmacotherapy of children and adolescents

Irma Moilanen

Basic rules

- The use of psychopharmacotherapy is not very common in the treatment of children and adolescents.

- If medication is used appropriately and combined with psychotherapeutic treatment, it can relieve a child's mental suffering and speed up recovery.
- Psychopharmacological treatment for children and, especially, the diagnosis and initiation of medication is the responsibility of specialists.
- The entire field of health care personnel should adopt a positive and unprejudiced attitude towards psychopharmaceuticals to motivate the children and families to accept needed medical treatment.
- Medical treatment is helpful, but never the only form of treatment for a child or adolescent with a psychological disorder.

Special characteristics of treatment

- Because of the special biochemical characteristics of children, medication affects children through different mechanisms than in adults.
- Because of children's rapid metabolism, medication must often be given more frequently than with adults.
- Many false and anxiety-arousing beliefs are associated with psychopharmaceuticals, which are often called tranquillizers even if sedation is only a part of their effects.
- Psychopharmaceuticals are also associated with narcotics. Especially adolescents link psychopharmaceuticals with insanity or with the fear of becoming mad and therefore have negative attitudes towards them.
- Both children and their parents must be carefully prepared for the medication by telling them why the medication is necessary, what the effects will be and what kind of side effects are possible. It is useful to discuss the general beliefs and fears that are connected with medical treatment.
- The symptoms of the psychiatric disorder and of the known adverse effects of the psychopharmaca should be recorded using symptom charts, to be filled in by the parents and by the children/adolescents, during hospitalisation by the staff nurses and, especially in case of ADHD, also by the teacher.

Examinations before treatment

- A clinical examination for somatic and neurological status.
- Recommendable: Complete blood count, serum AST, ALT, and creatinine, also others if needed, for example serum TSH and calcium.
- An ECG is necessary before medication is begun and also periodically during the treatment, especially, when tricyclic antidepressants, lithium or large doses of neuroleptics are administered.

Neuroleptic agents

- Neuroleptic agents are primarily needed for childhood and adolescent psychoses including schizophrenia. All neuroleptics have many adverse effects.
- The use of small doses of neuroleptics, especially haloperidol, has been studied also in the treatment of children and adolescents, and it can be used, for example, in cases of autism to reduce anxiety and restlessness and to improve the child's ability to make contact.
- Both haloperidol and pimozide have been proved effective in the treatment of tics.
- Atypical neuroleptics, clozapine risperidone, olanzapine and quetiapine have largely replaced the older neuroleptics in the psychopharmacotherapy of children and adolescents.
- Many open trial studies are suggesting an antiaggressive effect for atypical neuroleptics.

Antidepressants

Serotonin-specific reuptake inhibitors (SSRI)

- Serotonin-specific reuptake inhibitors have been used in pharmacotherapy of depression, panic disorder and obsessive-compulsive disorders in children and adolescents. However, they are not as effective as in adults.
- Because of serious adverse effects, including hostility and suicidality, all selective serotonin reuptake inhibitors, except fluoxetine, have been banned for use in patients under 18 years of age.
- SSRIs are less toxic and have milder adverse effects than tricyclic antidepressants.
- The long-term effects of SSRIs are not yet known.

Monoamine oxidase (MAO) inhibitor

- The use of moclobemide has been studied very little among children. The drug has been used in the treatment of severe depression, attention disorders, and hyperkinesia with moderate results among both children and adolescents.
- Combined pharmacotherapy with other serotonergic agents may produce serotonin syndrome, and is thus contraindicated.

Tricyclic antidepressants

- The results with children have been controversial, ranging from good to placebo-like.
- Imipramine has been found to affect severe depression in adolescents better than in children, but not as well as in adults.
- Tricyclic antidepressants have been used to treat attention disorders, hyperkinesia, obsessive-compulsive disorders, school phobia, separation anxiety and generalized anxiety. Imipramine is effective in treating sleepwalking and nightmares.
- Because of adverse effects the use of tricyclic antidepressants in child psychiatry has decreased.

Anxiety medication

- Little scientific knowledge is available of the use of anxiolytic medication in the treatment of children.
- Anxiolytic medication has mostly been used to treat such sleep disorders as nightly terror attacks and sleepwalking when the symptoms are severe and disturb sleep.

- Lorazepam and alprazolam have been used to treat school phobias and other states of fear.
- Long-term use of anxiolytic medication is not recommended. Such medication is primarily used for short-term "withdrawal" treatment.
- Open trials have demonstrated moderate response to 4 weeks of buspirone in children with anxiety disorders, but the efficacy seems to be lower than in treatment of adults.

Other medication that corresponds to psychopharmaceuticals

- Stimulants methylphenidate and D-amphetamine and noradrenergic–specific atomoxetine are effective in treatment of children and adolescents with ADHD.
- Carbamazepine has been effective in treating children's hyperactivity, aggressive conduct disorders and bipolar disorders. It is thought to be safer than neuroleptics because of the milder adverse effects.
- Also valproate has been effective in treatment of bipolar mood disorder and aggressive behaviour.
- Lithium is used to treat aggressive conduct disorders and affective illnesses. For the follow-up of lithium treatment, see 11.31.
- The effect of clonidine has been studied in treating both hyperkinetic children with attention deficit disorders and children who suffer from tics or Tourette's syndrome. The doses are smaller than when hypertonia is treated.

33.21 Psychotherapeutic forms of treatment for children and adolescents

Hanna Ebeling

Objectives

- The patient is helped to
  - come to terms with experiences that have caused anxiety and pain, and patient's development into a healthy and balanced direction is supported.
  - cope with problems concerning interaction in their relations with both adults and peers.
  - adopt a better concept of themselves and their relationships.

Prerequisites for treatment

- Before treatment can be initiated, a thorough diagnosis must be completed and the objectives of the treatment must be agreed upon with both the child and his/her family.
- Psychotherapeutic treatment not only requires the positive attitude of the child or adolescent but also the consent of the parents.
- With older adolescents the agreement of the therapy is done more clearly with the adolescent.
- The settings for psychotherapy should be clearly restricted. The place for therapy should remain the same throughout the therapy, as should the time. Therapy sessions last 45–50 minutes, and group therapy (A) [1 2] is even longer.
- Individual therapy is given at least once a week.
- Generally speaking, no psychotherapeutic treatment is sufficient by itself. It is common to combine individual psychotherapy with cooperation with the parents, and sometimes with family therapy, special school arrangements, medication etc.

Psychodynamic individual therapy

- Psychodynamic individual therapy is one of the most common forms of psychotherapy used with children, adolescents and adults.
- The objective is to
  - release the abilities and resources of the child or adolescent
  - help to experience and endure different emotions
  - support coping methods
  - build communication skills
  - reduce anxiety
  - build self-esteem
  - increase the ability to cope with disappointments
- Psychodynamic individual therapy is based on a psychoanalytical frame of reference. Transference, countertransference and verbalization play an important role in the therapy.

Cognitive-behavioural psychotherapies

- Cognitive psychotherapies are becoming increasingly common in the treatment of adults as well as children and adolescents.
- Cognitive psychotherapy focuses on distortions in the cognitive development and actions of a child or adolescent. According to behavioural and learning theories, the disorders are based on learning, and the conditioning process of learned models of behaviour or reactions.
- The objectives are that
  - the child or adolescent recognizes and names his or her feelings
  - the child changes his or her negative and distorted ideas of him/herself, others and environment
  - social and communication skills improve.

- The relationship with the therapist is important for the child, but the aim is not transference or interpretation.
- Cognitive therapy requires a certain level of maturity in cognitive skills. Therefore the therapy cannot be used for very young children, and it is often combined with medical treatment.
- Cognitive therapy can be used to treat, for example, depression, anorexia nervosa, and different fears or anxiety disorders.
- Therapy can be given once a week sometimes for 10–15 weeks, but children and adolescents are often treated longer.

Trauma therapy

- Trauma therapy focuses on traumatic experiences. It lasts often shorter period of time than other forms of psychotherapy. If the child has long-lasting traumatic experiences in his/her life, longer psychotherapy is usually needed.
- Playing is often used in children's psychotherapy and trauma therapy. The child can express his/her feelings and thoughts through play. Playing is a typical way for children to express themselves, and they handle different experiences through it. Playing itself is therapeutic.
- In play therapy the toys are either standardized or otherwise chosen so that the child can express different situations and emotions through play. For school-aged children, games fill the role that toys have for small children.
- In the therapy of adolescents discussion and verbalization are often used as well as different methods of trauma therapy.

Art therapy

- Art therapy combines artistic expression and the therapeutic process. The therapy concentrates on both the patient's artistic expression and the contact made through it with another person. The therapist acts as a receiver and an interpreter of the patient's inner images and helps the patient to face difficulties, fears and conflicts when they hinder the therapeutic process.
- Group art therapy treats the patient through a group process A [1] [2]. The process works between all group members, their pictures and the therapist.

Psychomotor therapy

- Psychomotor therapy combines therapy with physical exercises and supports social relations.
- The patient receives immediate and comprehensive feelings of well-being and pleasure through the individually chosen physical, relaxation and stretching exercises.
- In therapy sessions, excitement is released and relaxation is practised. Simultaneously, as the children or adolescents develop social skills and knowledge, they learn to express their feelings verbally and to listen to others.
- The best results have been achieved in the treatment of children or adolescents with
  - depression, attention disorders or motor disorders
  - low self-esteem
  - different phobias
  - symptoms manifested as asocial behaviour.
- Psychomotor therapy can be carried out through the use of individual therapy, group therapy A [1] [2], or both.

Riding therapy

- Riding therapy is used to treat and rehabilitate children and adolescents who are either physically handicapped or sick or who have behavioural or emotional disorders.
- The movement of the horse during riding and the contact with it can activate the communication skills of an inhibited or distressed patient.
- Riding therapy normalizes and improves physical reactions, perception, function of the senses and speech. It also improves the ability to concentrate and to inhibit oneself and also improves the social skills of the children and adolescents. The psychological objectives are to enable the children and adolescents to experience pleasure, feel success and trust their own skills. It is also meant to develop higher self-esteem through positive experiences.
- The therapy can be used to treat
  - conduct disorders and attention and eating disorders
  - disturbances in interactive relationships
  - autism.

Music therapy

- Music affects human beings in many different ways, from the lower levels of brain function (autonomic nervous system) to the higher levels.
- Music therapy has a positive effect on children
  - with difficulties in making contact
  - with mutistic, psychotic or aggressive conduct.
- Music therapy can be useful in situations when the child or adolescent is not able to verbally process his/her concerns.
- Music therapy can involve receiving, producing or performing. It can also be combined with art and psychomotor therapy. Because music makes people feel better and increases well-being, it also increases the effectiveness of other treatments.

Occupational therapy

- Supports the holistic functioning of a distorted child or adolescent. The objective is to improve the ability of the child or adolescent to express him/herself, to offer successful experiences and to develop learning abilities. Occupational therapy includes such creative activities as drama, music, and art or physical exercises.
- The intention is to use sensory integration to affect the way the brain processes, combines and uses the sensations sent by different senses.

- In occupational therapy patients also practice the activities needed in everyday life to increase independence. The objective of the treatment is to guide children and adolescents into recreational activities that would bring them joy and pleasure once the therapy has ceased.

Group therapy

- Group therapy (A) [1,2] involves psychotherapeutic methods, and the primary objective is to encourage the members of the group to create mutual and healing means of communication.
- Group therapy helps especially children with disturbances in their relations with their peers.
- For children, group therapy involves mainly playing and other activities; with adolescents the therapy often concentrates on discussion. In the therapy problems are handled in a direct manner. The task of the therapist or therapists is to guide the activities or discussions into constructive communication between the members of the group.
- A therapy group can consist of 3–5 children or adolescents at a time. Two therapists are needed to guide a bigger group. Group therapy generally lasts for 1–1.5 hours, and the group meets 1–2 times a week.
- Sometimes children's therapy sessions are combined with the sessions of their parents. These sessions deal with the behavioural problems of the children or adolescents and the means with which parents handle the problems. The objective is to find new ways to solve problems.

Cooperation with parents

- The behaviour of a child or adolescent is generally a result of many factors. Therefore many methods are needed for treatment. The success of all treatment requires working with the parents.
- For certain disorders the emphasis of the treatment is on the family. Parent training, family therapy and multisystemic therapy are generally more effective than individual therapy in the treatment of conduct disorders of children and adolescents.
- Sometimes it is also necessary to assess the parents' own need for psychotherapy and to refer them for treatment.
- The child psychotherapist may also meet the child's parents, but often someone other than the therapist of the adolescent deals with the adolescent's parents. The meetings with parents are aimed at informing them of the psychological development in childhood and adolescence as well as of the backgrounds of the child's disorders and, in this way, increase the parents' own understanding. The child's therapist gets also information from the parents about life events which the child may not inform about, but which are important and help the therapist to understand the child better. The meetings are not for "interrogating" the parents, nor are they for blaming them for their child's problems.
- It is possible to go through the child's or adolescent's problems during the meetings, to search for new ways of reacting to situations at home and to support the work the parents do in bringing up their child or adolescent. They should also be informed of the effects the therapy has on the development of the child or adolescent.

References

1. Hoag MJ, Burlingame GM. Evaluating the effectiveness of child and adolescent group: a meta-analytic view. J Clin Child Psychol 1997;26:234–246.
2. The Database of Abstracts of Reviews of Effectiveness (University of York), Database no.: DARE-983030. In: The Cochrane Library, Issue 4, 1999. Oxford: Update Software.

33.30 Bullying at school

Kirsti Kumpulainen

General information

- Bullying at school is often connected to traditional games of provocation and teasing, through which children were considered to practice skills of social interaction. Currently bullying at school has taken the form of violence rather than that of traditional play.
- Bullying includes both direct bullying like shoving, hitting or kicking as well as indirect bullying like social manipulation i.e. exclusion from the group or spreading rumours.
- Bullying at school can be paralleled to both physical and mental abuse which often affects school performance and also leads to absence from school or school phobia.
- Individuals being different in some respect like children with overweight, depression or learning difficulties as well as newcomers at school become more commonly the targets of bullying.

Prevalence

- According to various studies, 1/10–1/3 of all pupils are bullied at school.
- In a Finnish study in which one-third of the children reported being bullied at school, only one-fifth of the parents and 10% of the teachers had noticed the bullying. In other words, children who are bullied are often left alone.
- Adults are commonly unaware about the bullying and measures of intervention are found difficult to take. At early school age children tell about being bullied to adults more easily but older children often try to hide it.
- Children involved in bullying have many psychiatric problems. In particular, children who bully others in addition to being bullied themselves have many psychiatric symptoms and disturbances.

Treatment

- Early intervening in bullying is important. According to research other children gradually start to attribute repeatedly bullied children negatively in many respects.
- Bullies have been found to have more criminal convictions later in life, and they are also more likely to be involved in serious and recidivist crime as well as excessive use of alcohol.
- Victims are reported more likely to be depressed and to have poor self-esteem in later life. Long-term effects of being bullied at school affect personal relationships in general as well as lead to difficulties in later sexual relationships.
- School health care professionals along with teachers should actively observe if bullying exists at school, offer support to those involved in bullying and cooperate with all individuals at school in order to stop the bullying.
- Bullying is conducted between individuals and all present in the situation affect bullying through their own behaviour and therefore various educational campaigns, intervention programmes and mutual agreements between the pupils or the entire school can be effective.
- Many children need psychiatric treatment and support as a result of bullying.
- Often the bully needs professional help as well. Ending the bullying benefits also the bully.
- Discussions with the families of both the bully and the bullied have proven to be effective. Primarily these discussions are conducted by the teacher. Help and support for the teacher can be offered by the student welfare system at school. The student welfare group in which the school health care is taking part can also make a more comprehensive plan for the intervention, especially, if the child has definite psychiatric problems or earlier measures have proven ineffective. The school health nurse can for example take part in the discussions with the families as a partner of the teacher. Joint discussions with families of bullies and victims should handle bullying situations and aim to find a way to stop the bullying. The need for psychiatric consultation in children concerned is assessed separately and individually but the information given in previous discussions can help to assess the need for the consultation.
- It is the responsibility of the school health care to assess if psychiatric consultation is needed. Information concerning psychiatric symptoms and their duration as well as social skills of the child and the ability to perform at school should be gathered from the teacher for this assessment. If there seems to be the need for psychiatric consultation an appointment with the child and his/her parents should be organized in order to agree further measures. Youth mental health services and their organization are different in various countries and this is to be taken into account when planning further actions.
- The school health care personnel can consult child or adolescent psychiatric units.

33.32 Violence and abuse towards children and adolescents

Kirsti Kumpulainen

General information

- All violence experienced (e.g. being present during violent acts or being the target of violence) and in particular family violence, is harmful for the child although no physical damages can be seen.
- Violence between children, bullying (see 33.30), is faced by a substantial number of children.

Description of violence

- Violence can be divided into physical, chemical, psychological, sexual, socio-economical and contextual violence.
- Various forms of violence can further be divided into active and passive forms. For example hitting the child is active violence and neglecting proper care of the child is a passive form of violence. A child is considered to be neglected if his/her basic physical or mental needs are disregarded.
- The Münchhausen by proxy syndrome is a rare form of abuse that is directed towards a child. An adult, usually the child's mother, creates symptoms for the child to make him/her appear ill, which in turn, leads to unnecessary medical examinations. The symptoms found in the child do not seem to worry the parent at all.

PAE

Forms of violence most commonly seen in health care

Physical abuse

- Includes for example physical punishment (forbidden by law in Finland), spanking, kicking, dropping, throwing, burning and neglecting proper care.
- The origin of an injury does not generally refer to an accident or other mishap, and there is often a contradiction between the characteristics of the injury and the explanation how it happened.
- The child may have marks of bone fractures of different stages or bruises in atypical places.

Chemical violence

- Includes for example giving alcohol or other drugs for the crying child in order to calm him or her as well as not taking care of the adequate diet or not giving the medication the child needs.

Psychological violence

- Includes denying the child care, love or provision, frightening, black-mailing or threatening the child as well as mentally binding the child or restricting his/her independence. Psychological violence further includes treating the child as worthless or ridiculing him or her and discriminating against the child or showing hate.
- Psychological violence against children and adolescents is common and seen even during consultations in health care. Intervening is considered to be difficult by health care professionals.

Sexual violence

- Includes sexual harassment and abuse, leading the child to prostitution as well as exposing the child to the sexuality that is inappropriate at the age of the child or on his/her developmental level.

Epidemiology

- Violence and abuse directed towards children or adolescents is difficult to trace because only a small number of the cases are brought to the attention of the social and health authorities.
- 16-year-old pupils in Finnish comprehensive school answered a questionnaire concerning violence experienced. According to the responses 72% had faced mild forms of violence and 7–8% had been subjected to severe forms of violence.
- Sexual abuse has been reported (at the age of 15 to 16 years) by 7% of girls and by 3% of boys. The probability of sexual abuse increases with the age of the child.

Consequences of violence and abuse

- Symptoms related to abuse and neglect are variable and non-specific.
- The consequences can be physical
  - disturbances in growth
  - injuries (in some cases brain injuries can even result in retardation)
  - disturbances in biological rhythm (sleeping and eating rhythm and the excretion of growth hormones)
  - disturbances in self-regulation (attention, urination, defaecation)
- or psychological
  - mental disorders, depression, anhedonia
  - disturbances in social relations
  - underachievement
  - low self-esteem
  - inability to control oneself, aggressivity
  - withdrawal, running away from home, hypervigilance
  - in severe cases symptoms of post-traumatic stress disorder (PTSD) (35.36).

Background factors

- Abuse and neglect of a child or adolescent is associated both with the psychopathology of the parents and with social and environmental factors.
- Parents who abuse their children have commonly themselves been abused in childhood or adolescence.
- Abuse often takes place in situations in which a combination of disappointments and mental problems prohibit parents from acting in an adult way.
- Risk factors of family violence are the isolation of the family as well as poor social circumstances and financial problems.
- Depressed mothers rarely abuse their children physically, but their children are often neglected.
- The risk of abuse is also increased if the infant is premature, cries a lot, has a physical injury, is retarded, or is chronically ill.

Treatment

- Abuse of a child or adolescent demands co-operation between the authorities (child welfare, health care, police).
- Legislation concerning the treatment and mishandling of children varies in various countries.
- The duty of health care professionals to inform child welfare services about the abuse overrides the rule of confidentiality in most western countries. In Finland the child welfare authorities are responsible to contact the police if needed.
- Expert consensus guidelines for the need of further investigation of possible physical abuse have been given in Finland. According to them the investigation is recommended if following injures are found:
  - All fractures in children younger than 1 year.
  - Fractures of the rib, humerus, scapula or vertebrae in children younger than 5 years.
  - All skull fractures when
    - any damages inside the skull (contusion or hemorrhage etc)
    - the fracture fissure is more than 1 mm
    - the fracture is fragmented
    - the fracture is bilateral
    - the fracture is in the posterior part of the skull
  - If shaken baby syndrome is suspected.
  - All burns and scalds which are clear-cut or inflicted by hot objects.
  - If bruises are numerous and not located in typical places (legs, forearms or forehead)
  - All fractures and injures in children of any age when there is a discrepancy between the anamnestic information and findings in clinical examination or when the abuse seems to be a possibility.
- The abused child or adolescent also has to be referred for relevant psychiatric assessment and consultation.
- When assessing the risk of further abuse and neglect at least following factors are assessed: the duration of abuse and neglect, situational factors, psychological state of the

parents, family atmosphere, social relationships of the family and attachment relationships of the child.

- The goals of the treatment are related both to the parents as well as to the child.
- The treatment is commonly an individual combination of various therapy and support modalities. The authorities can also intervene by giving economical support for the family.
- Children and adolescents who are abused or neglected might need foster care either during the investigation or more permanently. Decision concerning the foster care is made by child welfare authorities.

Prevention

- It is essential to emphasize prevention along with treatment.
- Useful means include
  - promoting parental awareness about child abuse, neglect and psychoeducation
  - improving the economical and psychosocial environment of families with children
  - supporting parents and families in stressful situations.

33.33 Recognition and treatment of sexual abuse of a child

Sirpa Taskinen

Objectives

- Strive to improve the child's situation and provide mental support.
- Help the child and family rather than blame or judge.
- Ensure legal protection of the child, his/her family and the professionals. Guarantee objective handling of the situation, and control anxiety.
- Assist the police in investigating the crime.
- Consult a specialist (a child psychiatrist or other person with the proper expertise) before initiating measures.

Epidemiology

- Seven percent of girls and 4% of boys 15 years of age have been sexually harassed, generally by someone outside the family.
- The prevalence of father-daughter incest is approximately 0.3%.

Suspicion of sexual abuse

- The child him/herself tells about it.
  - Usually there is a good reason to believe the child, but it is essential to assess the reliability of the information.
- The abuse is revealed during other investigations.
  - Especially in these circumstances a team assessment of the situation as a whole is necessary to ensure that the investigating professional has not over-interpreted the situation.
- An adult concludes that abuse has taken place.
  - All reports and suspicions need to be investigated.
  - First it is necessary to observe the child (for example, at day care or at school) and gather information on the circumstances.
  - Excessive fears of sexual abuse have been found to be associated with divorces in particular.
- The behaviour and symptoms of the child are signals of problems (see below).

Symptoms

- The following symptoms can also be related to other problematic situations, but they should always be investigated:
- Physical observations
  - Venereal disease
  - Irritation, leucorrhoea, swelling or ulcerations of the genitals
  - Pregnancy
  - Bruises, contusions, cuts and the like in unusual places (for example, on arms, inner thighs)
- Psychosomatic symptoms
  - Constant, severe difficulties in eating
  - Disturbances in sleeping, nightmares
  - Encopresis
- Behavioural symptoms
  - Depression and withdrawal
  - Restlessness and anxiety
  - Seductive attitude towards adults
  - Over agitation
  - Sexually explicit behaviour, compulsive or public masturbation
  - The child seems to be afraid of either parent and is startled by touching
  - Running away from home
  - Sudden regression of behaviour (for example, thumb sucking, enuresis)
  - Self-punishment (for example self-mutilation), suicide at worst
- Not all sexually abused children show changes in behaviour. Some do their best keeping the abuse undetected.

Recognition

- Only 20%–50% of sexually abused children show clear physical signs.
- Bruises, signs of sperm, torn clothes, and the like are external signs.
- If the alleged abuse has occurred within 3 days, it is possible to detect signs of the abuser's sperm, secretions, fibres from clothes and the like in laboratory tests.

Immediate actions

- Acute cases are investigated as emergencies.
- Other than emergency cases should be investigated only after a request from the police.
- The investigation should be conducted by a minimum of two professionals to ensure
    - legal protection of clients and professionals
    - objective handling of the situation
    - control of professionals' anxiety.
    - The persons carrying out the investigations should be experienced in the field or they should have at least received proper guidance on how to conduct such investigations.

Child psychiatric and psychological examination of the child

- The objective of the psychological examination of the child is to
    - give the child mental support
    - determine his or her mental state
    - gather information of possible abuse for preliminary investigations by the police
    - assess the possibility of immediate danger at home.
- The investigation should be carried out according to the following guidelines:
    - A quiet place should be chosen to ensure against external disturbances or interruptions.
    - The interviewer should always be a person familiar with the development of children, such as a psychologist or child psychiatrist.
    - Anything the child might say and the investigators questions are recorded word for word in writing, with a tape recorder or on video.
    - The interviewer should not offer his or her opinion of what happened.
    - The interview can be supplemented by psychological tests, observations of the child's play, and drawings.

Somatic examination of the child

- The objective of the somatic examination is to
    - support the repair of the child's self-concept
    - examine the child's state of health
    - observe possible physical damage
    - verify possible venereal disease or pregnancy or both
    - refer the child for termination of pregnancy if needed
- It is important to build a positive relationship with the child before the somatic examination. A safe adult can accompany the child, not the suspected abuser, however. The examination can be an opportunity to support the child psychologically by commenting that his or her body parts are normal. It is often natural for the child to talk about the abuse during the examination. It can be useful to ask additional questions, but an atmosphere of interrogation should be avoided.
- The examination should be carried out according to the following procedures:
    - A normal paediatric examination is first carried out.
    - In addition the areas of the mouth, breasts, and buttocks are examined, and the body, for example, the shoulders and thighs, are inspected for marks of holding.
    - The genital and anal area are examined as follows:
        - Frog position with the child in the lap of an assisting adult is used or the child is on his or her hands and knees on the examination table
        - Inspection is enough.
        - The condition of the hymen is inspected.
        - If the alleged sexual abuse has occurred within 3 days, samples are taken from the vagina and anus with a dampened cotton swab.
    - Any injuries are photographed because they heal rapidly.

Additional measures

- If there is proof of sexual abuse or if the child needs child welfare actions for other reasons, the incident should be reported to the child welfare authorities. The authorities then evaluate the possibilities to support the family and the need for taking the child into custody. The need for treatment (C) [1 2] of the child and family is generally assessed in a cooperative effort between the representatives of several municipal bureaus.
- If abuse seems probable, child welfare must also report to the police.
- If a crime is suspected, the interrogations are always performed by the police.
- When incest is suspected, it should be kept in mind that even other children in the family might have been sexually abused.

References

1. Finkelhor D, Berliner L. Research on the treatment of sexually abused children: a review and recommendations. J Am Acad Child Adolesc Psychiatr 1995;34:1408–1423.
2. The Database of Abstracts of Reviews of Effectiveness (University of York), Database no.: DARE-963487. In: The Cochrane Library, Issue 4, 1999. Oxford: Update Software.

Adolescent Psychiatry

Evidence Based Medicine Guidelines. Edited by the Duodecim Editorial Team
 ISBN: 0-470-01184-X

34.10 Eating disorders among children and adolescents

Päivi Rantanen

Objectives

- Remember that eating disorders are very common among adolescent girls.
- One must remember to look for signs of an eating disorder; patients seldom report it themselves.
- The diagnosis and planning of treatment are the responsibility of special personnel.

Basic rules

- An eating disorder refers to states in which food and nourishment have an instrumental and manipulative role: food has become a way to regulate the appearance of the body.
- The spectrum of eating disorders is vast. The most common disorders are anorexia nervosa and bulimia nervosa. In addition, incomplete clinical pictures and simple binge eating have become more general.
- Even small children can have different kinds of eating disorders that relate to difficulties in the relationships between the child and his/her caretaker.

Aetiology

- Currently eating disorders are considered to be multifarious. Genetic and sociocultural factors and also individual dynamics all affect eating disorders.
- The typical age of onset is adolescence, when the body changes and grows.
- Anorexia nervosa typically emerges between 14 and 16 years of age or around the age of 18 years. Bulimia appears typically at the age of 19–20 years.
- Eating disorders are 10–15 times more common among girls than boys.
- Every 150th girl between the ages of 14 and 16 years suffers from anorexia nervosa.
- There is no epidemiological data on the occurrence of bulimia, but it is considered to be more common than anorexia nervosa.

Diagnostic criteria for anorexia nervosa

- The patient does not want to maintain his or her normal body weight.
- The patient's weight is at least 15% below that expected for age and height.
- The patient's body image is distorted.
- The patient is afraid of gaining weight.
- There is no other sickness that would explain the loss of weight.

Diagnostic criteria of bulimia nervosa

- Desire to be thin, phobic fear of gaining weight.
- Occasional binge eating, during which control over eating disappears. After the fit, the person seeks to get rid of the food consumed, for example, by inducing vomiting and by abusing laxatives and diuretics.
- A screening questionnaire is helpful in the assessment of patients with suspected eating disorder (each positive answer gives one point; 3 or more points suggests an eating disorder).
    - Do you try to vomit if you feel unpleasantly satiated?
    - Are you anxious with the thought that you cannot control the amount of food you eat?
    - Have you lost more than 6 kg of weight during the last 3 months?
    - Do you consider yourself obese although others say you are underweight?
    - Does food/thinking of food dominate your life?

Symptoms

- Anorexia nervosa generally starts gradually.
- Losing weight can either be very rapid or very slow. Generally the patients continue to go to school; they go on with their hobbies and feel great about themselves. Therefore the families are usually surprised to find that their child suffers from malnutrition.
- Anorectic adolescents deny their symptoms, and it takes time and patience to motivate them to accept treatment.
- Somatic symptoms include:
    - disappearance of menstruation
    - the slowing of metabolism, constipation
    - slow pulse, low blood pressure
    - flushed and cold limbs
    - reduction of subcutaneus fat
- Bulimic adolescents are aware that their eating habits are not normal, but the habit causes so much guilt and shame that seeking treatment is not easy.
- Bulimia also causes physical symptoms
    - disturbances of menstruation
    - disturbances in electrolyte and acid-alkali balances created by frequent vomiting and damage of the enamel of teeth (7.31)

Laboratory findings

- In anorexia nervosa
    - Slight anaemia
    - Blood glucose levels on the lower border of normal

- In bulimia
  - Hypokalaemia
  - Increased serum amylase

Differential diagnosis

- Severe somatic diseases, for example, brain tumours
- Psychiatric diseases–severe depression, psychosis, use of drugs

Treatment

- If the symptoms correspond to the diagnostic criteria of anorexia nervosa, the situation should be discussed with the family before treatment is arranged.
- The adolescent and his or her family should be made aware of the seriousness of the disorder.
- Sometimes it takes time to motivate the patient to participate in the treatment.
- The treatment is divided into
  - restoring the state of nutrition
  - psychotherapeutic treatment
- If the state of malnutrition is life threatening, the patient is first treated in a somatic ward, and thereafter the adolescent is guided into therapy if possible.
- The forms of psychotherapy vary: both individual and family therapy have brought results; in cases of bulimia cognitive therapy and medication C [1 2 3 4] have been successful.
- With adolescents between the ages of 14 and 16 years, positive results have been obtained by treating the entire family, because the adolescent's symptoms are often connected with difficulties to "cut loose" from the family.
- With older patients, individual, supportive and long-lasting treatment has been the best way to promote recovery.
- A prolonged state of malnutrition and insufficient outpatient care are reasons to direct a patient into forced treatment.

Medical treatment

- A specialist should start all drug treatment.
- Different psychopharmaceuticals, for example, neuroleptics and antidepressants A [5 6 7], have been tried in the treatment of anorexia nervosa. Controlled studies have proved them indisputably useful only if the disorder is linked to clear depression.
- Most research on the medical treatment of bulimia has concentrated on antidepressants, particularly fluoxetine, which has been found to decrease binge eating and vomiting for about two-thirds of bulimic patients A [5 6 7].

Prognosis

- Early intervention improves prognosis.
- Eating disorders comprise a severe group of diseases that are difficult to treat. The prognosis for the near future of anorectic patients is good, but for the long term the prognosis is worse. The percentage of mortality is still 5–16%.
- Not enough follow-up research has been carried out on the prognosis of bulimia, but the disease is thought to last years.
- Bulimia can be associated with depression, self-destructiveness, abuse of alcohol or drugs, and other psychological problems.

References

1. Meta-analysis of cognitive-behavioural treatment studies for bulimia. Clin Psychol Review 1997;17:703–718.
2. The Database of Abstracts of Reviews of Effectiveness (University of York), Database no.: DARE-983171. In: The Cochrane Library, Issue 2, 2000. Oxford: Update Software.
3. Whittal ML, Agras WS, Gould RA. Bulimia nervosa: a meta-analysis of psychosocial and pharmacological treatments. Behaviour Therapy 1999;30:117–135.
4. The Database of Abstracts of Reviews of Effectiveness (University of York), Database no.: DARE-999870. In: The Cochrane Library, Issue 2, 2001. Oxford: Update Software.
5. Bacaltchuk J, Hay P. Antidepressants versus placebo for people with bulimia nervosa. Cochrane Database Syst Rev. 2004;(2):CD003391.
6. Jimerson DC, Herzog DB, Brotman AW. Pharmacologic approaches in the treatment of eating disorders. Harward Review of Psychiatry 1993;1:82–93.
7. The Database of Abstracts of Reviews of Effectiveness (University of York), Database no.: DARE-983124. In: The Cochrane Library, Issue 3, 2000. Oxford: Update Software.

34.11 Depression of adolescents

Eila Laukkanen

General information

- Depressive feelings are common in adolescents: in the majority this is, however, a normative way of experiencing the growth and development of youth.
- In the evaluation of the depression of an adolescent, the present stage of development of the young person and events of life that could possibly affect mood should be taken into consideration.
- The depression of an adolescent may present by various symptoms, it can be masked, for example, by hobbies that are carried out fanatically or by disturbances of conduct (e.g., arguing, stealing, substance abuse). It is typical that the young person appears depressed only when he/she talks about the depression.
- Depressed adolescents smoke and use drugs and alcohol more often that other young people.

- The depression of an adolescent is a psychiatric disorder that must be taken seriously and treated appropriately.

Epidemiology

- According to population studies, the prevalence of severe depression (Major Depressive Disorder (current) in DSM-III-R) is 3.4%, the prevalence of mild long-lasting depression (Dysthymia DSM-III-R) is 3.2% and the life-time prevalence of severe depression is 13%. Depressive states are clearly more common in girls than in boys. According to various studies about 40% of the depressed manifest some other psychiatric comorbidity.
- The severe depression of an adolescent is associated with an increased risk of suicide. In post-mortem studies of adolescents who had committed suicide, 51–80% had been shown to have suffered from severe depression. The risk of self-destruction increases if substance abuse and asocial behaviour are associated with depression.

Aetiology

- The factors that affect the development of depression are not yet known in detail, but both sociedemographic factors and stressful life events have been shown to be associated with depression. Depressed adolescents have been observed to have poorer social skills that other young people and to have a more negative view of themselves than others.
- The risk of becoming clinically depressed is greater if some other member of the family has suffered from severe depression or bipolar affective disorder.

Symptoms

- Psychiatric symptoms associated with normal development are transient and not associated with direct or indirect self-destruction, and the ability of the young person to function is not impaired.
- It is important to differentiate between feelings of depression that are normative for the adolescence and pathological depression.

Normative depression in adolescence (or grief associated with loss)

- Sense of sadness and loss, crying
- Alternating moods: sadness–hate–joy
- Sudden changes in self-esteem
- Occasional worries about physical appearance
- Minor physical symptoms
- Occasional sleep disturbances
- Resorting alternatively to either primitive (e.g. denial, blaming others, splitting) or mature (e.g. rationalizing, rejection) defence mechanisms.
- Social relationships are intact, as is the ability to enjoy food and hobbies and to become infatuated.

Pathological depression

- Melancholiness, boredom, sense of emptiness or constant irritation
- Uncontrollable outbursts of feeling
- Difficulties in concentrating
- Feelings of worthlessness and shame, sometimes unrealistic feelings of guilt
- Thoughts of death, suicidal ideation, suicide plans
- Sleep disorders (difficulty in falling asleep, arousals, early morning insomnia, nightmares)
- Weight fluctuation
- Concern for own body to the point of hypochondria
- Pains and various somatic complaints
- Little ability to enjoy anything
- Fewer and poorer relationships with others
- Mainly primitive defence mechanisms

Examining and referring a depressed adolescent

- Somatic causes for tiredness, apathy etc. should be excluded.
- When examining a depressed adolescent it should be kept in mind that the young person may have a negative view of himself and may find it difficult to talk to a stranger. Reserve time for discussion and pose direct questions that allow you to determine the duration and nature of the symptoms and their effect on daily life. Questions concerning school, hobbies and time spent with friends are important. Questions concerning self-destructive thoughts should be asked separately as these may require immediate action.
- A structured questionnaire on symptoms, the Beck Depression Inventory (BDI) B [1], can be used to assess the severity of depression. BDI is a useful screening method for detecting depression although it produces some false-positive results.
- If the depression of an adolescent is prolonged or symptoms of severe depression or self-destruction are observed, the young person should be referred to a specialist adolescent psychiatry unit for examination.
- An adolescent should be referred immediately if there is a risk of suicide. Telephone consultation with a specialist unit may be helpful in the evaluation.
- Mild depressive states and grief reactions can be treated in primary health care.

Treatment of depression

- In primary health care the adolescent can be treated with supportive discussions. If necessary, medication can be used temporarily for alleviating symptoms, e.g. hypnotics or anxiolytics in very short courses; however, if the symptoms are not alleviated or the ability of the young person to function decreases, an evaluation by a specialist unit may be necessary (remember the possibility of telephone consultation).
- The diagnosis of severe depression, the planning and follow-up of treatment are carried out in a specialist unit. Because

a considerable portion of early-onset depressive states (<20 yrs) develop into severe states of depression, it is essential to arrange long-term treatment that covers also other existing mental disorders.

- Adolescents are primarily treated by individual therapy, however, close cooperation with the parents and measures supporting parenthood are an essential part of the treatment. Rehabilitation is also often necessary (e.g. education, social support).
- There is scientific evidence on the effectiveness of brief cognitive-behaviour therapies (B) [2 3 4 5 6 7 8] in the treatment of mild and moderately severe depression of adolescents, but not in that of severe depressive states.
- Also interpersonal psychotherapy has been shown to be effective in the treatment of adolescent's depression, it improves especially social functioning and self-esteem[10]. There are no controlled studies on long therapies.
- Unresolved conflicts in relations with parents affect recovery from severe depression.
- The treatment of adolescent depression may require medication in order to alleviate symptoms, restore the ability to function and in some cases to enable the initiation of other forms of treatment. Controlled studies have not been able to prove that tricyclic antidepressants are more efficient than placebo (B) [9], and they are not recommended for adolescents. On the contrary, serotonin-selective reuptake inhibitors have been shown to be beneficial at least in the treatment of severe depression, but further research data is warranted. When starting medication, careful monitoring of the effects and side-effects of the medication by the doctor is needed. It is recommended that the medication should be continued for at least 4–6 months. If the adolescent has had manic or hypomanic phases or there is a family history of bipolar affective disorder, SSRI medication cannot be started, or it must be done with concurrent antipsychotic medication. Initiation and follow-up of medication must be carried in a planned manner.

References

1. Roberts RE, Lewinsohn PM, Seeley JR: Screening for adolescent depression: A comparison of depression scales. J Am Acad Child Adolesc Psychiatry 1991;30:58–66.
2. Harrington R, Whittaker J, Shoebridge P, Campbell F. Systematic review of efficacy of cognitive behaviour therapies in childhood and adolescent depressive disorders. BMJ 1998;316:1559–63.
3. Marcotte D. Treating depression in adolescence: a review of the effectiveness of cognitive-behavioural treatments. A Youth Adolescence 1997;26:273–283.
4. The Database of Abstracts of Reviews of Effectiveness (University of York), Database no.: DARE-988532. In: The Cochrane Library, Issue 2, 2000. Oxford: Update Software.
5. Harrington R, Whittaker J, Shoebridge P. Psychological treatment of depression in children and adolescents: a review of treatment research. Br J Psychiatry 1998;173:291–298.
6. The Database of Abstracts of Reviews of Effectiveness (University of York), Database no.: DARE-981790. In: The Cochrane Library, Issue 2, 2000. Oxford: Update Software.
7. Reinecke MA, Ryan NE, DuBois DL. Cognitive-behavioural therapy of depression and depressive symptoms during adolescence: a review and meta-analysis. Journal of the American Academy of Child and Adolescent Psychiatry 1998; 37:26–34.
8. The Database of Abstracts of Reviews of Effectiveness (University of York), Database no.: DARE-983371. In: The Cochrane Library, Issue 1, 2000. Oxford: Update Software.
9. Hazell P, O'Connell D, Heathcote D, Robertson J, Henry D. Efficacy of tricyclic drugs in treating child and adolescent depression: a meta-analysis. BMJ 1995;310:897–901.
10. Asarnow JR, Tompson MC. Depression in Youth: Psychosocial Interventions. Journal of Clinical Child Psychology 2001;30:33–47.

34.12 Risk of suicide in adolescence

Mauri Marttunen

General

- Suicidal thoughts, attempted and completed suicides are rare in childhood but the incidence increases during adolescence.

Epidemiology

- The annual prevalence of suicidal thoughts among adolescents is approximately 10–15%, and that of attempted suicides approximately 2–5%.
- Suicidal thoughts and attempts are more common among girls, but about 80% of all suicides are committed by boys.

Risk factors for adolescent suicide

- One in three has previously attempted suicide.
- About 60% of adolescents who commit suicide had talked to someone about their suicidal thoughts; however, boys often only talk to their peers.
- Psychiatric disorders precede suicide in over 90% of the cases, mood disorder in at least half of the cases.
- At least one quarter have suffered from serious substance abuse.
- The most common precipitants to suicide and suicide attempts are a break-up of a relationship or an argument with someone close.

Symptoms

- Suicidal behaviour in adolescence is often associated with current psychosocial problems, such as arguments, bereavement and disappointment.

- Mood disorders, serious substance abuse and, particularly among males, antisocial behaviour is common.

Recognition and assessment

- Self-destructive behaviour in adolescence is strongly associated with depression and substance abuse.
- When depression is suspected in an adolescent, suicidal thoughts and suicide attempts should also be broached.
- Assess current living circumstances and family situation.
- Evaluate the type and severity of associated psychiatric disorder and/or substance abuse.
- Ask whether the patient has attempted suicide in the past
- Assess whether the patient really wants to die, has he/she made suicidal plans or arrangements.

Treatment

- Always agree on follow-up appointments and encourage the patient to carry on with the treatment.
- Facilitate easy access to treatment.
- If self-destructiveness is associated with severe depression, the treatment of depression should be instigated without delay.
- Selective serotonin reuptake inhibitors (SSRIs) are the first choice in the psychopharmacological treatment of a depressed adolescent with suicidal tendencies.
- Always refer an adolescent who has attempted suicide for psychiatric consultation, the quicker the better.
- Psychiatric hospitalization should be considered if the suicidal adolescent suffers from
  - psychotic disorder
  - major depression
  - bipolar disorder
  - severe aggressive behaviour
  - severe substance abuse or dependence
  - if care in the community after a previous suicidal episode has failed.
- Hospitalization is also justified after a serious suicide attempt (high lethality or high suicidal intent), if the adolescent has active suicidal thoughts, and if the adolescent's family cannot offer sufficient support.

34.13 Adolescent psychosis

Anders Sandqvist

Objectives

- Recognize an adolescent's psychosis when his or her functional capacity diminishes or typical symptoms of psychosis are apparent.
- Suspect a severe disorder when a teenager's behaviour is destructive even if there are no symptoms of psychosis.
- When the situation is acute, refer the patient directly to hospital care or organize sufficient supervision according to the principles applied in treating an adult.
- Attempt to establish such a contact with the adolescent or his or her family or both that would enable additional examinations by psychiatrists specialized in treating adolescents is possible.

Basic rules

- Adolescence refers to the age of 12–22-years (15–19 ±3 years), in practice a person is an adolescent for 10 years after the beginning of puberty.
- Both physical and mental development is rapid in adolescence, especially at the beginning. This rapid change burdens adolescents and exposes them to mental disorders, which is evident from the increase in disorders as children become adolescents.
- The special behaviour and ideas characteristic of the rapid development in adolescence and the myth of being "young and reckless" make the diagnosis of mental disorders among adolescents very difficult.
- Already in the 1970s, Offer and Offer proved that the mental health of adolescents has an inverse relation to conduct disorders and other symptoms.
- Laufer divides adolescent psychoses into the following three groups:
  - Acute psychotic states, which may, for example, result in suicide attempts
  - Psychotic states in which the disorder is mainly manifested as abnormalities of either the patient's conduct or his or her conception of the world, e.g. a life-threatening eating disorder in which the realities of the human body are denied
  - Psychotic personality, which resembles functional psychoses of adults, for example, syndromes such as schizophrenia.
- Generally adolescents are incapable of inhibiting strong emotions. Instead, they rid themselves of emotions in a symbolic, very concrete form of behaviour.
  - A young man, for example, who feels that he has been deprived of all good things because of his parents' alcoholism may indirectly express his fate by stealing and boozing. Respectively, a young girl who has been sexually abused may reflect it by pretending not to have any self-respect and by being at the disposal of any interested male.
- The same rules apply in principle to these psychoses as to those that can hide under conduct disorders for long periods of time. Someone who has attempted to commit suicide, for example, may have tried to rid him- or herself of his or her body as the cause of evil and problems without understanding the finality of the act at the time.
- Adolescents are generally "closer to psychosis" than adults because of their normatively weak mental defence mechanisms.

- The mental health of a young person cannot be addressed by the same criteria as those used for adults. A broad evaluation of the youth's development is central to the assessment of symptoms.
- Generally speaking it can be said that every long-lasting symptom or form of behaviour that is in conflict with the healthy development of an adolescent is worthy of a psychiatric evaluation because it may hide a mental illness.

Epidemiology

- Approximately 10–20% of adolescents suffer from a mental disorder that requires investigation or treatment.
- Estimations of the prevalence of psychoses vary. Approximately 0.5% of adolescents suffer from a schizophrenic-like psychosis, and about 1% have an affective psychosis. Affective psychoses are twice as common among girls as among boys.
- The figures are relative to the estimation that 55% of the population with schizophrenic symptoms show first signs of the illness before reaching 20 years of age and 14% have symptoms before the age of 14 years; 33% of persons with affective psychosis are below the age of 20 years.
- No estimations are available on the prevalence of toxic and other clearly organic psychoses.

Aetiology

- Genetic and somatic factors, as well as mental factors related to the individual and the family, are important in the aetiology of psychoses. When the aetiology is examined at the individual level, it is often found that a psychotic adolescent has suffered from multifarious disturbances of adaptation and behaviour throughout his or her lifetime.
- Epilepsy or other cerebral diseases such as a tumour or a metabolic disorder are possible, but rare causes of psychosis.
- Use of drugs may cause a toxic psychosis or trigger a latent psychosis.

High-risk groups for psychosis

- The following three groups are at a high (about 40%) risk to develop a psychosis within one year of follow-up:
  - adolescents who have had symptoms resembling those of mild psychosis, either repeatedly or for longer periods of time, but whose symptoms have not yet reached those of true psychosis
  - adolescents who have had clear but very brief, lasting only for some hours or a part of the day, psychoses
  - adolescents who have a family member with schizophrenia or some other psychotic disorder or who themselves have a schizotypal personality and whose functioning has decreased by 30 or more points on the GAF scale within the last year.

Initial symptoms of a schizophrenic disorder in an adolescent

- Symptoms of adolescents' in addition to the general criteria (DSM III R) of schizophrenia
  - increased passivity
  - stiff motor ability
  - tendency for withdrawal and suspiciousness
  - self-centeredness
  - compulsive symptoms
  - emotional instability
  - lack of control of impulses
  - antisocial actions
  - poor success in school despite good capacity
  - delusions and hallucinations
  - apathy and anhedonia
  - atypical neurological or neurovegetative symptoms
  - a diagnosis of schizophrenia in an adolescent is thought to be justified only after a year of follow-up.

Symptoms of affective syndrome in an adolescent

- In addition to the general criteria (DSM III R) of affective syndrome, there are symptoms of depression and mania
  - tiredness, lack of energy
  - insomnia/hypersomnia
  - headache, stomach trouble
  - irritation, hostility
  - melancholy, withdrawal
  - psychomotor inability
  - feelings of worthlessness
  - self-accusations and feelings of guilt
  - suicidal thoughts
  - antisocial, abnormal behaviour
  - escape into a world of fantasy.
- Symptoms of mania
  - euphoria
  - hyperactivity
  - fast, loose associations
  - excessive sexual activity
  - irritation, aggressiveness, threatening behaviour
  - neurovegetative symptoms such as hyperphagia, encopresis, sweating, excessive eating of sugar or salt.
- The symptoms of schizophrenia and affective psychoses are similar in adolescents and adults in principle, except for the fact that symptoms of delusions and auditory hallucinations can be hidden behind aggressive behaviour or anxiety.
- It is often especially difficult to differentiate between psychoses and deep depression in the case of an adolescent. Paranoid psychosis and related fears and suspicions can be manifest as the seeking of company of antisocial groups in which aggression and the excessive use of alcohol and drugs is accepted as a means of defence. Passivity, changes in emotional life and withdrawal are generally visible and recognizable symptoms, at least within the teenager's family.

- Diagnosing affective psychosis is especially difficult in the case of adolescence. A manic teenager channels his or her hyperactivity into direct action and attempts to relieve his or her unbearable feelings by drinking, using drugs or being otherwise reckless; for example, by being sexually overactive, aggressive or reckless in traffic.
- A depressive adolescent cannot stand his or her state of mind and feeling of emptiness and tries rid him- or herself of it by acting in a self-destructive manner. Suicidal thoughts or behaviour and self-blame in adolescents are similar to those in adults.

Treatment

- A psychotic adolescent is primarily sent for a psychiatric evaluation, or, if the situation is acute, directly to hospital care.
- The objective of the treatment is to help and support adolescents through an important developmental stage so that they can use their potential optimally in adulthood.
- The treatment is broad in scope and time consuming, and the relationships between the adolescent and his or her parents and other important adults are essential. Medication is used to minimize the psychotic symptoms so that positive contacts are possible and the ability to function is regained.

34.14 The adolescent and long-term illness

Pekka Ropponen

General information

- Experiencing puberty and long-term illness simultaneously is almost always problematic.
- An adolescent suffering from a long-term illness has more trouble than normal teenagers in facing the challenges of development in adolescence.

Developmental processes in adolescence

- Adolescence forms a developmental stage between childhood and adulthood that starts at puberty and lasts approximately 10 years. The changes that take place during this stage are both external and internal.
  - The reality of a person's own physical and sexual development places the adolescent's mind under a great deal of strain. The new sexually functioning body must be identified as part of one's permanent body image.
  - Separation from parents and mental re-identification should provide enough room for the growth and development of the adolescent.
  - The adolescent can start to perceive his- or her self in a new and more realistic way with the aid of friends of the same age and peer groups.
- The adolescent forms the identity of an adult in the aforementioned environment, and this identity is a combination of strengthened self-esteem, an ability to orientate towards the future and an ability to have a sex life.

Process of becoming ill

- Even a slight physical illness can mean surprisingly much to an adolescent. Many threats are linked to the developmental processes of adolescence: one's own body does not function and insecurity about recovery creates anxiety.
- An adolescent may be forced to become dependent on his or her parents and specialists, which fits poorly with the adolescent's stage of development. The adolescent's relationships to other adolescents of the same age may suffer as the experience of being different strengthens.

Long-term illness

- The possibility of an incurable illness or a permanent deviation is part of a long-term illness.
- A child is capable of understanding the actual nature of his or her illness only once he or she reaches adolescence. It also becomes possible for the adolescent to perceive the long-term illness as a part of him- or herself.
- Many of the problems between the cooperation of an adolescent and the nursing personnel are generated by a situation in which the adolescent perceives the illness to be an external enemy. The adolescent must adjust to such things as repeated treatment, possibly permanent medication and awkward restrictions of functioning. Long-term illnesses that hinder mental adaptation include diseases such as diabetes, rheumatism, epilepsy, asthma, malignancies, traumas that damage the body permanently, and other illnesses in which the adolescent is forced to encounter the fact that he or she is actively different from others.
- Mental reactions mainly include
  - problems in adjustment
  - depressive reactions (34.11).
- The severity of the reactions varies, and very severe psychological symptoms, even attempts to commit suicide can occur.
- Mental reactions can be influenced by
  - the adolescent's weak ability to analyse the factors that are associated with the illness
  - the adolescent's inability to anticipate things.

Views on treatment

- In addition to treating the basic sickness appropriately, one should talk to the adolescent realistically, emphatically, openly and considerately.
- The coping of the adolescent is promoted by
  - a possibility to speak about the threats that are associated with the illness
  - support of faith in the future
  - a realistic approach to the situation
  - perception of the illness as a part of one's self
  - interaction between the adolescent and personnel in organizing treatment.
- Courses on how to adapt to the situation may also help the adolescent learn to cope.
- When a basic illness is being treated, the adolescent is usually moved from the children's clinic to adult treatment facilities. The shift must be well planned and smoothly carried out. A permanent relation with a family physician is useful for adolescents who suffer from a long-term illness.
- An adolescent who suffers from a long-term illness is not mentally ill if he or she cries, becomes distressed or slightly depressed, or rebels against the treatment of the illness.
- If an adolescent endangers his or her health in one of the aforementioned ways, consultation with an adolescent psychiatrist may be in order. The referral to special care must take place discreetly, and the justification for the referral must be explained to the youth concretely.
- Medication should not be initiated in the case of crisis reactions until an adolescent psychiatrist has evaluated the situation.

34.15 Marginalization of adolescents

Matti Kaivosoja

General information

- Adolescents who become marginalized because of social or mental problems receive little attention in health care.
- Marginalization can be the end-result of many poor conditions: the adolescent becomes simultaneously worse off than others with respect to their economic situation, education, living conditions, and learn the skills needed in life.
- The marginalization process is complex, but it is often combined with considerable health problems.

Prevalence

- Marginalized adolescents are generally male.
- Most child psychiatric patients are boys, but at the age of 13–14 years more girls are affected.
- As the proportion of boys needing health care, the proportion of those needing child welfare services increases.

Reasons for marginalization

- Severe mental disorders (depression, psychosis, developmental disorders)
- Asocial behaviour
- Use of alcohol or drugs
- Disadvantageous living environment

Health problems of marginalized adolescents

- The following three important factors are associated with suicides: use of alcohol, asocial behaviour, and depression.
- The problems are often noted, but the means of helping are insufficient. In health care services, the adolescent may often be considered weakly motivated and to have a short attention span.
- The more differentiated the problem of the adolescent, the more holistic the help that he or she receives.

Encountering a marginalized adolescent and referral to treatment

- A possible mental disorder that has led to marginalization must be recognized and treated.
- The adolescent can be referred to an examination for rehabilitation.
- Vocational guidance must be supported, and the possibilities to arrange for vocational guidance must be looked into.
- Officials in different services need to cooperate in helping an adolescents with multifarious problems.
- One must be familiar with the autonomic development of the adolescent and know how to assess his or her actual readiness to take responsibility for both him- or herself and the treatment.

34.20 Psychiatric evaluation and referral to treatment of adolescents

Kari Pylkkänen

Need for treatment

- Adolescents need psychiatric care more often than children. About 20–30% of adolescents have psychiatric problems.

- Most mental problems that threaten the functional ability of adults begin in adolescence at about the age of 16.

Examination of an adolescent

- The adolescent himself is the most important source of information, but an interview of the parents may give vital additional information.
- School and school health care personnel often recognize a teenager's mental difficulties in their initial stages.
- Several interviews, reserving enough time and a free atmosphere aid in the examination of an adolescent.

Perspectives in encountering an adolescent

- Remember that adolescents are neither children nor adults.
- Respect the adolescent's pursuit for autonomy and independence.
- Encourage the adolescent to express his own experiences; show interest.
- Be neutral, avoid taking "sides" with instances that oppose the teenager.
- Make observations on the following
    - relationship with his self and parents; how he feels about his body; sense of reality
    - relationship with authorities
    - relationship with peers, does the adolescent have friends or does he withdraw from others
    - does the adolescent show signs of a severe mental disorder that would require a more thorough investigation.

Signs of severe mental disorder requiring consultation with a psychiatrist specialized in problems of adolescents

- Suicide attempt or self-destructive thoughts associated with a conscious will to die.
- Uncontrolled behaviour at home, assault of parents, breaking of furniture, locking oneself in room.
- Belief that one's body has changed or is changing.
- A physical reaction to an oral insult.
- Withdrawal from reality, for example, use of i.v. drugs, severe anorexia, self-mutilation.
- Withdrawal from social relationships.

Psychotic experience in adolescence

- Psychotic experiences in adolescence can be divided into the following three groups.
    - A psychotic episode can manifest itself as a suicide attempt, self-mutilation, or self-destruction. The adolescent's connection with reality is momentarily disturbed.
    - Psychotic actions can be manifested as, for example, anorexia, use of narcotics, addiction or severe depression.
    - The symptoms of actual psychosis resemble those of psychosis in adulthood (34.13).

Depression in adolescence

- See 34.11.

Aggression

- Is typical for this age–it is important to recognize situations in which the adolescents' aggressive behaviour or images hinder personal development.
- Signs of pathological aggression; see the section on signs of severe mental disorder.

Psychosomatic symptoms

- Are common in adolescents, occur in certain situations, and are temporary.
- Thoughts and images that are connected to the symptoms should be assessed (for example, fear of a serious illness or death).
- Generally discussion and providing the adolescent with realistic information help the symptoms disappear.
- Serious, long-lasting psychosomatic symptoms require consultation with a psychiatrist specialized in adolescents' problems.

Views of treatment

- Moderation is recommended in the medical treatment of adolescents.
- Assess the risk of dependence before issuing anxiolytic medication. (Dependence on alcohol and notable separation difficulties indicate a risk of developing dependence on medication).
- A psychotherapeutic examination is usually essential for adolescents. Their need for psychotherapeutic treatment is often short-term, however.
- Combining medication with psychotherapy is often necessary when more severe disorders are being treated.
- In the treatment of adolescents' psychoses a long period of hospital care in an adolescent unit that combines medication and psychotherapy is often necessary and often also proves successful.
- Adolescents' independence and autonomy from their parents creates an ethical problem with respect to treatment: Who has the authority to decide on matters concerning the developing adolescents' body and treatments? An attempt is generally made to respect the autonomy of the adolescent.

34.30 Substance abuse of adolescents

Pekka Aarninsalo

Objectives

- Identify adolescents' substance use and intervene, as even occasional use may result in serious health risks.
- Identify possible suicidal tendencies and refer a psychotic patient to psychiatric emergency care.
- Contact the parents of adolescents below 18 years of age even though the use of substances seems to be occasional.
- Evaluate the situation from the point of view of child protection and contact child protection authorities when needed.

Epidemiology

- The use of alcohol and drugs has increased among adolescents during the last 10 years.
- Only some experimenters develop actual substance dependence or start abusing alcohol or drugs.
- According to a Finnish school health survey from 1998–1999, 11% of 9th grade upper-level comprehensive school children reported having experimented with marihuana or cannabis (2% had used the substances 5 times or more). The respective figures were 15% and 5% for students at the 2nd level of the upper secondary school and 20% and 7% for 2nd-level vocational school students.

Identification of problem

- The adolescent is submitted directly to treatment in cases of toxication, incoherence or an accident due to intoxication.
- The adolescent seeks help for depression, anxiety or sleeping disorders.
    - The possible relation between substance use and symptoms is investigated. The youth may not have considered, for example, the possible connection between the continuous use of cannabis and depression.
    - Inquiries should be direct and neutral. Questions about symptoms should be asked with sympathy, because adolescents often interpret enquiries about substance use as accusations.
- Parents contact health care because of suspicions of drug use or drug-related problems, but the adolescent refuses to come in for discussions.
    - If it is a matter of suspicion, the parents should ask the adolescent directly about what they suspect. If the youth misuses drugs or alcohol and refuses to discuss it with experts, the parents can seek help from a substance treatment centre for adolescents.
        - According to family therapy, change is possible even though not all family members attend meetings.
- Adolescent seeks help to stop substance use.

Treatment

- The situation is viewed both from a somatic and a psychiatric point of view.
- Treatment concentrates more on therapy than on medication.
- The organisation of treatment varies by region and country. Larger urban centres have youth stations (age limit generally 13–25 years) or other treatment centres that specialize in substance abuse.
- Elsewhere adolescents' substance problems are handled as part of other health care and social services. Institutional care is generally arranged through child social services.
- Substance use is often only part of a larger set of problems among patients in youth psychiatric wards.
- The youth's family should be involved in the treatment. In cases in which the adolescent does not necessarily regard his or her substance use as a problem, family therapy sessions help to change the situation. According to research, family therapy has been more effective than individual treatment B [1,2,3].
- Many youth drug treatment centres are non-medication treatment facilities that replace medication with, for example, withdrawal acupuncture.

Co-morbidity

- Most young substance abusers also have other mental problems, most commonly a behavioural problem, an attention deficit–hyperactivity disorder or a mental disturbance (34.11), (34.12).
- The psychiatric situation of the youth should always be taken into consideration when substance problems of adolescents are treated.
- When a young person both abuses substances and has psychiatric problems, it is useful to concentrate first on terminating the substance use.
- Assess other problems in the family.

Medication

- The policy on medication is mainly determined by the other mental problems of the adolescent. Sometimes the use of a substance is a form of self-treatment with which the youth attempts to ease, for example, symptoms of depression.
- Patients most often seek medication for symptoms of anxiety and sleeping disorders. Benzodiazepines can be, or they can become, part of the problem, and their use as medication should be considered very carefully. Neuroleptic drugs can be used as medication in small dosages.
- Opiate substitution therapy is given by treatment centres that specialise in this method.

Co-operation with child protection services

- The legislation of each country determined how actively officials can intervene in problems related to substance use among adolescents.
- Health care and child protection services should agree on policies and cooperation.
- If the substance abuse is serious (e.g., intravenous use of drugs) or the adolescent has multiple problems or he or she is suicidal in addition to abusing substances, involuntary treatment in child protection institutions may be necessary (if stipulated in the law).
- Institutionalised treatment is recommended also for persons over 18 years of age in the aforementioned situations.

References

1. Stanton MD, Shadish WR. Outcome, attrition, and family-couples treatment for drug abuse. a meta-analysis and review of the controlled, comparative studies. Psychol Bull 1997;122: 170–91.
2. New Zealand Health Technology Assessment. Adolescent therapeutic day programmes and community-based programmes for serious mental illness and serious drug and alcohol problems: a critical appraisal of the literature. Christchurch: NewZealand Health Technology Assessment (NZHTA). 958374279. NZHTA Report 5. 1998. 56.
3. The Health Technology Assessment Database, Database no.: HTA-988953. In: The Cochrane Library, Issue 1, 2001. Oxford: Update Software.

Psychiatry

Evidence Based Medicine Guidelines. Edited by the Duodecim Editorial Team
 ISBN: 0-470-01184-X

35.1 Mental disorders due to organic disease

Editors

Aim

- To identify organic diseases causing psychiatric symptoms, particularly in the early phase. Many of these diseases are curable.

Basic rules

- The first symptoms of dementia (36.22) and delirium (22.2) are often interpreted as psychiatric. Most of the disorders presented here are also aetiological factors for dementia and delirium.
- Comorbidity is common: the patient may have organic and psychiatric problems. The knowledge of a serious disease and the limitations due to the disease predispose to mental disorders. Mentally retarded patients and patients with dementia are at risk of psychiatric disturbance.

When should an organic aetiology be suspected

- In delirium, especially if an elderly person without a psychiatric history develops an acute confusional state.
- In psychosis that is not functional by certainty, especially if the patient has not had a psychosis before.
- When there is suspicion of dementia
- If the patient also develops a neurological sign (paresis, epileptic seizure, cranial nerve sign).
- If the patient has symptoms of infection.
- If the patient has a significant organic disease (diabetes, hypertension, cardiac insufficiency, atrial fibrillation, renal or hepatic insufficiency etc.).
- If the psychiatric symptoms are atypical and an experienced clinician finds the clinical features extraordinary.

Organic disorders in which the patient may first be referred to psychiatric treatment

Intra-cranial expansions

- **A frontal lobe tumour** may cause a slow change in personality. Symptoms may include slowness and deterioration of thinking and behaviour, and loss of judgement and sometimes sense of smell.
- **A temporal lobe tumour** may also produce personality changes and often causes epileptic seizures.
- **Chronic subdural haematoma** (18.5) may cause slowness and deterioration of mental capacity that worsens gradually over weeks or months. It is often accompanied by nausea, headache and fluctuations in consciousness. The patients are often elderly people or alcoholics.
- If the history is imperfect (i.e. no information on possible traumas), **epidural haematoma** (18.5) and subacute subdural haematoma should be considered as causes of sudden confusion.

Infections

- **Infections** in the elderly and those in poor health (pneumonia, urinary tract infection, sepsis)
- **Infections of the central nervous system**
  - Encephalitis (36.57) may begin with a mental change that resembles acute psychosis.
  - Syphilis with symptoms in the nervous system is still seen (36.57). Initially it can produce non-specific mental symptoms that may be interpreted as depression. Later, the disease leads to personality changes, typically grandiosity and later dementia. The patient also has neurological symptoms: Argyll Robertson pupil (36.7), changes of deep sensation in the legs, and cerebral vascular disorders in neurovascular syphilis.
  - Borreliosis can affect the CNS.
  - Subacute sclerosing panencephalitis (SSPE) may start with symptoms resembling psychosis (36.57).
- **AIDS** may be accompanied by dementia, depression, personality changes, and even psychosis.

Metabolic disorders

- **Hypercalcaemia** (adenoma in the parathyroid gland) may result in symptoms interpreted as depression.
- **Hepatic coma** or hepatic failure causes changes of consciousness. The patient normally has a known history of liver disease or severe alcoholism.
- **Hypoglycaemia** can cause confusion, anxiety and other neuropsychiatric symptoms, e.g. aggressive behaviour.
- **Hyperglycaemia** may be accompanied by anxiety, agitation or delirium.
- **Thyroid disorders**: Hypothyroidism causes depression, and hyperthyroidism is characterized by agitation and insomnia.
- **Vitamin B_{12} deficiency** causes dementia and impairment of memory.

Dementia

- **Creutzfeldt-Jakob disease** (36.59) is characterized by rapidly progressing dementia accompanied by neurological signs (paralysis, extrapyramidal signs, myoclonus). In the early stage the disease can be interpreted as psychiatric disorder.
- **Huntington's disease** is often first diagnosed as psychosis, even as schizophrenia. These patients are lively and overactive. The development of choreiform movements and knowledge of similar disease in the family can lead to suspicion of Huntington's disease.

- **Vascular dementia** (36.23) may be characterized by depression and confusion before dementia and neurological signs can be detected.
- **Alzheimer's disease** (36.24) is associated with several psychiatric symptoms.
  - Depression is common in the early stages of disease when the patient is often aware of the memory impairment and loss of function.
  - The patient may deny or cover up symptoms of memory impairment and this may appear, for example, as paranoid symptoms. The patient explains memory gaps by confabulation or by saying that missing objects are stolen.
  - In the moderately severe phase many patients become anxious and restless. Various mental stimulations can arouse emotional memories and global anxiety for which the patient has no words. Many patients also suffer from insomnia, which is a considerable strain on the caregivers.
  - In the moderate to severe phases behavioural disorders, such as soiling, wandering, uncontrolled aggressivity, running, and constant dressing and undressing or eating disorders are often present.
- **Lewy body dementia** includes, in addition to memory impairment, also visual disturbances and rigidity, which may be confused with depression. The patients are sensitive to antiparkinson medications, which may trigger a state of confusion.
- **Pick's disease** and other frontal dementias.
- **Acute vascular stroke** (36.31) (in non-motor area)
  - An elderly person's stroke may present only with confusion without other signs.
  - Stroke in the right (non-dominant) hemisphere affects the sense of space. The patient may have a feeling that the environment is abnormal, giving an impression of a psychiatric disorder if the patient has no other signs of stroke.
  - Stroke in the left (dominant) hemisphere may cause only sensory dysphasia (inability to understand speech while the patient's speech is moderately normal), which may resemble a psychiatric disorder.

Confusion due to medication of Parkinson's disease

- In severe Parkinson's disease the patient may need abundant medication with dopaminergic drugs (levodopa, selegiline, dopamine agonists and COMT inhibitors) and anticholinergic drugs (classic Parkinsonian drugs) to maintain his or her ability to move. As a result of synergism a state of confusion may develop, possibly triggered by addition of a new drug.
- The confusion caused by levodopa is often accompanied by hallucinations in which the patient sees his or her relatives, dead or distant, and is aware that these sights are hallucinations.
- The treatment is a reduction of medication, which may lead to reduced ability to move. A balance must be sought in the level of medication: either the patient can move more easily but becomes confused or cannot move but avoids confusion.

Substance-related disorders and withdrawal symptoms

- Confusion can be related to abuse of medication or an abnormal susceptibility to medication (see also delirium 22.2, toxins and medication).
- **Alcohol abuse** may be well concealed, especially in women.
- If alcohol abuse is known, **Wernicke-Korsakoff's disease** (36.73) should be kept in mind and the patient should be given thiamine if he or she is hospitalized.

Epileptic dream state, temporal epilepsy, postictal state

- If the patient has unusual behaviour appearing as fits, the cause may be an epileptic dream state. An EEG taken during such a state may clarify the situation.
- Some patients with temporal epilepsy also have psychotic episodes.
- Certain epileptic patients have states of confusion after seizures lasting several hours during which they may act aggressively.

35.2 A patient with psychosomatic symptoms

Editors

Basic rules

- Psychosomatic symptoms seldom vanish entirely. The purpose of the therapy should therefore be to build a harmonious cooperative relation in which the patient does not require more help than the physician is capable of providing.
- The patient wishes to have his/her symptom named and acknowledged. Only after this he or she may be able to admit the symptom and receive treatment. The common goal to name the psychosomatic symptom is a kind of a deal between the physician and the patient. The patient is not satisfied until the explanation his physician gives for his symptoms correlates to his or her own views.
- Try to minimize unnecessary diagnostic testing and maximize the use of non-pharmacological therapies, such as psychological support and physical exercise.
- The physician should never doubt the existence of the symptom nor its subjective severity.
- The physician's ability to both listen and confront the patient during the interview is a requirement for understanding the psychological grounds of the somatic symptoms.

- It is essential that the physician can act as a "teacher" who helps the patient to understand how psychic stress and fears may naturally cause somatic symptoms and pain through the action of the autonomous nervous system and muscular tension. Calling the symptoms psychiatric is generally not recommended.

Chronic pain and psychosomatic syndrome

- It is important to treat psychogenic symptoms and pain as seriously as somatic ones.
- The patients typically have problems in understanding and expressing their emotions (alexithymia: no words for emotions).
- In order to learn about the patient's circumstances in life it may be easier to start by asking about the presence and severity of the symptom or pain in different situations in life.
- See also Chronic pain (17.40), Fatigued or tired patient (36.10) and Fibromyalgia (20.92).

Psychiatric disorders with somatic symptoms

- Major depressive disorder may present with symptoms of chronic pain syndrome or somatic exhaustion disorder (35.20), (35.21). One fourth of the patients with chronic pain syndrome also fill the criteria for major depressive disorder.
- Patients with panic disorder (35.29) have attacks with somatic sensations resulting from the activation of autonomous nervous system (hyperventilation, palpitations, chest pain, shortness of breath, dizziness, fainting, sweating, fear of dying). In generalized anxiety disorder, fear of social situations and phobias symptoms caused by activation of the autonomous nervous system are also common.
- In schizophrenia the somatic symptom is often strange and is a part of a larger paranoid system.
- In dissociative reactions (conversion disorder) the typical symptom is the loss of a physiological function (paralysis, blindness), which has an individual psychological meaning for the patient.
- Somatization disorder is a chronic disorder that begins in adolescence, in which the patient, most often female, has several somatic complaints.
- In grief reaction the patient often has symptoms of the disease that caused the loss of a loved person. The symptom may be activated on the anniversary of the loss, on the birthday of the deceased or during holiday festivities. If the patient has psychosomatic symptoms, it is useful to ask about the cause of death of his loved ones and examine the patient's attitude towards the loss.
- Hypochondria manifests as continuous fear of becoming sick or suspicion of a disease based on false interpretation of bodily symptoms. Triggering factors include the illness or death of a loved one, or own earlier illness.
- In Munchausen syndrome a person seeks the role of a patient purposefully, however, without the aim of obtaining immediate benefits, such as economic benefit or avoidance of certain tasks. Such a person may, for example, ingest or inject harmful substances or objects to cause somatic symptoms and thus gain the doctors attention.

Ordering diagnostic tests, medications, sick leaves and pensions

- Ordering diagnostic tests and writing out prescriptions may become a part of doctor–patient relationship, an unspoken and honourable compromise. The disadvantages of this practice are the costs of unnecessary diagnostic tests and treatments and possible dependence on or side effects of unnecessary drugs.
- The success of alternative medicine in psychosomatic disorders is largely based on this kind of a compromise, but also on empathy.
- A common mistake and often a fateful one for the doctor–patient relationship is to discuss the sick leave or pension as if the symptom were the decisive factor. If the doctor denies sick leave or pension pleading to the mildness of the symptoms he/she questions the patient's subjective experience and may insult the patient.
- When the doctor decides not to prescribe sick leave or recommend pension, he/she must convince the patient that he/she does not question the patient's symptom nor the severity of pain.
- If the psychosomatic symptom is associated with a life crisis or burnout, a sick leave is often indicated. A burnout often requires a 2–3-week and major depression a 2–3-month absence from work.
- When considering whether the patient is entitled to a pension it is important to pay attention to the patient's exhaustion, well-being in general, ability to express his feelings, personality and life situation. It is usually best to obtain the opinion of a psychiatrist or psychologist already at the beginning of possible retirement process.

The quality of the doctor–patient relationship

- Analytic and interpreting psychotherapies are seldom useful.
- The doctor–patient relationship has to be supportive and comforting.
- A regular long-term contact with a "somatic" physician gives the best possible support to a chronic psychosomatic patient, may improve the patient's functional capacity and save resources.
- The treatment should begin with building a confidential and protective doctor–patient relationship (active diagnostic strategy for symptoms, treatments to relieve symptoms, flexible attitude towards alternative therapies).

- Especially at the beginning it is better to avoid psychologizing the symptom or interpreting its meaning.
- It is important to convince the patient that the doctor–patient relationship may continue regardless of whether the symptom continues or disappears. The symptom should not be a ticket of admission to a doctor–patient relationship.
- It is not wise to give hope of a cure but rather offer realistic hope of the gradual smoothing or relieving of the symptom. Physician must know that sooner or later he will disappoint the dependent patient.
- After the acute phase the doctor–patient relationship may continue even throughout the patient's life, first as frequent consultations (e.g. once a month), later the contact may be more rare but regular.
- During the consultation the patient's current life situation rather than the symptom is discussed. Although the consultations may seem superficial and not planned and psychotherapeutic, such a doctor–relationship may provide the best possible psychotherapeutic support to patients with chronic pain and other psychosomatic symptoms.
- The aim of the doctor–patient relationship is to supply security and prevent the patient from drifting to a circle of different treatments and procedures which complicate the situation.
- If the physician is away on holiday or travels for a longer time, he/she should assign the patient to a colleague for urgencies and inform this physician of patient's symptoms and background. This arrangement is the best guarantee that the patient does not show up in the emergency room.

Other therapies

- Family therapy may be useful if the symptom is a part of a communication or a power struggle within the family. Systemic, strategic and solution-oriented family or network sessions may be the most effective and economic means to interfere with the communication within the family.
- Cognitive behavioural therapy **B** [1 2] has been proven useful in the treatment of unexplained somatic symptoms.
- It is essential that the psychosomatic symptom is taken seriously as a somatic symptom and unnecessary interpreting and psychologizing is avoided.
- Generally, it is recommendable to avoid pharmacological treatments. However, antidepressants appear to be effective for psychogenic pain and somatoform pain disorders **B** [3 4].
- Conditions are better for rehabilitation if the patient does not experience them as a threat to the safe doctor–patient relationship or as a means for the physician to get rid of a difficult patient.
- The physician's flexible attitude towards alternative medicine enables the patient to avoid very harmful and expensive treatment experiments.
- Some of the patients with chronic psychosomatic symptoms "need" their symptom or suffering. The chronic symptom is unconsciously sensed as a lesser evil than getting well and coping with the various consequences of being healthy.

References

1. Morley S, Eccleston C, Williams A. Systematic review and meta-analysis of randomized controlled trials of cognitive behaviour therapy and behaviour therapy for chronic pain in adults, excluding headache. Pain 1999;80:1–13.
2. The Database of Abstracts of Reviews of Effectiveness (University of York), Database no.: DARE-990758. In: The Cochrane Library, Issue 1, 2001. Oxford: Update Software.
3. Fishbain DA, Cutler RB, Rosomoff RS. Do antidepressants have an analgesic effect in psychogenic pain and somatoform pain disorder: a meta-analysis. Psychosomatic Medicine 1998;60:503–509.
4. The Database of Abstracts of Reviews of Effectiveness (University of York), Database no.: DARE-981319. In: The Cochrane Library, Issue 4, 2000. Oxford: Update Software.

35.3 Treatment of insomnia

Erkka Syvälahti

Basic rules

- Before starting medication find out whether the patient's insomnia could be eliminated by lifestyle changes.
- Identify depression, psychotic disorder or sleep apnoea as the underlying cause as their treatments differ significantly from the treatment of insomnia due to other causes.
- Occasional or short-term use of hypnotic should be encouraged, instead of regular use.
- The need for gradual withdrawal of the medication must be explained to the patient at the start of treatment.

PSY

Epidemiology

- Chronic insomnia is common in the general population (up to 10%).

Information needed

- How much the patient sleeps during the day, including afternoon naps (using a diary of sleep history, if necessary).
- Does the patient have difficulty falling asleep or remaining asleep during early hours?
- Does the insomnia cause daytime tiredness or other symptoms?
    - Patients with sleep apnoea (36.9), (6.71) do not normally complain of sleeplessness but of tiredness, narcolepsy during the daytime, irritability and amnesia. Avoid hypnotics!
- Is the insomnia temporary or every night?
- Dietary factors, especially the use of coffee and alcohol.

- Even 2–3 cups of coffee may affect the quality of sleep.
- Alcohol reduces the amount of REM and deep sleep periods.

♦ The medication the patient uses.

- Beta-blockers may cause nightmares.
- Diuretics taken in the evening may fill the bladder and lead to restless sleep.

Clinical features

♦ If the reason for insomnia is not clear, look for psychiatric and somatic disorders and medication that may cause insomnia, especially in elderly patients.

♦ Pollacisuria (prostate hyperplasia) may awaken the patient.

♦ Chronic heart failure can cause insomnia. ECG and chest x-ray are indicated if they have not been performed recently.

♦ Blood count and sedimentation rate can be examined to rule out anaemia and general medical conditions.

♦ Assess whether the patient is depressed.

General advice for the patient

♦ Always go to bed at the same time, including at the weekend C [1 2].

♦ Do not stay awake in bed but get up if you cannot go to sleep in half an hour and return when you get tired.

♦ Try to wake up regularly at the same time.

♦ Do not read, watch television or work in bed C [1 2].

♦ Avoid afternoon naps (longer than 20–30 minutes).

♦ Exercise regularly (at least 3–4 times per week) C [3] but do not exercise in the evening if this affects falling asleep.

♦ Reduce the consumption of alcohol, coffee, cigarettes and sleeping pills.

♦ Ensure that the bedroom is quiet, dark and pleasantly cool.

♦ Avoid intense thinking and emotions in the evening.

Pharmacotherapy

♦ The first-line treatment for temporary insomnia with difficulties in falling asleep is a small dose of short- or medium-acting benzodiazepines or non-benzodiazepine hypnotics A [4 5] (zaleplon, zolpidem C [6 7], zopiclone).

♦ If the patient wakes during early hours, oxazepam and nitrazepam are suitable drugs. Zaleplon can, if necessary, be taken up to 4 hours before the wake-up time.

♦ If the patient has not used sleeping pills before prescribe a small number of tablets (10–30) and ask the patient to make a new appointment if he needs more medication. Encourage the patient to take "days off" the medication, for example, on weekends.

Special cases

♦ If the patient with temporary insomnia has anxiety during the daytime, a long-acting benzodiazepine may be the drug of choice.

♦ If he patient is depressed and wakes up during the night the right treatment may be a small dose of a sedative antidepressant (doxepin, trimipramine, amitriptyline, mianserin, mirtazapine etc.) Unlike benzodiazepines, these drugs should be taken regularly every evening. Follow the patient up and assess the need for other forms of treatment for depression.

♦ In severe sleep disorders neuroleptics (levomepromazine, chlorprothixene) may be more effective than benzodiazepines. For example, confused and agitated patients may use neuroleptics. Neuroleptic as a treatment for insomnia is not adequate if the patient has incipient psychosis; a psychiatrist should be consulted if psychosis is suspected.

♦ If benzodiazepine-like drugs are contraindicated, sedative anti-histamines, e.g. hydroxyzine, are an alternative.

Adverse reactions of hypnotics

♦ When the effect of the medication disappears, rebound insomnia may develop. This comprises difficulties in falling asleep and waking up the night after the use of medication. Even short-term use of medication may lead to rebound insomnia. The symptom is seen particularly after the use of short-acting benzodiazepines and may appear early in the morning when the effect has worn out too abruptly. On the other hand, the symptoms may appear on the nights following withdrawal and vary according to the duration and dose of medication.

♦ Rebound anxiety is also possible, where the patient feel abnormally active and/or agitated the day after taking benzodiazepines.

♦ The use of long-acting benzodiazepines may cause problems in psychomotor and cognitive functions the day after using the medication.

♦ Benzodiazepines may also affect memory (antegrade amnesia).

♦ Confusion may also be seen if the sleep is interrupted. Dizziness and falls can occur. This may be a problem especially with the short-acting, high-raffinity benzodiazepines (midazolam and triazolam).

Dependence and withdrawal symptoms

♦ The benzodiazepines are best discontinued by halving the dose for 1 or 2 days before the end of treatment.

♦ Short periods of medication and moderate doses are the best way to prevent withdrawal symptoms.

♦ If the patient has taken high doses for long periods the discontinuation must be gradual.

♦ The withdrawal symptoms appear 5–7 days after discontinuation of long-acting drugs, and sooner (and are possibly more severe) after ending treatment with short-acting drugs.

♦ Changing to longer-acting benzodiazepines may sometimes help with discontinuation.

References

1. Morin CM, Culbert JP, Schwartz SM. Non-pharmacological interventions for insomnia: a meta-analysis of treatment efficacy. Am J Psychiatr 1994;151:1172–1180.
2. The Database of Abstracts of Reviews of Effectiveness (University of York), Database no.: DARE-940445. In: The Cochrane Library, Issue 4, 1999. Oxford: Update Software.
3. Montgomery P, Dennis J. Physical exercise for sleep problems in adults aged 60+. Cochrane Database Syst Rev. 2004;(2):CD003404.
4. Benzodiaxepines and zolpidem for chronic insomnia: a meta-analysis of treatment strategy. JAMA 1997;278:2170–2177.
5. The Database of Abstracts of Reviews of Effectiveness (University of York), Database no.: DARE-988111. In: The Cochrane Library, Issue 4, 1999. Oxford: Update Software.
6. Lobo BL, Greene WL. Zolpidem – distinct from triazolam? (review). Ann Pharmacother 1997;31:625–632.
7. The Database of Abstracts of Reviews of Effectiveness (University of York), Database no.: DARE-970668. In: The Cochrane Library, Issue 4, 1999. Oxford: Update Software.

35.4 A violent patient

Editors

The setting for interviewing a violent patient

People present at the interview

- The privacy of the patient is ensured by an interview behind closed doors and without others present. The doctor should sit closer to the door than the agitated patient.
- If an agitated patient is considered potentially dangerous the interview can be performed with the door open and with other personnel outside the room near the door. If this is not sufficient other personnel can be present in the room.
- In extreme cases the patient must be tied down in a wheelchair, stretchers or bed.

The interior of the interview room

- There should be no throwable objects or sharp instruments in the room.
- An emergency call button or another message system should be available.
- The receptionist or other personnel should have a warning sign or phrase to warn the doctor about an unexpected potentially dangerous patient.
- No sharp weapons should be available for the patients (knives in the staff coffee room!).

Encountering a violent patient

- Immediate assessment of the cause of violent behaviour
  - Drunkenness
  - Delirium
  - Narcotics
  - Acute confusion with an organic cause
  - Psychosis
  - Personality disorder
- Delirious, intoxicated or psychotic patients cannot usually be calmed by mere conversation.
- Talking often calms patients with personality disorders, but they can be extremely violent after drinking alcohol.

Medication before the interview

- Neuroleptics or benzodiazepines can be given to delirious or intoxicated patients (see below) C [1 2], however, the diagnosis may be more difficult to make after medication.
- Neuroleptic medication is usually necessary to calm a psychotic patient. However, the patient can be referred to a psychiatric hospital involuntarily and starting the drug treatment can be postponed until the patient is in the hospital. The referring physician can offer medication to the patient for anxiety.

Behaviour of the doctor

- Counter-aggressiveness must be avoided by all available means.
- Tones of conversation that embarrass, baffle, accuse, threaten or disapprove the patient may increase his/her violence.
- The voice must be calm and neutral.
- Patients with personality disorders should especially be given the impression that the doctor is able to put himself/herself in their position ("I understand that you are very nervous...").
- Do not get too close to the patient. Direct intensive eye-to-eye contact may also be perceived as threatening.

PSY

Self-defence

- Do not expose yourself to unnecessary risks. It is often reassuring if the personnel outnumber the patient.
- If possible remove spectacles, ties, and necklaces.
- Consider in advance how to protect your face, head, and neck.
- If the patient grasps your wrists, they can usually be released by rotating them against the patient's thumbs.
- If the patient grasps from the back, pressing the jaw against the chest and turning around quickly often loosens the grip.
- If the patient bites, push your arm deeper into his/her mouth and close the nostrils with your other hand.

Using restraints

- The purpose is to safeguard the patient and the personnel.

- If restraints are used temporarily, one of the personnel must be with the patient all the time.
- Remember the risk of thromboembolism in prolonged immobilization.

Medication for a violent patient

- The purpose of the medication is to calm a psychotic or excited patient if conversation is not successful.
- Antipsychotics and benzodiazepines and experienced staff are the means to manage imminent violence C [1 2].
- Haloperidol is the most effective drug C [1 2]. The dose is 2.5–5 mg perorally or intramuscularly, repeated at intervals of 30–60 min., if necessary. The patient is usually calmed after a few injections. The maximum daily dose is 100 mg.
- Diazepam can be administered simultaneously with haloperidol C [1 2]. The dose is 10–20 mg perorally or as a slow intravenous injection. Lorazepam 2–4 mg i.m. or i.v. is an alternative. Benzodiazepines can also be used alone without haloperidol.
- Beta-blockers may be effective in the management of agitation and aggression in people with acquired brain injury C [3].

Further assessment

- After the patient has been calmed assess whether
  - a somatic disease requiring treatment is present (injuries, infections such as encephalitis, intoxications)
  - the patient should be referred involuntarily to a mental hospital
  - the patient has committed such violence or crimes during the encounter or before it that a police hearing is indicated.
- According to the situation the patient can be referred to a hospital, ambulatory care, a clinic for alcoholics, a clinic for family problems, or allowed to go home without further treatment.
- If a patient is discharged home they should always be offered an appointment for assessment of their life situation with a suitable professional.

References

1. Wing J, Marriott S, Palmer C, Thomas V. Management of imminent violence: clinical practice guidelines to support mental health services. Occasional Paper OP41, March 1998, pp. 1–111.
2. The Database of Abstracts of Reviews of Effectiveness (University of York), Database no.: DARE-988469. In: The Cochrane Library, Issue 2, 2000. Oxford: Update Software.
3. Fleminger S, Greenwood RJ, Oliver DL. Pharmacological management for agitation and aggression in people with acquired brain injury. Cochrane Database Syst Rev. 2004;(2):CD003299.

35.5 A suicidal patient

Martti Heikkinen

Basic rules

- Suicidal plans and ideations should be asked about and discussed openly.
- The physician should help the patient to find other solutions than suicide and should give concrete advice on practical arrangements.
- It is important to ensure that the patient can get help at all times of the day.
- Family members should be invited to appointments if the patient agrees to this.

Identifying a patient at risk of suicide

Risk factors

- The severity of depression
  - Hopelessness associated with depression, concomitant anxiety symptoms, severe insomnia, considerable disturbance of concentration and memory, loss of pleasure, rapid alterations in mood and psychomotor agitation
- A suicide decision or plan, suicide note, recently made will or giving away of possessions
- Concomitant substance abuse
- Hopeless mood (strongest sign of danger), insomnia, self-disgust and memory problems in those with depression
- The availability of a means of suicide (weapons, drugs)
- Loneliness, lack of social support
- A somatic disorder, disability
- An earlier suicide attempt, especially using violent methods (hanging, etc.)
- Suicide of a relative or other close contact
- Males have a greater suicide risk than females. The risk of suicide increases with age.
- Suicide may be preceded by a precipitant factor: a life crisis, a recent loss (e.g. divorce), a situation that causes shame (drunk driving, unemployment, bankruptcy etc.)
- The patients considering suicide very often seek help in health care although they do not necessarily present their suicidal ideas.
- Biological factors have also been associated with suicide: persons who have committed suicide have been found to have lower concentrations of serotonin metabolites in CSF compared with controls.

Principles of treatment

- Before the treatment assess the following topics to learn about the severity of the situation and the risk of suicide:

- Is the patient psychotic?
- The patient's functional level: Is he capable of working? Capable of taking care of himself? Does he eat and drink sufficiently? Does he stay in bed all day?
- The patient's ability to make contact with people? Motivation for treatment?
- Social network: living alone, having a family, a spouse? What are the relationships like within the family? Is the family able to provide support?
- Does the patient have somatic problems that require treatment?
- Is the patient addicted? Is alcoholism a basic problem? A drunk patient who threatens with suicide must be brought under supervision. The risk of suicide should be assessed again when the patient is sober.

- Consider compulsory treatment if the patient has major or psychotic depression. The risk of suicide is greatest in these cases.
- If you decide to treat the patient in primary care, ensure that he has help available at all times.
- It is preferable that the patient always contacts the same professional or team. Options:
  - Primary care physician
  - Psychologist
  - Primary care mental clinic
  - Psychiatric outpatient clinic
  - A clinic for drug abusers.

Ensure that the patient is taken care of while he/she is waiting for secondary care treatment

- The people in charge of the patient should be active in contacting the patient and contact him/her themselves if the patient does not come to an appointment (C) [1 2 3 4]
- If the patient wants to be treated on a ward this should be organized. The crisis therapy on a ward should be arranged in cooperation with the primary care treatment team.

Medication for a patient at suicidal risk

- Before prescribing medication, any previous treatments and medications the patient possibly still has at home should be assessed (especially toxic products, e.g. psychotropics, toxic pain killers such as paracetamol and dextropropoxiphene, and beta-blockers).
- According to the latest research evidence, treating depression reduces the risk of suicide. The doses of medication should be adequate.
- When treating depression it should be kept in mind that the onset of the effect is delayed and the risk of suicide may be greater during the period of activation of the medication before the depression alleviates. The first signs of an effect of the medication are no reason for reducing the intensity of crisis therapy.
- Many patients cannot wait until the antidepressive treatment improves their mood but need treatment for anxiety with benzodiazepines or neuroleptics and sometimes also medication for insomnia.
- The medications should be prescribed only for 1 or 2 weeks at a time. The modern, less toxic antidepressants make the treatment safer.

Compulsory treatment

- Suicidal threat does not by itself justify compulsory treatment. Deep hopelessness and desire to die may be signs of psychosis that requires hospital treatment (sometimes against the patients will).
- If a doctor or a nurse is able to escort the patient safely to the hospital a referral for compulsory treatment may not be necessary in all cases.

References

1. van der Sande R, Buskens E, Allart E, van der Graaf Y, van Engeland H. Psychosocial interventions following suicide attempt: a systematic review of treatment interventions. Acta Psychiatr Scand 1997;96:43–50.
2. The Database of Abstracts of Reviews of Effectiveness (University of York), Database no.: DARE-970979. In: The Cochrane Library, Issue 4, 1999. Oxford: Update Software.
3. Linehan MM. Behavioural treatments of suicidal behaviours: definitional obfuscation and treatment outcomes. Ann N Y Acad Sci 1997;836:302–328.
4. The Database of Abstracts of Reviews of Effectiveness (University of York), Database no.: DARE-970979. In: The Cochrane Library, Issue 2, 2000. Oxford: Update Software.

35.11 Schizophrenia

Leea Muhonen

PSY

Aims

- To start the treatment before the first phase of psychosis.
- To identify the prodromal symptoms and the first symptoms of psychosis in time.
- Involving the patient's family and the other social network in the treatment reduces relapses (A) [1 2 3].

General points

- The aetiology of schizophrenia includes biological, psychological, and social factors.
- The symptoms of schizophrenia are due to cognitive and emotional dissolution of varying severity that leads to the patient's isolation, apathy and emotional problems.
- Disorders of thought appear as thought blocking, bizarre associations and concrete thinking.

- The emotional problems are characterized by incoherence, lack of consistency between thoughts and emotions. Flat or blunt affects are typical. The patient may also have bizarre feelings that are difficult to understand.

Symptoms

- In the acute phase, the patient almost always has hallucinatory experiences, most often auditory hallucinations. Somatic hallucinations are also possible, for example, the patient may feel that he/she has a machine in the brain, or he/she may have olfactory or gustatory hallucinations.
- Visual hallucinations are less common and may also be a symptom of an organic brain disease.
- Paranoid delusions are also common. The patients may believe the newspapers or television are making references about them. They may feel that other people are controlling them in a telepathic manner. At worst the delusions are paranoid and the patient may attempt to escape the threat he constantly feels or start to defend himself aggressively.
- Catatonic posture is possible, and earlier it used to be a typical sign.
- The patients with schizophrenia are often depressed and many commit suicide.

Aetiology

- Biological factors may predispose to schizophrenia and psychosocial factors may initially trigger the beginning of the disease and maintain it.
- Schizophrenia has a genetic component. There is also evidence that influenza during the second trimester of pregnancy elevates the risk of schizophrenia in the offspring.
- The patients with schizophrenia have a reduced ability to filter sensory and emotional impulses. This leads to a lower capacity to tolerate stress and symptoms of psychosocial stress during normal life crisis.
- The structural weakness makes the patients especially vulnerable to disturbances of early interaction, e.g., excessive binding, parental conflicts and unreliability of parenteral response. The personality of the patient does not develop normally, and the patient lacks a sense of reality, which is why stressful situations may lead to psychotic dissolution.

Epidemiology

- The prevalence of schizophrenia is approximately 1%. The incidence of first time schizophrenia is 0.2% annually. The symptoms of schizophrenia differ depending on the culture: for example, catatonic schizophrenia is widely seen in African cultures while in the industrialized world the paranoid form is commonly seen.

Diagnosis

- Based on the symptoms, with disturbances continuing for at least 6 months and on a change in the functional capacity.
- Often the patient starts to isolate him-/herself from other people before falling ill. He/she may have had a strange feeling of altering of the self, and the patient may experience severe anxiety and unreal sensations.
- Active treatment and rehabilitation should be started for both the patient and the closest relatives in this phase.
- The clinical interview should be performed without haste, with empathy and interest. A neutral attitude towards the patient's answers is best. Somatic clinical examination is necessary to rule out, for example, hallucinations caused by neurological diseases. See (35.1).

Treatment

- The forms of treatment include medication, psychotherapy, B [4] family-oriented and group therapy, and rehabilitation. A combination of these is tailored individually according to a treatment protocol.
- An acute psychosis does not always require hospitalization. If the patient is cooperative the treatment can be given in an outpatient unit.
- If necessary the patient is referred for involuntary treatment.
- Community mental health teams (CMHT) can take responsibility for outpatient treatment C [5].

Medication

Acute phase

- Neuroleptics are the most effective drugs for relieving active psychotic symptoms; however, they are also intended for relieving depression and anxiety.
- In acute psychotic state of anxiety the drugs of choice are haloperidol 2.5–5 mg i.m. or i.v. B [6], zuclopenthixol 100 mg i.m. D [7] combined with clonazepam for a normal weight adult D [7]. The effect lasts a couple of days.
- The patients earlier experience is important in choosing the medication because different patients are predisposed to different side effects.
- Elevating the dose gradually is helpful in finding the smallest effective dose and avoiding the unpleasant side effects that may cause the patient to refuse medication.

Long-term therapy

- The drug doses are normally smaller in long-term treatment compared with the acute situation. The dose of chlorpromazine A [8] and other so-called large-dosage neuroleptics is 200–400 mg/day in acute treatment and 100–200 mg/day in continuous treatment B [9 10 11 12].
- The new, atypical neuroleptics (risperidone B [13 14 15 16 17], olanzapine B [18 19 20], quetiapine A [21] and ziprasidone) have fewer side effects than the traditional neuroleptics B [18 19 20].
- Olanzapine increases the risk of diabetes C [22].

- Clozapine is more effective than 'typical' neuroleptic medication in reducing symptoms and recurrences A [23].
- The efficacy of newer atypical neuroleptics is equal to that of clozapine C [24].
- The doses of small-dosage neuroleptics are usually: haloperidol 4–12 mg/day, perphenazine 8–32 mg/day, risperidone 3–6 mg/day, and olanzapine 20 mg/day A [25].
- Because of side effects thioridazine A [26] is a second-line drug B [27]. It is used only if no response is obtained with other antipsychotics. The maximum daily dose is 400 mg/day due to possible cardiac complications B [27].
- After the psychotic state the dose of medication is gradually reduced and the patient is followed up frequently. When the minimum effective dosage is found, the medication can be continued either as oral regimen or long-acting depot injections C [28 29].
- Continuing the medication for up to 2 years after the psychotic phase reduces recurrences A [30]. After a relapse it is recommend to continue the medication for 5 years.

Adjuvant drugs

- Benzodiazepines are a valuable addition to the medication for patients in anxiety or panic. For example, diazepam may be combined with neuroleptic treatment starting with a small dose and increasing it if necessary to 10 mg × 3. This medication must be reduced gradually as soon as the psychotic anxiety is relieved.
- In the acute phase schizophrenia is often complicated with depression, hopelessness and an increased risk of suicide. Many patients with chronic schizophrenia are also depressed. Antidepressive medication (35.41) is necessary for a schizophrenic patient with depression.
- Mood-stabilizing drugs combined with a neuroleptic have been found useful to be in some cases.

Side effects

- A general practitioner may be confronted with the side effects of neuroleptic medication: high-dosage neuroleptics may cause orthostatic hypotension and collapses, high values in a liver function test, and the patient may even have jaundice. In such cases the medication must be changed. Allergic drug reactions are possible.
- Some patients taking chlorpromazine develop a photosensitive reaction resembling sunburn. Use in the summertime is not recommended.
- Neurological adverse effects include Parkinsonism and extrapyramidal signs. Any involuntary movements in the jaw, tongue or neck in particular should be noted. Side effects are an indication for a specialist consultation.
- Traditional neuroleptics, particularly thioridazine, may cause cardiac complications B [27].

Family

- Involving the family and close acquaintances of the patient with schizophrenia in the treatment from the beginning reduces relapses A [1 2 3]. It also makes eventual rehabilitation easier and helps family members to overcome their own crisis.
- It is important to help the family to understand the patient's need for isolation and protection as a positive reaction and to help the family to avoid critical, intrusive attitude towards the patient.
- A patient who needs long-term care and his/her family and social network can be supported by means of family intervention and by education and guidance. The aim is to create a supportive network that allows the patient enough time alone but is still warm and encouraging. The expectations and requirements set on the patient should be modest.

Individual psychotherapy

- Individual psychotherapy may help the patient to control his/her disease better, to recognize his/her strengths and weaknesses and to find new solutions for stressful situations.
- Cognitive therapy for patients with schizophrenia reduces the risk of relapses B [4].

Primary vs specialist care

- The responsibility for care is determined by local practices.
- A schizophrenic patient presenting with the first episode must be referred to specialist care.
- Patients with a labile disease need specialist level care, but can also be managed by a general practitioner who has the possibility of consulting a specialist.
- Clozapine therapy (35.42) is started in specialized care but can be followed up in primary care.

Prognosis

PSY

- Schizophrenia is a severe disease but the prognosis is not always negative. According to follow-up data 25–30% of patients with a first episode of schizophrenic psychosis are cured and free from symptoms after 5–10 years. Only 10–20% remain ill to the extent that they need daily help. Other patients recover sufficiently to be socially capable.
- The on-going symptoms of schizophrenia vary: the patient may have repeated episodes of psychosis but may be almost free of symptoms at other times.

References

1. Pharoah FM, Rathbone J, Mari JJ, Streiner D. Family intervention for schizophrenia. Cochrane Database Syst Rev. 2004;(2):CD000088.
2. Barbato A, D'Avanzo B. Family interventions in schizophrenia and related disorders: a critical review of clinical trials. Acta Psychiatrica Scandinavica 2000:102;81–97.
3. The Database of Abstracts of Reviews of Effectiveness (University of York), Database no.: DARE-20001547. In: The Cochrane Library, Issue 1, 2002. Oxford: Update Software.

4. Cormac I, Jones C, Campbell C, Silveira da Mota Neto J. Cognitive behaviour therapy for schizophrenia. Cochrane Database Syst Rev. 2004;(2):CD000524.
5. Tyrer P, Coid J, Simmonds S, Joseph P, Marriott S. Community mental health teams (CMHTs) for people with severe mental illnesses and disordered personality. Cochrane Database Syst Rev. 2004;(2):CD000270.
6. Joy CB, Adams CE, Lawrie SM. Haloperidol versus placebo for schizophrenia. Cochrane Database Syst Rev. 2004;(2): CD003082.
7. Fenton M, Coutinho ESF, Campbell C. Zuclopenthixol acetate in the treatment of acute schizophrenia and similar serious mental illnesses. Cochrane Database Syst Rev. 2004;(2):CD000525.
8. Thornley B, Rathbone J, Adams CE, Awad G. Chlorpromazine versus placebo for schizophrenia. Cochrane Database Syst Rev. 2004;(2):CD000284.
9. Barbui C, Saraceno B, Liberati A, Garattini S. Low-dose neuroleptic therapy and relapse in schizophrenia: meta-analysis of randomized controlled trials. European Psychiatry 1996;11: 306–313.
10. The Database of Abstracts of Reviews of Effectiveness (University of York), Database no.: DARE-961859. In: The Cochrane Library, Issue 4, 1999. Oxford: Update Software.
11. Bollini P, Pampallona S, Orza MJ, Adams MR, Chalmers TC. Antipsychotic drugs: Is more worse? A meta-analysis of the published randomized controlled trials. Psychological Medicine 1994;24:307–316.
12. The Database of Abstracts of Reviews of Effectiveness (University of York), Database no.: DARE-940125. In: The Cochrane Library, Issue 4, 1999. Oxford: Update Software.
13. Hunter RH, Joy CB, Kennedy E, Gilbody SM, Song F. Risperidone versus typical antipsychotic medication for schizophrenia. Cochrane Database Syst Rev. 2004;(2):CD000440.
14. de Oliveira IR, Miranda-Scippa AM, de Sena EP, Pereira EL, Ribeiro MG, de Castro-e-Silva E, Bacaltchuk J. Risperidone versus haloperidol in the treatment of schizophrenia: a meta-analysis comparing their efficacy and safety. J Clin Pharmal Therap 1996;21:349–358.
15. The Database of Abstracts of Reviews of Effectiveness (University of York), Database no.: DARE-970218. In: The Cochrane Library, Issue 4, 1999. Oxford: Update Software.
16. Bech P, Peuskens JC, Marder SR, Chouinard G, Hoyberg OJ, Huttunen MO, Blin O, Claus A. Meta-analytic study of the benefits and risks of treating chronic schizophrenia with risperidone or conventional neuroleptics. European Psychiatry 1998;13:310–314.
17. The Database of Abstracts of Reviews of Effectiveness (University of York), Database no.: DARE-981993. In: The Cochrane Library, Issue 1, 2001. Oxford: Update Software.
18. Leucht S, Pitschel-Walz G, Abraham D, Kissling W. Efficacy and extrapyramidal side effects of the new antipsychotics olanzapine, quetiapine, risperidone and sertindole compared to conventional antipsychotis: a meta-analysis of randomized controlled trials. Schizophrenia Research 1999;35:51–68.
19. The Database of Abstracts of Reviews of Effectiveness (University of York), Database no.: DARE-993710. In: The Cochrane Library, Issue 2, 2001. Oxford: Update Software.
20. Rummel C, Hamann J, Kissling W, Leucht S. New generation antipsychotics for first episode schizophrenia. Cochrane Database Syst Rev 2003(4):CD004410.
21. Lawrie S. Quetiapine in schizophrenia. Clinical Evidence 2000;4:564–565.
22. Koro CE, Fedder DO, Lítalien GJ, Weiss SS, Magder LS, Kreyenbuhl J et al. Assessment of independent effect of olanzapine and risperidone on risk of diabetes among patients with schizophrenia: population based nested case-control study. BMJ 2002;325:243.
23. Wahlbeck K, Cheine M, Essali MA. Clozapine versus typical neuroleptic medication for schizophrenia. Cochrane Database Syst Rev. 2004;(2):CD000059.
24. Tuunainen A, Wahlbeck K, Gilbody SM. Newer atypical antipsychotic medication versus clozapine for schizophrenia. Cochrane Database Syst Rev. 2004;(2):CD000966.
25. Duggan L, Fenton M, Dardennes RM, El-Dosoky A, Indran S. Olanzapine for schizophrenia. Cochrane Database Syst Rev. 2004;(2):CD001359.
26. Sultana A, Reilly J, Fenton M. Thioridazine for schizophrenia. Cochrane Database Syst Rev. 2004;(2):CD001944.
27. Glassman AH, Bigger JT Jr. Antipsychotic drugs: prolonged QTc interval, torsade de pointes, and sudden death. Am J Psychiatry 2001;158:1774–82.
28. Quraishi S, David A. Depot haloperidol decanoate for schizophrenia. Cochrane Database Syst Rev. 2004;(2): CD001361.
29. David A, Adams CE, Quraishi SN. Depot flupenthixol decanoate for schizophrenia or other similar psychotic disorders. Cochrane Database Syst Rev. 2004;(2):CD001470.
30. Lawrie S. Continued treatment with antipsychotic drugs in schizophrenia. Clinical Evidence 2000;4:568–569.

35.12 Delusional disorder

Martti Heikkinen

- For a geriatric patient with delusional disorder, see 22.3.

General points

- The primary, although certainly not the only, symptom of delusional disorder is a resistant, unshakable delusion. However, the delusions are not always persecutory in nature. They may also be, for example, jealousy-based, somatic, erotomanic or grandiose.

Epidemiology

- The prevalence of delusional disorder is estimated at 0.03%, but it may be higher, as patients often do not seek help voluntarily.
- The disorder is slightly more frequent in women than in men.
- The mean age at onset of disease is 40 years.

Aetiology

- The aetiology of delusional disorder is not known. Many psychosocial factors are connected with the disorder, such as an environment during childhood which did not support the development of normal trust, deafness, visual problems, isolation, recent immigration and old age.

Symptoms

- The delusions are constant, and unlike in schizophrenia, clear and structured. The patient adapts to his delusion but his personality remains unchanged. The patients are often excessively sensitive and cautious, which may lead to social isolation.
- The patient's functional capacity may remain good and often he may hide his disease effectively.

Diagnosis

- A concrete delusion for at least one month (for example the patient feels he/she is being followed, poisoned, loved or hurt by somebody, often a well-known person).
- Auditory or visual delusions may exist but they are not dominant. The criteria for schizophrenia are not fulfilled.
- Apart from the delusions, the behaviour of the patient is normal.
- A mood disorder occurring together with delusions lasts for a clearly shorter time than the delusions.
- The symptoms are not caused by organic disease, medication, or substance abuse.

Differential diagnosis

- General medical conditions (Parkinson's disease, vascular dementia, Alzheimer's disease, Huntington's disease, hypo- and hyperthyroidism, basal ganglia disorders) and certain medications (amphetamine derivatives, anticholinergics, Parkinson's medications, cimetidine, disulfiram, corticosteroids and isoniazid) may provoke delusions.
- Paranoid personality disorder
- Schizophrenia with paranoid features
- Serious depression, with psychotic symptoms
- Bipolar disorder

Treatment

- Delusional disorder is treatment resistant and chronic in 30–50% of cases.
- Patients seldom seek help themselves, normally the family brings the patient for treatment.
- Hospitalization is indicated if the patient is openly psychotic or cannot control his suicidal or other violent impulses. Sometimes the differential diagnosis requires hospital-based examinations.
- Psychotherapy is seldom effective because of lack of trust on the part of the patient. Supportive psychotherapy and a working patient–doctor relationship may help the patient cope with the symptoms.
- The paranoid attitude may also be a barrier to the medication. A small dosage of antipsychotics (e.g. haloperidol 2 mg/day) may be tried, increasing the dosage slowly.

Psychotherapeutic aspects

- Do not deny the delusion because it may be strengthened if the patient feels he/she or she has to defend his or her view. Illogical rationales cannot be altered by debates that appeal to logic.
- Do not pretend you believe the delusion because the patient needs support for his sense of reality.
- Listen to the worries the patient has and help him/her make his/her life more comfortable with the delusion.
- Take into account that the delusion may be a means of coping with severe feelings of shame or inadequacy, resulting in oversensitive behaviour.
- Be straight with the patient. Carefully explain the medication you prescribe, the indication, for example anxiety, irritability or sleeplessness, and the side-effects. Be punctual with the appointments and follow-up the patient regularly.
- Investigate whether there were stressful life events or other experiences that triggered the delusions. Help the patient to deal with these experiences with other ways than delusions.

35.13 Postpartum psychosis and other postpartum mental disorders

PSY

Antti Perheentupa

Aims

- Remember that postpartum depression is common.
- Learn to identify the risk groups and to suspect postpartum depression.
- Diagnose the onset of postpartum psychosis as early as possible.

Epidemiology

- As many as 80% of mothers experience depressed mood ("baby blues") after childbirth, and this is a normal phenomenon.

- After childbirth approximately 10–20% of mothers fulfill the diagnostic criteria for postpartum depression.
- The incidence of postpartum psychosis requiring hospitalization is 1–2 per 1000 childbirths.

General points

- The risk of a woman developing depression during the first month after childbirth is three-fold compared with other women of the same age.
- If the mother has suffered from depression before the pregnancy, the risk of postpartum depression is 25%. If the mother has suffered from postpartum depression before, the risk of recurrence is 40%.
- Other risk factors for postpartum mental disorders include first childbirth, relationship difficulties, being unmarried, caesarean section and a family history of mood disorders.
- A history of bipolar mood disorder is the greatest known risk factor for postpartum psychosis.

Depressed mood after childbirth

- Up to 80% of all mothers experience postpartum melancholy of some degree, and the symptoms are at their strongest 3–5 days after childbirth. This phenomenon is common, and is therefore often considered as a normal reaction to childbirth. However, it does increase the risk of the mother developing postpartum depression.
- Symptoms include tearfulness, mood changes, headache, irritability, occasional loss of appetite and sleep disturbances.
- The condition usually resolves spontaneously and does not need treatment other than a supportive attitude from the family and physician.

Postpartum depression

- Appears most often within the first three months after delivery, but the incidence remains increased for up to 6 months after childbirth.
- Predisposing factors include a history of severe depression, stress, negative experiences during the perinatal period and insufficient social support. The prevalence of postpartum depression is lower in cultures where the family or the community offer the new mother a great deal of support.
- Typical symptoms are sleep disturbances, anhedonia, inability to concentrate, feelings of inadequacy, excessive concern and fear about the infant. The symptoms may be as severe as in psychosis.
- Thyroiditis and hypothyroidism may also be the cause of maternal depression.
- A mother's depression affects her ability to care for the infant and may jeopardize the development of a normal mother–child relationship. Furthermore, maternal postpartum depression increases the child's, and the entire family's, subsequent risk of psychiatric disorders. The incidence of sudden infant death syndrome is higher in the children of mothers with postnatal depression than in controls.

Treatment

- Treatment of postnatal depression does not differ from treatment of any other depression (35.21). A specialist consultation is often indicated. Possible treatment forms include pharmacotherapy (35.41) C [1], social support, help in child care and psychotherapy. Sometimes hospitalization is indicated.
- If the symptoms of depression persist, the situation needs re-assessment, by a psychiatrist if necessary, in order to avoid harmful consequences for the child and the family.

Postpartum psychosis

- The rarest but the most severe of the psychiatric disorders after childbirth.
- The symptoms most often start 3–14 days after childbirth. At this stage the mother and child have usually been discharged home, and the family members notice the mother's strange behaviour.
- The first symptoms include restlessness, insomnia, agitation and mood changes which develop into confusion and usually into manic psychosis.
- Postpartum psychosis is a **psychiatric emergency** and requires hospitalization. Suicidal risk is considerable and the newborn may also be at risk.
- Treatment consists of antipsychotics, psychotherapy and social support for the mother and the family.
- In psychotic depression, electrotherapy can bring faster relief than drugs.
- Oestrogen therapy has also given promising results.
- The prognosis is good after the first episode, but the psychosis often recurs after subsequent childbirths and this should be explained to the patient and her family.
- The patient should be referred for psychiatric consultation during any subsequent pregnancies. Antidepressive medication started early enough may prevent the condition from developing.

Reference

1. Hoffbrand S, Howard L, Crawley H. Antidepressant treatment for post-natal depression. Cochrane Database Syst Rev. 2004;(2):CD002018.

35.14 Neuroleptic malignant syndrome (NMS)

Hannu Koponen

Aim

- To recognize and treat neuroleptic malignant syndrome in patients with
  - fever
  - extrapyramidal symptoms
  - autonomic disturbances
  - altered consciousness.

Epidemiology

- Estimated to occur in 0.2–1.4% of patients receiving neuroleptics.
- NMS is usually seen with low-dose neuroleptics (among others haloperidol), but it may also result from the use of high-dose neuroleptics. It has also occurred with atypical antipsychotic drugs.
- Often develops soon after initiation of neuroleptics or after a major change in their dosage.
- In addition to neuroleptics, NMS may be related to metoclopramide treatment or sudden discontinuation of a dopaminergic drug such as levodopa.

Clinical picture

- Probable NMS can be diagnosed if the patient has two of the main symptoms together with clouding of consciousness, leucocytosis or an increased serum creatine kinase level
  1. Hyperthermia: body temperature over 37.5°C without an alternative explanation
  2. Severe extrapyramidal symptoms:
     - rigidity (often the dominant symptom in addition to fever)
     - oculogyric crisis (dystonia of the eye muscles)
     - opisthotonus
     - retrocollis
     - trismus
     - choreoathetotic movements
     - dyskinesias
     - failure to eat, inability to swallow
     - salivation
  3. Disturbances of the autonomic nervous system:
     - elevation or changes in blood pressure
     - tachycardia
     - tachypnoea
     - profuse perspiration
     - incontinence or urinary retention

Additional criteria

- changes in the level of consciousness
- leucocytosis
- elevated serum creatine kinase

Laboratory investigations

- Changes in laboratory parameters are not diagnostic. The most commonly seen changes are:
  - elevated levels of serum creatine kinase (in about two thirds of cases)
  - leucocytosis
  - elevation of the haematocrit due to dehydration.
- In addition, the patients may have electrolyte or acid-base imbalance.
- Serum creatine kinase monitoring is advisable, as normalization of the level indicates a favourable treatment response.

Differential diagnosis

- It is important to exclude other disorders featuring clouding of consciousness, confusion and elevation of body temperature.
  - Meningitis, encephalitis (cerebrospinal fluid tap, computerized tomography of the head)
  - Malignant hyperthermia (related to anaesthesia)
  - Lethal catatonia in a schizophrenic patient. The condition is preceded by extreme agitation and hallucinations. Muscle rigidity, abnormal postures and stupor develop later. The condition is often difficult to distinguish from NMS. Electroconvulsive therapy is beneficial.
  - Thermal paralysis in patients receiving anticholinergics. There is no sweating, rigidity or rise in serum creatine kinase.
  - Central anticholinergic syndrome is a condition brought on by excessive use of anticholinergic drugs and some psychopharmaceuticals. Symptoms include confusion, agitation, convulsions and mild elevation of body temperature. The pupils are wide, skin dry and reddened, mouth dry. Tachycardia, urinary retention and dull bowel sounds are typical.
- Serotonin syndrome is a condition resembling NMS caused by concurrent use of serotonin-specific antidepressants and MAO inhibitors. Symptoms include fever, tremor, confusion, restlessness, rigidity, myoclonus, and epileptic seizures. The condition is managed by stopping serotonergic drugs.

Treatment

- Mild cases can be managed in primary care if laboratory follow-up can be arranged.
  - Cessation of neuroleptics
  - Attention to fluid intake and renal functioning (observe for rhabdomyolysis (10.41) and renal failure)

- Body temperature control by giving antipyretics and by mechanical means
- Treatment of secondary infections (aspiration pneumonia may be present)
- Respiratory support
- Laboratory follow-up
- Drug treatment with bromocriptine (or dantrolene)
  - The recommended starting dose of bromocriptine is 5 mg 3 times daily. The response to the 15mg/day dose is followed (alleviation of muscle rigidity, fall in body temperature and serum creatine kinase level) and the dose is increased to a level at which the symptoms have alleviated (up to 20 mg 3 times daily). After the symptoms have disappeared the medication is continued for 10 days and thereafter tapered down.
- ♦ During the syndrome, restlessness can be treated with benzodiazepines. If catatony is suspected, electroconvulsive therapy should be considered. Anticholinergics have not been proven effective.

Treatment after NMS

- ♦ Restarting neuroleptics after NMS is the responsibility of a specialist. Neuroleptics should not be restarted within 2–4 weeks of NMS. An antipsychotic compound of another type from another chemical class should be used.
- ♦ NMS is a severe treatment complication that should be reported to the national drug authority.

35.20 Recognition and diagnostics of depression

Editors

General principles

- ♦ Evaluate the severity of the depression; this step is decisive in choosing the appropriate form of treatment.
- ♦ Note psychotic symptoms and evaluate the risk of committing suicide, if needed arrange for involuntary care.
- ♦ Rule out the possibility of an organic affective disorder (35.1).
- ♦ Note other concurrent syndromes that may require treatment and attention:
  - anxiety disorder (35.31)
  - substance abuse (40.1)
  - personality disorder
  - somatic disease (35.27).

Definition

- ♦ Depression may be
  - a normal emotional reaction that is often associated with situational changes and loss,
  - a symptom, syndrome or
  - a difficult, symptomatically complex and, at worst, life threatening psychological disorder.
- ♦ In ICD-10 diagnostic classification depression is divided to
  - major depression (F32)
  - recurrent depression (F33) where long-term treatment needs to be considered.
- ♦ The symptoms of depression are different in children, the elderly, men and women.
- ♦ The diversity of depression makes it difficult for the patient and clinician to recognize, and it also makes the disorder difficult to treat.

Risk factors of depression

- ♦ Previous episode of depression
- ♦ Depressive disorders in the family
- ♦ Female gender
- ♦ Young adulthood or middle-age
- ♦ Postpartum period
- ♦ Somatic long-term diseases
- ♦ Low socio-economic status
- ♦ Divorce, widowhood or living alone
- ♦ Long-term unemployment
- ♦ Alcohol or drug abuse

Recognition of depression

- ♦ Clinical interview is the most effective method for determining depression. Recognition can be facilitated by conducting the examination in an unhurried, safe and free atmosphere, which permits questions concerning mood to be presented.
- ♦ During consultation the patient often brings up only somatic complaints. Questions such as "How is your family life" or "How are things at work?" may help to direct the discussion to mood.
- ♦ During the interview proceed from open questions to more closed ones with the aim of identifying specific symptoms of depression.
- ♦ There is a 24-hour variation in the severity of the symptoms of depression, with mornings typically being worse.
- ♦ The interview concentrates on
  - disorders of the patient and the family
  - the patient's life history
  - changes in family setting and other personal relationships; changes in studies and at work
  - the patient's experiences of loss
  - changes in capacity to function
  - feelings of anxiety.

Evaluation scales

- Various validated evaluation scales can be used to assist in recognising depression (such as, BDI – Beck Depression Inventory or Ham-D – Hamilton depression scale). There are no significant differences in accuracy between these scales.

Symptoms and diagnosis

- The core symptoms of depression include
  - depressed mood
  - loss of feelings of pleasure and interest
  - fatigue
  - loss of self-confidence and self-respect
  - unreasonable self-criticism or unwarranted feelings of guilt
  - recurrent thoughts concerning death or suicide or suicidal behaviour
  - lack of initiative, feelings of indecision or inability to concentrate
  - psychomotor slowness or excitement
  - sleep disorder
  - change in appetite and weight.
- A diagnosis of depression (F32–F33) calls for the simultaneous existence of four of the aforementioned symptoms for a period of at least two weeks; in addition, at least two of the three first-mentioned symptoms must exist.
- Other concurrent mental disorders (anxiety or personality disorder, substance abuse) or medication for these disorders can conceal the symptoms of even severe depression.
- It is typical that patients of general practitioners describe somatic feelings that relate to depression but fail to describe or even seek to conceal the changes in mood they have experienced.

Severity of symptoms and functional capacity of the patient

- A diagnosis of depression (F32–F33) conveys that the patient suffers from severe depression syndrome.
- States of depression can be divided into categories according to the severity and quality of the symptoms.
- Mild depression: 4–5 symptoms:
  - Patient is often capable of work.
- Moderate depression: 6–7 symptoms:
  - Patient is often not capable of work and cannot cope with routine tasks.
- Severe depression: 8–10 symptoms:
  - Patient is in need of continuing surveillance, often in a hospital environment.
- Psychotic depression:
  - In addition to the signs of severe depression, the patient has psychotic symptoms (depressive stupor, delusions, hallucinations).

Differential diagnosis

- Has the patient ever experienced extensive lifts in mood, which would indicate a bipolar affective disorder (35.22)?
- Has the patient experienced delusions or hallucinations characteristic to schizophrenia, which would indicate a schizoaffective disorder?
- An organic affective disorder can be caused by a somatic disease, medication or other chemical substance (35.1).

35.21 Major depressive disorder

Editors

Basic rules

- Assess functional capacity, ability to manage situations at work and at home, and the need for sick leave, supportive measures or hospitalization.
- Evaluate the risk of suicide and arrange for frequent follow-up in outpatient care or for hospitalization (voluntary or involuntary care).
- Depression is a multi-factorial condition; the use of both biological and psychological therapies is justified. The best result is often obtained by combining them.

Prevalence and the course of the disease

- Major depressive disorder is a common disease with a prevalence of 4–5% in population studies and with a lifetime prevalence of 15%.
- Hereditary factor and predisposing personality traits are associated with the onset of depression, with psychosocial stress as the triggering factor in many cases.
- Severe depression often begins after a negative life event (divorce, unemployment, loss).
- Recurrent episodes are common.
- The risk of suicide is remarkably high and suicidal thoughts are common. In men the risk is higher than in women.

Diagnosis

- See 35.20.

Clinical features

- More than half of the patients have cognitive impairment and difficulties with concentration and memory.
- Up to half of the patients may deny depression or may not have a depressive appearance.

Table 35.21.1 Severity of depression and choice of acute phase treatment

Treatment	Mild	Moderate	Severe	Psychotic
Psychotherapy	+	+	(+)	−
Antidepressants	+	+	+	+
Antipsychotics	−	−	−	+
Electroconvulsive therapy (ECT)	−	−	+	+

- Many depressed patients speak at a slowed rate and give delayed and short responses to questions.
- The patient may have perceptual disturbances, or sometimes psychotic or catatonic symptoms (the patient is speechless and does not take care of him/herself).

Treatment

- The treatment options for major depression include:
  - empirically supported psychotherapies
  - pharmacotherapy
  - combined psychotherapy and pharmacotherapy
  - in certain cases other somatic therapies (e.g. bright light therapy or electroconvulsive therapy)
- Choice of acute phase treatment, see Table 35.21.1.
- See also articles 35.5, 35.41, 35.51.
- Follow up response to therapy and change the treatment at a few weeks' interval until the patient no longer has symptoms.

Acute treatment

- Assess whether the patient needs acute hospitalization.
  - Refer the patient to hospital, immediately and involuntarily if needed, if he or she
    - is unable to take care of him/herself
    - clearly has lost his/her sense of reality
    - is suicidal or unable to cooperate (35.5).
  - Ensure treatment until the patient is in the hospital.

Pharmacotherapy

- If the patient can be treated in primary care, start medication.
  - Consider whether the patient also needs treatment for anxiety (35.43) or possibly neuroleptics for psychotic symptoms.
  - Arrange for a rapid control visit or ask the patient to call the next day. If the patient does not call you, try to contact him/her somehow.
  - Inform the patient and the family sufficiently of depression, its course and treatment.

Psychotherapies

- Psychological interventions are used particularly in mild and moderate depressive disorder.
- Alternatives:
  - cognitive psychotherapy B [1 2]
  - psychodynamic psychotherapy B [3]
  - interpersonal therapy
  - problem-solving therapy.
- Referring the patient to therapy, see 35.51.

Electroconvulsive therapy (ECT)

- Indicated in severe, psychotic or melancholic depressive disorders.
- Equally or even more efficient than pharmacotherapy.

Bright light therapy

- Has been shown to be effective in winter depression (seasonal affective disorder).
- Bright light at an intensity of 2500 lux is given for 30–60 minutes.
- The effect can be evaluated after approximately one week.

Treatment after the acute phase

- Continue the medication for 6 months after the patient is symptomless.
- Advise the patient about the risks of recurrence and inform how to seek care.
- If the patient has had recurrent episodes of major depressive disorder, consider preventive antidepressive treatment for 2–3 years. Some patients need continuous medication.

Table 35.21.2 Staging the treatment of depression

Primary care	Psychiatric outpatient care	Psychiatric hospital
Uncomplicated, mild and traumatic crises	Crises that threaten mental health or development	Serious crises
Mild or moderate acute depression	Severe acute depression Risk of suicide Bipolar depression	Psychotic depression, acute phase Mania
Chronic, life-style or personality-related depression	Acute phase in long-term depression (medication, re-evaluation of diagnosis)	Anxious or prolonged depressive disorders Treatment-resistant depressions
Adjustment disorder manifesting as depression	Depression in a child or adolescent	
Depression in the aged		
Somatization disorder	Evaluation of the ability to work	

- Utilize the general psychotherapeutic approaches at control visits
  - Help the patient to clarify his or her life situation
  - Support the patient's self-esteem
  - Help in the bereavement process
  - Help in altering the distorted depressive thinking
  - Cooperate with the patient's social network
  - Inform the patient and his/her family of depression and its treatment
- When needed, organize social support in cooperation with social workers.

Staging of treatment and criteria for specialist consultation

- The patient is in danger of suicide.
- Problems with diagnosis or treatment
  - Severe problems in co-operation with the patient.
  - Absence from work threatens to last for more than 3 months.
- For staging of treatment, see Table 35.21.2.

References

1. Gloaguen V, Cottraux J, Cucherat M, Blackburn IM. A meta-analysis of the effects of cognitive therapy in depressed patients. Journal of Affective Disorders 1998;49:59–72.
2. The Database of Abstracts of Reviews of Effectiveness (University of York), Database no.: DARE-983865. In: The Cochrane Library, Issue 1, 2000. Oxford: Update Software.
3. Brown C, Schulberg HC. The efficacy of psychosocial treatments in primary care: a review of randomized clinical trials. General Hospital Psychiatry 1995;17:414–424.

35.22 Bipolar disorder (manic-depressive disorder)

Editors

Basic rules

- The main aim of therapy is to prevent recurrences of manic and depressive episodes to decrease the associated morbidity and mortality.
- Assess the patient's safety and functional disability to decide about the optimal treatment setting.
- Arrange for the immediate hospitalization of a manic patient.
- Recognize possible substance abuse, which may cause problems in differential diagnosis or be a secondary problem.

Prevalence and classification

- The lifetime incidence of bipolar disorder is approximately 1.3–1.6%.
- Of patients with bipolar disorder, 10–20% commit suicide and one third is estimated to make at least one attempt.
- The disorder is classified into two categories:
  - Type I disorder includes both manic and depressive episodes
  - In type II disorder, episodes of hypomania and depression alternate.

Symptoms and diagnosis

- The patient usually has episodes of both major depression and mania or hypomania, rarely only manic episodes.

Hypomania

- Mild, but clearly perceivable rise in mood that differs clearly from the patient's normal psychological functioning.
- Duration varies from days to weeks.
- At least three of the following symptoms are present:
  - increase in activity and physical restlessness
  - increase in talkativeness
  - difficulties in concentrating and distractibility
  - reduction in the need for sleep
  - increase in sexual interest and drive
  - money spending spree or other irresponsible behaviour
  - increase in sociability or familiarities.

Mania

- The symptoms are much the same as in hypomania but stronger and thus result in social harm and loss of functional ability.
- If the symptoms develop slowly, they are not necessarily identified as abnormal right away.
- The patient may also pull himself together during consultation and behave normally giving good explanations for his behaviour. History should be taken from other people in addition to the patient.
- For diagnosis, three (four if the mood is irritated) of the following symptoms must have been present for at least one week:
  - increase in activity and physical restlessness
  - increase in talkativeness or flood of words
  - flow of thoughts or feeling of accelerated thinking
  - lack of inhibitions
  - reduced need for sleep (the patient typically sleeps only a few hours a night)
  - heightened self-esteem or delusions of grandiosity
  - distractibility or constant changes in actions or plans
  - reckless of irresponsible behaviour with risks that the patient does not recognize
  - increased sexual drive and promiscuity.
- In psychotic mania the patient also has either delusions or hallucinations.

- Sometimes the condition can develop into a delirium-type state of confusion that necessitates immediate treatment.

Episodes of depression

- The depression phases of bipolar disorder to not differ from severe states of depression (35.20), (35.21).

Mixed episodes

- Episodes of mania and depression are present at the same time or alternate rapidly (rapid cycling)
- The mood can be depressed but activity may be accelerated.
- Typically, the patients condition varies and both extreme moods and periods on concurrent symptoms occur.

Differential diagnosis

- Certain medications (amphetamines, corticosteroids, levodopa and isoniazid) and hyperthyroidism and certain intracranial processes may cause mania, although very seldomly.
- For alcohol or substance abuse, see 40.10.

Treatment

- If the patient does not have a confirmed diagnosis of bipolar disorder, a psychiatric consultation is required.
- After acute phase preventing new episodes and functional impairment is essential. Monitor patient's psychiatric status, provide education on bipolar disorder to the patient and his closest to identify new episodes early and to avoid risk factors, such as stress and lack of sleep.
- Psychosocial interventions may have effect in bipolar disorder **C** [1 2].
- Treatment options in the different phases of the disorder are listed in Table 35.22.

Acute mania

- Manic patients need hospitalization, compulsory treatment if the patient does not consent.
- Lithium is the therapy of choice in mania. In severe mania, an antipsychotic can be combined to it, e.g. haloperidol p.o. or i.m. at 5 mg doses administered every 30–60 minutes. More than 40 mg per day is seldom needed. For elderly patients the dose is 1–2 mg. See also 35.40.
- Extrapyramidal side-effects should be monitored, especially akathisia (subjective feeling of muscular tension due to medication which may cause restlessness, pacing, agitated behaviour) as they may easily be mixed with mania.
- If the patient is restless, benzodiazepines can be combined with neuroleptics at the beginning.
- Carbamazepine, valproate, olanzapine and electroconvulsive therapy have also been used in the treatment of acute mania.

Table 35.22 Summary or treatment options in type I bipolar disorder in the various phases of the disorder.

Acute mania
lithium (concentration 0.80–1.20 mmol/l)
valproate
carbamazepine
antipsychotics (stop within 6–12 weeks after remission)
clonazepam (stop within 6–12 weeks after remission)
the above drugs in combination
electroconvulsive therapy (in therapy-resistant cases)
Depressive episode
lithium (concentration 0.80–1.20 mmol/l)
lamotrigine
carbamazepine
the above drugs in combination
antidepressants (only in combination with one of the above, stop gradually within 6–12 weeks of remission
electroconvulsive therapy
Mixed episode
valproate
lithium (0.80–1.20 mmol/l)
carbamazepine
lamotrigine
the above drugs in combination
electroconvulsive therapy
Rapic cycling
valproate
carbamazepine
lithium
the above drugs in combination
Maintenance therapy
lithium (concentration 0.60–1.00 mmol/l)
carbamazepine
valproate
the above drugs in combination.

Lithium treatment

Initiation

- Lithium can be started immediately when the diagnosis of mania has been confirmed.
- Starting dose is 600–1200 mg/day in two doses.
- 80% of the patients feel better in 2–3 weeks **A** [3 4].
- Neuroleptic treatment can be stopped when the effect of lithium is clearly visible.
- Valproate **B** [5 6] and carbamazepine **D** [7 8] are alternatives to lithium.
- Long-term lithium therapy has been found to reduce the risk of suicide in bipolar disorder **C** [9].
- The following initial examinations should be performed before treatment:
  - Erythrocyte sedimentation rate

- Blood count (lithium often causes benign leucocytosis, leucocyte count 11–15 × 10^9/l, which may mask infection)
- ECG
- Thyroid function test (if elevated, lithium contraindicated)
- Urine test for protein (if clear proteinuria, lithium contraindicated)
- Serum sodium and potassium and creatinine (renal function)
- Creatinine clearance in cases of verified or suspected renal dysfunction
- Pregnancy test if pregnancy is not otherwise excluded
- Weight

Follow-up

- Thyroid function should be monitored once a year and always when there is clinical suspicion of hypothyroidism. The thyroid function of women more than 40 years of age should be examined twice a year. The incidence of hypothyroidism is 2–5% in patients on lithium therapy.
- If there is a suspicion of renal failure, creatinine and creatinine clearance should be determined (lithium does not cause renal failure).
- Lithium may cause changes on the ECG: reversible T-wave flattening or inversion, seldom sinus node depression and arrhythmias.

Plasma concentrations

- A serum concentration of 0.8–1.2 mmol/l is required for effect. In the elderly a lower concentration may be sufficient.
- Plasma concentration is assessed from a sample taken 12 h after the last dose of lithium and should be examined:
  - In the beginning of the treatment once a week until the patient achieves the steady state (two measurements giving the same concentration).
  - If the dosage is changed assess the concentration after one week.
  - In the treatment of mania when the lithium doses are large the concentration should be tested every other day.
  - If intoxication is suspected
  - In certain risk conditions the lithium treatment should be discontinued and the concentration examined (fever, gastroenteritis, delivery, surgical interventions, dehydration, unconsciousness).
  - The lithium levels should be examined regularly
    - if the patient is treated with diuretics
    - during reduced salt intake or dieting (sodium deficit may cause lithium intoxication)
    - during NSAID therapy.
  - The patient and his family should be familiar with the signs of intoxication and how changes in the body's water and salt content can affect lithium excretion.
  - Lithium levels need not be examined regularly in otherwise stable life situations. However, the patient should be in regular clinical follow-up to guarantee compliance.

Cyclothymia

- Cyclothymia (F34.0) is a mental disorder in which hypomanic and mild depressive episodes alternate. Severe depressions do not occur.
- The estimated life-time prevalence is 0.4–1%.
- Up to half of the patients later develop bipolar disorder.
- Lithium, valproate and carbamazepine are options for pharmacotherapy; however, most patients do not seek treatment because of the mildness of the symptoms.
- The patients should be informed of the risk of bipolar disorder, particularly if family history suggests a high risk.

References

1. Huxley NA, Parikh SV, Baldessarini RJ. Effectiveness of psychosocial treatments in bipolar disorder: state of the evidence. Harvard Review of Psychiatry 2000, 8(3), 126–140.
2. The Database of Abstracts of Reviews of Effectiveness (University of York), Database no.: DARE-20004135. In: The Cochrane Library, Issue 2, 2002. Oxford: Update Software.
3. Zornberg GL, Pope HG. Treatment of depression in bipolar disorder: new directions for research. J Clin Psychopharmacol 1993;13:397–408.
4. The Database of Abstracts of Reviews of Effectiveness (University of York), Database no.: DARE-940175. In: The Cochrane Library, Issue 4, 1999. Oxford: Update Software.
5. Macritchie KAN, Geddes JR, Scott J, Haslam DRS, Goodwin GM. Valproic acid, valproate and divalproex in the maintenance treatment of bipolar disorder. Cochrane Database Syst Rev. 2004;(2):CD003196.
6. Macritchie K, Geddes JR, Scott J, Haslam D, de Lima M, Goodwin G. Valproate for acute mood episodes in bipolar disorder. Cochrane Database Syst Rev. 2004;(2):CD004052.
7. Dardennes R, Even C, Bange F, Heim A. Carbamazepine and lithium in the prophylaxis of bipolar disorders. Br J Psychiatr 1995;166:378–381.
8. The Database of Abstracts of Reviews of Effectiveness (University of York), Database no.: DARE-952092. In: The Cochrane Library, Issue 4, 1999. Oxford: Update Software.
9. Goodwin FK, Fireman B, Simon GE, Hunkeler EM, Lee J, Revicki D. Suicide risk in bipolar disorder during treatment with lithium and divalproex. JAMA 2003;290(11):1467–73.

PSY

35.23 Chronic depression (dysthymia)

Editors

Basic rules

- Dysthymia is a chronic disorder, which is characterized by tiredness, depressed mood, fatigue, and lack of interest.

- Chronically depressed patients often present with somatic complaints and they tend to underestimate the severity of their psychiatric symptoms.
- Treatment of dysthymia helps to prevent long-term decrease in functional ability and later periods of severe depression (double depression, see 35.25), which are common in these patients.

Epidemiology and progress of the disease

- The prevalence of chronic depressive disorder is 3–5%. Women have a higher prevalence than men.
- Comorbidity is very often seen with dysthymia and anxiety disorder, personality disorders, substance abuse and, in young female patients, also eating disorders are often seen.

Symptoms and diagnosis

- Half of the patients have their first symptoms before the age of 25.
- When the symptoms begin at a young age, the patient may consider them as a natural part of life and may not seek help for years.

Core diagnostic criteria

- Depressive mood most of the time for at least two years and at least two of the following attached symptoms:
  - Reduced energy or activity
  - Insomnia
  - Decreased self-esteem or feelings of insufficiency
  - Difficulty in concentrating
  - Frequent crying
  - Loss of interest in sex or other sources of pleasure
  - Feelings of hopelessness or despair
  - Feeling that coping with daily life is too much
  - Pessimistic thoughts about the past or continued grieving over the past
  - Withdrawal from social contacts
  - Decrease in talkativeness.

Findings

- In distinction from major depressive disorder the symptoms of dysthymia are present most of the time and separate periods of disease do not exist.
- The dysthymic patient is pessimistic, sarcastic or demanding, very often "a difficult patient" for whom no treatments are effective.
- Dysthymia often causes deterioration of functional ability because of its long-lasting nature. Working capacity is often decreased and social problems are common.

Treatment

- See also 35.41.
- Around half of the patients benefit from long-term (>6 months) treatment with antidepressive medication (there is evidence on e.g. imipramine, fluoxetine, moclobemide and sertraline) A [1,2].
- Most of the patients benefit from a stable, supportive physician–patient relationship.
- Psychotherapies, especially in combination with pharmacotherapy, have also proved to be useful.

References

1. Lima MS, Moncrieff J. Drugs versus placebo for the treatment of dysthymia. Cochrane Database Syst Rev. 2004;(2):CD001130.
2. Lima MS, Hotopf M. Pharmacotherapy for dysthymia. Cochrane Database Syst Rev. 2004;(2):CD004047.

35.25 Depression and other psychiatric disorders

Editors

Depression and substance abuse disorders

- Depression is common in patients with substance abuse or dependence. Substance abuse may also cause depressive disorders.
- Co-morbid substance dependence or abuse (most often alcohol abuse), exists in 10–30% of patients with major depression. In women the depression most commonly precedes substance disorder, while in men the order is most often the opposite.
- A co-morbid substance abuse disorder increases the risk of suicide.
- Treatment choices, see Table 35.25.
- See also 40.2, 40.6.

Depression and anxiety disorders

- The coexisting of depression and anxiety disorder is a common clinical problem and the aim is to control the symptoms of both disorders.
- Antidepressants are effective both for depression and for most anxiety disorders (except specific phobias). They are effective also for the symptoms of anxiety in depressive patients when depression and anxiety disorders coexist.
- Selective serotonin reuptake inhibitors are effective in almost all anxiety disorders and are the recommended drugs (see Table 35.25).
- Panic disorder patients are sensitive to overstimulation and increased anxiety caused by SSRIs and the dosages of the SSRIs must be increased slowly in these patients.

Table 35.25 Treatment of patients with co-morbid conditions

Co-morbid conditions	Selective serotonin reuptake inhibitors	Other antidepressants	Brief psychotherapy	Other treatments
Depression and substance abuse disorders	++	–	–	Substance withdrawal therapies
Depression and anxiety disorders (generalized anxiety, panic disorder, social phobia)	++	+	+	
Depression and personality disorders (borderline personality)	++	–	–	Small dose of antipsychotic, long term psychotherapy

- When considering the need and form of psychotherapy it is important to assess the possible co-existing of anxiety disorders.
- See also 35.31.

Depression and personality disorders

- Depression in patients with co-morbid borderline personality disorder usually requires specialist treatment.
- The use of SSRIs is recommended if the patient has a co-morbid borderline personality disorder (see Table 35.25).
- Long term psychotherapy is warranted if available and if the patient is motivated and capable to benefit from psychotherapy. See also 35.33.

Adjustment disorder with depressed mood

- Adjustment disorders are emotional states associated with stressful experiences or demanding life-experiences. See also 35.34.
- Adjustment disorder with depressed mood is characterized by depressed mood, tearfulness and hopelessness.
- Crisis intervention is often an adequate treatment. The patients benefit from discussing the situation, and from the physician's empathy and support.
- Medication is not necessary.

Double depression

- Approximately 40% of patients with major depressive disorder also fulfill the criteria for chronic dysthymic disorder (35.23).
- Double depression is a negative prognostic factor.
- The treatment should aim at relieving both conditions.

Postpartum depression

- See 35.13

Winter seasonal affective disorder (SAD)

- The patient has episodes of major depressive disorder especially during autumn and winter.
- In addition to symptoms of major depression, symptoms include hypersomnia, daytime tiredness, increased appetite and weight again.
- Bright light **B** [1] [2] has been used for prevention and treatment (green/blue/yellow wavelengths are essential **C** [3] [4]). A dose-response relationship has been observed in typical SAD **C** [5] [6].

References

1. Tam EM, Lam RW, Levitt AJ. Treatment of seasonal affective disorder: a review. J Psychiatry – Rev Can Psych 1995;40:457–466.
2. The Database of Abstracts of Reviews of Effectiveness (University of York), Database no.: DARE-953129. In: The Cochrane Library, Issue 4, 1999. Oxford: Update Software.
3. Lee TM, Chan CC, Paterson JG, Janzen HL, Blaschko CA. Spectral properties of phototherapy for seasonal affective disorder: a meta-analysis. Acta Psychiatr Scand 1997;96:117–121.
4. The Database of Abstracts of Reviews of Effectiveness (University of York), Database no.: DARE-971044. In: The Cochrane Library, Issue 4, 1999. Oxford: Update Software.
5. Lee TM, Chan CC. Dose-response relationship of phototherapy for seasonal affective disorder: a meta-analysis. Acta Psychiatrica Scandinavica 1999;99:315–323.
6. The Database of Abstracts of Reviews of Effectiveness (University of York), Database no.: DARE-991049. In: The Cochrane Library, Issue 1, 2001. Oxford: Update Software.

35.27 Depression, drugs and somatic diseases

Editors

Essentials

- Depression is a common disorder related to other psychiatric and somatic diseases, and it often complicates the diagnosis and treatment.

- According to various studies 20–60% of patients with general medical conditions have symptoms of depression and 15–45% fulfil the criteria of a mood disorder.
- Remember somatic diseases that may cause depression (Table 35.27).
- Rule out possible drugs and narcotic substances that may cause mood disorders (Table 35.27).
- The role of somatic differential diagnosis is especially emphasized:
  - in elderly patients with no previous mood disorders
  - in patients with atypical symptoms of depression
  - in patients who do not benefit from traditional treatment of depression
- In a patient with somatic disease it is not always easy to differentiate the somatic symptoms from those of depression.

General medical conditions

- Depression is especially related to:
  - stroke, dementia and Parkinson's disease
  - hypothyroidism, hyperparathyroidism
  - diabetes and coronary heart disease
  - cancer
  - exhaustion and fibromyalgia.

Table 35.27 Medical conditions, drugs and substances that may cause mood disorders.

Medical conditions	Pharmacological agent	Psychoactive substance
Stroke	Anabolic steroids	Alcohol
B_1-, B_2-, B_6- ja B_{12}-vitamin deficiencies	Psychosis drugs	Amphetamine (during withdrawal)
Folic acid deficiency	Beta-blockers	Ecstasy (MDMA)
Diabetes mellitus	Estrogens	Cocaine (during withdrawal)
Hypothyroidism	Digitalis	
Hyperthyroidism	Clonidine	
Hypoadrenalism (Addison's disease, hypopituitarism)	Corticosteroids	
Hyperadrenalism (Cushing's syndrome)	Methyldopa	
Hyperparathyroidism	Ranitidine	
Hypoparathyroidism		
Parkinson's disease		
Porphyria		
Coronary artery disease		
Status post infarctum		
Neoplasms (especially pancreatic cancer)		
Temporal lobe epilepsy		
Uraemia		

- Depressive patients have an increased risk of myocardial infarction. After myocardial infarction, depression as a comorbid disorder increases mortality from heart diseases.
- Depression may also predispose to cancer. There is a small but clinically significant association with depression and incidence of cancer.

35.29 Panic disorder

Ulla Lepola, Gérard Emilien

Highlights

- Panic disorder is associated with a relatively chronic course and a high risk of relapse for those individuals whose symptoms do remit.
- Cognitions during panic attacks play an important role in the patient's levels of fear and anxiety.
- Both pharmacological and cognitive behavioral therapies (CBT) are more effective than placebo or control treatment.
- The combination of antidepressants with exposure in vivo is superior to other therapies for the short-term treatment of patients with panic disorder with agoraphobic avoidance

Aims

- To properly diagnose panic disorder.
- To recognize depression, and suicide risk or abuse of alcohol that often co-occur with panic disorder.
- To treat panic disorder and reduce symptoms as much as possible.

Epidemiology

- The prevalence of panic disorder is estimated to be 3–4%.
- Panic disorder is often related to agoraphobia.
- The prevalence of panic disorder is two times higher in women than in men.
- The onset is often in adolescence or young adulthood, sometimes even in childhood.
- About 30% of the patients recover completely, but recurrences are common. Some residual symptoms will be present in 40–50%. About 20% of the patients remain severely and chronically affected.
- 25% of adult panic patients have had school phobia in childhood.

Symptoms

- The patient has at least four panic attacks in a 4-week period.

- The panic attacks are not associated with a specific situation or certain circumstances and they are unpredictable.
- The panic attacks are not related to a physical disorder.
- The symptoms reach maximum intensity in 10 min.
- At least four of the symptoms listed below must be present, one of which must be from items (a) to (d):
  - (a) palpitations, a pounding heart, or an accelerated heart rate
  - (b) sweating
  - (c) trembling or shaking
  - (d) a dry mouth
  - (e) difficulty in breathing
  - (f) a feeling of choking
  - (g) chest pain or discomfort
  - (h) nausea or abdominal distress
  - (i) feeling dizzy, unsteady, faint, or light-headed
  - (j) feelings of derealization or depersonalization
  - (k) fear of losing control, "going crazy" or passing out
  - (l) fear of dying
  - (m) hot flushes or cold chills
  - (n) numbness or tingling sensations

Differential diagnosis

- Other psychiatric illnesses
  - Phobic disorders, generalized anxiety disorder, depression
- Cardiovascular disorders
  - Anaemia, tachyarrhythmia, angina pectoris
- Endocrine disorders
  - Hyperthyroidism, hyperglycaemia (23.10), menopause
- Respiratory disorders
  - Asthma, hyperventilation, pulmonary embolism, pulmonary oedema
- Neurological disorders
  - Cerebral vascular disorders (36.4), epilepsy, TIA
- Withdrawal symptoms
  - Alcohol, caffeine, amphetamines
- A panic attack may be provoked by excessive doses of beta2-sympathomimetics used for asthma.
- Phaeochromocytoma: the attacks are characterized by flushing, palpitation and a markedly increased blood pressure.

Examinations

- Physical examination
- Serum TSH, ECG
- Other examinations (blood count, blood glucose, serum calcium) if needed, or neurological consultation

Treatment strategies

- It is important to estimate the suicide risk
- A combination of drug treatment (A) [1 2 3 4] and psychotherapy (A) [5 6 7 8 9 10 11 12] is often needed.
- A supportive approach, encouragement and discussion of the situation (and benign nature of the somatic symptoms) with the patient are useful.
- Possible comorbid alcohol abuse needs management, for example with mini-intervention (40.3). Alcohol worsens panic symptoms.
- The effects of treatment are long-lasting (C) [13 14].

Drug treatment

Selective serotonin uptake inhibitors (SSRIs)

- SSRIs are the drugs of choice (B) [15 16]; they are effective and safe (A) [1 2 3 4]
- Drugs of choice include citalopram, escitalopram, fluoxetine, fluvoxamine, paroxetine, and sertraline.
- They are used as in the treatment of major depression, but are started with a half dose (e.g. citalopram 10 mg/day) because panic patients are sensitive to the possible side effects.
- For recurrent symptoms longer prophylactic treatment is indicated.

Tricyclic antidepressants

- Clomipramine (A) [1 2 3 4]
  - The starting dose is 10 mg × 1, increased stepwise.
  - The dosage is the same or smaller than in the treatment of major depression: 100–200 mg/day.
  - An effect is seen after 2–4 weeks.
  - At the start of the treatment the symptoms may increase.
  - Anticholinergic side effects or weight gain are common.

Benzodiazepines

- Not suitable for alcoholics. They can be used early in the treatment, for example combined with SSRIs. They should be tapered and stopped later.
- Alprazolam (B) [15 16]
  - Starting dose 0.25 mg × 3
  - Maintenance treatment 1.5–4 mg
  - Taper slowly: 0.25 mg/week
  - If tapering is not successful, change to clonazepam, which may be easier to taper.
- Clonazepam
  - Starting dose 0.5 mg × 2
  - Maintenance treatment 1–4 mg

MAO inhibitor

- Moclobemide
  - Starting dose 75 mg × 2
  - Maintenance treatment 300–600 mg

Duration of drug treatment

- Long-term treatment is often needed, as in major depression.
- 8–12 months with effective dosage

PSY

Psychotherapy

- Cognitive psychotherapy is effective (A) [1 2 3 4], including cognitive restructuring (D) [17 18 19 20].
- Exposure in vivo (A) [1 2 3 4]
- Self-help groups, relaxation, education
- Rehabilitation courses

References

1. van Balkom AJ, Bakker A, Spinhoven P, Blaauw BM, Smeenk S, Ruesink B. A meta-analysis of the treatment of panic disorder with or without agoraphobia: a comparison of psychopharmacological, cognitive-behavioural, and combination treatments. J Nerv Ment Dis 1997;185:510–516.
2. The Database of Abstracts of Reviews of Effectiveness (University of York), Database no.: DARE-971064. In: The Cochrane Library, Issue 4, 1999. Oxford: Update Software.
3. Gould RA, Otto MW, Pollack MH. A meta-analysis of treatment outcome for panic disorder. Clin Psychol Rev 1996;15:819–844.
4. The Database of Abstracts of Reviews of Effectiveness (University of York), Database no.: DARE-968034. In: The Cochrane Library, Issue 4, 1999. Oxford: Update Software.
5. van Balkom AJ, Bakker A, Spinhoven P, Blaauw BM, Smeenk S, Ruesink B. A meta-analysis of the treatment of panic disorder with or without agoraphobia: a comparison of psychopharmacological, cognitive-behavioural, and combination treatments. J Nerv Ment Dis 1997;185:510–516.
6. The Database of Abstracts of Reviews of Effectiveness (University of York), Database no.: DARE-971064. In: The Cochrane Library, Issue 4, 1999. Oxford: Update Software.
7. The Database of Abstracts of Reviews of Effectiveness (University of York), Database no.: DARE-968034. In: The Cochrane Library, Issue 4, 1999. Oxford: Update Software.
8. Oei TP, Llamas M, Devilly GJ. The efficacy and cognitive processes of cognitive behaviour therapy in the treatment of panic disorder with agoraphobia. Behavioural and Cognitive Psychotherapy 1999;27:63–88.
9. The Database of Abstracts of Reviews of Effectiveness (University of York), Database no.: DARE-20008184. In: The Cochrane Library, Issue 1, 2002. Oxford: Update Software.
10. Clark DM. Anxiety disorders: why they persist and how to treat them. Behaviour Research and Therapy, 37, S5–S27, 1999.
11. Clark D & Salkovskis PM. Cognitive treatment of panic: therapist's manual. UK: Department of Psychiatry, University of Oxford, 1986.
12. Clark DM. A cognitive approach to panic. Behaviour Research and Therapy, 24, 461–470, 1986.
13. Bakker A, van Balkom AJ, Spinhoven P, Blaauw BM, van Dyck R. Follow-up on the treatment of panic disorder with or without agoraphobia: a quantitative review. J Nerv Ment Dis 1998;186:414–419.
14. The Database of Abstracts of Reviews of Effectiveness (University of York), Database no.: DARE-981282. In: The Cochrane Library, Issue 4, 1999. Oxford: Update Software.
15. Boyer W. Serotonin uptake inhibitors are superior to imipramine and alprazolam in alleviating panic attacks: a meta-analysis. Int Clin Psychopharmacol 1995;10:45–49.
16. The Database of Abstracts of Reviews of Effectiveness (University of York), Database no.: DARE-920019. In: The Cochrane Library, Issue 4, 1999. Oxford: Update Software.
17. Taylor S. Meta-analysis of cognitive-behavioural treatments for social phobia. J Behav Ther Exp Psych 1996;27:1–9.
18. The Database of Abstracts of Reviews of Effectiveness (University of York), Database no.: DARE-973122. In: The Cochrane Library, Issue 4, 1999. Oxford: Update Software.
19. Stravynski A, Greenberg D. The treatment of social phobia: a critical assessment. Acta Psychiatr Scand 1998;98:171–181.
20. The Database of Abstracts of Reviews of Effectiveness (University of York), Database no.: DARE-981694. In: The Cochrane Library, Issue 2, 2000. Oxford: Update Software.

35.31 Anxiety disorder

Editors

Basic rules

- Anxiety is a normal, fear-like emotional state.
- The condition can be called anxiety disorder when anxiety is intense, long lasting and restricts both psychological and social functioning.
- If the anxiety becomes intensive or chronic, it warrants evaluation including its probable causes. Thorough evaluation and treatment of anxiety includes the careful assessment of the patient and his or her situation, reconstruction of the cause and effect pattern, giving the patient more information and helping the patient to understand his problem. Intellectual and emotional analysis of the situation together with the patient is essential.
- In acute anxiety temporary medication may be indicated if the patient's functional capacity is impaired. However, in severe chronic anxiety long-term pharmacotherapy may be required (35.43).

Epidemiology

- Anxiety disorders are some of the most common mental disorders and affect more than men.

Pathogenesis

- The sensation of anxiety is commonly experienced in everyday situations and it is often related to worrying about common every day problems including unfinished tasks.

- Long continuing feeling of anxiety may lead to secondary avoidance or adjustment by using psychological defence mechanisms or behaviour. The anxiety and its possible causes include childhood untoward experiences and recent stresses and these may remain unnoticed or subconscious.
- The difference between normal and pathological anxiety is not always clear. Functional ability is an important criterion.

Symptoms

- Paroxysmal or continuous anxiety which may be related to context.
- Apprehension, fear, difficulties in concentration, agitation, difficulties in falling asleep.
- Peripheral somatic complaints are typical: palpitation, tremor, dizziness, sweating, nausea, urinary frequency, upset stomach, sense of suffocation, trembling voice, blushing.
- Continuous tension-like tension in the neck and back, headache, sense of a lump in the throat, tiredness.

Main forms of anxiety disorder

Panic disorder

- See 35.29.

Social phobias

- Intense anxiety and associated avoidance behaviour in social situations is central.
- The phobia is frequently associated with:
  - eating or drinking in public
  - meeting superiors or strangers
  - situations where the persons performs in front of others (speeches etc.)
  - working or doing something with others present
  - use of the telephone.

Specific phobias

- Typical situations involve high places, darkness, enclosed places, snakes and insects.
- The role of pharmacotherapy is not as significant as with other anxiety disorders.
- If the patient is motivated, exposure therapy can be used.

Generalized anxiety disorder

- The life time prevalence is 5.1% (according to DSM-IIIR criteria) and 8.9% (according to ICD-10 criteria) but only 20–30% of patients receive treatment for their symptoms.
- The symptoms include continuous unrealistic anxiety including fearfulness and worrying regarding the future and every day concerns.
- Often the patient has internal tension and motor restlessness.
- The person reacts with symptoms of anxiety to stressful situations, such as setbacks, stress, social situations and deterioration of health.
- The condition is often co-morbid with depression, phobias or hypochondriasis.

Post-traumatic stress disorder

- See 35.36.

Obsessive-compulsive disorder

- See 35.32.

Differential diagnosis

- Many somatic conditions may simulate anxiety and vice versa (for example, anaemia, many heart conditions, chronic pulmonary embolism, asthma, hyperthyroidism and other endocrine diseases, infections, etc.).
- Certain drugs and medications may cause generalized anxiety or panic attacks (sympathomimetic agents, caffeine intoxication, drug intoxications, alcohol and sedative drug withdrawal symptoms).
- Differentiating between anxiety and depression is not always simple. Very often both disorders are seen in the same patient. A continuum is often thought to exist between the conditions with variation from anxiety to depression and from agitation to retardation.

Basic rules of treatment

- The treatment is based on identification of symptoms and making correct diagnosis, adequate patient information including defining the patient's problem and emotions, helping the patient's situation.
- Medication is temporarily necessary in intensive anxiety. In severe chronic anxiety a long-lasting treatment e.g. by antidepressants **A** [1] may be required (35.43).
- Autogenic training may have some effect for stress and anxiety, but evidence for its effectiveness is inconclusive **C** [2 3].

PSY

References

1. Kapczinski F, Lima MS, Souza JS, Cunha A, Schmitt R. Antidepressants for generalized anxiety disorder. Cochrane Database Syst Rev. 2004;(2):CD003592.
2. Kanji N, Ernst E. Autogenic training for stress and anxiety: a systematic review. Complementary Therapies in Medicine 2000, 8(2), 106–110.
3. The Database of Abstracts of Reviews of Effectiveness (University of York), Database no.: DARE-20004019. In: The Cochrane Library, Issue 2, 2002. Oxford: Update Software.

35.32 Obsessive-compulsive disorder (OCD)

Ulla Lepola, Hannu Koponen, Esa Leìnonen, Gérard Emilien

Introduction

- Age of onset is usually approximately 20 years; however, in one third of the patients OCD first appears in adolescence.
- OCD is usually a chronic condition.
- Effective treatment forms include cognitive behaviour therapy, selective serotonin reuptake inhibitors (SSRIs) and clomipramine.

Aims

- Be aware of this moderately common disorder. Ask about compulsive behaviour and obsessive thoughts, particularly if the patient has depression or anxiety.
- Treat patients with OCD with clomipramine or SSRIs, using fairly large doses. Monitor response for a sufficient length of time.

Epidemiology

- According to cross-sectional studies, the prevalence of OCD in the general population is 1.6%. The lifetime prevalence rate for OCD is approximately 2.5%.
- The prevalence of OCD shows no gender variation.

Aetiology

- Genetic studies, the latest imaging techniques as well as the results achieved with psychosurgery suggest that OCD has a biological origin.
- The serotonergic system has become the focus of the studies, because good treatment responses have been achieved in OCD with serotonin-selective drugs.
- Experimentally, OCD symptoms can be exacerbated with serotonin agonists.
- No specific OCD genes have yet been identified but some studies suggest that genetic predisposition may sometimes be associated with the disorder. Childhood onset OCD appears to be inherited (sometimes in association with tic disorders).

Clinical picture

- OCD is classified as an independent disorder in ICD-10.
- The patient has either obsessive thoughts (obsessions) or compulsive behaviour (compulsions). Obsessions and compulsions are repetitive, and the patient finds them disturbing.
- Patients with OCD recognize that their obsessions are a creation from within their own minds.
- Common obsessions include:
  - fear of contamination, avoidance of dirt, fear of germs
  - imagining having harmed oneself or others
  - fear of losing control
  - intrusive sexual thoughts
  - excessive religious or moral doubt
  - forbidden thoughts
  - a need to keep things a certain way
  - a compulsive need to talk, ask questions or confess.
- Common compulsions include:
  - washing, repeating things, checking, counting
  - organising possessions, hoarding or keeping things.
- Compulsions are often performed and repeated according to strict rituals. The aim is to obtain relief from something that is perceived to be unpleasant. Patients usually recognize that their behaviour is unreasonable.
- OCD symptoms cause distress, take time (more than an hour a day) or significantly interfere with the person's everyday life.
- The onset of the disorder usually occurs at about 20 years of age, but starts in childhood in one third of patients.
- OCD is usually a long-term condition, even life long. The symptoms often improve over time, and they vary from being almost insignificant to symptoms causing severe distress.
- OCD is an underdiagnosed and undertreated disorder, because patients either hide their symptoms or do not perceive them as a sign of an illness.

Differential diagnosis

- Obsessive thoughts occur in many psychiatric illnesses, but not usually compulsive behaviour. The existence of compulsive behaviour therefore supports the diagnosis of OCD.
- Tic disorders (Tourette's syndrome and other tic disorders) (33.11) may resemble OCD. Tics and OCD often occur together, particularly in childhood onset disorders.
- In the general anxiety disorder the patient sees the reason for his/her anxiety as realistic, whereas there is no realistic reasoning behind the OCD symptoms.
- OCD patients sometimes have panic attacks but they are secondary to obsessive fears.
- OCD and depression often occur together in adults, but less commonly in children and adolescents.
- Eating disorders and schizophrenia are common comorbid disorders with OCD. Typical schizophrenia is no more common than in general population – but some patients may present delusion-like ideas in relation to their obsessions invoking a diagnosis of a psychotic disorder. However usually unlike psychotic individuals, people with OCD continue to have a clear idea of what is real and what is not.

- In children and adolescents, OCD may worsen or cause disruptive behaviour as well as cause problems with attention and concentration.
- Although stress can exacerbate OCD, symptoms do occur regardless of stress.
- OCD patients usually seek treatment because of depression or anxiety, and not obsessions or compulsions per se. Short questions relating to repetitive hand washing, the need to check things or obsessive thoughts lead to the recognition of OCD in 80% of cases.
- Only a small number of people with OCD suffer from Obsessive Compulsive Personality Disorder (OCPD). This refers to a personality pattern that involves a preoccupation with rules, time tables, perfectionism, rigidity and inflexibility.

Comorbidity

- Psychiatric conditions that may co-exist with OCD include:
  - Anxiety disorders (such as panic disorder or social phobia)
  - Depression/dysthymia
  - Behaviour and attention disorders (e.g. attention-deficit hyperactivity disorder, ADHD)
  - Learning disorders
  - Tic disorders
  - Trichotillomania (hair pulling)
  - Body dysmorphic disorder (imagined ugliness).

Treatment

- Education is crucial in helping patients and families learn how best to manage OCD and prevent its complications.
- Cognitive behaviour therapy is effective in OCD (A) [1 2].
- SSRIs are the most effective treatment form (A) [1 2]. The response is not related to possible depression.
- SSRIs are used in higher doses than in depression, and the dose is increased gradually. The most often used SSRIs:
  - fluvoxamine (25–250 mg/day)
  - fluoxetine (5–60 mg/day)
  - paroxetine (10–40 mg/day)
  - citalopram (20–60 mg/day)
  - sertraline (50–150 mg/day)
- Clomipramine is most studied: it is effective in 50–85% of patients in controlled studies. The starting dose is 25 mg. The dose may be increased up to 150–200 mg/day, which is a higher dose than used in depression.
- An effect may appear slowly (within 2–3 months) and the efficacy may continue to increase for up to 1 year.
- Drug treatment should be continued for at least 1.5 years, sometimes lifelong.
- Relapse is very common when medication is withdrawn, particularly if the person has not had the benefit of cognitive behaviour therapy (CBT). It is recommended that patients continue medication, particularly if they do not have access to CBT.
- Other tricyclic antidepressants or neuroleptics are not effective. However, neuroleptics can be used to alleviate tic symptoms.
- A combination of drug treatment and behaviour therapy is often beneficial.

References

1. Abramowitz JS. Effectiveness of psychological and pharmacological treatments for obsessive-compulsive disorder: a quantitative review. J Consult Clin Psychol 1997;65:44–52.
2. The Database of Abstracts of Reviews of Effectiveness (University of York), Database no.: DARE-973326. In: The Cochrane Library, Issue 4, 1999. Oxford: Update Software.

35.33 Antisocial personality disorder

Martti Heikkinen

Definition and classification

- Personality disorder signifies deeply rooted and persistent behavioural patterns that are inflexible and appear harmful in various circumstances and situations in life.
- In the DSM-IV, personality disorders are classified into three main clusters.
  - Cluster A includes the paranoid, schizoid and schizotypal personality disorders. People with these disorders often appear odd or eccentric.
  - Cluster B consists of antisocial and narcissistic personality disorders. Persons suffering from these disorders are often dramatic, emotional and erratic.
  - Cluster C includes avoidant, dependent and obsessive-compulsive disorders. Persons suffering from them are often anxious or phobic.

PSY

Antisocial personality disorder

Description

- Disregard to social responsibilities and indifference to other persons' feelings are characteristic to the disorder.
- Discrepancy between the person's behaviour and social norms is often large.
- Behaviour is characterized by poor tolerance of frustrations, low threshold of irritation, aggressiveness, and impulsivity.
- The inner world of the patient is devoid of feelings and the patient lacks the ability to feel guilt or empathy, or the patient has very strong emotions, anxiety, and impulsiveness.

- Not all the patients are criminals, and even chronic offenders do not always fulfill the criteria of antisocial personality disorder.
- According to the DSM-IV classification the symptoms usually commence around the age of 15 years, often before puberty.
- As more secondary benefit is obtained the situation becomes more complicated.
- The cumulative prevalence is about 3%.
- About 80% will be cured from their problematic behaviour before the age of 45 years.

Principles of treatment

- Aim at description of problems in concrete terms and suggest practical solutions.
- Cope with your own negative transference evoked by the patient's aggression and antisocial behaviour.

During the consultation

- Although there is no scientific evidence of the benefit of any particular intervention, pessimism should not be allowed to prevail.
- Due to their behaviour, antisocial patients often encounter other people's loss of temper and blame. Therefore, attempts at tuition are not helpful.
- The most important means are empathetic calmness, flexibility, and a practical approach.
- For the physician it is useful to be aware of his/her own countertransference. Professional counselling may give the physician insight into these feelings.
- Try to define the patient's problem as clearly as possible: always ask the following five questions:
  - What made you come?
  - Why did you come now?
  - What do you expect me to do?
  - What do you think is the cause of your problems?
  - If you had not come to me now what would have happened?
- Is the presenting symptom an excuse for contact that reveals something more essential (so that unnecessary examinations can be avoided)?
- Treating and excluding somatic diseases may alleviate irritability and impulsiveness.
- The incidence of psychiatric disorders (mania, schizophrenia, alcoholism, and drug addiction) is increased in patients with antisocial personality disorder. Treatment of these disorders may be of help in behavioural problems.
- Normal life crises, problems with human relationships or unemployment may be the cause of changes in mood. The feeling that somebody understands is as important to these patients as to anybody else.
- The opportunity to share the problems in an emphatic (but professional) human relationship is often the best means of reducing self-destructive impulsiveness and of letting time cure the behavioural disorder.

35.34 Adjustment disorders

Editors

Basic rules

- Adjustment disorders are reactive and usually short-lasting states associated with life situations. They manifest as anxiety, depression or behavioural symptoms and appear after a major change in life or a psychologically straining experience.
- The diagnosis of adjustment disorder is made by excluding other disorders: stressors may trigger several psychological disorders, particularly severe states of depression (35.21).
- Although adjustment disorders are mostly mild and transient they should not be underestimated. An adjustment disorder may develop into a more severe disorder, and particularly in the young it may be associated with self-destructive behaviour.

Diagnosis

- Although adjustment disorders are some of the most common disorders in patients presenting to primary care physicians, making a diagnosis requires the exclusion of other disorders. The presence of a stressor does not automatically mean that the patient has adjustment disorder.

Diagnostic criteria

- Emotional or behavioural symptoms develop within three months of the appearance of a stressor.
- Symptoms or behavioural characteristics are clinically significant
  - The stressor causes more suffering than expected or
  - Impairs considerably the patient's social and occupational functioning
  - The disorder does not fulfil the criteria of some other psychological disorder that could be pertinent to the patient's life situation nor is it the aggravation of an earlier disorder.
- The symptoms are not grief caused by a loss.
- When the stressor has ceased to affect the patient, the symptoms resolve within 6 months.

Diagnoses based on the major symptom

- Reactive depression
  - The principal symptoms are depressed state, crying and hopelessness.
- Reactive anxiety

- The principal symptoms are nervousness, worry and tension.
- Reactive behavioural disorders
  - The principal manifestations are behaviour that violates the rights of other people and breaks central age-associated social norms and rules (e.g. vandalism, reckless driving, fighting).
- Reactive emotional and behavioural disorder
  - The principal manifestations are both emotional symptoms and those associated with behaviour disorder.

Treatment

- The treatment of adjustment disorder is carried out according to the principles of crisis psychotherapy (35.50).
- The patient needs to be heard and understood. The person providing care should both accept the psychological malaise associated with the patient's life situation and at the same time calmly help the patient to see that the situation can be overcome or that it can be alleviated.
- Typically, one or two meetings alleviate the condition, and the patient begins to see how he/she could function in this new life situation.
- The need for sick leave varies from a few days to a few weeks.
- The role of pharmacotherapy is secondary. Benzodiazepines can be used to alleviate severe anxiety and difficulty in falling asleep can be treated with short-acting hypnotics.

35.36 Acute stress reaction and post-traumatic stress disorder

Matti Ponteva

Introduction

- The psychological responses to highly traumatic events are usually divided into two main categories, i.e. stress reactions and stress disorders.
  - A **stress reaction** is in principle a normal reaction to an excessively traumatic event and does not always require medical attention.
  - A **stress disorder** usually requires medical intervention.
- Consider the possibility of **post-traumatic stress disorder (PTSD)** if the patient has experienced an exceptionally stressful and psychologically traumatic incident or event within the past six months.

Epidemiology

- After a major disaster 50–90% of those involved will experience at least a brief stress shock, which usually fulfils the criteria for an acute stress reaction. Symptoms in the acute phase do not necessarily predict the development of long-term disorders.
- It has been estimated that, depending on the population, 1–8% will experience PTSD at some time during their lifetime. In addition, up to 15% of the population will experience milder forms of the condition. The proportion of affected individuals may be considerably higher in predisposed populations.
- Stress disorders occur among people of all ages, including children.
- Typical causes for the disorder include major accidents, acts of war and terrorism, witnessing or experiencing violence and, among women, rape.
- A clear majority of the patients with PTSD will also be affected by another mental health disorder during their lifetime, e.g. alcoholism or affective disorders.

Acute stress reaction

Symptoms

- Physical and emotional symptoms of generalized anxiety disorder emerge within an hour of the stressful experience, possibly including symptoms associated with social behaviour or mood. After the exposure to a stressful event the symptoms should begin to subside within 8 hours. If the exposure to the stressful event is prolonged the symptoms may persist for up to 48 hours.
- Symptoms have generally disappeared altogether within 72 hours.

Differential diagnosis and investigations

- Similar acute symptoms may also be attributable to a somatic illness, poisoning or a complication of an injury.
- Panic disorder
- Diagnosis is based on observing and listening to the patient.

Treatment

- In the case of a major incident the general guidelines detailed below are to be followed.
- Short-acting benzodiazepines or hypnotics may be prescribed for a couple of days to treat anxiety or sleep disorders.

Psychological first aid and mental care after a major incident

Basic principles

- Proximity
- Immediacy

- Expectancy
- Simplicity

Guidelines for psychological first aid

- Consider the possibility of multiple injuries.
- Make sure that the survivors can rest, keep warm and have access to hot drinks.
- Initiate psychological support at the scene or in its immediate vicinity to enable the survivors to participate in helping others where necessary and develop a feeling of solidarity with them. Avoid transferring anyone to unfamiliar surroundings.
- Ensure that all survivors are given support together and no one is left alone.
- Delegate the psychological first aid to trained layman members of the rescue team as much as possible.
- Initiate crisis intervention immediately to avoid fixation on the psychological trauma. Offer opportunities to talk and express emotions during the initial shock phase, but make no attempt to forcibly shorten this phase.
- Be aware of the differences between psychological first aid and subsequent support (referral to various care facilities, when this becomes appropriate).
- Whenever seriously disturbed and disturbing panic-prone victims cannot be calmed with first aid measures, transfer them to special treatment facilities to be cared for by a stress management team.
- Restrain from using psychopharmacological drugs, and consult a psychiatrist if possible. If tranquillisers have been administered, the patient must rest and be evacuated on a stretcher.
- Pay special attention to those who had a somatic or mental illness at the time of the disaster.
- Give accurate and responsible information to survivors, relatives and the mass media. Disprove false rumours immediately.
- Pay attention to the relatives and other secondary victims.
- Allow survivors access to their deceased relatives, should they so wish, for a final farewell. Often this practice is beneficial for the person's own crisis management.

Organizing mental after-care

- Social as well as medical and psychological intervention is necessary immediately after a major incident; the arrangement of the mental after-care is the responsibility of the medical personnel. Voluntary lay members may continue to offer some of the psychological support.
- To promote the self-directed coping of the victims, written and electronic information should be freely available, meetings and discussions should be arranged etc.
- Those with severe stress-related symptoms at the onset should be referred to the care of their health center or to their occupational health crisis management team or similar.
- A **stress defusing session** should be arranged for the rescue and medical personnel who have been exposed to severe psychological stress, usually on the same day or within 24 hours.
- A **psychological debriefing session** can be arranged for primary and secondary victims, usually within 1 to 3 days after the incident. The following should be taken into consideration:
  - The psychological trauma experienced by the group members should be of similar type and severity.
  - Individuals who show open symptoms of re-experience or avoidance are not to be included in a group debriefing session. They should be offered individual crisis intervention.
  - The person in charge of a psychological debriefing session must have adequate training in crisis therapy and in controlling of group dynamics as well as be well versed in the practice of referring individuals for further care.
  - Psychological debriefing is most suitable for groups who are going to work together in the future, such as rescue and medical personnel. Debriefing may contribute towards enhanced future work capacity.
  - Group debriefing sessions do not replace the need for individual crisis intervention. There is no current evidence that single individual psychological debriefing is a useful treatment form for the prevention of PTSD.
  - Participation in psychological debriefing must be entirely voluntary.
  - Debriefing should not be considered as the primary form of mental care after more commonplace disturbing events. Adequate information, counselling and an opportunity to talk with a professional should usually be considered as adequate support.
  - Those who need guidance or care provided by the social services should be referred to the care of appropriate personnel.

Post-traumatic stress disorder (PTSD): symptoms and diagnosis

Symptoms

- Persistent re-experiencing of the traumatic event
  - Recurrent distressing recollections of the event
  - Nightmares of the event
  - Dissociative flashback episodes and a sense of reliving the event
  - Intense distress when exposed to reminders of the traumatic event
  - Physiological reactions when exposed to stimuli resembling an aspect of the traumatic event
- Avoidance of stimuli associated with the trauma and numbing of general responsiveness
  - Efforts to avoid thoughts, feelings, activities, places or people associated with the trauma
  - Inability to recall important aspects of the trauma
  - Diminished interest in significant activities, feeling of detachment, restricted range of mood, sense of foreshortened future
- Persistent symptoms of autonomic hyperarousal

- Difficulty falling or staying asleep
- Irritability or outbursts of anger
- Concentration difficulties
- Hypervigilance
- Exaggerated startle response

♦ The diagnosis of PTSD is justifiable when the duration of symptoms exceeds one month. Generally, the delay between the event and the onset of symptoms should not exceed six months because the causal connection is usually doubtful thereafter.

♦ The criteria for PTSD diagnosis specify that the person must have been exposed to an event which is likely to cause pervasive distress in anyone. Furthermore, the criteria set by the American Psychiatric Association (DSM-IV) further stipulate that the person's subjective response was marked by intense fear, helplessness or horror.

Differential diagnosis

♦ Adjustment disorders and other reactions to severe stress

♦ Prolonged depressive reaction after trauma

♦ Relapse of a mental disorder following exposure to stress

♦ Generalised anxiety disorder without a preceeding traumatic event

♦ Personality change after a catastrophic experience

Diagnostic examination

♦ Careful interview with the patient and detailed history of the symptoms, possibly with the aid of standardized questionnaires

♦ Psychological examination

♦ Exclusion of physical causes of autonomic hyperactivity (e.g. hyperthyroidism, factors causing excessive adrenalin secretion, use of stimulants)

Post-traumatic stress disorder: treatment

Psychotherapy

♦ Supportive contact therapy carried out by the general practitioner, often combined with pharmacotherapy.

♦ Personal or group therapy organized through a primary care crisis team (stress management team).

♦ Crisis intervention or short focused psychodynamic psychotherapy at a mental health unit.

♦ Brief treatment and investigation period either as an inpatient in a psychiatric ward of a general hospital or in an open ward of a psychiatric hospital.

♦ In chronic cases, cognitive-behavioural psychotherapy in specialized units or by a private therapist.

Pharmacotherapy

♦ For lowering initial anxiety and improving sleep: normal doses of benzodiazepines with the aim to reduce and withdraw medication rapidly.

♦ Antidepressants. Suggested order:

- selective serotonin reuptake inhibitors (SSRI)
- serotonin-noradrenaline reuptake inhibitors
- conventional tricyclic antidepressants.

♦ If indicated, it is recommendable to start an antidepressant with a small dose which is gradually increased. The patient should be monitored for possible adverse effects. The correct medication is usually found by trial and error. Significant response may be achieved with antidepressants, even in cases where the patient has no obvious symptoms of depression.

♦ For prolonged sleep disorders a sedating antidepressant at bedtime is preferable.

♦ Beta-blockers (particularly propranolol), clonidine or other drugs that lower sympathetic activity can be tried when symptoms of autonomic hyperactivity are prevalent.

♦ The PTSD patient's proneness to self-treatment with alcohol should be kept in mind.

35.40 Drugs used in psychiatric emergencies

Heikki Rytsälä

Antipsychotic drugs in acute psychosis

♦ The management of an aggressive patient may be initiated with:

- Olanzapine 10 mg i.m. If necessary, the dose can be repeated after 2 hours, and again after 4 hours. The maximum dose is 30 mg daily, or
- Risperidone 2 mg liquid concentrate and lorazepam 2 mg orally, or
- Zuclopenthixol acetate 50–150 mg i.m. The earliest the dose needs to be repeated is 24 hrs, but usually 2–3 days after the initial dose (extrapyramidal symptoms are the most common adverse effects, for management see section Adverse effects), or
- Haloperidol 2.5–5 mg i.m. The dose can be repeated several times per day. It can be administered once per hour i.m. until the patient calms down (extrapyramidal symptoms are the most common adverse effects).

♦ Diazepam 5–10 mg 3–4 times daily p.o., or lorazepam 1–2.5 mg p.o. or i.m., during the first days of acute psychosis will relieve anxiety.

Antidepressants

- For depressive patients with insomnia and anxiety a good choice of medication is a sedative antidepressant taken in the evening (mirtazapine, mianserin, trazodone, or a tricyclic antidepressant such as amitriptyline or doxepin).

Starting a tricyclic antidepressant

- The patient starts the treatment with a tricyclic antidepressant by taking 25–50 mg at 8 p.m. If he/she does not feel tired at all at 10 p.m., he/she may take an additional 25 mg dose and repeat this again at midnight, if necessary.
- If the patient has fallen asleep only after taking 100 mg of the medicine and has not been too drowsy in the morning, next evening he/she should take 100 mg, 1–2 hours before his/her usual bed-time. This allows the quick introduction of the maintenance dose of a tricyclic antidepressant, which normally is at least 150 mg/day.

Starting a selective serotonin reuptake inhibitor (SSRI)

- A SSRI is usually started with the therapeutic dose.

Mania

- Medication is usually warranted when the patient suffers from sleep disorders, as extreme insomnia may trigger mania.
- A sedating antipsychotic drug is the drug of choice (chlorpromazine, chlorprothixene, levomepromazine). If necessary, a hypnotic can be added for a brief period.
- Dose titration: Initially 100–200 mg (levomepromazine 25–50 mg) at 7 p.m. If the patient does not feel tired at 9 p.m., an additional dose of 100 mg (50 mg) may be administered. The dose may be repeated twice more with a two hour interval, i.e. at 11 p.m. and 1 a.m.
- If the patient sleeps at least 5 hours and is not too drowsy the next morning, the next evening he/she should take the entire dose of the first evening (100–500 mg), approximately 2 hours before his/her usual bed-time.

Delirium

- The main aim is to establish the cause of delirium and, if possible, to treat it.
- Haloperidol 5 mg i.m. is the drug of choice, repeated every 30–60 minutes. Severely disturbed patients may require doses up to 5–100 mg daily.

Agitated patient with dementia

- Haloperidol 0.5–5 mg or lorazepam 0.5–1 mg

Adverse effects

- Neuroleptic malignant syndrome, see (35.14)
- Dystonia and akathisia (extrapyramidal symptoms)
  - The primary treatment is to reduce the dose of the drug causing the symptoms or to change to a drug with fewer symptoms.
  - Symptoms occur most frequently with haloperidol, perphenazine, fluphenazine, flupenthixol and zuclopenthixol.
  - Acute dystonia may be treated with biperiden 2 mg three times daily orally or 2.5–5 mg i.m.
- In akathisia the dose of the antipsychotic should be reduced. The symptoms can be alleviated temporarily with propranolol with a dose up to 40–120 mg daily.
- Anticholinergic adverse effects
  - Large doses of sedating antipsychotic drugs and tricyclic antidepressants co-administered with antiparkinsonian and other anticholinergic drugs may cause anticholinergic syndrome, which is characterised by confusion, irritability and delirium.
  - Constipation, urinary retention, elevated intraocular pressure.
- All antidepressants may produce akathisia during the first days of treatment.
  - Patients with panic disorder are particularly susceptible.
  - Treatment is important because akathisia can contribute to an elevated risk of suicide.
  - Benzodiazepines are a suitable treatment.
- Decrease of seizure threshold
  - Chlorpromazine and clozapine are more epileptogenic than thioridazine and fluphenazine.
  - Amitriptyline, imipramine, clomipramine and nortriptyline are the most epileptogenic of tricyclic antidepressants, while doxepin is the least epileptogenic.
  - Caution should be exercised with other antidepressants when prescribing for an epileptic patient.
- Agranulocytosis may result from the use of clozapine (1:100–1:1000), mianserin (1:4. 000–1:10 000) as well as mirtazapine.
- Clozapine may cause myocarditis and cardiomyopathy
- Priapism may be induced by trazodone (1:1000–1:10 000), sometimes also by thioridazine and chlorpromazine. The patient should have emergency urological consultation.
- Changes in blood concentration of other drugs
  - Carbamazepine induces liver enzymes and decreases the blood concentrations of many other medications.
  - Fluoxetine and fluvoxamine inhibit metabolizing enzyme activity, and may lead to elevated concentrations of other drugs.
- Monoamine oxidase inhibitors (moclobemide) may in conjunction with tricyclic antidepressants and selective serotonin reuptake inhibitors cause hypertensive crisis or the serotonin syndrome. These drugs should not be used together concomitantly.

35.41 Antidepressants from the General Practitioner's viewpoint

Heikki Rytsälä

Aims

- Choose the correct antidepressant.
- Ensure the dose is large enough to produce a beneficial effect.
- Treatment should be of sufficient duration.
- Medication should support other treatments (psychotherapeutic support).
- Prophylaxis is necessary in recurrent depression.

When to start antidepressants

- Most patients with depression A [1,2] or dysthymia A [3,4] benefit from antidepressants. However, medication must be tailored individually by trying and changing drugs as necessary.
- The benefit gained from antidepressants is not directly proportional to the severity of depression.
- If depression becomes prolonged, the physician should, regardless of the degree of severity, be prepared to start an antidepressant.
- Antidepressants are effective also in patients with depression caused by a physical illness.
- According to some research, medication is sometimes beneficial in prolonged bereavement reaction.
- The effectiveness of medication always also depends on other simultaneous treatment. In the treatment of depressed patients, maintaining contact is essential, even if it is only occasional. It is easier for the patient to keep an appointment that has been agreed upon in advance.
- An anxiolytic is often necessary at the beginning of treatment, in addition to an antidepressant, in order to relieve the most intense anxiety (remember the dangers associated with long-term use!) B [5]. Benzodiazepines alone do not have antidepressant effect B [6,7].

Duration of treatment

- Continue full dosage for at least 6–9 months after depression is in remission (if possible without any symptoms of depression).
- Dosage should be adjusted individually; too small a dose is ineffective, too large a dose does not enhance the effect but exaggerates the adverse effects (mainly related to tricyclic antidepressants).
- Medication should be withdrawn gradually.
- Even short-term medication may bring relief, e.g. to sleep disorders, in chronic depression (dysthymia).
- If a patient has a history of depressive disorder (F33.x) that has previously responded favourably to medication, a maintenance therapy even lasting several years may be necessary A [8,9,10,11]. After three episodes of depression a long maintenance treatment is always indicated.

Choice of medication

- Choose a small number of antidepressants and become thoroughly familiar with them.
- Major groups
  - Tricyclics
  - Tetracyclics
  - Selective serotonin reuptake inhibitors (SSRIs) A [12,13]
  - Selective serotonin and noradrenaline reuptake inhibitors (SNRI)
  - Noradrenergic and specific serotonergic antidepressants (NaSSA)
  - Selective reversible MAO-A inhibitors
- The drugs differ more in their side effects A [14,15] than in their actual effects C [16,17,18,19,20,21,22,23,24].
- Serotonin reuptake inhibitors are often the primary choice because they are easy to use, have few adverse effects and are relatively harmless B [25,26,27,28,29,30,31,32].
- Drug tolerance becomes a major issue with elderly patients. Tricyclic antidepressants should therefore be prescribed for the elderly only when there is no alternative B [25,26,27,28,29,30,31,32].
- Mirtazapine, mianserin, trazodone or tricyclic drugs are suitable for depressed patients with sleep disorders or anxiety A [33,34].

Selective serotonin reuptake inhibitors

- Are as effective as tricyclic antidepressants.
- Are not sedative (a hypnotic is often needed).
- An effect is seen 2–3 weeks from start of treatment.
- Are considerably more expensive than older antidepressants.
- Cause fewer adverse effects than tricyclic drugs, resulting in better drug compliance A [35].
- When switching to MAO inhibitors a "wash out" period of 2–5 weeks is needed.

Fluoxetin

- Dose for depression is 20–40 mg per 24 h, divided into 1–2 doses to be taken in the morning and during the day. The dose for bulimia is 60 mg per 24 h, generally as a single dose in the morning.
- Half-life is 2–4 days; the half-life of the active metabolites is considerably longer.
- Renal or hepatic insufficiency can increase the half-life of fluoxetine.

- When switching to MAO inhibitors a "wash out" period of at least 5 weeks is needed.
- Adverse effects are those typical for this drug group, i.e. are nausea, vertigo and sleep disorders.
- Increases considerably the concentrations of many drugs that are metabolized by in the liver, e.g. tricyclic antidepressants, long-acting benzodiazepines, carbamazepine and valproate.

Fluvoxamine

- Dose is 100–200 mg, up to 300 mg per 24 h (A) [36 37].
- Doses exceeding 150 mg are usually divided into 2–3 doses. The starting dose is taken in the evening.
- Average half-life is 20 h.
- Adverse effects are those typical for this drug group, i.e. nausea, vomiting, insomnia or drowsiness, headache, tremor and vertigo.
- Slows the clearance of drugs that are metabolized by the liver. Has significant interactions with beta-blockers, haloperidol and warfarin.
- May increase the plasma concentrations of tricyclic drugs.
- Raised liver enzymes and creatinine have been documented.
- Caution should be exercised in the treatment of epileptics as susceptibility to seizures may increase.

Paroxetine

- The first dose is 20 mg in the morning. The dose may be increased in increments of 10 mg up to 50 mg. Maximum of 40 mg for patients over 65 years of age. Safe dose for those with liver or renal malfunction is about 20 mg per 24 h.
- Half-life averages at 24 h but varies individually.
- Adverse effects are nausea, sweating and sleep disorders; in men, decreased libido and ejaculation disturbances.
- Interactions with tricyclic antidepressants, phenothiazine-type neuroleptics, warfarin, cimetidine, antiarrhythmic drugs belonging to class 1C (flecainide), phenytoin and other anticonvulsants.

Sertraline

- The first dose is 50 mg once a day, morning or evening. If necessary, the dose may be increased gradually over several weeks up to 200 mg.
- Half-life averages at 26 h.
- No particular effect on psychomotor performance; however, patients should always be cautioned against driving and using dangerous machinery.
- Adverse effects are headache, nausea, sleep disorders, vertigo and dry mouth.
- Does not significantly affect the clearance of drugs metabolized by the liver.
- May have minor interactions with some drugs, e.g. the dose of lithium should be kept as small as possible; also, prothrombin time should be monitored during warfarin treatment as it may increase.
- Caution should be exercised in the treatment of epileptics.

Citalopram

- Dosage is 20–60 mg once daily, generally taken in the morning. The initial dose for the elderly is 10 mg.
- Half-life is about 36 h.
- There are no significant interactions with other drugs, although when used concomitantly with some neuroleptics an increase in citalopram concentration has been observed, which is of no apparent clinical significance.
- Adverse effects are nausea, sleep disorders and sweating.
- Caution should be exercised in the treatment of epileptics.

Escitalopram

- Escitalopram is the S-enantiomer of citalopram, and it is a highly specific inhibitor of serotonin reuptake.
- Dose is 10–20 mg once daily, generally taken in the morning.
- Half-life is about 30 h.
- There are no significant interactions with other drugs, although when used concomitantly with some neuroleptics an increase in citalopram concentration has been observed, which is of no apparent clinical significance.
- Adverse effects are nausea, sleep disorders and sweating.
- Caution should be exercised in the treatment of epileptics.

Selective serotonin and noradrenaline reuptake inhibitors

Venlafaxine

- Start with the smallest possible dose, usually 37.5 mg twice daily. If the response is insufficient after 2–4 weeks, the dose is increased gradually up to 75 mg twice daily. The maximum recommended dose is 125 mg three times daily. Often the dose may be reduced and even halved when the patient has been symptomless for one month, provided that the symptoms do not recur. Particular caution and care should be exercised in the treatment of the elderly.
- Treatment should be withdrawn cautiously and with decreasing doses over at least 2 weeks. Withdrawal symptoms may include nausea, vertigo, headache, sleep disorders, general malaise, anxiety and muscle spasms.
- Do not use together with MAO inhibitors.
- May raise blood pressure, which is why routine blood pressure monitoring is recommended for all patients on venlafaxine. Particular caution should be exercised with cardiac patients.
- Regular check-ups are necessary for patients with disturbances in micturition, acute angle-closure glaucoma, raised intraocular pressure, low blood pressure or cardiac complaints. The depressive period of manic-depressive psychosis may change to mania during venlafaxine treatment.
- Possible adverse effects are vertigo, insomnia, drowsiness, nervousness, GI-tract symptoms, headache, cardiovascular symptoms (including increased blood pressure), increased

appetite and weight gain, CNS symptoms, accommodation disturbances, increased voiding frequency, sexual disturbances, sweating and weakness.
- Venlafaxine should be stopped at least 1 week before switching to MAO inhibitors.
- There are interactions with many drugs that are metabolized by in the liver, such as quinidine, paroxetine, ketoconazole, erythromycin, verapamil and cimetidine.

Noradrenergic and specific serotonergic antidepressants (NaSSA)

Mirtazapine

- Starting dose is 15 mg, which is then slowly increased as needed. 15–45 mg is the average effective dose. The dose for the elderly is the same as that for adults, but the response and possible adverse effects should be closely monitored.
- The drug is usually taken as a single dose at bedtime or sometimes in equally divided doses in the morning and the evening.
- The treatment response Ⓐ [38 39] is likely to be best when the symptoms include features of the somatic syndrome of depression: anhedonia, psychomotor inhibition, sleep disorders, lack of interest, suicidal thoughts and a better mood in the evening than in the morning.
- Half-life, which is 20–40 h, is lengthened by renal or hepatic insufficiency.
- May increase the effects of alcohol and benzodiazepines.
- Must not be used with MAO inhibitors.
- May impair concentration and alertness.
- Adverse effects are: increased appetite and weight, fatigue, (orthostatic) hypotension, mania, seizure attacks, tremor, myoclonus, oedema, acute bone marrow depression, increased serum level of transaminases and exanthema.

Tricyclic antidepressants

- Products: amitriptyline, amoxapine, clomipramine, dosulepin, doxepin, imipramine, lofepramine, nortriptyline, trimipramine
- Have been on the market for a long time; abundant research and practical experience are available.
- The usual adult dose is 75–150 mg per 24 h. In most cases the effective daily dose is 150–300 mg. However, there is evidence on the efficacy of low-dose therapy Ⓐ [40]. Determination of the plasma concentration is beneficial for treatment monitoring. With the daily dose of 150 mg the concentration is still too low in 30% of the patients.
- May be administered as a single dose each evening.
- Anticholinergic side-effects are most common, i.e.:
  - dry mouth
  - constipation
  - urinary retention.
- Other common adverse effects:
  - Weight gain, sedation, orthostatic hypotension
- Take into account:
  - Cardiovascular diseases require caution.
  - Slightly increased risk of arrhythmias
  - Patients with compensated cardiac insufficiency may use tricyclic drugs.
  - The seizure threshold is lowered in epileptics.
  - With local anaesthesia etc. the potency of epinephrine and norepinephrine may increase markedly.
  - Must be avoided in alcohol abusers (danger of intoxication).

Tetracyclic antidepressants

Maprotiline

- A drug developed from tricyclic antidepressants with adverse effects that are similar but somewhat milder than those of the tricyclics.
- Lowers the seizure threshold.

Mianserin

- Causes fewer adverse effects than tricyclic drugs.
- Usually taken in the evening.
- Considerable but transient fatigue, which sometimes presents at the early stages of treatment, may discourage compliancy.
- Has not caused lethal intoxications.
- Adverse effects:
  - Because of reports of bone marrow depression, which were mainly cases of agranulocytosis and granulocytopenia, patients are advised to see their physician immediately should signs of infection appear. Previous recommendation was to routinely check leucocytes on weeks 4 and 6 after starting treatment.

Other antidepressants

PSY

Moclobemide

- Selective reversible MAO-A inhibitor that may be used without dietary restrictions.
- Is used for all forms of depression.
- Starting dose is 150 mg twice daily.
- Take into account:
  - Well tolerated
  - Activates the patient.
  - Suitable also for the elderly
  - May be combined with anxiolytics and neuroleptics if necessary; combination with benzodiazepines may be advisable at the beginning of treatment (the activating effect may cause insomnia).
  - Should not be used with serotonin reuptake inhibitors; remember both the new selective serotonin reuptake inhibitors as well as clomipramine and trazodone.
  - A "wash out" period of at least 2 weeks is necessary when switching over from a selective serotonin reuptake inhibitor to moclobemide.

- When switching over to any other antidepressant, no "wash out" period is required.
- When used in combination with cimetidine, caution should be exercised and at least the dose of moclobemide should be halved.
- May increase and prolong the effect of a systemically administered sympathomimetic.

Milnacipran

- Serotonin and noradrenaline reuptake inhibitor
- Usually administered 50 mg twice daily.
- Dose should be decreased in renal insufficiency.
- Half-life about 8 h. Steady state will be achieved after 2–3 days.
- Eliminated mainly unchanged, via the renal route. Hepatic insufficiency does not significantly affect the pharmacokinetics of the drug.
- In sleep disorders and anxiety, symptomatic treatment is generally needed.
- It always is important to be careful with suicidality. Patient's psychomotor activity may increase before depression has alleviated.
- Do not use
  - with MAO-inhibitors, triptanes (especially sumatriptan), digoxin, epinephrine, norepinephrine, clonidine and similar drugs
  - in prostatic hyperplasia and other urogenital diseases
  - during pregnancy and lactation.
- The most usual adverse effects include dizziness, hyperhidrosis, anxiety, hot flushes and dysuria. Also nausea, vomiting, anticholinergic adverse effects, tremor, palpitations and agitation may occur. Cardiovascular adverse effects occur more often in those with coexisting cardiovascular diseases or relevant medication.

Trazodone

- Indicated for patients with mild to moderate depression who cannot use tricyclic antidepressants.
- Cardiovascular effects are milder compared with tricyclic antidepressants.
- Adverse effects include orthostatic hypotension and priapism.
- Maximum dose is 600 mg per 24 h divided into three doses.

Nefazodone

- A $5HT_2$-receptor blocker as well as serotonin and noradrenaline reuptake inhibitor
- The initial dose is 50–100 mg twice daily. The dose is increased over one week to 200 mg twice daily, or even up to 300 mg twice daily, if necessary.
- If another antidepressant is replaced by nefazodone, a pause of a few days to one week should be held in medication, and nefazodone is then started at a dose of 50 mg twice daily.
- The drug has no anticholinergic or antihistamine effects and it does not affect REM sleep.
- The clinical profile of nefazodone resembles that of SSRIs but the adverse effects on sexuality are less frequent.
- The most common adverse effects are dryness of mouth, nausea, constipation, somnolence and orthostatic hypotension.
- Severe interactions related to prolonged QT interval are possible. Caution is warranted if used simultaneously with digoxin or drugs that are metabolized via the CYP_3A_4 and CYP_2D_6 isoenzymes. There are no interactions with alcohol.

Reboxetine

- Selective and potent noradrenaline reuptake inhibitor. The drug also acts as a very weak serotonin reuptake inhibitor.
- The initial dose for adults is 4 mg twice daily. The daily dose can be increased up to 10 mg after 3–4 weeks. The maximum daily dose is 12 mg. The drug is not recommended for the elderly.
- The drug is activating rather than hypnotic.
- Adverse effects include dryness of mouth, constipation, insomnia and hyperhidrosis.
- The drug is not suitable for patients with epilepsy or those with severe somatic diseases. Caution is warranted if used for patients with benign prostatic hyperplasia, glaucoma and cardiac diseases.
- The drug should be used cautiously with drugs that are metabolized through enzymes other than CYP_2D_6.
- Should not be combined with MAO inhibitors.
- Contraindicated during pregnancy and lactation.

Sulpiride

- A neuroleptic with an antidepressant effect.
- The most effective adult dose is between 50–400 mg daily.
- Administered in the morning and daytime because an evening dose may cause sleep disorders.
- Adverse effects are milk secretion caused by increased prolactin secretion, and occasional motor restlessness (akathisia).
- Tardive dyskinesia may develop during long-term use, particularly in the elderly. If it persists for a prolonged period it may become permanent. Smacking of the lips is usually the first sign of tardive dyskinesia. It is usually reversible upon immediate discontinuation of sulpiride.

St. John's wort

- Extracts of hypericum are more effective than placebo for the short-term treatment of mild to moderately severe depressive disorders (A) [41 42 43]. The current evidence is inadequate to establish whether hypericum is as effective as other antidepressants.
- The extract may lower the serum concentration, and thus the efficacy of concomitantly used drugs such as ciclosporin, digoxin, oral contraceptives, theophylline, warfarin, and indinavir.

Combining antidepressants

- In psychotic depression a neuroleptic should be combined with an antidepressant, e.g. perphenazine, risperidone or olanzapine if the patient has delusions or hallucinations.
- Lithium may be combined if the response to a suitable dose of a tricyclic antidepressant is inadequate. If the response still remains inadequate, small but slowly increasing doses of thyroid hormone may be further added. Response is usually seen in a few weeks.
- Tricyclic antidepressants may also be combined with selective serotonin reuptake inhibitors (or vice versa).
- Selective serotonin reuptake inhibitors, selective serotonin and noradrenaline reuptake inhibitors as well as noradrenergic and specific serotonergic antidepressants must not be combined with selective reversible MAO-A inhibitors.
- Fluoxetine and fluvoxamine may more than double the plasma concentration of tricyclic antidepressants by slowing down liver metabolism.

References

1. Joffe R, Sokolov S, Streiner D. Antidepressant treatment of depression – a meta-analysis. Canadian J Psychiat 1996;41: 613–616.
2. The Database of Abstracts of Reviews of Effectiveness (University of York), Database no.: DARE-970163. In: The Cochrane Library, Issue 4, 1999. Oxford: Update Software.
3. Lima MS, Moncrieff J. Drugs versus placebo for the treatment of dysthymia. Cochrane Database Syst Rev. 2004;(2): CD001130.
4. Lima MS, Hotopf M. Pharmacotherapy for dysthymia. Cochrane Database Syst Rev. 2004;(2):CD004047.
5. Furukawa TA, Streiner DL, Young LT. Antidepressant and benzodiazepine for major depression. Cochrane Database Syst Rev. 2004;(2):CD001026.
6. Birkenhager TK, Moleman P, Nolen WA. Benzodiazepines for depression? A review of the literature. Int Clin Psychopharmacol 1995;10:181–195.
7. The Database of Abstracts of Reviews of Effectiveness (University of York), Database no.: DARE-964063. In: The Cochrane Library, Issue 4, 1999. Oxford: Update Software.
8. Viguera AC, Baldessarini RJ, Friedberg J. Discontinuing antidepressant treatment in major depression. Harvard Review of Psychiatry 1998;5:293–306.
9. The Database of Abstracts of Reviews of Effectiveness (University of York), Database no.: DARE-983602. In: The Cochrane Library, Issue 2, 2000. Oxford: Update Software.
10. Blacker D. Maintenance treatment of major depression: a review of the literature. Harvard Review of Psychiatry 1996;4:1–9.
11. The Database of Abstracts of Reviews of Effectiveness (University of York), Database no.: DARE-983291. In: The Cochrane Library, Issue 2, 2000. Oxford: Update Software.
12. Selective serotonin reuptake inhibitors (SSRIs) for major depression: evaluation of the clinical literature. Canadian Coordinating Office for Health Technology Assessment 1997;Part 1:1–73.
13. The Database of Abstracts of Reviews of Effectiveness (University of York), Database no.: DARE-978514. In: The Cochrane Library, Issue 1, 2000. Oxford: Update Software.
14. Trindade E, Menon D, Topfer LA, Coloma C. Adverse effects associated with selective serotonin reuptake inhibitors and tricyclic antidepressants: a meta-analysis. Can Med Ass J 1998;159:1245–1252.
15. The Database of Abstracts of Reviews of Effectiveness (University of York), Database no.: DARE-989726. In: The Cochrane Library, Issue 3, 2000. Oxford: Update Software.
16. SSRIs versus tricyclic antidepressants in depressed inpatients: a meta-analysis of efficacy and tolerability. Depression and Anxiety 1998;7(suppl 1):11–17.
17. The Database of Abstracts of Reviews of Effectiveness (University of York), Database no.: DARE-983856. In: The Cochrane Library, Issue 1, 2000. Oxford: Update Software.
18. Selective serotonin reuptake inhibitors (SSRIs) for major depression: evaluation of the clinical literature. Canadian Coordinating Office for Health Technology Assessment 1997;Part 1:1–73.
19. The Database of Abstracts of Reviews of Effectiveness (University of York), Database no.: DARE-978514. In: The Cochrane Library, Issue 1, 2000. Oxford: Update Software.
20. Steffens DC, Krishnan KR, Helms MJ. Are SSRIs better than TCAs? Comparison of SSRIs and TCAs: a meta-analysis. Depression and Anxiety 1997;6:10–18.
21. The Database of Abstracts of Reviews of Effectiveness (University of York), Database no.: DARE-983110. In: The Cochrane Library, Issue 3, 2000. Oxford: Update Software.
22. Hirschfeld RM. Efficacy of SSRIs and newer antidepressants in severe depression: comparison with TCAs. Journal of Clinical Psychiatry 1999;60:326–335.
23. The Database of Abstracts of Reviews of Effectiveness (University of York), Database no.: DARE-991201. In: The Cochrane Library, Issue 1, 2001. Oxford: Update Software.
24. Guaiana G, Barbui C, Hotopf M. Amitriptyline versus other types of pharmacotherapy for depression. Cochrane Database Syst Rev. 2004;(2):CD004186.
25. Menting JE, Honing A, Verhey FR, Hartmans M, Rozendaal N, de Vet HC, van Praag HM. Selective serotonin reuptake inhibitors (SSRIs) in the treatment of elderly depressed patients. Int Clin Psychopharmacol 1996;11:165–175.
26. The Database of Abstracts of Reviews of Effectiveness (University of York), Database no.: DARE-973205. In: The Cochrane Library, Issue 2, 2000. Oxford: Update Software.
27. Anderson IM, Tomenson BM. Treatment discontinuation with selective serotonin reuptake inhibitors compared with tricyclic antidepressants: a meta-analysis. BMJ 1995;310: 1433–1438.
28. The Database of Abstracts of Reviews of Effectiveness (University of York), Database no.: DARE-978082. In: The Cochrane Library, Issue 4, 1999. Oxford: Update Software.
29. Selective serotonin reuptake inhibitors (SSRIs) in the treatment of elderly depressed patients: a qualitative analysis of the literature on their efficacy and side-effects. International Clinical Psychopharmacology 1996;11:165–175.
30. The Database of Abstracts of Reviews of Effectiveness (University of York), Database no.: DARE-973205. In: The Cochrane Library, Issue 1, 2000. Oxford: Update Software.
31. Mittmann N, Herrmann N, Einarson TR, Busto UE, Lanctot KL, Liu BA, Shulman KI, Silver IL, Narango CA, Shear NH.

The efficacy, safety and tolerability of antidepressants in late life depression: a meta-analysis. Journal of Affective Disorders 1997;46:191–217.
32. The Database of Abstracts of Reviews of Effectiveness (University of York), Database no.: DARE-983425. In: The Cochrane Library, Issue 1, 2000. Oxford: Update Software.
33. McCusker J, Cole M, Keller E, Bellavance F, Berard A. Effectiveness of treatments of depression in older ambulatory patients. Arch Intern Med 1998;158:705–712.
34. The Database of Abstracts of Reviews of Effectiveness (University of York), Database no.: DARE-988580. In: The Cochrane Library, Issue 4, 1999. Oxford: Update Software.
35. Barbui C, Hotopf M, Freemantle N, Boynton J, Churchill R, Eccles MP, Geddes JR, Hardy R, Lewis G, Mason JM. Treatment discontinuation with selective serotonin reuptake inhibitors (SSRIs) versus tricyclic antidepressants (TCAs). Cochrane Database Syst Rev. 2004;(2):CD002791.
36. Ware MR. Fluvoxamine: a review of the controlled trials in depression. J Clin Psychiatr 1997;58(suppl 5):15–23.
37. The Database of Abstracts of Reviews of Effectiveness (University of York), Database no.: DARE-970788. In: The Cochrane Library, Issue 4, 1999. Oxford: Update Software.
38. Holm KJ, Markham A. Mirtazapine: a review of its use in major depression. Drugs 1999;57:607–631.
39. The Database of Abstracts of Reviews of Effectiveness (University of York), Database no.: DARE-990980. In: The Cochrane Library, Issue 1, 2001. Oxford: Update Software.
40. Furukawa T, McGuire H, Barbui C. Low dosage tricyclic antidepressants for depression. Cochrane Database Syst Rev. 2004;(2):CD003197.
41. Linde K, Mulrow CD. St John's wort for depression. Cochrane Database Syst Rev. 2004;(2):CD000448.
42. Linde K, Ramirez G, Mulrow CD, Pauls A, Weidenhammer W, Melchart D. St John's wort for depression: an overview and meta-analysis of randomised clinical trials. BMJ 1996;313:253–258.
43. The Database of Abstracts of Reviews of Effectiveness (University of York), Database no.: DARE-968370. In: The Cochrane Library, Issue 4, 1999. Oxford: Update Software.

35.42 Clozapine therapy

Virpi Raitasuo

Background

- Clozapine is an antipsychotic agent that has proved to be effective in treatment-resistant schizophrenia. It lacks many adverse effects of several other antipsychotics, such as extrapyramidal symptoms, tardive dyskinesia or elevation of serum prolactin concentration.
- Severe adverse effects of clozapine include **granulocytopenia or agranulocytosis** (in 0.8% of patients) and, according to recent reports, also **myocarditis and cardiomyopathy** that occur in 0.29% of patients C [1].
- In treatment-resistant schizophrenia, clozapine should only be prescribed by psychiatrists or physicians well versed in the use of clozapine therapy. In psychosis associated with Parkinson's disease, clozapine may also be prescribed by a neurologist.
- When treated with clozapine many schizophrenic patients can be managed in the community. Primary care doctors should therefore be familiar with the principles of monitoring clozapine therapy (frequent laboratory testing, recognition of adverse effects).
- High doses of clozapine, in particular, may cause epileptic seizures in 2–5% of patients.
- Constipation is a common adverse effect. If left untreated it may lead to paralytic ileus.
- Several drugs, smoking and consumption of coffee may cause clinically significant changes in clozapine concentrations.
- If it is necessary to abruptly withdraw the therapy (e.g. due to granulocytopenia), the psychotic symptoms may return within a few days. Most patients will also suffer from withdrawal symptoms due to the cholinergic rebound effect.

Dosing

- The recommended maximum dose of clozapine is 600 mg/day. The dose can be divided into 2–3 doses so that a larger portion is given at bedtime.
- A primary care physician should not change the dose without first consulting with the specialist who has started the medication.

Administration and monitoring of therapy

- Clozapine should not be used concomitantly with drugs that are likely to cause myelosuppression. The use of long-acting depot injections of antipsychotics should also be avoided.
- Arrange cooperation with the investigating laboratory so that the white blood cell (WBC) count of the patient is immediately reported to the physician treating the patient and that the count is recorded in the patient's notes. Monitoring charts are available from the manufacturer of the drug.
  - Before starting clozapine therapy (usually in hospital), a WBC count with a differential count must be carried out.
  - After the therapy has been initiated, a WBC count and an absolute neutrophil count (ANC) must be carried out weekly for the first 18 weeks of treatment.
  - After 18 treatment weeks, a WBC count must be carried out at least monthly for as long as the patient is taking clozapine.
- At each consultation, the patient should be reminded to contact the treating physician immediately if any kind of infection begins to develop, e.g. fever or sore throat.

Action in leucocytopenia/granulocytopenia

- In case of infection, or if the WBC count is below 3.5×10^9 or the ANC is below 2.0×10^9.

- WBC count with differential count must be repeated immediately.
- If the WBC count is 3.0–3.5 × 10^9, OR if the granulocyte count is 1.5–2.0 × 10^9, both counts must be repeated at least twice weekly until the values have returned to normal.

♦ If the WBC count is below 3.0 × 10^9 or the granulocyte count below 1.5 × 10^9

- Clozapine therapy must be discontinued immediately and the patient's WBC count checked daily until the values begin to rise (if monitoring cannot easily be arranged over the weekend the measurements can be postponed until the next weekday with instructions to the patient to seek emergency care if symptoms of infection appear).

♦ If clozapine therapy has been discontinued and the WBC count continues to fall to below 2.0 × 10^9 or if the granulocyte count is below 1.0 × 10^9

- Management of this condition must be guided by an experienced haematologist.
- The patient must be admitted to a general ward for monitoring.
- **If clozapine therapy has been discontinued for haematological reasons the patient must not be re-exposed to clozapine.**

Reference

1. Kilian JG, Kerr K, Lawrence C, Celermajer DS. Myocarditis and cardiomyopathy associated with clozapine. Lancet 1999;354:1841–1845.

35.43 Drug treatment of anxiety and related disorders

Erkka Syvälahti

Aims

♦ To specify the nature of the disorder.
♦ To estimate the factors contributing to the disorder and evaluate the need for medication.
♦ To try to avoid continuous anxiolytic medication.
♦ To consider alternatives to benzodiazepine medication and the possibilities for psychotherapy.

Various anxiety disorders

♦ Choose the treatment according to the nature of the disorder.

- There are differences in e.g. drug treatment for generalized anxiety, panic disorder, social phobias and mixed anxiety-depression disorder.
- Benzodiazepine treatment of short duration is possible in adaptation disorder that manifests as anxiety, and in the acute phase of traumatic stress reaction.

Generalized anxiety

♦ The most common anxiety disorder
♦ Drug treatment is often indicated if it clearly supports psychosocial management. Predisposing factors (stress, overuse of drugs, coffee etc.) must be considered.
♦ Antidepressants (A) [1] (venlafaxine, amitriptyline, doxepin, mianserin, selective serotonin reuptake inhibitors, etc.) may be more useful than benzodiazepines (C) [2 3] in the long-term treatment of anxiety.
♦ The most important differences between the various benzodiazepines are pharmacokinetic. Use long-acting benzodiazepines (diazepam, chlordiazepoxide, chlorazepate) especially in chronic disorders, and when reducing and stopping the medication. Oxazepam and lorazepam have an intermediate duration of action, and because of their minimal liver metabolism they are also suitable for old people and patients with liver disease.
♦ The most common adverse effects of benzodiazepines include sedation, worsening of psychomotor functions and transient disturbances of memory.
♦ Benzodiazepines should be used at low doses and the treatment should be of short duration (2–6 weeks), if possible. Before discontinuation of the drug the daily doses are slowly decreased to avoid possible withdrawal symptoms.
♦ Buspirone is a non-benzodiazepine (azapirone) compound whose therapeutic action emerges in 1–3 weeks after beginning treatment (as with antidepressants). The indications are chronic anxiety disorders where immediate relief of symptoms is not necessary. Neither withdrawal symptoms, nor disturbances of psychomotor or cognitive functions have been reported.
♦ Beta-receptor antagonists decrease symptoms caused by stimulation of the sympathetic nervous system in connection with anxiety. Antihistamines or carbamazepine or, in special cases, alpha-2-agonists (clonidine), or low doses of neuroleptics may be beneficial.

PSY

Panic disorders

♦ See article 35.29.
♦ Repeated, sudden attacks of fear and anxiety are characteristic of panic disorder. A panic attack may lead to avoidance behaviour (panic disorder with agoraphobia). The fear of a panic attack is often associated also with generalized, anticipating anxiety.
♦ An acute panic attack, in particular, may be treated with benzodiazepines, e.g. alprazolam (occasional or short-term use). In long-term treatment the antidepressants imipramine and clomipramine and serotonin selective antidepressants

(SSRI) are the first-line therapy. At the start of treatment the drugs may, however, augment panic symptoms, and the doses must be increased slowly. Buspirone is probably not effective in panic disorder.

Social phobia

- Manifests in social situations, when the patient feels he or she is being observed by other people. The symptoms may include an increase in the heart rate, palpitation, tremor, speech impairment and flushing.
- Beta-receptor antagonists can be tried for the symptoms of sympathetic nervous stimulation in social phobia.
- Benzodiazepines may be used for occasional treatment of severe symptoms.
- MAO inhibitors and SSRIs may be effective in extensive fear symptoms that may sometimes warrant continuous medication.

Obsessive-compulsive disorder

- Manifests as repeated compulsive thoughts or actions. The patient understands the futility of his or her actions and tries to restrain the compulsive action, but this often leads to increased anxiety.
- Clomipramine and SSRIs have been effective in this disorder. The dosage is the same as in the treatment of depression. The therapeutic effect usually becomes evident only weeks or months after starting the medication.

Mixed anxiety–depression disorder

- Is a rather new diagnostic entity in the ICD classification. Neither condition is clearly dominant.
- Antidepressants are often indicated, and buspirone is also an alternative in drug treatment.

Basic rules

- In the treatment of anxiety disorder the use of drugs may not be appropriate, and the special features of each disorder not taken into account. Skilful drug therapy can greatly reduce many symptoms of anxiety disorders.
- The best results in the treatment of anxiety disorders are obtained by combining psychopharmacological and psychotherapeutic treatment. Cognitive therapies, behavioural therapies and dynamic psychotherapies are useful, especially in the treatment of prolonged anxiety disorders.

References

1. Kapczinski F, Lima MS, Souza JS, Cunha A, Schmitt R. Antidepressants for generalized anxiety disorder. Cochrane Database Syst Rev. 2004;(2):CD003592.
2. Casacalenda N, Boulenger JP. Pharmacologic treatments effective in both generalized anxiety disorder and major depressive disorder: clinical and theoretical implications. Canadian Journal of Psychiatry 1998;43:722–730.
3. The Database of Abstracts of Reviews of Effectiveness (University of York), Database no.: DARE-981749. In: The Cochrane Library, Issue 4, 2000. Oxford: Update Software.

35.50 Psychotherapy in general practice

Pekka Larivaara

Need for psychotherapy in general practice

- Only half the patients in general practice have a clear, traditional medical diagnosis. The others have complaints and symptoms that are related to psychological distress, problems in the family or other relationships. A psychotherapeutic approach would be beneficial in the treatment of these patients in general practice.
- General practitioners see many patients with psychosomatic disorders. Very often attention is paid mainly to the somatic complaints and patients are directed to specialist clinics where the efficacy of the treatment may even be worse than it would be in the hands of a skilled GP.

Practical points

- All treatments based on the doctor–patient relationship have psychotherapeutic effects.
- The stronger the relationship, the easier it is for the physician to assess whether the patient needs psychotherapy and what therapy to choose.
- In general practice, a specific psychiatric diagnosis is not always necessary. It is more important to get a good picture of the patient, his family and other social circumstances. It is also essential to assess the patient's anxiety, mood, sense of guilt or shame, zest for life or lack of it, and possible suicidal ideation.
- If the physician widens his approach to include also the family, his work can be defined as family-oriented with the therapeutic effect extending beyond the patient treated.

Choices of therapy available to a GP

Supportive psychotherapy

- The best form of treatment if the patient has symptoms of current distress and conflicts that are presumed to need only temporary help.

- Aims at strengthening the patient's normal functions and suits a GP who has not had special training in psychotherapies.
- Although transference and countertransference are not dealt with in supportive psychotherapy, the physician should be aware of these psychological phenomena.
- In supportive therapy the attitude of the physician is empathic, humane, understanding and respecting, and at the same time encouraging and reassuring.
- Sufficient time must be reserved for therapy patients in order to avoid an atmosphere of hurry.
- The physician must be able to control his own negative or aggressive feelings so as not interfere with the therapy. It is important to remember that initial dislike for a patient may change as the physician comes to understand him/her better.
- In long-lasting therapy a dependency relationship between the doctor and patient is a possible danger. In such cases the therapy should be aimed at encouraging the patient to become independent. In practice, this means that the therapy sessions should become less frequent. The patient is encouraged to make his/her own decisions and an authoritative approach is avoided.

Crisis intervention

- The basic rules of crisis intervention are much the same as in supportive therapy. However, solutions must be found more quickly.
- The treatment often starts in an emergency situation; a typical case is a patient in a panic state of anxiety or irresolution, or at suicidal risk. The suicidal ideas should be discussed openly to help the patient to find hope, realistic optimism and new solutions to solve the anxiety.
- In the acute crisis it is essential that the physician stays calm, reassuring, and empathic. If the patient feels the physician is interested in his or her situation, is understanding and not in a hurry, it is easier for him or her to find a way out of the crisis. Giving the patient the possibility of reaching the physician by telephone may also help him feel more secure.
- At the start of the therapy it may be worthwhile to combine psychotherapy and short-term pharmacotherapy.
- Crisis intervention should take into account all family members or other individuals affected by the crisis.

Family-oriented therapy

- Family therapy may be beneficial if one family member has severe mental problems, psychosomatic problems or if there are illnesses or symptoms in the family that may be related to the family's difficult life situation.
- The aim is to help the family relations develop in such way that the problems or the disease may become milder or cured. Another goal is to prevent further problems and disease in the family. Therapeutic family discussions may also help the family to become more functional and help to create better relations in the family.
- In practice family therapy consists of empathy, facing bereavement, finding the strengths and resources in the family and enhancing problem-solving skills. The aim is to start a process that leads to healing without a long-lasting therapy.
- The results are best if the whole multidisciplinary team accepts the importance of family-oriented work and if some of the team have special training in family medicine and family therapy.

Counselling as an aid in general practice psychotherapy

- It is best that the general practitioner uses the kind of psychotherapy he feels he knows best. The more the physician gives psychotherapy the more he receives patients who benefit from it. There is a lot of incipient need for psychotherapy. Very often this may also be a burden to the physician. Signs of exhaustion should be recognized and the physician should have the possibility of receiving education or counselling in psychotherapy, for example in Balint groups or individually.

35.51 Psychotherapies for adults

Kari Pylkkänen

Aims

- To identify and eliminate barriers to psychological development and maturity.
- To help the patient find insight to his own thinking and actions, and evaluate whether they are appropriate.
- To help the patient to find new ways of coping with human relationships.

PSY

Referring to psychotherapy

- It is estimated that approximately 2% of the population might benefit from psychotherapy.
- Assessing the need and reasons for psychotherapy requires specialist consultation.
- A general practitioner should keep psychotherapy in mind, especially when a patient starts to have psychiatric symptoms A [1 2 3]. Psychotherapy is more effective if the diagnosis and treatment are early-phase.
- Psychotherapy should be considered
  - if the patient has a non-psychotic mental disorder with symptoms of anxiety, depression or personality disorder that affects working capacity or social relations
  - in psychiatric disorders in youth

- when medication and crisis interventions have no effect and the medication seems to have become long-term
- when the patient feels more need to change him/herself than modify his/her environment.

♦ Combining psychotherapy and medication is often effective but psychotherapy can be carried out as the only form of treatment.

Forms of psychotherapy

♦ More than 400 different psychotherapy techniques have been described in literature. Most of these are applications of the six following main forms of psychotherapy:
- psychodynamic psychotherapy
- cognitive psychotherapy
- interpersonal psychotherapy
- systemic psychotherapies and family therapies
- group therapies
- supportive psychotherapy.

Psychoanalytic (psychodynamic) psychotherapies

♦ Objective
- To assess the effect of earlier experiences on the current models of functioning (thoughts, feelings, images, actions).

♦ Goal
- To help the patient to understand his way of outlining the world and to find alternatives that would work better and give more autonomy.

♦ Method
- Therapeutic alliance
- Free association
- Defence analysis and interpretation of transference, especially in relation to the therapist.
- The emphasis is based on the psychoanalytic school.

♦ Indications
- Psychotherapies are most effective in neurotic disorders, e.g., obsessive-compulsive, anxiety, and dissociative disorders, in psychiatric symptoms due to somatic disease, in dysthymic and adjustment disorders, in mild and moderate mood and personality disorders.
- Personality disorders and comorbid states in which the traits of personality disorder play a significant role are a particularly important indication for psychotherapy. Comorbidity occurring with personality disorders is very common in most psychiatric diagnoses: 56% in anxiety disorder, 41% in phobia, 41% in severe depression, 22% in social phobia. In mental disorders that threaten the ability to work, comorbidity associated with personality disorders is significant and should be taken into account when rehabilitation is planned. Randomized studies have shown that psychoanalytical psychotherapy is efficient in treating borderline personality disorder in particular.

♦ Duration of treatment
- From months to several years
- The sessions must be sufficiently frequent.

♦ Forms of treatment
- Psychoanalysis: 3–5 sessions a week for 4–6 years
- Psychoanalytical/psychodynamic-oriented individual psychotherapy: 1–3 sessions a week for 2–4 years
- Psychodynamic brief psychotherapy: limited number of sessions (12–40), restricted focus

Cognitive therapy

♦ Object
- Cognitive distortions (thoughts) and related emotions

♦ Goal
- To identify and alter personal cognitive distortions that cause symptoms.

♦ Method
- Therapeutic sessions normally 1–2 a week for 1–3 years
- In brief therapies the number of sessions is restricted (15–20).

♦ Indications
- Primarily used in depressive disorders. Other indications are anxiety, nervousness, panic disorder and substance abuse.

♦ In the recent years the development of cognitive therapy has been characterized by a strong tendency to develop a systematic therapy process that fulfils the following three criteria:
- The therapy is based on an extensive theory that is supported by research evidence.
- The therapy is operationalized and the therapy process is linked to theoretical concepts.
- The effect of the therapy has been proven by studies.

♦ Cognitive therapy is the most extensively studied form of therapy, and its efficacy has been shown more clearly than that of other therapies in controlled, randomized studies. Studying the effect is made easier by standardized manuals that allow to repeat the therapy process in a controlled manner.

Family therapy

♦ The roots of family therapy are in psychodynamic theory, cognitive theory and system-oriented family research.

♦ Object
- Disorders in the family interaction or in an individual family member.

♦ Goal
- To modify interaction within the family, to find the strengths of the family.

♦ Indications
- Indicated especially in severe psychiatric disorders where problems of dependency are central.

- In crisis interventions family therapy may solve a locked situation (e.g., crisis of divorce or child independence)

Interpersonal psychotherapy

- Object
  - The basic idea is that mental disorders occur in a psychosocial, interpersonal setting. Interpersonal psychotherapy focuses on current interaction relationships. Transference and childhood experiences are not included in the therapy process, although their importance is not neglected. Current relationships are considered as the most essential ones and are thus in focus.
- Indications
  - Developed initially only for the treatment of acute depression. The method has, however, been adjusted for use in other mental disorders.
- Methods
  - Four main problem areas are emphasized
    - conflicts in roles
    - interpersonal insufficiency
    - prolonged reaction to grief and
    - changes in roles.
- Aim
  - To help the patient to develop coping strategies for social and interaction problems.
- Duration
  - Usually limited to 12–16 weeks.

Group psychotherapy

- Many techniques used in individual therapy have been applied in groups. The methods used in group therapy can be psychodynamic, interpersonal and cognitive. Psychodrama is a special form of group therapy in which internal conflicts are processed in play-like processes.

Supportive psychotherapy

- Object
  - Psychodynamic supportive psychotherapy is especially utilized in the treatment of patients with severe personality disorders.
- Aim
  - Better control of the symptoms and a more realistic attitude towards the disease. Main themes include finding solutions to every-day problems: living, housekeeping, work. Solving acute family conflicts and sorting out age-specific developmental problems, such as relationships, sexuality, loneliness, hobbies, religious questions, is equally important.
- Method
  - The main therapeutic element is the continuity of a supportive therapy relationship and regarding the patient primarily as a person. The theoretical foundation of supportive therapy can rise from several frameworks. The psychodynamic experience is probably most significant in understanding the patient and supervising the therapy process. Cognitive approach is also always important.
- The process described here is a special clinical application of supportive psychotherapy that has a significant role in the treatment of psychoses.

Brief psychotherapies

- Brief psychotherapy is a common name for a group of different techniques of psychotherapy restricted in time (5–20 sessions) that may be based on different theoretical backgrounds.
- The most well known are:
  - psychodynamic-focused brief psychotherapy
  - crisis intervention
  - cognitive brief psychotherapy
  - cognitive-analytical therapy
  - problem solving oriented brief psychotherapy
  - interpersonal therapy.

Effectiveness of psychotherapies

- Meta-analyses have shown that psychotherapy is highly effective. On average, more than 90% of patients who have received psychotherapy improve significantly compared with controls not receiving psychotherapy. The effect remains after 5 years.
- Efficacy studies with long-term follow-up are lacking
  - Comparison of different psychotherapy techniques using the methodology of effectiveness studies is a much more complicated research problem than, for example, the comparison of pharmacotherapies. Thus far, usable and reasonably priced methods for comparing psychotherapies are not available. Most mental disturbances are long lasting. Unfortunately, efficacy studies have not been able to address the question of effect in the long term. The majority (99%) of studies on the effectiveness and efficacy of therapies assess brief therapies, and the effectiveness estimates are limited to the short-term results. Several dozens of meta-analyses assessing the effectiveness of psychotherapies by combining the results of hundreds of trials have been made. According to these studies the effectiveness of psychotherapy compared with a no-treatment group equals that of patients treated with psychopharmacological drugs.
- Comparison of long and short therapies has not been possible
  - Problems related to research methods are particularly complicated when a controlled trial of long psychotherapy processes is attempted, as using a randomized study design in long psychotherapies is extremely difficult. Thus far, there are no controlled trials that would have succeeded in comparing long psychoanalytic therapy with short psychotherapies.

Prioritizing in psychotherapy

- As the resources are limited, decisions must be made concerning whom to refer for psychotherapy. Johan Cullberg from Sweden (1995) presented a model for prioritizing in psychotherapy that also takes into account preventive and societal factors.

First priority

- Treatment of diagnosed psychiatric disorders or symptoms or barriers to normal psychological development. For example,
  - Personality disorders with risk of suicide
  - Anxiety, mood and eating disorders
  - Obsessive-compulsive disorders and restricted disorders such as phobia or compulsive gambling
  - First time psychosis and the family members of these patients
  - Long-term psychosis (supportive psychotherapy)
  - Long-term personality disorders that cause personal suffering and reduced ability to live or work
  - Anxiety and depression related to traumatic experiences

Second priority

- Preventive treatment for employees in health care and in occupations where a high self-knowledge is needed
  - People who take care of the mentally ill
  - People in educational work and in leading positions
  - People in creative tasks, for example, art or scientific research where using imagination and developing ideas is essential

Third priority

- People with no general indications who have a special reason for psychotherapy
  - Long-term psychosis
  - Psychotherapy in certain cases that have been traditionally considered as contraindicated for psychotherapy.

References

1. Brown C, Schulberg HC. The efficacy of psychosocial treatments in primary care: a review of randomized clinical trials. Gen Hosp Psychiatr 1995;17:414–424.
2. The Database of Abstracts of Reviews of Effectiveness (University of York), Database no.: DARE-960172. In: The Cochrane Library, Issue 4, 1999. Oxford: Update Software.
3. Huibers MJH, Beurskens AJHM, Bleijenberg G, Schayck CP van. The effectiveness of psychosocial interventions delivered by general practitioners. Cochrane Database Syst Rev. 2004;(2):CD003494.

35.62 Transsexualism

Eila Sailas

Definition

- Transsexualism is defined as a gender identity disorder that belongs to the category of mental disorders. The central feature of transsexualism is a contradiction between the sensed sexual identity and anatomical gender. The transsexual person considers him/herself to belong to the other gender permanently and invariably and wishes to change his/her gender both socially and anatomically to correspond with his/her own image of him/herself. Transsexualism is the ultimate form of gender identity disorder in a continuum of disorders.

Prevalence

- In the Netherlands the estimated prevalence of transsexualism is 1:11 900 in men and 1:34 000 in women.
- The underlying cause of transsexualism is not known, although several different theories arising from various bases have been put forward.

Diagnosis

- A patient with suspected gender identity disorder should be referred for evaluation by a multi-professional team.
- Before referral for special investigations the possibility of a psychotic disorder should be excluded. Extensive psychiatric examinations are not necessary.
- The diagnosis of transsexualism requires a thorough psychiatric examination that lasts for at least six months and consists of frequent contacts with the patient.

Treatment

- After the diagnosis has been made the patient and the team that has examined him/her together draft a treatment and rehabilitation plan that may include different treatment options, such as psychotherapy, treatment of possible psychiatric comorbidities, and progression towards partial or total social and anatomical gender reassignment. The treatment plan is always tailored individually.
- If the decision to reassign the gender of the patient is made, the treatment is given in three phases.
- This three-phase treatment consists of hormone therapy after the diagnosis and the so-called real life test. If these are successful, the process may be progress to gender reassignment surgery. Hormone therapy and surgery can be implemented only if the patient meets the aptitude and maturity requirements.

Real life test

- The patient begins to live according to the role of the desired gender.
- The decision on gender assignment is not made before this phase, as it is important to see how the change affects the family, work and future perspectives of the patient.
- In most cases the patient changes his/her first name at this point.
- How satisfied the patient is with his/her life and how he/she copes in professional and social relationships is evaluated.

Hormone treatment

- Hormone treatments can be started only after the diagnostic phase if the patient meets the requirements of aptitude and maturity. The patient must be at least 18 years of age and thoroughly acquainted with the social and medical risks of hormone treatment. His/her gender identity must be clear and he/she may not show, for example, severe antisocial or psychotic behaviour, self-destructiveness or have problems with substance abuse.
- The psychiatrist of the multi-professional team that has evaluated the patient writes the referral for hormone treatment. A gynaecologist or internist who is familiar with endocrinology may give the hormone treatment.
- Many of the effects of hormone treatment are partially reversible even after years of treatment.
- The follow-up of treatment may be the responsibility of a GP or a specialist after appropriate guidance.

Surgical treatment

- The decision to start surgical treatments is made by a multi-professional team after a successful fulltime real life test that has continued for at least 12 months.
- At this point the patient may seek permission to be castrated.
- In woman-to-man reassignment surgical procedures include hysterectomy, salpingo-oophorectomy, vaginectomy, meto-idoplasty, scrotoplasty, urethroplasty, and falloplasty. Man-to-woman reassignment includes orchiectomy, penectomy and vaginoplasty. Several surgical techniques are used.

Rehabilitation

- The transsexual patient may need referral for consultation with a specialist in phoniatry, and he/she may need speech therapy or surgery of the thyroid cartilage and vocal cords.
- Removal of body hair, i.e. epilation, is also necessary for rehabilitation in man-to-woman transsexuals.
- The patients may need social or psychiatric support in the gender reassignment process.

Neurology

Evidence Based Medicine Guidelines. Edited by the Duodecim Editorial Team
 ISBN: 0-470-01184-X

36.1 Evaluation of a neurological patient

Markku Ellonen

Typical cases requiring urgent treatment

- Acute stroke
- Impaired consciousness or state of confusion
- Loss of consciousness in an individual not known to suffer from epilepsy (after first aid, neurological diagnostic tests may usually be performed by appointment in the outpatient clinic)
- Severe acute headache, especially when accompanied by symptoms of infection, nuchal rigidity or impaired consciousness.
- Gait disturbance or sphincter malfunction

History

- For a neurological diagnosis, patient history is the most significant investigative element. It is often determinant and sometimes the only tool, e.g. in the assessment of pain (headache) and paroxysmal symptoms.
- If necessary, elicit the history also from family members or accompanying persons (emergency room situations, unconsciousness, dementia).
- Note
    - Onset of symptoms, their manifestation and progression
    - Description of current symptoms
    - Are the present symptoms paroxysmal or continuous?
    - Previous neurological examinations
    - Other diseases (hypertension, atrial fibrillation)
    - Patient's current medications
    - Use of alcohol; possible drug abuse?

Neurological examination

- Usually the general practitioner performs a neurological examination based on the symptoms. (If the patient is able to walk, communicate, undress and dress correctly, he/she has already managed very demanding neurological tasks.)
- Pay attention to the following factors:
    - whether the patient comes alone or accompanied by other person
    - level of consciousness described verbally (36.5)
    - memory and ability to logical thinking
    - speech production and comprehension
    - how the patient moves (walks, needs aid devices, bedridden)
    - neck rigidity (potential source for diagnostic error)
    - muscle tone, muscle appearance (atrophy, fasciculation)
    - dyskinesia (tremors, involuntary movements)
    - paresis or muscle weakness
    - ataxia
    - tendon reflexes (in the elderly, nonsignificant defects are often found)
    - Babinski's sign
    - evident sensory impairment (the patient often spontaneously discloses this; possible sensory level)
    - Motor skills: Can the patient lift his/her limbs, walk on toes and heels (distal strength in lower extremities); can he/she stand up from a chair without pushing with arms (proximal strength in lower extremities); how he/she uses hands while undressing. The grip may be weak because of poor cooperation. An assessment of weakness in individual muscles is necessary mainly when a disorder affecting peripheral nerves is suspected, e.g. triceps strength in spinal cord syndrome affecting C7.
- Cranial nerves
    - Pupils, eye movements and nystagmus, also, if necessary, the fundi and visual fields
    - Facial movements, wrinkling up the forehead
    - Tongue and pharynx
    - Patients with vertigo should have their hearing, ears, and provoked nystagmus examined (38.70).
- General condition
    - Blood pressure measured also in standing position if the patient had a syncope. Cardiac arrhythmias (especially atrial fibrillation), carotid arteries
    - When there is weakness in the lower extremities, probe for back pain, tenderness on percussion, circulation in lower extremities, and Babinski's test.

Tests

- **Blood tests** are helpful in detecting the non-neurological causes of symptoms (such as anaemia or infection as the cause of dizziness) and use of alcohol. When the patient is unconscious, blood tests of metabolic disorders are important (36.5).
- **Skull and neck x-ray** is indicated only in cases of trauma.
- **A CSF examination** is advisable in an emergency room situation if meningitis is suspected. It should be performed only in well-equipped units (hospitals). A cerebral haemorrhage should be diagnosed by using a CT scan. Taking a sample of CSF with a fine needle is permissible if SAV is not probable but needs to be excluded.

36.2 Paralysis–muscle weakness

Kiti Müller

Aetiology

- The underlying causes of paralysis or muscle weakness may include

- upper motor neurone disorders
- lower motor neurone disorders
- myoneural junction disorders
- myopathy
- psychosocial factors (psychogenic paralysis).

Neurological findings in upper motor neurone disorders or pyramidal tract lesion

- Paralyses not confined to the nerve root or peripheral nerve area; their symptoms include clumsiness and ataxia.
- In the acute variant (shock phase), muscle tone is decreased and tendon reflexes may be lacking.
- Frequently includes an extensor plantar sign (Babinski +)
- Increased tendon reflexes, clonus
- Increased muscle tone or spasticity.

Causes originating in the brain

- Cerebral infarction (36.31)
- TIA (36.30)
- Cerebral haemorrhage (36.33)
- Brain tumours (36.99)
- Intracranial haemorrhage (18.5)
- Symptoms
  - Unilateral muscle weakness, often with dysaestesia
  - Increased reflexes
  - Extensor plantar sign (Babinski +)
  - Cranial nerve abnormalities and neuropsychological symptoms are seen frequently.

Disorders of the spinal cord

- See 36.82.
- Trauma
- Tumour
- Circulatory disorder
- Spondylomyelopathy
- Syringomyelia, myelitis, etc.
- Symptoms
  - Indications of damage to the spinal cord tracts are:
    - paraparesis: muscle weakness in lower extremities
    - tetraparesis: muscle weakness in upper and lower extremities
    - paraplegia
    - tetraplegia
    - also, limb spasticity, dysaesthesia, bladder and erectile dysfunction.
  - Indications of localized injury to the spinal cord, such as with syringomyelia or intramedullary tumour, are:
    - muscle weakness and atrophy of the hands or shoulder area
    - abnormal sensory responses to cold and heat, even when the sense of touch and vibration remain intact (dysaesthesia).

Diseases causing damage to several areas of the central nervous system

- For example, demyelinating disorders (36.75)
- Symptoms are: dysaesthesia, limb coordination disorder, spasticity, muscle weakness, and fatigue.

Neurological findings in lower motor neurone disorders

- Decreased or absent tendon reflexes
- Decreased muscle tone
- Muscle atrophy
- Paralyses follow the distribution of nerve roots or peripheral nerves, or are located in distal parts of the extremities.
- A flexor or absent plantar sign.

Polyneuropathies

- See 36.90.
- Muscle strength and tendon reflexes decrease symmetrically, progressive sensory deficits (sock or glove type of distribution), later development of muscle atrophy.

Polyradiculites

- See 36.92.
- Generally symmetrical muscle weakness, progressing from the distal to the proximal direction, developing within a few days or over a few weeks' time. Frequently there is myalgia in the extremities, and tendon reflexes decrease or disappear.

Radiculopathies, damage to one or more nerve roots

- See 36.91.
- Symptoms include paraesthesia, numbness, and radiating pain in the dermatome innervated by the nerve root.
- Increasing muscle weakness in the muscles innervated by the affected nerve and decreased segmental tendon reflexes. When the condition has become chronic, muscle atrophy develops.

Damage to neural plexus, plexus injury, plexus neuritis

- Symptoms include myalgia, sensory deficits, muscle weakness, decreased tendon reflexes, and muscle atrophy, which appear in one or more segments of the peripheral nerves involved in the plexus.

Nerve entrapment or compression injuries

- See 36.88.
- Symptoms include muscle weakness in the region innervated by a single peripheral nerve, and related sensory deficit.

Upper and lower motor neurone disorders

Motor neurone diseases

- Amyotrophic lateral sclerosis (36.84)
- Symptoms are progressive muscle weakness in voluntary muscles with muscle atrophy and involuntary muscle twitching or fasciculation.
- However, muscle tone may be increased (spastic) and the plantar response may be extensor.

Neurological findings of myoneural junction disorders

- A typical presentation is muscle fatigue intensified by strain.
- Reflex and sensory functions appear normal.
- The plantar sign may be flexor or absent.

Myasthenia gravis

- See 36.86.
- Typically, voluntary muscles tire easily, and the weakness is relieved by rest.

Myasthenic syndrome

- See 36.86.
- The myasthenia is more pronounced in proximal muscles.

Congenital myasthenias

- These are extremely rare.

Neurological findings in myopathies

- Muscle weakness
- Muscle atrophy, occasionally hypertrophy
- In some diseases: myalgia, muscle hypotonia
- Reflexes are often normal.
- The plantar sign is flexor or absent.

Myopathies

- These include congenital muscular dystrophies, metabolic myopathies, inflammatory myopathy or myositis, as well as toxic and endocrine myopathies (36.85).

Periodic paralyses: sporadic attacks of flaccid paralysis

- Hypokalaemic: teenage onset
- Hyperkalaemic: childhood onset
- Normokalaemic
    - The myasthenic attack is often preceded by muscle strain or a meal high in carbohydrates.

36.3 Gait disturbances

Editors

Non-neurological causes of gait disturbance

- Fracture of lower extremity
- Joint symptoms, arthritis
- Poor general health
- Orthostatic hypotonia (measure blood pressure with the patient standing; review all medications!)
- Arterial insufficiency in lower extremities (claudication pain, absent pulses, skin changes)
- Localized leg/foot pain (calluses, toe misalignment, fallen plantar arch, etc.)
- Old traumas

Neurological causes of gait disturbance

- A neurological aetiology of gait disturbance is the more likely the younger the patient.
- Compression of the spinal cord, paraparesis (36.82)
    - **A history of acute weakness in the lower extremities is significant. This is an emergency and the patient should immediately be referred to a hospital.**
- Compression of lumbar nerve roots and cauda equina
    - Especially in a young patient, the main symptom is back pain radiating down the leg. This condition is not called gait dysfunction, but sciatica.
    - Difficulty in walking is a description used by the elderly, in whom the symptoms of chronic stenosis of the lumbar spine have become acute.
    - Cases where the condition is accompanied by sphincter dysfunction and sensory deficits in the buttocks, i.e. cauda equina syndrome, **are emergencies and the patient should immediately be referred to a hospital.**
- Subdural haematoma (especially if bilateral)
    - Symptoms include weakness of the lower extremities, impaired or fluctuating consciousness, and possible signs of increased intracranial pressure or mild hemiparesis.
    - The history may include (even a slight) head injury.
    - Risk groups: the elderly, alcoholics, and patients receiving anticoagulant medication.
- Multiple lacunar infarcts
    - Among the most common causes of a slowly or gradually developing gait abnormality in the elderly.

- Apraxic gait (the feet are strong enough, but the patient is unable to take any steps or the steps are short; legs are "glued to the floor") is a typical presentation.
- Tendency to fall (22.1)

♦ Normal-pressure hydrocephalus (NPH) triad
- Dementia
- Ataxic gait
- Urinary incontinence
- The underlying cause is a disorder in CSF flow, NPH (36.22).

♦ Parkinson's disease or secondary parkinsonism (36.72)
- Rarely diagnosed on the basis of gait disturbance, because the symptom does not develop until a later stage in the disease, although the patients's steps may become shorter also in the beginning of the disease.

♦ Alcoholism (36.73)
- Cerebellar degeneration (widened gait, poor balance, ataxia predominantly in the lower extremities)
- Polyneuropathy with such severe pain in the feet (hyperalgesia) in the acute stage that it prevents walking
- Myopathy (rare).

♦ Polyradiculitis (36.92)
- Causes increasing weakness in the lower limbs accompanied by sensory disturbances within a few days, and later on also upper extremity symptoms. Tendon reflexes are decreased or absent.

♦ Myelitis (36.91) and MS (36.75)
- Spinal plaques cause lower extremity weakness and sensory loss developing within a few days. The presentation often includes sphincter dysfunction.

♦ Several other neurological disorders (brain or spinal canal tumour, slow infection, polyneuropathy, myopathy, ALS, etc.) may cause gait disturbance. Whenever the cause of the deteriorated ability to walk is unclear, neurological examination should be considered.

36.4 Differential diagnostics of paroxysmal loss of consciousness

Editors

Basic rules

♦ Benign vasovagal syncope does not require further examinations.
♦ Benign positional vertigo does not call for further procedures.
♦ Vertebrobasilar insufficiency in the elderly can usually be managed only with ASA and by caution in bending the neck.
♦ In other cases, differential diagnosis of the seizure symptoms may require referral to the following specialty units for further diagnostic workup:
- Neurology: epilepsy, TIA
- Internal medicine: cardiogenic symptoms (C) [1 2]
- ENT: vertigo of vestibular origin
- Psychiatry: severe panic attacks.

Diagnostic clues

♦ If the patient has been unconscious, the description provided by a witness to the seizure is helpful.
♦ Further information is provided by the patient's age, other illnesses, and medications.
♦ The examination should include
- cardiac auscultation
- pulse
- blood pressure (both arms, if VBI is suspected; measured with the patient standing, if orthostatism or collapse are suspected)
- neurological examination: look for findings pointing to a central nervous system disorder.

Generalized epileptic seizures

♦ See 36.45.
♦ Patient becomes stiff and falls.
♦ Tonic-clonic contractions (a few jerks are possible also in other aetiologies).
♦ The patient bites his/her tongue during the seizure.
♦ The patient sustains other injuries.
♦ The patient voids during the seizure.
♦ The seizure is followed by long sleep or confusion.
♦ The patient does not remember the events during the seizure.
♦ Short loss of consciousness, absence

Partial epileptic seizures

♦ Jerky movements of the extremities (on one side), other unusual movement
♦ Local temporary sensory disturbance
♦ Taste sensation
♦ Smell sensation
♦ Déjà-vu, repeated thought pattern

Transient ischaemic attacks (TIA)

♦ See 36.30.
♦ The patient often has a history referring to vascular disease.
♦ Symptoms endure from a few minutes to 24 hours.
♦ TIA in the carotid region: weakness or sensory loss in one extremity or both extremities ipsilaterally, amaurosis fugax, i.e. temporary loss of vision in one eye. Symptoms arising from the dominant side may include speech impediment (dysphasia).
♦ Vertebral TIA (VBI): dizziness, diplopia, blurred vision in both eyes, slurred speech (dysarthria), weakness or

numbness in the extremities, drop attack (legs giving way without loss of consciousness).

Global amnesia

- An attack lasting a few hours, during which the patient cannot store anything in his/her memory.
- The patient's behaviour is otherwise normal, but he/she continues to repeat the same questions and cannot recall anything that happened during the attack.
- There are no other symptoms.
- Global amnesia is not likely to recur, and it is associated with a lesser risk of cerebral infarction than TIA episodes in general.

Other causes

- Cardiogenic (arrhrythmia, ischaemia, aortic stenosis) (4.35)
- Collapse (4.36)
- Vertigo (38.70).

Migraine

- See 36.67.
- Typical migraine attacks are not a diagnostic problem.
- Atypical attacks with prodromal symptoms of migraine without the subsequent headache may be difficult to identify. Often the patient has also had typical migraine attacks and is in "migraine age". Further tests may be necessary to differentiate these attacks from TIA and focal epilepsy.
- In basilar migraine the attack may include brainstem symptoms and loss of consciousness.

Panic attack

- See 35.29.
- A sensation of suffocation, gasping respiration, numbness or tingling in the hands and face
- Palpitations, tremors, perspiration
- A sensation of impaired consciousness or dizziness
- Anxiety, fear of death

Other psychogenic or pseudoepileptic attacks

- These may clinically resemble an epileptic seizure: differential diagnosis is possible only with further diagnostic workup.
- The attack occurs in the presence of other people.
- The patient is not unconscious and reacts to pain even during an attack. Reflexes (pupils reacting to light, Babinski's sign, corneal reflex) are normal.

Sleep disorders

- See 36.9.
- Narcolepsy, episodes of cataplexy, and certain parasomnia-related conditions

Initial laboratory tests

- ECG and blood glucose, other tests if deemed necessary

References

1. Linzer M, Yang EH, Estes M, Wang P, Vorperian VR, Kapoor WN. Diagnosing syncope part 1: value of history, physical examination, and electrocardiography. Ann Intern Med 1997;126:989–996.
2. The Database of Abstracts of Reviews of Effectiveness (University of York), Database no.: DARE-978219. In: The Cochrane Library, Issue 4, 1999. Oxford: Update Software.

36.5 An unconscious patient

Kati Juva

- An unconscious patient is always an emergency case.
- First check ventilation and circulation. Tracheal tube and lying in lateral recumbent position help to keep the airways open. If there is no pulse, resuscitate (see 17.1).

Assessing the level of consciousness

1. Conscious, oriented
2. Somnolent but can be waken by talk and is then able to cooperate.
3. Very somnolent, difficult to waken, confused
4. Reacts to pain adequately (withdrawal).
5. Reacts to pain stereotypically (e.g. extension).
6. Does not react to pain, spontaneous respiration maintained.
7. Does not react to pain, no spontaneous respiration.
8. Always report the findings thoroughly; a general comment "the patient is unconscious" is not enough. See Table 36.5.

Revealing the cause of unconsciousness

- After securing the vital functions one should quickly proceed to discover the cause of unconsciousness. The history is very important; do not allow family members or other witnesses to leave before all available information has been obtained.
  - Was the loss of consciousness sudden? Were there any convulsions, trauma, pre-existing symptoms?
  - Has the patient suffered from any major disease (epilepsy, diabetes, etc.) and did they receive medication?
- Always bear in mind the potentially treatable causes of unconsciousness. Remember the MIDAS rule:
  - Meningitis

Table 36.5 Glasgow coma score

Criteria		Score
Best eye response	Eyes open spontaneously	4
	Eye opening to verbal command	3
	Eye opening to pain	2
	No eye opening	1
Best motor response	Obeys commands	6
	Localizing pain	5
	Withdrawal from pain	4
	Flexion to pain	3
	Extension to pain	2
	No motor response	1
Best verbal response	Orientated	5
	Confused	4
	Inappropriate words	3
	Incomprehensible sounds	2
	No verbal response	1
		Total 3–15

- Intoxication
- Diabetes
- Anoxia
- Subdural haematoma.

♦ There is no time to waste when
- you suspect a treatable infection. Treatment of bacterial meningitis must be started immediately after the lumbar puncture without waiting for the laboratory test results, if the cerebrospinal fluid is cloudy or there is otherwise very strong suspicion of bacterial meningitis.
- the unconsciousness is deepening and there are progressive signs, e.g. a dilatating, non-reactive pupil. This can mean an expansion needing quick neurosurgical intervention.

♦ Treating and examining an unconscious patient usually requires the resources of a regional hospital. If there are inadequate resources, immediately refer the patient further to an appropriate unit, providing it is certain that the patient can withstand the transfer (Figure 36.5.1).

♦ At a health centre or health post always measure the blood sugar. Other tests may be performed, if their results will be ready before or during the transfer.

♦ Pulse oximetry is useful in assessing hypoxia.

♦ When bacterial meningitis is suspected and the transfer time will be long, a lumbar puncture should be taken and the treatment started immediately. The CSF sample can be sent to the hospital with the patient, and it must be preserved at body temperature (e.g, in an inside pocket). Part of the CSF sample can be put directly into a blood culture bottle.

♦ Intravenous infusion should usually be started before the transfer, especially if there are signs of shock.

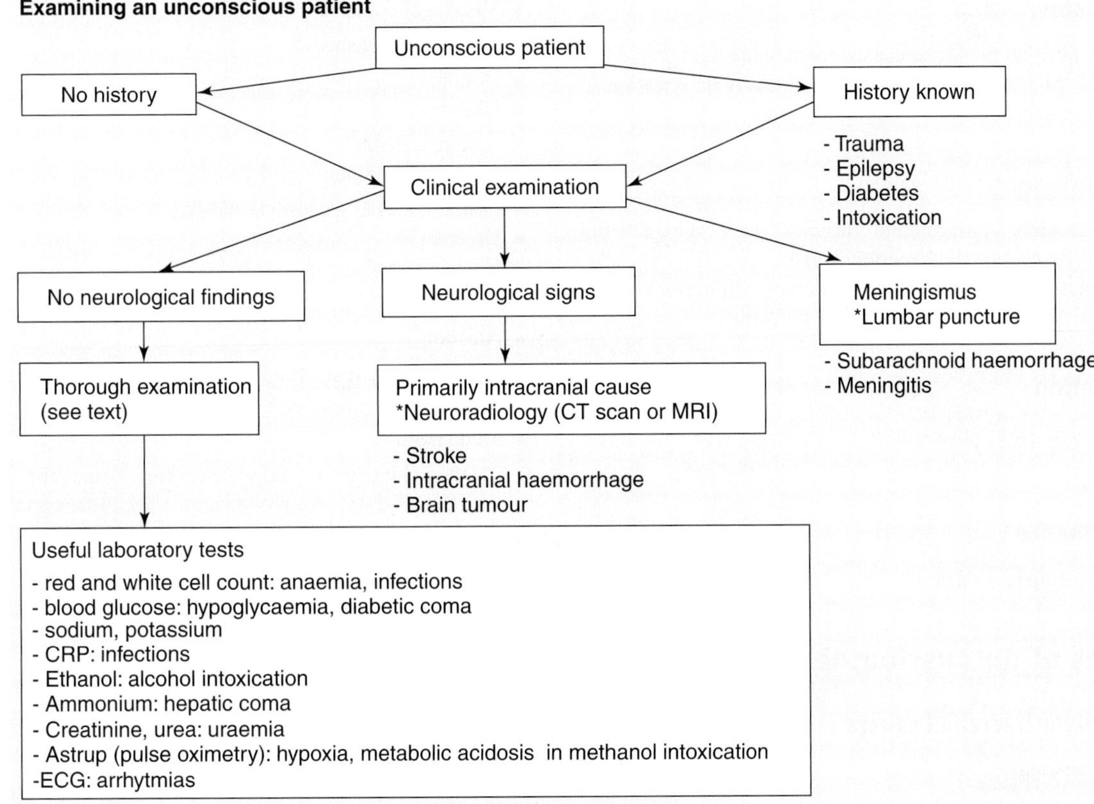

Figure 36.5.1 Investigations of an unconscious patient

Aetiological clues in the status of an unconscious patient

Skin

- Signs of trauma (bruises, scratches): intracranial trauma
- Pallid, sweaty: hypoglycaemia, hypovolaemic shock
- Dry, red: diabetic coma
- Cyanotic: retention of carbon dioxide
- Spider naevi: alcohol intoxication, hepatic coma
- Scarlet: carbon monoxide intoxication

Tongue

- Signs of biting: epilepsy

Smell of breath

- Ethanol: alcohol intoxication
- Acetone: diabetic coma
- Urine: uraemia

Body temperature

- Hypothermia: freezing, severe brain damage or intoxication
- Hyperthermia: infection (meningitis, sepsis), severe brain damage

Heart rate

- Atrial fibrillation: stroke caused by an embolism
- Bradycardia: atrioventricular block, digitalis intoxication
- Tachycardia: infection, shock, arrhythmia

Blood pressure

- Hypertension: intracerebral haemorrhage, subarachnoid haemorrhage, anoxia, hypertonic crisis
- Hypotension: shock (bleeding, myocardial infarction), intoxication, severe brain damage, diabetic coma

Respiration

- Superficial, fast: intoxication
- Cheyne–Stokes respiration: severe brain damage

Incontinence

- Faecal: epileptic seizure

Causes of unconsciousness

Primarily intracranial causes

- Brain trauma
    - In chronic subdural haematoma there is not always any known trauma.
- Intracranial haematomas
    - Subarachnoid haemorrhage
    - Intracerebral haematoma
- Stroke
- Brain tumours
    - If the tumour begins to bleed acutely, there may not be any preceding neurological symptoms.
- Epileptic seizure and postictal state
    - Convulsions are usually seen.
    - There may be bite signs on the tongue and incontinence.
    - A person suffering from epilepsy is prone to head trauma. Keep this is mind if there are neurological signs or the recovery from the seizure is exceptionally slow.
- Infections in the central nervous system
    - Meningitis
    - Encephalitis
    - Brain abscess

Systemic diseases that can cause unconsciousness

- Circulation disturbances
    - Shock (hypovolaemic, cardiogenic, anaphylactic)
    - Hypertensive crisis
    - Arrhythmia
        - Tachycardia
        - Bradycardia
        - Adams–Stokes
    - Vasovagal collapse
- Metabolic disturbances
    - Hypoxia
    - Diabetes
        - Ketoacidosis
        - Hypoglycaemia
    - Disturbances in electrolyte balance
    - Uraemia
    - Hepatic coma
- Intoxications
    - Alcohol
        - Remember that drunken people are also prone to traumas.
    - Medication
        - Often known or suspected. Test urine for drugs (dipstick test), take blood sample for further analysis
- Infections
    - Sepsis, pneumonia
- Freezing or heatstroke.

Flow chart for examining an unconscious patient

- See Figure 36.5.1

36.6 Involuntary movements

Seppo Kaakkola

Introduction

- Involuntary movements are often caused by an injury or altered metabolism in the extrapyramidal system, or are associated with degenerative brain disease.
- Their aetiology is often unknown. Recently, however, some genetic causes have been identified.
- Involuntary movements are often resistant to treatment.

Focal dystonia

- Cervical dystonia, i.e. wryneck (spasmodic torticollis)
  - Adult onset
  - The head twists, leans or jerks initially to one direction; gradually leading to a constant abnormal position of the neck.
  - Treatment consists of botulinum toxin injected in small doses into the overactive muscles. Occasionally the identification of the affected muscles requires EMG diagnostics. Possible adverse effects of the injections include muscle weakness, e.g. dysphagia. The effect of the injection lasts for 3–6 months; repeated injections are therefore necessary.
  - Neurosurgical procedures, directed to reduce the innervation of the neck muscles, are indicated in rare cases.
- Mogigraphia or writer's cramp
  - Muscle cramps in the writing hand usually inhibit writing with a pen, sometimes also using a keyboard. Similar symptoms may be seen in musicians, e.g. in piano or guitar players (musician's cramp).
  - The condition often develops in circumstances where the patient has been forced to do much writing under stress. The hand functions otherwise normally, and no nerve damage is evident.
  - The condition often forces the patient to abandon the work that provokes the cramps. Botulinum toxin may be tried for treatment; EMG monitoring is required.
- Blepharospasm
  - Compulsive closing of the eyelids
  - Good results have been obtained with botulinum toxin treatment.
- Facial spasms
  - Involuntary spasms of facial muscles, sometimes involving one half of the face (not formally classified as dystonias).
  - Possible aetiological factors include the sequelae of facial paresis (36.93), degeneration of the facial nerve or its compression (hemifacial spasms).
  - Botulinum toxin treatment is the most effective. Other therapies include phenytoin, carbamazepine (frequently with unsatisfactory results) and surgical decompression of the facial nerve.

Generalized dystonia

- Often hereditary
- Childhood onset

Hemiballismus

- Caused by damage to the subthalamic nucleus, most commonly as a result of cerebral infarction. In such cases, the onset of symptoms is acute, and the patient is usually elderly.
- The involuntary movements affect the proximal muscles of the upper and lower extremities; the limbs are flung in a wide motion.
- Treatment: haloperidol 1–2 mg t.d.s. will provide reasonable relief. Sodium valproate 800–1200 mg/day might be effective in some cases. Generally, hemiballismus subsides within a few weeks; however, symptoms may also be continuous.

Chorea and athetosis

- Chorea denotes rapid jerky movements and athetosis denotes distal writhing, "wormlike" involuntary movements. When they occur together, the condition is called choreoathetosis.
- Choreoathetosis may be associated with cerebral palsy with basal ganglia involvement. In infancy these patients are flaccid.
- Sydenham's chorea occurs as a sequela of streptococcal infection and is an arteritis affecting the minor arteries of the basal ganglia region. The patients are children or adolescents. The disorder may be accompanied by rheumatic fever or carditis.
- Huntington's disease (formerly Huntington's chorea, see 36.25) is a dominantly inherited disease, causing dementia with onset typically at middle age. The involuntary movements vary in severity.

Restless legs

- See also 20.80.
- Restless legs cause an unpleasant sensation or pain in the lower limbs, particularly at bedtime. The patient often needs to get out of bed to walk around.
- The symptoms may be associated with iron deficiency, uraemia, pregnancy or neuropathy.
- Treatment consists of correcting possible iron deficiency, small doses of dopaminergic drugs (e.g. pramipexole, ropinirole, levodopa), gabapentin, tramadol or clonazepam.

Involuntary movements caused by medications

Levodopa

- In patients with long-standing Parkinson's disease levodopa may cause choreoathetoid movements (36.72) and painful muscle cramps (dystonias).

Antipsychotic drugs

- The use of antipsychotics, i.e. neuroleptics, (including antivertigo drugs) is associated with several types of movement disorders.
- Acute dystonia develops at the beginning of the drug treatment. Contortion of the extremities, head and face into unusual, even painful positions is characteristic. The condition is most common in young males.
    - Treatment
        - Anticholinergic medication; slow intravenous infusion of 5 mg of biperiden provides rapid relief; diazepam 5–10 mg i.v. will have a more delayed effect.
        - The patient should avoid the drug that caused the condition.
- Drug-induced parkinsonism (36.72) typically occurs when large doses of antipsychotics are used. The condition is dose-dependent and generally reversible.
- Akathisia is drug-induced motor restlessness; there is a compulsive need to move. Legs are particularly affected.
    - The most common agents to induce akathisia are antipsychotics (one in five users of classical neuroleptics), metoclopramide and sometimes antidepressants.
    - Akathisia must be differentiated from restless legs (see above), where the patient finds it difficult to lie down and sleep. In akathisia the patient typically walks on the spot and finds it difficult to remain in a sitting posture.
    - Reducing the dose or changing medication will relieve the symptoms. Alternative medication includes the atypical antipsychotics (risperidone, olanzapine, quetiapine, clozapine) and, of antidepressants, mirtazapine and nefazodone.
- Tardive dyskinesia is the most difficult movement disorder associated with antipsychotics, because it may become permanent. In general, the syndrome develops after years of treatment with an antipsychotic agent, but it has been described after six months of treatment. The most typical manifestations are involuntary movements around the mouth, but the limbs and trunk can also be affected. Typically, the symptoms appear or increase when the dose of the antipsychotic is decreased. The elderly and female patients are at greater risk.
    - Treatment
        - If possible, antipsychotic medication should be withdrawn. The involuntary movements will initially increase but may (C) [1] gradually disappear over several weeks.
        - The most effective treatment of tardive dyskinesia is an antipsychotic with dopamine-receptor blocking action, such as haloperidol. In long-term use, however, this drug will exacerbate the condition. Other possible treatments include reserpine, sodium valproate, propranolol, clonidine and tetrabenazine, but their effect is often unsatisfactory.
        - Botulinum toxin may be considered in some cases.
        - The most important remedy is prevention: avoidance of prolonged treatment with antipsychotics.

Other involuntary movements

- Myoclonia denotes brief muscle contractions. They may be physiological, for example jerks in the limbs at the point of falling asleep and hiccoughs (36.95). They may be familial and they may accompany several neurological disorders, such as progressive myoclonal epilepsy and Creutzfeldt-Jakob's disease. Piracetam is an effective treatment in some cases.
- A tic is a brief, compulsive movement, most often in the face or neck. It may be associated with Tourette's syndrome.
- Tremor (36.71) is also classified as a movement disorder.

Reference

1. McGrath JJ, Soares-Weiser KVS. Neuroleptic reduction and/or cessation and neuroleptics as specific treatments for tardive dyskinesia. Cochrane Database Syst Rev. 2004;(2):CD000459.

36.7 Size difference between pupils

Kati Juva

Basic rules

- First check the patient's medication, especially any eyedrops used.
- If both pupils react to light normally, a small difference in size has no clinical importance.
- Isolated size difference without any other neurological symptoms or signs does not usually require further neurological examinations.
- If you are not sure whether the difference is a new or old phenomenon, ask for old photographs for reference.
- Remember eye injury as a possible cause of size difference.

Factors causing size difference between pupils

- Adie's pupil is normal sized or slightly larger than average and reacts very slowly to light and convergence. This is a benign finding. It is often associated with the absence of several tendon reflexes (Adie syndrome).

- Paralysis of the third cranial (oculomotor) nerve causes a large pupil that does not react to light. When found in an unconscious patient it usually suggests an increase of the intracranial pressure that compresses the third cranial nerve, indicating a risk for brain herniation.
- Argyll Robertson pupil is small and does not react to light but diminishes at convergence. It is nearly always associated with syphilis.
- In Horner's syndrome the pupil is small (miosis), the upper eyelid droops (ptosis), the eye may be drawn inwards, and the perspiration of the same side of the face can be absent (anhidrosis). This is caused by a lesion of the sympathetic nerve fibres in the central nervous system: in the upper part of the thorax (e.g. apical tumour), near the carotid artery (e.g. carotid dissection) or near the eye.

36.8 Double vision (diplopia)

Kati Juva

Basic rules

- Determine
  - whether diplopia is permanent or transient, e.g. appearing only in the evenings when the patient is tired
  - whether there is double vision in all gaze positions or only when the patient is looking in a certain direction
  - are the doubled pictures besides each other or partly underneath each other?
  - are there any other symptoms or signs, e.g. ptosis?
- Patients with permanent or recurrent diplopia should often be referred to a neurologist.

Reasons for double vision

Covert strabismus

- Covert strabismus can cause double vision especially when the patient is tired.

Paresis of individual ocular muscles

- Paresis of individual ocular muscles may cause double vision when the other eye does not move normally in all gaze directions. In mild cases the doctor is not necessarily able to observe any clear paresis even though the patient reports double vision.
- The oculomotor nerve (third cranial nerve) innervates most of the muscles moving the eye and the muscles raising the upper lid and constricting the pupil.
  - In total oculomotor paresis there is
    - drooping of the upper lid (ptosis)
    - a large pupil not reacting to light
    - the eye turned downwards and outwards.
  - If there is partial paresis caused by a process compressing the nerve, the main phenomenon is a large, non-reactive pupil.
  - If the partial paresis is due to diabetic neuropathy, the pupil is usually preserved but there are difficulties in gaze movements, with double vision.
  - Doubled pictures in oculomotor paresis are partly underneath each other.
- The trochlear nerve (fourth cranial nerve) innervates the superior oblique muscle of the eye.
  - When the nerve is paralysed the patient has difficulty in looking downwards and has double vision, especially when walking down the stairs. Doubled pictures are partly on top of each other.
- The abducent nerve (sixth cranial nerve) innervates the lateral rectus muscle, and its paralysis hinders the eye from moving directly outwards.
  - The eye is turned inwards, and double vision is enhanced when looking towards the injured side.
  - The doubled pictures are beside each other.
- Aetiology of ocular muscle pareses
  - Lesions in the brain stem at the nuclei of the nerves (stroke, tumour, MS, etc.)
  - Tumour or aneurysm compressing the nerve.
  - Trauma or meningitis
    - The eye socket and sinus cavernosus are common locations for lesions.
    - Raised intracranial pressure often leads to lesions in the oculomotor and abducent nerves.
    - Mononeuropathy of the oculomotor nerve is not uncommon. Often the reason is diabetes.
  - In internuclear ophthalmoplegia there is a disconnection between the nuclei of the nerves innervating the ocular muscles. The sick eye does not move inwards, but instead makes twitching movements. In total internuclear ophthalmoplegia neither eye can move inwards from the middle line and thus the double vision is enhanced as the gaze is directed more and more laterally. Possible reasons for this can be vascular lesions or MS.

NEU

Muscle diseases

- Double vision may occur in certain muscle diseases (36.85). Seeing double pictures when one is tired can be the first symptom of myasthenia gravis (36.86). Often this is associated with drooping of the lid (ptosis). You can try to provoke myasthenia by asking the patient to look up. Normally people can do this easily for about 1.5 minutes, while in myasthenia the ptosis usually appears within a minute.

36.9 Sleep disorders

Unto Nousiainen, Esa Mervaala

Objectives

- To recognize sleep disturbances as a cause of daytime fatigue
- To exclude secondary causes of fatigue before special examinations
- To prevent health hazards or accidents caused by sleep disorders

Prevalence

- About 5% of adults suffer from chronic insomnia and about 3% from daytime fatigue.

Classification

- Insomnia (35.3)
- Excess daytime fatigue, narcolepsy
  - Fatigue caused by insomnia
  - Narcolepsy
  - Other hypersomnias
  - Sleep deprivation
- Disturbances of sleep–wake rhythm
  - Jet lag syndrome
  - Stress caused by shift work
- Parasomnias
  - Somnambulism
  - Night terrors
  - Nocturnal enuresis
  - Other parasomnias (nightmares, bruxism)

Age dependence

- Typical parasomnias in childhood include e.g. somnambulism, night terrors (pavor nocturnus) and swinging of the head (jactatio capitis).
- In adults, the most common parasomnias are snoring, nightmares and speaking in sleep (often psychological background).
- Sleep apnoea (6.71) can occur at any age, but it is most common in middle age.
- Fragmentary sleep and insomnia are problems of aged persons.

Examinations

- First-line examinations
  - Patient history about the length and quality of sleep, daytime tiredness and occurrence of sleep paralysis (sleep diary) (29.5).
  - Most sleep disturbances can be "diagnosed" on the basis of clinical symptoms.
- Sleep studies
  - Pathological abrupt sleep onset (narcolepsy) can be diagnosed in EEG. Daytime fatigue can be quantified in mean sleep latency (Multiple Sleep Latency Test) examination. The ability to sustain vigilance (i.e. full alertness) may be of crucial importance in some occupations (e.g. drivers). This can objectively be tested by Multiple Wakefullness Test (MWT).
  - In university hospitals or other specialized hospitals, sleep polygraphias and other special examinations (video telemetry, sleep profile analysis) may be performed.
  - Specific disturbances of sleep, such as narcolepsy, should be diagnosed and treated in specialized hospitals or units.

Narcolepsy

- Narcolepsy is a rare disturbance in the regulation of REM sleep. It usually begins in adolescence or early adult age, has strong association with a certain haplotype, and possibly autoimmune aetiology.
- Symptoms
  - Daytime fatigue, compulsive falling in sleep
  - Sudden loss of muscle tone (cataplexy)
  - Sleep paralysis (when falling asleep or on awakening, the patient is unable to move)
  - Hypnagogic hallucinations (auditory or visual hallucinations at the onset of sleep or on awakening); the patient knows that the phenomena are unrealistic (in contrast to a psychotic patient).
- Diagnosis
  - Clinical picture
  - Mean sleep latency (MSL) (36.16) examination confirms the diagnosis, showing shortened sleep onset with REM sleep.
- Treatment
  - Initiated in special units.
  - Psychostimulants: prolintan or phencamphamine 10–30 mg/day.
  - For cataplexy, tricyclic antidepressants may be effective (e.g. clomipramine 75–150 mg/day).
  - If possible, working conditions should be arranged so that the patient can take a short nap during the day (e.g. farmers).
  - The possibility of narcolepsy-related accidents must be taken into account e.g. in the traffic.

Jet lag

- Melatonin in the dose range 0.5–5 mg taken close to the target bedtime at the destination is effective in reducing the symptoms of jet lag (A) [1].

Reference

1. Herxheimer A, Petrie KJ. Melatonin for the prevention and treatment of jet lag. Cochrane Database Syst Rev. 2004;(2):CD001520.

36.10 Fatigued or tired patient

Markku Ellonen

Aims

- Clarify what the patient means by fatigue.
- Exclude somatic diseases.
- Recognize sleep disorders (6.71) and depression as possible causes.
- Recognize the mental problems of a person suffering from burnout.
- Encourage a patient who is recovering slowly from an infectious disease, but do not neglect follow-up.
- Temporary stress, tiredness and depression belong to the normal course of life.
- Be alert when a patient who is "always well" presents with fatigue –the underlying cause can be a serious disease.

Basic rules

- Physical illness or recovery from it can cause fatigue exhaustion, or lack of energy but usually more specific symptoms are also associated with it. Fatigue correlates with the psychosocial trouble caused by an illness.
- Stress is the attempt to adjust to loading. If adjustment is unsuccessful, burnout follows.
- Burnout (44.25) is caused by experienced stress at work. Burnout does not usually result from much work, but from poor control over one's work or from work that conflicts with the employee's personality.
- Chronic fatigue syndrome is a descriptive name for a syndrome affecting functional capacity that likely has several causes, both physical and mental.
- A depressed patient may talk of "tiredness/fatigue" but actually means that he/she is depressed. Other symptoms of depression include apathy, melancholic state of mind, sleep disturbances, anxiety and eating disorders.
- Normal ageing alone does not cause fatigue. Performance levels of the ageing individuals must be compared with others of the same age.

Common diseases and situations causing fatigue or tiredness

- Assess whether the fatigue symptom is caused by
    - a physical illness or convalescence
    - a psychological disturbance, or psychosocial problem
    - tiredness during the day resulting from sleep disorders
    - burnout
    - effects of drugs, both normal and adverse.
- Inquire important disease-specific symptoms, as subsequent investigations will be based on them. (Fatigue is such a common symptom that when present alone it is an almost useless symptom in diagnostics.)
    - Hypothyroidism: chill, slowness, dryness of skin (changes in these properties) and mental lethargy
    - Hyperthyroidism: sweating, weight loss, muscle fatigue, physical weakness
    - Diabetes: thirst, polyuria, weight loss
    - Anaemias: reduced tolerance for physical strain, if severe
    - Infections: fever, weight loss, focal symptoms
    - Malignancies: weight loss, pain, focal symptoms; sometimes paraneoplastic fatigue without other symptoms (e.g. hyponatraemia)
    - Heart failure: fatigue following physical exercise, dyspnoea on exertion, tachycardia
    - Fibromyalgia: chronic, diffuse pain and tender points, disturbed sleep, mild depression, etc.
    - Side effects of drugs: medications for neurological and psychiatric illnesses, hypnotics. Always bear in mind that a psychiatric patient can also have a somatic disease.
    - Metabolic effects of medications: hypokalaemia, hyponatraemia, dehydration

Laboratory examinations

- Benefits are limited when fatigue is the only symptom. The aim is to exclude physical diseases.
- Blood count, ESR, serum TSH, free T4, ALT, creatinine, basic urine tests, blood glucose, electrolytes. If haemoglobin and ESR values are borderline, compare them with the patient's earlier values; the change may be significant.
- If a somatic illness still seems possible, the scope of examinations may be expanded: e.g. serum creatinine, ECG, chest x-ray.
- Explain to the patient that examinations are ordered to exclude diseases, and that negative findings should not be considered a disappointment. Ask your patient if the cause of tiredness could be something else than a disease and what disease he/she would suspect. Continue the evaluation of the psychosocial context if the results are all normal.

Chronic fatigue syndrome (CFS) and principles of therapy

- Chronic fatigue syndrome is a poorly understood and unspecific diagnostic entity, and its existence continues to be debated.
- The preceding event is often an infection that the patient does not recover from, and the fatigue continues for more than 6 months. After that the symptoms are mainly somatic.

- The diagnosis can be made when at least four of the following symptoms are present:
  - Experienced memory impairment
  - Throat pain
  - Tender lymph nodes
  - Muscle pain
  - Joint pain
  - Headache
  - Unrefreshing sleep
  - Malaise after physical activity lasting for more than 24 hours.
- Diagnosis requires the exclusion of physical and psychotic mental diseases. Also the patient must not have dementia, alcoholism, anorexia, bulimia or severe obesity.
- A specific infectious aetiology or endocrinological explanation for the syndrome has been sought. The phenomenon is heterogeneous, often mood-associated and debated.
- Cognitive behavioural therapy B [1 2 3 4 5 6 7 8 9 10 11] combined with medical follow-up and patient education has been effective.
- Physical activity has also abolished fatigue.
- Starting therapy with antidepressive medication readily for a tired patient may be a tempting alternative; however, this approach may lead to neglect in the assessment of the patient's life situation and somatic symptoms. On the other hand, endless examinations for excluding diseases may prevent the treatment of fatigue and depression.
- A working group report on CFS that appeared in 2002, has been criticized for being unscientific; however, patient organizations have been pleased ("finally it is acknowledged that CFS is a real disease that can affect anyone").
- The common concept, however, is that it is a problem with multiple aetiologies, mostly psychosocial. The danger in medicalizing the condition is that the patient's real problems are not solved. Endless investigations should be stopped, and the consultation should become a positive, supportive meeting, as has been the practice with fibromyalgia patients. Patient organizations have reservations regarding straightforward application of cognitive psychotherapy and physical exercise.

Examination strategy

- Fatigue/tiredness alone is a general symptom and does not usually help in diagnostics. The absence of fatigue may be an important piece of information.
- If tiredness is the only symptom, exclusion of the most common diseases is an adequate approach.
- If disease seems unlikely, ask the patient to consider if the cause of fatigue could lie somewhere else; with this you can begin to evaluate the patient's psychosocial situation.
- Patients who are always tired and often visit the doctor should be examined carefully once and then supported to live their difficult circumstances. Tonics may help, although medical evidence of their effectiveness is limited.
- Follow-up is a practical way of managing patients who recover slowly from viral infections.
- Always consider carefully the personality of the patient complaining of fatigue/tiredness, and try to evaluate what is his/her way of coping with changes in life. Be particularly careful with patients who rarely visit a doctor, as even vague symptoms should be considered potential signs of a serious disease.

References

1. Price JR, Couper J. Cognitive behaviour therapy for chronic fatigue syndrome in adults. Cochrane Database Syst Rev. 2004;(2):CD001027.
2. NHS Centre for Reviews, Dissemination. Interventions for the management of CFS/ME. York: Centre for Reviews and Dissemination. 2002. 12. Centre for Reviews and Dissemination (CRD).
3. Defining and managing chronic fatigue syndrome. Rockville, MD: Agency for Healthcare Research and Quality (AHRQ). 2001. Agency for Healthcare Research and Quality (AHRQ).
4. NHS Centre for Reviews, Dissemination. The effectiveness of interventions used in the treatment/management of chronic fatigue syndrome and/or myalgic encephalomyelitis in adults and children. York: Centre for Reviews and Dissemination. 2002. 118. Centre for Reviews and Dissemination (CRD).
5. Dolors Estrada M. Chronic fatigue syndrome. Barcelona: Catalan Agency for Health Technology Assessment and Research (CAHTA). 2001. 62. Catalan Agency for Health Technology Assessment and Research (CAHTA).
6. Health Technology Assessment Database: HTA-20020386. The Cochrane Library, Issue 1, 2004. Chichester, UK: John Wiley & Sons, Ltd.
7. Health Technology Assessment Database: HTA-20020325. The Cochrane Library, Issue 1, 2004. Chichester, UK: John Wiley & Sons, Ltd.
8. Health Technology Assessment Database: HTA-20030028. The Cochrane Library, Issue 1, 2004. Chichester, UK: John Wiley & Sons, Ltd.
9. Health Technology Assessment Database: HTA-20010129. The Cochrane Library, Issue 1, 2004. Chichester, UK: John Wiley & Sons, Ltd.
10. Ross S D, Levine C, Ganz N, Frame D, Estok R, Stone L, Ludensky V. Systematic review of the current literature related to disability and chronic fatigue syndrome. Rockville, MD: Agency for Healthcare Research and Quality (AHRQ). 2002. Agency for Healthcare Research and Quality (AHRQ).
11. Health Technology Assessment Database: HTA-20030464. The Cochrane Library, Issue 1, 2004. Chichester, UK: John Wiley & Sons, Ltd.

36.15 Clinical use of neuroradiological imaging

Editors

Skull x-ray

- No longer used for imaging skull injuries, as it does not rule out cerebral pathology.

- In children skull x-ray reveals craniosynostosis, the premature fusion of the sutures.

Plain x-ray of the spine

- In neurological diseases significant findings include
  - narrowing of the spinal canal (most commonly posterior osteophytes)
  - narrowing or enlargement (neurinoma) of intervertebral foramen and destruction of vertebral bone.
- Determination of postural faults, such as scoliosis, continues to be based on plain radiographs.
- Plain chest x-rays do not rule out spinal canal processes, but they are necessary for planning further tests: magnetic resonance imaging (MRI) and computed tomography (CT). Myelography is no longer used routinely.

Computed tomography

- This is the primary examination for most brain processes.
  - CT is the best and most rapid method for identifying or excluding intracranial haemorrhages and for differential diagnosis between haemorrhage and infarction.
- Contrast medium enhancement adds accuracy to the diagnosis, if the disease process involves blood-brain barrier damage or abnormal neovascularisation (neoplasms, etc.).
- The CT scan is suitable for studying spinal canal processes only if the exact level of the lesion is known.
- CT is not useful for longitudinal imaging of the vertebral canal: it lasts too long, the radiation exposure is too high, and the lesion may be located between the scanned layers.

Magnetic resonance imaging (MRI)

- Does not cause ionizing radiation.
- Produces image planes of different orientations. The procedure is suitable for longitudinal examination of the vertebral canal, and often yields more information on the brain than CT.
- MRI is suitable for
  - brain stem and occipital lobe imaging
  - verifying demyelination changes
  - verifying neoplasms.
- Magnetic angiography can be used to visualize blood vessels C [1,2]. It is suited for screening for aneurysms in SAH families.
- Contraindications
  - Pacemaker and other implanted electronic devices
  - Intracorporeal magnetizing metal objects (older aneurysm clips), metallic inner ear prostheses
  - Claustrophobia

Digital subtraction angiography (DSA) and traditional angiographies

- DSA is the method of choice in both neuro- and other angiographies.
- Contrast medium is administered into the artery.
- Conventional film-based (cine) angiography is used only in hospitals where DSA equipment is not available.
- Most neuroradiological angiographies require admitting the patient to the hospital.
- Indications for carotid artery angiography:
  - When endarterectomy is planned due to the stenosis of carotid artery.
  - SAH, suspected aneurysm
  - Suspected arteritis or other cerebrovascular disease
  - Investigation of the vascularisation of a known brain tumour or arterio-venous (AV) malformation before surgery.
- Indications for vertebral angiography
  - In principle these are the same as those for carotid angiography, when the lesion is located in the region of vertebrobasilar circulation in the occipital fossa.
  - The risk of complications is clearly greater than with carotid angiography, and the examination can only be performed on young patients (ca 50 years or less).
- Indications for aortic arch angiography
  - Investigating carotid artery stenoses (often detected by ultrasound) in patients with TIA or cerebral infarction in cases where the patient is eligible for operative treatment. For criteria, see TIA 36.30.
  - Suspected Takayasu's disease or subclavian steal syndrome.
- All mentioned angiography examination carry ca 1% risk of stroke.

Ultrasound and Doppler examination of carotid arteries

- Non-invasive procedure for detecting carotid artery stenoses and changes in the arterial walls.

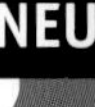

- When the examination is performed by an experienced practitioner, the results correlate well with angiographic findings.
- The procedure is used
  - to select patients for aortic arch angiography
  - to provide orientation into the status of the carotid arteries in patients in whom angiography is contra-indicated
  - before coronary surgery.

Echoencephalography

- In infants with open fontanels, real-time echography is a frequently used method of brain structure imaging.
- Used to detect peri- and intraventricular haemorrhages in neonates and to evaluate the amount of CSF in cerebral ventricles in case of hydrocephalus suspicion.

Radioisotope investigations

Single photon emission computed tomography (SPECT imaging)

- Based on identifying circulatory variations in different sections of the brain with radioisotopic markers (IMP, HM-PAO).
- This method is in a developmental stage, but can be utilized
  - to identify early cerebral infarctions
  - to differentiate between Alzheimer's disease (bilateral degeneration in the temporal and parietal lobes) and vascular dementia (uneven isotope distribution)
  - to identify early Herpes simplex encephalitis.

Positron emission tomography (PET)

- The clinical applications of this method are mainly Alzheimer's disease and epilepsy.
- Allows to measure quantitatively the location and amount of metabolites in the brain, and print out 2-dimensional images.

References

1. Kallmes DF, Omary RA, DIx JE, Evans AJ, Hillman BJ. Specificity of MR angiography as a confirmatory test in carotid artery stenosis. Am J Neuroradiol 1996;17:1501–1506.
2. The Database of Abstracts of Reviews of Effectiveness (University of York), Database no.: DARE-961623. In: The Cochrane Library, Issue 4, 1999. Oxford: Update Software.

36.16 Clinical use of neurophysiological tests

Editors

Basic rules

- The methods used are objective, functional tests of the various levels of the nervous system.
- There are no contraindications or age limitations.
- Some neurophysiological tests are painful and relatively expensive. Their use for screening is not justified.
- Most often, a sensible selection of tests for the neurological patient is a combination of neurophysiological, neuroradiological, and other tests, after the neurological malfunction has been initially localized and characterized through history taking and physical examination.

EEG, electroencephalography

- Indications for use are
  - seizures, suspected epilepsy
  - encephalitis
  - delirium, dementia (rarely).
- Sleep EEG is indicated if the patient's EEG is normal when awake, but there is a clinically strong suspicion of epilepsy (e.g. temporal epilepsy). In sleep deprivation EEG the patient is kept awake through the preceding night, which may activate epileptic phenomena.
- QEEG (quantitative EEG): The signal is processed with a computer.
- Antiepileptic medication is not discontinued for the EEG test. Benzodiazepines, however, should be avoided before the test.

ENMG, electroneuromyography

- ENMG is a test designed for the peripheral nervous system, myoneural junction, and muscle cells. It is not applicable for the central nervous system (with the exception of tremor analysis).
- The test includes measuring nerve conduction velocity and spinal reflexes during stimulation with electrodes as well as examining electric muscle activity with a needle inserted in the muscle.
- In order to avoid excessive patient discomfort, the number of muscles to be tested should be reasonable, and the referral should include a clear clinical question or diagnostic hypothesis, such as the location of the suspected nerve entrapment.
- Denervation changes in the muscle develop in ca. 2–3 weeks from the injury to the peripheral nerve. An ENMG is generally not advisable before that time. ENMG is not a primary examination for conditions requiring urgent care, such as increasing weakness in the lower extremities. If muscle disease is suspected, the muscle enzyme levels should be measured before the ENMG examination, because the test will increase the enzyme levels.
- Indications for the test
  - Motor neurone diseases (ALS)
  - Nerve root injury, polyradiculitis
  - Nerve plexus injury, such as plexus neuritis
  - Polyneuropathy, mononeuropathy
  - Pressure injury, transection, or entrapment of a peripheral nerve
  - Myasthenia gravis, myasthenic syndrome (require tetanization and single-fibril EMG or both, the need for which should be disclosed in the referral)
  - Muscle diseases

Evoked potential tests

SEP (Somatosensory Evoked Potential)

- Obtained by averaging neural responses generated by sensory stimuli.

- Usually the saphenus nerve SEP is measured in the lower extremity and the median nerve SEP in the upper extremity.
- Test indications are of the CNS diseases such as MS and certain degenerative conditions and spinal chord injuries.

BAEP (Brainstem Auditory Evoked Potential)

- Obtained by averaging the responses generated by auditory stimuli, describes the auditory pathway.
- Nowadays this investigation is largely being replaced by MRI.
- Test indications are
  - suspected acoustic neurinoma
  - suspected brain stem injury.

VEP (Visual Evoked Potential)

- Obtained by averaging the responses generated in the visual cortex by displaying a varying chessboard image.
- Test indications are
  - suspected visual pathway injury
  - suspected inflammation of the optic nerve and MS.

Long-term recording

Long-term recording of the EEG (ambulatory EEG, EEG tape recorder)

- Recorded on a portable tape recorder over a longer period, for example at the patient's home.
- The purpose of the test is to obtain a recording of the seizure as it occurs.

EEG videotelemetry

- The electric activity of the patient's brain and other biosignals (such as the ECG and EMG) are recorded on multiple channels with simultaneous video image of the patient seen on the same screen.
- The test enables to analyse the symptoms accurately on the basis of biosignals recorded in relation to time and place.

Sleep studies

- The polygraphic MSLT (Multiple Sleep Latency Test) is designed for studying the daytime sleepiness of a subject who is allowed to fall asleep 4 times at 2-hour intervals.
- Static charge sensitive bed for recording the patient's movements, such as breathing, during the night; suitable for screening for the sleep apnoea syndrome.
- Polysomnography includes, in addition to the static charge sensitive bed, monitoring blood oxygen with oxymetry, EEG, ECG, and possibly other recordings.

36.17 Lumbar puncture, examination of cerebrospinal fluid and findings

Editors

On duty examination of CSF

- A general practitioner usually has to perform a lumbar puncture only in an emergency setting.

Indications

- Bacterial meningitis (36.56) (necessary)
  - If the patient has neurologic deficit symptoms or impaired consciousness, neurological imaging should be performed before lumbar puncture. If necessary, antibiotic treatment can be commenced after a blood culture sample has been obtained.
- Viral meningitis (36.56)
- Neuroborreliosis (1.29)
- Other infectious or inflammatory CNS diseases
- CT is the primary diagnostic procedure for SAH. Lumbar puncture is indicated if the CT is negative and there is a clinical probability of SAH (5% of cases). A normal finding on CT does not rule out SAH.
- Lumbar puncture may be performed in order to rule out SAH in a situation where a CT scan is not available and the patient's condition is good.

Contraindications

- Suspected **increased intracranial pressure** (risk of cerebellar herniation!)
  - Papilloedema
  - Symptoms such as morning headache, vomiting, impaired consciousness (36.96)
- In unclear situations, such as lack of patient cooperation that prevents the examination of eye fundi, CT of the head is indicated before lumbar puncture.

Relative contraindications

- If the patient is scheduled to undergo myelography shortly (although myelography is rarely performed nowadays), the CSF specimen may be taken in connection with it. Lumbar puncture performed before myelography may cause a haematoma, which may affect the performance and interpretation of myelography.
- Anticoagulant therapy or other bleeding tendency.

On duty lumbar puncture, consider the following:

- If meningitis is suspected, culture the sample in a special dish (procure the necessary dish in advance) or, in a case

NEU

of emergency, in a blood culture bottle, and keep part of the sample for bacterial staining.

- Take an extra tube of CSF to be stored in the laboratory refrigerator for possible further tests.
- Time of the lumbar puncture and its performance need to be documented in the medical records as also any problems and artefact blood, as the latter may lead to a false suspicion of SAH and consequent unnecessary examinations.
- If the patient is sent home soon after the lumbar puncture, he/she must be told to anticipate possible post-puncture headache and how to treat it.

Suggestions for technical performance of lumbar puncture

- The puncture is normally made between L3–L4 or L4–L5, either above or below the level of the iliac crest.
- Check the patient's position yourself.
- The most common error is to have the spine twisted instead of only being bent forward.
- Palpate carefully and make sure where to puncture.
- Local anaesthesia helps also the person performing the puncture: the anaesthesia needle can be used to find the correct location and direction of the puncture. A patient who does not feel pain will remain still during the lumbar puncture.
- If there is scar formation from a previous back operation, the tissue will be harder than normal, and a thicker needle should be used to avoid bending.
- The puncture may be technically impossible to perform if the patient is very obese, has a history of lumbar bone grafting or has severe spinal stenosis.

Herniation of the cerebellum after lumbar puncture

- Extremely rare.
- Immediately or a few hours after the puncture the patient loses consciousness, his/her respiration becomes irregular and ceases.
- Maintain vital functions, usually respiration; the heart will function.
- Adjust the bed into the steep Trendelenburg's position (supine position with pelvis higher than the head).
- Administer mannitol intravenously.
- Consult a neurosurgeon.

Post-punctional headache

- Probably caused by loss of CSF pressure in the head.
- The onset of headache is more related to the amount of fluid leaking extradurally after the puncture than the amount of fluid withdrawn as a sample. Bedrest after puncture does not prevent headache (A) [1 2].
- Patients with a history of headache or MS are more susceptible to prolonged (1–2 weeks) postpunctional headaches.
- Post-punctional headache occurs less often if a Pencil-point needle is used; however, its use needs some training.
- Caffeine i.v. infusion is normally tried at hospital before the application of blood patch.

Treatment

- Bed rest relieves the pain and is generally all that is needed (sick leave is necessary).
- Pain medications are fairly ineffective.
- For nausea, prochlorperazine is suitable.
- Blood patch: The patient's own blood is injected into the puncture area following a codeine infusion. This procedure requires sterile operating-room conditions and is generally effective (consult an anaesthesiologist or a neurosurgeon if severe pain persists for more than 3 weeks).

HSF analysis

- Normally colourless, clear
- Opaque → bacterial meningitis
- Evenly bloody, liquid, yellow after centrifugation (xanthochromia) → haemorrhage
- Yellow → old haemorrhage, very high protein concentration. Occasionally this kind of spinal fluid is coagulated. It can be examined by heating to 37°C.
- The fluid is coagulated, streaked with blood; bloody, but later clear, colourless after centrifugation → artefact blood
- CSF findings are listed in Table 36.17.

Cells

Erythrocytes

- See 36.32.
- Normal: 0
- 0–1000: frequently artefact, but may be caused by a disorder involving slight haemorrhage (infarct, encephalitis, etc.)
- 1000 → 100 000: haemorrhage

Relative concentrations of albumin in spinal fluid and serum

- Measure the blood-brain barrier function.
- The spinal fluid/serum antibody concentration ratio related to the spinal fluid/serum albumin ratio measures antibody synthesis within the central nervous system.

CSF IgG index

- Increased in MS, but may also rise in many inflammatory and infectious conditions.

Oligoclonal IgG bands

- Present in ca. 90% of MS patients and in nearly all patients with subacute sclerosing panencephalitis (SSPE) or meningovascular syphilis.

Table 36.17 CSF findings

	Normal CSF	Pathological findings	Other comments
Erythrocytes	0	0–1000 in mildly haemorrhagic disturbance (infarction, encephalitis, etc.) 1000 → 100 000 in haemorrhage	The result 1–1000 is often an artefact
Leucocytes	0–3/mm^3	4–100/mm^3 in MS, tumour, slow CNS infarctions, sarcoidosis, meningeal irritation from general infection, viral meningitis (beginning) 100–1000/mm^3 in virus meningitis or other serous meningitis, listeria meningitis, slow CNS infection >1000 mm^3 in bacterial meningitis	Laboratory states the percentage of polymorphonuclear and mononuclear leucocytes. In cell count malignant cells can be interpreted as leucocytes. Their accurate interpretation requires pathoanatomical diagnosis.
Glucose	2.2–4.2 mmol/l (about half of blood glucose level)	**Elevated in**: diabetes, during glucose-containing infusion. **Diminished in**: infection, (bacteria, tuberculosis, fungus), sarcoidosis.	
Protein	150–450 mg/l	**Diminished**: no practical implications. **Elevated**: high blood protein concentration (e.g. myeloma), damage of the blood–brain barrier (e.g. CSF blockage), increased CNS antibody synthesis (e.g. MS); diabetes. In the elderly, protein concentration can be increased without pathology; infarction of the brain; haemorrhage, tumours, polyradiculitis, meningitis, encephalitis, disturbance in the circulation of CSF, several degenerative diseases.	

TPHA (treponemal haemagglutination assay)

- Most frequently used test for identifying syphilis from CSF.

Exfoliated cells in CSF (PAD)

- Provides somewhat varying information depending on the laboratory techniques used.
- Findings
  - Malignant cells are found in meningeal carcinomatosis (several samples may be required) and in CNS leukaemia, but rarely in connection with primary brain neoplasms.
  - Post-haemorrhage: the first to appear are erythrophages followed by siderophages (even up to 6 months).
  - Plasma cells indicate immune response within the CNS as, for example, in MS; a more common finding in MS is the so-called lymphoid reaction.
  - Lipophages indicate brain tissue damage.
  - With CNS infections, independent of the cause, there are three phases in the cellular representation of CSF:
    - neutrophilic or exudative phase
    - lymphocytic or proliferative phase
    - mononuclear or phagocytic phase.

References

1. Allen C, Glasziou P, Del Mar C. Bed rest: a potentially harmful treatment needing more careful evaluation. Lancet 1999;354:1229–1233.
2. The Database of Abstracts of Reviews of Effectiveness (University of York), Database no.: DARE-999726. In: The Cochrane Library, Issue 2, 2001. Oxford: Update Software.

36.20 Memory disorders and dementia

Timo Erkinjuntti

NEU

- Examination of a patient with memory impairment (36.21).

Definition

- Dementia is cognitive impairment due to an organic cause that limits the patient's social and professional activities.
  - Dementia is a clinical diagnosis made on the basis of adequate examination by a physician who knows the patient.
  - Dementia may be progressive (e.g. Alzheimer's disease), permanent sequela (e.g. brain damage), or treatable (36.22).

Symptoms

- Memory impairment (inability to acquire new information and to recall previously learned)

- Cognitive impairment manifested by at least one of the following:
  - Aphasia (language disturbance)
  - Apraxia (inability to carry out motor activities despite intact sensory function)
  - Agnosia (failure to recognize or identify objects despite intact sensory function)
  - Disturbance in executive functioning (i.e. planning, organisation, sequencing, abstracting).
- In dementia consciousness is not impaired, although patients with dementia have a higher risk of delirium. Delirium is vital in differential diagnosis, as it requires urgent treatment.

Dementia classified by severity

- **Mild**
  - Although the ability to work and social competence are markedly deteriorated, the patient is still capable of independent living and moderate judgment.
- **Moderate severity**
  - The patient's ability to function independently is threatened, and some degree of supervision is necessary.
  - In most patients the ability to drive a car has deteriorated.
  - Legal competence is compromized.
- **Severe**
  - The patient's daily activities are affected to such an extent that continuous supervision is required.

The epidemiology of dementia

Occurrence

- An individual may have a dementing illness at any age after maturation, but its prevalence increases with age.
- Among people aged 65–74, 4% suffer from moderate or severe dementia; in the 75–84 age group, 11%; and among those 85 and older, 35%.
- Among all people aged 65 or over, 30% are affected by a mild memory impairment.

Types

- Alzheimer's disease, 60–70% (36.24)
- Alzheimer's disease and vascular factors, 10%
- Vascular dementias, 15–20% (36.23)
- Other causes of dementia, 10% (36.22) (36.25)
- Treatable causes of dementia, 5–10%; these are most prevalent in younger age groups.

Survival

- Alzheimer's disease, 10–12 years
- Vascular dementia, 5–7 years

Normal ageing and memory

- In individuals free of disorders affecting the central nervous system age-related changes in cognitive functions are minor, and they have an insignificant impact on the patient's activities of daily living or social interactions.
- A normal elderly person is capable of learning, albeit more slowly, and thus is not "senile".
- The normal ageing process involves slight deterioration in functions such as
  - learning
  - speed of cognitive processes
  - abstract thinking requiring flexibility
  - memory capacity.

Differential diagnostics of memory disorders

- Normal ageing
- Isolated memory disorders (amnesias)
- Other neuropsychological disorders (such as aphasia or apraxia) (36.28)
- Psychiatric disorders
- Acute confusional state (delirium)
- Mental retardation
- Dementia

Causes of memory disorders

- Causes of transient memory disorders
  - Transient ischaemic attack–TIA
  - Global amnesia (36.4)
  - Minor brain injuries
  - Epileptic seizures
  - Medications
  - Stimulants
  - Psychiatric causes
  - Acute confusional state (delirium)
- Treatable causes of memory disorders are mostly identical to those of treatable dementia (36.22). Progressive memory disorders are caused by
  - Alzheimer's disease (36.24)
  - vascular dementias (36.23)
  - other conditions leading to dementia (36.25).

Psychiatric disorders and memory

- Memory impairment is associated with several psychiatric disorders. These include
  - mood disorders: depression, anxiety
  - burnout
  - schizophrenic and other psychoses.
- Depression, anxiety, and other psychiatric factors may also aggravate memory disorders with other causes.
- Memory disturbances associated with functional psychiatric disorders are generally minor: impaired attention and concentration, increased interference, and diminished capacity

for memory overload. Depression, however, may be associated with more severe memory disturbances, although these are rarely as widespread and incapacitating as in dementia (so-called pseudo-dementia).

- Depression with obvious memory impairment often includes the following characteristics that differentiate it from dementia:
  - Previous psychiatric disorders
  - The onset of symptoms can often be determined.
  - The symptoms are of brief duration, and they progress rapidly.
  - The patient's awareness of illness and emotional sensitivity are heightened.
  - The patient gives answers such as "I don't know" and has selective memory gaps with both recent and earlier memories forgotten.
- Treatment trial should be initiated as soon as depression or any other mood disorder is suspected.

36.21 Examination of patients with memory disorders and dementia

Timo Erkinjuntti

When should dementia be suspected?

- Dementia should be suspected in the following circumstances:
  - The patient or family members express concern about his/her impaired memory or other mental capacities, even when his/her social skills are unchanged.
  - The patient's independence is diminishing, and his/her need for assistance is growing.
  - The patient repeatedly forgets appointments, clearly has difficulty following treatment instructions, or is using available health services more often or inappropriately.
  - The patient is depressed or anxious and complains of cognitive symptoms.
  - The patient feels acutely confused.
  - During the consultation, a change in the patient's mental acuity arouses the physician's or nurse's suspicion ("a peculiar, strange patient").

Scheduling of tests for the patient with memory disorder

1. Symptom diagnosis (Does the patient really have a memory disorder or dementia?)
2. Identifying treatable causes
3. Identifying secondary factors contributing to the patient's performance

Assessment of functional capacity

- In symptom diagnostics, the assessment of functional capacity is crucial.

Mental or cognitive capacity

- Mini-Mental State Examination (MMSE) is a brief tool for measuring intellectual capacity. It should be noted, however, that the results can be affected by the patient's level of education and linguistic problems.
- For the assessment of mental capacity a more comprehensive neuropsychological examination is useful (36.28). Specific indications for this examination include evaluation of work disability or rehabilitation, differential diagnostics (specific disorder, depression), and assessment of legal competence in problem situations involving new, particularly younger patients. In mild and incipient disorders, repeating the examination in 6–12 months often helps to establish the diagnosis.

Social skills

- Among the daily activities to be assessed are bathing, feeding, dressing, walking, using the toilet, and continence (ADL or Activities of Daily Living). More complicated activities (IADL or Instrumental Activities of Daily Living) include the ability to use the telephone, shopping, cooking, housework, going out, and managing medications and personal finances. Several brief tests have been developed for the assessment of ADL and IADL functions (22.21).
- The assessment of the patient's social skills is often based on interviews with the patient and a family member as well as on reports from housekeeping or home health service staff.

Mood factors

- Depression can be identified by interviewing and observing the patient. Occasionally, the depression is "masked", in which case the symptoms consist of mental impairment or somatic symptoms. In such cases certainty is possible only through trial treatment and monitoring. In unclear cases the patient should be directed to a psychiatric examination.

Basic tests for patients with memory disorders

- Elicit history, interview family members, and obtain medical records.
- Assess mental capacity clinically: brief screening test, e.g. Mini-Mental State Examination (MMSE).
- Evaluate social skills and mood factors.
- Perform a general and neurological examination
  - Normal neurological status is common at the onset of Alzheimer's disease.
  - Unilateral symptoms (weakness on one side, abnormal Romberg test, increased tendon reflexes, positive Babinski's sign), and bulbar findings (dysarthria, dysphagia,

compulsive crying and laughter), as well as extrapyramidal symptoms (increased muscle tone, short-step gait) are indications of vascular dementias.
  - Extrapyramidal symptoms, frequently accompanied by tremor, indicate Parkinson's disease.
  - Apraxic gait is an indication of normal-pressure hydrocephalus or subcortical vascular dementia.
  - Myoclonus, frequently in connection with other status abnormalities, is an indication of Creutzfeldt–Jakob's disease.
  - Involuntary movements indicate Huntington's disease. These are also found in Parkinson's disease patients on drug treatment.
- Basic tests
  - Blood tests, serum potassium, serum sodium, blood glucose, serum calcium, serum creatinine, serum ALT, serum TSH, serum vitamin B_{12}
  - Basic brain imaging: CT scan (or MRI) of head
  - Complementary tests as needed in each case
    - Erythrocyte sedimentation rate, serum glutamyl transferase, serum alkaline phosphatase, serum cholesterol, free serum thyroxine, folate, TPHA, HIV antibodies, Borrelia antibodies, urinalysis, heavy metals in urine, drug screening.
- If the cause of the memory disorder is not evident the patient should be referred to a neurology clinic for further tests.

36.22 Treatable causes of dementia and memory disorder

Timo Erkinjuntti

Aims

- Identify incipient dementia and treatable causes of dementia in time, recognize dementia caused by drugs (benzodiazepines) and alcohol.
- Treat these patients before their mental capacity reaches a stage of permanent impairment.

Pseudodementia

- Bear in mind the possibility of depression as the cause of dementia-like symptoms (36.20). Trial of treatment should be readily undertaken.

Hypothyroidism

- Dementia in the elderly may disguise other symptoms of hypothyroidism.

Hyper- and hypocalcaemia

- Serum calcium concentration may be only slightly higher even when the patient is profoundly demented. Ionised calcium is a better marker of the body's calcium balance.
- The rate of occurrence of hyperparathyroidism in the elderly is ca. 4%.
- An increase in serum parathyroid hormone concentration is a sign of parathyroid adenoma.
- Some patients will benefit from surgery.
- Manifestations of hypoparathyroidism include, in addition to memory impairment and dementia symptoms, also epileptic seizures, ataxia, and muscle spasms.

Vitamin B_{12} deficiency

- Mental capacity impairment has been found in 25% of patients.
- Symptoms may precede changes in blood tests or appear without any changes in blood tests.

Chronic subdural haematoma

- The majority of these patients are elderly.
- One-half of them present with symptoms of memory impairment or confusion.
- The trauma may have occurred several months earlier. Some of the patients may not be aware of any head injury.
- Bilateral subdural haematoma in particular does not necessarily include unilateral neurological symptoms, nor is it always visible in the CT scan.
- Treatment consists of neurosurgical removal of the haematoma; however, if the haematoma is less than 1 cm in thickness, monitoring of resorption is frequently sufficient.

Normal-pressure hydrocephalus (NPH)

- Partial disruption in the circulation of the cerebrospinal fluid. The condition may develop as a delayed complication of meningitis, encephalitis, subarachnoidal haemorrhage, brain injuries, and brain surgery. In some cases the cause is unclear.
- NPH symptoms include progressive memory impairment and dementia, apractic gait, urinary incontinence, rigidity, and occasionally spasticity and increased tendon reflexes.
- Surgical shunting can relieve the symptoms in some patients.

Vitamin B_1 (thiamine) deficiency

- Thiamine deficiency can cause Wernicke's syndrome, which includes eye movement dysfunction, ataxia, and memory impairment (36.73).

Infections

- Even today, cases of dementia caused by tertiary syphilis are found (12.3).
- Dementia may occur as a sequela of suppurative or tuberculous meningitis.
- Memory impairment and dementia may be symptoms of immune deficiency disorders.
- The Borrelia burgdorferi spirochete may cause chronic encephalitis and dementia (36.57) (1.29).

Uraemia

- In addition to memory impairment, personality changes, apathy, flapping tremor, muscle twitching, and spasms are typical to uraemia.

Liver diseases

- The accumulation of toxic substances in the brain is a generally recognized cause of hepatic encephalopathy.
- The blood ammonia concentration is increased.
- Symptoms include diminished mental capacity and also impaired consciousness and flapping tremor, among others.

Chronic pulmonary diseases

- These may cause cerebral insufficiency related to oxygen deprivation and carbon dioxide retention; however, only extremely severe pulmonary disease will cause actual dementia.

Hypoglycaemia

- Repeated and prolonged hypoglycaemic attacks may lead to permanent brain damage, memory impairment, and dementia.

Tumours

- Symptoms related to malignant tumours (e.g. gliomas and metastases) usually progress rapidly; thus the patient should be examined with appropriate urgency.
- Symptoms related to benign tumours may progress insidiously, which can cause difficulties in their differentiation from Alzheimer's disease, psychiatric conditions, or other disorders. In such cases, the tumour often resides in the frontal lobe or falx.
- With malignant tumours, dementia may also be expressed as a paraneoplastic phenomenon. In such cases the symptom is most often an indication of lung or breast cancer.

36.23 Vascular dementia

Timo Erkinjuntti

Definition

- Dementias due to various vascular factors (risk factors, stroke) affecting the brain are called vascular dementias. It is not one distinct disease, but a syndrome with various causes and clinical manifestations.
- Vascular dementia has also been called multi-infarct dementia.

Cerebrovascular disorders related to vascular dementia

- Atherothrombotic stroke
- Cardiac embolic stroke
- Lacunar infarcts
- Haemodynamic causes
- Ischaemic white matter lesions (WMLs)
- Intracranial haemorrhage
- Distinct diseases of brain vessels
- Certain haematological diseases

Clinical symptoms and signs

- Cognitive impairment emerges relatively rapidly (in days to weeks).
- Often stepwise worsening and fluctuating course of symptoms
- In a number of cases onset is insidious and symptoms progress gradually.
- Clinical findings indicating focal brain damage are often seen even in mild dementia.
  - Unilateral weakness or clumsiness
  - Bulbar signs: dysarthia and dysphagia
  - Gait disorder: hemiplegic or apraxic–ataxic
  - Often urinary incontinence
- Personality and insight are preserved relatively long. Emotional disturbances are common: anxiety, affective lability.
- The patient often has a cardio- or cerebrovascular disease.
- Abnormal laboratory findings may be related to the underlying diseases, e.g. hyperlipidaemia, diabetes.
- Brain CT and MRI show infarct(s) and/or ischaemic WMLs.
- In advanced cases slowing of EEG, and often focal abnormality.

Subtypes of vascular dementia

- Cortical vascular dementia (multi-infarct dementia) suggests atherothrombotic and cardiac embolic infarcts. In cortical

NEU

subtype, aphasia and hemiplegia with associated impairment of gait are typical.

- In subcortical (small vessel) dementia, changes in the small vessels of the brain, lacunar infarctions and ischaemic changes in the white matter dominate. Typical symptoms include speech disorder (dysarthria) and sole motor or sensory hemiplegia.

Treatment

- Impact of the treatment of risk factors (i.e. hypertension, hypotension, cardiac arrhythmias, disturbances of glucose and lipid metabolism) of cerebrovascular disorders is not fully established. However, it is likely that such treatments are of preventive significance.
- Treatment of risk factors of cerebrovascular disorders as well as secondary prevention follow the treatment guidelines of stroke. The effect of specific drugs (acetosalicylic acid (D) [1 2], dipyridamole, anticoagulants) in vascular dementia has not been ascertained in clinical studies.

References

1. Meyer JS, Rogers RL, McClintic K, Mortel KF, Lotfi J. Randomized clinical trial of daily aspirin therapy in multi-infarct dementia. A pilot study. J Am Ger Soc 1989;37:549–555.
2. Rands G, Orrel M, Spector A, Williams P. Aspirin for vascular dementia. Cochrane Database Syst Rev. 2004;(2):CD001296.

36.24 Alzheimer's disease

Raimo Sulkava

Symptoms

- Usually begins with memory disturbances: acquisition of new skills is impaired.
- Symptoms usually progress slowly and steadily, although periods of slower and faster deterioration may occur.
- Duration of the disease from first symptoms to death is approximately 12 years (range 2–20 years).

Diagnosis

- Physical findings are at first normal. Later on, the tonus of the limbs increases, the patient walks with a stoop, the gait is shuffling, and the patient loses weight.
- Laboratory values are normal.
- Head CT and MRI can be normal in the early stages; later, unspecific atrophy is found on CT. MRI may show more marked atrophy in the entorhinal cortex and the hippocampus compared with other areas.
- EEG is normal or slowed.
- The clinical diagnosis is correct in about 90% of cases. No specific laboratory marker has been found yet.
- In familial cases ApoE typing and gene analysis (presenilin genes PS1 and PS2) may be considered.

Progression of Alzheimer's disease

Mild degree

- Memory impairment (impaired ability to learn new information or to recall previously learned information)
- Perceiving the surroundings becomes difficult, and the patient gets lost easily, especially in strange surroundings.
- Sense of time is lost.
- Finding of words becomes difficult.
- Understanding complicated and abstract ideas becomes difficult.
- The patient is inactive and withdrawn.
- Sometimes the patient is depressive, paranoid or aggressive.
- Complicated household chores create problems (e.g. cooking).

Moderate degree

- Insight into the illness is lost.
- Orientation is lost.
- The patient gets lost even in familiar surroundings.
- Visual hallucinations, which are more common in dementia with Lewy bodies.
- The patient loses weight.
- There are difficulties in activities of daily living (e.g. dressing).

Severe degree

- The ability to speak and understand speech is lost.
- The limbs become stiff and the ability to walk is lost.
- The patient is incontinent.
- Epileptic seizures may occur.
- Activities of daily living are lost (dressing, bathing, toileting, feeding).

Therapy

- Preventive or curative therapy is not available.
- Donepezil (A) [1], rivastigmine (A) [2], and galantamine (A) [3] give some benefit in mild or moderate Alzheimer's disease for functional improvement and for cognitive and behavioural symptoms.
- Memantine is beneficial in moderate and severe Alzheimer's disease (B) [4].
- The combination of memantine with donepezil appears to be both useful and safe (B) [5].
- The aim of the therapy is to preserve functional capacity and delay the need for hospital treatment.
- Depression has been treated with paroxetine or citalopram 5–10 (–20) mg once daily. Antidepressants may sometimes

improve the situation, but adverse effects should be avoided. In studies, risperidone at the dose 0.25–0.5 mg × 2 has proven effective for behavioural symptoms. However, risk of stroke is increased in elderly patients with dementia.

- The functional capacity of a patient with Alzheimer's disease can often be improved for a while with surroundings that offer a suitable amount of stimulus. The supporting care of those responsible for the patient is an essential part of the therapy.
- Hormone replacement therapy (B) [6] or anti-inflammatory drugs appear not to be effective in maintaining cognitive function in Alzheimer's disease.

References

1. Birks JS, Harvey R. Donepezil for dementia due to Alzheimer's disease. Cochrane Database Syst Rev. 2004;(2):CD001190.
2. Birks J, Grimley Evans J, Iakovidou V, Tsolaki M. Rivastigmine for Alzheimer's disease. Cochrane Database Syst Rev. 2004;(2):CD001191.
3. Olin J, Schneider L. Galantamine for dementia due to Alzheimer's disease. Cochrane Database Syst Rev. 2004;(2): CD001747.
4. Areosa Sastre A, Sherriff F. Memantine for dementia. Cochrane Database Syst Rev. 2004;(2):CD003154.
5. Tariot PN, Farlow MR, Grossberg GT, et al; Memantine Study Group. Memantine treatment in patients with moderate to severe Alzheimer disease already receiving donepezil: a randomized controlled trial. JAMA 2004 Jan 21;291(3):317–24.
6. Hogervorst E, Yaffe K, Richards M, Huppert F. Hormone replacement therapy to maintain cognitive function in women with dementia. Cochrane Database Syst Rev. 2004;(2):CD003799.

36.25 Other conditions leading to dementia

Timo Erkinjuntti, Raimo Sulkava

- Slow infections of the central nervous system (36.59).

Dementia with Lewy bodies (DLB)

- Causes 10–15% of all cases of dementia.
- Lewy bodies are typically found in basal nuclei in Parkinson's disease. In DLB they are also found in the cerebral cortex. Half of the patients with DLB also exhibit cerebral changes typical to Alzheimer's disease.
- Symptoms include gradually worsening rigidity, akinesia, Parkinson-like difficulties in walking, fluctuating memory disturbances, confusion and visual hallucinations.
- Mean duration of the disease is 8 years.
- Patients with DLB are sensitive to neuroleptics and already very low doses may cause confusion and gait disturbances. Low doses of L-dopa (150–300 mg/day) may reduce these symptoms. Atypical neuroleptics (clozapine, risperidone, quetiapine) can diminish visual hallucinations and confusion. Acetylcholinesterase inhibitors (donepezil, galantamine, rivastigmine) seem to be effective for behavioral disturbances in DLB.
- Physiotherapy and walking exercises must be initiated early to maintain motor functions.

Frontotemporal dementia

- In frontotemporal dementia convolutional atrophy affects mainly the frontal and temporal lobes.
- Clinical picture resembles that of Alzheimer's disease, but frontal psyche, especially loss of inhibitions and early aphasia, are typical in frontotemporal dementia.
- Memory loss is less severe than in Alzheimer's disease.
- The disease often begins before the age of 65 years and frequently has a familial occurrence.
- Prognosis and course of disease are similar to those in Alzheimer's disease.

Huntington's disease

- Huntington's disease is an autosomal dominant hereditary disease with progressive intellectual deterioration.
- Diagnosis can be made by genetic testing.
- Symptoms usually begin in the middle age (30–50 years).
- Ataxia, choreiform movements, dementia and changes of character. The patient is often diagnosed as psychotic.

Hakola's disease

- Polycystic lipomembranotic osteodysplasia–sclerosing leucoencephalopathy is an autosomal recessive hereditary disease.
- Diagnosis can be made by genetic testing.
- The patient has cavities in e.g. ankle and wrist bones and consequent pathological fractures.
- Progressive intellectual deterioration leads to dementia. The patients have no inhibitions.
- Symptoms begin at the age of 30–40 years.

Creutzfeldt-Jakob disease

- A potentially infectious dementia caused by a prion (36.59).

Parkinson's disease

- In Parkinson's disease, especially in late phases, 15–30% of patients have dementia.

- Symptoms are usually not as widespread and severe as in Alzheimer's diseases.
- It may be difficult to distinguish dementia from depression and bradykinesia.

36.27 Treatment of dementia

Raimo Sulkava

Supportive measures in ambulatory care

- It is most important to support those who care for the patient at home. Patients with progressive dementia who live alone soon need institutionalized care (hospital or a home for the aged) if not supported adequately (22.30).
- Regular visits to the health centre or home visits, e.g. every third month, are necessary to solve problems as they rise.
- Arrange for visits by a nurse and other essential services.
- Arrange short-term or daytime care according to the needs of the family member responsible for care at home.

Transferral of the patient from home to an institution

- The most common reasons for permanent institutionalization are
  - behavioural disturbance, aggression in particular (the most common cause)
  - stress or illness of the care-giver
  - loss of motor functions
  - loss of activities of daily living (toileting, washing)
  - incontinence (modern diapers are good)
  - inability to recognize relatives and home environment
  - restlessness at night (appropriate drug therapy in the evening often helps).
- When a family member wishes to stop home care, the reasons for his/her intention should be discussed. If these reasons cannot be overcome, long-term institutional treatment must be arranged. A care-giver with knowledge of the support available (and experience in the use of available services) is the best expert when the possibility of continuing home care is being evaluated.
- Daily visits by a nurse and night patrol prolong the home treatment period of a patient who lives alone. Electronic surveillance methods may be used in some cases. A demented person is not able to use personal alarm devices. Accidental fire and getting lost present the biggest dangers. When the disease progresses, a home for the aged or a housing unit with night patrol is the next solution.

Factors that worsen the symptoms of dementia

- Factors that impair the functional capacity of the patient must be determined and, if possible, removed. Things to be avoided include:
  - strange places (travel only with a familiar relative)
  - being alone for a prolonged time
  - too many stimuli (e.g. occasions with too many strange people)
  - darkness (suitable lighting also at night-time)
  - all infections (urinary infection is the most common)
  - operations and anaesthesia: only when unavoidable (spinal anaesthesia is not necessarily safer than general anaesthesia)
  - hot weather (heat, fluid loss)
  - extensive medication.

Principles of drug therapy

- Sedative drugs should be used only in low doses and only when needed. In the evening the dose may be higher, as restlessness at night is harmful.
- In Alzheimer's disease and vascular dementia, antidepressant therapy should be tried when depression or anxiety is suspected C [1]. Restlessness and aggression may be caused by anxiety, in which case antidepressants may be effective.
- Most benzodiazepines and neuroleptics may be used but initial doses must be very low. New atypical antipsychotics (risperidone, quetiapine) should be favoured because they have fewer adverse effects. The response is individual and to achieve the best effect it may be useful to test several drugs. On the other hand, in acute situations, higher doses are naturally advisable.
- Donepezil, rivastigmine, galantamine and memantine in Alzheimer's disease (36.24).

Examples of drug therapy

- **Benzodiazepines**
  - Oxazepam 7.5–30 mg for the night, also during the day if needed.
  - Temazepam 10–30 mg for the night, if needed; for treatment of anxiety, also 5–10 mg during the day; rapid effect.
- **Neuroleptics** A [2] [3]
  - Risperidone for aggression and psychotic symptoms 0.25–0.5 mg two times daily
  - Haloperidol for aggression, anxiety and restlessness 0.25–0.5 mg × 2–3 daily; effective at least for aggression C [4], but extrapyramidal adverse effects are common.
- **Antidepressive drugs** C [1]
  - Paroxetine 5–10 mg once daily; activates.
  - Citalopram 10–20 mg once daily; activates.
  - Sertraline 25–50 mg × 1
  - Mirtazapine 15–30 mg × 1 in the evening (sedating).

References

1. Bains J, Birks JS, Dening TR. Antidepressants for treating depression in dementia. Cochrane Database Syst Rev. 2004;(2):CD003944.
2. Lanctot KL, Best TM, Mittman N, Liu BA, Oh PI, Einarson TE, Naranjo CA. Efficacy and safety of neuroleptics in behavioural disorders associated with dementia. J Clin Psychiatr 1998;59:550–561.
3. The Database of Abstracts of Reviews of Effectiveness (University of York), Database no.: DARE-981935. In: The Cochrane Library, Issue 2, 2000. Oxford: Update Software.
4. Lonergan E, Luxenberg J, Colford J. Haloperidol for agitation in dementia. Cochrane Database Syst Rev. 2004;(2):CD002852.

36.28 Neuropsychological disorders

Marja Hietanen

General

- Damage or injury to the brain may cause temporary or permanent changes in the patient's cognitive, emotional and behavioral capacity.
- The severity of these so-called neuropsychological symptoms is variable, and their characteristics are related to the location of the brain damage.

Damage to the dominant hemisphere

- In right-handed individuals and in many left-handed ones, the left hemisphere of the brain is dominant.
- Cognitive impairments may be manifest in
  - speech production
  - speech comprehension
  - writing, reading or calculation
  - visuoconstructive abilities
  - verbal memory.
- Emotional reactions may include depression and anxiety.

Damage to the non-dominant hemisphere

- The following abilities may be impaired:
  - spatial perception
  - visuoconstructive perception
  - visual memory
  - attention to stimuli presented to one side of the body or one side space
  - symptom recognition, awareness of illness
  - perception and expression of emotional communication.
- Emotional reactions may consist of euphoria or indifference, but also anxiety.

Crucial manifestations of neuropsychological disorders

Verbal dysfunction or aphasia

- See 36.40.

Disorders in reading, calculation, and writing

- Varying degrees of dysfunction that are not the result of decline in visual acuity, impaired motor control or limited education. They may be associated with brain damage or appear as primary learning disabilities.

Disorders in stimulus recognition or agnosia

- Agnosia means difficulty in recognising familiar stimuli despite adequate perception of the stimuli, that is when the patient's nerve pathways and consciousness remain normal.
  - Visual agnosia = inability to recognise what is seen
  - Auditive agnosia = inability to recognise acoustic stimuli sound
  - Tactile agnosia = inability to recognise objects by touch

Disorders in perception of spatial relationships

- Deficits in the ability to determine the position, orientation and direction of stimuli in space.
- Manifestations include problems in spatial and topographical orientation.
- Other possible manifestations are difficulties in accuracy in making a drawing of a model or in constructing a three-dimensional representation of a model.

Disorders of voluntary apraxia

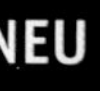

- Manifestations involve difficulties in performing voluntary movements even when the motor pathways and consciousness are normal.
- Inaccuracy of skilled movements, difficulties in using objects.
- So-called dressing-apraxia is seen mostly in connection with generalized functional disorder (such as dementia).

Memory disorders or amnesia

- See 36.20.
- Memory disturbances are among the most common neuropsychological disorders resulting from brain damage; with a wide variety of cerebral pathologies as possible aetiology.

Disorders of attention and concentration

- Difficulties in attention and concentration, in addition to memory impairment, are among the most common neuropsychological disorders.

Stimulus neglect

- The condition manifests itself as a failure to notice or defect a stimulus in the absence of a sensory deficit.
- Usually in the one side of the body or one side of space.
- Can occur in one sensory modality or in several sensory modalities simultaneously.
- Denial of deficits resulting from brain damage, i.e. anosognosia.

Emotional changes

- These may include an appropriate reaction to the illness (e.g. depression) or as a part of the neuropsychological symptomatology.
- Heightened good mood, or euphoria
- Depression or anxiety
- Indifference
- Cf. frontal lobe injury

Neuropsychological disorders of frontal lobe injury

- Crucial among these are disorders of executive functions, including deficits in initiation, planning purposive action, self-regulation and variation. Manifestations include
  - diminished creativity and productivity
  - diminished persistence
  - diminished fluency and flexibility
  - impulsiveness
  - impaired social adaptability
  - personality changes.

Diseases often accompanied by neuropsychological symptoms

- Cerebrovascular disorders
- Brain trauma
- Degenerative brain diseases (including Alzheimer's disease and Parkinson's disease)
- Alcoholism
- Brain tumours
- Psychiatric diseases (depression and schizophrenia)

Indications for neuropsychological examination

- A diagnostic question, particularly for the differentiation of psychological factors from brain-related causes
- Symptom mapping and testing mental capacity (information on functions impaired and preserved)
- Assessment of the patient is cognitive performance for rehabilitation purposes or in the course of vocational and educational planning
- Assessment of the patient's cognitive performance in order to evaluate the working ability
- Special cases such as the need to assess the patient's legal competency or driving license

Neuropsychological rehabilitation

- Neuropsychological rehabilitation is based on neuropsychological examination.
- Neuropsychological rehabilitation is part of medical rehabilitation.
- Neuropsychological rehabilitation includes retraining of impaired function, functional adaptation compensation.
- Rehabilitation is carried out in accordance with each individual patient's neuropsychological disorders, personality, education, occupation, etc.
- Neuropsychological rehabilitation is carried out in tertiary (central, university) hospitals, most regional hospitals, rehabilitation units, and private outpatient clinics.

36.30 Transient ischaemic attack (TIA)

Risto O. Roine

Basic rules

- A transient ischaemic attack (TIA) has conventionally been defined as a transient disturbance of cerebral blood circulation, with symptoms lasting less than 24 hours. Its aetiology is the same as that of an ischaemic cerebral infarction, i.e. embolisation from atheromatous large vessels, microangiopathy or cardiogenic embolism. TIA may also have a haemodynamic origin and it can be mimicked by several other cerebral illnesses.
- The definition of a TIA is currently being revised. It is now considered that cerebral imaging is the only way to differentiate between a TIA and a cerebral infarction with transient symptoms.
- If the transient ischaemic symptoms last for more than 1–2 hours the patient has, in practice, usually suffered a cerebral infarction and not a TIA.
- Up to 9% of patients will suffer a cerebral infarction within a week of their first TIA, and 30% of patients who present to a casualty department with a TIA will suffer an adverse event (stroke, myocardial infarction, death) within 3 months
- A patient with a TIA must be referred immediately to a hospital for investigation, particularly in cases where the aetiology remains undisclosed or treatment guidelines are unclear.

Diagnosis

- Based on patient history
- With carotid artery involvement, the symptoms generally consist of hemiparesis or hemiparaesthesia predominantly in the upper extremity with associated weakness in the lower branch of the facial nerve.
- Ischaemia of the dominant hemisphere causes dysphasia, which may sometimes be the only sign of a TIA.
- Loss of vision in one eye (amaurosis fugax) is indicative of ipsilateral retinal ischaemia. It is usually associated with an embolus originating from the carotid artery or central circulation.
- A typical symptom of vertebrobasilar system involvement is vertigo, which is accompanied with brainstem or cerebellar symptoms (diplopia, dysphagia, dysarthria as well as numbness and paresis, involving one or both sides of the body). Vertigo alone is not suggestive of disturbed cerebral circulation.
- Transient loss of muscle tone in the lower limbs (drop attack), binocular blindness and scintillating visual disturbances also are symptoms of vertebrobasilar TIA.

Clinical examination and signs indicating TIA

- A TIA warrants imaging of the head (CT or MRI), particularly at first presentation. The characteristics of the attack and the site of vascular involvement may be suggestive of the aetiology. The establishment of the correct aetiology is imperative for the provision of successful prophylactic treatment. A patient with a TIA has a significantly increased risk of suffering cerebral infarction and other vascular end events.
- The aetiological investigations of a TIA should be carried out urgently at an appropriate hospital. The clinical investigations include a non-invasive examination of the carotid arteries, at the very least by duplex ultrasound scanning. The state of the entire circulatory system should be clinically evaluated in order to identify other manifestations of atherosclerosis and to diagnose any potentially embolic heart diseases.
    - Atrial fibrillation is the most significant cardiogenic cause of a TIA, but the following should also be given consideration: valvular disease, artificial valves, myocardial infarction, dilated cardiomyopathy, endocarditis and aortic atheromatosis.
- The clinical examination should encompass the palpation of peripheral pulses and the measurement of blood pressure in both arms.
- The blood tests of interest are blood picture, ESR, CRP, glucose and lipid profile.
- An ECG and chest x-ray should always be carried out.
- For rare causes of a TIA see Cerebral infarction 36.31.

Differential diagnosis

- Migraine
- Epilepsy
- Ménière's disease, vestibular neuronitis, benign positional vertigo
- Syncope

Treatment

Urgency of treatment

- A self-caring patient who warrants active treatment must be sent immediately to a casualty department of an appropriate hospital or to a neurological unit.
- However, if the patient presents for the first time several weeks after the attack the investigations may be carried out at an outpatient clinic. Should the patient suffer a new TIA, immediate investigations are to be instigated.
- If the aetiology of the TIA is known and the treatment has already been instigated, a neurological unit should be consulted before referring the patient.

Aspirin

- Aspirin should be administered even if a TIA is only suspected, unless there are contraindications (A) [1 2].
    - The dose of aspirin is 100 mg/day.
    - Dipyridamole 200 mg b.d. may be added; a combination product with aspirin is usually used (A) [3].
- Clopidogrel should be considered as a second-line treatment should the patient suffer a new vascular event (e.g. a TIA) during aspirin or aspirin+dipyridamole treatment. A concomitant peripheral arterial disease may act as a further indication for the introduction of clopidogrel. The indications of clopidogrel in the treatment of coronary artery disease should also be considered.
- If the patient has coronary artery disease or other symptomatic arterial disease a statin should be prescribed, even if the lipid values are normal.

Anticoagulant therapy

- A TIA of cardiac origin requires warfarin therapy, which should preferably be introduced during heparin therapy in order to avoid the prothrombotic state associated with the instigation of warfarin therapy (A) [1 2].
- If the origin of a TIA is not cardiac warfarin might be of benefit during the first three months, but there are no evidence-based indications.
- A CT scan of the head must always be carried out before the initiation of an anticoagulation therapy, which may only take place in a hospital setting preferably under specialist care.

Surgical management (endarterectomy)

- Surgical management is beneficial if the operating surgeon's total perioperative complication (stroke and death) rate is lower than 6%.
- Surgical approach is indicated in severe stenosis (70–99%) if the patient has suffered a TIA, retinal infarction or a

non-disabling stroke in the distribution area of the stenosed artery (surgery is not indicated if there has been, for example, a severe occlusion of the middle cerebral artery) Ⓐ [4 5 6].

- Surgical approach is not cost-effective in asymptomatic carotid stenosis, excluding some special subgroups.
- However, asymptomatic carotid stenosis denotes an increased risk of stroke and is indicative for the introduction of effective primary and secondary prevention. Asymptomatic carotid stenosis alone does not warrant a specialist referral.
- Surgery is contraindicated if
  - the intracranial vessels are more stenotic than the carotid artery
  - the carotid occlusion is complete.
  - the patient has suffered a major disabling cerebral infarction with a major neurological deficit
  - the patient is in an unstable acute phase.
- If the patient belongs to a particularly high risk category (uncontrolled hypertension, uncontrolled diabetes, unstable coronary artery disease or serious general disease) the benefit expected to be gained from surgery must be individually weighed against possible risks.
- A patient's eligibility for surgery should be judged by a neurologist, who will also consult a vascular surgeon.

Secondary prevention

- Active treatment of hypertension
- A statin in symptomatic carotid disease or in coronary artery disease Ⓐ [7 8]
- Statins, ACE inhibitors and angiotensin-II receptor blockers have been shown to effectively prevent strokes and TIAs, therefore offering much improved medical treatment Ⓐ [9 10 11 12].
- Smoking cessation
- Obesity must be treated and the exercise level increased.

References

1. Matchar DB, McCrory D, Barnett HJM et al. Medical treatment for stroke prevention. Ann Intern Med 1994;121:41–53.
2. The Database of Abstracts of Reviews of Effectiveness (University of York), Database no.: DARE-948039. In: The Cochrane Library, Issue 4, 1999. Oxford: Update Software.
3. De Schryver ELLM, Algra A, van Gijn J. Dipyridamole for preventing stroke and other vascular events in patients with vascular disease. Cochrane Database Syst Rev. 2004;(2): CD001820.
4. Cina CS, Clase CM, Haynes RB. Carotid endarterectomy for symptomatic carotid stenosis. Cochrane Database Syst Rev. 2004;(2):CD001081.
5. Crouse JR, Byington RP, Hoen HM, Furberg CD. Reductase inhibitors and stroke prevention. Archives of Internal Medicine 1997;157:1305–1310.
6. The Database of Abstracts of Reviews of Effectiveness (University of York), Database no.: DARE-989051. In: The Cochrane Library, Issue 3, 2000. Oxford: Update Software.
7. Crouse JR, Byington RP, Hoen HM, Furberg CD. Reductase inhibitors and stroke prevention. Archives of Internal Medicine 1997;157:1305–1310.
8. The Database of Abstracts of Reviews of Effectiveness (University of York), Database no.: DARE-989051. In: The Cochrane Library, Issue 3, 2000. Oxford: Update Software.
9. Hebert PR, Gaziano JM, Chan KS, Hennekens CH. Cholesterol lowering with statins and risk of stroke. JAMA 1997;278:313–321.
10. The Database of Abstracts of Reviews of Effectiveness (University of York), Database no.: DARE-978231. In: The Cochrane Library, Issue 4, 1999. Oxford: Update Software.
11. Bucher HC, Griffith LE, Guyatt GH. Effect of HMGcoA reductase inhibitors on stroke. Ann Intern Med 1998;128: 89–95.
12. The Database of Abstracts of Reviews of Effectiveness (University of York), Database no.: DARE-988130. In: The Cochrane Library, Issue 4, 1999. Oxford: Update Software.

36.31 Cerebral infarction

Risto O. Roine

Epidemiology

- Cerebral infarction is the cause of approximately 85% of all strokes. One in three patients are adults in working age.

Aetiology

- Atherosclerosis of the large vessels, microangiopathy and cardiogenic embolism each account for approximately one third of all cerebral infarctions. Their proportion varies according to patient age group.
- The most common risk factors for cerebral infarction are advanced age, hypertension, diabetes, smoking, known disorder of cerebral circulation and other vascular disease.
- Approximately one in three cerebral infarctions, with some age-related variation, are attributed to cardiogenic embolism, where aetiological factors include atrial fibrillation, myocardial infarction, heart failure, mitral valve prolapse, endocarditis, atrial myxoma and artificial valves. In patients aged over 80 years, atrial fibrillation is the causative factor in one out of four cases.
- In young patients the underlying cause is rarely atherosclerosis. The infarction is most commonly attributed to arterial dissection or paradoxical embolism associated with hereditary or acquired prothrombotic state particularly in patients with patent foramen ovale.
- Screening for prothrombotic states should be considered particularly for young patients whose cerebral embolism is potentially of venous origin.
- Migraine with aura may be a significant predictor particularly in smokers and in women taking the contraceptive pill or hormone replacement therapy.

- The use of illegal drugs is a significant risk factor for cerebral infarction. Other triggering factors are dehydration, surgery, pregnancy, immobilisation, the instigation and cessation of anticoagulant therapy, acute excessive alcohol intake and acute infection.

Clinical presentation

- Cerebral infarction will generally lead to acute hemiplegia and/or sensory disturbance and expressive language impairment. The patient may also present with hemiparesis, a drooping mouth, visual disturbances and disturbed eye movements, dysphagia, vertigo, balance problems, or tetraplegia. An acute neuropsychological deficit, e.g. dyspraxia, memory loss or confusion, may also be indicative, of cerebral infarction.
- **Carotid (hemispheral) infarction** typically presents with hemiparesis and/or sensory disturbance, often accompanied by weakness in the lower branch of the facial nerve.
  - Occlusion of the middle cerebral artery is the most common site; paralysis is more pronounced in the upper extremity.
  - Occlusion of the anterior cerebral artery, which is a rare condition, leads to paralysis mainly involving the lower extremity and to urinary incontinence.
  - An infarction in the dominant hemisphere often involves expressive and receptive language impairment as well as reading and writing difficulties.
  - An infarction in the non-dominant hemisphere may include impairment in the sense of direction and spatial orientation as well as anosognosia (lack of a sensation of illness) and sensory neglect (ignoring the affected side of the body).
- **Vertebrobasilar (brainstem) infarction** typically presents as acute and severe vertigo, nausea, diplopia, dysphagia, dysarthria and sensory disturbance, weakness or paresis in the contralateral extremities. The symptoms are caused by the progressive (often lasting for several days) occlusion of vertebral artery, basilar artery and cerebellar arteries. Homonymous hemianopia without paralysis is most often caused by the occlusion of the posterior cerebral artery.
- **Lacunar infarctions** are small infarctions occurring secondary to the occlusion of small terminal arteries. Their location is either subcortical or they occur in the basal ganglia or the brainstem. The most common cause of lacunar infarctions is hypertension; often causes include type 2 diabetes, vasculitis and hyperhomocysteinaemia. The clinical manifestation is often typical: pure, often fluctuating, motor or sensory hemiparesis, ataxia and hemiparesis or dysarthria—clumsy hand syndrome. See also Vascular dementia 36.23.
- **Sinus thrombosis** (cerebral venous thrombosis) may occur during pregnancy or puerperium, in association with hormone therapy, dehydration, coagulopathies, or malignancy. Sinus thrombosis causes symptoms of increased intracranial pressure: headache, lowered consciousness, or seizures with associated unconsciousness as well as paralysis inconsistent with the arterial distribution areas.
- Cerebral infarctions rarely involve a headache, particularly at the initial stage. A large infarction may cause increased intracranial pressure, headache, nausea and lowered consciousness.

Diagnostic work-up

1. Is the condition caused by disturbed cerebral circulation or some other illness (brain tumour, chronic subdural haematoma, epilepsy, migraine, MS, encephalitis etc.)?
2. Does the patient suffer from an ischaemic disturbance of cerebral circulation or haemorrhage? The two conditions need to be differentiated with the use of a CT scan.
3. If the condition is an infarction, was the occlusion caused by an embolism?
   - An acute onset (e.g. whilst getting out of bed or straining), loss of consciousness, seizures, and a history of a potentially embolic cardiac disorder suggest cardiogenic embolism. A CT scan may show, for instance, a haemorrhagic infarction or multiple infarctions. Anticoagulant therapy should be intigated.
4. Has recanalisation taken place? Is the patient's condition during examination stable, progressive or recurring?
   - The stroke is considered to be progressing if carotid symptoms progress within 24 hours or vertebrobasilar symptoms within 48 hours. An unstable phase usually persists until recanalisation has taken place, either spontaneously or through thrombolysis. Improved symptoms do not always translate to reduced risk. An unstable phase often warrants the introduction of urgent anticoagulant therapy.
5. Other aetiologies?
   - Neck pain, Horner's syndrome, and neck trauma prior to the stroke are suggestive of carotid dissection, in which case anticoagulant therapy must be instigated D [1].
   - Autoimmune disease may suggest vasculitis, which requires treatment according to its aetiology.
   - Previous venous thromboses or miscarriages in a young patient may be suggestive of hederitary coagulopathy.

NEU

Treatment

- All previously self-catering patients should be referred to the care of a specialist team at an appropriate hospital where the patient should primarily be cared for in dedicated wards (stroke units) A [2].
- Care in a stroke unit is cost-effective, reduces mortality and improves the patient's chances of regaining independence A [2].
- General treatment
  - Airways must be open, if necessary with the aid of an oral airway or the patient must be intubated. Oxygen therapy is instigated in the casualty department and continued, should there be problems with ventilation or oxygenation.

  - Intravenous fluids should always be administered during the acute phase. The patient must be kept nil by mouth. Continuous ECG and blood pressure monitoring are commenced.
- Temperature
  - Temperature reduction is the most effective neuroprotective treatment in cerebral ischaemia. Fever increases the ischaemic damage, promotes bleeding and swelling and increases mortality. The aim is to achieve normal body temperature. Therapeutic hypotermia in cerebral infarction is still at an investigational stage, but is current practise in cardiac arrest.
  - Oedema following cerebral infarction is a life-threatening condition which can be treated with temperature reduction, blood glucose control, osmotic preparations, positional therapy, prevention of restlessness and seizures, maintenance of optimal blood gas values or hemicraniectomy.
- Blood pressure
  - Cerebral infarction is often accompanied by an acute reactive increase in blood pressure, which acts as a defence mechanism and, therefore, a reduction of blood pressure is not generally advisable.
    - If the diastolic pressure is below 120 mmHg and the systolic pressure below 220 mmHg, no antihypertensive medication is needed. If, however, thrombolytic or anticoagulant therapy is instigated the upper limit should be around 185/110 mmHg.
    - The first-line antihypertensive agents are intravenous labetalol or enalapril. Vasodilators and other forms of abrupt blood pressure reduction should be avoided (no chewable nifedipine) C [3].
    - If systolic pressure exceeds 220 mmHg, blood pressure should be reduced during the acute stage, and also whenever necessary from the cardiovascular viewpoint.
- Any signs of heart failure must be treated.
- Arrhythmias
  - Patients with cerebral infarction often suffer from arrhythmias and myocardial ischaemia during the acute phase, including ST changes in an ECG. These are suggestive of myocardial damage, secondary to increased catecholamine concentrations. Beta-blockade is often indicated.
- Management of blood glucose and fluid balance.
  - Hyperglycaemia should be treated however slight (>8 mmol/l), at the acute phase; hyperglycaemia will worsen cerebral ischaemia and increase mortality.
  - An increased haematocrit value suggests dehydration, which should be corrected by intravenous fluids. The majority of stroke patients are dehydrated on admission, which compromises prognosis.
- Prevention of pneumonia
  - The risk of aspiration is high and fluids are to be administered orally only after a careful swallow test. Any patient who has vomited or was found on the floor or unconscious is presumed to have aspirated and prophylactic intravenous antibiotics should be instigated before the emergence of chest-related symptoms or a rise in CRP.
- Prevention of deep venous thrombosis and pulmonary embolism
  - Low molecular weight heparins: dalteparin 5,000 IU o.d. or b.d. subcutaneously or enoxaparin 40 mg o.d. or b.d. subcutaneously B [4].
- Anticoagulant therapy
  - Either unfractionated heparin with APTT monitoring or low molecular weight heparin according to anti-FXa activity (dalteparin approximately 50 IU/kg b.d. or enoxaparin approximately 0.5 mg/kg b.d.)
  - Indications for anticoagulant therapy: cardiogenic embolism, arterial, sinus thrombosis, progressing thrombosis of the basilar or other artery or frequently recurring TIA.
  - Warfarin is introduced under heparin cover, and oral anticoagulation is usually continued for 6 months in carotid artery dissection. The treatment of cardiogenic embolism is continued until the source of the embolism no longer exists.
  - If warfarin is instigated without heparin cover the risk of thrombotic complications increases.
  - If the anticoagulant therapy was prescribed for dissection, and a check-up examination (ultrasound or MR angiography) shows a totally patent or recanalised artery, warfarin is substituted by aspirin. In other cases warfarin is continued, and in special cases vascular surgery could be considered.
  - The instigation of anticoagulant therapy calls for the consideration of contradictions and indications.
- Thrombolysis with recombinant tissue plasminogen activator (rt-PA) B [5]
  - In 2002, thrombolysis with rt-PA was approved in the EU countries for the treatment of ischaemic stroke if administered within three hours from symptom onset and under detailed selection criteria.
  - Different selection criteria and a longer time window apply in basilar artery occlusion.
  - The centres offering this form of treatment have introduced relevant treatment guidelines which also cover, for example, the emergency services.
- Rehabilitation
  - Introduced at an early stage and is most effective if carried out by a multidisciplinary team at a stroke unit. Mobilisation of patients is introduced gradually after the unstable phase (36.34).
- Secondary prevention following cerebral infarction is commenced during the acute phase, after individual risk factors have been evaluated.
  - Blood pressure reduction is the most effective treatment form, and diabetics seem to derive most benefit from it.

- ACE inhibitors and AT receptor antagonists appear to have prophylactic properties, irrespective of their antihypertensive effect.
- Statins are indicated in symptomatic arteriopathy, irrespective of the patient's cholesterol values.
- See 36.30.

References

1. Lyrer P, Engelter S. Antithrombotic drugs for carotid artery dissection. Cochrane Database Syst Rev. 2004;(2): CD000255.
2. Stroke Unit Trialists' Collaboration. Organised inpatient (stroke unit) care for stroke. Cochrane Database Syst Rev. 2004;(2): CD000197.
3. Gubitz G, Sandercock P. Stroke management. Clinical Evidence 2002;7:161–174.
4. Counsell C, Sandercock P. Low-molecular-weight heparins or heparinoids versus standard unfractionated heparin for acute ischaemic stroke. Cochrane Database Syst Rev. 2004;(2): CD000119.
5. Wardlaw JM, del Zoppo G, Yamaguchi T, Berge E. Thrombolysis for acute ischaemic stroke. Cochrane Database Syst Rev. 2004;(2):CD000213.

36.32 Subarachnoid haemorrhage (SAH)

Editors

Aims

- SAH is diagnosed using CT scanning, whenever available. Lumbar puncture is not included in routine SAH diagnostics.
- Screening family members for aneurysms is advisable, at least if there have been two cases of SAH in the family.

Basic rules

- A significant proportion of SAH cases are aneurysmal haemorrhages–surgical treatment requires early diagnostics. The complications and possible recurrence of the haemorrhage are the main risks.

Incidence

- The incidence is 5–30/100 000 and increases with age.

Symptoms and findings

- Symptoms of subarachnoid haemorrhage are: acute intensive headache and impaired consciousness, followed by deterioration of the patient's general condition, nausea and vomiting and later nuchal rigidity.
- Neurological deficiency symptoms (paralyses) are possible; 20–25% of patients die as a direct consequence of the haemorrhage.
- Ophthalmoscopic examination reveals, in some patients (less than 10%), haemorrhage between the retina and vitreous body.

Causes of blood in the cerebrospinal fluid

- Primary SAH
  - Arterial aneurysm
  - Arteriovenous malformation
- Secondary SAH
  - Cerebral haemorrhage rupture into the cerebral ventricles. Clinical differential diagnosis is difficult.
- Trauma
  - Even a mild contusion brings blood into the spinal fluid.
  - With a history of trauma, lumbar puncture is contraindicated as having no diagnostic value.
- Conditions leading to haemorrhagic disease:
  - Thrombocytopenia, leukaemia, aplastic anaemia, Hodgkin's disease, coagulation disorders, liver diseases, haemophilia, idiopathic conditions
  - The disease is frequently in its late stages and the underlying diagnosis is known.
- Anticoagulant therapy
  - Anticoagulant therapy alone does not usually cause SAH; there must be attendant causes–trauma?
- Brain tumour
  - Haemorrhage can be the first symptom of an intraventricular brain tumour.
- Inflammation
  - Inflammatory diseases
  - Sepsis (meningococcal)
  - Mycotic aneurysms
- Vascular diseases
  - Collagenoses, polyarteritis
  - Purpura
- Spinal haemorrhage
  - AV malformation
  - Tumour
- No evident cause
  - 15–20% of SAH patients; the prognosis is good.
  - There may be an underlying small thrombosed aneurysm or haemorrhage in the region of the brainstem.
- Artefact blood
  - Usually caused by a technically difficult lumbar puncture (36.17)
  - Venal puncture

CT scanning in SAH diagnostics

- SAH is diagnosed using CT scanning, which should be performed as soon as haemorrhage is suspected. If obtained within the first three days, the accuracy of the CT scan will be more than 95%, but after two weeks from the haemorrhage less than 50%. In the majority, the causes of the haemorrhage, its extent and quantity, can be determined. The differential diagnosis of primary and secondary haemorrhages can be established clearly by using CT scanning; also the location can often be determined. The existence of an intracerebral haemorrhage can be determined at the same time.
- When CT scanning is available, the indications for lumbar puncture in SAH are distinguishing between SAH and inflammation, mild symptoms of a suspected haemorrhage or differential diagnosis in the case of a patient with multiple disorders. A thin needle and a few drops of spinal fluid are sufficient. A clinically distinct SAH suspicion that appears negative in the CT scan should be confirmed by a lumbar puncture (a normal finding on CT does not rule out SAH).

Prognosis of aneurysmal haemorrhage

- 30% die directly from the haemorrhage; 30–35% within three months of a recurrent haemorrhage.
- Thereafter, the risk of recurrence will diminish, with the probability of getting a new SAH being 3% per year. Their susceptibility to illness and mortality increase at every occurrence.

Treatment in the acute phase

- Treat the symptoms of increased intracranial pressure (36.96), headache and vomiting.
- An unconscious patient needs intensive care. A respirator may be required.
- After a SAH diagnosis, angiographic confirmation is needed–preferably within one day of the onset of haemorrhage. Both carotid and vertebrobasilar territories should be examined. It is most important, however, to determine the pathology in the vascular area involved in the localized findings.

Timing of surgical intervention

- Today, early surgical intervention is considered important to prevent recurrent haemorrhages and vascular spasm C [1].
- The patient should be operated on within the first few days or as soon as angiography findings have been obtained.
- Emergency surgery is required for temporal haematoma and occasionally for acute hydrocephalus.
- For some patients, endovascular aneurysm obliteration is a good alternative to surgery. The results are as good as those of surgery, or even better for aneurysm of the posterior cranial fossa.

Aneurysm surgery

- The primary procedure is microsurgical ligation of the aneurysmatic neck.
- In 30% of patients the aneurysm may be multiple, and in 6% its size may be gigantic, in excess of 25 mm.
- The risk that a non-bleeding aneurysm will rupture may be as great as the risk of recurrent bleeding from an aneurysm that has bled previously. A non-bleeding aneurysm should, as a rule, be repaired surgically.

Results of aneurysm surgery

- Surgical intervention in young, healthy patients hardly ever results in death.
- Total mortality in patients with early-stage surgery is less than 10%, and 80% will return to normal, independent living.

Complications

- Cerebral vasospasm is a feared complication of SAH, which occurs in 6–10 days after the bleeding. The spasm is a contraction of the vessels that can be seen in angiographs; it later develops into an actual structural lesion.
- There are symptoms in 30% of patients. In 15% of them the ischaemic symptoms are permanent.
- Spasm can be prevented by using the calcium channel blocker nimodipine A [2 3].
- Acute hydrocephalus, which usually disappears, is a possible complication of SAH, and especially aneurysmal haemorrhage at the early stage.
- Hydrocephalus, which is often caused by impaired resorption after two weeks, requires a shunt.
- Cardiac symptoms, haemorrhage into the vitreous body.
- Oculomotor dysfunction will complicate treatment of an aneurysm in the posterior cerebral artery and basilar aneurysms.
- Technical problems associated with the surgery are highly probable in aneurysm surgery. Complications C [4 5] such as infections and haemorrhages are ever-present risks in all craniotomies.
- **Epileptic** symptoms occur at later stages in 12% of patients.

Screening of relatives

- Magnetic angiography is a safe method for screening family members of SAH patients for aneurysms. Screening family members is indicated if there have been at least two cases of SAH in the family. 10% of all aneurysm cases have such a family history. The screening will reveal a symptomless aneurysm in ca. 10% of family members aged 30–60 years.

References

1. Whitfield PC, Kirkpatrick PJ. Timing of surgery for aneurysmal subarachnoid haemorrhage. Cochrane Database Syst Rev. 2004;(2):CD001697.

2. Barker FG, Ogilvy CS. Efficacy of prophylactic nimodipine for delayed ischaemic deficit in subarachnoid haemorrhage: a meta-analysis. J Neurosurg 1996;84:405–414.
3. The Database of Abstracts of Reviews of Effectiveness (University of York), Database no.: DARE-960515. In: The Cochrane Library, Issue 4, 1999. Oxford: Update Software.
4. Raaymakers TW, Rinkel GJ, Limburg M, Algra A. Mortality and morbidity of surgery for unruptured intracranial aneurysms: a meta-analysis. Stroke 1998;29:1531–1538.
5. The Database of Abstracts of Reviews of Effectiveness (University of York), Database no.: DARE-981374. In: The Cochrane Library, Issue 2, 2000. Oxford: Update Software.

36.33 Intracerebral haemorrhage

Risto O. Roine

Epidemiology

- Intracerebral haemorrhage is the cause of ca. 15% of strokes.
- The incidence has fallen as the result of improved management of hypertension.
- Acute phase mortality is higher in intracerebral haemorrhage than in cerebral infarction. In subarachnoid haemorrhage (SAH) mortality is almost 50%; one third of the patients die within the first 24 hours.

Aetiology

- Hypertension is the most common cause of intracerebral haemorrhage. Hypertension leads to changes at the walls of small cerebral blood vessels. Hypertension-associated haemorrhage usually occurs in the area of the basal ganglia, thalamus, cerebellum or the brainstem. Such haemorrhage usually leads to massive hemiparesis and impaired consciousness. The bleed may also occur within the cerebrospinal fluid space.
- SAH is usually (80%) caused by a rupture of a cerebral artery aneurysm. Other causes include arteriovenous malformation or head injury.
- The more rare underlying causes of intracerebral haemorrhage include arteriovenous malformation, cerebral amyloid angiopathy, cavernous haemangioma and malignant brain tumours. Factors suggesting a tumour include an unusual location of the haemorrhage and the absence of hypertension. The tumour is not always identifiable on the CT scan taken at the acute phase due to the quantity of blood present. An MRI scan, or a CT scan with contrast medium, is usually diagnostic when carried out a few weeks after the event.
- Haemorrhage at the temporal lobe often originates from an aneurysm of the middle cerebral artery, in which case the haemorrhage can be considered to be subarachnoid in nature (36.32).
- For other causes of blood in the cerebrospinal fluid, see 36.32.

Symptoms

- Progressive hemiplegia which may be associated with impaired consciousness, vomiting or focal seizure with associated unconsciousness. Intracerebral haemorrhage is not always associated with headache, particularly in the early stages.
- The neurological signs and symptoms are the same as seen in cerebral infarction, but usually develop more slowly and are dependent on the site and extent of the bleed. Intracerebral haemorrhage may also cause transient symptoms similar to those seen in TIAs.
- Cerebellar haemorrhage: dizziness, vomiting, ataxia and disturbances in eye movements are the most common symptoms. The level of consciousness may deteriorate rapidly and a patient with few symptoms may suffer respiratory arrest due to the sudden disturbances in the flow of the cerebrospinal fluid.
- The typical symptoms of pontine haemorrhage are unconsciousness and contracted pupils.
- If the haemorrhage is extensive or located in the brainstem or cerebellum, there is a risk of increased intracranial pressure (36.96).
- In almost 50% of patients, the intracerebral bleeding will continue for the next 24 hours. It is therefore appropriate to attempt to correct any spontaneous or iatrogenic bleeding tendencies if the chances of recovery are still present. Measures should be taken to reduce blood pressure to below 180/100 mmHg, but hypotonia should be prevented to ensure adequate tissue perfusion.

Symptoms of SAH

- Sudden, intense headache, unconsciousness, often nuchal rigidity, photophobia, nausea and paralysis depending on the site and extent of the haemorrhage.

Diagnosis and treatment

- All previous self-caring patients should be treated at a stroke or neurological unit.
- CT scan is the diagnostic investigation of choice. Lumbar puncture is contraindicated on very ill patients. If the CT scan is negative a lumbar puncture should be carried out to exclude a warning bleed (often seen prior to SAH) and other causes.
- A neurosurgical team must always be consulted in cases of SAH. Neurological unit is not that important in the beginning.
- The treatment of a patient with intracerebral haemorrhage differs little from that of a patient with cerebral infarction, see 36.31. The patient is kept at bed rest during the acute phase, and any bleeding tendencies (INR > 1.3) must be corrected promptly with the administration of clotting factor

concentrates. Particular caution should be exercised in the administration of anticoagulants after the acute phase.

- Rehabilitation should be started early (36.34).
- In the early phase of intracerebral haemorrhage the mortality rate is high, but the prognosis of surviving patients is better than that of patients with cerebral infarction.

Neurosurgical management of intracerebral and subarachnoid haemorrhage

- A neurosurgeon should always be consulted in cases of intracerebral haemorrhage. However, surgical approach is only rarely indicated, except in cerebellar haematoma.
- The management of a SAH includes the maintenance of vital functions during the acute phase, the identification of the bleeding point with cerebral imaging (primarily with a CT angiography or digital subtraction angiography) and the prevention of a rebleed through immobilising the patient and blood pressure reduction (<160/100 mmHg). Furthermore, arterial spasm should be prevented by the administration of i.v. nimodipine and fluids.

36.34 Rehabilitation of the stroke patient

Mervi Kotila

- Many people who have suffered a stroke continue to experience symptoms that interfere with their daily life. Most significant among these are
  - paralysis of extremities (at the acute stage, three out of four have these)
  - defects in the visual field
  - disorders of higher brain functions
    - aphasia, or difficulty in producing and understanding speech (36.40)
    - apraxia, or movement dysfunction (36.28)
    - agnosia, or cognitive dysfunction (36.28).

Aims of stroke patient rehabilitation

- Extensive long-term therapy is aimed at correcting or alleviating the consequences of the disease.
- Support the patient in adapting to the situation.

Forms of rehabilitation

- **Physiotherapy**
  - Promotes spontaneous recovery.
  - Prevents misalignment in posture and movements.
  - Normalizes muscle tone.
  - The effectiveness of physiotherapy has been improved by new techniques
    - Functional electric stimulation is useful in activating voluntary muscle function, and cutaneous electric stimulation may improve sensation in the limb and reduce spasticity.
    - Forced training of the upper extremity may generate new active movement and enhance functional skills.
    - Gait training with partial body weight support increases the efficiency of learning to walk and the learning may take place faster.
- **Occupational therapy**
  - Skills acquired in physiotherapy are taken into use in daily activities.
  - The patient's need for aids is determined and training in their use is given.
- **Speech therapy** (36.40)
  - The nature of aphatic or (infrequently in stroke victims) dysarthric speech impairment is defined and the course of individualized speech therapy is planned.
  - Family members are given information on and instruction in alternative methods of communication.
- **Neuropsychological rehabilitation**
  - Only some stroke patients need neuropsychological rehabilitation. The availability of neuropsychological rehabilitation services is limited.
  - Neuropsychological tests are used to establish the nature and extent of cognitive impairment.
  - Rehabilitation is aimed at correcting the functional impairment and providing means of compensating for them by utilising retained abilities.

Implementation of rehabilitation

- The best results are obtained by starting rehabilitation early (A) [1 2].
- Rehabilitation involves teamwork (A) [3 4]. Where the available resources are adequate, a rehabilitation team should consist of:
  - a physician
  - a nurse
  - a social worker
  - a physiotherapist
  - an occupational therapist
  - a speech therapist
  - a neuropsychologist.
- Organised inpatient care is effective; patients treated in stroke units are more likely to be alive, independent and living at home one year after the stroke (A) [5].
- Irrespective of the extent of resources available, the most important aspect is real interest in the rehabilitation of the stroke patient.
- Responsibilities of the rehabilitation team:

- Assign specific rehabilitation objectives (e.g. return to work or independent living at home).
- Create a plan for achieving the objectives, which should be reviewed and changed when necessary.

Scheduling of rehabilitation therapy

1. Intensive rehabilitation **B** [6 7 8] in the hospital ward
   - Physiotherapy should be started on the day of the stroke or the following day, initially with postural therapy and later with increasingly active exercises. Especially the paralysed side should be trained, and the unaffected side should not be allowed to compensate for the functions of the paralysed side. At the early stage assistive devices should not be provided. The evaluation of the need for assistive devices should be postponed until the patient's situation has stabilised.
   - Efforts to initiate other forms of rehabilitation as well (such as speech therapy) in the hospital should be made as soon as possible.
   - All attending staff and the patient's family members should participate in the rehabilitation.
   - Acute illness is often accompanied by reactive depression. Recognition and treatment of this condition will enhance the motivation for rehabilitation and improve the results.
   - Initially, therapy should be provided daily.
   - The patient should be discharged as soon as he/she is able to manage at home **B** [9 10].
   - Should the patient after the acute stage be unable to function at home, but there still is potential for rehabilitation, continued intensive rehabilitation in a specialised facility should be considered.
2. Post-discharge intensive rehabilitation
   - Intensive rehabilitation **B** [6 7 8] should continue after hospital discharge on an outpatient basis 2–3 times weekly.
   - Intensive rehabilitation should continue until no further progress is seen.
3. Maintenance rehabilitation
   - The shift to maintenance rehabilitation occurs after the intensive phase of rehabilitation, generally in six months to a year after the stroke.
   - The purpose of maintenance rehabilitation is to retain the results of rehabilitation.
   - Maintenance rehabilitation usually consists of:
     - annually 2–3 courses of physiotherapy, as needed in each individual case
     - other therapy (such as speech therapy), a few visits annually, or follow-up visits
     - group therapy (e.g. group speech therapy, groups for memory enhancement, etc.), as needed
     - Severely disabled patients in home care may, if necessary, be referred to therapy in a rehabilitation facility for 3–4 weeks at a time. The aim is to maintain the patient's independence and enhance the motivation of family members for home care.
   - Maintenance rehabilitation therapy is a distinct responsibility of primary health care.

Adaptation training

- After the intensive phase of rehabilitation, when the long-term consequences of the stroke are evident, the patient often becomes depressed and suffers from other adaptation problems (such as having to retire). Adaptation training is often helpful at this stage.

References

1. Cifu DX, Stewart DG. Factors affecting functional outcome after stroke: a critical review of rehabilitation services. Archives of Physical Medicine and Rehabilitation 1999;80:S35–S39.
2. The Database of Abstracts of Reviews of Effectiveness (University of York), Database no.: DARE-991088. In: The Cochrane Library, Issue 1, 2001. Oxford: Update Software.
3. Evans RL, Connis RT, Hendricks RD, Haselkorn JK. Multidisciplinary inpatient rehabilitation for geriatric and stroke patients versus standard medical care. Soc Sci Med 1995;40:1699–1706.
4. The Database of Abstracts of Reviews of Effectiveness (University of York), Database no.: DARE-968169. In: The Cochrane Library, Issue 4, 1999. Oxford: Update Software.
5. Stroke Unit Trialists' Collaboration. Organised inpatient (stroke unit) care for stroke. Cochrane Database Syst Rev. 2004;(2):CD000197.
6. Kwakkel G, Wagenaar RC, Koelman TW, Lankhorst GJ, Koetsier JC. Effects of intensity of rehabilitation after stroke: a research synthesis. Stroke 1997;28:1550–1556.
7. The Database of Abstracts of Reviews of Effectiveness (University of York), Database no.: DARE-971047. In: The Cochrane Library, Issue 4, 1999. Oxford: Update Software.
8. University of York. NHS Centre for Reviews and Dissemination. Stroke rehabilitation. Effective Health Care 1992;1:12.
9. Britton M, Andersson A.: reviewing the scientific evidence on effects and costs. International Journal of Technology Assessment in Health Care 2000, 16(3), 842–848.
10. The Database of Abstracts of Reviews of Effectiveness (University of York), Database no.: DARE-20008619. In: The Cochrane Library, Issue 2, 2002. Oxford: Update Software.

36.40 Aphasia and dysphasia

Editors

Aphasia, dysphasia

- The term refers to impairment of the ability to process, produce, and comprehend spoken and written language resulting from disease or trauma. The damage is often located in the left hemisphere.

- Associated with these are disturbances in other cortical brain functions:
  - articulation (dysarthria)
  - memory functions (amnesia)
  - perception (agnosia)
  - voluntary movements (apraxia).

Main types

- Non-fluent (motor, Broca's aphasia)
  - Laboured and halting speech; the patient's comprehension is often not as extensively impaired as his/her speech.
- Fluent (sensory, Wernicke's aphasia)
  - Effortless speech with an abundance of malformed words (jargon); marked limitations in comprehension.

Degrees of severity

- Slight
  - May escape diagnosis; however, the patient may be aware of the impairment, which may interfere with his/her work and thus cause a secondary mental health risk.
- Moderate
  - Significant difficulties in linguistic functions; the patient is capable of only limited expression and speech reception.
- Severe
  - All linguistic functions are greatly impaired.

Aims of rehabilitation

- Restoration of lost capacities as far as possible (restorative rehabilitation).
- Training in the maximal use of remaining communication skills (compensatory rehabilitation).
- Promoting the patient's adaptation to the disability and life change.
- Team rehabilitation is most effective. Rehabilitation needs time; optimum progress is achievable during the first year of disability. Best results are obtained when the disability is mild (C) [1 2 3 4].

Rehabilitation methods

- Slight impairment
  - Examination and rehabilitation performed by speech therapist and neuropsychologist. Intensive and restorative rehabilitation bring the best results.
- Moderate impairment
  - Both restorative and compensatory rehabilitation by a speech therapist and an occupational therapist aimed at optimal communicative capacity.
- Severe impairment
  - Rehabilitation by a speech therapist and an occupational therapist aimed at finding some means of communication; guidance and training given to others in the patient's environment with the goal of creating a positive communication capacity.
- Difficulty in swallowing may be associated with non-fluent forms of aphasia in particular. Observe whether the patient is able to drink a glass of water without difficulty. Refer patients with problems to a speech therapist for swallowing training.
- The long-term prognosis is highly dependent on the patient's ability to adapt to the life change brought on by the disability. A supportive caregiver relationship, encouragement for the grief process, and possible treatment of depression will bring relief. Do not forget support and training of family members. Adaptation training provided by patient organisations can contribute to long-term adjustment.

Communication tips

- Set aside ample time; it will be needed.
- Address the patient, not the person accompanying her.
- Speak clearly but naturally, facing the patient.
- Use informal everyday language; do not raise your voice.
- Bring up one topic at a time; repeat if necessary using other words (additional clues will improve comprehension).
- Do not forget the potential of gestures, facial expressions, drawings, etc., that are part of full expression.
- Give the patient enough time to answer; do not guess. You may explain and ask whether you understood correctly. Give feedback; if you do not understand, say so.
- Formulate your questions unambiguously (not "Do you smoke or use alcohol and how much?", but "Do you smoke? How much? Do you drink alcohol?", etc.).
- Provide all instructions in written form as well as orally.
- It is a good idea to inquire about the coping ability of family members.
- Remember: depression is common in aphasic patients, but the diagnosis is difficult. "Listening" to one's own emotional reactions may help in recognizing the signs.
- A calm and relaxed atmosphere is beneficial for communication.

References

1. Robey RR. The efficacy of treatments for aphasic persons: a meta-analysis. Brain and Language 1994;47:582–608.
2. The Database of Abstracts of Reviews of Effectiveness (University of York), Database no.: DARE-920021. In: The Cochrane Library, Issue 4, 1999. Oxford: Update Software.
3. Robey RR. A meta-analysis of clinical outcomes in the treatment of aphasia. J Speech, Language, and Hearing Research 1998;41:172–187.
4. The Database of Abstracts of Reviews of Effectiveness (University of York), Database no.: DARE-983563. In: The Cochrane Library, Issue 2, 2000. Oxford: Update Software.

36.45 Examination of patients with epileptic symptoms

Esa Mervaala, Reetta Kälviäinen

- See Diagnostics of seizure symptoms 36.4.

Basic rules

- The first physician describes and records the course of the seizure, including preceding and subsequent postictal signs and symptoms.
- Patients should be referred to comprehensive neurological testing for confirmation of the diagnosis and for aetiological studies (in adult-onset epilepsy, brain tumour as a possible cause should be considered). The patient's first alcohol-withdrawal seizure should be approached in the same way as a suspected non-provoked epileptic seizure.
- If the seizure is not clearly epileptiform, a cardiologic examination is often crucial.

Epidemiology

- The incidence in patients aged over 15 is 24/100 000 per year, and the prevalence is 700/100 000.

Aetiology

- Brain trauma, 10%
- Perinatal injuries, 10%
- Cerebrovascular disorders, 6%
- Central nervous system infections, 5%
- Brain tumours, 3%
- Other organic causes, 5%
- Unknown, 61%

Types of seizures

- **Partial (focal, localized) seizures**. Symptoms point to damage in a localized area of the brain and reflect dysfunction of that area.
  - Twitching or somatosensory dysfunction in one limb, the limbs on one side, or the face (Jacksonian convulsions)
  - Visual disturbances or other symptoms typical of temporal epilepsy (e.g. abdominal discomfort, olfactory or gustatory sensation, déjà-vu) (36.4)
  - A partial seizure may become secondarily generalized.
- **Generalized seizures**. The initial symptom is loss of consciousness; convulsions are symmetrical from onset. Among these are:
  - Generalized seizures without prodromal symptoms (tonic-clonic seizures)
  - Brief absence seizures

History

- Predisposing factors (e.g. sleep-deprivation, fasting, alcohol ingestion–especially alcohol withdrawal, medications, flickering light) (36.49)
- What was the patient doing at the onset of the seizure?
- Prodromal symptoms and sensations (e.g. nausea, numbness in the arm/hand, dizziness)
- Did the patient remain conscious during the seizure?
- Description of the attack by observers
- Recovery from the attack (rapid or gradual, orientation, memory impairment)
- Urinary or faecal incontinence
- Skin colour

Clinical findings

- If the physician is able to examine the patient during the attack or immediately thereafter, it is important to note
  - possible injuries
  - whether the patient has bitten his/her tongue
  - whether there are unilateral neurological symptoms (Todd's paralysis following the seizure indicates epilepsy of focal origin)
  - pupillary reaction, positive Babinski's sign
  - whether there is evidence of recent use of alcohol or other intoxicants
  - blood pressure, pulse, indications of cardiovascular aetiology.
- If the physician does not see the patient until several days after the seizure, there are often no significant clinical findings. However, it is advisable to look for unilateral neurological symptoms and signs of increased intracranial pressure.

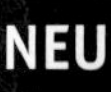

Laboratory tests

- Blood count, serum calcium, sodium, potassium, creatinine, creatinine kinase, and blood glucose
- TSH
- ECG (conduction times must be measured)

Additional tests to be performed in a neurology unit

- EEG (electroencephalogram)
  - The optimal timing is as soon as feasible after the seizure, initial waking EEG, followed by sleep EEG if needed. Epileptiform EEG findings (spikes, sharp waves, spike-slow-wave complexes) are strongly associated to epilepsy, a focal slow-wave finding points to cerebral trauma.
- Computerised tomography of the head (CT) or magnetic resonance imaging (MRI) must be performed in order to

determine the aetiology of epilepsy (as permitted by current resources: evident withdrawal convulsions).

- Special tests required in problem cases, such as in connection with therapy-resistant epilepsy, diagnostics of atypical seizures, and when surgical therapy is being considered:
    - Long-term EEG monitoring (ambulatory EEG) aimed at obtaining an EEG during the seizure itself (36.16)
    - EEG videotelemetry (36.16) aimed at obtaining EEG with simultaneous video picture.

Cardiological tests

- The increased use of long-term Holter-monitoring and the tilt test has revealed that arrhythmia or acute variations in blood pressure often are the cause of seizures.
- If the seizure is not epileptiform, the probable cause is cardiovascular.

36.46 Treatment of status epilepticus

Reetta Kälviäinen

Basic rules

- A generalized seizure is considered to be prolonged if convulsions continue for 5–10 minutes.
- The seizure should be terminated as soon as possible to avoid irreversible brain damage, at least within 30 minutes of the beginning of convulsions.
- Hypoglycaemia must always be recognized and treated.
- Potential thiamine deficiency is corrected (alcoholics and persons on a poor or restricted diet are a risk group).
- Diazepam is the drug of choice in status epilepticus. It should be administered intravenously, as the effect of rectal dosing may be poor if the drug is retained in faecal mass. Lorazepam is an alternative. It has a longer duration of action, but poorer availability than diazepam.
- If the seizure lasts for more than 10 minutes, or if several diazepam doses have already been given, or if the seizure recurs three times within a day, a saturation dose of phenytoin is administered. Fosphenytoin is the prodrug of phenytoin that is transformed into phenytoin in the body. It is water soluble and thus causes less irritation of the veins. ProEpanutin® should be diluted to a maximum concentration of 25 mg phenytoin equivalents (PE)/ml (1.5–25 mg PE/ml) before use.
- Status epilepticus requires follow-up in a hospital and investigation of the aetiology (brain imaging, CSF, further laboratory studies) and treatment also after the seizure has ended.

The first 10 minutes

1. Secure and monitor vital functions
    - Open airways, give oxygen, and, if necessary, intubate after relaxation
    - ECG monitoring, pulse oximetry
    - Careful follow-up is necessary also during and after drug administration.
2. Thiamine 100 mg i.v.
3. Examine blood glucose (rapid test) and treat hypoglycaemia.
4. Diazepam is given preferably i.v. (or rectally) in boluses of 5–10 mg, or lorazepam 4 mg in 2 minutes.
5. History and clinical examination
6. Laboratory tests: blood count, serum CRP, sodium, potassium, creatinine, antiepileptic drug concentrations, a blood sample to evaluate intoxication.

10–40 minutes of convulsions

1. Give fosphenytoin 18 mg phenytoin equivalents (PE)/kg diluted to 25 mg of PE/ml at an injection speed of 150 mg PE/min.
2. Repeat diazepam in doses of 5 mg, if the convulsions do not cease. The maximum dose is 30 mg i.v., or repeat lorazepam as a dose of 4 mg after 5–10 min has elapsed from the first dose. The action of both drugs starts in 2–3 min. The duration of action is only 15–30 min with diazepam, but 12–24 h with lorazepam.
3. If necessary, give additional fosphenytoin 7–10 mg PE/kg i.v. If the patient is sensitive to phenytoin, give i.v. valproate as a bolus of 15–20 mg/kg (200 mg/min) and thereafter 1–2 mg/kg/hour.

Convulsions lasting over 40 minutes

- The patient is transferred to intensive care where general anaesthetics can be used.
    - The starting dose of midazolam is 0.2 mg/kg i.v.; the extra boluses (if necessary) are 0.2–0.4 mg/kg every 5 minutes, the maintenance dose as an infusion is 0.1 mg/kg/h.
    - Propofol (Diprivan®, Propofol, Recofol®) as a starting dose of 2 mg/kg, the extra boluses (if necessary) every 3–5 min are 1–2 mg/kg, the maintenance dose as an infusion is 2 mg/kg/h (range 1–15 mg/kg/h).
    - Thiopental is given 5 mg/kg as an initial bolus, the extra boluses (if necessary) are 1–2 mg/kg every 3–5 min, the maintenance dose as an infusion is 5 mg/kg/h (range 4–7 mg/kg/h).

36.47 Treatment of epilepsy in adults

Reetta Kälviäinen

Basic rules

- Epilepsy requires regular, long-term pharmacotherapy, and the indications should be considered carefully.

- Antiepileptics should be started as soon as the diagnosis has been made and the risk of recurrences has been established.
- Brain imaging is important already after the first seizure to identify processes that can be treated surgically.

General

- In untreated epilepsy, the seizures begin to appear with an increasing frequency, and with time disturbances in brain function may begin to appear also between seizures (e.g. cognitive disturbances).
- The seizures involve an increased risk of accidents and trauma.
- Patients with epilepsy have a 2–3-fold risk of death compared with the normal population.
- With modern medications, 80% of the patients become seizure-free or achieve a satisfactory control over the disease. There are no significant differences in the efficacy of new antiepileptic drugs Ⓒ [1 2].

Chain of treatment

- Epilepsy is diagnosed and treatment is initiated at a neurology clinic.
- Working aged patients are followed up by a neurologist.
- Follow-up can also be carried out in primary care if the disease is in good control, particularly if the patient is elderly or has multiple diseases.
    - When the follow-up is transferred to primary care, a treatment plan and instructions on follow-up are drafted by a neurologist individually for each patient.
    - If the control of seizures deteriorates or new adverse effects or something else alarming appears, the patient is referred to a neurologist.
    - A neurologist should follow-up and treat all patients whose disease is poorly controlled (would new medication or surgery Ⓒ [3 4] give benefit?) or whose medication has caused adverse effects Ⓒ [5 6]. Decisions on stopping medication Ⓒ [7 8], determining the ability to drive a car or to work, and follow-up during pregnancy are always the responsibility of a neurologist.

Choice and implementation of drug therapy

Initiation, dosage, determination of the concentration and follow-up

- Medication is usually initiated when the patient has had two or more epileptic seizures within a year without obvious predisposing factors.
- Medications should be started already after the first seizure if there is no doubt about the diagnosis and the risk of recurrences is high.
    - Symptomatic epilepsy in connection with cerebral infarction, brain injury, dementia in an elderly or other obvious aetiological factor.
- The drug is chosen according to the type of seizure, and treatment is started with only one drug.

Dosing and choice of drug

- The aim is to find the lowest effective dose that controls seizures.
- In newly diagnosed patients the aim is to achieve a state in which the patient does not need to fear new seizures and impose restrictions on living because of fear.
- Carbamazepine, oxcarbazepine, lamotrigine, topiramate or gabapentin are used for the treatment of partial seizures.
- Valproate is the drug of choice if the patient has several types of seizures:
    - generalized epilepsy with tonic-clonic seizures and no prodromal signs
    - typical absence seizures
    - myoclonic seizures
    - atonic seizures.
- Of the new drugs, lamotrigine and topiramate are effective also in generalized epilepsy.
- The dose is always tailored individually. However, steady-state concentrations can be used to determine the dose. The time to steady state is at least 3–5 times the half-life of the drug.

Determining the concentration and adjusting medication

- The concentration is usually determined from a blood sample taken before the morning dose.
- If seizures continue when the concentration is in the therapeutic range (see Table 36.47), the dose is increased to the highest tolerated level.
- Remember that concentrations and half-lifes are mean values obtained in studies and that a considerable part of the patients differ from the average. When the dose is escalated within the treatment range, it is more meaningful to monitor the patient's possible dose-dependent side effects rather than only the laboratory values (with the exception of phenytoin).
- The patient is informed of the dose-dependent side effects so that he/she knows to contact his/her physician when the highest tolerated dose has been exceeded. The dose is then reduced to the highest tolerated dose, and the patient is followed up to see if this dose controls the seizures without having to add another drug.
- If the patient continues to have random seizures when on medication, the therapy usually needs to be intensified even if an obvious predisposing factor is known (with the exception of non-compliance and alcohol abuse).
- Although prophylactic antiepileptics reduce seizures after acute brain injury, they have no effect on mortality and they do not prevent the occurrence of late seizures Ⓐ [9].

Laboratory follow-up

- For follow-up, see the drugs listed below.

NEU

Table 36.47 Pharmacokinetics of antiepileptic drugs

Drug	Therapeutic concentration µmol/l	Half-life (hours)	Days to steady state
Carbamazepine	20–50	10–30	15–30
Valproate	350–700	8–20	3–5
Phenytoin	40–80	9–20(–140)	7–14(–60)
Phenobarbital	50–150	50–100(–160)	10–30
Primidone	30–50	4–12	10–30
Ethosuximide	300–600	40–70	10–15
Clonazepam	0.05–0.2	22–33(–60)	5–7(–13)
Clobazam	–	20	–
Oxcarbazepine	30–120	5–8	15–21
Vigabatrin	–	8–10	2
Lamotrigin	–	29	–
Gabapentin	–	5–7	–

- When the medication has been used for a long time without adverse effects, routine laboratory follow-up can be reduced considerably.
- With some of the newer drugs, follow-up of blood values is not necessary even on initiation.

Adverse effects

- Sometimes medication has to be changed because of intolerable adverse effects.
- Idiosyncratic reactions, such as eczema, always necessitate changing the drug.
- In the starting and escalating phases, drugs may cause CNS adverse effects that usually subside in 1–2 months.

Drugs used for treatment of epilepsy

Phenytoin

- Used for partial epilepsy and for generalized tonic–clonic seizures.
- One advantage of phenytoin, in addition to efficacy, is parenteral administration (fosphenytoin). However, administration is quite complicated because of interactions and saturation kinetics.
- Phenytoin also causes acute CNS adverse effects and long-term adverse effects such as gingival hyperplasia and osteoporosis. Because of these effects, the use of phenytoin is declining.
- Starting dose 50 mg/2 days; 100 mg × 2/day is a common initial dose.
- Saturation kinetics: necessitates careful dosing with dose escalation up to 25 mg/day. The concentration must be monitored.
- Metabolized by the liver (cytochrome P450)
- Enzyme inducer
- Blood count and ALT follow up over the first year
- Alkaline phosphatase (ALP) in long-term use
- Remember that the drug is sometimes effective already at concentrations below the therapeutic range.

Carbamazepine

- Carbamazepine is effective in preventing all types of seizures with focal onset (B) [10]. Problems associated with its use include CNS adverse effects that are common particularly in the initiation phase, idiosyncratic reactions (morbilliform rash), complicated pharmacokinetics, and drug interactions.
- The drug is metabolized by the liver (cytochrome P450 enzyme inductor)
- Depot tablets must be used.
- The initial dose is 100 mg × 2/day, usually up to 300 mg × 2.
- The dose is raised by 200 mg increments.
- The efficacy correlates well with the therapeutic concentration.
- Lower concentrations (below 20 µmol/l) are not effective.
- Blood count and ALT must be followed up over the first year.
- Mild leucocytopenia (up to 2 × 10^9/l) or elevated liver enzymes (ALT up to 150–200) do not predict more severe side effects.
- Lower leucocyte levels or higher ALT levels necessitate changing the drug.
- Indicated for partial epilepsy and tonic-clonic seizures.

Valproate

- Used for generalized epilepsy and partial epilepsy.
- Adverse effects include weight gain and hormonal changes, tremor and hair loss. Valproate is also somewhat more teratogenic than carbamazepine. Valproate causes less adverse effects than carbamazepine or phenytoin, but it may rarely cause quite severe liver reactions.
- Metabolized by the liver (cytochrome P450)
- Enzyme inhibitor
- Depot tablets, dosing 1–2 times a day
- The initial dose for adults is 1000 mg/day, elevations with 500 mg increments
- Maximum dose 2000–(3000) mg/day
- The efficacy does not correlate very well with the therapeutic concentration.
- Follow-up: blood count and ALT over the first year (NOT amylase)
- Vomiting is the most common initial symptom of rare acute liver damage. The combination of vomiting and weight loss occurs in 82%. Routine liver function tests do NOT necessarily show anything abnormal.

Clobazam

- Used only as an add-on drug, mainly in partial epilepsy.
- Dose: 10–20 mg/day, up to 80 mg/day.
- The dose is adjusted according to response; determination of concentration is not necessary.

Lamotrigine

- Used for all types of seizures.

- Use involves the risk of eczema, which occurs more seldom when the dose is elevated slowly. Instructions on dose escalation must be followed carefully and the patient must be advised about possible eczema. If necessary, the drug is discontinued.
- The drug increases the concentration of carbamazepine epoxide by up to 45%: if adverse effects occur, reduce the dose of carbamazepine.
- Metabolized by the liver.
- When combined with valproate, the initiation must be slower (weeks 1–2: 25 mg every other day, weeks 3–4: 25 mg × 2; thereafter 100–200–(300) mg/day in 1–2 doses)
- When combined with enzyme inhibitors, such as carbamazepine, initiation: weeks 1–2: 50 mg × 1, weeks 3–4: 50 mg × 2; thereafter 100–200 mg × 2 (up to 700 mg/day)
- Monotherapy: weeks 1–2: 25 mg × 1, weeks 3–4: 50 mg × 1; thereafter 100–200–500 mg/day in 1–2 doses.

Gabapentin

- Used for partial epilepsy and also as an analgesic.
- Excreted by the kidneys, no interactions.
- Effective as an add-on drug in drug-resistant partial epilepsy A [11].
- Dose escalation 300–600 mg/day up to 900–2400–3600 (4800) mg/day.

Oxcarbazepine

- Used for partial epilepsy and generalized tonic-clonic seizures.
- Oxcarbazepine A [12] causes fewer adverse effects and interactions with other drugs than carbamazepine but is equally effective. Its use is thus increasing.
- However, in the elderly in particular, oxcarbazepine causes hyponatraemia that requires changing the drug if symptoms appear.
- Dose increments of 300 mg to a maximum of 600–1200 mg/day, if necessary up to 3000–4000 mg/day.
- The concentration need not be determined.
- Serum sodium is followed up if symptomatic hyponatraemia is suspected.

Tiagabine

- Indicated for partial epilepsy.
- Metabolized by the liver (cytochrome P450)
- Initial dose 50–10 mg/day with weekly increments.
- Dosing twice daily, high doses 3–4 times daily.
- When combined with an enzyme inducer the minimum dose is 30 mg/day, without enzyme inducer 10 mg/day.
- Maximum dose 70 mg/day.

Topiramate

- Indicated for partial and generalized epilepsy.
- Metabolized partially by the liver.
- Enzyme inducers lower the concentration of topiramate.
- Rapid titration causes cognitive adverse effects, which is why the dose must be raised gradually.
- Weight loss (follow-up)
- Risk of renal calculi (advise to drink amply)
- Initiated slowly: weeks 1–2: 25 mg in the evenings, weeks 3–4: 25 mg × 2, further increments 25–50 mg/day, up to 200–400–(1000) mg/day.

Vigabatrin

- Indicated for partial epilepsy only if other drugs have not been effective. Drug of choice for infantile spasm.
- Excreted by the kidneys, no drug interactions.
- Dose increments of 500 mg to a maximum of 2–3–(4) g/day.
- Determination of concentration is not needed.
- One third of patients develop a concentric visual field defect, the risk of which must always be considered when assessing the benefits against adverse effects.
- Initiated only by an specialist. Requires follow up by an ophthalmologist.

Levetiracetam

- Used as add-on for drug-resistant partial epilepsy A [13].

Managing treatment-resistant epilepsy

- About 35% of patients need several drugs, and 20% suffer from recurring seizures despite the combined use of modern drugs.
- A patient with treatment-resistant epilepsy should always be followed up by a neurologist. In partial epilepsy gabapentin, lamotrigine A [14], topiramate or levetiracetam can be used as a combination in addition to traditional drugs. In generalized epilepsy lamotrigine or topiramate are suitable.
- Some patients with treatment-resistant partial epilepsy benefit from surgery. A neurologist makes the necessary assessment.

NEU

References

1. Chadwick DW, Marson T, Kadir Z. Efficacy and tolerability of new antiepileptic drugs. Epilepsia 1996;37(suppl 6):17–22.
2. The Database of Abstracts of Reviews of Effectiveness (University of York), Database no.: DARE-973055. In: The Cochrane Library, Issue 4, 1999. Oxford: Update Software.
3. Chilcott J, Howell S, Kemeny A, Rittey CD, Richards C. The effectiveness of surgery in the management of epilepsy. Working Group on Acute Purchasing. Sheffield: University of Sheffield, Trent Institute for Health Services Research. Guidance Notes for P. 1999. 1–54.
4. The Database of Abstracts of Reviews of Effectiveness (University of York), Database no.: DARE-20008004. In: The Cochrane Library, Issue 1, 2001. Oxford: Update Software.
5. Vermeulen J, Aldenkamp AP. Cognitive side-effects of antiepileptic drugs. Epilepsy Research 1995;22:65–95.
6. The Database of Abstracts of Reviews of Effectiveness (University of York), Database no.: DARE-964224. In: The Cochrane Library, Issue 4, 1999. Oxford: Update Software.

7. Berg AT, Shinnar S. Relapse following discontinuation of antiepileptic drugs: a meta-analysis. Neurology 1994;44:601–608.
8. The Database of Abstracts of Reviews of Effectiveness (University of York), Database no.: DARE-940235. In: The Cochrane Library, Issue 4, 1999. Oxford: Update Software.
9. Schierhout G, Roberts I. Anti-epileptic drugs for preventing seizures following acute traumatic brain injury. Cochrane Database Syst Rev. 2004;(2):CD000173.
10. Marson AG, Williamson PR, Hutton JL, Clough HE, Chadwick DW; on behalf of the epilepsy monotherapy trialists. Carbamazepine versus valproate monotherapy for epilepsy. Cochrane Database Syst Rev. 2004;(2):CD001030.
11. Marson AG, Kadir ZA, Hutton JL, Chadwick DW. Gabapentin add-on for drug-resistant partial epilepsy. Cochrane Database Syst Rev. 2004;(2):CD001415.
12. Castillo S, Schmidt DB, White S. Oxcarbazepine add-on for drug-resistant partial epilepsy. Cochrane Database Syst Rev. 2004;(2):CD002028.
13. Chaisewikul R, Privitera MD, Hutton JL, Marson AG. Levetiracetam add-on for drug-resistant localization related (partial) epilepsy. Cochrane Database Syst Rev. 2004;(2): CD001901.
14. Ramaratnam S, Marson AG, Baker GA. Lamotrigine add-on for drug-resistant partial epilepsy. Cochrane Database Syst Rev. 2004;(2):CD001909.

36.48 Epileptic patients in traffic and at work

Mikael Ojala

Traffic

- Even one epileptic seizure or induced convulsions permanently prevents the patient driving heavy vehicles or taxi.
- A driving licence may be granted for non-professional driving after consultation with a neurologist, if at least one year has passed without seizures, including nightly seizures and even short disturbances of consciousness.
- After the first seizure, driving must be prohibited for 3 months if all investigations are normal. If epilepsy or other brain pathology is diagnosed, the patients should not drive for one year.
- Antiepileptic medication does not usually prevent driving. Other possible (e.g. neuropsychological) disturbances are more important with regard to driving ability.
- Usually, professional secrecy cannot be broken; the patient will be told not to drive but the authorities are not informed.

Working life

- If the seizures are not completely controlled with medication, the patient should not work in transportation or a job where he or she is prone to accidents (high scaffolding, use of dangerous machinery).
- Seizures hamper work only in severe epilepsy, as long as the tasks have been chosen taking the risk of seizures into account. The neuropsychological problems common in epileptic patients influence the choice of profession more often than the seizures. A thorough assessment of the rehabilitation needs of an epileptic patient may be in place.
- Adequate antiepileptic medication does not impair working capacity.
- Negative attitudes in the working environment often limit working capacity more than the patient's disease.

36.49 Alcohol and epilepsy

Matti Hillbom

Basic rules

- When the excessive use of alcohol or some other substances that act on the central nervous system (barbiturates, benzodiazepines, etc.) is stopped, transient over-excitability in the brain often causes signs of a typical withdrawal syndrome.
- Drugs (heroin, cocaine, amphetamine) do not cause seizures after excessive use, but only in association with intoxication (over-dosage).
- About 25% of acute seizure problems brought to the emergency room of general hospitals may be provoked by alcohol or drug abuse (Finnish figure) (C) [1]. In alcoholics the risk of epileptic seizure is 10-fold compared with a control population.

Withdrawal seizures

- The seizures are primarily generalized grand mal (GM) seizures that occur along with other signs of withdrawal syndrome when long-term excessive use of alcohol or medications is stopped.
- The diagnosis is based on a temporal connection between seizures, other signs of the alcohol withdrawal syndrome, and cessation of long-term and excessive use of alcohol.
- Hangover is the mildest condition of withdrawal and is usually not associated with seizures unless some other cause (scar, tumour, etc.) lowers the seizure threshold.
- Abrupt discontinuation of prolonged heavy drinking often leads to a typical alcohol withdrawal syndrome starting with a seizure or a short burst of seizures within a couple of hours. This usually occurs within 1–2 days of the last drink.
- If convulsions occur after a longer period of time, the cause may be either the cessation of the effect of a sedative drug or an organic brain disease (e.g. subdural haematoma).

Examination and treatment

- A patient with a withdrawal seizure is examined as any other patient with an acute seizure problem (36.45). If there are no signs indicating local brain disease, the probability of a disease that requires treatment (intracranial bleeding, trauma, stroke) is about 6% C [2 3]. Check the serum electrolytes, blood glucose and the acid-base balance (respiratory alkalosis suggests alcohol withdrawal).
- Alcohol withdrawal seizures may lead to status epilepticus (36.46). Therefore, give a rapidly acting drug (e.g. diazepam) rectally or intravenously (not i.m.) immediately after the first seizure.
- Do not prescribe antiepileptic drugs to a patient who consumes excessive amounts of alcohol, because he/she is not capable of using the drug regularly D [4]. Often the patient stops the medication during the drinking period. Alcohol affects drug metabolism. In epileptic patients irregular use of drugs increases the frequency of seizures, which should be kept in mind if the patient is an alcoholic with post-traumatic epilepsy.

Epilepsy provoked by alcohol

- Focal epilepsy or a focal neurological defect usually indicates brain disease C [2 3] and always warrants brain imaging after the first seizure. In post-traumatic epilepsy, or in epilepsy caused by a stroke or other lesion in brain, alcohol withdrawal seizures usually manifest as focal convulsions C [5].
- If moderate alcohol drinking provokes a first-ever seizure in a subject without epilepsy, a careful neurological examination is always warranted C [2 3].

Alcohol, epilepsy and a driving licence

- Subjects with recent alcohol withdrawal seizures should not be granted a driving licence. The successful treatment of alcoholism is the prerequisite for granting a driving licence. This should be explained to the patient.

Can epileptics use alcohol?

- Moderate occasional use of alcohol (1–2 drinks) together with a meal does not increase the frequency of seizures, nor does it affect the metabolism of antiepileptic drugs. A couple of drinks daily (<30 g of alcohol) may be allowed for epileptic patients. However, drinking for intoxication clearly increases the frequency of seizures in epileptic patients.

References

1. Hillbom M, Pieninkeroinen I, Leone M. Seizures in alcohol-dependent patients: epidemiology, pathophysiology and management. CNS Drugs. 2003;17(14):1013–30.
2. Earnest MP et al. Intracranial lesions shown by CT scans in 259 cases of first alcohol-related seizures. Neurology 1988;38:1561–1565.
3. Shoenenberger RA, Heim SM. Indication for computed tomography of the brain in patients with uncomplicated generalised seizures. Br J Med 1994;309:986–989.
4. Hillbom M, Hjelm-Jäger M. Should alcohol withdrawal seizures be treated with anti-epileptic drugs. Acta Neurol Scand 1984;69:39–42.
5. Bråthen G, Brodtkorb E, Helde G. ym. The diversity of seizures related to alcohol use. A study of consecutive patients. European Journal of Neurology 1999:6;697–703.

36.55 Infection and central nervous system manifestation

Jussi Kovanen

Basic rules

- Infections may cause central nervous system manifestations
  - when the pathogens spread directly into the central nervous system or
  - indirectly, e.g. as a result of toxic factors, fever, or electrolyte disorders, in which case inflammatory reactions are not found in the cerebrospinal fluid.
- When a patient with infection also presents with neurological symptoms, he or she should be referred to a hospital for adequate testing and treatment.
- A patient under neuroleptic treatment may present with neuroleptic malignant syndrome (36.6), including high fever, confusion, and muscle rigidity.

NEU

Most common symptoms

Headache

- Often of vascular type, felt as a pulsating throb. No neck stiffness is present. Causes:
  - infections in the head (sinuitis, dental infections)
  - pyelonephritis
  - bronchopneumonia
  - sepsis
  - various virus infections.
- Treatment consists of treating the underlying disease and, if symptoms so indicate, prescribing a prostaglandin inhibitor.

Nausea and vomiting

- Treatment of the underlying disease, intravenous hydration, metoclopramide or prochlorperazine suppositories.

Confusion

- High fever is often the only cause. Sepsis is possible, especially in the elderly. Confusion is also frequently found in connection with respiratory infections and pyelonephritis. Differential diagnoses are meningitis and encephalitis.
- Consider lumbar puncture if you suspect central nervous system infection.
- Avoid excessive sedation in order not to interfere with the monitoring of the patient's state of consciousness.

Epileptic seizures

- Especially in epileptics, but also in others, seizures may be provoked by fever, electrolyte disturbances, or toxic factors.
- Treatment consists of intravenous diazepam, lowering the fever, and treating the underlying disease or electrolyte disorder.

36.56 Meningitis

Jussi Kovanen

Aims

- The cause of acute meningitis should be established quickly, and the disease should be treated according to the aetiology.
- Slowly progressing meningitis can be the cause of general symptoms and impaired consciousness, even when neck stiffness is absent.

Acute bacterial meningitis

- In adults the most significant causes are Neisseria meningitidis and Streptococcus pneumoniae.

Symptoms

- High fever
- Headache
- Neck stiffness
- Impaired consciousness
- Meningococcal disease is often associated with petechiae and endotoxin shock.

Diagnosis

- CRP level is elevated.
- A cerebrospinal fluid (36.17) and blood sample should be obtained for bacterial culture before starting treatment.
  - Cerebrospinal fluid is opaque, drips under pressure.
  - Cell count, glucose, protein, a stained smear, and culture must be examined (36.17).

Typical cerebrospinal fluid findings

- Polymorphonuclear leucocytes, 1000–10 000 × 10^6/l.
- Glucose concentration low, <2 mmol/l.
- Protein concentrations increased to >1000 mg/l.
- At the initial stage, the cell reaction may not have fully developed; therefore, a new sample should be obtained in a few hours.

Treatment

- Initially, G-penicillin 4 million IU × 6 i.v.; for patients allergic to penicillin, cefotaxime 2 g × 4 i.v. or ceftriaxone 2 g × 1 i.v.
- The above initial treatment is appropriate for meningitis caused by meningococci and pneumococci. If haemophilus is the suspected cause, the preferred initial medication is ceftriaxone 2 g × 1 i.v, with ampicillin 2 g × 6 i.v. as a secondary alternative. The final selection of an antibiotic occurs when the causing agent is known.
- Dexamethasone 10 mg × 4 i.v. for 3 days, started 15 min before the antibiotic, is recommended **A** [1,2,3,4,5,6].
- There are reports suggesting that perorally administered glycerol may reduce complications. The optimal dosage is not known, but 5 ml/kg ad 30 ml/dose 3 times a day can be used.
- If the aetiology is meningococcal, preventive medication is advisable for
  - family members
  - other children and staff at any day care site, child care center and in the child's school class
  - individuals who have been exposed to the patient's saliva.
- Preventive medication **D** [7]
  - For both children and adults, rifampicin 10 mg/kg × 2 for 2 days is appropriate.
  - For adults, an alternative is ciprofloxaczin 500 mg as a single dose.
- If feasible, vaccination against the specific type of meningococcus may be considered.

Acute viral meningitis

- 3–4 times as common as bacterial meningitis. The predominant causative agents are the Coxsackie, ECHO and herpes viruses.
- Mumps has become rare due to vaccination programmes.
- Onset is most common in late summer or early autumn.
- The possibility of HIV infection should be kept in mind in acute, spontaneously healing meningitis.

Symptoms

- These develop more slowly than in bacterial meningitis, and the patient's general condition is clearly better.
  - Headache
  - Nausea and vomiting
  - Fatigue
  - Neck stiffness is common, but not necessarily present.

Diagnosis

- Lumbar puncture should be performed in order to rule out bacterial meningitis.
- Even if the cerebrospinal fluid is clear, it is advisable to take samples for bacterial stain and culture, possibly including tuberculosis stain and culture.
- In addition, 2 ml of spinal fluid should be stored for later virological testing.
- Obtain a serum sample for antibody testing and repeat in 10–14 days.

Typical cerebrospinal fluid findings

- Leucocytes, predominantly mononuclear, $20–200 \times 10^6$/l
- Glucose concentration over 2 mmol/l
- Proteins generally under 1000 mg/l

Treatment

- Depending on symptoms, initially with fluid therapy.
- For nausea, methoclopramide; for headache, a prostaglandin inhibitor.
- A decision about the appropriate treatment facility should be based on the final diagnosis and the general condition of the patient. Home care may also be considered, depending on the circumstances and the condition of the patient.
- If symptoms persist or become more severe, repeated diagnostic evaluation is necessary.

Subacute and chronic meningitis

Causes

- Tuberculosis
- Fungi
- Borrelia
- Syphilis
- Sarcoidosis
- Malignant tumours
- These patients should always be hospitalized for adequate testing and evaluation.

Symptoms

- Fever, headache, fatigue
- Neck stiffness may not be present.

Tuberculous meningitis

- Today this condition tends to be rare; however, it is important to bear in mind, because early treatment is crucial for the prognosis.
- A history of recent of previously treated tuberculosis may be elicited.
- Symptoms develop slowly in 1–2 weeks.
- Treatment must be initiated no later than at the point when the patient's consciousness begins to become impaired.

Cerebrospinal fluid findings

- The findings are the same as in viral meningitis; except the glucose concentration is decreased, <2 mmol/l.
- Initially the glucose concentration may even be normal, especially if the patient has a glucose infusion.
- Diagnostic problems are caused by the unreliability of the acid-fast stains, or if the confirmation based on the culture will be too late to be of use in treatment decisions.

Other investigations

- Tuberculosis stains and culture are also performed on the sputum and urine; chest radiographs are taken with tuberculosis in mind.

Treatment

- Pyrazinamide, rifampicin, initially possibly INH and a combination (up to 2 months) of streptomycin and ethambutol
- Treatment duration is 9–12 months; in cases of tuberculoma a minimum of 18 months. Adjunctive steroids may be beneficial C [8].

Fungal meningitis

- The condition is rare, unless there are underlying factors that compromise the immune system.
- Causes include Candida albicans, Cryptococcus, and frequently in association with diabetes, mucormycosis of sinus origin.
- The manifestation of the disease resembles meningeal tuberculosis.

Cerebrospinal fluid findings

- Similar to those in tbc meningitis, but the cellular content may also include some polymorphonuclear leucocytes.
- Diagnosis is based on a positive fungus culture.

NEU

Borrelia meningitis

- Associated with Lyme disease (1.29), a possible manifestation of neuroborreliosis.
- Onset of symptoms generally in 1–2 months from the tick bite, which may have been followed by an erythema migrans skin rash.
- The bite may often be ignored, or a rash is not always present.

Symptoms

- Slowly developing neck and back pain
- Headache and fatigue
- Some patients have distinct neck stiffness
- Cranial nerve pareses are common, most likely facial paralysis.
- Neuralgia and/or motor pareses in the nerve roots or peripheral nerves.

Cerebrospinal fluid findings

- Cell counts are similar to those in viral meningitis, and glucose concentration is mostly normal.
- Protein concentrations in the cerebrospinal fluid are often increased, >1000 mg/l.
- The IgG index of the cerebrospinal fluid is elevated (normal value < 0.60).
- Borrelia antibodies (1.29) are usually elevated both in the serum and in the cerebrospinal fluid, occasionally in only one of them. False positive borrelia antibodies are found in connection with syphilis, recurrent fever (Borrelia recurrentis), and tuberculosis.

Treatment

- In most cases, the symptoms disappear with no treatment in a few weeks or months, but may also become chronic. Even after a long asymptomatic period (several years), new manifestations of chronic borreliosis may appear, which is why effective treatment is indicated as early as possible.
- The most effective treatment of chronic borreliosis consists of ceftriaxone 2 g × 1 i.v. for 14 days.

Other chronic types of meningitis

- Most important of these are the meningitis possibly associated with secondary syphilis and neurosarcoidosis, as well as a carcinoma and lymphoma that has spread into the meninx. The most appropriate test for syphilis is serum and spinal fluid TPHA. The presence of malignant cells can only be determined by cytological examination of the cerebrospinal fluid.

References

1. Prasad K, Haines T. Dexamethasone treatment for acute bacterial meningitis: how strong is the evidence for routine use. J Neurol Neurosurg Psych 1995;59:31–37.
2. The Database of Abstracts of Reviews of Effectiveness (University of York), Database no.: DARE-951931. In: The Cochrane Library, Issue 4, 1999. Oxford: Update Software.
3. McIntyre PB, Berkey CS, King SM, Schaad UB, Kilpi T, Kanra GY, Perez CM. Dexamethasone as adjunctive therapy in bacterial meningitis: a meta-analysis of randomized clinical trials since 1988. JAMA 1997;278:925–931.
4. The Database of Abstracts of Reviews of Effectiveness (University of York), Database no.: DARE-978360. In: The Cochrane Library, Issue 2, 2000. Oxford: Update Software.
5. de Gans J, van de Beek D; European Dexamethasone in Adulthood Bacterial Meningitis Study Investigators. Dexamethasone in adults with bacterial meningitis. N Engl J Med 2002 Nov 14;347:1549–56.
6. van de Beek D, de Gans J, McIntyre P, Prasad K. Corticosteroids in acute bacterial meningitis. Cochrane Database Syst Rev 2003(3):CD004305.
7. Hart C. Prophylactic antibiotics in contacts of patients with meningococcal disease. Clinical Evidence 2000;4:404–405.
8. Prasad K, Volmink J, Menon GR. Steroids for treating tuberculous meningitis. Cochrane Database Syst Rev. 2004;(2): CD002244.

36.57 Encephalitis

Jussi Kovanen

Aims

- Encephalitis should be suspected in patients with acute-onset confusion or stupor when no other causative factor is evident.
- If encephalitis is suspected, the patient should be hospitalised immediately for adequate testing.

Aetiology

- The most common form of encephalitis is meningoencephalitis, where the disease has spread from the meninges also to brain tissue.
- The incidence of viral encephalitis is 3/100 000 per year.
- The most important causes are:
  - herpes simplex virus
  - enteroviruses in late summer
  - tick-borne encephalitis
  - Japanese encephalitis.
- Other causes include:
  - cytomegalovirus, Ebstein–Barr virus, varicella virus, adenovirus, and influenza viruses.
- HIV infection may be accompanied by chronic encephalitis caused by the HI virus itself, or, in an immunosuppressed patient, by some other microbe, especially toxoplasma.
- Bacterial diseases with encephalitic manifestations:
  - Listeriosis
  - Mycoplasma infections
  - Borreliosis
  - Syphilis

Differential diagnosis

- A polymorphonuclear leucocyte reaction in the cerebrospinal fluid, developing a few days after subarachnoid or cerebral haemorrhage, and a concurrently low glucose level, may complicate differential diagnosis.

Herpes encephalitis

- A disease caused by the HSV-1 virus, where fever, fatigue, and headache are usually associated with symptoms indicating damage to the temporal lobe:

- confusion and hallucinations
- epileptic seizures
- dysphasia
- impaired consciousness.

Diagnosis

- The cerebrospinal fluid is typical of viral meningitis, and the glucose level is also likely to be normal.
- Encephalitis is unlikely if the patient has no fever and the cerebrospinal fluid is found to be normal.
- In the acute stage, the virus may be demonstrated in the spinal fluid by using the PCR method.
- The EEG is abnormal and shows evidence of damage in one or both temporal lobes. A typical periodic change is an occasional manifestation.
- Changes seen in the CT scan of the head are generally slight at the initial stage, but in about a week changes can be observed in the affected temporal region. Abnormal findings usually appear earlier in MRI and SPECT.
- The diagnosis is later supported by an increase of CSF herpes antibodies. Changes in serum antigens or positive results from pharyngeal culture should not be regarded as significant. A viral culture of the cerebrospinal fluid is rarely positive.

Treatment

- In practice, treatment should be initiated upon clinical suspicion, because mortality in untreated cases is ca. 70%, and survivors often suffer severe sequelae.
- Acyclovir 10 mg/kg × 3 i.v. for 10 days
- If herpes encephalitis is suspected or treated, it is important to make sure that treatable bacterial diseases have been ruled out. In unclear cases it is advisable to provide simultaneous treatment, e.g. for meningeal tuberculosis.

Prognosis

- Even among treated patients mortality is ca. 20%, and 50–60% will recover well or satisfactorily.

Encephalitis following chickenpox

- One of the most common forms of paediatric encephalitis.
- Typically appears 2–4 weeks after other symptoms of infection.
- Antiviral treatment is administered only to immunosuppressed patients.

Tick-borne encephalitis

- The disease is caused by a virus infection via tick bite.

Symptoms

- 10–30% of those infected will be afflicted with the clinical disease.
- The incubation period is 7–14 days.
- The disease manifests itself in two stages:
  - Initial common cold-like illness lasting up to a week
  - After the cold, the patient is asymptomatic for about a week, followed by the late stage lasting from one week to two months when typical symptoms of meningeal encephalitis are present.

Prognosis, treatment, and prevention

- Mild irritability and other neuropsychiatric symptoms are common after the disease has run its course. Permanent damage, such as paralysis, is possible.
- Treatment is symptomatic. Bed rest and hospitalisation are recommended in the meningeal stage.
- A vaccine containing inactivated whole viruses is available. The inoculation series includes two injections at one-month intervals and a booster in one year. The vaccine provides good protection, and side effects are minor (B) [1].

Chronic neuroborreliosis

- See 1.29.
- Possible manifestations include:
  - progressing dementia
  - MS-like clinical presentation
  - ataxia
  - cranial nerve pareses
  - chronic paroxysmal vertigo
  - loss of hearing
  - myelitis
  - polyradiculitis
  - polyneuropathy
  - various psychological symptoms.
- Serological diagnostics and treatment are the same as in borrelia meningitis.

Nervous system syphilis

- The possibility of syphilis should be noted in association with:
  - meningitis
  - differential diagnosis of myelitis or spinal meningitis
  - diagnostics of progressing vascular symptoms.
- Dementia paralytica is the classic manifestation of dementia associated with late-stage syphilis.
- Dorsal tabes involves sensory loss caused by damage to the dorsal column system and ataxia as well as neuralgic pain sensations.
- Serum TPHA can be used as a diagnostic screening test.

NEU

Reference

1. Demicheli V, Graves P, Pratt M, Jefferson T. Vaccines for preventing tick-borne encephalitis. Cochrane Database Syst Rev. 2004;(2):CD000977.

36.58 Brain abscess

Jussi Kovanen

Basic rules

- If an abscess is suspected, the patient should be sent to the hospital emergency room. The patient usually presents with a focal neurological symptom.
- Lumbar puncture is contraindicated because of the risk of brain herniation.

Aetiology

- Previous infections as starting points for diagnosis:
  - Dental infections and treatment
  - Skin infections
  - Respiratory infections
  - Endocarditis
- The propagation of the infection is mostly haematogenic, usually caused either by streptococci, staphylococci, or anaerobes; mixed infections are also frequent. Several abscesses may occur simultaneously.

Symptoms

- Principally caused by the local effect of the abscess on brain tissue, i.e. symptoms point to specific sites.
- Symptoms of infection are often slight or even absent.
- Neurological symptoms are typically progressing.
  - Hemiparesis
  - Dysphasia
  - Visual field defects
  - Changes in personality
  - Epileptic seizures
  - Headache
  - Papilloedema is common.

Diagnosis

- A CT scan generally shows a typical circular lesion with surrounding oedema. Differentiation from a malignant brain tumour is often uncertain until a neurosurgical puncture has been performed.

Treatment

- Choice of treatment is determined by the causing organism; usually penicillin or chloramphenicol combined with metronidazole i.v.
- Referral to a neurosurgeon.

36.59 Slow viral infections of the central nervous system

Jussi Kovanen

SSPE – Subacute Sclerotic Panencephalitis

- Encephalitis caused by the measles virus in children and young adults. Measles vaccination programs have rendered this disease extremely rare.
- Slowly progressing; symptoms include deterioration of psychological capacity, motor disturbances, and muscle twitches.
- Mostly fatal; usually results in death in less than two years.

Diagnosis

- The cerebrospinal fluid sample usually shows slight mononuclear pleocytosis, increased protein concentration (>1000 mg/l), increased IgG index and rubeola antibodies.
- EEG shows a typical finding of periodic wave complexes.

PML – Progressive Multifocal Leukoencephalopathy

- A progressing infection caused by the papovavirus that results in white matter lesions.
- This rare infections occurs in patients with lymphoma, carcinoma, sarcoidosis, or immunosuppression.
- Progressing motor disorder and deterioration of psychological capacity are typical findings.
- The disease is generally fatal within 3–6 months.

Creutzfeldt–Jakob disease (CJD)

Sporadic CJD

- A subacute dementing prion disease in patients aged 50–70 years with progressing motor disorders and myoclonic twitching.
- Incidence of the sporadic disease is 1/1000 000 per year. Usually fatal within 3–12 months.

Variant CJD

- Bovine spongiform encephalopathy (BSE), a prion disease of cattle ("mad cow disease") was first identified in Great Britain in 1986.
- In 1996 BSE was confirmed to infect man and cause variant CJD that affects young persons.
- In the years 1995–2000, approximately 100 persons have developed variant CJD in Britain, most of the patients have been 15–35-year-olds.

- Symptoms initially include depression and sensory defects, later also dementia, cerebellar symptoms, myoclonus, involuntary movements and other neurological manifestations.
- Unlike the sporadic form, the disease lasts for more than a year and EEG changes are not observed.
- The incubation time is not known, but it has been proposed to be as long as 20–30 years.
- BSE can be transmitted by blood transfusion. Many countries have prohibited persons who have resided in Great Britain in 1980–1996 from donating blood.
- BSE has since been found in cattle in several European countries.

Diagnosis

- Routine cerebrospinal fluid tests and CT findings are normal, but in the sporadic form EEG shows a progressive change consisting of triphasic sharp wave complexes at intervals of one second.
- MRI and some special CSF tests may also show pathological changes.
- The infectious nature of the disease has been demonstrated by inoculating diseased central nervous tissue into laboratory animals that contract the disease after a long asymptomatic latency period.
- Even though the only confirmed methods of transmission of sporadic CJD are by central nervous tissue and the cornea, it is advisable to maintain so-called blood–barrier isolation when the patient is being treated.
- The causal agent is resistant to several common disinfectants, but not to sodium hydroxide.

36.60 Poliomyelitis and post-polio syndrome

Jussi Kovanen

Acute poliomyelitis

Infection

- Infection is possible in those regions of Asia and Africa where the disease is endemic if vaccine protection is inadequate.
- Incubation period is 1–2 weeks.

Manifestation

- At the onset, muscle pains and paraesthetic sensations are typical.
- Of those infected, 1% will get aseptic meningitis; of these 1–2% also develop paralyses.
- Rapidly developing flaccid paralyses are often asymmetrical.
- 10–15% of patients with paralyses develop bulbar symptoms, most commonly pharyngeal paresis.
- In addition to muscle weakness, respiratory distress may be caused by damage to the respiratory centre.
- Recovery will begin within a few weeks from the onset of symptoms and can be expected to be complete in about 6 months.
- Functional recovery is fairly good in those muscles that were not completely paralysed.

Diagnosis of acute poliomyelitis

- Serological tests and faecal virus isolation
- Cerebrospinal fluid
  - A finding of 20–300 mononuclear leucocytes, some of which may initially be polymorphonuclear.
  - Protein concentration may increase to up to 2000 mg/l.
  - Glucose concentration is normal.

Differential diagnosis

- Coxsackie and echo viruses may cause a mild condition resembling poliomyelitis.
- In polyradiculitis (36.92) the symptoms are generally symmetrical, and the cell findings of the cerebrospinal fluid are normal, while the protein concentration is increased.

Post-polio syndrome

- Some patients afflicted with poliomyelitis develop increased weakness and fatigue in the muscles affected by the disease, or varying degrees of muscle and joint pain many years or even decades after their acute illness.
- The origin of the syndrome is still undetermined; however, the most likely explanation of the pain symptoms is the chronic stress associated with the muscle weakness.
- Neurophysiological test results suggest that the cells of the anterior horn must take over the supply of an increased number of muscle cells–a task that, as the patient ages, overwhelms the cells.
- Muscle weakness usually progresses rather slowly.
- Treatment consists of maintaining muscle activity and avoiding overexertion; the need for assistive devices should also be assessed.

36.65 Headache

Markus Färkkilä

Epidemiology and classification

- Headache is experienced by 70–95% of all people at some point in their life.

- Headache is most common in 20–45-year-olds, and its incidence decreases steadily with ageing.
- According to international criteria, headaches are divided into 14 different classes. Classes 1–4 cover primary, classes 5–12 cover secondary headaches and classes 13–14 cover cranial neuralgias and facial pain. According to the International Headache Society (IHS) classification, each headache of a patient is classified separately, i.e. a patient may have several concurrent headache diseases.

Primary headaches

- Migraine (36.67)
- Tension-type headache (36.66)
- Cluster headache and other trigeminal autonomic cephalalgias (36.68)
- Other primary headaches

Secondary headaches

- Headaches associated with cerebrovascular disorders
- Headaches associated with pressure changes in cerebrospinal fluid or the brain (expanding lesions, hydrocephalus, headache caused by either spontaneous or lumbar puncture-induced lowering of CSF pressure)
- Traumatic headaches
- Headaches associated with infections
- Withdrawal headaches (e.g. analgesics D [1,2], caffeine, alcohol)
- Headaches associated with disorders of homeostasis (electrolyte disturbances etc.)
- Headaches associated with structures of the skull, e.g. the ears, eyes, sinuses and teeth
- Headaches attributed to psychiatric disorders

Cranial neuralgias and facial pain

- Cranial neuralgias and central causes of facial pain (36.94)
- Other headache, cranial neuralgia or primary facial pain

Examining the headache patient

- On the basis of history, the examination follows one of the two main lines
  - Acute pain
  - Subacute, chronic pain

Causes of acute headache

- Migraine attack
- Subarachnoid haemorrhage (SAH) (36.32) and cerebral haemorrhages (36.33)
- Meningitis/other infection
- Skull traumas
- Neuralgias
- Vasodilatating drugs, nitrate
- Headache associated with physical exertion, coital headache
- Sudden rise in blood pressure, pheochromocytoma (24.68)
- Elevated intracranial pressure
- Cluster headache (36.68)

Causes of subacute or chronic headache

- Tension-type headache
- Addiction to analgesics D [1,2]
- Traction headache (tumours)
- Post-traumatic headache
- Sinusitis, otitis
- Chronic meningitis (sarcoidosis, fungus, tuberculosis)
- Headache caused by malocclusion and teeth
- Hyperthyroidism
- Hyperparathyroidism
- Hypoglycaemia, hypoxia, hypercapnia
- Vasculitis, thrombosis of dural venous sinuses

Chronic daily headache

- Daily or almost daily headache caused by several concurring different headaches, such as chronic migraine, chronic tension-type headache, excessive use of analgesics, etc. It is most important to stop the excess use of analgesics D [1,2] and to start to treat each headache disease separately.

Diagnostic work-up of the headache symptom

- Analyse the origin of the headache symptom.
- Examine the patient carefully for general and neurological status.
- Evaluate the need for possible (differential) diagnostic examinations.
- Explain to the patient the mechanisms underlying headache.
- Consider treatment options.

History and status of the headache patient

- Duration of ache
  - 1–3 days, as in migraine, or more continuous pain as in tension type headache, etc.
  - Very short-term pain, as in an episode of cluster headache (30–180 min) or an attack of neuralgic pain (seconds)
- Onset of symptoms
  - Sudden as in SAH, migraine or cluster headache
  - Gradual as in tension-type headache or expanding lesion, infection, etc.
- Rate of occurrence, recurrence
  - Recurring, long-term ache is often a migraine or tension headache.
  - Episodes of cluster headache occur daily.
- Location of the pain
  - Tension headache is often occipital and temporal occurring either unilaterally or bilaterally.

- Migraine is almost always and cluster headache is invariably unilateral.
- Causes underlying unilateral temporal headache may include e.g. tension headache, bruxism, sinusitis, temporal arteritis (21.46) or disorders of the temporomandibular joint or malocclusion

♦ Nature of the pain

- Vascular pain is often throbbing or pulsating; tension headache is vice-like, pressing or tightening.
- Migraine and headache caused by an increase in intracranial pressure (36.96) begin early in the morning
- A cluster headache attack often begins after a couple of hours of sleep.

♦ Symptoms associated with the headache

- Prodromal symptoms, such as tiredness, yawning, craving for sweets, etc. suggest migraine.
- The aura symptom of migraine may be an expanding, bright scintillating visual disturbance, rarely also hemilateral numbness, difficulty of speech, etc.
- In an episode of TIA (36.30) the visual field or parts of it become blurred, and there is no bright scintillation; however, numbness and speech symptoms may also suggest ischaemic cerebrovascular disturbance. A TIA episode is not followed by headache.
- An aura may sometimes also be epileptic and associated with a tumour, etc.
- There is no nausea or vomiting in tension-type headache. If these symptoms occur, a migraine attack is also present or the nausea may be associated with increased intracranial pressure.

♦ Provocating and alleviating factors

- A migraine attack may be triggered by a change in the amount of mental stress or by alcohol; odours and bright lights may also trigger the attack.
- A patient with migraine seeks rest in a darkened place; whereas tension-type headache may be alleviated by alcohol or a walk.

♦ History of medications

- Daily use of analgesics is associated with the risk of withdrawal headache.
- Triptans are effective only against migraine and cluster headache.

Status examination

♦ A headache patient is given a neurological status examination interictally; the results are often normal.

♦ The fundi of the eyes should be examined from all headache patients. Irregularity of the edge of the papilla and the absence of venous pulsation may suggest elevated intracranial pressure.

♦ In cases of headache in the area of the eyes,

- intraocular pressure should be measured
- blood pressure should be measured.

Further investigations

♦ Primary headache diseases, such as migraine and tension headache, are diagnosed on the basis of history and status examination.

♦ If necessary for differential diagnosis, test selectively the following parameters

- Blood count
- Erythrocyte sedimentation rate
- Serum TSH and/or free T_4
- Fasting blood glucose
- Serum sodium, potassium, calcium
- Serum creatinine.

♦ Patients with symptoms of infection are examined by ultrasonography or x-ray of the maxillary and frontal sinuses.

♦ Lumbar puncture should be performed when SAH, meningitis or other CNS infection is suspected (36.17). In SAH suspicion head CT is considered the primary examination (of choice), because in SAH patients lumbar puncture may increase the risk of herniation. If brain CT scan is normal in a patient with suspected SAH, the condition must be excluded by performing a lumbar puncture.

Indications of referral to further examinations

♦ Headache is associated with an abnormal status

- Nuchal rigidity, personality change, diplopia, papillary stasis, asymmetrical reflexes, etc.

♦ Headache is continuous even though the patient's status is normal.

♦ Headache occurs in connection with physical strain or coughing.

♦ When a CNS infection or SAH is suspected.

♦ There are indications (see 36.66) for performing a head CT scan or MRI and the patient needs a referral to a neurology specialist unit for the examination.

♦ The patient needs withdrawal treatment for analgesics or ergotamine.

♦ A headache attack that does not respond to medication is encountered in primary care.

♦ The headache causes inability to work.

Treatment of headache

♦ Treatment of headache is discussed separately in the articles on different types of headache.

- Tension-type headache (36.66)
- Migraine (36.67)
- Lumbar puncture headache (36.17)
- Headache in children (29.1)

References

1. Medication-induced headache: overview and systematic review of therapeutic approaches. Annals of Pharmacotherapy 1999; 33:61–72.
2. The Database of Abstracts of Reviews of Effectiveness (University of York), Database no.: DARE-990346. In: The Cochrane Library, Issue 4, 2000. Oxford: Update Software.

36.66 Tension-type headache

Markus Färkkilä

Basic rules

- Tension-type headache is the most common cause of headache, head pain; however, the underlying mechanism remains unclear.
- According to the definition of an international classification committee (ICHD 2004) headaches are divided to episodic (<15 headache days/month) and chronic (>15 headache days/month) types.
- Tension-type headache includes headaches caused by both muscle tension and mental stress.
- Findings on muscle palpation do not correlate with the occurrence of headache.
- In complicated cases, tension headache occurs often concomitantly with migraine.

Symptoms

- A steady, vice-like, pressing and tightening pain that worsens gradually towards the evening.
- Localized to the temples, occiput or the skullcap; usually bilateral, but may also be unilateral.
- The scalp may be tender locally, and stabbing, excruciating pains are felt on the skullcap.
- Occasionally night-time numbness of the upper extremities occurs.
- Dizziness when sitting or standing up, with a sense of momentary loss of balance.
- Depression-type sleep disturbance often associated.

Diagnosis

- Based on history and clinical examination.
- Neurological status is normal.
- On palpation some patients have temporal or occipital tenderness as well as tension of the neck and shoulders.
- An x-ray of the cervical vertebrae often reveals straightened lordosis.

Differential diagnosis

- Migraine without aura (includes: prodromal symptoms, nausea/vomiting, aggravated by strain)
- Malocclusion (localization of pain, bruxism)
- Sinusitis (radiograph or ultrasound of the maxillary sinuses)
- Glaucoma (tonometry)
- Temporal arteritis (elevated erythrocyte sedimentation rate, often unilateral)
- Hyperthyroidism
- Hyperparathyroidism
- Compression of the N. occipitalis major (follows the boundaries of the region innervated, unilateral)
- Brain tumour (morning nausea, progressively worsening headache, other relevant symptoms)

Indications for head computed tomography or magnetic resonance imaging in headache

- Suspicion of subarachnoidal haemorrhage
- Progressively worsening headache
- Abnormal neurological status in association with headache
- Headache occurs only in connection with coughing or physical exertion.
- An episode of unconsciousness is associated with the headache.
- An endocrine disturbance is associated with the headache.
- The patient or a member of his/her family has neurofibromatosis.
- Recurring/continuous vomiting is associated with the headache.

Treatment

Episodic tension headache

- Exercise, stretching, physical training
- Short-term (5 days) course of paracetamol or NSAIDs, combined with a muscle relaxant or benzodiazepine, if necessary.

Chronic tension headache

- Stopping excess use of analgesics
- Massage, physical training, exercise, sauna (not form-building exercise or jogging)
- Ergonomics
- Relaxation
- Physiotherapy, acupuncture
- Injections of local anaesthetics to trigger points
- Medication
  - Amitriptyline 10–25 mg in the evening, flupenthixol 0.5–1.5 mg, doxepin 10–25 mg alone or combined with a muscle relaxant or tizanidine 2–6 mg/day.
  - Medication is continued for 1–6 months depending on the case.

36.67 Migraine

Markus Färkkilä

Basic rules

- The therapy for mild migraine consists of paracetamol, aspirin or NSAIDs either alone or combined with metoclopramide.
- In severe or disabling attacks, triptan should be taken as primary treatment, not after the NSAID taken at the onset of the attack has proven inefficient (B) [1].

Definition and epidemiology

- Migraine is a hereditary paroxysmal disease with its origin in the brainstem nuclei.
- Average prevalence in the general population is 10%, in men 4.8% and in women 14.6%. It occurs mainly in persons of working age.
- Migraine attacks are classified into the form with aura (15%), in which the attack is preceded by prodromal symptoms, i.e. aura (e.g. visual disturbance) before the headache, and the form without aura (85%), which begins directly with the headache.
- Factors precipitating migraine attacks include disturbances of the sleep–wake rhythm, hypoglycaemia and changes in the amount of stress. The effect of nutritional factors, with the exception of alcohol, varies greatly between individuals.

Symptoms

- Prodromal symptoms on the day before the attack: yawning, desire for sweets, tiredness, and change of personality
- Aura symptoms: enlargening visual disturbance, scintillating scotomas, zigzag-shaped fortification line, numbness, speech disturbance, paraesthesia lasting for 5–60 min.
- At the end of the aura phase or after it, a pulsating, unilateral severe or moderate headache begins, which is followed by nausea and vomiting.
- Migraine without aura begins with the headache.
- A migraine aura can also occur without the following headache (NB: differential diagnosis).
- The attack is associated with disturbances of the autonomous nervous system, pale skin, disturbed motility of the bowel, etc.

Diagnosis

- Based on patient history and normal neurological status between attacks. In adult patients with typical migraine neuroimaging is not warranted if neurological status is normal (C) [2 3].

Diagnostic criteria of migraine with aura (ICHD 2004)

- The patient has had at least two attacks during which the following symptoms have occurred:
  - The aura symptom
  - The duration of the aura is more than 4 minutes or the patient has had two consecutive auras
  - The aura is followed by a headache within 60 minutes.
- The headache fulfils the criteria of migraine without aura.

Diagnostic criteria of migraine without aura (ICHD 2004)

- The patient has had at least five headache attacks lasting for 4–72 hours with at least two features from group A and at least one feature from group B associated with it.
  - A. Symptoms
    - The headache is pulsating.
    - The headache is unilateral.
    - The headache is moderate or severe and interferes with normal daily activities.
    - Physical activity aggravates the headache.
  - B. Symptoms
    - Nausea and/or vomiting
    - Photophobia and phonophobia

Differential diagnosis

- Tension headache (no prodromal symptoms, exercise improves the condition)
- Subarachnoid haemorrhage
- Transient ischaemic attack (TIA) (dark visual field deficiency, no bright visual sensations, no subsequent headache)
- Acute glaucoma
- Meningitis (fever)
- Temporal lobe epilepsy seizure
- Cluster headache (typically no aura, no vomiting)

Treatment of migraine attack

- Rest in a quite, dark room
- During a migraine attack, drugs are best absorbed rectally or as effervescent tablets or in powdered form.
- Combining metoclopramide (A) [4 5] to other migraine drugs improves their absorption.

Non-steroidal anti-inflammatory drugs

- Aspirin acid at 1000 mg or paracetamol 1000 mg either alone or combined with metoclopramide 10–20 mg or some other peroral nonsteroidal anti-inflammatory drug (A) [4 5]: tolfenamic acid 200 mg, ketoprofen 50–100 mg, naproxen 500–1000 mg, ibuprofen 800 mg, etc.

Triptans

- Triptans are drugs of first choice in severe or incapacitating migraine attacks B [1].
- Sumatriptan 50–100 mg p.o A [6], 25 mg suppository, 6 mg s.c. A [7 8 9 10], 20 mg intranasally
- Zolmitriptan 2.5–5 mg p.o., 5 mg intranasally
- Naratriptan 2.5–5 mg p.o.
- Rizatriptan 5–10 mg p.o. A [11]
- Almotriptan 12.5 mg p.o.
- Eletriptan 40–80 mg p.o. A [12]
- Contraindications for triptans
  - Ischaemic heart disease, prinzmetal angina, recent TIA, subarachnoid haemorrhage, stroke, untreated or otherwise high blood pressure and severe renal failure B [1].

Ergotamine derivatives

- Ergotamine tartrate 1–2 mg p.o. or rectally
- Dihydroergotamine 1.0 mg i.m. or 0.5 mg i.v.

Other drugs

- Pitofenone-metamizol 5 ml i.m.
- Diazepam 2–10 mg p.o./rectally
- Tramadol 50–100 mg p.o./rectally/s.c.

Medication during pregnancy and lactation

- Paracetamol can be used throughout pregnancy. Tolfenamic acid and naproxen can be used in early pregnancy.
- Triptans and ergotamine are contraindicated. Sumatripan is known to be excreted in breast milk, as probably also other triptans.

Preventive therapy

- Maintaining a steady sleep–wake rhythm and taking meals regularly, avoiding precipitating factors.
- Consider preventive medication if there are three or more attacks in a month.
- Beta-blockers
  - Propranolol 20–40 mg × 2–3, 160 mg × 1/day
  - Metoprolol 47.5–200 mg/day
  - Atenolol 100 mg × 1/day
  - Timolol 10 mg/day
- Amitriptyline 10–25 mg/day, especially if tension headache is associated with the migraine
- Sodium valproate 300–500 mg × 2–3/day (see also follow-up treatment of epilepsy 36.47)
- Topiramate up to 50 mg × 2/day

Intervention in chronic daily headache

- Chronic daily headache, which is frequently a combination of chronic migraine and tension headache, can be treated by stopping all the previous overused pain medication, and starting headache prophylaxis, possibly combined with amitriptyline.

References

1. Lipton RB, Stewart WF, Stone AM, Lainez JA, Sawyer JPC. Stratified care vs. step care strategies for migraine: the disability in strategies of care (DISC) study: a randomised trial. JAMA 2000;284:2599–2605.
2. Frishberg BM. The utility of neuroimaging in the evaluation of headache in patients with normal neurological examination. Neurology 1994;44:1191–1197.
3. The Database of Abstracts of Reviews of Effectiveness (University of York), Database no.: DARE-940437. In: The Cochrane Library, Issue 4, 1999. Oxford: Update Software.
4. Chabriat H, Danchot J, Hugues FC, Joire JE. Combined aspirin and metoclopramide in the acute treatment of migraine attacks: a review. Headache Quarterly, Current Treatment and Research 1997;8:118–121.
5. The Database of Abstracts of Reviews of Effectiveness (University of York), Database no.: DARE-975265. In: The Cochrane Library, Issue 2, 2000. Oxford: Update Software.
6. McCrory DC, Gray RN. Oral sumatriptan for acute migraine. Cochrane Database Syst Rev. 2004;(2):CD002915.
7. Harrison DL, Slack MK. Meta-analytic review of the effect of subcutaneous sumatriptan in migraine headache. J Pharm Technol 1998;12:109–114.
8. The Database of Abstracts of Reviews of Effectiveness (University of York), Database no.: DARE-988407. In: The Cochrane Library, Issue 2, 2000. Oxford: Update Software.
9. Theft-Hansen P. Efficacy and adverse events of subcutaneous, oral and intrnasal sumatriptan used for migraine treatment: a systematic review based on number needed to treat. Cephalalgia 1998;18:532–538.
10. The Database of Abstracts of Reviews of Effectiveness (University of York), Database no.: DARE-982039. In: The Cochrane Library, Issue 3, 2000. Oxford: Update Software.
11. Oldman AD, Smith LA, McQuay HJ, Moore RA. Rizatriptan for acute migraine. Cochrane Database Syst Rev. 2004;(2):CD003221.
12. Smith LA, Oldman AD, McQuay HJ, Moore RA. Eletriptan for acute migraine. Cochrane Database Syst Rev. 2004;(2):CD003224.

36.68 Cluster Headache (Horton's syndrome)

Markus Färkkilä

Definition and epidemiology

- This headache, which differs from migraine, begins at the age of 30–40 years and affects mainly (80%) men. The prevalence is about 0.3 per mille, with 10% suffering from the continuous, chronic form.

Symptoms and diagnostics

- Only unilateral severe pulsating, excruciating, burning and stabbing severe pain around the eye that lasts for 30–180 min.
- Attacks occur in 3–4-week periods that can be followed by symptomless periods lasting from 2 months to several years.
- Attacks of pain occur daily, often at night after a couple of hours of sleep and some are associated with REM sleep.
- During attacks lacrimation, conjunctival irritation, miosis and ptosis occur ipsilaterally.
- There are no prodromal symptoms.
- There is no vomiting.
- Diagnosis is based on the symptoms.

Differential diagnosis

- Migraine (36.67) (onset at a younger age, longer and more rarely occurring attacks, prodromal symptoms, nausea)
- Trigeminal neuralgia (36.94) (attacks are electric shock-like, shorter in duration and are set off by touching the skin and teeth on the side of the ache)
- Atypical facial pain (milder, continuous pain, often following dental or facial surgery)
- Unilateral, temporal tension headache (milder, continuous pain)
- Chronic, paroxysmal hemicrania (occurs mainly in women, more than 5 attacks per day that last for minutes at a time, indomethasin cures the attacks completely)

Treatment

Acute attack

1. Sumatriptan 6 mg s.c. (B) [1 2]
2. Ergotamine 2 mg rectally, fast-acting triptans p.o. and NSAIDS can also be tried (often without any effect at all)
3. Breathing 100% oxygen through a face mask for 15–20 min at a flow of 7 l/min. Treatment can be repeated after a 5-min pause. The patient could also have an oxygen supply at home.

Prophylaxis

1. Verapamil starting with 80 mg × 3 daily up to 480 mg/day or even more, if no cardiovascular contraindications are present.
2. Prednisone 80 mg for 5 days, thereafter 60 mg for a couple of weeks after which the steroid is discontinued over a period of one week (consider the adverse effects of long-term use of steroids).
3. Propranolol 40 mg × 3 daily, sotalol 80 mg × 2 daily, atenolol 100 mg × 1 daily may be tried if previous treatments fail or are contraindicated.
4. Lithium (requires monitoring of concentration in blood as even a short-term overdosage may cause renal damage; aim at the lowest effective dose).

References

1. Ekbom K, Monstad I, Prusinski A, Cole JA, Pilgrim AJ, Noronha D. Subcutaneous sumatriptan in the acute treatment of cluster headache: a dose comparison study. The Sumatriptan Cluster Headache Study Group. Acta Neurol Scand 1993;88:63–9.
2. The Sumatriptan Cluster Headache Study Group (see comments). Treatment of acute cluster headache with sumatriptan. N Eng J Med 1991;325:322–6.

36.70 Tremor

Heikki Teräväinen

Basic rules

- The most important diseases with tremor are essential tremor (36.71) and Parkinson's disease (36.72).
- Various types of tremor are differentiated by clinical examination. Characterising the type of tremor makes differential diagnosis easier.

Tremor at rest

- Occurs in the absence of voluntary movement.
- Exhibits low frequency and wide amplitude.
- "Pill-rolling" tremor subtype is characterised by minute rolling movements of thumb and forefinger against each other with concomitant small supination-pronation movements of the forearm.
- Lower jaw and lips may tremble, but the head hardly ever.
- Tremor diminishes or disappears during movement, e.g. when the arm is lifted to vertical position, but is intensified by mental stress and anxiety.

NEU

Aetiology

- The most common cause is Parkinson's disease.
- Other causes include
  - Excessive dosage of neuroleptic drugs.
  - Certain extrapyramidal disorders that resemble Parkinson's disease
  - Rarely caused by a variant of essential tremor.

Intention tremor

- Manifests only when the muscles are voluntarily contracted, either in active movement or when a fixed position is maintained (sustention tremor), and disappears when the muscles are relaxed.

- Occurs in fingers and upper limbs, but also in head, oral region, larynx (voice) and in lower limbs.
- The amplitude of the tremor increases in accurate performance and during stress or anxiety.
- Ataxia is the most important differential diagnostic sign.
- Common causes
  - Alcoholism
  - Benign essential tremor
  - Intensified physiological tremor
  - Metabolic tremor, e.g. caused by hyperthyroidism
- Uncommon causes
  - Cerebellar lesions
  - Symptomatic tremor
  - Toxic tremor
  - Psychogenic tremor

Physiologic tremor

- Occurs in all people, e.g. as sustention tremor, may intensify to symptomatic because of many causes
- Can be treated with various non-selective beta-blockers (propranolol, timolol)
- Aetiology
  - Increased secretion of catecholamines; stress, exercise, fatigue, abstinence
  - Caffeine, nicotine
  - Hyperthyroidism, pheochromocytoma
  - Hypoglycaemia, hypothermia
  - Drugs: levodopa, lithium, sodium valproate, neuroleptic drugs, pindolol, cimetidine, sympathomimetic drugs (isoprenaline, salbutamol etc.), tricyclic antidepressants, mexiletine, thyroxine

Metabolic tremor

- Aetiology
  - Parenchymal lesions of the liver
  - Uraemia, hypokalaemia, hypomagnesaemia
  - Polycythaemia
  - Hypercapnia
  - Steatorrhoea, malabsorption
- Tremor is often mainly distal and usually irrelevant when the underlying disease is considered.

Cerebellar disorders

- Aetiology
  - Alcoholism
  - Multiple sclerosis
  - Brain tumours and infarctions
- In addition to sustention or action tremor there may be manifestations of ataxia, disturbances of equilibrium, nystagmus, speech disturbances and muscular hypotonia.
- Tremor is accentuated in distal parts of the body, in upper limbs the frequency is faster than in lower limbs.

Toxic tremor

- Especially in heavy metal poisonings tremor in sustained position or action tremor is evident (e.g. mercury, lead, arsenic and phosphorus, but also certain chemicals, such as dioxine).
- Myoclonic jerks and compulsive movements may occur in addition to tremor, and tremor may be present also in rest.

Symptomatic tremor

- In the following neurological disorders, action tremor may be present in addition to the symptoms of the underlying disease:
  - Myoclonus
  - Dystonies
  - Roussy-Levy syndrome
  - Certain neuropathies (e.g. Charcot–Marie–Tooth disease or peroneal muscular atrophy)
  - Brain injuries
  - Tourette's syndrome
  - Wilson's disease.
- Also in Parkinson's disease the patient may have action tremor in addition to resting tremor.

36.71 Essential tremor

Heikki Teräväinen

Objective

- To differentiate essential tremor on the basis of the clinical picture from Parkinson's disease and other diseases causing tremor.

Symptoms

- Tremor is initiated by movement and is rarely present at rest.
- It is most intense in a static sustained position, e.g. in extended arms.
- Tremor may be seen also in the tongue, the head may be turned from side to side ("no-no"-movement; not Parkinson's disease).
- Psychological stress intensifies tremor which is worst in social situations, e.g. in the bank or when holding a cup of tea or coffee.
- Tremor is intensified when skilled acts should be performed (e.g. signature) and is relieved by ingestion of small amounts of alcohol.
- Tremor can be quite incapacitating.

Diagnosis

- Is based on physical examination and patient history.

- Essential tremor is more common than tremor caused by Parkinson's disease with a prevalence of approx. 5%.
- In about half of the patients, the condition is hereditary. Genetic defects have been located in chromosomes 2p and 3q13.
- About half of the patients are under 40 years of age.
- Alcohol relieves the symptoms.

Differential diagnosis

- There are no symptoms typical to Parkinson's disease, such as
  - hypokinesia
  - rigidity.
- In essential tremor
  - the patient's face is expressive
  - speed of movements is normal
  - muscular tone is normal
  - gait is normal.
- It may be more difficult to differentiate essential tremor clinically from enhanced physiological tremor in metabolic-toxic conditions (36.70).
- Risk of Parkinson's disease is higher in patients with essential tremor; sometimes both types of tremor are concomitant.

Treatment

- Non-selective beta-blockers
  - Propranolol 20–80 mg × 2–3, timolol
  - Beta-blockers are first used daily, later as needed, because in long-term treatment tolerance may develop.
  - All patients do not respond to medication.
- Beta-blockers with intrinsic sympathomimetic activity (ISA) (e.g. pindolol) may aggravate the symptoms.
- In selected cases, primidone, benzodiazepines. Some patients benefit from acetazolamide, gabapentin, or nimodipine.
- Botulinum injections are used in some cases (tremor of the head, rarely hand).
- Neurosurgery (thalamic stimulation or thalamotomy) may be considered in drug-resistant and incapacitating cases. Thalamic stimulation is safer and probably more effective than thalamotomy.

36.72 Parkinson's disease

Heikki Teräväinen

Aetiology

- Age at onset is typically 50–70 years, on average 62 years.
- The disease is caused by destruction of the neurones of the nigrostriatal neural pathway and consequent diminishing of dopamine in the basal nuclei.
- The aetiology is unknown in most cases.
- Rare causes of parkinsonism include
  - poisoning (carbon monoxide, manganese, MTPT)
  - brain infarction, brain tumour or injury
  - hereditary factors.
- Parkinsonism is a common adverse effect of neuroleptic drugs.

Symptoms

- Usually unilateral in the beginning. Suspect other causes if the patient has bilateral symptoms without tremor.
- Most common
  - Resting tremor
  - Hypokinesia
  - Increase in muscle tone (rigidity)
- Other
  - Muscle pain
  - Abnormal posture
  - Tendency to fall
  - Disturbances of autonomic nervous system (constipation, impotence, orthostatic hypotension)
  - Drooling
  - Greasy skin
  - Depression (in about 40% of cases)
  - Dementia in late phases of the disease (15–25% of cases)
- Unlike in Alzheimer's disease, mild disturbances of memory are more common than dementia.
- The tremor is coarse and diminishes during movement.
- The mouth may tremble, whereas the head usually does not ("no-no" movement = Parkinson's disease is unlikely).
- Rigidity may be felt as an even (lead-pipe rigidity) or as a rhythmically fluctuating resistance (cogwheel rigidity) depending on the type of tremor.
- Hypokinesia is expressed as scarceness of movements (akinesia) and slowness of movement (bradykinesia).
- Expressions and blinking of the eyes are reduced, the face becomes mask-like, and speech may be monotonous.
- Writing becomes slower and handwriting is small (micrographia).
- The arms are held flexed to the waist and fail to swing with the stride, the steps shorten and the gait becomes shuffling and slow.
- With time the posture becomes stooped.
- Tendency to fall may be associated with both motor problems and orthostatic hypotension.
- Psychological and physiological stress aggravates all the symptoms.
- All patients do not have all the symptoms.

Diagnosis

- Consider Parkinson's disease if the patient has two out of three major symptoms (tremor, hypokinesia, rigidity).

- The symptoms do not start rapidly within days or a week.
- Falling and dementia are not present in the initial phase.
- The signs do not include hyperreflexia or positive Babinski's sign.
- Most incorrect diagnoses are, in fact, cases of essential tremor.
- Exclude diseases where symptoms or signs additional to those seen in Parkinson's disease are found:
  - Progressive supranuclear ophthalmoplegia (restricted movements of the eye)
  - Shy-Drager syndrome (marked orthostatic hypotension)
  - Hydrocephalus with normal pressure (ataxia in the lower limbs, incontinence)
  - Multi-infarction syndrome (memory and emotional disturbances, spasticity and/or positive Babinski's sign, no resting tremor).
  - Alzheimer's disease (severe dementia)
  - Drug-induced Parkinson's disease.
- Some diseases causing parkinsonism (Lewy body parkinsonism, striatonigral degeneration) cannot be distinguished with certainty from Parkinson's disease in the early years.

Treatment

- Consists of voluntary exercise, drugs, and sometimes surgery.
- Exercise (D) [1] aims at preservation of functional capacity and freedom of movement in the joints.
- A specialist in neurology should design the treatment, especially for younger patients (e.g. those still at work) in order to minimize the adverse effects of long-term treatment.
- Drug treatment is chosen individually, according to age and other illnesses.
- Total freedom from symptoms is not the aim, as long-term results are better in patients who have been slightly undermedicated.
- Patients should be informed of the effects of drugs. They should also be encouraged to keep a diary of medication, meals and drug effects for 2–3 days before a follow-up visit.

Levodopa

- Dopaminergic cells transform levodopa into dopamine.
- Used concomitantly with a decarboxylase inhibitor (carbidopa, benserazide), which inhibits the metabolism of levodopa outside the central nervous system and thus diminishes peripheral adverse effects.
- Initial doses are low (50 mg three times daily), and the dose is increased stepwise at 3–5-day intervals up to 100–200 mg three times daily, depending on the response and adverse effects.
- Absorption varies between individuals, and even higher doses may be needed.
- In the early stages of the treatment (the first few years) the drug should be taken around 7 a.m., at noon, and at 5 p.m. (at about five-hour intervals) if the patient is awake from 7 a.m. to 10 p.m.
- For the first 1–2 months of treatment, the drug is taken with food (adjustment period), later into an empty stomach, e.g. about 30 min before meals to ensure better and more reliable onset of action and absorption (bioavailability). Some depot preparations are an exception to this rule, as they are absorbed slightly better when the patient has eaten a little.
- The efficacy of depot preparations is approximately 60–70% of that of standard drugs, the plasma peak concentrations are lower, duration of effect is longer and onset of action is slower (within 2 hours). The effect of standard preparations begins in 45 minutes, unless they are chewn before swallowing. Water-soluble preparations (Quick®) have the most rapid onset of action.
- The drug is usually effective for rigidity and mobility disorders and the adverse effects are tolerable in the beginning.
- Adverse effects
  - Gastrointestinal (gastric pain, heartburn)
  - Increased sweating
  - Confusion
  - Cardiac arrhythmias (infrequent)
  - In rare cases, disorders of the sense of smell (olfactory hallucinations)
- Patients with recent myocardial infarction should not use levodopa because of the risk of arrhythmias.
- Phenothiazines decrease the efficacy.
- Long-lasting treatment with levodopa causes dyskinesia or dystonia in many patients. Decreasing the dose diminishes these symptoms, but often the symptoms of Parkinson's disease are simultaneously aggravated.
- Younger patients are more susceptible to dyskinesia. As the expected treatment time in these patients is long, the aim is to start therapy with drugs that do not cause dyskinesia when used alone (e.g. selegiline and dopamine agonists). The initiation of levodopa can often be postponed or at least the daily dose can be reduced.

Selegiline

- Is a MAO-B inhibitor and potentiates the action of levodopa. The drug is usually given in the morning, 5–10 mg.
- Concomitant use of MAO-A inhibitors is contraindicated (risk of hypertensive crisis).
- Selegiline aggravated orthostatic hypotension.
- May cause sleep disturbances.
- Used to prevent progression of the disease. Results from studies are contradictory: there is some evidence that the drug may slow down the progression of the disease.

Entacapone

- Entacapone is a cathecol-O-methyltransferase (COMT) enzyme inhibitor. As levodopa is a substrate of the COMT enzyme, entacapone slows the metabolization of levodopa in the body and thus prolongs its effect.
- One tablet (200 mg) is taken concomitantly with levodopa.

- Beneficial for patients suffering from on–off fluctuations.
- Entacapone does not affect the maximal plasma concentration of levodopa when standard levodopa preparations are used, but with depot levodopa it may increase the concentration.
- The drug is well tolerated and has not caused severe organic adverse effects.
- Entacapone may aggravate dopaminergic adverse effects, such as the duration of dyskinesia. With depot levodopa the severity of dyskinesia may also increase. In these cases the single dose of levodopa should be reduced.
- May cause diarrhoea and abdominal pain.

Dopamine agonists

- Stimulate dopamine receptors, i.e. act like dopamine.
- Some drugs (bromocriptine, cabergoline and pergolide) are ergot derivatives, while some of the newer drugs (pramipexole, and ropinirole) are not.
- These drugs are also used in levodopa-induced motor complications; pergolide may be slightly more effective than bromocriptine C [2].
- The patient must get used to the medication slowly.
- Medication is started at low doses (e.g. bromocriptine C [3] 1.25 mg twice daily, increased stepwise ad 5–10 mg three times daily).
- Dopamine agonists are not as effective as levodopa but more effective than amantadine or anticholinergic drugs.
- The advantage of these drugs compared with levodopa is their longer duration of action; the half-lifes of these drugs are several hours (levodopa 1 hour).
- Adverse effects are similar to those of levodopa, but more common. The elderly tolerate the drugs less well than younger patients.
- Falling asleep is a special adverse effect. The patient may fall asleep quite suddenly. This phenomenon has been described with all dopamine agonists.
- Ergot derivatives may cause pleurisy and fibrosis, which occurs particularly in the lungs and stomach. Accumulation of fluid in the pleura and elevated ESR and CRP are associated. The pleural fluid disappears when the drug is stopped; however, pulmonary fibrosis may be irreversible and lead to permanent impairment in respiratory function.
- When ergot derivatives are used, follow-up of ESR and CRP at 6-month intervals is indicated. Elevated values predict ergotism.
- Patients who have developed pleurisy can use a non-ergot agonist. Changing to another ergot-agonist would result in a recurrence.
- A significant number of pergolide-treated patients has been reported to have some degree of valvular insufficiency. This may be an class effect of ergot agonists.
- Apomorphine is an old dopamine-receptor agonist, which is liver toxic when ingested but not when the enterohepatic circulation is passed. An apomorphine self-injector (for i.m. administration) and an infusion device resembling an insulin pump are available in Europe.
- The effect of apomorphine begins in minutes and lasts a short time (1–2 hours).

Anticholinergic drugs

- All patients benefit from anticholinergic drugs, but adverse effects are also common.
- Treatment is initiated at a low dose, which is increased stepwise until an acceptable response is attained or adverse effects prevent further increase.
- Adverse effects of anticholinergic drugs include worsening of narrow angle glaucoma (untreated), impairment of memory even in patients with otherwise normal memory, visual disturbances, confusion (to be remembered if the patient has memory deficits), dryness of the mouth, constipation, urinary retention (to be remembered if the patient has prostatic hypertrophy).

Amantadine

- Originally developed for influenza A.
- The drug's beneficial effect on the symptoms of Parkinson's disease was discovered accidentally.
- The mechanism of action remained poorly known for long, until blocking of a receptor (N-methyl-D-aspartate, NMDA) was identified as one mechanism of action.
- NMDA receptors are associated with dyskinesia, the reduction of which has become one of the indications of amantadine.
- The efficacy is comparable to anticholinergics, although there is little evidence from randomized controlled trials D [4].
- Treatment can be started at therapeutic doses and adverse effects are uncommon.
- Tolerance may sometimes develop.
- The most harmful adverse effect is livedo reticularis.

Stereotactic surgery

- Thalamotomy can be performed to treat unilateral, drug-resistant incapacitating tremor.
- Pallidotomy also relieves other symptoms C [5] [6]. Reduction of dyskinesia has become one of the main indications of use.
- Electrical stimulation is also used successfully. It does not cause permanent tissue damage like other surgical procedures and has proven effective in the treatment of dyskinesia.

Special treatment-related problems

- Dystonia
  - Dystonia is a long-lasting and sometimes quite painful muscle contraction.
  - Levodopa is beneficial; however, the intensity of dystonia may also increase with the rise and fall of plasma drug concentration.
  - Dystonia occurring in the morning or at nights can be managed with dopamine-receptor agonists, as these drugs have a long duration of action. Diazepam (5 mg) should be taken at bedtime.

- In the morning, the most rapid levodopa effect is achieved with the Quick® preparation form.
- Confusion associated with antiparkinsonian medications
  - Frequently a severe problem.
  - In younger patients confusion occurs usually with dopamine-receptor agonists. The dose must be reduced or the drug stopped and compensated for by increasing the dose of levodopa.
  - In long-enduring disease and in the elderly, confusion correlates in most cases with the decline in cognitive function and occurs also with levodopa.
  - Classic neuroleptics cannot be used, as these drugs block dopamine receptors and aggravate the symptoms of Parkinson's disease.
  - So-called atypical neuroleptics, such as quetiapine, can be considered if the drug is started with low doses (sedation may prevent use).
- Treatment of end-stage akinetic patient
  - Total destruction of neurones
  - Levodopa no longer effective
  - Dopamine-receptor agonists have only a mild effect.
  - Treatment is unrewarding (basic care).

References

1. Deane KHO, Jones D, Playford ED, Ben-Shlomo Y, Clarke C E. Physiotherapy versus placebo or no intervention in Parkinson's disease. Cochrane Database Syst Rev. 2004;(2):CD002817.
2. Clarke C E, Speller J M. Pergolide versus bromocriptine for levodopa-induced complications in Parkinson's disease. Cochrane Database Syst Rev. 2004;(2):CD000236.
3. Ramaker C, Hilten JJ van. Bromocriptine versus levodopa in early Parkinson's disease. Cochrane Database Syst Rev. 2004;(2):CD002258.
4. Crosby N, Deane KHO, Clarke CE. Amantadine in Parkinson's disease. Cochrane Database Syst Rev. 2004;(2):CD003468.
5. Kottler A, Hayes S. Stereotactic pallidotomy for treatment of Parkinson's disease. Technology Assessment Program 1998;8:1–17.
6. The Database of Abstracts of Reviews of Effectiveness (University of York), Database no.: DARE-989084. In: The Cochrane Library, Issue 3, 2000. Oxford: Update Software.

36.73 Neurological complications of alcoholism

Matti Hillbom

- This guideline discusses alcohol-related neurological diseases requiring therapy. For treatment of alcohol withdrawal symptoms, see 40.5.

Basic rules

- Alcohol passes to the brain and always causes neurological symptoms. Most frequently the symptoms are attributed to ethanol.
- A long-lasting drinking bout is followed by a withdrawal syndrome, which is more severe than a hangover and may be accompanied by epileptic seizures or delirium tremens.
- Differential diagnosis of withdrawal symptoms should take into account brain contusion, intracranial haemorrhage, and infections of the central nervous system; particular attention should be paid to the potential of incipient Wernicke's disease.
- Thiamine (vitamin B_1) deficiency causes Wernicke's disease.
- Thiamine deficiency can also cause polyneuropathy, beriberi and Marchiafava–Bignami disease (necrosis of the corpus callosum).

Wernicke's disease

- Groups at risk include, in addition to undernourished alcoholics, undernourished elderly, all who suffer from long-lasting vomiting, patients on parenteral feeding therapy, cancer patients, and those with chronic intestinal disease.
- Thiamine is required for carbohydrate metabolism; administration of glucose, for example, will increase the need for it.

Symptoms

- Complete manifestation of the deficiency is rare, and many mild cases remain undiagnosed. Therefore, suspicion of the disease is important.
- Eye symptoms: nystagmus, abducens paresis, conjugated gaze paresis, slow pupillary reflex, anisocoria, ptosis, retinal haemorrhage, papilloedema.
- Mental symptoms: Korsakoff's syndrome (loss of short-term memory, disorientation, amnesia and transient confabulation), euphoria, delusions, lack of concentration, lack of initiative, depression, agitation.
- Gait and balance dysfunction (ataxia and polyneuropathy)
- Impaired consciousness: somnolence, unconsciousness.
- Hypothermia or hyperthermia
- Hypotension

Treatment

- The disease is often fatal; therefore, treatment must be initiated on suspicion alone.
- In ambiguous cases, the alcoholic should be given 50–100 mg thiamine i.v. before any food or infusion rich in carbohydrates. Therapy should be continued daily for 2 weeks. Thiamine is not readily absorbed in the intestine.

Pellagra

- A deficiency disease rare among alcoholics in Western countries; caused by deficiency of nicotinic acid or its precursor, tryptophan.

Symptoms

- Eczema, dementia, and diarrhoea (or constipation), possibly also spastic paresis or polyneuropathy, primitive reflexes, loss of appetite, incontinence, tongue pain, epilepsy and delirium.

Cerebral atrophy in alcoholics

- Diminished intellectual capacity is approximately four times as common in alcoholics as in the normal population. Permanent abstinence may, however, correct the condition.
- A diagnosis of alcoholic dementia should not be made until other causes of dementia have been ruled out.

Alcoholic cerebellar atrophy

- The most common cause of alcoholic gait dysfunction; it is more common than, e.g. significant polyneuropathy.

Clinical manifestations

- Symptoms develop subacutely in connection with heavy drinking and are most clearly evident during a hangover.
- Wide-based gait, difficulty in walking a straight line
- Heel-knee tap yields symmetrical oscillation
- Low-frequency (3 Hz) tremor of lower limbs appears when the supine patient raises his/her leg with the knee bent at a 90-degree angle.

Differential diagnosis

- The symptoms of alcoholic cerebellar degeneration are typically limited to the lower limbs. Other disorders causing cerebellar symptoms include also symptoms involving the upper limbs and the cranial nerve region (multiple sclerosis, paraneoplastic cerebellar atrophy, hereditary diseases of the cerebellum).

Treatment

- Discontinuation of alcohol use

Central nervous system myelinolysis (central pontine myelinolysis)

- Iatrogenic disorder caused by rapid correction of significant hyponatraemia (Na < 120 mmol/l).
- Most patients are alcoholics, but the disease may develop in connection with hyponatraemia arising from other causes.
- Contrary to earlier assumptions, myelinolysis is not limited to the pons region alone.

Clinical manifestation

- Mild forms of the disease are almost unnoticeable or findings are few, but the severe forms result in tetraparesis, diminished consciousness, neurological brain disturbances (difficulty in swallowing, dysarthria, nystagmus, gaze paresis). Severe forms may be fatal.

Treatment

- Alcoholic hyponatraemia should not be treated by infusions. A suggested safe rate of normalising the serum sodium level is <0.5 mmol/l/hour, but even this may lead to myelinolysis D [1].
- If the patients clinical condition worsens during normalisation, sodium administration must be stopped and lowering of the sodium level should be attempted.

Other

- Polyneuropathy (36.90) and compression neuropathies (36.88) are fairly common among alcoholics; as is mild myopathy (36.85), whereas severe myopathy is rare.
- Alcoholics are obviously more subject to the following neurological disorders:
  - Brain injuries are three times as common in alcoholics as in the general population on average. Mild injuries often go undetected.
  - Chronic subdural haematoma
  - Cerebral circulatory disorders
    - Continuous excessive use of alcohol (>60 g of ethanol/day) has been proven a risk factor for spontaneous intracerebral haemorrhage, subarachnoid haemorrhage and ischaemic stroke C [2].
  - Hepatic encephalopathy is caused by hepatic insufficiency. Symptoms include loss of attention, postural tremor, asterixis and myoclonia. The EEG displays slow-wave activity, and MRI shows typical hyperintense lesions in the area of globus pallidus, which are probably due to the increased manganese concentration of this brain structure.
  - Movement disorders
    - Alcohol withdrawal status includes supporting tremor that resembles essential tremor. The alcohol withdrawal status sometimes involves symptoms resembling those of Parkinson's disease (36.72), but these do not lead to the development of the actual disease.
    - Cerebellar degeneration and hepatic encephalopathy also involve tremors (see above).
  - Sleep disorders
    - Intoxication compounds sleep apnoea.
  - Infections
    - Listeria and pneumococcal meningitis in particular, are common among heavy consumers of alcohol.

Foetal alcohol syndrome (FAS)

- Alcohol penetrates the placenta and readily damages the developing nervous system of the foetus.

- The risk of spontaneous abortion during the second trimester of pregnancy is threefold if alcohol is consumed at the rate of four servings per day.
- FAS (29.15) symptoms include small overall size and small head, abnormal facial features, developmental impairment, and epilepsy.

References

1. Brunner JE, Redmond JM, Haggar AM, Kruger DF, Elias SB. Central pontine myelinolysis and pontine lesions after rapid correction of hyponatremia: a prospective magnetic resonance imaging study. Ann Neurol 1990;27:61–6.
2. Kiyohara Y, Kato I, Iwamoto H, Nakayama K, Fujishima M. The impact of alcohol and hypertension on stroke incidence in a general Japanese population. The Hisayama Study. Stroke 1995;26:368–72.

36.75 Multiple sclerosis (MS)

Juhani Wikström

Aims

- Symptoms of multiple sclerosis (MS) should be identified and the patient referred for relevant tests.
- MS patients should be appropriately monitored and rehabilitated.

Epidemiology

- In high risk zones (Scandinavia, North America, Canada and South Australia) the prevalence is 30–120/100 000 and there MS is the most common disease of the nervous system causing disability in young individuals; it is also the most common demyelinising disorder.
- MS is twice as common in females as in males. Their average age at onset is 30. The youngest patients are 13 to 14 years old. The disease is extremely rare before puberty.

Aetiology

- The aetiology is unknown.
- Childhood viral infections may affect the immune system in a way that turns the natural human defence mechanisms against the nerve tissue. Among leucocytes, the numbers of T-cells are reduced, and the B-cells of the central nervous system produce large amounts of antibodies against a factor as yet unknown.
- Hereditary factors also play a role: MS patients possess tissue types HLA-A3, B7, and DR2 more frequently than expected. MS occurs 25 times more often among the siblings of Finnish MS patients than in the rest of the population.
- Most recent research has demonstrated that the myelin structure in these patients is abnormal, exposing them to the disease.

Clinical manifestations

- Demyelination occurs in foci in the brain, optical nerve, and spinal cord. Symptoms are related to the location and size of the foci. Usually there are several foci at various sites in the white matter of the central nervous system; thus the symptoms are multiform.

Most common symptoms

- Blurred vision in one or both eyes (optic neuritis)
- Spastic paresis of one or more limbs
- Ataxic gait
- Intention tremor
- Various somatosensory disorders
- Bladder and bowel dysfunction
- Impotence
- Double vision caused by eye muscle paresis or internuclear ophthalmoplegia (36.8)
- Vertigo and nausea
- Speech dysfunction, normally dysarthria
- Fatigue tendency
- Less frequent symptoms:
  - Cognitive disturbances
  - Trigeminal neuralgia (36.94)
  - Epilepsy is somewhat more common in MS patients than in the general population.
  - Polyneuropathy of no other proven aetiology.
- The disease progresses in episodes, as old foci become inactive and others are formed. Both the symptoms and the course of the disease are idiosyncratic. Various factors that activate the immune system, such as infections, inoculations, surgery, pregnancy, traumas, and stress will exacerbate MS.

Diagnostics

- The diagnosis is based on the patient's description of his/her symptoms and a clinical examination by a neurologist.
- The most important distinctive characteristic of this disease is the episodic symptomatology. The diagnosis cannot be confirmed until the symptoms again become worse.
- The diagnosis is confirmed by:
  - an increase in the cell count of the cerebrospinal fluid and immunoglobulin (IgG index and oligoclonal zones) (36.17)
  - abnormalities in neurophysiological evoked response tests of the optic, auditory, and somatosensory pathways (36.16).
- The inflamed foci in the brain and spinal cord indicating MS are more readily revealed by MRI than CT (36.15).

- It is important to rule out other, treatable diseases. If symptoms are limited to one location, tumour or medullary compression should be suspected.
- The diagnosis should not be disclosed to the patient until it has been confirmed.

Treatment and prognosis

- There is no medicinal cure for MS. Even so, there have been steady improvements in the prognosis.
- The best results are achieved with a combination of drug management, rehabilitation, and appropriate lifestyle.
- Methylprednisolone i.v. is most effective in an acute phase of a relapse B [1]. Treatment should not be attempted at the start of the exacerbation, because in some patients the symptoms will improve spontaneously. If the relapse is associated with a viral or bacterial infection, steroid therapy should not be administered.
- Optic neuritis and a drastic exacerbation of the disease are always treated with methylprednisolone.
- Beta interferon has been shown to reduce the number of MS relapses B [2] and prevent the formation of new foci. The treatment is indicated for patients with repeated acute relapses of the disease C [3 4].
- Glatiramer acetate may prevent exacerbations.
- Adequate attention should be paid to the treatment of individual symptoms
  - Spasticity is not always harmful; it may be an important support for the lower extremity with its weak muscles and for facilitating movement. Medications for the relief of spasticity include baclofen, tizanidine, and diazepam D [5] (36.83).
  - Physiotherapy is an essential form of treatment for the patients' movement disorders.
  - Bladder function disorders come in several forms; their successful treatment should be based on a urological examination. The diminished function of the urinary bladder exposes the patient to urinary tract infections; symptoms of infections should be actively monitored. Intermittent catheterisation is indicated for some patients.
  - Constipation may be medically treated.
- MS is a chronic, lifelong illness, in which psychological factors are of crucial importance. Treatment of depression improves the prognosis. At the onset, the patient finds it difficult to accept the disease and to understand the prescriptions for treatment. It is essential to create the correct mental images in the patient and his/her closest family members. The family's presence is recommended at the visit when treatment and rehabilitation is prescribed. Counselling and rehabilitation should be correctly timed.
- Find out the possibilities for adaptation training in your region. Periods of institutional rehabilitation, operational therapy, and appropriate assistive devices contribute to the handicapped patient's ability to manage at home.
- An MS patient needs a personal physician, who knows the patient and his/her life situation and its problems.

References

1. Filippini G, Brusaferri F, Sibley WA, Citterio A, Ciucci G, Midgard R, Candelise L. Corticosteroids or ACTH for acute exacerbations in multiple sclerosis. Cochrane Database Syst Rev. 2004;(2):CD001331.
2. Rice G PA, Incorvaia B, Munari L, Ebers G, Polman C, D'Amico R, Filippini G. Interferon in relapsing-remitting multiple sclerosis. Cochrane Database Syst Rev. 2004;(2): CD002002.
3. Parkin D, Miller P, McNamee P, Thomas S, Jacoby A, Bates D. A cost-utility analysis of interferon beta for multiple sclerosis. Health Technology Assessment. The national Coordinating centre for Health Technology Assessment (NCCHTA)13665278. Vol.2:No.4.1998.pp58.
4. The Health Technology Assessment Database, Database no.: HTA-999898. In: The Cochrane Library, Issue 1, 2001. Oxford: Update Software.
5. Shakespeare DT, Boggild M, Young C. Anti-spasticity agents for multiple sclerosis. Cochrane Database Syst Rev. 2004;(2): CD001332.

36.81 Rehabilitation in spinal cord injuries

Antti Dahlberg

Initial rehabilitation

- After acute care rehabilitation at a specialized unit lasts about 3 months in paraplegia and 4–5 months in tetraplegia.
- Rehabilitation should ideally be given in specialized units where the personnel has acquired extensive experience in the treatment.
- Meeting and receiving support from other patients with spinal cord injury is one of the benefits of rehabilitation at a specialized unit.
- The aim of early rehabilitation is to manage the unavoidable sequelae, to prevent complications and to approach or attain the targeted functional capacity, which depends on the injury. Rehabilitation includes the following components:
  - Psychological help in the acute crisis following the injury taking into account family members
  - Prevention of joint contractures; however, in tetraplegia the aim is to achieve a functional position for the upper extremities (initial position therapy)
  - Exercise for preserved muscular function
  - Exercises for independent locomotion
  - Exercises in the upright position and standing are usually a part of the rehabilitation programme.
  - Prevention of pressure sores and care of the skin

- Rehabilitation of the urinary bladder and care of the urinary tract
  - Individualized bladder training and rehabilitation according to urodynamic studies. The method of bladder emptying, medication, and urinary aids must be planned individually.
  - Repeated catheterization for bladder emptying and learning self-catheterization if needed.
  - Prevention, treatment and follow-up of urinary tract infections and other urological complications by regular assessment.
- Bowel function is trained and the method of emptying is chosen.
- Rehabilitation and counselling of sexual C [1 2] function
- Assessment of the need for and training in the use of aids (wheelchair, appliances to control the environment)
- Changes in housing
- Peer support and readjustment rehabilitation
- Psychological support C [3 4]
- Training and support for independence during home leaves
- Training and counselling of the family
- Financial arrangements
- Training and mechanical aids for driving
- Career choice counselling and rehabilitation

♦ After the initial rehabilitation nearly all patients with spinal cord injury return to life at home. Even patients with severe disability can live at home with a personal assistant.

♦ Planned rehabilitation and follow-up can considerably relieve the disability caused by the injury. Because of effective initial treatment and rehabilitation, the prognosis of spinal cord injury has greatly improved, and the life expectancy approaches that of the general population.

Follow-up and maintenance rehabilitation

♦ In order to detect and treat severe sequelae and threatening complications (18.11) annual comprehensive assessment is needed. The assessment is best accomplished at a specialized unit dedicated to spinal cord injuries.

♦ The primary health care team must be involved in rehabilitation.

♦ To maintain their functional ability the patients may need regular institutional rehabilitation.

- The aim of such rehabilitation is to maintain or improve independence of locomotion, treatment of musculoskeletal problems, and improvement of general physical performance.
- A need for a holiday for the family members can be considered as an indication for rehabilitation at an institution.

♦ The need for ambulatory physiotherapy must be assessed individually.

- Tetraplegics usually need regular physiotherapy 1–2 times weekly or periodical courses of physiotherapy. Ambulatory physiotherapy includes functional exercises, preservation of movement of the joints, relief of spasticity, and muscle care.
- Paraplegics may also need ambulatory physiotherapy, particularly for muscle care.

♦ Occupational rehabilitation and counselling for adjustment are needed during the first few years after the injury. Adjustment training may be needed even later. Sometimes occupational rehabilitation is only possible after the situation has become sufficiently stable over a period of years.

References

1. Beckerman H, Becher J, Lankhorst GJ. The effectiveness of vibratory stimulation in anejaculatory men with spinal cord injury: review article. Paraplegia 1993;31:689–699.
2. The Database of Abstracts of Reviews of Effectiveness (University of York), Database no.: DARE-940145. In: The Cochrane Library, Issue 4, 1999. Oxford: Update Software.
3. McAweeney MJ, Tate DG, McAweeney W. Psychosocial interventions in the rehabilitation of people with spinal cord injury: a comprehensive methodological inquiry. SCI Psychosocial Process 1997;10:58–66.
4. The Database of Abstracts of Reviews of Effectiveness (University of York), Database no.: DARE-985185. In: The Cochrane Library, Issue 1, 2000. Oxford: Update Software.

36.82 Diseases of the spinal cord

Kati Juva

Basic rule

♦ Lesions in the spinal cord should be assumed to be due to compression until proven otherwise.

Situations needing urgent attention

♦ A patient with a suspected compression of the spinal cord should be referred immediately to a neurological or neurosurgical unit, when

- the lesion is caused by a trauma
- paraparesis or tetraparesis has developed over a short period of time (a few days)
- the paresis progresses in such a way that the patient can no longer stand or walk or is incontinent.

♦ If the compression has caused a total paraparesis the spinal cord must be liberated in 24 hours. Otherwise the paralysis will remain permanent.

Symptoms of a spinal cord lesion

♦ The spinal cord is part of the central nervous system. Lesions in it cause an upper motor neurone lesion.

- Symptoms: below the level of the lesion there is weakness and paresis of the muscles, and numbness of the skin. There can also be paresis of the bladder and bowel.
- When the lesion progresses slowly the para- or tetraparesis will be spastic. Typical symptoms are
  - increase of the muscle tonus (spasticity)
  - heightened tendon reflexes
  - positive Babinski's sign
  - the function of the bladder is by micturition reflex; the bladder empties often and the reflex causes an urge-type incontinence.
- When the lesion progresses quickly (e.g. in traumas or with metastases in the spine) there may be a spinal shock. This appears as a flaccid paresis resembling paresis of the lower motor neurone.
  - Muscle tone is flaccid.
  - The reflexes are alleviated or absent and the Babinski's sign is negative.

Determining the level of the lesion

- Some spinal cord diseases are local, others are disseminated. Try to assess the level and location of the lesion.
  - Is it really an upper motor neurone lesion? (see above)
  - Exclude diseases of the brain. Spinal cord diseases do not affect cranial nerves, consciousness or higher mental functions (speech, memory). In brain damage at least some of these symptoms are usually present. A parasagittal tumour expanding between the hemispheres can cause a spastic paraparesis without any other symptoms.
  - In assessing the level of the lesion it is most important to distinguish between para- and tetraparesis. If there are no symptoms or signs in the upper extremities, the lesion is below the Th1 segment.
  - Try to determine the sensory level. In diffuse spinal cord diseases there is no sensory level, but in spinal cord compression it can usually be found. The lesion in the cord is usually higher than the sensory level. Tenderness on percussion can reveal a lesion in the spine. Saddle block anaesthesia can indicate a tumour in the conus medullaris, which is the lowest part of the spinal cord.
  - An x-ray of the spine may reveal fractures, spondylosis or erosions. A normal spine x-ray does not rule out spinal cord compression.
  - Lesions in the lumbar spine do not cause compression of the medullary cord but a lesion of the lower motor neurone.

Causes of spinal cord lesions

Spinal cord compression

- Spinal cord traumas
  - Usually known when the patient comes to the hospital.
  - Should be referred to an orthopaedic or neurosurgical unit.
- Tumours in the spinal canal
  - Extradural (25%)
    - Usually metastases, progress fast, usually painful.
    - The primary tumour may or may not be known.
  - Intradural (50%)
    - Meningiomas or neurinomas; progress slowly. The prognosis may be very good.
  - Intramedullary (25%)
    - Gliomas
    - The prognosis has been poor but operative results are improving.
- Epidural abscess
  - Symptoms and signs of infection can be absent.
  - The primary source is usually spondylitis or osteomyelitis.
- Spinal extradural haematoma
  - Can be a complication of anticoagulant treatment.
  - Sometimes appears after an operation or other procedures in the area.
- Mechanical compression
  - Spondylosis (most common in the cervical area)
  - Medial intervertebral disc herniation.

Infectious and inflammatory diseases

- Myelitis
  - Can be diffuse, transverse (lesion in a narrow area, symptoms come from below this level) or ascending.
  - Causes:
    - Viral infections (HSV2, HIV)
    - Specific microbes (borreliosis, syphilis)
    - MS
    - Connective tissue diseases, such as SLE
    - Sarcoidosis
  - Often the cause can not be determined.
- Abscesses
  - Extradural (tuberculosis, bacteria)
  - Intradural (protozoa)

Vascular lesions of the spinal cord

- Haematomas
  - Extradural (compressions: see above)
  - Intramedullary
    - Usually caused by arteriovenous malformations.
- Infarction of the arteria spinalis anterior

Metabolic spinal cord diseases

- Vitamin B_{12} deficiency
  - A diffuse spinal cord lesion, progresses slowly.

NEU

36.83 Treatment of spasticity

Juhani Wikström

Basic rules

- Spasticity does not necessarily require treatment. It may function as support for a limb with weakened muscle strength and facilitate movement.
- Drug therapy is indicated when muscle strength is adequate but spasticity is pronounced.
- Drug therapy is always indicated for spastic limbs in a completely non-ambulatory patient.
- Other possible treatments to be considered are the regional anaesthesia of a nerve or nerve roots with alcohol or phenol, and certain neurosurgical procedures.

General information

- Damage to the central nervous system causes muscle stiffness that presents as spasticity or rigidity. Spasticity is caused by damage to the pyramidal (motor) tract. Rigidity that appears when the muscle is quickly stretched is typical. This initially meets strong resistance, which is released as the stretching continues. The "jackknife" spasticity characteristic of motor tract damage differs from the "lead-pipe" rigidity of extrapyramidal tract disease.
- The most common causes of damage to the motor tract are cerebrovascular events (36.31), (36.32), tumours (36.99), and brain and spinal cord injuries (36.82) and MS (36.75).

Motor tract symptoms

- In addition to spasticity, damage to the motor tract also causes
  - muscle weakness
  - increased tendon reflexes
  - positive Babinski's sign
  - spasms in the extensor or flexor muscles.
- Damage to the motor tracts of the lower extremities may also cause symptoms involving bladder and bowel functions:
  - urinary frequency caused by detrusor hyperreflexia
  - incontinence.

Drug therapy

- Baclofen **C** [1] and diazepam are more effective in spinal cord injury than in brain injury. The most significant adverse effect of both of these drugs is drowsiness; large doses also cause confusion, restlessness, and hypotension. Abrupt discontinuation of drug therapy may trigger epileptic seizures. Tizanidine is effective in both brain and spinal cord injuries **C** [1].

Baclofen

- Normal initial dosage is 5 mg × 2–3.
- Average dosage is 20 to 30 mg/day.
- The maximum daily dose is 75 mg.
- Overdose causes muscular hypotonia, experienced by the patient as increased muscle weakness.
- Baclofen can also be administered intrathecally **A** [2 3].

Diazepam

- The dose is adjusted individually, initially 2.5–5 mg × 2–3.
- Side effects appear before the therapeutic level has been reached.
- Diazepam is used in combination with baclofen. Diazepam is initially administered only in the evening.

Tizanidine

- A sufficient dose to reduce spasticity is 4–6 mg × 3–4. Maximum dosage is 12 mg × 3.
- Side effects include drowsiness, fatigue, and dry mouth. If used in combination with antihypertensive medications, tizanidine may cause hypotension and bradycardia.

Anticonvulsants

- Spasticity is occasionally associated with muscle cramps in the lower extremities and trunk. These spasms are of short duration but painful. They can be treated with anticonvulsants, e.g. clonazepam 0.5–2.0 mg for the night.

Surgical treatment

- Surgery is indicated only in severe paresis of the lower extremities resulting from damage to the spinal cord. The reflex arch maintaining spasticity is interrupted by ablating the anterior nerve roots at level L1 to S1.
- The reflex arch can also be interrupted by regional anaesthesia of the nerve roots with alcohol or phenol. This procedure will damage the sacral nerve roots and may cause bladder and bowel dysfunction.
- In myelotomy the reflex arch is interrupted at level L1 to S1 between the anterior and posterior horns. The effect is long lasting.
- Pain and spasticity in the lower extremities can also be treated by electrical stimulation. Electrodes are placed on the spinal cord in a surgical procedure. This procedure is performed only on patients who benefit from transcutaneous test stimulation.

General measures

- Spasticity can be relieved by continuous and regular physiotherapy. Ice therapy enhances the efficacy of physiotherapy.
- The extent of the spasticity depends on posture. For example, spasticity of the extensors is less pronounced in the upright position than in the supine position.

- Bladder function should be closely monitored, because sensory stimuli of the lower abdomen may trigger spasms in the paralysed muscles. Detrusor hyperreflexia is treated with anticholinergic drugs.
- Special attention should be paid to the prevention and treatment of urinary tract infections.
- Skin care is important for a non-ambulatory patient, because painful pressure sores increase spasticity.

References

1. Taricco M, Adone R, Pagliacci C, Telaro E. Pharmacological interventions for spasticity following spinal cord injury. Cochrane Database Syst Rev. 2004;(2):CD001131.
2. Creedon SD, Dijkers MP, Hinderer SR. Intrathecal baclofen for severe spasticity: a meta-analysis. International Journal of Rehabilitation and Health 1997;3:171–185.
3. The Database of Abstracts of Reviews of Effectiveness (University of York), Database no.: DARE-985160. In: The Cochrane Library, Issue 1, 2000. Oxford: Update Software.

36.84 Amyotrophic lateral sclerosis (ALS)

Hannu Laaksovirta

Basic rules

- The terms ALS and motor neurone disease (MND) are often used interchangeably. ALS is the most common form of MND.
- ALS is a progressive neurodegenerative disorder involving motor neurones in the brain and spinal cord, which leads to progressive weakness and atrophy of the voluntary muscles without sensory deficit.
- The functions of the autonomic nervous system and the sphincters remain intact.
- There is no significant cognitive impairment.
- The diagnosis should be based on investigations in a neurological unit by exclusion of other diseases.

Aetiology

- The aetiology of ALS remains unknown.
- 5–10% of cases are familial (FALS); however, the mechanism of inheritance is not straightforward.
- The disease is not contagious.

Epidemiology

- Incidence: 1–2.5/100 000
- Prevalence: 2.5–8.5/100 000 (higher prevalence in certain areas of the Western Pacific)
- Median age of onset 55 years.

Symptoms

- The most common primary symptoms is distal weakness of the upper or lower extremity in functions requiring normal muscle strength.
- Leg cramps are typical.
- In bulbar involvement, the initial symptom is deterioration of speech and swallowing.
- 10–25% of patients may complain of mostly slight distal numbness, paraesthesiae or mild pain.

Clinical course

- Muscle weakness and atrophy progress proximally starting in the distal parts and spread to other limbs, respiratory muscles and to the bulbar area. The weakness can also begin in the bulbar area and progress distally.
- Upper motor neurone involvement leads to spasticity (not always detected) and to accelerated tendon reflexes. Babinski's sign is positive in about 50%.
- Lower motor neurone damage weakens muscle tonus and reflexes, which is why the tonus can vary between individuals.
- As the disease progresses, muscle atrophy and paresthesia become dominant.
- The cardiac muscle is not involved.
- Ocular muscle functions are spared until the final stage of the disease.

Clinical findings

- Atrophy of the small thenar and palmar muscles is the most prominent finding.
- Weight loss is mainly result of muscular atrophy.
- Fasciculations in the muscles and the tongue. Fasciculations alone are not a sign of a pathological situation.
- True and persistent sensory symptoms should prompt a search for an alternative diagnosis.
- Subtle frontal type dementia may occur in some cases, a typical case being an older female with bulbar onset of disease.

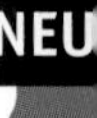

Laboratory tests

- There is no specific laboratory test for ALS.
- Routine laboratory studies should be performed to exclude other treatable conditions (suggested by a neurologist).
  - Serum CK and CSF protein level may be slightly increased.
  - Lumbar puncture should be undertaken in atypical cases.
  - In about 5% of patients immune electrophoresis may show paraproteinaemia, but the clinical significance is uncertain.

- ENMG (electromyography and nerve conduction studies) is essential for the diagnosis and should be requested by a neurologist (who poses relevant questions). In definite ALS ENMG shows:
  - fibrillation and fasciculation.
  - reduction in the number of motor unit action potentials and polyphasia.
  - normal motor nerve conduction velocity or, in more severely affected muscles, not less than 70% of the average normal value. A motor conduction block may suggest a possibly treatable condition such as multifocal motor neuropathy.
- CT or MRI imaging of the head and neck is recommended to exclude other CNS disorders, cervical spondylotic myelopathy and neoplasm.

Prognosis

- Refrain from predicting survival time.
  - Median survival is about 3.5 years from onset of symptoms, but 10% may live over 10 years.
  - Older age at onset, and bulbar and/or respiratory dysfunction early in the clinical course indicate poorer prognosis.
  - The basic cause of death is ALS, but in most cases the immediate cause is pneunomia.

Therapy

- Therapy is symptomatic.
- Riluzole (50 mg × 2) has been shown in two placebo-controlled trials to prolong survival by a mean of 3 months B [1 2 3 4 5], but it does not slow the rate of progression of muscle dysfunction. The drug is generally well tolerated, but mild nausea and asthenia may occur. All of the adverse effects can be reversed by decreasing the daily dosage or discontinuing it. Fatal adverse effects or significant interactions have not been described. Blood count and serum aminotransferases should be measured before and during riluzole therapy. Treatment should be discontinued if ALT levels increase to five times the upper limit of normal. Treatment is initiated by a specialist in motor neurone diseases.

Asthenia

- Physiotherapy for maintaining muscle function. The exercises must be adjusted to the patient's performance. The muscles cannot be made stronger by training. Contractures are prevented.
- Occupational therapist should help with the acquisition of supports and assistive devices.

Cramps and spasticity

- Quinine chloride + meprobamate, quinine chloride + diazepam, phenytoin or carbamazepine help.
- Treatment of spasticity (36.83).

Salivation and mucus production

- Scopolamine patches placed at the submandibular angle
- Amitriptyline 25–50 mg × 2–3 p.o. (the drug of choice)
- Benzhexol (trihexylphenidyl) initially 2 mg × 1, thereafter up to 2 mg × 3–4
- ALS patients rarely benefit from antitussives.
- Correct head positioning and emptying
- Portable suction device for use at home (use needs to be instructed).

Difficulty with speech

- Early referral to a speech therapist for acquisition of swallowing and communication aids.
- Paroxysmal involuntary crying and laughter are caused by pseudobulbar paresis. Imipramine derivatives may help.

Dysphagia

- Semi-solid food
- Instructions given by a speech therapist
- Nasogastric tube (NG) feeding only temporarily
- Percutaneous endoscopic gastrostomy (PEG) most helpful. The possibility of PEG should be discussed early in the disease.
- The carers should be taught the Heimlich manoeuvre (Figure 6.60.1).

Ventilatory failure

- Elevations for the bed
- Oxygen nasal cannulas
- Nasal BiPAP (Bilevel Positive Airway Pressure) or other therapy (for use at home)
- Assisted ventilation with tracheostomy is considered only after serious discussion of the implications with the family, and the neurological and respiratory care team. The decisions made together with the patient about the eventual use of respirator therapy are recorded in the medical chart and acute care teams are informed of the decision.
- In the terminal phase (aspiration pneumonia, CO_2 narcosis) analgesics are given.

References

1. Miller RG, Mitchell JD, Lyon M and Moore DH. Riluzole for amyotrophic lateral sclerosis (ALS)/motor neuron disease (MND). Cochrane Database Syst Rev. 2004;(2):CD001447.
2. Wagner ML, Landis BE. Riluzole: a new agent for amyotrophic lateral sclerosis. Ann Pharmacother 1997;31:738–744.
3. The Database of Abstracts of Reviews of Effectiveness (University of York), Database no.: DARE-970803. In: The Cochrane Library, Issue 4, 1999. Oxford: Update Software.
4. Bensimon G, Lacomblez L, Meininger V, ALS/Riluzole Study Group. A controlled trial of riluzole in amyotrophic lateral sclerosis. N Engl J Med 1994;330:585–91.

5. Lacomblez L, Bensimon G, Leigh PN, Guillet P, Powe L, Durrleman S, Delumeau JC, Meininger V, ALS/Riluzole Study Group-II. A confirmatory dose-ranging study of riluzole in ALS. Neurology 1996;47(Suppl. 4):S242–S250.

36.85 Myopathies

Hannu Somer

Basic rules

- The majority of patients with myopathies have an inherited disease.
- The diagnostic work-up should be centralised in larger hospitals and in special outpatient clinics for neuromuscular disorders.

Examination of patients with muscular disorders

- History of presenting complaint, family history, physical examination and laboratory investigations
- Serum creatine kinase and serum aldolase levels are increased in many myopathies.
  - Note that the levels are also increased by traumas, intramuscular injections, and previous ENMG.
- Electroneuromyography (ENMG)
- Muscle biopsy
  - Suitable for differential diagnosis between myopathy and neuropathy. Due to the specialist techniques required, biopsies should only be carried out in facilities with relevant experience.
- DNA studies
  - Suitable for verifying the diagnosis of certain mitochondrial myopathies as well as for prenatal screening of certain diseases.

When should a myopathy be suspected?

- Symptoms alone are not usually enough to diagnose myopathy, but they may warrant further neurological examinations.
- Typical symptoms include
  - Slowly progressive muscle weakness
  - Muscular atrophy
  - Muscle stiffness or cramps associated with exercise
  - Ptosis
  - Dysphagia
  - Speech impairment
  - Erythematous facial rash
  - Positive family history supports the suspicion.

Treatment and rehabilitation

- Treatment should be provided under the supervision of a specialist unit.
- Many myopathies hinder mobilisation and coping with daily activities. Physiotherapy, alterations to the patient's home and various aids and equipment are often necessary. Patients may also benefit from adaptation training and occasional rehabilitation at an appropriate facility.
- The patient should also be provided with information about the heritability of the disease. If appropriate, the patient should be referred for genetic counselling for further tests and information.

Myopathies in early childhood

- Symptoms include
  - muscle hypotonia and weakness in a neonate or infant, presenting as difficulty in holding the head upright, lack of facial expressions, immobility, breathing difficulties, or recurrent respiratory tract infections.
  - hip joint luxation, joint contractures, and scoliosis.
- Nemaline myopathy appears at this age. Dystrophia myotonica and myasthenia gravis may also be congenital.

Spinal muscular atrophies

- These diseases have a pathognomonic lesion in the anterior horn of the spinal cord. They are usually inherited as an autosomal recessive trait.
- Symptoms include muscular flaccidity, weakness and atrophy. Fasciculation may also occur.

Werdnig–Hoffman's disease

- Onset generally during the first weeks of life; the prognosis is poor. There is also an intermediate form of the disease with less severe symptoms and with disease onset at around 12 months of age.

(Wohlfart -) Kugelberg–Welander's disease (chronic proximal spinal muscular atrophy, PSMA)

- Onset in childhood or young adulthood. The severity and rate of progression of this disease vary, and the symptoms may be unilateral or limited to one limb.

Inherited neuropathies and disorders of the neuromuscular junction

- Inherited neuropathies (36.90) and disorders of the neuromuscular junction, such as myasthenia gravis (36.86) and the myasthenic syndrome (36.86), also cause weakness of the muscles; muscles tire and become weak during repetitive exercise. These conditions should be considered in differential diagnostics.

Progressive muscular dystrophies

- There are various forms of dystrophies that differ in their clinical picture and the way in which they are inherited. Muscle biopsy will reveal a characteristic histopathological finding, i.e. the diameter of muscle fibres will show great variability. Some of the fibres will be atrophied and replaced by fibrous tissue and fat. ENMG is applicable for these myopathies. In the active stage, serum creatine kinase is greatly increased.

Duchenne's muscular dystrophy

- Most common of all muscular dystrophies; the pattern of inheritance is X-chromosomal recessive. About one third of the cases are new mutations. The underlying cause is dystrophin deficiency in the skeletal muscle surface membrane, which is apparent on muscle biopsy.
- The patients are boys whose symptoms appear around the age of 5 years.
  - Initial symptoms include gait dysfunction and weakness in the proximal muscles (difficulty in getting up from a squat).
  - Calves are thick (pseudohypertrophy).
  - The muscle weakness increases and the patient is confined to a wheelchair at around 12 years of age.
  - Other disease manifestations include joint contractures and deformity of the back (scoliosis) as well as breathing difficulties that predispose the patient to infections.

Becker's muscular dystrophy

- Inheritance is X-chromosomal recessive.
- The dystrophin level is reduced, but not as much as in Duchenne's dystrophy.
- Severity is variable.
- Time of onset varies from childhood to adulthood.

Limb-girdle dystrophy

- The muscle weakness is localised to the proximal muscles of the extremities (difficulty in ascending stairs and holding arms raised).
- Onset in childhood or early adulthood.
- Inheritance is usually autosomal recessive, rarely autosomal dominant.

Facioscapulohumeral muscular dystrophy

- Causes muscular atrophy in the affected regions; however, the disorder is fairly benign. Its inheritance is autosomal dominant.

Myotonic dystrophy

- A disease of variable incidence and severity with autosomal dominant inheritance.
- Age of symptom onset ranges from neonate to old age.
- Clinical manifestations include:
  - muscular atrophy and weakness especially distally in the extremities, facial muscles and eyelids
  - myotonia, e.g. prolonged muscle contraction when the patient is attempting to open his/her fist is evident in electromyography
  - endocrine disturbances
  - cardiac arrhythmias
  - cataracts.
- Congenital forms of the disease may include mental retardation.

Polymyositis

- Inflammatory, relatively rare disorder
- Most common age of onset is 50–70 years. However, may occur in children when the typical manifestation is dermatomyositis.
- May be associated with cancer (most commonly ovarian cancer) or autoimmune disorders.
- Symptoms include muscle weakness and tenderness.
- Laboratory findings: serum creatine kinase and aldolase levels are increased; ESR and gamma globulin are also increased in some patients.
- Muscle biopsy shows the presence of inflammatory cells, particularly in the perivascular muscle tissue.
- Treatment consists of corticosteroids. Possible co-existing cancer or autoimmune disease must also be diagnosed and treated. Steroids are given for extended periods of time; therapy should never be discontinued without consulting a specialist.

Metabolic myopathies

- These are rare myopathies that manifest themselves as reduced muscular endurance and increased tendency for cramps. The underlying cause is a disturbance in muscle metabolism.

Secondary myopathies

- A disorder of muscle tissue may be associated with a systemic disease.
  - Hyperthyroidism
  - Hypothyroidism
  - Hyperparathyroidism, hypercalcaemia
  - Cushing's disease
  - Alcoholism

Distal myopathies

- Myopathies with symptoms predominantly in the distal parts of the hands and feet. Welander distal myopathy is an autosomal dominant myopathy which is almost only seen in Sweden and some parts of Finland. Symptom onset is around the age of 40.
- In 1993 a new phenotype of distal myopathy, tibial muscular dystrophy, was described in Finland, where at least 300 cases have been confirmed so far.
- The symptoms emerge in middle age; the patient develops a slapping and unsteady gait. Electromyography will show characteristic changes of muscle damage and magnetic resonance imaging will reveal the location and severity of the disease.
- The disease progresses slowly. There is no pain or sensory loss. The patient benefits from physical therapies and walking aids. No curative treatment is available.

36.86 Myasthenia gravis and myasthenic syndrome

Kiti Müller

Myasthenia gravis

- A rare disease; the annual incidence is about 2–8/1 000 000.
- Treatment is the domain of a specialist in neurology.
- Two main types:
    - Limited to the eye muscles, or ocular
    - Generalised

Aetiology

- Autoimmune disease, in which the function of the myoneural junction of the voluntary muscles is impaired.
- The patients frequently have antibodies to the myoneural acetylcholine receptors.
- Associated with tissue types HLA B8 and Dr3.
- Thymic hyperplasia is found in ca. 70–80% of patients; ca. 10% have a benign thymoma. The onset of the disease may not occur until several years after the discovery of the thymoma.

Symptoms

- Variable degrees of fatigue and weakness in voluntary musculature, which is aggravated by strain and relieved by rest.
    - Double vision, ptosis
    - Bulbar symptoms, nasal tone of speech and tiredness when speaking
    - Facial muscle weakness: hypomimia, grimacing/whistling are not possible
    - Muscle fatigue in neck, limbs, and hips.
- Clinical symptoms vary from patient to patient.

Accompanying disorders

- The patient is more likely than average to have other autoimmune diseases.
    - Thyreoiditis, arthritis, SLE, pernicious anaemia, coeliac disease, Sjögren's syndrome.

Diagnostics

- Tensilon-test
- Serum acetylcholine receptor antibodies; neurophysiological tests: EMG-tetanisation, single-fibril EMG

Differential diagnostics

- Myopathies, myositis, myasthenic syndrome, congenital myasthenia, Guillain–Barré polyneuritis, tumours in the brainstem (when ocular and bulbar symptoms are present), MS, amyotrophic lateral sclerosis, hypokalaemia, hypocalcaemia, hypomagnesaemia, hypothyroidism, burn-out, depression, congenital strabismus/heterophoria.
- Penicillamin can trigger acetylcholine receptor antibody production and MG symptoms.

Treatment

- Symptomatic medication: anticholinesterases (Mestinon®, Mytelase®, Ubretid®), ephedrine, theophyllamine, potassium preparations
    - Anticholinesterase overdose may cause a cholinergic crisis, whose differential diagnosis from a myasthenic crisis is difficult.
    - Symptoms of overdose: muscle twitches, muscle cramps, increased salivation, and muscle weakness, which is aggravated after taking the medication
- Thymectomy (in generalized MG, not in ocular disease)
- Immunosuppressive medications: rule out infection foci before initiation
- Cortisone
- Azathioprine
- Plasmapheresis (primarily in myasthenic crisis); the effectiveness is questionable C [1].
- Sometimes i.v. immunoglobulin

Myasthenic crisis

- The symptom is pronounced muscle weakness, most importantly weakness of the respiratory muscles and bulbar symptoms.
- Treatment

- Respiratory therapy, do not rely on arterial acid-base balance values
- Parenteral anticholinesterase medication (administered subcutaneously or intramuscularly)
- As needed, plasmaphaeresis and immunosuppressive medication

♦ Look for a triggering factor, such as infections (pneumonia, sinusitis, UTI, dental root infection).

Prognosis

♦ Following thymectomy, the disease is relieved in ca. 70% of all patients.

♦ Remission is achieved in about 25%.

Special problems

♦ Infections

- These often aggravate the disease symptoms
- Influenza vaccination is indicated in the absence of immunosuppressive treatment.
- Do not use expectorants or respiratory centre-depressing antitussives. Teophylline or ephedrine often relieves bulbar and respiratory muscle weakness during infections.

♦ Other medicines

- Absolutely contraindicated: morphine, penicillamine, procainamide, aminoglycoside antibiotics
- To be used with caution (because they may aggravate symptoms): beta blockers, calcium blockers, diazepam, contraceptives, sulfa, tetracyclines, chloroquine, gold, short-acting hypnotics, centrally acting analgesics.
- Safe to use: erythromycin, ibuprofen, paracetamol
- Safest sleep aids: antihistamines.

♦ Pregnancy and parturition require monitoring by a specialist. Breastfeeding can be undertaken in the normal manner.

♦ MG must be know to staff when anaesthesia is planned.

Dental care

♦ Anticholinesterase medication should be taken one hour before a dental procedure.

♦ Local anasthesia suits most patients.

♦ A patient with severe symptoms should receive dental care in hospital.

Myasthenic syndrome – Eaton-Lambert's syndrome

♦ Extremely rare

♦ Two forms:

- Autoimmune disease with no related malignancy
- Paraneoplastic (often microcellular carcinoma of the lungs), which may be manifest before tumour development.

Reference

1. Gajdos P, Chevret S, Toyka K. Plasma exchange for myasthenia gravis. Cochrane Database Syst Rev. 2004;(2):CD002275.

36.87 Peripheral neuropathies: examination of the patient

Esa Mervaala

Aims

♦ Determine whether

- the patient's symptoms are caused by damage to the peripheral nerve system
- only one nerve is affected, i.e., mononeuropathy
- the patient has systematic peripheral nerve damage, i.e., polyneuropathy.

Symptoms

♦ Motor symptoms:

- Weakness, fatigue, cramps, fasciculation ("tic").

♦ Sensory symptoms:

- Sensory deficits, dysaesthesia, pain, burning sensation, ataxia.

♦ Autonomic nerve system symptoms:

- Postural hypotension
- Disturbances in the alimentary canal, urinary system, or perspiratory function
- Impotence

History

♦ Many neuropathies are caused by systemic diseases.

♦ Risk groups:

- Diabetics
- Heavy alcohol users

♦ Determine:

- previous illnesses
- medications (36.90)
- exposure to environmental toxins (36.90)
- history of alcohol use
- symptoms experienced by other family members and relatives (36.90)
- whether the neuropathy is associated with some systemic disease (36.90)
- course of the disease: acute, subacute (several weeks, a few months), chronic (months, years), or recurrent.

Crucial clinical findings

- Examination of a neurological patient (36.1).
- Muscle weakness or atrophy
- Sensory deficits and dysaesthesia (for all sensory modalities)
- Weak or absent tendon reflexes, weakened muscle tone
- Trophic skin changes
- Clinical findings indicating abnormalities in the autonomic nerve system
    - Pupillary abnormalities
    - Dry socks (anhidrosis)
    - Bradycardia associated with respiration

Types of neuropathy

Polyneuropathy

- See 36.90.
- Most common presentation: sensorimotor, characterised by ascending and symmetrical distal dysaesthia ("sock-and-glove" type), flaccid muscle weakness, muscle fatigue, and absence of tendon reflexes.
- Exclusively sensory or motor polyneuropathies are rare.
- Aetiology (36.90).

Multiple mononeuropathy

- Two or more nerves in several extremities are affected (e.g. n. ulnaris and n. peroneus)
- The classic manifestation is associated with periarteritis nodosa and collagen diseases as well as diabetes.

Mononeuropathy

- Certain mononeuropathies are typical of certain aetiologies:
    - Paresis of the femoral nerve and the oculomotor nerve: diabetes
    - Paresis of the facial nerve: sarcoidosis, borreliosis
- See also Nerve entrapment and compression disorders 36.88.

Differential diagnostics

- In disorders of the upper motoneuron, tendon reflexes may be initially weaker, but later increased, and the muscle tone may be increased. The patient may also present with other indications of damage related to the brain (36.31), (36.91) or the spinal cord (36.82).
- In muscle disorders (36.85) and motoneuron disorders (ALS) (36.84) dysaesthesia is not present.
- Diseases of the musculoskeletal system (arthritis, osteoarthritis, tendinitis, etc.) are not associated with reflex changes or dysaesthesia. Joint or tendon pain is a frequent presentation.
- Polyradiculitis (36.92) is a disease of the peripheral nerves with rapid and severe progression, which is why it must be identified.

36.88 Nerve entrapment and compression disorders

Esa Mervaala

Compression neuropathy

- Peripheral nerve compression (entrapment neuropathy) is caused by external pressure on the nerve that is often a one-time occurrence (e.g., a night's drunken sleep with the upper arm pinched), or occasionally intermittent (e.g., leaning on the elbow while on the telephone).
- Compression is most likely to injure nerves that have no surrounding protective soft tissue.
- Compression neuropathy usually recovers spontaneously once the external pressure is removed.

Entrapment neuropathy

- Peripheral nerve entrapment means that the nerve is compressed between surrounding anatomical structures. The pressure is usually persistent, although its severity may vary according to the extent of tissue oedema and strain on the limb.
- In order to recover completely, entrapment neuropathies generally require treatment (reduction of the oedema, surgical release of the nerve, etc.).
- Peripheral nerve entrapments are common causes of pain and numbness. Less often, in chronic cases, there is also motor weakness or atrophy in the muscles supplied by the compressed nerve, distal to the site of the entrapment.

Symptoms of nerve entrapment and compression

Sensory symptoms

- Numbness, stinging or tingling sensations, increased or decreased sensation, pain. Symptoms are usually more disturbing at night.
- Sensory symptoms usually occur distal to the entrapment; however, they may be referred all the way to the root level (e.g. carpal tunnel syndrome → neck pain).

Motor symptoms

- Distally to the damage site the muscles lack strength, function clumsily, or may be atrophied.
- In entrapment neuropathy, the motor symptoms require timely surgical treatment, because if not operated, muscle atrophy is usually irreversible.

- Tinel's sign
  - The site of the nerve lesion is tender when palpated; tapping it causes a distally radiating sensation.
  - As the compression is released, the site where Tinel's sign is elicited moves distally along the nerve. This will assist in assessing the prognosis after the release.

Most common disorders caused by nerve entrapment and compression

- Carpal tunnel syndrome
- Entrapment of the ulnar nerve at the condylar groove
- Compression paresis of the radial nerve
- Entrapment of the ulnar nerve at the wrist
- Peroneal paresis
- Other conditions caused by nerve entrapment and compression are evidently more rare.

Medial nerve

Entrapment at wrist level (carpal tunnel syndrome, or wrist nerve pain symptoms)

- See 20.61.
- The typical patient is a middle-aged female who uses her hands at work a great deal.
- Symptoms and clinical findings
  - Numbness in the thumb, index and middle fingers, weakness and clumsiness of thumb opposition
  - Occasionally sensory symptoms extending all the way to the neck
  - A typical symptom is night-time numbness of the upper limb.
  - Often bilateral, even when symptoms are unilateral.
- Treatment is conservative or operative, see 20.61.

Nerve entrapment at the proximal end of the forearm below the pronator muscle (pronator syndrome)

- An over-diagnosed rarity.
- Symptoms and clinical findings
  - As above; in addition, the pain is provoked and radiates distally at resisted pronation of the forearm; occasionally flexion of the elbow and wrist is also weak.

Ulnar nerve

Entrapment of the ulnar nerve at the condylar groove (cubital tunnel syndrome)

- Symptoms and clinical findings
  - Sensory symptoms in the ring and little fingers
  - Weak flexion of ring and little fingers
  - Weak scissors movement
- If the symptoms are caused by luxation of the ulnar nerve from the groove, the symptoms are provoked by elbow flexion, and the luxation can simultaneously be palpated or felt.
- Simple decompression is the treatment of choice 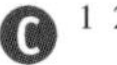 [1 2].

Entrapment at wrist level (ulnar tunnel syndrome)

- See 20.62.
- Symptoms and clinical findings
  - As above, ring and little fingers
  - Weak scissors movement

Entrapment in the hollow of the palm (the motor branch leading to the first interosseal muscle)

- Rare; typical history includes, e.g. floor-tile work, competitive bicycling, local injuries
- More often a local compression injury than a true entrapment.
- Symptoms and clinical findings
  - Weak adduction of thumb and index fingers, pain in the region of the ulnar metacarpal bones
  - No sensory impairment

Radial nerve

Compression posteriorly in the upper arm ("Saturday night palsy")

- Alcohol is a contributing factor (sleeping on the hand/arm).
- Symptoms and clinical findings
  - Weakness or paresis in extension of wrist and fingers
  - Sensory symptoms on the radial side of the back of the hand
  - Extension of the elbow joint is usually normal.
- Treatment
  - Generally spontaneous recovery with monitoring over a few months
  - Failing the above, consider further consultation.

Entrapment at the proximal end of the radial nerve below the supinator muscle (supinator syndrome)

- Ca. 1% of clinical suspicions are actually confirmed; the symptoms are mostly caused by local tendinitis or other painful conditions.
- Symptoms and clinical findings
  - Exclusively motor weakness in extension of wrist and fingers with normal sensations.

Common peroneal nerve

Entrapment at the end of the fibula

- Berry pickers, alcoholics
- Symptoms and clinical findings

- Sensory symptoms anterior to the fibula and over the metatarsal area.
- Paresis or weak dorsiflexion of ankle and foot.
- The foot is dangling, gait consists of short steps, the patient cannot walk on his/her heels.

♦ Treatment
- Generally spontaneous recovery with possible monitoring over a few months
- Failing the above, consider further consultation.

♦ Note: Differentiate from the L5 root symptoms.

Posterior tibial nerve

Entrapment at the level of the medial malleolus (tarsal tunnel syndrome)

♦ Symptoms and clinical findings
- Sensory impairment in the plantar area, pain in the plantar and medial malleolar area
- Motor symptoms are rare: atrophy of small plantar muscles.
- Rising on tiptoe is difficult.

Lateral femoral cutaneous nerve

Entrapment at the inguinal ligament ("meralgica paresthetica")

♦ See 20.63.

♦ Frequently nerve irritation without an actual entrapment (symptoms are not persistent).

♦ Symptoms and clinical findings
- Exclusively sensory symptoms
- Burning pain and numbness on the lateral side of the thigh

♦ Treatment
- Weight-loss programme, avoidance of tight clothing
- Injection of local anaesthetic into the medial area of the lateral attachment site (about two centimeters medially and slightly caudally from the anterior superior iliac spine)
- In persistent cases, the treatment is surgical release of the nerve, or neurolysis.

Diagnostics of nerve entrapments

♦ Electroneuromyography (ENMG) is a necessary addition to the clinical tests when the compression neuropathy does not seem to resolve as expected, or when surgical treatment of the entrapment neuropathy is being considered. This will also reveal polyneuropathy, which increases the risk of nerve injury.

♦ Specialist consultation is always advisable when the clinical symptoms of nerve damage are atypical.

♦ The decision to operate on an entrapped nerve should be made by an expert in the field.

References

1. Bartels RH, Menovsky T, Van Overbeeke JJ, Verhagen WI. Surgical management of ulnar nerve compression at the elbow. Journal of Neurosurgery 1998;89:722–727.
2. The Database of Abstracts of Reviews of Effectiveness (University of York), Database no.: DARE-990432. In: The Cochrane Library, Issue 1, 2001. Oxford: Update Software.

36.89 Quick diagnostics of peripheral nerve disorders

Editors

Typical symptoms and clinical findings in the most common disorders of the peripheral nerves

♦ See Table 36.89.

NEU

Table 36.89 Typical symptoms and clinical findings in the most common peripheral nerve disorders

Nerve	Impairment	Atrophy	Sensory impairment
Medianus	Opposition of the thumb	Thenar	Palmar side of thumb, index and middle fingers
Radialis	Extension of wrist and fingers	Radial side of forearm	Dorsal side of the hand, base of thumb
Ulnaris	Adduction and abduction of fingers	Interosseal, hypothenar muscles	Little finger and ulnar side of ring finger (IV)
Femoralis	Extension of knee, straight leg lifting	Quadriceps femoris muscle	Front thigh
Peroneal	Extension of toes and foot	Anterior tibial muscle (tibial bone "sharp")	Lateral side of leg, base of toes I–II
Tibial	Flexion of foot, rising on toes	Small plantar muscles	Sole of foot
Lateral cutaneous femoral	–	–	Lateral anterior surface of thigh

Note: Exaggerated reflexes, spasticity, clumsiness and pareses and sensory impairment not consistent with peripheral nerve or root territories indicate a disorder of the central nervous system.

36.90 Polyneuropathies

Esa Mervaala, Juhani Partanen

Definition

- Symmetrical disease of (motor and sensory) peripheral nerves and the autonomic nerve system.
- The aetiology includes an agent causing damage to the peripheral nerves.

Diagnosis

- Some patients can be examined and treated in the primary care clinic; some require referral to a specialty hospital.
- Diagnosis can be confirmed with an ENMG (electroneuromyography). This will also provide information on the type and severity of the polyneuropathy. Examination of thresholds for hot and cold stimuli can be used in the diagnosis of polyneuropathy of fine nerve fibers.
- In ca. 25% of patients even a thorough clinical examination will leave the aetiology unknown.

Investigations

- The following tests can be performed in primary care: glucose tolerance, blood count, serum vitamin B_{12}, ESR, serum glutamyl transferase, serum TSH, and serum creatinine.
- If the aetiology cannot be determined on the basis of the history and the initial tests, the patient should be referred to a neurologist.
- DNA analysis is helpful in the diagnostics of hereditary motor and sensory neuropathy (HMSN) and hereditary neuropathy with liability for pressure palsies (HNPP).
- The most common causes of polyneuropathy are diabetes, hypothyroidism, alcohol and vitamin B_{12} deficiency. Other causes are rare.

Toxic neuropathies

Alcohol polyneuropathy

- The most common toxic neuropathy
- Clinically confirmed in ca. 20% of alcoholics; in addition, ca. 30% are subclinical (i.e. abnormalities revealed only with ENMG)
- Typical sensorimotor polyneuropathy, in which mild cases have primarily sensory symptoms (burning feet and painful paraesthesia), while more severe conditions include also motor impairment.
- In chronic polyneuropathy, disease progression and recovery are slow.
- Acute polyneuropathy develops during heavy drinking binges in the distal parts of the extremities, usually first in the legs. Symptoms include severe hyperalgesia, erythema, and occasional oedema, that may prevent walking.
- Treatment
  - The symptoms of polyneuropathy will improve over a sufficiently long period of alcohol abstinence (ca. 6 months). After an acute drinking binge, vitamin B therapy is indicated.

Polyneuropathy caused by heavy metals and solvents

- Exposure to arsenic, lead, thallium, mercury, and gold can produce clinical polyneuropathy.
- Solvents such as hexane in glues, MBK (methyl butyl ketone) in paints and shellacs, and acrylamide used for coating paper can cause polyneuropathy as a result of occupational exposure, and occasionally deliberate sniffing. Other causes are carbon disulphide and organophosphates.

Drug-induced polyneuropathy

- Many cytotoxic drugs (especially cisplatin and vincristine) may cause peripheral neuropathy.
- Polyneuropathies caused by nitrofurantoin and isonicotinic acid hydrazide (INH) are relatively common problems. Onset of INH polyneuropathy usually involves pain.
- Disulfiram (antabus) may cause a neuropathy which may be attributed to alcohol abuse.
- Pyridoxine (vitamin B_6) in large doses may cause polyneuropathy (sensory symptoms dominate). This may lead to diagnostic problems as vitamin B supplements have been prescribed for polyneuropathy patients without taking regard into the specific aetiology.
- Other causes include chloramphenicol, clioquinol, dapsone, metronidazole, certain antiarrhythmic drugs (amiodarone, propafenone), ethionamide, glutethimide, hydralazine, and chlorprothixene. New causes are statins and zalcitabine (an antiretroviral drug).

Metabolic neuropathies

Diabetic neuropathy

- Described under Diabetes (23.42).

Uraemic polyneuropathy

- Common complication of renal failure that occurs in approximately 25% of the patients. Haemodialysis has a clearly resolving effect.
- This condition differs from other metabolic neuropathies in that motor and sensory impairment are equally severe (i.e. sensory symptoms are not dominant).

Polyneuropathy associated with vitamin deficiency

- Vitamin B_{12} deficiency (pernicious anaemia) is often associated with polyneuropathy in clinical practice.
- B_{12} therapy partially resolves the symptoms in about a year's time.
- Pellagra, which is caused by nicotine acid or tryptophan deficiency, has been found among alcoholics in Western countries. In addition, deficiency of pyridoxine (B_6), thiamine (B_1) or tocopherol (E) can on rare occasions cause polyneuropathy. Neuropathy following gastroplasty can be caused by a vitamin deficiency.

Polyneuropathy associated with hypothyroidism

- This condition is mostly expressed as mononeuropathy (= carpal tunnel syndrome, which is often bilateral).
- Sensory polyneuropathy is the next most common peripheral nerve disorder associated with hypothyroidism.
- Medication for hypothyroidism may completely resolve clinical neuropathy.

Polyneuropathy associated with acute porphyria

- Clinical presentations include acute abdominal pain, psychiatric symptoms, and peripheral neuropathy.
- The patient typically has an acute flaccid motor paralysis and absence of tendon reflexes.

Paraneoplastic polyneuropathy

- In males, the condition is usually associated with lung cancer, in females, with breast cancer.
- If subacute sensory polyneuropathy is detected, look for signs of cancer.
- In paraneoplastic neuropathies the protein concentration in the cerebrospinal fluid is often increased.
- Motor neuropathies may also be involved with leukaemias and myelomas.

Hereditary neuropathies

- Some polyneuropathies are hereditary; however, their heritability may remain undetected if genetic family studies are not performed. A major proportion of hereditary neuropathies are autosomal dominant. Molecular genetic methods have become central in the diagnosis of hereditary polyneuropathies.

Hereditary motor and sensory neuropathy (HMSN)

- Type 1: Demyelinating Charcot–Marie–Tooth disease
  - Muscle weakness accentuated in the peroneal region typically presents with distal atrophy and prominent plantar arch.
  - These symptoms frequently have their onset in childhood and manifest as a tendency to sprain the ankles.
  - Later symptoms appear in the distal parts of upper limbs.
  - The mode of inheritance is autosomal dominant; the severity of the symptoms may vary, but they rarely cause ambulatory disability.
  - Diagnosis
    - ENG findings are typical: motor conduction velocity is greatly reduced, and sensory response is usually absent.
    - Confirmation through nerve biopsy (often performing the biopsy on one relative will suffice).
    - Molecular genetic testing is also available and may replace nerve biopsy.
- Type 2: Neuronal Charcot–Marie–Tooth disease
  - Differential diagnosis of demyelinating or hypertrophic and neuronal syndromes is clinically challenging, but in Type 2 the average onset of symptoms is later. Charcot–Marie–Tooth disease (peroneal muscle atrophy) can easily be confused with tibial muscle dystrophy, which is a primary autosomal dominant hereditary muscular disease.
  - Diagnosis
    - ENG reveals that nerve conduction velocities are only slightly reduced or normal.
    - Muscle ENMG, however, reveals chronic denervation.
    - Nerve biopsy
- There are some rare genetic sensorimotor polyneuropathies and hereditary sensory neuropathies.
- Brittle nerve -syndrome
  - There are some families in several countries who carry an autosomal dominant disease of the myelin sheath. This condition renders the nerve susceptible to myelin sheath damage. "Hereditary pressure sensitive neuropathy" and "Hereditary neuropathy with liability to pressure palsies" are also often used determinants for this condition.
  - Symptoms include intermittent pareses and sensory impairment, frequently in the region of the brachial plexus or peroneal nerve.
  - The ENMG findings are typical. An asymptomatic carrier may also be identified by nerve conductivity measurements.

Polyneuropathies associated with immunological disorders

Acute polyradiculitis = Guillain–Barré–syndrome

- Ascending muscle weakness and numbness develop acutely within a few days to a few weeks. If this condition is suspected, the patient should be referred to a hospital immediately (36.92).
- There are several types of chronic inflammatory polyneuropathies; demyelinating and axonal, and motoric or sensory. Diagnosis is based on ENMG and antibody tests, done in specialist care.

Neuropathy associated with HIV infection

- The initial symptoms in 10–30% of HIV patients originate either from the central or the peripheral nervous system.
- Neuropathies of various kinds found in association with HIV infection and AIDS include:
  - Distal, painful sensory polyneuropathy
  - Multiple mononeuropathies
  - Progressive polyradiculitis (Guillain-Barré).
  - Chronic disorders of the Guillain-Barré–type
- In addition, many other viruses (cytomegalo, herpes, hepatitis B and C) may cause neuropathies.

Neuropathy in Lyme disease

- See 1.29.
- Initial symptoms, such as paresis or a painful radiculitis, may derive from the peripheral nervous system.
- This is usually a subacute, sensorimotor polyneuropathy.
- Occasionally there are mononeuritis-related symptoms (most common of these is facial paralysis, but they may also include peroneal paresis).
- Painful radiculopathy or polyradiculitis
- In addition, many other bacteria and parasites (diphtheria, leprosy, trypanosome) may cause neuropathies.

Polyneuropathy associated with paraproteinaemias

- Benign paraproteinaemia or myeloma may be associated with a sensorimotor polyneuropathy caused by protein binding in the peripheral nerve.
- If this condition causes significant symptoms, the treatment consists of immunosuppression (corticoids or cytotoxic drugs) or, in severe cases, plasmapheresis.

Polyneuropathies associated with vasculitis and systemic diseases

- Neuropathies caused by vasculites often present with unilateral symptoms mainly in the lower limbs.
- SLE can be associated with many types of neuropathies, a Guillain-Barré-resembling or a distal sensorimotor polyneuropathy.
- In addition to mononeuropathies, Sjögren's syndrome can be associated with a distal sensorimotor polyneuropathy.
- MCTD (mixed connective tissue disease) or sarcoidosis can also be associated with neuropathies.

Treatment, prognosis, and follow-up of polyneuropathies

- The aetiology is of crucial importance in the treatment and prognosis. Treatment is directed at the basic cause.
- Symptomatic medication

Treatment of neuropathic pain

- In nociceptive pain, which is caused by damage in the tissue sensing the pain, the nerves themselves are healthy. Treatment directed at the cause relieves the pain, which can be managed with anti-inflammatory analgesics.
- Neurogenic pain indicates damage in the nerve tissue itself.
  - Pain resembling electric shocks or shooting pain: carbamazepine up to 200 mg × 2–3 (increasing the dose incrementally)
  - Aches, hyperalgesia, pain interfering with sleep: amitriptyline, initially 10–25 mg per day (in the evening), increased over 2–3 weeks to up to 100 mg per day. Alternative medications include clomipramine and imipramine.

36.91 Radiculopathies

Editors

Symptoms

- Most root disorders are associated with pain radiating from the spine to the territory innervated by the affected root. This type of pain is typical in root compression, where increased compression intensifies the pain and reduced compression relieves it. In mild cases there may be radiating paraesthesia instead of pain.
- Sensory impairment in the territory innervated by the root. The variations and overlap between territories innervated by separate roots should be taken into account. Even a complete loss of one root may not result in complete anaesthesia.
- Weakness in muscles innervated by a root and atrophy in chronic states. Chronic root lesions may involve fasciculations.
- The reflexes innervated by the root are diminished or absent.

Checklist

- See Table 36.91.

Causes of radiculopathies

Compression

- Prolapsed disc
  - Most common cause in the lumbar region
  - In root-related conditions with weakness in the lower extremities, pain is usually felt in the back and lower

Table 36.91 Clinical findings in nerve root lesions

CERVICAL NERVE ROOTS			
Root	**Radiates to**	**Affected muscles**	**Reflex**
♦ C2–C3	♦ Occiput		
♦ C4	♦ Neck		
♦ C5	♦ Shoulder, upper arm	♦ Shoulder, upper arm	♦ Biceps
♦ C6	♦ Thumb	♦ Upper arm, forearm	♦ Biceps
♦ C7	♦ Middle finger	♦ Forearm, hand	♦ Triceps
♦ C8	♦ Little finger	♦ Intrinsic muscles of the hand	♦ Triceps
THORACIC NERVE ROOTS			
Root		**Sensory level**	
♦ Th1		♦ Below the clavicle	
♦ Th5		♦ Nipples	
♦ Th10		♦ Navel	
♦ Th12		♦ Groin	
LUMBAR NERVE ROOTS			
Root	**Radiates to**	**Weakness**	**Reflex**
♦ L2	♦ Base of the thigh	♦ Lumbar flexion	
♦ L3	♦ Front of the thigh	♦ Knee extension	
♦ L4	♦ Front of the thigh and lower leg	♦ Knee extension	♦ Patella
♦ L5	♦ Big toe	♦ Big toe and toe extension	
SACRAL NERVE ROOTS			
Root	**Radiates to**	**Impairment**	**Reflex**
♦ S1	♦ Heels and soles of the feet	♦ Rising on toes	♦ Achilles tendon
♦ S2	♦ Back and inside of the thigh	♦ Lower sacral roots: "saddle" denervation, bladder, bowel, sexual function	

limbs. If there is no pain associated with the weakness, other causes than radiculopathy should be suspected (spinal cord disorders (36.82) or gait disturbances (36.3)).

- Prolapsed disc in the cervical spine
  - Symptoms usually begin as acute neck pain, often in connection with moving the head.
  - The pain radiates down the upper limb and intensifies when the head is inclined toward the side of the pain.
  - The neck is often stiff.
  - The most common site is C5–C6; next most common are C4–C5 and C6–C7.
  - A medial prolapse may compress the spinal cord and cause weakness in the lower extremities; in such cases treatment is urgently required.
  - Treatment for mild conditions is conservative. Surgical treatment: pareses, severe sensory disturbances, persistent pain.
- Tumours
  - Symptoms progress slowly and may extend to several roots.
  - If the tumour is located in the neck or the thoracic spine, there are also symptoms of spinal cord compression.
  - Neurinoma causes a widening in the root canal of the nerve, evident in plain x-rays (the C2 root canal is normally wider than the others; thus both sides must be compared).
- Degenerative changes
  - Especially in the cervical spine region, narrowing of the root canal may cause symptoms of root irritation.
  - It should be noted whether the radiographic and clinical findings indicate the same segmental level.
  - Imaging often reveals asymptomatic narrowed canals.

Inflammation

- Herpes zoster (1.41)
- Radiculitis
  - Radiculites affecting one or more roots whose aetiology often remains unknown occur in both the cervical and the lumbar regions. Conditions such as Lyme disease may be a possible cause.
- Polyradiculitis
  - Develops within a few days and causes ascending symmetrical muscle weakness. Treatment is urgent (36.92).

Diabetes

- Diabetic radiculopathy of the thoracic region causes unilateral encircling pain, sensory impairment, and localized muscle weakness (23.42).

Urgency of treatment

- Emergencies:
  - Cauda equina syndrome
  - Spinal cord compression symptoms.
- Urgent:
  - Root-related paralytic symptoms
  - Intolerable pain.

Referral

- Conservative treatment:
  - Primary health clinic, physiatry.
- Surgical treatment:
  - Orthopaedics or neurosurgery.
- Diagnostics of indistinct conditions:
  - Neurology.

Diagnosis

- ENMG is helpful in differentiating between root and other peripheral nerve disorders and provides information about the duration of the disorder
- Denervation does not develop until after 2–3 weeks; therefore ENMG is not helpful in conditions requiring urgent treatment (36.16).
- Neuroradiology is often necessary. The method of choice for the lumbar region is CT or MRI, for the cervical or thoracic region only MRI.

36.92 Guillain-Barré syndrome (polyradiculitis)

Markus Färkkilä

Aim

- Remember the possibility of polyneuritis in a patient presenting with limb weakness or numbness.

Basic rules

- Polyneuritis is an inflammation of the nerve roots, that affects mainly the motor nerves and has an ascending course.
- Aetiology is unknown.
- In 70% of patients, the condition is preceded by infection (e.g. Campylobacter jejuni), vaccination or immunomanipulation.
- The incidence is 1.0–1.9/100 000 inhabitants/year worldwide.
- Presents in two clinical forms: an acute idiopathic form (95% of cases) and a rare chronic or relapsing form.

Symptoms

- Ascending, symmetrical symptoms of pins and needles, numbness and muscle weakness starting in the lower limbs and moving upwards.
- Muscle weakness dominates the clinical picture.
- The disease may progress to respiratory paralysis in hours.
- Often associated with peripheral pareses of cranial nerves, of which facial paresis is the most common.
- No disturbance of bladder function
- Often neck and low back pain

Diagnosis

- The tendon reflexes are weak or absent.
- Sensory disturbances are only minor.
- Symmetric muscle weakness
- Normal cell count in CSF, although leucocytes may be present, up to 50/mm^3.
- Increased protein concentration of CSF, even up to 6000–7000 mg/l (sometimes a rise in protein content is not seen until the end of the second week of illness).
- ENMG findings may confirm the diagnosis but no earlier than three weeks after the onset of illness.
- There is no diagnostic benefit from blood tests.

Differential diagnosis

- Acute paralytic poliomyelitis (asymmetrical, more leucocytosis in CSF)
- Acute myelitis (upper motor neurone lesion, bladder paralysis)
- Polyneuropathy associated with diphteria
- Botulism
- Myasthenia gravis
- Acute polyneuropathy (36.90)

Treatment

- The patient is transferred to hospital with facilities for respirator treatment and, if needed, an intensive care unit.
- Early intubation of the patient, if there are signs of respiratory failure.
- Steroids have shown no benefit in the treatment of acute forms of polyneuritis (B) [1].

- I.v. immunoglobulin therapy (B) [2] or plasma exchange (B) [3] in severe cases (loss of walking ability, threat of need for a respirator) that should be carried out during the first two weeks of the illness.
- Physiotherapy is recommended, when the progression has stopped.
- Thrombosis prophylaxis for the severely paralysed.
- Steroids are recommended in chronic and relapsing forms of the disease.

Prognosis

- Complete recovery in more than 90% of acute idiopathic cases in 1–2 years.
- Mortality 5–10%
- The progressive phase lasts about four weeks, the stable phase about two weeks, and recovery takes about six weeks.

References

1. Hughes RAC, van der Meché FGA. Corticosteroids for Guillain-Barré syndrome. Cochrane Database Syst Rev. 2004;(2):CD001446.
2. Hughes RAC, Raphaël JC, Swan AV, van Doorn PA. Intravenous immunoglobulin for Guillain-Barré syndrome. Cochrane Database Syst Rev. 2004;(2):CD002063.
3. Raphaël JC, Chevret S, Hughes RAC, Annane D. Plasma exchange for Guillain-Barré syndrome. Cochrane Database Syst Rev. 2004;(2):CD001798.

36.93 Facial paralysis

Kati Juva, Sirpa Asko-Seljavaara

Basic rules

- Patients with facial paresis due to a lesion in the central nervous system should be referred for neurological investigations, if the cause (usually stroke, trauma, or surgical intervention) is not apparent.
- Peripheral paresis can be idiopathic, but potentially treatable causes should be borne in mind.
- When the peripheral paresis has had an acute onset, involves all the branches of the facial nerve and is occasionally accompanied with mild ear pain, an examination by a GP is usually sufficient. This should include neurological and otolaryngological status, TSH and Borrelia antibodies.

Anatomy

- The facial nerve innervates the facial muscles, taste in the front part of the tongue, the lacrimal glands and the sublingual and submandibular salivary glands.
- The innervation of the upper part of the face crosses partly so that the innervation to both halves of the forehead and to muscles surrounding the eyes comes from both hemispheres.
- The innervation of the lower part of the face comes only from the opposite hemisphere.

Paresis of central origin

- A lesion in the central nervous system causes drooping of the contralateral side of the mouth.
- Usually appears with other neurological symptoms (hemiparesis etc.) and common causes include
  - stroke
  - intracerebral haemorrhage
  - brain tumour
  - cerebral contusion.
- The patient should normally be sent for neurological investigations.

Peripheral facial palsy

- Causes paralysis of one half of the face: the forehead cannot be wrinkled, the eye cannot be closed and half of the mouth does not function. Sometimes there is also weakening of the sense of taste, cessation of tear secretion and hyperacusia (sounds are heard too loud because of the abnormal function of the stapedius muscle).
- Known causes of peripheral facial palsy are:
  - borreliosis (1.29) and sarcoidosis (6.43) (often cause a bilateral facial palsy)
  - diabetes
  - fracture at the base of the skull
  - tumour (usually with a slowly progressive paresis) (7.14) or operation of a tumour at the base of the skull (vestibular schwannoma)
  - operation and radiotherapy for tumours of the parotid gland.

NEU

Bell's palsy

- Idiopathic facial palsy (Bell's palsy) usually recovers spontaneously. Sometimes permanent weakness or tendency to hemifacial spasms remains.
- There is no evidence of the efficacy of prednisolone treatment and it is not recommended (B) [1 2 3].
- If the eye does not close properly, there is a risk of drying of the cornea. In this case the eye should be covered at night. In problematic cases the patient can be referred to an ophthalmologist, who can narrow the palpebral fissure by suture or place a gold weight in the upper lid.

- When there is suspicion of a process near or in the ear (e.g. acute or chronic otitis, parotid tumour) the patient should be referred to an otolaryngologist.
- Idiopathic Bell's paresis is often preceded by ear pain without any infection.
- Facial palsy that does not recover normally can sometimes be treated by liberating the nerve surgically.
- Electroneuromyography (ENMG) helps in assessing the severity and recovery of the palsy.

Treatment with plastic surgery

Background

- The facial nerve innervates 16 different muscles in both sides of the face.
- The most problematic consequence is lagophthalmus, where the eye does not close properly and there is a risk of drying. Paresis of the forehead causes drooping of the skin over the eye, and paresis of the side of the mouth causes mumbling of speech and difficulties in eating.

Plastic surgical procedures

- If the facial palsy is permanent, a plastic surgeon should be consulted. The following corrective measures can be used:
- When the forehead hangs over the visual field, endoscopic frontal lift can be performed.
- Lagophthalmos can be closed in the acute phase by using a gold weight or by performing lateral tarsorrhaphy. Both procedures are minor operations that are performed under local anaesthesia either by an ophthalmologist or a plastic surgeons. In severe lower lid ectropion, transposition of the temporal muscle is usually performed.
- Cheek. A static procedure for the correction of a hanging cheek and side of the mouth is elevation of the cheek with a fascia sling. Masseter muscle transposition is a dynamic method of correction.
- Microsurgical methods of correction. In permanent facial paresis (the patient is usually below 60 years of age) cross-over nerve transplantation following by microvascular muscle transplant is the method used for restoring function. This method involves two long microsurgical operations and the recovery time is more than one year.

References

1. Salinas RA, Alvarez G, Alvarez MI, Ferreira J. Corticosteroids for Bell's palsy (idiopathic facial paralysis). Cochrane Database Syst Rev. 2004;(2):CD001942.
2. Williamson IG, Whelan TR. The clinical problem of Bell's palsy: is treatment with steroids effective? Br J Gen Pract 1996;46:743–747.
3. The Database of Abstracts of Reviews of Effectiveness (University of York), Database no.: DARE-978205. In: The Cochrane Library, Issue 4, 1999. Oxford: Update Software.

36.94 Trigeminal neuralgia

Kati Juva

Symptoms

- Trigeminal neuralgia is characterized by paroxysms of intense, stabbing pain on the other half of the face in the area of one of the branches of the trigeminal nerve.
- Between the attacks the pain is totally absent and may be provoked by touching certain areas of the face (trigger zones) or by eating.
- The pain attacks are very short and resemble electrical shock.
- There are no permanent neurological deficiency symptoms.

Differential diagnosis

- So-called atypical facial pain is much more common than trigeminal neuralgia.
  - The pain is usually constant and deep and is not restricted to one half of the face.
  - There is often underlying depression.
- See also cluster headache 36.68.

Treatment

Trigeminal neuralgia

- The drug of choice is carbamazepine (A) [1]. The dose is increased until a response is seen (or until there are unbearable side-effects). Oxcarbazepine is probably as effective (C) [2] [3] [4], and can be tried especially if carbamazepine causes adverse effects (fatigue, dizziness).
- The initial dose of carbamazepine is 100 mg × 2. The dose can be increased slowly up to 300 mg × 2.
- In the beginning follow-up of blood cell counts and liver function tests is recommended. Carbamazepine concentration can be measured if there are signs of overdose (dizziness, tiredness, diplopia or nystagmus).
- If carbamazepine does not help or there are unbearable side effects, operative treatment should be considered. The trigeminal ganglion can be electrocoagulated, or the compression of the nerve by a small nearby artery can be released by microsurgery.

Atypical facial pain

- Atypical facial pain is treated with painkillers or by antidepressants. Tricyclic antidepressants are used in small dosages.

References

1. Wiffen P, Collins S, McQuay H, Carroll D, Jadad A, Moore A. Anticonvulsant drugs for acute and chronic pain. Cochrane Database Syst Rev. 2004;(2):CD001133.
2. Lindström 1987, reported in brief.
3. Zakrzewska JM, Patsalos PN. Oxcarbazepine: a new drug in the management of intractable trigeminal neuralgia. Journal of Neurology, Neurosurgery & Psychiatry 1989;52:472–6.
4. Farago F. Trigeminal neuralgia: its treatment with two new carbamazepine analogues. European Neurology 1987;26:73–83.

36.95 Hiccup

Mikael Ojala

Causes

- Physiological hiccup
  - Over-eating
  - Drinks with carbon dioxide
  - Changes in temperature
- Toxic and metabolic causes
  - Alcohol
  - Uraemia
- Brain stem diseases
  - Bleeding
  - Infarction
  - Tumour
  - Infection
  - Multiple sclerosis
- Mediastinal processes
  - Lymphoma
- Diseases of the upper abdomen
  - Hiatus hernia
  - Gastric carcinoma
  - Subphrenic abscess
  - Ileus
  - Postoperative condition
- Other causes
  - Psychiatric causes
  - "Essential hiccup" with no discernible cause

Treatment

- Treatment according to aetiology
- Physiological hiccup
  - A spoonful of fine dry sugar
  - Breathing into a paper bag
  - Drinking from the opposite brim of a glass
- Drug treatment
  - Chlorpromazine, e.g. 25 mg orally or i.m.
  - Sodium valproate 1 g/day orally
  - Metoclopramide 40 mg/day per rectum
  - Droperidol 2.5 mg i.v.
- Phrenectomy is rarely indicated.

36.96 Increased intracranial pressure

Editors

Objectives

- The possibility of intracranial pressure must be considered in a patient whose symptoms include headache, nausea, and vomiting.
- Direct ophthalmoscopy should be performed for the presence of papilloedema; normal pupils do not rule out an acute increase in intracranial pressure.
- Increased intracranial pressure must be treated aggressively if it has a negative effect on the patient's prognosis.

Basic rules

- In adults, the brain is enclosed in a rigid skull. If something causes an increase in the volume of the tissues inside the skull, pressure will increase. Variable factors in this volume are cerebral tissue, amount of blood in the brain, and cerebrospinal fluid. A foreign mass can increase the volume: tumour, blood clot, or infection.
- It is not the pressure itself that is harmful, but the resulting ischaemia.

NEU

Symptoms

- These are dependent on the rate of increase in the volume–it is difficult to compensate for a rapid change.
- Progressive impairment in the level of consciousness generally indicates cerebral herniation and ischaemia.
- Headache, nausea, and vomiting
- Symptoms related to pupillary reactions and eye movements:
  - Symptoms related to the third cranial nerve are pupillary dilatation and ptosis.
  - Symptoms related to the sixth cranial nerve may be limited to paresis of the lateral movement of the eye and double vision.
- Pressure symptoms developing more slowly cause less dramatic changes in the level of consciousness. The patient

is somnolent and sluggish, and the pressure may cause changes in intuition and memory as well as indifference.

- Prolonged pressure may be indicated by papilloedema, which is always diagnostic of increased intracranial pressure. It is rarely seen today, as patients usually receive care at an early stage.

Diagnosis

- The diagnosis is based on medical history, basic neurological examination findings, and neuroradiological tests.
  - A CT scan performed at the acute stage will nearly always both confirm the increased intracranial pressure and provide an aetiological diagnosis.
  - **Lumbar puncture is contraindicated** (36.17).
- Magnetic resonance imaging is often needed in order to arrive at a precise aetiology.

Aetiology

- Of all intracranial disorders, oedema is a crucial cause for increased pressure; it is a typical reaction in the brain after a mechanical, chemical, or vascular injury. It is more difficult to treat than to prevent.
- Changes in blood volume are the most rapidly occurring causes of increased pressure, and also most rapidly responsive to treatment. The level of carbon dioxide and, to some extent, that of partial pressure of oxygen regulate pressure in the cerebral vessels. Hypoventilation and hypoxia increase the pressure, while hyperventilation is the quickest way to reduce the pressure. Chronic pulmonary disease and hypoventilation may be the cause of increased intracranial pressure.
- Hydrocephalus generally presents as a steady increase in the pressure, even though the final-stage symptoms may be violent. In children, enlargement of the head is a typical symptom of hydrocephalus; papilloedema does usually not develop. The cause of hydrocephalus may be tumour-related disturbances in the circulation of the cerebrospinal fluid or a resorption dysfunction.
- Chronic hydrocephalus (normal-pressure hydrocephalus) triad: gait dysfunction, urinary incontinence, and dementia (36.22)
- Pressure symptoms due to an expanding mass are classic presentations of increased pressure.
- The pressure effect of haemorrhage always occurs rapidly.
- In inflammations, other symptoms of infection may aid in the diagnosis.

Treatment

- Treatment of increased intracranial pressure is directed at its cause:
  - Removal of the tumour or haematoma
  - Anti-inflammatory therapy
  - Surgical treatment of the hydrocephalus with a temporary stoma or permanent shunt.
- Most challenging is the treatment of oedema.
  - Hyperventilation
  - Osmotic diuretics (mannitol)
  - Corticoids (dexamethasone)
  - Correction of the fluid and electrolyte balance
  - Correct positioning of the patient
- In the unconscious patient, maintaining the airways unobstructed is crucial.

36.98 Sequelae of traumatic brain injury

Mikael Ojala

Basic rules

- All primary data on the trauma are documented carefully as they are useful in the treatment of sequelae and planning of rehabilitation.
- Permanent sequelae can be evaluated one year after the trauma at the earliest.
- A neuropsychological examination is often needed to determine the degree of disability and to plan rehabilitation.

General observations

- The assessment and treatment of acute brain injuries is presented in another article (18.3).
- One year from the trauma the sequelae can be considered permanent, and changes in the condition can no longer be expected. However, in some cases social and occupational problems may become apparent only later.
- Sequelae of brain injury involve problems related to diagnosis, insurance medicine, and also therapy that are usually greater in milder injuries.
- Mild injuries are also much more common than severe injuries.

Evaluating the severity of brain injury

- In the evaluation of the severity of the injury, primary information is taken into account, i.e. mechanism of trauma, duration of possible unconsciousness, and post-traumatic amnaesia (PTA) (18.3), level of consciousness when brought to the hospital, and findings on neurological examination.

- The following factors are also considered: health status prior to the trauma, CT and MRI findings, neuropsychological observations, and follow-up of social and occupational functioning.
- If the patient did not experience primary unconsciousness and was conscious when hospitalized, and if the duration of PTA was less than one hour and head CT and MRI findings are normal, it is unlikely that the trauma would cause permanent brain damage.
- However, the patient may continue to have symptoms for weeks or months.
- In more severe cases than that described above the most common sequelae are neuropsychological in nature.

Neuropsychological examination

- Useful for planning rehabilitation and assessing the degree of disability.
- Unspecific: there are no pathognomonic findings that are typical to the injury.

Brain injury and rehabilitation

- Some patients with a moderate to severe brain injury recover enough to resume working.
- The medical and occupational rehabilitation of a patient with brain injury follows the principles of stroke rehabilitation (36.34).
- Management of post-traumatic epilepsy is an important medical intervention. It is worthwhile to remember that the most common form of vertigo following a blow to the head is benign positional vertigo, which responds well to treatment (38.72).

36.99 Brain tumours

Editors

Basic rules

- Brain tumours occur at all ages.
- Peak occurrence is in early childhood and from middle age upward.

Aetiology

- The cause of most brain tumours is unknown. Immunosuppression and immunological deficiencies (AIDS) increase the incidence of e.g. primary cerebral lymphoma.
- Neurofibromatosis type 2 and tuberous sclerosis carry an increased risk of brain tumours.

Most common brain tumours

- Approximately one-half of all brain tumours are gliomas. They are classified according to the stem cell and increasing grade of malignancy.
  - Astrocytomas (grades I–IV) occur in adults. They grow inside the brain tissue and infiltrate the surrounding tissue without a margin. Grades I and II grow fairly slowly. In grade III astrocytoma the patient's survival outcome is a couple of years. Patients with grade IV glioblastoma multiforme, generally do not survive for more than a year, regardless of treatment.
  - Oligodendrogliomas (grades I–IV) grow slower than astrocytomas; therefore their prognosis is better. They often contain calcifications.
  - Ependymoma (grades I–IV) originates from ependymic tissue and is located in the lining of cerebral ventricles, most commonly in the region of the fourth ventricle. The tumour is relatively sensitive to radiation. When the tumour is located in the supratentorial region the prognosis is fairly good; however, an ependymoma in the fourth ventricle is seldom completely removed, and its prognosis is poorer.
  - Medulloblastoma (grades I–IV) is a paediatric tumour located infratentorially; it may metastasize in the spinal canal. It is malignant, but sensitive to radiation.
  - Pilocytic astrocytoma (cerebellar astrocytoma, spongioblastoma) (grades I–II) is the most common tumour in children. It is located infratentorially or in the optic chiasm. Successful surgical treatment of cerebellar astrocytoma is curative.
- Neurinoma or schwannoma is benign and slowly growing. Neurinomas may be located in several parts of the nervous system. In the intracranial space they originate in the cranial nerves, most commonly in the acoustic nerve.
- Colloid cyst is a rare benign tumour located in the third ventricle.
- Meningeoma is a benign, encapsulated, circumscribed tumour originating in the cerebral meninges. Anaplasia is rarely found in meningeomas. Meningeoma is slowly growing, and occurs more commonly in females and middle-aged or older individuals. It is often totally excisable.
- The majority of hypophyseal tumours are hypophyseal adenomas (24.67). Also located in the same region is craniopharyngioma, an inborn tumour that can cause pituitary insufficiency and/or visual impairment.
- Primary cerebral lymphoma is being diagnosed in increasing numbers nowadays.
- Dermoid tumour is benign, contains structural elements of the skin, and is usually located at the cerebral midline.
- Epidermoid tumour is benign and consists of a mass containing cholesterol.
- Metastases.
  - Approximately one-fourth of all brain tumours are metastases of tumours located elsewhere in the body.
  - Many neoplasms may metastasize in the brain; most common of these are lung and breast cancers.

- In meningeal carcinosis, malignant neoplastic cells proliferate along the meninges without forming a distinct neoplasm. The manifestation of the disease resembles chronic meningitis (36.56). Meningeal carcinosis is associated with melanoma, leukaemias, breast cancer, and lung cancer.

Symptoms of brain tumours

- These are either general symptoms caused by an intracranial mass or local symptoms caused by localized tissue damage, pressure, or irritation.
- Symptoms progress slowly. Haemorrhage into the tumour may cause an acute symptom manifestation.
- With slowly growing tumours the brain accommodates to the extra mass, and therefore the tumour may be quite large by the time pressure symptoms appear. When the reserve space within the skull has been exceeded, the symptoms rapidly worsen.

General symptoms

- Epilepsy is the initial symptom of a brain tumour in ca. 15% of patients; it occurs in ca. 30% of all tumour patients. The possibility of a tumour should always be considered in the case of adult-onset epilepsy, particularly of the focal type (36.45).
- Headache is not an early symptom. It will develop when the tumour causes hydrocephalus by blocking the CSF flow or by growing so large that its mass increases intracranial pressure (36.96). Characteristics of a neoplastic headache are the following:
  - Grows progressively more severe.
  - Occurs while lying down, in the morning, and interrupts the patient's sleep.
  - Causes nausea and vomiting.
  - Increased pressure (coughing or straining) increases severity.
- False localized symptoms: the oculomotor and abducent nerves are easily damaged as the intracranial pressure increases (36.96), even if the tumour is not located in their vicinity. The brainstem may be pressed against the margin of the tentorium cerebelli, causing symptoms of hemiparesis.

Local symptoms

- A tumour in the anterior frontal lobe causes a personality change: general slowing down, performance impairment, and loss of self-criticism. The sense of smell may be lost. A tumour in the posterior frontal lobe may compress the optic nerve and cause a unilateral loss of vision and atrophy of the optic nerve. If the tumour extends into the precentral gyrus, a slowly progressing hemiparesis or epilepsy of the Jackson type may develop (focal attacks where the twitching occurs in the limbs on one side). A tumour in the dominant hemisphere may cause dysphasia.
- A tumour in the parietal lobe may cause unilateral sensory and motor impairment as well as neuropsychological disturbances; if deeply seated, it may cause homonymous hemianopia.
- Tumours in the temporal lobe readily cause temporal epilepsy (36.45). In addition, there may be memory loss and personality changes. A tumour in Wernicke's area causes impairment in speech and comprehension. Visual field defects are also possible.
- A tumour in the occipital lobe causes visual field defects or seizure-like visual disturbances.
- In its initial stage, a tumour in the cerebellum often causes symptoms of increased intracranial pressure, and localized symptoms may be slight. These include loss of balance, dysarthria, and ataxia.
- Tumours in the brainstem cause brainstem syndromes, which include cranial nerve disorders associated with symptoms of long tracts. CSF flow is also easily disturbed.
- Acoustic neurinoma is the most common tumours at the cerebellopontine angle. The initial symptom is slow sensory-neural hearing loss. A later manifestation is dizziness and damage to adjacent cranial nerves: facial paresthesia and motor disturbances. Subsequently, the tumour causes compression of the brainstem and symptoms in the extremities as well as hydrocephalus.
- Tumours in the sella turcica (24.67) cause hormonal disturbances and visual field defects due to the compression of the optic chiasm.
- Symptoms of central tumours:
  - Colloid cyst causes periodic disturbances of CSF flow, and the patient has attacks of headache, nausea, and weakness.
  - Tumours in the area of the pineal gland cause Parinaud's syndrome: The patient is unable to raise his/her gaze above the horizontal level.
  - A tumour in the area of the internal capsule causes pareses, and a tumour in the basal ganglia may cause extrapyramidal symptoms.

Diagnosis

- History and neurological examination are crucial. Objective abnormalities are significant. Papilloedema is rare today, as tumours are usually detected before it develops.
- A tumour is often not evident as the cause of symptoms; on clinical examination the patient is found to have brain-related symptoms that require additional tests: CT or MRI of the brain (36.15).
- When necessary, angiography or MR angiography should be performed before surgery.
- A CSF examination is not part of the diagnostics of brain tumours. Sometimes PAP of liquor is investigated. In case of lymphomas, surface markers are examined.
- Early symptoms of acoustic neurinoma are found in otological tests. BAEP (= brainstem auditory evoked potential) is abnormal already in the early stages (36.15).

- In preparation for radiation therapy, an open or stereotactic biopsy may be performed.

Treatment

Treatment of increased intracranial pressure

- Increased intracranial pressure (36.96).
- When the patient presents with symptoms of increased intracranial pressure or significant neurological deficits, his/her condition can be alleviated in 6–24 hours with dexamethasone, which helps to reduce the oedema surrounding the tumour.
- Dexamethasone may be administered orally or intravenously, in doses up to 5 mg × 4. For life-threatening symptoms (unconsciousness, pupillary dilation), mannitol may be administered in doses of 1.5–2 g per kg of weight i.v. This will improve the patient's condition for ca. 3 hours, during which time he/she may be transferred to a neurosurgical unit.

Surgical and radiation treatment

- Consulting a neurosurgeon is mandatory in order to determine the treatment of brain tumour patients. Even if the tumour is inoperable, it is important for the patient and his/her family to know that a specialist has considered all treatment alternatives.
- Surgical success depends primarily on the location of the tumour. The size and type of neoplasm and the patient's age and general condition are also significant factors.
- The treatment of benign tumours is aimed at their complete removal.
- Total removal of gliomas is rarely successful. Gliomas have a general tendency to recur. A partial resection is often performed to relieve symptoms and gain extra time. Resection is usually followed by radiotherapy.
- Cerebral lymphoma responds well to radiation. The biopsy is followed by radiotherapy.
- A solitary metastasis should be surgically removed.
- Certain inoperable tumours cause hydrocephalus. In such cases the patient may benefit from a shunt operation. Hydrocephalus may also develop postoperatively.
- Radiotherapy for brain tumours is generally non-curative. As a rule, it requires a preceding brain biopsy. In order to counteract oedema, dexamethasone must be administered during cranial radiotherapy.
- New forms of therapy include stereotactic radiation administered externally with a "gamma knife" C [1 2] or with a stereotactic linear accelerator, or internally through an implanted radioisotope. Boron-neutron capture, cytotoxic gene therapy and cytostatic treatments are still in the experimental stages.

Follow-up

- Initial follow-up of brain tumour patients is often scheduled to take place in the neurosurgery or neurology outpatient clinic. In the terminal stage, the responsibility for palliative treatment may be transferred to the primary health care clinic.
- Follow-up blood tests or chest x-rays are not significant in the evaluation of a brain tumour. Primary brain tumours do not metastasize beyond the central nervous system.

Problems

- The tumour or its treatment has left residual symptoms of neurological deficits. If the prognosis, even for the short term, is good, the patient should have access to rehabilitation.
- Epilepsy is common. Medication should be continued after tumour removal, if the patient had epilepsy before the operation.
- Shunt dysfunction should be suspected if the patient develops headaches, nausea, drowsiness, deterioration of mental capacity, or gait dysfunction. A radiograph of the skull and thorax verifies the integrity of the shunt. When the shunt is palpated, the valve is usually felt behind the right ear. It should be flexible. A hard or indented valve indicates dysfunction. Suspicion of shunt dysfunction usually requires a brain CT.

When to suspect recurrence?

- Symptoms of neurological deficits aggravate. The physician must be familiar with this patient's earlier symptoms and findings.
- Symptoms of increased intracranial pressure appear.
- Epileptic seizures occur more frequently, or their symptomatology changes.
- The patient's general performance is impaired.
- If recurrence is suspected, a neurologist or neurosurgeon must be consulted. The treatment possibilities for a recurrent tumour vary from patient to patient. Occasionally, progressive symptoms are caused by radiation encephalopathy.

References

1. Anderson D, Flynn K. Stereotactic radiosurgery for metastases to the brain: a systematic review of published studies of effectiveness. Techn Assess Program 7, 1997:1–16.
2. The Database of Abstracts of Reviews of Effectiveness (University of York), Database no.: DARE-988592. In: The Cochrane Library, Issue 4, 1999. Oxford: Update Software.

Ophthalmology

Evidence Based Medicine Guidelines. Edited by the Duodecim Editorial Team
 ISBN: 0-470-01184-X

37.1 Assessment of vision

Lea Hyvärinen

- Basic functions of vision can be accurately assessed in primary health care provided that the test methods are known and the instructions followed.
- Vision is composed of more than ten simultaneous functions that may be disturbed independent of each other. Damage to the visual pathways may cause symptoms that may even seem neurasthenic to an unexperienced examiner. It is essential to interpret visual symptoms correctly. With the increase in work requiring accurate vision, such as office work, the importance of the assessment of vision will grow in the future.
- So far there is little evidence that community-based screening of asymptomatic older people would lead to improvements in vision C [1]. However, vision, spectacle correction and visual devices should be considered in the care of elderly persons. Quality of life and independence are related to the quality of sensory functions, both vision and hearing. Such simple things as having correct glasses on when eating/reading or watching TV and having batteries in hearing aids should be routinely checked in the care of elderly persons.

Visual pathways

- The rod and cone cells in the outer retina absorb light energy and transform it into electrical signals. The parvocellular pathway (80% of fibres in the optic nerve) transfers all colour information and high-contrast information. The magnocellular pathway transfers all motion-related and low-contrast visual information (transient information).
- Visual information is transferred via the optic nerve to the lateral geniculate nucleus (LGN) and from there to the primary visual cortex in the occipital lobe, where parts of the pictures of the left and right eye are fused. In the associative cortical areas visual information is combined with information from other sensory modalities and with memory. Subcortical visual information is related to balance and motor functions. When in a familiar place, we rarely stop to think of our whereabouts, whereas in a strange environment we use our cortical analysis of space. The orientation of a visually impaired person to space and moving in it must be assessed separately in a familiar and strange environment.
- Vision is a cerebral function. The peripheral part of the visual system gives us information like a camera. In work and traffic low-contrast visual information and motion perception are important.

Methods of assessing vision

- The clinical evaluation of visual function has traditionally included the following functions: visual acuity, binocularity, colour vision and visual field. In addition, accommodation (particularly in presbyopic persons), night vision, contrast sensitivity and glare sensivity are significant.

Visual acuity

- Visual acuity depicts the size of the smallest figures that can be correctly recognized. According to the international recommendation, visual acuity should be measured with a chart where the distance between the figures (optotypes) is equal to their width and the space between the lines is equal to the height of the lower line. The old Snellen E chart is substituted by letter, number and symbol charts.
- The use of tests on lightboxes with standard, even luminance removes the problem of non-standardized illumination.
- Visual acuity should be measured at a distance of 4 meters in adults and at a distance of 3 meters in children. (Note that there are charts for 5 and 6 meters still in use in many countries.) The patient is asked the first or last optotype on each line until s/he hesitates. Then all the optotypes of that line are read. If less than 3 out of 5 optotypes are correctly named, the patient is asked to read the line above. Visual acuity is the value of the line where at least 3 out of 5 optotypes were correctly identified. The most accurate way of documenting the result is to write, for example, 0.8 (-2) [20/25 (-2); 6/9 (-2)] if the subject had two wrong answers on line 0.8 [20/25; 6/9].
- Near vision is assessed with a near vision card at a distance of 40 cm or, if the patient uses reading glasses, at the clearest vision of the glasses. The result is written down either as, for example, "reads line 0.8 at a distance of 52 cm". Visual acuity can then be calculated by dividing the measured value by 40 and multiplying it by the distance used $(52/40) \times 0.8 = 1.0$.

Contrast sensitivity

- Contrast sensitivity depicts the ability to perceive small differences in luminance between adjacent surfaces. The fainter a shadow a person can see the better the contrast sensitivity.
- Contrast sensitivity can be assessed by using an optotype test or a grating test. Testing is useful in the follow-up of vision in diabetics (low-contrast function is affected before high-contrast function), in occupational health care (some nerve toxins affect contrast sensitivity), and in the investigation of vague visual symptoms (incipient optic nerve infection, some intoxications).

Visual fields

- Visual field depicts the area that a person can see without moving his/her eyes. The functional visual field is wider because of the continuous movement of the eyes. Central visual field is important in demanding near and distance vision tasks, the peripheral part of the visual field is important in moving around and in observing the surroundings.

- Visual fields can be measured by finger perimetry, with the Vice Versa (VV) perimeter or by using a small ball on a thin stick. The person examined sits looking straight ahead and responds when and from which side he/she detects the fingers, the VV test rod or the ball. The person examining may not follow the movement of the fingers or the rod or ball with his eyes, but watches that the eyes of the person examined stay fixed in the midline.
- Constriction of visual fields (particularly homonymous) can be detected by the above methods but not small scotomas. Changes in the central visual field can be assessed by using a text of proper size at 57 cm distance from the patient's eyes. The patient looks at a certain word and describes whether there are any distortions or shadows, dim spots or change of tone in the text. At this distance 1 cm on the paper corresponds to one degree of visual angle.

Colour vision

- Colour vision can be screened in primary care (C) [2 3] with Ishihara (B) [4 5], Velhagen or HRR tests. Typical red-green colour defects can be detected with these tests, but some persons with normal vision are also caught in the screen. Abnormal results need to be confirmed with sorting tests, such as the Farnsworth Panel D-15 test. Of these tests, the Good-Lite Panel 16 test is suitable for primary health care. The type and severity of the disorder can be determined when the results are drawn on the recording form.
- Colour vision is measured "at a window facing north at noon on a day with light overcast" and, as this is difficult to arrange, a blue "daylight" lamp (colour temperature > 6000 K) should be used.

Night vision

- Cone cells function in daylight (photopic vision) and rod cells function in dim light (scotopic vision). There is a large area at lower luminance levels where both cell types function (mesopic vision). The speed of adaptation and visual acuity in dim light are singificant in some occupations and in daily activities.
- The speed of cone adaptation can be measured by comparing the patient's ability to detect colours of the red and blue pieces in the CONE Adaptation test to that of the examiner, who must have normal speed of cone adaptation. The assessment of threshold values of visual acuity in darkness is important when, for example, security personnel is tested.

Accommodation and presbyopia

- Presbyopia is such a common problem at workplaces that it requires special attention.
- The effect of presbyopia on the working position is emphasized in office and visual display work and in monitoring tasks as well as in jobs where the worker must be able to clearly see objects above the eye level (technicians, nurses, librarians). Inadequate ergonomics, such as placing the computer screen too high, causes nodding of the head, chin-up posture and leaning forwards resulting in pain in the neck, shoulders and lower back.
- In order to prevent neck and back problems, visual ergonomics, design of workstations and illumination of the workplace should be given special consideration in the health care of presbyopic workers.
- See www.lea.test.fi

References

1. Smeeth L, Iliffe S. Community screening for visual impairment in the elderly. Cochrane Database Syst Rev. 2004;(2):CD001054.
2. New Zealand Health Technology Assessment. Colour vision screening: a critical appraisal of the literature. Christchurch: New Zealand Health Technology Assessment. New Zealand Health Technology Assessment (NZHTA). NZHTA Report 7. 1998. 59.
3. The Health Technology Assessment Database, Database no.: HTA-989043. In: The Cochrane Library, Issue 1, 2001. Oxford: Update Software.
4. New Zealand Health Technology Assessment. Colour vision screening: a critical appraisal of the literature. NZHTA 1998 (report 7, pp. 1–59).
5. The Database of Abstracts of Reviews of Effectiveness (University of York), Database no.: DARE-989721. In: The Cochrane Library, Issue 4, 2000. Oxford: Update Software.

37.2 Assessment of visual impairment and disability

Lea Hyvärinen

OPH

- A great majority of people with visual impairment are elderly persons who also have many other impairments and chronic diseases. Totally blind persons can easily be classified as visually impaired. In persons with a less than total visual impairment, the significance of the impairment varies in different situations. The following two cases depict this problem: Mr. A. has normal size of visual field and a central scotoma. Mr. B. has tunnel vision with an intact central visual field.
    - Mr. A. has no problems in orientation as his peripheral vision is intact, whereas Mr. B. uses the white cane.
    - In daily activities both use varyingly techniques typical to the blind, to low vision and to persons with normal sight.
    - Mr. A. cannot see facial expressions or recognize acquaintances across the street. Mr. B. does not notice gestures or the reactions of people in group communication.

- Mr. A. uses talking books because of his very slow reading speed while Mr. B. can easily read even newspapers.

- It is obvious that both these individuals cannot be classified with one common label that would depict the level of vision loss. Neither is blind but both need to use techniques typical to the blind in some tasks while performing like a normally sighted person in other situations.
- For statistical purposes visual impairment is defined as visual acuity less than 6/18 (0.3, 20/60) or visual field less than 10 degrees from the fixation point. As was pointed out by the WHO/ICEVI expert group in 1992, these values should not be used for assessment of eligibility for services.
- Planning of services in (re)habilitation and special education is based on disability. Its assessment requires thorough evaluation of all visual functions and their effect on communication, daily living skills, orientation and mobility and sustained near vision tasks like reading and writing. Services are given in areas where they are needed independent of visual acuity or visual field size. The national organizations for the visually impaired have their representatives at the county/district level and can help the local health care officers in the evaluation of need for rehabilitation and devices.
- The new ICF (International Classification of Functioning, Disabilities and Health) proposes that nine different aspects should be evaluated: learning and applying knowledge, general tasks and demands, communication, mobility, self care, domestic life, interpersonal interactions and relationships, major life areas, community, social and civic life.
- ICF is not applicable to children or persons with multiple disabilities, which is an obvious shortcoming, as more than 50% of persons with visual impairment have some other impairment, abnormality or chronic disease that affects their life.

37.3 Refractive errors

Paula Summanen

Aims

- To understand the basic function of the eye as an optical system and disturbances in it.

Definition

- An imbalance between the refractive power of the optical system of the eye and its axial length (i.e. the position of the retina, the "film" of the eye). Patients in whom these factors are in balance are emmetropic. If they are unbalanced (ametropia), optical correction is needed to achieve emmetropia.

Basic rules

- The most important refractive elements of the eye are the cornea (43 diopters, D) and the lens (23 D), together 65 D. They cause parallel rays of light coming from far away objects to converge so that a sharp image falls on the retina, which is located 23–24 mm behind the cornea in an emmetropic eye.
- The refractive power of the cornea cannot be changed.
- The refractive power of the lens can be increased by active work of the ciliary muscle (accommodation).When looking into the distance, the ciliary muscle is at rest, the suspensory fibres of the lens, the zonules, are tight and the lens is thin and stretched and its refractive power at its lowest. During close-up work, accommodation is needed. The ciliary muscle contracts and the zonules relax, the convexity of the lens increases due to the elasticity of the lens material, and its refractive power increases. Accommodation decreases gradually, causing symptoms (presbyopia) at the age of 40–45 years.
- Ametropia is usually due to abnormal axial length of the eye rather than to altered refractive power of the cornea and the lens (short eyes, long eyes). Therefore, some eye diseases are more common in myopes (retinal detachment), some in hyperopes (angle closure glaucoma, branch vein occlusion, age-related macular degeneration). However, the cornea may be steeper than normal, which increases its refractive power (e.g. keratoconus). Similarly the refractive power of the lens may be increased, for example as it becomes thicker with age due to nuclear sclerosis.

Hyperopia (farsightedness)

- Most children are hyperopic at birth, i.e. the eye is too short in relation to the lens system. This may be compensated for by accommodation, the capacity for which is excellent in children (about 20 diopters). By the age of 7 years, the eyeball reaches the length of 23–24 mm of an adult emmetropic eye.
- A hyperopic child may develop convergent strabismus (esotropia), particularly if one eye is more hyperopic than the other (anisometropia) and has to accommodate more. Convergence associated with accommodation pulls the eye to esotropia.
- Strong hyperopia is rarer than myopia, but more unpleasant, as it prevents from seeing objects clearly at any distance. Mild hyperopia is easily compensated with accommodation (latent hyperopia), but as the accommodation capacity decreases with age, patients will eventually get eyestrain (asthenopia), first in close-up work where the need for accommodation is greatest, but later also when looking far away.
- Symptoms are variable:
  - Frontal headache, pain around the eyes, headache
  - Stomach problems
  - Burning of the eyes, foreign body sensation, the eyes feel tired (asthenopia).
  - Possibly also redness of the eyes.

- In differential diagnosis, remember dry eye syndrome (the Schirmer test and artificial tears) and latent strabismus.
- Sometimes diabetic maculopathy, age-related macular degeneration and central serous retinopathy cause macular oedema and decrease the effective axial length of the eye, making it hyperopic.

Treatment

- On examination the patient is seen to accommodate also when looking at a distance.
- When accommodation is corrected with convex spectacles (plus power) that allow the patient to see far with the eyes at rest, younger patients are first able to do any close-up work with the same glasses without any problems. Later the patient will need bifocal, trifocal or multifocal (progressive addition) lenses that correct both distance vision and compensate for the weakened accommodation reserve in near vision.

Myopia (nearsightedness)

- Every third adolescent or young adult is myopic.
- The eye is too long for its refractive power. Light rays from infinity are focused in front of the retina. One millimetre excess in length corresponds to 2–3 diopters of myopia (axial myopia). With concave spectacles (minus power) the rays of light are diverged so that when they enter the eye its own lens system converges them and a sharp picture falls on the retina.
- In emmetropic eyes, the far point plane of the eye is at infinity (6 metres for practical purposes). In -3 diopter myopia the eye sees clearly at a distance of 33 cm (the power of a lens, in diopters, is 1/focal length in metres). In this example the focal length is 0.33 m, and 1/0.33 m = 3 D). The eyes of a person with a -3 diopter myopia are at rest when reading text that is 33 cm away. Any objects beyond this far point plane are not sharp. Screwing up one's eyes makes the object sharper. The narrow palpebral fissure works like the aperture in a camera: the smaller the aperture, the greater the depth of focus. Objects closer than the far point plane are seen sharply with accommodation.
- When examining vision a so-called stenopic hole can be used to distinguish between refractory error and organic cause of visual impairment, as in the latter case looking through a hole does not improve vision, but often makes it even poorer. A hole made on a piece of paper with a needle serves as a stenopic hole.
- Distance vision is blurred. Children prefer to watch TV closer than usual, school children cannot see the blackboard, especially if they are tall and thus sit at the back of the classroom. Problems recur when glasses become weak.
- Drivers notice difficulties seeing in the dark or they do not see traffic signs even in broad daylight.

Differential diagnosis

- Keratoconus and increased refractive power of the lens associated with cataract may cause myopia. A presbyopic person with cataract may be able to read again without spectacles (so-called "second sight").
- Acute swelling of the lens in diabetic hyperglycaemia or epidemic nephropathy causes transient myopia.

Treatment

- Concave (minus power) spectacles or contact lenses.
- Currently, refractive surgery is popular. The refractive power of the cornea may be weakened by relaxing incisions (less common) or by flattening its surface with an excimer laser and related techniques.
- Surgery involves the risk of permanent injury to the cornea: scar formation leading to haze that disturbs vision C [1 2]. Therefore it is not the treatment of choice for myopia that can be treated totally risk-free with spectacles.

Astigmatism

- The refractive power of the cornea is not uniform, because it often has an uneven curvature, it is steeper in one direction and flatter in the other (regular astigmatism) or even its surface is uneven (irregular astigmatism). In regular astigmatism there are two main different radii of the curvature of the cornea: smaller and larger.
- The steeper surface refracts the rays of light more than the flatter one, so that the image of an object is never sharp on the retina.

Symptoms

- Patients may experience that the vertical and horizontal elements of the text or pictures are not sharp at the same time, part of it being sharp and the other part not.
- May cause headache and eye strain.

Treatment

- Cylinder lenses in which the refractive power is present only at an angle of 90 degrees towards its axis (regular astigmatism).
- Irregular astigmatism cannot be corrected with spectacles. It occurs in keratoconus and scarred corneas and can be corrected with rigid contact lenses, as long as the cornea itself is clear. If not effective, penetrating keratoplasty is indicated.

Presbyopia

Basic rules

- Accommodative amplitude is almost 20 diopters in children but decreases gradually during the subsequent decades. By the age of 45 years, the loss of accommodative power begins to cause symptoms, since one third of it should be unused. Virtually no accommodation is left by 60 years of age.

Treatment

- Plus correction, which is added to the glasses needed to correct far vision. The amount of this "addition" is about +1.0 D for those aged 45, and a maximum of +2.5 D for those aged 60 years or more.
- Stronger additions act as near vision aids for the visually handicapped. The need for magnification is determined with a simple formula of 1/visual acuity at distance (e.g. for a distance acuity of 0.2, the addition needed is 5 D).

References

1. Jain S, Azar DT. Eye infections after refractive keratotomy. J Refractive Surgery 1996;12:148–155.
2. The Database of Abstracts of Reviews of Effectiveness (University of York), Database no.: DARE-960363. In: The Cochrane Library, Issue 4, 1999. Oxford: Update Software.

37.4 Work with visual display terminals (VDTs) and health

Editors

Problems associated with VDTs

- Strain of the neck, shoulders, and upper extremities
- Fatigue of the eyes
- Psychological and psychosocial problems

Prevention

- Good ergonomics of the workstation
- Correctly planned visual ergonomics
- Adequate work organization
- Optimal job requirements
- Training in use of information technology and of the equipment
- Rhythmicity of work
- Versatile work
- There is a EU directive on visual display work (90/270).

Examining vision and the eyes

- The employer must organize examination of vision and the eyes for employees using VDTs at work (EU 90/270).
- The employee has the right to have his vision and the eyes examined by a professional
  - before starting work with the VDT
  - at regular intervals thereafter
  - if the employee has problems with vision that may be related to the VDT.
- Employees have the right to have an examination by an ophthalmologist if indicated by the result of a screening examination.
- At the pre-employment examination
  - An occupational health nurse performs the screening examination of the vision. The visual acuity must be sufficient either without or with glasses.
  - If necessary, an optician or an ophthalmologist examines the worker's eyes.
- The aim of the periodical examinations is to identify the need for changes in spectacles or other aids related to normal ageing as a part of health promotion at work.

Special spectacles

- The employer has an obligation to provide the employee with special spectacles or other corrective appliances if necessary specifically for work with VDTs. Special spectacles differ from ordinary spectacles in refractivity, lens type, or installation of the lenses.
- Principles and actions to be taken
  - The workstation and the equipment should be constructed in a way that allows the employee to use his or her ordinary spectacles.
  - The spectacles should allow the employee to see accurately to all distances needed at work.
  - The occupational health personnel should always inform the optician/ophthalmologist about the visual requirements of the work and the ergonomics of the workstation.
  - If the employee has problems with vision, the occupational health personnel first evaluates whether the workstation can be reconstructed and whether the employee's vision is optimally corrected.
  - If necessary, the employee is referred to the examination by an optician/ophthalmologist.
  - The occupational health personnel decide on the need for special spectacles based on the written statement from the optician/ophthalmologist.

37.5 Impaired vision

Paula Summanen, Kirsi Setälä

- See Table 37.5.

Basic rules

- The cause of impaired vision must always be determined.
- If the cause of acute visual disturbance remains unknown, refer urgently.

Table 37.5 Causes of impaired vision

	Laterality[1)]	Pain	Redness	Generalized symptoms
Sudden, in minutes–hours				
Central artery occlusion	uni	no	no	possible, TIA
Temporal arteritis	uni-bi	no	no	Essential: weight loss, fatique, pains and aches = polymyalgia rheumatica
Angle closure glaucoma	uni	yes	yes	yes
Anterior ischaemic optic neuropathy	uni-bi	no	no	cardiovascular diseases
Central vein occlusion	uni	no	no	no (DM, hypertension, coagulation disorders)
Vitreous haemorrhage	uni	no	no	no (DM)
Haemorrhage in the fovea	uni	no	no	no (myopes)
Retinal detachment	uni	no	no	no (myopes)
Intoxication: methanol*, alcohol, quinine*, ethambutol, thioridazine, chloroquine	bi	no	no	yes, *loss of vision is sudden
Periodic (with typical duration)				
Papilloedema (seconds, attacks of loss of vision less than one second long)	uni-bi	no	no	associated with increased intracranial pressure
Ocular TIA, amaurosis fugax (minutes)	uni-bi	no	no	cardiovascular morbidity, other TIA symptoms
Migraine (ca. 15–20 min, up to 1–2 hours)	uni-bi	no	no	migraine
Gradual (speed of development) [2)]				
Keratitis (days)	uni	yes	yes	no
Corneal oedema (hours)	uni-bi	no/yes	no/yes	possible (angle closure glaucoma)
Endophthalmitis (hours–days)	uni	yes	yes	no
Iridocyclitis (days)	uni[3)]	yes	yes	possible
Cataract (hours–days)	uni-bi	no	no	no
Open closure glaucoma (months, years)	uni-bi	no	no	no
Optic neuritis (one day–days)	uni[3)]	no	no	possible (MS)
Compressive lesion of the optic nerve/ optic pathway	uni-bi	no	no	possible
Chorioretinitis (days–weeks)	uni[3)]	no	no	possible
Macular oedema (hours–days)	uni-bi	no	no	possible (DM)
Age-related macular degeneration (days–weeks)	uni-bi	no	no	no
Macular hole and preretinal fibrosis resulting from vitreous detachment (days–months)	uni	no	no	no
Hereditary retinal degeneration e.g. retinitis pigmentosa (years)	bi	no	no	possible (syndromes)

1. uni = unilateral, bi = bilateral
2. in seconds, minutes, hours, days, weeks, months, years
3. Both eyes may be affected at different times and recurringly.

History

- Is the vision impaired in one or both eyes?
- Did the vision become impaired in seconds, minutes, hours, days, months or years?
- Preceding or accompanying symptoms (local and systemic):
  - redness of the eye
  - pain in the eye
  - pain in the temple region, headache or jaw claudication
  - fever, fatigue, generalized ache
  - weight loss
  - Other changes in visual function (floaters, flashing, micropsia, diplopia, changes in the visual field)
- Other diseases and medication: diabetes, hypertension, blood dyscrasias, polymyalgia rheumatica and other connective tissue diseases, infections (e.g. HIV, Lyme boreliosis), etc. The causes vary according to geographical location (e.g. onchocerciasis, malaria). Therefore ask about possible journeys to the tropics.

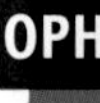

Examination

- Visual acuity
- Visual field (finger perimetry)
- Eye movements
- Pupillary reactions
- Ophthalmoscopy: red fundus reflex, vitreous body, optic nerve, retina, and particularly the macula.

Sudden visual loss or impairment: transient, painless, lasting for seconds

Papilloedema

- Aetiology

- Increased intracranial pressure that spreads via the subarachnoidal space in the optic nerve sheath causing stasis of the axonal flow.
- The cause is a brain tumour, subdural or subarachnoidal haemorrhage, meningitis, encephalitis, brain abscess or hydrocephalus.

♦ Symptoms and findings
- Occasionally diplopia (abducens paresis)
- Vertigo, headache, nausea and vomiting, especially in the morning.
- Tinnitus
- Blind spots enlarged, otherwise visual fields normal
- Papilloedema is often visible on ophthalmoscopy.
  - Early: blurred margins, central cupping is present, no venous pulsation is observable (distinguishing it from intrapapillary drusen)
  - Definite: optic disc head raised, very blurred margins, haemorrhages, veins dilated, retinal infarctions
  - Chronic: dilated capillaries
  - Atrophic: optic atrophy, impaired vision

♦ Differential diagnosis
- Hypertensive retinopathy
  - Bilateral
- Central vein occlusion
  - Unilateral
- Papillitis
  - Unilateral, in children often (70%) bilateral
- Pseudopapilloedema (hyperopic eye, drusen and other disc anomalies); refer to an ophthalmologist if the diagnosis is uncertain.

♦ In case of bilateral papilloedema, refer to a department of neurology or neurosurgery.

♦ NB: one optic disc may be atrophic (visual acuity decreased) and no longer reacts to oedema, although the underlying cause is increased intracranial pressure.

Sudden visual loss (in seconds), painless

Central retinal artery occlusion

♦ See 37.40.

♦ Aetiology
- Embolus or thrombus may originate from vegetation on the valves of the heart, mural thrombus in an infarction, calcified plaques of the aorta or, more commonly, the carotid artery.
- Transient ischaemic attacks (TIA) often precede occlusion. Ocular TIA (amaurosis fugax) refers to sudden blindness lasting for a few minutes (3–5) up to half an hour. They are usually caused by cholesterol emboli. Circulation disturbance in the vertebrobasilar region is associated with blurred speech and loss of vision lasting less than one minute.
- The typical patient is an elderly with cardiovascular morbidity, rarely a young patient with valvular disease.
- Always rule out temporal arteritis (the vision of the other eye can be saved with steroid therapy!)

♦ Findings
- Visual acuity ranges from hand movement to light perception
- Afferent pupillary defect
- The fundus is initially normal, but within 60 minutes becomes pale and oedematous, with "cherry red spot" fovea.
- Sometimes glittering plaques of cholesterol (Hollenhorst plaques) or calcified emboli are seen intravascularly.

♦ First aid
- Firm, intermittent pressure on the globe using the fist for about one minute at a time and sudden release of the pressure (instruct the patient on the phone) may cause the emboli to proceed from the central retinal artery into its branch when the intraocular pressure suddenly decreases when pressing is stopped. This procedure often restores circulation at least to a part of the central retina. The patient may continue pressing the eye on the way to the doctor.
- Check first that the eye has not been operated for cataract!
- In the emergency room, one tablet of acetazolamide can be given orally, whereafter the patient is referred urgently to an ophthalmology unit. The efficacy of the drug is uncertain; it may even be harmful.
- Anterior chamber puncture to rapidly reduce the intraocular pressure (paracentesis) is possible in the eye department.
- Thrombolysis is still experimental.

Anterior ischaemic optic neuropathy (AION)

♦ Aetiology
- May be the cause of sudden loss of vision in an elderly person. Occurs also in younger persons with predisposing factors:
  - dyslipidaemia
  - diabetes
  - smoking
  - small discs.
- The circulatory disturbance often affects the actual optic nerve.

♦ Findings
- Pupillary reaction to light is decreased or absent (relative afferent pupillary defect, i.e. positive Marcus Gunn).
- Pale and oedematous optic disc
- Horizontal visual field defect

♦ Differential diagnosis
- Papilloedema (bilateral, normal or only slightly impaired vision).

♦ Treatment
- Seek and treat the predisposing factors if possible.
- Aspirin
- Corticosteroids to prevent the visual loss in the other eye if temporal arteritis cannot be ruled out.

Sudden visual loss with headache or general symptoms

Temporal arteritis, polymyalgia rheumatica

- See 21.46.
- Symptoms and signs:
  - The patient is usually older than 45 years of age
  - Pain in the temple, headache, jaw claudication (ischaemia of the jaw muscles) and difficulties with eating
  - Tenderness of the temples on palpation
  - Decreased visual acuity
  - Fever, weight loss, muscle pain for weeks or months
- The most important investigation:
  - ESR without any delay: usually high (over 40, frequently 80–100 mm/h)
- Confirming the diagnosis
  - Temporal artery biopsy, if readily available. Treatment is started before the biopsy.
- Treatment
  - Prednisolone, initially in high doses intravenously.

Sudden visual impairment associated with consumption of toxic substances

- Methanol intoxication
  - Even a small amount of methanol causes toxic optic neuropathy and acute visual impairment.
  - The optic disc is hyperaemic.
  - Diagnosis is based on patients history suggesting methanol ingestion.
  - Refer immediately to the intensive care unit: treat the acidosis.
  - Quinine-induced blindness (37.46).
    - A large dose of quinine may cause a severe and only partly reversible visual impairment within 6–24 hours of drug ingestion.
  - Ethambutol may cause toxic optic neuropathy, thioridazine and chloroquine may cause toxic retinopathy.

Painless visual impairment over several hours

Hypertensive retinopathy

- Aetiology
  - High blood pressure causes acute arterial constriction in the retina (autoregulation) and over a prolonged time hypertrophy of the smooth muscle in the arterial walls, narrowing the lumen.
  - Hypertensive retinopathy occurs in connection with pre-eclampsia and malignant hypertension and in chronic hypertension in elderly patients, when the hypertension is poorly controlled.
- Findings
  - In the acute type: extremely narrow arterioles in the retina, oedema of the optic nerve head and retina, retinal haemorrhages (flame, spot or patch-shaped) and lipid exudates, oedema of the retina.
  - In the chronic type: general and topical sclerosis of the retinal arterioles: narrowing (artery/vein $< 2/3$), thickened walls seen as marked reflexes (copper and silver thread-like arteries), abnormal arteriovenous crossing, retinal haemorrhages and lipid exudates
- Treatment
  - The acute form is an emergency; refer to a internal medicine unit.
  - Visual recovery is good.

Central retinal vein occlusion

- See 37.41.
- The typical patient is diabetic or hypertensive and aged above 50 years.
- Frequently the underlying cause is untreated glaucoma or a disease predisposing to venous thrombosis (polycythaemia vera, use of oral contraceptives).
- Visual acuity ranges from near normal to hand movement.
- Fundus: "blood and thunder"–widespread dot and blot haemorrhages in the retina, oedema, veins congested and tortuous, optic disc oedematous, retinal microinfarcts ("cotton wool spots")
- Investigations
  - Blood pressure
  - Intraocular pressure
  - Glucose
  - Lipids
- Treatment
  - No direct treatment for the thrombosis itself. Admission to the eye department within 1 month to assess the need of laser treatment to prevent neovascular glaucoma.

Vitreous haemorrhage

- See 37.42.
- May cause sudden impairment of vision.
- The patient complains of a sudden onset of smoke- or dust-like particles (floaters, "cobwebs") in the visual field that may move when moving the eyes or the head.
- In most cases the cause is so-called posterior vitreous detachment or diabetic proliferative retinopathy.
- Other causes include untreated retinal central or branch vein occlusion, senile macular degeneration, retinal detachment with damage to transversing vein, and even intraocular tumours (malignant uveal melanoma), or blunt or penetrating trauma.
- Ophthalmoscopy shows a red reflex with dark moving shadow in the vitreous body.

- Refer to the ophthalmologist within one day, especially if associated with flashing lights and in the absence of diabetes (to rule out retinal detachment).

Visual impairment within hours accompanied by a headache and gastrointestinal symptoms

Acute angle closure glaucoma

- See 37.34.
- The patient has eye pain and/or headache, sometimes a rainbow halo around lights due to corneal oedema.
- Nausea and vomiting is common.
- The eye is usually intensely red, the cornea (often) dim, pupil mid-dilated, vertically oval, non-reactive to light, and the anterior chamber is shallow.
- Intraocular pressure is greatly elevated (generally > 60 mmHg).
- In differential diagnosis consider acute abdomen and the aetiology of headache, such as subarachnoid haemorrhage.
- First aid
  - Acetazolamide 500 mg i.v. or per os only if the patient is not allergic to sulphonamides.
  - Refer the patient without delay to the ophthalmology unit.

Visual impairment within days accompanied with initially slight ocular pain

Iridocyclitis

- See 37.32.

Chorioretinitis

- Caused, for example, by Toxoplasma, Toxocara, tuberculosis, and cytomegalovirus in HIV or otherwise immunocompromized patients.
- The most frequent symptoms are decreased vision and floaters.
- The diagnosis requires fundus examination under mydriasis. Treated at an ophthalmology unit.

Retinitis

- Seen in, for example, Lyme borreliosis
- Herpes viruses can cause so-called acute retinal necrosis syndrome.

Endophthalmitis

- Infection inside the eye caused by bacteria (acute: Staphylococcus epidermidis, aureus, streptococci, Pseudomonas; chronic: Propionibacter acnes) or fungi.
- Predisposing factors include recent cataract surgery ($\leq$ 0.1% of operated eyes), penetrating trauma, perforating corneal ulcer, systemic diseases such as diabetes, immunosuppression, abuse of narcotics.
- Symptoms and signs include lid oedema, hyperaemia, pain, decreasing vision, white blood cells in the anterior chamber (hypopyon) and loss of the red reflex.
- The patient must be referred immediately to an ophthalmic unit to save vision (intravitreal and local antibiotics, paraocular and systemic steroids).

Sympathetic ophthalmia

- Autoimmune granulomatous inflammation of the other eye (the sympathizing eye) several days to decades after a severe penetrating injury. Cells and flare in the anterior chamber.
- Refer the patient to an ophthalmology unit.

Visual impairment over days and a shadow in the visual field

Retinal or vitreous body detachment

- See 37.43.
- The patient is often myopic, has undergone surgery for cataract or has previously had a blunt eye injury or has vitreous body detachment.
- Posterior vitreous detachment usually occurs after the age of 60 years, but in myopes as early as at 30 years. Causes annoying but usually harmless floaters and flashing lights (photopsia), indicating that the collapsed vitreous body causes traction on the retina that may lead to a retinal break (usually horseshoe-shape) and/or haemorrhage.
- The patient sees flashes, floaters and a dark shadow at the edge of the visual field. Central vision is spared until the detachment reaches the fovea.
  - When the patient enters a dimly lit space, he/she sees a flash of light always at the same area of the visual field in one eye (in migraine the picture is disturbed as in a bad television picture, in migraine the symptoms usually affect both eyes).
- Ophthalmoscopy shows lack of red reflex from the detached retina and a floating, greyish, curtain-like retina with folds and curled vessels within the vitreous cavity if the detachment is large and central enough to be seen by direct ophthalmoscopy; small peripheral detachments may be difficult to see with a direct ophthalmoscope.
- Treatment
  - Refer the patient to an ophthalmology unit for the next morning (surgery is scheduled within one week, and even more urgently if the macula is still attached).
  - NB: In myopics, retinal detachment may develop from small peripheral retinal breaks within months without acute symptoms. Only when a large part of the retina is detached does the patient notice narrowing of the visual field; when the macula is detached, vision is suddenly impaired.

Visual impairment over a few days with dull pain aggravated by eye movements

Retrobulbar optic neuritis, papillitis

- Aetiology
  - Often unknown
  - Occurs more often in women than in men
  - The patient may have been diagnosed with multiple sclerosis (MS), or retrobulbar neuritis may be the first manifestation of MS already years before other manifestations of the disease. In such cases the prognosis of MS is better than usual.
  - Viral infections
  - Onchocerciasis, Lyme borreliosis
- Impairment of visual acuity with a central visual field defect. Sometimes vision is reduced to seeing only hand movement.
- Altered colour vision and contrast sensitivity
- A relative afferent pupillary defect is present even if visual acuity is almost normal (Marcus Gunn positive).
- The optic disc may be swollen and hyperaemic if the neuritis is anterior (papillitis) or pale and atrophic after a neuritis.
- Otherwise the eye is normal.
- Differential diagnosis
  - Early papilloedema (usually invariably bilateral)
  - Brain tumour (meningioma) or other cause of compression of the optic nerve (neuro imaging is always indicated in atypical patients).
  - Optic disc drusen – does not impair vision
  - Anterior ischaemic optic neuropathy (usually elderly patients)
  - Temporal arteritis (elderly patients)
- Treatment
  - In mild cases follow-up and possibly vitamin B, although the efficacy is unproven.
  - In case of obvious visual deterioration, a large dose of cortisosteroids i.v. (1 g, 3 days) should be given in a hospital setting **B** [1 2].

Visual impairment and/or metamorphopsia, micropsia, macropsia

- Symptoms appear within days or weeks.
- Oedema or traction in the centre of the macula causes distortion of the images (metamorphopsia) and changes the size of image (most often micropsia). These symptoms can be very confusing to the patient.
- Usually the symptoms are unilateral.
- Aetiology can be variable:
  - If the patient has diabetes the cause is most probably leakage from the capillaries to the fovea (diabetic macular oedema).
  - Age-related macular degeneration.
  - Macular hole or preretinal fibrosis caused by "unsuccessful" posterior vitreous detachment.
  - Cataract extraction may cause leakage from the macular capillaries in diabetics and patients with retinitis or several uveites (cystic macular oedema).
  - Severe myopia may lead to rupture of the structures underneath the macula (Bruch's membrane) and growth of new leaky vessels from the choroid.
  - So-called central serous chorioretinopathy is seen in working-aged stressed and busy persons, mostly men or in pregnant women. The condition may heal spontaneously over months.
  - Retinal macroaneurysms may leak within the retinal layers
- Metamorphopsia always necessitates referral to an ophthalmologist within 1–2 weeks. Especially diabetics and some patients with age-related macular degeneration require laser therapy – the latter group is more urgently in need of therapy.

Painless, impaired vision developing slowly over months or years

Cataract

- See 37.33.
- Sometimes uniocular diplopia or polyopia
- Glare, especially from the car lights
- Red reflex is uneven, locally invisible or totally absent. The fundus of the eye may be impossible to see.
- In diabetics and patients on corticosteroids, cataract may develop early and rapidly, but it is mostly seen after the age of 60 years.
- The timing of surgery is determined by the patients occupation and daily activities.

Refractive errors

- See 37.3.

Myopia

- The patient screws up his/her eyes when looking to a distance, whereas seeing close up is normal. The patient may have problems watching TV from the same distance as others or does not see the blackboard at school.
  - Examine both distance vision (impaired) and near vision (normal) separately. Stenopic (pin) hole improves distance vision.

Hyperopia

- Headache, especially as a band around the forehead, the eyes are tired, eye strain (asthenopia), even a foreign body sensation in the eyes. The symptoms are caused by excessive accommodation.
- According to the amount of hyperopia, distance vision may be good without glasses, but difficulties and symptoms occur

in close-up work, or there is impairment of both distance and near vision. Hyperopia may be accompanied by esotropia during attempts to look at close objects.

Astigmatism

- Text is occasionally unclear and there may be asthenopia.

Visual impairment over months or years associated with a progressive visual field defect

Chronic open-angle glaucoma

- May be asymptomatic almost to the end.
- The optic disc is pale, and central cupping is enlarged (either in one or both eyes).
- The patient does not necessarily have other symptoms.
- Intraocular pressure is measured (not always elevated, may be normal).
- Finger perimetry may reveal a far advanced visual field defect, often in the lower temporal field.
- The diagnosis is made by an ophthalmologist.
- Differential diagnosis: brain tumour, vascular diseases of the optic nerve.

Hereditary degenerations of the retina

- A group of progressive diseases that are often part of a syndrome.
- Retinitis pigmentosa is the most common cause of visual impairment in working age people in industrialized countries.
- Symptoms include glare and photophobia (intolerance to light), night blindness, nyctalopia and progressive narrowing of the visual fields. Central vision may remain for a long time or deteriorate in early adulthood.
- Findings include narrowed visual field, pale optic disck, narrow retinal arterioles and pigment clumpings.
- Refer the patient to an ophthalmologist for the diagnosis, to discuss the prognosis, and for the treatment of possible associated diseases (myopia and astigmatism, cataract and glaucoma, macular oedema) and for fitting of assistive devices and rehabilitation.

References

1. Kaufman DI, Trobe JD, Eggenberger ER, Whitaker JN. Practice parameter: the role of corticosteroids in the management of acute monosymptomatic optic neuritis. Report of the quality standards subcommittee of the American Academy of Neurology. Neurology 2000, 54(11), 2039–2044.
2. The Database of Abstracts of Reviews of Effectiveness (University of York), Database no.: DARE-20003848. In: The Cochrane Library, Issue 3, 2002. Oxford: Update Software.

37.6 Red, wet, or sore eye

Editors

Conjunctival erythema

- Most prominent at the conjunctival sac
- The vessels can be seen moving with the conjunctiva
- Often bilateral
- Conjunctivitis (37.22)

Pericorneal erythema

- Bluish red, circular zone around the cornea
- Often unilateral
- Acute iritis (37.32)
  - Sensitivity to light, eye pain
  - Small and irregular pupilla
  - Visual acuity may be impaired.
  - Pain on pressure
  - Wet eye
- Acute angle closure glaucoma 37.34
  - Severe pain in the ocular region
  - Nausea and vomiting
  - Impaired visual acuity
  - Opacity of the cornea
  - Mid-sized, non-responding pupilla
  - The patient may see a coloured halo around a lighted object.
- Corneal ulcers (37.24)
  - Pericorneal erythema near the ulcer
  - Mild sensitivity to light
  - Variable pain in the ocular region, sometimes feeling of a foreign body
  - An ulcer in the cornea that can be stained with fluorescein
- Marginal ulcer of the cornea (37.25)
  - Red and painful eye
  - No impairment of visual acuity
  - Fluorescein-adsorbing ulcer at the corneal margin
- Episcleritis (37.31)
  - Tear-flow is not increased.
  - Pain and feeling of a foreign body, sometimes sensitivity to light
  - Local tenderness on palpation
  - Spontaneous recovery within 1–2 weeks

Wet eye with irritation or feeling of a foreign body

- Hordeolum at the lid margin (37.13)
- Chalazion in the tarsus (37.13)

- Foreign body in the cornea or on the conjunctiva (37.26)
- Corneal ulcers
- Trichiasis
- Entropion and ectropion

37.7 Pain in and around the eye

Lea Hyvärinen

Basic rule

- Pain can be referred to the eye from many structures in the skull and neck. The characteristics and localization of the pain help in the diagnosis.

Causes and treatment

Musculoskeletal pain from the neck and shoulders

- Pain in the deep muscles of the neck radiates to the lateral side of the eye.
- Pain from the superficial muscles of the neck and from the trapezius muscle radiates to the temporal region.
- Pain from the sternocleidomastoid muscle can radiate to the eyebrow.
- If pain in the eye originates from muscles of the skull or neck, physiotherapy may be helpful, but a permanent cure usually requires changes in ergonomics at work.
- Pain may disappear while stretching the muscles in hot shower, which is diagnostic.

Inflammation of the supraorbital nerve

- Pain is felt in the eyebrow.
- The orifice of the nerve canal in the upper border of the orbita is tender on palpation.

Malocclusion of the teeth

- Ask the patient about orthodontic treatments; a small change in dental alignment may cause the pain.

Inflammation or allergic swelling in the ethmoidal and sphenoidal sinuses

- Symptoms
  - Negative pressure in the paranasal sinuses results in typical pain behind and in the eye.
  - The pain is often located behind the eye, even causing the feeling of the eye bulging out. No exophthalmos is present.
  - The patient feels a need to clear his/her throat as the discharge in the larynx irritates the vocal cords.
  - Focusing on objects may be difficult although visual acuity is normal.
  - Pressing the painful eye with the palm alleviates the pain as long as the pressing is continued.
- Treatment
  - Following treatment may help to set the diagnosis: nasal spray in the nostril on the side of the painful eye, breathing vapour for a quarter of an hour, cleaning the nose, and repeating the nasal spray.
  - Vasoconstrictors as tablets and electric pillow on the face can be used as an adjunct treatment.
  - The diagnosis is supported by good response to treatment.

37.10 Entropion and ectropion

Anna-Maija Paakkala

Basic rules

- Treat ectropion before conjunctival hypertrophy develops.
- Treat entropion before corneal ulcers develop.

Symptoms and signs

- The lower lid is more frequently affected. With advancing age the connective tissue in the lids becomes loose, the amount of adipose tissue decreases, the skin becomes thin, and its flexibility decreases.

Entropion

- The lid is inverted. The eyelashes rub the cornea, causing a feeling of a foreign body, tear-flow, and erythema of the conjunctiva.
- As the irritation continues, opacities and ulcers develop on the cornea.

Ectropion

- The eyelid is everted. Either the lid margin or the whole tarsus of the lid may be malpositioned. As the conjunctiva is exposed it becomes irritated, erythematous, and hypertrophic.
- At a later phase ulcers develop on the exposed conjunctiva.
- Senile ectropion of the lower lid is the most common lid abnormality.
- M. orbicularis oculi, which is responsible for closing the eyelids, is innervated by the facial nerve. Facial palsy may cause paralytic ectropion of the lower lid.

Treatment

- Traction with tape can alleviate the symptoms of entropion temporarily: a butterfly tape is applied on the lid to keep it in the correct position.
- Both entropion and ectropion should be treated surgically at an early phase. Ectropion should be treated before conjunctival hypertrophy develops. The operation can always be performed under local anaesthesia.

37.11 Ptosis

Anna-Maija Paakkala

Basic rule

- Refer the patient to a specialist (ophthalmologist or neurologist) for the identification of the cause of the condition.

Aetiology and clinical features

- If the muscles elevating the upper lid (m. levator palpebrae, m. tarsalis) do not function properly the upper lid becomes ptotic. The ptosis may be associated with paralysis of the ocular muscles. It can be an independent disease or part of a syndrome.
- The most common cause of ptosis is congenital ptosis.
  - It is usually unilateral and constantly present from birth.
  - Whether the cause is a muscular or neurological abnormality is not known.
  - The severity of the condition varies from hardly detectable to ptosis totally obscuring the pupilla. If the pupilla is covered, visual ability does not develop normally and the eye becomes amblyopic.
- Secondary ptosis may be a symptom of a muscle disease (myasthenia gravis (36.86), ophthalmoplegia progressiva externa, or myotonia dystrophica (36.85)). The symptom may be associated with paresis of the oculomotor nerve because the nerve to m. levator palpebrae superioris is derived from n. oculomotorius. In this case the patient always has other symptoms in addition to the ptosis.

Examining the patient

- The asymmetry is usually easily visible. When the patient looks up, a ptotic upper lid does not rise normally and the cornea slides under the lid.
- Examine the pupillar reaction (miosis is observed in oculomotor palsy).
- Examine eye movements (external strabismus is common in oculomotor palsy).

Treatment

- Mild ptosis needs no treatment if it does not cause cosmetic problems.
- Cosmetically unacceptable ptosis should be treated surgically.
- If the pupillar opening is free, allowing vision to develop normally, the operation should be postponed until school age. If the pupillar opening is covered, the operation should be performed in early infancy to prevent amblyopia.

37.12 Lagophthalmos

Tero Kivelä

Aims

- To recognize the danger of inadequate lid closure and to prevent corneal drying and subsequent complications.

Background and symptoms

- If the eyelids do not close to cover the eye when blinking and sleeping, the cornea will rapidly dry out and become inflamed. It may then perforate spontaneously.
- The conjunctiva is red, irritated and swollen.
- The cornea may become cloudy.

Aetiology

- Unconsciousness (e.g. patients in intensive care units)
- Facial nerve paresis or facial injury (orbicular muscle paralysed or injured)
- Orbital tumour (mechanical factors, exophtalmos)

Management

- Treatment must be initiated as soon as lagophthalmos is noted, otherwise good vision may be permanently lost from a previously good eye.
- Copious and frequent instillation of artificial tears and ointments. Initially an antibiotic ointment may be used to combat secondary infection.
- The eyelid can be closed with adhesive at night time or a special small, moist chamber made from plastic can be used in front of the eye when sleeping.
- If failure to close the eyelids is expected to continue for longer that a few weeks, consult an ophthalmologist to have

the eyelids temporarily or permanently partly fused to each other (tarsorrhaphy). They can easily be separated again when the patient can close the eyelids.

37.13 Chalazion and hordeolum

Anna-Maija Paakkala

Aims

- Differentiate hordeolum from more severious infections in the ocular region.
- Relieve symptoms by means of antibiotic eye drops and, if necessary, by incising the hordeolum with a needle.

Definition and aetiology

- A chalazion develops in the eyelid as a result of an obstruction of a meibomian gland and the consequent accumulation of secretions within the gland. A chalazion may develop into a hordeolum.
- A hordeolum (also called a stye or sty) is an infection of the external glands (of Zeis and Moll) or of the deeper (meibomian) glands of the eyelid.
- The causative agent is usually Staphylococcus aureus.

Symptoms

- A chalazion develops slowly and causes no other symptoms than slight erythema on the eyelid. It is most common in the age group of 20–40 years.
- With a hordeolum the entire eyelid becomes swollen, erythematous and painful. A tender spot can be palpated within the lid.
- After a couple of days a purulent abscess develops. The pain will ease if the hordeolum bursts.

Differential diagnosis

- The possibility of dacryocystitis, dacryoadenitis and orbital phlegmon should be considered. All these conditions are more rare and more painful than hordeolum.
    - In dacryoadenitis the painful spot is in the lateral corner of the eye socket, and in dacryocystitis in the medial corner of the eye.

Treatment

- A chalazion nearly always heals spontaneously. However, it may grow initially and then remain static for several months. Eye drops containing an antibiotic and hydrocortisone may be used for a short time. If the chalazion remains annoyingly large for a long time, an ophthalmologist can remove the contents of the gland and excise the capsule. An intralesional injection of triamcinolone may also be tried.
- The treatment of a hordeolum consists of local antibiotic eye drops. An abscess can be incised with an injection needle or a foreign body remover.

37.15 Blepharitis

Lea Hyvärinen

Basic rules

- Identify the condition that tends to become chronic.
- Support the patient to prevent chronicity.

Aetiology

- The basic abnormality is probably in the structure of the lid margin or the composition of the sebaceous secretions. Scaled skin remains at the root of the eyelashes, promoting bacterial growth beneath. Infections spread into the sebaceous glands and change the composition of the secretions of the meibomian glands, finally resulting in obstruction of the ducts (meibomitis).
- Over the course of several years so many glands are destroyed that the tear layer becomes disrupted, and the eye becomes dry and irritated.

Diagnosis

- The lid margin is red, scaly, and sometimes crusty.

Treatment

- Clean the lid margin with a moistened cotton swab to remove the scales.
- Rub an eye drop (hydrocortisone + antibiotic) on the lid margin with a fingertip.
- Apply the drug every night at first. After the lid margin looks normal continue with the treatment once a week for a lengthy period. If the inflammation recurs the patient needs to start using the drug again.

37.16 Preseptal cellulitis and eyelid wounds

Paula Summanen

Definition and aetiology

- Preseptal cellulitis is a severe purulent infection and inflammation of the eyelid(s).
- In distinction to a usual wound infection, the entire eyelid is infected. It does not, however, extend to the orbit as in orbital cellulitis (i.e. preseptal) and is thus not life-threatening.
- It almost invariably develops from an untreated wound of the lid that has become infected (for example alcoholics are susceptible). The wound is caused by the patient falling and hitting the orbital region on the ground.

Diagnosis

- Infected purulent and often wide wound in the lid that can result in marked necrosis of the skin.

Differential diagnosis

- Orbital cellulitis causes forward displacement of the eye, diplopia and often pain. See 37.20.
- Acute dacryocystitis causes redness and swelling (abscess) in the medial region of the lower eyelid in place of the lacrimal sac and sometimes also fever.

Treatment

- Admission to hospital where the situation is assessed, wound debridement is performed and systemic antibiotics are started.
- If an eyelid wound has not developed into preseptal cellulitis, it can be managed in primary health care. Systemic antibiotics are indicated, as the infection spreads easily.
- Cephalosporin is the antibiotic of choice (e.g. cephalexin); chloramphenicol ointment and eye drops are used topically. The wound should be showered three times daily, and it can be covered with mesh.
- Acute dacryocystitis requires antibiotics and usually dacryocystorhinostomy at a later phase.

37.20 Orbital cellulitis

Paula Summanen

Aim

- To recognize this life- and vision-threatening condition without delay and refer the patient urgently.

Definition and aetiology

- Infection inside the orbit (postseptal).
- A severe condition that threatens both vision and life.
- Aetiology
  - Infection in the paranasal sinuses (pansinusitis)
  - Mastoiditis
  - Trauma to the orbit, occasionally unknown foreign bodies
  - Preseptal cellulitis (37.16)
  - Haematogenic spread (sepsis)

Symptoms and findings

- Hyperaemia and oedema in the eyelids, the conjunctiva and the eye.
- Severe pain, forward displacement of the bulbus (proptosis), eye movements limited, diplopia. (The diagnosis is based on these findings.)
- Damage to the optic nerve caused by infection and oedema impairs vision and may rapidly lead to loss of vision.
- The infection can also spread intracranially leading to CNS symptoms and death.

Treatment

- Suspicion of orbital cellulitis is an indication for urgent referral to a hospital with emergency radiographic facilities (CT, MRI) and eye and ENT specialists.
- Treatment consists of i.v. antibiotics, per oral corticosteroids and careful follow-up. Possible abscesses are drained.
- In case of pansinusitis, an ENT specialist drains the affected sinuses.

37.21 Subconjunctival haemorrhage (suggillation)

Anna-Maija Paakkala

Aim

- To identify elevated blood pressure (remember to measure!) and other underlying causes.

Aetiology

- Suggillation usually develops spontaneously.
- Elevated blood pressure, anticoagulant therapy, conjunctivitis, ocular trauma, and epidemic nephropathy are possible underlying conditions.

Symptoms

- The patient is usually asymptomatic and recognizes the suggillation incidentally. Sometimes the eye may feel stiff.

Treatment

- Medicines do not help. Normalization of conjunctival colour takes at least a couple of weeks.
- Diagnose and treat the underlying condition.

37.22 Conjunctivitis

Editors

Basic rules

- Differentiate conjunctivitis from the following conditions requiring investigation and treatment by an ophthalmologist:
  - Iritis
  - Keratitis
  - Mild attack of glaucoma
- Examine the ears in all small children who present because of discharge from the eyes. Many of them also have otitis media.
- Identify allergic conjunctivitis and avoid unnecessary local antibiotics.

Aetiology

- Bacteria
  - Pneumococci, Haemophilus, Chlamydia, meningococci, gonococci, staphylococci, Moraxella, E. coli, etc.
- Viruses
  - Adenovirus, herpes simplex virus, molluscum contagiosum
- Fungi
  - Candida albicans
- Atopy
- Chemical conjunctivitis
  - Local medications, other exposures
- Dry eyes

Symptoms

- Discharge from the eyes
- Feeling of a foreign body
- Smarting
- Itching, usually associated with an allergic reaction
- Rarely photophobia (usually a symptom of iritis)

Diagnostics

- If the patient has a purulent discharge in the eye, the diagnosis is almost certainly bacterial or viral conjunctivitis.
- If there is no purulent discharge or a very small amount of discharge the differential diagnosis is more difficult, and the following should be observed:
  - If the patient has concomitant upper respiratory infection he/she probably has viral or bacterial conjunctivitis.
  - If the patient has atopy with other simultaneous allergic (clear rhinorrhoea, prolonged cough, atopic eczema) the patient probably has allergic conjunctivitis. Exposure to pollen or animals is not always evident from the history. Mucus occurs in narrow ribbons only in allergic conjunctivitis.
- A slightly purulent or non-discharging inflammation can be considered as conjunctivitis if the patient does not have any of the following symptoms suggesting keratitis, iritis, episcleritis, or acute glaucoma:
  - Severe pain or ache
  - Sensitivity to light (occurs in iritis and sometimes in allergic conjunctivitis)
  - Tenderness on pressure
  - Impaired visual acuity
  - Opacified, spotty, or ulcerating cornea
  - Small or distorted pupil
- If the patient has one or more of the above-mentioned symptoms, the eye must be examined more thoroughly:
  - Inspection of the cornea before and after fluorescein staining
  - Visal acuity
  - Measuring intraocular pressure with a tonometer (in cases where a corneal ulcer is not suspected).

OPH

Treatment

- An acute conjunctivitis associated with viral respiratory infection can be treated with artificial tears.
- Even slightly purulent conjunctivitis (caused by a virus or bacteria) should be treated with antibiotic drops for 3–7 days B [1]. An oculentum is recommended for the night and even daytime use at home if there is a lot of discharge.
  - Chloramphenicol drops (4–)6–8 times a day
  - An ointment containing fucidinic acid is given only twice a day. The drops are viscous and they may be more difficult to apply in the eye than water- or fat-soluble chloramphenicol drops.

    • Norfloxacin drops can be used as first-line drugs but preferably they should be reserved for therapy-resistant cases.
- Allergic conjunctivitis can be treated with:
    • Sodium cromoglicate drops that prevent the allergen from adhering to the mucosal cells is the basic drug. Drops containing 40 mg/ml sodium cromoglicate can be used for acute symptoms.
    • Local antihistamines (e.g. levocabastine, nedocromil)
    • Do not use vasoconstrictor drops.
    • Severe conjunctival allergy is an indication for specialist investigations.

Special problems

- If the eye drops fail after one week, discontinue the antibiotics and reconsider the case. The patient may have
    • a viral infection
    • an infection caused by resistant bacteria (remember gonococci in patients with a lot of purulent discharge)
    • a chlamydial infection that manifests as neonate conjunctivitis commencing at the end of the first week of life or, in an adult, inclusion conjunctivitis with small yellow or translucent nodules
    • lacrimal stenosis (28.12) is a common cause for recurrent conjunctivitis in children below six months of age
    • an incorrect diagnosis.
- If the neonate has typical symptoms of chlamydial conjunctivitis, take chlamydial specimens both from the patient and the mother (using the same equipment as in cervical sampling) and start peroral erythromycin for both.
- If an adult patient has typical inclusion conjunctivitis give the patient and his/her partner doxycycline or erythromycin perorally. Local tetracycline drops supplement the treatment.
- In other cases, especially with atypical or very severe symptoms, an ophthalmologist should be consulted.

Indications for bacterial culture

- Severe conjunctivitis
- Corneal injuries

Dacryocystitis

- Chronic dacryocystitis is a rare cause of discharge from the eye.
    • The disease most frequently occurs in middle-aged and elderly women.
    • Pressure on the lacrimal sac triggers the flow of inflammatory secretions from the lacrimal ducts.
    • The treatment consists of local antimicrobials, and later surgery where the obstructed connection of the lacrimal sac to the nasal cavity is restored.

Reference

1. Sheikh A, Hurwitz B, Cave J. Antibiotics versus placebo for acute bacterial conjunctivitis. Cochrane Database Syst Rev. 2004;(2):CD001211.

37.23 Pterygium

Anna-Maija Paakkala

Basic rule

- A pterygium should be treated surgically only if it causes symptoms.

Symptoms and signs

- A pterygium is defined as the growth of a triangular wedge of vascular conjunctiva on the surface of the cornea. It is situated in the lid space, usually on the nasal side of the eye.
- A hot, dry, and dusty environment promotes the development of a pterygium.
- It grows over months and years towards the central cornea and finally affects vision. The growth may also cease spontaneously.
- In some patients the pterygium becomes irritated, causing daily inconvenience and tear-flow.

Treatment

- Surgery is the treatment of choice.
- A pterygium often recurs after resection **A** [1 2 3 4].

References

1. Sanchez-Thorin JC, Rocha G, Yelin JB. Meta-analysis on the recurrence rates after bare sclera resection with and without mitomycin C use and conjunctival autograft placement in surgery for primary pterygium. Br J Ophthalm 1998;82:661–665.
2. The Database of Abstracts of Reviews of Effectiveness (University of York), Database no.: DARE-981109. In: The Cochrane Library, Issue 2, 2000. Oxford: Update Software.
3. Tan DT, Chee SP, Dear KB, Lim AS. Effect of pterygium morphology on pterygium recurrence in a controlled trial comparing conjunctival autografting with bare sclera excision. Arch Ophthalmol 1997;115:1235–40.
4. Panda A, Das GK, Tuli SW, Kumar A. Randomized trial of intraoperative mitomycin C in surgery for pterygium. Am J Ophthalmol 1998;125:59–63.

37.24 Corneal ulcers and erosions

Anna-Maija Paakkala

Basic rules

- Identify a corneal ulcer as a cause of ocular symptoms (use fluorescein in the clinical examination).
- The general practitioner can treat an erosion caused by mechanical trauma.
- The aetiological diagnosis and treatment of other corneal ulcers should be left to a specialist.

Aetiology

- Corneal ulcers may be sterile or infected. An intact cornea and normal tears protect the eye well from infections. If they are not normal, susceptibility to infections increases.
- An infected corneal ulcer (ulcus corneae serpens) is rare nowadays, and it usually develops only on previously affected cornea (trauma, contact lens injury, keratoconjunctivitis sicca etc.)

Symptoms and signs

Ulcus corneae serpens

- Pain, redness, discharge, impaired vision, and sensitivity to light.
- A grey, opaque, abnormal area is visible on the cornea
- In severe cases a collection of leukocytes (hypopyon) is visible in the anterior chamber. The irritation may spread to the internal parts of the eye and cause secondary iritis.
- The patient should be hospitalized. A specific infectious agent should be identified.

Keratitis dendritica

- An ulcer caused by the Herpes simplex virus can be seen as a typical twig-like opacity with fluorescein staining.
- The symptoms include slight redness, sensation of a foreign body, sensitivity to light, and impaired vision. A history of earlier episodes of Herpes simplex infection can often be elicited.
- The treatment consists of acyclovir ointment (A) [1] five times a day.
- The patient should be referred to an ophthalmologist because the ulcer may remain open for a long time and healing should be followed up by microscopy.

Corneal erosions

- A corneal erosion usually develops after trauma; rarely spontaneously. The patient has a strong sensation of a foreign body, and tear-flow.
- The erosion is clearly visible with fluorescein staining.
- The eye is painful as long as epithelialization is not complete, usually for 1–3 days.
- The treatment consists of oil-based antibiotic drops or ointment to prevent infection and adhesion of the eyelid to the cornea.
- If the erosion is situated centrally in the cornea, vision is temporarily impaired. Restoration of normal vision takes longer than the epithelialization, which should be explained to the patient to prevent unnecessary consultations.
- Advise the patient not to rub the eye.
- For the treatment of an erosion see also article 37.26.

Reference

1. Wilhelmus KR. Interventions for herpes simplex virus epithelial keratitis. Cochrane Database Syst Rev. 2004;(2):CD002898.

37.25 Marginal ulcer of the cornea

Anna-Maija Paakkala

Basic rule

- Treat marginal ulcers with antibiotic–corticosteroid drops until the symptoms alleviate.

Symptoms

- Conjunctival erythema, pain and feeling of a foreign body.

Causes

- Probably bacterial toxins.

Diagnosis

- A marginal ulcer becomes visible with fluorescein staining in the lateral part of the cornea. The cornea is opaque in this area.
- The most important differential diagnostic condition is marginal keratitis caused by scleritis associated with e.g. rheumatoid arthritis.

Treatment

- Antibiotic–corticosteroid drops can be used locally after assessment by an opthtalmologist. A follow-up visit is not necessary. The patient should contact a doctor if the symptoms recur.

37.26 A foreign body on the cornea

Anna-Maija Paakkala

Basic rule

- Remove all foreign bodies, including the rust ring caused by a metal foreign body.

Symptoms

- A foreign body on the cornea is felt as if it were under the upper lid.
- A metal foreign body rapidly corrodes. All the rust must be removed because it causes irritation.
- After the foreign body has been removed, the feeling of a foreign body continues for 1–2 days until the epithelium of the cornea has regenerated.
- If the foreign body was situated in the central part of the cornea, the restoration of normal visual acuity takes longer than epithelization because the new epithelium is not as transparent as mature epithelium.

Techniques for foreign body removal

- The patient lies supine.
- Two drops of a local anaesthetic are dropped into the eye with an interval of a couple of minutes.
- Use a magnifying glass. Use the blunt tip of a foreign body needle to remove the foreign body and rust.
- If a corneal drill is available it is recommended for removal of the rust. If a piece of metal has been in the eye for a long time the cornea around the foreign body is stained. The stained cornea need not be removed. Rust, however, is a foreign body that needs to be removed.

Further treatment

- If no significant erosion remains, a single dose of an oculentum is sufficient. If the recovery of the cornea is delayed, local antibiotics should be used.
- Use antibiotic (e.g. chloramphenicol) drops or an oculentum (3–4 times a day for 3–4 days) for the treatment of an erosion.
- Patching the eye is usually not indicated (A) [1,2].
- Delayed healing of the original ulcer with failing attachment of the new epithelium is the most common cause of recurrence. Healing of the erosion may be slowed by blinking and the use of local anaesthetic eye drops.

Indications for referral to a specialist

- If a foreign body or a rust ring cannot be removed the patient should be referred to an ophthalmologist within 1–2 days (not necessarily in the evening or during the weekend).
- The rust is easier to remove if an oculentum is used which is why it should be administered amply for first aid.

References

1. Flynn CA, Damico F, Smith G. Should we patch corneal abrasions? A meta-analysis. Journal of Family Practice 1998;47: 264–270.
2. The Database of Abstracts of Reviews of Effectiveness (University of York), Database no.: DARE-981808. In: The Cochrane Library, Issue 4, 2000. Oxford: Update Software.

37.27 Ocular injuries

Editors

Suspicion of a penetrating eye injury

- Typical history: While hammering a metal object a foreign body hits the eye, or a sharp object, for example, a piece of broken glass stabs the eye.
- The patient should be transported to an ophthalmological unit supine with both eyes covered. Children can sit in the arms of a parent with both eyes covered. However, if covering the eyes causes fear, only the injured eye is covered.

An irritating or corrosive substance in the eye

- Irrigate the eye immediately at the site of the accident, or if this has not been done, as soon as the patient arrives, for at least ten minutes, preferably 30 minutes (or even 60 minutes if the substance was alkaline).
- Do not use old bottles of stored water for eye irrigation because they may be unsterile. Disposable bottles of saline are recommended as first aid at workplaces where

dangerous substances are used. Tap water is also suitable for irrigation.

- 0.9% saline should first be poured into the eye. The irrigation should then continue from an infusion set (without the needle) during transportation. Local anaesthesia of the cornea facilitates the irrigation.
- Tear gas is best expelled from the eye by ventilating with flowing air for at least ten minutes. Irrigation is usually not helpful.
- Examine the eye with a magnifying glass and fluorescein. Small erosions can be treated in primary care. If the erosions are large or they are continuous to the limbus (risk of slow recovery) or the cornea is opaque refer the patient to an ophthalmologist immediately.

Eyelid injuries

- Avoid removal or revision of lacerated skin. Foreign material can be removed by irrigation.
- Do not use local ointments.
- Immediately refer patients with injuries interrupting the lid margin and patients with a deep lid injury.

A ball or fist hitting the eye

- Check the pupillary reactions, eye movements, ocular fundus, intraocular pressure, and sense of touch in the lower lid.
  - Limitation of eye motion, diplopia, or paraesthesia of the lower lid suggest an impact fracture of the orbita, and is an indication for immediate referral.
  - Asymmetric pupillary reaction suggests a contusion injury. Such patients may have significant bleeding in the anterior chamber even if no blood streak is seen at the bottom of the anterior chamber. Refer patients with ocular contusion to an ophthalmologist.
  - There may be haemorrhages or choroidal tears in the ocular fundi necessitating hospital treatment.
- If the patient does not have diplopia, the anterior chamber looks clear, the visual acuity is not impaired, and the pupillary reactions are normal, the patient does not need a referral.

Blood in the anterior chamber (hyphaema)

- An ophthalmologist should examine the eye urgently (the patient should be transported with both eyes covered).

Slight impairment of vision in an injured eye without other symptoms or signs

- Follow up the visual acuity on the next day.
  - If the visual acuity is not improved, refer the patient to an ophthalmologist the next working day.
  - If the visual acuity has decreased consult an ophthalmologist immediately.

A foreign body in the eye

- See 37.26.

37.28 Photophthalmia

Anna-Maija Paakkala

Basic rules

- Treat symptomatic patients with antibiotic ointments or eye drops.
- Avoid local anaesthetics.

Causes

- The cornea absorbs ultraviolet radiation from the sun. The higher the altitude the more UV radiation is absorbed because the radiation traverses thin air.
- Snow reflects 85% of UV radiation, increasing the radiation exposure of the cornea. The welding arc also radiates in the UV range.

Symptoms

- Tear flow
- Intense sense of a foreign body in the eye
- Pain
- Sensitivity to light
- Blepharospasm
- The latency from exposure to the onset of symptoms is usually 6–8 hours. The symptoms disappear in 1–2 days.

Clinical signs

- Conjunctival erythema and spotted staining of the cornea with fluorescein (keratitis)
- In severe cases the epithelium of the cornea is detached, resulting in an erosion.

Treatment

- Prophylaxis with protective glasses absorbing UV radiation.
- Antibiotic eye drops or oil-based antibiotic ointments are used to alleviate symptoms.

- Do not prescribe local anaesthetics because their effect is short-lived and they may impede the healing of the corneal erosion. They can be used at the doctor's office to facilitate the clinical examination. Pain is alleviated by compressive dressings and analgesics.

37.29 Eye problems in contact lens users

Osmo Kari

General information

- Eye drops should not be used whilst contact lenses are in the eye (with the exception of preservative-free sodium cromoglicate or preparations indicated for moistening the eye).
- Many ophthalmic preparations and their preservatives (e.g. benzalkonium chloride) are absorbed by contact lenses, resulting in toxic or allergic reactions. Furthermore, contact lenses, being a foreign body, delay healing.
- Corneal lesions can be prevented by early treatment.
- Users who are allergic to pollen should avoid using contact lenses when they have eye symptoms.
- The use of contact lenses should also be avoided during other allergic ocular manifestations.
- Dry eyes are a relative contraindication to the use of contact lenses when the condition is mild; in severe cases dry eyes are an absolute contraindication.
- Contact lenses should not be used in a very dusty environment, or when the air is particularly dry or hot. Intensive computer work is also a relative contraindication.
- When swimming or diving in unclean water (e.g. swimming pool) contact lenses should not be worn (if single-use lenses are used, they should be removed immediately after swimming and replaced with a new fresh pair).
- Contact lenses should not be used during coughs and colds.
- All people using contact lenses should see an ophthalmologist regularly: young (<20 years) patients with allergies twice a year, other users once a year.
- An ophthalmologist should individually ensure the suitability of continuously worn contact lenses.
- The 24 h use of permanent contact lenses should be avoided and the use of 24 h is recommended only in exceptional cases.
- Regular ophthalmologic controls are needed 2 times a years in persons using continuous wear lenses.
- An ophthalmologist should always verify the suitability of contact lenses after laser or other surgical procedures for refractive errors.

Examining the eye and treatment

- The lenses should be removed and their use should be avoided as long as the symptoms persist.
- Examine the eye with a magnifying lens using blue light and a fluorescein stain. If a corneal lesion is detected (a fluorescein-absorbing area in the cornea), consult an ophthalmologist.
- If the patient has conjunctivitis, prescribe antibiotic drops or ointment, or both. Before the treatment is recommenced take a specimen for bacterial culture from the conjunctiva for an antibiotic sensitivity test. Also take a sample for bacterial culture from the contact lens solution and from the lens itself.
- If the symptoms and visual acuity do not improve after a few days, repeat the examination with a fluorescein stain and consult an ophthalmologist (iritis and keratitis must be ruled out).
- If the eye is painful and discharging, and the visual acuity is impaired, refer the patient immediately to an ophthalmologic unit.
- In primary care, corticosteroid drops should not be prescribed for a contact lens user to treat an inflamed eye.
- Persistent problems (however small) in the eyes of a contact lens user warrant a referral to an ophthalmologist.
- Allergic conjunctivitis is often associated with itchy and dry eyes which may continue after the contact lenses have been removed. Contact lenses should not be worn whilst the eyes remain itchy or painful. A variety of eye drops not containing corticosteroids may be used to treat allergic conjunctivitis, i.e. mast cell stabilisers (e.g. sodium cromoglicate), antihistamine drops (e.g. olopatadine, ketotifen). These drops are always safe. If they are not effective, allergic conjunctivitis is probably not the correct diagnosis and the contact lenses should not be worn before an ophthalmologic examination. Antihistamine eye drops are not recommended during the use of contact lenses.
- Do not use vasoconstrictive drops for the treatment of a red eye.
- When using moisturing or other drops with contact lenses, use always preservative free ones.

Replacing contact lenses and the solution

- The contact lenses should be replaced as instructed by the manufacturer. The containers should be replaced at least every 6 months.
- Oxygen-permeable hard contact lenses are replaced at 2 year intervals.
- People with allergies or those with sensitive eyes for other reasons, should use short-term (one-month) or one-day lenses.
- The contact lens solution may cause toxic reactions if, for example, the hydrogen peroxide in the solution has not neutralised sufficiently.
- Contact lens solutions, as well as protein-absorbing tablets, may cause allergic reactions.

- If the contact lenses have been in a container for some time after disinfection with hydrogen peroxide they should be rinsed well before being placed in the eyes.

37.30 Dry eye syndrome

Tero Kivelä

Aims

- To recognize typical symptoms and signs of dry eye syndrome.
- To recognize and manage underlying diseases.
- To alleviate symptoms and prevent complications.

Symptoms and signs

- A burning and gritty sensation in the eyes, paradoxically accompanied by intermittent lacrimation (reflex lacrimation due to increasing irritation).
- The symptoms are worse in the morning (tear secretion diminishes at night time), in windy weather (evaporation), and in a smoky or dusty atmosphere (tears do not protect the eye).
- The conjunctiva becomes easily irritated and bloodshot.
- Otherwise asymptomatic patients may have symptoms in an air-conditioned environment (office eye syndrome, evaporation).

Aetiology

- Tear secretion diminishes with increasing age.
- Connective tissue diseases such as rheumatoid arthritis damage the lacrimal glands (keratoconjunctivitis sicca) and salivary glands (Sjögren's syndrome (21.43)).
- Skin diseases such as psoriasis, atopic dermatitis, seborroeic dermatitis, acne rosacea, erythema multiforme, ocular pemphigoid, and Lyell's syndrome.
- Several medications, especially beta-blockers. Check your patient's medication.
- Endocrinological factors (menopause, Graves' disease, anti-oestrogen therapy).

Diagnosis

- A typical history is often diagnostic.
- The tear meniscus (tears collecting at the rim of the lower eyelid) is poor or absent and the eye appears dry.
- The corneal light reflex may be irregular, and filaments, strands of dried epithelial cells may be found on the corneal surface in severe cases.
- The Schirmer test result is less than 5–10 mm in 5 minutes.

Schirmer test

- Use specially manufactured filter paper strips.
- When looking for dry eye syndrome, measure basal tear secretion by performing the test a couple of minutes after administering anaesthetic oxybuprocain eye drops to prevent reflex lacrimation.
- The test strip is bent at its notch and the strip is then inserted in the lower conjunctival cul-de-sac at the border of the middle and outer third of the eyelid, so that the strip hangs down. The patient may keep the eyes open or closed.
- After 5 minutes remove the strip and measure the distance in millimetres from the notch to the moistened tear front.

Management

- Remove known predisposing factors if possible.
- Advise the patient to avoid wind, dust and air-conditioned environments.
- An air moistener may help and in severe cases evaporation can be minimized by using swimming goggles.
- Instruct the patient not to wash his/her eyes with water in the morning. Although this may feel good, it aggravates dry eye syndrome in the long run.
- Various types of artificial tears are available over the counter. It is advisable that every patient tries out several types and selects the one that alleviates the symptoms most effectively, as this is very individual. Start with one viscous and one fluid alternative. Artificial tears are not equivalent to natural ones. In long-term use, try to avoid artificial tears that contain benzalkonium chloride as a preservative.
- If artificial tears are not enough, consult an ophthalmologist regarding possibilities of temporary or permanent punctal occlusion.

37.31 Episcleritis

Anna-Maija Paakkala

Basic rules

- Differentiate the disease from iritis.
- Alleviate symptoms.

Aetiology and pathology

- Episcleritis is rare because blood vessels are sparse in the sclera and the conjunctiva protects it from external irritants. The inflammation is nearly always endogenous, and scleral diseases resemble connective tissue diseases.
- The outer, vascular, and loose layer of sclera is called episclera. Episcleritis is more common than scleritis.

- Episcleritis may be a symptom of a connective tissue disease or it may be associated with allergies.

Symptoms and signs

- The patient is asymptomatic, or has mild ocular pain.
- The distribution of episcleritis can be nodular, sectorial or diffuse. In nodular inflammation a red node appears under the conjunctiva, in sectorial episcleritis the erythema spreads sectorially to the corneal margin, and in the diffuse form the episclera is erythematous around the cornea.
- Mild iritis associated with diffuse episcleritis may cause differential diagnostic problems. Consider iritis as the diagnosis if the eye is sensitive to light or if visual acuity is impaired.
- Episcleritis is cured without sequelae, but scleritis results in a scleral scar that can be seen as bluish atrophy of the sclera under the conjunctiva.

Treatment

- Episcleritis should be treated with non-steroidal anti-inflammatory drugs, e.g. indomethacin (25–50 mg × 3). Local NSAID drops, e.g. diclofenac, can also be used. NSAIDs speed recovery.
- The patient should avoid draught and heat, which delay healing.
- Patients with prolonged inflammation should be referred to an ophthalmologist for consideration of steroid treatment.
- A specialist should treat patient with scleritis.

37.32 Iridocyclitis (iritis)

Paula Summanen

Aims

- To learn to suspect iridocyclitis in patients with a painful red eye or with local tenderness in the eye or photophobia and to refer these patients to an eye specialist.
- To remember the possibility in children with chronic juvenile arthritis (sometimes only one joint, for example a finger, is affected), even if the eyes appear unaffected.
- To recognize and treat the predisposing factors of iridocyclitis (upper respiratory, dental and gingival infections, sarcoidosis, juvenile chronic arthritis, ankylosing spondylitis and other seronegative spondylarthropathies, intestinal infections and diabetes mellitus).
- To control healing in order to prevent chronicity and complications (glaucoma, cataract).
- To encourage the patient to treat the eye condition and to treat and prevent the predisposing factors (HLA-B27 positive patients and infections) to prevent complications.

Epidemiology and aetiology

- Incidence of acute iridocyclitis: 12/100 000/year (all uveitis 20/100 000/year).
- Mainly affects young adults.
- Uncommon in children (except with chronic juvenile arthritis) and the elderly (except with herpes zoster infection, vasculitis, lymphoma).
- Acute iridocyclitis tends to recur. It often occurs in one eye at a time, but changes from one eye to another.
- Active infection focus elsewhere may trigger iridocyclitis, (especially in HLA-B27 positive persons Yersinia enterocolitica, Salmonella, Campylobacter, Klebsiella, Shigella or Chlamydia (immunotypes D and E)) or iridocyclitis may be the manifestation of one of the following systemic diseases:
    - ankylosing spondylitis
    - sarcoidosis
    - juvenile chronic arthritis, particularly oligoarthritis of small children (chronic, asymptomatic iridocyclitis)
    - Behcet's disease (HLA-B51 individuals)
    - systemic infections, such as herpes viruses, Lyme disease (Borrelia burgdorferi), Toxoplasma, Toxocara, HIV, syphilis
    - sinusitis
    - dental root infection
    - intestinal infections
    - diabetes mellitus, types 1 and 2.
- May be associated with anterior segment infection, e.g. keratitis or trauma such as a longstanding corneal foreign body or ocular contusion.
- Many patients are otherwise healthy and no cause is identified (idiopathic).
- In diabetes, iridocyclitis can be one of the first symptoms leading to the diagnosis. In patients with type 2 diabetes fundus changes often present, indicating the importance of examination of the fundi with pupils dilated.

Symptoms and findings

- Dull pain in the eye
- Photophobia (tearing, blepharospasm)
- Pericorneal injection (may also be absent)
- Impaired vision (may be normal at the beginning)
- No discharge or foreign body sensation
- Almost invariably unilateral (except when associated with a systemic disease)
- Often miotic pupil
- In longstanding inflammation the iris may adhere to the anterior surface of the lens (posterior synechiae).

Examination of the patient and initiation of treatment

- Any of the three symptoms (pain, photophobia or pericorneal injection) justifies the suspicion of iridocyclitis.
- Such a patient needs to be referred to an ophthalmologist within 24 hours. Diagnosis is confirmed with microscopic examination (cells and flare in the anterior chamber), because treating unspecific irritation with steroid eye drops may cause permanent damage (concurrent herpes keratitis!).
- Patients with recurrent iridocyclitis, knowing their disease well, may start mydriatic therapy independently, but they are advised to visit an ophthalmologist within 24 hours. As prompt mydriatic as well as steroid therapy is beneficial and may shorten the duration of the disease. The patient could have mydriatic drops available all times.
- In special cases (e.g. long distance to an ophthalmologist) a general practioner may start the therapy in patients with recurring iridocyclitis. Consult an ophthalmologist and check the cornea with a loupe for possible staining with fluorescein to rule out corneal ulcer or keratitis (see keratitis dendritica). Arrange a consultation with an ophthalmologist within a few days.
- Laboratory investigations are performed according to the patient history; there are no routine tests.
    - Chest x-ray if sarcoidosis is suspected (bilateral acute iridocyclitis)
    - Paranasal sinus x-ray if there are symptoms of sinusitis
    - Tests for Chlamydia and intestinal infections
    - In case of joint symptoms or back pain refer the patient to a rheumatologist.

Treatment

- Started after confirmation of the diagnosis.
    - Local steroid therapy, e.g. dexamethasone drops, one drop every 1–2 hours at the beginning, later 4–6 times a day. Steroid ointment for the night.
    - Long-acting cycloplegic medication, e.g. atropine or scopolamine one drop 1–2 times daily.
- The treatment is continued at the same frequency (steroid drops) until the first check up, usually within a week, and after that according to the response.
- In severe iridocyclitis (fibrin, even hypopyon in the anterior chamber, high intraocular pressure, posterior synechiae) admission to hospital and paraocular steroid injections or peroral steroids may be indicated.
- In frequently recurring iridocyclitis, sulphasalazine may be tried as a prophylaxis for patients with a rheumatoid disease.

37.33 Cataract

Editors

Basic rule

- A cataract should be operated on when the harm caused by impaired vision is significant. Significant harm is determined by the patient's work and leisure-time activities. In working-aged people cataract should be operated on early.

Investigations

- The visual acuity is determined without spectacles or with the spectacles the patient normally wears (both minus and plus lenses).
- On examination with a slit lamp the pupil is pale, greyish, or greenish brown.
- The pupil reacts to light.
- At ophthalmoscopy the red reflex is weakened, extinct, or shady.
- The visibility of the ocular fundi is poor or absent.
- The intraocular pressure is normal. (However, a mature, swelling cataract may cause an acute increase in intraocular pressure.)

Urgency of referral

- **Referral is urgent if all the following conditions are fulfilled:**
    - The patient can only see hand movements or light.
    - The pupil is light grey.
    - The anterior chamber is lower than in the other eye, or the intraocular pressure is increased.
- In other cases a normal referral is made.

OPH

Treatment

- The cataract can be replaced by an artificial lens in a day-surgery procedure performed under local anaesthesia A [1 2]
- The patient is operable if he/she is able to lie supine (without e.g. significant dyspnoea).
- Tremor of the head or restlessness may be an indication for general anaesthesia.

After the operation

- Eye drops are used as local treatment for 3–4 weeks. Applying the drops can be made easier by making a hole for the tip of the bottle in old spectacles.

- Refer the patient to an ophthalmologist if there is a feeling of a foreign body (caused by the sutures: nowadays sutures are used only rarely).
- Refer the patient to a hospital immediately if the visual acuity has been impaired rapidly or if the patient has pain in the eye (the patient may have endophthalmitis or high intraocular pressure).
- Painless gradual impairment of visual acuity several months or years after cataract surgery is usually caused by secondary opacification of the lens capsule B [3 4]. The red reflex is blurred. The condition is treated by laser surgery.

References

1. Powe NR, Schein OD, Gieser SC, Tielsch JM, Luthra R, Javitt J, Steinberg EP. Synthesis of literature on visual acuity and complications following cataract extraction with intraocular lens implantation. Arch Ophthalmol 1994;112:239–252.
2. The Database of Abstracts of Reviews of Effectiveness (University of York), Database no.: DARE-940022. In: The Cochrane Library, Issue 4, 1999. Oxford: Update Software.
3. Schaumberg DA, Dana MR, Christen WG, Glynn RJ. A systematic overview of the incidence of posterior capsule opacification. Ophthalmology 1998;105:1213–1221.
4. The Database of Abstracts of Reviews of Effectiveness (University of York), Database no.: DARE-981267. In: The Cochrane Library, Issue 2, 2000. Oxford: Update Software.

37.34 Glaucoma

Anja Tuulonen

Aims

- A general practitioner should primarily be able to recognize the symptoms of an acute glaucoma attack, master the diagnostics and the principles of acute care.
- The diagnostics and follow-up of open-angle glaucoma require the equipment and special skills of an ophthalmologist.

Acute angle-closure glaucoma

- It is vital that the diagnosis and treatment of acute glaucoma are not delayed.
- In atypical cases a GP should readily consult an ophthalmologist on call at the nearest hospital with an ophthalmology unit for the appropriate treatment and referral.

Symptoms

- Headache and eye pain
- Often nausea and vomiting
- Redness of the eye
- Occasionally rainbow halo around lights (cause: corneal oedema)
- Visual impairment

Primary diagnostic procedure

- Measuring intraocular pressure (usually over 50–80 mmHg)

Other findings

- Impaired visual acuity
- Conjunctival erythema
- Middle-sized, non-responding pupil
- Greyish colour of the cornea
- The eyeball feels hard on palpation through the lid.

Treatment

1. Lower the intraocular pressure with 500 mg of acetazolamide (i.m., i.v. or p.o.).
   - Intravenous administration is fastest and most effective.
   - A vomiting patient cannot take tablets.
   - Intramuscular injection may be painful.
   - Allergy to sulphonamides is a contraindication.
2. After acetazolamide pilocarpine can be dropped on the eyes at 10–15-minute intervals.
3. Timolol drops can also be used if the patient does not have
   - asthma
   - bradycardia or
   - II–III-degree AV block.
4. Refer the patient immediately to an ophthalmological unit where medication to lower intraocular pressure is continued and laser peripheral iridotomy is performed.

What a general practitioner should know about open-angle glaucoma

- In most patients primary open-angle glaucoma is a slowly progressing disease in which changes may take years to be noticed.
- Open-angle glaucoma is a progressive neuropathy of the optic nerve leading to typical structural and functional defects of the optic disk, the nerve fibre layer and visual field.
- Glaucoma requires life-long follow-up.

Findings

- Visual acuity and intraocular pressure:
- Normal central visual acuity and statistically normal intraocular pressure (10–21 mmHg) do not exclude open-angle glaucoma.

- The risk of glaucoma defects increases when intraocular pressure rises (particularly when it exceeds 30 mmHg).
- Often the intraocular pressure may be elevated to 21–30 mmHg but the optic disk remains normal and visual field defects do not appear (so-called ocular hypertension).
- Typical fundoscopic finding in glaucoma:
  - The optic disk is asymmetric between the right and the left eye.
  - The central cup may be enlarged or drop-like in shape or paler than in the other eye.

- Finger confrontation perimetry
  - Finger confrontation perimetry only reveals visual field defects caused by advanced glaucoma.

Risk groups

- The general practitioner should remember the possibility of glaucoma in risk group patients (Table 37.34) and refer them to an ophthalmologist for further examinations.

Medications and other diseases

- It is worthwhile to ask the patient about the use of eye drops in addition to asking about other medicines, as some patients do not remember to mention them.
- Drugs used for other diseases may raise intraocular pressure (e.g. corticosteroids, parasympatholytics).
- Topically used glaucoma drugs may also cause systemic adverse effects.
  - Alpha antagonists (apraclonidine, brimonidine)
    - Drying of the mucosa of the mouth and nose, taste disturbances, slowing of the heart rate and hypotension, fatigue
  - Non-selective beta-blockers (timolol, carteolol):
    - bradycardia, hypotension, aggravation of asthma, dizziness, nausea, depression, sleep disturbances
    - non-selective beta-blockers should not be prescribed to patients with asthma, slow heart rate, low blood pressure, untreated cardiac insufficiency or II–III-degree AV block.
  - Selective beta-blockers (betaxolol):
    - systemic adverse effects are the same as those of non-selective agents, but rarer.
  - Systemic carbonic anhydrase inhibitors (acetazolamide)
    - Fatique, dizziness, GI tract disturbances, metabolic acidosis, depression, tingling of the extremities, hypersensitivity reactions, hypokalaemia, renal stones
  - Topical carbonic anhydrase inhibitors (dorzolamide, brinzolamide)
    - Disturbances of taste, drying of the mouth. Other adverse effects of sulphonamides and carbonic anhydrase inhibitors are also possible.
  - Prostaglandin derivatives (latanoprost, travoprost, bimatoprost, unoprostone)
    - No common systemic adverse effects have been observed
  - Parasympathomimetics (pilocarpine, carbachol)
    - Headache in the beginning of the treatment, but other systemic effects are rare.

Table 37.34 Risk factors for glaucoma

Risk factors[1]	The size of the risk	Level of evidence
Age	Doubled every 10 years	A
Intraocular pressure		
22–29 mmHg	10–13-fold	A
>30–35 mmHg	40-fold	
Myopia	2–4-fold	A
Exfoliation	5–10-fold[2]	A
Family history	3–9-fold	A
Lowered perfusion pressure together with age	3-fold	B

1. Ethnic background has also been found to be a risk factor. The role of diabetes as a risk factor is uncertain.
2. The size of risk in persons aged 65–70 years or more.

37.40 Occlusion of the central retinal artery

Anna-Maija Paakkala

Basic rule

- Try to restore circulation by massage of the eye and by lowering the intraocular pressure if the patient consults on the day of loss of vision.

OPH

Symptoms

- The history is typical: sudden, painless loss of vision in a previously healthy eye.

Clinical picture and course of the disease

- Visual acuity is at the level of being able to count fingers in front of the eye, or worse. About 20% of patients are able only to detect light.
- The pupillar light reaction is impaired.

Fundoscopic findings

- The findings vary with age of the occlusion.
- Immediately after the occlusion only slight oedema can be seen in the retina. The oedema increases over the next few hours, with the retina appearing pale, and the foveal area red. (In the foveal area the retina is very thin and the colour of the choroid is visible through the retina.) The arteries of the retina are narrow and spastic.
- During the next few weeks the retinal oedema disappears, and the necrotic internal layers of the retina are substituted by transparent scar tissue. The arteries remain narrow, but the veins have their normal appearance restored.
- Complete optic atrophy usually develops as a result of the occlusion.

Other investigations

- The following examinations should be performed on a patient with retinal artery occlusion:
  - ESR (temporal arteritis)
  - Blood lipid and glucose concentrations at least from patients of working age.
  - ECG (atrial fibrillation)
  - Chest x-ray (cardiac insufficiency)
  - Carotid artery auscultation and ultrasonography (atherosclerotic plaque)
- Coagulation studies are not indicated if the patient has not also had thromboses at other sites.
- Central artery occlusion is usually caused by an embolus. Artery spasm is rare. Atherosclerosis predisposes the patient to occlusion. Most patients have a pre-existing atherosclerotic disease, usually carotid stenosis. The assessment of the cardiovascular status and a neurology consultation are therefore necessary for the planning of treatment for the primary disease.

Treatment

- The occlusion cannot usually be opened.
- An embolus may pass further peripherally in the artery by massage of the eye, which results in a smaller area of retinal damage. The retinal circulation may be improved by pressing the eye with the palm for about one minute at a time, releasing the pressure suddenly for a moment (see 37.5). This procedure lowers the intraocular pressure.
- The intraocular pressure can also be lowered by drugs (acetazolamide, 500 mg i.v. or p.o.).
- These treatments should be tried if no longer than 8 hours have passed since loss of vision.
- Aspirin (100–250 mg/day) can be used if the patient has other atherosclerotic symptoms or diseases.
- Intra-arterial fibrinolytic therapy of the central retinal artery is experimental, and not in routine use C [1 2].
- Because there is no effective treatment for central artery occlusion there is no hurry as regards an ophthalmological consultation; however, consultation is often needed for verifying the diagnosis and for assessment of working ability.

References

1. Schumacher M, Schmidt D, Wakhloo AK. Intra-arterial fibrinolytic therapy in central retinal artery occlusion. Neuroradiology 1993;35:600–5.
2. Vulpius K, Hoh H, Lange H, Maercker W, Ruhle H. Selective percutaneous transluminal thrombolytic therapy with rt-PA in central retinal artery occlusion. Ophthalmology 1996;93:149–53.

37.41 Retinal venous thrombosis

Paula Summanen

Aim

- To identify and treat predisposing factors (diabetes, hypertension, glaucoma, susceptibility to venous thrombosis).

Definition

- Occlusion of the central retinal vein by thrombosis usually at the level of the lamina cribrosa.
- Branch vein occlusion occurs at the arteriovenous crossing.

Frequency and risk factors

- Branch vein occlusion is about three times more common that central vein occlusion.
- The most frequent vascular disorder of the ocular fundus after diabetic retinopathy.
- The patients are typically aged 50 years or more.

Predisposing factors

- Diabetes, hypertension, arteriosclerosis are the most common.
- Untreated glaucoma in about 20% of patients with central retinal vein thrombosis
- Hyperviscosity states: polycythaemia, macroglobulinaemia, myeloma
- Infections
- In young patients defects in the coagulation system: APC resistance, vasculitis or hormonal substitution.

Symptoms and findings

- Painless unilateral visual impairment over a period of hours, often during the night (noticed first in the morning).

- Visual acuity varies from almost normal to counting fingers according to the location and severity of the occlusion.
- In a complete occlusion ophthalmoscopy shows
  - an oedematous retina and optic disc
  - widespread dot and blot haemorrhages in the retina
  - veins congested and tortuous
  - retinal microinfarcts ("cotton wool spots")
- In partial occlusion the findings are less severe and in branch vein occlusion the changes are only in the affected quarter of the fundus, most commonly in the upper temporal quadrant and often with oedema and haemorrhages also in the macula.

Treatment

- Effective emergency medication does not exist.
- Anticoagulants are used only if a coagulation defect is found: repeated thrombosis, positive family history. See article 5.41. Consult an ophthalmologist or an internist.
- It is important to find out and treat the predisposing factors (see aetiology).

Investigations

- General examination (general practitioner, internist)
- Blood pressure, blood glucose, lipids, blood count
- Intraocular pressure
- Special examinations in young individuals and those with a family history or repeated thrombi (e.g. factor V Leyden)
- Within 2 months, an ophthalmological examination; laser treatment may be indicated.

Prognosis

- Up to one third of central vein and almost all branch vein occlusions are of ischaemic type (capillary closure). These may lead to angiogenesis in the retina, iris and the anterior chamber angle. New vessels cause vitreous haemorrhages and neovascular secondary glaucoma refractory to treatment that may develop in 3 months.
- After ischaemic central vein occlusion more than two thirds of the patients develop new vessels and more than half develop neovascular glaucoma.
- Prompt laser treatment of the retina (panretinal photocoagulation) stops the angiogenesis, as shown in randomized controlled studies.

37.42 Vitreous haemorrhage (VH)

Paula Summanen

Aim

- To identify the condition and underlying cause.

Aetiology

- VH is not a disease entity itself but a symptom of an eye disease. The prevalence of VH is about 7/100 000/year and the average age of patients is about 60 years. The most common causes are
  - Posterior vitreous detachment sometimes with tears of the retina
  - Proliferative diabetic retinopathy
  - Central or branch retinal vein occlusion
  - Retinal arterial macroaneurysms
  - The exudative type of senile macular degeneration
  - Other vaso-occlusive diseases with proliferative retinopathy (e.g. sickle cell anaemia, vasculitis), a vascular anomaly of the retina (e.g. Coats' retinitis, an angioma of the retina, von Hippel-Lindau disease) or e.g. subarachnoid haemorrhage
  - Malignant choroidal melanoma
  - Ocular trauma: blunt (contusion) or perforating trauma may both cause retinal breaks

Symptoms and findings

- A fog suddenly appears in the visual field, impairing the vision. In the early stage floaters and flashes of light may appear.
- Coagulated blood (clots) may be seen as individual moving shadows in the visual field (specific to vitreous haemorrhage).
- Dense vitreous haemorrhage impairs the vision down to light perception.
- On ophthalmoscopy, moving dark shadows are seen in the red reflex and the details of the fundus are cloudy – details might not be seen at all (neither the red reflex).

Referral

- Urgent consultation, same or next day, is needed if the cause of bleeding is not known. Ultrasonography is important to detect retinal detachment if the fundus is not visible.
- Diabetic patients with known proliferative retinopathy are advised to contact their own ophthalmologist.

Treatment

- Most VH clear up spontaneously without specific treatment. Tranexamic acid is not indicated (it may not be given).
- Initially the patient can be instructed to sleep using a higher pillow than usual or in a sitting position to settle the blood by gravity and thus speed the recovery of vision.
- The underlying cause of VH may require laser therapy, which is given as soon as the vitreous body is sufficiently clear.
- Laser treatment is given in proliferative retinopathy irrespective of the cause; diabetes and retinal vein occlusions being

the most common causes and to seal retinal breaks caused by posterior vitreous detachment or trauma.

- Vitrectomy is indicated if the vitreous humour does not clear up and always promptly in case of retinal detachment.

37.43 Detached retina

Anna-Maija Paakkala

Basic rule

- Detached retina should be identified and treated surgically.

Epidemiology, symptoms, and signs

- The cumulative incidence of detached retina in the population is 0.1%. The incidence is 8-fold in patients with myopia compared with patients with normal refraction or hyperopia. The incidence is also increased after cataract surgery and after contusion and perforation injuries of the eyes.
- As a result of retinal degeneration and the traction of vitreous adhesions a hole develops in the retina, the vitreous humour leaks under the retina, and detaches it from the choroid.
- The initial symptoms consist of visual disturbances, moving shadows, and "swarms of flies" in the visual field associated with small retinal haemorrhages, and "lightning". The initial symptoms are not specific. The same symptoms can be a result of "innocent" vitreous opacities and circulatory disturbances.
- As retinal detachment progresses a visual field defect develops. Note that the defect is on the contralateral side of the detachment.
- In young persons with myopia, retinal detachment progresses insidiously and remains asymptomatic for a long period. Regular ophthalmological examinations are therefore recommended.

Clinical examination

- The retina should be examined after dilatation of the pupil.
    - The ophthalmoscopic appearance is nearly always abnormal: the detached retina is greyish, folded and mobile. The retinal vessels are dark and tortuous at the site of detachment.
    - The retinal reflex may show a greenish grey, oscillating shadow.
- A shallow peripheral detachment may be difficult to detect. Consult an ophthalmologist if there is even a slight suspicion of retinal detachment.

Treatment

- Surgery is the treatment of choice. The operation should be performed as soon as possible, but usually not in the evening or during the weekend; refer the patient for the next working day or on the first weekday, as agreed locally with the department of opthalmology.
- Advise the patient to lie on the side of the detachment.

37.44 Age-related macular degeneration (ARMD)

Paula Summanen

Aim

- Identify this most important cause of visual impairment in the elderly and consider the significance of the handicap it causes in the patients' daily life.

Epidemiology

- The most common cause of visual impairment in patients aged over 65 years in all industrialized countries.
- Changes are seen in 2–23% of the population aged 43–64 years, an in 27–37% of persons aged 75 years or more. The prevalence of more severe ARMD is 1% in persons older than 60 years. It is bilateral in two out of three patients.
- One fifth have the exudative form of ARMD, and four-fifths the "dry" non-exudative form.

Pathogenesis

- The pigment epithelium and photoreceptor cells grow old causing macular degeneration, i.e. affecting the retinal area of central vision.
- Changes in the circulation of the fundus may also contribute.

Types

Atrophic or dry form

- Pigment epithelium and photoreceptor cells degenerate (a type of degenerative change).
- Because of the uneven distribution of pigment in the pigment epithelium, pigment clumps and depigmented areas are seen in the fundus as well as yellowish, rather regular round pale degenerative deposits often of varying size (drusens).
- The degeneration progresses slowly over years and decades.

Exudative or wet form

- May develop from the dry form.

- New vessels grow from the choroid through breaks in Bruch's membrane under the retinal pigment epithelium and the retina. These vessels are fragile, progress rapidly, and easily bleed and leak serum into the subretinal space impairing vision.
- In addition to atrophic changes, oedema, (yellowish) lipid exudates and varying sites of bleeding are seen in the fundus.
- The bleeding may sometimes spread to the vitreous space.
- The condition usually progresses rapidly over weeks and months.
- Differential diagnosis: transient macular oedema and diabetic maculopathy, see article on impaired vision and there under metamorphopsia 37.5.

Symptoms

- Elderly patients most often notice the symptoms only when the second, better eye is affected (when the non-dominant eye was first affected). The first eye may have already lost vision without being noticed.
- Typical experience: distortion of objects and lines (metamorphopsia) and disappearance of letters or changes in their size (micropsia, macropsia) (caused by fluid accumulation under and within the retina).
- The patient may notice that his/her colour vision has changed (blue and yellow being affected first) and see a grey patch (relative scotoma).
- The blind central area (central scotoma) makes communication difficult as the face of a person in front is not seen, but the hands and torso are well visible.
- Both near and distance vision progressively deteriorates, being eventually typically 0.3 to 0.1 in the non-exudative form of ARMD, and count finger in the exudative form.

Diagnosis

- Based on fundus findings.
- Refer the patient to an ophthalmologist for confirmation of the diagnosis. Patients with exudative ARMD need a rapid referral to a centre where fluorescein angiography (FAG) and laser treatment are available.

Treatment

- There is no known treatment for the atrophic form of ARMD.
- Antioxidative therapies have been evaluated with inconclusive results C [1].
- About one fifth to one tenth of patients with exudative macular degeneration are amenable to laser treatment that aims to destroy the new vessels growing under the retina and retinal pigment epithelium.
  - The need for laser treatment is assessed with fluorescein angiography: i.v. injection of fluorescent dye and photographing the ocular fundus through suitable filters.
  - In the exudative form new vessels and fluorescein leakage are visualized. If they do extend under the fovea, laser treatment would mean immediate loss of central vision and is generally not given. If a well-defined neovascular membrane is found outside the fovea, closure of the vessels with a laser may stop their progression. Studies have shown that laser therapy helps to keep the central scotoma smaller and the visual acuity better than in eyes without laser therapy B [2]
- It is important to know that in more than half of the patients with exudative ARMD the second eye becomes affected within 5 years if there are both large drusens and retinal pigment epithelial hyperpigmentation and that the disease may progress in the treated eye at a later date.
- Moreover, special irradiation techniques (photodynamic therapies) are being evaluated for patients unsuitable for laser treatment, but these are still experimental.

Visual rehabilitation

- Very important for most patients with severe ARMD due to lack of effective treatment.
- Optical and electronical means of image magnification may help in the reading of the most important papers.
- Everyday household aids may improve the ability to function at home.
- Since the peripheral visual field is unaffected, patients have ambulatory vision, at least in familiar places.

References

1. Evans JR, Henshaw K. Antioxidant vitamin and mineral supplementation for preventing age-related macular degeneration. Cochrane Database Syst Rev. 2004;(2):CD000253.
2. Wormald R, Evans J, Smeeth L, Henshaw K. Photodynamic therapy for neovascular age-related macular degeneration. Cochrane Database Syst Rev. 2004;(2):CD002030.

37.45 Retinoblastoma

Tero Kivelä

OPH

Aims

- To recognize retinoblastoma in an early phase, usually on the basis of a white pupillary reflex (leucokoria) reported by the parents or relatives.

Epidemiology and prognosis

- The most frequent eye cancer in children.
- Most common before the age of 3 years, very rare after the age of 8 years.
- One third of children with retinoblastoma have tumours in both eyes.

- Almost one half of retinoblastoma is inherited as an autosomal dominant trait. However, most hereditary retinoblastomas are due to new germline mutations and only every tenth child has a previously affected relative. The disease will be transmitted to the patient's children.
- Unless treated promptly, the eye will rapidly become blind and the tumour can metastasize and kill the child. Early diagnosis is vital to save vision.

Symptoms

- The most common symptom is leucokoria, a white reflex seen in the pupillary aperture. It is best seen in dim light when the pupil is large, and the parents are usually the first to notice it. Leucokoria reported by parents is always a reason for emergency consultation with an ophthalmologist, even if its presence cannot be confirmed.
- In obvious cases, a shadow or an abnormal white area may be noted in the fundus reflex.
- The second most common symptom is strabismus. Typically, a child who has previously had straight eyes begins to squint. For this reason, every child that develops an obvious squint should always be referred to an ophthalmologist without delay.
- As a rule an eye with retinoblastoma is not injected or otherwise abnormal in its outward appearance.

Treatment

- Conservative therapies that save the eye and remaining eyesight are preferred: cryocoagulation, plaque radiotherapy, and laser therapy.
- Advanced tumours necessitate enucleation of the affected eye. Orbital extension must be treated with chemotherapy and radiotherapy, which can also be used to salvage some eyes with advanced tumours.
- Treatment results are best when management of retinoblastoma is centralized in one national centre.

Screening

- If there is a family history of retinoblastoma, the fundi of a newborn child must be examined under general anaesthesia within the first 2 weeks of life and regularly thereafter.

37.46 Quinine amblyopia

Tero Kivelä

Aims

- To recognize the signs, symptoms and long-term consequences of quinine poisoning.
- To provide emergency care.

Background and aetiology

- Pills combining quinine with anxiolytic drugs are widely used to treat nocturnal leg cramps.
- Children and elderly people can accidentally take an overdose, whereas young adults may misuse these drugs for their presumed narcotic effect.
- Quinine is toxic to the neuroretina (quinidine does not have this effect).

Symptoms and signs

- An overdose first causes nausea and lethargy.
- Due to its quinidine-like properties, quinine prolongs the QT time and serious tachycardias may ensue (torsade-de-pointes).
- Vision deteriorates profoundly within 6–24 hours after an overdose. Light perception may even be lost. Central vision recovers during the next few days, usually to normal levels, but the visual fields, colour vision, and night vision are permanently damaged. The patient may be incapacitated and unable to continue to work due to his or her visual handicap.
- Tinnitus is also a typical symptom of quinine overdose.

Diagnosis

- Suspect quinine poisoning when your patient suddenly becomes blind, his or her ears are ringing, and the QT time is prolonged on the ECG.
- A careful history of drugs ingested and determination of plasma quinine levels confirm the diagnosis.
- In the acute stage, the ocular fundus frequently resembles that seen in occlusion of the central retinal artery, with a generally swollen white retina and a cherry red spot on the macula. It may, however, appear entirely normal in spite of marked loss of vision. During the following months, atrophy of the retina and optic nerve ensue.

Management

- Immediate, repeated administration of copious amounts of active charcoal reduces the amount of quinine absorbed from the gut. When the visual symptoms commence, the full dose has already been absorbed and the symptoms cannot be reversed with any known therapy. Repeated dosing of active charcoal may absorb quinine back to the gut from the blood circulation.

Otorhinolaryngology

Evidence Based Medicine Guidelines. Edited by the Duodecim Editorial Team
 ISBN: 0-470-01184-X

38.1 Upper respiratory tract infections in adults

Editors

Basic rules

- Diagnose viral infections by ruling out:
  - streptococcal tonsillitis (30–65/1000 persons/year) (38.20)
  - maxillary sinusitis (10–25/1000 persons/year) (38.31)
  - other bacterial diseases (otitis media, pneumonia, peritonsillar abscess etc).
- Avoid unnecessary antibiotics (A) [1]
  - A cough or bronchial rales (symptoms and signs of bronchitis) are not an indication for antibiotics (6.10).
  - Antibiotics are not beneficial in common cold (A) [1].
- Identify recurrent or chronic infections.
- Advise the patient to stop smoking.

Investigations

History

- Earlier episodes of sinusitis or bronchitis
- Smoking
- Fever

Lungs

- Rales, wheezing, sputum
- If the patient has wheezing or dyspnoea, measure the peak expiratory flow and perform a bronchodilator test if necessary.

Mouth and pharynx

- Peritonsillar swelling is a sign of an abscess (about 2 cases/1000 patients with sore throat).
- Other findings are not helpful in the differential diagnosis of viral and bacterial diseases.
- If streptococcal infection is suspected take a throat bacterial smear.

Neck

- Enlarged lymph nodes (adenovirus, mononucleosis, streptococci)
- Tender thyroid gland (subacute thyroiditis is an uncommon cause of a sore throat 24.32)

Maxillary sinuses

- Local symptoms, prolonged symptoms, and earlier episodes of sinusitis are indications for ultrasonography (38.30).

Ears

- In adult patients the ears are examined only if the patient has ear symptoms.
- The most common cause of ear pain is referred pain from the pharynx and the lymph nodes of the jaw angles.

Laboratory tests

- Take a test only if the result influences your treatment decision.
- In suspected tonsillitis take a throat bacterial smear (preferably a streptococcal culture) (38.21).
- In suspected mononucleosis take a rapid test or Epstein-Barr virus serology (1.42).

Treatment

Symptomatic treatment

- Analgesics for pain (paracetamol is the safest)
- Nasal decongestants can be used temporarily (A) [2].
- There is some evidence that zinc lozenges may be effective in reducing duration and severity of cold symptoms (C) [3] [4]. Adverse effects limit the use of the treatment.
- Long-term daily supplementation with vitamin C in large doses does not appear to prevent colds, but it may provide a modest reduction in the duration of cold symptoms (C) [5].
- There is little support from published literature for the use of antihistamines in common cold (A) [6] [7]. Most trials show that combinations of antihistamines and decongestives have beneficial effect on general recovery as well as on nasal symptoms in older children and adults. It is however not clear whether these effects are clinically significant.

Bacterial diseases

- Also bacterial diseases can be self-limiting. The treatment effects of antibiotics on tonsillitis (A) [8] and acute maxillary sinusitis (A) [9] [10] [11] are marginal: symptoms may be shortened at best by one day.
- To avoid adverse effects on both patient and population level, be cautious with the prescription of antibiotics for upper respiratory tract infections.
- If the antibiotic is considered necessary, the selection is influenced by
  - epidemiological knowledge of the most probable aetiology
  - the effectiveness and safety of the drug
  - the price of the drug.
- The first choice is usually penicillin or amoxicillin, and macrolides should be used only for those with penicillin allergy.

Follow-up

- A positive streptococcal test need not be followed up after treatment.

- A follow-up visit is indicated only if the symptoms persist or recur.
- In recurrent sinusitis a follow-up examination is indicated for the planning of further treatment.

References

1. Arroll B, Kenealy T. Antibiotics for the common cold and acute purulent rhinitis Cochrane Database Syst Rev. 2004;(2):CD000247.
2. Taverner D, Bickford L, Draper M. Nasal decongestants for the common cold. Cochrane Database Syst Rev. 2004;(2): CD001953.
3. Garland ML, Gagmeyer KO. The role of zinc lozenges in treatment of common cold. Ann Pharmacother 1998;32: 63–69.
4. The Database of Abstracts of Reviews of Effectiveness (University of York), Database no.: DARE-980225. In The Cochrane Library, Issue 2, 2000. Oxford: Update Software.
5. Douglas RM, Chalker EB, Treacy B. Vitamin C for preventing and treating the common cold. Cochrane Database Syst Rev. 2004;(2):CD000980.
6. Luks D, Anderson MR. Antihistamines for the common cold: a review and critique of the literature. J Gen Int Med 1996;11:240–244.
7. The Database of Abstracts of Reviews of Effectiveness (University of York), Database no.: DARE-960816. In: The Cochrane Library, Issue 4, 1999. Oxford: Update Software.
8. Del Mar CB, Glasziou PP, Spinks AB. Antibiotics for sore throat (Cochrane Review). In: The Cochrane Library, Issue 2, 2004. Chichester, UK: John Wiley & Sons, Ltd.
9. Williams Jr JW, Aguilar C, Cornell J, Chiquette E. Dolor RJ, Makela M, Holleman DR, Simel DL. Antibiotics for acute maxillary sinusitis. Cochrane Database Syst Rev. 2004;(2): CD000243.
10. de Ferranti SD, Ioannidis JP, Lau J, Anninger WV, Barza M. Are amoxycillin and folater inhibitors as effective as other antibiotics for acute sinusitis? A meta-analysis. BMJ 1998;317:632–637.
11. The Database of Abstracts of Reviews of Effectiveness (University of York), Database no.: DARE-989022. In: The Cochrane Library, Issue 2, 2000. Oxford: Update Software.

38.2 Hoarseness, laryngitis and dysphonia

Leenamaija Kleemola

Basic rules

- In the treatment of laryngitis the most important advice to the patient is voice rest, to avoid coughing, clearing one's throat and whispering. Voice rest does not necessitate total avoidance of talking, only significant restriction. Antibiotics are not indicated. It is important to keep the mucosa of the vocal cords moist (inhalation of a humidifying aerosol).
- People in professions needing the voice should have one week of sick leave in acute hoarseness.
- Indirect laryngoscopy must always be performed if the hoarseness is not associated with a respiratory infection, and in all patients with hoarseness lasting for more than two weeks. If the vocal cords cannot be fully visualized at indirect laryngoscopy the patient should be referred to a phoniatrician or an ENT specialist.
- Hoarseness in children is an indication for consultation by a phoniatrician or an ENT specialist (indirect laryngoscopy is difficult to perform).

Hoarseness in children

- Causes
  - Nodules
  - Papilloma (condyloma)
  - Laryngitis
  - Functional voice disorders
  - Congenital structural anomalies (laryngomalacia, stenoses)
- Examine hearing in children who talk loudly and have a hoarse voice.
- Indirect laryngoscopy is difficult to perform.
- Refer the patient to a phoniatrician or an ENT specialist.
- The vocal cords of a hoarse child must always be examined.

Acute hoarseness starting with symptoms of a respiratory tract infection

Laryngitis

- The vocal cords are erythematous and swollen.
- The treatment consists of voice rest, vapour breathing, antitussives, and avoidance of coughing, clearing one's throat and whispering.
- Antibiotics may be indicated because of other respiratory infections, not just because of laryngitis.
- People in professions needing the voice (teachers, kindergarten teachers, telephonists, etc.) should have a sufficiently long (at least one week) sick leave.

Prolonged hoarseness (>2 weeks) starting with symptoms of infection

Laryngitis

- The vocal cords are erythematous, swollen, and sometimes dry, or covered with crusts or mucus.
- Detect eventual prolonged infections, professional and toxic factors, allergies (take a thorough history!) and possible gastropharyngeal reflux.

- Oesophageal reflux is probably one of the most important causes of prolonged hoarseness.
- The treatment consists of voice rest, vapour breathing, antitussives, and possibly a trial of antibiotics according to other respiratory symptoms or even because of the laryngitis alone.
  - Amoxicillin
  - Doxycycline

Functional voice disorder

- Often starts after a respiratory tract infection, and continues even if the infection is cured (see below).

Prolonged hoarseness without symptoms of infection

Functional voice disorder

- Symptoms: hoarseness, fatigue of the voice, or hoarseness after talking; sometimes laryngeal pain, or a globus sensation. Patients with voice disorders are not always hoarse!
- The vocal cords look structurally normal.
- Organic causes should be excluded (thyroid or cervical surgery, pareses, tumours, infections).
- Underlying causes should be identified (excessive talking, an excited way of talking, hobbies requiring use of the voice, bad acoustics in the work environment (background noise, high reverberation)).
- Refer the patient to a phoniatrician (or an ENT specialist) if indirect laryngoscopy cannot be performed adequately or if you need advice on treatment.
- The patient often needs voice therapy.
  - All patients who are referred to voice therapy should also be seen by a phoniatrician or an ENT specialist (the therapy can be started while the patient is waiting for the consultation).
- Principles of treatment: relaxation, avoiding talking loudly, and breathing, postural and vocal exercises.

Vocal cord paralysis

- Symptoms
  - The motion of the vocal cords is defective or the vocal cord is totally paralytic.
  - The vocal cord is abnormally situated during inspiration or asymmetric.
  - The patient is always hoarse (a "whispering", breathy voice).
  - Finding the cause
    - A complication of surgery
    - Tumours (base of the skull, the neck, mediastinum, including the lungs)
    - Viral infections ("idiopathic")
    - Neurological diseases
- Always refer the patient to a phoniatrician or an ENT specialist.
- Refer the patient to voice therapy as early as possible (the therapy first consists of "gymnastics" for the primary weakness, and later avoidance of incorrect compensation).
- Voice amplification
- Voice-enhancing surgery (thyroplasty, injection methods). Surgery should already be considered when 6 months have passed from the onset of paresis.

Chronic laryngitis

- The vocal cords are red, dry, crusty or covered with mucus. The epithelium is thickened and hyperkeratotic.
- Occupational, toxic, and allergic exposure should be considered (take a good history!).
- The causative factors may also include upper and lower respiratory tract infections, drugs (inhaled corticosteroids for asthma), irradiation, oesophageal reflux or functional factors.
- Refer the patient to an ENT specialist of phoniatrician.
- The condition is often therapy-resistant.
- The treatment consists of vocal hygiene and vapour breathing.

Tumours

- Benign tumours (nodules, polyps, granulomas)
- Malignant tumours
- Always refer the patient to an ENT specialist or phoniatrician.
- Functional voice disorder may be associated with benign tumours, and the patients need voice therapy.

Hoarseness associated with neurological disease

- Myasthenia gravis, multiple sclerosis, Parkinson's disease, amyotrophic lateral sclerosis
- Hoarseness is rarely the initial symptom (with the exception of myasthenia).
- The voice is hoarse and quiet. The loudness, pitch, or rhythm may be altered. Loading the voice makes the symptoms worse.
- The movement or apposition of the vocal cords may be defective on indirect laryngoscopy, but the findings may also be quite normal.
- Refer the patient to a phoniatrician, an ENT specialist, or a neurologist.

Indications for indirect laryngoscopy in patients with hoarseness

- Indirect laryngoscopy should be performed at least
  - if the hoarseness has lasted for more than two weeks
  - if the hoarseness is not associated with a "flu"
  - in all children (ruling out papilloma)
  - in smokers aged 30 years or above.
- If indirect laryngoscopy cannot be performed reliably, the patient should be referred to a specialist. A "glance" is not enough.

Length of sick leave

- If talking is not necessary at work, sick leave is prescribed according to the general condition.
- If the work mainly involves talking, the sick leave should last for 1–4 weeks.
- Total avoidance of talking is not necessary, but voice rest, and avoidance of coughing, clearing one's throat and whispering is indicated.

38.3 Ear pain in an adult

Jukka Luotonen

Basic rules

- Identify the origin of local pain by taking a careful history and by physical examination.
- Consider the possibility of referred ear pain from any structure in the pharynx or neck.

Primary ear pain

- Primary ear pain originates from the ear or adjacent structures.
- The pain may be caused by inflammation or injury of the ear canal (38.37) or middle ear (38.35).
- Pain in chronic otitis media (38.36) often indicates a complication.
- Pain may be the first symptom of a malignant tumour in the ear canal (38.60) (or middle ear). Tumours of the ear canal are not always evident on normal inspection. Otomicroscopy and possibly also biopsy are needed.
- Cold air and wind may cause pain, particularly in a wide ear canal. Such pain rapidly subsides in a warm room.
- Negative pressure: infection, barotitis or barotrauma (38.41).
- Neuralgias are rare but may occur in the ear.

Referred (secondary) pain

- The pain is referred from distant processes.
- The most common cause of referred ear pain is a masticatory dysfunction or abnormality (7.17). Temporomandibular pain is often felt in the ear rather than in the joint itself. Dental pain may radiate to the ear. Examine the teeth of a patient with unexplained ear pain and palpate the masticatory muscles and temporomandibular joints.
- Diseases in the parotid gland (7.14) may also cause ear pain.
- Pain originating from the neck is commonly referred to the ear. Tension neck (20.1) often causes pain in the insertion of the sternocleidomastoid muscle. Ear pain is also common in cervical syndrome. Palpation of the muscles of the neck is important in the assessment of a patient suffering from ear pain.
- Diseases of the pharynx are the most common causes of referred ear pain. The pain caused by tonsillitis (38.20) or a peritonsillar abscess (38.22) may be reflected to the ear by the glossopharyngeal nerve.
- Pain originating from the pharynx, tongue, or palate may be caused by a barely visible abnormality, e.g. a small tumour.
- The vagus nerve may mediate pain from the oesophagus, thyroid gland or bronchi. The most common cause of vagal ear pain is a benign ulcer of the vocal cords, but cancer of the larynx may also be detected.
- Dissection or other disorders of the large arteries of the chest and neck may also cause ear pain through the sympathic nervous system.

Primary investigations of a patient with ear pain

- Otorhinolaryngological examination
  - Otoscopy
  - Laryngoscopy
  - Anterior and posterior rhinoscopy and indirect laryngoscopy
  - Palpation of the temporomandibular joints (examine the joint with the little finger while the patient opens and closes his/her mouth repeatedly)
  - Palpation of the neck
- Radiological investigations
  - Paranasal sinuses
  - Orthopantomography
  - X-rays of the cervical spine (if cervical syndrome is suspected)

Further investigations

- If the cause is not detected with careful history taking and clinical examination it is essential to rule out malignant causes by follow-up and consultation. Symptomatic treatment of pain is a secondary target.

38.4 Tinnitus

Seppo Savolainen

Introduction

- Establish the aetiology. In some cases, the cause may be eliminated (noise, otosclerosis, acoustic neurinoma).
- Remember the possibility of Ménière's disease.

- No cure is available in the majority of cases. Explain to the patient that the condition is harmless despite it being annoying.

Definition and epidemiology

- Tinnitus refers to an auditory perception in the absence of external auditory signal.
- Subjective tinnitus is heard only by the patient. Objective tinnitus is also audible to the examiner, either with or without the use of a stethoscope. Objective tinnitus is rare. If tinnitus is pulsating it might be caused by a vascular anomaly, and the patient should be referred for further investigation.
- 5% of the population experience tinnitus at some time during their lives. The prevalence of severe tinnitus is 0.5–1%.

Aetiology

- The most common cause is noise (noise at workplace, music, explosion, fireworks, gunshot).
- Tinnitus is often associated with sensorineural or conductive hearing impairment irrespective of its aetiology.
- Tinnitus is usually caused by inner ear damage which leads to increased automatic activity of the cochlear nerve and erroneous perception of noise by the brain.

Clinical picture

- The quality of the perceived noise varies (ringing, fluctuating, whistling, whining, hissing, humming, buzzing etc.)
- A low pitch noise may often be associated with a middle ear disease or Ménière's disease.
- The pitch of the noise is not enough to determine the aetiology.
- The degree of disturbance caused by tinnitus also varies; from tinnitus only heard in noiseless surroundings to tinnitus interfering with the quality of life.
- Tinnitus may lead to sleep disturbance, poor concentration and depression.

Investigations and indications for referral

- Ask whether tinnitus is associated with vertigo (for diagnosis and treatment of vertigo see article 38.70).
- Ask about possible exposure to noise and drug history (e.g. aspirin, valproate, ototoxic medication).
- Inspect the eardrum and test its mobility
- Weber's and Rinne's tuning fork tests
- Audiogram
- In unilateral cochlear (sensorineural) hearing impairment further investigations to rule out acoustic neurinoma are always indicated. Refer the patient to an ENT specialist.
- If the patient has conductive hearing loss with a normal eardrum, refer the patient for investigations to verify possible otosclerosis (38.17).
- If the patient's hearing is not impaired or the impairment is bilateral the indications for consultation are determined by the need for treatment of tinnitus. Usually a referral is not necessary.

Treatment

- In most cases there is no effective treatment.
- In otosclerosis, surgery usually cures tinnitus.
- In patients who need a hearing aid, the amplification of sound will help to mask tinnitus.
- The disturbance caused by the symptoms can be decreased by
    - counselling the patient (and explaining the commonness and benign nature of the symptom)
    - keeping a radio on or using personal stereos
    - treatment of concomitant depression.
- In severe cases betahistine can be tried.
- Peer support (tinnitus associations).

38.5 Ear wax

Jukka Luotonen

Basic rules

- Ear wax protects the ear canal from infection.
- Do not remove ear wax unless it
    - impairs hearing or causes other symptoms
    - prevents the investigation of the ear canal and tympanic membrane.

Symptoms

- In addition to a feeling of blockedness, wax can cause a humming noise, impairment of hearing and sometimes even dizziness.

Removal of ear wax

- Soft ear wax is usually easy to remove with a suction tip or a small cotton wool probe through an ear speculum.
- Harder wax can often be removed with an alligator forceps. An ordinary ear forceps is often too clumsy.
- Hard earwax can be difficult to remove. If the wax cannot be removed with an ear probe or by inserting a wax curette behind the wax lump and pulling, or with small alligator forceps, the ear should be irrigated with body-warm saline (or water). Direct the tip of the syringe towards the posterior upper wall of the ear canal and straighten the ear canal by pulling the auricle with fingers.
- **Irrigating is contraindicated in cases of perforated tympanic membrane.**

- Sometimes it is necessary to soften the wax prop before irrigating with a surface-active substance, saline or water C [1].
- Patients with a tendency for blocking ear wax should have ear wax removed 1–2 times a year.

Reference

1. Cheng AC, Stephens DP, Currie BJ. Granulocyte colony stimulating factor (G-CSF) as an adjunct to antibiotics in the treatment of pneumonia in adults. Cochrane Database Syst Rev. 2004;(2):CD004400.

38.6 Disturbances of the sense of smell

Editors

Basic rules

- Identify "conductive" disorders caused by obstructed nostrils that can be relieved by self-help measures and medication.
- Remember the possibility of a tumour adjacent to the olfactory tract.

Definition

- Disorders of the taste of smell include an-, hyp-, hyper-, and dysosmia (parosmia). They can be caused by central (intracranial) disorders of the olfactory tract or peripheral (intranasal) ventilatory disorders of the nose.
- Remember that the patient often first complains of a weakened sense of taste!

Investigations

- A bottle of tar should be available for the general practitioner in the clinical examination.

Aetiology

- Intranasal mucosal swelling
  - Viral or bacterial infection, allergic rhinitis (38.50)
  - A fluctuating disturbance of the sense of smell is often associated with chronic rhinitis (38.55) and particularly with nasal polyps (38.54).
- Injuries and tumours
  - Blows on the head (particularly on the back of the head) may cause a rupture of the olfactory bundle and a permanent deficit of the sense of smell.
  - Tumours adjacent to the olfactory tract are rare.

Differential diagnosis

- The history (of infection or injury) is diagnostic in most cases of acute onset.
- Other causes include
  - Toxic substances
  - Drugs causing allergic rhinitis (local anaesthetics, antibiotics)
  - Neurological diseases
    - Frontal lobe tumour: disappearance of the sense of smell
    - migraine: hypersensitization to olfactory stimuli
    - temporal epilepsy: paroxysmal sensations of strange odours
  - Endocrine diseases or functional states (hypopituitarism, diabetes, menstrual cycle)
  - Psychological causes (hysteria, cancerophobia)

Treatment

- Causal treatment may be helpful in nasal diseases.
- There is no generally accepted treatment for injuries of the olfactory tract.

Indications for specialist consultation

- Unilateral disorders and dysosmia (erratic sense of smell) without evident intranasal cause and olfactory hallucinations may suggest a tumour indicating investigation by a neurologist.

38.8 A lump on the neck

Editors

Risk of malignancy of neck lumps

Children

- See also article 32.3.
- About one in every ten abnormal lumps that differs from a normal lymph node is malignant.
- The most common causes of malignant neck lumps are Hodgkin's disease and lymphoma. Other causes include rhabdomyosarcoma, fibrosarcoma, thyroid tumours, neuroblastoma, and epidermoid carcinoma.
- A solitary nodule in the thyroid gland is malignant in 70% of the cases.
- Of benign masses, cysts, lymphangiomas and haemangiomas are usually visible from the first months after birth.

Adults above 40 years of age

- A large proportion of lumps situated outside the thyroid gland (24.31) are malignant.
- Most malignant lumps are metastases of tumours in the neck or head.

Investigations

- A solitary lump exceeding 2 cm is an indication for investigations.
- Bilateral enlargement of submandibular glands can be followed for a month without further investigations if they are clearly associated with a pharyngeal infection.
- Lumps under 2 cm in diameter can be followed up until their size is clearly reduced or they have disappeared.

Questions to the patient

- Pain in the ear
- Dysphagia
- Pain during swallowing
- Hoarseness
- Earlier removed tumours of the skin or lips
- General symptoms (fever, fatigue, weight loss, night sweats, loss of appetite, nausea)
- Travelling history (tuberculosis, some fungal diseases)
- Animal contacts (tularaemia, atypical mycobacteriae)
- Infected mosquito bite (tularaemia)

Physical examination

- Palpation of the neck and face (also the mouth with a glove-covered finger)
- Indirect laryngoscopy
- Anterior and posterior rhinoscopy
- Ear examination

Further investigations

- Ultrasonography + fine-needle biopsy

38.9 Globus syndrome (sensation of a lump in the throat)

Antti Mäkitie

Basic rules

- Rule out physical disorders (gastro-oesophageal reflux, thyroid nodule, thyroiditis tumours of the head and neck).
- Possible causes also include long uvula, long styloid process, or cervical spine osteophyte.
- Treat symptomatically.

Definition

- The patient has the feeling of a lump in the middle of the laryngeal area.
- There is usually no pain or dysphagia.

Epidemiology

- More common in young people and in women.
- Often associated with stressful psychological conditions (e.g. anxiety about possible cancer)

History

- Globus sensation is usually felt only when the patient swallows with the mouth empty, and is alleviated by swallowing food.
- There is no pain or weight loss.
- Ask about gastro-oesophageal symptoms (i.e. reflux)
- Ask about thyroid symptoms.
- Ask about psychologically distressing events.

Investigations and treatment

- Phase I
  - Underlying psychological disorders.
  - Inspection of the mouth and pharynx, palpation of the floor of the mouth, tongue and tonsils
  - Palpation of the neck
  - Indirect laryngoscopy of the lower pharynx and larynx is important.
  - Tendency for reflux
  - Thyroid function tests
  - Therapeutic trial: H2-receptor antagonist or proton pump inhibitor D [1]. Convince the patient of the functional origin of the symptom.
- Phase II
  - Consultation with an ENT specialist if the symptoms continue
  - X-rays of the hypopharynx and oesophagus
  - Ultrasonography of the neck
  - Chest x-ray
  - Hypopharyngo-oesophagoscopy if necessary
- For chronic pharyngitis, see 38.24.

Reference

1. Wilson JA, Pryde A, Piris J ym. Pharyngoesophageal dysmotility in globus sensation. Arch Otolaryngol Head Neck Surg 1989;115:1086–90.

38.15 Interpretation of an audiogram: impaired hearing

Martti Sorri

Quality requirements of hearing examinations

- Reliable hearing examinations require adequate equipment and surroundings as well as qualified personnel.
- The examinations should be performed in acoustically isolated conditions; a diagnostic or clinical audiometer is required.
- The examiner should be familiar with air and bone conduction measurements and the use of a masking noise. A speech unit (e.g. a CD player, ROM of a computer) for speech audiometry is often needed.
- For international guidelines, see standards ISO 6189 and ISO 8253-1, 8253-2, 8253-3.

Grade of hearing impairment

- According to a WHO classification, hearing impairment is classified according to the average hearing level in the so called speech frequencies, i.e. better ear hearing level over the frequencies 0.5–2kHz = $BEHL_{0.5-2kHz}$ (Table 38.15). A more recent and recommendable classification by an EU working group is based on the frequencies 0.5–4 kHz ($BEHL_{0.5-4kHz}$) (Table 38.15).
- The grade of hearing impairment is usually classified according to the hearing thresholds in the better ear. However, unilateral profound hearing impairment causes a considerable disability even if this is not considered in any of the above classifications. Hearing, and particularly perception of speech, is difficult, particularly in a noisy environment. According to the Finnish assessment guidelines, unilateral deafness may be defined as a class 3 disability (15% disability). When the difference of the average hearing levels in the frequency range from 0.5 to 2 kHz exceeds 35 dB between the ears, the patient is placed one class higher than what the better ear would suggest.

Conductive or sensorineural hearing impairment?

- Conductive and sensorineural hearing impairment can only be defined by audiometry if both air and bone conduction thresholds are measured. The patient has conductive hearing impairment if bone conduction thresholds are 20 dB or better and air conduction thresholds at 0.5 to 2 kHz are at least 15 dB worse than bone conduction thresholds. Bone conduction thresholds can never be greater (i.e., worse) than air conduction thresholds! Because the maximal output levels of audiometers are always smaller (softer) for bone conduction measurements than for air conduction measurements, the contribution of conductive impairment cannot be assessed in severe or profound hearing impairments. Tuning fork tests are often highly valuable.
- In sensorineural hearing impairment, bone conduction thresholds are worse than 20 dB and the difference between air and bone conduction thresholds is less than 15 dB.
- In combined hearing impairment both components are present. Bone conduction thresholds are worse than 20 dB and the gap between air and bone conduction thresholds exceeds 15 dB.

Table 38.15 Grade of hearing impairment according to two classifications

Grade of hearing impairment	WHO (1991)	EU working group (1996)
Mild hearing impairment	20–40 dB	20 dB $< BEHL_{0.5-4kHz} <$ 40 dB
Moderate hearing impairment	41–60 dB	40 dB $\leqslant BEHL_{0.5-4kHz} <$ 70 dB
Severe hearing impairment	61–80 dB	70 dB $\leqslant BEHL_{0.5-4kHz} <$ 95 dB
Profound hearing impairment	>80 dB	$BEHL_{0.5-4kHz} \geq$ 95 dB

Causes of conductive hearing impairment

- In a conductive hearing impairment, the Weber test is lateralizing towards the defective ear and the Rinne test is abnormal (negative). The Rinne test will be negative, when the conductive gap is 20 dB or greater at the frequency of the tuning fork used.
- Conductive hearing defects are practically always of the stiffness type, with the greatest impairment at low frequencies.
- Otitis media
  - See article 38.35.
  - The most common cause of hearing impairment
  - Acute otitis media or secretory otitis media ("glue ear") usually causes a 10–25 dB conductive hearing impairment (or even less, but never more than 30 dB).
- Perforation of the tympanic membrane
  - The hearing impairment is usually greatest at low frequencies.
  - If conductive hearing impairment (air-bone gap) is greater than 30 dB in chronic otitis media, the ossicular chain is also damaged (fixed or disrupted).
  - The audiogram of a chronically discharging ear may also show sensorineural component as a result of cochlear injury.
  - A totally adhesive tympanic membrane causes a conductive hearing impairment of about 60 dB (a pure conductive hearing impairment cannot be greater than 60 dB).

- Otosclerosis
  - See article 38.17.
  - Initially conductive hearing impairment is evident at low frequencies, later the hearing impairment spreads to higher frequencies.
  - Conductive hearing impairment may reach 60 dB. Particularly in severe cases, a sensorineural component may also be present.
- Mass type conductive hearing impairment (at high frequencies) is rare. It may be caused by, for example
  - an atrophic tympanic membrane
  - a disruption of the ossicular chain.

Causes of sensorineural hearing impairment

- Presbyacusis
  - Always a sensorineural hearing impairment
  - Usually, the audiogram slopes more or less steeply towards high frequencies.
  - The speed of progression varies.
  - Discrimination of speech may be disproportionately poor in relation to pure tone thresholds.
- Noise-induced hearing loss (NIHL)
  - See article 38.42.
  - In mild NIHL, the hearing impairment is generally greatest at 4 kHz (3–6 kHz; the so-called 4 kHz dip).
  - An audiogram sloping steadily towards high frequencies ("ski slope") is also quite common. Double dips may also occur.
  - An advanced NIHL may spread to the mid frequencies, but pure chronic NIHL never affects the low frequencies.
  - No audiometric findings confirm the diagnosis of NIHL without a history of sufficient noise exposure.
- Ménière's disease
  - See article 38.71.
  - The hearing impairment is usually sensorineural and fluctuates in the early phase.
  - Initially the impairment is seen at the low frequencies, and at times the hearing may be quite normal.
  - A transient hearing impairment at the low frequencies observed during an acute attack may be a valuable clue to the diagnosis.
  - At a later phase, a flat or even a high frequency hearing impairment develops. The flat hearing impairment at the later stage does not usually fluctuate or the fluctuation is very limited.
- Sudden deafness
  - The aetiology is unknown. There are probably many causes.
  - The audiogram may show several types of sensorineural hearing impairment.
  - Mild acute hearing loss confined to low frequencies has the best prognosis. Dexamethasone treatment may be beneficial **C** [1 2]. The role of other medical treatment is more controversial.
  - An indication for immediate referral.
  - If the symptoms have started after, for example, diving, blowing one's nose, physical exercise, or air travel, the patient may have a rupture of the round window (requires an urgent operation).
- Chronic otitis media
  - See otitis media above.
  - If an acute hearing deterioration develops in a patient with chronic otitis media or cholesteatoma, the patient may have a cochlear complication requiring urgent treatment.
- Acoustic neuroma (tumour of the 8th cranial nerve)
  - The usual finding is a slowly progressing unilateral sensorineural hearing impairment.
  - The hearing impairment is often greatest at high frequencies.
  - However, any type of unilateral sensorineural hearing impairment (even acute or fluctuating) may be associated with acoustic neuroma.

Reliability of an audiogram

- Audiograms are not always totally reliable, particularly if economic profit, e.g., in the form of insurance benefits or job security are associated with a certain grade of hearing impairment. Malingery is common, and approximately one fifth of reimbursed hearing impairments have been exaggerated.
- As a rule of thumb, the hearing deterioration is significant or genuine if the worsening of pure tone thresholds at follow-up is at least 15 dB at one frequency, or at least 10 dB at two adjacent frequencies. However, changes in hearing thresholds even greater than this are not always genuine.
- Assessment of audiometry results
  - The more qualified the examiner, the more reliable the results
  - The distance from the examiner during conversation gives a good impression of hearing.
  - The behaviour of the patient gives clues about possible exaggerated hearing impairment.
  - Air and bone conduction thresholds must be in accordance with each other (the hearing impairment entitling the patient to financial support to be reimbursed is usually sensorineural).
  - Speech audiometry is particularly valuable to confirm the results of pure tone audiometry.
- Despite air and bone conduction measurements it is sometimes difficult to distinguish a conductive component in the hearing impairment. Tuning fork tests are often useful in such cases.

Indications for specialist consultation

- The result of audiometry is an indication for referral in the following cases:
  - There is a need for rehabilitation (38.16). As a rule of thumb, the average threshold in speech frequencies

(0.5–2 kHz) is 30 dB or worse in the better ear (25 dB in children, 35–40 dB in the elderly).
- There is a possibility of a serious disease (complication of chronic otitis media, acoustic neuroma, etc.).
- The patient has an ear disease requiring treatment (secretory otitis media, otosclerosis, acute loss of hearing).

References

1. Stokroos RJ, Albers FW. Therapy of idiopathic sudden sensorineural hearing loss: a review of the literature. Acta Oto-Rhino-Laryngologica Belgica 1996;50:77–84.
2. The Database of Abstracts of Reviews of Effectiveness (University of York), Database no.: DARE-964082. In: The Cochrane Library, Issue 4, 1999. Oxford: Update Software.

38.16 Technical rehabilitation of hearing impairment

Martti Sorri

Requirement for hearing rehabilitation

- The prevalence of hearing impairment requiring rehabilitation (usually a hearing aid) is approximately 5% of the population in Western European countries.
- In Finland, 3% of individuals aged 55 years and 22% of individuals aged 75 years are considered to need hearing rehabilitation.

Hearing aids

Principles of operation

- Types of hearing aids
  - Behind-the-ear hearing aids (or hearing spectacles)
  - In-the-ear hearing aids may be used in mild or moderate hearing impairment (38.15). Flexible fingers and a good visual acuity are required.
  - Body-worn hearing aids (approximately 1%) may be used in severe hearing impairment and in patients who are not able to handle the smaller instruments.
- For all types of hearing aids, digitally programmable models or models with digital signal processing will lead the market in the next few years.
- Usually the sound is conducted into the ear by air conduction. If the patient has ear canal atresia or chronic middle ear infection with discharge from the ear, a bone conduction vibrator or a bone-anchored hearing aid may be used.
- Using a hearing device always requires practice. As many as 10–25% of patients do not use the hearing aid because of poor motivation or lack of skills in handling the instrument.
- Hearing aids need regular inspection and maintenance. The batteries must be changed as required. All primary health care units should be able to help patients with their hearing aids.

Common causes of hearing aid dysfunction

- Displacement of the ear mold or the in-the-ear hearing aid → whistling (acoustic feedback). Correct the position of the instrument.
- The earpiece is loose → whistling. Replace the ear mold.
- The sound channel of the ear mold (or the shell of the in-the-ear hearing aid) is obstructed by ear wax → the hearing aid is mute. Clean the channel. The ear mold may be cleaned with mild soap or special detergent. Always remember to dry the mold as waterdrops may also block it. The sound channel of an in-the-ear hearing aid is cleaned with a special instrument and/or the wax shield is replaced with a new shield.
- The battery is empty or incorrectly inserted → the hearing aid is mute. Replace the battery correctly.
- The battery is unsuitable → zinc-air batteries may cause a humming noise in some hearing aids. Try to replace the battery with another type of battery (or consult a hearing centre).
- The tube of a behind-the-ear hearing aid is stiff or broken → whistling. Wrong length of the tube may result in the same problem. Change the tube.
- The cord of a body-worn hearing aid is broken or the contact is poor → the hearing aid is mute or the sound is interrupted. Change the cord.
- M-T switch is in the wrong position → the hearing aid is mute. Correct the position: M for microphone, T for induction (telephone) coil of the hearing aid. In some instruments, both functions may be used at the same time (MT position of the switch).

Testing the functioning of a hearing aid

- Use the checklist above.
- Acoustic feedback (whistling) may be induced in a properly functioning aid by turning the instrument on and turning the volume switch to maximum. Close your fist around a behind-the-ear or in-the-ear instrument. If no acoustic feedback is induced (and the battery is in order), the hearing aid does not work and it needs to be checked by a hearing aid technician. Body-worn aids may be tested in the same way by bringing the microphone close to the receiver (earpiece).
- The quality of the sound may be tested by listening to the hearing aid with an ear mold fitted for tester's ear canal. Another possibility is to use special stethoscope earpieces. Note that the sound of a hearing aid is far from linear high fidelity output.

Assistive listening devices

Communication amplifiers

- Suited for the elderly who are unable to use even a body-worn hearing aid.
- Used instead of a hearing aid to amplify speech and environmental sounds.

Alarm equipment

- Doorbells
- Telephone alarms
- Vibration alarm clocks
- Light indicators for telephone and doorbell
- Cry alarms

Aids for telephone communication

- Telephone amplifiers
- Portable amplifying telephone adapter (most adapters may also be used to change the acoustic signal from the telephone to an inductive signal which is received by the hearing aid switched into the T-position).
- Induction loops for mobile phones (to be used with the T-switch on).
- Text telephone (in severe hearing impairment). The short message function of cellular phones, or fax and e-mail may also be used for communication.

Entertainment electronics, inductive listening

- Accessory head or earphones (wireless infrared earphones also exist; some infrared devices produce an acoustic signal and some an inductive signal to be received with the person's hearing aid in the T-position).
- A portable induction loop to be attached to an accessory output of a radio or a television, or a loop with its own amplifier installed in the room (to be used with the hearing aid switch in the T-position).
- Induction loops are often available in public buildings (churches, meeting rooms, theatres) and offices. They should also be installed in health care institutions.

Equipment for education

- Toys, recorders, and other equipment for hearing training in children with hearing impairment
- Special equipment in schools (usually radio-frequency communication between the teacher and the hearing impaired child)

Cochlear implants

- Cochlear implants are hearing instruments for profoundly impaired hearing. The instrument transmits an electric signal directly to the cochlear nerve by-passing the nonfunctioning inner ear.
- Cochlear implants may be considered for both postlingually deaf children and adults as well as for pre- or perilingually deaf children. Perlingually deaf adult subjects are not suited for implant candidacy.
- After implantation, the device has to be programmed individually and hearing must be trained. Pre- and perilingually deaf children need the same kind of hearing rehabilitation as other children with profound early childhood hearing impairment.
- The implantees need follow-up for the rest of their lives.

Indications for hearing aid assessment

- Technical hearing rehabilitation should be considered if the better ear hearing level over the frequencies 0.5–2 kHz ($BEHL_{0.5-2\ kHz}$) is 30 dB or worse (current Finnish guidelines). In children, the corresponding limit is 25 dB or sometimes even 20 dB, whereas in the elderly the limit is often set at 35–40 dB. Children usually are fitted with two hearing aids, and adults often with only one. In adults, two instruments may also be indicated if needed for work or study.
- The motivation of the patient and his/her social needs are of great importance. Note that hearing impairment in an elderly person living alone may result in social isolation.
- Assessment of the need and selection of the hearing aid and assistive listening devices may require several home or workplace visits.
- The rehabilitation plan includes assessment of the hearing impairment, other medical problems, and the social situation.

Indications for referral for hearing aid assessment

- A rule of thumb
  - In a child, the better ear hearing level over the frequencies 0.5–2 kHz ($BEHL_{0.5-2\ kHz}$) is 25 (20) dB or worse.
  - In an adult, the better ear hearing level over the frequencies 0.5–2 kHz ($BEHL_{0.5-2\ kHz}$) is 30 dB (35–40 dB in the elderly) or worse.
- Ask about the patient's problems and record them in the referral.

38.17 Otosclerosis

Hans Ramsay

Basic rule

- Suspect otosclerosis in a patient with conductive hearing impairment and a normal eardrum.

Definition

- Otosclerosis is a primary focal disease of the labyrinth capsule occurring in otherwise healthy people. It has no association with known skeletal diseases with the exception of osteogenesis imperfecta.

Epidemiology

- According to one study the prevalence of clinical otosclerosis was about 3% and, in addition, 4% of the population has foci of otosclerosis in the labyrinth capsule without clinical disease.
- The age of onset is usually between 15 and 30 years. The disease only rarely commences earlier, but a later onset is possible.

Symptoms and signs

- The most important symptom is a gradually progressing hearing impairment that rarely affects both ears at once. The better ear usually becomes affected years after the first one.
- A typical symptom is an impression of improved hearing in a noisy environment (Willis' paracusis). This is explained by the fact that people speak louder in a noisy environment, and environmental noise that consists of low frequencies is less disturbing for people with conductive hearing impairment caused by otosclerosis than for persons with normal hearing.
- Tinnitus is common at an early stage of the disease but it gradually disappears. Sometimes the tinnitus may remain and severely annoy the patient. The tinnitus is typically low-pitched. Mild disturbances of equilibrium may occur.
- An intact, pale eardrum with normal mobility is observed at otoscopy. Sequelae of otitis media from childhood may be visible in the eardrum and make the diagnosis more difficult.
- Findings typical of a conductive hearing impairment are detected in functional examination.
  - Identification of spoken and whispered words is impaired. Words containing low-pitched syllables (vowels like a, o, u) are particularly difficult to hear.
  - The Weber' tuning fork test lateralizes to the more severely affected ear, and the Rinne's test is abnormal (negative).
  - The typical audiogram shows a flat air conduction that may be impaired to the conductive maximum of 60 dB. In pure stapedial fixation with a normal internal ear the bone conduction may be nearly normal.
  - The bone conduction typically shows Carhart's notch, with a hearing impairment at 2000 Hz.
  - A combined hearing impairment is common, affecting both air and bone conduction. At low frequencies there is, however, a marked difference between air and bone conduction.
  - In speech audiometry the speech threshold is impaired as much as the air conduction threshold. Speech discrimination is good in pure stapedial fixation, but it may be affected in combined hearing impairment.
  - Acoustic impedance testing reveals a normal middle ear pressure and absence of the stapedial reflex.

Treatment

- There is no pharmacological or other treatment that prevents the formation of otosclerotic foci.
- In progressive hearing impairment of inner ear type large doses of fluoride can be used to slow the progression of the impairment.

Alleviation of hearing impairment

- Hearing aids are well suited for patients with otosclerosis and they usually restore hearing to a socially adequate level.
- The indications for surgery are the following:
  - The hearing must be markedly impaired, usually to 40–60 dB at speech range (500–2000 Hz).
  - Bilateral otosclerosis in most cases. The worse ear is operated on first.
  - Unilateral otosclerosis can be operated on if the symptoms are annoying.

38.20 Sore throat and tonsillitis

Marjukka Mäkelä, Jouko Suonpää

Basic rules

- Antibiotics are indicated in infections caused by group A streptococci or gonococci and in severe infections caused by group C or G streptococci. Symptomatic treatment is sufficient for infections caused by other agents.
- A peritonsillar abscess should be identified and treated immediately.
- The following diseases should be recognized:
  - mononucleosis
  - pharyngeal gonorrhoea
  - subacute thyroiditis
  - granulocytopenia (in patients receiving drugs that affect the bone marrow)
- The source of infection should be identified in recurrent tonsillitis.
- Epidemics should be recognized and controlled (even those caused by non-A streptococci).

Aetiology of tonsillitis

- Group A streptococci cause 5–20% (during epidemics 40%) of all cases of tonsillitis. Prevalence of tonsillitis is lowest in the summer.
- Other streptococci may cause epidemics but no sequelae.
- Neisseria gonorrhoeae is a rare cause of tonsillitis (1%).
- Mycoplasma and chlamydia are detected equally in asymptomatic and symptomatic patients, and need not be searched for.
- Mononucleosis is diagnosed in 1–2% of the patients.
- Arcanobacterium is the causative agent in less than 1% of the cases. The clinical picture resembles scarlet fever. No therapy is indicated.
- In the majority, sore throat has a viral aetiology. Viruses can also cause high fever, rash and pharyngeal exudate.

Risk groups

- Streptococci: children above 3 years and young adults (15–24 years)
- Mononucleosis: children and young adults.
- Gonorrhea: sexually active individuals.

Investigations

- Examination of the pharynx: peritonsillar oedema, exudate, trismus
- Palpation of the neck
  - Enlarged lymph nodes in other locations than the jaw angle–mononucleosis?
  - Enlarged, tender thyroid gland: thyroiditis?
- Rash: viruses, erythrogenic strains of group A streptococci, arcanobacterium?
- Oedema of the eye lids: mononucleosis? (1.42)
- Other focuses of infection: sinuses, ears, teeth, lower respiratory tract
- Streptococcal culture or rapid test is the most important investigation. Clinical assessment is not accurate in determining the microbial aetiology.
  - Culture of a throat swab is the most accurate and least expensive method, provided that notification of the result to the patient and delivery of the prescription to the pharmacy are organized effectively.
    - Streptococcal culture also reveals non-A streptococci (no inhibition of haemolysis around a bacitracin disk).
  - If a rapid test is used, a negative result should be confirmed by culture (confirmation of a negative test is not necessary in children under the age of 3 years, as streptococcal disease is uncommon in this age group).
- Rapid test for mononucleosis and culture for Neisseria gonorrhoeae as required.

Organizing the treatment

- The physician should see all children and those adults who have an underlying disease, pain in the sinuses or in the ear, productive cough, or trismus.
- Adult patients can usually be examined by a nurse, who takes a streptococcal test.
- Antibiotics are indicated only for patients with a positive culture or rapid test for either
  - group A streptococci or
  - any streptococci if the symptoms are severe, particularly during an epidemic.
- If the patient has severe symptoms, a one-day dose of antibiotic can be given while waiting for the result of the bacterial culture. If the result is negative, the antibiotic should be discontinued.

Drug therapy in streptococcal disease

- Penicillin V 1.5 million units × 2 × 10
- In case of penicillin allergy: oral cephalexin 750 mg × 2 or cephadroxil 1 g × 1 (A) [1 2].
- It is not necessary to start antibiotics immediately: a delay of 1 (-3) day(s) does not increase complications or delay the resolution of acute disease.
- Antibiotics shorten the duration of symptoms somewhat (A) [3] and reduce the risk of rheumatic fever (C) [4].
- An analgesic (B) [5 6] (paracetamol and ibuprofen are the safest) is more effective than antibiotics against symptoms. Pain at swallowing can even be treated with lidocaine spray or gargling solution.
- Non-A streptococci: in patients with severe symptoms and during epidemics, the same medication as for group A streptococci.
- Repeated throat culture is not necessary unless the symptoms recur.
- The patient is no longer infective after 1 day on antibiotics.

Drug therapy for other causative agents

- Pharyngeal gonorrhea often causes only mild symptoms. Remember the provision of free antibiotics for STD and tracing of the contacts.
- Mononucleosis should not be treated with antibiotics. Particularly ampicillin should be avoided (rash!).

Peritonsillar abscess

- Trismus (difficulty and pain in opening the mouth)
- Difficulty in swallowing and increased salivation.
- Oedema around and above the tonsils, deviation of the uvula, asymmetry and forward displacement of the soft palate.
- Treatment consists of drainage of the abscess (often immediate tonsillectomy) and antibiotics.

Recurrent tonsillitis

- Recurrent sore throat, with positive test for group A streptococci

- Reinfection is the most common cause.
- Throat cultures should be taken from the patient and all family members.
- Other symptomatic patients at the work place should be traced.
- In recurrent infection first-line therapy is cephalexin or cephadroxil that erase group A streptococci even more efficiently than penicillin Ⓐ [1 2]. Clindamycin (300 mg × 2 for 10 days) also erases group A streptococci and prevents recurrent tonsillitis caused by other bacteria as well.

Indications for tonsillectomy

- Recurrent, confirmed bacterial tonsillitis (>4 x/year), irrespective of the type of bacteria Ⓒ [7 8]
  - Dates and results of bacterial cultures and rapid tests should be included in the referral
- Complications of acute tonsillitis: peritonsillar abscess, septicaemia originating from the tonsils.
  - A peritonsillar abscess in a patient under 40 years of age is treated by acute tonsillectomy without prior incision.
- Suspicion of malignancy (marked asymmetry or ulceration)
- Airway obstruction caused by tonsils (which may almost touch each other), sleep apnoea, disorder of dental occlusion
- Chronic tonsillitis is a relative indication for tonsillectomy. The operation is indicated if the patient continuously suffers from bad breath, sore throat and gagging, and if the symptoms do not diminish during follow-up.

Streptococcal epidemics

- A streptococcal epidemic should be suspected if
  - there are several patients from the same location OR
  - the same patient has recurrent streptococcal disease.

References

1. Deeter RG, Kalman D, Rogan M, Chow SC. Therapy for pharyngitis and tonsillitis by group A beta-hemolytic streptococci: a meta-analysis comparing the efficacy and safety of cephadroxil monohydrate versus oral penicillin V. Clin Therap 1992;14:740–754.
2. The Database of Abstracts of Reviews of Effectiveness (University of York), Database no.: DARE-953519. In: The Cochrane Library, Issue 4, 1999. Oxford: Update Software.
3. Del Mar CB, Glasziou PP, Spinks AB. Antibiotics for sore throat Cochrane Database Syst Rev. 2004;(2):CD000023.
4. Manyemba J, Mayosi BM. Penicillin for secondary prevention of rheumatic fever. Cochrane Database Syst Rev. 2004;(2):CD002227.
5. Thomas M, Del Mar C, Glasziou. How effective are treatments other than antibiotics for acute sore throat? British Journal of General Practice 2000, 50, 817–820.
6. The Database of Abstracts of Reviews of Effectiveness (University of York), Database no.: DARE-20018156. In: The Cochrane Library, Issue 3, 2002. Oxford: Update Software.
7. Marshall T. A review of tonsillectomy for recurrent throat infection. Br J Gen Pract 1998;48:1331–1335.
8. The Database of Abstracts of Reviews of Effectiveness (University of York), Database no.: DARE-988675. In: The Cochrane Library, Issue 4, 1999. Oxford: Update Software.

38.21 Throat bacterial swab

Marjukka Mäkelä

Basic rules

- Group A beta-haemolytic streptococci are detected or excluded.
- Other types of streptococci (groups C and G) are also tested for during epidemics.
- Other microbes are only tested for if there are special indications
  - Gonorrhoea or pertussis can be diagnosed by bacterial cultures, and mononucleosis by serology.
  - Chlamydiae and mycoplasmae need not be tested for.

How to organize testing

- Become familiar with sampling and interpretation.
- Ensure availability of the equipment out-of-hours.
- Local guidelines are recommended.
- A nurse or a medical laboratory technologist can also take culture samples.

Taking a throat smear

- A headlamp, a good chair, and for children someone to hold them.
- Use a carbon stick, or the stick included in the test pack for rapid tests.
- Press the tongue firmly with a wooden spatula.
- Take the sample from both tonsils, and the palatal arches, preferably from areas with exudate.

Culture

- Culture immediately on a special plate (blood agar) (remember bacitracin disk) or send the specimen in a Stuart tube.

- Keep the specimen in a warm incubator for 18–24 hours. A positive result can often be read earlier (ask the patient to phone the next morning).
- A clear (not greenish) zone around an inoculation of bacteria indicates beta-haemolytic streptococci.
- Group A streptococci are identified by an inhibition ring (absence of haemolysis) around a bacitracin disk.

Rapid test

- Perform the test according to the instructions on the test pack.
- Use a positive control regularly.
- The test can only identify group A streptococci.

Other aetiological agents

- Gonococci: special culture
- Mononucleosis: rapid test, Epstein-Barr virus serology or blood smear (lymphocytosis and atypical lymphocytes)
- Pertussis: special culture. Consult the laboratory in advance.

38.22 Drainage of a peritonsillar abscess

Antti Mäkitie

- Peritonsillar abscess is the most common deep infection of the head and neck and usually a complication of acute tonsillitis. It always warrants immediate therapy.
- Most cases can be managed in primary health care.
- Refer to an ENT specialist:
  - a paediatric patient
  - a severely ill patient
  - a patient with difficulty in breathing
  - a bilateral abscess
  - a patient with a large abscess (pharynx is obstructed or a parapharyngeal abscess is suspected)
  - if the abscess cannot be drained, trismus does not alleviate or a suspicion of another cause for symptoms (malignancy) arises.

Instruments

- An ENT examination chair, a nurse to hold the patient's head still and a headlight
- 10% xylocaine for topical anaesthesia
- 1% lidocaine-adrenaline for local anaesthesia (25 Gauge needle and 2 ml syringe)
- tongue blade, a long 18 Gauge needle and 10 ml or 20 ml syringe, a No. 11 scalpel blade, angulated forceps
- suction equipment
- I.v. rehydration kit if the patient is dehydrated.

Procedure

1. If necessary the patient is administered i.v. fluids and analgesics before the procedure.
2. The patient is placed in a sitting upright position with his head supported against a headrest. Explain the procedure to the patient and ask him/her to open the mouth. Depress the tonque with tonque depressor (trismus often compromises an adequate intraoral examination). Hypopharynx and larynx are inspected with a mirror to exclude lower oedema and bulging of the tissues and possible airway obstruction.
3. The most prominent area of the mucous membrane overlying the abscess is sprayed with topical anaesthetic.
4. Local anaesthetic is infiltrated into the palatoglossal arch at the location of the abscess, first intraepithelially into the mucous membrane and then deeper. Ensure that the needle is not in a vein. Try to localize the abscess by using the three-point method: needle aspirations from the superior, middle and lower regions of the peritonsillar space (Figure 38.22.2).
5. The abscess can be emptied by draining the pus with a large needle. The patient should come for a check up next day and the procedure can be repeated. If this does not bring relief, a larger incision is needed (see point 6).
6. Under local anaesthesia make a 1–1.5 cm incision in the mucous membrane parallel to the palatal arch at the site with the largest bulge.

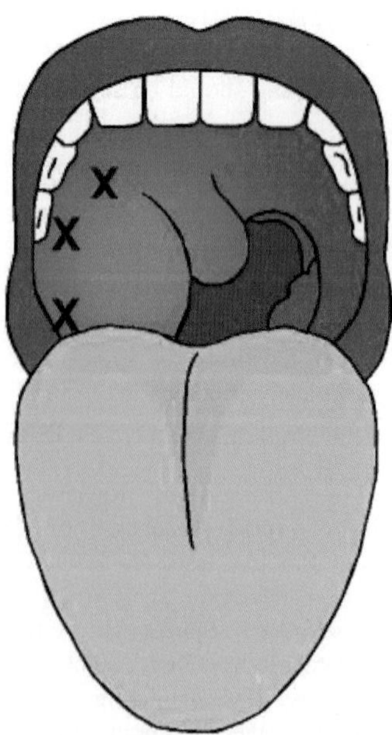

Figure 38.22.1 A peritonsillar abscess can be effectively drained by aspirating pus from three different points with a thick needle and syringe, after first infiltrating the points of aspiration with local anaesthetic.

7. Dissect along the capsule of the tonsil with angulated forceps until the abscess cavity is found. Spread the forceps only when in the abscess cavity. You should find your way to the back of the tonsil and not get mixed up in the tonsillar tissue. Work in sagittal plane and avoid posterolateral aspect of the tonsil (carotid artery).
8. Remove all pus by suction and take a sample for bacterial culture.
9. The patient should sit leaning forward until bleeding stops and should rinse his mouth with cool mouth wash.
10. Give a sufficient dose of analgesics (e.g. ibuprofen 400–600 mg × 3 as necessary)
11. Antimicrobial therapy for adults: penicillin 1.5 million IU × 2 for 10 days. Can be started by giving benzyl penicillin (penicillin G) 1.2–1.5 million IU intramuscularly. Add metronidazole if no response within the first 24 hours.
12. Sick leave is usually needed for one week.
13. The patient should come for a follow-up visit 1 to 2 days after the incision. The abscess cavity is opened with angular forceps (local anaesthesia) and drained. If necessary, the procedure is repeated after 2 days. Patients whose abscess has been drained with a needle should be followed up more frequently (daily). Incision is performed if necessary.

Tonsillectomy

- Peritonsillar abscess is an indication for tonsillectomy if the patient has had recurrent episodes of tonsillitis.
- In children, tonsillectomy is usually performed immediately (in the "hot" phase).

38.24 Chronic pharyngitis

Jouko Suonpää

Basic rule

- Chronic pharyngitis is rarely a disease in itself; try to eliminate factors maintaining the inflammation.

Causes of chronic pharyngitis

- External causes
  - Dry and dusty air
  - Smoking and passive smoking
  - Mucosal irritation
  - Industrial chemicals and dusts
  - Drugs (including topical drugs)
  - Alcohol
  - Allergens
  - Radiotherapy
  - Excessive use of voice (noisy environment)
- Internal causes
  - Infections of the nasal and paranasal cavities
  - Postnasal drip
  - Chronic nasal obstruction
  - Oral and dental infections
  - Chronic or recurrent tonsillitis
  - Chronic inflammatory lung diseases
  - Diseases of the oesophagus and stomach (gastro-oesophageal reflux)
  - Hormonal causes
  - Incorrect use of voice
  - Structural factors (wide pharynx etc.)
  - Systemic diseases

Findings

- The clinical signs are variable.
- Mucosal swelling and erythema prevail in the catarrhal form. The uvula may be elongated and swollen. This often suggests tendency to snore and possible sleep apnoea syndrome (6.71).
- In hypertrophic pharyngitis the amount of lymphatic tissue is increased in the entire pharynx. Sometimes accessory streaks of lymphoid tissue can be seen behind the palatal arches.
- In dry pharyngitis the mucosa is attenuated and sometimes keratinized. The pharynx is wide, and dried foul-smelling mucus may be present.

Treatment

- The need for treatment depends on the patient's symptoms: pain, a feeling of tightness or a globus sensation, need to swallow, clear one's throat, snoring, hoarseness and foul-smelling breath.
- Examine the patient carefully to eliminate the fear of cancer, which is often associated with the symptoms.
- Identifying the factors that maintain the pharyngitis requires time and cooperation with the patient.
- Irritation caused by foci of infection, nasal obstruction and gastric secretions should be eliminated.
- Continuous throat-clearing and cough irritation can be treated by drugs.
- Humidification of air reduces the drying of the pharynx that is made worse by central heating.
- Stopping smoking is a must without which all other measures are futile.
- Tonsillectomy may be of benefit. However, it should not be performed as a treatment for dry pharyngitis.
- Nose drops containing vitamin A or a humidification nose spray are often beneficial in dry pharyngitis.
- Gargling helps to remove mucus adhering to the pharynx and reduces the bad odour of the breath.

38.30 Diagnosis of sinusitis

Helena Varonen

Basic rules

- Acute rhinosinusitis is most often a self-limiting disease where antibiotics are not helpful **A** [1 2 3]. Clinical examination can be used to rule out severe sinusitis and to select the mild cases for symptomatic treatment only.
- If prolonged bacterial sinusitis is suspected, sinus ultrasound performed by clinician is the method of choice because of its safety (no irradiation) and low costs **B** [4].
- Focusing antibiotic treatment only on patients with symptom duration of more than one week and with fluid retention in sinus ultrasound reduces the number of unnecessary antibiotic prescriptions for sinusitis in primary care.
- A sinus x-ray should be taken if the symptoms persist or recur, suggesting chronic sinusitis.
- The results of sinus ultrasound or x-ray should influence the choice of therapy: no antibiotics are indicated if the findings are negative.
- Severe cases (patients with suspected frontal sinusitis or bacterial pansinusitis) should be treated with antibiotics on clinical grounds to avoid complications.
- Sinusitis in children, see 31.11.

Sinus ultrasound

- In experienced hands the sensitivity and specificity of a properly performed sinus ultrasound examination are comparable to those of a sinus x-ray when compared with maxillary sinus puncture findings **B** [4].
- Fluid retention is common in maxillary sinuses in the first days of common cold **C** [5]. Sinus ultrasound should only be used to examine patients with symptoms lasting more than one week.
- Even frontal sinusitis can be diagnosed by sinus ultrasound devices.

How to perform sinus ultrasound

- The probe should not cross the line between the outer corner of the eye and the mouth angle. The lower border of the probe should not cross the line level with the tip of the nose. Examining outside these boundaries may give false positive findings.
- The examination is started near the nose, with the lower border or the probe level with the tip of the nose. The probe is held in place while its axis is turned from one side to another so that the sound beam is certain to hit the posterior wall of the maxillary sinus perpendicularly. If the findings are negative, the position of the probe is changed until the entire allowed area has been examined.

Interpreting the results

- A single echo at least 3 cm from the baseline (back wall echo) is a clearly positive result.
- Multiple echoes near the baseline suggest thickened mucosal lining and are not diagnostic.
- Low echoes repeated with regular intervals are usually so called multiplied echoes. There is probably no fluid and the finding is interpreted as negative.

Sinus x-ray

If sinus ultrasound is available, the indications for sinus x-ray are as follows:

- An asymptomatic patient repeatedly has a positive ultrasound finding (the patient may, for example, have a cyst, which is worth knowing when later findings are interpreted).
- Suspicion of chronic sinusitis as the cause of asthmatic symptoms. The mucosal lining of the sinus may be thick and inflamed without fluid visible as an echo.
- Before sending the patient to specialized care.
- Multiple echoes (possibly suggesting a neoplasm) from some other location than only the lower part of the sinus.

If sinus ultrasound is not available, a sinus x-ray should be taken in the following cases:

- Sinusitis should be ruled out in order to avoid unnecessary antibiotics (particularly in patients with repeated antibiotic regimens on clinical grounds).
- The patient has high fever or his general condition is affected (if there is no opacity or fluid level in the maxillary sinus, a more serious bacterial infection should be suspected).
- Maxillary sinus puncture is planned, but an unnecessary procedure is to be avoided (if no imaging is available, the puncture can be performed on the basis of the clinical presentation).

References

1. Williams Jr JW, Aguilar C, Cornell J, Chiquette E. Dolor RJ, Makela M, Holleman DR, Simel DL. Antibiotics for acute maxillary sinusitis. Cochrane Database Syst Rev. 2004;(2): CD000243.
2. de Ferranti SD, Ioannidis JP, Lau J, Anninger WV, Barza M. Are amoxycillin and folater inhibitors as effective as other antibiotics for acute sinusitis? A meta-analysis. BMJ 1998;317: 632–637.
3. The Database of Abstracts of Reviews of Effectiveness (University of York), Database no.: DARE-989022. In: The Cochrane Library, Issue 2, 2000. Oxford: Update Software.
4. Varonen H, Mäkelä M, Savolainen S, Läärä E, Hilden J. Comparison of ultrasound, radiography, and clinical examination in the diagnosis of acute maxillary sinusitis: a systematic review. J Clin Epidemiol 2000;53(9):940–8.

5. Puhakka T, Mäkelä MJ, Alanen A, Kallio T, Korsoff L, Arstila P, Leinonen M, Pulkkinen M, Suonpää J, Mertsola J, Ruuskanen O. Sinusitis in the common cold. J Allergy Clin Immunol 1998;102(3):403–8.

38.31 Acute maxillary sinusitis

Jouko Suonpää

Principles

- Antibiotics or diagnostic imaging for diagnosing sinusitis is not indicated during the first 7 days of a common cold.
- Sinusitis is diagnosed by sinus ultrasound in adults and in children above 7 years of age.
- Antibiotics are indicated only for patients with fluid in the maxillary sinus.
- Sinusitis is recognized as a reason for the worsening of asthma symptoms.
- In recurring sinusitis search for a predisposing factor.

Definition and epidemiology

- Usually maxillary sinusitis is referred to as "sinusitis", although the infection may affect other sinuses too. In practice acute sinusitis is diagnosed when fluid retention is detected in the maxillary sinus of a symptomatic patient.
- Sinusitis is preceded by a viral upper respiratory tract infection. A common cold is complicated by sinusitis in less than 5% of cases.
- Allergic or vasomotor rhinitis and structural abnormalities predispose to sinusitis. Obstruction of the ostium and dysfunction of the cilia are the most important factors in pathophysiology.
- Because of developmental anatomy, a sinusitis can rarely be considered a disease entity in children below 3 years of age.

Symptoms

- Facial pain above the infected sinus
- Purulent nasal discharge
- Prolonged cough and rhinitis
- Headache
- Impaired sense of smell
- Often symptomless

Causes

- Haemophilus: 30–40%
- Pneumococci: about 20–30%
- Others: Moraxella, streptococci, viruses, anaerobes, other bacteria

Diagnosis

- Sinus ultrasound (38.30) is quite reliable in adults and children above 7 years of age, but performing the examination needs experience (31.11). Accuracy in the detection of acute fluid retention is at best 80–95%. Performing sinus ultrasound routinely before the decision to treat with antibiotics reduces the number of unnecessary antibiotic regimens. If no fluid is detected in a patient with symptoms suggesting sinusitis, do not prescribe antibiotics but ask the patient to return after a few days if the symptoms persist.
- In problematic cases an x-ray can be taken. A fluid level and clear sinuses are reliable findings. Mucosal swelling is common in children and may conceal fluid retention. The probability of retention is increased as the mucosal swelling becomes thicker.
- If no investigations are available, antibiotics can be prescribed to a patient with severe symptoms, or a diagnostic and therapeutic lavage can be performed. Another course of antibiotics should not be given without confirming the diagnosis.

Therapy

- The therapy of choice is an antibiotic regimen for 5–7 days. If the patient has severe pain or he has frequently recurring episodes of sinusitis, a lavage can be suggested at the first encounter.
- The preferable drugs are **A** [1 2 3]
  - amoxicillin 500–750 mg × 2 for adults, 40 mg/kg daily for children divided in two doses, or
  - penicillin V 2 million units × 2 for adults, 100 000 units/kg daily for children divided in two doses.
- Alternative drugs
  - doxycycline (some pneumococcal strains may be resistant.
  - macrolides **C** [4 5] (some strains of Haemophilus influenzae are resistant).
  - amoxicillin-clavulanic acid
  - cephalosporins
  - trimethoprim-sulphamethoxazole (only modest effect against pneumococci)
- Conservative therapy of the functional disturbance consists of local decongestants for a maximum of 7 days.
- Steroids are beneficial in recurring and chronic sinusitis **B** [6].
- Preparations containing pseudoephedrine and antihistamine can be used in addition.
- Flushing with saline brings subjective relief.
- The patient is asked to return if the symptoms persist after the antibiotic treatment. If there is fluid in the sinus according to sinus ultrasound or x-ray, a maxillary lavage can be performed.

Maxillary lavage

- 4% lidocaine solution is used for local anaesthesia. 2–3 drops of adrenaline (1:1000) are added for each 5 ml. The anaesthetic is placed under the concha inferior. Anaesthesia is sufficient after 20 minutes.

- The puncture is performed with a straight needle with a mandrin. The site of puncture is at the insertion of concha inferior 2–3 cm from the nasal orifice.
- Physiological, body-temperature saline solution is carefully injected into the sinus, from where it flows into the nasal cavity through the ostium. Strong resistance for the injection may be due to viscous mucus or obstruction of the ostium. Increasing the pressure with force may result in complications. Do not inject air into the sinus.

Follow-up

- If secretions are detected, the lavage can be repeated after one week and a specimen can be taken for bacterial culture. The presence of fluid should be confirmed by sinus ultrasound before the puncture.

Detecting predisposing factors in recurrent sinusitis

- Allergic rhinitis (history, nasal eosinophilia)
- Mucosal swelling, polyps, septum deviation (anterior rhinoscopy)
- Condition of the teeth (sinusitis of dental origin)
- Enlargement of the adenoids (snoring, oral breathing)

Indications for specialist consultation

- If treatment has not brought relief in 4–6 weeks.
- Children with persistent sinusitis after two antibiotic courses.
- Adults with more than 3 recurrences within 6 months, or a chronic sinusitis (persistent secretions despite 5 repeated lavages)
- Insertion of lavation tubes is a specialist procedure. The tubes should not be kept in place for more than 3 weeks. A new consultation is indicated in cases of persistent secretions.

Surgical treatment

Indications

- Recurrent acute sinusitis
- The decision to operate is based on diagnostic endoscopy and computed tomography of the sinuses.

The operation

- Endoscopic fenestration (FES): Inflamed mucosa is removed from the anterior ethmoid sinuses and the natural maxillary sinus orifice is widened.

Results

- Healing of the mucosa promotes ciliar activity and breaks the vicious circle.
- Sinusitis may recur even after FES.

Treatment of sinusitis after an operation

- Lavage under the concha inferior is not usually necessary, but prior surgery is no contraindication for this procedure.

References

1. Williams Jr JW, Aguilar C, Cornell J, Chiquette E. Dolor RJ, Makela M, Holleman DR, Simel DL. Antibiotics for acute maxillary sinusitis. Cochrane Database Syst Rev. 2004;(2): CD000243.
2. de Ferranti SD, Ioannidis JP, Lau J, Anninger WV, Barza M. Are amoxycillin and folater inhibitors as effective as other antibiotics for acute sinusitis? A meta-analysis. BMJ 1998;317:632–637.
3. The Database of Abstracts of Reviews of Effectiveness (University of York), Database no.: DARE-989022. In: The Cochrane Library, Issue 2, 2000. Oxford: Update Software.
4. Cooper BC, Mullins PR, Jones MR, Lang SDR. Clinical efficacy of roxithromycin in the treatment of adults with upper and lower respiratory tract infection due to Haemophilus influenzae: a meta-analysis of 12 clinical studies. Drug Investment 1994;7:299–314.
5. The Database of Abstracts of Reviews of Effectiveness (University of York), Database no.: DARE-953422. In: The Cochrane Library, Issue 4, 1999. Oxford: Update Software.
6. Dolor RJ, Witsell DL, Hellkamp AS, Williams JW, Califf RM, Simel DL for the Ceftin and Flonase for Sinusitis (CAFFS) Investigators. Comparison of cefuroxime with or without intranasal fluticasone for the treatment of rhinosinusitis. JAMA 2001;286:3097–3105.

38.32 Acute frontal sinusitis

Jouko Suonpää

Basic rule

- Identify acute frontal sinusitis, provide initial care, and identify patients needing immediate treatment.
- Fluid retention visible on x-ray strongly suggests frontal sinusitis, and clear sinuses rule out frontal sinusitis.
- If the sinuses are entirely opaque on the x-ray they may be interpreted as undeveloped. In such cases, clinical condition is decisive in choosing therapy.

Aetiology

- Frontal sinusitis is defined as retention of inflammatory secretions in the frontal sinuses.

- Frontal sinusitis usually follows an acute viral respiratory infection. About two thirds of the patients also have maxillary sinusitis.
- The infection spreads to the frontal sinus from the anterior ethmoidal sinuses through the nasofrontal duct. The narrow duct is easily obstructed by infection, allergy or other mucosal irritation.
- The most common causative agents include Streptococcus pneumoniae and Haemophilus influenzae.
- In children frontal sinuses are only formed at the age of 8–10 years.

Symptoms and diagnosis

- Frontal sinusitis should be suspected always if rhinitis or maxillary sinusitis is accompanied by a frontal headache.
- Other symptoms are similar to those of maxillary sinusitis.
- Morning headache and impairment of general condition are common in frontal sinusitis.
- The diagnosis cannot be made on the basis of symptoms or laboratory investigations alone.
- A fluid level in sinus x-rays is diagnostic. Clear frontal sinuses in x-ray rule out frontal sinusitis. In problematic cases an x-ray taken with the head tilted sideways helps to detect fluid.
- Ultrasonographically detected back wall echo is sufficient for diagnosis, but x-rays are also indicated if the symptoms persist for more than 3 days.
- In some patients the symptoms are severe. The risk of complications (meningitis, orbital abscess, etc.) is higher than in maxillary sinusitis. **Intensive headache, eyelid oedema, or meningism are signs of an incipient complication, and the patient should be referred immediately to a hospital.**

Treatment

- Remember appropriate therapy for maxillary sinusitis.
- Maxillary lavage helps to clear the medial conchal area and improves the evacuation of fluid from the frontal sinus.
- Antibacterial treatment is indicated for all patients. If the causative agent is not known the following drugs (in this order) are recommended: ampicillins, penicillin, tetracycline, trimethoprim-sulfamethoxazole, and cephalosporins.
- Decongestive nose drops should always be used as a part of conservative treatment. The maximum duration of treatment is 10 days.

Follow-up and further treatment

- If secretions are obtained in maxillary lavage, the procedure should be repeated after 2–3 days.
- If frontal headache continues and there is fluid retention in the frontal sinus the patient should be referred to a specialist clinic where the frontal sinus can be drained surgically.

38.33 Chronic sinusitis

Jouko Suonpää

Basic rule

- Identify patients with chronic sinusitis and select those who need treatment by an ENT specialist.

Definition and aetiology

- Sinusitis is defined as chronic if an acute infection is not cured by 1–2 months of active treatment.
- Probable causes of the condition include permanent changes in the partial pressures of gases in the sinuses resulting in enzyme imbalances in the mucosa and irreversible changes in the mucous membrane.
- There is no clear evidence that indoor air contaminants would cause chronic sinusitis.

Symptoms and diagnosis

- The symptoms of chronic sinusitis usually result from rhinitis and inflammation of the pharynx, larynx and bronchi caused by the sinusitis.
- Local pain may be present occasionally.
- Chronic frontal sinusitis may cause continuous pain and eyelid oedema.
- Headache and vertigo are common in chronic sphenoidal sinusitis.
- It is essential to differentiate chronic sinusitis with pus retention from that with mucosal oedema filling the sinuses. In the latter the secretions may be eliminated sufficiently, and surgical treatment is not indicated. Such mucosal thickening may be caused by allergy, however, unspecific mucosal irritation is a more common cause.
- Diagnostic methods in primary care are x-ray and sinus ultrasound of the sinuses, complemented by maxillary puncture in problematic cases.

Treatment

- Conservative treatment aims at opening the ostium, avoiding aggravating factors, and treating the symptoms.
- Intranasal steroids prompt recovery from an episode of acute rhinosinusitis in selected patients with recurrent or chronic sinusitis B [1].
- Surgical treatment aims at removing the anatomical problem causing retention of secretions, opening a drainage outlet, resecting inflamed mucosa or eliminating the whole sinus.
- Chronic sinusitis should be treated by a specialist, however, repeated lavations and continued follow-up are often delegated to primary care.

OTO

Reference

1. Dolor RJ, Witsell DL, Hellkamp AS, Williams JW, Califf RM, Simel DL for the Ceftin and Flonase for Sinusitis (CAFFS) Investigators. Comparison of cefuroxime with or without intranasal fluticasone for the treatment of rhinosinusitis. JAMA 2001;286:3097–3105.

38.35 Acute otitis media in adults

Hans Ramsay

Aetiology

- Usually no other cause can be found than Eustachian tube obstruction caused by an upper respiratory infection.
- Nasopharyngeal tumours, although rare, should be remembered as a possible cause of otitis media in adults. If the infection becomes prolonged the patient should be referred to an ENT specialist for ruling out a tumour.
- Barotrauma (38.41) leads to serous otitis media.
- Radiotherapy of the pharynx may result in Eustachian tube obstruction and acute otitis media.

Symptoms

- Ear pain and feeling of blockedness are typical symptoms.

Clinical signs

- The eardrum is opaque or cloudy and usually red.
- The mobility of the eardrum is impaired when examined with a pneumatic otoscope. Tympanometry **B** [1 2] or acoustic reflectometry (31.43) are reliable aids in diagnosis.

Treatment

- The most common causative bacteria in purulent otitis media are Streptococcus pneumoniae, Haemophilus influenzae, and Moraxella catarrhalis. Antibiotic treatment should be directed against these bacteria.
  - Penicillin V is the drug of choice: 2 million IU × 2 for one week.
  - Alternative drugs include amoxicillin 750 mg × 2 or 500 mg × 3, amoxicillin-clavulanic acid, trimethoprim-sulfamethoxazole, second-generation cephalosporins or macrolides.
- Complications are rare. Tympanocentesis can be performed on the first encounter if the patient has severe pain. Tympanocentesis is usually indicated in prolonged or severe otitis media.
- Serous otitis media caused by barotrauma can be treated with vasoconstrictor drugs and by aeration of the middle ear (38.41) and, if necessary, by tympanocentesis. Antibiotics are indicated only if a secondary infection is suspected.

Follow-up

- No routine follow-up visits are indicated in adult patients. The patient is asked to contact the doctor if the ear feels blocked or is paroxysmally painful after 3–4 weeks.

References

1. van Balen FAM, de Melker RA. Validation of a portable tympanometer for use in primary care. Int J Pediatr Otorhinolaryngol 1994;29:219–25.
2. Koivunen P, Alho O-P, Uhari M, Niemelä M, Luotonen J. Minitympanometry in detecting middle ear fluid. J Pediatr 1997;131:419–22.

38.36 Chronic otitis media

Hans Ramsay

Basic rules

- Patients with a cholesteatoma or chronic perforation should be referred to an ENT specialist. Elderly patients and those whose general condition is poor can be treated conservatively.
- Adequate local treatment should be provided while the patient is waiting for the appointment with the ENT specialist.

Definition

- The patient is considered to have chronic otitis media if the infection has lasted for more than 2 months. The activity of the infection may vary and the infection may even subside, but a permanent injury or functional impairment may result.

Active chronic otitis media

- A yellowish or greenish discharge through a permanent perforation in the tympanic membrane.
- The middle ear can be seen through the perforation as wet and glistening, or there is profuse discharge requiring several daily changes of cotton wool tampons in the ear canal.

Cholesteatoma

- The keratinized epithelium of the ear canal and tympanic membrane grows into the middle ear and into the mastoid bone resulting in an osteolytic, tumour-like process.

Causative bacteria

- The bacteria are different than in acute otitis media, and several species can be isolated simultaneously.
- The prevailing bacteria are Pseudomonas aeruginosa (greenish sweet-smelling discharge) and Staphylococcus aureus. Proteus species, Klebsiella, E. coli and many other aerobic bacteria are also common. In one third of cases anaerobic bacteria are also detected (bad odour).

Symptoms and signs

- A perforation in the Shrapnell's membrane is almost invariably a sign of a cholesteatoma.
- A marginal perforation of the pars tensa also signifies a cholesteatoma, and a keratinized mass can often be seen in the tympanic cavity. If the ear is rinsed with saline, a white sediment (keratin from the cholesteatoma) is often visible in the out coming fluid.
- The ear can be further examined at a specialized clinic by computed tomography.

Conservative treatment of chronic otitis media

- The appearance of the tympanic membrane is important in the assessment of the disease.
  - If the ear is dry and a central perforation in the pars tensa is present, no treatment is indicated. Myringoplasty should be planned later.
  - If the ear is dry but a perforation is seen in the Shrapnell's membrane the patient most probably has a cholesteatoma and an operation is indicated.

Treatment of an ear with discharge

First consultation

1. If there is discharge from the ear take a bacterial culture. If antibiotics have already been administered also take a fungal culture, because yeasts, Candida, Penicillium, or Aspergillus may be present, and further antibiotic treatment makes the symptoms worse.
2. Rinse the ear with sterile, 37°C saline, dry the ear canal with a piece of cotton wool, and record the status of the tympanic membrane.
3. Rinsing and drying is essential before installation of drugs. If suction is used remember the possibility of a caloric reaction caused by flowing cold air, and discontinue the suction immediately if the patient has vertigo.
4. Before the antibiotic resistance assay has been performed, preferably use antibiotic-free eardrops. If the process is in the Shrapnell's membrane, 3% borate solution or 1–2% acetic acid spirit solution are recommended. If the middle ear mucosa is widely exposed do not use surgical spirit stronger than 50%. Alternatively, other non-ototoxic drops (a combination of local antiseptics and corticosteroids) can be used (4–5 drops 3 times a day). Warm the bottle by keeping it in the palm before administration of the drops to avoid vertigo caused by the caloric reaction. During the administration the patient should lie for 5 minutes with the ear upwards. Thereafter excess fluid is allowed to flow out into a piece of cotton wool at the ear canal orifice.
5. Systemic antimicrobials are indicated only in patients with temporary discharge from the ear during an upper respiratory infection or if the discharge has become more profuse than before. The antibiotics are the same as for acute otitis media.

Second and third consultation

- The second consultation after about 10 days may show that the ear is already dry.
- Repeat clinical examination, as the disappearance of the swelling may result in altered findings.
- If there is still discharge, rinse the ear with saline.
- At this stage antibiotic drops (not systemic antibiotics) can be prescribed according to the result of the antibiotic resistance test (A) [1].
  - Antibiotic drops, particularly those containing aminoglycosides (e.g. neomycin, gentamicin, framycetin) may cause cochlear injury in addition to their tendency to sensitize the skin of the ear canal.
  - Ototoxicity need not be considered in the treatment of a profusely discharging ear because the swollen mucous membrane near the round window prevents contact of the drug with the membrane and absorption into the cochlea.
- If fungal culture is positive, fungicides can be administered in the ear (e.g. 3% borate spirit or 1–2% acetic acid diluted in spirit). Corticosteroid drops should be avoided in fungal otitis. The ear canal and the tympanic membrane can be wiped with a piece of cotton wool moistened with 0.5–1% methyl rose solution.
- After the third consultation the patient should be referred to a specialist for eventual surgery. Conservative treatment should be continued if necessary until the operation is performed.

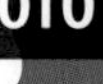

Reference

1. Acuin J, Smith A, Mackenzie I. Interventions for chronic suppurative otitis media. Cochrane Database Syst Rev. 2004;(2): CD000473.

38.37 Otitis externa

Jukka Luotonen

Basic rules

- Use effective local medication.
- Inform the patient about factors causing or exacerbating the condition.
- Consider malignancies and malignant external otitis as a cause of prolonged inflammation.

Predisposing factors

- Avoid incubating water in the ear canal (acute diffuse external otitis is common in summer).
- A hot and humid climate
- Atopy and other allergies, seborrhoeic eczema and other skin diseases, some systemic diseases (diabetes), and some psychosocial problems
- Chronic and sometimes acute otitis media
- External otitis may also be associated with some skin infections such as erysipelas and herpes zoster.

Investigations

History

- Duration and earlier recurrences of the symptoms
- Self-manipulation of the ear canal preceding the symptoms, other injuries, and water in the ear canal.
- Allergies and other skin diseases as well as systemic diseases should be enquired about.
- Medicines and cosmetic preparations applied in the ear or its surroundings can be the cause of external otitis.

Clinical findings

- In acute otitis externa the skin of the ear canal is red, moist, swollen, and very tender. Sometimes a small abscess is present in the outer part of the ear canal. The tympanic membrane may not be visible at all because of massive swelling of the ear canal skin.
- In chronic inflammation the skin of the ear canal is not tender but itching is the main symptom. The skin is thickened and scaly.

Clinical examination

1. Clean the ear canal: possible foreign bodies, scaling, and secretions should be removed mechanically with care.
2. Rinse the ear canal with hand-warm saline (not in a perforated ear) and dry it with suction or cotton wool.
3. Examine the tympanic membrane to detect chronic or acute otitis media. A pneumatic otoscope is necessary. Also tuning fork tests are often useful.

Laboratory and radiological investigations

- Differentiation between acute, fulminant otitis externa and mastoiditis may be difficult.
- In acute infection, gram-positive cocci are usually predominant. Gram-negative rods and sometimes fungi are also detected in chronic infection. In fungal otitis externa the ear canal may seem mouldy and be covered by a grey membrane. Bacterial or fungal cultures are only indicated in prolonged, chronic cases.

Treatment

- Thorough and frequent cleaning of the ear canal (rinsing with saline and drying thereafter) is the most important treatment for otitis externa.
- An ethanol-water (30/70) solution can be used to rinse a seborrhoeic ear canal.
- A severely swollen ear canal is treated with a gauge tampon infiltrated with a topical preparation. An antibiotic-steroid-solution or 3% borate in spirit are suitable (C) [1].
- If no tampon is needed, topical eardrops are prescribed.
- An abscess in the ear canal can be incised, for example with a tympanocentesis lancet using topical lidocaine/prilocaine (e.g. Emla®) as an anaesthetic.

Topical medication

- Topical preparations should be selected according to common dermatological principles: wet for acute inflammation, greasy for chronic inflammation. A low pH value of the ointment is beneficial.
- The preparations used should be as simple as possible to avoid contact allergy. Topical neomycin and bacitracin should especially be avoided.
- Topical antifungal preparations should only be used in confirmed fungal infections.
- A local corticosteroid preparation is the best treatment for itching and swelling of the ear canal skin.

Systemic drugs

- NSAIDs can be used in acute inflammation.
- Systemic antimicrobials are usually not indicated.

Recurrent or chronic external otitis

- Advise the patient to avoid manipulating his/her ear canals.
- Prescribe a corticosteroid ointment or liniment for alleviating the itch.
- Water should be avoided (showering or swimming without protection of the ear canal). Patients with frequent recurrences of otitis externa should always avoid water in the ear canal.

Indications for specialist consultation

- Chronic or recurrent otitis externa despite microbiological investigations and therapeutic trials.
- Granulation tissue in the ear canal may be a sign of malignant otitis externa.
- Unilateral otitis externa in the elderly may be a symptom of a malignant tumour. Refer the patient to a specialist if the response to treatment is poor.

Reference

1. Hirsch BE. Infection of the external ear. Am J Otolaryngol 1992;13:145–55.

38.38 Acute mastoiditis

Hans Ramsay

Basic rule

- Refer patients with a retroauricular or neck abscess associated with otitis media to hospital as emergencies.

Symptoms

- Purulent otitis media predisposes to mastoiditis.
- The clinical picture consists of
  - high fever
  - marked tenderness of the ear and tenderness on percussion of the retroauricular area
  - impaired general condition.
- If antibiotics are administered the disease may be milder but results in secretory or chronic otitis media with discharge.

Investigations

- Laboratory findings
  - Marked leucocytosis
  - Increased ESR and CRP
- A normal x-ray shows clear septa between the cavi of the mastoid bone, and the air in the cavi is dark. In mastoiditis the septa are poorly visible and the cavi are shaded. An x-ray interpreted normal by a radiologist practically excludes mastoiditis in a patient above 3 years of age.

Differential diagnosis

- Otitis externa with swelling of the outer auditory canal. The symptoms are not as severe as in mastoiditis, the results of the laboratory tests are only slightly abnormal, and the mastoid x-ray is normal.
- If a patient has lymphadenitis of the neck, always examine the ears.

Treatment

- Refer the patient to a specialist unit without delay. If treatment with antibiotics (e.g. cefuroxim) is not successful within 1–2 days, mastoidectomy should be performed.
- Tympanocentesis is indicated to evacuate infectious secretions, to relieve the pressure, and to prevent necrosis of the tympanic membrane.
  - Take a sample for bacterial culture from the aspirate to identify the cause of infection.

38.40 Injuries of the auricle

Jukka Luotonen

Basic rules

- Treat the injury so that
  - the cosmetic result is satisfactory
  - no functional harm remains (in users of spectacles and hearing aids).

Principles of treatment

- Strictly aseptic techniques should be used in the treatment of injuries.
- If cartilage or a perichondrium is exposed it should be covered with skin. Save as much skin as possible.

Types of injury

- Small clean incision wounds can be sutured with a 5–0 monofilament thread. In small wounds the cartilage is supported by the skin, in large wounds the cartilage must sometimes be sutured with a 4–0 resorbable thread.
- Contusions and contaminated incision wounds must first be cleaned mechanically and then rinsed with saline. If parts of the auricle have to be excised this is best performed by a wedged incision so that the sharp edge of the wedge is directed towards the centre of the auricle. When the margins of the incision are sutured together the auricle remains in its original shape but becomes smaller. More skin can be transplanted on the auricle using a pedunculated flap.

- A totally detached auricle must not be disposed of. Replantation may be successful, or at least the cartilage can be transplanted under the skin for reconstructive surgery to be performed later in a specialized hospital.

Further treatment

- After suturation the auricle is supported in its natural position with cotton wool and dressings.
- Prophylactic antibiotics are indicated in contaminated wounds (betalactamase-resistant penicillins, first-generation cephalosporins).
- Make sure that the patient has been vaccinated against tetanus.
- Skin sutures can be moved after 5 days.

Haematoma

- A blunt wound may cause a haematoma between the cartilage and the perichondrium. A fluctuating, non-tender mass can be felt in the auricle.
- Evacuate the haematoma aseptically by aspirating with a needle and a syringe. After the procedure apply a compressive, well-aligned dressing. Sometimes the aspiration must be repeated several times over the next few days.
- An old haematoma that cannot be aspirated with a needle and a syringe can be evacuated through a small incision (aseptically).
- An untreated auricular haematoma results in deformation of the cartilage and the whole auricle.

Frostbite and burns

- There is no specific treatment for frostbite of the auricle. Secondary infection should be prevented by aseptics and prophylactic antibiotics, if necessary. Mild frostbite tends to heal spontaneously. Severe frostbite may result in auricle necrosis that requires resection of a part of the auricle (in a specialized hospital).
- Burns should be treated according to the same principles as burns elsewhere.

Perichondritis of the auricle

- Infection can result from injuries to the external ear.
- Severe pain is the first symptom. After a few hours the skin over the inflamed area becomes red, tender, and swollen. Pus accumulates between the perichondrium and the cartilage.
- The condition must be treated surgically and antibiotics should be administered intravenously in a specialized hospital.
- If left untreated the infection may result in widespread destruction of the cartilage and a severe deformity of the auricle.

38.41 Barotitis and barotrauma

Editors

Mechanism

- As atmospheric pressure decreases (e.g. when an aircraft takes off) the higher pressure in the middle ear usually passes out through the Eustachian tube.
- As the pressure increases (e.g. when an aircraft is landing) swallowing and manoeuvres to decrease pressure (see below) allow the air to flow into the middle ear.
- If the pressure gradient between the outer air and the middle ear is greater than 80 mmHg the Eustachian tube does not open. Barotitis or barotrauma results.
- Factors predisposing to the development of barotitis include
  - respiratory tract infection
  - allergic or chronic rhinitis
  - nasal septum deviation
  - sinusitis
  - adenoid hyperplasia.

Symptoms

- Feeling of blocked ears, humming, and sometimes mild vertigo
- Ear pain (present when the pressure difference is more than 60 mmHg)
- Severe pain and rupture of the tympanic membrane, which alleviates the pain to some extent. Bloody discharge may be visible from the ear.

Findings

- Retracted, stiff, or poorly mobile tympanic membrane
- Clear fluid in the middle ear
- Redness of the shaft of the malleus and small petechiae on the tympanic membrane
- If there is a perforation it is usually situated in the anterior part of the pars tensa.

Prophylaxis

- Manoeuvres to distribute the pressure evenly
  - Swallowing with the nose and mouth closed
  - Valsalva's manoeuvre: increase the pressure in the nasopharynx by forced expiration with the nose and mouth closed.
- Nasal decongestants applied locally before landing starts and during landing
- A combination of antihistamine and sympathomimetic may be effective.

Treatment

- Constricting the nasal and Eustachian tube mucosa with decongestant drops or spray
- The patient opens the Eustachian tube with a nasal balloon (31.44).
- The patient uses a Politzer balloon.
- If symptomatic treatment does not help in a couple of days and the symptoms are annoying, tympanocentesis should be considered. If necessary, consult a specialist.

38.42 Noise-induced hearing loss

Seppo Savolainen

Noise as the cause of hearing loss

- Long-term exposure to noise can cause chronic cochlear-type hearing loss.
- Sudden exposure to extensive noise (such as a percussion drilling machine, gunshot, explosion, fireworks, music etc.) can cause mechanical injury to the middle or inner ear.
- The incidence of noise-induced hearing loss may be reduced by providing information about the harmful effects of noise and by advocating the use of hearing protectors (earmuffs).

Decibel scale

- The energy of noise intensity (decibels) = 10 × log I/i where
  - I = observed noise intensity
  - i = default comparison intensity (0 decibels): average hearing threshold that has been agreed upon internationally (20 micropascals = 20 μPa).
- A 3-decibel increase in noise intensity corresponds to a doubling of the noise energy.

Safe exposure times (steady noise)

- See Table 38.42.1
- The safe noise exposure limit for steady noise is considered to be a sound pressure level of 85 dB (A). Exposure to impulse noise must not exceed 140 dB (A) peak sound pressure level.

Table 38.42.1 Safe noise exposure times

Maximum noise intensity dB (A)	Safe daily exposure time
85	8 hours
88	4 hours
91	2 hours
94	1 hour
97	30 min
100	15 min
106	4 min
112	1 min
115	Less than 30 seconds

Clinical picture

- A temporary threshold shift is a physiological protective mechanism. If after an 8-hour working day the full recovery of hearing takes longer than 16 hours, a permanent threshold shift may be anticipated. A temporary hearing loss appears over the same frequency range (around 3000–6000 Hz) as do the first signs of permanent noise injury.
- Chronic noise-induced hearing loss is cochlear-type and usually symmetrical. The decrease (a dip) in hearing starts at 4000 Hz and advances to the speech frequency range (500–2000 Hz).
  - The most important differential diagnoses include presbyacusis and congenital hearing defects.
  - The diagnosis of noise-induced injury is based on demonstration of exposure to noise and a plausible correlation between the level of noise exposure and the severity of the injury.

Health check-ups

- Health check-ups are indicated if the safe noise levels and exposure times described above are exceeded.
- The purpose of a pre-employment check-up is to identify workers who have pre-existing hearing injury or who are not suitable for work involving noise exposure. Decisions on unsuitability must be based on evaluation by an ENT specialist.
- At the pre-employment check-up the hearing thresholds are determined covering the whole frequency range of the audiometer (250–500–1000–2000–3000–4000–6000–8000 Hz).
- Periodical check-ups are performed annually for the first 4 years of noise exposure, and thereafter once every three years. The purpose of the frequent early check-ups in the beginning is to identify persons who are particularly inclined to suffer from noise injury.
- The periodical check-ups consist of a screening examination where the hearing threshold is examined at the screening level of 20 dB. According to the screening results the workers are divided into hearing categories.

Hearing categories

- See Table 38.42.2.
- Hearing threshold is determined separately for both ears. The threshold of the worse ear determines the hearing category. The categories can be reported separately for both ears.

Table 38.42.2 Hearing categories

Hearing category	Hearing threshold [1)]
I	20 dB or better in both ears over all frequencies. If one of these criteria is not fulfilled the actual thresholds should be determined over all frequencies.
II	20 dB or better over speech frequency (0.5–1–2 kHz), up to 40 dB at 3 kHz and up to 65 dB at 4 kHz.
III	Hearing impairment over speech frequency, but average threshold better than 20 dB or threshold exceeds 40 dB at 3 kHz or 65 dB at 4 kHz.
IV	Average hearing threshold over speech frequency 20 dB or worse.

[1)] Hearing threshold is determined separately for both ears. The threshold of the worse ear determines the hearing category. The categories can be reported separately for both ears.

Prophylaxis and prognosis

- The aim is to prevent the development of hearing impairment that hampers speech recognition.
- Information supplied to workers regarding the risks associated with noise at work is of utmost importance.
- Noise levels can be reduced by technical means.
- Hearing protectors can be used as additional protection.
  - Instruction in the correct use of hearing protectors will increase their efficacy.
- The progression of noise injury stops when noise exposure is withdrawn.

38.43 Fracture of the nose

Jouko Suonpää

Basic rules

- Repair a nose fracture by immediate reposition (within one week of the accident at the latest).
- Refer patients with associated fractures of other facial bones or unsuccessful repositioning after several attempts.

Clinical examination

- Palpation and inspection are the most important examinations.
- Possible oedema can be reduced by squeezing the nose for a while.
- Suspect a fracture if the nose is swollen or dislocated, there is blood in the nostrils, or a crepitation is felt. The upper meatus is often obstructed.
- The diagnosis is made difficult by
  - swelling
  - earlier fractures or distortions
  - old deviations of the nasal septum.

Treatment

- Fractures confined to the outer nasal pyramid can be treated in ambulatory care.
- Local anaesthesia is necessary for repositioning. The same anaesthetic can be used as for maxillary puncture (38.31). A piece of cotton wool soaked with the anaesthetic is inserted in the upper meatus, and another in the meatus between the inferior and medial conchae. Both gauzes should be placed as posteriorly as possible. The anaesthesia is completed by infiltration anaesthesia on the sides and back of the nose with 1% lidocaine.
- A slightly curved elevator or a special instrument, the Walsham forceps, can be used for repositioning. The purpose of the repositioning is to detach the fragments from each other. This is usually best accomplished by pushing the nose in the direction of the dislocation. After the fragments have been mobilized with the elevator they can be lifted into place keeping the fingers on the nose to control the procedure.
- The position is usually maintained by the periosteum holding the fragments in place. External fixation by tape on the nose secures the position.
- A fracture in the base of the nasal bone usually requires surgical correction. The fracture is seen as an impression at the base of the nose.
- If fractures of the cartilaginous parts of the nose are present the patient should be referred.
- X-rays are not always indicated in isolated nasal fractures. The repositioning can be performed on the basis of the clinical presentation. A crepitation is the most reliable sign of a fracture.
- Small fractures of the tip of the nasal bone need not be repaired if there is no distortion of the shape of the nose.

38.44 Foreign body in the ear canal

Jukka Luotonen

- Foreign bodies in the ear canal are usually found in children. In adults a piece of cotton wool or an instrument used for cleaning the ear can sometimes be found.
- A foreign body left in the ear canal for a long time causes local inflammation that makes removal difficult. (This is particularly the case with parts of plants that swell when absorbing moisture.)

Removal of a foreign body

- Small foreign bodies can be easily removed with an ear forceps, small alligator forceps or suction.
- A foreign body next to the eardrum is best removed by rinsing.
- Living insects are the most annoying foreign bodies. Water or cooking oil can be dropped into the ear canal as first aid.
- Large foreign bodies can often be pulled out with an ear sound with a twisted tip that is passed behind the foreign body carefully protecting the sensitive skin of the ear canal. The procedure may be painful.
- If removal seems difficult it can be left to an ENT specialist who uses local or (for children sometimes) general anaesthesia.

Aftercare

- After the removal of a foreign body the skin of the ear canal is often irritated or injured. Spontaneous healing in a few days is the rule.
- If the skin is infected, a few days' treatment with eardrops containing a disinfectant and a corticosteroid is indicated.
- If the skin has been rolled out from the bony ear canal it should be set in place with a tampon containing an antibiotic cream.
- In cases of skin injury a follow-up examination is indicated after one week.

38.45 Foreign body in the nose

Erkki Virolainen

Basic rules

- Typical foreign bodies in the nose include pearls, plastic toy parts, coins, peas, nuts and pieces of rubber or foam rubber.
- Water-absorbing foreign bodies swell in the nose. Adjacent mucous membranes become irritated and swollen. The swollen mucosa and increased secretions retain the foreign body in place.
- Foreign bodies are usually located between the upper and middle conchae, rarely on the bottom of the nasal meatus.

Symptoms

- Unilateral obstruction
- Purulent and often foul-smelling secretions

Diagnosis

- Clinical examination is usually sufficient. X-rays are indicated in problematic cases. Remember radiolucent foreign bodies.

Differential diagnosis

- Sinusitis
- Acute or chronic rhinitis
- Nasal tumours

Treatment

- Parent's kiss (using mouth-to-mouth blowing with the child's other nostril pressed closed by parent's finger) appears to be safe and effective in removing nasal foreign bodies in children (B). It is successful in approximately 80% of cases.
- If the foreign body cannot be removed by blowing, local anesthesia is needed.
- Apply a cotton wool soaked with lidocaine-adrenalin solution to shrink the nasal mucous membrane. This reduces pain and swelling and makes the removal easier.
- After local anaesthesia and removal of secretions by suction, the foreign body is best removed by suction, with an ear probe, or small forceps. Pieces of foam rubber may be difficult to distinguish from surrounding secretions. When removing hard foreign bodies the probe should be passed behind it, and then pulled back with the foreign body. Getting a good hold of, for example, a pearl can be difficult.
- In adults, pushing a foreign body into the pharynx is usually safe, but this should be avoided in children.

38.46 Epistaxis

Henrik Malmberg

OTO

Basic rules

- Identify the site of bleeding and stop the bleeding.
- Identify the cause of bleeding by taking a good history.
- Assess the need for further investigations.

Causes and diagnostic assessment

- Dry mucosa of the anterior part of the nasal cavity
- Injuries: nose fracture, contusion, manipulation by finger
- Respiratory tract infections (particularly in children)
- Drugs predisposing to bleeding (aspirin, sometimes other NSAIDs, anticoagulants)

- ♦ Hypertension (remember to measure blood pressure!)
- ♦ Atherosclerosis and advanced age
- ♦ Rarely bleeding disorders, haematological diseases (that should be suspected if the patient has petechiae, other bleedings, or the bleeding is very difficult to control)

Recurrent or chronic epistaxis

- ♦ Consider
  - a foreign body in children
  - a tumour in the elderly, particularly if there is unilateral bloody discharge from the nose.

Initial examination and treatment

1. Clean the nose: remove tampons, use suction or ask the patient to blow out the clots.
2. Identify the site of bleeding by anterior rhinoscopy: from which side does the bleeding originate; is the site of bleeding the nasal septum (Locus Kiesselbach), the upper part of the nose or lower posterior part of the nose.
3. Constrict the mucous membranes with an anaesthetic-vasoconstrictor solution (lidocaine 4 mg/ml with adrenalin 1:1000 three drops per 5 ml of the solution)
   - Soak a piece of cotton wool with the solution
   - Place the piece on the supposed site of bleeding for about 3 minutes.
   - If the bleeding is profuse soak a tampon with the same solution and insert it in the bleeding nostril.
4. If the bleeding site is visible as a small pinhead-like clot (or at least the superficial feeding vessels) cauterize it with a pearl of silver nitrate (first choice), or alternatively, chromium trioxide or electrocauterization.
   - To prepare a pearl of silver nitrate, heat one end of a metal stick and touch (a piece) a powder of silver nitrate so that it adheres to the stick. Place the stick in a flame so that the silver nitrate melts and forms a droplet. Let the droplet cool in the air.
   - Apply the silver nitrate pearl on the site of bleeding so that a pale coagulated area 2–4 mm in diameter appears. The surroundings must be immediately rinsed with 0.9% saline applied repeatedly with a piece of cotton wool. Finally the nose is dried gently with dry cotton wool.
5. If the bleeding site cannot be seen and the bleeding has stopped, and if the bleeding has not been profuse, insertion of a tampon is not necessary. Provide the patient with written instructions on what to do if the bleeding recurs.
   - If the bleeding continues or it was profuse insert an anterior tampon.
     - ◘ Apply lidocaine-adrenalin solution locally (see above).
     - ◘ Soak a long gauze tampon with 0.9% saline or tranexamic acid solution, and lubricate the gauze with white Vaseline. The length of the narrow gauze should be at least 50 cm.
     - ◘ Tamponate the nostril by filling the posterior and upper parts first under visual control using a nasal speculum. Finally, fill the anterior part of the nose.
     - ◘ Leave the tampon in place for at least one day (maximum 3 days). Remove the tampon gradually by pulling as much as can be easily detached. If there is bleeding cut the tampon and insert the end into the nostril to continue with extraction later.
   - Alternatively, pieces of gelatin (e.g. Spongostan®) can be inserted into the nostril. The gelatin is usually resolved or removed by itself.
6. Posterior tamponation should be performed if the bleeding does not stop with anterior tamponation.
   - Apply lidocaine-adrenalin solution (see above).
   - As an alternative to the traditional gauze tampon (not explained here) a ready-made silicon tampon with two separate air-inflatable balloons can be used (a Foley urine catheter can be used if a nasal silicon tampon is not available).
     - ◘ Insert the empty tampon into the nose so that the tip is visible in the posterior pharynx.
     - ◘ The posterior balloon is filled with a specified amount of air (usually about 10 cc) and pulled into the choanal opening. Thereafter fill the anterior balloon with a sufficient amount of air so that it aligns in the nostril tightly. If a Foley catheter is used, insert anterior tamponation and tie the catether in front of it.
     - ◘ Leave the tampon in place for 2–4 days. The patient must always be treated in a hospital.
     - ◘ Penicillin V or erythromycin for 4–5 days is given as antibiotic prophylaxis.
7. Determine blood haemoglobin (haematocrit) if bleeding has been profuse.

Home instructions for patients

1. Calm down.
2. Sit leaning forward so that you do not swallow the blood.
3. Blow out clots from your nose and close the bleeding nostril by pressing your nose from the side for at least 5 minutes. Take the pressing finger off slowly.
4. Place a cold package on your neck or forehead.
5. If the bleeding has not stopped in 5 minutes, blow your nose again and put a piece of cotton wool in the bleeding nostril. Press the nostril from the side again, this time for 15 minutes. If the bleeding does not stop contact a doctor. When you go to see a doctor you should sit (in the car), not lie down.

Indications for specialist consultation

Immediate referral

- ♦ The bleeding cannot be stopped by tamponation. Infuse physiological saline during transportation if the bleeding has been profuse or prolonged. Place the patient in a sitting position or on his/her side to prevent the blood from being swallowed.
- ♦ If a patient with a posterior tampon cannot be followed up in a primary care hospital, refer him to a specialist unit.

Elective referral

- The bleeding recurs persistently despite local treatment (rare causes such as tumours should be ruled out).

38.50 Allergic rhinitis

Pirkko Ruoppi

Aims

- Identification of atopic allergic rhinitis (Table 38.50.1)
- Identification and treatment other causes of rhinitis than allergy and aggravating factors (polyps, septum deformation, adenoids in children, etc).
- Instructions to patients with allergic rhinitis on how to minimize exposure to allergens.
- Identification of non-specific irritants in ambient air (smoking, dusts, fumes) in the patient's environment.
- Evaluation of the need for special investigations (occupational rhinitis, planning of immunotherapy).
- Choosing and implementing the treatment (medication, immunotherapy).

Epidemiology

- About 15% of adults in Western Europe have atopic IgE-mediated rhinitis. In about 10% of them the rhinitis is caused by pollen allergy. Additionally, about 10% of adults have non-allergic hypersensitivity rhinitis, which means that about 25% of the adult population has sometimes in their life suffered from hypersensitivity rhinitis.

Investigations

- Carefully compiled patient history (a questionnaire). Sinus x-ray, particularly if the symptoms have continued for long (months, years).
- Rhinoscopy with topical decongestion of the nasal mucosa (on first visit a thorough ENT examination is indicated).
- Possibly also nasal smears/eosinophil count in smear (particularly if the symptoms are perennial)
- RAST and skin prick tests, if available.

Further investigations

- Referral to a specialist in allergology is necessary when
  - occupational rhinitis is suspected
  - immunotherapy is considered
  - the patient has therapy-resistant rhinitis.

ARIA guidelines

- ARIA (Allergic rhinitis and its impact on asthma) guidelines, which have been drafted by an expert panel together with WHO, are research and treatment guidelines for general practitioners and specialists (http://www.whiar.com). The emphasis is on the concept "one airway, one disease". The main message of the working group is that the connection and inter-relatedness of rhinitis and asthma symptoms must be kept in mind and that examinations and treatment should be combined, when possible. The ARIA classification of rhinitis (Figure 38.50.1), has been defined on the basis of the duration of the symptoms and their impact on quality of life.

Treatment

- Careful removal of allergens (pets, house dust) is the basic action in all forms of allergic rhinitis (C) [1].
- Antihistamines are effective for sneezing and nasal discharge in atopic rhinitis. Adding a sympathomimetic will give relief also from stuffiness.
- Local steroids are effective against all symptoms of allergic rhinitis and they are the only drugs that significantly diminish the growth of polyps (A) [2 3].
- Cromones show some effect against all symptoms of allergic rhinitis, but their efficacy is clearly weaker than that of corticosteroids.
- Antileukotrienes have been recently introduced to relieve all symptoms of allergic rhinitis.

Table 38.50.1 Symptoms and findings in different forms of hypersensitivity rhinitis.

	Allergic rhinitis	Non-allergic rhinitis	
		Eosinophilic	Non-eosinophilic (vasomotor)
Genetic predisposition	Yes (tendency for atopy)	No	No
Age at onset	Childhood	Middle-age (30–50 yrs)	Middle-age (often > 40 yrs)
Occurrence of symptoms	Seasonal, may also be perennial	Perennial	Perennial
Asthma	In about 20%	In 30–40%	Rare
Polyps	Occasionally	Often	Rarely
Prick/RAST tests positive	Yes	No	No
Secretory eosinophilia	Often	In all patients at some point (diagnostic criterion)	No

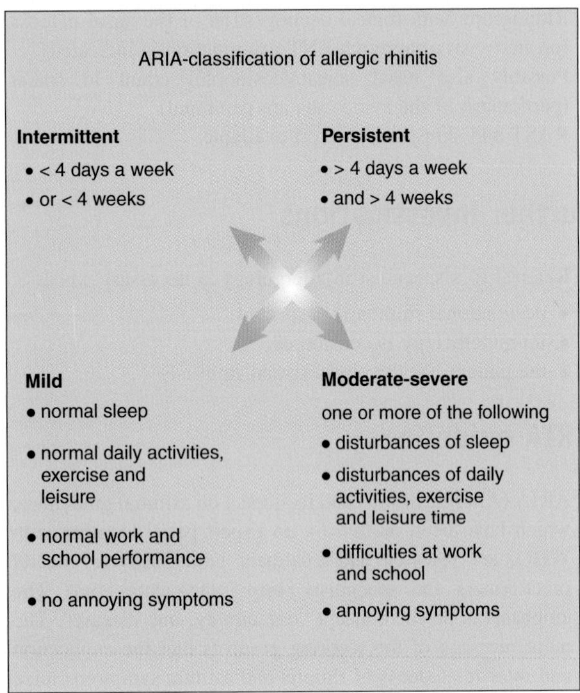

Figure 38.50.1 ARIA-classification of allergic rhinitis

- Immunotherapy (hyposensitization, desensitization) (14.9) is mainly for pollen-induced rhinitis. A specialist designs the course of the therapy. A general practitioner can administer the therapy to an adult patient in co-operation a specialists.

Drug treatment

Seasonal rhinitis

- Antihistamines alone may suffice as long as pollen counts remain low. They should be used as a complement to topical therapy for pollen allergy (local steroids) when need arises. Local antihistamines, levocabastine and azelastine are an alternative to tablets. Antihistamines are also available as eyedrops.
- Local steroids are most effective against nasal symptoms when treatment is started before and continued through the pollen season. Patients can regulate the dosage depending on exposure (pollen count) and symptoms. Local steroids are recommended to consider in moderate and severe intermittent and even in mild persistent symptoms (ARIA classification).
- Cromone treatment is also commenced before the pollen season and onset of symptoms. In addition to nasal spray eye drops are also available. The treatment is continued through the pollen season.

Perennial rhinitis

- Local steroids can be used either intermittently or continuously (for example in patients with nasal polyps). The starting dose is generally two sprays daily (in the evening) in both nostrils. The maintenance dose is usually smaller, e.g. one spray every or every other day in both nostrils.
- Antihistamines can be used as needed for sneezing and nasal discharge, and concomitantly with a sympathomimetic drug to relieve mild stuffiness of the nose.
- Cromones can be used preventively to alleviate symptoms caused by house dust, for example before cleaning the house.

NARES (non-allergic rhinitis with eosinophilia syndrome)

- Antihistamines, local steroids and other drugs used in allergic rhinitis are effective in this type of hypersensitivity rhinitis.

Vasomotor rhinitis

- An anticholinergic agent, ipratropiumbromide, is effective for nasal discharge. Antihistamines combined with sympathomimetic drugs may also relieve symptoms.

References

1. Sheikh A, Hurwitz B. House dust mite avoidance measures for perennial allergic rhinitis. Cochrane Database Syst Rev. 2004;(2):CD001563.
2. Weiner JM, Abramson MJ, Puy RM. Intranasal corticosteroids versus oral H1 receptor antagonists in allergic rhinitis: systematic review of randomised controlled trials. BMJ 1998;317:1624–1629.
3. The Database of Abstracts of Reviews of Effectiveness (University of York), Database no.: DARE-989737. In: The Cochrane Library, Issue 3, 2000. Oxford: Update Software.

38.51 Examination of a nasal smear

Pirkko Ruoppi

Basic rule

- Microscopy of a nasal smear is one of the routine examinations of a patient with symptoms of chronic rhinitis. The smear does not give information for a specific diagnosis but it indicates whether to suspect allergy or hypersensitivity as the underlying factor. Nasal smear can also confirm the diagnosis of vasomotor rhinitis.

Collection of a nasal secretion sample

- Wipe the surface of the middle or the inferior nasal concha as far back as possible very gently with a cotton swab.

Table 38.51 Interpretation of nasal smear test.

Finding	Interpretation
♦ Neutrophils	♦ Irritation rhinitis
♦ Neutrophils accompanied by virus inclusions and/or bacteria	♦ Virus/bacterial Infection
♦ Eosinophils ♦ Basophils	♦ Allergy or NARES (non-allergic rhinitis with eosinophilia syndrome), Aspirin-induced rhinitis
♦ Columnar cells ♦ Goblet cells	♦ Vital mucosa
♦ Metaplastic cells ♦ Squamous cells	♦ Atrophic mucosa

- For the study of inflammatory cells alone (i.e. neutrophils, eosinophils, basophils, lymphocytes), the sample can be obtained by asking the patient to blow his nose to a plastic film.
- Spread out the secretion sample on a glass slide and let it air dry.
- Staining with eosin-methylene blue is sufficient for demonstration of inflammatory cells.

Interpretation

- Nasal smears can be examined for inflammatory cells in primary care. Microscopy is then limited to determining the number of neutrophils and eosinophils.
- To study morphological changes in the epithelium of the nasal mucosa, the specimen must be taken by using a special technique and the microscopist should be well trained in cytology. The information obtained by more extensive cytological examination of the nose is summarized in table 38.51.

38.53 Occupational rhinitis

Kari Reijula

Objectives

- The relationship between rhinitis and occupational exposure should be established in order to reduce exposure and prevent new cases of the disease.
- The concurrent development of occupational asthma should be prevented, or an already developed asthma should be diagnosed as early as possible.

Prevalence

- In Northern Europe, occupational rhinitis appears most often among farmers and bakers.

Clinical outcome

- The patient develops sneezing, a runny nose or rhinorrhoea soon after arriving at the workplace.
- Sore throat, mucous fluid in the pharynx or dry secretion in anterior parts of the nose, itching or stinging of the eyes and lacrimation may also be present.
- In early stages the symptoms disappear when patient leaves the workplace for weekends or during vacation. If the exposure continues the symptoms become chronic and no recovery can be seen while the patient stays out of work.

Examinations

- The history of exposure and symptoms is important, especially the relationship between the symptoms and exposure at work. Do the symptoms also appear while out of work?
- Anterior rhinoscopy. Does the patient have infections, polyps, or disturbing structural obstruction?
- Sinus ultrasound scan or x-ray to rule out chronic sinusitis
- Measuring serum IgE to verify atopy if the history or nasal fluid did not reveal any allergy

Further examinations

- Skin prick tests (SPT) to verify immediate allergy to specific allergens. The basic series usually includes pollens and animal danders, house mites, etc. Other test series include occupational irritants, such as other animal danders, flour, indoor plants, wood dusts, several types of molds and various chemicals.
- Specific IgE (RAST) is performed when the suspicion of a specific exposure factor is strong but SPT is negative or is not available. If necessary, serum IgE can be used to determine the total IgE level to support the interpretation of specific IgE or SPT results.
- Peak flow measurements are performed at home and at work if the patient reports respiratory symptoms.
- Nasal provocation with relevant allergens is performed by an ENT or sometimes by a pulmonary specialist.
- If nasal provocation, SPT and/or specific IgE with a relevant allergen are positive, the diagnosis of occupational rhinitis is confirmed. Certain chemicals can cause occupational rhinitis without IgE-mediated hypersensitivity.

Further actions

- If the patient cannot be transferred to another position at the workplace, respiratory devices should be used to prevent the exposure. For example, farmers with occupational rhinitis

and asthma have used motorized helmet-type devices while working. Devices may protect the person from developing asthma after occupational rhinitis.
- If the symptoms are mild and the conditions at work cannot be adjusted, the patient may try to continue at work under medical therapy provided that the occupational health care is closely controlling the situation.

38.54 Nasal polyposis

Pirkko Ruoppi

Aims

- To identify polyps and distinguish them from swollen middle nasal concha (and tumours).
- To start therapy (removal of polyps/local steroids).
- To treat sinusitis, which may be associated with polyposis.
- To determine the need for further specialist-level therapy (ethmoidectomy)

Pathology

- Nasal polyps usually arise from ethmoidal cells but may also develop from the maxillary sinus mucosa (so-called choanal polyps), although this is much less frequent. It has been estimated that approximately 4% of chronic rhinitis patients suffer from nasal polyposis.
- The pathogenesis and aetiology of nasal polyposis are largely unknown. The presence of polyposis is associated with chronic mucosal inflammation and sometimes also with allergy. Aspirin intolerance may be the underlying cause of rapidly recurring, treatment-resistant nasal polyposis. In children nasal polyps are extremely rare (choanal polyps may sometimes occur) and are usually associated with cystic fibrosis (31.23).

Symptoms

- The dominant symptom is permanent obstruction of the nose, whereas obstruction caused by mucosal swelling of conchae is variable.

Examination

- History. Has acetylsalicylic acid (ASA, aspirin) intolerance occurred?
- Rhinoscopy
  - Palpation of the polyp with a cotton applicator (moves, not painful).
  - If a polyp is suspected, examine the nose again after mucosal decongestion (see 38.55 for examination of the obstructed nose).
  - Choanal polyps are usually seen only in posterior rhinoscopy.
- X-ray of the nasal and paranasal sinuses (only CT gives reliable information about the ethmoidal cells)
- Possibly nasal smear (eosinophils, neutrophils)
- Histological examination of the removed polyps is always indicated (differential diagnosis: papilloma)

Treatment

- Corticosteroids are the only drugs that have an effect on polyp growth. A local steroid is the therapy of choice for nasal polyposis (B) [1].
- Local therapy has little effect, however, if the nose is blocked by large polyps. The polyps must first be removed surgically.

Removal of nasal polyps

- The primary care physician can extirpate a solitary polyp.
  - Apply anaesthetic-containing cotton swabs (4% lidocaine + adrenaline 1:1000 diluted 2 gtt/5 ml) to the base of the polyp. Wait for 20 minutes. In case there are several polyps, nerve block anaesthesia of the nasal mucosa can be applied with cotton swabs: a swab soaked with the anaesthetic is inserted in the upper meatus, and another between the inferior and medial conchae placed in the nasal cavity as posteriorly as possible. Wait at least 30 minutes.
  - Slide an open polyp loop along the floor of the nose underneath the polyp and around it. See that the sling is at the very base of the polyp. Tighten the loop firmly around the polyp and jerk it out so that the base of the polyp extending into the ethmoidal cells is also extirpated.
  - Follow the patient up until the anaesthetic effect has worn out (ca. one hour). Possible bleeding will stop quickly on application of a Spongostan® tampon.

Specialist consultation and treatment

- Patients with frequently recurring polyps should be referred to a specialist for evaluation of the need for ethmoidectomy and endoscopic surgery.

Prognosis

- Polyposis tends to recur easily in patients with aspirin (ASA) intolerance. Many of these patients have asthma, which must be treated adequately.

Reference

1. Filiaci F, Passali D, Puxeddu R, Schrewelius C. A randomized controlled trial showing efficacy of once daily intranasal budesonide in nasal polyposis. Rhinology 2000;38:185–90.

38.55 Nasal obstruction

Jouko Suonpää

Basic rules

- Detect the causative foci of infection, polyps, and tumours.
- Identify structural anomalies of the nasal cavities and possible allergens or irritants.
- Deviation of the nasal septum should be remembered as a potential cause for nasal and even lower respiratory tract disorders, particularly infections.
- Diagnose septum deviation by anterior rhinoscopy.

Common causes of nasal obstruction

- Nonperennial allergic rhinitis (38.50), nasal polyps (38.54), and subtle sinusitis (38.33).
- Frequently also long-term use of topical vasoconstrictors and some antihypertensive drugs.
- In children, enlarged adenoids or sometimes a foreign body.

Nasal septum deviation

- Few people have a completely straight nasal septum.
- Deviation of the nasal septum is significant if it interferes with normal functioning of the nose such as nasal breathing, evacuation of secretions from the nose and paranasal sinuses, or the ability to smell. The symptoms may be uni- or bilateral.
- Congenital septum deviation may be associated with other developmental abnormalities of the central face such as choanal atresia or cleft palate.
- Septum deviation acquired during growth may be caused by the septum growing asynchronously from many sites at the same time.
- Acquired "congenital" septum luxation occurs in 5% of normal vaginal deliveries.
- Septal fracture associated with nasal fracture is suggested by mucosal lacerations of the septum, haematomas and thickening. A fracture of the cartilaginous part of the septum may occur without a nasal fracture, but the risk for septum injury is increased with increasing severity of a nasal injury.

History

- Duration, time and place of occurrence, a history of atopy in the family, and evident allergens or irritants are clues to an allergic aetiology.
- A preceding infection suggests sinusitis.
- Ask about drugs, smoking, and type of work.
- Disturbances of the sense of smell may be associated with even mild septum deviation.
- Facial pain may be associated with large septal prominences.

Clinical signs

- Tenderness on pressure or percussion of the face suggests a focus of infection.
- Itching, a watery discharge, and sneezing suggests allergens or irritants as the cause for the symptoms.
- Nasal septum deviation, foreign bodies, and tumours cause unilateral symptoms.

Primary investigations

- Careful inspection of the nose and upper pharynx with a good light source together with a good history are the most important diagnostic methods. Observe structural abnormalities, musocal swelling, polyps, and tumours (which should be looked for in the upper part of the nasal cavity and under the medial concha. Two drops of adrenalin (1:1000) soaked in a cotton wool stick are effective in constricting the mucous membrane to allow visualization of the nasal cavity.
- Obstructing septal deviation may be diagnosed on the basis of nasal breathing sounds which can be listened to separately by closing one snare at a time by pressing with a finger from the side.
- Maxillary sinusitis can be diagnosed with ultrasonography or x-ray. Sinus radiographs should always be taken if the symptoms are prolonged.
- An increased number of eosinophils in nasal secretions suggests allergy.

Treatment

- Avoiding drugs or specific irritants of ambient air.
- Cessation of smoking is essential before other treatments are attempted.
- Topical treatment for allergic rhinitis can be started after allergy has been established.

Indications for specialist consultation

- Assessment of several allergens, occupational exposure, chronic sinusitis, and severe structural anomalies.
- A reddish, bleeding tumour in the nasal cavity.
- Indications for surgery for nasal septum deviation

- Obstruction of nasal breathing is the main indication.
- Other indications include recurrent epistaxis, recurrent sinusitis, headache and facial pain.

38.56 Atrophic rhinitis and ozaena

Pirkko Ruoppi

Aim

- Atrophic changes in the nasal mucosa should be identified in their early stage.
- Ensure that the patient is seen at regular intervals for cleansing of the nose and administration of topical therapy.
- Evaluate the need for antibiotics.
- Evaluate the need for treatment by an ENT specialist.

Occurrence

- Atrophy of the nasal mucosa is either primary or the consequence of e.g. nasal surgery, trauma or irradiation. The advanced stage of primary atrophic rhinitis, ozaena, is becoming rare in developed countries. Only a few new cases are diagnosed each year. Mild atrophy associated with ageing is common.

Symptoms

- Mild atrophy of the nasal mucous membrane leads to disturbed mucus transport. As a result, viscous secretion and crusts are accumulated in the nasal cavities.
- Typical symptoms are nasal obstruction, headache and a strong foul smell that the patient does not sense but that can be detected at a distance of several metres from the patients. Greenish scale-like smelling crusts are formed, under which the mucous membrane is irritated and bleeding. Swelling of the mucous membrane is usually not seen.
- As the disease progresses the nasal cavities become very wide. Even then the patient usually complains of nasal obstruction.

Investigations

- Rhinoscopy
- Nasal smear (squamous cells, metaplastic cells)
- Bacterial culture (verifies the diagnosis of ozaena, Klebsiella ozaenae grows in the sample accompanied often with other rod-shaped bacteria).
- X-ray of the nasal sinuses, if sinusitis is suspected.

Treatment

- Frequent lavage of the nasal cavities with physiological saline
- Humidifying nasal aerosols
- Oil sprays and drops
- Remember: no steroid sprays for atrophic rhinitis even if the patient complains of nasal obstruction!
- Culture-based antibiotic therapy may be considered if the symptoms are aggravated.

Further investigations and treatment

- Each new ozaena patient should be referred to a specialist for the planning of treatment and follow-up.

Follow-up

- Patients requiring treatment (lavages, removal of crusts) should be seen 2–4 times a year, depending on the severity of the symptoms.

38.60 Tumours of the ear canal

Jukka Luotonen

Basic rules

- Identify malignant tumours as early as possible because the prognosis of advanced cancer in the ear canal is poor.
- Suspect a malignant tumour particularly in elderly people with prolonged, unilateral otitis externa.

Benign tumours

- Benign tumours of the ear canal originate from the skin, its glands, cartilage, or bone. They are very rare.

Exostosis of the bony ear canal

- The most common benign tumour of the ear canal
- A convex, bony prominence is felt under the skin near the tympanic membrane.
- Usually asymptomatic unless it obstructs the ear canal.
- Cold water in the ear canal may predispose to exostosis (swimmer's lump).
- Most exostoses need no treatment, but those causing symptoms can be removed surgically.

Osteoma

- Far more infrequent than an exostosis
- Usually pedunculated

- There are no symptoms unless the tumour obstructs the ear canal.

Polyps

- Associated with otitis media, and sometimes with chronic otitis externa.
- Purulent secretion is often present.
- Usually grows from the middle ear through a perforation in the tympanic membrane, sometimes filling the whole ear canal.
- Removal of polyps is the task of an ENT specialist. The polyp must be examined histologically.

Cholesteatoma

- If migration of the ear canal epithelium is prevented, scaling and cerumen may develop into an ear canal cholesteatoma. This mass consisting of scaling skin enlarges and may destroy bone from the bony ear canal or injure the tympanic membrane and the structures of the middle ear.
- Removal of a cholesteatoma may be difficult because it is firmly attached to the sensitive skin of the ear canal.
- Refer the patient to an ENT specialist if the cholesteatoma is large or causes symptoms.

Malignant tumours

- Most malignant tumours of the ear canal are squamocellular carcinomas. Basaliomas are much more infrequent.
- Pain is the predominant symptom.
- The differential diagnosis between cancer and chronic otitis externa is difficult. Basalioma is the most difficult to diagnose because it may grow under normal skin and become widespread before the diagnosis is made.
- Suspect a malignant tumour particularly in elderly people with prolonged, unilateral otitis externa.

38.61 External tumours of the nose

Antti Mäkitie

Aims

- Excise a suspected small basal cell carcinoma (BCC) including a large margin of healthy tissue, and send it for histological analysis.
- Refer patients with large basal cell carcinomas, tumours near the nostrils (possibly squamous cell carcinoma) or a strongly suspected melanoma to an ENT specialist or a plastic surgeon, without taking a biopsy in primary care.

Benign tumours

Naevus

- The most common external tumour of the nose.
- Manifests as a raised, discoloured lesion.
- Excision is indicated if the naevus
  - grows rapidly
  - is ulcerated or bleeds.

Haemangioma

- Fairly common in the newborn and infants.
- Manifests as a congenital bluish, bulging lesion which grows rapidly during the first few months of life.
- Later on, the growth ceases, the colour fades, the tumour decreases in size spontaneously and sometimes totally disappears.
- Treatment
  - Monitor without intervention during the first few years of life.
  - Laser surgery.

Other tumours (rare)

- Fibroma
- Lipoma
- Chondroma
- Osteoma
- Lymphangioma

Malignant tumours

- The incidence of malignant tumours is on the increase.
- Prevention and early diagnosis are of utmost importance as is skin self-examination carried out by the patient.
- Primary treatment usually involves surgery.

Basal cell carcinoma (BCC)

- The most common external malignant tumour of the nose.
- A small, pearly, reddish nodule develops on the nose. A central ulceration appears later on with scab formation. This gives rise to a lesion with a rolled border. The lesion appears to remain the same size, but tissue destruction continues underneath the lesion.
- The tumour is always localized, but in 20–30% of the cases there are multiple BCCs on the face and head.
- Treatment
  - A suspected small BCC should be removed with a wide margin. Cryotherapy is an alternative to surgical excision, particularly if the BCC affects the eyelids.
  - If the diagnosis is uncertain or the lesion is large, a biopsy can be taken from the margin of the tumour.
    - If the diagnosis of a BCC is confirmed the patient should be referred to a specialist unit since cosmetic reconstruction may be required for the excisional site.
    - The patient should be followed up.
  - If the removal of a suspected BCC is not indicated in elderly patients or in patients in very poor health topical

silver nitrate or cryotherapy may be used on bleeding tumours (caused by scratching).
- A specialist should treat BCCs in the cartilaginous part of the nose because the tumour may have caused extensive destruction of the cartilage.

Squamous cell carcinoma (SCC)

- Incidence on the external nose is less frequent than that of BCC. The site of predilection is the vicinity of the nostrils. The site of predilection is the vicinity of the nostrils.
- Initially a small nodular lump will develop on the skin. May also present as a cauliflower lesion. A central, persistent ulcerative crater appears later.
- The tumour is more aggressive than a BCC with respect to speed of growth, tissue destruction and metastasis.
- Any tumour situated in the nasal vestibule should therefore be removed at a specialist unit.
- If the history of an excised lesion reveals a SCC, an ENT specialist should be consulted even if the tumour has been totally removed.

Melanoma

- In case of a strong clinical suspicion of a melanoma the patient should be referred to the care of a specialist team. If the histological examination of an excised tumour reveals a melanoma, the patient must always be referred to a specialist. Ensure that the patient receives an appointment and is treated promptly.

38.62 Tumours of the nasal and paranasal cavities

Antti Mäkitie

Aim

- Remember the possibility of a paranasal tumour in recurrent sinusitis in the elderly patients, particularly if there is no previous history of sinusitis.

Osteoma

- Bony outgrowth of tissues.
- Often detected as an incidental finding in sinus x-rays (visible as roundish, solid radiolucent area which resembles a tumour).
- Osteomas are most commonly seen in the frontal sinuses.
- Initially monitored with x-rays.
- They need no treatment unless they grow or cause problems through pressure.

Papilloma

- The most common tumour of the nasal cavities and more common in men.
- In an exophytic papilloma the connective tissue beneath the surface epithelium increases along with the epithelium giving rise to mushroom-like tumours that are visible in the nasal vestibule and the septum.
  - Local excision is usually sufficient (cryotherapy or laser surgery after biopsy).
- Transitional cell papilloma usually occurs in the conchal region and in the paranasal sinuses.
  - Symptoms
    - Nasal breathing becomes difficult as the tumour obstructs the nasal cavities
    - Epistaxis
    - A papilloma in the ethmoid region may cause lacrimation, obstruct the lacrimal duct or cause bulging of the medial part of the eye socket after the bony structures have been destroyed.
  - Refer the patient to a specialist unit since the type of papilloma tends to recur, and it may undergo malignant transformation. Patients also warrant a long follow-up period.

Malignant tumours

Epidemiology

- The annual incidence is about 1 in 100 000. Males are more commonly affected than females.
- Squamous cell carcinoma is the most common type of tumour.
- Mucous membrane melanoma is rare but aggressive.

Symptoms

- There are no early signs or symptoms.
- Tumours in the nasal cavities usually cause obstruction, secretions and bleeding.
- Tumours in the paranasal sinuses may cause recurrent sinusitis. X-rays are indicated in recurrent sinusitis in the elderly.
- Abnormalities in the surrounding tissues.
  - Deviation of an eye laterally or outwards
  - Limitation in eye movements, visual disturbances
  - Bulging of the cheek, lacrimation
  - Erosion of the hard palate: loosening of teeth, loose dentures
  - Pain in the upper teeth and cheek is a late symptom.

Diagnosis

- Anterior and posterior rhinoscopy, imaging and, if needed, antroscopy and a biopsy.

Treatment and prognosis

- Treatment at specialist facilities.
- The chance of a cure at 5 years is about 30%.

38.70 Vertigo

Mikael Ojala

Aims

- To recognize benign postural vertigo, cervical vertigo, orthostatic hypotension and vestibular neuronitis without further examination.
- TIA in the elderly presenting as vertigo is treated with aspirin. Younger patients are referred to hospital examinations.
- Further examinations are indicated in cases of frequently recurring or prolonged spinning dizziness as well as in cases involving impairment of hearing or other findings possibly combined with nystagmus. Learn to suspect Ménière's disease, acoustic neurinoma, temporal epilepsy and multiple sclerosis.
- The use of vertigo-inducing medication is either stopped or the dose is reduced.
- Prescribing medication for vertigo should be avoided with the elderly.

Causes of vertigo

- Vertigo is mainly caused by organic malfunction: The vertigo patient should not be considered a neurotic. The following list includes the most common causes of vertigo, not necessarily in the order of importance:
  - Benign postural vertigo (38.72)
  - Ménière's disease (38.71)
  - Otogenic vertigo without aetiological basis
  - So-called vestibular neuronitis
  - Tension neck
  - Circulatory disturbances of the brain stem or cerebellum
  - Cerebellar atrophy
  - Vertigo related to the ageing process in the elderly (brain, eyes, organs of equilibrium, peripheral sense of posture, orthostatism)
  - Panic attack (hyperventilation)
  - Undefined vertigo despite extensive examinations
- Only about 10% of vertigo cases can be placed in the last group.
- Vertigo induced by excessive medication is common in patients seeing a general practitioner.

Case history

- A thorough interview is the most important part of diagnostics.
  - Is spinning involved? Does the vertigo create a sense of falling? Is there a certain direction to the falling sensation?
  - The association of vertigo with various situations (change in posture, head rotation, physical exertion)
  - Paroxysmal nature (short duration in postural vertigo and TIA, longer if caused by Ménière's disease). Continuous and violent vertigo that has lasted for more than a week is often caused by vestibular neuronitis or cerebellar infarction. Continuous but mild vertigo is of cervical origin.
  - Accompanying symptoms indicating brain or ear involvement
  - Hearing impairment or tinnitus (Ménière's disease, acoustic neurinoma)
  - Paralysis involvement (TIA)
- Regular medication

Status

- Evidence of nystagmus in various positions
  - Occurs in vestibular neuronitis, Ménière's disease and postural vertigo.
  - Rarely occurring vertical nystagmus indicates a cerebral disorder.
- Neurological, otological and circulatory examination
  - In the Unterberger's marching test the patient marches 40 paces on the spot with eyes closed. The finding is abnormal if the patient rotates to either side more than 45 degrees. This test allows easy to determination of one-sided dysfunction, eg in cases of vestibular neuronitis or acoustic neurinoma rotation occurs to the involved side.
  - The Romberg test evaluates objectively the degree of disturbance in equilibrium.
  - Gait
  - Coordination tests
  - Cranial nerves, tendon reflexes
  - Tympanic membranes (otitis or perforation)
  - Tuning fork test
  - An audiogram is indicated if the patient has persistent spinning dizziness (>1 min), tinnitus, or if a hearing impairment is suspected.
  - Blood pressure sitting and standing
  - Auscultation of the heart and jugular veins
- The neck should also be examined (muscular tension, compression test).

Typical signs and symptoms

Benign postural vertigo

- See 38.72

- The dizziness spell often begins in the morning.
- It is exacerbated as the patient reclines from a sitting position or turns in the bed a few seconds after the change in position. A new change in position will cause a milder spell.
- A spell can often be provoked during the patient visit.
- Nystagmus may often be observed during the spell (usually rotatory).
- In 90% of the patients spells usually subside within 3 months, but relapses may occur.

Acute vestibulopathy (vestibular neuronitis)

- Rapid onset, violent spinning vertigo and nausea
- Normal (symmetrical) audiogram
- Spontaneous horizontal nystagmus towards the healthy ear
- Severe vertigo passes in 1–2 weeks. Mild difficulty with equilibrium lasts longer.
- The attack does not recur.

Ménière's disease

- See 38.71
- Symptom triad: spinning vertigo, tinnitus, variable hearing impairment.
- Attacks last 2–5 h (10 min–48 h).
- Often a sensation of pressure in the ears.
- The initial transient loss of hearing is later followed by a permanent hearing impairment of inner ear type beginning with the lower frequencies. Differentiation of speech diminishes.

Panic-related vertigo (hyperventilation)

- Usually affects younger people and presents either as continuous vertigo or is related to circumstances (queues, shops, theatre). Diagnosis can be made after organic causes have been excluded with sufficient certainty.
- No findings of rotatory vertigo or nystagmus.

Vertigo of cervical origin

- The sense of movement and position in the cervical region is impaired.
- Caused by muscle tension or the cervical syndrome.
- Findings are either taut neck and shoulder musculature or a positive compression test.
- Nystagmus is not a usual finding.

Vertigo related to the ageing process in the elderly

- Evolves as the result of a combination of several factors, particularly the weakening of the senses. See 22.1.

Vertigo caused by medication and alcohol

- Drugs causing orthostatic hypotension (drugs for hypertension and Parkinson's disease, tricyclic antidepressants, phenothiazines)
- Anticonvulsants: carbamazepine and phenytoin can cause cerebellar vertigo accompanied by ataxia and nystagmus.
- Benzodiazepines
- Alcohol causes
  - cerebellar degeneration in chronic use: ataxia and tremor
  - polyneuropathy that weakens the sense of position.

TIA

- In most cases also other CNS symptoms besides vertigo can be found (diplopia, dysarthria, paralysis symptoms in the extremities).
- Individual attacks of spinning vertigo accompanied by nystagmus (rarely observed because the attack is usually over by the time the patient is seen by the physician).
- Drop attack–legs suddenly give way
- The risk factors of stroke (hypertension, atherosclerosis) increase both the likelihood of the diagnosis and the risk of reccurrence.

Acoustic neurinoma

- Gradually progressive hearing impairment is the major symptom.
- Tinnitus
- Feeling of uncertainty in walking, generally without spinning vertigo.

Multiple sclerosis

- Sometimes the initial symptoms are a feeling of dizziness and uncertainty in walking.
- Other neurological findings lead to the diagnosis.

Vertigo of cardiac origin

- In orthostatic hypertension, the symptoms are worst in the morning and after a meal.
- Arrhythmias may be accompanied by attacks of vertigo (non-spinning type) and collapses.
- Vertigo may be related to physical exertion.

Auxiliary examinations

- Basic general examinations
  - ECG, blood count, ESR
  - Audiogram if an ear disorder is suspected
  - A cervical x-ray is generally not useful.
- Specialist examinations
  - ENG (electronystamograph) in most cases; scan or MRI if a brain dysfunction is suspected.
  - BAEP to exclude acoustic neurinoma (36.16).
  - EEG only if epilepsy is suspected.
- Consultations
  - The need for consultation is evaluated on the basis of the case history and status. Generally consultation is not necessary.
  - Depending on the observed signs and symptoms, the patient may be referred to an ENT specialist, neurologist or cardiologist.

Treatment of vertigo

- Acute vertigo possibly accompanied by vomiting: prochlorperazine in tablet or suppository form
- Postural vertigo: positional treatment, no medication
- In patients with acute stage of vestibular neuritis, methylpredisolone with decreasing doses, starting with 100 mg/day p.o., for three weeks, appears to improve the recovery of peripheral vestibular function. However, results on clinical outcomes, such as vertigo and imbalance, are lacking
- Undefined vertigo or vertigo associated with one ear: betahistine
- Antihistamines may be tried, however there is little evidence of their effectiveness.
- Brain disorders: only epileptic vertigo can be treated. TIA can be partly prevented (aspirin).
- Cervical origin: physiotherapy and acupuncture, physical training by the patient
- Panic attack: selective serotonin reuptake inhibitor (SSRI), tricyclic antidepressants, alprazolam, clonazepam.
- Self-care training to improve control of equilibrium is beneficial for all patients with recurrent vertigo.

38.71 Ménière's disease

Jouko Suonpää

Aetiology

- Ménière's disease is characterized by an increased amount of endolympha in the internal ear. The aetiology is unknown.

Diagnosis on the basis of history and symptoms

- The diagnosis is based on three symptoms:
  - paroxysmal tinnitus followed by
  - vertigo and
  - impaired hearing.
- The patient often has several bouts lasting 0.5–6 hours in succession, followed by an asymptomatic period.
- The disease commences at the age of 20–60 years unilaterally but later affects both ears in 15–20% of the patients.
- The history and course of the disease are important in the diagnosis. The diagnosis can often be made only after months of follow-up. A consultation by an ENT specialist is indicated at this stage at the latest. Overdiagnosis is common: continuous symptoms caused by circulatory disorders of the internal ear are labelled Ménière's disease.

Symptoms and signs

- Vertigo causing nausea and vomiting is usually the most annoying symptom.
- A feeling of pressure in the affected ear
- At the initial stage there is a transient hearing impairment of the cochlear type, but as the disease advances the impairment becomes permanent and deteriorates to deafness in some patients.
- Levelling of hearing and unpleasant sensations caused by noise are often associated with the hearing impairment.
- The appearance and mobility of the eardrum and the performance in equilibrium tests are normal.
- A flat, cochlear-type hearing impairment is detected on the audiogram. Low frequencies are most affected. However, the shape of the audiogram is not diagnostic of the disease.
- During an attack a nystagmus directed towards the affected ear can be observed.
- The caloric response of the affected ear is continuously diminished.

Differential diagnosis

- Vestibular neuronitis
  - No hearing impairment
  - One or just a few severe attacks of vertigo
- Acoustic neuroma (schwannoma)
  - The vertigo can be paroxysmal at first, but the hearing is not improved between attacks.
  - Discrimination of words is particularly poor on the affected side.

Treatment

- The initial treatment is conservative.
- Betahistine is the drug of choice C [1], starting with a dose of 16 mg × 3 and continuing with a maintenance dose of 8 mg × 3. If no attacks occur for 3 months the drug can be discontinued and restarted if symptoms recur. If the patient has attacks during medication the dose should be increased for 2–4 weeks.
- Betahistine counteracts the effect of antihistamines.
- Patient information and counselling, avoidance of stress and a regular lifestyle are as important as drug treatment. The patients need a personal doctor.
- Reduced salt intake can be recommended, although firm scientific evidence of its effect is lacking.
- Patient organisations can provide counselling and help in coping with the disease.
- In severe cases with impaired hearing and incapacitating attacks the treatment options include local anaesthetics and aminoglycosides injected in the middle ear, surgical decompression of the endolymphatic sac, or transection of the vestibular nerve.

Driving licence

- As the attacks are nearly always preceded by warning symptoms the disease does not prevent driving. Drugs used for the treatment of nausea (but not those for circulation) may impair driving performance.

Reference

1. James AL, Burton MJ. Betahistine for Menière's disease or syndrome. Cochrane Database Syst Rev. 2004;(2):CD001873.

38.72 Benign positional vertigo

Mikael Ojala

Basic rules

- Recognize benign paroxysmal positional vertigo (BPPV) as the most common cause of vertigo.
- Avoid unnecessary investigations, consultations, and ineffective drugs.
- Cure the patient with positioning manoeuvres.
- Both diagnosis and treatment of the condition are carried out in primary care.
  - The diagnosis is easier to make at the first consultation than later on because the diagnostic nystagmus may no longer be present when the patient is eventually examined by a specialist after referral.
- The disease is so common that general practitioners have experience of it.

Epidemiology

- About 20% of all patients with vertigo have positional vertigo. It is the most common single cause of vertigo.
- The disease occurs in all age groups, but middle-aged and elderly people are most frequently affected.

Aetiology

- The disease is probably caused by sludge in the posterior semicircular canal of one ear (rarely of both ears) causing an intensive attack of vertigo on change of body posture.
- Sometimes a minor injury or stretching may be a triggering factor, but in most cases no predisposing factors can be found.
- The treatment is based on removing the sludge from the semicircular canal.

Clinical picture and diagnosis

Symptoms

- The symptoms often start in the morning when the patient is still in bed or has just sat up.
- The vertigo is of the rotatory or tilting type and severe. The patient often has nausea.
- The patient can usually walk normally after he/she has recovered from the first shock, but certain postures (lying down, sitting up, twisting the neck forwards, for example when washing the face, or simultaneous extension and rotation of the neck while standing) trigger the vertigo again.
- Patients tend to avoid the posture causing vertigo and they tend to sleep in a partly sitting position.

Diagnosis

- The diagnosis is suspected on the basis of the patient's history and is confirmed by clinical examination.
- A tilting provocation test is the key to the diagnosis. Other findings are normal.
  - Ask the patient to keep his eyes open. Tilt the patient rapidly on the examination couch to the supine position so that the neck is extended and rotated on one side. Intensive vertigo and a rotatory nystagmus develop after a delay of 2–20 s. The nystagmus gradually wanes. When the patient sits up the vertigo recurs. If the tilting is repeated the vertigo recurs with less intensity. The vertigo is more severe on right rotation of the neck (or while lying on the right side) if the right ear is affected.
- No instruments are necessary for diagnosis. ENG does not show properly the rotatory nystagmus that is typical of benign positional vertigo.

Differential diagnosis

- The most common false diagnoses include:
  - transient ischaemic attack (acute vertigo in an elderly patient)
  - cervical vertigo (also position-dependent, but there is no nystagmus)
  - vestibular neuronitis (which also affects standing equilibrium)
- In atypical cases (nystagmus is not evident, poor habituation on repeated tilting, prolongation of the symptoms despite treatment) consider consultation with an otorhinolaryngology specialist or a neurologist.

Prognosis

- The symptoms last on average 10 weeks if untreated, but the duration varies greatly.
- The symptoms tend to recur in many patients.

Treatment

- Drug treatment is ineffective.

- Explain to the patient the benign nature of the symptom and advise self-treatment by positional exercises:
  - The patient should perform a series of 5 repetitive tiltings 5 times a day for 1 week to the position where the symptom is provoked.
- A single effective manoeuvre can also be used (either with the Semont or Epley methods **B** [1 2 3]) but they require an experienced professional (often a physiotherapist).

References

1. Hilton M, Pinder D. The Epley (canalith repositioning) manoeuvre for benign paroxysmal positional vertigo. Cochrane Database Syst Rev. 2004;(2):CD003162.
2. van der Velde GM. Benign paroxysmal positional vertigo part II: a qualitative review of non-pharmacological, conservative treatments and a case report presenting Epley's "canalith repositioning procedure", a non-invasive bedside manoeuvre for treating BPPV. Journal of Canadian Chiropractic Association 1999;43:41–49.
3. The Database of Abstracts of Reviews of Effectiveness (University of York), Database no.: DARE-995387. In: The Cochrane Library, Issue 4, 2000. Oxford: Update Software.

OTO

Alcohol and Drugs

Evidence Based Medicine Guidelines. Edited by the Duodecim Editorial Team
 ISBN: 0-470-01184-X

40.1 Recognition of alcohol and drug abuse

Antti Holopainen

Basic rules

- In addition to social dysfunction the abuse of alcohol and drugs may cause health problems that make the user seek medical care. Doctors, especially those working in primary care, are in a key position to detect harmful use at its early stages when interventions are more feasible and simple.
- In particular the readiness to detect alcohol and drug-associated problems is mandatory in primary, occupational and school and student health care.
- The best way to address problems caused by alcohol and drugs is to ask the patients directly and clearly about the use. This gives the patient the feeling that problems related to alcohol or drug abuse can be dealt with.
- A primary care physician can take care of the treatment of an alcohol or drug problem or the patient may be referred to a specialized unit.

Direct detection of alcohol or drug use

- Use of alcohol can be detected from the typical odour of respiration, by using a breath analyser, or by assessing blood alcohol concentration.
- Toxicological analyses are needed for detecting the use of other drugs in a urine sample. Some of the major groups of commonly misused psychotrophics can be detected by using readily available commercial kits based on immunochemical methods (about intoxications, see 17.20). An informed consent from the patients is needed prior to analysing the urine sample.

Symptoms and signs typically associated with alcohol and drug abuse

- Drugs influence the level of consciousness and mood, and some drugs may induce hallucinations.
- Neurological disorders in particular and other psychiatric disorders must be considered and ruled out.
- Drug abuse may be complicated by a concurrent medical disorder such as a head injury, diabetes or an infection.
- Several unspecific signs are associated with drug abuse:
    - absenteeism from school, impairment in academic performance
    - behavioural disturbances in children and adolescents
    - a decline in general or occupational performance, inability to concentrate
    - sleeplessness and depression
    - unexplained absence from work
    - increased risk of accidents
    - vague abdominal complaints and unexplainable pain
    - problems with close relations or work team
    - financial problems
    - housing problems
    - demanding and manipulative conduct of the patient

Applying a semistructured interview for detecting harmful alcohol use

- Requires some extra time, and the patient must be cooperative.
- AUDIT (Alcohol Use Disorders Identification Test) is the most recommended measure of abuse with a sensitivity of approximately 90% (the limit of risk use is 8–11 points, see Table 40.1.1).
- Several other tests are available, the majority of which are based on the Michigan Alcoholism Screening Test (MAST) C [1] [2]. An abridged version of this is called Veterans Administration Screening Test (VAST).

Laboratory tests for detecting heavy alcohol use

Serum glutamyltransferase (GGT)

- Elevated values in 30–90% of alcoholics
- Values normalize slowly (half-life about a month) after drinking is stopped.
- Increased values are associated with the following diseases:
    - hepatobiliary diseases
    - diabetes
    - obesity
    - medicines, such as amitriptyline, barbiturates, phenytoine, contraceptives and warfarin, may increase values.

Other liver enzymes

- Abnormal liver enzyme values, see 9.12.

MCV

- Increased values in 34–89% of alcoholics
- During abstinence normal values are reached within a period of several months
    - Not a suitable indicator for detecting a violation of abstinence
    - For other possible causes of pathological values, see 15.8 (increased MCV).

Table 40.1.1 AUDIT (Alcohol Use Disorders Identification Test) by WHO

FOR EACH QUESTION SELECT YOUR ANSWER AND FILL IN THE SCORE GIVEN IN BRACKETS [ ] IN THE BOX

One unit of alcohol is: $\frac{1}{2}$ pint average strength beer/lager OR one glass of wine OR one single measure of spirits. Note: a can of high strength beer or lager may contain 3–4 units.

1. How often do you have a drink containing alcohol?

[0] Never
[1] Monthly or less
[2] 2–4 times a month
[3] 2–3 times a week
[4] 4 or more times a week

2. How many units of alcohol do you drink on a typical day when you are drinking?

[0] 1 or 2
[1] 3 or 4
[2] 5 or 6
[3] 7, 8 or 9
[4] 10 or more

3. How often do you have six or more units of alcohol on one occasion?

[0] Never
[1] Less than monthly
[2] Monthly
[3] Weekly
[4] Daily or almost daily

4. How often during the last year have you found that you were not able to stop drinking once you had started?

[0] Never
[1] Less than monthly
[2] Monthly
[3] Weekly
[4] Daily or almost daily

5. How often during the last year have you failed to do what was normally expected from you because of drinking?

[0] Never
[1] Less than monthly
[2] Monthly
[3] Weekly
[4] Daily or almost daily

6. How often during the last year have you needed a first drink in the morning to get yourself going after a heavy drinking session?

[0] Never
[1] Less than monthly
[2] Monthly
[3] Weekly
[4] Daily or almost daily

7. How often during the last year have you had a feeling of guilt or remorse after drinking?

[0] Never
[1] Less than monthly
[2] Monthly
[3] Weekly
[4] Daily or almost daily

Table 40.1.1 (*continued*)

8. How often during the last year have you been unable to remember what happened the night before because you had been drinking?

[0] Never
[1] Less than monthly
[2] Monthly
[3] Weekly
[4] Daily or almost daily

9. Have you or someone else been injured as a result of your drinking?

[0] No
[2] Yes but not in the last year
[4] Yes, during the last year

10. Has a relative or friend or doctor or another health worker been concerned about your drinking or suggested you cut down?

[0] No
[2] Yes but not in the last year
[4] Yes, during the last year

Record total of specific items here

Table 40.1.2 Severity of Dependence Scale – SDS

During the past year...	Never (0)	Sometimes (1)	Often (2)	Always (3)
1. Did you think your alcohol or other drug use was out of control?				
2. Did the thought of not being able to get any alcohol or other drug make you anxious or worried?				
3. Did you worry about your alcohol or other drug use?				
4. Did you wish you could stop?				
5. How difficult would you find it to stop or go without?	Not at all (0)	A little (1)	Quite difficult (2)	Impossible (3)

Think about your alcohol or other drug use. In particular, answer the following about the substance(s) you mostly use.

CDT (carbohydrate deficient transferrin)

- Serum concentration increases when daily alcohol consumption exceeds 50–80 g.
- CDT can be used to detect heavy alcohol use in cases where clinical history, MCV, and GGT have not given clarity (also in cases in which the GGT value is elevated for some other cause).
- The upper limit is 20 U/l in men and 26 U/l in women. Even small differences are significant clinically.
- Pathological values can also be found in multiple sclerosis, primary biliary cirrhosis, chronic active hepatitis, and in a rare syndrome of carbohydrate deficient glycoprotein.

Applying a structured interview for recognizing drug addiction

- Several tests have been developed for assessing harmful use of drugs, some of which are quite extensive and others more limited and suitable for application in primary health care.
- The use of more extensive questionnaires in particular, such as the EuropASI (European Addiction Severity Index), require basic instruction and training in their use from the person administering the test.
- EuropASI can be applied to assess the patient's need for treatment and rehabilitation in a holistic manner. The test is used increasingly for example in units where the need for substitution therapy for opioid dependence is evaluated.
- Less extensive tests that the patient can apply himself are, for example, the DAST (Drug Abuse Screening Test) and the SDS (Severity of Dependence Scale), see Table 40.1.2
- Both tests are well applicable in primary health care, as the patient can fill in the questionnaire in a few minutes.
- Many centres where drug dependence is managed use the questionnaire of the Pompidou Group of the Council of Europe for epidemiological studies. The questionnaire assesses the history of drug abuse and risk behaviour in a structured manner. The Pompidou questionnaire can also be used in primary health care when the number of drug abusers is high among the patient population. The questionnaire is also used by the European Monitoring Centre for Drugs and Drug Addiction.

References

1. Storgaard H, Nielsen SD, Gluud C. The validity of the Michigan Alcoholism Screening Test (MAST). Alcohol Alcoholism 1994;29:493–502.
2. The Database of Abstracts of Reviews of Effectiveness (University of York), Database no.: DARE-940827. In: The Cochrane Library, Issue 4, 1999. Oxford: Update Software.

40.2 Providing care for an alcohol or drug abuser

Antti Holopainen

Basic rules

- The threshold for seeking help is low in primary care: the possibilities offered for early detection and referral to therapy should be utilized.
- In cases of overdosing, the patient is followed up and treated.
- Information and other services regarding injection and sexual hygiene should be made available to those drug users who are otherwise not within the reach of health care services. This is a way of encouraging drug users to seek medical services without requiring them to stop abuse or seek help as a condition to receiving help.

General comments on the drug problem

- Infectious viral diseases (hepatites and HIV) as well as tuberculosis and STDs whose spread is associated with drug use are an increasing health risk for the entire population.
- The use of and dependence on hard drugs (amphetamine, heroin, cocaine) spreads like disease epidemics among regular drug users.
- Chronically dependent daily users distribute addicting drugs (benzodiazepines, buprenorphine, other opioids) for abuse. Furthermore, they seek new users to fund their own drug use. The use of i.v. drugs is common in this group with the aim of maximizing the effect of the expensive drug.

How to arrange emergency care and withdrawal

First aid services

- Managing heroin overdosing is becoming a major new task in emergency rooms, as respiratory failure follows i.v. heroin injection immediately. Naloxone is the specific therapy, see 17.20.
- Following successful resuscitation the patient should be offered the possibility of follow-up in a specialized unit for drug addicts, if such service is available.
- Psychosis caused by amphetamine or other stimulants or hallucinogenics should be referred to psychiatric care as emergencies when the criteria of involuntary care are met.
- The psychosis is often transient. Referral to further treatment is the responsibility of the treating psychiatric unit.
- Management of acute withdrawal symptoms may be necessary in opioid-dependent persons who are hospitalized for a medical problem such as septicaemia, hepatitis or some other condition. In such cases substitution therapy may be administered according to the legislation of the country in question.
- Opioid withdrawal and substitution therapy should be the responsibility of specialized units.

Health counselling services

- In many countries health counselling services have been established for users of i.v. drugs with needle exchanging services.
- These services are offered anonymously. The clients can bring dirty injection syringes and needles and get clean ones in exchange.
- The service offers counselling on infectious diseases, vaccinates against hepatitis A and B, performs HIV tests, gives out condoms and information on sexually transmitted diseases and refers those interested in withdrawal to further therapy.
- The staff is usually trained health care personnel and social workers, previous drug users and consultant doctors.

Withdrawal therapies

- Patients dependent on stimulants or opioids need withdrawal to break the habit.
- Many such patients have used overdoses of benzodiazepines to manage their dependence, which is why the problems caused by benzodiazepines, such as strong need for drugs and seizures with unconsciousness and convulsions, must be taken into account when planning the therapy.
- Sometimes persons dependent on high doses of cannabis may also need withdrawal, or cannabis dependency is one aspect when planning therapy for other dependencies.
- Opioid dependency often requires specific drug therapy that is administered in specialist units (40.10).

Rehabilitation for drug addiction

- Rehabilitation of a drug addict often requires long-term therapy in a special programme. In the initial stages of the therapy the setting must be institutional with the capability of supporting the patient's struggle to rid himself/herself of the group of active users.
- This early remission usually takes 3–6 months. Some patients may need medication for psychiatric symptoms in this phase.

- The withdrawal therapy for benzodiazepine dependency often takes place in this stage. Some patients are then referred to non-pharmacological withdrawal programmes after this phase. Therapy in such units may take from 6 months to one year.
- Even after this time many patients continue to need a supportive network that consists of former users (AA groups).

Referral of alcoholics

- Options
  - In outpatient care (C) [1 2]: brief intervention (40.3), disulfiram (40.6), naltrexone (40.6)
  - On ward in a local health care centre: diazepam loading (40.5)
  - A-clinics (specialized community alcohol and drug teams)
  - Withdrawal in delirious patients should be carried out in a psychiatric hospital or an intensive care unit
- The basic social and health services should provide facilities for the emergency treatment of alcohol or drug abusers.
- The services should be arranged in cooperation with the various providers in order to avoid inefficiency and to ensure that no one is left without proper services. Collaboration with psychiatric services is necessary as patients attending alcohol and drug treatment programmes often have psychiatric problems.

Special treatment services for alcohol and drug abusers

Alcoholism clinics and youth clinics run by communities or foundations

- Provide ambulatory services for alcohol or drug abusers and their families. The employees of these units are professionals in medicine, nursing or social work. The services consist of:
  - individual, family or group therapy
  - counselling in social problems
  - treating minor health problems
- The services are provided free of charge. Usually an appointment must be made in advance.
- At some clinics an appointment with a nurse can be made without prior reservation.

Detoxification units

- The aim of the treatment is:
  - to help the patient stop the use of alcohol or drugs within a short period (5–12 days) in an inpatient setting
  - to enable physical rehabilitation and the solving of social problems.
- This treatment can also be provided on ward at a health care centre.

Patients' associations/guilds

- Registered associations run by clients of alcoholism clinics. The guilds provide aftercare and support after other treatment has been completed.

AA groups

- Anonymous groups founded by alcoholics
- A similar group for relatives or friends of alcoholics is called Al Anon.
- The groups accept all alcoholics or members of their families or friends.
- The groups provide a place for discussing problems associated with alcohol and support efforts to remain abstinent.
- Some aspects of AA may be effective (C) [3 4].

Psychotherapies

- Different modes of psychotherapies (cognitive, behavioural, brief or family therapy) are used at some clinics or institutions.

Occupational health

- Occupational health care units are often active in referring alcohol or drug abusing employees to treatment by making arrangements and planning the treatment and rehabilitation.

References

1. Mattick RP, Jarvis T. In-patient setting and long duration for the treatment of alcohol dependence? Out-patient care is as good. Drug Alcohol Review 1994;13:127–135.
2. The Database of Abstracts of Reviews of Effectiveness (University of York), Database no.: DARE-948068. In: The Cochrane Library, Issue 4, 1999. Oxford: Update Software.
3. Kowenacki RJ, Shadish WR. Does Alcoholics Anonymous work: the results from a meta-analysis of controlled experiments. Substance Use and Misuse 1999;34:1897–1916.
4. The Database of Abstracts of Reviews of Effectiveness (University of York), Database no.: DARE-992138. In: The Cochrane Library, Issue 1, 2001. Oxford: Update Software.

40.3 Brief interventions for heavy use of alcohol

Antti Suokas

Rationale

- It is often possible to influence the patient's drinking by guidance and advice (A) [1 2 3 4 5 6 7 8]. Brief intervention is a tool for health care personnel.

Epidemiology

- Excessive use of alcohol for men is more than 24 drinks and for women more than 16 drinks per week.
- 10% of the heaviest drinkers account for more than half of the total consumption of alcohol. In practice, this means 7–8 bottles of beer every day or four bottles of vodka per week.
- 90% of heavy drinkers are men, the majority of them between 20 and 39 years of age. Up to 20% of men and 10% of women in working age are heavy drinkers.
- The majority of heavy drinkers are employed.
- The risk of alcohol-induced problems is high in heavy drinkers. About 20–25% of them are clearly dependent on alcohol.

Recognition of heavy drinking

- See article on recognition of alcohol and drug abuse 40.1.
- Heavy drinking is recognized by combining the patient history with the clinical picture and laboratory tests. Multiple choice questionnaires may also be used.

Brief intervention

- Mini-intervention consists of questions, discussions, and guidance to urge the individual to reduce his/her alcohol consumption to a safer level.
- Moderate alcohol consumption is often a more realistic goal than abstinence. However, abstinence is recommended during the first few weeks.
- Mini-intervention includes 3–4 sessions at intervals of 2–4 weeks.
- Mini-intervention is successful only if the patient admits his/her excessive use of alcohol.
- In addition to spoken and written instructions, the outcome of laboratory tests and general physical inspection are a valuable means of influencing the patient.
- During the sessions the following subjects may be discussed:
  - How does the patient feel about his or her drinking?
  - Analysis of the situation (amount of alcohol consumed weekly, impact on health, alcohol-related problems at home and at work, development of tolerance).
  - Results of the laboratory tests (liver enzymes, MCV, other if necessary). Emphasize that the changes are reversible.
  - The patient's consumption of alcohol compared with average consumption.
  - The patient's consumption of alcohol compared with that of his/her friends.
  - The risks of alcohol (obesity, hypertension, liver diseases, headache, hangover, insomnia, sexual dysfunction, accidents).
  - Benefits of reduced alcohol consumption (tolerance and risk of dependence decrease, safety aspects, economic benefit).
  - Written information (risks of heavy drinking, how to estimate one's own drinking, limits of safe drinking, how to reduce drinking).
  - Guidelines and limits: guidelines can be regarded as a prescription. Set clear limits with the patient: a limit of daily use and a limit of days per week and month when alcohol is consumed. The patient must not drink on consecutive days.
  - Further sessions at about two week intervals (a drinking diary if necessary, new laboratory tests). Tell the patient that drinking will be discussed again at the next meeting.
  - Motivate the patient to change his/her drinking habits.
  - Emphasize the patient's personal responsibility and encourage him with optimism.

Who benefits from brief intervention?

- Heavy drinkers (and those approaching the limits of heavy drinking) who do not yet have severe problems caused by alcohol abuse. They may not yet have noticed their excessive use of alcohol, or looked for help to reduce their drinking.
- The patients are identified by family doctors, in outpatient clinics and at health check-ups when the doctor pays attention to symptoms or laboratory test results that indicate alcohol abuse, and when heavy drinking is recognized as a possible cause of symptoms.
- Carefully consider whether it is useful to start talking about alcohol abuse when the patient has come for some other reason than alcohol abuse. The motivation of the patient may be insufficient.
- In case of emergency situations it is not very realistic to try to influence the patient's drinking habits, especially if he/she is intoxicated. It is better to offer a new appointment time. When testing a driver's blood for alcohol, inform the individual where to find professional help. Interventions for drunken drivers have been shown to be moderately effective B [9 10].
- A heavy drinker with clear dependence seldom benefits from mini-intervention. If they cannot reduce alcohol consumption during, for example, three months' intervention, they should be forwarded to a unit specialized in alcohol-related diseases.

References

1. University of York. Centre for Reviews and Dissemination. Brief interventions and alcohol use. Effective Health Care 1993;1:13.
2. The Database of Abstracts of Reviews of Effectiveness (University of York), Database no.: DARE-950035. In: The Cochrane Library, Issue 4, 1999. Oxford: Update Software.
3. Kahan M, Wilson L, Becker L. Physician-based interventions with problem drinkers. Can Med Ass J 1995;152:851–859.
4. The Database of Abstracts of Reviews of Effective ness (University of York), Database no.: DARE-954003. In: The Cochrane Library, Issue 4, 1999. Oxford: Update Software.
5. Poikolainen K. Effectiveness of brief interventions to reduce alcohol intake in primary health care populations. Preventive Medicine 1999;28:503–509.
6. The Database of Abstracts of Reviews of Effectiveness (University of York), Database no.: DARE-999258.

In: The Cochrane Library, Issue 1, 2001. Oxford: Update Software.
7. Freemantle N, Song F, Sheldon T, Long A. Brief interventions and alcohol use. York: NHS Centre for Reviews and Dissemination. NHS Centre for Reviews and Dissemination (NHSCRD). ISBN: 0965 0288. Effectiv Health Care 1993. 13.
8. The Health Technology Assessment Database, Database no.: HTA-950035. In: The Cochrane Library, Issue 1, 2001. Oxford: Update Software.
9. Wells-Parker E, Bangert-Drowns R, McMillen R, Willians M. Final results from a meta-analysis of remedial interventions with drink/drive offenders. Addiction 1995;90:907–926.
10. The Database of Abstracts of Reviews of Effectiveness (University of York), Database no.: DARE-950357. In: The Cochrane Library, Issue 4, 1999. Oxford: Update Software.

40.5 Treatment of alcohol withdrawal

Editors

Aims

- To help the patient to adjust physically to function without alcohol and to avoid seizures, cardiac arrhythmia or delirium tremens associated with withdrawal.
- To provide a calm, non-judgemental environment that will motivate the patient to continue to deal with the problem of alcohol abuse.
- To prevent irreversible brain damage associated with thiamine deficiency (Wernicke encephalopathy).

Pathology

- At least 80 g/day of pure alcohol must be consumed on several days before clinically significant symptoms of alcohol withdrawal can occur.
- Severe withdrawal symptoms indicate consumption of more that 180 g/day of alcohol over one or several weeks.

Pharmacological treatment

- All patients suffering from symptoms of alcohol withdrawal are given thiamine.
  - Intramuscularly 50 mg
  - The absorption of vitamins given orally is uncertain.
- Measured with the CIWA-Ar scale, a score below 20 indicates minor withdrawal symptoms and does not necessitate the use of sedative medication.
  - Prescription medication should be avoided during withdrawal as mixed patterns of drug use and abuse are common.
  - Medication is given only to a patient whose identity is known. Never prescribe for an unknown person.
  - The patient can be given the daily medication at one time, e.g. chlordiazepoxide (A) [1 2 3 4 5 6] 25–50 (–75) mg.
  - Medication can be tapered over a period of a few days. The patient is expected to be sober when collecting the medication on a daily basis.
- If the CIWA-Ar score is above 20, diazepam (A) [1 2 3 4 5 6] loading is indicated.

Diazepam loading

Basic rule

- The patient is given a loading dose of diazepam during the course of less than 12 hours. The elimination of the drug and its active metabolites takes several days.

To observe

- Prior to starting the medication rule out the possibility of skull injury, infection, diabetes or drug intoxication.

Dosing

- A dose of 20 mg of diazepam is given orally every 90 to 120 minutes until the patient falls asleep peacefully. If the breath analyser measures more than 0.1 % alcohol, the starting dose is 10 mg.
- The mean total dose of diazepam needed for loading is 80–120 mg (4–5 doses over 8–10 hours). A dose below 180 mg is sufficient in more than 90% or the patients. If necessary, the sedative effect of diazepam can be boostered by giving 5 mg of haloperidol orally.

Aftercare

- The patient must be observed for 2 days on ward from the onset of the loading dose treatment. The initial dose of diazepam is sufficient to ensure sleep during several following nights. In case the patient suffers from sleep disturbances, 20 mg temazepam can be given on the first 5–10 evenings.
- On leaving the ward, the patient is given (preferably written) a warning stating that the medication influences adversely the ability to perform and drive a vehicle during the following 5 days. Drinking alcohol is not recommended during this period.
- The use of neuroleptics is not recommended in alcohol withdrawal as they lower the threshold of seizures (A) [1 2 3 4 5 6] and may cause hypotension.

References

1. Mayo-Smith MF. Pharmacological management of alcohol withdrawal: a meta-analysis and evidence-based practice guideline. JAMA 1997;278:144–151.

2. The Database of Abstracts of Reviews of Effectiveness (University of York), Database no.: DARE-978228. In: The Cochrane Library, Issue 4, 1999. Oxford: Update Software.
3. Williams D, McBride AJ. The drug treatment of alcohol withdrawal syndrome: a systematic review. Alcohol and Alcoholism 1998;33:103–115.
4. The Database of Abstracts of Reviews of Effectiveness (University of York), Database no.: DARE-980796. In: The Cochrane Library, Issue 2, 2000. Oxford: Update Software.
5. Holbrook AM, Crowther R, Lotter A, Cheng C, King D. Meta-analysis of benzodiazepine use in the treatment of acute alcohol withdrawal. Canadian Medical Association Journal 1999;160:649–655.
6. The Database of Abstracts of Reviews of Effectiveness (University of York), Database no.: DARE-998514. In: The Cochrane Library, Issue 1, 2001. Oxford: Update Software.

40.6 Drugs used in alcohol dependence

Editors

Basic rules

- Alcohol dependence is a chronic illness the prognosis of which may be improved with drug therapy.
- The best results have been achieved by combining pharmacological agents with therapy aimed at controlling alcohol use and preventing relapses. Alcoholism clinics have experience in adapting these cognitive methods into the care of patients with alcohol dependence.

Naltrexone

- Naltrexone is an opiate antagonist and its use in alcohol dependence is based on the hypothesis that addiction is a dysfunction of the reward-regulating centres within the central nervous system. The dysfunctioning may be relieved by blocking the opioid-mediated activity of the centres.

Dose

- The recommended daily dose is 50 mg.
- However, the bioavailability shows great variability and the daily dose required to achieve adequate opiate blockade may vary from 25 mg to 100 mg. The individual dose should be decided according to clinical response.

Clinical efficacy

- In clinical trials, alcohol-dependent patients have been treated with daily naltrexone for 12 weeks as an adjunct to other psychosocial rehabilitation B [1 2 3].
- During a three month follow-up period over half of the subjects treated with naltrexone avoided relapse if they received concomitant therapy for relapse prevention and coping skills. The study subjects were followed for a six month period, and some but not all of the benefits resulting from naltrexone treatment persisted after discontinuation of treatment. Continued treatment of more than three months duration may, however, be beneficial for some patients. To induce abstinence the initial treatment period should be uninterrupted and of sufficient duration.

Adverse effects

- Naltrexone may cause disturbances in hepatic function, and serum transaminases (ALT and AST) should be checked every 2–3 weeks after the therapy has been initiated.

Disulfiram

- Disulfiram is used as a "brief intervention" to offer support and to prevent impulsive relapses in motivated patients, who have undergone successful detoxification.
- Disulfiram inhibits the enzyme aldehyde dehydrogenase. The inhibition gives rise to the accumulation of acetaldehyde in the body after the ingestion of alcohol.
- Aceltadehyde causes very unpleasant systemic reactions (an "Antabuse reaction"), the fear of which stops the person from ingesting alcohol.
  - The symptoms include: flushing of the face, hypotension, reflectory tachycardia, palpitations, anxiety, headache, nausea and vomiting.
- **Disulfiram may induce liver damage** 2–3 months after treatment onset. Even though the liver damage will not become chronic upon discontinuation of treatment, it may rarely prove to be fatal.

Dose

- The treatment is started with a dose of 800 mg on 3 consecutive days, thereafter the dose is 400 mg twice a week. Alternatively, a 100–200 mg dose can be administered daily.
- The patient takes the medicine under supervision.
- Even small amounts of alcohol may precipitate a reaction up to 2 weeks after the last dose.
- In some patients the above-mentioned doses are insufficient to induce a reaction. In these patients the dose can be doubled.
- The medication should be taken for 6–12 months. During this period the risk of relapse diminishes. If the patient does relapse after discontinuing the medication, disulfiram can be introduced again.
- The pharmacological efficacy of disulfiram implants has not been proven.

Follow-up

- In order to avoid adverse effects, liver enzymes (ALT and gamma-GT) should be checked before the treatment is introduced and every two weeks thereafter for two months.
- Laboratory markers of alcohol consumption, such as gamma-GT and MCV, should be checked on the regular follow-up visits, e.g. every 3–6 months. Favourable changes in the markers support abstinence.
- Close monitoring is important at the beginning of the treatment because disulfiram may also cause neurological and psychiatric adverse effects as well as cutaneous eruptions.
- Disulfiram has interactions with phenytoin, theophylline and warfarin. The dose of these drugs should be adjusted accordingly.
- The concomitant use of metronidazole, isoniazid and amitriptyline can induce confusion which may lead to psychosis.

Other drugs

- Selective serotonin re-uptake inhibitors have been studied in the treatment of alcohol dependence, particularly in depressive patients. No strong evidence has been gained of their efficacy. On the other hand, many psychoactive drugs, anxiolytics in particular, may help to alleviate the symptoms of alcohol dependence.
- Acamprosate is an alternative to naltrexone. Both drugs are superior to placebo B [4 5 6 7 8 9 10 11]. Long-term studies have been carried out with acamprosate; its effect may last for some time after treatment discontinuation.
- Topiramate is an antiepileptic drug which might antagonise the rewarding effects of alcohol and thus be of use in the treatment of alcohol dependence B [12].

References

1. Srisurapanont M, Jarusuraisin N. Opioid antagonists for alcohol dependence. Cochrane Database Syst Rev. 2004;(2): CD001867.
2. Agency for Health Care Research and Quality (AHCR). Pharmacotherapy for alcohol dependence. Rockville, MD: Agency for Health Care Research and Quality (AHQR). Agency for Health Care Research and Quality (AHCR). Evidence Report/Tech. 1999.
3. The Health Technology Assessment Database, Database no.: HTA-200082420. In: The Cochrane Library, Issue 1, 2001. Oxford: Update Software.
4. Hoes MJ. Relapse prevention in alcoholics: a review of acamprosate versus naltrexone. Clinical Drug Investigation 1999;17:211–216.
5. The Database of Abstracts of Reviews of Effectiveness (University of York), Database no.: DARE-990792. In: The Cochrane Library, Issue 1, 2001. Oxford: Update Software.
6. Agency for Health Care Research and Quality (AHQR). Pharmacotherapy for alcohol dependence. Rockville, MD: Agency for Health Care Research and Quality (AHQR). Agency for Health Care Research and Quality (AHQR). Evidence Report/Tech. 1999.
7. Health Technology Assessment Database: HTA-200082420. In: The Cochrane Library, Issue 1, 2001. Oxford: Update Software.
8. Bouza Alvarez C, Magro de la Plaza MA, Romero Martinez JJ, Amate Blanco JM. Assessment of therapeutic strategies for alcohol dependence: opioid antagonists and acamprosate. IPE-02/35. Madrid: Agencia de Evaluacion de Tecnologias Sanitarias (AETS). 2002. 114. Agencia de Evaluacion de Tecnologias Sanitarias (AETS).
9. Health Technology Assessment Database: HTA-20030481. The Cochrane Library, Issue 1, 2004. Chichester, UK: John Wiley & Sons, Ltd.
10. Berglund M, Andreasson S, Franck J, Fridell M, Hakanson I, Johansson B-A. Treatment of alcohol and drug abuse – an evidence-based review. Stockholm: Swedish Council on Technology Assessment in Health Care (SBU). 2001. 850. Swedish Council on Technology Assessment in Health Care (SBU).
11. Health Technology Assessment Database: HTA-20010980. The Cochrane Library, Issue 1, 2004. Chichester, UK: John Wiley & Sons, Ltd.
12. Johnson BA, Ait-Daoud N, Bowden CL, DiClemente CC, Roache JD, Lawson K, Javors MA, Ma JZ. Oral topiramate for treatment of alcohol dependence: a randomised controlled trial. Lancet 2003;361(9370):1677–85.

40.10 Encountering a drug addict in ambulatory care

Editors

Objectives

- An addict characteristically uses any means to increase the dose of the drug beyond recommendations. Addiction is clearly different from usual drug dependence, where abstinence symptoms prevent discontinuation of medication.
- A certain degree of mistrust is needed to identify a drug addict. However, when a physician encounters an addict, he/she should be capable of empathizing, being direct and should have a sincere desire to understand and help the patient.

Drugs commonly available on the street

- Buprenorphine
- Methadone
- Dextromethorphane (used both orally and intravenously)
- Ethyl morphine
- Codeine
- Psychostimulating drugs

- Antitussives containing opioids
- Benzodiazepines
- Drugs that cause intoxication in combination with alcohol
  - Atropine-containing drugs for diarrhoea
  - Biperiden
- Anticholinergic drugs
- Barbiturates

Addicts' strategies for acquiring drugs

- Target
  - Young physicians
  - Physicians who, because of personal problems or lack of professional skills, prescribe unnecessary medications
  - Naive, empathetic physicians.
- A patient trying to obtain drugs
  - Knows the indications of narcotic drugs and is able to tell the physician "the correct patient history and symptoms".
  - May say that they are an addict, but are trying to give up drug abuse and now need the drug only temporarily to get through the worst period.
  - Is able to appeal with many touching stories.
  - Often complains of pain in the neck, migraine or urethral colic pain. Prescribing a strong opioid for an unknown patient, at least at the first visit, is hardly ever justified.
  - Often has various credentials concerning his/her disease, for example medical reports, statements and prescriptions from well-known physicians. Some of the addicts really have had the disease they claim to have.
  - Often shows a scar as evidence of pain.
  - Seldom, but regularly, visits many physicians, and in each instance pretends to be a patient who uses the medication only as prescribed.
  - May threat with violence, suicide or blackmail, for example by writing to the newspaper.
  - A "drug hunter" may be a clean, nice guy or an attractive young woman.

How to act when suspecting drug abuse

- The physician should state that although abstinence symptoms may be troublesome, they are seldom life threatening. By so doing the physician introduces some discipline into the situation.
- Calmness of the physician shows that he is in control of the situation and is not easily fooled.
- The physician may say that he can contact a specialized drug abuse centre to provide the patient with proper care.
- The physician may prescribe other analgesics than opioids for pain treatment, and sedative neuroleptics (chlorpromazine 50–200 mg, levomepromazine 25–100 mg for the night) to alleviate anxiety. The patient can refuse this symptomatic treatment; the physician should not.
- Do not prescribe opioids, psychostimulants or barbiturates to people who clearly want these drugs in particular.
- Do not prescribe benzodiazepines to unknown patients, or to those inclined to addictive behaviour; do not prescribe high doses and large amounts, especially at the first visit and without a regular, firm psychotherapeutic treatment relationship.
- You may use various proper examinations (thorough somatic examination for a patient with pain) or consultations to clarify the situation. This gives you more time and the possibility of warding off drug seekers and dealers in a friendly but pertinent way.
- Do not succumb and write a prescription if an addict threatens you. Tell them that you will call the police immediately or report blackmail to the authorities. For a violent patient, see 35.4.
- A doctor-patient relationship can begin if the physician is able to understand the poor somatic, psychological or social situation of an addict, and is willing to help these patients according to the possibilities.
- Finally, it is important to remember that most of the patients who use benzodiazepines regularly are not drug addicts but need constant drug therapy to alleviate long-lasting and severe anxiety symptoms.

40.11 Treatment of drug addicts

Antti Holopainen

General

- A physician may encounter a drug addict in any situation. It is important to recognize addiction (alcohol, drugs) and always act professionally and pertinently, see 40.2.
- An addict may try to obtain addictive drugs, see 40.10. They may have acute psychosis with anxiety and hallucinations, acute hepatitis, endocarditis, any severe disease from pneumonia to sepsis, an epileptic attack, etc.
- An addict may also seek withdrawal or substitution therapy. The physician should not trust that withdrawal in ambulatory care with the help of codeine, ethylmorphine, dextropropoxyphene or tramadol that the patient may have requested could be successful. The use of buprenorphine and methadone in withdrawal substitution or maintenance therapy is limited to specialized clinics or to be carried out under their supervision.
- Because of the threat of spreading HIV and hepatitis C and B, the risks associated with intravenous drug use should be discussed in all contacts with addicted persons.

Common somatic diseases, symptoms and signs

- Central nervous system complications, rhabdomyolysis and peripheral compression damage resulting from overdosage and unconsciousness have become more common.

- Epidemics of hepatitis A occur among drug users.
- Viral infections.
- Hepatitis C is very common in patients who use i.v. drugs (approximately 40%), sometimes concomitantly with hepatitis B. In acute cases, symptoms include icterus, poor general condition and hepatomegaly. The majority of cases are asymptomatic carriers of the disease.
- Infections ranging from infected needle punctures to endocarditis.
- Needle punctures can be found anywhere in addition to the cubital area. Patients who have used injected drugs for a long time often inject between the fingers and toes.
- Patients who use injected dextropropoxyphene may have deep necrotized cavities in the skin.
- Cannabis users often have erythematous conjuctivae and buccal mucous membranes.
- Opioid users have small, non-reactive pupils.
- Amphetamine users are often hyperkinetic and have hypertension and tachycardia.
- There are increasing numbers of pregnant young women who are addicted to heroin, amphetamine or use a mixture of substances and who are unable to break the habit without treatment (26.18).

Psychiatric diseases, symptoms and signs

- Anxiety, poor impulse control, and change of mood are common.
- Most patients have a personality disorder in addition to alcohol or drug abuse.
- There are increasing numbers of drug-dependent persons with a chronic psychiatric disorder (schizophrenia).
- Pay particular attention to psychotic symptoms.
    - Massive paranoid or hallucinatory symptoms warrant treatment in a psychiatric hospital in a closed ward.
    - Milder paranoid symptoms (feeling of being observed) and auditory hallucinations (patient hears his/her name being called or a phone ringing) often subside even without neuroleptic treatment, and the patient is familiar with these symptoms.
- Acute depression is typical when the effect of amphetamine or cocaine ceases; a more chronic depression and apathy can be associated with any drug either primarily or secondarily.
- Most patients who abuse drugs are also heavy drinkers.
- Anxiety, sleep disorders and adverse effects of the abused drugs have made many drug addicts additionally dependent on benzodiazepines.

Examination in a health centre

- Blood count, CRP, hepatic enzymes, serum HbsAg, hepatitis C antibodies, HIV antibodies and a urine test for drugs are basic tests.
- A qualitative urine test for drugs
    - reveals e.g. cannabis, opioids (except buprenorphine, tramadol and dextropropoxyphene), amphetamine, benzodiazepines and cocaine. If a buprenorphine test is deemed necessary, it should be requested separately.
- Codeine (antitussives containing codeine) and paracetamol-codeine combinations may give positive results.
- Other laboratory tests and x-ray as indicated by clinical signs.

Vaccinations

- All persons who use i.v. drugs and those in close contact with them should be given a hepatitis B vaccination. The need for a vaccination should be brought up whenever the clinical findings give grounds for it.

Drug therapy

- Benzodiazepines should be avoided; on the other hand, it is important to diagnose possible benzodiazepine dependence and arrange treatment.
- If there is a risk of convulsions (barbiturate or benzodiazepine dependence, previous convulsions), carbamazepine and, for patients with hepatitis C, oxcarbazepine should be used. These drugs can also be used in the treatment of aggression problems and mood changes.
- Psychosis and anxiety caused by amphetamine or other stimulants may be treated with, for example, melperone 25 mg three times daily or flupenthixol 0.5–1 mg three times daily. If the symptoms are severe, haloperidol in small doses is effective.
- Prefer short courses maximally 3 to 5 days of short-acting benzodiazepines. If insomnia is long lasting, prescribe promazine or sedative tricyclic antidepressants if there is good and stable patient-doctor relationship.
- In prolonged depression citalopram and sulpiride, for example, are safe alternatives. Concomitant use of serotonin uptake inhibitors and amphetamine derivatives may lead to dangerous adverse effects that should be avoided.
- Withdrawal and substitution therapy in opioid-dependence, see below.

Referring to further treatment

- If the somatic condition requires acute attention at the specialist unit level, refer the patient according to normal criteria; however, it is useful to discuss the possibilities of treating addiction already in this initial phase.
- Consider referral to psychiatric care if the patient is psychotic.
- In minors, serious cases of substance abuse justify compulsory care.
- Find out the possibilities for treatment in your own area and distribute this information at your workplace; this will reduce anxiety and feelings of hate and helplessness, and resources can be directed towards treating the patients.

Withdrawal, substitution and maintenance treatment of opioid addiction

Withdrawal therapy

- Buprenorphine is the drug of choice for withdrawal in opioid dependency (C) [1].
- In withdrawal treatment the medication is started under supervision with a single dose of 2–4 mg when at least 6 hours have elapsed from the last dose of heroin. If the patient has used methadone, the time gap must be at least 24–48 hours depending on the dose. The maximum dose during the first 24 hours is 8 mg.
- The dose is raised during the first 3 days of therapy to 10–12 mg and the drug is discontinued over 5–8 days with dose tapering if the aim is to stop heroin use.
- If the person seeking withdrawal has used buprenorphine for a long time, the treatment should be implemented over 1–2 months with gradual dose tapering. Buprenorphine can be started to control withdrawal symptoms and it can be used at a sufficient dose for the necessary time during the course of a somatic disease if the withdrawal symptoms aggravate the patient's clinical condition and impede therapy (refer to local legislation).
- Clonidine chloride or lofexidine (C) [2] [3] can be used to control opioid withdrawal symptoms in mild opioid dependency, for example, in adolescents aged below 18 years with a short history of opioid use. Other indications of clonidine and lofexidine are
  - withdrawal symptoms triggered by buprenorphine on initiation of the medication when the patient has been using methadone or some other long-acting opioid agonist,
  - the discontinuation phase of withdrawal using buprenorphine if the symptoms become too aggravated, and also
  - the possible activation of withdrawal symptoms when the patient transfers from buprenorphine to naltrexone.
- The starting dose of clonidine is 75–200 $\mu g \times 2$–4. The maximum daily dose is 1–1.2 mg. Monitoring of blood pressure is essential.
- Lofexidine is used increasingly for opioid withdrawal as the drug does not lower blood pressure as easily and the patients appear to approve the drug better. The dose is 1–2 tablets administered 2–3 times daily up to a dose of 12 tablets daily (2.4 mg). The medication can be continued for 7–10 days in heroin withdrawal. The therapy is continued for 2–3 weeks for the symptoms of the tapering phase of buprenorphine. With both clonidine and lofexidine additional drugs are needed: anti-inflammatory analgesics, levomepromazine in low doses, often also loperamide for diarrhoea and low doses of benzodiazepines.
- Rapid and successful withdrawal of opioids without substitution or maintenance therapy is highly unlikely if the dependency has become chronic. Instead of quick withdrawal, buprenorphine can be used for long-term (one month) withdrawal or for short-term (less than a year) substitution therapy where the aim is withdrawal. This treatment option is suitable for those patients who have used buprenorphine for years for self-medication and are motivated to try withdrawal. If withdrawal even with a slow schedule fails, the drug can be continued as substitution therapy.

Substitution therapy

- Buprenorphine (B) [4] or methadone can be used for substitution (B) [5]. Good compliance is achieved with daily buprenorphine doses of 16–24 mg. In routine therapy 32 mg is considered the maximum daily dose. Moderate doses of methadone have been found to be equally effective as high doses of buprenorphine. If high-dose buprenorphine (16–32 mg/day) is not sufficient to abolish the craving for opioids or withdrawal symptoms, methadone is a better alternative.
- When used for substitution, buprenorphine is started as in withdrawal (see above). The dose is raised according to response by 2–4 mg per day up to the optimal treatment range of 12–24 mg. The patient's graving for opioids, withdrawal symptoms before the next dose and possible concominant use of injected substances are followed up. Possible benzodiazepines use that has accumulated over time is gradually discontinued when the optimal range of substitution has been achieved. If benzodiazepines have been used in very high doses, they may cause sedation when the buprenorphine dose is raised, and the speed of dose increments must be reduced.
- Methadone medication is started with 10–20 mg following up the patient's condition. During the first 24 h the maximum dose is 30–40 mg. The dosage is raised by 5 mg per day up to the daily dose of 50 mg, whereafter the interval between dose increments is prolonged to 3–7 days according to response. Remember that unlike buprenorphine, methadone is a toxic substance and the dose increments lead to stabilization level only in one week. With methadone, the level of medication corresponding to high-dose buprenorphine is reached with 60–80 mg. However, in the majority of patients methadone tolerance develops gradually over the first treatment weeks after the stable phase has been achieved, causing withdrawal symptoms and necessitating dose increments. In long-term therapy the dose of methadone is tailored individually, however, a large group of patients manages well with 80–120 mg daily (A) [6].
- Substitution is usually given under supervision. Depending on the legislation of each country, the patient may also be given doses for administration at home. This requires good compliance. With buprenorphine, the patient can move on to supervised less frequent dosing (every other day or 3 times per week with twice or three times the daily dose given at the place of care). A maximum of eight daily doses can be given to a compliant patient at one time. The patient should have a medical form confirming his/her right to have the medicines in question for therapy. This form should contain dosing and storage instructions. Methadone must be stored in a locked container, as one daily dose is already lethal to an adult without tolerance to methadone.
- At the end of 2002 FDA approved a combination preparation containing buprenorphine (8 mg) and naloxone (2 mg)

for use in primary care B [7]. Injecting the drug is unpleasant for heroin addicts, which is expected to prevent misuse by injecting. Buprenorphine – naloxone – combination has been in a trial use also in Finnish specialized clinics, and their experience suggests decreased risk of injecting and distribution to the streets. Prospective official acceptance of the preparation enables more flexible substitution and maintenance practise in future. Buprenorphine implants and depot preparation are in clinical trial. Their future utilization may enable even safer substitution and maintenance treatment.

- Naltrexone is an option for patients who wish to stop agonist substitution therapy given under supervision but who are at risk of relapse because of late withdrawal symptoms and opioid craving C [8]. The medication is started after withdrawal with buprenorphine at a low dose (e.g. 12.5 mg) and is raised gradually. If withdrawal symptoms appear when the drug is changed, clonidine or lofexidine can be used for alleviation (see withdrawal symptoms above). Naltrexone should be given under supervision for the first 3 months so that the patient adjusts to the decrease in opioid craving caused by the drug. Naltrexone can be prescribed for self-medication. However, an intensive doctor-patient relationship should continue also after the first 3 months for early detection and prevention of possible relapses.

References

1. Gowing L, Ali R, White J. Buprenorphine for the management of opioid withdrawal. Cochrane Database Syst Rev. 2004;(2):CD002025.
2. Gowing L, Farrell M, Ali R, White J. Alpha2 adrenergic agonists for the management of opioid withdrawal. Cochrane Database Syst Rev. 2004;(2):CD002024.
3. Gowing L, Ali R, White J. Opioid antagonists and adrenergic agonists for the management of opioid withdrawal. The Cochrane Database of Systematic Reviews, Cochrane Library number: CD002021. In: The Cochrane Library, Issue 2, 2002. Oxford: Update Software.
4. Mattick RP, Kimber J, Breen C, Davoli M. Buprenorphine maintenance versus placebo or methadone maintenance for opioid dependence. Cochrane Database Syst Rev. 2004;(2):CD002207.
5. Mattick RP, Breen C, Kimber J, Davoli M. Methadone maintenance therapy versus no opioid replacement therapy for opioid dependence. Cochrane Database Syst Rev. 2004;(2):CD002209.
6. Faggiano F, Vigna-Taglianti F, Versino E, Lemma P. Methadone maintenance at different dosages for opiod dependence. Cochrane Database Syst Rev. 2004;(2):CD002208.
7. Fudala PJ, Bridge TP, Herbert S, Williford WO, Chiang CN, Jones K, Collins J, Raisch D, Casadonte P, Goldsmith RJ, Ling W, Malkerneker U, McNicholas L, Renner J, Stine S, Tusel D. Office-based treatment of opiate addiction with a sublingual-tablet formulation of buprenorphine and naloxone. N Engl J Med 2003;349(10):949–58.
8. Kirchmayer U, Davoli M, Verster A. Naltrexone maintenance treatment for opioid dependence. Cochrane Database Syst Rev. 2004;(2):CD001333.

40.12 Steroid doping

Editors

Aims

- Remember the possibility of anabolic steroid use when a young competitive athlete or a recreational power athlete seeks medical treatment for acne. The physician should be particularly alert if the patient has, in addition to acne, a strong musclature and other side effects of anabolic steroids visible on the skin. Rule out the use of anabolic steroids before starting therapy for acne.

Preparations

- All steroids used for doping have both androgenic and anabolic properties. The range of non-medically used anabolic substances on the black market includes, for example, the following:
- Methandrostenolone
  - The most widely used, injectable anabolic steroid
  - The names of methandrostenolone preparations sold on the black market include Silabolin, Deca-Durabolin, Retabolin and Laurobolin.
  - Methandrostenolone is detectable for long periods in doping tests.
- Testosterone and derivatives
  - The most frequently confiscated anabolic substance
  - There are several preparations of East European origin on sale on the street. Commercial injectable preparations include Androxon, Estandron Prolongatum, Primodian-Depot, Primoteston-Depot, Restandol, Sustanon, Panteston, Testoviron depot and Undestor. The most popular preparation is Sustanon 250 of which there is a wide range of bogus products.
  - Orally administered testosterone derivatives include methyltestosterone and testosterone undecanoate (Panteston). Nicknamed "chocolate raisins", Panteston is used especially towards the end of a course of steroids because it is not evident in doping tests for very long.
- Trenbolone
  - An injectable derivative of nandrolone, sold on the street as Parabolan and Finajet. Trenbolone does not cause gynaecomastia.
- Stanozolol
  - Strongly virilizing.
  - The most familiar trade names are Stromba and Winstrol.
- Tamoxifen
  - Tamoxifen is an oestrogen receptor antagonist used to prevent gynaecomastia during use of anabolic steroids.

Common side effects

Subjective

- Increased aggressiveness
- Mood fluctuations
  - Euphoria (omnipotence)
  - Depression
  - Delusions
  - Sleep disturbances
- Increased libido, later impotence
- Spasticity
- Headache
- Dizziness
- Nausea

Urogenital

- In men
  - Dysuria
  - Testicular pain
  - Oligozoospermia or azoospermia
  - Prostatic hypertrophy
  - Prostatic cancer
  - Gynaecomastia
- In women
  - Dimished size of breasts
  - Deepening of voice
  - Menstrual irregularities, amenorrhoea
  - Clitoral enlargement
  - Uterine atrophy
  - Teratogenic effects (pseudohermaphroditism, foetal death)

Hepatic

- Elevations in transaminases
- Cholestasis
- Increase in LDL-cholesterol concentration
- Decrease in HDL-cholesterol concentration
- Peliosis hepatis (blood-filled cysts in the liver)
- Benign tumours
- Ruptures of hepatic tumours
- Cancers

Musculoskeletal

- Increased susceptibility to injuries
- Premature epiphyseal closure (these young people will never achieve their full growth potential)

Cardiovascular and vascular

- Increased blood pressure
- Cardiomyopathy
- Direct toxic effect (cardiovascular accident)
- Atherosclerotic heart disease

Endocrine

- Impaired glucose tolerance and insulin resistance
- Changes of thyroid function

Dermatological

- Seborrhoea, greasy skin and hair
- Comedones, sebaceous cysts
- Papulopustular or cystic acne or rosacea
- Furunculosis, folliculitis, pyoderma, abscesses (from contaminated needles)
- Male-type alopecia (permanent in women)
- Hirsutism of face and body (in women)
- Striae

Immunological

- Reduced immunoglobulin A concentration can lead to increased susceptibility to infections.

Investigations

- Serum ALT, serum AST
- Serum cholesterol, serum HDL-cholesterol
- Serum triglycerides
- Liver ultrasound

Withdrawal

- Warning about the risks of steroid abuse
- The patient should be informed that giving up steroids after many weeks of use may cause tiredness, depression and impotence.

Follow-up

- Serum SHBG, serum LH
- Monitoring of liver function as required
- Referral to a sports physician

40.20 Smoking cessation

Marina Erhola, Heidi Alenius

- Fourteen percent of all deaths are caused by illnesses related to smoking, and 50% of smokers will die of an illness caused by smoking (Figure 40.21.1).
- The majority of smokers (80%) see their doctor annually, but only about 20% are advised to stop smoking.
- Seven out of ten smokers would like to stop smoking. Smoking cessation usually needs 3–4 attempts to succeed.

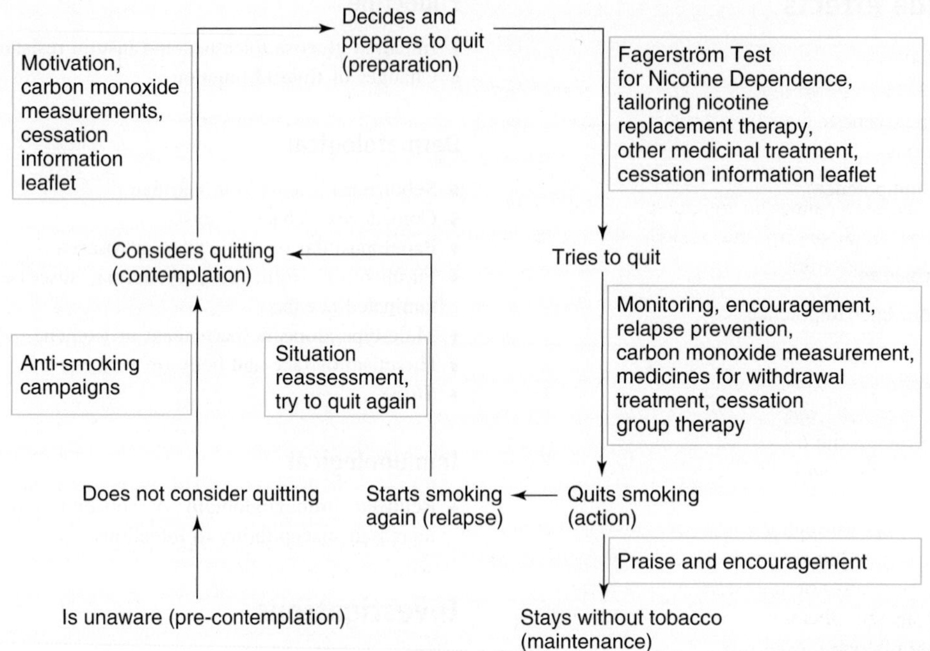

Figure 40.20.1 The process of cessation in stages and the various interventions used during the process (adapted from Prochaska JO, DiClemente CC. Stages and processes of self-change in smoking: towards an interactive model of change. J Consult Clin Psychol 1983;51:390–5).

- A simple encouragement by a doctor to stop smoking is effective (A) [1 2 3], but a three minute counselling session is even more effective. Use the Six A's Approach (ask, assess, account, advise, assist, arrange).
- Nicotine quickly causes physical dependence.
- Nicotine replacement therapy increases the success rate of smoking cessation 1.5–2 fold (A) [4 5 6].
- Smoking cessation should form a part of public health activities (C) [7 8].

Nicotine dependence and other factors

- The pharmacological and behavioural processes that determine nicotine addiction are similar to those that determine other substance dependencies.
- Propensity to dependence, personality and living surroundings all contribute towards starting and continuing to smoke.
- In the western countries the average age to start smoking is 14 years, and there are a multitude of social factors involved in starting smoking.
- Attempts should be made to stop a young person's smoking when smoking is still experimental and only occasional.

Smoking cessation

Stages of Change Model

- Motivation to lifestyle change has been described with a Stages of Change Model by Prochaska and DiClemente, see Figure 40.20.1:
    - Precontemplation (apathy, denial)
    - Contemplation
    - Preparation, decision making
    - Action (cessation) and
    - Maintenance (permanent non-smoker)
- Determine your patient's present stage in order to be able to support and motivate him/her in the best way possible.
- Accept that smoking cessation is a long process.

Positive effects of smoking cessation

- Circulation starts to improve within weeks, and cough and dyspnoea will improve within 3–9 months.
- Subjective stress will decrease, and both the quantity and quality of sleep will improve.
- The risk of myocardial infarction will halve within five years, and that of lung cancer within ten years.
- In chronic obstructive pulmonary disease, smoking cessation at any stage will have a beneficial effect on prognosis.

Withdrawal symptoms

- Most people will experience some withdrawal symptoms which usually are caused by the decreased concentration of nicotine in the body:
    - Irritability
    - Impatience
    - Craving for a cigarette
    - Restlessness
    - Difficulty in concentrating

- Insomnia
- Headache
- Increased appetite

♦ Symptoms will emerge within 2–12 hours after stopping smoking, peak at days 1–3 and last on average from 3 to 4 weeks.

♦ The duration of symptoms show great interindividual variation. The duration cannot be anticipated by the number of cigarettes smoked or by the results of a nicotine dependence test (Fagerström).

Weight gain

♦ Weight gain should be expected after stopping smoking.

♦ In men, the average weight gain is 2.8 kg and in women 3.8 kg during the 6–12 months following stopping. However, 10% of men and 13% of women will gain more than 13 kg.

♦ Weight management through dietary measures and exercise should be advocated, but the main focus should remain on giving up smoking and not on weight management.

♦ Nicotine replacement therapy, particularly chewing gum, may prevent weight gain.

Guidance and management

♦ The opportunity to discuss smoking should be offered to all smokers.

♦ A three minute counselling session is more effective than simple encouragement as an aid to smoking cessation.

♦ **The Six A's Approach**

- ASK about the patient's smoking status at least once a year
  - This is easy to achieve in connection with medical examinations or when instigating treatment or prophylaxis for an illness.
- ASSESS the patient's readiness and willingness to stop. Ask about previous attempts (how successful, how relapsed etc.)
- Keep ACCOUNT on smoking status
  - Preferably on the same sheet in the medical notes (e.g. a dedicated sheet)
  - Smoking habits: cigar, cigarette, snuff, pipe
  - Quantity
  - Duration
    - * Total pack-years of smoking (e.g. 20 years of $\frac{1}{2}$ pack per day = 10 pack-years)
- ADVISE the patient to stop smoking and instigate treatment where necessary.
  - If you feel that stopping smoking will improve the prognosis of a particular illness, make this clear to the patient.
  - Explain to the patient how to prepare for situations where temptation to smoke is great, and about possible withdrawal symptoms.
  - Discuss the treatment options available.
- ASSIST and help the patient in his/her attempt to stop smoking
  - Positive feedback is essential for success
  - Each smokeless day is an achievement and warrants further encouragement
  - Where necessary, guide the patient towards further intervention (an organized group, smoking cessation nurse, regional centres).
- ARRANGE monitoring of progress at follow-up appointments.

♦ Regular visits. The effect of intervention is directly proportionate to the total time spent on the intervention process.

♦ Counselling by a nurse alone also has a positive effect.

♦ Successful cessation seems to be best predicted by the number of contacts with the patient, the duration of the intervention process, the type of contact (multiprofessional) and the mode of contact (individualized). Telephone counselling provides additional benefit B [9].

♦ Individually planned programmes are more effective than using standard models A [10].

♦ Neither acupuncture B [11] nor hypnosis are effective treatment forms. There is no adequate evidence of the benefit of physical exercise alone D [12].

♦ An organized, gradual smoking reduction might be a beneficial treatment form.

♦ Group work. A suitable size of a group is 8–12 persons.

- A session should last about $1\frac{1}{2}$ hours, and the group should meet 6–10 times over 6–10 weeks, according to a planned group programme which should
  - be versatile and flexible
  - progress in stages and
  - take into account the needs of the group.
- Group work which uses behavioural scientific techniques has been shown to be more effective than self-help or short-term counselling A [13].
- The Stages of Change Model can be applied in group work.
- The group leader must carefully prepare the sessions and be appropriately trained.

Drug treatment

Nicotine replacement therapy

♦ Nicotine replacement therapy significantly alleviates withdrawal symptoms.

♦ All forms of nicotine replacement therapy (chewing gum, transdermal patches, nasal spray, inhalator, sublingual tablets and lozenges) are effective and increase the success rate of smoking cessation 1.5–2 fold A [4 5 6].

♦ Nicotine replacement therapy should be recommended to smokers who smoke more than 10 cigarettes per day. Dependence can be assessed by using the Fagerström Test for Nicotine Dependence, Table 40.20.

♦ The dose of nicotine replacement must be sufficiently high and the duration of treatment long enough (3–6 months).

Table 40.20 Fagerström Two Question Test for Nicotine Dependence

Question	Time/Amount	Points
How soon after waking up do you smoke your first cigarette?	within 6 minutes	3
	6–30 minutes	2
	31–60 minutes	1
	after 60 minutes	0
How many cigarettes do you smoke each day?	Fewer than 10	0
	11–20	1
	21–30	2
	more than 3	3

Interpretation: Total number of points 0–1 point = minor nicotine dependence, 2 points = moderate nicotine dependence, 3 points = heavy nicotine dependence, 4–6 points = very heavy nicotine dependence

- A suitable product(s) is chosen individually according to the degree of dependence as well as the patient's situation and preference. For example:
  - For a smoker with a heavy nicotine dependence, 8–12 pieces of 4 mg nicotine chewing gum per day.
  - The strongest patch initially for 3 months, followed by a medium strength patch for 3 weeks and finally the mildest patch.
  - Inhalator or lozenges for denture wearers.
- The combination of a patch with either chewing gum or nasal spray is more effective than any of the products alone.
- Nicotine replacement therapy, even when used for a long time, is less harmful to health than smoking.
- Nicotine chewing gum should be withdrawn gradually or be replaced by patches, because people occasionally become addicted to nicotine chewing gum, but this has not been observed with patches.
- Nicotine replacement therapy is also safe in patients with coronary heart disease. Nevertheless caution should be exercised for two weeks after myocardial infarction, in unstable angina and serious arrhythmias.
- Nicotine replacement therapy is a better alternative than smoking for pregnant and breastfeeding women. Short-acting preparations are recommended.

Bupropion

- Bupropion is effective in smoking cessation (A) [14] [15].
- The dose for the first week is 150 mg o.d. From the second week onwards the dose is 150 mg b.d. Target stop date is agreed for the first or second treatment week. The duration of treatment is 7–9 weeks.
- Support and monitoring form a part of the treatment.
- It is possible to combine bupropion and nicotine replacement therapy.
- Bupropion is associated with a dose-dependent risk of seizure. It is contraindicated in patients with a history of seizures. Particular caution should be exercised in concomitant administration of drugs that can lower the seizure threshold (antipsychotics, antidepressants, antimalarials, quinolones, sedating antihistamines, tramadol, theophylline, systemic corticosteroids or hypoglycaemia inducing antidiabetic drugs), as well as in patients with alcohol abuse or a history of head trauma.

Nortriptyline, other drugs

- The effectiveness in smoking cessation is likely to be based on the occurrence of depression either as a withdrawal symptom or as latent depression activated by smoking cessation.
- Nortriptyline appears to be effective (A) [14] [15]. It is recommended as second-line medication, where nicotine replacement therapy or bupropion cannot be used or where cessation therapy has been unsuccessful.
- Anxiolytics are of no benefit in cessation therapy (A) [14] [15].
- There is no evidence of the effectiveness of naltrexone in the long-term abstinence from smoking (C) [16].
- It has been shown that smoking induces a clinically significant decrease in the concentration of the following drugs: theophylline, tacrine, flecainide, propoxyphene, propranolol, atenolol, nifedipine, benzodiazepines, chlordiazepoxide, heparin, tricyclic anti-depressants, haloperidol and clozapine. Once smoking ceases, plasma concentrations may alter.

References

1. Silagy C, Stead LF. Physician advice for smoking cessation. Cochrane Database Syst Rev. 2004;(2):CD000165.
2. Ashenden R, Silagy C, Weller D. A systematic review of promoting life-style change in general practice. Family Practice 1997;14:160–175.
3. The Database of Abstracts of Reviews of Effectiveness (University of York), Database no.: DARE-970628. In: The Cochrane Library, Issue 4, 1999. Oxford: Update Software.
4. Silagy C, Lancaster T, Stead L, Mant D, Fowler G. Nicotine replacement therapy for smoking cessation. Cochrane Database Syst Rev. 2004;(2):CD000146.
5. Ling Tang J, Law N, Wald N. How effective is nicotine replacement therapy in helping people to stop smoking? BMJ 1994;308:21–26.
6. The Database of Abstracts of Reviews of Effectiveness (University of York), Database no.: DARE-948006. In: The Cochrane Library, Issue 4, 1999. Oxford: Update Software.
7. Sowden AJ, Arblaster L. Mass media interventions for preventing smoking in young people. The Cochrane Database of Systematic Reviews, Cochrane Library number: CD001006. In: The Cochrane Library, Issue 4, 2001. Oxford: Update Software. Updated frequently.
8. Sowden A, Arblaster L, Stead L. Community interventions for preventing smoking in young people. Cochrane Database Syst Rev. 2004;(2):CD001291.
9. Stead LF, Lancaster T, Perera R. Telephone counselling for smoking cessation. Cochrane Database Syst Rev. 2004;(2): CD002850.
10. Lancaster T, Stead LF. Individual behavioural counselling for smoking cessation. Cochrane Database Syst Rev. 2004;(2): CD001292.

11. White AR, Rampes H, Ernst E. Acupuncture for smoking cessation. Cochrane Database Syst Rev. 2004;(2):CD000009.
12. Ussher MH, West R, Taylor AH, McEwen A. Exercise interventions for smoking cessation. Cochrane Database Syst Rev. 2004;(2):CD002295.
13. Stead LF, Lancaster T. Group behaviour therapy programmes for smoking cessation. Cochrane Database Syst Rev. 2004;(2): CD001007.
14. Hughes JR, Stead LF, Lancaster T. Anxiolytics for smoking cessation. Cochrane Database Syst Rev. 2004;(2):CD002849.
15. Hughes JR, Stead LF, Lancaster T. Anxiolytics and antidepressants for smoking cessation. The Cochrane Database of Systematic Reviews, Cochrane Library number: CD000031. In: The Cochrane Library, Issue 43 2003. Oxford: Update Software. Updated frequently.
16. David S, Lancaster T, Stead LF. Opioid antagonists for smoking cessation. Cochrane Database Syst Rev. 2004;(2): CD003086.

40.21 The most common health risks of smoking

Editors

Smoking and risk of disease

- Men who smoke have a 1.7-fold risk of premature death compared with those who do not smoke. In women who smoke, the risk is 1.3–1.9 -fold **A** [1]. The increase in risk is correlated to the quantity of cigarettes and duration of smoking. The risk diminishes after stopping smoking **B** [2].
- The risk of lung cancer is on average 12-fold, but it rises with increased consumption of cigarettes. Smoking increases the risk of cancer of mouth, oesophagus, bladder, kidney and pancreas. Smoking also decreases the efficacy of antineoplastic drugs.
- The risk of myocardial infarction and cerebrovascular diseases increases. In women who use oral contraceptives, smoking increases synergistically the risk of thromboembolic complications.
- The risk of stroke increases.
- The risk of dementia may increase.
- Smoking can act additively or synergistically with chemicals at work and increase the risk of occupational diseases.
- Perinatal mortality and the risk of sudden infant death is higher if the mother smokes.

Smoking and impairment of health

- Smoking causes atherosclerosis and therefore e.g. intermittent claudication. Smoking also may cause impotence by impairing blood circulation in the penis.
- Smoking causes constant irritation in the airways. Chronic bronchitis, COPD and emphysema are much more common in smokers compared with non-smokers.
- Smokers have acute respiratory infections more often than non-smokers.
- Ulcer is more common in smokers. Non-smoking prevents recurrence of ulcer as efficaciously as effective drug therapy.

Exposure to tobacco smoke (passive smoking)

Risk of cancer

- Passive smoking increases the risk of lung cancer by approximately 25%. The risk of lung cancer has also been shown at the individual level.

Cardiovascular diseases

- Exposure to tobacco smoke increases the risk of coronary artery disease. According to recent studies, the risk of coronary events at the population level is 25–30% higher compared with non-exposed indivuals. The risk of all persons exposed to environmental tobacco smoke is about half of the additional risk that active smokers have. The risk is dose-dependent, i.e. it grows with increasing exposure. The risk has not been proven at the individual level as it has been for lung cancer. From the public health point of view the risk of coronary artery disease is more significant than that of lung cancer because of the higher prevalence of the disease.
- Although evidence on the association of passive smoking with stroke is scant, the association appears to be of a similar magnitude as that of smoking and coronary artery disease.

Other respiratory tract effects than lung cancer

- Passive smoking causes inflammatory changes in the respiratory tract that may lead to the development of respiratory symptoms and alterations in lung function as well as to the appearance of asthma. Exposure to tobacco smoke also suppresses the immune response and function of the pulmonary epithelium cilia, leading to increased susceptibility to respiratory infections.
- In children, exposure increases susceptibility to respiratory infections and the risk of asthma. In children with asthma, exposure can exacerbate the disease.
- Also in adults, exposure may be associated with an increased risk of asthma and COPD. There is also some evidence that passive smoking would increase the risk of invasive pneumococcal infection.

Other harmful effects of smoking

- Nicotine causes strong dependence that can be compared to that of narcotic substances.

- Growth of the foetus is slowed if the mother smokes. Children born to smoking mothers weigh about 200 g less at birth than children of non-smoking mothers.
- Nicotine is excreted in mother's milk in correlation to the quantity of cigarettes smoked.
- Smoking can alter the clinical effects of various drugs. Histamine H2 blockers prevent recurrence of ulcer much less in smokers than in those who do not smoke. Smoking decreases the efficacy of angina pectoris medication and diuretics, and induces metabolism of at least theophylline, coffeine, imipramine, pentazocine and vitamin C.
- Cessation of smoking may decrease deaths from injury, although the reduction is not statistically significant C [3 4].

References

1. Nicholas JJ. By how much does smoking cessation, or avoidance of starting smoking, reduce risk. In: Primary prevention. Clinical Evidence 2002;7:91–123.
2. Nicholas JJ. How quickly do risks diminish when smokers stop smoking. In: Primary prevention. Clinical Evidence 2002;7:91–123.
3. Leistikow BN, Shipley MJ. Might stop smoking reduce injury death risks: a meta-analysis of randomized controlled trials. Preventive Medicine 1999;28:255–259.
4. The Database of Abstracts of Reviews of Effectiveness (University of York), Database no.: DARE-998458. In: The Cochrane Library, Issue 1, 2001. Oxford: Update Software.

Forensic Medicine

Evidence Based Medicine Guidelines. Edited by the Duodecim Editorial Team
 ISBN: 0-470-01184-X

41.2 Determining the time of death

Kari Karkola

- Determining the time of death may be important for
  - medicolegal criminal cases
  - insurance, compensation, and pension
  - the assessment of reliability of the stated cause of death.
- All observations should be recorded systematically. Conclusions can be drawn later on. If the determination of the time of death is particularly important, as in homicide, several methods should be used together.

Cooling down of the corpse

- The temperature is measured at a depth of 10 cm per rectum without moving the body or changing the clothing. In important cases the temperature should be followed for about 2 hours.
- The estimated time should be adjusted on the basis of body build, clothing, and the thermal conduction of the surface on which the body lies. The margin of error is ± 2 hours during the first 10 hours after death, and thereafter ± 3–4 hours.

Methods of estimation

- James and Knight's equation
  - (37°C–measured temperature) × K = time (hours) since death.
  - The value of K depends on the surrounding temperature
  - See Table 41.2.
- Graphic method
  - The temperature is recorded on the vertical axis and the times of the day on the horizontal axis.
  - Two recorded temperatures are placed on the graph and a line is drawn through them to the level of 37°C.
  - The intersection of the line and the level of 37°C shows the time from which two hours are subtracted.
- Marshall's method
  - The body temperature falls 85% of the difference between the body temperature (37°C) and the surrounding temperature in an average time of 19 hours (lean, naked), of 28 hours (normal weight, dressed), or of 41 hours (overweight, dressed).
- Henssge's method
  - Based on temperature measurements
  - The body temperature, the ambient temperature, and the weight of the body are taken into account.
  - A nomogram is used.
- Rough estimation
  - The skin on the stomach feels warm <10 hours from death, and cold thereafter.

Table 41.2 Value of K in relation to surrounding temperature according to James and Knight

Surrounding temperature	0 °C	5 °C	10 °C	15 °C	20 °C
Value of K	1.00	1.25	1.50	1.75	2.00

Rigor mortis

- All joints should be examined systematically. At room temperature
  - the jaw and neck become stiff in 2–4 hours
  - the fingers and toes become stiff next
  - the large joints are the last to become stiff.
- Rigor mortis is fully developed in 6–8 hours. It disappears in the opposite order when putrefaction starts, after about 2 days at room temperature.
- Fever, hot weather and exercise before death accelerate the process, and cold weather and a well-developed musculature delay the process.

Post-mortem livores

- Blood discolours the lower body parts, with the exception of the parts pressed against the ground. In a supine position the livores are
  - visible on the sides of the thorax after 15–20 min
  - visible on the neck and ears after 20–40 min
  - united after 2–3 hours
  - fully developed 10–12 hours after death.
- The livores disappear on pressure or move when the position of the body is changed if no more than 4–6 hours have elapsed since death.
- The skin of bodies that have been in water after drowning is usually evenly pink all over.
- Patients who have died of blood loss do not usually have livores.
- Putrefaction destroys the livores.

Potassium concentration of the vitreous humour

- A sample is drawn with a large injection needle from the outer corner of the eye (the needle is directed towards the centre of the eye ball). The sample is centrifuged immediately, and the potassium concentration is determined at the nearest hospital laboratory.
- The potassium concentration rises steadily within about 100 hours from 5 to 25 mmol/l.

Other methods

- Attention should be paid to
  - drying (eyes, fingers, lips)
  - putrefaction (the first sign is the green colour of the stomach skin)
  - eggs or larvae of insects.
- The gastric contents and the condition of the chyle in the abdominal cavity can be examined during the autopsy.

FOR

Radiology

Evidence Based Medicine Guidelines. Edited by the Duodecim Editorial Team
© 2005 John Wiley & Sons, Ltd ISBN: 0-470-01184-X

42.1 Opacity in chest x-ray

Ossi Korhola

Basics of chest x-ray interpretation

- Use an adequate light table. Do not examine x-rays, for example, against a window.
- Always compare present abnormalities with findings in earlier x-rays if they are available.
  - Was the abnormality present already in the earlier x-ray?
  - Has it become larger or declined?
- Interpretation of the chest x-ray is not simple. Ask for interpretation by a radiologist if necessary.
- A chest x-ray that appears normal at first sight may hide significant pathology, e.g. behind the heart, mediastinum or diaphragm.

Make sure that the x-ray is technically adequate

- The lung parenchyma is difficult to see in an overexposed (too dark) x-ray.
- Abnormalities behind the heart are not visible in an underexposed (too light) x-ray.
- The picture must be straight because, for example, the hiluses cannot be assessed properly if the x-ray has been taken in an oblique position.
- The costophrenic sulcuses should be visible.
- A supine x-ray looks different from an erect x-ray. The heart looks bigger and the mediastinum wider.

Examples of eventual findings

Inflammatory changes

- In acute bronchitis the chest x-ray is normal.
- In pneumonia the chest x-ray shows one or more ill-demarcated infiltrates, or sometimes an increased peri-bronchial enhancement in viral pneumonia.
- Tuberculotic changes are usually seen in the apex of the lungs. Caverns may also be visible.
- Pneumonia may be caused by a specific abnormality (lung tumour, bronchiectasis, aspiration, foreign body or immunological disorder).

Atelectasis

- A local infiltrate confined to one lobe that is caused by the occlusion of a branch of the bronchus because of a tumour, foreign body or viscous mucus. The aetiology should always be determined.

Lung cancer

- The radiographic findings are varying. The most common abnormalities are opacity (from 1–2 cm to 10 cm and either well or poorly demarcated) atelectasis, unilateral hilar enlargement or widening of the mediastinum.
- If the tumour is small or situated intrabronchially or behind the mediastinum or the diaphragm the x-ray may be normal.
- If a long-time smoker has pneumonia the x-ray should be controlled after treatment to rule out lung cancer.

Pulmonary metastases

- One or more round opacities of varying size. Sometimes plenty of small densities or linear enhancement are visible all over the lungs.

Sarcoidosis

- The hilar lymph nodes are symmetrically enlarged. The lung parenchyma may show linear or nodular opacities.

Hodgkin's disease and other lymphomas

- Mediastinal widening, hilar enlargement

Heart failure

- In mild left ventricular failure the upper zone vessels are enlarged.
- In interstitial oedema the vascular pattern becomes dizzy, the lobar interspaces become clearly visible, horizontal 1–2 cm lines, and pleural effusion (usually first on the right side) are observed.
- Alveolar oedema is seen as poorly demarcated patchy infiltrates.
- In patients with emphysema the findings may be atypical and resemble pneumonia.

Pleural effusion

- The costophrenic sulcuses are usually, but not always, rounded. If there is a clinical suspicion of pleural effusion, the fluid can be diagnosed by a x-ray taken in the lateral recumbent position with horizontal beams: the fluid is seen as a layer between the lung and the chest wall (the translateral view).

Spontaneous pneumothorax

- Air (a dark area without lung structures) is visible between the lung and the chest wall. The lung may be totally collapsed.
- Sometimes the pressure in the pleural cavity exceeds atmospheric pressure (tension pneumothorax). The mediastinum shifts to the contralateral size. Tension pneumothorax must be treated immediately by puncture or pleural suction.

Other pulmonary opacities

- Pulmonary opacities are seen in many diseases (eosinophilic pneumonia, allergic alveolitis such as farmer's lung, and fibrotizing alveolitis).

Pulmonary embolism

- Even large pulmonary emboli may not cause abnormalities in the chest x-ray, and the eventual findings are often atypical. Clinical presentation is essential in primary diagnosis.
- Further investigations, if available, include spiral CT or pulmonary angiography.

42.2 Urography and pyelography

Editors

Safety precautions

- The result of a recent serum creatinine determination must be available
  - Consider the indications for the investigation if serum creatinine is 150–200 µmol/l.
  - The investigation is contraindicated if serum creatinine exceeds 200 µmol/l.
- Stop metformin medication 3 days before the investigation.

Excretory urography

- Has been a the basic investigation when urinary tract calculi are suspected, but is now being replaced by spiral computed tomography, which can be performed without contrast media.
- If Omnipaque® 300 is used as the contrast medium, the dose for an adult is 40 ml. The contrast medium is injected over 1–2 minutes.
- Imaging scheme: plain x-ray (including the urinary bladder), injection of contrast medium, 5-min x-ray (showing the kidneys), 20-min, 45-min etc. x-rays (showing the whole urinary tract) as long as renal excretion and the ureters are visible. At the end of the examination a picture is taken showing the urinary bladder after bladder emptying. If one kidney excretes very slowly the last picture may be taken as late as 6–12 hours after the injection of the contrast medium.

Intravenous pyelography (with ureteral compression)

- Use the same contrast medium as in excretory urography.
- Imaging scheme: plain x-ray, injection of contrast medium, 5-min x-ray, ureteral compression, 10-min x-ray, and final picture after the compression has been relieved.

42.3 Ultrasonographic examinations: indications and preparation of the patient

Editors

Abdominal ultrasonography

Upper abdomen

- Includes the liver, gallbladder, biliary tract, pancreas, spleen, kidneys, aorta and retroperitoneal space (for details see below).
- The patient should not eat for 6 hours and drink for 2 hours before the examination.

Ascites

- A clinically suspected ascites can be confirmed in patients with, for example, heart failure, cirrhosis of the liver, nephrotic syndrome or abdominal tumour who would probably benefit from the treatment of the condition.
- No preparations are needed.

Abdominal infections

- Ultrasonography may be helpful in detecting acute infection or peritonitis when the indications for surgery are determined.
- When intra-abdominal abscess as a complication of abdominal surgery or appendicitis (B) [1 2] is suspected.
- Ultrasonography is NOT a routine examination in suspected acute appendicitis (although the sensitivity of a negative examination is not sufficient to exclude appendicitis an inflamed appendix can often be seen) (B) [1 2].

Pancreas

- Included in the upper abdominal examination
- Indications
  - Suspicion of moderate or severe pancreatitis
  - Suspicion of a pancreatic pseudocyst
  - Suspicion of pancreatic carcinoma
- Pancreatic ultrasonography is rather insensitive and has many sources of error.
- The patient should not eat for 6 hours and drink for 2 hours before the examination.

Liver

- Included in the upper abdominal examination
- All liver diseases: hepatomegaly, cirrhosis, tumours and metastases, cysts and abscesses, biliary obstruction, abdominal trauma, jaundice.

- The patient should not eat for 6 hours and drink for 2 hours before the examination.

Kidneys and adrenal glands

- Included in the upper abdominal examination
- Renal tumours, cysts, polycystic disease, hydronephrosis, trauma and urologically silent kidney
- Adrenal adenomas can often be diagnosed (but not excluded) by ultrasonography.
- Primary examination in children with urinary tract infection to exclude structural abnormalities
- No preparations are needed,
- In the assessment of recurrent abdominal pain in children the patient should not eat for 6 hours and drink for 2 hours before elective examination.

Spleen

- Included in the upper abdominal examination
- Splenomegaly, ruptured spleen in abdominal trauma
- The patient should not eat for 6 hours and drink for 2 hours before the examination.

Gallbladder

- Included in the upper abdominal examination
- Primary examination in the diagnostics of gallstone disease and cholecystitis.
- Cancer of the gallbladder cannot be ruled out by ultrasonography.
- The patient should not eat for 6 hours and drink for 2 hours before the examination.

Urinary bladder and prostate

- Investigation of haematuria, diagnosis of urinary retention
- Residual urine after voiding (42.4)
- Size of the prostate, prostatic nodules
- Preparations: the patient should have a full bladder during the examination.
- Transurethral ultrasonography of the prostate is a basic examination by urologists in the assessment of prostatic disease.

Pelvic ultrasonography and ultrasonography during pregnancy

- See 25.2, 26.3.

Ultrasonography of blood vessels

Aorta

- Aortic aneurysm and dissection
- Preparations: the patient should not eat for 6 hours and drink for 2 hours before the examination (with the exception of emergencies).

Vascular prostheses

- Surgical complications: haematoma, aneurysm or abscess
- Preparations: the patient should not eat for 6 hours and drink for 2 hours before the examination.

Compression and doppler examination of the lower extremities

- Arterial obstruction and occlusion of the lower extremities (B) [3,4]
- Deep venous thrombosis of the femoral and popliteal veins (B) [5,6] (5.40). Ultrasonography is insensitive in the examination of calf veins (A) [7,8].
- The function of superficial veins can be assessed when planning surgery for varicose veins.
- No preparations are needed.

Carotid arteries

- Carotid stenosis, follow-up after endarterectomy
- No preparations are needed.

Thoracic ultrasonography

Pleural and pericardial cavity

- Suspected pleural or pericardial effusion
- No preparations are needed.
- Echocardiography (by cardiologists) see 4.8.

Thyroid and parathyroid ultrasonography

- Primary examination of a thyroid nodule
- No preparations are needed.

Soft tissues and joints of the extremities

- Assessment of the need of surgical treatment for muscle and tendon injuries (e.g. rotator cuff, achilles tendon, patellar tendon)
- Baker's cyst, bursal fluid, peritendinitis
- Diagnosis of synovitis
- Confirmation of the diagnosis of a ganglion
- A limp or hip pain in children (effusion of the hip joint).
- No preparations are needed.

Maxillary and frontal sinuses

- Diagnosis of sinusitis, follow-up the therapy.
- No preparations are needed.
- See 38.30.

Testis and epididymis

- Enlarged or painful scrotum (differential diagnosis of testis torsion and epididymitis, varicocoele, hydrocoele, spermatocoele, scrotal hernia, haematoma, or contusion)

- Always when testicular tumour is suspected.
- Investigation of male infertility
- No preparations are needed.

Ultrasonographically guided biopsies and punctures

- Evacuation of cysts, haematomas and abscesses
- Cytological and histological specimens of suspected tumours (e.g. breast, thyroid gland)

Ultrasonographic examinations by general practitioners

- Ultrasonography is a dynamic examination that must be interpreted during the examination. The interpretation cannot usually be reliably performed from printouts afterwards.
- A doctor performing ultrasonographic examinations should be trained by a specialist.
- Some ultrasonographic examinations are suitable to be performed by any doctors, and some for non-radiologists with a special training.
- A positive finding is significant (be careful not to harm the patient with false positive findings): a negative finding in ultrasonography performed by an inexperienced examiner should not be used to rule out a treatable disease.

Any doctor can perform the following examinations after local training

- Determination of the size and position of a fluid cavity before puncture (urinary bladder, pleural space, ascites, abscess)
- Determination of residual urine volume and size of the prostate (42.4).

A doctor with special training in ultrasonography can perform the following examinations

- Search for gallstones and signs of acute cholecystitis (thickened gallbladder wall and/or halo) in a patient with upper abdominal pain
- Search for hydronephrosis or dilated urinary tract in patient with urinary symptoms
- Diagnose or exclude abdominal aortic aneurysm
- Detect ascites or intra-abdominal bleeding (e.g. in a patient with mild, blunt abdominal trauma that does not require referral on the basis of the history or clinical presentation)
- Estimate the size of the spleen (a length exceeding 10–12 cm can be considered abnormal)
- Differentiate between a fluid collection or abscess from other subcutaneous masses (confirmation by puncture can be performed after ultrasonography)
- Some ultrasonographic examinations during pregnancy (26.3).

References

1. Orr RK, Porter D, Hartman D. Ultrasonography to evaluate adults for appendicitis: decision making based on meta-analysis and probabilistic reasoning. Acad Emerg Med 1995;2:644–650.
2. The Database of Abstracts of Reviews of Effectiveness (University of York), Database no.: DARE-951712. In: The Cochrane Library, Issue 4, 1999. Oxford: Update Software.
3. Koelemay MJ, Denhartog D, Prins MH, Kromhout JG, Legemate DA, Jacobs MJ. Diagnosis of arterial disease of the lower extremities with duplex ultrasonography. Br J Surg 1996;83:404–409.
4. The Database of Abstracts of Reviews of Effectiveness (University of York), Database no.: DARE-960604. In: The Cochrane Library, Issue 4, 1999. Oxford: Update Software.
5. Kearon C, Julian JA, Math M, Newman TE, Ginsberg JS. Noninvasive diagnosis of deep venous thrombosis. Ann Intern Med 1998;128:663–677.
6. The Database of Abstracts of Reviews of Effectiveness (University of York), Database no.: DARE-988578. In: The Cochrane Library, Issue 2, 2000. Oxford: Update Software.
7. Wells PS, Lensing AWA, Davidson BL, Prins MH, Hirsh J. Ultrasound for the diagnosis of deep vein thrombosis in asymptomatic patients after orthopaedic surgery. Ann Intern Med 1995;122:47–53.
8. The Database of Abstracts of Reviews of Effectiveness (University of York), Database no.: DARE-959305. In: The Cochrane Library, Issue 4, 1999. Oxford: Update Software.

42.4 Determining the volume of residual urine by ultrasonography

Editors

Principles

- Any doctor can determine the volume of residual urine after brief education.

Indications

- Urinary incontinence (to rule out overflow)
- Urinary symptoms in elderly men
- Urinary tract infection in the male
- A palpable mass in the lower abdomen

Techniques

- The patient voids.
- Keep the ultrasonography probe in a transverse position and find a view that shows the bladder in its maximum size.

Freeze the view and measure the horizontal (a) and vertical (b) dimensions of the bladder.

- Move the probe to a longitudinal position, find the maximum longitudinal dimension (c) of the bladder and measure it.
- The (minimum estimate of) residual urine volume = $0.6 \times a \times b \times c$ B [1 2]. If the dimensions are given in cm, the result is in ml.
  - A volume exceeding 100 ml is abnormal, and a volume exceeding 200 ml is usually an indication of treatment.
- The volume of the prostate can be measured by using the same formula.

Examining the full bladder

- If you intend to determine the position and depth of the bladder before bladder puncture or percutaneous cystostomy, do not ask the patient to void, but perform ultrasonography with a full bladder.

References

1. Nwosu CR, Khan KS, Chien PF, Honest MR. Is real-time ultrasonic bladder volume estimation reliable and valid? A systematic review. Scand J Urol Nephrol 1998;32:325–330.
2. The Database of Abstracts of Reviews of Effectiveness (University of York), Database no.: DARE-981930. In: The Cochrane Library, Issue 2, 2000. Oxford: Update Software.

Administration

Evidence Based Medicine Guidelines. Edited by the Duodecim Editorial Team
 ISBN: 0-470-01184-X

43.53 Health care for refugees arriving in Northern Europe

Heli Siikamäki

Aims

- Infectious diseases that are either treatable or require protective measures are screened on the first visit.
- Ensure that the person has received all necessary vaccinations.
- Prevent, identify and treat psychiatric problems.
- An American cost-benefit analysis showed that giving a 5-day course of albendazole to all persons coming from developing countries without screening is the most cost-effective measure for treating parasitic diseases. It reduced costs, hospital stays, DALYs and even deaths. This is not, however, necessarily applicable in Northern Europe.

Health check for refugees (recommendations in Finland)

- With the refugee's permission the following tests are recommended:
  - Chest x-ray for all persons aged 7 years or more
  - Serum HBsAg (all persons)
  - Serum cardiolipin (all persons)
  - Serum HIV antibodies (all persons)
- Other investigations are planned on an individual basis, after examination by a nurse. Investigations are based on information about the epidemiological situation in the country of origin.
- After an interview by a nurse, a physician should examine all children, pregnant women and persons with symptoms. For all others, an interview by a nurse is sufficient; physician's examination is indicated only if a screening test result is positive.
- The decision on immigration permission should not be dependent on the results of the health check, and the results of the check should not be handed over to the immigration officers.
- The most serious problems of the refugees are psychosocial, related to the circumstances leading to leaving their own country, a different cultural background, and change of environment. The health professionals performing the interviews and health checks should know something about the culture of the refugees' native country, and about the ways of thinking and beliefs concerning health and disease.

The immigrant as patient

- Reserve ample time for the visit.
- Use a qualified interpreter.
- Take a careful history
  - Areas of residence and conditions prior to immigration
  - Physical and psychological traumas
  - Possible exposure to contagious diseases
  - Earlier diseases and treatment
  - History of tuberculosis and given treatment and exposure to tuberculosis in close contacts
  - Vaccinations, BCG scar
- Thorough examination
  - In children measure height and weight, assess nutritional status.
  - Careful examination of the skin for detection of scabies and skin diseases, assessment of anaemia
  - Condition of the teeth
  - Palpation of lymph nodes, liver and spleen
  - Auscultation of the heart and lungs
- In addition to basic investigations (chest x-ray, HBsAg, cardiolipin, HIV antibodies) a more thorough examination should also include
  - Complete blood count
    - Anaemia: iron insufficiency, chronic infection, thalassaemia, haemoglobinopathy
  - Eosinophilia: parasitic worms
  - Erythrocyte sedimentation rate (ESR)
    - Tuberculosis
    - Other chronic infection
  - ALT
    - Hepatic diseases
  - Hepatitis C antibodies
  - HBcAb
    - Assess the need for vaccination if there is a hepatitis B carrier in the family
  - Urine sedimentation
    - Haematuria: schistosomiasis, tbc
    - Pyuria: tbc
  - Faecal parasites × 2–3
  - A Mantoux test (2 TU/0.1 ml) is performed on all children below 7 years for assessing the need for BCG vaccination

Most common infections in immigrants

- Knowledge of the epidemiology of infections in the country of origin is helpful in the diagnosis of acute and chronic infections.
- In the investigations of an acute febrile disease, malaria must be excluded if exposure is possible.
- Weight loss and fatigue may result from tuberculosis or advanced HIV infection or both.

Tuberculosis

- In many countries tuberculosis is still a common disease. Multi-resistant tuberculosis occurs in Eastern Europe.
- Information on BCG vaccination, exposure to infection, earlier tuberculosis and its treatment should be found during the first health check.
- A Mantoux test (2 TU/0.1 ml) is performed on all children below 7 years with no BCG scar. The test is considered negative (and BCG vaccination is indicated) if the diameter of the reaction is less than 5 mm. If the reaction is strong (> 10 mm), consider active tuberculosis.
- Symptoms of tuberculosis may appear several years after infection and this possibility should be kept in mind.
- Only patients with sputum-positive tuberculosis spread the disease. All persons living in the same household are considered exposed.
- A considerable part of tuberculosis cases among immigrants are non-pulmonary with the disease affecting lymph nodes, bone, joint, or kidneys. These patients are not contagious.
- An immigrant with respiratory problems should be referred to chest radiograph readily. If the finding suggests tuberculosis
  - take sputum samples for staining and culture on three consecutive mornings
  - refer the patient to a specialist unit for pulmonary diseases, internal medicine, or paediatrics.
- Tuberculosis should be suspected in all patients arriving from endemic areas who suffer from weight loss, fever, anaemia and hypersedimentation.
- Enlarged lymph nodes, particularly in the region of the neck strengthen suspicion and a biopsy should include, in addition to histology, also tuberculosis staining, culture and PCR.
- In many areas where HIV is endemic, tuberculosis also prevails and often these occur together. Both conditions should be remembered in the diagnosis, particularly as the symptoms may be very similar.

Hepatitis B

- Countries with a high prevalence (more than 8% of the population as carriers) are found in Africa, Asian, tropical America and Eastern Europe. Some immigrants arriving from these countries are hepatitis B carriers.
- Patients should be given verbal and, if possible, written instructions in their own language on how to reduce the risk of transmission via blood or sexual contact.
- Vaccination is recommended for persons living in the same household as the hepatitis B carrier as well as his or her regular sex partners who are HBsAg negative.
- Children of HBsAg-positive women should receive hepatitis B immunoglobulin immediately after birth, and a series of vaccinations should be started as soon as possible.
- Responsible day care or school personnel working with HBsAg-positive children should be informed of the risks involved with blood contact.
- In cases of exposure, hepatitis B infection can be prevented by vaccination and immunoglobulin administration.
- Health care personnel working mainly in refugee health care should be vaccinated against hepatitis B. The vaccination is recommended for other personnel in refugee centres, if they work in close contact with small children.

HIV

- An HIV test is part of a voluntary immigration health check. The person to be tested or his guardian should be allowed to refuse the test.
- A nurse can report a negative test result, but a doctor should report a positive result.
- HIV-positive refugees are referred to a specialist unit for internal medicine.
- The test result should not be given to immigration officers, refugee centre workers or schools.

Faecal bacteria

- Bacteria should be sought for in patients with diarrhoea or other cause suggesting infection.
- Shigella is more contagious than salmonella, and deserves stricter hygienic measures. Symptomatic shigella infection should be treated with antimicrobial drugs.

Intestinal parasite infections

- Parasites should, accordingly to recommendations, only be sought for primarily in patients who have symptoms. Faecal parasite examination should be carried out in children under 7 years of age who have a history or signs of anaemia or chronic health problems.
- In practice, if is often sensible to take at least two parasite samples in connection with a more thorough health check and treat actively.
- The most common findings are Trichuris, Ascaris, hookworm (Ancylostoma), Strongyloides and Giardia.
- Strongyloides infection, which is associated with considerable eosinophilia, may lead to a life threatening general infection in immunosuppressed persons.
- Other intestinal parasites should also be eradicated because of possible sequelae or risk of transmission.

Vaccinations

- If background information on the person is scarce, the aim should be to ensure at least basic protection from diseases. If a person arriving from developing countries is known to have received vaccinations, it can be assumed that the Expanded Programme for Immunization (EPI) recommended by the WHO has been followed (Table 43.53.1)
- For unvaccinated children, the so-called accelerated programme is used. If a BCG vaccination scar is not found (left thigh, left arm, more rarely right thigh or arm), the Mantoux test is first performed to ensure that the child is not a tuberculosis carrier. BCG vaccination is given only to

Table 43.53.1 Basic vaccination programme recommended for developing countries by the WHO (EPI). The times are minimum intervals between vaccinations; longer periods can be applied.

Vaccination	Schedule
Children	
BCG	1 shot before the age of 6 weeks
PDT	3 shots: at the ages of 6, 10, and 14 weeks
OPV (oral polio vaccination)	4 doses: at the ages of <2, 6, 10, and 14 weeks
Measles	1 shot at the age of 9 months
Hepatitis B	3 shots: one after birth and boosts at the ages of 1 and 6 months in endemic areas
Fertile and pregnant women	
Tetanus (T)	5 shots: 1st shot (T1) on any visit to a health care unit; 2nd shot 4 weeks from T1; 3rd shot 6 months from T2; 4th shot 1 year from T3 or during the next pregnancy; 5th shot 1 year from T4 or during the next pregnancy.

children under 7 years of age with a negative Mantoux test. After the BCG vaccination other vaccinations should not be given within 6 weeks. Other live and inactivated vaccinations can, however, be given simultaneously with BCG.

Table 43.53.2 Accelerated vaccination programme.

Age group	Vaccination
Under 6-year-olds	
1st visit	PDT, polio, Hib[1], and MMR; BCG if the Mantoux test is negative
2 months later	PDT, polio, Hib
2 months later	PDT and thereafter the child follows the national vaccination programme for children of his/her age
Over 6-year-olds	
1st visit	PDT/DT/Td, polio, MMR; PDT for under 7-year-olds, DT for 7–9-year-olds[2]
2 months later	PDT/DT/Td, polio
6–12 months later	PDT/DT/Td, polio and thereafter according to the national vaccination programme
Adults	
1st visit	Td, polio
2 months later	Td, polio
6–12 months later	Td, polio

1. Hib vaccination is given according to the following scheme: under 12-month-olds are given three doses; 12–17-month-olds two doses; 18-months to 4-year-olds one dose. Over 5-year-olds do not need a Hib vaccination.
2. Ten-year-olds and older are given Td instead of PDT.

- Unvaccinated adults should be immunized against diphtheria, tetanus and polio (Table 43.53.2).

Occupational Health Service

Evidence Based Medicine Guidelines. Edited by the Duodecim Editorial Team
 ISBN: 0-470-01184-X

44.20 Physical hazards at work

Mari Antti-Poika

Noise

Exposure

- It has been estimated that noise at the level of 85 dB for 40 hours per week is safe for approximately 95% of the population.
- Noise exposure occurs not only in industrial work but also in teaching, childcare, industrial kitchens, cleaning work etc.
- Exposure to the more harmful impulse noise occurs in the armed forces, mines and the metal industry.
- Noise-induced hearing loss, see 38.42.

Prevention

- The purpose of a medical examination carried out before noise exposure commences is to identify individuals who are not suitable for work involving noise exposure. This group particularly includes young persons with any hearing loss of the cochlear type.
- Noise-induced hearing loss as such does not prevent work involving noise exposure.
- Periodical hearing tests should be carried out for employees whose work exceeds safe noise levels (38.42). Periodical hearing tests should be performed annually for the first four years and thereafter once every three years.
- The purpose of the annual testing is to identify persons who are particularly inclined to suffer from temporary hearing loss, in order to enhance their hearing protection.
- Employees with category III hearing impairment should be referred for further investigations, unless their hearing loss has been investigated previously, see 38.42.

Radiation

Exposure

- **Ionizing radiation**. Those at risk of exposure include workers at nuclear power stations, radiographers, radiologists and industrial radiographers.
- Ionizing radiation may cause cancer in all organs.
- **Nonionizing radiation** is classified according to wavelength:
  - optic radiation (ultraviolet radiation (UV), visible light and infrared radiation)
  - radio frequency radiation (microwaves and radio waves)
  - low frequency, electromagnetic fields.
- Nonionizing radiation mainly causes acute adverse effects (UV radiation also predisposes to skin cancer).
  - The most common occupational eye disease is radiation-induced corneal or conjunctival damage (welder's eye) (37.28).

Prevention

- The proper functioning of equipment must be ensured and relevant safety instructions must be followed.
- Exposure to ionizing radiation is monitored with radiation decimeters.
- National guidelines should be consulted regarding periodic medical examinations of employees exposed to ionizing radiation in their work.

Vibration

- Hands are exposed to vibration when using tools driven by compressed air, chain saws, nailers or other vibrating tools or machines.
- Vibration may lead to Raynaud's phenomenon (white fingers, see 21.4) and peripheral polyneuropathy, predominantly in the upper limbs.
- Vibration syndrome, see 5.62.
- The aim of an initial medical examination should be to identify individuals with pre-existing Raynaud's phenomenon, poor peripheral circulation, carpal tunnel syndrome or other illnesses involving the hands, which may deteriorate when exposed to vibration.
- In periodical examinations emerging symptoms should be identified as early as possible.

44.21 Chemical hazards at work

Mari Antti-Poika

Exposure to chemicals

- Occupational health and safety measures, as well as statutory regulations, have contributed towards a reduced risk of exposure to chemicals at the workplace, particularly to the most dangerous substances.
- Lack of information, particularly in small workplaces, may lead to the neglect of occupational safety.

Estimating exposure

- Exposure alone does not signify an illness. Whether a person becomes ill or not is determined by many factors, e.g. the effect of the substance, absorption into the body, exposure time and level, work methods and individual factors.
  - Most substances encountered at the workplace enter the body via the respiratory system.

- Cyanides, chlorophenols, some organic solvents and several herbicides and pesticides are absorbed through the skin.
- Substances, as liquids or gases, may also irritate and corrode the skin, mucous membranes or the conjunctiva of the eyes.
- Reactive airways dysfunction syndrome (RADS) is an asthma-like condition which develops after sudden exposure to irritating gases or fumes. The condition is not involved with sensitization or a latency period and develops within 24 hours of exposure.

♦ The degree of hazard posed by various particles is influenced by their size and form (dust or fumes) as well as the biological activity of the dust (ability to irritate or sensitize, fibrogenicity).

- The particle size of dust will determine how far down the respiratory tract the dust is able to be driven.

Risk assessment

♦ The main stages of a risk assessment of chemical substances include the recognition of chemical hazards, evaluation of the level of exposure and assessing the risk of exposure to health.

♦ In Finland the manufacturer of chemicals is legally obliged to list chemicals hazardous to health and the environment, to label packages appropriately to indicate hazard and the need for protection as well as to provide relevant Safety Data Sheets.

♦ If an occupational disease is suspected both the employer and employee should be interviewed regarding possible exposure. If necessary workplace visits and industrial (hygienic measurements may be indicated).

- Exposure to air impurities is evaluated by measuring the concentration of the substance in the workplace air industrial hygienic measurements.
- Exposure to some substances can be measured from a sample of blood, urine or expiratory air supplied by the employee (biological monitoring).
- Most metals with health risk implications can be detected with biological measurements, but only some tens of organic compounds can be reliably detected.
- Results obtained from industrial hygienic measurements are evaluated by comparing them to official occupational exposure limits.

Illnesses caused by chemicals

♦ A multitude of chemicals are used at workplaces, and occupational health personnel deal with problems relating to a great variety of chemicals.

♦ Skin diseases are the most common group of occupational diseases, see Table 44.21.1.

♦ Many chemicals may sensitize employees to respiratory tract allergies (e.g. chemicals used in the plastics industry, natural resins, detergents and disinfectants), see 6.33.

- Symptom onset is preceded by an asymptomatic latency period of varying duration.

Table 44.21.1 The most common agents causing occupational skin diseases

Type of rash	Most common agents
Irritant contact dermatitis	• detergents • work involving wet and dirty conditions • mineral oils, lubricating oils and mineral waxes • organic solvent mixtures • food handling
Allergic contact dermatitis	• rubber and rubber chemicals • plastic chemicals (e.g. epoxy compounds, acrylates, synthetic resins) • metals and their compounds (e.g. nickel, chrome compounds, cobolt) • formaldehyde and antimicrobial agents) • organic dusts and materials (e.g. ornamental plants, trees, vegetables)
Protein contact dermatitis	• organic dusts and materials (e.g. animal epithelium, flour, grains, animal feed, ornamental plants) • natural rubber

Table 44.21.2 The most common carcinogenic chemicals according to the Finnish Register of Employees Exposed to Carcinogens

Agent	Mode of exposure	Increased risk of
Hexavalent chrome compounds, nickel	Manufacture of chromates and dichromates, chrome and nickel plating, welding and grinding of stainless steel, manufacture of chrome and nickel products	cancer of the lungs and paranasal sinuses
Asbestos	Demolishing of old buildings and maintenance work, insulation work, ship building	lung cancer, mesothelioma, possibly cancer of the larynx, intestinal tract and kidneys.
Acrylamide	Laboratory work, chemical processes	possibly carcinogenic
Polycyclic aromatic hydrocarbons	Exposure to exhaust gas, smoke, soot and coal tar	lung cancer
Benzene	Machine and engine repair work, chemical processes, laboratory work	leukaemia, possibly lymphoma

- Nasal and conjunctival symptoms may precede pulmonary symptoms.

♦ Lung cancer and mesothelioma caused by asbestos are the most well known occupational cancers.

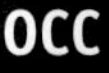
OCC

- The most common carcinogenic chemicals according to the Finnish Register of Employees Exposed to Carcinogens are presented in Table 44.21.2.

44.23 Occupational exposure to viral agents

Editors

Basic rules

- Occupational exposure to viruses is prevented by adequate training and protection of the personnel.
- The risk of infection is assessed immediately after the accident, and necessary precautions to prevent infection are taken.
- All emergency rooms and on-call units must have clear instructions on how to act in case of exposure.

Accidents involving risk of infection

- A needle or other instrument contaminated by blood, bloody secretions or tissue fluids causes a penetrating skin wound.
- Blood spurts into the eyes or mouth, or on erythematous or broken skin.
- Bite wounds

First aid

- Do not squeeze the wound but rinse it with ample water.
- In punctures, allow the wound to bleed.
- Remove possible foreign bodies.
- Wash the injured area with water and soap.
- If blood contaminates broken skin, a wound or a puncture, place an alcohol-containing compress on the site of the injury for 2 minutes or rinse the wound with alcohol.
- Rinse mucous membranes with ample water.

Laboratory samples

- The following blood samples are taken from the source of possible infection with the person's consent: HIV antibodies, hepatitis B surface antigen (HBs-Ag), hepatitis B core antibody (HBc-Ab), hepatitis C antibody (HCV-Ab).
- Corresponding samples are taken from the exposed person (zero sample). These zero samples are sent to the laboratory immediately if the suspected source of infection does not comply with testing. If the tests from the source are obtained, the zero samples can be frozen while waiting for the results for the source of infection. If the test results are negative, the zero samples of the exposed person need not be examined and further samples are not necessary. If the source is found to have HIV, hepatitis B or C, the zero samples are sent for examination.
- In accidents occurring during off-hours, the samples can be collected in 7-ml serum tubes (2/person) and stored in a refrigerator until the next working day.
- If the source of infection is not known, does not cooperate or is found to be HIV, HBV or HCV positive, further samples are taken from the exposed person at 1, 3 and 6 months.

Course of action when the source is a verified or strongly suspected hepatitis B carrier

- The exposed person has had hepatitis B earlier
  - No action
  - Further samples for hepatitis B are not taken, however, hepatitis C and HIV samples are taken as usual.
- The exposed person has been vaccinated against hepatitis B
  - If the vaccinations have been given within 5 years, HBs-Ab is taken to verify that the exposed person is protected by the vaccination.
  - If more than 5 years have elapsed from the vaccination a booster is given.
  - Further actions depend on the result of the HBs-Ab test: if protection is not verified or does not develop, HBsAg and HBcAb are examined as usual.
- The exposed person has not had hepatitis B and has not been vaccinated
  - Anti-HBV-immunoglobulin (1 ampoule, 5 ml) is injected intramuscularly (buttock or upper arm, not at the site of the hepatitis B vaccination) and the first hepatitis B vaccination is given to the muscle of the upper arm.
    - If more than 24 hours but less than 7 days have elapsed from exposure, the benefit of immunoglobulin is uncertain, however, it is still considered worthwhile.
    - When more than 7 days have elapsed, immunoglobulin is no longer given, however, the vaccination series can be started.
    - In obvious exposure the vaccination series is given immediately to boost immune response, with further doses at 1 and 2 months and a booster at 12 months.

Exposure to hepatitis C

- When the risk is obvious, an HCV PCR test can be performed on the source of infection to evaluate infectivity.
- Hepatitis C antibodies are investigated from the exposed at 1, 3 and 6 months from exposure.
- If hepatitis C antibodies are detected during follow-up, interferon treatment can be started.
- There is no vaccination.

Table 44.23 Occupational exposure to viral agents

Virus	Penetrating wound	Bite	Infective material		
			Certain	Probable	Unprobable
HBV	5–25%	Proven	Blood, blood products	Semen, body fluids, vaginal secretion, sputum	Urine, faeces
HCV	1–5%	Not proven	Blood	Blood products, bloody body fluids, semen, vaginal secretion	Sputum, urine
HIV	0.3–0.4%	Proven (2 cases)	Blood, blood products	Semen, vaginal fluid, liquor, breast milk, exudates, serous fluids, amniotic fluid, sputum, dental procedures	Sputum, urine, faeces

Occupational exposure to HIV

- Investigate HIV serology immediately after exposure and repeat the test at 2 month intervals for 6 months.
- Condom use is recommended during the follow-up period.
- Inform the insurance company about accidental exposure.
- If the risk of infection is evident, prophylactic medication should be considered (1.45). Treatment should be started within 2 hours of exposure. Find out from the nearest hospital treating HIV patients what drugs should be used and have this information readily available in your practice.

Risk of infection following exposure

- See Table 44.23

Protection for personnel treating HIV-positive and hepatitis patients

- Use gloves and a face mask when treating patients with injuries. Avoid stitch wounds.
- Use gloves during blood sampling. A face mask is not necessary (if vacuum bottles are used).
- Ensure that sharp objects are handled carefully and disposed off safely.

44.25 Burnout

Aki Rovasalo

- See also 36.10

Objectives

- Burnout is not an illness but a syndrome. It should not be medicalized.
- Burnout is identified, and other illnesses, especially psychological problems, are assessed.
- Depression and burnout overlap. Depression is actively treated as in other cases (35.21). Fatigue may be the symptom of a somatic disease (36.10).

Epidemiology

- Burnout does not appear overnight. Instead, it develops gradually through the interaction of one's personality, work and work community.
- Burnout is not the same as work stress. Stress is created when a person tries to adapt to his or her workload, and it is not entirely negative. Burnout develops when mere adaptation does not suffice, normalisation is not achieved, and the state of stress is prolonged.

Symptoms and diagnosis

- The basic symptoms of burnout are
  - intense, overwhelming fatigue
  - cynical relationship to work
  - diminished professional self-esteem.
- Common psychiatric differential diagnoses are (clinical clues given in parentheses)
  - severe depression (especially when feelings of worthlessness or guilt are associated)
  - alcohol and drug abuse problem (for example, recurring short absence from work)
  - so-called atypical depression (for example, getting emotionally hurt at workplace triggers strong fluctuations in mood)
  - stress disorders (a distinct external triggering factor must be identified)
  - generalized anxiety disorder (worry over one's performance, constant restlessness)
  - social anxiety disorder (fatigue in social situations)
  - somatization disorder (several somatic symptoms)
  - personality disorder (functioning may vary, but problems have continued throughout adulthood)
  - adjustment disorders (identifiable external stress factor that impairs functioning unexpectedly)
- According to the present classification of diseases, burnout is a symptom diagnosis that does not require compensation on the part of the employer. Health insurance requires that the loss of work ability must be a result of an illness.

- If the patient is unable to work because of burnout, his or her state can be considered a disease, and the main diagnosis is some sort of mental disorder (e.g., state of depression, adjustment disorder, somatoform disorder). Burnout can be recorded as an additional diagnosis.

Treatment

- The situation can be mitigated by sick leave, if the patient is unable to work.
  - It usually requires a few days and nights to normalize a patient's sleep rhythm.
  - Severe burnout that diminishes functional capacity requires a sick leave of 2–3 weeks.
  - A severe state of depression often requires even longer sick leave because it takes longer to regain functional capacity than it does for symptoms to disappear.
  - Sick leave does not substitute for treatment and follow-up. Book regular appointments with the patient.
- Treatment is planned individually and can include, for example, stress management, medication or psychotherapy.
- Mental problems, such as depression, must be actively treated.
- It is important to take into consideration the subjective experience of the patient and to familiarize oneself with his or her life conditions.
- The patient should be referred to a psychiatric outpatient care if his or her situation does not improve notably in 2–3 months or if the diagnosis remains uncertain.
- If occupational health care services believe that burnout is prevalent at a specific workplace, actions can be planned to influence it.

Prevention of burnout

- Burnout can be prevented by
  - the ability to say "no"
  - the ability to plan one's work in advance
  - taking care of one's physical condition
  - admitting one's own limits
  - good relationships at home
  - working relationships at work
  - an open work climate
  - consistent career development
  - a supportive employer
  - clear definitions of work assignments
  - perception of one's job as meaningful
  - maintenance of expertise.
- Work supervision may prevent burnout of at least health care and teaching personnel.

Pollution and Health

Evidence Based Medicine Guidelines. Edited by the Duodecim Editorial Team
 ISBN: 0-470-01184-X

45.1 Adverse health effects of ambient air pollution

Antti Pönkä

- With the exception of malodorous sulphur compounds, adverse health effects of ambient air impurities are experienced only in built-up areas where the most hazardous compounds are respirable particles, nitrogen oxide and carbon monoxide.

Sources of emissions

- Traffic is the most important source in cities and towns (nitrogen dioxide, respirable particles, hydrocarbons, carbon monoxide).
- Energy production (nitrogen dioxide, sulphur dioxide, respirable particles)
- Industry (sulphur dioxide, nitrogen dioxide, respirable particles, hydrocarbons, malodorous sulphur compounds, heavy metals)

Health effects

- Respirable particles are nowadays considered by far the most hazardous air impurities, and are the only factor known to reduce life expectancy at the population level. Their short-term adverse effects include a higher prevalence of cough, respiratory tract infections and symptoms of asthma and COPD and the risk of hospitalization in person with cardiac problems or cerebrovascular disturbances.
- Nitrogen dioxide, sulphur dioxide, and ozone (formed in air in reactions of nitrogen dioxide and hydrocarbons) irritate the respiratory tract.
  - The acute effects are a cough, asthma attacks and infections of the respiratory tract.
  - Other effects are exacerbation of symptoms of chronic bronchitis and asthma.
- Increased concentrations of carbon monoxide are associated with increased hospitalization among people with cardiac diseases and increased mortality among people with underlying serious diseases.
- Genotoxic compounds, such as polyaromatic hydrocarbons originating from traffic and energy production, increase the risk of lung cancer. Air pollution is estimated to cause 2–3 cases of lung cancer per 100 000 inhabitants annually in cities.
- Malodorous sulphur compounds, for example mercaptanes and hydrogen sulphide cause acute health effects, such as dyspnoea when occurring in sudden, high concentrations. Long-term effects include irritation of the eyes and respiratory tract, headache, tiredness, depression and nausea.
- Lead emissions are no longer a significant health problem in countries in which lead-containing fuels for cars have been forbidden. Blood levels below 5–10 μg/100 ml are not believed to cause disturbances in the development of the central nervous system. The lead blood concentrations among children in the Nordic Countries are below 3–5 μg/100 ml. In the vicinity of foundries and industrial plants using metal the concentrations of lead in vegetables (lettuce, parsley, dill) may be elevated due to contamination by dust emissions.
- Cadmium mainly originates from the metal industry. Cadmium accumulates in the liver and kidneys of cows and moose. Therefore, abundant use of these organs as food is not recommended.

Guidelines

- There are national guidelines for the concentrations of sulphur dioxide, nitrogen dioxide, carbon monoxide and particulates. These are measured in major cities continuously.
- Council Directive 1999/30/EC gives health based short and/or long-term limit values for mean concentrations of nitrogen dioxide (200 μg/m^3; 1 h), respirable particles (50 μg/m^3, 24 h), sulphur dioxide and lead in ambient air.

45.2 Epidemics due to contaminated drinking water

Antti Pönkä

Monitoring drinking water

- Drinking water distributed by water plants is monitored by taking water samples for chemical, microbiological and physical analyses regularly.
- In the EU countries, presence of E. coli and enterococci are used as microbiological indicators of contamination. A 100 ml sample should be free of these bacteria. Since the end of the year 2003, all water distributed within the EU must meet these criteria.
- If the above-mentioned bacteria are found in samples, control samples must be taken immediately. Simultaneously, necessary action has to be taken: prohibition of the use of water, disinfection of water pipes or recommending that users boil water before consumption.

Causes of water-borne epidemics

- The most common causes of water-borne epidemics are contamination of drinking water by pathogenic faecal microbes of human or animal origin, insufficient treatment of water, or both.

The most common pathogens in Northern Europe

- Viruses (noro-, adeno- and rotaviruses)
- Bacteria (Campylobacter jejuni, Yersinia enterocolitica, Salmonella, E. coli including enterohaemorrhagic E. coli (EHEC) O157, Plesiomonas shigelloides, Aeromonas)
- Parasites, especially in cases of traveller's diarrhoea (Giardia lamblia, Cryptosporidium, Entamoeba histolytica).
- Toxins of moulds may rarely cause allergic or toxic general or respiratory symptoms transmitted by drinking or bathing water.

Laboratory investigations and differential diagnosis

- In epidemics, samples have to be taken from at least 5–10 ill people for the following investigations:
  - bacterial stool cultures for the above-mentioned bacteria and for Clostridium perfringens, Bacillus cereus and Staphylococcus aureus
  - viral stool culture, PCR (to detect noro-, astro- or rotaviruses), electron microscopy of stools and rapid diagnostic viral tests (rota- and adenoviruses)
  - microscopic examination for parasites
  - paired serum samples for viral antibodies.
- Consultation with the specialist of infectious diseases in the central hospital is advisable.
- Take food-borne infections and poisoning, as well as viral infection spreading via personal contact, into consideration in the differential diagnosis.

45.3 Indoor air pollution

Antti Pönkä

- See also 45.4.

Causes and sources

- Building materials, furnishing materials, human activities, especially smoking, domestic animals and outdoor air are the most important sources of indoor air pollutants. The adverse health effects may be caused by physical, chemical or biological factors, or due to irradiation.
- Radon is the most harmful indoor source of radioactivity. Radon originates from soil and ground as a fission product of uranium.
- The most important physical factors are temperature, rate of ventilation, moisture, fibres (asbestos, man made mineral fibres) and dust.

Biological factors

- These include viruses, bacteria, moulds, house mites and scales from human beings and animal dander.
- The main source of indoor air bacteria is human beings.
- Increased concentrations of moulds are most often due to water damage, possibly associated with insufficient ventilation.
- The main allergenic factors in indoor air are the epithelium and excretions from animals, mould fungi, and to a lesser extent house dust mites and their excretions, and plants.

Chemical factors

- The most important chemical factors include tobacco smoke due to active or passive smoking, organic volatile compounds (VOC), polycyclic aromatic hydrocarbons (PAH) and formaldehyde, as well as many inorganic gases such as carbon monoxide, ozone, nitrogen dioxide, nitrites and ammonia.
- Building materials, varnishes, glues, upholstery materials and burning processes emit organic chemicals.

Health effects

- An increase in the amount of moulds or their metabolites induced by a moisture damage in the building causes symptoms generally known as the sick building syndrome. People living in moisture damaged houses suffer more frequently from symptoms of respiratory tract irritation and infection and from allergic diseases.
- Allergic reactions caused by indoor pollutants either have a delayed pathogenetic mechanism (farmers' lung, humidifier

Table 45.3 The most frequent symptoms and causes of sick building syndrome according to the US National Institute for Occupational Safety and Health.

Symptoms	Percentage
Eye irritation	81
Throat irritation	71
Headache	67
Tiredness	53
Stuffy nose	51
Rashes, dry skin	38
Dyspnoea	33
Cough	24
Vertigo	22
Nausea	15
Observed causes	
Deficient ventilation	50
Indoor chemicals	19
Outdoor pollutants	11
Indoor microbes	5
Fibres	4
Unknown	11

POL

fever) or (usually) are IgE-mediated (asthma, atopic rhinitis, atopic excema). The most common cause of an immediate allergic reaction is an exposure to epithelium or excretions from animals, to mould fungi or to house dust mites.
- Chipboard, some furnishing materials and varnish emit formaldehyde, which irritates mucosae of the eyes, nose and respiratory tract. The smell of formaldehyde is typically pungent.
- The syndrome caused by the increased amount of mould and/or their metabolites due to moisture damage of buildings is presented in detail in the chapter (45.4).
- The exact causes of the sick building syndrome are unknown. However, according to current opinion the syndrome is multifactorial, and due to various chemical and microbiological indoor pollutants, unsatisfactory physical indoor conditions and psychological problems. This syndrome may occur among as many as 30% of the employees in new office buildings.
- For symptoms, see Table 45.3.

45.4 Exposure to microbes in water-damaged buildings

Kari Reijula

Background

- In this article the word mould covers moulds, yeasts and bacteria (e.g. Actinomycetes).
- The most important task in water-damaged buildings is to repair the damage as soon as possible to prevent growth of microbes and exposure to moulds.
- Assessment of exposure to moulds is in most cases the responsibility of primary health care. Patients with a suspicion of asthma, extrinsic allergic alveolitis or ODTS (organic dust toxic syndrome) should be sent to special clinics.
- Symptoms associated with an exposure to moulds in water-damaged buildings can appear as an irritation in eyes, skin or respiratory tract (symptoms), or as rhinitis, asthma or even allergic alveolitis (diseases).
- Diagnosis of mould-induced diseases is based on the confirmation of exposure, clinical findings and differential diagnosis.
- It is important to investigate the damaged building and symptomatic individuals at the same time.

Epidemiology of mould-induced disorders

- Moisture problems may appear in more than 50% of buildings in many parts of Europe. The problems seem to affect all kinds of buildings including single houses, apartments, school buildings, hospitals and day care centers.
- Flat roof frequently cause problems. Even newer buildings can be damaged because of faulty building techniques or leaking pipes.

Symptoms caused by moulds and clinical picture of the diseases caused by them

- Irritation symptoms occur in about half of the affected
  - Eye symptoms
  - Blockage and itching of nose, watery discharge
  - Sore throat, hoarse voice
  - Cough
  - Mucus secretion
  - Itching and redness of skin

General symptoms

- Fatigue, headache, nausea, fever, pain in joints and muscles
- Organic dust toxic syndrome (ODTS)

Diseases

- Allergy to moulds is rarely the cause for the symptoms
- Rhinoconjunctivitis
- Asthma
- Extrinsic allergic alveolitis (farmer's lung)
- ODTS

Secondary infections

- Sinusitis, bronchitis, middle ear infection

Strategies for investigation of mould exposure at home or in the workplace

History

- Extent of the water damage
- Prevalence of symptoms among exposed persons
- Nature of symptoms
- Temporal relation between the symptoms and exposure
- At the workplace the extent of the problem can be assessed by e.g. a questionnaire survey.

Clinical manifestation

- Eyes, nose, skin and respiratory tract should be examined clinically.
- Symptoms of asthma, alveolitis and ODTS should be registered.

Differential diagnosis

- Allergic disorders caused by house pets, pollen or other inhaled allergens

- Sinusitis, prolonged bronchitis (mycoplasma or chlamydia, etc.)
    - Repeated infections may also be a sign of exposure to moulds!
- Smoking
- Psychosocial problems

Actions to be taken

- Repairment of water-damaged materials as quickly as possible to prevent further exposure to moulds.
- If the extent of the problem is limited, the number of symptomatic persons is low and there are no cases of severe mould-induced diseases, the construction repairs and follow-up of patients can be performed under the control of local health care unit.
- If the extent of the problem is large and severe cases of diseases appear (asthma, allergic alveolitis, ODTS, recurring infections), local authorities should inspect the building technically, and the local health care unit should consult indoor air specialists who should carry out microbiological examinations in the damaged buildings.
- When the building is inspected, material samples are collected for microbiological analysis. Surface dust and air samples are collected when no damage is detected in the material samples but the suspicion of water damage is strong (for example, the smell of mould is strong).
- If the inspection of the building reveals mibrobes indicating water damage and if there are many persons with symptoms or the symptoms are those commonly associated with allergy, skin prick tests with mould extracts and measurement of IgE class antibodies to moulds should be performed on the exposed persons. IgG class antibodies show mainly that the person has been exposed to microbes.
- Suspicion of asthma, allergic alveolitis and ODTS warrants further investigations in a specialist clinic.

Microbiology of a moisture-damaged building

- Following microbes require plenty of water: Aspergillus fumigatus, Exophiala, Phialophora, Trichoderma, Ulocladium, Stachybotrys, Fusarium, Actinomycetes, yeasts, gram-negative bacteria (e.g. Pseudomonas).
- Microbes requiring moderate or small amounts of water: Aspergillus versicolor, Eurotium, Penicillium (P. chrysogenum, P. auratiogriseum), Wallemia.
- Some microbes can produce mycotoxins, e.g. Stachybotrys chartarum (atra), Aspergillus versicolor and Trichoderma viride.

Index

Evidence Based Medicine Guidelines. Edited by the Duodecim Editorial Team

 ISBN: 0-470-01184-X

Mobile EBM Guidelines includes more than 900 guidelines on practical medical topics. The unique feature of the mobile EBM Guidelines is the evidence summaries that support the given recommendations and are graded from A to D with links to the corresponding Cochrane abstracts. The concise structure of EBM Guidelines suits perfectly the small screens of the portable PDAs and literally brings the quidelines into the physician's pocket.

EBM Guidelines is available for the Nokia 9200/9300/9200 Series, Palm and Pocket PC (Windows Mobile). For further information, please refer to www.ebm-guidelines.com/mobile.html.